ARTHRITIS
AND ALLIED CONDITIONS

A TEXTBOOK OF RHEUMATOLOGY

DANIEL J. McCARTY, M.D.

Will and Cava Ross Professor and Chairman
Department of Medicine
The Medical College of Wisconsin
Milwaukee, Wisconsin

WILLIAM J. KOOPMAN, M.D.

Howard L. Holley Professor of Medicine
Director, Division of Clinical Immunology and Rheumatology
University of Alabama at Birmingham
Birmingham, Alabama

Foreword By
Joseph Lee Hollander, M.D.

ARTHRITIS

AND ALLIED CONDITIONS

A TEXTBOOK OF RHEUMATOLOGY

VOLUME **2**

Twelfth Edition

LEA & FEBIGER ▪ Philadelphia ▪ London ▪ 1993

Lea & Febiger
PO Box 3024
200 Chester Field Parkway
Malvern, Pennsylvania 19355
U.S.A.
(215) 251-2230

Executive Editor—R. Kenneth Bussy
Production Manager—Samuel A. Rondinelli
Project Editor—Susan L. Hunsberger

First Edition, 1940
Second Edition, 1941
Third Edition, 1944
Fourth Edition, 1949
Fifth Edition, 1953
Sixth Edition, 1960
Seventh Edition, 1966
Eighth Edition, 1972
Ninth Edition, 1979
Tenth Edition, 1985
Eleventh Edition, 1989
Twelfth Edition, 1993

Library of Congress Cataloging-in-Publication Data

Arthritis and allied conditions / a textbook of rheumatology. — 12 ed. / [edited by] Daniel J. McCarty, William J. Koopman; foreword by Joseph Lee Hollander.
p. cm.
Includes bibliographical references and index.
ISBN 0-8121-1430-2
1. Arthritis. 2. Rheumatism. 3. Rheumatology. I. McCarty, Daniel J., 1928– . II. Koopman, William J.
[DNLM: 1. Arthritis. WE 344 A7866]
RC933.A64 1993
616.7′22—dc20
DNLM/DLC
for Library of Congress
91-33513
CIP

PRINTED IN THE UNITED STATES OF AMERICA

Print Number 3 2 1

Reprints of chapters may be purchased from Lea & Febiger in quantities of 100 or more. Contact Sally Grande in the Sales Department.

Foreword

More than fifty years have elapsed since Dr. Bernard Comroe, recognizing early the need for a comprehensive textbook on the budding field of arthritis and allied conditions, gathered together what had been written both from his own careful notes and from the early Rheumatism Reviews. These Reviews of American and other English language papers on rheumatic diseases had been collected and edited by a small group of pioneer rheumatologists headed by Phillip Hench, M.D., and published at intervals in the *Annals of Internal Medicine* since 1935.

Having myself studied Comroe's first edition when it appeared in 1940, and now having the opportunity to contrast it with the current twelfth edition, I have watched the tremendous development of rheumatology from its infancy to maturity during my lifetime. This progress is also well documented in *The History of Rheumatology in the United States*, by Charley J. Smyth, M.D., Richard H. Freyberg, M.D., and Currier McEwen, M.D., three of my collaborating editors of previous editions of the textbook, and published by the Arthritis Foundation in 1985.

The authors and editors whose combined efforts have augmented and perpetuated Dr. Comroe's original production of 1940 can pride themselves that they have refined, improved, and greatly expanded the work he began more then a half century ago. While watching the Penn Relays a short time ago, the thought came to me that this time-honored tradition at my medical alma mater symbolizes the repeated collaborative efforts of the many clinicians and scientists working together on *Arthritis and Allied Conditions* over the years. None could have accomplished the final product alone, but the separate efforts added together over these many years have established a tradition of repeated excellence never yet duplicated.

Dan McCarty's superb organizing and editing accomplishments in producing the ninth, tenth, and eleventh editions of this book are well appreciated and this new twelfth edition will cap the pinnacle of his editorship. Comroe, dying after only the third edition, passed the baton to me, and I passed it to Dan after my five editions, but now it startles me, in my eighty-second year, that the time will soon arrive when he will pass the baton to a younger successor. The Relay goes on and on! *Semper fidelis!*

Joseph Lee Hollander, M.D., M.A.C.P., M.A.C.R.

Preface

The twelfth edition of *Arthritis and Allied Conditions—A Textbook of Rheumatology* faithfully records the results of the ever-growing clinical and laboratory studies germane to its field. The eleventh edition was as well received as its predecessors, but a recurring lament was its size and weight, attributable to a change in format, namely larger pages and more of them! This upward creep in the book's size has occurred despite ruthless editing and constant scrutiny to minimize duplication of material in overlapping subjects. Thus, although the twelfth edition contains only three chapters more than the eleventh, we have decided to offer it as a two-volume set.

All major texts benefit from a periodic infusion of new blood, both authorial and editorial. To this end, William J. Koopman, M.D., was recruited as editor. The organization of the thirteenth edition will be largely his responsibility. Twenty-four new authors have contributed to the current edition. As the number of comprehensive textbooks of rheumatology has begun to proliferate, we feel strongly that ours should remain both authoritative and unique. We have adopted a policy that none of our authors may henceforth write on the same subject for competing textbooks. This is only fair to our readership. One competing text, for example, once invited 29 of our authors to contribute chapters identical to those they had written for *Arthritis and Allied Conditions*! Although imitation is the sincerest form of flattery, it seems fair to expect each textbook to develop its own character and viewpoint. There is now sufficient talent in our field to permit such diversity.

Our unique chapters on paleopathology of humans and animals have been retained and expanded. The field of rheumatic disease epidemiology, so important for health planning and in providing insights into disease etiology and definition, has also retained its pre-eminent position in this edition. We address the applications of magnetic resonance (MR) imaging in an expanded chapter by skeletal radiologists, who have been at the cutting edge of this field since its inception. MR has literally blown computed tomography (CT) out of the water. This is reflected by deletion of the CT chapter. We expanded the chapter on bone mineral assessment because many rheumatologists have become interested in the clinical practice of bone and mineral metabolism. Osteopenia will become a larger problem in the populations of developed countries, as these will contain an increasing percentage of aged persons. The field of clinimetrics has matured rapidly in the past few decades. It is addressed here by an innovative senior clinician who has made many of the original advances in this field, working closely with a master statistician. The chapter on joint fluid analysis has been thoroughly revised and interdigitated with the chapters dealing with arthritis related to particulate matter.

Advances in understanding of the structure and function of the joint and its constituent molecules, the mechanisms underlying the inflammatory response, and the molecular basis of the diversity of the immune response have been truly remarkable since the last edition. All chapters covering the scientific basis for the study of the rheumatic diseases have been authored by leaders in their respective fields who are well positioned to interpret the significance of these advances.

Following succinct discussions of the structure of joints and of synovial physiology, new chapters on collagen, proteoglycans, and chondrocyte function provide authoritative treatments of these rapidly developing subjects. The molecular basis of immunoglobulin and T-cell receptor diversity are clearly presented. Several chapters convey exciting new insights concerning the role of immune complexes in disease and the biology of cellular participants in the inflammatory response including macrophages, neutrophils, eosinophils, mast cells, and platelets. It has become clear that adhesion molecules play a critical role in cellular communication and migration; a new chapter provides authoritative insights concerning the structure and function of the molecules and their likely role(s) in rheumatic diseases. Progress in the molecular characterization of several complement component receptors and elucidation of their functional properties has altered thinking concerning the roles of the complement system in inflammation and autoimmunity. A completely rewritten chapter by two experts in this field clearly conveys these new ideas. Recent insights concerning the likely physiologic roles of acute-phase proteins are presented in a new chapter authored by an innovator in the field. The contributions of arachidonic acid metabolites to the inflammatory response are masterfully communicated in a revised chapter. Solution of the three-dimensional structure of human major histocompatibility (MHC) molecules offers hope that precise understanding of the mechanisms underlying the association of some of these molecules with susceptibility to several rheumatic diseases will be achieved; a new chapter concisely describes these exciting advances. The association between some MHC molecules and disease susceptibility likely reflects altered host responses to an infectious agent(s); a re-written chapter provides a detailed discussion of the possible role of infectious agents in chronic rheumatic disease. Animal models offer the best hope for ultimately delineating the pathogenesis of their human disease counterparts. New insights gained from the intensive study of animal models of rheumatic disease are delineated in a new chapter.

Although remarkable progress has occurred in understanding the mechanisms contributing to the pathogenesis of several rheumatic diseases, therapy has lagged. Nonetheless, growing experience with the use of sulfasalazine and methotrexate in treatment of several rheumatic diseases prompted addition of separate chapters for these agents. Expanded indications for the use of cytotoxic agents have become apparent and are clearly described in a substantially rewritten chapter. This chapter also presents a scholarly discussion concerning the controversial use of combination drug therapy in rheumatoid arthritis (RA). Although corticosteroids have been a mainstay of rheumatic disease therapy for four decades, a new chapter provides fresh insights regarding the mechanisms underlying the efficacy of these agents and advances the provocative notion that defects in regulation of glucocorticoid homeostasis may contribute to the pathogenesis of rheumatic disease, a concept pioneered by the authors. Finally, improved understanding of the mechanisms underlying immune responses and chronic inflammation has fostered the development of a host of promising biologic agents destined to be tested in the clinic. Early experience with the use of these agents is described in a completely rewritten chapter.

Rheumatoid arthritis remains the prototypic rheumatic disease, and as such retains its place as the focus of the first clinical section of this edition. Newly recognized syndromes that superficially resemble it are discussed in the context of its clinical picture. The drug treatment of RA has undergone rapid recent conceptual changes, as discussed in the chapter devoted to this subject. Newer developments that have led to successful elbow and shoulder joint surgery have resulted in these now being considered in separate chapters.

The exciting new developments in reactive arthritis and enteropathic arthritis are addressed by investigators who have played major roles in these fields. Understanding of the immunologic aspects of systemic lupus has continued to expand; interest in humeral autoantibodies and in cellular immunoregulation continues apace, as discussed by authors who have long been at the forefront of these topics. The antiphospholipid antibody syndromes continue to exhibit more clinical signs and symptoms, as discussed by the originator of this exciting new area of lupus research. The chapter on scleroderma and related syndromes has been shortened by discussing pathogenesis in a separate chapter. A chapter on cerebral vasculitis has been added, providing a focused discussion on this important, underemphasized topic that comes up so frequently in rheumatologic consultation. The advent of ever more precise imaging techniques has injected this subject with new importance.

The enigmatic field of fibromyalgia and related syndromes has been critically addressed by new authors who have long provided thoughtful studies on these subjects. Recent insights into the etiology and pathogenesis of osteoarthritis (OA) have been profound, as discussed by authors who have been very much responsible for them. Therapy has not yet caught up with these developments, and it is conceivable that some current drugs may actually be harmful. As in OA, elegant studies at the cellular and molecular level have expanded the frontier of the arthritic diseases associated with the deposition of microcrystals. Apart from gout, successful drug therapy again lags. The field of metabolic muscle disease is developing rapidly, as discussed by a rheumatologist expert in this arena. Rheumatologists must be aware of these conditions in the differential diagnosis of patients presenting with weakness. The osteopenic bone diseases are also discussed by a rheumatologist who has contributed much to their understanding, and this complements the introductory chapter on bone mineral assessment.

A chapter on the basic biology of borreliosis has been added to complement that on Lyme disease. Although this disease is potentially curable, many diagnostic and therapeutic problems remain to be solved. Last, an overdue chapter has been written on the diverse rheumatic syndromes that may accompany infection with retroviruses such as the human immunodeficiency viruses (HIV-1 and HIV-2) and human T-cell lymphotrophic virus 1(HTLV-1).

In conclusion, we believe that the 12 editions of this textbook covering the period of 53 years from 1940 to 1993 have recorded the countless small steps that have advanced rheumatology as a respected scientific medical specialty. As always, we are grateful to our hard-working authors and remain open to suggestions from our readers as to how we can make this book even better.

Daniel J. McCarty, M.D.

Milwaukee, Wisconsin

William J. Koopman, M.D.

Birmingham, Alabama

Contributors

GRACIELA S. ALARCON, M.D., M.P.H.
Professor of Medicine and Associate Director
Alabama Multipurpose Arthritis and Musculoskeletal Diseases Center
University of Alabama at Birmingham
Birmingham, Alabama

ROY D. ALTMAN, M.D.
Professor of Medicine
University of Miami School of Medicine
Chief, Arthritis Section
Miami VA Medical Center
Miami, Florida

PAUL A. BACON, M.D.
Professor of Rheumatology and Head of Department
Department of Rheumatology
University of Birmingham Medical School
Birmingham, England

GENE V. BALL, M.D.
Jane Knight Lowe Professor of Medicine in Rheumatology
University of Alabama at Birmingham
Birmingham, Alabama

JOHN BAUM, M.D.
Professor of Medicine, Pediatrics and Orthopedics
Director, Arthritis/Immunology Unit
Monroe Community Hospital
Co-Director Pediatric Rheumatology Clinic
University of Rochester
Strong Memorial Hospital
Rochester, New York

MICHAEL A. BECKER, M.D.
Professor of Medicine
Department of Medicine
Section of Rheumatology
University of Chicago
Chicago, Illinois

NICHOLAS BELLAMY, M.D., M.Sc., F.R.C.P.(Glas.), F.R.C.P.(Edin.), F.R.C.P.(C), F.A.C.P.
Associate Professor of Medicine, Epidemiology, and Biostatistics
University of Western Ontario, London, Ontario
Associate Professor of Clinical Epidemiology and Biostatistics
McMaster University
Hamilton, Canada

J. CLAUDE BENNETT, M.D.
Professor and Chairman
Department of Medicine
University of Alabama at Birmingham
Birmingham, Alabama

ROBERT M. BENNETT, M.D., F.R.C.P., F.A.C.P.
Professor of Medicine
Director, Arthritis and Rheumatic Diseases Division
Oregon Health Sciences University
Portland, Oregon

W. WATSON BUCHANAN, M.D.
Professor of Medicine
Director of Rheumatic Disease Unit
McMaster University Health Sciences Center
Hamilton, Ontario, Canada

GRANT W. CANNON, M.D.
Associate Chief of Staff for Education
VA Medical Center
Associate Professor of Medicine
Division of Rheumatology
University of Utah School of Medicine
Salt Lake City, Utah

JUAN J. CANOSO, M.D.
Professor of Medicine
Tufts University School of Medicine
Director, Clinical Rheumatology
New England Medical Center
Boston, Massachusetts

C. WILLIAM CASTOR, M.D.
Professor of Internal Medicine
Rackham Arthritis Research Unit and Rheumatology Division
Associate Director
Multipurpose Arthritis Center
University of Michigan Medical Center
Ann Arbor, Michigan

DANIEL O. CLEGG, M.D.
Associate Professor of Medicine
Associate Chief, Division of Rheumatology
University of Utah School of Medicine
Salt Lake City, Utah

ALAN S. COHEN, M.D.
Director, Thorndike Memorial Laboratory, Boston City Hospital
Chief of Medicine
Boston City Hospital
Conrad Wesselhoeft Professor of Medicine
Boston University School of Medicine
Boston, Massachusetts

LESLIE J. CROFFORD, M.D.
Senior Clinical Investigator—Arthritis and Rheumatism Branch
National Institute of Arthritis and Musculoskeletal and Skin Diseases
National Institutes of Health
Bethesda, Maryland

MARY E. CRONIN, M.D.
Assistant Professor of Medicine
Division of Rheumatology
Medical College of Wisconsin
Milwaukee, Wisconsin

BRUCE N. CRONSTEIN, M.D.
Assistant Professor of Medicine
New York University Medical Center
New York, New York

JOHN J. CUSH, M.D.
Assistant Professor of Internal Medicine
The University of Texas Southwestern Medical Center
Dallas, Texas

PAUL DIEPPE, M.D., B.Sc., F.R.C.P.
ARC Professor of Rheumatology
University of Bristol
Bristol Royal Infirmary
Bristol, England

JOSEPH DUFFY, M.D.
Department of Internal Medicine
Division of Rheumatology
Mayo Clinic
Rochester, Minnesota

MICHAEL J. EBERSOLD, M.D.
Associate Professor of Neurological Surgery
Mayo Medical School
Consultant, Department of Neurological Surgery
Mayo Clinic and Foundation
Rochester, Minnesota

MICHAEL H. ELLMAN, M.D.
Director, Division of Rheumatology
Humana Hospital—Michael Reese
Associate Professor of Clinical Medicine
College of Medicine, Department of Medicine
University of Illinois at Chicago
Chicago, Illinois

EDGAR G. ENGLEMAN, M.D.
Professor of Pathology and Medicine
Stanford University Medical Center
Palo Alto, California

LUIS R. ESPINOZA, M.D.
Professor of Medicine
Chief, Section of Rheumatology
School of Medicine in New Orleans
Louisiana State University
New Orleans, Louisiana

ANTHONY S. FAUCI, M.D.
Director, National Institute of Allergy and Infectious Diseases
National Institutes of Health
Bethesda, Maryland

DOUGLAS T. FEARON, M.D.
Professor of Medicine
Director, Division of Molecular and Clinical Rheumatology
Director of the Graduate Program in Immunology
Johns Hopkins University School of Medicine
Baltimore, Maryland

DAVID T. FELSON, M.D., M.P.H.
Associate Professor of Medicine and Public Health
Boston University School of Medicine
Boston, Massachusetts

ADRIAN E. FLATT, M.D.
Chairman
Department of Orthopaedics
Baylor University Medical Center
Clinical Professor
University of Texas Southwestern Medical Center
Dallas, Texas

ROBERT I. FOX, M.D., Ph.D.
Adjunct Associate Member
Department of Immunology
Scripps Clinic and Research Foundation
La Jolla, California

DANIEL E. FURST, M.D.
Clinical Professor of Rheumatology/Medicine
University of Medicine and Dentistry of New Jersey
Robert Wood Johnson Medical School
New Brunswick, New Jersey

ROBERT A. GATTER, M.D.
Associate Clinical Professor of Medicine
University of Pennsylvania School of Medicine
Philadelphia, Pennsylvania
Physician-in-Chief, Division of Rheumatology
Abington Memorial Hospital
Abington, Pennsylvania
Director, Center for Arthritis and Back Pain
Willow Grove, Pennsylvania

HARRY K. GENANT, M.D.
Professor of Radiology, Medicine, and Orthopaedic Surgery
Chief of Skeletal Radiology
Director, Osteoporosis Research Group
University of California
San Francisco, California

MARK H. GINSBERG, M.D.
Committee on Vascular Biology
Scripps Clinic and Research Foundation
La Jolla, California

EDWARD J. GOETZL, M.D.
Robert L. Kroc Professor of Rheumatic Diseases
University of California
San Francisco, California

DON L. GOLDENBERG, M.D., P.C.
Chief of Rheumatology
Newton-Wellesley Hospital
Newton, Massachusetts
Professor of Medicine
Tufts University School of Medicine
Boston, Massachusetts

IRA M. GOLDSTEIN, M.D.
Professor of Medicine
University of California, San Francisco
School of Medicine
San Francisco, California

JOHN S. GOULD, M.D.
Professor and Chairman
Department of Orthopaedic Surgery
Medical College of Wisconsin
Director, Orthopaedic Surgery
Milwaukee County Medical Complex
Milwaukee, Wisconsin

BARRY L. GRUBER, M.D.
Assistant Professor of Medicine
Department of Medicine
State University of New York at Stony Brook
Stony Brook, New York

NORTIN M. HADLER, M.D.
Professor of Medicine and Microbiology/Immunology
Department of Medicine
University of North Carolina at Chapel Hill
Chapel Hill, NC

BEVRA HANNAHS HAHN, M.D.
Professor of Medicine
Chief of Rheumatology
University of California, Los Angeles
UCLA School of Medicine
Los Angeles, California

JAMES T. HALLA, M.D.
Private Practice
Abilene, Texas

PAUL B. HALVERSON, M.D.
Associate Professor of Medicine
Medical College of Wisconsin
Milwaukee, Wisconsin

JOE G. HARDIN, M.D.
Professor of Medicine
Department of Internal Medicine
University of South Alabama College of Medicine
Mobile, Alabama

E. NIGEL HARRIS, M.PHIL., M.D., D.M.
Associate Professor of Medicine
Department of Medicine
University of Louisville
Louisville, Kentucky

LOUIS A. HEALEY, M.D.
Clinical Professor of Medicine
University of Washington
Head, Section of Rheumatology
The Mason Clinic
Seattle, Washington

GEORGE HO, JR., M.D.
Associate Professor of Medicine
Division of Rheumatology
The Miriam Hospital
Brown University
Providence, Rhode Island

DAVID A. HORWITZ, M.D.
Professor of Medicine and Microbiology
Chief, Division of Immunology/Rheumatology
School of Medicine
University of Southern California
Los Angeles, California

AUBREY J. HOUGH, JR., M.D.
Professor and Chairman, Department of Pathology
University of Arkansas College of Medicine
Little Rock, Arkansas

DAVID S. HOWELL, M.D.
Director, Arthritis Division
Professor of Medicine
Medical Investigator/VAMC
Department of Medicine
University of Miami
Miami, Florida

GRAHAM R. V. HUGHES, M.D., F.R.C.P.
Consultant Rheumatologist and Head, Lupus Arthritis Research Unit
The Rayne Institute
St. Thomas Hospital
London, England

ERNST B. HUNZIKER, M.D.
Professor of Biomechanics
University of Bern
Bern, Switzerland

ROBERT D. INMAN, M.D.
Professor of Medicine and Immunology
Director of Rheumatic Disease Unit
University of Toronto
Toronto, Ontario, Canada

JOHN N. INSALL, M.D.
Professor of Orthopaedic Surgery
Cornell University Medical College
Director, Insall Scott Kelly Institute for Orthopaedic and Sports Medicine
Attending Orthopaedic Surgeon
Beth Israel Hospital North
New York, New York

RUSSELL C. JOHNSON, PH.D.
Professor of Microbiology
Department of Microbiology
University of Minnesota
Minneapolis, Minnesota

JOHN PAUL JONES, JR., M.D.
Medical Research Director
Diagnostic Osteonecrosis Center and Research Foundation
Kelseyville, California

LAWRENCE J. KAGEN, M.D.
Professor of Medicine
Cornell University Medical College
Attending Physician
The Hospital for Special Surgery
Attending Physician
The New York Hospital
New York, New York

HOIL KANG, M.D., PH.D.
Research Fellow
The Scripps Research Institute
La Jolla, California

GEOFFREY S. KANSAS, PH.D.
Research Associate, Division of Tumor Immunology
Dana Farber Cancer Institute and Department of Pathology
Harvard Medical School
Boston, Massachusetts

ALLEN P. KAPLAN, M.D.
Chairman, Department of Medicine
School of Medicine
Health Sciences Center
State University of New York at Stony Brook
Stony Brook, New York

MUNTHER A. KHAMASHTA, M.D., PH.D.
Deputy Director, Lupus Arthritis Research Unit
The Rayne Institute
Honorary Consultant Physician and Senior Lecturer
St. Thomas Hospital
London, England

WILLIAM J. KOOPMAN, M.D.
Howard L. Holley Professor of Medicine
Director, Division of Clinical Immunology and Rheumatology
University of Alabama at Birmingham
Birmingham, Alabama

FRANKLIN KOZIN, M.D.
Division of Rheumatology
Scripps Clinic Medical Group, Inc.
La Jolla, California

STEPHEN M. KRANE, M.D.
Persis, Cyrus and Marlow B. Harrison Professor of Medicine
Harvard Medical School
Physician and Chief, Arthritis Unit
Massachusetts General Hospital
Boston, Massachusetts

NANCY E. LANE, M.D.
Assistant Professor of Medicine and Rheumatology
Division of Rheumatology
University of California San Francisco Medical School
San Francisco, California

SANFORD J. LARSON, M.D., PH.D.
Professor and Chairman, Department of Neurosurgery
Medical College of Wisconsin
Milwaukee, Wisconsin

RANDI Y. LEAVITT, M.D., PH.D.
Assistant Chief
Laboratory of Immunoregulation
National Institute of Allergy and Infectious Diseases
National Institutes of Health
Bethesda, Maryland

JAMES M. LEIPZIG, M.D.
Assistant Professor of Orthopedic Surgery
The Ohio State University
Columbus, Ohio

E. CARWILE LeROY, M.D.
Rheumatology Division
Medical University of South Carolina
Charleston, South Carolina

DAVID B. LEVINE, M.D.
Hospital for Special Surgery
New York, New York

DENNIS J. LEVINSON, M.D.
Clinical Associate Professor of Medicine
Division of Rheumatology
University of Illinois
Chicago, Illinois

ROBERT W. LIGHTFOOT, JR., M.D.
Professor of Medicine
Director, Division of Rheumatology
University of Kentucky Medical Center
Lexington, Kentucky

PETER E. LIPSKY, M.D.
Professor of Internal Medicine and Microbiology
Director, Rheumatic Diseases Division
Director, Harold C. Simmons Arthritis Research Center
University of Texas, Southwestern Medical Center
Dallas, Texas

ALBERT LoBUGLIO, M.D.
Director, Comprehensive Cancer Center
Professor of Medicine
Division of Hematology-Oncology
University of Alabama at Birmingham
Birmingham, Alabama

STEPHEN E. MALAWISTA, M.D.
Professor of Medicine
Department of Medicine
Yale University School of Medicine
New Haven, Connecticut

HENRY J. MANKIN, M.D.
Chief of the Orthopaedic Service
Massachusetts General Hospital
Edith M. Ashley Professor of Orthopaedics
Harvard Medical School
Boston, Massachusetts

ROGER A. MANN, M.D.
Director, Foot Fellowship
Oakland, California
Associate Clinical Professor of Orthopedic Surgery
University of California Medical School
San Francisco, California

MART MANNIK, M.D.
Professor of Medicine
Head, Division of Rheumatology
University of Washington
Seattle, Washington

ALFONSE T. MASI, M.D., DR.P.H.
Professor, Department of Medicine
University of Illinois College of Medicine at Peoria
Peoria, Illinois

DANIEL J. MCCARTY, M.D.
Will and Cava Ross Professor
Department of Medicine
Director, Arthritis Institute
Medical College of Wisconsin
Milwaukee, Wisconsin

THOMAS A. MEDSGER, JR., M.D.
Professor of Medicine
Chief, Division of Rheumatology and Clinical Immunology
University of Pittsburgh School of Medicine
Pittsburgh, Pennsylvania

RONALD P. MESSNER, M.D.
Professor of Medicine
Director, Section of Rheumatology
University of Minnesota
Minneapolis, Minnesota

HERMAN MIELANTS, M.D.
Professor of Rheumatology
Department of Rheumatology
University Hospital
Ghent, Belgium

ROLAND W. MOSKOWITZ, M.D.
Professor of Medicine
Case Western Reserve University
Director, Division of Rheumatic Diseases
University Hospitals
Cleveland, Ohio

SHAWN W. O'DRISCOLL, M.D., PH.D., FRCS (C)
Director, Cartilage and Connective Tissue Research Laboratory and Orthopedic Consultant
Upper Extremity Reconstructive Service
St. Michael's Hospital
Assistant Professor of Orthopaedic Surgery
University of Toronto
Toronto, Canada

J. DESMOND O'DUFFY, M.D.
Department of Internal Medicine
Division of Rheumatology
Mayo Clinic
Rochester, Minnesota

LAUREN M. PACHMAN, M.D.
Professor of Pediatrics
Northwestern University Medical School
Head, Division of Immunology/Rheumatology
Children's Memorial Hospital
Chicago, Illinois

RICHARD S. PANUSH, M.D.
Chairman, Department of Medicine
Saint Barnabas Medical Center
Livingston, New Jersey
Professor of Medicine
University of Medicine and Dentistry of New Jersey
Newark, New Jersey

HAROLD E. PAULUS, M.D.
Professor of Medicine
Division of Rheumatology
University of California, Los Angeles
Los Angeles, California

JEAN-PIERRE PELLETIER, M.D., F.R.C.P.C.
Associate Professor of Medicine
University of Montreal
Head, Arthritis Division
Director, Cartilage Research Laboratory
Notre Dame Hospital
Montreal, Quebec, Canada

ROSS E. PETTY, M.D., Ph.D., F.R.C.P.C.
Professor, Department of Pediatrics
Head, Division of Pediatric Rheumatology
The University of British Columbia and British Columbia's Children's Hospital
Vancouver, British Columbia, Canada

PAUL E. PHILLIPS, M.D., FACP, FACR
Professor of Medicine and Pediatrics
Chief, Division of Clinical Immunology
SUNY Health Science Center
Syracuse, New York

MARILYN C. PIKE, M.D., Ph.D.
Assistant Professor of Medicine
Massachusetts General Hospital
Boston, Massachusetts

ROBERT S. PINALS, M.D.
Professor of Medicine
Associate Chairman, Department of Medicine
UMDNJ—Robert Wood Johnson Medical School
New Brunswick
The Medical Center at Princeton
Princeton, New Jersey

SETH H. PINCUS, M.D.
Expert, Laboratory of Microbial Structure and Function
N.I.A.I.D. Rocky Mountain Laboratories
Hamilton, Montana
Adjunct Associate Professor
Division of Rheumatology
University of Utah School of Medicine
Salt Lake City, Utah

A. ROBIN POOLE, Ph.D., DSc
Director, Joint Disease Laboratory
Professor, Department of Surgery
McGill University
Montreal, Quebec, Canada

ANDREW K. POZNANSKI, M.D.
Professor of Radiology
Northwestern University Medical School
Radiologist-in-Chief
The Children's Memorial Hospital
Chicago, Illinois

DARWIN J. PROCKOP, M.D., Ph.D.
Professor and Chairman
Department of Biochemistry and Molecular Biology
Director, Jefferson Institute of Molecular Medicine
Thomas Jefferson University
Philadelphia, Pennsylvania

REED E. PYERITZ, M.D., Ph.D.
Professor of Medicine and Pediatrics
Clinical Director, Center for Medical Genetics
The Johns Hopkins University School of Medicine
Baltimore, Maryland

ERIC L. RADIN, M.D.
Director, Bone and Joint Center
Henry Ford Hospital
Clinical Professor of Surgery
University of Michigan
Detroit, Michigan

DANIEL W. RAHN, M.D.
Associate Professor of Medicine
Department of Internal Medicine
Yale University School of Medicine
New Haven, Connecticut

ANTONIO J. REGINATO, M.D.
Professor of Medicine
Head, Division of Rheumatology
UMDNJ—Robert Wood Johnson Medical School at Camden
Camden, New Jersey

MORRIS REICHLIN, M.D.
Head, Arthritis/Immunology
Oklahoma Medical Research Foundation
Oklahoma City, Oklahoma

JULIET M. ROGERS, M.D., Ch.B.
Lecturer, Paleopathology
Rheumatology Unit
Bristol Royal Infirmary
Bristol, England

THEODORE W. ROONEY, D.O., F.A.C.P.
Medical Director
Mercy Arthritis Center
Des Moines, Iowa

LAWRENCE ROSENBERG, M.D.
Professor of Orthopaedic Surgery
Albert Einstein College of Medicine
Director of Orthopaedic Research
Montefiore Medical Center
Bronx, New York

NAOMI F. ROTHFIELD, M.D.
Professor of Medicine
Chief, Division of Rheumatic Diseases
University of Connecticut Health Center
Farmington, Connecticut

BRUCE M. ROTHSCHILD, M.D.
Professor and Director
Northeastern Ohio Universities College of Medicine
Professor and Director
The Arthritis Center of Northeast Ohio
Youngstown, Ohio

LORNE A. RUNGE, M.D.
Clinical Associate Professor
State University of New York
Health Science Center at Syracuse
Syracuse, New York

DORAN E. RYAN, D.D.S., M.S.
Associate Professor and Chairman
Oral and Maxillofacial Surgery
Medical College of Wisconsin
Clinical Professor
Marquette University School of Dentistry
Milwaukee, Wisconsin

LAWRENCE M. RYAN, M.D.
Professor and Chief, Rheumatology
Medical College of Wisconsin
Milwaukee, Wisconsin

MANSOOR SALEH, M.D.
Assistant Professor of Medicine
Division of Hematology-Oncology
Associate Scientist
Comprehensive Cancer Center
University of Alabama Medical Center
Birmingham, Alabama

FRANK R. SCHMID, M.D.
Professor of Medicine
Arthritis-Connective Tissue Disease Section
Northwestern University Medical School
Chicago, Illinois

THOMAS J. SCHNITZER, M.D., PH.D.
Willard L. Wood, M.D., Professor of Medicine
Director, Sections of Rheumatology and Geriatric Medicine
Medical Director, Johnston R. Bowman Health Center for Elderly
Rush-Presbyterian St. Luke's Medical Center
Chicago, Illinois

HARRY W. SCHROEDER, JR., M.D., PH.D.
Assistant Professor of Medicine and Microbiology
Division of Developmental and Clinical Immunology
The University of Alabama at Birmingham
Birmingham, Alabama

RALPH E. SCHROHENLOHER, PH.D.
Professor of Medicine
Division of Clinical Immunology and Rheumatology
The University of Alabama at Birmingham
Birmingham, Alabama

H. RALPH SCHUMACHER, JR., M.D.
Professor of Medicine and Acting Chief Rheumatology
University of Pennsylvania School of Medicine
Director, Arthritis-Immunology Center
Veterans Administration Medical Center
Philadelphia, Pennsylvania

BENJAMIN D. SCHWARTZ, M.D., PH.D.
Director, Immunology
Montsanto Corporate Research
Saint Louis, Missouri

GORDON C. SHARP, M.D.
Einbender Professor of Medicine and Pathology
Director, Division of Immunology and Rheumatology
University of Missouri-Columbia School of Medicine
Columbia, Missouri

WILMER L. SIBBITT, JR., M.D.
Associate Professor, Rheumatology
Director of Medical Research
Center for Non-Invasive Diagnosis
University of New Mexico School of Medicine
Albuquerque, New Mexico

LEONARD H. SIGAL, M.D.
Associate Professor, Department of Medicine
Adjunct Assistant Professor, Department of Molecular Genetics and Microbiology
Acting Chief, Division of Rheumatology
UMDNJ—Robert Wood Johnson Medical School
New Brunswick, New Jersey

PETER A. SIMKIN, M.D.
Professor of Medicine
Adjunct Professor of Orthopaedics
Department of Medicine
University of Washington
Seattle, Washington

BERNHARD H. SINGSEN, M.D., M.P.H.
Professor, Department of Pediatrics
Thomas Jefferson University
Chief, Division of Rheumatology
Alfred I. Dupont Institute
Wilmington, Delaware

JOHN L. SKOSEY, M.D., PH.D.
Professor of Medicine
Chief, Section of Rheumatology
University of Illinois at Chicago
Chicago, Illinois

RALPH SNYDERMAN, M.D.
Chancellor for Health Affairs
Duke University Medical Center
Durham, North Carolina

RICHARD N. STAUFFER, M.D.
Robinson Professor and Director
Orthopaedic Surgeon-in-Chief
Johns Hopkins Medical Institutions
Baltimore, Maryland

ESTHER M. STERNBERG, M.D.
Chief, Unit on Neuroendocrine Immunology and Behavior
National Institutes of Health/NIHM
Bethesda, Maryland

JAMES B. STIEHL, M.D.
Assistant Professor, Orthopaedic Surgery
Medical College of Wisconsin
Milwaukee, Wisconsin

DAVID W. STOLLER, M.D.
Assistant Clinical Professor, Skeletal Radiology
University of California, San Francisco
Medical Director
California Advanced Imaging
San Francisco, California

NOBORU SUZUKI, M.D.
Institute of Medical Science
St. Marianna University School of Medicine
Kawasaki City, Japan

ROBERT L. SWEZEY, M.D., FACP, FACR
Clinical Professor of Medicine, U.C.L.A.
Medical Director
The Arthritis and Back Pain Center
The Swezey Institute Building
Santa Monica, California

NORMAN TALAL, M.D.
Professor of Medicine and Microbiology
Head, Division of Clinical Immunology
University of Texas Health Science Center at San Antonio
San Antonio, Texas

ENG M. TAN, M.D.
Director, Autoimmune Disease Center
Scripps Clinic and Research Foundation
La Jolla, California

ANGELO TARANTA, M.D.
Professor of Medicine
New York Medical College
Director of Medicine
Cabrini Medical Center
New York, New York

ROBERT A. TERKELTAUB, M.D.
Assistant Professor of Medicine in Residence
University of California, San Diego
Chief, VA Rheumatology Section
Veterans Administration Hospital
San Diego, California

DAVID E. TRENTHAM, M.D.
Chief, Division of Rheumatology
Beth Israel Hospital
Associate Professor of Medicine
Harvard Medical School
Boston, Massachusetts

PHILIPP VANDENBERG, M.D.
Research Associate
Department of Biochemistry and Molecular Biology
Thomas Jefferson University
Philadelphia, Pennsylvania

ERIC M. VEYS, M.D.
Professor of Rheumatology
Ghent University Hospital
Ghent, Belgium

JOHN E. VOLANAKIS, M.D.
Anna Lois Waters Chair of Medicine in Rheumatology
Professor of Medicine, Microbiology and Pathology
University of Alabama at Birmingham
Birmingham, Alabama

JOHN R. WARD, M.D.
Professor of Medicine, Department of Internal Medicine
University of Utah School of Medicine
Salt Lake City, Utah

MICHAEL H. WEISMAN, M.D.
Professor of Clinical Medicine
Division of Rheumatology, Department of Medicine
University of California Medical Center
San Diego, California

GERALD WEISSMANN, M.D.
Professor of Medicine
Director, Division of Rheumatology
New York University Medical Center
New York, New York

PETER F. WELLER, M.D.
Associate Professor of Medicine
Harvard Medical School
Boston, Massachusetts

RONALD L. WILDER, M.D., PH.D.
Senior Investigator
Arthritis and Rheumatism Branch
National Institute of Arthritis and Musculoskeletal and Skin Diseases
National Institutes of Health
Bethesda, Maryland

CHARLENE J. WILLIAMS, PH.D.
Research Assistant Professor
Department of Biochemistry and Molecular Biology
Thomas Jefferson University
Philadelphia, Pennsylvania

RUSSELL E. WINDSOR, M.D.
Associate Professor of Surgery
Cornell University Medical College
Associate Attending Physician, Associate Chief, Knee Surgery
The Hospital for Special Surgery
New York, New York

ROBERT L. WORTMANN, M.D.
Professor and Chief, Medical Services
Veterans Administration Medical Center
Vice Chairman, Medicine
Interim Chairman, Department of Medicine
Medical College of Wisconsin
Milwaukee, Wisconsin

STEVEN R. YTTERBERG, M.D.
Rheumatology Section
Veteran Administration Medical Center
Minneapolis, Minnesota

MUHAMMAD B. YUNUS, M.D.
Associate Professor of Medicine
Section of Rheumatology
Department of Medicine
University of Illinois College of Medicine at Peoria
Peoria, Illinois

MORRIS ZIFF, M.D., PH.D.
Ashbel Smith Professor Emeritus of Internal Medicine
Morris Ziff Professor Emeritus of Rheumatology
The University of Texas Southwestern Medical Center
Dallas, Texas

NATHAN J. ZVAIFLER, M.D.
Professor of Medicine
Division of Rheumatology
University of California Medical Center, San Diego
San Diego, California

SAMUEL H. ZWILLICH, M.D.
Assistant Professor of Medicine
University of Rochester School of Medicine and Dentistry
Rochester, New York

Contents

VOLUME 1

Introduction Joseph Lee Hollander, M.D.

I INTRODUCTION TO THE STUDY OF THE RHEUMATIC DISEASES

II SCIENTIFIC BASIS FOR THE STUDY OF THE RHEUMATIC DISEASES

V OTHER INFLAMMATORY ARTHRITIC SYNDROMES

VOLUME 2

VI SYSTEMATIC RHEUMATIC DISEASES

IX OSTEOARTHRITIS

X METABOLIC BONE AND JOINT DISEASES

SECTION VI

Systemic Rheumatic Diseases

66

Introduction to Systemic Rheumatic Diseases: Nosology and Overlap Syndromes

MORRIS REICHLIN

The diffuse connective tissue diseases are a group of syndromes of unknown origin whose classification often presents formidable clinical problems. One cause of this classification problem is the large number of "overlap syndromes," which exist among and between what are manifestly uncommon conditions. Dubois stated that as many as 25% of all patients with diffuse rheumatic disease will have overlapping features.[1] These findings include coexistent systemic lupus erythematosus (SLE) and scleroderma; an overlap of SLE, scleroderma, and polymyositis (PM), which has been called mixed connective tissue disease (MCTD); scleroderma-PM; coexistent SLE and rheumatoid arthritis (RA); and the relationship that lymphocytic infiltration of the lacrimal and salivary glands bears to all of the diffuse connective tissue diseases in what is recognized as Sjögren's syndrome.

Two current areas of investigation show promise for identifying specific biologic or biochemical markers that could be tightly linked with specific disease processes. These areas are (1) immunogenetics and (2) the identification of individual antigen-antibody reactions that exhibit disease specificity. The former subject is covered in Chapter 28, whereas the latter subject is discussed in many other chapters. Some specific aspects of this latter approach are explored here.

CLASSIFICATION OF POLYMYOSITIS

These problems are best illustrated by considering the classification of one group of these diseases, the PM syndromes. A clinical diagnosis of PM depends on the recognition of a pattern of proximal muscle weakness, on characteristic histopathologic findings in muscle biopsy specimens, on electromyography (EMG), and on the presence of elevated serum muscle enzyme levels, notably creatine phosphokinase (CK), transaminases, and aldolase (see Chapter 72). Further study could also suggest the presence of another of the connective tissue diseases, such as RA, SLE, scleroderma, or Sjögren's (sicca) syndrome. If no features of another connective tissue disease are present, one views the patient as simply having PM or, if a characteristic dermatitis accompanies the muscle involvement, dermatomyositis (DM). This group of patients has long been believed to carry an increased risk for various carcinomas, although questions have been raised about the extent of this relationship.[2]

Nosology is often complicated by the variable presence in the diffuse rheumatic diseases of shared clinical features. Polyarthritis and Raynaud's phenomenon can appear in PM patients without other clinical or serologic features that suggest the presence of other connective tissue diseases. In early evaluations, one might be erroneously led to the diagnosis of either SLE or scleroderma. Opportunities for confusion abound.

Is PM one or many diseases with one or many pathogenetic mechanisms and one or many causes? PM occurring by itself is not distinguishable on clinical grounds from PM coincident with another connective tissue disease, and no solid clinical clues exist to differentiate the various forms of PM. Although nothing is known of the causes of these diseases, something is known of their pathogenesis.[3] Evidence for humoral mechanisms, either immune complex–mediated or organ-specific, is sparse, whereas evidence supporting a cell-mediated immune attack on muscle is strong.[3] Lymphocytes found in patients with PM are specifically cytotoxic for muscle cells and do not require serum factors for their activity. The presence and intensity of the activity of such cells correlates roughly with clinical disease activity. It is likely that such muscle-specific cytotoxic lymphocytes constitute the immunopathogenetic mechanism leading to muscle destruction and weakness in PM.

In the future, identification of the precise muscle antigens responsible for the activation of lymphocytes might shed light on the identity or nonidentity of immunopathogenetic pathways in different patients with PM. If lymphocytes are activated by a single, unique, muscle-specific antigen, considerable importance will be given to the idea that a unitary immune mechanism exists in all PM patients. If, however, a group of lymphocytes from patients with PM, DM, or PM associated with another connective tissue disease reacts to a specific but different antigen, the alternative idea that PM is a collection of separate diseases in which the original sensitization process is characteristic for each case would be more attractive. Finally, if such investigations reveal no pattern of antigenic specificity, such studies will have failed to improve our ability to classify these diseases. So far the detection of relatively specific "marker" antibodies for the various connective tissue diseases is encouraging.

The rest of this chapter will describe a group of specific antigen antibody reactions that show in some instances an exquisite specificity for patients with myositis in overlap with interstitial lung disease and in other instances with other systemic rheumatic diseases, particularly SLE and progressive systemic sclerosis (PSS). The autoantibody specificities that are strongly associated with PM and DM are listed in Table 66–1.

TABLE 66–1. MYOSITIS-SPECIFIC AUTOANTIBODIES AND THEIR CLINICAL SUBSETS

AUTOANTIGENIC TARGET	DISEASE-SPECIFIC ASSOCIATIONS
Jo_1—histidyl tRNA synthetase PL-7—threonyl tRNA synthetase PL-12—alanyl tRNA synthetase alanyl tRNA OJ—isoleucyl tRNA synthetase EJ—glycyl tRNA synthetase KJ—unknown translation factor	Polymyositis with interstitial lung disease
Signal recognition particle	Polymyositis without interstitial lung disease
Mi_2 nuclear protein	Dermatomyositis
PM-Scl nucleolar protein	PM/DM, PSS, PM/PSS overlap
U_2RNP, U_1RNP	PM overlap with SLE, PSS

ANTIBODIES TO tRNA SYNTHETASES

The first antibody that was found to be a marker for PM was the anti-Jo_1 system demonstrated by the precipitin reaction of sera with calf thymus extract. This precipitin was found in about 30% of patients with PM and was rarely found in DM patients.[4] Rosa et al. showed that anti-Jo_1 sera bound only histidyl tRNA, but that an unidentified protein was the antigenic target because the histidyl tRNA did not bind directly to the antibody.[5] Mathews and Bernstein suggested that the antigenic target was the cognate enzyme histidyl tRNA synthetase because anti-Jo_1 effectively inhibited the aminoacylation of histidine but not any of the other 19 amino acids.[6] Subsequent work directly proved this point because the Jo_1 antigen eluted from anti-Jo_1 IgG affinity columns had aminoacylation activity only for histidine.[7]

Subsequent work has shown that the threonyl and alanyl tRNA synthetases are less frequent targets of autoantibodies in polymyositis patients and that a few PM patients with anti-alanyl tRNA synthetase also produce antibodies to the alanyl tRNA.[8,9] Production of antibodies to the tRNA itself is thus far unique to the alanyl tRNA. PM patients rarely produce antibodies to either the isoleucyl or the glycyl tRNA synthetases.[10]

The clinical correlates of these autoantibodies are an increased frequency of interstitial lung disease (ILD), Raynaud's phenomenon, and polyarthritis. This has been referred to as the *Jo_1 syndrome* in which the major clinical manifestations are PM and ILD and, less frequently, Raynaud's phenomenon plus polyarthritis.[11–13]

ANTIBODY TO THE TRANSLATION FACTOR KJ

Antibodies to a translation factor KJ, which is not a tRNA synthetase, have been found in two patients with PM with interstitial lung disease, that is, the Jo_1 syndrome.[14] Thus the clinical picture relates not only to antibodies to tRNA synthetases but to other biochemical components of the translation apparatus. These findings have stimulated speculation that an RNA virus is the etiologic trigger in these diseases because RNA viruses parasitize host cells by commandeering their translation apparatus to produce viral rather than host proteins. No RNA virus has yet been found that can be held responsible for these diseases, however.

ANTIBODY TO SIGNAL RECOGNITION PARTICLE

A second cytoplasmic target for autoimmunity is the *signal recognition particle*, or SRP. This particle binds the signal sequence of nascent secretory, membrane, and lysosomal proteins and directs them to the endoplasmic reticulum.[15] SRP is a ribonucleoprotein particle with a unique RNA (7SL) and a series of six proteins of molecular weights 9, 14, 19, 54, 68, and 72 kd. It is the 54-kd protein component that is the most frequent target of autoimmunity, but the 68- and 72-kd components are also reactive with some sera. The clinical interest is that antibodies to SRP occur in patients with PM but without interstitial lung disease.[16] Thus, this antibody is not associated with the Jo_1 syndrome, and its occurrence is associated with a different clinical subset of the disease.

ANTIBODIES TO NUCLEAR COMPONENTS

There are four important myositis-specific autoantibody specificities in which the antigenic target resides in the nucleus. These are the PM-Scl, Ku, U_2RNP, and Mi_2 antigens. Three of these are proteins and U_2RNP is a ribonucleoprotein particle related to the other URNP particles (U_1, U_4, U_5, and U_6).

ANTIBODIES TO PM-Scl

PM-Scl is a complex of proteins that are nucleolar in origin; all sera with anti–PM-Scl bind the nucleolus in indirect immunofluorescent assay (IFA). The proteins are not reactive by Western blotting and are defined in immunoprecipitation with ^{35}S methionine labeled Hela cell extracts in which a complex of 11 proteins are seen. The specific polypeptides that are antigenic are unknown.

Sera with precipitins designated anti–PM-Scl stain both the nucleus and the nucleolus in IFA. Either there is a second antibody in these sera or PM-Scl is represented in both the nucleus and the nucleolus. Interestingly, specific antibody isolated from immune precipitates made with sera that stain both the nucleus and the nucleolus bind only the nucleolus in IFA.[17] This result favors the first hypothesis.

These antibodies occur most frequently in patients with scleroderma-myositis overlap, but they also occur in isolated DM and PM.

ANTIBODIES TO Ku AND U_2RNP

Two other antigen antibody reactions are also seen in scleroderma-polymyositis overlap patients: these are the Ku and the U_2RNP systems. Ku is a complex of nuclear proteins with 70- and 80-kd components that bind internucleosomal segments of DNA.[18–19] Antibodies to Ku occur more commonly in Japanese patients with scleroderma myositis overlap than in caucasians from the United States, in whom this reactivity is rare.[20] Antibodies to Ku probably occur more frequently in SLE patients than in patients with myositis. Complementary DNAs (cDNAs) for the 70- and 80-kd proteins have been cloned and sequenced, and the epitopes are being defined.[21,22] The human proteins are the preferred targets, and this species specificity is strong evidence for the immune response being antigen-driven by the human protein.[23]

A small group of sera have been recognized that immunoprecipitate only U_1 and U_2 RNAs but not U_4, U_5, and U_6 RNAs. These sera are directed at two proteins, the A′ and B″ components of the U_2 particle, and are thus referred to as antibodies to the U_2RNP particle. Because the B″ protein of U_2RNP and the A protein of the U_1RNP particle are structurally related, such sera invariably immunoprecipitate U_2 and U_1 RNAs. Almost all patients with antibodies to U_2RNP have scleroderma-myositis.[24,25] The association of anti-U_1RNP in patients with various combinations of PM, PSS, and SLE will be discussed later.

It is unclear why the overlap syndrome of scleroderma-myositis should be so serologically heterogeneous and found to have antibodies to either PM-Scl, Ku, U_2RNP, or U_1RNP. A possible hint is that antibodies to PM-Scl, Ku, and U_1RNP have strong distinctive class II associations. Antibodies to Pm-Scl are associated with HLA-DR_3,[26] anti-U_1RNP with HLA-DR_4,[27] and anti-Ku with HLA-DQ_1.[28]

ANTIBODIES TO Mi_2

In the original studies of sera with anti-Mi, two precipitins were found, designated Mi_1 and Mi_2.[29] Mi_1 proved to be bovine IgG, and antibodies to the antigen were also found in SLE. Anti-Mi_2 has strong specificity for DM, and the antigen is a nuclear complex of proteins of molecular weights 205, 196, 151, 54, and 50 kd.[30] The protein has been found in the nucleus of all cells thus far examined, including HEp2 cells, Hela cells, mouse kidney and liver, rat liver, and bovine liver, spleen, and thymus. Its function is unknown.

Anti-Mi_2 occurs in about 20% of DM patients and in all clinical subsets of DM including adult and juvenile forms, DM with malignancy, and DM overlapped with other connective tissue diseases.[31]

AUTOANTIBODIES TO THE U_1RNP PARTICLE

Antibodies to nRNP or U_1RNP constitute the only constant serologic feature of patients with MCTD,[32–34] and the definition of this entity as distinct from its component diseases SLE, PM, and PSS remains controversial.[35–37] The nosologic problem can be illustrated by the following considerations. Many SLE patients lacking "overlap" features such as myositis and sclerodactyly show anti-nRNP as their sole precipitating serum antibody. Many such patients fulfill the American Rheumatism Association (ARA) criteria for the diagnosis of SLE. If these patients are classified as having MCTD, the clinical criteria for this diagnosis are meaningless, because overlap features are absent. Yet these patients share with the MCTD patients a low frequency of serious renal disease and a relatively favorable prognosis.[38] In my experience such "SLE" patients with anti-nRNP outnumber those showing the overlap features of MCTD by four or five to one.

Later studies have shown a strong correlation between antibodies to the U_1RNP specific 68-kd polypeptide and MCTD.[39] Other studies, however, that show a high correlation of antibodies to the 68-kd U_1RNP specific polypeptide also show that such anti–68-kd antibodies are also common in SLE patients with no overlap features.[40]

CONCLUSION

The demonstration that myositis-specific autoantibodies have a strong association with overlapping diseases should help define the mechanism of overlap syndromes. Because these antigen-antibody reactions are disease-specific probes, it is reasonable to believe that they relate to the nature of the etiologic agents, all of which are presently unknown in the systemic rheumatic diseases. Autoantibodies to Jo_1 might result from an RNA virus infection that has affinity for receptors on both muscle and lung, accounting for initiating inflammatory events that result in myositis and interstitial lung disease, respectively. Antibodies to different tRNA synthetases might result from infection with different RNA viruses. The strong association of PSS and PM with an assortment of antibodies to defined nuclear antigens (i.e., Ku, U_1RNP, U_2RNP, and PM-Scl) could reflect an inciting agent that has a nuclear locus of interaction (i.e., a DNA virus) in which the autoimmune response is strongly dictated by class II restriction. These hypotheses are speculative, but could serve as a basis for future study.

On a more generic level, the presence of frequent overlap of distinct diseases raises the possibility that the presence of one disease promotes the development of a second. For example, in an SLE patient who produces multiple autoantibodies that mediate tissue damage via an immune complex mechanism, the chronic release of large amounts of autoantigens might promote the development of PSS or PM in a host with the appropriate genes for the second disease. In another scenario, the various autoimmune diseases might already share predisposing factors (genetic or otherwise) insufficient in themselves to mediate disease expression but rendering the host susceptible to several of the connective tissue diseases once one of the component diseases is triggered. This latter idea draws support from the observation that in many families, multiple distinct autoimmune diseases can be observed, and it is common knowledge that these diseases frequently occur sequentially in a given patient.

Given the pace of molecular biology and biochemical work in this area, these issues should be further clarified in the coming decade.

REFERENCES

1. Dubois, E.L.: The relationship between systemic lupus erythematosus, progressive systemic sclerosis and mixed connective tissue disease. *In* Systemic Lupus Erythematosus. Edited by E.L. Dubois. Los Angeles, University Southern California Press, 1974.
2. Bohan, A., and Peter, J.R.: Polymyositis and dermatomyositis. N. Engl. J. Med., *292*:344–347, 1975.
3. Dawkins, R.L.: Experimental autoallergic myositis, polymyositis, and myasthenia gravis. Clin. Exp. Immunol., *21*:185–201, 1975.
4. Nishikai, M., and Reichlin, M.: Heterogeneity of precipitating antibodies in polymyositis and dermatomyositis. Characterization of the Jo_1 antibody system. Arthritis Rheum., *23*:881–888, 1980.
5. Rosa, M.D., et al.: A mammalian tRNA histidyl-containing antigen is recognized by the polymyositis specific antibody anti-Jo-1. Nucleic Acids Res., *11*:853–870, 1983.
6. Mathews, M.B., and Bernstein, R.M.: Myositis autoantibody inhibits histidyl tRNA synthetase: A model for autoimmunity. Nature, *304*:177–179, 1983.
7. Targoff, I.N., and Reichlin, M.: Enzymatic activity of purified Jo-1 antigen (abstract). Arthritis Rheum., *27*:S45, 1984.
8. Mathews, M.B., et al.: Antithreonyl tRNA synthetase, a second myositis-related autoantibody. J. Exp. Med., *160*:420–434, 1984.
9. Bunn, C.C., Bernstein, R.M., and Mathews, M.B.: Autoantibodies against alanyl tRNA synthetase and $tRNA^{Ala}$ coexist and are associated with myositis. J. Exp. Med., *163*:1281–1291, 1986.
10. Targoff, I.N.: Autoantibodies to aminoacyl-transfer RNA synthetases for isoleucine and glycine: Two additional synthetases are antigenic in myositis J. Immunol., *144*:1732–1743, 1990.
11. Yoshida, S., Akizuki, N., Mimori, T., et al.: The precipitating antibody to an acidic nuclear protein antigen, the Jo_1, in connective tissue disease. A marker for a subset of polymyositis with interstitial pulmonary fibrosis. Arthritis Rheum., *26*:604–611, 1983.
12. Bernstein, R.M., Morgan, S.H., and Chapman, J.: Anti-Jo_1 antibody: A marker for myositis with interstitial lung disease. Br. Med. J., *289*:151–152.
13. Wasicek, C.A., Reichlin, M., Montes, M., and Raghu, G.: Polymyositis and interstitial lung disease in the patient with the anti-Jo_1 prototype. Am. J. Med., *76*:538–544, 1984.
14. Targoff, I.N., Arnett, F.A., Berman, L., et al.: Anti-KJ—A new antibody associated with the myositis/lung syndrome that reacts with a translation related protein. J. Clin. Invest., *84*:162–172, 1990.
15. Reeves, W.H., Nigaw, S.K., and Blobel, G.: Human autoantibodies reactive with the signal recognition particle. Proc. Nat. Acad. Sci. U. S. A., *83*:9507–9511, 1986.
16. Targoff, I.N., Johnson, A.E., and Miller, F.W.: Antibody to signal recognition particle in polymyositis. Arthritis Rheum., *33*:1361–1370, 1990.
17. Targoff, I.N., and Reichlin, M.: Nucleolar localization of the PM-Scl antigen. Arthritis Rheum., *28*:226–230, 1985.
18. Reeves, W.H.: Use of monoclonal antibodies for the characterization of novel DNA-binding proteins recognized by human autoimmune sera. J. Exp. Med., *161*:18–39, 1985.
19. Mimori, T., Hardin, J.A., and Steitz, J.A.: Characterization of the DNA binding protein antigen Ku recognized by autoantibodies from patients with rheumatic disorders. J. Biol. Chem., *261*:2274–2278, 1986.
20. Mimori, T., Akizuki, M., Yamagata, H., et al.: Characterization of a high molecular weight acidic nuclear protein recognized by autoantibodies in sera from patients with polymyositis scleroderma overlap. J. Clin. Invest., *68*:611–620, 1981.
21. Mimori, T., Hama, N., Suwa, A., et al.: Molecular cloning of the human antigen Ku (p70/p80) (abstract). Arthritis Rheum., *31*:513, 1988.
22. Reeves, W.H., and Sthoeger, Z.M.: Molecular cloning of the cDNA encoding the p70 (Ku) lupus autoantigen. J. Biol. Chem., *244*:5047–5082, 1989.
23. Porges, A., and Reeves, W.H.: Autoepitopes of p70/p80 (Ku) antigen are in regions of evolutionary instability (abstract). Arthritis Rheum., *32*:S81, 1989.

24. Mimori, T., Hinterberger, M., Petterson, I., and Steitz, J.A.: Autoantibodies to the U_2 small nuclear ribonucleoprotein in a patient with scleroderma-polymyositis overlap syndrome. J. Biol. Chem., *259*:560–565, 1984.
25. Craft, J., Mimori, T., Olsen, T.L., and Hardin, J.A.: The U_2 small nuclear ribonucleoprotein particle as an autoantigen. Analysis with sera from patients with overlap syndromes. J. Clin. Invest., *81*:1716–1724, 1988.
26. Genth, E., Mieraw, R., Genetzky, P., et al.: Immunogenetic associations of scleroderma-related antinuclear antibodies. Arthritis Rheum., *33*:657–665, 1990.
27. Harley, J.B., Sestak, A.L., Willis, L.G., et al.: A model for disease heterogeneity in systemic lupus erythematosus: Relationships between histocompatibility antigens, autoantibodies and lymphopenia or renal disease. Arthritis Rheum., *32*:826–836, 1989.
28. Yaneva, M., and Arnett, F.C.: Antibodies against Ku protein in sera from patients with autoimmune diseases. Clin. Exp. Immunol., *76*:366–372, 1989.
29. Nishikai, M., and Reichlin, M.: Purification and characterization of a nuclear non-histone protein (Mi-1) which reacts with anti-immunoglobulin sera and the sera of patients with dermatomyositis. Mol. Immunol., *17*:1129–1141, 1980.
30. Nilasena, D., and Targoff, I.N.: Biochemical analysis of the dermatomyositis associated Mi-2 autoantigen (abstract). Clin. Res., *38*:550, 1990.
31. Targoff, I.N., and Reichlin, M.: The association between Mi-2 antibodies and dermatomyositis. Arthritis Rheum., *28*:796–803, 1985.
32. Sharp, G.C., et al.: Association of antibodies to ribonucleoprotein and Sm antigens with mixed connective tissue diseases, systemic lupus erythematosus, and other rheumatic diseases. N. Engl. J. Med., *295*:1149–1154, 1976.
33. Sharp, G.C., et al.: Mixed connective tissue disease. An apparently distinct rheumatic disease syndrome associated with a specific antibody to an extractable nuclear antigen. Am. J. Med., *52*:148–159, 1972.
34. Sharp, G.C., et al.: Association of autoantibodies to different nuclear antigens with clinical patterns of rheumatic disease and responsiveness to therapy. J. Clin. Invest., *50*:350–359, 1971.
35. Reichlin, M.: Mixed connective disease. *In* Modern Topics in Rheumatology. Edited by G.R.V. Hughes. London, Heinemann Ltd., 1976.
36. Reichlin, M.: Problems in differentiating SLE and mixed connective tissue disease. N. Engl. J. Med., *295*:1194, 1976.
37. Maddison, P.J., Mogavero, H., and Reichlin, M.: Patterns of clinical diseases associated with antibodies to nuclear ribonucleoprotein. J. Rheumatol., *5*:407:411, 1978.
38. Reichlin, M., and Mattioli, M.: Correlation of a precipitin reaction to an RNA-protein antigen and a low prevalence of nephritis in patients with systemic lupus erythematosus. N. Engl. J. Med., *286*:908–911, 1972.
39. Petterson, I., Wang, G., Smith, E.I., et al.: The use of immunoblotting and immunoprecipitation of (U) small nuclear ribonucleoproteins with mixed connective tissue disease and systemic lupus erythematosus. Arthritis Rheum., *29*:986–996, 1986.
40. Reichlin, M., and van Venrooij, W.J.: Autoantibodies to the URNP particles: Relationship to clinical diagnosis and nephritis. Clin. Exp. Immunol., *83*:286–290, 1991.

67

Systemic Lupus Erythematosus: Clinical Aspects and Treatment

NAOMI F. ROTHFIELD

Systemic lupus erythematosus (SLE) is a disease of unknown cause that affects many organ systems and is characterized by the presence of multiple autoantibodies that participate in immunologically mediated tissue injury.

HISTORICAL ASPECTS

During the nineteenth century, the term "lupus" described a skin disease that consisted of spreading ulcerations of the face. Acute and chronic types were distinguished in 1872 by Kaposi.[1] The concept of a systemic form of the disease was formulated by Osler in 1895 when he suggested that the basis of the disease was vasculitis.[1] He described a systemic disease with a variety of skin manifestations and recognized the involvement of joints, intestinal tract, serosal surfaces, and kidney. Osler also described the characteristic periods of exacerbation and remission. The pathologic abnormalities were later described by Libman and Sacks,[1] Gross,[1] and Baehr, Klemperer, and Schrifrin,[1] who emphasized that changes in many organs occurred even in the absence of the typical skin lesions.

In 1948, Hargraves et al. described the lupus erythematosus (LE) cell.[1] This major advance soon led to an increased interest in the disease, to an increased frequency of diagnosis, and eventually to our understanding of the mechanism of the LE cell phenomenon and to the concept that antibodies were directed against nuclear antigens. Soon after the discovery of the LE cell, corticosteroids and antimalarials were used for treatment. It became possible to prolong the life of patients and to follow the course of successfully treated patients. The discovery of antinuclear antibodies by means of the indirect fluorescent technique led to the recognition of a wide variety of antibodies and to an understanding of their clinical significance (see Chapter 68). The concept of SLE as an immune complex–mediated disease evolved, and the role of complement in producing tissue damage was elucidated. More recently, various abnormal B cell, T cell, and macrophage functions have been noted in patients with active SLE (see Chapter 69). Genetic factors have been elucidated (Chapter 28). An abnormality of estrogen metabolism has been described. No single abnormality can totally explain the disease, however. Additional environmental factors appear to be necessary for disease expression.

INCIDENCE AND PREVALENCE

SLE affects individuals of all races, but its prevalence varies in different countries (see Chapter 3). In France, the disease appears to be more common among immigrants from Portugal, Spain, North Africa, and Italy than among natives. In Hawaii, the disease is more common in Orientals or Polynesians than among whites.[1] The disease has only recently been described in black Africans and appears to be more prevalent in China than in the United States.[1]

The average annual incidence in the United States has been estimated to be 27.5 per million population for white females and 75.4 per million population for black females. The incidence of SLE among hospitalized patients was 4.6 per 100,000 per year in a Baltimore, Maryland, study,[1] and 1.8 per 100,000 per year for patients living in Rochester, Minnesota.[1] The 1.8 annual incidence rate is similar to that observed in Sweden, in New York, and in Jefferson County, Alabama, between

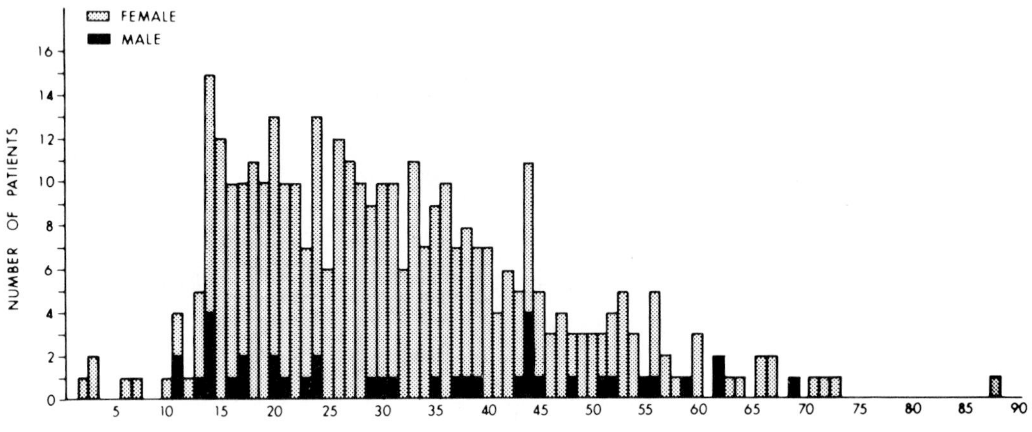

FIGURE 67–1. Sex and age at diagnosis in 356 SLE patients. From Tan, E., and Rothfield, N.: Lupus erythematosus. *In* Immunologic Disease. 3rd Ed. Edited by M. Samter. Boston, Little Brown, 1979.

1955 and 1965. The incidence rates showed a steady increase beginning in early 1960, but they have stabilized since then, probably because of a greater appreciation of milder cases and improvement of diagnostic tests during the 1960s. The prevalence of SLE in a prepaid health plan for 125,000 patients indicates that SLE affects approximately 1 in 1000 women.[1] In the Rochester, Minnesota study, which included all patients in a white population, the prevalence of definite SLE per 100,000 population on January 1, 1980, was 40.0 (53.8 for women and 19.0 for men). This figure is somewhat lower than 51 per 100,000 reported for a prepaid health group in San Francisco from 1965 to 1973.

SLE occurs in children and in the elderly, but the peak age at the onset of the first symptom is between 15 and 25 years. The mean age at diagnosis is 30 years (Fig. 67–1). In our own series of 433 patients, 90% are females. A higher percentage of males is affected among children and among the elderly SLE patients.

GENETIC FACTORS

Several factors of SLE can occur within a family (see Chapters 3 and 28).[1] Families with members who have chronic discoid lupus and others who have SLE have been reported. Family members of some SLE patients have isolated laboratory abnormalities such as false-positive tests for syphilis, antinuclear antibodies, hypergammaglobulinemia, antiphospholipid antibodies, and deposits of immunoglobulins in their skin.[1] Relatives of SLE patients have an increased frequency (5%) of the disease.[1] The frequency of HLA-DR2 (human leukocyte antigen DR2) and -DR3 in white patients is increased.[2] HLA-DR2, -DQw1, and especially a rare allele, -DQB1, AZH confer a high risk for lupus nephritis.[3] The association with DR3 may be due to C4A null allele because the C4A gene deletion is linked to B8-DR3 haplotypes. C4A deficiency is associated with poor clearance of immune complexes. In addition, some autoantibodies are associated with certain class II major histocompatibility complex (MHC) specificities.[2] An association of SLE with hereditary deficiencies of several complement proteins exists, also.

HORMONAL FACTORS

Both male and female SLE patients have increased hydroxylation of estrone to 16-hydroxyestrone, a metabolite that is a potent estrogenic hormone.[1] The onset of SLE frequency occurs at menarche, during pregnancy, during the postpartum period, or with the use of oral contraceptives containing estrogen.[1] Testosterone metabolism also is different in women with SLE.[1] The association of Klinefelter's syndrome with SLE has been well documented and suggests that X chromosomes may be a predisposing factor for human SLE as well as for murine lupus.[1]

ENVIRONMENTAL FACTORS

A history of sun exposure before onset of the disease is obtained in about 36% of patients. The number of new cases of SLE usually is increased during the late spring and summer months in southern New England and in New York. In other parts of the country with persistent year-round sunny weather, the incidence of new cases may not vary in this fashion. The relative lack of sunlight in England has been postulated as an explanation of the rarity of SLE in that country.

SLE patients develop exacerbations of their disease during episodes of infection. Bacterial products such as lipopolysaccharides (polyclonal B-cell activators) can induce antibodies to single- and double-stranded DNA in various strains of mice.[1] During infection bacterial products might produce similar changes in individuals with the appropriate genetic background and thereby lead to the development of SLE. A variety of drugs have been implicated as capable of producing all or some of the clinical and serologic features of SLE.

CLINICAL FEATURES AND PATHOLOGY

GENERAL FEATURES

Fatigue is present in nearly all SLE patients during periods of disease activity. It is frequently an early manifestation and can precede the appearance of objective findings such as rash or joint swelling. Corticosteroid treatment leads to a feeling of well-being and disappearance of fatigue. During subsequent periods of clinical exacerbation, fatigue usually reappears and may be the first symptom of an impending flare. The fatigue of SLE is similar to that felt by patients with viral hepatitis and may be the patient's major symptom.

Fever is present in about 90% of patients at the time of diagnosis. In some patients, fever is low-grade, whereas in others it is spiking. It responds rapidly to corticosteroid therapy if the drug is given every 6 hours. A single daily dose of prednisone is usually not adequate to control the fever, which will return 6 to 8 hours after the daily dose has been ingested. During the course of the disease, recurrence of fever is viewed with concern because it may result from infection. *Fever in a treated SLE patient should be attributed to infection until proved otherwise.*

Weight loss has occurred in about 85% of patients at the time of diagnosis unless the nephrotic syndrome is present. Subsequent exacerbations may be preceded by either a gradual or a rapid loss of weight and accompanying fatigue.

DERMATOLOGIC MANIFESTATIONS

Abnormalities of the skin, hair, or mucous membranes are the second most common manifestations of SLE. Whereas arthralgia or arthritis occurs in 95% of patients, dermatologic abnormalities occur in 85%.

A rash after sun exposure (photosensitivity) is common, occurring in 33% of SLE patients. The onset of the disease frequently occurs after significant sun exposure and, in most patients, a rash will recur after sun exposure during the course of the disease. Sun exposure may exacerbate systemic manifestations of the disease.[4]

The classic *butterfly blush* was present at the time of diagnosis in 52% of our patients and is nearly always located on both cheeks and across the bridge of the nose. It may be preceded by sun exposure and is initially considered by the patient to be sunburn. The blush can also occur without a history of sun exposure. The lesions heal well and leave no scars. They may be confused with the erythematous rash of acne rosacea or seborrheic dermatitis, but the erythema of seborrheic dermatitis is located mainly in the nasolabial folds, whereas the butterfly rash of SLE *characteristically spares the nasolabial folds.* Acne rosacea is characterized by the presence of papules and pustules, but pustules are not found in the facial rash of SLE unless secondary infection is present.

The second most common lupus erythematosus rash is a nonspecific maculopapular rash resembling a drug eruption. This rash may occur after sun exposure and may be located anywhere on the body, although it is most often found on the face and chest. Occasionally, scattered macules may also occur on the palms and fingers and less often on the soles of the feet. The rash usually heals without scarring or hyperpigmentation, but lesions occasionally persist; they become crusted and the skin may show hyperpigmentation and atrophy, although no scarring is noted. The persistent lesions with central atrophy of the skin without true scarring has been called *subacute cutaneous lupus.*

Acute or subacute lesions differ from discoid lesions in that they do not lead to scarring. They are erythematous at the edge and tend to be annular and widespread on the chest, back, arms, and occasionally legs. Subacute lesions usually begin as small erythematous, slightly scaly papules and may evolve into either annular lesions or a papulosquamous lesion with a scaly surface, resembling psoriasis. Such subacute lesions are more common in patients with antibodies to Ro (SSA) who have the HLA antigens B8 and DR3.[1]

Lesions of *chronic discoid lupus* occurred in 19% of our patients. In about 40% of these patients, the lesions preceded the development of SLE by 2 to 35 years. About half the lesions developed around the time of the initial diagnosis of SLE, and only 10% of the patients developed discoid lesions after the diagnosis of SLE. Discoid lesions commonly involve the scalp and may also be seen on and in the external ear. Discoid lesions begin as erythematous plaques or papules and spread outward, leaving central areas of hyperkeratosis, follicular plugging, and atrophy.[5] The edge of an active lesion is edematous and erythematous, whereas a healed lesion may show central depigmentation with scarring and hyperpigmentation at the margin.

Alopecia occurs in about 70% of patients. The alopecia is usually diffuse, but can appear as patches of hair loss (Fig. 67–2). In about 20% of SLE patients, the diffuse

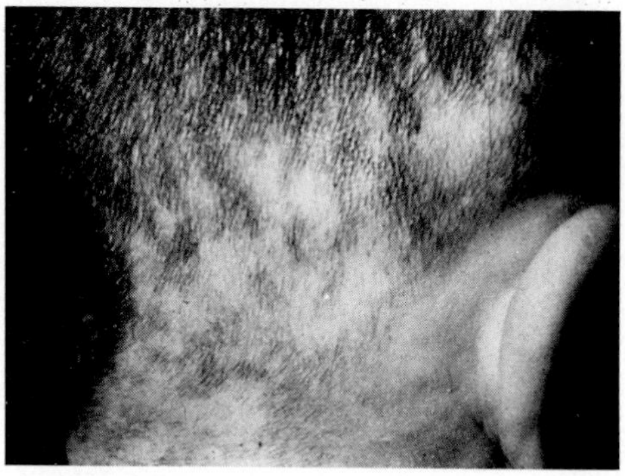

FIGURE 67–2. Patchy alopecia in a man with systemic lupus erythematosus.

alopecia is so extreme that the patients are compelled to buy wigs. The hair slowly regrows as the disease becomes inactive. It is important to reassure the patient that the loss of hair is not permanent. Alopecia usually recurs with disease exacerbation and, in some patients, can be an excellent first sign of an impending flare. Tufts of hair are easily pulled out in a patient with alopecia, and the severity of the alopecia can be followed quantitatively by serial attempts to pull the hair out. As the new hair grows in, the patient's scalp develops a stubbled look. Patches of alopecia can occur temporarily when maculopapular lesions occur in the scalp. Lesions of discoid lupus in the scalp heal with atrophy and scarring. The permanent loss of hair follicles results in permanent areas of alopecia.

Vasculitic skin lesions are not uncommon in SLE patients and usually occur in the setting of significant disease activity in other organ systems. Vasculitic lesions with ulceration may occur on the extensor surface of the forearm. Palpable purpuric lesions might be observed, especially on the lower extremity; on biopsy, these lesions reveal leukocytoclastic angiitis. Less commonly, vasculitic lesions may be noted on the backs of the hands, on the palms as blotchy and slightly purpuric lesions, near the small joints of the fingers, and on the finger pads as tender erythematous nodules. Periungal erythema is noted in about 10% of patients, and palmar erythema is noted in 20%. Splinter hemorrhages or nailfold thrombi are occasionally found. Atrophic "blanche" lesions similar to those seen in Degos' disease consist of erythematous papular or infiltrated lesions that gradually develop pearly white centers and telangiectasis at the margins.[1]

Livido reticularis is common in SLE patients, especially those with active disease, and is noted on the lower extremities, particularly around the knees and ankles. When the legs are dependent, the toes may take on a purplish hue. Livido reticularis is due to vasculitis of small vessels and precedes gangrene in some patients. Livido may involve not only all four extremities, but the trunk as well. Livido reticularis has recently been associated with the presence of anti-phospholipid antibodies (see Chapter 70).

Mucosal ulcers are common (40%) in SLE patients.[1] These are most commonly found on the hard or soft palate and are asymptomatic (Fig. 67–3). Occasionally, a patient complains of pain when eating spicy foods or notes a tender area on the roof of the mouth. These palatal ulcers are present in patients with active disease and disappear within a few days of institution of corticosteroid therapy. Nasal septal ulcerations are less common. These lesions are seen on the anterior aspect of the nasal septum and will be missed if the otoscope is inserted too far into the nares. Nasal septal perforations occur in some of these patients.[1] Patients with nasal ulcerations might complain of epistaxis and nasal stuffiness caused by secretions or crusts over the ulcerated areas.

Leg ulcers are similar to those seen in patients with rheumatoid vasculitis. They are most frequently located about the malleoli. The leg ulcers are punched-out lesions that are exquisitely tender. In a few of our patients, these leg ulcers preceded the recognition of SLE by many years.

Less common dermatologic abnormalities occur in many patients. *Bullous* lesions may be present.[1] In patients who are thrombocytopenic, the bullae can be hemorrhagic. *Periorbital edema, urticaria, or erythema multiforme* might be noted. *Ecchymoses and petechiae* may be observed in patients with severe thrombocytopenia. Many patients complain of easy bruising prior to diagnosis of SLE and treatment with corticosteroids. *Gangrene* of the fingers or toes is uncommon and may be preceded by severe Raynaud's phenomenon or by severe livido reticularis. Occlusion of the medium-sized vessels of the legs has been noted in one such patient who eventually had a midcalf amputation because of gangrene.

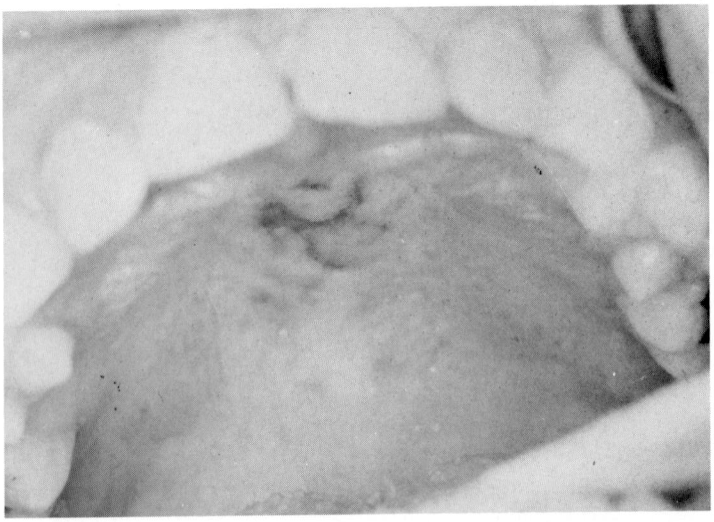

FIGURE 67–3. Mucosal ulcer in hard palate.

Lupus profundus or *panniculitis* is occasionally noted and, in some patients, these lesions calcify. Soft-tissue calcification occurs rarely in SLE.[6] *Rheumatoid nodules* are present in about 10% of patients, usually, but not always, in patients with non-erosive deforming arthritis. The association of SLE with *porphyria cutanea tarda* has been reported,[1] and about 5% of our SLE patients have psoriasis. *Dystrophic nail changes*, usually affecting only a few nails, may be found in about 10% of patients, especially those with long-standing disease. In the most extreme form, the nails are totally lost. Nail bed erythema is found in most of these patients earlier in the course of the disease. *Hypermelanosis* of the skin, mucous membranes, or both is observed rarely in patients treated for prolonged periods with antimalarial drugs.[1]

Histopathology of the skin lesions varies greatly. Biopsies of the typical rash of acute SLE usually show thinning of the epidermis, liquefaction degeneration of the basal layer of the epidermis with disruption of the dermal-epidermal junction, and edema of the dermis with a scattered infiltrate of lymphocytes throughout the dermis but concentrated around the upper dermal capillaries. Some biopsies reveal only a nonspecific vasculitis, however. In some patients, the histologic picture lies between that of chronic discoid lupus and systemic lupus. The histologic picture of subacute lupus may be indistinguishable from that of chronic discoid lupus.[7] Leukocytoclastic angiitis may be seen histologically in patients with palpable purpuric vasculitic lesions or with urticaria.

Immunopathologic studies of skin lesions reveal deposits of immunoglobulins and complement components at the dermal-epidermal junction in 80 to 100% of patients (Fig. 67–4).[1] This finding is not specific for lesions of SLE. Similar deposits may be found in lesions of lepromatous leprosy, telangiectatic lesions from scleroderma patients, lesions of rosacea, and lesions of active porphyria cutanea tarda.[1] Lesions from patients with chronic discoid lupus and without clinical or serologic evidence of SLE also have deposits of immunoglobulins and complement proteins in the dermal-epidermal junction.[1] Thus, *the diagnosis of SLE should not depend on the demonstration of deposits at the dermal-epidermal junction of skin lesions.* Because rosacea is commonly confused with the butterfly blush of SLE, the finding of deposits in 70% of lesions of rosacea is of particular importance.[1]

Immunopathologic studies of nonlesional skin from SLE patients also reveals the presence of immunoglobulins and complement proteins.[1] These deposits are more common in biopsies obtained during periods of clinical and serologically active disease.[1] Repeated biopsies of SLE patients have revealed that the deposits present during active disease may no longer be found later in the course when the patient has been in a sustained remission.[1] Similar deposits in normal skin have been found in patients with rheumatoid arthritis, Sjögren's syndrome, scleroderma, Raynaud's phenomenon, polydermatomyositis,[1] and lepromatous leprosy.[1] We have found intermittent deposits in nonlesional skin of some patients with chronic discoid lupus and without evidence of SLE. Similarly, deposits are found in nonlesional skin from one third of patients with rosacea.[1]

Granular focal deposits have been noted in the normal skin of some relatives of SLE patients, including spouses,[1] and deposits have been found in the skin of technicians handling SLE sera. The latter observation is similar to that of increased lymphocytotoxic antibodies, antinuclear antibodies, and positive LE cell preparations

FIGURE 67–4. Immunoglobulin deposits in the dermal-epidermal junction of the nonlesional skin from a patient with clinically active SLE (anti-IgG fluorescein isothiocyanate ×500).

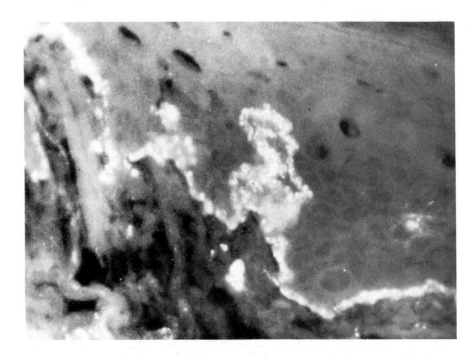

found among workers in laboratories handling SLE sera.

MUSCULOSKELETAL MANIFESTATIONS

Involvement of the joints is the most frequent manifestation of SLE.[1] Objective evidence of pain on motion, tenderness, effusion, or periarticular soft-tissue swelling was present at the time of diagnosis of SLE in 88% of 209 patients. Additional patients later developed objective evidence of joint disease so that fully 86% of all patients had arthritis at some time. Although other patients have joint pain without objective evidence of arthritis, 95% of SLE patients have either arthralgia or arthritis.

In some patients, arthralgia or arthritis precedes the onset of multisystem disease by many years. At the time of diagnosis, arthritis or arthralgia of the proximal interphalangeal joints was present in 82% of our patients; this was symmetric in all but two patients. The knees were the next most commonly involved joints (76%), followed by the wrists and metacarpophalangeal joints. Ankles, elbows, and shoulders were involved less frequently (55%, 54%, and 45%, respectively). The metatarsophalangeal joints and hips were involved in 20% of patients, and the distal interphalangeal joints of the hands in 14% of patients. Involvement was symmetric in nearly all patients. Inflammation of the temporomandibular joints is rare, although several malocclusions occurred in one patient because of involvement of this joint.

Knee effusions are moderately severe in some patients, and joint aspiration usually reveals a clear (group 1) fluid. The leukocyte count is less than 3000/μl, and most of the cells are small lymphocytes. Antinuclear antibodies and LE cells may be found in the synovial fluid. Serum complement proteins and total hemolytic complement levels are usually low, reflecting similar low levels in the serum. Occasionally, opaque fluids with a higher leukocyte count and a greater percentage of neutrophils (group 2 fluid) may be found. *Inflammatory joint fluids should be cultured, especially if the arthritis is monoarticular*, and a special culture should always be performed to rule out gonococcal arthritis. A single swollen or painful joint should be suspected as not resulting from SLE and should always be aspirated for cultures. If a bland fluid is present and cultures are negative, a diagnosis of aseptic (avascular) necrosis should be considered.

The histologic examination of the synovium reveals a fibrous villous synovitis. Typical pannus formation and erosions of bone and cartilage are extremely rare.[1] Arthritis disappears completely within a few days when patients are treated with corticosteroids for their systemic disease.

Although uncommon, deformities certainly do occur in some SLE patients. The revised criteria do not exclude deformities as long as these are due to nonerosive disease (Table 67–1).[1] Typical swan-neck deformities and ulnar deviation of the fingers developed in about 10% of our SLE patients after 3 to 4 years of disease. Intermittent mild joint pains had been noted by many patients in this group, but in others no joint pain had been present since the time of diagnosis. Radiographs of the hands revealed no bony erosions or loss of joint space, although osteoporosis and joint subluxation occurred. Surgical repair of the deformities has been performed on some of these patients, and normal cartilage has been noted in the affected joints. The joint deformities are thought to be related to chronic inflammatory involvement of the tendons of the hands and fingers and spasm of the intrinsic muscles. The presence of radiographic erosions excludes the use of "arthritis" in the revised criteria, however.

Morning stiffness is present in 50% of patients. Typical subcutaneous nodules occur in 10% of patients with active disease and disappear after treatment with corticosteroids. Tenosynovitis occurs in about 7% of patients. Rupture of the infrapatellar and Achilles tendons may occur, and may relate to corticosteroid therapy or to SLE itself because histologic findings include chronic inflammatory changes.[8]

It is extremely important to rule out two causes of joint pain that can occur in SLE patients, i.e., infectious arthritis and avascular necrosis of bone. The latter may involve the knees, elbows, shoulders, and carpal bones, and typically involves the hips. I have seen both acute and chronic tophaceous gouty arthritis in SLE patients. Monoarticular arthritis developing in a patient with SLE should be considered to be caused by a condition other than the primary disease.

Involvement of muscles is not uncommon. Myalgia was present in 30% of patients and abnormalities of serum glutamic-oxaloacetic transaminase (SGOT) and serum glutamate pyruvate transaminase (SGPT) were also present in 30% of patients before any treatment. The enzyme abnormalities probably reflect liver disease. The myalgia occurs with arthritis and, in some patients, the pain is "all over" and difficult to localize. These patients have pain in and between their joints. The muscles may be tender to palpation. Muscle pain and tenderness are more common proximally than distally. Such muscle involvement rapidly disappears with corticosteroid doses needed to control the more significant systemic manifestations. Severe and prominent muscle involvement was noted in 8% of 228 patients studied by Psokas et al.[1] Biopsy usually reveals a nonspecific perivascular mononuclear infiltrate, but polymyositis with muscle necrosis can occur.[1] True polymyositis with muscle weakness, electromyographic changes typical of polymyositis, vacuolar myopathy, and necrosis has been reported in untreated SLE patients.[1] These abnormalities improved with corticosteroid therapy.

CARDIOVASCULAR MANIFESTATIONS

Clinically evident pericarditis occurs in about 35% of patients. Most often, an intermittent friction rub is heard, though massive pericardial effusions and tam-

TABLE 67–1. THE 1982 REVISED CRITERIA FOR CLASSIFICATION OF SYSTEMIC LUPUS ERYTHEMATOSUS

CRITERION*	DEFINITION
1. Malar rash	Fixed erythema, flat or raised, over the malar eminences, tending to spare the nasolabial folds.
2. Discoid rash	Erythematous raised patches with adherent keratotic scaling and follicular plugging; atropic scarring may occur in older lesions.
3. Photosensitivity	Skin rash as a result of unusual reaction to sunlight, by patient history or physician observation.
4. Oral ulcers	Oral or nasopharyngeal ulceration, usually painless, observed by a physician.
5. Arthritis	Nonerosive arthritis involving two or more peripheral joints, characterized by tenderness, swelling, or effusion.
6. Serositis	a) Pleuritis—convincing history of pleuritis pain or rub heard by a physician or evidence of pleural effusion. OR b) Pericarditis—documented by ECG or rub or evidence of pericardial effusion.
7. Renal disorder	a) Persistent proteinuria greater than 0.5 per day or greater than 3+ if quantitation not performed. OR b) Cellular casts—may be red cell, hemoglobulin, granular, tubular, or mixed.
8. Neurologic disorder	a) Seizures—in the absence of offending drugs or known metabolic derangements: e.g., uremia, ketoacidosis, or electrolyte imbalance. OR b) Psychosis—in the absence of offending drugs or known metabolic derangements, e.g., uremia, ketoacidosis, or electrolyte imbalance.
9. Hematologic disorder	a) Hemolytic anemia—with reticulocytosis. OR b) Leukopenia—less than 4000/mm total on two or more occasions. OR c) Lymphopenia—less than 1500/mm on two or more occasions. OR d) Thrombocytopenia—less than 100,000/mm in the absence of offending drugs.
10. Immunologic disorder	a) Positive LE cell preparation. OR b) Anti-DNA; antibody to native DNA in abnormal titer. OR c) Anti-SM: presence of antibody to Sm nuclear antigen: OR d) False-positive serologic test for syphilis known to be positive for at least 6 months and confirmed by Treponema pallidum immobilization or fluorescent treponemal antibody absorption test.
11. Antinuclear antibody	An abnormal titer of antinuclear antibody by immunofluorescence or an equivalent assay at any time and in the absence of drugs known to be associated with "drug-induced lupus syndrome."

* The proposed classification is based on 11 criteria. For the purpose of identifying patients in clinical studies, a person shall be said to have systemic lupus erythematosus if any 4 or more of the 11 criteria are present, serially or simultaneously, during any interval of observation.

ponade rarely occur. Echocardiography revealed pericardial thickening in 29% of patients.[1] LE cells are found frequently in pericardial fluid, and a markedly acidic pH has been reported to distinguish SLE effusions from those resulting from uremia, bleeding, or unknown cause.[1] Transient electrocardiographic abnormalities caused by myocardial ischemia may be seen, and tachycardia may persist for many months after the subsidence of the acute episode. Myocardial disease accompanies pericarditis. Death caused by myocardial infarction from arteritis has been reported early in the course of the disease in young patients.

Pathologically, SLE heart involvement is characterized by a pancarditis with involvement of pericardium, myocardium, endocardium, and coronary arteries.[1] Studies of hearts of patients dying from SLE has revealed a high incidence of coronary atherosclerosis in the patients treated for more than 1 year with corticosteroids.[1] Myocardial infarction late in the course of the disease in corticosteroid-treated patients is an important cause of late death.[1] One of our patients died suddenly of a myocardial infarction while in remission in the eighth year of disease. On the other hand, studies of the hearts of young SLE patients revealed not only severe atherosclerotic coronary narrowing but also more extensive and severe lupus carditis.[1] Coronary arteritis may cause myocardial infarction. Segmental myocardial perfusion abnormalities found in 39% of asymptomatic patients did not correlate with disease duration or the amount of corticosteroid received, but did correlate with a history of pericarditis.[1]

Aortic and mitral insufficiency caused by scarring of leaflets and thickened or ruptured chordae tendineae have been reported.[1] Valve replacement has been used to correct these conditions.[1] Verrucous endocarditis is present at autopsy in nearly all patients. The lesions are usually microscopic, but macroscopic vegetations are observed in nearly half the cases. Typical verrucous endocarditis is a pathologic diagnosis and does not correlate with the presence of cardiac murmurs. A recent report of Spanish patients revealed a higher prevalence of echocardiographically proven vegatations in patients who had received a smaller cumulative dose of corticosteroids than in those without vegetations.[9] Both subacute and acute bacterial endocarditis have occurred on valves affected by lupus endocarditis.

Raynaud's phenomenon was present in 18% of our 365 patients and may precede the development of multisystem disease by many years. Cryoglobulinemia was commonly present in patients with an onset of Raynaud's phenomenon at the time of diagnosis, and such patients also often had nephritis. Unlike Raynaud's phenomenon in systemic sclerosis, the Raynaud's phenomenon in SLE may gradually disappear after institution of corticosteroid therapy. Pulmonary hypertension can develop many years later in patients with Raynaud's syndrome.[10] Thrombophlebitis occurs in about 10% of patients. Large vein thrombosis is less common. Thrombosis with occlusion of the femoral artery occurred in one of our patients, necessitating midthigh amputation. The presence of the antiphospholipid antibodies (false-positive Venereal Disease Research Laboratory [VDRL] test, lupus anticoagulant, anticardiolipin antibodies) is common in these SLE patients with thombosis (see Chapter 70), but the level of the antibodies can fall at the time of thromboocclusive episodes.[11]

Thrombotic episodes clearly occur more often in patients with the lupus anticoagulant than in those without this abnormality.[1] We have found the lupus anticoagulant in our three patients with cerebral infarctions and in patients with venous and arterial thrombosis of other vessels.

Thrombotic thrombocytopenic purpura (TTP) occurs rarely in patients with SLE. We have observed this catastrophic event in 2 of 443 patients. In one patient, TTP occurred in the fourth month of pregnancy and resulted in massive brain infarcts. In the other, TTP was recognized earlier, and the patient responded to corticosteroid therapy and plasmapheresis.

PULMONARY MANIFESTATIONS

SLE in elderly patients may present with pulmonary disease in the absence of skin and joint findings. Pleural involvement is even more common than pericardial disease. Pleural effusions occur in 40% of patients. Most pleural effusions are small to moderate, but massive effusions occur occasionally. LE cells may be seen in those transudates that contain the same immunoglobulin and complement proteins as the peripheral blood. Occasionally, effusions persist for months after the institution of corticosteroid therapy, leading to concern regarding cause. "Lupus pneumonitis," characterized by dyspnea, rales, and areas of platelike atelectasis associated with elevation and fixation of the diaphragm, occurs in about 10% of patients. Infiltrates may be bilateral and associated with pleural effusions.[1] A study of the pathology of the lungs in SLE patients revealed that the most common cause of pulmonary infiltrates was infection.[1] Pneumonias caused by bacterial and fungal agents are particularly common in corticosteroid-treated SLE patients. *The diagnosis of lupus pneumonitis should be made only after a rigorous search for an infectious agent.*

Abnormalities of pulmonary function are common even in patients without respiratory symptoms.[12] Tests reveal a combination of pulmonary restriction, vascular obstruction, and airway obstruction.[1]

Pathologic abnormalities are extremely common in autopsied lungs and are most often nonspecific. All patients show evidence of pleural thickening, and intra-alveolar hemorrhage is not uncommon. Miller et al. found interstitial fibrosis in one third of 18 autopsied lungs.[1]

"Shrinking" lung syndrome is an unusual abnormality caused by weakness of the respiratory muscles; it is seen in dyspneic patients with elevation of the diaphragm and progressive or stable loss of lung volume. This abnormality has been reported as a major presenting feature of SLE but may be found in patients with otherwise inactive disease.[13]

Pulmonary hemorrhage caused by pulmonary vasculitis is a rare but life-threatening manifestation of SLE. Pulmonary hypertension rarely occurs; it is associated with Raynaud's phenomenon and may be associated with the presence of the lupus anticoagulant.[1]

RENAL DISEASE

Clinical evidence of renal disease occurs in about 50% of patients; pathologic abnormalities recognized by light microscopy are present in additional patients. Immunofluorescent studies of biopsy or autopsy material from nearly all patients reveal deposits of immunoglobulins or complement proteins. Therefore, the definition of lupus nephritis is unclear. Persistent proteinuria is the most common clinical sign of lupus nephritis.

The most characteristic pathologic abnormality is the variability of glomerular lesions and the patchy distribution of the various changes. Thus, lesions vary from one glomerulus to the other, and different structural abnormalities occur within a single glomerulus. Mesangial immune deposits are present in nearly all SLE patients. These deposits occur in all patients with clinical evidence of lupus nephritis (unless there is sclerosis of all glomeruli) and in most SLE patients without urinary abnormalities. At present, the World Health Organization (WHO) classification is used by most investigators.[1] This classification includes six distinctive morphologic patterns based on light, immunofluorescence, and electron microscopic findings, as briefly described below. *The type and severity of the renal disease bears no relation to the presence of other manifestations of the disease, which may be either mild or severe.*

Normal

Tissue in this classification cannot be distinguished from kidney tissue of a normal healthy person.

Mesangial Lupus Nephritis

The glomeruli either appear normal or show a slight irregular increase in mesangial cells and matrix (Fig. 67–5). The diagnosis depends on the demonstration of IgG and C3 in the mesangium. Electron-dense deposits may be noted in the mesangium. Patients have normal urinary findings, transient minimal proteinuria, or minimal hematuria. All biopsies of 11 consecutive SLE patients without clinical renal abnormalities showed mesangial lupus nephritis.[1] A few instances of progression from the mesangial to the diffuse proliferative form have been described.[1] *It is unlikely that the condition of patients with little or no clinical evidence of renal disease at the time of diagnosis will progress if the disease is adequately treated and initial normalization of the serologic abnormalities is sustained over time.* The presence of IgG in the mesangium is analogous to the finding of IgG in the nonlesional skin of patients with clinically active disease. Deposits of immunoglobulins in the dermal-epidermal junction and in the mesangium of the glomeruli both occur without inflammation.

Focal Proliferative Lupus Nephritis

This condition is characterized by segmental proliferation of some glomerular tufts while others appear normal (Fig. 67–6). Mesangial proliferation may be present, but segmental proliferation is present in less than 50% of glomeruli. The glomerular abnormalities used for the index of activity score described in the section on diffuse proliferative lupus nephritis may be present, but less than 50% of glomeruli will be affected. *Thus, it is important to note the index of activity and the extent of sclerosis as well as the classification of the lesion.* For example, focal lupus nephritis with a high activity index is not uncommon, whereas diffuse proliferative lupus nephritis can have a low activity index and significant sclerosis.

In focal proliferative lupus nephritis, immunofluorescence reveals immunoglobulins and C3 in the mesangium of all glomeruli. Fine, scattered granules may be present along the capillary loops, especially in the areas of proliferation. The deposits are scattered and not evenly distributed along all capillary loops. Electron-dense deposits are noted by electron microscopy in the mesangium, and occasional deposits are also found in the subendothelial, subepithelial, and intrabasement membrane areas. Proteinuria occurs, but the nephrotic syndrome is uncommon.[1] Mild hematuria is usual, but renal insufficiency is either mild or absent.

FIGURE 67–5. Minimal (mesangial) lupus nephritis (hematoxylin and eosin stain ×500).

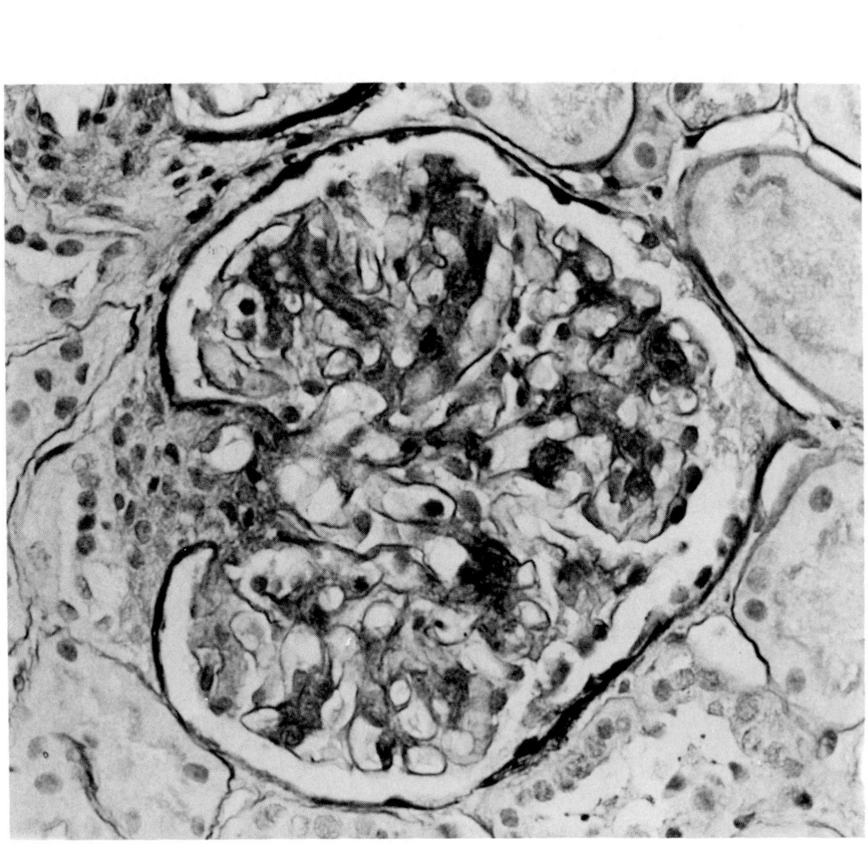

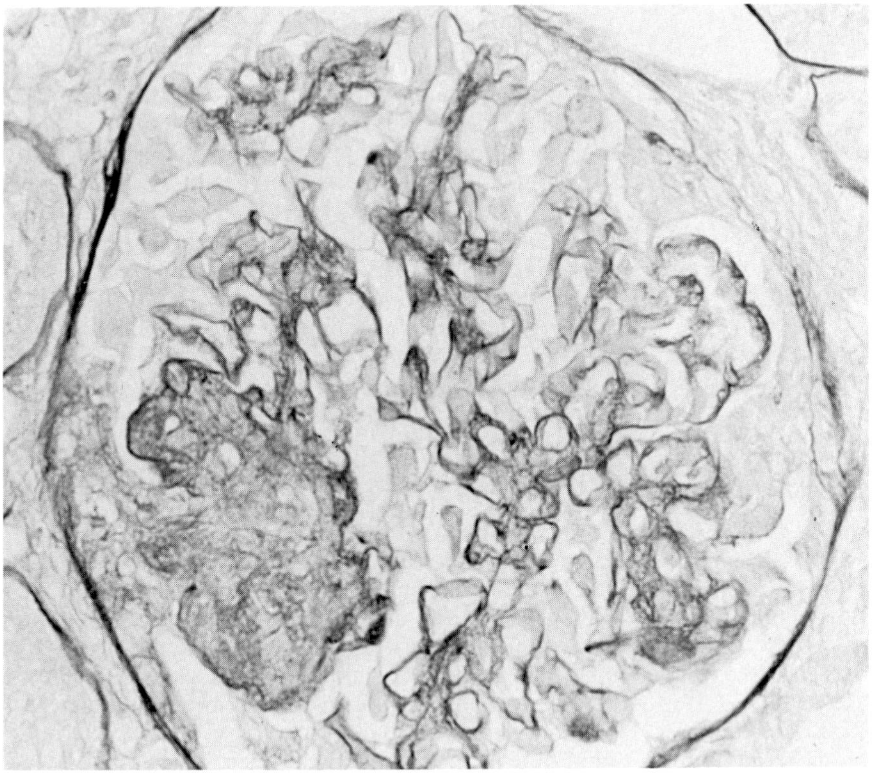

FIGURE 67–6. Focal proliferative lupus nephritis (hematoxylin and eosin stain ×500).

Patients with mild (focal) lupus nephritis usually do not have mild systemic disease. They may be acutely ill with high fevers and severe extrarenal disease, including central nervous system disease. Antinative DNA antibodies and low serum complement levels may be present in those patients with active systemic disease. Treatment with corticosteroids in doses adequate to control the systemic manifestations of the disease usually leads to a clearing of the renal insufficiency, if present, and to clearing of the hematuria.[1] Proteinuria may persist for several months, but it gradually clears, and the urinalysis becomes normal. Such patients do not usually develop severe renal disease later, nor do they develop renal insufficiency if the serologic abnormalities return to the normal range with initial therapy and if the patient remains in serologic and clinical remission.[1] If an exacerbation of the disease does occur, the same focal lesion is again found. Prompt treatment leads to remission. Death from renal disease or from other causes in the presence of renal insufficiency does not occur in these patients if no serologic or clinical disease activity occurs.

Progression from focal to diffuse lupus nephritis has been reported[1] but is uncommon in our experience. In a review of 22 patients with focal nephritis, the 5-year cumulative survival rate from the first sign of renal involvement was 82%, which is similar to the rate found in an earlier study.[1] Deaths occurred in patients who had normal renal function.[1] Progression to diffuse lupus nephritis was more frequent in the patients described by Ginzler et al.[1] and by Zimmerman et al.[1] Progression occurred in 9 of 31 patients (29%) in the former study and in 6 of 17 patients (38%) in the latter study (Table 67–2). Sclerosis occurs occasionally in patients with focal lupus nephritis, but its degree is minimal.[1] Minimal to mild sclerosis was noted in 8 of 16 patients with focal nephritis who had a stable course, and mild sclerosis was noted in the initial biopsy in half of the patients who later progressed to diffuse proliferative nephritis.[1]

Diffuse Proliferative Lupus Nephritis

In this condition there are abnormalities of more than 50% of the total area of the glomerular tufts. Although the proliferation is irregular, all glomeruli are involved, and usually most of each glomerulus is abnormal (Fig. 67–7). Sclerosis may or may not be present in the initial biopsy. The activity of the proliferative lesion may be graded on a semiquantitative basis as originally suggested by Pirani, et al.[1] The 5-year survival rate of patients with diffuse proliferative nephritis appears to be improving. The 5-year survival rate was 41% of 24 patients treated before 1968,[1] and 86% of 22 patients who were followed thereafter. It is clear that the renal biopsy provides useful information in addition to the type of lupus nephritis present. The prognosis in patients with diffuse proliferative lupus nephritis might depend greatly on the degree of activity and of sclerosis noted in the biopsy.

The immunofluorescence findings in diffuse proliferative lupus nephritis are usually striking, with granules

TABLE 67–2. MINIMAL GLOMERULAR AND FOCAL LUPUS NEPHRITIS: CLINICAL AND HISTOLOGIC COURSE

	MOREL-MAROGER ET AL.	GINZLER ET AL.	ZIMMERMAN ET AL.
Number of patients	81	32	17
Stable course	77*	20†	11‡
Renal deterioration GN	4	11	5
Progression to diffuse GN	6 (7.4%)	9 (29%)	6 (35%)

GN, glomerular nephritis.

* GN remained focal in 16 of 18 patients in which biopsy was repeated (mean time between first and second biopsy was 28 months); GN progressed to a diffuse GN in the other patients.

† GN remained focal in the two patients in whom biopsy was repeated.

‡ GN remained focal in the five patients in whom biopsy was repeated.

From Morel-Maroger, L. et al.: The course of lupus nephritis: Contribution of serial renal biopsies. *In* Advances in Nephrology, Vol. 6. Edited by J. Hamburger. Chicago, Year Book, 1976.

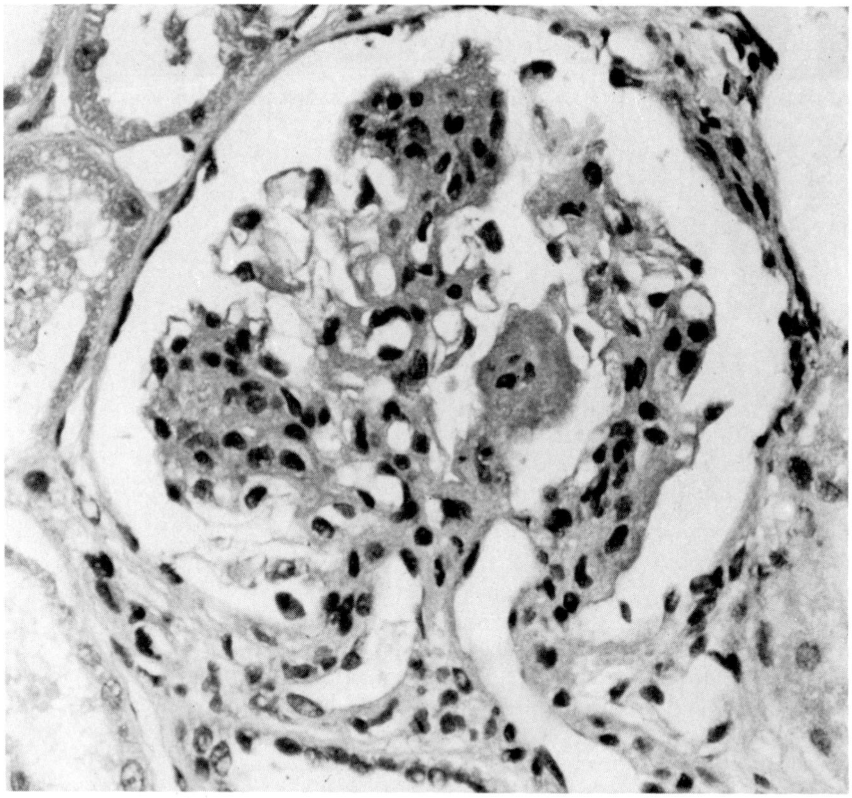

FIGURE 67–7. Diffuse proliferative lupus nephritis (hematoxylin and eosin stain ×500).

or bumps of immunoglobulins and complement proteins, as well as mesangial deposits, noted along the peripheral capillary wall. Infiltrates and deposits of immunoglobulins and complement proteins might also be noted along the tubular basement membrane, within the walls of the peritubular capillaries, or in the interstitium.[1] Electron-dense deposits are noted in the mesangium, in the subendothelial and subepithelial areas, and within the basement membrane. The deposits are located all over the glomeruli, but are not evenly distributed.

The clinical picture is one of moderate to heavy proteinuria with nephrotic syndrome, hematuria, and mild to severe renal insufficiency. Red cell casts are not infrequent. Antibodies to native DNA and low serum C3 are usual unless the lesion is inactive, with a predominance of sclerotic glomeruli. Many patients with severe sclerosis and inactive nonsclerotic glomeruli are in clinical

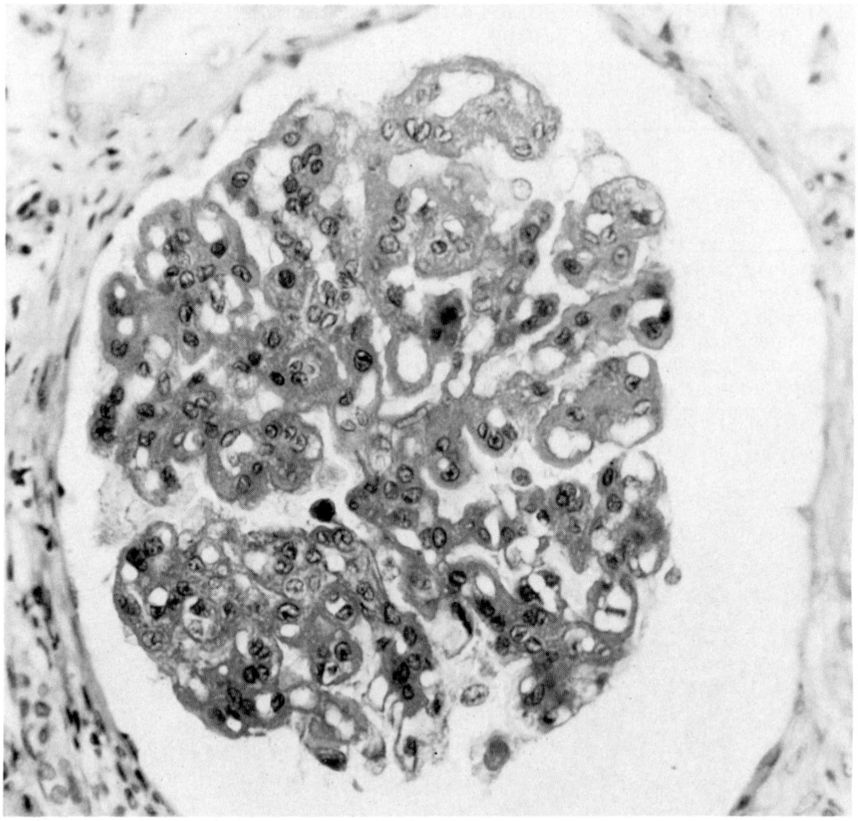

FIGURE 67–8. Membranous lupus nephritis (hematoxylin and eosin stain ×500).

remission and should be treated with small doses of corticosteroids, if at all. These individuals seem to experience a prolonged serologic and clinical remission and do not require treatment for the SLE, although hemodialysis has been required in some.

Membranous Lupus Nephritis

The histologic appearance of this condition is similar to that of idiopathic membranous glomerulonephritis (Fig. 67–8). Although no proliferation is noted, slight, irregular increases in mesangial cells and matrix may be present. Immunofluorescence is striking in that the immunoglobulins are located in a regular fashion along all the basement membranes (Fig. 67–9). It is even possible to observe the spikes of the IgG that protrude on the epithelial side of the capillary loop. Electron microscopy confirms the presence of subepithelial deposits. Patients with this form of lupus nephritis have proteinuria and might have hematuria. The nephrotic syndrome is always present at onset or during the course of the disease.[1] Serologic evidence of disease activity is absent. Normal C3 levels and absence of antibodies to native DNA have been found in these patients when the renal disease was noted and the biopsy was performed, but we have observed some patients with hematuria, low serum C3 levels, and high titers of anti-DNA antibodies. The prognosis is variable but usually is good. We have noted some patients with persistent nephrotic syn-

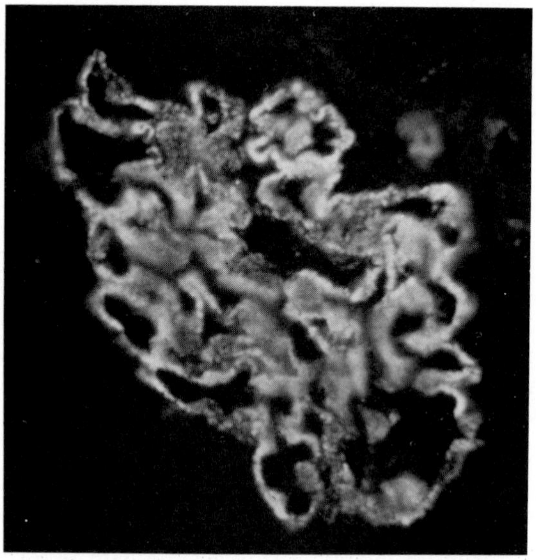

FIGURE 67–9. Membranous lupus nephritis with granular deposits on all capillary loops. Anti-IgG fluorescein isothiocyanate (hematoxylin and eosin stain ×500).

drome and slowly progressive renal insufficiency for as long as 10 years, and we have observed progression to severe renal insufficiency 14 years after the first biopsy. We observed transition to diffuse proliferative lupus nephritis in a patient who refused increased corticosteroid therapy despite clinical evidence of disease activity, persistently normal complement levels, but high levels of complement fixing anti-DNA antibody levels. The onset of severe renal disease was heralded by a severe headache, and the patient was found to be extremely hypertensive with an active urinary sediment, low C3 and C4, and elevation of serum creatinine. Renal biopsy showed very active diffuse proliferative lupus nephritis. This patient, like others, has done extremely well with intravenous cyclophosphamide therapy added to daily corticosteroids. (See also the section on treatment.)

Sclerosing Lupus Nephritis

This is seen in patients with end-stage kidneys, but as already described sclerosis may be present to a greater or lesser extent in patients with either proliferative or membranous lupus nephritis.

Interstitial Nephritis

This condition has been described in approximately 50% of patients.[1] Focal or diffuse infiltrates of inflammatory cells, tubular damage, and interstitial fibrosis are observed. Immunoglobulins, complement, or both can be found in the peritubular capillaries, the interstitium, or the tubular basement membrane in a granular pattern. The interstitial abnormalities are more severe and frequent in patients with diffuse proliferative lupus nephritis, but severe interstitial nephritis with few or no glomerular abnormalities has been noted occasionally. *Renal tubular acidosis* occurs in some patients.

Activity and Sclerosis Index

The renal biopsy can provide information in addition to the WHO classification. The extent of activity and sclerosis can be estimated. Fibrinoid necrosis, endocapillary proliferation, epithelial crescents, nuclear debris, hematoxylin bodies, wire loops, and hyaline thrombi are considered to represent active disease. Markers of active interstitial disease include interstitial cell infiltration and acute tubular epithelial lesions.[1] Necrotizing angiitis is also considered to be an active lesion. The pathologic index of activity is particularly useful if successive biopsies on the same patient are to be evaluated or if groups of patients with lupus nephritis are to be compared. Similarly, the amount of sclerosis in each biopsy can also be graded. Studies of repeated sequential biopsies in 40 patients with diffuse lupus nephritis found that the presence of extensive sclerotic lesions indicated a poor prognosis and that high doses of prednisone given to 14 patients after the first biopsy did not prevent progression of the sclerosis in eight of the patients, even though active lesions diminished.[1] Patients with active lesions had a good prognosis, however, responding to high doses of corticosteroids. In 19 of 25 patients with only moderate glomerular sclerosis, the initially active lesions were considerably decreased in the biopsies repeated after treatment. These conclusions are similar to those reported by Stricker, et al.[1]

Prognosis

In general, most investigators agree that maleness and a serum creatinine level greater than 1.3 predict renal failure.[14] In our own series, most of the deaths from renal disease have occurred in our male patients. These individuals have been particularly noncompliant, refusing to take significant doses of corticosteroids, or refusing intravenous cyclophosphamide. Patients with persistent or recurrent hypocomplementemia have been shown to have significantly worse chances of survival (at 5 or more years) than patients with normal CH_{50} assay levels.[15] Esdaile et al. found that low C3 was a predictor of poor prognosis and renal death in their group of lupus nephritis patients, the majority of whom had diffuse proliferative disease.[16] The WHO class of diffuse proliferative nephritis suggests a poor prognosis, as does a high activity index. The use of renal biopsy information in the treatment of lupus nephritis is discussed below.

NERVOUS SYSTEM

Involvement of neural tissue is common in SLE.

Peripheral Neuropathy

This condition has occurred in 14% of our patients, an incidence similar to that reported by Feinglass.[1] The most common defect is sensory disturbance, but a mixed sensory-motor disturbance is seen in about 5% of patients with the typical asymmetric involvement of mononeuritis multiplex. These episodes occur most often at the time of diagnosis along with evidence of active disease in other systems. In most patients, treatment of the systemic disease with corticosteroids leads to a gradual return of function of the affected extremities. Other less common abnormalities consist of a picture suggesting the Guillain-Barré syndrome and myelopathy. Some patients with peripheral neuropathy also have evidence of cranial neuropathy.

Cranial Nerve Signs

These signs were noted in only 16 of the 140 SLE patients reported by Feinglass et al.[1] We have noted facial weakness, ptosis, diplopia, and other evidence of cranial nerve involvement. Optic neuritis might be the first manifestation of SLE.[1] These abnormalities frequently occur with other neuropsychiatric features. Feinglass et al. described one patient with optic neuritis who had transverse myelitis at the same time.[1] We have a patient with thrombosis of the opthalmic artery and mononeuritis multiplex. Peripheral neuropathy is common in patients with cranial neuropathy.

Long tract involvement occurred in 16 of 140 SLE patients described by Feinglass et al.[1] Five of their patients with long tract signs had cerebrovascular accidents. Long tract signs also usually occur along with other evidence of neuropsychiatric disease.

Central Nervous System

More common and more serious than peripheral nervous system involvement, central nervous system (CNS) disease occurs in two major forms, organic psychosis and seizures. Seizures in the absence of renal insufficiency, hypertension, or infection occur in about 15% of SLE patients[1] and are usually present at the time of the original diagnosis, accompanying active systemic disease. We have noted the onset of seizures in two of our patients late in the course of the disease. Grand mal seizures are most common, but we have also seen patients with chorea, Jacksonian fits, petit mal, and temporal lobe seizures. Pseudotumor cerebri can also occur with acute disease. Nearly all of these manifestations occur at the time of disease onset and in many cases are accompanied by other neuropsychiatric abnormalities.[1] Chorea and petit mal seizures sometimes begin at the time of diagnosis of SLE, along with other evidence of disease activity, and can persist for many years, even when no clinical evidence of disease activity elsewhere can be documented.

CNS involvement can also be manifested by organic brain disease.[1] Organic syndromes are characterized by impairment of orientation, perception, and the ability to calculate. Memory deficits are common, and the patients might have difficulty remembering the names of their own physicians. In our series of patients studied at the Bellevue Medical-Psychiatric wards, 21% of the total group of 209 patients had episodes of CNS disease during the first year of diagnosis. These patients were acutely ill with multisystem disease and fever; 15% had CNS disease during the first year after diagnosis, but only 2% showed CNS findings during the fifth through the sixth years. No episodes of CNS disease occurred in 43 patients in their eighth year or in 24 patients during their ninth year. No episodes of psychosis occurred in 25 patients during their tenth through twelfth years, although two patients had cerebrovascular accidents, one in the eleventh year and one in the twelfth year after diagnosis. Thus, CNS disease is a manifestation of severe active lupus, occurs early in the course of the disease, and coincides with evidence of disease activity in other systems.[1]

Complete recovery from the organic brain disease is usual, but some patients have residual impairment of mental processes, such as an inability to calculate as rapidly as they could before the disease episode. SLE patients with CNS disease are more likely to have evidence of vasculitis than those without such findings.[1] The 5-year survival rate of our 82 patients with organic brain disease at the time of diagnosis was 71%, compared to a 77% survival rate of the 274 patients without organic brain disease.[1] All of the patients with CNS disease were treated with high doses of corticosteroids.

Severe Headaches

At the time of diagnosis, 21 of our 209 SLE patients in New York complained of severe headaches. In five of these patients, the headache was associated with organic brain disease; in eight others it was associated with seizures. Brandt and Lessel described 11 patients with severe throbbing headaches or with wavy or zigzag line scotomata typical of the fortification specters of migraine.[1] These phenomena either occurred for the first time after the diagnosis of SLE or occurred as an initial feature along with other manifestations of systemic disease. Migraine headaches or fortification specters have also occurred as an isolated symptom prior to the development of other clinical manifestations of SLE, but at a time when serologic abnormalities of SLE were found. Classic migraine headaches have an increased prevalence in SLE patients.[1] It is important to recognize these headaches as a manifestation of SLE because they disappear when prednisone is administered or when the dose of corticosteroid is increased, and they occur along with other manifestations of the disease during periods of exacerbation.

Cerebrovascular Accident

This occurs rarely in SLE patients. Classic strokes secondary to cerebral infarction or intracranial hemorrhage have been seen in 1 of 204 patients in my Bellevue series and in 3 of 583 patients I have seen in Connecticut. In all instances, patients had active SLE at the time, and the majority of accidents occurred at onset or within 1 year of the time of diagnosis. Polyarteritis-like lesions in cerebral vessels have been documented by angiography, and embolization from Libman-Sacks vegetations on heart valves has been reported.[1] The presence of the lupus anticoagulant in patients with cerebral infarcts has been noted in our patients and reported in the literature. We have treated these patients with long-term anticoagulant therapy.

Psychologic Problems

Most SLE patients have major psychologic problems coping with their disease and with side effects of the therapy they are receiving. They become depressed and anxious. The disfigurement caused by high doses of corticosteroids is especially difficult in young women and adolescents and may lead to a major depression. Such mental abnormality is not part of the disease itself and should not be called "CNS lupus." The corticosteroid dose should not be increased in such patients. These individuals need reassurance and may require psychotherapy.

Laboratory Findings

Abnormalities of the cerebrospinal fluid (CSF) were present in 32% of episodes of neuropsychiatric illness in 37 patients studied by Feinglass et al.[1] Protein elevation was noted in about half the fluids, and in a few patients, both protein and white cells were increased. Elevation of CSF pressure may be associated with papilledema. Protein elevation may be absent, modest, or even insignificant. Elevation of CSF IgG is relatively specific for active CNS lupus but is not a very sensitive measure. Rarely, the cerebrospinal fluid suggests an infectious process. Feinglass et al. noted that death correlated with CSF abnormalities.[1] A test for the presence of antibodies to neuronal cell membranes correlated with the presence of neuropsychiatric lupus, but this test is not readily available.[1]

The electroencephalogram (EEG) is frequently abnormal during an episode of neuropsychiatric disease. An abnormal EEG can also be noted in patients without CNS abnormalities, but EEGs are more frequently abnormal in patients with CNS disease. Diffuse slow-wave activity is the most common abnormality, but focal changes may also be observed.

The use of computed tomography (CT), magnetic resonance imaging, auditory evoked potentials, cerebral blood flow measurement with oxygen-15, and positron emission tomography have been claimed to detect subclinical disease or generalized central nervous system disease.[17–21] At present most researchers agree that computed tomography is able to detect focal lesions most successfully. Future longitudinal studies are needed for thorough evaluation of the newer techniques. The search for a serologic marker for CNS lupus has not yet been successful.

Pathology

Pathologic abnormalities in patients with seizures usually consist of microinfarcts.[1] Vasculitis is found in 35% and intracerebral hemorrhages in 22% of patients. Focal motor seizures are associated with findings of subarachnoid hemorrhage. Pathologic changes in 12 patients with hemiparesis were similar to the changes associated with seizures, except that intracerebral hemorrhage was present in six patients and the hemorrhage was related to the presence of brain vasculitis.[1] Vasculitis was also present in one-third of patients with subarachnoid hemorrhage and in 25% of those patients with microhemorrhages. Patients dying with lupus psychosis show microinfarcts, vasculitis, and cerebral hemorrhages.[1] Immunofluorescence studies have revealed deposits of immunoglobulins and C3 in the choroid plexus of SLE patients.[1]

GASTROINTESTINAL MANIFESTATIONS

The most common gastrointestinal manifestation is abdominal pain. The pain may be accompanied by nausea and less often by diarrhea. In most patients, abdominal pain occurs in association with evidence of disease activity in other systems. The cause of abdominal pain usually is not clear. Mesenteric arteritis may be noted on arteriography. Patients with mesenteric arteritis have ileal and colonic ulcers, and ileal and colonic perforations can occur.[1] In addition, necrosis of the large and small bowel may be present. We have observed three deaths from intestinal perforation in our 365 patients. Zizic et al. described colonic perforations as the cause of 4 of 15 deaths (27%) occurring in 197 patients with SLE.[1]

The pain in patients with perforations is colicky and well-localized to the lower abdomen or infraumbilical area. Abdominal pain in SLE patients without perforations is less well localized or might be localized to the epigastrium or upper quadrants. It may be either sharp or colicky. Both rebound and direct tenderness were present in our patients with perforations and in four of the five patients reported by Zizic et al.[1] Neither rebound tenderness nor localized direct tenderness was present in SLE patients with abdominal pain without perforations. Abdominal pain is much more common in children with SLE than in adults, but perforations have not been observed. The abdominal pain in children is crampy and occurs during periods of disease activity, disappearing as other manifestations of the disease resolve.

Patients with colonic perforation usually have evidence of severe active SLE in other systems. Both our patients and those described by Zizic et al. had highly active SLE. The only surviving patient received early surgical intervention before radiologic evidence of perforation was apparent, even though she was considered a poor surgical risk because of lupus nephritis with uremia.[1] Thus, early surgical intervention is strongly suggested if the diagnosis of perforation is suspected.

Some SLE patients had regional enteritis with erosions and ulceration of the intestinal mucosa at the time of operation for abdominal pain.[1]

In our series, abdominal pain of acute onset with evidence of peritonitis occurred in 17 patients. The pain was due to massive ascites, ruptured ovarian cyst, perforated gastric ulcer, appendicitis, diverticulitis, and abscess of the fallopian tubes. It is wise to consider early surgical intervention in SLE patients.

Ascites is present in about 10% of SLE patients and can persist for months.

PANCREATITIS

Pancreatitis occurred in 7 of our 365 SLE patients when the disease was active in other systems. In our patients, pancreatitis was associated with organic brain disease as well as with other clinical and serologic evidence of active SLE. In one analysis, elevated serum amylase was found in 26 SLE patients, and pancreatitis caused by SLE was present in four patients, all of whom recovered with corticosteroid treatment.[1]

LIVER AND SPLEEN

Hepatomegaly occurs in about 30% of patients, more commonly among children than among adult-onset patients.[1] Clinically evident jaundice occurred in 1 of 365 patients, and hepatic insufficiency was the cause of death in one 8-year-old girl. Autopsy revealed acute fatty degeneration of the liver. Four of our 365 SLE patients had biopsy evidence of chronic active hepatitis, and all four met the American Rheumatism Association (ARA) Criteria for the Classification of SLE.[1] Skin manifestations, CNS lupus, and mild lupus nephritis were present in these patients. Liver enzyme elevations are noted in about 30% of patients at the time of diagnosis, when active disease is evident in many systems. In addition, aspirin can cause elevations of transaminase levels in patients with SLE. Liver biopsies from SLE patients who had either clinical liver disease or liver enzyme abnormalities revealed findings only of chronic active hepatitis, granulomatous hepatitis, cirrhosis, acute hepatitis, fatty change, or cholestasis.[1]

Slight to moderate splenomegaly is present in 20% of patients and is more common in children.[1] Splenomegaly is not usually associated with hemolytic anemia. Asplenism has been reported in SLE patients, including two of 65 patients whose functional asplenism was only detected by CT scan.[1] The onion-skin appearance of the splenic arterioles is present in 15% of patients. This change is due to concentric periarterial fibrosis, thought to be the end stage of an earlier focal arteritis.

LYMPH NODES

Lymph nodes enlargement occurs in about half of all SLE patients with active disease. Lymphadenopathy is more common in children than in adults.[1] Adenopathy is usually generalized but may be limited, and the enlarged nodes are usually nontender. One of our patients had two severe episodes of active disease, each associated with massive nontender enlargement of the occipital nodes. Microscopic changes in lymph nodes are nonspecific. They consist of follicular hyperplasia, which may be associated with areas of necrosis resembling giant follicular lymphoma.

OCULAR MANIFESTATIONS

Conjunctivitis or episcleritis occurred in 15 of our patients and appeared to be more common in patients with extensive cutaneous manifestations. Periorbital edema and subconjunctival hemorrhages have also been reported. Occlusion of the central retinal artery has been reported during periods of disease activity, but is a rare occurrence. Active retinal arteritis and arteriolar occlusion have been reported.[1] Blindness may be the first symptom of the disease.[1] Cytoid bodies, which occurred in 8% of our patients and in 7% of 550 SLE patients followed prospectively every 3 months, are retinal exudates appearing as hard, white lesions adjacent to retinal vessels during periods of disease activity.[23] They can be associated with organic brain disease and seizures. These exudates disappear gradually as the disease becomes inactive.

PAROTID GLAND ENLARGEMENT

Enlarged parotid glands occurred in 8% of our patients, most of whom did not have xerostomia. Typical keratoconjunctivitis sicca is uncommon. Unilateral enlargement of a parotid gland may be observed during periods of disease activity in a small number of patients. One prospective study reported a high incidence of associated Sjögren's syndrome, including a positive Schirmer's test in 21%, positive parotid scan in 58%, and positive lip biopsy in 50% of patients.[1]

MENSTRUAL ABNORMALITIES AND PREGNANCY

Cessation of menses during the initial 3 to 6 months of treatment occurs frequently, but menstrual periods return as the disease goes into remission and the dose of corticosteroids is reduced. Menorrhagia occasionally occurs, possibly because of thrombocytopenia or an inhibitor of one of the clotting factors. A small percentage of SLE patients experience a monthly flare-up of the disease just prior to or at the onset of menses. This usually is manifested by a transient facial rash, joint pain, or pleuritic chest pain.

Stillbirths and spontaneous abortions are common in untreated patients with active disease. Normal deliveries are the rule in well-controlled patients taking low doses of corticosteroids for at least 6 months prior to conception.[1] Normal deliveries may be due to the suppression of maternal lupus anticoagulant.[1] Slight exacerbations of the disease are common in the immediate prepartum and postpartum periods, however.[1] The impact of pregnancy on SLE has recently been reviewed.[24]

We have not observed congenital abnormalities in the children of our patients, with the exception of complete heart block. This was present in two children of one of our patients, who was one of three patients in the first report describing the association of congenital heart block and SLE.[1] We recently tested her banked serum and found that she had very high levels of anti-Ro. Congenital heart block is clearly associated with anti-Ro antibody passively transferred to the infant from the mother, although mothers with SLE and anti-Ro antibodies usually give birth to normal infants.

ALLERGIC REACTIONS

SLE patients do not have a higher than normal incidence of allergic dermatitis, rhinitis, asthma, or food or drug allergies. Instances of severe exacerbations of the disease have been observed after treatment of urinary infections with sulfasoxazole, however. Hives are not uncommon and are probably a manifestation of the disease rather than of allergy.

LABORATORY FINDINGS

HEMATOLOGIC ABNORMALITIES

One or more hematologic abnormalities are present in nearly all SLE patients with active disease. Most common is a mild-to-moderate normocytic, normochromic *anemia* caused by retarded erythropoiesis. Hematocrit values of less than 30% occur in about half the patients during periods of clinical disease activity. On the other hand, Coombs' test–positive hemolytic anemia occurred in only 10% of our 365 patients, although positive Coombs' tests occur more frequently as an isolated abnormality owing to the presence of C3 or C4 on the erythrocyte surface without evidence of hemolysis or reticulocytosis.

Mild to moderate *leukopenia* is less common than anemia. Leukopenia of less than 4000 cells/cmm was present in 17% of our patients. Usually both lymphocyte and neutrophil numbers are decreased. Lymphopenia is usually present during periods of disease activity.[1] *Leukocytosis* is occasionally noted during episodes of active disease and can be a confusing finding if spiking fever is also present. Leukocytosis resulting from corticosteroid therapy also occurs in SLE patients. White blood counts of 30,000, nearly all mature neutrophils, have occasionally been observed in corticosteroid-treated, noninfected patients.

Mild *thrombocytopenia* of between 100,000 and 150,000/cmm is present in about one-third of patients, but severe thrombocytopenia with purpura has occurred in only 5%. Thrombocytopenia might occur for the first time late in the course of the disease. It occurred as an isolated event in the last trimester of pregnancy in two well-controlled SLE patients taking low doses of prednisone. An antiplatelet factor on the surface of the platelets occurs in most patients even without thrombocytopenia and is found during periods of remission as well as during disease activity. Qualitative thrombocyte defects are also common.[1]

The *lupus anticoagulant* (see also Chapter 70) can be identified by the presence of a slight prolongation of the prothrombin time and more marked prolongation of the partial thromboplastin time, which is not corrected by the addition of equal volumes of normal plasma to the patient's plasma at dilutions of 1:50, 1:100, and 1:500. Anti-cardiolipin (antiphospholipid) antibody can be detected using an enzyme-linked immunosorbent assay (ELISA) technique. The false-positive VDRL is also due to this or to an associated antibody. The lupus anticoagulant is not clinically related to increased bleeding; bleeding and clotting times are normal. Renal biopsies have been performed on individuals with the lupus anticoagulant without any bleeding. There is a significant relationship between the lupus anticoagulant and thrombosis. Arterial and venous thrombosis, placental infarction, cerebral infarction, and thrombocytopenia are all more common in patients with the lupus anticoagulant. The lupus anticoagulant disappears with high-dose corticosteroid therapy, but usually recurs as the dose is lowered. If a patient has had a major thrombosis, I use anticoagulants.

Inhibitors that specifically inactivate clotting factors are significant clinically. These are most frequently directed at Factors II, VIII, IX, and XII and must be identified, because major bleeding episodes can result from renal biopsies or operative procedures. The action of these specific anticoagulants is also reversed by corticosteroid therapy. In general, bleeding problems in SLE patients occur in individuals with active disease, especially in those with vasculitis.

False-positive serologic tests for syphilis were present in 25% of our patients and are frequently, but not always, associated with the lupus anticoagulant (see Chapter 70).

The erythrocyte sedimentation rate (ESR) is elevated in nearly all SLE patients and, in most patients, falls to normal when the disease becomes inactive. Some patients, however, maintain a markedly elevated ESR for years in the absence of clinical or serologic evidence of active disease.

Serum C-reactive protein (CRP) levels are elevated in infections and in rheumatoid arthritis but rarely in uncomplicated SLE.[1] CRP levels above 60 mg/L were found in 8 of 18 SLE patients with infection and in only 3 of 42 patients without infection (sensitivity = 39%; specificity = 93%).

Cryoglobulins of the mixed IgG-IgM type are found in about 11% of patients. They are usually associated with clinical and serologic disease activity, lower serum complement levels, and clinical nephritis.

A diffuse elevation of serum γ-globulin is observed in about 80% of patients with clinically active disease. Rheumatoid factor is present in 14% of SLE patients.

Serum complement levels are usually depressed in active disease. The most sensitive test for disease activity is C4, but a low level can be due to a C4 null allele, as already discussed. The association of SLE-like conditions with complement component deficiencies has been discussed already.

DIFFERENTIAL DIAGNOSIS

The ARA Preliminary Criteria for the Classification of SLE[24] have been used since 1971 and are sensitive.[1] These criteria have helped remind physicians of the major laboratory and clinical manifestations of SLE, but they were established prior to the common availability of useful serologic tests such as complement levels, antinuclear antibodies, anti-DNA, and anti-Smith antibodies. The Revised Criteria were published in 1982 (Table 67–1).[1] Although not included in the Revised Criteria, serum C3 levels are of major importance in the diagnosis of an individual patient with SLE. We have shown that a low serum C3 in the presence of antibodies to native DNA is highly specific for SLE.[1] The sensitivity of the anti-DNA antibody test was 72%, and the specificity was 96%. The sensitivity of a low serum C3 level was 38%, and the specificity was 90%. Thus, in addition to studies of serum antibodies to nuclear antigens, a serum C3 level should be performed in all individuals for whom a diagnosis of SLE is considered. The most common diagnosis made in patients before a definitive diagnosis of SLE is rheumatoid arthritis or "nonspecific" arthritis. Approximately one quarter of our SLE patients had this diagnosis for at least 1 year prior to the diagnosis of SLE. Young women presenting with a history of arthritis or arthralgia should be studied carefully for SLE. The onset of arthritis or arthralgia during pregnancy or postpartum should particularly alert the physician to the possibility of SLE. Diagnoses that can predate a definitive diagnosis of SLE by 2 to 10 years include rheumatic fever, chronic discoid lupus, idiopathic thrombocytopenic purpura, seizure disorder, Raynaud's phenomenon, psychosis, and hemolytic anemia.

SLE does occur in elderly persons in whom the diagnosis is frequently missed early in the course of their disease.

Other diseases to consider in patients with multisystem findings include subacute bacterial endocarditis, infected atrioventricular shunts, gonococcal or meningococcal septicemia with arthritis and skin lesions, serum sickness, lymphoma and leukemia, thrombotic thrombocytopenic purpura, sarcoidosis, secondary syphilis, bacterial septicemia, and acquired immunodeficiency disease (AIDS).

MANAGEMENT

At the time of diagnosis, the severity of the disease should be determined using the history, physical examination, and laboratory. With rapid disease onset, the patient should be considered to have a more severe condition. The presence of both anti-DNA antibodies and low serum complement (especially C3) levels suggests active disease as well as more severe disease. Patients in whom these two abnormalities persist have a poorer prognosis[16]; therefore it is important to monitor the C3 and anti-DNA and to treat these abnormalities.

RENAL BIOPSY

Urinary abnormalities should lead to complete study for renal disease. Renal biopsy provides information regarding prognosis and potential degree of reversibility, which is needed to select the appropriate type of therapy.[25] Serum creatinine levels should be obtained on two occasions to determine whether renal insufficiency is present or impending. Patients with proteinuria and red cells in the urine should have a renal biopsy to determine the following: (1) the *type* of lupus nephritis, as discussed already; (2) the *activity* of the glomerular lesion; (3) the presence and extent of glomerular, tubular, or both types of *sclerosis*; and (4) the presence and extent of tubular and interstitial disease. The presence of sclerosis early in the course of the disease is a sign of a poor prognosis. Extensive sclerosis does not respond to any kind of aggressive therapy. The management of the various forms of lupus nephritis with corticosteroids is described in the section on renal disease. The use of other forms of therapy for lupus nephritis will be described.

Management of SLE is divided into four sections: (1) general measures that should be applied to most patients; (2) management of active disease, particularly at the onset of the illness; (3) management of the period between control of the initial episode of active disease and clinical remission; and (4) management of the patient over an extended clinical remission. An additional section covers the use of specific agents.

GENERAL MEASURES

Both patient and physician should become familiar with the signs and symptoms present during the time of disease onset. The early clinical recurrence of disease activity may then be recognized by the patient, who should alert the physician. For example, some patients develop an erythematous rash as the first sign of an impending serious systemic exacerbation. If the patient merely waits until the next appointment to inform the physician of the rash, the delay may result in the appearance of more serious, additional manifestations, such as hematuria or pericarditis.

The physician should be familiar with the laboratory evidence of active disease in each patient and with the response of each laboratory abnormality to corticosteroid therapy. Thus, if the ESR is initially elevated and rapidly returns to normal after therapy, a future significant increase in the ESR may be viewed with concern because it might signal exacerbation of the disease. Similarly, initial low C3 or C4 levels, which return to the normal range as the disease becomes inactive, usually fall again either just before or as the clinical disease activity recurs. Prior to treatment, the physician should know which laboratory tests were *not* abnormal during the initial episode of disease activity. Other patients have abnormal laboratory findings that do not resolve with treatment and clinical remission. For example, elevated antinative DNA antibodies have been noted over the course of 5 years in patients who are clinically well. Abnormal test results that do not respond initially to adequate treatment should probably be ignored in most patients. Patients with persistently high anti-DNA antibody levels but who are clinically well and have otherwise normal laboratory tests become acutely ill when their C3 levels fall.

All SLE patients initially need reassurance from their physician, adequate rest when the disease is active, and avoidance of sun exposure. Sunscreen creams and ointments, wide-brimmed hats, and long sleeves should be used by all SLE patients. Exercise should be encouraged at each visit after the patient has initially responded to corticosteroids with loss of fatigue, disappearance of arthritis or arthralgia, and an increase in sense of well being.

Birth Control

Pregnancy should be avoided during the first few years of disease. Oral contraceptives should be avoided. Pregnancy has been well tolerated in our patients who have no evidence of active renal disease or sclerotic glomeruli and who are in clinical remission while taking less than 15 mg of prednisone daily for at least 1 year. Exacerbations of disease during pregnancy should be managed by vigorous treatment with corticosteroids rather than by therapeutic abortion.[1]

Infections

All SLE patients should be observed carefully for infections. Patients should be instructed to inform the physician immediately if any symptoms occur or if a fever is present. Urinalysis should be performed and cultures should be performed on specimens that show bacteria. Patients should be treated prophylactically with antibiotics if scaling of the gums, teeth extraction, or major dental surgery is performed.

Hypertension

Patients should be treated as aggressively as necessary to lower their blood pressure. One factor that may explain the better prognosis of severe lupus nephritis today as compared with that reported during the 1950s is the current use of antihypertensive agents to control blood pressure elevations.[1]

Disease Severity

Treatment depends not only on the target organs involved but on the severity of the disease. Renal disease can be minimal or mild. Anemia may be slight or a severe hemolytic anemia. Mildly ill patients frequently are diagnosed at a time when arthritis and a butterfly rash are the only signs and symptoms of the disease. The laboratory evidence of severe disease is of great importance in such patients. A low serum C3 and high titers of antinative DNA antibodies are considered by many, although not all, investigators to indicate that severe clinical or renal disease (or both) might ensue unless the patient is treated aggressively.

Other laboratory parameters that may be present in patients whose signs and symptoms are mild include thrombocytopenia, hemolytic anemia, renal disease with more than mild proteinuria, seizures, organic brain disease, and vasculitis of the skin or other organs. If present, these parameters indicate that the disease is severe and should be treated aggressively. In our experience, pericarditis and pleuritis are also considered "severe," but others do not agree.

MANAGEMENT OF ACTIVE DISEASE, PARTICULARLY AT ONSET OF ILLNESS

Patients with severe disease should be treated with corticosteroids (see Chapter 37). Most patients respond to 60 mg of prednisone given in doses of 15 mg every 6 hours. Many severely ill patients without CNS or active renal disease require a similar high dose of prednisone initially. In most patients, evidence of disease activity disappears rapidly. Large pericardial or pleural effusions, hematuria and, occasionally, CNS manifestations might respond more slowly and might require a higher daily dose of prednisone. In an analysis of 67 neuropsychiatric episodes, 84% had a favorable outcome, usually associated with initiation or increase in steroid dose.[1]

The use of pulse-therapy corticosteroids (intravenous infusion of large doses, usually 1 g methylprednisolone daily for 3 days) has been advocated in the management of severe SLE patients with rapidly advancing renal failure who have not responded to oral doses.[1] Although some investigators have described a rapid fall of "nephrotic range" proteinuria, we have not found this to occur in a small number of patients so treated. Improvement has been described in one of three patients with lupus cerebritis, in all three patients with lung disease, and in one patient with thrombocytopenia.[1]

In patients with pulmonary hemorrhage not caused by infection, pulse therapy and plasmapheresis may be the treatment of choice because these patients need as rapid a therapeutic effect as possible. It is important to continue with high-dose oral corticosteroid therapy after the 3-day pulse therapy in such acutely ill patients. There are still no definitive studies to determine whether pulse therapy provides better long-term management. The question regarding possible long-term side effects, such as aseptic necrosis, is not clear at present. Acute side effects resulting from intravenous pulse therapy include bacteremia and sudden death, the latter presumably owing to electrolyte effects on the myocardium. In addition, hyperglycemia, hypokalemia or hyperkalemia, sodium retention, hypotention or hypertension, and acute psychosis have been described. In some centers, intravenous pulse therapy is administered only to inpatients with continuous cardiac monitors. Infusion over at least 30 minutes is recommended.[1]

Plasmapheresis is still an experimental treatment and, in general, should be restricted to centers where controlled protocol studies are being conducted. Recorded data strongly suggest that plasmapheresis is followed by a serious rebound of both immunologic and clinical activity.[1] In addition, many of the reports in the literature describe a short-lived remission. Plasmapheresis together with corticosteroid therapy appears to be effective, but the response is also short-lived, as is the response to plasmapheresis and azathioprine. The most prolonged response follows plasmapheresis combined with both corticosteroids and cyclophosphamide. Patients so treated responded and had no rebound, and the improvement lasted for at least 4 months. Thus, if plasmapheresis is to be used, it should be given with corticosteroids and cyclophosphamide. Patients with pulmonary hemorrhage have responded to a combination of pulse intravenous corticosteroids, plasmapheresis, and intravenous cyclophosphamide.

Less severely ill patients respond to 20 to 40 mg of prednisone given in a regimen of 5 to 10 mg four times daily. The response is usually prompt (i.e., within 1 to 2 weeks), with disappearance of symptoms and a change in abnormal laboratory tests toward a normal range.

SLE patients with mild disease and without significantly abnormal laboratory tests may be treated with a combination of aspirin and hydroxychloroquine sulfate (Plaquenil). Aspirin is used in anti-inflammatory doses (see Chapter 32), and 200 mg of hydroxychloroquine is given twice daily (see Chapter 34). This regimen is adequate for most patients in whom arthritis and dermatologic abnormalities are the only clinical signs and symptoms and in whom laboratory test results are not "severe"—for example, in patients with subacute cutaneous lupus.

Experimental therapies such as cyclosporin and total nodal irradiation are reserved for patients who do not respond to the above therapies.

MANAGEMENT AFTER INITIAL RESPONSE

Most SLE patients respond initially to high doses of oral corticosteroids. As the clinical disease responds, resolution of laboratory abnormalities is observed. The corticosteroid dose can then be lowered. Gradual tapering with frequent monitoring of laboratory values is usually successful until the daily dose of prednisone reaches 10 to 20 mg. At this dosage, there may be evidence of serologic or clinical flare of the disease, and the prednisone dose should then be held constant temporarily or should be slightly increased.

MANAGEMENT DURING EXTENDED CLINICAL DISEASE INACTIVITY

In patients controlled on small doses of prednisone, repeated attempts should be made to further reduce the dose. It might be necessary to lower the dosage by small increments (e.g., by 1 mg per week). In most patients, a daily dose of 10 mg or less is adequate to control the disease and to allow the patients to feel totally free of symptoms. Even in these individuals, the primary goal should be administration of no medication or of the lowest possible dose. Alternate-day therapy has been used successfully in some patients. In my experience, daily small doses (2.5 to 10 mg) lead to better prolonged control. As always, the dose should be given early in the morning to avoid suppression of the nocturnal adrenocorticotropic hormone (ACTH) secretion.

SPECIFIC AGENTS

Antimalarials

Antimalarials are effective in patients with dermatologic manifestations of SLE.[1] A randomized study revealed a significant increase in the relative risk of a clinical flare-up or an increase in disease severity during the 6 months after hydroxychloroquine was withdrawn from patients with SLE.[26] This multicenter study extends our previous findings of increase in skin and mucous membrane manifestations as well as malaise and generalized complaints after drug withdrawal. The new information strongly suggests that hydroxychloroquine should be used in all SLE patients. Retinal toxicity occurs in some SLE patients who have taken antimalarial drugs for a significant length of time in high doses.[1] The incidence of retinopathy is related to the total ingested dose of the antimalarial drugs. Patients should be seen by an ophthalmologist before treatment and every 6 months while receiving therapy (see Chapter 33). Hydroxychloroquine, 400 mg daily, can be used initially with eventual decrease in daily dose to 200 mg when skin lesions are no longer present. An attempt should be made to further reduce the dosage to alternate days, or three or two times per week, or to discontinue the drug. In some patients, however, relapses occur and the drug must be restarted.

Aspirin and Nonsteroidal Anti-inflammatory Drugs (NSAIDs)

Anti-inflammatory doses of aspirin or other NSAIDs are of value in controlling arthritis in patients whose symptoms are not satisfactorily controlled by low doses of corticosteroids. Rapid dramatic control of pleural effusions, pericardial effusions, or both is sometimes achieved with indomethacin, 25 mg t.i.d. If NSAIDs are used, the physician should be aware of the reports of aseptic meningitis caused by ibuprofen, tolmetin, and sulindac.[1] These agents may cause either a rapid or a slow fall in renal function, and thus should not be used without monitoring serum creatinine levels. It is wise to withhold these agents in patients with renal disease. In patients with the lupus anticoagulant or antiphospholipid antibodies, a baby aspirin daily or an adult aspirin every other day is indicated to help prevent thrombosis.

Cyclophosphamide

The use of immunosuppressive agents in the treatment of SLE has been generally accepted as indicated in specific situations. The National Institutes of Health studies strongly suggest that patients with diffuse proliferative nephritis with active lesions do better when they are treated with a combination of intravenous cyclophosphamide and oral prednisone.[27] McCune et al. have also shown the clear benefit of intravenous cyclophosphamide when used monthly.[28] The need for a renal biopsy prior to using this therapy is clear, and treatment with corticosteroids is continued as necessary. The toxicity and long-term side effects of these drugs and their use in the management of SLE have been reviewed in Chapter 38. Oral daily cyclophosphamide is of great value in patients with medium- or small-vessel necrotizing vasculitis. Its efficacy is similar to that in patients with Wegener's vasculitis or periarteritis nodosa (see also Chapters 36 and 75).

Azathioprine

Azathioprine is helpful in patients whose disease is difficult to control when the dose of prednisone is reduced below 15 mg daily. In some patients, the addition of azathioprine, 75 to 150 mg daily, is definitely followed by remission, allowing the patient to remain on very small daily prednisone doses.

Other Measures

The use of other agents has been reviewed recently.[29] Methotrexate has been reported to be of value in patients in whom large doses of prednisone are required for clinical remission.[30] We have treated four such SLE patients with methotrexate, and three are currently taking it with significantly lower doses of prednisone. Cyclosporine might be of value in the treatment of lupus nephritis, although the drug is very nephrotoxic in the doses used thus far.[31] Intravenous immunoglobulin is of value in the treatment of thombocytopenia, but its value for other manifestations of SLE is unclear.[29] C2-deficient SLE has been treated successfully with plasma infusions.[32]

Severe or Refractory Cutaneous Manifestations

Retinoids and their metabolites have been successfully used in the treatment of refractory subacute and discoid lesions. We have treated SLE patients with discoid or subacute lesions refractory to antimalarials who required high doses of corticosteroids with isotretinoin (Accutane). Most patient's lesions became less erythematous, and pruritic, and healed; the corticosteroid dose could be lowered, but relapses occurred rapidly after drug withdrawal.[33] The use of these agents must be accompanied by effective contraception because they are associated with fetal abnormalities. Dapsone and thalidomide have also been used for severe skin lesions.[34]

PROGNOSIS

Studies on the survival of SLE patients have shown improvement over time (Table 67–3).[1]

Corticosteroid-treated patients have shown 5-year survival rates of 93% and 94% in two reports.[1] It is important to consider the period of observation when patients treated recently with immunosuppressive therapy are compared with patients treated 15 to 20 years ago with corticosteroids. The improved survival rate could be due to better use of serologic parameters, more effective antihypertensive agents and antibiotics, an increased awareness of the disease on the part of both patient and physician, or a change in the natural history of the disease.

RELATED OR ASSOCIATED CONDITIONS: RHEUMATOID ARTHRITIS AND OTHER CONNECTIVE TISSUE DISEASES

Related or associated conditions are also discussed in Chapter 66. Only a small percentage of individuals fulfilling the ARA Preliminary or Revised Criteria have definite coincident rheumatoid nodules, erosive arthritis, and rheumatoid factor.[1] Such individuals have at least 4 of the 14 manifestations of the Preliminary Criteria, excluding arthritis. Patients with classic or definite rheumatoid arthritis occasionally develop typical multisystem SLE, including lupus nephritis. An occasional patient has typical SLE along with one or more manifestations of another connective tissue disease. SLE patients with a typical violaceous rash of the V area of the chest and edematous violaceous upper eyelids have been observed. Necrotizing vasculitis typical of polyarteritis and plaques of scleroderma have also been observed occasionally in SLE patients, and full-blown CREST syndrome (calcinosis, Raynaud's phenomenon, esophagial dysfunction, sclerodactyly, and telangiectasia) has been noted in some of our SLE patients along with anticentromere antibodies.

TABLE 67–3. REPORTED SURVIVAL IN CORTICOSTEROID-TREATED SLE PATIENTS*

SERIES	NO. OF CASES	YEARS OF OBSERVATION	YEARS AFTER DIAGNOSIS				
			1	3	5	7	10
Johns Hopkins	99	1949–1953	78	62	. .	. .	. .
Cleveland Clinic	299	1949–1959	89	75	69	59	54
University of Southern California	57	1950–1955	42	12	4	2	. .
Sweden	54	1955–1961	82	72	70	63	51
University of Southern California	100	1956–1962	63	32	16	12	4
Group 1	209	1957–1967	89	79	70	67	63
Columbia University	150	1963–1971	98	90	77	68	59
University of Southern California	92	1963–1973	98	91	79	65	41
Group 2	156	1968–1975	99	97	93	90	84
Johns Hopkins	140	1970–1975	. .	. .	94	. .	82

* For whom life-table analysis was employed.

From Urman, J.D., and Rothfield, N.F.: Corticosteroid treatment in systemic lupus erythematosus: Survival studies. JAMA, *238*:2272–2276, 1977.

Myasthenia Gravis. SLE has been reported in association with myasthenia gravis either before or after thymectomy.[1]

Porphyria Cutanea Tarda. This condition has been reported in association with SLE.[1]

Chronic Discoid Lupus. This benign skin disease is not rare and is thought to be more common than SLE itself. Discoid lupus has been reported in infants and in the elderly, but most patients are between the ages of 25 and 45 years at the time of onset. Although women are affected more often than men, the sex ratio is only 2:1.[1] The disease occurs in all races. Family studies have revealed more than one case in the same family, and studies of relatives of SLE patients have revealed other family members with discoid lupus.[1] Studies of anti–native DNA antibodies and complement proteins in discoid lupus patients show no increases compared to age-, sex-, and race-matched controls.[1] Complement proteins were normal in these studies except for increased levels of properdin found in nearly half the patients studied. It is of interest that a number of individuals with a hereditary deficiency of C2 have lesions of discoid lupus as their only clinical abnormality.

It is clear that some patients with discoid lupus develop SLE but the percentage that does so is unknown. No serologic markers identifying patients who eventually develop systemic disease have been found.

Drug-Induced Lupus. This syndrome is caused by the chronic ingestion of several drugs and has been reviewed.[1] Prospective studies have revealed that procainamide-induced antinuclear antibodies develop in about 50% of individuals, about half of whom develop a lupus-like illness. Procainamide is, therefore, the most common drug that induces a lupus syndrome. Patients with this syndrome typically have joint pains and swelling, rashes, pleurisy, pericarditis, and pulmonary atelectasis. The disease clinically resembles the non–drug-induced disease in elderly individuals. In both the procainamide-induced syndrome and in SLE in elderly individuals, renal disease is uncommon, and antibodies against native DNA are usually absent. Withdrawal of procainamide gradually leads to disappearance of the clinical syndrome and eventual disappearance of the serum antinuclear antibodies.

Although drug-induced clinical disease has been described rarely after isoniazid use, the drug did induce antinuclear antibodies in 20% of individuals who received it.[1]

A prospective study on the immunologic effects of hydralazine was completed in a group of black patients. The results after 2 years revealed that antinuclear antibodies developed in 15 of the 25 patients. The antinuclear antibodies were detected in undiluted sera in 12 patients, and a titer of 1:10 or greater occurred in three patients. Clinical symptoms of SLE developed in only one of the 25 patients.[1]

REFERENCES

1. Rothfield, N.F.: Systemic lupus erythematosus: Clinical aspects and treatment. *In* Arthritis and Allied Conditions: A Textbook of Rheumatology. 11th Ed. Edited by D.J. McCarty. Philadelphia, Lea & Febiger, 1989, pp. 1022–1048.
2. Reveille, J.D.: Molecular genetics of systemic lupus erythematosus and Sjögren's syndrome. Curr. Opin. Rheum., *2*:733–739, 1990.
3. Fronek, Z., Timmerman, L.A., Alper, C.A., et al.: Major histocompatibility complex genes and susceptibility to systemic lupus erythematosus. Arthritis Rheum., *33*:1542–1553, 1990.
4. Wysenbeck, A.J., Block, D.A., and Fries, J.F.: Prevalence and expression of photosensitivity in systemic lupus erythematosus. Ann. Rheum. Dis., *48*:461–463, 1989.
5. Hymes, S.R., and Jordon, R.E.: Chronic cutaneous lupus erythematosus. Med. Clin. North Am., *73*:1055–1071, 1989.
6. Rothe, M., Grant-Kels, J., and Rothfield, N.F.: Extensive calcinosis cutis with systemic lupus erythematosus. Arch. Dermatol., *126*:1060–1063, 1990.
7. Jerdan, M.S., Hood, A.F., Moore, G.W., and Callen, J.P.: Histopathologic comparison of the subsets of lupus erythematosus. Arch. Dermatol., *126*:52–55, 1990.
8. Furie, R.A., and Chartash, E.K.: Tendon rupture in systemic lupus erythematosus. Semin. Arthritis Rheum., *18*:127–133, 1988.
9. Galve, E., Candell-Riera, J., Pigrau, C., et al.: Prevalence, morphologic types, and evolution of cardiac valvular disease in systemic lupus erythematosus. N. Engl. J. Med., *319*:817–823, 1988.
10. Simonson, J.S., Schiller, N.B., Petri, M., and Hellman, D.B.: Pulmonary hypertension in systemic lupus erythematosus. J. Rheumatol., *16*:918–925, 1989.
11. Drenkard, C., Sanchez-Guerrero, J., and Alarcon-Segovia, D.: Fall in antiphospholipid antibody at the time of thromboocclusive episodes in systemic lupus erythematosus. J. Rheumatol., *16*:614–617, 1989.
12. Andronopoulos, A.P., Constantopoulos, S.H., Galanopoulou, V., et al.: Pulmonary function of nonsmoking patients with systemic lupus erythematosus. Chest, *94*:312–315, 1988.
13. Stevens, W.M.R., Burdon, J.G.W., Clemens, L.E., and Webb, J.: The "shrinking lungs syndrome"—An infrequently recognized feature of systemic lupus erythematosus. Aust. N. Z. J. Med., *20*:67–70, 1990.
14. Kaufman, L.D., Gomez-Reino, J.J., Heinicke, M.H., and Gorevic, P.D.: Male lupus: Retrospective analysis of the clinical and laboratory features of 52 patients, with review of the literature. Semin. Arthritis Rheum., *18*:189–197, 1989.
15. Laitman, R.S., Glicklich, D., Sablay, L.B., et al.: Effect of long-term normalization of serum complement levels on the course of lupus nephritis. Am. J. Med., *87*:132–138, 1989.
16. Esdaile, J.M., Levinton, C., Federgreen, W., et al.: The clinical and renal biopsy predictors of long term outcome in lupus nephritis: A study of 87 patients and review of the literature. Q. J. Med., *269*:779–833, 1989.
17. Sewell, K.L., Livneh, A., Aranow, C.B., and Grayzek, A.I.: Magnetic resonance imaging versus computed tomographic scanning in neuropsychiatric lupus erythematosus. Am. J. Med., *86*:625–626, 1989.
18. Fradis, M., Podoshin, L., Ben David, J., et al.: Brainstem auditory evoked potentials with increased stimulus rate in patients suffering from systemic lupus erythematous. Laryngoscope, *99*:325–329, 1989.

19. Kushner, M.J., Tobin, M., Fazekas, F., et al.: Cerebral blood flow variations in CNS lupus. Neurology, *40*:99–102, 1990.
20. Stoppe, G., Wildhagen, K., Seidel, J.W., et al.: Positron emission tomography in neuropsychiatric lupus erythematosus. Neurology, *40*:304–308, 1990.
21. McCune, W.J., MacGuire, A., Aisen, A., and Gebarski, S.: Identification of brain lesions in neuropsychiatric systemic lupus erythematosus by magnetic resonance scanning. Arthritis Rheum., *31*:159–166, 1988.
22. Schousboe, J.T., Koch, A.E., and Chang, R.W.: Chronic lupus peritonitis with ascites: Review of the literature with a case report. Semin. Arthritis Rheum., *18*:121–126, 1988.
23. Stafford-Brady, F.J., Urowitz, M.B., Gladman, D.D., and Easterbrook, M.: Lupus retinopathy: Patterns, association, and prognosis. Arthritis Rheum., *31*:1105–1109, 1988.
24. Buyon, J.P.: Systemic lupus erythematosus and the maternal-fetal dyad. *In* Pregnancy and the Rheumatic Diseases. Edited by A.L. Parke. Baillieres Clin. Rheumatol., *1*:53–68, 1990.
25. Hahn, B.H.: Lupus nephritis: Therapeutic decisions. Hosp. Pract. [Off.], 89–104, 1990.
26. The Canadian Hydroxychloroquine Study Group: A randomized study of the effect of withdrawing hydroxychloroquine sulfate in systemic lupus erythematosus. N. Engl. J. Med., *324*:150–154, 1991.
27. Balow, J.E., Austin, H.A., Tsokos, G.C., et al.: Lupus nephritis. Ann. Intern. Med., *106*:79–94, 1987.
28. McCune, W.J., Golbus, J., Zeldes, W., et al.: Clinical and immunologic effects of monthly administration of intravenous cyclophosphamide in severe systemic lupus erythematosus. N. Engl. J. Med., *318*:1423–1431, 1988.
29. Miller, M.L.: Treatment of systemic lupus erythematosus and adults and children. Curr. Opin. Rheumatol., *2*:712–716, 1990.
30. Rothenberg, R.J., Graziano, F.M., Grandone, J.T., et al.: The use of methotrexate in steroid-resistant systemic lupus erythematosus. Arthritis Rheum., *31*:612–615, 1988.
31. Geutren, G., Querin, S., Noel, L.H., et al.: Effects of cyclosporine in severe systemic lupus erythematosus. J. Pediatr., *111*:1063–1068, 1987.
32. Steinsson, K., Erlendsson, K., and Valdimarsson, H.: Successful plasma infusion treatment of a patient with C2 deficiency and systemic lupus erythematosus: Clinical experience over forty-five months. Arthritis Rheum., *32*:906–913, 1989.
33. Shornick, J.K., Formica, N., and Parke, A.L.: Isotretinoin for refractory lupus erythematosus. J. Am. Acad. Dermatol., *24*:49–52, 1991.
34. Lo, J.S., Berg, R.E., and Tomecki, K.J.: Treatment of discoid lupus erythematosus. Int. J. Dermatol., *28*:497–507, 1989.

68

Autoantibodies in Systemic Lupus Erythematosus

ENG M. TAN

Systemic lupus erythematosus (SLE) is a disease of multiple pathogenetic mechanisms affecting many organs of the body and characterized by abnormalities of the immune system. These abnormalities are manifested primarily by the presence of many autoantibodies in the serum. The autoantibodies of greatest clinical significance are those directed against nuclear antigens (ANA). In recent years, there has been an increasing awareness of the complexity of serum ANAs in SLE and a better understanding of how these play a role in pathogenetic mechanisms. The cumulative work of several investigators has shown that some autoantibodies participate in immune complex–mediated tissue injury. Such injury may occur as immune complexes forming in the circulation or as immune complexes occurring at sites of tissue-fixed antigens (Fig. 68–1) (see Chapter 27).

ABNORMALITIES OF HUMORAL IMMUNITY

The types of autoantibodies encountered were discussed in a review by Kunkel, a pioneer in the study of immunologic aberrations in SLE (Table 68–1).[1] Autoantibodies in SLE can be divided into two classes. The first includes those antibodies that are not tissue specific but react with antigens present in many tissues and organs. This class is exemplified in the autoantibodies to nuclear and cytoplasmic antigens. A second class of autoantibodies includes those that are tissue specific, that is, those directed against cellular elements in the hematopoietic system, such as red cells, white cells, and platelets, and antibodies to tissue-specific antigens (thyroid, liver, muscle, stomach, and adrenal gland).

ANAs have received the most intensive scrutiny in SLE and can be classified in great detail (Table 68–2). ANAs can be divided into four main groups: (1) those directed against double-strand DNA; (2) those directed against single-strand DNA; (3) those directed against histones, a family of basic proteins present within the nucleus; and (4) those directed against nonhistone nuclear proteins or nucleic acid–protein complexes.[2]

Antibodies to DNA were first reported in 1959.[3] Antibody to double-strand DNA reacts with an antigenic determinant present on both double-strand and single-strand DNA. This antibody is present in 50% of patients with SLE. It is generally agreed that antibody to double-strand DNA, when present in significant titer, is a diagnostic marker for SLE. It is rarely, if ever, present in other diseases. Antibody to single-strand DNA is antibody reactive with antigenic determinants that are related to the exposed purines and pyrimidines in single-strand DNA. This antibody is present in 60 to 70% of patients with SLE but may also be present in other rheumatic diseases as well as in nonrheumatic diseases. In the nonrheumatic diseases, antibody to single-strand DNA is most often seen in patients with chronic infections. Because antibody to single-strand DNA is not restricted to SLE, it is not a useful serologic marker for diagnostic purposes. However, this should not be interpreted to mean that antibody to single-strand DNA is not pathogenetically important. Indeed, it has been shown that single-strand DNA antibody can be eluted from the glomeruli of patients with SLE and that it is present in the form of immune complexes in such tissues.[4,5]

Antibodies to histones are present in approximately 70% of patients with SLE. The use of enzyme-linked immunosorbent assay (ELISA) can demonstrate that antibodies to histones are reactive with all the classes of histones, including H1, H2A, H2B, H3, and H4, as well as H2A/H2B and H3/H4 complexes.[6] Of great interest is the demonstration that patients with certain drug-induced lupus syndromes have antibodies to histones to the exclusion of other types of ANAs.[6,7]

Antibodies to nonhistone antigens have been reported with increasing frequency in SLE. Antibody to Sm antigen was the first such antibody reported.[8] Over the years, it has been confirmed repeatedly that this antibody is present almost exclusively in SLE and is a useful diagnostic marker, but it is present only in 30 to 40% of patients with SLE. Antibody to nuclear ribonucleoprotein (RNP) was reported by Sharp et al.[9] as a characteristic feature of patients with mixed connective tissue disease (MCTD) (see Chapter 71). It was soon apparent that this antibody was similar to an antibody described by Mattioli and Reichlin in patients with SLE.[10] Studies have elucidated the chemical nature of this antigen and have shown that it is a complex of U1-RNA and proteins.[11] Hence, the current designation for nuclear RNP is U1-RNP. Antibody to U1-RNP is present in 35 to 45% of patients with SLE and in more than 95% of patients with MCTD.

Two classes of ANAs in patients with SLE are related to ANAs seen in patients with Sjögren's syndrome.

TABLE 68–1. AUTOANTIBODIES IN SLE

TISSUE REACTIVITY	ANTIBODY SPECIFICITY
Nuclear antigens	DNA, nucleoprotein, histones, nonhistone (acidic) proteins
Cytoplasmic antigens	RNA, ribosomes and other RNA-protein complexes, cytoplasmic protein and liquid antigens
Clotting factors	Lupus anticoagulants
Red cell antigens	
White cell antigens	T-lymphocyte cell surface antigens, B-lymphocyte cell surface antigens
Platelet antigens	
Other tissue-specific antigens (thyroid, liver, muscle, stomach, adrenal gland)	

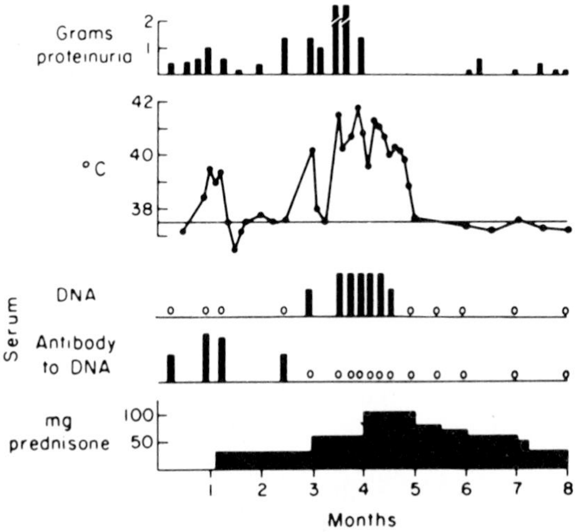

FIGURE 68–1. Antibody to native DNA but no free DNA was detected in four consecutive serum samples of a patient with SLE. A relapse characterized by high fever and increased proteinuria coincided with disappearance of the antibody and the appearance of excess DNA antigen in the serum. The temporal sequence of DNA antibody followed by antigen strongly suggested immune complex formation during the period of relapse. (From Tan, E.M.[1a])

TABLE 68–2. CELLULAR ANTIGENS IN SYSTEMIC LUPUS ERYTHEMATOSUS

CLINICAL/ IMMUNOLOGIC DESIGNATION	STRUCTURE/ FUNCTION	MOLECULAR CHARACTERISTICS	ASSOCIATED RNAs	PREVALENCE (%)
Native DNA	Nucleic acid	Double-strand DNA	None	SLE (50%)
Denatured DNA	Nucleic acid	Single-strand DNA	None	SLE (60–70%)
Histones	Chromatin/ nucleosome	H1, H2A, H2B, H3, H4	None	SLE (70%)
Sm	RNA processing	Proteins 28KD(B), 29KD(B′), 16KD(D), 13KD(E)	U1, U2, U4, U5, U6	SLE (30%)
Nuclear-RNP	RNA processing/ splicing	Proteins 68KD, 33KD(A), 22KD(C)	U1	SLE (35%)
SSA/Ro	RNA processing	Protein 60KD, 52KD	Y1–Y5 (human)	SLE (30%)
SSB/La	RNA polymerase III transcription	Phosphoproteins 46KD, 48KD	Pol III transcripts, pre-tRNA, 5S RNA, 4.5S, RNA, VA-RNA, EBER RNAs	SLE (15%)
Ribosomal RNP	Protein translation	Phosphoproteins 38KD, 16KD, 15KD	None reported	SLE (10%)
PCNA/cyclin	DNA replication	Protein 36KD	None	SLE (3%)
Ku	(Nuclear protein)	Protein 86KD, 66KD	None	SLE (10%)

EBER = Epstein-Barr Encoded RNA; RNP = ribonucleoprotein; SLE = systemic lupus erythematosus.

These ANAs are antibodies to SS-A/Ro and SS-B/La. Anti-SS-A/Ro is present in 30 to 40% of patients with SLE but in approximately 70% of patients with Sjögren's syndrome. Of great interest is the demonstration that anti-SS-A/Ro is related to neonatal lupus. The presence of anti-SS-A/Ro autoantibodies in maternal sera has been correlated with increased risk of skin rash and congenital complete heart block.[12] Antibody to SS-B/La is present in only 15% of patients with SLE but in 45 to 60% of patients with Sjögren's syndrome.

Antibody to ribosomal RNP is the antibody that most often accounts for cytoplasmic staining in immunofluorescence. The antigens are three proteins of 38,000, 16,000, and 15,000 MW, which are components of the large ribosomal subunit. These antibodies are present in 10% of patients.[13] The Ku antibody reacts with a doublet protein of 66,000 and 86,000 MW and is present in 10% of patients.[14] Finally, antibody to proliferating cell nuclear antigen (PCNA) is present in 3% of patients. This autoantibody reacts with a cell cycle-regulated proliferation–associated protein of 36,000 MW.[15] The antibody is useful in cell biology as a probe for identifying proliferating cells; the antigen is the auxiliary protein of DNA polymerase-δ.[16]

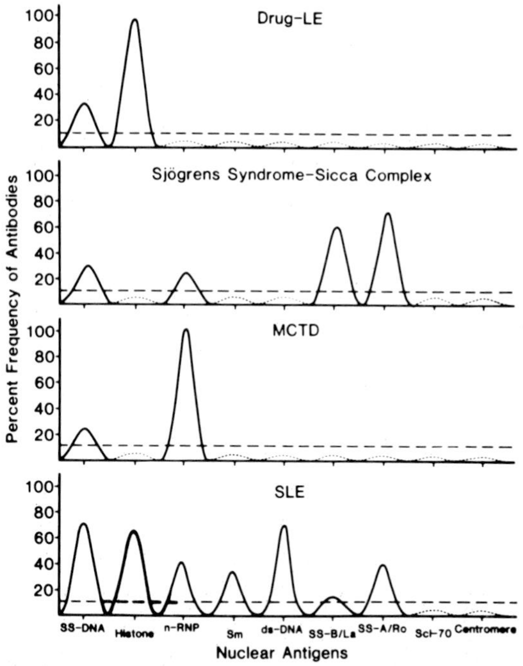

FIGURE 68–2. Distinctive profiles of ANAs occur in various autoimmune diseases. SLE is characterized by a multiplicity of ANAs occurring in different frequencies. This is in contrast to other diseases, such as MCTD, Sjögren's syndrome, and drug-induced LE, in which the ANA profile is more restricted in heterogeneity. The dotted lines below 10% indicate relative absence of antibodies. ANA = antinuclear antibody; MCTD, mixed connective tissue disease; SLE, systemic lupus erythematosus. (From Tan, E.M.[1a])

PROFILES OF ANAs IN SLE AND OTHER SYSTEMIC RHEUMATIC DISEASES

SLE is characterized by a multitude of ANAs (see also Chapter 66). A striking feature of the profile of ANAs in SLE, which contrasts it with other systemic rheumatic diseases, is the simultaneous presence of three or four different types of ANAs in the same serum (Fig. 68–2).[17] In contrast, other systemic rheumatic diseases have two features that are different from SLE. One is the presence of antibodies of other specificities and the other is the presence of fewer types of ANAs in each individual serum. Table 68–3 describes the ANA profiles characteristic of MCTD, Sjögren's syndrome, scleroderma, and dermato- or polymyositis. It is important to compare Table 68–3 with the profile of SLE in Table 68–2 and Fig. 68–2. In certain syndromes, such as MCTD, antibody to U1-RNP is present in most patients, but this feature alone does not differentiate it from SLE, where it is present in 35 to 45% of patients. An equally important feature in MCTD is the absence of other ANAs, such as antibody to double-strand DNA, antibody to Sm antigen, and antibody to histones. Similarly, in Sjögren's syndrome, antibodies to SS-A/Ro and SS-B/La, characteristic of this disease, are also present in some patients with SLE. However, in Sjögren's syndrome as in MCTD, antibodies to double-strand DNA, Sm, and nuclear histones are absent.

The importance of ANAs in the clinical characterization and classification of SLE was recognized in the 1982 revised criteria for the classification of SLE.[18] In this scheme, ANA was recognized as an independent criterion, and anti-double-strand DNA and anti-Sm were included with the LE cell test and the biologically false-positive test for syphilis (anticardiolipin antibody—the "lupus anticoagulant") as four subitems in a second immunologic criterion. (See Chapter 70 for a discussion of anticardiolipin antibodies.)

IDENTIFICATION AND CHARACTERIZATION OF NUCLEAR ANTIGENS

There have been significant advances in the characterization of some of the nuclear antigens reactive with serum ANAs. Both Sm antigen and U1-RNP antigen are proteins, as demonstrated by the transfer of electrophoretically separated antigens to nitrocellulose paper and the demonstration that specific polypeptide bands react with antibodies, a process called Western blotting. Several polypeptides are reactive with anti-Sm and anti-U1-RNP, and these vary from 8,000 to 70,000 Daltons in MW.[11,19] The observation that anti-Sm antibody and anti-U1-RNP antibody immunoprecipitated highly specific sets of small nuclear RNAs was interesting.[11] Anti-U1-RNP immunoprecipitated only U1-RNA, whereas anti-Sm precipitated U1 as well as four other species of small nuclear RNAs: U2, U4, U5, and U6 (Fig. 68–3). These antibodies are not reactive with the small nuclear

TABLE 68–3. ANA PROFILES IN CERTAIN AUTOIMMUNE DISEASES

ANTIBODIES TO	PERCENT FREQUENCY IN SLE	MCTD	Sjögren's Syndrome	Scleroderma	Dermatopolymyositis
dsDNA	50	<5*	<5	<5	<5
ssDNA	60–70	10–20	10–20	10–20	10–20
Histones	70	<5	<5	<5	<5
Sm	30–40	<5	<5	<5	<5
UI-RNP	35–45	95–100	<5	20	<5
SS-A/Ro	30–40	<5	60–70	<5	<5
SS-B/La	15	<5	45–60	<5	<5
Scl-70	<5	<5	<5	20–30	<5
Centromere/kinetochore	<5	<5	<5	25–30	<5
Nucleolar antigens	<5	<5	5–10	50–60	5–10
PM-1	<5	<5	<5	<5	50†
Jo-1	<5	<5	<5	<5	30
Ku	<10	<5	<5	<5	55†

MCTD, mixed connective tissue disease; SLE, systemic lupus erythematosus.
* <5% frequency is used to signify that the antibody is rarely observed.
† These reported frequencies are present in polymyositis-scleroderma overlap syndrome.

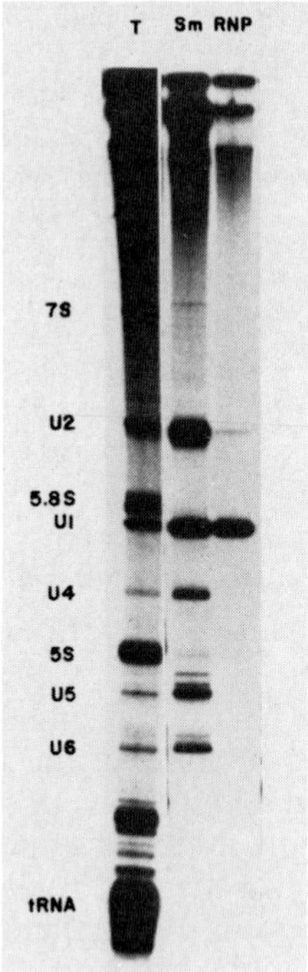

FIGURE 68–3. Profiles of small nuclear RNAs immunoprecipitated by anti-Sm and antinuclear RNP sera. HeLa cells were labeled with phosphorus-32 and cell extract reacted with sera. The immunoprecipitates were solubilized and run on polyacrylamide gels to identify precipitated RNAs. Left lane represents total cellular RNA. Middle lane shows five major RNA bands precipitated by anti-Sm serum: U1, U2, U4, U5, and U6 RNAs. Right lane shows that only U1 RNA is precipitated by anti-RNP serum.

RNAs per se but are reactive with polypeptides complexed to these small nuclear RNAs in highly specific associations. Such studies on the molecular biology of the nuclear antigens have clarified the nature of nuclear antigens and have also shown that ANAs can be used as probes to aid in identification of the structure and function of cellular constituents. Some studies have indicated that U1-RNA associated with its protein components (U1 ribonucleoprotein) is involved in processing heterogeneous nuclear RNA, the primary transcript of genomic DNA.[20] A comprehensive review of the molecular and cell biology of ANAs and nuclear antigens was published in 1991.[21]

ANTI-SS-A/RO AND NEONATAL LUPUS

The relationship between anti-SS-A/Ro and neonatal lupus was studied in three infant–mother pairs.[22] All three infants and their mothers had serum anti-SS-A/Ro antibodies. Three months later, anti-SS-A/Ro antibody had disappeared from the sera of the children but was still present in the mothers, strongly suggesting transplacental passage of antibody from mother to infant. An interesting observation was the presence of a complete heart block in one of the infants. Following this initial study, several groups of investigators confirmed these findings.[23–25] Clinical features include typical SLE skin lesions in the infants and a high association of congenital complete or partial heart block. It has been correctly pointed out that pregnant mothers with known SLE should be screened for the presence of anti-SS-A/Ro to promote awareness of the possibility of cardiac problems in the infant. However, some of the mothers with anti-SS-A/Ro antibody may not have overt clinical disease at the time of gestation or delivery.

TABLE 68–4. TYPES OF ANTIHISTONE ANTIBODIES INDUCED BY PROCAINAMIDE AND HYDRALAZINE

ANTI-BODY CLASS	DRUG	ANTIBODIES TO H2A	H2B	H2A/H2B	H3
IgM	Procainamide	0	0	+ +	0
	Hydralazine	+ +	+/−	+/−	+ +
IgG	Procainamide	+ +	+/−	+ + +	+/−
	Hydralazine	0	0	+/−	+/−

DRUG-INDUCED LUPUS AND ANTIHISTONE ANTIBODIES

A close association exists between antihistone antibodies and drug-induced lupus, particularly those antibodies linked with ingestion of procainamide and hydralazine.[6,7] Owing to the increased use of sustained-release types of procainamide, the incidence of drug-induced lupus has increased.

Differentiation between drug-induced lupus and the idiopathic form of systemic lupus can be made serologically. In drug-induced lupus, ANAs are characterized by the presence of antihistone antibodies, and the absence of anti-double-strand DNA, anti-Sm, or the other SLE-related ANAs listed in Table 68–2. Differentiation between drug-induced lupus and SLE has been notoriously difficult, although serologic analysis has helped to clarify the situation. Although both procainamide and hydralazine are characterized by antihistone antibodies, there is a difference in the classes of histones that are reactive in the two conditions. Table 68–4 shows that procainamide-induced antihistone antibodies are different from hydralazine-induced anti-histone antibodies. The former are more reactive with the H2A/H2B complex of histones. This involves both the immunoglobulin G (IgG) and IgM classes of antibodies. In contrast, hydralazine-induced antihistone antibodies are characterized by IgM antibodies against histone H3 and H2A. In addition, hydralazine-induced antihistone antibodies are primarily of the IgM class with few IgG antibodies. *Drug-induced ANAs are almost exclusively of the antihistone type, and there are different antihistone antibodies in procainamide- and hydralazine-induced ANAs.*

ANA-NEGATIVE LUPUS

There has been some controversy concerning ANA-negative lupus. This controversy is probably associated with two features: (1) ANA as detected with the immunofluorescence technique varies in sensitivity from one laboratory to the next; and (2) many ANA-negative lupus patients have anti-SS-A/Ro.[26] Recent studies may have clarified some of these discrepancies. The SS-A/Ro antigen, unlike Sm and U1-RNP antigens, varies remarkably in concentration in cells from one animal species to the next.[27] SS-A/Ro antigen is present in higher concentrations in man, monkey, and dog than in the mouse, rat, and hamster. Therefore, when tissues from species such as rat or mouse are used as substrates in indirect immunofluorescence, a serum containing anti-SS-A/Ro may not show nuclear staining. When rabbit, human, or dog tissues are used as the substrate, however, this serum is positive for ANAs. Some patients with anti-SS-A/Ro antibodies have been classified into a subset of lupus called *subacute cutaneous lupus.*[28] These individuals are highly photosensitive and have prominent skin lesions but have less involvement of other organ systems[28] (see Chapter 67).

REFERENCES

1. Kunkel, H.G.: The immunologic approach to SLE. Arthritis Rheum., *20*:S139, 1977.

1a. Tan, E.M.: The LE cell and antinuclear antibodies. A breakthrough in diagnosis. *In* Landmark Advances in Rheumatology ARA Golden Anniversary synposium. Edited by D.J. McCarty. Atlanta, GA, Arthritis Foundation, 1984, pp. 43–52.

2. Tan, E.M.: Autoantibodies to nuclear antigens. Their immunobiology and medicine. Adv. Immunol., *33*:167, 1982.

3. Deicher, H.R.G., Holman, H.R., and Kunkel, H.G.: The precipitin reaction between DNA and a serum factor in systemic lupus erythematosus. J. Exp. Med., *109*:97, 1959.

4. Andres, G.A. et al.: Localization of fluorescein-labeled aminonucleoside antibodies in glomeruli of patients with active systemic lupus erythematosus. J. Clin. Invest., *49*:2106, 1971.

5. Koffler, D. et al.: The occurrence of single stranded DNA in the serum of patients with systemic lupus erythematosus and other diseases. J. Clin. Invest., *52*:198, 1973.

6. Totoritis, M.C. et al.: Association of antibody to histone complex H2A-H2B with symptomatic procainamide-induced lupus. N. Engl. J. Med., *318*:1431, 1988.

7. Fritzler, M.J., and Tan, E.M.: Antibodies to histones in drug-induced and idiopathic lupus erythematosus. J. Clin. Invest., *62*:560, 1978.

8. Tan, E.M., and Kunkel, H.G.: Characteristics of a soluble nuclear antigen precipitating with sera of patients with systemic lupus erythematosus. J. Immunol., *96*:464, 1966.

9. Sharp, G.C. et al.: Mixed connective tissue disease—An apparently distinct rheumatoid disease associated with a specific antibody to an extractable nuclear antigen (ENA). Am. J. Med., *52*:148, 1972.

10. Mattioli, M., and Reichlin, M.: Physical association of two nuclear antigens and mutual occurrence of their antibodies: The relationship of the Sm and RNA protein (Mo) systems in SLE sera. J. Immunol., *110*:1318, 1973.

11. Lerner, M.R., and Steitz, J.A.: Antibodies to small nuclear RNAs complexed with proteins are produced by patients with systemic lupus erythematosus. Proc. Natl. Acad. Sci. U. S. A., *765*:5495, 1979.

12. Buyon, J.P. et al.: Acquired congenital heart block: Pattern of maternal antibody response to biochemically defined antigens of the SSA/Ro-SSB/La systems in neonatal lupus. J. Clin. Invest., *84*:627, 1989.

13. Francoeur, A.M. et al.: Identification of ribosomal protein autoantigens. J. Immunol., *135*:2378, 1985.

14. Francoeur, A.M., Peebles, C.L., Gomper, P., and Tan, E.M.: Identification of Ki (Ku p70/p80) autoantigens and analysis of anti-Ki autoantibody. J. Immunol., *136*:1648, 1986.

15. Miyachi, K., Fritzler, M.J., and Tan, E.M.: Autoantibody to a nuclear antigen in proliferating cells. J. Immunol., *121*:2228, 1978.

16. Prelich, G. et al.: Functional identity of proliferating cell nuclear antigen and a DNA polymerase delta auxiliary protein. Nature, *326*:517, 1987.
17. Notman, D.D., Kurata, N., and Tan, E.M.: Profiles of antinuclear antibodies in systemic rheumatoid diseases. Ann. Intern. Med., *83*:464, 1975.
18. Tan, E.M. et al.: The 1982 revised criteria for the classification of systemic lupus erythematosus. Arthritis Rheum., *25*:1271, 1982.
19. Conner, G.E. et al.: Protein antigens of the RNA-protein complexes detected by anti-Sm and anti-RNP antibodies found in serum of patients with systemic lupus erythematosus and related disorders. J. Exp. Med., *156*:1475, 1982.
20. Yang, V.W. et al.: A small nuclear ribonucleoprotein is required for splicing of adenoviral early RNA sequences. Proc. Natl. Acad. Sci. U. S. A., *78*:1371, 1981.
21. Tan, E.M.: Antinuclear antibodies and autoimmunity. Encyclopedia Hum. Biol., *1*:331, 1991.
22. Franco, H.L. et al.: Autoantibodies directed against sicca syndrome antigens in the neonatal lupus syndrome. J. Am. Acad. Dermatol., *4*:67–72, 1981.
23. Kephart, D.C., Hood, A.F., and Provost, T.T.: Neonatal lupus erythematosus: New serologic findings. J. Invest. Dermatol., *77*:331–333, 1981.
24. Lockshin, D.D. et al.: Neonatal lupus erythematosus with heart block: Family study of a patient with anti-SS-A and anti-SS-B antibodies. Arthritis Rheum., *26*:210–213, 1983.
25. Scott, J.S. et al.: Connective tissue disease, antibodies to ribonucleoprotein, and congenital heart block. N. Engl. J. Med., *309*:209–212, 1983.
26. Provost, T.T. et al.: Antibodies to cytoplasmic antigens in lupus erythematosus. Arthritis Rheum., *20*:1457, 1977.
27. Harmon, C.E. et al.: The importance of tissue substrates in the SS-A/Ro antigen-antibody system. Arthritis Rheum., *27*:166–173, 1984.
28. Gilliam, J.N., and Sontheimer, R.D.: Distinctive cutaneous subsets in the spectrum of lupus erythematosus. J. Am. Acad. Dermatol., *4*:471, 1981.

69

Systemic Lupus Erythematosus: Generalized Autoimmunity Arising From Disordered Immune Regulation

DAVID A. HORWITZ

Systemic lupus erythematosus (SLE) includes several syndromes in which autoantibodies either by themselves or in the form of immune complexes are responsible for tissue injury and inflammation. These autoantibodies are directed against a variety of nuclear structures including double-stranded DNA, cytoplasmic antigens, and cell surface antigens. Individual patients vary in the number of autoantibodies expressed, and the presence of specific autoantibodies may correlate with the pattern of clinical disease.[1]

With the exception of antineuronal antibodies, the autoantibodies in SLE are not tissue specific. Thus, SLE is characterized by B cells producing a wide variety of autoantibodies resulting in *generalized autoimmunity*. SLE differs from other autoimmune diseases such as multiple sclerosis or insulin-dependent diabetes mellitus, in which a restricted group of self-reactive T-lymphocytes attack a specific target organ, or myasthenia gravis or pemphigus, in which highly specific autoantibodies are responsible for localized tissue injury.

The most consistent finding in SLE is an imbalance between the humoral and cellular components of the immune response.[2–4] Coinciding with B-cell hyperactivity, there is T-cell hypoactivity. For this reason, SLE was once considered to be a "B-cell" disease. T cells, however, have a primary role in the initiation of SLE and other autoimmune diseases. Depletion of CD4-positive cells in murine SLE, for example, prevents the development of the disease.[5]

The pathogenesis of SLE is multifactorial and involves the influence of genetic, environmental, and hormonal factors on the immune response. To comprehend generalized autoimmunity, one must understand the mechanisms involved in the development and maintenance of "tolerance" (nonresponsiveness to self-antigens). Current views on this topic will be discussed. On the basis of clinical and experimental observations, one can propose the following scenario: In a genetically predisposed individual exposed to the appropriate trigger factor, T-cell tolerance to self-antigens is broken, and auto-reactive T cells provide help for the induction and expansion of autoantibody-producing memory B cells. An integral part of this process is the disruption of regulatory mechanisms normally preventing pathologic autoimmunity in resistant individuals. Both the trigger factors and the regulatory T cells that prevent autoimmunity are poorly understood but have been the subject of intensive investigation. Current views are summarized here.

Once SLE has become established, other pathologic immune circuits involving both CD4- and CD8-positive lymphocytes perpetuate autoantibody production, resulting in one of the several syndromes clinically recognized as SLE. Thus, in a discussion of the pathogenesis of SLE, the factors that initiate the disease should be separated from those responsible for its perpetuation.

Formerly, it was generally believed that an intrinsic abnormality of T cells or B cells was responsible for the abnormalities described in SLE. However, after two decades of intensive research, there is still no convincing evidence of a primary T-cell defect in human SLE and only suggestive evidence of a B-cell or stem cell defect. Moreover, it has become clear that both foreign and self-antigens are recognized similarly. For these reasons, diseases that were classified as "autoimmune" must now be considered to be disorders of immune regulation.

TABLE 69–1. PHYSIOLOGIC SELF-RECOGNITION IN IMMUNE REGULATION

T cells recognize peptide in the antigen-binding groove of self-MHC molecules
CD4-positive cells recognize self-MHC class II (HLA-DR, DP, DQ) on an antigen-presenting cell
CD8-positive cells recognize self-MHC class I (HLA-A,B,C) on target cells
T cells and B cells can mount responses against structures on their antigen-binding receptors (anti-idiotypic responses)
Anti-idiotypic antibodies regulate antibody production
T-cell anti-idiotypic responses may be important in the regulation of autoimmunity

HLA = human leukocyte antigen; MHC = major histocompatibility complex.

MECHANISMS CONTROLLING ANTI-SELF-IMMUNE RESPONSES

PHYSIOLOGIC SELF-RECOGNITION

Anti-self-responses were once believed to be caused by "forbidden clones" of lymphocytes that should have been eliminated from the immune system. We now understand, however, that unlike B cells, T-lymphocytes cannot recognize bound foreign antigens directly but recognize peptides fixed to class I (HLA-A, -B, -C) or class II (HLA-DR, -DP, -DQ), molecules of the major histocompatibility complex (MHC). Foreign proteins are taken up by various antigen-presenting cells are broken down by protogses. The digested peptides are fixed to the antigen-binding cleft of class II MHC molecules and translocated to the surface. CD4-positive T cells recognize both the peptide and self-MHC class II molecules. Correspondingly, CD8-positive cells recognize foreign peptide complexed to self-MHC class I molecules (Table 69–1).

A second physiologic anti-self-immune response is directed against sites on antigen-binding receptors of lymphocytes. The sites recognized are called "idiotypes," and anti-idiotypic antibodies or T cells constitute a feedback regulatory mechanism. At times anti-idiotypic responses can become pathologic. The formation of antibodies against acetylcholine choline receptors in myasthenia gravis is one such example.

B cells with receptors for self-antigens such as DNA or and anti-IgG (rheumatoid factor) must have an important role in host defense because the genes encoding these autoantibodies are highly conserved in phylogeny.[6] A protective role for natural autoantibodies has been proposed.[7] However, it is unlikely, because anti-single-stranded DNA or rheumatoid factor bind antigen with low affinity these IgM autoantibodies are useful in host defense. Alternatively, B cells with these antigen receptors are numerous in the mantle region of lymph nodes, and it has been proposed that they bind filtered bacterial or viral antigens complexed to host DNA or IgG.[8] These B cells, therefore, may serve as an important source of antigen-presenting cells in the induction of T-cell responses against infectious agents.

Because this mechanism may be important in mounting an immune response against infectious agents, this defect could lead to the persistence of viruses or other intracellular parasites that require a vigorous T cell response for their elimination.

CLONAL DELETION AND CLONAL ANERGY

If T cells only recognize self-MHC molecules, an elaborate mechanism is needed for the selection of these highly restricted antigen-binding receptors. This selection takes place in the thymus. The thymic cortex contains T cells with a wide diversity of receptors, but only those T cells that recognize self-MHC class II or class I molecules are allowed to survive by a mechanism called *positive selection*.[9] These T cells become CD4- or CD8-positive cells, respectively. In the thymic medulla T cells where those that bind strongly to self-peptide-MHC complexes presented by stromal cells are eliminated by a mechanism called *negative selection*.[9] Thus, some potentially autoaggressive T cells are eliminated in the thymus by clonal deletion (Table 69–2).

Studies with transgenic mice reveal that in both the thymus and the periphery, some potentially autoaggressive T cells are not deleted but are rendered anergic or nonresponsive by the manner with which they recognize antigen.[10] T cells require at least two signals for complete activation: To proliferate or develop an effector function, they need a co-stimulatory signal such as interleukin-1 (IL-1) in addition to antigen. If T cells bind antigen, but do not receive a proper co-stimulatory signal, they not only fail to proliferate but also undergo a series of events preventing them from becoming activated by antigen at some subsequent time.[11] This is called *clonal anergy* and is probably the principal mechanism accounting for immunologic nonresponsiveness after birth. Unfortunately, anergy is not always irreversible. T-cell anergy can be reversed by IL-2.[12] Interleukin-2 produced by T cells stimulated by foreign antigens could convert anergic autoreactive T-lymphocytes

TABLE 69–2. MECHANISMS RESPONSIBLE FOR SELF-TOLERANCE

Clonal deletion of self-reactive T and B cells in central lymphoid organs
Principal mechanism for eliminating strongly autoreactive T cells
May eliminate very immature B cells with receptors for multivalent self-antigens
Clonal anergy: Results of binding antigen to receptor without a second co-stimulatory signal
Principal mechanism for achieving nonresponsiveness in the periphery
Predominantly involves T cells
Anergy may be reversed by interleukin-2
Suppressor mechanisms: Remain poorly understood
Suppressor cells may down-regulate immune responses nonspecifically
Memory CD45RA-RO-positive anti-idiotypic T cells may suppress autoimmunity
Self-reactive CD3-positive CD4-negative CD8-negative T cells may regulate autoimmunity

to cells capable of responding to self-antigens (Table 69–2).

T-SUPPRESSOR CELLS

Because antibody-forming B-cell precursors can be detected in healthy individuals, the relatively uncommon occurrence of autoantibody production must be due to suppressor cells or suppressive mechanisms. There is clear evidence that some autoreactive T cells escape both clonal deletion and clonal anergy.[13] These T cells can initiate autoimmune diseases if they are activated appropriately. The existence of true antigen-specific suppressor cells is a hotly debated topic. Many workers consider "suppression" to be the mopping up of cytokines released by activated T cells, or an idiotypic antiself response. There are few examples, however, of cloned antigen-specific CD8-positive suppressor cells. It is likely that self-regulatory suppressor cells minimize the opportunity for the clonal expansion of autoreactive T cells that trigger autoimmune disease.

Both CD4- and CD8-positive cells can develop suppressor activity. In addition there are small numbers of T cells that lack both CD4 and CD8 that are called CD3-positive "double-negative" cells. These T cells may have an especially important role in autoimmune disease because they may develop outside the thymus and thereby may escape the mechanisms that delete lymphocytes with high binding affinity for self-peptides. Most of the CD3 double-negative T cells bear T-cell receptor (TCR) with γ- and δ-chains (γδ), but some bear αβ-TCR. Those with TCRs displaying γδ-chains are characterized by autoreactive cytotoxicity,[14,15] and those expressing αβ-chains can up-regulate[16] or down-regulate[17] autoimmunity (Table 69–2).

POST-THYMIC T-CELL MATURATION

After they leave the thymus, potentially autoreactive T cells presumably undergo further maturation before they can provoke autoimmunity. Almost all T cells in newborn infants are considered to be "naive."[18] These cells have a limited capacity to recognize antigen and stimulated they produce few cytokines. After antigenic stimulation, however, naive cells undergo a transition in their ability to respond to antigens and in their functional properties.[19] They are then called "memory" cells because they can bind antigen more easily because of the high concentrations of various adhesion molecules displayed on their cell surface. When stimulated these memory cells can produce a wide variety of cytokines that facilitate B-cell differentiation.[20] CD4-positive memory cells function can function as antigen-specific helper cells but in the proper environment can also function as antigen-specific suppressor–inducer cells. CD8-positive memory cells become antigen-specific T killer cells.

Both CD4- or CD8-positive naive and memory cells can be recognized by reciprocal expression of CD45 isoforms on their cell surface. CD45 is a membrane tyrosine phosphatase that has a crucial role in T-cell activation. Various isoforms of CD45 are expressed on the cell surface of all leukocytes. Naive T cells display the high molecular weight CD45RA isoform, and memory cells reciprocally express the low molecular weight CD45RO isoform.[21] In SLE, it is likely that naive, autoreactive CD4-positive T cells undergo clonal expansion and become memory cells. Because memory cells have a much lower threshold for activation than naive cells, help for autoantibody-forming B cells would be relatively easy to sustain. Therefore, mechanisms retaining autoreactive T cells in the naive state are important in preventing autoimmunity.

GENETIC FACTORS LEADING TO INCREASED SUSCEPTIBILITY TO SLE

The importance of genetic factors in the pathogenesis of SLE was revealed in studies of identical twins among whom a high concordance was reported. It was believed that the concordance rate of SLE in identical twins was 60 to 62%.[22] This figure was revised downward to 24% in a later study,[23] a figure similar to those reported in other disorders of immune regulation such as rheumatoid arthritis (RA),[24] juvenile diabetes mellitus,[25] and multiple sclerosis.[26] The concordance of SLE in dizygous twins is only 2%, a figure that is surprising because the concordance rate in subjects with cancer does not differ greatly between identical and nonidentical twins.[23]

FAMILIAR STUDIES

These have revealed further evidence of a genetic predisposition to SLE. Nonaffected family members of lupus patients have decreased suppressor T-cell function,[39] hyper-γ-globulinemia, and antinuclear antibodies,[39–42] suggesting that abnormalities of immune regulation have a primary role in disease pathogenesis rather than merely being epiphenomena. Genetic factors, by themselves, will not result in one of the clinical lupus erythematosus (LE) syndromes.

MAJOR HISTOCOMPATIBILITY COMPLEX GENES

There are several associations between the presence of certain MHC alleles on chromosome 6 and SLE. These associations principally involve class II MHC genes, which are important in immune response recognition and regulation. Class II MHC alleles regulate T-cell reactivity to tetanus toxoid,[27] mumps,[28,29] and Coxsackie B virus.[28,29] T cells from DR3-positive subjects are hyporesponsive to these antigens, while those from DR4-positive subjects are hyperresponsive. The proliferative response of lymphocytes from healthy DR3-positive women to phytohemagglutinin is decreased. MHC alleles correlate with suppressor T-cell activity and/or lymphokine production. DR3 is associated with decreased suppressor cell activity,[30] and DR2 regulates the

TABLE 69–3. GENETIC FACTORS RESPONSIBLE FOR INCREASED SUSCEPTIBILITY

MAJOR HISTOCOMPATIBILITY COMPLEX GENES
HLA-DR2, DQ1 correlate with anti-double-stranded DNA antibody, decreased production of tumor necrosis factor-α, and lupus nephritis
HLA-DR3, DQw2, HLA-B8 correlate with anti-Ro and anti-La, subacute cutaneous lupus, mothers of neonatal lupus syndrome, and lupus/Sjögren's syndrome overlap
C4A* QO null allel correlates with increased incidence of SLE
T-CELL RECEPTOR GENES
Correlation between an α-chain constant region gene and increased incidence.
B-CELL RECEPTOR GENES
Correlation between deletion of a germ-line gene encoding anti-IgG (rheumatoid factor) and anti-DNA and increased incidence.

HLA = human leukocyte antigen; SLE = systemic lupus erythematosus.

production of tumor necrosis factor-α (TNF-α).[31] DR3-positive individuals also have impaired reticuloendothelial Fc receptor function.[32] All these abnormalities are found in patients with SLE.

Although HLA-DR2, DR3, and the nearby C4A null allele were once believed to be associated with an increased risk for SLE, it is now evident that MHC alleles correlate even more strongly with particular autoantibodies and related syndromes. HLA-DR2 and DQw1 correlate with anti-double-stranded DNA autoantibody, decreased production of TNF-α and lupus nephritis.[1] The increased risk has been localized to amino acid sequences encoded by the DQ β_1-chain gene.[33] The phenotype human leukocyte antigen (HLA)-DR3, DQw2, and HLA-B8 correlates with anti-Ro (SSA), anti-LA/SSB, and the following syndromes: subacute cutaneous lupus, neonatal lupus erythematosus syndrome, and lupus/Sjögren's overlap syndrome.[34,35] (See Table 69–3). HLA-DR3 is associated by linkage disequilibrium with the C4A*QO null gene and C4A gene deletion.[36]

The class III MHC genes include those encoding C2 and C4. Besides an association with C4A gene deletion two thirds of individuals with a homozygous C2 deficiency have SLE or a lupus-like disorder.[37] One of the principal roles of serum complement is to remove immune complexes. Persistence of potentially pathogenic immune complexes could lead to their deposition in tissues with subsequent injury.

T-CELL RECEPTOR GENES

With the ability to identify families of immunoglobulin genes of B cells and genes encoding the variable region of the T-cell antigen receptor, there has been a considerable effort to look for an association between certain families of antigen-recognition receptors and SLE. So far, these efforts have been largely unsuccessful. Because certain T-cell clones preferentially recognize certain MHC alleles, there should be preferential selection of T cells involved in autoimmunity. An association between a framework gene encoding the constant region of the T-cell receptor α-chain gene and SLE has been reported.[38] Although the β-chain of the T-cell receptor is even more polymorphic than the α-chain, there is still no evidence of oligoclonal T-cell selection. Definitive studies have yet to be performed.

The T-cell receptor repertoire is determined by random rearrangement of the genes encoding the two chains of the receptor molecule. Because of the random nature of events, the receptor repertoire selected may not be identical in monozygotic twins. Moreover, the number of T cells expressing a given receptor will be determined by responses to environmental antigens. These factors probably explain why the concordance rate in monozygotic twins is only 25%. Environmental factors are required for the triggering of SLE.

ROLE OF INFECTIONS IN THE PATHOGENESIS OF SLE

ADJUVANT-LIKE EFFECTS

The factors believed to be important in the initiation of SLE include ultraviolet light, drugs, pregnancy, stress, and infections. Notwithstanding intensive efforts, there is still no conclusive evidence that specific bacteria or viruses trigger SLE. Nonetheless, there is increasing evidence that infectious agents are involved in the pathogenesis of this disease because of their known effects on the immune system. Infectious agents have adjuvant-like effects that enhance lymphocyte reactivity. A failure to clear infectious agents rapidly from the host will lead to sustained polyclonal B-cell activation and the appearance of rheumatoid factors and antinuclear antibodies. Autoantibodies produced by such nonspecifically activated B cells are predominantly of the IgM isotype.

Because IgG autoantibodies occur in human SLE, T cells must be involved. T cells are required for the switch from the IgM to IgG isotype, and there is considerable evidence of direct T-cell–B-cell (cognate) interactions in the induction of autoantibody formation.[43] This means that antigen-specific CD4-positive cells must directly interact with autoantibody-forming B cells in the production of autoantibodies. Therefore, if infectious agents participate in the pathogenesis of SLE, they must be involved in the breakdown of mechanisms sustaining self-tolerance. Viruses can induce or alter self-derived peptides or may be directly involved with self recognition (Table 69–4).

MOLECULAR MIMICRY

Certain epitopes displayed by infectious agents are sufficiently similar to those of host origin that the immune response elicited cross-reacts with self-antigens. Moreover, bacteria or viruses may share peptides in common with the infected host. Many instances have been documented of a foreign antigen sharing a sequence of at

TABLE 69–4. ROLE OF INFECTIONS IN TRIGGERING SLE

Bacteria and Viruses Can Alter Self-Reactivity by Several Mechanisms
Adjuvant-like effects on the immune system.
Molecular mimicry: Infectious agent shares structural characteristics in common with the MHC molecule
Superantigens: Microbial toxins that cause intense T-cell activaton by coupling antigen-presenting cells to T cells. This is achieved by binding to both MHC molecules and the Vβ-region of the T-cell receptor.
Consequences of Altered Self-Reactivity by Infectious Agents
The failure to respond to immunodominant peptides because of molecular mimicry may result an inability to mount an effective immune response with persistence of the infection and chronic inflammation.
Persistence of the infectious agent may lead to the production of pathogenic autoantibodies via molecular mimicry because an immune response to a shared determinant results in antibodies that cross-react with tissues of the host.
Superantigens can initiate autoantibody formation. In healthy individuals, SLE-like autoantigens (repetitive, charged self-peptides) would induce clonal anergy because of the lack of co-stimulatory signal. By contrast, microbial superantigens would trigger autoantibody formation because of cytokines provided by activated T cells.

MHC = major histocompatibility complex; SLE = systemic lupus erythematosus.

least 5 amino acids in common with a self-antigen. Steinberg has calculated that there is a 1% chance that a foreign and a human protein each 300 amino acids long which have at least a pentapeptide in common.[44] This homology is sufficient to induce an immune response through what is called *molecular mimicry*. The antigen-binding groove of MHC molecules binds up to eight amino acids, and this complex is presented to T cells. The adjuvant-like effects of infectious agents also increases the chances that foreign antigens shared by self can activate T cells. Cytokines such as interferon-γ released by T cells during infections can induce epithelial cells of various tissues to display class II MHC gene products. Circulating autoreactive CD4-positive T cells now have the opportunity to recognize and respond to these elements. Autoreactive T cells can only be activated if an appropriate so-stimulatory signal is provided.

Molecular mimicry and increased self-immunogenicity can possibly explain the stimulation of one or more autoreactive T cell clones and emergence of clones with a memory phenotype. These mechanisms are sufficient to explain the development of local (tissue-specific) autoimmunity. Other explanations are needed, however, to explain the generalized autoimmunity characteristic of SLE.

ROLE OF SELF-REACTIVE B CELLS

As stated previously, it is likely that B cells with receptors for self-IgG and DNA have a physiologic protective role in host defense against infections. These cells can bind infectious agents complexed to IgG antibodies or DNA-binding proteins. B cells internalize these complexes and present foreign peptide fixed to class II MHC to CD4-positive T cells initiating a response against the foreign invader. However, cytokines released from the activated T-helper cells and direct cell to cell interactions could stimulate the antigen-presenting B cells to produce anti-IgG (rheumatoid factor) or anti-DNA. Thus, it is possible for B cells with receptors for IgG and DNA to become autoantibody-producing cells as part of a normal immune response. This mechanism may explain the low titers of rheumatoid factor and antinuclear antibodies that appear transiently following infections. That pathogenic autoantibodies appear only infrequently is believed to be due to a poorly understood regulatory network. Dysregulation of this network could, therefore, lead to pathologic autoimmunity.

CHRONIC GRAFT VERSUS HOST DISEASE AND GENERALIZED AUTOIMMUNITY

In experimental animals, the development of chronic graft versus host disease leads to generalized autoimmunity similar to SLE.[45,46] In this disorder, donor CD4-positive T cells recognize foreign class II MHC expressed by recipient B cells. These cognate interactions and the cytokines produced by the activated CD4-positive cells induce the B cells to become antibody-producing cells. In chronic graft versus host disease, T killer cells are not activated, and lupus-like autoantibodies appear. Thus, self-reactive B cells can be induced to become autoantibody-producing cells.

The autoantigens are highly charged, repetitive structures such as DNA or RNA that cross-link immunoglobulin receptors on self-reactive B cells and trigger autoantibody production. These autoantigens probably interact with self-reactive B cells continuously, but in the absence of the appropriate co-stimulatory signals, these B cells are rendered anergic. It is only with the help provided by activated CD4-positive cells that these B cells become autoantibody-secreting cells. Once clones of autoantibody-forming cells have expanded, the potential for further autoantibody production is greatly increased.

MICROBIAL SUPERANTIGENS AND GENERALIZED AUTOIMMUNITY

Certain bacteria such as streptococci, staphylococci, and mycoplasma bear structures that bind to both the T cells and class II MHC expressed by B cells. These structures are microbial toxins and have been called *superantigens* because they promote T-cell–B-cell interactions and antibody formation.[47–49] Superantigens bind to designated β-chains of the T-cell receptor, and this selectivity is a function of genes encoding the variable region or Vβ-elements. Therefore, T cells with receptors belonging to certain Vβ-gene families will bind to specific superantigens.

Analogous to chronic graft versus host disease, microbial superantigen-dependent T-helper–B-cell interactions do induce polyclonal IgM and IgG production.[50] The T-cell–B-cell interactions resulting from bacterial superantigens could possibly trigger autoantibody formation if there is extensive cross linking of immunoglobulin receptors on B cells by autoantigen. If it is correct, a selective increase in the number of T cells expressing specific Vβ genes in SLE should be present.

IMMUNE DYSREGULATION IN SLE

LYMPHOCYTE SUBSETS

Patients with active SLE may be neutropenic and are usually lymphopenic as well.[51] The total numbers of T cells, B cells, and natural killer cells are decreased. Presently, T cells are divided into subsets by developmental and maturation criteria. Almost all T cells exiting from the thymus have acquired antigen receptors (TCR) comprising α- and β-chains complexed to CD3 and displaying either CD4 or CD8 molecules, which associate with the antigen receptor. The usual 2:1 ratio of CD4-positive cells to CD8-positive cells in peripheral blood is frequently abnormal in SLE, and decreased percentages of CD4-positive cells may often be observed in patients with very active disease[51] or with renal disease.[52] Other individuals with SLE may have decreased percentages of CD8-positive cells.[53,54]

CD3-positive, CD4-negative, and CD8-negative T cells usually account for less than 5% of total lymphocytes. Approximately three quarters of CD3 double-negative T cells bear TCR with γ- and δ-chains and one quarter bear αβ-TCR. Reportedly, αβ-CD3 double-negative cells are increased in SLE and provided specific help for the production of pathogenic anti-DNA antibodies.[16] γδCD3 double-negative cells are not increased in SLE. CD3 double-negative cells may also bear natural killer cell markers such as CD11b or CD56. Increased numbers of CD3-positive CD11b-positive cells have been reported in active SLE.[55]

As stated previously, T cells can be divided into naive or memory cells. Using reciprocal isoforms of CD45 to assess these subsets, researchers found that patients with lupus nephritis had an apparent maturation arrest of both CD4-positive and CD8-positive cells. In some patients, there were markedly decreased naive and memory lymphocytes populations and a corresponding increase in CD45RA-positive CD45RO-positive "transitional cells."[56] In SLE, but not in other controls with chronic diseases, T cells were unable to complete the transition from naive to memory cells.

Percentages of B cells are not usually increased in SLE and may be decreased. Some B cells display the T-cell marker CD5 (Leu 1), and a significant percentage of these cells can produce anti-DNA or anti-IgG autoantibodies. But they are predominantly IgM with low binding affinities for antigen. Although it was proposed that CD5-positive B cells may make up a separate lineage, the presence of CD5 on the B-cell surface most likely reflects a differentiation stage. CD5-positive B cells are not increased in SLE.[57]

SPONTANEOUS B CELL HYPERACTIVITY

Increased activity of B cells in SLE has been demonstrated both in vivo and ex vivo. There is spontaneous B-cell proliferation,[58] and immunoglobulin (Ig) secretion is increased in patients with either active[59–63] or inactive[64] disease. Moreover, nonaffected family members of SLE patients have increased numbers of Ig-secreting cells.[65]

Many factors appear to be contribute to B-cell hyperactivity. In murine SLE, a defect in bone marrow stem cells has been described, and human SLE B-cell colony formation is increased.[66,67] Unlike healthy controls, resting SLE B cells proliferate following cross linking of their surface immunoglobulin receptors[68] and are hyperresponsive to T-cell–derived growth factors.[69,70] Two groups have reported that purified B cells can differentiate by themselves and become antibody-forming cells.[71,72] Others, however, have found that T cells are needed for sustained antibody production by SLE B cells.[73–75] T-cell help is required for the IgM to IgG switch. Nuclear autoantibody production is increased out of proportion to that of total IgG, providing evidence of a specific T-cell–dependent response.[76,77]

Increased antibody production could result from defective feedback regulation. IgG immune complexes normally shut off antibody production by an Fc receptor-dependent mechanism.[78] Although circulating immune complexes are increased in SLE, they do not down-regulate antibody production, and the Fc receptor-bearing natural killer cells appear to contribute to the loss of this feedback loop (see following discussion).

T-cell dysregulation with the production of cytokines with B-cells stimulating activity could be a major factor in sustaining B-cell hyperactivity. As stated, depletion of CD4-positive T cells in murine SLE ameliorates the disease,[5] and in human SLE we have shown that total immunoglobulin and specific autoantibody production by B cells depend on help provided by other regulatory cells.[75] There is a dichotomy between the spontaneous activity of B cells in SLE and their response to specific antigens or mitogens. The antibody response of SLE patients to influenza vaccine or tetanus toxoid is not increased and may even be decreased.[79] Antibody production by cultured SLE mononuclear cells stimulated with pokeweed mitogen is decreased.[80] This is because lymphocytes that have already been activated are refractory to further stimulation, and there is considerable evidence for sustained activation of T cells as well as B cells in patients with active SLE (see following).

T CELL HYPOACTIVITY

Since the early 1970s, B-cell hyperactivity in SLE has been associated with T-cell hypoactivity (Table 69–5). In patients with active SLE, there is impaired delayed hypersensitivity,[2–4] decreased T-cell proliferative re-

TABLE 69–5. IMMUNE DYSREGULATION IN SLE

Lymphocyte Subsets
Decreased numbers of circulating T-cells, B-cells, and natural killer cells in patients with active disease
Postthymic maturation arrest of CD4-positive and CD8-positive T cells
B-Cell Hyperactivity in Patients With Active and Inactive Disease
B-cell colony formation in the bone marrow is increased
Increased proliferation and antibody formation by unstimulated B cells
B cells are hyperresponsive to T-cell–derived growth factors
T-Cell Function in Patients With Active Disease
Impaired delayed skin test reactions to recall antigens
Decreased T-cell proliferative responses to mitogens, soluble antigens, and MHC class II antigens
Generation of antigen-specific T-killer cells is decreased
By contrast, there is considerable evidence of persistent T-cell activation
Activated T cells cannot respond to further stimulants
Natural Killer Cell Activity
Decreased
Monocytes
Have phagocytic defects and decreased accessory cell function
Cytokines
Increased spontaneous production of cytokines such as IL-1, IL-2, IL-6, IFN-γ and decreased cytokine production following stimulation in vitro
Antilymphocyte Antibodies
Alter T-cell subsets and function
Estrogens
Depress cell-mediated immunity

IFN-γ = inteferon-γ; IL-1 = interleukin-1; MHC = major histocompatibility complex.

sponses to mitogens,[81–85] to soluble antigens,[86] and to MHC class II antigens on both allogeneic[87–89] and autologous antigen-presenting cells.[90–93] Generation of antigen-specific T-killer cells is decreased.[94,95] Although considerable efforts have been undertaken to define an intrinsic defect in T cells from SLE patients, these have been largely unsuccessful.

The prevailing paradigm during the 1970s was that B-cell hyperactivity in SLE was due to decreased numbers of activated T suppressor cells. This concept was based on many reports of decreased suppressor cell activity generated by stimulating lymphocytes with concanavalin A.[95–104] The biologic significance of this phenomenon, however, is now questionable and, as stated already, the existence of true antigen-specific suppressor cells is a hotly debated topic. It is clear, however, that CD8-positive cells can down-regulate antibody production and that in subjects with active SLE, CD8-positive lymphocytes lack this ability.[75]

Although there are many examples of decreased T-cell function in SLE, it is evident that T-cell activation is persistent in SLE in vivo. This is probably due to the breakdown of feedback control mechanisms occurring after disease onset (see following discussion). T-cell activation in SLE is manifested by (1) increased spontaneous proliferation,[105] (2) increased percentages of both CD4-positive cells and CD8-positive cells in patients with active SLE that express MHC class II antigens;[106,107] (3) increased spontaneous production of cytokines (see following), and (4) markedly increased levels of soluble IL-2 receptors in the serum that had been released by activated cells;[108,109] The depressed capacity of SLE lymphocytes to respond to various stimuli in vitro may be explained simply by the fact that cells previously activated in vivo are refractory to further stimulation. The various abnormalities in T and B cell in SLE are summarized in Table 69–5.

NATURAL KILLER CELLS

Natural killer cells lack antigen receptors and, therefore, cannot undergo clonal expansion. They are CD3-negative lymphocytes, which display the CD56 surface marker. Most exhibit Fc receptors for IgG (CD16), which they use for antibody-dependent cellular cytotoxicity. The percentage of circulating CD16-positive natural killer cells is frequently decreased in active SLE. This lymphocyte subset can kill infected cells and certain tumor cells, and their cytotoxic activity is decreased in SLE, especially in subjects with active disease.[110–116] Natural killer cell activity is increased by interferon and IL-2, but these lymphokines may only partially correct the cytotoxic defect in SLE.[112,114,115]

Besides their cytotoxic activity, natural killer cells from healthy subjects act synergistically with CD8-positive cells in down-regulating B-cell activity. In SLE, however, these cells have the opposite effect, enhancing antibody production.[75]

MONOCYTE FUNCTION

Proliferation of monocyte precursors is increased in patients with active SLE,[117] but the phagocytic capacity of monocytes is decreased.[118] Accessory cell function of monocytes is also decreased.[119,120] Decreased proliferative responses to mitogens and anti-CD3 has been attributed to a monocyte defect.[83,121,122] Factors responsive for this defect include excessive prostaglandin production[121] and decreased expression of MHC class II molecules.[123,124]

Again, there is a dichotomy between spontaneous and induced antibody production. Although monocytes cannot support lymphocyte responses in vitro, adherent cell-derived factors potentiate polyclonal immunoglobulin and anti-DNA synthesis.[125,126]

CYTOKINE PRODUCTION AND LYMPHOCYTE RESPONSES TO CYTOKINES

Cytokines are soluble molecules that regulate the growth and/or effector function of immune cells. Unlike hormones, they exert their effects at short distances from the cells that produce them. Some cytokines such as IL-2 are produced only by lymphocytes, but others such as IL-1 and IL-6 are produced by macrophages and other cells such as epithelial or endothelial cells. The properties of a given cytokine vary but depend on the composition and the state of activation of the cells exposed to them. Thus, IL-2 produced by CD4-positive cells can up-regulate antibody production. However, if CD8-positive cells and natural killer cells are also present, IL-2 will stimulate these cells to down-regulate antibody production.

As discussed, in considering cytokine production in SLE, it is important to consider separately spontaneous production by blood mononuclear cells from production by cells stimulated in vitro. Spontaneous production reflects the properties of cells previously activated in vivo.

Interleukin-1 release by freshly isolated blood mononuclear cells is increased in SLE,[71,126,127] although IL-1 production by *stimulated* cells is decreased in comparison with healthy controls.[128,129] B cells in SLE secrete IL-1.[71] Increased IL-1α and IL-1β secretion correlates with anti-nRNP antibody production.[127] Monocytes produce both IL-1 and IL-1 antagonists.[130] Decreased production of the latter has been reported.[131]

Interleukin-2 is produced primarily by CD4-positive cells, but CD8-positive cells also have the capacity to produce this lymphokine.[132] IL-2 production by lymphocytes stimulated in vitro is decreased.[128,133–136] Some investigators found that this defect correlated with disease activity, but others found decreased IL-2 production in patients with inactive disease as well.[128] In patients with active SLE, this defect could not be explained by passive absorption of this cytokine. Decreased IL-2 activity has also been reported on stimulation of lymphocytes from relatives of subjects with SLE.[137] We have confirmed this observation. This defect, however, was largely explained by passive absorption of newly released IL-2 by activated mononuclear cells rather than by a decreased capacity to produce it.[138]

There is increasing evidence that defective IL-2 production in SLE is explained by immune dysregulation and persistent T-cell activation rather than by an intrinsic abnormality of CD4-positive cells. We found activated CD8-positive cells inhibited IL-2 production by CD4-positive cells.[75] Huang, Miescher, and Zubler found that after "resting" for a few days in culture, blood mononuclear cells from SLE patients that produce IL-2 as well as those from normal controls.[139] These workers also detected IL-2 in the serum of patients with active disease,[140] suggesting that production of IL-2 is increased in vivo in SLE patients. We found that a neutralizing anti-IL-2 monoclonal antibody inhibited spontaneous antibody synthesis in SLE,[75] and using the polymerase chain reaction, we documented IL-2 gene activation in freshly isolated lymphocytes from most patients with active SLE, but not in controls.[141] Consistent with sustained T-cell activation in vivo, expression of the IL-2 receptor α-chain (Tac or CD25)[56,142] and the p70/75 β-chain[143] is decreased after T-cell stimulation in vitro.

Interferon-γ regulates the expression of MHC products on immune cells, inhibits lymphocyte proliferation, and has mixed effects on antibody production.[144] In SLE, decreased or normal production of this lymphokine has been reported in vitro.[145–147] Serum levels of an acid-labile interferon-α are increased in SLE.[148]

SLE lymphocytes produce increased levels of growth factors that promote B-cell growth and differentiation.[149,150] Until recently, however, these cytokines were not characterized. Increased levels of IL-1[71,126,127] and IL-6[151,152] have now been reported. IL-6 is increased in the cerebral spinal fluid in SLE.[153] Moreover, SLE B cells are hyperresponsive to certain B-cell growth factors, suggesting up-regulation of cytokine receptors. IL-6, by itself, can enable activated B cells in SLE to become antibody-forming cells.[64] This finding indicates either an intrinsic B-cell defect or that B cells from subjects with SLE have received a priming signal in vivo.

EFFECTS OF ANTILYMPHOCYTE ANTIBODIES ON LYMPHOCYTE FUNCTION

SLE sera may contain autoantibodies reactive with CD4-positive, CD8-positive, and natural killer cells.[53,100,154–159] There is evidence that cold-reactive, IgM antilymphocyte antibodies react preferentially with CD4-positive lymphocytes.[159] Such autocytotoxicity could contribute to the decreased percentages of CD4-positive cells found in some patients with active disease. Cold-reactive IgM antibodies can be found in almost all SLE sera regardless of disease activity.[160] Autoantibodies reactive with the CD45, membrane tyrosine phosphatase CD45 molecule have been found in SLE.[161,162] These antibodies characteristically react with the high molecular weight CD45RA isoform. As stated, this surface marker is displayed by naive T cells.[21] Autoantibodies against the MHC class I-associated β_2-microglobulin[163] and MHC class II molecules[164] have also been described. Autoantibodies reacting with signal transducing molecules could alter T-cell function.

In contrast to cold-reactive IgM antilymphocyte antibodies, warm-reactive IgG antibodies in SLE serum inhibit the lymphocyte-proliferative response to mitogens,[165,166] autologous,[164,166–170] allogeneic,[169,171,172] and soluble antigens.[173] IgG antibodies react with resting and even more strongly with mitogen-activated lymphocytes.[173,174] IgM and IgG antilymphocyte antibodies inhibit the generation of suppressor cells[103,175] and natural killer activity[110,176,177] and inhibit antibody-dependent cellular cytotoxicity (ADCC).[178,179] IgG antilymphocyte antibodies can sensitize cells for ADCC.[180–184] In addition to antilymphocyte antibodies, SLE serum may contain antibodies to IL-2.[185] Moreover, anti-double-stranded DNA antibodies inhibit lymphocyte function.[186] This agrees with our findings that many of the abnormalities of lymphocyte function reported in SLE can be reproduced by incubating normal lymphocytes with SLE serum.[165,166] Therefore, it is very likely that antilymphocyte antibodies contribute to the persistence of immune dysfunction in SLE.

HORMONAL FACTORS

SLE affects females predominantly, and it is well known that sex hormones have important roles in immune regulation.[187] Estrogens increase and androgens reduce spontaneous and induced antibodies to single-stranded DNA in mice.[188] Estradiol impairs T-cell responsiveness[189–191] and significantly decreases natural killer cell activity.[193] Estrogens generally depress cell-mediated immunity in parallel with an increase in autoantibody production.

CONSEQUENCE OF IMMUNE DYSREGULATION

Abnormalities in T-cell subsets, functional properties of T cells, and cytokine production are chiefly observed in patients with active disease. Because of the abnormalities of CD4-positive T cells described previously, these cells are unable to provide the necessary help for CD8-positive cells to down-regulate antibody production. Under these conditions, both CD8-positive T cells and natural killer cells support instead of suppress antibody production in SLE.[75] This pathologic immune circuit is illustrated in Fig. 69–1. Perturbation of normal regulatory pathways, therefore, can sustain B-cell hyperactivity and autoantibody production.

Fortunately, these regulatory abnormalities can be reversed in SLE. Spontaneous remissions occur, and complete remissions have been observed with the judicious use of cyclophosphamide. Patients with SLE require lower doses than those with RA, and remission can occur on low-dose therapy, providing patients have received an appropriate loading dose.[194] One such case is

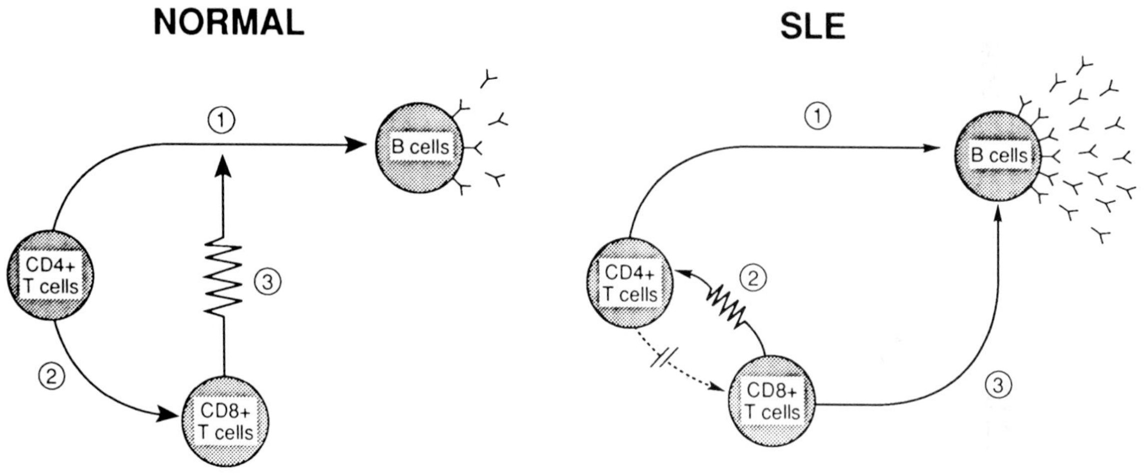

FIGURE 69–1. Regulation of antibody production in normals and subjects with systemic lupus erythematosus (SLE). In healthy individuals, antigen-stimulated CD4-positive lymphocytes provide help for antibody production and also provide help for CD8-positive cells to down-regulate the antibody response. In subjects with active SLE, CD4-positive T cells become abnormal for reasons summarized in the text and are unable to provide help for CD8-positive cells. In the absence of the proper inductive influence of CD4-positive cells, CD8-positive cells become helper cells for B cells and, paradoxically, down-regulate CD4-positive cells. This pathologic circuit sustains B-cell activity. (Summarized from references 56, 75, 106 and 192).

TABLE 69–6. REVERSAL OF IMMUNOLOGIC ABNORMALITIES AFTER CLINICAL REMISSION

MONTH	HCT	ESR	$CH5_0$	ANTI-DNA	CRYO	PHA	CYCLOPHOSPHAMIDE (mg)	PREDNISONE (mg)
0	25	107	low	2+	3+	82	150	10
2	30	112	nl	0	3+	31	50	7.5
4	36	110	nl	0	0	454	50 q4d	7.5
6	39	70	nl	0	0	190	50 q4d	7.5
12	41	36	nl	0	0	910	50 q2d	2.5

This 21-year-old woman was treated with cyclophosphamide at age 19 for severe SLE. Her disease included episodes of cerebritis with nephritis, and after 5 years she developed deterioration of renal function. She had received high-dose prednisone for several years and had developed bilateral aseptic necrosis of the femoral heads. The starting dose of cyclophosphamide was 2 mg/kg, and this was reduced as the total lymphocyte count decreased by 50%. Before therapy, the proliferative response of her blood mononuclear cells to phytohemagglutinin (expressed as counts per minute) was markedly decreased. Within 4 months of treatment, renal function normalized, all serologic evidence of SLE activity disappeared, and lymphocyte function returned to normal. Her remission has lasted for more than 8 years.

$CH5_0$ = serum complement level; Cryo = cryoglobulins; ESR = erythrocyte sedimentation rate; Hct = hematocrit; PHA = phytohemagglutinin; SLE = systemic lupus erythematosus.

described in Table 69–6. The mechanism of action of cyclophosphamide is not understood, but almost all the abnormalities of T-cell function disappear with clinical remission.

In conclusion, both genetic and environmental factors are involved in the pathogenesis of SLE. Although family studies have shown evidence of B-cell hyperactivity such as hyper-γ-globulinemia and autoantibody formation in relatives, the onset of clinical disease is likely to be T-cell dependent with failure of memory self-regulatory T cells to prevent the development of clones of T-helper cells and B cells capable of making IgG autoantibodies. Once the disease has become fully established, disruption of homeostatic regulatory circuits sustain B-cell hyperactivity and the perpetuation of SLE. The aim of therapy should be to interrupt these pathologic circuits. Unlike the other human autoimmune diseases with a female predisposition, SLE is usually most severe during early childbearing years, and in some patients long-term remissions have been observed.

REFERENCES

1. Harley, J.B., Sestak, A.L., Willis, L.G., et al.: A model for disease heterogeneity in systemic lupus erythematosus. Arthritis Rheum., *32*:826, 1989.
2. Horwitz, D.A.: Impaired delayed hypersensitivity in systemic lupus erythematosus. Arthritis Rheum., *15*:353, 1972.
3. Hahn, B.H., Babgy, M.D., and Osterland, C.K.: Abnormalities of delayed hypersensitivity in systemic lupus erythematosus. Am. J. Med., *55*:25, 1973.
4. Paty, J.G. et al.: Impaired cell-mediated immunity in systemic lupus erythematosus. A controlled study of 23 untreated patients. Am. J. Med., *59*:769, 1975.
5. Wofsy, D., and Seaman, W.E.: Reversal of advanced murine lupus in NZB/NZW F_1 mice by treatment with monoclonal antibody to L3T4. J. Immunol., *138*:3247–3253, 1987.
6. Sanz, I., and Capra, J.D.: The genetic origin of human autoantibodies. J. Immunol., *140*:3283–3285, 1988.
7. Cohen, I.R., and Cooke, A.: Natural autoantibodies might prevent autoimmune disease. Immunol. Today, 7:363–364, 1986.
8. Carson, D.A., Chen, P.P., and Kipps, T.J.: New roles for rheumatoid factor. J. Clin. Invest., *87*:379–383, 1991.
9. Blackman, M., Kappler, J., and Marrack, P.: The role of the T cell receptor in positive and negative selection of developing T cells. Science, *248*:1335–1341, 1990.
10. Burkly, L.C., Lo, D., and Flavell, R.A.: Tolerance in transgenic mice expressing major histocompatibility molecules extrathymically on pancreatic cells. Science, *248*:1364–1368, 1990.
11. Schwartz, R.H.: A cell culture model for T lymphocyte clonal anergy. Science, *248*:1349–1356, 1990.
12. DeSilva, D.R., and Jenkins, M.K.: Role of proliferation in T cell clonal anergy. (Abstract.) FASEB J., *5*:5831, 1991.
13. Ohashi, P.S., Oehen, S., Buerki, K., et al.: Ablation of "tolerance" and induction of diabetes by virus infection in viral antigen transgenic mice. Cell, *65*:305–317, 1991.
14. Brenner, M.B., McLean, J., Scheft, H., et al.: Two forms of the T-cell receptor τ protein found on peripheral blood cytotoxic T lymphocytes. Nature, *324*:689–694, 1987.
15. Bluestone, J.A., Cron, R.Q., Cotterman, M., et al.: Structure and specificity of T cell receptor τ/σ on major histocompatibility complex antigen-specific $CD3^+$, $CD4^-$, $CD8^-$ T lymphocytes. J. Exp. Med., *168*:1899–1916, 1988.
16. Shivakumar, S., Tsokos, G.C., and Datta, S.K.: T cell receptor α/β expressing double-negative ($CD4^-/CD8^-$) and $CD4^+$ T helper cells in humans augment the production of pathogenic anti-DNA autoantibodies associated with lupus nephritis. J. Immunol., *143*:103–112, 1989.
17. Van Vlasselaer, P., and Strober, S.: α β TCR^+ $CD3^+$ $CD4^-$ $CD8^-$ cloned natural suppressor (NS) cells produce an immunosuppressive factor which is different from IFN-τ and TGF-β. Transplant. Proc., *23*:200–202, 1991.
18. Bradley, L.M., Bradley, J.S., Ching, D.L., and Shiigi, S.M.: Predominance of T cells that express CD45R in the $CD4^+$ helper/inducer lymphocyte subset of neonates. Clin. Immunol. Immunopathol., *51*:426, 1989.
19. Smith, S.H., Brown, M.H., Rowe, D., et al.: Functional subsets of human helper-inducer cells defined by a new mAb, UCHL1. Immunology, *58*:63, 1986.
20. Ehlers, S., and Smith, K.A.: Differentiation of T cell lymphokine gene expression: The in vitro acquisition of T cell memory. J. Exp. Med., *173*:25–36, 1991.
21. Beverley, P.: Immunological memory in T cells. Curr. Opin. Immunol., *3*:355–360, 1991.
22. Block, S.R., Winfield, J.B., Lockshin, M.D., et al.: Studies of twins with systemic lupus erythematosus. Am. J. Med., *59*:533–552, 1975.
23. Deapen, D., Escalante, A., Weinrib, L., et al.: A revised estimate of twin concordance in SLE, (in press), 1991.
24. Aho, K., Koskenvuo, M., Tuominen, J., and Kaprio, J.: Occurrence of rheumatoid arthritis in a nationwide series of twins. J. Rheumatol., *13*:899–902, 1986.
25. Olmos, P., A'Hern, R., Heaton, D.A., et al.: The significance of the concordance rate for type 1 (insulin-dependent) diabetes in identical twins. Diabetologia, *31*:747–750, 1988.
26. Kinnunen, E., Koskenvuo, M., Kaprio, J., and Aho, K.: Multiple sclerosis in a nationwide series of twins. Neurology, *37*:1627–1629, 1987.
27. Feehally, J. et al.: Impaired IgG response to tetanus toxoid in human membranous nephropathy: Association with HLA-DR3. Clin. Exp. Immunol., *63*:376–384, 1986.
28. Bruserud, O., Jervell, J., and Thorsby, E.: HLA-DR3 and -DR4 control T-lymphocyte responses to mumps and Coxsackie B4 virus: Studies on patients with type 1 (insulin-dependent) diabetes and healthy subjects. Diabetologia, *28*:420–426, 1985.
29. Bruserud, O., Stenersen, M., and Thorsby, E.: T lymphocyte responses to Coxsackie B4 and mumps virus: II. Immunoregulation by HLA-DR3 and -DR4 associated restriction elements. Tissue Antigens, *26*:179–192, 1985.
30. Ambindery, M. et al.: Special characteristics of immune function in normal individuals of the HLA-DR3 Type. Clin. Immunol. Immunopathol., *23*:269–274, 1982.
31. Jacob, C.O., Fronek, Z., Lewis, G.D., et al.: Heritable major histocompatibility complex class II-associated differences in production of tumor necrosis factor alpha: relevance to genetic predisposition to systemic lupus erythematosus. Proc. Natl. Acad. Sci. USA, *87*:1233–1237, 1990.
32. Lawley, T.J. et al.: Defective Fc-receptor functions associated with the HLA-B8/DRw3 haplotype: Studies in patients with dermatitis herpetiformis and normal subjects. N. Engl. J. Med., *304*:185, 1981.
33. Fronek, Z., Timmerman, L.A., Alper, C.A., et al.: Major histocompatibility complex genes and susceptibility to systemic lupus erythematosus. Arthritis Rheum., *33*:1542–1553, 1990.
34. Alexander, E.L., McNicholl, J., Watson, R.M., et al.: The immunogenetic relationship between anti-Ro (SS-A)/La (SS-B) antibody positive Sjoegren's/lupus erythematosus overlap syn-

drome and the neonatal lupus syndrome. J. Invest. Dermatol., *93*:751–756, 1989.

35. Arnett, F.C., Bias, W.B., and Reveille, J.D.: Genetic studies in Sjoegren's syndrome and systemic lupus erythematosus. J. Autoimmunol., *2*:403–413, 1989.
36. Kemp, M.E., Atkinson, J.P., Skanes, V.M. et al.: Deletion of C4A genes in patients with systemic lupus erythematosus. Arthritis Rheum., *30*:1015–22, 1987.
37. Schur, P.H.: Complement and lupus erythematosus. Arthritis Rheum., *25*:793, 1982.
38. Tebib, J.G., Alcocer-Varela, J., Alarcon-Segovia, D., and Schur, P.H.: Association between a T cell receptor restriction fragment length polymorphism and systemic lupus erythematosus. J. Clin. Invest., *86*:1961–1967, 1990.
39. Miller, K.B., and Schwartz, R.S.: Familial abnormalities of suppressor-cell function in systemic lupus erythematosus. N. Engl. J. Med., *3011*:803, 1979.
40. Larsson, O., and Leonhardt, T.: Hereditary hypergammaglobulinaemia and systemic lupus erythematosus: I. Clinical and electrophoretic studies. Acta Med. Scand., *165*:371, 1959.
41. Holman, H.R., and Deicher, H.R.: The appearance of hypergammaglobulinemia, positive serological reactions for rheumatoid arthritis and complement fixation reactions with tissue constituents in the sera of relatives of patients with systemic lupus erythematosus. Arthritis Rheum., *3*:244, 1960.
42. DeHoratius, R.J., Pillarisetty, R., Messner, R.P., and Talal, N.: Anti-nucleic acid antibodies in systemic lupus erythematosus patients and their families. Incidence and correlation with lymphocytoxic antibodies. J. Clin. Invest., *56*:1149, 1975.
43. Morris, S.C., Cheek, R.L., Cohen, P.L., and Eisenberg, R.A.: Autoantibodies in chronic graft versus host result from cognate T-B interactions. J. Exp. Med., *171*:503–517, 1990.
44. Steinberg, A.D.: Mechanisms of disordered immune regulation. *In* Basic and Clinical Immunology. Edited by D.P. Stites and A.I. Terr. Norwalk, CT, Appleton & Lange, 1991, pp. 432–437.
45. Gleichmann, E., Van Elven, E.H., and Van der Veen, J.P.W.: A systemic lupus erythematosus (SLE)-like disease in mice induced by abnormal T-B cell cooperation. Preferential formation of autoantibodies characteristic of SLE. Eur. J. Immunol., *182*:129, 1982.
46. Gleichmann, E. et al.: Graft-versus-host reactions: Clues to the etiopathology of a spectrum of immunological diseases. Immunol. Today, *5*:324, 1984.
47. White, J., Herman, A., Pullen, A.M., et al.: The V beta specific superantigen staphylococcal enterotoxin B: Stimulation of mature T cells and clonal deletion in neonatal mice. Cell, *56*:27–35, 1989.
48. Tomai, M., Kotb, M., Majumdar, G., and Beachey, E.H.: Superantigenicity of streptococcal M protein. J. Exp. Med., *172*:359–362, 1990.
49. Atkin, C.L., Cole, B.C., Sullivan, G.J., et al.: Stimulation of mouse lymphocytes by a mitogen derived from Mycoplasma arthritidis: V. A small basic protein from culture supernatants is a potent T cell mitogen. J. Immunol., *137*:1581–1589, 1986.
50. Friedman, S.M., Posnett, D.N., Tumang, J.R., et al.: A potential role for microbial superantigens in the pathogenesis of systemic autoimmune disease. Arthritis Rheum., *34*:468, 1991.
51. Bakke, A.C. et al.: T lymphocyte subsets in systemic lupus erythematosus. Arthritis Rheum., *26*:745, 1983.
52. Smolan, J.S. et al.: Heterogenicity of immunoregulatory T-cell subsets in systemic lupus erythematosus. Am. J. Med., *72*:783, 1982.
53. Morimoto, C. et al.: Alteration in T cell subsets in active systemic lupus erythematosus. J. Clin. Invest., *66*:1171, 1980.
54. Tsokos, G.C., and Balow, J.E.: Phenotypes of T lymphocytes in systemic lupus erythematosus: Decreased cytotoxic/suppressor subpopulation is associated with deficient cytotoxic responses rather than with concanavalin A-induced suppressor cells. Clin. Immunol. Immunopathol., *26*:267, 1983.
55. Gray, J.D. et al.: Studies on human blood lymphocytes with iC3b (type 3) complement receptors: Abnormalities in patients with active systemic lupus erythematosus. Clin. Exp. Immunol., *67*:556, 1987.
56. Horwitz, D.A., Basin, K., and Gray, J.D.: Evidence for a postthymic T-cell developmental defect in SLE. (Abstract.) Clin. Res., *39*:249A, 1991.
57. Suzuki, N., Sakane, T., and Engleman, E.G.: Anti-DNA antibody production by $CD5^+$ and $CD5^-$ B cells of patients with systemic lupus erythematosus. J. Clin. Invest., *85*:238–247, 1990.
58. Glinski, W. et al.: Study of lymphocyte subpopulations in normal humans and patients with systemic lupus erythematosus by fractionation of peripheral blood lymphocytes on discontinuous Ficoll gradient. Clin. Exp. Immunol., *26*:228, 1976.
59. Blaese, R.M., Grayson, J., and Steinberg, A.D.: Elevated immunoglobulin secreting cells in the blood of patients with active systemic lupus erythematosus: Correlation of laboratory and clinical assessment of disease activity. Am. J. Med., *69*:345, 1980.
60. Fauci, A.S.: Immunoregulation in autoimmunity. J. Allergy Clin. Immunol., *66*:5, 1980.
61. Ginsburg, W.W., Finkelman, F.D., and Lipsky, P.E.: Circulating and pokeweed mitogen-induced immunoglobulin-secreting cell in systemic lupus erythematosus. Clin. Exp. Immunol., *35*:76, 1979.
62. Fauci, A.S., and Moutsopoulos, H.M.: Polyclonally triggered B-cells in the peripheral blood and bone marrow of normal individuals and patients with systemic lupus erythematosus and primary Sjögren's syndrome. Arthritis Rheum., *24*:577, 1986.
63. Dar, O., Salaman, M.R., Seifert, M.R., and Isenberg, D.A.: B lymphocyte activation in systemic lupus erythematosus: Spontaneous production of IgG antibodies to DNA and environmental antigens in cultures of blood mononuclear cells. Clin. Exp. Immunol., *73*:430, 1988.
64. Kitani, A. et al.: Heterogeneity of B cell responsiveness to interleukin 4, interleukin 6 and low molecular weight B cell growth factor in discrete stages of B cell activation in patients with systemic lupus erythematosus. Clin. Exp. Immunol., *77*:31, 1989.
65. DeHoratius, R.J., and Levinson, A.I.: Increased circulating immunoglobulin secreting cells in asymptomatic family members with systemic lupus erythematosus. (Abstract.) Arthritis Rheum., *24*:S92, 1981.
66. Kumagai, S. et al.: Defective regulation of B lymphocyte colony formation in patients with systemic lupus erythematosus. J. Immunol., *128*:258, 1982.
67. Kumagai, S. et al.: Possible different mechanisms of B cell activation in systemic lupus erythematosus and rheumatoid arthritis: Opposite expression of low affinity receptors tor IgE (CD23) on their peripheral B cells. Clin. Exp. Immunol., *78*:348, 1989.
68. Suzuki, N., and Sakane, T.: Induction of excessive B cell proliferation and differentiation by an in vitro stimulus in culture in human systemic lupus erythematosus. J. Clin. Invest., *83*: 937–944, 1989.
69. Delfraissy, J.F. et al.: B cell hyperactivity in systemic lupus erythematosus: Selectively enhanced responsiveness to a high molecular weight B cell growth factor. Eur. J. Immunol., *16*:1251–1256, 1986.
70. Ueda, Y., Sakane, T., and Tsunematsu, T.: Hyperreactivity of activated B cells to B cell growth factor in patients with systemic lupus erythematosus. J. Immunol., *143*:3988–3993, 1989.
71. Tanaka, T., Saito, K., Shirakawa, F., et al.: Production of B cell-

stimulating factors by B cells in patients with systemic lupus erythematosus. J. Immunol., *141*:3043–3049, 1988.

72. Pelton, B.K., Speckmaier, M., Hylton, W., et al.: Cytokine-independent progression of immunoglobulin production in vitro by B lymphocytes from patients with systemic lupus erythematosus. Clin. Exp. Immunol., *83*:274–279, 1991.
73. Cohen, P.L., Litvin, D.A., and Winfield, J.B.: Association between endogenously activated T cells and immunoglobulin-secreting B cells in patients with active systemic lupus erythematosus. Arthritis Rheum., *25*:168, 1982.
74. Takeuchi, T. et al.: In vitro immune response of SLE lymphocytes. The mechanism involved in B-cell activation. Scand. J. Immunol., *16*:369, 1982.
75. Linker-Israeli, M., Quismorio, F.P., Jr., and Horwitz, D.A.: $CD8^+$ lymphocytes from patients with systemic lupus erythematosus lymphocytes sustain rather than suppress spontaneous polyclonal IgG production and synergize with $CD4^+$ cells to support autoantibody synthesis. Arthritis Rheum., *33*: 1216–1225, 1990.
76. Bizar-Scheebaum, A., O'Dell, J.R., and Kotzin, B.L.: Anti-histone antibody production by peripheral blood cells in SLE. Arthritis Rheum., *30*:511, 1987.
77. Gharavi, A.E., Chu, J., and Elkon, K.B.: Autoantibodies to intracellular proteins in human systemic lupus erythematosus are not due to random polyclonal B cell activation. Arthritis Rheum., *31*:1337, 1988.
78. Sinclair, N.R.: Regulation of the immune response: I. Reduction in ability of specific antibody to inhibit long-lasting IgG immunological priming after removal of the Fc fragment. J. Exp. Med., *129*:1183, 1969.
79. Brodman, R., Gilfillan, G., Glass, P., and Schur, P.H.: Influenzal vaccine response in systemic lupus erythematosus. Ann. Intern. Med., *88*:735, 1978.
80. Bobrove, A.M., and Miller, P.: Depressed in vitro B-lymphocyte differentiation in systemic lupus erythematosus. Arthritis Rheum., *20*:1326, 1977.
81. Horwitz, D.A., and Garret, M.A.; Lymphocyte reactivity to mitogens in subjects with systemic lupus erythematosus, rheumatoid arthritis and scleroderma. Clin. Exp. Immunol., *27*:92, 1977.
82. Lockshin, M.E. et al.: Cell mediated immunity in rheumatic diseases. Mitogen responses in RA, SLE and other illnesses: Correlation with T and B lymphocyte populations. Arthritis Rheum., *18*:245, 1975.
83. Markenson, J.A. et al.: Suppressor monocytes in patients with systemic lupus erythematosus. Evidence of suppressor activity associated with cell free soluble product of monocytes. J. Lab. Clin. Med., *95*:40, 1980.
84. Rosenthal, C.J., and Franklin, E.C.: Depression of cellular-mediated immunity in systemic lupus erythematosus. Relation to disease activity. Arthritis Rheum., *18*:207, 1975.
85. Utsinger, P.D., and Yount, W.J.: Phytohemagglutinin response in systemic lupus erythematosus. Reconstitution experiments using highly purified lymphocyte subpopulations and monocytes. J. Clin. Invest., *60*:626, 1977.
86. Gottlieb, A.B. et al.: Immune function is systemic lupus erythematosus. Impairment of in vitro T-cell proliferation and in vivo antibody response to exogenous antigen. J. Clin. Invest., *63*:885, 1979.
87. Suciu-Foca, N. et al.: Impaired responsiveness of lymphocytes in patients with systemic lupus erythematosus. Clin. Exp., *18*:295, 1974.
88. Tsokos, G.C., and Balow, J.E.: Cellular immune response in systemic lupus erythematosus. J. Clin. Immunol., *1*:208, 1981.
89. Kumagai, S., Steinberg, A.D., and Green, I.: Immune responses to hapten-modified self and their regulation in normal individuals and patients with systemic lupus erythematosus. J. Immunol., *127*:1643, 1981.
90. Kuntz, M.M., Innes, J.B., and Weksler, M.E.: The cellular basis of the impaired autologous mixed lymphocyte reaction in patients with systemic lupus erythematosus. J. Clin. Invest., *63*:151, 1979.
91. Sakane, T., Steinberg, A.P., and Green, I.: Failure of the autologous mixed lymphocyte reactions between T cells and non T cells in patients with systemic lupus erythematosus. Proc. Natl. Acad. Sci. USA, *75*:3464, 1978.
92. Sakane, T. et al.: Studies of immune functions of patients with systemic lupus erythematosus: III. Characterization of lymphocyte subpopulations responsible for defective autologous mixed lymphocyte reactions. Arthritis Rheum., *22*:770, 1979.
93. Takada, S. et al.: Abnormalities in autologous mixed lymphocyte reaction-activated immunologic processes in systemic lupus erythematosus and their possible correction by interleukin 2. Eur. J. Immunol., *15*:262–267, 1985.
94. Charpentier, B., Carnoud, C., and Bach, J.F.: Selective depression of the xenogeneic cell-mediated lympholysis in systemic lupus erythematosus. J. Clin. Invest., *64*:351, 1979.
95. Alarcon-Segovia, D., and Palacios, R.: Differences in immunoregulatory T cell circuits between diphenylhydantoin-related and spontaneously occurring systemic lupus erythematosus. Arthritis Rheum., *24*:1086, 1981.
96. Bresnihan, B., and Jasin, H.E.: Suppressor function of peripheral blood mononuclear cells in normal individuals and in patients with systemic lupus erythematosus. J. Clin. Invest., *59*:106, 1977.
97. Fauci, A.S., Steinberg, A.D., Haynes, B.F., and Whalen, G.: Immunoregulatory aberrations in systemic lupus erythematosus. J. Immunol., *121*:1473, 1978.
98. Ilfeld, D.N., and Krakauer, R.S.: Suppression of immunoglobulin synthesis of systemic lupus erythematosus patients by concanavalin A-activated normal human spleen cell supernatants. Clin. Immunol. Immunopathol., *17*:196, 1980.
99. Morimoto, C.: Loss of suppressor T lymphocyte function in patients with systemic lupus erythematosus. Clin. Immunol. Immunopathol., *32*:125, 1978.
100. Morimoto, C., Abe, T., and Homma, M.: Altered function of suppressor T lymphocytes in patients with active systemic lupus erythematosus. Clin. Immunol. Immuopathol., *13*:161, 1979.
101. Newman, B. et al.: Lack of suppressor cell activity in systemic lupus erythematosus. Clin. Immunol. Immunopathol., *13*:187, 1979.
102. Ruiz-Arguelles, A., Alarcon-Segovia, D., Llorente, L., and del Gindice-Knipping, J.A.: Heterogeneity of the spontaneously expanded and mitogen-induced generation of suppressor cell function of T cells on B cells in systemic lupus erythematosus. Arthritis Rheum., *23*:1004, 1980.
103. Sagawa, A., and Abdou, N.I.: Suppressor-cell dysfunction in systemic lupus erythematosus. Cells involved and in vitro correction. J. Clin. Invest., *62*:789, 1978.
104. Sakane, T., Steinberg, A.D., and Green, I.: Studies of immune functions of patients with systemic lupus erythematosus: I. Dysfunction of suppressor T-cell activity related to impaired generation of, rather than response to, suppressor cells. Arthritis Rheum., *21*:657, 1978.
105. Horwitz, D.A., Stastny, P., and Ziff, M.: Circulating DNA-synthesizing mononuclear leukocytes: I. Increased numbers of proliferating mononuclear leukocytes in inflammatory disease. J. Lab. Clin. Med., *76*:391–402, 1970.
106. Linker-Israeli, M., Bakke, A.C., Quismorio, F.P., and Horwitz, D.A.: Correction of interleukin 2 production in patients with systemic lupus erythematosus by removal spontaneously activated suppressor cells. J. Clin. Invest., *75*:762–768, 1985.

107. Inghirami, G., Simon, J., Balow, J.E., and Tsokos, G.C.: Activated T lymphocytes in the peripheral blood of patients with systemic lupus erythematosus induce B cells to produce immunoglobulin. Clin. Exp. Rheumatol., *6*:269–276, 1988.
108. Campen, D.H., Horwitz, D.A., Quismorio, F.P., Jr., et al.: Serum levels of interleukin-2 receptor and activity of rheumatic diseases characterized by immune system activation. Arthritis Rheum., *31*:1358–1364, 1988.
109. Ter Borg, E.J., Horst, G., Limburg, P.C., and Kallenberg, C.G.: Changes in plasma levels of interleukin-2 receptor in relation to disease exacerbations and levels of anti-dsDNA and complement in systemic lupus erythematosus. Clin. Exp. Immunol., *82*:21–26, 1990.
110. Silverman, S.L., and Cathcart, E.S.: Natural killing in systemic lupus erythematosus. Inhibitory effects of serum. Clin. Immunol. Immunopathol., *17*:219, 1978.
111. Hoffman, T.: Natural killer function in systemic lupus erythematosus. Arthritis Rheum., *23*:30, 1980.
112. Katz, P. et al.: Abnormal natural killer cell activity in systemic lupus erythematosus: An intrinsic defect in the cytolytic event. J. Immunol., *129*:1966, 1982.
113. Tsokos, G.C., Rook, A.H., Diej, J.Y., and Balow, J.E.: Natural killer cells and interferon responses in patients with systemic lupus erythematosus. Clin. Exp. Immunol., *5*:239, 1982.
114. Tsokos, G.C. et al.: Interleukin-2 restores the depressed alogeneic cell-mediated lympholysis and natural killer cell activity in patients with systemic lupus erythematosus. Clin. Immunol. Immunopathol., *34*:379, 1985.
115. Sibbitt, W.L., Jr., Matthews, P.M., and Bankhurst, A.D.: Defects in effector lytic activity and response to interferon and interferon inducers. J. Clin. Invest., *10*:71, 1983.
116. Oshimi, K., Sumiya, A., Gond, N., et al.: Natural killer cell activity in systemic lupus erythematosus. Lancet, *2*:1023, 1979.
117. Horwitz, D.A.: The development of macrophages from large lymphocyte-like cells in the blood of patients with inflammatory diseases. J. Clin. Invest., *51*:760–769, 1972.
118. Boswell, J., and Schur, P.H.: Monocyte function in systemic lupus erythematosus. Clin. Immunol. Immunopathol., *52*: 271–278, 1989.
119. Yu, C.L., Chang, K.L., Chiu, C.C., et al.: Alteration of mitogenic responses of mononuclear cells by anti-ds DNA antibodies resembling immune disorders in patients with systemic lupus erythematosus. Scand. J. Rheumatol., *18*:265–276, 1989.
120. Muryoi, T., Sasaki, T., Sekiguchi, Y., et al.: Impaired accessory cell function of monocytes in systemic lupus erythematosus. J. Clin. Lab. Immunol., *28*:123–128, 1989.
121. Markenson, J.A. et al.: Responses of fractionated cells from patients with systemic lupus erythematosus and normals to plant mitogen: Evidence for a suppressor population of monocytes. Proc. Soc. Exp. Biol. Med., *158*:5, 1978.
122. Martorell, J., Font, J., Rojo, I., et al.: Responsiveness of systemic lupus erythematosus T cells to signals provided through LCA T200 (CD45) and T1 (CD5) antigens. Clin. Exp. Immunol., *78*:172–176, 1989.
123. Nagai, H. et al.: Diminished peripheral blood moncyte DR antigen expression in systemic lupus erythematosus. Clin. Exp. Rheumatol., *2*:131, 1984.
124. Shirakawa, F., Yamashita, U., and Suzuki, H.: Decrease in HLA-DR monocytes in patients with SLE. J. Immunol., *134*:3560, 1985.
125. Jandl, R.C. et al.: The effect of adherent cell-derived factors on immunoglobulin and anti-DNA synthesis in systemic lupus erythematosus. Clin. Immunol. Immunopathol., *42*:344–359, 1987.
126. Sasaki, T., Shibata, S., Hirabayashi, Y., et al.: Accessory cell activity of monocytes in anti-DNA antibody production in systemic lupus erythematosus. Clin. Exp. Immunol., *77*:37–42, 1989.
127. Aotsuka, S., Nakamura, K., Nakano, T., et al.: Production of intracellular and extracellular interleukin-1 alpha and interleukin-1 beta by peripheral blood monocytes from patients with connective tissue diseases. Ann. Rheum. Dis., *50*:27–31, 1991.
128. Linker-Israeli, M., Bakke, A.C., Kitridou, R.C., et al.: Defective production of interleukin 1 and interleukin 2 in patients with systemic lupus erythematosus (SLE). J. Immunol., *130*: 2651–2655, 1983.
129. Alcocer-Varela, J., Laffon, A., and Alarcon-Segovia, D.: Defective monocyte production of, and T lymphocyte response to, interleukin-1 in the peripheral blood of patients with systemic lupus erythematosus. Clin. Exp. Immunol., *54*:125, 1983.
130. Arend, W.P., Joslin, F.G., and Massoni, R.J.: Effects of immune complexes on production by human monocytes of interleukin 1 or an interleukin 1 inhibitor. J. Immunol., *134*:3868, 1985.
131. Schur, P.H., Chang, D.M., Baptiste, P., et al.: Human monocytes produce IL-1 and an inhibitor of IL-1 in response to two different signals. Clin. Immunol. Immunopathol., *57*:45–63, 1990.
132. Luger, T.A. et al.: Human lymphocytes with either OKT4 or OKT8 phenotype produce interleukin 2 in culture. J. Clin. Invest., *70*:470–473, 1982.
133. Alcocer-Varela, J., and Alarcon-Segovia, D.: Decreased production and response to interleukin 2 by cultured lymphocytes from patients with systemic lupus erythematosus. J. Clin. Invest., *69*:1388, 1982.
134. Murakawa, Y. et al.: Characterization of T lymphocyte subpopulations responsible for deficient interleukin-2 activity in patients with systemic lupus erythematosus. J. Immunol., *134*:187, 1985.
135. Warrington, R.J., Sauder, P.J., Homik, J., and Ofosu-Appiah, W.: Reversible interleukin 2 response defects in systemic lupus erythematosus. Clin. Exp. Immunol., *77*:167, 1989.
136. Sierakowski, S., Kucharz, E.J., Lightfoot, R.W., and Goodwin, J.S.: Impaired T cell activation in patients with systemic lupus erythematosus. J. Clin. Immunol., *9*:469, 1989.
137. Sakane, T., Murakawa, Y., Suzuki, N., et al.: Familial occurrence of impaired interleukin-2 activity and increased peripheral blood B cells actively secreting immunoglobulins in systemic lupus erythematosus. Am. J. Med., *86*:385–390, 1989.
138. Escalante, A., Rivera, J., Stohl, W., and Horwitz, D.A.: Unpublished observations.
139. Huang, Y.P., Miescher, P.A., and Zubler, R.H.: The interleukin 2 secretion defect in vitro in systemic lupus erythematosus is reversible in rested cultured T cells. J. Immunol., *137*:3515, 1986.
140. Huang, Y.P., Perrin, L.H., Miescher, P.A., and Zubler, R.H.: Correlation of T and B cell activities in vitro and serum IL-2 levels in systemic lupus erythematosus. J. Immunol., *141*:827–833, 1988.
141. Wang, H., and Horwitz, D.A.: Unpublished observations.
142. Ishida, H., Kumagai, S., Umehara, H., et al.: Impaired expression of high affinity interleukin 2 receptor on activated lymphocytes from patients with systemic lupus erythematosus. J. Immunol., *139*:1070–1074, 1987.
143. Tanaka, T., Saiki, O., Negoro, S., et al.: Decreased expression of interleukin-2 binding molecules (p70/75) in T cells from patients with systemic lupus erythematosus. Arthritis Rheum., *32*:552–559, 1989.
144. Oppenheim, J.J., Ruscetti, F.W., and Faltynek, C.R.: Cytokines. *In* Basic and Clinical Immunology. Edited by D.P. Stites and A.I. Terr. Norwalk, CT, Appleton & Lange, 1991, pp. 78–100.
145. Tsokos, G.C. et al.: Deficient gamma-interferon production in

patients with systemic lupus erythematosus. Arthritis Rheum., *29*:1210, 1986.

146. Stolzenburg, T., Binz, H., Fontana, A., et al.: Impaired mitogen-induced interferon-gamma production in rheumatoid arthritis and related diseases. Scand. J. Immunol., *27*:73–81, 1988.
147. McKenna, R.M., Wilkins, J.A., and Warrington, R.J.: Lymphokine production in rheumatoid arthritis and systemic lupus erythematosus. J. Rheumatol., *15*:1639–1642, 1988.
148. Prebble, O.T. et al.: Systemic lupus erythematosus: Presence in human serum of unusual acid labile leukocyte interferon. Science, *216*:429, 1982.
149. Hirose, T. et al.: Abnormal production of and response to B cell differentiation factor in patients with systemic lupus erythematosus. Scand. J. Immunol., *21*:141, 1985.
150. Martinez-Cordero, E., Alcocer-Varela, J., and Alarcon-Segovia, D.: Stimulating and differentiation factors for human B lymphocytes in systemic lupus erythematosus. Clin. Exp. Immunol., *65*:598–604, 1986.
151. Klashman, D.J., Martin, R.A., Martinez-Maza, O., and Stevens, R.H.: In vitro regulation of B cell differentiation by interleukin-6 and soluble CD23 in systemic lupus erythematosus B cell subpopulations and antigen-induced normal B cells. Arthritis Rheum., *34*:276–286, 1991.
152. Linker-Israeli, M., Deans, R.J., Wallace, D.J., et al.: Elevated levels of endogenous IL-6 in systemic lupus erythematosus. A putative role in pathogenesis. J. Immunol., *147*:117–123, 1991.
153. Hirohata, S., and Miyamoto, T.: Elevated levels of interleukin-6 in cerebrospinal fluid from patients with systemic lupus erythematosus and central nervous system involvement. Arthritis Rheum., *33*:644–649, 1990.
154. Morimoto, C. et al.: Studies of antilymphocyte antibody of patients with active systemic lupus erythematosus. Scand. J. Immunol., *10*:213, 1979.
155. Sakane, T., Steinberg, A.D., Reeves, J.P., and Green, I.: Studies of immune functions of patients with systemic lupus erythematosus: Complement-dependent immunoglobulin-M anti-thymus derived cell antibodies to T-cell subsets. J. Clin. Invest., *64*:1260, 1979.
156. Morimoto, C. et al.: Relationship between systemic lupus erythematosus T cell subsets, anti-T cell antibodies and T cell functions. J. Clin. Invest., *73*:689, 1984.
157. Yamada, A., Shaw, M., and Winfield, J.B.: Surface antigen specificity of cold reactive IgM antilymphocyte antibodies is systemic lupus erythematosus. Arthritis Rheum., *28*:44, 1985.
158. Yamada, A., Cohen, P., and Winfield, J.B.: Subset specificity of antilymphocyte antibodies in systemic lupus erythematosus: Preferential reactivity with cells bearing the T4 and autologous erythrocyte receptor phenotypes. Arthritis Rheum., *28*: 262–270, 1985.
159. Winfield, J.B., Shaw, M., Yamada, A., and Minota, S.: Reactivity with T4$^+$ cells is associated with relative depletion of autologous T4$^+$ cells. Arthritis Rheum., *30*:162–168, 1987.
160. Winfield, J.B. et al.: Nature of cold-reactive antibodies to lymphocyte surface determinants in systemic lupus erythematosus. Arthritis Rheum., *18*:1–8, 1975.
161. Tanaka, S., Matsuyama, T., Steinberg, A.D., et al.: Antilymphocyte antibodies against CD4$^+$ 2H4$^+$ cell populations in patients with systemic lupus erythematosus. Arthritis Rheum., *32*: 398–405, 1989.
162. Mimura, T., Fernsten, P., Jarjour, W., and Winfield, J.B.: Autoantibodies specific for different isoforms of CD45 in systemic lupus erythematosus. J. Exp. Med., *172*:653–656, 1990.
163. Messner, R.P., De Horatius, R., and Ferrone, S.: Lymphocytotoxic antibodies in systemic lupus erythematosus patients and their relatives. Arthritis Rheum., *23*:265, 1980.
164. Okudaira, K., Searles, R.P., Goodwin, J.S., and Williams, R.C., Jr.: Antibodies in the sera of patients with systemic lupus erythematosus that block the binding of monoclonal anti-Ia positive targets also inhibit the autologous mixed lymphocyte response. J. Immunol., *129*:582, 1982.
165. Horwitz, D.A., and Cousar, J.B.: A relationship between cellular immunity, humoral suppression of lymphocyte function and severity of systemic lupus erythematosus. Am. J. Med., *58*:829, 1975.
166. Horwitz, D.A., Garrett, M.A., and Craig, A.H.: Serum effects on mitogenic reactivity in subjects with systemic lupus erythematosus, rheumatoid arthritis and scleroderma. Clin. Exp. Immunol., *27*:100, 1977.
167. Hahn, B.H., Pletcher, L.S., Muniain, M., and MacDermott, R.P.: Suppression of the normal autologous mixed lymphocyte reaction by sera from patients with systemic lupus erythematosus. Arthritis Rheum., *25*:381, 1982.
168. Sakane, T. et al.: A defect in the suppressor circuits among OKT4$^+$ cell population in patients with systemic lupus erythematosus occurs independently of a defect in the OKT8$^+$ suppressor T cell function. J. Immunol., *131*:753, 1983.
169. Stephens, H.A.F., Fitzharris, P., Knight, R.A., and Snaith, M.L.: Inhibition of proliferative and suppressor responses in the autologous mixed lymphocyte reaction by serum from patients with systemic lupus erythematosus. Ann. Rheum. Dis., *41*:495, 1982.
170. Suciu-Foca, N., Buda, J.A., Thiem, T., and Reemtsa, K.: Impaired responsiveness of lymphocytes in patients with systemic lupus erythematosus. Clin. Exp. Immunol., *18*:295, 1974.
171. Wernet, P., and Kunkel, H.G.: Antibodies to a specific surface antigen of T cells in human sera inhibiting mixed leukocyte culture reactions. J. Exp. Med., *138*:1021, 1973.
172. Williams, R.C., Jr., Lies, R.B., and Messner, R.P.: Inhibition of mixed leukocyte culture responses by serum and gamma globulin fractions from certain patients with connective tissue disorders. Arthritis Rheum., *16*:597, 1973.
173. Yamada, A., and Winfield, J.B.: Inhibition of soluble antigen-induced T cell proliferation by warm-reactive antibodies to activated T cells in systemic lupus erythematosus. J. Clin. Invest., *74*:1948, 1984.
174. Litvin, D.A., Cohen, P.L., and Winfield, J.B.: Characterization of warm-reactive IgG anti-lymphocyte antibodies in systemic lupus erythematosus. Relative specificity for mitogen-activated T cells and their soluble products. J. Immunol., *13*:181–186, 1983.
175. Morimoto, C. et al.: Studies of antilymphocyte antibody of patients with active systemic lupus erythematosus. Scand. J. Immunol., *10*:213, 1979.
176. Goto, M., Tanimoto, K., and Horiuchi, Y.: Natural cell mediated cytotoxicity in systemic lupus erythematosus. Suppression by antilymphocyte antibody. Arthritis Rheum., *23*:1274, 1980.
177. Rook, A.H. et al.: Cytotoxic antibodies to natural killer cells in systemic lupus erythematosus. Clin. Immunol. Immunopathol., *24*:179, 1982.
178. Scheinberg, M.A., and Cathcart, E.S.: Antibody-dependent direct cytotoxicity of human lymphocytes: I. Studies on peripheral blood lymphocytes and sera of patients with systemic lupus erythematosus. Clin. Exp. Immunol., *24*:317, 1976.
179. Schneider, J. et al.: Reduced antibody-dependent cell-mediated cytotoxicity in systemic lupus erythematosus. Clin. Exp. Immunol., *20*:187, 1975.
180. Dasgupta, M.D. et al.: Antibody-dependent cellular cytotoxicity against Raji cells ADCC (Raji): Evaluation of false positives in the detection of circulating immune complexes by Raji-cell assay. J. Clin. Immunol., *2*:197, 1982.
181. Feldmann, J.L. et al.: Antibody-dependent cell-mediated cytotoxicity in Hashimoto's thyroiditis. Clin. Exp. Immunol., *14*:153, 1973.

182. Mahowald, M.L., and Dalmasso, A.P.: Lymphocyte destruction by antibody-dependent cellular cytotoxicity mediated in vitro by antibodies in serum from patients with systemic lupus erythematosus. Ann. Rheum. Dis., *41*:593, 1982.
183. Wright, J. et al.: Serum-induced enhancement of peripheral blood mononuclear cell mediated cytotoxicity towards human targets in systemic lupus erythematosus. J. Clin. Lab. Immunol., *11*:81, 1983.
184. Kumagai, S., Steinberg, A.D., and Green, I.: Antibodies to T cells in patients with systemic lupus erythematosus can induce antibody-dependent cell-mediated cytotoxicity against human T cells. J. Clin. Invest., *67*:605, 1981.
185. Miyagi, J., Minato, N., Sumiya, M. et al.: Two types of antibodies inhibiting interleukin-2 production by normal lymphocytes in patients with systemic lupus erythematosus. Arthritis Rheum., *32*:1356–1364, 1989.
186. Yu, C.L., Chang, K.L., Chiu, C.C., et al.: Alteration of mitogenic responses of mononuclear cells by anti-ds DNA antibodies resembling immune disorders in patients with systemic lupus erythematosus. Scand. J. Immunol., *18*:265–276, 1989.
187. Steinberg, A.D. et al.: Approach to the study of the role of sex hormones in autoimmunity. Arthritis Rheum., *22*:1170–1176, 1979.
188. Steinberg, A.D. et al.: Studies of immune abnormalities in systemic lupus erythematosus. Am. J. Kidney Dis., *2*:101–110, 1982.
189. Wyle, F.A., and Kent, J.R.: Immunosuppression by sex steroid hormones. The effect upon PHA- and PPD-stimulated lymphocytes. Clin. Exp. Immunol., *27*:407–415, 1977.
190. Luster, M.I. et al.: Estrogen immunosuppression is regulated through estrogenic responses in the thymus. J. Immunol., *133*:110–116, 1984.
191. Kolland, T., Strand, O., and Forsberg, J.G.: Long-term effects of neonatal estrogen treatment on mitogen responsiveness of mouse spleen lymphocytes. J. Natl. Cancer Inst., *63*:413–421, 1979.
192. Takahashi, T., Gray, J.D., and Horwitz, D.A.: Human $CD8^+$ lymphocytes stimulated in the absence of $CD4^+$ cells enhance IgG production by antibody-secreting B cells. Clin. Immunol. Immunopathol., *58*:352–365, 1991.
193. Seaman, W.E. et al.: Beta-estradiol reduces natural killer cells in mice. J. Immunol., *121*:2193–2198, 1978.
194. Horwitz, D.A.: Selective depletion of Ig-bearing lymphocytes by cyclophosphamide in rheumatoid arthritis and systemic lupus erythematosus. Arthritis Rheum., *17*:363–374, 1974.

70

Antiphospholipid Antibody Syndrome

E. NIGEL HARRIS
MUNTHER A. KHAMASHTA
GRAHAM R. V. HUGHES

Evidence shows that some patients with antibodies to phospholipids are subject to repeated episodes of venous and arterial thrombosis, repeated fetal loss, and thrombocytopenia.[1–3] Enough patients have been identified with these features[4–16] to warrant use of the term *antiphospholipid syndrome (APS)*.[17a] The term *antiphospholipid* seems justified because its specific associated serologic feature is the production of antibodies cross-reacting with cardiolipin and a variety of other negatively charged phospholipids.[17–21] The term *syndrome* is used because of the constellation of clinical features, particularly thrombosis, fetal loss, and thrombocytopenia, that can occur in association with these antibodies, often in the absence of any other clinical manifestations.[17a] The term *primary APS* has been introduced as a means of categorizing and studying these patients who do not have any features of systemic lupus erythematosus (SLE) or any other well-defined disease.[22–26]

APS overlaps to some extent with other connective tissue disorders, in particular SLE; many APS patients have one or more of the clinical or serologic features associated with the connective tissue disorders.[17a,22–26] Because of this overlap, the true clinical and serologic boundaries of APS are vague and will probably remain so until these patients are studied over time. Some clinicians have already proposed that livedo reticularis,[27,28] migraine headaches,[27,29–33] chorea,[34,35] endocardial lesions,[36–39] and transverse myelopathy[40] might be features of APS.

Current data show that only a minority of patients with antiphospholipid antibodies are subject to thrombosis, fetal loss, or thrombocytopenia. Approximately 30% of patients with the lupus anticoagulant appear to develop thrombosis.[12,13] Because of the high sensitivity of anticardiolipin antibody tests, the actual percentage of patients who develop thrombosis may be small. The association of clinical complications with antiphospholipid antibodies appears to depend on specificity, isotype, level, and probably the time during which these antibodies are present.[41–43]

Antiphospholipid antibodies are detected by one or more of three groups of tests. The oldest tests are the standard tests for syphilis (STS), which include the Venereal Disease Research Laboratories (VDRL) (agglutination) and Wasserman (complement fixation) tests. STS levels are usually strongly positive in patients with syphilis but are either weakly positive or negative in APS patients. Patients who have a positive STS but a negative fluorescent treponema antigen-antibodies (FTA-ABS) or treponema pallidum immobilization (TPI) test are defined as having a biologic false-positive test for syphilis (BFP-STS).[44]

The more useful tests for detecting antiphospholipid antibodies in APS patients are the lupus anticoagulant and the anticardiolipin antibody tests. The lupus anticoagulant test relies on the ability of some antiphospholipid antibodies to inhibit in vitro clot formation.[3,19] These antibodies probably inhibit the assembly of clotting factors on a phospholipid surface at the prothrombin activator complex stage of the clotting cascade (Fig. 70–1).[45–48] APS patients are first identified because of a prolonged partial thromboplastin time (PTT), Russell Viper Venom Time (RVVT), or prothrombin time (PT), not corrected by the addition of normal plasma.

The most sensitive test for antiphospholipid antibodies is the anticardiolipin antibody test, introduced in 1983[49] and extensively improved since that time.[50,51] This test uses enzyme-linked immunoabsorbent assay

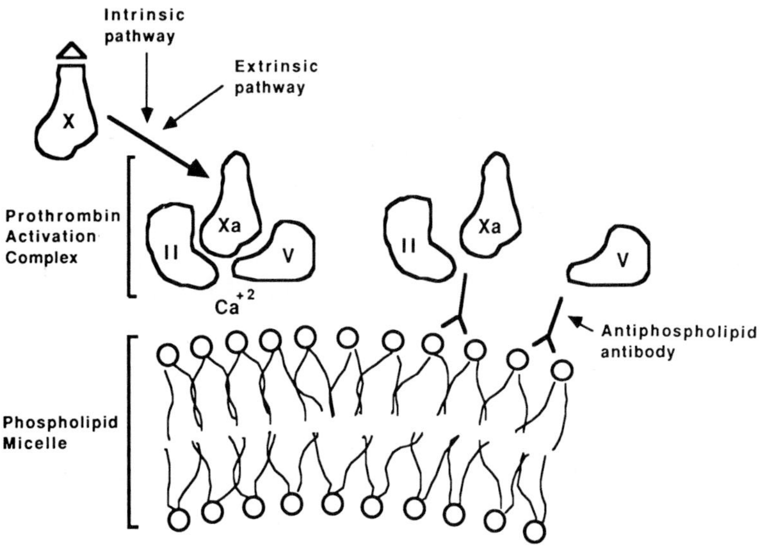

FIGURE 70–1. Diagrammatic representation of *prothrombin activation complex* and proposed mechanism by which antiphospholipid antibodies can interrupt formation of the complex. The *prothrombin activation complex* (left) is believed to be formed by factor Xa (factor X is converted to Xa either by activation of the intrinsic or extrinsic coagulation pathways), prothrombin, and factor V interacting the presence of Ca^{+2} on a phospholipid template. By binding the template, antiphospholipid antibodies may interrupt formation of the complex (right) and prolong in vitro clotting.

(ELISA)[52–57] or solid-phase radioimmunoassay techniques[17] to determine antibody binding to solid plates coated either with cardiolipin or with other negatively charged phospholipids.[21,51] It is likely that the lupus anticoagulant and anticardiolipin antibody tests detect antibodies with overlapping specificities,[2] but some investigators believe that *the results of these two tests differ frequently enough*[58–61] *to recommend that both tests be performed in patients with APS.*

OCCURRENCE

Antiphospholipid antibodies are detected in patients with a variety of autoimmune, infectious, malignant, and drug-induced disorders, as well as in some apparently healthy individuals.[2,62–64] Other than patients with APS, the single disorder in which these antibodies have been reported most frequently is SLE, in which false-positive tests for syphilis are reported in 10% of cases, lupus anticoagulant in 6 to 10% of cases, and anticardiolipin antibodies in 15 to 40% of cases.[2,65] The specificities of antiphospholipid antibodies probably differ in various disorders. An example of these differences was demonstrated in a study of antiphospholipid antibodies in patients with autoimmune disorders or with syphilis.[66] Antiphospholipid antibody specificity, isotype, and level of positivity and the period of time during which these antibodies are present may all determine clinical complications,[2] irrespective of the underlying disease in which these antibodies occur.

CLINICAL FEATURES

THROMBOSIS

Although some antiphospholipid antibodies prolong in vitro clotting tests, hemorrhage is rare in patients with these antibodies, even if the patients undergo surgery.[19,67] When hemorrhage does occur, other causes such as thrombocytopenia[68] or clotting factor resulting from the presence of other clotting factor inhibitors, should be excluded.[68] The reason antiphospholipid antibodies with lupus anticoagulant activity do not cause hemorrhage is still unknown. Although these antibodies can interrupt clotting factor interactions on phospholipid micelles in vitro, they may be unable to interrupt similar interactions on platelet surfaces in vivo.[19] Others have questioned this explanation, arguing that the in vitro lupus anticoagulant reaction is observed even in the presence of plasma with high platelet counts.[12,14]

Instead of being associated with hemorrhage, antiphospholipid antibodies are paradoxically associated with thrombosis. The occurrence of venous and arterial thrombosis in a significant minority of patients with lupus anticoagulant activity has been recognized by centers throughout the world.[4–17] Of reported patients whose plasma contained lupus anticoagulant activity, about 25 to 36% have had a history of venous or arterial thrombosis.[12,13] If patients are grouped according to anticardiolipin antibody isotype and level, the frequency of thrombosis in patients with moderate to high IgG anticardiolipin levels may exceed 50%.[41] Most figures, however, have been based on retrospective studies, and the true frequency of thrombosis in these patients must await prospective studies with properly standardized assays.[50,69,70]

Thrombosis can occur anywhere in the venous or arterial circulation and involves vessels of all sizes. In the venous circulation, thrombosis of the deep and superficial veins of the lower extremities has been reported most frequently.[4–15] Other reported venous sites of thrombosis include the axillary,[9,10,14] renal,[71–73] and hepatic veins[74,79] and the inferior vena cava. Some patients with lupus anticoagulant activity also have pulmonary hypertension,[80–82] perhaps caused by recurrent pulmonary emboli or intravascular thromboses.

In the arterial circulation, occlusion of the intracranial arteries has been reported most frequently, with the majority of patients presenting with stroke.[6,8–15,32,33,83–88] A few of our patients with high anticardiolipin antibody levels have dementia, perhaps caused by multiple small cerebral infarcts secondary to occlusion of intracranial vessels.[89] Other thromboses have involved the coronary,[90,91] retinal,[92,93] and mesenteric arteries,[94] adrenal gland,[95,96] and peripheral arteries.[94,97]

Small vessels of the placenta may be affected, causing placental infarction[98–100] and fetal loss. Thrombosis of placental vessels and fetal loss are probably part of the generalized thrombotic diathesis present in some patients with antiphospholipid antibodies. Thrombosis of the renal glomeruli has been associated with the presence of lupus anticoagulant activity in patients with SLE, but similar histologic findings were found in tissue from SLE patients who did not have lupus anticoagulant activity in their plasma.[101]

Only a few case reports have recorded thrombosed vessels in patients with antiphospholipid antibodies. Although data are limited, because thrombosis occurred without cellular infiltration of blood vessel wall, it is unlikely that thrombotic occlusion of blood vessels in patients with antiphospholipid antibodies was due to vasculitis, which may be seen in other patients with connective tissue disorders.[97–103]

The hemostatic profile of patients with lupus anticoagulant activity has been documented in only a few series.[10,14,104] In these patients, no measurable parameters are apparent suggesting ongoing thrombosis or fibrinolysis. Because many of these patients have recurrent episodes of thrombosis after cessation of anticoagulant therapy, however,[7,12–15,105] it is likely that there is an ongoing thrombotic process, features of which may be undetectable using currently available analytic methods. Because of the persistent risk of thrombosis, it would seem advisable to treat affected patients with oral anticoagulants for as long as antiphospholipid antibodies are present. Because thrombosis occurs only in a minority of patients with antiphospholipid antibodies, there is no justification for prophylactic treatment of patients with these antibodies who have no history of thrombosis. We recommend that patients with moderate to high IgG anticardiolipin antibody levels and no history of thrombosis be monitored carefully because they have the greatest risk of thrombosis.[106–109]

The role of steroids and immunosuppressive drugs in treatment of patients with antiphospholipid antibodies and thrombosis is uncertain. Such drugs have severe side effects when given for prolonged periods, and we and others[10,58] have found that antiphospholipid antibodies are not always suppressed by these agents. Such treatment is probably justified only in patients with repeated episodes of thrombosis despite adequate anticoagulant therapy.

The association of antiphospholipid antibodies with thrombosis appears strong enough to justify proposals that antiphospholipid antibodies play a direct role in causation of thrombosis. Demonstration of such a role may be difficult, but many postulates, based on fragmentary evidence, have been advanced.[3] Thrombosis involves an interplay of clotting factors and their physiologic inhibitors, fibrinolytic proteins, platelets, and endothelial cells. One or more of these systems have been reported to be abnormal in patients with these antibodies. Immunoglobulin fractions from sera of patients with lupus anticoagulant activity inhibited prostacyclin release from the endothelium of umbilical veins and from cultured endothelial cells.[110] Inhibition of prostacyclin production was found in four of seven patients with lupus anticoagulant activity, but only two of these with prostacyclin inhibitor activity had a history of thrombosis.[10] Other studies, however, have shown only a minority of antiphospholipid antibody-positive sera binds endothelial cells,[111–113] and such sera did not consistently inhibit prostacyclin production.[111–112]

An alternative explanation is based on the finding that plasminogen activator activity was reduced or absent after venous occlusion in 24 of 28 SLE patients, 12 of whom had the lupus anticoagulant.[114] Francis, McGehee, and Fenstein repeated this study in 11 patients with the lupus anticoagulant and thrombosis, failing to find any difference from healthy controls.[104] More encouraging data linking antiphospholipid antibodies to thrombosis was obtained by Cariou et al.,[115] who found that IgG fractions and Fab fragments, isolated from sera of patients with lupus anticoagulant activity, produced a decrease in the rate of activation of purified protein C by human endothelial cells in the presence of thrombomodulin. Anionic phospholipids neutralized this inhibitory effect on protein C activation.

Other proposals include inhibition of prekallikrein activity and inhibition of antithrombin III activity.[116,117] Because thrombocytopenia occurs frequently in patients with APS,[14,118,119] it has been postulated that these antibodies might bind phospholipids in platelet membranes, causing their activation, aggregation, and thrombosis.[2,118,120] Two groups of investigators, working independently, found that affinity-purified antibodies to negatively charged phospholipids do not bind to cardiolipin in ELISA plates unless there is plasma or serum in the system.[121–122] A serum cofactor was therefore sought and identified as β_2-glycoprotein I (apolipoprotein H). Interestingly, apolipoprotein H has a strong affinity for anionic phospholipids and behaves as a natural anticoagulant.[123] An antibody interfering with the interaction of apolipoprotein H with phospholipids could have thrombogenic effects. These findings are likely to open new avenues of research on the mechanisms of thrombosis associated with antibodies to phospholipids.

FETAL LOSS

Most women with antiphospholipid antibodies and/or lupus anticoagulant activity appear to have high-risk pregnancies, with fetal loss being a frequent result.[5,8–15,41,56,99,100,124–142] In 1980, reports of four women with lupus anticoagulant activity and recurrent fetal loss[124] and three women with lupus anticoagulant activity, thrombosis, and fetal loss were published.[5] Several additional series of women with lupus anticoagulant activity and fetal loss have since been reported.[8–11,56,99,100,124,132,140–141] The introduction of solid-phase assays for detection of anticardiolipin antibodies has provided a more sensitive means of identifying women with antiphospholipid antibodies who may be prone to recurrent fetal loss.[41,56,100,132] A study of 40 women with SLE and related autoimmune disorders showed that 23 had a history of fetal loss. Anticardiolipin antibodies were present in 16 of 23 women with fetal loss but in only 3 of the 17 women with normal deliveries ($p < .01$).[100] In a prospective study of 21 pregnant women with SLE, all 9 patients with midpregnancy fetal distress had elevated anticardiolipin antibody levels.[56] The anticardiolipin antibody test has a sensitive and specific indicator for fetal loss.[56] In another study of 121 patients, IgG anticardiolipin antibody level was found to be highly predictive for fetal loss.[41] An analysis of sera from women with recurrent fetal loss showed that the anticardiolipin antibody test was a more sensitive method of identifying women with antiphospholipid antibodies than were tests for the lupus anticoagulant.[132]

Although most women with plasma lupus anticoagulant activity have a poor obstetric outcome, some have normal pregnancies. In a survey of literature on women with lupus anticoagulant activity who had become pregnant, 89% of 43 women had one or more fetal losses.[128] In a series of 28 women with the lupus anticoagulant, there was a perinatal survival rate of only 14%.[128] In another series, fetal loss occurred in 73% of lupus anticoagulant-positive women.[15] In still another series, only 1 of 26 pregnancies in 7 women with the lupus anticoagulant had a successful outcome.[10] None of 36 pregnancies in 12 women with lupus anticoagulant activity had a successful outcome without prednisone and aspirin therapy in another report.[99] However, not all investigators found that lupus anticoagulant activity is uniformly associated with a poor obstetric outcome. One report showed that only 3 of 10 pregnant women with the lupus anticoagulant had between one and three spontaneous abortions[11] Our own experience and that of other clinicians[133,143–145,146] is that some patients with lupus anticoagulant activity can have uncomplicated pregnancies.

Because normal pregnancy outcome can occur in women with lupus anticoagulant activity, there appears to be no justification for prophylactic treatment with steroids during pregnancy unless the patient already has a history of fetal loss.

Fetal loss can occur at any stage of pregnancy; of 60 fetal losses in 23 women, 22 occurred in the first trimester, 31 in the second trimester, and 7 in the third trimester.[110] Of 36 episodes of fetal loss in 12 women, 24 occurred in the first trimester and 12 occurred in the second and third trimesters of pregnancy.[99] In a series of 28 women with the lupus anticoagulant, 51% of fetal losses occurred in the first trimester and 29% in the second trimester.[128] Because fetal loss can occur at any stage of pregnancy, treatment should be instituted *early* in the course of pregnancy if these women are to be treated at all.

Antiphospholipid antibodies with lupus anticoagulant activity are responsible for fetal loss, and platelets may be involved; consequently, steroids and aspirin have been used. Live births occurred in five of six women with histories of fetal loss who were treated during a subsequent pregnancy with doses of prednisone sufficient to suppress lupus anticoagulant activity (40 mg/day) and with aspirin (75 mg/day).[125] This experience has been extended to 16 treated pregnancies in 12 women, with live births in 10.[99] Subsequently, various combinations of high-dose corticosteroids and low-dose aspirin have been reported.[146] Such regimens, however, regularly produce severe cushingoid effects, hypertension, and diabetes, and their beneficial effects are questionable.[147]

Protocols using various combinations of steroids, aspirin, and subcutaneous heparin are currently being evaluated.[148] If one form of therapy fails, it may be worthwhile to try another. We have managed a patient with features of APS who had a fetal loss despite treatment with prednisone and aspirin. In a subsequent pregnancy, the use of aspirin and dipyridamole alone, as well as careful supervision, resulted in a live baby at 32 weeks' gestation. Fetal loss can and does occur in women with autoimmune disorders other than APS, especially SLE.[130,137,138,142] Consequently, obstetricians and rheumatologists should consider other causes of fetal loss in women with autoimmune disorders. These women must be monitored carefully during pregnancy, whatever their treatment. They often benefit from close observation in a hospital during the final weeks of pregnancy.[144]

Thrombosis of placental vessels resulting in placental infarction is the most popular explanation given for fetal loss in women with antiphospholipid antibodies;[8] however, thrombosis of placental vessels was not a uniform finding in one report, and placental infarction was not thought to be extensive enough to account for fetal loss.[56]

Because prostacyclin is a potent vasodilator, it is possible that if the lupus anticoagulant inhibits prostacyclin production by the endothelial cells of placental vessels, constriction of these vessels might occur, resulting in placental insufficiency and fetal growth retardation or death.[8]

THROMBOCYTOPENIA

Thrombocytopenia occurs frequently in patients with antiphospholipid antibodies.[5–14,41,118,119] First recognized as a complication in patients with lupus anticoagulant activity[5–14] it is now frequently noted in patients with high IgG anticardiolipin levels.[41] A survey of sera from patients presenting with idiopathic thrombocytopenic purpura found a small percentage with high anticardiolipin antibody levels.[119] This finding raises the possibility that patients with APS may present only with severe thrombocytopenia and will later develop fetal loss or thrombosis.[119]

When thrombocytopenia occurs in patients with APS, it is in the 50 to 150 × 10^6/L range and not severe enough to cause a hemorrhage. If a hemorrhage occurs in a patient with antiphospholipid antibodies, however, severe thrombocytopenia should be excluded as a cause of bleeding.[19]

The association of antiphospholipid antibodies with thrombocytopenia has prompted proposals that antiphospholipid antibodies might cause thrombosis by causing platelet activation and aggregation.[2] The platelet membrane is made up of phospholipids, which in some circumstances might be bound by antiphospholipid antibodies. Although an IgM monoclonal antiphospholipid antibody caused inhibition of factor Xa binding to phospholipid micelles in one study, it did not inhibit binding of factor Xa to platelet membranes,[18,19] leading to the statement that antiphospholipid antibodies could not attach to platelet membrane phospholipids because of steric hindrance. Others have found that partially disrupted platelets can bypass lupus anticoagulant activity[48,149,150] and that platelet membrane phospholipids can inhibit lupus anticoagulant activity.[150] We found that incubation of anticardiolipin-positive sera with freeze-thawed platelets inhibited binding to cardiolipin.[120] Crude phospholipid extracts of platelets also inhibited cardiolipin binding activity; such inhibition was probably due to negatively charged phospholipids in the extract.

Admittedly, none of these studies proves that antiphospholipid antibodies mediate thrombosis through platelet activation, but the demonstrated binding of antibodies to platelet membranes raises the possibility that they might mediate platelet activation and even their destruction.[118,119] Such a mechanism must include a process by which the negatively charged phospholipid, located primarily on the inner leaflet of platelet membranes, flips to the outer leaflet, becoming available to the antiphospholipid antibody. We could not show inhibition of cardiolipin binding activity by platelets unless the platelet membranes were first disrupted, perhaps exposing the inner-leaflet phospholipids.

OTHER POSSIBLE CLINICAL FEATURES OF APS

Sufficient data regarding patients have been published from diverse sources[5-16] to postulate the existence of the discrete clinical entity that we have labeled APS.[17a] Minimal criteria for this syndrome should be the presence of antiphospholipid antibodies, proven by the lupus anticoagulant test and/or by solid-phase anticardiolipin antibody test, together with one or more of the following clinical features: thrombosis, fetal loss, and thrombocytopenia (Table 70–1). Because neither of these serologic or clinical features is confined to these particular patients, there is certain to be debate as to the appropriateness of the term *antiphospholipid syndrome*, but it seems useful to designate this group of patients to promote future clinical and laboratory studies. Several patients with APS also have other autoimmune disorders, in particular SLE, but as greater numbers of these patients are becoming identified, the proportion with clinically evident SLE is decreasing.

TABLE 70–1. CLINICAL AND SEROLOGIC FEATURES OF ANTIPHOSPHOLIPID ANTIBODY SYNDROME (APS)*

CLINICAL FEATURES	SEROLOGIC FEATURES
Venous thrombosis	IgG anticardiolipin antibody (moderate/high levels)
Recurrent fetal loss	IgM anticardiolipin antibody (moderate or high levels)
Arterial thrombosis	Positive lupus anticoagulant test
Thrombocytopenia	

* Patients with APS are defined as having at least one clinical and one serologic feature at some time in their disease course. An antiphospholipid test, performed more than 8 weeks apart, should be positive on at least two occasions.

Given that antiphospholipid antibodies occur frequently, particularly when sensitive tests are used, and given the degree of overlap with other autoimmune diseases, the attribution of additional clinical or serologic features to APS must be done cautiously. Some clinicians who have examined patients with APS have suggested that transverse myelopathy,[1,40] leg ulcers,[4,40] splenomegaly,[10] migraine headaches,[27,29-33] pulmonary hypertension,[80-82] livedo reticularis,[27,28] chorea,[34,35] cardiac valvular lesions,[36-39] a Coombs' positive test,[40,41] and antimitochondrial antibodies (M5 pattern)[17,53] may all be features of this disorder. This list will undoubtedly grow. Prospective evaluation of a well-defined population of patients (Table 70–1) will enable us to determine whether these additional clinical and serologic features are truly part of the proposed syndrome.

IMMUNOLOGIC CHARACTERISTICS

LUPUS ANTICOAGULANT AND ANTICARDIOLIPIN ANTIBODIES

The possibility that lupus anticoagulant (LA) activity is attributable to antiphospholipid antibodies is based largely on deductive reasoning and was first suspected because patients with a positive LA test often had a false-positive serologic test for syphilis. Several groups have shown that phospholipids can inhibit LA activity in patient plasma,[48,151,152] and it is known that the LA test is most sensitive when phospholipid concentration and platelets (platelets presumably as a source of phospholipid) are low.[151,152] In 1980, Thiagarajan and coworkers isolated a monoclonal IgM antibody with LA activity from a patient with Waldenström's macroglobulinemia and showed that this antibody bound negatively charged phospholipids.[18] In subsequent studies, they showed that IgG fractions from several patients with LA activity cross-reacted with cardiolipin and other negatively charged phospholipids.[19,153]

The introduction of solid-phase assays to detect antiphospholipid antibodies has provided another means of examining antibodies with LA activity. Most, but not all, patients with LA activity have been found to have a positive anticardiolipin antibody test.[2] In a study of 20 LA-positive patients, a statistically significant correlation was found between the degree of prolongation of the activated partial thromboplastin time and positivity of the anticardiolipin antibody test.[154] Antiphospholipid antibodies that were purified using cardiolipin liposomes[21,155] or phosphatidylserine-diacetyl phosphate-cholesterol liposomes[19,153] were shown to have LA activity. Preincubation of anticardiolipin antibody-positive sera with negatively charged phospholipids (e.g., phosphatidylserine, phosphatidic acid, and phosphatidylinositol) inhibited cardiolipin binding activity.[20] Affinity-purified anticardiolipin antibody preparations and sera from patients with anticardiolipin antibodies bound ELISA plates coated with a variety of negatively charged phospholipids.[21]

Taken together, the data suggest that LA activity is attributable to antiphospholipid antibodies that cross-react with negatively charged phospholipids. Antiphospholipid antibodies with LA activity also have specificities in common with a subgroup of antibodies detected by the anticardiolipin antibody test[2]

Increasing numbers of reports show discordance between the LA and anticardiolipin antibody tests, however.[59–61] Derksen and colleagues reported a small series of pregnant women with a history of fetal loss in whom LA activity normalized with steroid therapy without significant decrease in anticardiolipin antibody levels.[58]

One possible explanation is that antiphospholipid antibodies responsible for a positive LA test are a subset of the antiphospholipid antibody population detected by the anticardiolipin antibody assay. In most solid-phase anticardiolipin assays, at high levels there may be a twofold to fourfold decrease in antibody levels with little measurable change in absorbance readings.[50] Therefore, significant decreases may occur in anticardiolipin antibody concentration that may escape detection in the anticardiolipin assay. Proper dilutions of high-positive sera to the sensitive range of the assay may solve this problem.[50] We recommend, however, that both tests be performed, particularly because high IgG anticardiolipin antibody levels appear to be more predictive than the LA test for thrombosis[41] and fetal loss.[41,56,132] On the other hand, the LA test may be a more sensitive indicator of response to steroid therapy.[58]

The reason some LA-positive patients show a negative anticardiolipin antibody test is more difficult to explain. More than 90% of LA-positive patients are also positive with the anticardiolipin antibody test, but there are clearly instances in which LA-positive plasma gives a negative anticardiolipin test. Because the antiphospholipid antibody response in patients with autoimmune disorders is polyclonal, it is possible that some clones of antiphospholipid antibodies are not detected in the anticardiolipin assay.[153] The LA test is nonspecific, so it is also possible that antibodies other than antiphospholipid antibodies sometimes cause prolongation of the PTT. Nearly all patients we have seen with APS have been identified by using the anticardiolipin antibody test. We believe that solid-phase assays for detection of antiphospholipid antibodies represent a more sensitive means of detecting these antibodies than does the LA test.

REAGIN

Although the antibodies produced in syphilis (reagin[2]) bind cardiolipin,[19–21,66,156,157] evidence shows that these antiphospholipid antibodies differ from those produced in patients with APS.[2] Unlike antiphospholipid antibodies in APS, reagin does not appear to cause LA activity,[158] and there is no correlation between binding to cardiolipin-coated plates and VDRL titers.[21,52,54]

Reagin is usually detected by agglutination or complement fixation tests in which the antigen (the VDRL antigen) is a mixture of cardiolipin, phosphatidylcholine (PC), and cholesterol. Although some reports suggest that reagin binds the PC portion of the VDRL antigen, evidence accumulated over 40 years suggests that reagin binds cardiolipin.

Demonstration of differences in binding properties between reagin and anticardiolipin antibodies has recently been made possible using an ELISA assay with VDRL-coated carbon particles as antigen.[66] Reagin bound both VDRL-coated and cardiolipin-coated plates, but binding to VDRL was always greater, a finding that was confirmed by inhibition studies.[66] Significantly less binding to plates coated with negatively charged phospholipids other than cardiolipin took place, however. Inhibition studies showed that negatively charged phospholipids caused less inhibition of reagin binding to VDRL than did cardiolipin. There was no significant binding of reagin to PC-coated plates and to phosphatidylethanolamine (PE)-coated plates. In contrast, APS sera did not bind VDRL-coated plates and, unlike reagin, APS sera bound plates coated with negatively charged phospholipids to the same extent as they did plates coated with cardiolipin.[21,51,66]

These experiments suggest that reagin binds cardiolipin best, particularly when cardiolipin is mixed with auxiliary lipids, but antiphospholipid antibodies in APS bind negatively charged phospholipids to an extent similar to cardiolipin. Mixing cardiolipin with auxiliary lipids probably alters its physical characteristics[157,159,160] in such a way that reagin binding is enhanced, whereas APS binding is decreased.[66]

The differences between reagin and APS antiphospholipid antibodies may have both clinical and immunologic significance. Cardiolipin is largely confined to mitochondrial membranes, but other negatively charged phospholipids are also present in cell membranes. Cross-reacting antiphospholipid antibodies from APS patients may be more likely to bind cell membranes and to affect cell function than reagin, which may explain why patients with APS develop complications such as thrombocytopenia and thrombosis while patients with syphilis are largely free from these complications. In addition, phospholipids used in the LA test probably contain negatively charged phospholipids but little or no cardiolipin, which might explain why LA activity is seen in APS but not in syphilis plasma.[158] These differences in specificities of reagin and APS antiphospholipid antibodies also suggest that the genes coding for the variable regions of these two groups of antibodies may differ, although both groups of antibodies bind cardiolipin. Support for this possibility comes from a study by Valesini and co-workers, who showed that two monoclonal anti-idiotypic antibodies to an anticardiolipin antibody preparation cross-reacted with anticardiolipin and anti-ss DNA antibodies from patients with SLE but did not bind anticardiolipin antibodies from patients with syphilis.[161]

THE PHOSPHODIESTER GROUP

Antiphospholipid antibodies bind a variety of negatively charged phospholipids that have only a phosphodiester group in common; thus, most investigators believe that the phosphodiester group is the epitope recognized by antiphospholipid antibodies.[18–21,156,157,162–165] Because phospholipids form micelles in aqueous solution with the glyceride portion of the molecule directed inward to the core of the micelle and with the phosphodiester groups directed outward, it is the phosphodiester group or substituted group (X) that is accessible to antibody binding (Fig. 70–2). If the epitope is the phosphodiester group, one must explain why antiphospholipid antibodies from APS patients do not bind phosphodiester groups of zwitterionic phospholipids and why they do not bind the phosphodiester-linked ribose backbone of DNA.[20,21,166] We propose that positively charged substituted groups (e.g., choline or ethanolamine) block antibody access to the phosphodiester group because of an electrostatic interaction between these two oppositely charged groups (Fig. 70–2). If the enzyme phospholipase D is used to remove the positively charged choline moiety from phosphatidylcholine so that the phosphatidic acid is formed, it can be demonstrated that antiphospholipid antibodies not able to bind phosphatidylcholine will bind avidly the resulting phosphatidic acid.[66] This suggests that it is the choline moiety that blocks antibody access to the phosphodiester group of phosphatidic acid.

Although repeating negatively charged phosphodiester groups are present in the backbone of DNA, polyclonal antiphospholipid antibodies from patients with APS do not seem to bind DNA,[20,21,166] and it appears that polyclonal anti-DNA antibodies from patients with SLE do not bind cardiolipin.[20,21,166,167] In contrast to these findings, some investigators have found that polyclonal antiphospholipid antibodies raised in rabbits do bind DNA,[166] and monoclonal anti-DNA antibodies raised in mouse–mouse hybridomas[162,163] and in human–human hybridomas[164] bind cardiolipin. Moreover, monoclonal anticardiolipin antibodies raised in mouse–mouse hybridomas bind DNA.[165] The apparent polyspecificity of these monoclonal autoantibodies and the relatively restricted specificities of polyclonal antibodies in humans with APS and syphilis seem to be the opposite of what might be expected.[168,169] Several

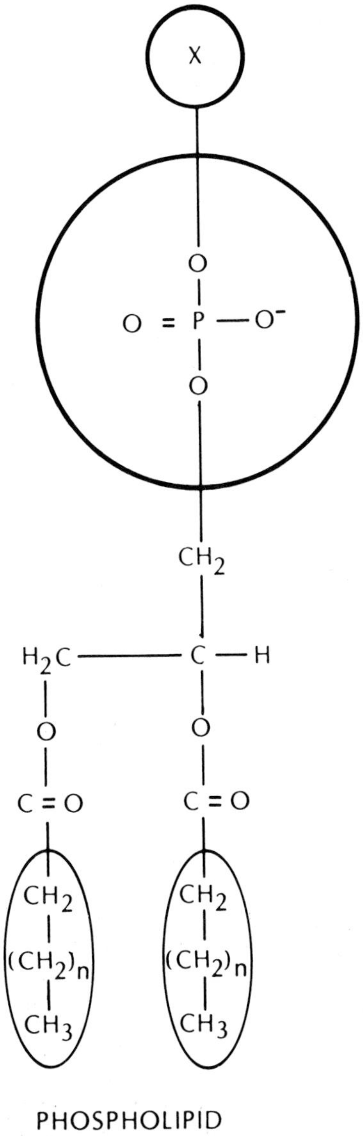

FIGURE 70–2. A phospholipid molecule as it may be oriented in aqueous solution. Phospholipid molecules align themselves so that the phosphodiester groups and substituted moiety (X) are directed toward the aqueous phase, while the glyceride portion of the molecule forms the *hydrophobic core* of the micelle or membrane.

groups of investigators are currently addressing this fascinating paradox.[169,170]

SUMMARY

Since 1980, there has been an exponential growth in publications about antiphospholipid antibodies. Although knowledge about these antibodies will increase, there will inevitably be greater confusion as claims and counter-claims are made. To minimize such confusion, we propose that patients with APS be defined as in Table 70–1. To fulfill minimal criteria for this "syndrome," patients must have both a positive antiphospholipid test and a related clinical complication. This will avoid mistreatment of patients whose sera contain antiphospholipid antibodies alone or of patients with related clinical features who may have no antiphospholipid antibodies or only slight transient increases of these antibodies, the significance of which is still uncertain. The use of one of the more recently introduced anticardiolipin antibody ELISA tests,[50,51] calibrated with standard sera,[171] may enable more specific patient identification and management.

REFERENCES

1. Hughes G.R.V.: Thrombosis, abortion, cerebral disease and the lupus anticoagulant. Br. Med. J., *287*:1088, 1983.
2. Harris, E.N., Gharavi, A.E., and Hughes, G.R.V.: Anti-phospholipid antibodies. Clin. Rheum. Dis., *11*:591, 1985.
3. Vermylen, J., Blockmans, D., Spitz, B., and Deckmyn, H.: Thrombosis and immune disorders. Clin. Haematol., *15*:393, 1986.
4. Johansson, E.A., Niemi, K.M., and Mustakallio, K.K.: A peripheral vascular syndrome overlapping with systemic lupus erythematosus. Dermatologica, *155*:257, 1977.
5. Soulier, R.P., and Boffa, M.C.: Avortements a repetition, thromboses et anticoagulant circulant antithromboplastine. Nouvelle Presse Medicale, *9*:859, 1980.
6. Mueh, J.R., Herbst, K.D., and Rapaport, S.I.: Thrombosis in patients with the lupus anticoagulant. Ann. Intern. Med., *92*:156, 1980.
7. Williams, H., Laurent, R., and Gibson, T.: The lupus coagulation inhibitor and venous thrombosis: A report of four cases. Clin. Lab. Haematol., *2*:139, 1980.
8. Carreras, L.O., and Vermylen, J.G.: "Lupus" anticoagulant and thrombosis—Possible role for inhibition of prostacyclin formation. Thromb. Haemost., *48*:28, 1982.
9. Boey, M.L., Colaco, C.B., Gharavi, A.E. et al.: Thrombosis in SLE: Striking association with the presence of circulating "Lupus anticoagulant." Br. Med. J., *287*:1021, 1983.
10. Elias, M., Eldor, A.: Thromboembolism in patients with the "lupus-like" circulating anticoagulant. Arch. Intern. Med., *144*:510, 1984.
11. Jungers, P., Liote, F., Dautzenberg, M.D. et al.: Lupus anticoagulant and thrombosis in systemic lupus erythematosus. Lancet, *1*:574, 1984.
12. Gastineau, D.A., Kazmier, F.J., Nichols, W.L., and Bowie, E.J.W.: Lupus anticoagulant: An analysis of the clinical and laboratory features of 219 cases. Am. J. Hematol., *19*:265, 1985.
13. Lechner, K., and Pabinger-Fasching, I.: Lupus anticoagulants and thrombosis. A study of 25 cases and review of the literature. Haemostasis, *15*:254, 1985.
14. Glueck, H.I., Kant, K.S., Weiss, M.A. et al.: Thrombosis in systemic lupus erythematosus: Relation to the presence of circulating anticoagulants. Arch. Intern. Med., *145*:1389, 1985.
15. Derksen, R.H., Kater, L.: Lupus anticoagulant: Revival of an old phenomenon. Clin. Exp. Rheumatol., *3*:349, 1985.
16. Gardlund, B.: The lupus inhibitor in thromboembolic diseases and intrauterine death in the absence of systemic lupus. Acta Med. Scand., *215*:293, 1984.
17. Harris, E.N.: Syndrome of the black swan. Br. J. Rheumatol., *26*:324, 1987.

17a. Tincani, A., Meroni, P.L., Brucato, A. et al.: Anti-phospholipid and anti-mitochondrial type M5 antibodies in systemic lupus erythematosus. Clin. Exp. Rheumatol., *3*:321, 1985.

18. Thiagarajan, P., Shapiro, S.S., and De Marco, L.: Monoclonal immunoglobulin M coagulation inhibitor with phospholipid specificity—Mechanism of a lupus anticoagulant. J. Clin. Invest., *66*:397, 1980.
19. Shapiro, S.S., and Thiagarajan, P.: Lupus anticoagulant. Prog. Hemost. Thromb., *6*:263, 1982.
20. Harris, E.N., Gharavi, A.E., Loizou, S. et al.: Cross-reactivity of anti-phospholipid antibodies. J. Clin. Lab. Immunol., *16*:1, 1985.
21. Harris, E.N. et al.: Affinity purified anticardiolipin and anti-DNA antibodies. J. Clin. Lab. Immunol., *17*:155, 1985.
22. Asherson, R.A: A primary antiphospholipid syndrome? J. Rheumatol., *15*:1742, 1988.
23. Mackworth-Young, C.G., Loizou, S., and Walport, M.J.: Primary antiphospholipid syndrome: Features of patients with raised anticardiolipin antibodies and no other disorder. Ann. Rheum. Dis., *48*:362, 1989.
24. Asherson, R.A., Khamashta, M.A., Ordi-Ros, J. et al.: The primary antiphospholipid syndrome: Major clinical and serological features. Medicine (Baltimore), *68*:366, 1989.
25. Alarcon-Segovia, D., and Sanchez-Guerrero, J.: Primary antiphospholipid syndrome. J Rheumatol., *16*:482, 1989.
26. Font, J., Lopez-Soto, A., Cervera, R. et al.: The primary antiphospholipid syndrome: Antiphospholipid antibody pattern and clinical features of a series of 23 patients. Autoimmunity, *9*:69, 1991.
27. Hughes, G.R.V.: The anticardiolipin syndrome. Clin. Exp. Rheumatol., *3*:285–286, 1985.
28. Asherson, R.A., Mayou, S.C., Merry, P. et al.: The spectrum of livedo reticularis and antiphospholipid antibodies. Br. J. Dermatol., *120*:215, 1989.
29. Levine, S.R., Joseph, R., D'Andrea, G., and Welch, K.M.A.: Migraine and antiphospholipid antibodies. Cephalalgia, *7*:93, 1987.
30. Hogan, M.J., Brunet, D.G., Ford, P.M., and Lillicarp, D.: Lupus anticoagulant, antiphospholipid antibodies and migraine. Can. J. Neurosci., *15*:420, 1988.
31. Shuaib, A., Barklay, L., Lee, M.A., and Suchowersky, O.: Migraine and antiphospholipid antibodies. Headache, *29*:43, 1989.
32. Briley, D.P., Coull, B.M., and Goodnight, S.H.: Neurological disease associated with antiphospholipid antibodies. Ann. Neurol., *25*:221, 1989.
33. Levine, S.R., Deegan, M.J., Futrell, N., and Welch, K.M.A.: Cerebrovascular and neurologic disease associated with antiphospholipid antibodies: 48 cases. Neurology, *40*:1181, 1990.
34. Asherson, R.A. et al.: Chorea in sytemic lupus erythematosus and "lupus-like" disease: Association with antiphospholipid antibodies. Semin. Arthritis Rheum., *16*:253, 1987.
35. Khamashta, M.A., Gil, A., Anciones, B. et al.: Chorea in sytemic lupus erythematosus: Association with antiphospholipid antibodies. Ann. Rheum. Dis., *47*:681, 1988.

36. Chartash, E.K., Lans, D.M., Paget, S.A. et al.: Aortic insufficiency and mitral regurgitation in patients with systemic lupus erythematosus and the antiphospholipid syndrome. Am. J. Med., *86*:407, 1989.
37. Khamashta, M.A., Cervera, R., Asherson, R.A. et al.: Association of antibodies against phospholipids with heart valve disease in systemic lupus erythematosus. Lancet, *335*:1541, 1990.
38. Nihoyannopoulos, P., Gomez, P.M., Joshi, J. et al.: Cardiac abnormalities in systemic lupus erythematosus. Association with raised anticardiolipin antibodies. Circulation, *82*:369, 1990.
39. Cervera, R., Khamashta, M.A., Font, J. et al.: High prevalence of significant heart valve lesions in patients with the primary antiphospholipid syndrome. Lupus, (in press), 1991.
40. Alarcon-Segovia, D., Deleze, M., Oria, C.V. et al.: Antiphospholipid antibodies and the antiphospholipid syndrome in systemic lupus erythematosus. A prospective analysis of 500 consecutive patients. Medicine (Baltimore), *68*:353, 1989.
41. Harris, E.N. et al.: Thrombosis, recurrent fetal loss, and thrombocytopenia: Predictive value of the anticardiolipin antibody test. Arch. Intern. Med., *146*:2153, 1986.
42. Alving, B.M., Barr, C.F., and Tang, D.B.: Correlation between lupus anticoagulants and anticardiolipin antibodies in patients with prolonged activated partial thromboplastin times. Am. J. Med., *88*:112, 1990.
43. Ishii, Y., Nagasawa, K., Mayumi, T., and Niho, Y.: Clinical importance of persistence of anticardiolipin antibodies in systemic lupus erythematosus. Ann. Rheum. Dis., *49*:387, 1990.
44. Moore, J.E., and Mohr, C.F.: Biologically false positive serologic tests for syphilis: Type, incidence, and cause. J. Am. Med. Assoc., *150*:467, 1952.
45. Shapiro, S.S., Thiagarajan, P., and De Marco, L.: Mechanism of action of the lupus anticoagulant. Ann. NY Acad. Sci., *370*:359, 1981.
46. Coots, M.C., Miller, M.A., and Glueck, H.I.: The lupus inhibitor: A study of its heterogeneity. Thromb. Haemost., *46*:734, 1981.
47. Exner, T.: Similar mechanism of various lupus anticoagulants. Thromb. Haemost., *53*:15, 1985.
48. Triplett, D.A., Brandt, J.T., Kaczor, D., and Shaeffer, J.: Laboratory diagnosis of lupus inhibitors: A comparison of the tissue thromboplastin inhibition procedures with a new platelet neutralization procedure. Am. J. Clin. Pathol., *79*:678, 1983.
49. Harris, E.N. et al.: Anticardiolipin antibodies: Detection by radioimmunoassay and association with thrombosis in systemic lupus erythematosus. Lancet, *2*:1211, 1983.
50. Harris, E.N., Gharavi, A.E., Patel, S.P., and Hughes, G.R.V.: Evaluation of the anti-cardiolipin antibody test: Report of an international workshop held April 4, 1986. Clin. Exp. Immunol., *68*:215, 1987.
51. Gharavi, A.E., Harris, E.N., Asherson, R.A., and Hughes, G.R.V.: Anticardiolipin antibodies: Isotype distribution and phospholipid specificity. Ann. Rheum. Dis., *46*:1, 1987.
52. Koike, T. et al.: Anti-phospholipid antibodies and biological false positive serological tests for syphilis in patients with systemic lupus erythematosus. Clin. Exp. Immunol., *56*:193, 1984.
53. Norberg, R. et al.: Further immunological studies of sera containing anti-mitochondrial antibodies, type M5. Clin. Exp. Immunol., *58*:639, 1984.
54. Colaco, C.B., and Male, D.K.: Anti-phospholipid antibodies in syphilis and a thrombotic subset of SLE: Distinct profiles of epitope specificity. Clin. Exp. Immunol., *59*:449, 1985.
55. Meyer, O., Cyra, L., Borda-Iriarte, O. et al.: Anticorps antiphospholipids, thromboses et maladie lupique: Interet du dosage des anticorps anticardiolipine per la methode ELISA. Revue du Rhumatisme, *52*:297, 1985.
56. Lockshin, M.D. et al.: Antibody to cardiolipin as a predictor of fetal distress or death in pregnant patients with systemic lupus erythematosus. N. Engl. J. Med., *313*:152, 1985.
57. Loizou, S. et al.: Measurement of anticardiolipin antibodies by an enzyma-linked immunosorbent assay (ELISA): Standardization and quantitation of results. Clin. Exp. Immunol., *62*:738, 1985.
58. Derksen, R.H.W.M. et al.: Discordant effects of prednisone on anticardiolipin antibodies and the lupus anticoagulant. Arthritis Rheum., *29*:1295, 1986.
59. Lockshin, M.D.: Anticardiolipin antibody. Arthritis Rheum., *30*:471, 1987.
60. Exner, T., Sahman, N., and Trudinger, B.: Separation of Anticardiolipin antibodies from lupus anticoagulant on a phospholipid coated polystyrene column. Biochem. Biophys. Res. Commun., *155*:1001, 1988.
61. McNeil, H.P., Chesterman, C.A., and Krilis, S.A.: Anticardiolipin antibodies and lupus anticoagulants comprise separate antibody subgroups with different phospholipid binding characteristics. Br. J. Haematol., *73*:506, 1989.
62. Harris, E.N.: Antiphospholipid antibodies. Br. J. Haematol., *74*:1, 1990.
63. Mackworth-Young, C.: Antiphospholipid antibodies: More than just a disease marker? Immunol. Today, *11*:60, 1990.
64. Sammaritano, L.R., Gharavi, A.E., and Lockshin, M.D.: Antiphospholipid antibody syndrome: Immunologic and clinical aspects. Semin. Arthritis Rheum., *20*:81, 1990.
65. Love, P.E., and Santoro, S.A.: Antiphospholipid antibodies: Anticardiolipin and the lupus anticoagulant in systemic lupus erythematosus (SLE) and in non-SLE disorders. Ann. Intern. Med., *112*:682, 1990.
66. Harris, E.N., Gharavi, A.E., Wasley, G., and Hughes, G.R.V.: Use of an enzyme-linked immunosorbent assay and of inhibition studies to distinguish between antibodies to cardiolipin from patients with syphilis or autoimmune disorders. J. Infect. Dis., *157*:23, 1988.
67. Manoharan, A., and Gottlieb, P.: Bleeding in patients with lupus anticoagulant. (Letter.) Lancet, *2*:171, 1984.
68. Triplett, D.A., and Brandt, J.: Laboratory identification of the lupus anticoagulant. Br. J. Haematol., *73*:139, 1989.
69. Exner, T., Triplett, D.A., Taberner, D.A. et al.: Comparison of test methods for the lupus anticoagulant: International survey on lupus anticoagulants-1 (ISLA-1). Thromb. Haemost., *64*:478, 1990.
70. Harris, E.N.: The Second International Anticardiolipin Standardisation Workshop/The Kingston Antiphospholipid Antibody Study (KAPS) Group. Am. J. Clin. Pathol., *94*:476, 1990.
71. Asherson, R.A. et al.: Rental vein thrombosis in SLE: Association with the lupus anticoagulant. Clin. Exp. Rheumatol., *2*:75, 1984.
72. Kleinknecht, D., Bobrie, G., Meyer, O. et al.: Recurrent thrombosis and renal vascular disease in patients with a lupus anticoagulant. Nephrol. Dial. Transplant., *4*:854, 1989.
73. Liano, F., Mampaso, F., Garcia Martin, F. et al.: Allograft membranous glomerulonephritis and renal vein thrombosis in a patient with a lupus anticoagulant factor. Nephrol. Dial. Transplant., *3*:684, 1988.
74. Pomeroy, C. et al.: Budd-Chiari syndrome in a patient with the lupus anticoagulant. Gastroenterology, *86*:158, 1984.
75. Hughes, G.R.V., Mackworth-Young, C.G., Harris, E.N., Gharavi, A.S.: Veno-occlusive disease in SLE: Possible association with anti-cardiolipin antibodies. (Letter.) Arthritis Rheum., *27*:1017, 1984.
76. Bernstein, M.L. et al.: Thrombotic and hemorrhagic complications in children with the lupus anticoagulant. Am. J. Dis. Child., *138*:1132, 1984.

77. Roudot-Thoraval, F. et al.: Budd-Chiari syndrome and the lupus anticoagulant. (Letter.) Gastroenterology, *88*:605, 1985.
78. Averbach, M., and Levo, Y.: Budd-Chiari syndrome as the major thrombotic complication of systemic lupus erythematosus with the lupus anticoagulant. Ann. Rheum. Dis., *45*:435, 1986.
79. Asherson, R.A., Khamashta, M.A., and Hughes, G.R.V.: The hepatic complications of the antiphospholipid antibodies. Clin. Exp. Rheumatol., (in press), 1991.
80. Asherson, R.A. et al.: Pulmonary hypertension in systemic lupus erythematosus. Br. Med. J., *287*:1024, 1983.
81. Anderson, N.E., and Ali, M.R.: The lupus anticoagulant, pulmonary thromboembolism, and fetal pulmonary hypertension. Ann. Rheum. Dis., *43*:760, 1984.
82. Asherson, R.A., Higenbottam, T.W., Dinh Xuan, A.T. et al.: Pulmonary hypertension in a lupus clinic: Experience with twenty-four patients. J. Rheumatol., *17*:1292, 1990.
83. Landi, G., Calloni, M.V., and Sabbadini, M.G.: Recurrent ischemic attacks in young adults with lupus anticoagulant. Stroke, *14*:377, 1983.
84. Hart, R.G., Miller, V.T., Coull, B.M., Bril, V.: Cerebral infarction associated with lupus anticoagulant—Preliminary report. Stroke, *15*:114, 1984.
85. Harris, E.N. et al.: Cerebral infarction in systemic lupus: Association with anticardiolipin antibodies. Clin. Exp. Rheumatol., *2*:47, 1984.
86. Asherson, R.A., Khamashta, M.A., Gil, A. et al.: Cerebrovascular disease and antiphospholipid antibodies in systemic lupus erythematosus, "lupus-like" disease and the primary antiphospholipid syndrome. Am. J. Med., *86*:391, 1989.
87. Brey, R.L., Hart, R.G., Sherman, D.G., and Tegeler, C.H.: Antiphospholipid antibodies and cerebral ischemia in young people. Neurology, *40*:1190, 1990.
88. Montalban, J., Codina, A., Ordi, J. et al.: Antiphospholipid antibodies in cerebral ischemia. Stroke, *22*:750, 1991.
89. Asherson, R.A., Mercy, D., Philips, G. et al.: Recurrent stroke and multi-infarct dementia in systemic lupus erythematosus associated with antiphospholipid antibodies. Ann. Rheum. Dis., *46*:605, 1987.
90. Asherson, R.A., Khamashta, M.A., Baguley, E. et al.: Myocardial infarction and antiphospholipid antibodies in SLE and other disorders. Q. J. Med., *73*:1103, 1989.
91. Hamsten, A. et al.: Antibodies to cardiolipin in young survivors of myocardial infarction: An association with recurrent cardiovascular events. Lancet, *1*:113, 1986.
92. Asherson, R.A., Merry, P., Acheson, J.F. et al.: Antiphospholipid antibodies: A risk factor for occlusive ocular vascular disease in systemic lupus erythematosus and primary antiphospholipid syndrome. Ann. Rheum. Dis., *48*:358, 1989.
93. Hall, S., Buettner, H., and Harvinder, L.S.: Occlusive retinal vascular disease in systemic lupus erythematosus. J. Rheumatol., *11*:846, 1984.
94. Asherson, R.A. et al.: Large vessel occlusion and gangrene in systemic lupus erythematosus and "lupus-like" disease: A report of 6 cases. J. Rheumatol., *13*:740, 1986.
95. Levy, E.N., Ramsey-Goldman, R., and Kahl, L.E.: Adrenal insufficiency in two women with anticardiolipin antibodies. Arthritis Rheum., *33*:1842, 1990.
96. Asherson, R.A., and Hughes, G.R.V.: Hypoadrenalism, Addison's disease and antiphospholipid antibodies. J. Rheumatol., *18*:1, 1991.
97. Jindal, B.K., Martin, M.F., and Gayner, A.: Gangrene developing after minor surgery in a patient with undiagnosed systemic lupus erythematosus and lupus anticoagulant. Ann. Rheum. Dis., *42*:347, 1983.
98. De Wolf, F. et al.: Decidual vasculopathy and extensive placental infarction in a patient with thromboembolic accidents, recurrent fetal loss and a lupus anticoagulant. Am. J. Obstet. Gynecol., *142*:829, 1982.
99. Lubbe, W.F., Butler, W.S., Palmer, S.J., and Liggins, G.C.: Lupus anticoagulant in pregnancy. Br. J. Obstet. Gynaecol., *91*:357, 1984.
100. Derue, G.J., Englert, H.J., Harris, E.N., and Hughes, G.R.V.: Fetal loss in systemic lupus: Association with anticardiolipin antibodies. J. Obstet Gynaecol., *5*:207, 1985.
101. Kant, K. et al.: Glomerular thrombosis in systemic lupus erythematosus: Prevalence and significance. Medicine, *60*:71, 1981.
102. Lie, J.T.: Vasculopathy in the antiphospholipid syndrome: Thrombosis or vasculitis, or both? J. Rheumatol., *16*:713, 1989.
103. Asherson, R.A. et al.: Multiple venous and arterial thrombosis associated with the lupus anticoagulant and antibodies to cardiolipin in the absence of SLE. Rheumatol. Int., *5*:91, 1985.
104. Francis, R.B., McGehee, W.G., and Fenstein, D.I.: Endothelial dependent fibrinolysis in subjects with the lupus anticoagulant and thrombosis. Thromb. Haemost., *59*:412, 1988.
105. Asherson, R.A. et al.: Anti-cardiolipin antibody, recurrent thrombosis, and warfarin withdrawal. Ann. Rheum. Dis., *44*:823, 1985.
106. Harris, E.N.: A reassessment of the antiphospholipid syndrome. J. Rheumatol., *17*:733, 1990.
107. Hughes, G.R.V.: The antiphospholipid antibody syndrome. Semin. Clin. Immunol., *1*:5, 1991.
108. Khamashta, M.A., and Wallington, T.: The management of the antiphospholipid syndrome. Ann. Rheum. Dis., (in press), 1991.
109. Hughes, G.R.V., and Khamashta, M.A.: Anticardiolipin antibody. A cause of a tendency to thrombosis. Br. Med. J., *299*:1414, 1989.
110. Carreras, L.O. et al.: Arterial thrombosis, intrauterine death and the lupus anticoagulant: Detection of immunoglobulin interfering with prostacyclin formation. Lancet, *1*:244, 1981.
111. Hasselaar, P., Derksen, R.H.W.M., Blokzikl, L., and DeGroot, P.G.: Thrombosis associated with antiphospholipid antibodies cannot be explained by effects on endothelial cells and platelet prostanoid synthesis. Thromb. Haemost., *59*:80, 1988.
112. Rustin, M.H.A., Bull, H.A., Machin, S.J. et al.: Effects of the lupus anticoagulant in patients with systemic lupus erythematosus on endothelial cell prostacyclin release and procoagulant activity. J. Invest. Dermatol., *90*:744, 1988.
113. Vismara, A., Meroni, P.L., Tincani, A. et al.: Relationship between anticardiolipin and antiendothelial cell antibodies in systemic lupus erythematosus. Clin. Exp. Immunol., *74*:247, 1988.
114. Angles-Cano, E., Sultan, Y., and Clauvel, J.P.: Predisposing factors to thrombosis in systemic lupus erythematosus: Possible relation to endothelial cell damage. J. Lab. Clin. Med., *94*:315, 1979.
115. Cariou, R., Tobelin, G., Bellucci, S. et al.: Effect of the lupus anticoagulant on antithrombogenic properties of endothelial cells—Inhibition of thrombomodulin dependent protein C activation. Thromb. Haemost., *60*:54, 1988.
116. Sanfelippo, M.J., and Drayna, C.J.: Prekallikrein inhibition associated with the lupus anticoagulant. Am. J. Clin. Pathol., *77*:275, 1982.
117. Cosgriff, T.M., and Martin, B.A.: Low functional and high antigenic anti-thrombin III level in a patient with the lupus anticoagulant and recurrent thrombosis. Arthritis Rheum., *24*:94, 1981.
118. Harris, E.N. et al.: Thrombocytopenia in SLE and related autoimmune disorders: Association with anticardiolipin antibodies. Br. J. Haematol., *59*:227, 1985.
119. Harris, E.N. et al.: Anticardiolipin antibodies in autoimmune thrombocytopenic purpura. Br. J. Haematol., *59*:231, 1985.
120. Khamashta, M.A., Harris, E.N., Gharavi, A.E. et al.: Immune

medicated mechanism for thrombosis: Antiphospholipid antibody binding to platelet membranes. Ann. Rheum. Dis., *47*:849, 1988.
121. Galli, M., Comfurius, P., Maasson, C. et al.: Anticardiolipin antibodies (ACA) directed not to cardiolipin but to a plasma protein cofactor. Lancet, *335*:1544, 1990.
122. McNeil, P.H., Simpson, R.J., Chesterman, C.N., and Krilis, S.A.: Antiphospholipid antibodies are directed against a complex antigen that include a lipid binding inhibitor of coagulation: beta 2 glycoprotein I (apolipoprotein H). Proc. Natl. Acad. Sci. USA, *87*:4120, 1990.
123. Schousboe, I.: Beta 2 glycoprotein I: A plasma inhibitor of the contact activation of the intrinsic blood coagulation pathway. Blood, *66*:1086, 1985.
124. Firkin, B.G., Howard, M.A., and Radford, N.: Possible relationship between lupus inhibitor and recurrent abortions in young women. Lancet, *2*:366, 1980.
125. Lubbe, W.F. et al.: Fetal survival after prednisolone suppression of maternal lupus anticoagulant. Lancet, *1*:1361, 1983.
126. Ros, J.O. et al.: Prednisone and maternal lupus anticoagulant. (Letter.) Lancet, *2*:576, 1983.
127. Prentice, R.L. et al.: Lupus anticoagulant in pregnancy. (Letter.) Lancet, *1*:464, 1984.
128. Branch, W.D. et al.: Obstetric complications associated with the lupus anticoagulant. N. Engl. J. Med., *313*:1322, 1985.
129. Farquharson, R.G., Pearson, J.F., and John, L.: Lupus anticoagulant and pregnancy management. (Letter.) Lancet, *2*:228, 1984.
130. Clauvel, J.P. et al.: Spontaneous recurrent fetal wastage and autoimmune abnormalities: A study of fourteen cases. Clin. Immunol. Immunopathol., *39*:523, 1986.
131. Cowchock, S., Smith, J.B., and Gocial, B.: Antibodies to phospholipids and nuclear antigens in patients with repeated abortions. Am. J. Obstet. Gynecol., *155*:1002, 1986.
132. Lockwood, C.J., Reece, E.A., Romero, R., and Hobbins, J.C.: Antiphospholipid antibody and pregnancy wastage. (Letter.) Lancet, *2*:742, 1986.
133. Lockshin, M.D., and Druzin, M.L.: Antiphospholipid antibodies and pregnancy. (Letter.) N. Engl. J. Med., *313*:1351, 1985.
134. Lubbe, W.F., Pattison, N., and Liggins, G.C.: Anti-phospholipid antibodies and pregnancy. N. Engl. J. Med., *313*:1350, 1986.
135. Gregorini, G., Setti, G., and Remuzzi, G.: Recurrent abortion with lupus anticoagulant and pre-eclampsia: A common final pathway for two different diseases? (Case report.) Br. J. Obstet. Gynaecol., *93*:94, 1986.
136. Chan, J.K.H., Harris, E.N., and Hughes, G.R.V.: Successful pregnancy following suppression of anticardiolipin antibody and lupus anticoagulant with azathioprine in systemic lupus erythematosus. J. Obstet. Gynaecol., *7*:16, 1986.
137. Hull, R.G., Harris, E.N., Morgan, S.H., and Hughes, G.R.V.: Anti-Ro antibodies and abortions in women with SLE. (Letter.) Lancet, *2*:1138, 1983.
138. Cowchock, S., De Horatius, R.D., Wapner, R.J., and Jackson, L.G.: Subclinical autoimmune disease and unexplained abortion. Am. J. Obstet. Gynecol., *150*:367, 1985.
139. Lockshin, MD., Qamar, T., Druzin, M.L., and Goei, S.: Antibody to cardiolipin lupus anticoagulant and fetal death. J. Rheumatol., *14*:259, 1987.
140. Howard, M.A., Firkin, B.G., Healy, D.L., and Choong, S.S.C.: Lupus anticoagulant in women with multiple spontaneous miscarriage. Am. J. Hematol., *26*:175, 1987.
141. Lubbe, W.F., and Liggins, G.C.: Role of lupus anticoagulant and autoimmunity in recurrent pregnancy loss. Semin. Reprod. Endocrinol., *6*:181, 1988.
142. Cowchock, S., Smith, J.B., and Gocial, B.: Antibodies to phospholipids and nuclear antigens in patients with repeated abortions. Am. J. Obstet. Gynecol., *155*:1002, 1986.
143. Stafford-Brady, F.J., Gladman, D.D., and Urowitz, M.B.: Successful pregnancy in systemic lupus erythematosus with an untreated lupus anticoagulant. Arch. Intern. Med., *148*:1647, 1988.
144. Trudinger, B.J., Stewart, G.J., Cook, C.M. et al.: Monitoring lupus anticoagulant positive pregnancies with umbilical artery flow velocity waveforms. Obstet. Gynecol., *72*:215, 1988.
145. Triplett, D.A., and Harris, E.N.: Antiphospholipid antibodies and reproduction. Am. J. Reprod. Immunol., *21*:123, 1989.
146. Walport, M.J.: Pregnancy and antibodies to phospholipids. Ann. Rheum. Dis., *48*:795, 1989.
147. Lockshin, M.D., Druzin, M.C., and Qamar, T.: Predisone does not prevent recurrent fetal death in women with antiphospholipid antibody. Am. J. Obstet. Gynecol., *160*:439, 1989.
148. Harris, E.N.: Need for a prospective treatment trial. Am. J. Obstet. Gynecol., *162*:1121, 1990.
149. Firkin, B.G., Booth, P., Hendrix, L., and Howard, M.A.: Demonstration of a platelet by-pass mechanism in the clotting system using an acquired anticoagulant. Am. J. Hematol., *5*:81, 1978.
150. Howard, M.A., and Firkin, B.G.: Investigations of the lupus-like inhibitor by-passing activity of platelets. Thromb. Haemost., *50*:775, 1983.
151. Exner, T., Rickard, K.A., and Kronenberg, H.: Studies on phospholipids in the action of a lupus coagulation inhibitor. Pathology, 7:319, 1975.
152. Exner, T., Rickard, K.A., and Kronenberg, H.: A sensitive test demonstrating lupus anticoagulant and its behavioural patterns. Br. J. Haematol., *40*:143, 1978.
153. Shapiro, S., Thiagarajan, P., and McCord, S.: Immunological specificity and mechanism of action of IgG lupus anticoagulants. Blood, *70*:69, 1987.
154. Harris, E.N. et al.: Anticardiolipin antibodies and the lupus anticoagulant. Lancet, *2*:1099, 1984.
155. Violi, F. et al.: Anticoagulant activity of anticardiolipin antibodies. Thromb. Res., *44*:543–547, 1986.
156. Costello, P.B., and Green, F.A.: Reactivity patterns of human anticardiolipin and other antiphospholipid antibodies in syphilitic sera. Infect. Immun., *51*:771, 1986.
157. Alving, C.R.: Antibodies to liposomes, phospholipids and phosphate esters. Chem. Phys. Lipids., *40*:303, 1986.
158. Shoenfeld, Y. et al.: Circulating anticoagulant and serological tests for syphilis. Acta Derm. Venereol. (Stockh.), *60*:365, 1980.
159. Takashi, T., Inoue, K., and Nojima, S.: Immune reactions of liposomes containing cardiolipin and their relation to membrane fluidity. J. Biochem., *87*:679, 1980.
160. Rauch, J. et al.: Human hybridoma lupus anticoagulants distinguish between lamellar and hexagonal phase lipid systems. J. Biol. Chem., *261*:9672, 1986.
161. Valesini, G. et al.: Use of monoclonal antibodies to identify shared idiotypes on anticardiolipin and anti-DNA antibodies in human sera. Clin. Exp. Immunol., *70*:18, 1987.
162. Lafer, E.M. et al.: Polyspecific monoclonal lupus autoantibodies reactive with both polynucleotides and phospholipids. J. Exp. Med., *153*:897, 1981.
163. Koike, T. et al.: Specificity of mouse hybridoma antibodies to DNA II. Phospholipid reactivity and biological false positive serological test for syphilis. Clin. Exp. Immunol., *57*:345, 1984.
164. Shoenfeld, Y. et al.: Polyspecificity of monoclonal lupus autoantibodies produced by human-human hybridomas. N. Engl. J. Med., *308*:414, 1983.
165. Rauch, J., Tannenbaum, H., Stoller, B.D., and Schwarz, R.S.: Monoclonal anticardiolipin antibodies bind DNA. Eur. J. Immunol., *14*:529, 1984.
166. Eilat, D., Zlotnick, A.Y., and Fischell, R.: Evaluation of the cross-

reaction between anti-DNA and anti-cardiolipin antibodies in SLE and experimental animals. Clin. Exp. Immunol., *65*:269, 1986.
167. Edberg, J.C., and Taylor, R.P.: Quantitative aspects of lupus anti-DNA autoantibody specificity. J. Immunol., *136*:4581, 1986.
168. Eilat, D.: Anti-DNA antibodies: Problems in their study and interpretation. Clin. Exp. Immunol., *65*:215, 1986.
169. Emlen, W., Pisetsky, D.S., and Taylor, R.P.: Antibodies to DNA: A perspective. Arthritis Rheum., *29*:1417, 1986.
170. Smeenk, R.J.T., Lucassen, W.A.M., and Swaak, T.J.G.: Is anti-cardiolipin activity a cross-reaction of anti-DNA or a separate entity? Arthritis Rheum., *30*:607, 1987.
171. Harris, E.N., Gharavi, A.E., and Hughes, G.R.V.: Anticardiolipin antibody testing: the need for standardization. Arthritis Rheum., *30*:835, 1987.

71

Mixed Connective Tissue Disease

GORDON C. SHARP
BERNHARD H. SINGSEN

Some patients have features of more than one rheumatic disease and thus do not fit into traditional classifications. Patients with a combination of clinical findings similar to those of systemic lupus erythematosus (SLE), progressive systemic sclerosis (PSS), polymyositis, and rheumatoid arthritis (RA), and with unusually high titers of a circulating antinuclear antibody with specificity for a nuclear ribonucleoprotein antigen, are considered to have *mixed connective tissue disease* (MCTD).[1]

Initial observations of MCTD suggested infrequent renal disease, a good response to corticosteroids, and a favorable prognosis.[1,2] Further study has shown, however, that renal disease occurs in 10 to 20% of patients, that some patients may require aggressive or prolonged pharmacologic intervention, and that pulmonary involvement is common. Pulmonary hypertension, associated with proliferative vascular lesions, may be a serious complication. The prognosis, therefore, is not always favorable.[3–7]

SEROLOGIC ALTERATIONS

All patients in the original study of MCTD had high hemagglutination titers of antibody to a nuclear antigen extractable in isotonic buffers (ENA).[1,8] Antibodies to ENA were also detected in about half of a series of patients with SLE, although usually at reduced titers, and the reported incidence of ENA antibodies was very low in other rheumatic disorders.[1,8] Treatment of ENA-coated red blood cells with ribonuclease (RNase) reduced or eliminated the agglutination reaction in serum from patients with MCTD but had little or no effect on serum from patients with SLE.[1]

Immunodiffusion studies subsequently revealed that ENA consisted of at least two distinct antigens, one sensitive to RNase and trypsin, which appeared to be a nuclear ribonucleoprotein (nRNP), and the previously described Sm antigen,[2,9,10] which is resistant to RNase and trypsin. Sera that reacted with either the nRNP antigen or the Sm antigen produced a speckled, fluorescent antinuclear antibody pattern.[1,9,11] Treatment of the tissue substrate with RNase eliminated the antinuclear antibody reaction due to anti-nRNP, however.[1,9,11]

Sera containing nRNP antibodies in high titer and no Sm antibodies are usually found in patients with MCTD, are uncommon in patients with SLE or PSS, and are rare in patients with polymyositis, RA, or other rheumatic diseases.[1,2,11–14] That some patients with high nRNP antibody titers initially appear to have another rheumatic disorder and then in several years develop additional clinical features typical of MCTD suggests a predictive value of this serologic pattern for evolving MCTD.[1,6,11,13]

The typical serologic pattern in MCTD includes high titers of speckled antinuclear antibodies, usually greater than 1 : 1000, high levels of antibody to RNase-sensitive ENA by hemagglutination, frequently greater than 1,000,000, and nRNP antibody by immunodiffusion. Sm antibodies and high antinative DNA titers are infrequent in MCTD, and their appearance usually correlates with a severe flare of SLE-like features.[3,6,15] Rheumatoid agglutinins occur in over half the patients with MCTD, and titers are often high.[11] Diffuse hyper-γ-globulinemia, ranging from 2 to greater than 5 g/dL, may be present.[1,11,16] Serum complement levels are usually normal or only modestly reduced.[1,11,17]

Rarely, patients with clinical features of MCTD have no nRNP antibody initially.[1,3,11,18] This test may subsequently become positive, sometimes after corticosteroid therapy.[1,11,18] Once present, high titers of circulating anti-nRNP usually persist during periods of active and inactive disease, but antibody levels may fall or become undetectable in 5 to 11 years in association with remission.[6]

Several laboratories have further elucidated the nature of the nRNP and Sm antigens. Antibodies to nRNP immunoprecipitate U1 snRNA-protein complexes, whereas anti-Sm antibodies immunoprecipitate snRNA-protein complexes containing U1, U2, U4, U5, and U6 snRNAs.[19] Immunoblotting studies have shown that anti-U1 RNP antibodies react with RNP antibodies react with polypeptides designated 70K (previously referred to as 68K), A, and C, whereas anti-Sm antibodies react with the B/B′ and D polypeptides. Several reports indicate that anti-70K antibodies are associated with anti-U1 RNP antibodies in MCTD but rarely occur in SLE.[20–24] A longitudinal study demonstrated the serologic persistence of U1 snRNP polypeptide autoantibody patterns over many years and their subsequent disappearance in patients who were in prolonged remission.[20]

TABLE 71–1. CHARACTERISTICS OF 34 PATIENTS WITH MIXED CONNECTIVE TISSUE DISEASE

CHARACTERISTIC	NUMBER	PERCENTAGE
Raynaud's phenomenon	31	91
Polyarthritis	29	85
Swollen hands or sclerodactyly	29	85
Pulmonary disease	29	85
Inflammatory myositis	27	79
Esophageal hypomotility	25	74
Lymphadenopathy	17	50
Alopecia	13	41
Pleuritis	12	35
Malar rash	10	29
Renal disease	9	26
Cardiac disease	9	26
Anemia	8	24
Leukopenia	7	21
Diffuse scleroderma	7	21
Sjögren's syndrome	4	12
Trigeminal neuropathy	2	6
Positive antinuclear antibody	34	100
Positive ribonucleoprotein antibody	34	100
Positive rheumatoid agglutinins	20	59
Hypergammaglobulinemia	18	53
Hypocomplementemia	11	32

(From Sullivan, W.D., et al.[6])

CLINICAL FEATURES

These features include prevalence, course, and specific clinical manifestations.

PREVALENCE AND CLINICAL COURSE

MCTD occurs in patients ranging from 4 to 80 years, with a mean of 37 years; approximately 80% of patients are female.[11,13] MCTD may occur as frequently as scleroderma, more commonly than polymyositis, and less frequently than SLE. Typical clinical features of MCTD (Table 71–1) include polyarthritis, Raynaud's phenomenon, swollen hands or sclerodactyly, pulmonary disease, muscle disease, and esophageal hypomotility.[6] Lymphadenopathy, alopecia, malar rash, serositis, and cardiac and renal disease are less frequent findings. No particular racial or ethnic distribution has been noted.

In some patients, the typical overlapping pattern is fully expressed when they are first evaluated. As physicians appreciate more fully the association of anti-U1 RNP antibody with MCTD, however, larger numbers of cases are identified at an early phase of disease. Initially, minimal symptoms such as Raynaud's phenomenon, arthralgias, myalgias, and swollen hands may be insufficient to make a definitive diagnosis. This constellation of clinical findings has been referred to as *undifferentiated connective tissue disease*.[6,25] Long-term followup study reveals that this pattern may persist for years in some patients; in others it may progress to PSS, whereas yet other patients develop additional manifestations resulting in MCTD.[3,6,13,17] In one prospective study, 60% of patients were initially thought to have RA, PSS, SLE, polymyositis, or undifferentiated connective tissue disease[6] (Table 71–2). At their most recent evaluation, 91% demonstrated typical overlapping features of MCTD, while 9% maintained their undifferentiated status. Thus, MCTD is an evolving disease in which the overlapping features typically occur sequentially.

DIAGNOSTIC CRITERIA AND CLASSIFICATION

The 1986 International Symposium on MCTD and Antinuclear Antibodies introduced three sets of diagnostic criteria.[26–28] Major criteria included myositis, pulmonary involvement, Raynaud's phenomenon, swollen hands or sclerodactyly, and high titer anti-U1 RNP antibody. Preliminary evaluation of these criteria showed a very high sensitivity and specificity.[29,30] However, more detailed testing is needed.

SPECIFIC MANIFESTATIONS

Skin

Swelling of the hands and fingers occurs in over two thirds of patients with MCTD, resulting in a "sausage" appearance[1,2,11,13,17] (Fig. 71–1). The skin may be taut and thick, with histologic changes of marked edema and increased dermal collagen content.[1] Scleroderma-like changes are occasionally extensive, but diffusely involved or tightly bound skin with contractures is rare.[1,11] In 40% of patients, lupus-like rashes occur, including malar eruptions; diffuse, nonscarring erythematous lesions; and chronic, scarring discoid lesions.[1,11,13,17] (Fig. 71–2). Other findings include alopecia, areas of hyper and hypopigmentation, periungual telangiectasia, "squared" telangiectasia over the hands and face, violaceous discoloration of the eyelids, and

TABLE 71–2. TRANSITIONS IN MIXED CONNECTIVE TISSUE DISEASE IN LONGITUDINAL STUDY

DISEASE CLASSIFICATION	NO. CLASSIFIED AT INITIAL MEDICAL EVALUATION	NO. CLASSIFIED AT LATEST MEDICAL EVALUATION
Polymyositis	1	0
Progressive systemic sclerosis	2	0
Adult or juvenile rheumatoid arthritis	4	0
Systemic lupus erythematosus	6	0
Undifferentiated connective tissue disease	7	3
Mixed connective tissue disease	14	31

(From Sullivan, W.D., et al.[6])

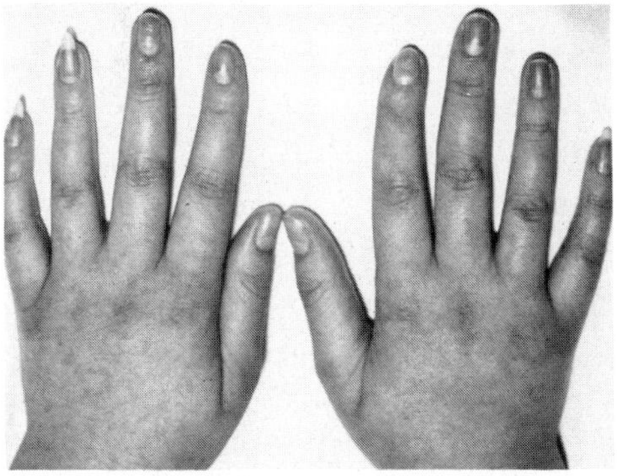

FIGURE 71–1. Hands of a patient with mixed connective tissue disease demonstrating the sausage appearance of fingers and erythematous discoloration over the metacarpophalangeal, proximal interphalangeal, and distal interphalangeal joints.

erythema over the knuckles, elbows, or knees.[1,11,13,17] Severe necrotic and ulcerative skin changes are seen only rarely.[1,11] Immunoglobulin deposits at the dermal-epidermal junction have been noted in some patients.[1,17]

Raynaud's Phenomenon

Paroxysmal vasospasm of the fingers and, less often, the toes occurs in approximately 85% of patients with MCTD and may precede other manifestations of the disease by months to years.[1,2,11,13,17] Severe vasospasm and ischemic necrosis or ulceration of the fingertips, common in PSS, are rare in MCTD.[1,17,31] However, two reports showed dilated capillary changes, with avascular areas, in 50 to 90% of MCTD patients,[31,32] and a study using hand angiography revealed organic obstruction in 60% of ulnar arteries, 87% of superficial arches, and 65% of digital arteries.[31] These findings provide further evidence for vasculopathy in some patients with MCTD.

Joints

Polyarthralgias occur in most patients, and frank arthritis is seen in about three quarters of those affected.[1,11,13,33,34] Although the arthritis is often non-deforming, its features may be similar to those of RA with flexion contractures, ulnar deviation, and swan-neck deformities.[1,33–35] The metacarpophalangeal, proximal interphalangeal, and carpal joints are frequently affected. Subcutaneous nodules and roentgenographic evidence of erosive changes are sometimes observed.[1,35] Tightness of the extrinsic flexors of the hands related to volar tenosynovitis may be particularly prominent in MCTD.[36]

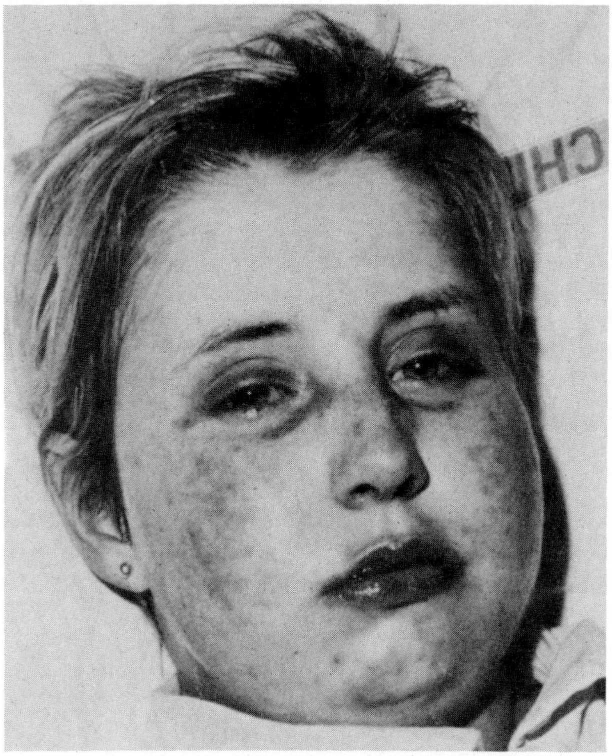

FIGURE 71–2. Facial rash of MCTD; the violaceous periorbital rash is suggestive of dermatomyositis; the malar rash is more commonly seen in systemic lupus erythematosus.

Muscles

Proximal muscles are commonly tender and weak, and serum levels of creatine kinase and aldolase may be elevated at some point in the course of MCTD.[1,2,11,37]

Electromyographic findings are typical of inflammatory myositis, and biopsies reveal muscle fiber degeneration and perivascular and interstitial infiltration of plasma cells and lymphocytes.[1,5,11,13,37] Even in patients with only mild muscular weakness, histochemical and immunofluorescent analyses reveal perifascicular atrophy, type I fiber predominance, and immunoglobulin deposition within normal-appearing vessels, within normal fibers, around or on the sacroplasmic membrane, or within the perimysial connective tissues.[37]

Esophagus

Esophageal abnormalities are frequent in MCTD.[1,11,38,39] Systematic studies of 35 patients by cine-esophagram or manometry revealed dysfunction in 80%, but 70% of these patients had no history of esophageal problems.[38] Heartburn and dysphagia are the most common symptoms.[39] Decreased peristaltic amplitude in the distal two thirds of the esophagus and reduced upper and lower esophageal sphincter pressures are characteristic changes.[39] Abnormal function of the upper sphincter may occur less frequently in PSS[40–42] and may represent a distinguishing feature of MCTD. The severity of measured esophageal dysfunction appears to correlate with the duration of the disease but not necessarily with the expression of symptoms.[13,38,39] Reflux esophagitis, sometimes leading to ulceration and stricture, may occur.

Lungs

Pulmonary dysfunction is usually clinically silent in the early phases of MCTD and may go undetected unless detailed evaluations are performed. One prospective study showed that 80% of patients with MCTD had pulmonary disease, but 69% were asymptomatic.[43] Serial followup of those treated with corticosteroids revealed clinical and physiologic improvement in 12 of 14. It has become apparent that pulmonary involvement in MCTD may lead to serious exertional dyspnea or to pulmonary hypertension, particularly in the later stages of the disease.[6] Hemoptysis and dysfunction of the diaphragm have also been reported.[44,45]

Pulmonary hypertension associated with proliferative pulmonary vascular lesions was frequent and serious in a longitudinal evaluation of 34 individuals with MCTD.[6] The most common clinical finding was dyspnea, followed by pleuritic pain and bibasilar rales. Of 11 asymptomatic patients, 8 (73%) had abnormal pulmonary function tests or chest roentgenograms. Single-breath diffusing capacity (DLCO) was abnormal in 73%, and the vital capacity was reduced in 33%. These findings have been confirmed.[46] Total lung capacity was low in 41%, and forced expiratory volume in 1 second (FEV_1) was abnormal in 17%; resting hypoxemia was present in 21% of patients. *Radiographic abnormalities* consisting of small, irregular opacities predominantly in the bases and middle regions occurred in 30%.[6] These findings underscore the fact that pulmonary involvement in MCTD is common and may be clinically inapparent until far advanced.

Right-heart catheterization was performed on 15 of the 34 patients in our longitudinal study.[6] Ten had elevated pulmonary vascular resistance, and 10 had increased pulmonary artery pressure; wedge pressure was only abnormal in one patient. This study suggested that MCTD patients with features similar to those of PSS are more likely to develop pulmonary hypertension. Additionally, nailfold capillaroscopy in three of these patients showed severe capillary loop changes before pulmonary symptoms were present. All three patients subsequently developed pulmonary vascular disease. Thus, *nailfold changes may predict pulmonary hypertension in MCTD.*

Heart

Cardiac involvement is less common than pulmonary disease in adult MCTD, but it may be frequent in children.[1,11,13] Pericarditis is the most common cardiac abnormality reported.[13,47,48] In a prospective study of 37 adults with MCTD, pericarditis or pericardial effusion occurred in 10 patients, pulmonary hypertension was present in 10 of 15, and mitral valve prolapse occurred in 9 patients. Electrocardiographic abnormalities include arrhythmias, chamber enlargement, and conduction defects.[47] A subsequent study comparing MCTD with a control group confirmed that mitral valve prolapse occurs with unusually high frequency in MCTD.[49] The prognostic significance of these cardiac findings is unclear.

Kidneys

Longer followup suggests that renal disease is more frequent in MCTD than initially thought. When isolated case reports are excluded, published studies give a combined incidence of renal involvement of 28%, including children.[13,50–52] Glomerular deposition of immune complexes may be observed, although the patterns differ from those of SLE.[53,54] Patients with MCTD occasionally die of progressive renal failure.[50]

In a longitudinal study of MCTD, six patients had evidence of renal disease manifested by proteinuria or hematuria: one developed the nephrotic syndrome.[6] Two renal biopsies showed focal glomerulonephritis. The kidney disease responded well to corticosteroid therapy, and renal failure did not occur. At autopsy, three patients without clinical evidence of renal disease had proliferative vascular lesions similar to those noted in other organs; the glomeruli were normal in two of these patients, and mesangial thickening and hypercellularity were noted in the third. In a report of children with MCTD,[5] 7 of 15 had clinical or histologic evidence of renal disease, and a patient in another study had died of "scleroderma kidney."[3] Comparable levels of circulating immune complexes in MCTD and SLE are observed,[15,55] but the clinical and histologic findings suggest that vascular lesions may represent a more serious problem than immune complex nephritis in MCTD.

Nervous System

Neurologic abnormalities, noted in only 10% of patients with MCTD, are not usually major management problems.[11,13,35,56] Trigeminal neuropathy is the most frequent finding.[11] Other observed problems include organic mental syndromes, "vascular" headaches, aseptic meningitis, seizures, encephalopathy, multiple peripheral neuropathies, and cerebral infarction or hemorrhage, probably related to hypertension and atherosclerosis.[11,13,56–58]

Blood

Anemia and leukopenia are found in a third of patients with MCTD.[1,11] Coombs-positive hemolytic anemia and significant thrombocytopenia are rare;[1,11,59] however, in a report of 14 children with MCTD, 6 had severe thrombocytopenia.[13] Two of these required splenectomy because persistent, severe thrombocytopenia, which had previously responded to corticosteroids, could only be controlled by 2 mg/kg/day prednisone. One child with thrombocytopenia died of an intracranial hemorrhage. Diminished granulocyte chemotaxis also occurs in children and adults with MCTD and may be associated with the sudden onset of unexpectedly severe infections, often with encapsulated organisms such as pneumococcus or meningococcus.[60]

Other Findings

Sjögren's syndrome occurs frequently in MCTD.[61] Hashimoto's thyroiditis and persistent hoarseness are observed occasionally in both children and adults.[5] Fever and lymphadenopathy occur in about one third of patients.[1,11,17] Lymph nodes may be massively enlarged and may suggest a lymphoma, but biopsy reveals only lymphoid hyperplasia. In addition to the esophageal abnormalities previously described gastrointestinal manifestations may include hypomotility, pseudosacculation, dilatation, malabsorption, secretory diarrhea, sclerosis, perforation of the intestinal tract,[13,39,62–66] acute pancreatitis and pancreatic pseudocyst,[39] and chronic active hepatitis.[39]

CHILDHOOD DISEASE

Since 1973, 15 reports of pediatric MCTD have been published.[13,67–69] These studies encompass 59 children, with an additional 20 patients, <16 years of age, briefly mentioned in other reports but whose clinical features and treatment responses could not be isolated from the larger groups of adults. In a large pediatric rheumatic disease service, MCTD was 10% as frequent as SLE and occurred once for every 100 children with juvenile RA (JRA). The median age of onset of MCTD in children is 10.8 years (range: 4 to 16 years); 45 girls and 14 boys have been reported.[35,69–72]

MCTD in children has several distinguishing features: (1) dermatomyositis and SLE-like rashes more common than in adults[13,53] (Fig. 71–2); (2) thrombocytopenia in about 20%; (3) a higher frequency of cardiac disease, especially pericarditis (41%), than in adults;[13,73,74] and (4) clinical and histologic evidence of renal disease, more frequent in pediatric MCTD.[13,73,75] In our experience, 6 of 19 children developed significant renal disease, including 2 who eventually required long-term hemodialysis. In all childhood cases, 18 of 42 (43%) eventually developed clinically evident renal involvement.

Deforming, painless arthritis and the presence of rheumatoid factor are common in childhood MCTD.[13,53,75] Synovitis is moderate, but complaints of discomfort are usually not marked in children; thus, responses to treatment may appear better than they actually are. Erosive disease is uncommon in children, but flexion contractures and deformity may occur.

Because Sjögren's syndrome is rare in children with rheumatic diseases, it is infrequently or incompletely sought in pediatric MCTD. At least half of carefully assessed children with MCTD have xerostomia, parotid gland enlargement, or keratoconjunctivitis sicca.[5,61] These findings suggest that salivary gland evaluation, Schirmer's test, and lip biopsy should be considered in all children with possible MCTD.

MCTD in children is frequently a sequential disease. The majority initially manifest Raynaud's phenomenon (85%) and polyarthritis (95%). They then develop other features of MCTD, progressively but not in any particular order. Serologic findings may also change over time, commensurate with the clinical situation. Thus, the absence of antinuclear antibodies and the presence of rheumatoid factor may be associated with early polyarthropathy, whereas anti-Sm antibodies may appear along with renal disease, hypocomplementemia, and other features of SLE.[5]

Many of the features of MCTD in children are initially silent and may remain undetected unless carefully sought. The limited verbal skills, memory, and experiential understanding of children may magnify this observation. These asymptomatic features include the following: (1) minimal muscle disease with mild atrophy, moderate serum muscle enzyme elevations, and perhaps electromyographic changes, but with no significant proximal weakness; (2) esophageal dysfunction; (3) minimal alterations in bowel habits, related to early gastrointestinal tract involvement; and (4) pulmonary function test abnormalities found before complaints or roentgenographic changes. Children do not usually complain of dyspnea or shortness of breath. Thus, *pulmonary function testing should be part of the routine evaluation of any child in whom a diagnosis of MCTD is considered.* Overall, 28 of 43 children (65%) with MCTD have showed radiographic and pulmonary function abnormalities; 30% developed pulmonary hypertension. Pulmonary hypertension and idiopathic fibrosis must be recognized as potentially life-threatening.[13,73,76]

HISTOLOGIC AND IMMUNOPATHOLOGIC FEATURES

HISTOLOGIC MANIFESTATIONS

The first comprehensive histologic investigation of MCTD reviewed material from three autopsies and from five additional renal biopsies.[5] The study group included 15 children with MCTD with a median age of disease onset of 10.7 years; the three who died had had the disease for 5.4 years before histologic evaluation. The age of these patients, the short duration of their disease, the absence of systemic or pulmonary hypertension, and the lack of corticosteroid treatment are relevant because, in adult patients, all would be variables that could cause, or reduce, the observed vasculopathy.

Widespread proliferative vascular lesions were the most prominent histopathologic features in the patients studied. All three children had diffuse vasculopathy; in combination, 9 organs (16%) revealed medial vessel wall thickening, and 31 of 58 organs (53%) had intimal proliferation (Fig. 71–3). These abnormalities occurred in large vessels such as the renal artery and aorta and within small arterioles. This vasculopathy has been shown angiographically in digital, radial, and ulnar arteries as well.[31]

The frequency and severity of vascular compromise in organs without overt evidence of clinical involvement was striking and included coronary vessels, myocardium, aorta, lungs, intestinal tract, and kidney (Fig. 71–4). Inflammatory infiltration of vessels was not a prominent feature.[5] Similar obstructive vascular lesions, particularly in the lungs, have now been described in MCTD in adults.[6,7,77] Thus, the presence of pulmonary hypertension in MCTD appears to be related to marked luminal vessel narrowing, rather than to interstitial fibrosis.[6,77]

Other pathologic alterations in MCTD include prominent lymphocytic and plasmacytic infiltration of salivary glands, liver, and gastrointestinal tract, and a widespread inflammatory myopathy. Cardiac myopathy has been found in a few patients with MCTD,[5,47,78] but its prevalence is not yet known.

Our histopathologic understanding of MCTD is developing slowly. The absence of fibrinoid change, a predilection for large-vessel involvement, and minimal fibrosis all suggest fundamental differences from scleroderma. Evidence suggests a widespread but largely silent vasculopathy, cardiac and skeletal myopathy, membranoproliferative nephropathy, and pulmonary and gastrointestinal involvement in MCTD. Prospective histopathologic studies with serial treatment observations are necessary to determine whether current expectations of MCTD morbidity and mortality are overly optimistic.

IMMUNOPATHOLOGIC FINDINGS

The immunologic aberrations identified in MCTD suggest that immune injury mechanisms are involved in the pathogenesis of the disease. The persistence of high

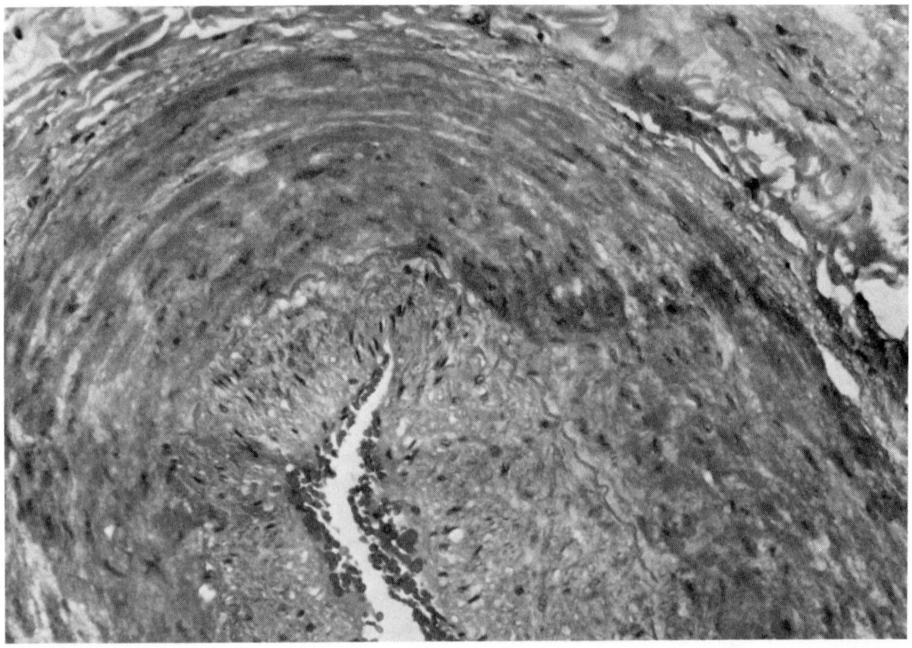

FIGURE 71–3. Photomicrograph of a section of coronary artery from a 14-year-old boy with mixed connective tissue disease, showing intimal thickening, medial proliferation, and luminal narrowing (hematoxylin-eosin stain ×566).

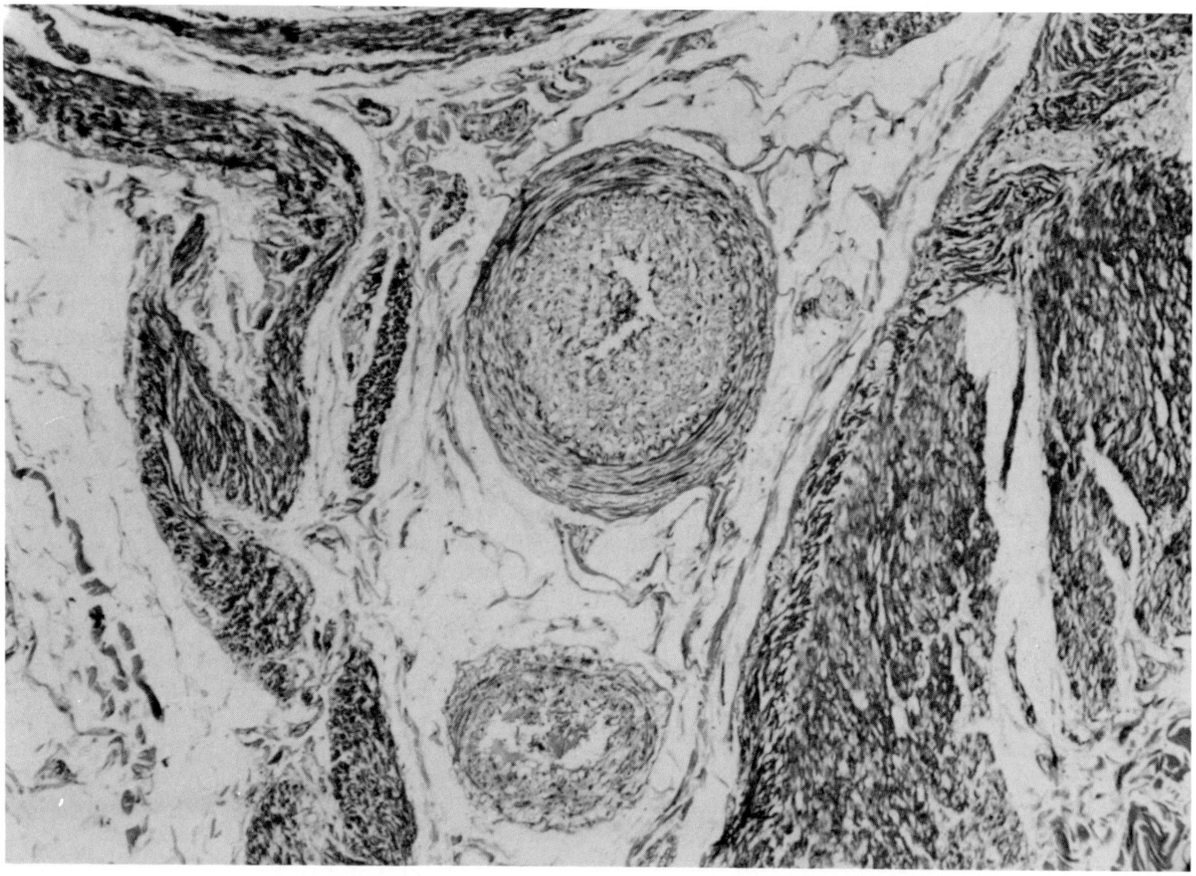

FIGURE 71–4. Small serosal artery from the ileocecal region; this child with mixed connective tissue disease had no signs or symptoms of gastrointestinal disturbance. There is striking intimal proliferation and luminal occlusion, but no inflammatory infiltrate (hematoxylin and eosin stain ×466).

titers of ribonucleoprotein antibody for many years and a marked polyclonal hyper-γ-globulinemia indicate B-cell hyperactivity. Epitope mapping studies have shown that most MCTD sera containing antibodies to the U1 snRNP-associated 70K polypeptide react with a region of the polypeptide (amino acid-residues 94-194) that specifically binds to U1 snRNA.[79–82] Interestingly, MRL/Mp mice also develop circulating autoantibodies to U1 RNP and Sm antigens, and their anti-70K reactivity is with this same RNA binding epitope region.[79] Pulmonary vascular lesions previously reported in the MRL mice[83] were particularly severe in mice demonstrating very high autoimmune responses to the 70K antigen (unpublished data, Sharp, G.C. et al., 1991), raising the possibility of analogies to patients with MCTD. Human[84] and murine[85] monoclonal antibodies that have been produced to the 70K antigen react with a different epitope region of the polypeptide.[79]

Alarcon-Segovia has compared the immunoregulatory characteristics of MCTD and other connective tissue diseases.[86] MCTD patients frequently had lymphopenia and diminished total T-lymphocytes. Subpopulations of T-lymphocytes that may be diminished include T4 (helper-inducer), T8 (cytotoxic-suppressor), or both, and Tγ cells. Despite increased numbers of post-thymic precursor cells (which suggests normal serum thymic factor), concanavalin-A-induced suppression and spontaneously expanded suppression functions were both diminished. Natural killer cell function may be normal (although less responsive to interleukin-2 [IL-2] induction), and production of IL-1, IL-2, B cell growth factor (BCGF), and B cell differentiation factor (BCDF) was either normal or increased in MCTD. Stimulation of T-cell circuits toward increased help could result in B-cell stimulation and anti-U1 RNP antibody production. Differences in these immunoregulatory functions among MCTD and SLE, Sjögren's syndrome, PSS, and RA support the concept of MCTD as a distinct entity.[16,86]

Other observations in MCTD include reduced serum complement levels in about 25% of patients,[1,11,17] circulating immune complexes during active disease,[15,55,87] and deposition of IgG, IgM, and complement within muscle fibers, in the sarcolemmal-basement membrane region, in vascular walls, and along the glomerular basement membrane.[37,54]

Frank et al. studied 18 patients with MCTD. Most had active disease; only 4 had defective reticuloendothelial system Fc-specific immune clearance, although 17 had circulating immune complexes detected by Raji cell and C1q binding assay.[15] The 4 patients with defective clearance had an illness that, at that time, more closely resembled typical SLE, with antibodies to Sm or DNA, higher levels of immune complexes, glomerulonephritis, and severe skin lesions. Renal disease was absent in the 14 patients with normal clearance of the reticuloendothelial system. The maintenance of normal reticuloendothelial function in classic MCTD may enable these patients to clear immune complexes and thus to avoid serious renal damage.

A solid-phase radioimmunoassay for the detection of U1 RNP immune complexes[88] showed many U1 RNP immune complexes in the pericardial fluid, but not in the serum, of an MCTD patient with acute hemorrhagic pericarditis.[89] These data suggest that locally formed U1 RNP immune complexes may have played an important role in the development of pericarditis.

Immunogenetic studies of MCTD patients showed associations between disease susceptibility and both specific HLA and immunoglobulin genes.[24,90,91] In serologic studies of human leukocyte antigen (HLA), association was found between the presence of anti-70Kautoantibody-positive MCTD and the presenceof HLA-DR4/DRw53 or HLA-DR2.[24,92] MCTD patients typically possessed the HLA-DR4/Dw4 (DRB1*0401)/DQw3 (DQB1*0301, *0302 or *0303); DR4/Dw14 (DRB1*0407); or DR2/Dw2 (DRB1*1510) /DQw1 (DQB1*0602) genotypes. Specific human T-cell clones can be generated in vitro for individual 70K snRNP polypeptides that are restricted in their recognition of the 70K antigen by HLA-DR on antigen presenting cells,[93] further evidence for a direct role of HLA-DR contribution to disease susceptibility (also Hsu, K.-C. et al., unpublished data). Studies of immunoglobulin allotypes among MCTD patients found an association with the Gm (1,2;5, 21) allotype.[90,91,94] Disease susceptibility appears to be independently affected by both HLA and immunoglobulin genes (Hoffman, R.W., and Pandey, J.P., 1991, unpublished data).

TREATMENT AND PROGNOSIS

Treatment recommendations have been based largely on anecdotal information because no controlled, long-term evaluations exist. Because MCTD is a progressive disease, different therapies may be appropriate for the same patient over a period of several years. For example, some children and adults initially respond to intramuscular gold or methotrexate for RA-like or JRA-like features, then improve with corticosteroids when proximal muscle weakness develops, and finally require cytotoxic agents for renal disease.[13]

Originally, MCTD was described as responsive to corticosteroids, although a few patients who did not respond to high doses of corticosteroids improved after the addition of cyclophosphamide. Further observations do not support a uniformly optimistic outlook, however. In extended investigations, almost two thirds of patients have responded favorably to treatment.[6] Patients with scleroderma-like features are the least likely to improve. A potentially good long-term prognosis for MCTD is demonstrated by the 13 of 34 (38%) patients studied who have inactive disease, including 10 who have not required therapy for 1 to 8 years (mean 5 years). Inflammatory changes are likely to respond to corticosteroids, whereas pulmonary and sclerodermatous lesions are less likely to respond.

Of our patients, 36% have had less corticosteroid-responsive and more severe illness; 4 patients died. Pulmonary hypertension and widespread proliferative vasculopathy are major complications of MCTD that have emerged from several investigations. The pulmonary hypertension may or may not respond to corticosteroids or immunosuppressive agents, but without controlled studies, the most appropriate therapies remain uncertain.

Patterns of organ system involvement may be a useful guide to therapy. Arthritis may occur well before other overlapping manifestations suggest MCTD.[34] As the erosive and deforming potential of MCTD has been better recognized, so has the value of the early use of agents such as gold and penicillamine. The arthritis has responded to nonsteroidal anti-inflammatory drugs in some centers,[33] but others have not had similar success.[95] Rash, serositis, anemia, leukopenia, fever, and lymphadenopathy commonly improve within days to weeks of adding low-to-moderate doses of corticosteroids.[1] An inflammatory myopathy may require 1 to 2 mg/kg of prednisone or the addition of methotrexate.

The therapeutic response of other organ systems is more difficult to characterize. Pericarditis and pleuritis in MCTD apparently respond well to corticosteroids.[63] Pulmonary disease in general may improve with corticosteroids;[6,43] interstitial and restrictive lung disease may improve,[70] or it may not.[58] In addition, pulmonary hypertension does not uniformly respond to combinations of corticosteroids and cytotoxic agents.[6,7,73,76] Renal involvement that is due to MCTD may lead to the use of high doses of corticosteroids, possibly in association with cytotoxic agents. Most patients show at least some response to corticosteroids, but the outcome is not uniformly predictable among the few patients treated with cytotoxic agents.

Studies of 10 patients before and after treatment for other manifestations of the disease suggested that esophageal function in MCTD may be responsive to corticosteroids.[39] One patient had marked upper esophageal sphincter hypotension and recurrent aspiration, which resolved with corticosteroid therapy.[39] Histopathologic studies in MCTD and PSS suggest differences in pathophysiology between these diseases that make the former disorder more likely to respond to corticosteroid therapy.[5] Several descriptions of the intestinal manifestations of MCTD exist, but indications of treatment response are lacking.[62,64,66]

Initial estimations of the prognosis of MCTD suggested a mild disease.[1] A more severe prognosis was first mentioned in the pediatric literature,[5,13] of particular concern were cardiac disease, life-threatening thrombocytopenia, and renal involvement. The proximate causes of death were infection in three, and cerebral hemorrhage in one patient. The infections, caused by encapsulated organisms (pneumococcal in two patients and meningococcal in one), were rapidly fatal, may have been associated with chemotactic abnormalities and were not related to significant corticosteroid doses.[60]

The current prognosis for MCTD can be projected from the data in five studies with long-term, sequential assessment.[3–6,11] Nimelstein et al. observed that six of eight deaths were not directly related to a rheumatic disorder.[4] Pulmonary hypertension, other lung disease, and heart failure were major factors in another four reported deaths;[3] a fifth death was due to squamous cell carcinoma of the lung. In another investigation, four deaths were related to MCTD; contributing factors included pulmonary hypertension and cor pulmonale in three patients, pericardial tamponade in one, perforated bowel in two, and sepsis in three. The combined mortality rate from these five reports (194 patients) was 13%, with the mean disease duration varying from 6 to 12 years.

These observations of MCTD morbidity and mortality suggest that our early predictions must be modified. In both adults and children, the prognosis of MCTD is generally similar to that of SLE but better than that of scleroderma. Our understanding of ideal therapy for MCTD, morbidity, and outcome all remain uncertain. Treatment protocols and longitudinal prospective assessments of this illness should all improve the care of patients with MCTD.

CONCLUSION

The International Symposium on Mixed Connective Tissue Disease and Antinuclear Antibodies determined that "on the basis of clinical, serologic, and immunologic data, mixed connective tissue disease seems to be a distinct entity."[96] Recent investigations tend to support the unique nature of this disease. Features that appear to distinguish MCTD include (1) immunoregulatory abnormalities in MCTD that differ from those found in other rheumatic diseases; (2) high titers of nuclear ribonucleoprotein antibody, usually in the absence of significant titers of other antibodies; (3) strong reactivity of nuclear ribonucleoprotein antibodies with the U1 RNP 70K polypeptide in MCTD, in contrast to infrequent U1 RNP 70K reactivity in SLE; (4) normal clearance by the reticuloendothelial system of immune complexes in most patients with MCTD, in contrast to SLE; (5) immunogenetic association of MCTD with HLA-DR4 and DR2, in contrast to SLE and PSS; (6) frequent pulmonary hypertension and a unique proliferative vasculopathy; and (7) other pathologic changes that may be restricted to MCTD, such as widespread plasmacytic and lymphocytic infiltration of tissues, an absence of fibrosis, and a distinctive hyalinization of the esophagus.

From our perspective, the status of MCTD as a distinct entity is not the most critical issue. As clinical, serologic, and pathologic characteristics of these patients have become known, and as reports of prognosis have begun to appear, certain repetitive patterns have emerged. First, the initially limited, undifferentiated connective tissue disease frequently becomes more widespread and typical of MCTD, and clinical and serologic transitions are observed during longitudinal study. Second, MCTD usually evolves gradually and, during the early phases, biopsies of tissues and functional tests often reveal abnormalities before the advent of clinical symptoms. Third, certain organs and tissues, such as the lung, the esophagus, and muscle, are at higher risk for pathologic involvement. Fourth, many manifestations of this disease initially respond to corticosteroids, but the scleroderma-like findings, which are the most resistant to treatment, may become the dominant clinical features later in the course of MCTD. Finally, although the prognosis remains favorable, a significant percentage of MCTD patients develop serious and sometimes fatal complications of pulmonary hypertension, proliferative vascular lesions, or overwhelming infections.

The most significant outcome of the continuing controversy surrounding MCTD is the stimulus to further investigation. The numerous immunopathologic abnormalities of MCTD indicate that immune-injury mechanisms may play an important role. Environmental, genetic, hormonal, and immunologic factors probably determine whether patients will continue to have a prolonged, benign undifferentiated rheumatic disorder or will develop major organ-system involvement typical of MCTD, or whether the disease will become more typical of SLE or PSS. The MRL mouse model, which has some features in common with MCTD, may permit incisive investigation of some of these factors.

Finally, an unexpected but remarkable consequence of the investigations stimulated by MCTD has been the demonstration that Sm, U1 RNP, and other nonhistone nuclear antigens may have central roles in cell biology, such as in the processing of messenger RNA.[97,98] Thus, just as the monoclonal proteins of multiple myeloma stimulated an elucidation of immunoglobulin structure and function, recognition of unique autoantibodies to antigens occurring in MCTD and other rheumatic diseases has facilitated their purification, biochemical characterization, and study of their biologic roles.

REFERENCES

1. Sharp, G.C. et al.: Mixed connective tissue disease. An apparently distinct rheumatic disease syndrome associated with a specific antibody to an extractable nuclear antigen (ENA). Am. J. Med., *52*:148–159, 1972.
2. Parker, M.D.: Ribonucleoprotein antibodies: frequencies and clinical significance in systemic lupus erythematosus, scleroderma and mixed connective tissue disease. J. Lab. Clin. Med., *82*:769–775, 1973.

3. Grant, K.D., Adams, L.E., and Hess, E.V.: Mixed connective tissue disease—A subset with sequential clinical and laboratory features. J. Rheumatol., *8*:587–598, 1981.
4. Nimelstein, S.H. et al.: Mixed connective tissue disease: A subsequent evaluation of the original 25 patients. Medicine, *59*:239–248, 1980.
5. Singsen, B.H. et al.: A histologic evaluation of mixed connective tissue disease in childhood. Am. J. Med., *68*:710–717, 1980.
6. Sullivan, W.D. et al.: A prospective evaluation emphasizing pulmonary involvement in patients with mixed connective tissue disease. Medicine, *63*:92–107, 1984.
7. Wiener-Kronish, J.P. et al.: Severe pulmonary involvement in mixed connective tissue disease. Am. Rev. Respir. Dis., *124*:499–503, 1981.
8. Sharp, G.C. et al.: Association of autoantibodies to different nuclear antigens with clinical patterns of rheumatic disease and responsiveness to therapy. J. Clin. Invest., *50*:350–359, 1971.
9. Northway, J.S., and Tan, E.M.: Differentiations of antinuclear antibodies giving speckled staining patterns in immunofluorescence. Clin. Immunol. Immunopathol., *1*:140–154, 1972.
10. Reichlin, M., and Mattioli, M.: Correlation of a precipitin reaction to an RNA protein antigen and low prevalence of nephritis in patients with systemic lupus erythematosus. N. Engl. J. Med., *286*:908–911, 1972.
11. Sharp, G.C. et al.: Association of antibodies to ribonucleoprotein and Sm antigens with mixed connective tissue disease, systemic lupus erythematosus and other rheumatic diseases. N. Engl. J. Med., *295*:1149–1154, 1976.
12. Notman, D.D., Kurata, N., and Tan, E.M.: Profiles of antinuclear antibodies in systemic rheumatic diseases. Ann. Intern. Med., *83*:464–469, 1975.
13. Singsen, B.H. et al.: Mixed connective tissue disease in childhood. A clinical and serologic survey. J. Pediatr., *90*:893–900, 1977.
14. Tan, E.M. et al.: Diversity of antinuclear antibodies in progressive systemic sclerosis. Arthritis Rheum., *23*:617–625, 1980.
15. Frank, M.M. et al.: Immunoglobulin G Fc receptor-mediated clearance in autoimmune disease. Ann. Intern. Med., *98*:206–218, 1983.
16. Alarcon-Segovia, D.: Mixed connective tissue disease—a decade of growing pains. (Editorial). J. Rheumatol., *8*:535–540, 1981.
17. Gilliam, J.N., and Prystowsky, S.D.: Mixed connective tissue disease syndrome: The cutaneous manifestations of patients with epidermal nuclear staining and high titer antibody to RNase sensitive extractable nuclear antigen (ENA). Arch. Dermatol., *113*:583–587, 1977.
18. Alarcon-Segovia, D.: Mixed connective tissue disease: Appearance of antibodies to ribonucleoprotein following corticosteroid treatment. J. Rheumatol., *6*:694–699, 1979.
19. Pettersson, I. et al.: The structure of mammalian small nuclear ribonucleoproteins: identification of multiple protein components reactive with anti-(U1) ribonucleoprotein and anti-Sm autoantibodies. J. Biol. Chem., *259*:5907–5914, 1984.
20. Pettersson, I. et al.: The use of immunoblotting and immunoprecipitation of (U) small nuclear ribonucleoproteins in the analysis of sera of patients with mixed connective tissue disease and systemic lupus erythematosus. A cross-sectional, longitudinal study. Arthritis Rheum., *29*:986–996, 1986.
21. Habets, W.J. et al.: Antibodies against distinct nuclear matrix proteins are characteristic for mixed connective tissue disease. Clin. Exp. Immunol., *54*:265–276, 1983.
22. Habets, W.J. et al.: Quantitation of anti-RNP and anti-Sm antibodies in MCTD and SLE patients by immunoblotting. Clin. Exp. Immunol., *59*:457–466, 1985.
23. Takeda, Y. et al.: Enzyme-linked immunosorbent assay using isolated (U) small nuclear ribonucleoprotein polypeptides as antigens to investigate the clinical significance of autoantibodies to these polypeptides. Clin. Immunol. Immunopathol., *50*:213–230, 1989.
24. Hoffman, R.W. et al.: Human autoantibodies against the 70-kd polypeptide of U1 small nuclear RNP are associated with HLA-DR4 among connective tissue disease patients. Arthritis Rheum., *33*:666–673, 1990.
25. LeRoy, E.C., Maricq, H.R., and Kahaleh, M.B.: Undifferentiated connective tissue syndromes. Arthritis Rheum., *23*:341–343, 1980.
26. Sharp, G.C.: Diagnostic criteria for classification of MCTD. *In* Mixed Connective Tissue Disease and Anti-nuclear antibodies. Edited by R. Kasukawa and G.C. Sharp. Amsterdam, Elsevier Science Publishers B.V., 1987.
27. Alarcon-Segovia, D.A., and Villarreal, M.: Classification and diagnostic criteria for mixed connective tissue disease. *In* Mixed Connective Tissue Disease Disease and Anti-nuclear Antibodies. Edited by R. Kasukawa and G.C. Sharp. Amsterdam, Elsevier Science Publishers B.V., 1987.
28. Kasukawa, R. et al.: Preliminary diagnostic criteria for classification of mixed connective tissue disease. *In* Mixed Connective Tissue Disease and Anti-nuclear Antibodies. Edited by R. Kasukawa and G.C. Sharp. Amsterdam, Elsevier Science Publishers B.V., 1987.
29. Porter, J.F. et al.: The AI/RHEUM knowledge-based computer consultant system in rheumatology: Performance in the diagnosis of 59 connective tissue disease patients from Japan. Arthritis Rheum., *31*:219–226, 1988.
30. Alarcón-Segovia, D., and Cardiel, M.H.: Comparison between 3 diagnostic criteria for mixed connective tissue disease. Study of 593 patients. J. Rheumatol., *16*:328–334, 1989.
31. Peller, J.S., Garbor, G.T., Porter, J.M., and Bennett, R.M.: Angiographic findings in mixed connective tissue disease. Arthritis Rheum., *23*:768–774, 1985.
32. Maricq, H.R. et al.: Diagnostic potential of in vivo capillary microscopy in scleroderma and related disorders. Arthritis Rheum., *23*:183–189, 1980.
33. Bennett, R.M., and O'Connell, D.J.: The arthritis of mixed connective tissue disease. Ann. Rheum. Dis., *37*:397–403, 1978.
34. Halla, J.T., and Hardin, J.G.: Clinical features of the arthritis of mixed connective tissue disease. Arthritis Rheum., *21*:497–503, 1978.
35. Bennett, R.M., and O'Connell, D.J.: Mixed connective tissue disease: a clinicopathologic study of 20 cases. Semin. Arthritis Rheum., *10*:25–51, 1980.
36. Lewis, R.A. et al.: The hand in mixed connective tissue disease. J. Hand Surg., *3*:217–222, 1978.
37. Oxenhandler, R. et al.: Pathology of skeletal muscle in mixed connective tissue disease. Arthritis Rheum., *20*:985–988, 1977.
38. Winn, D. et al.: Esophageal function in steroid treated patients with mixed connective tissue disease (MCTD). Clin. Res., *24*:545A, 1976.
39. Marshall, J.B. et al.: Gastrointestinal manifestations of mixed connective tissue disease. Gastroenterology, *98*:1232–1238, 1990.
40. Stentoft, P., Hendel, L., and Aggestrup, S.: Esophageal manometry and pH-probe monitoring in the evaluation of gastroesophageal reflux in patients with progressive systemic sclerosis. Scand. J. Gastroenterol., *22*:499–504, 1987.
41. Weihrauch, T.R., and Korting, G.W.: Manometric assessment of oesophageal involvement in progressive systemic sclerosis, morphoea and Raynaud's disease. Br. J. Dermatol., *170*:325–332, 1982.
42. Hamel-Roy, J. et al.: Comparative esophageal and anorectal motility in scleroderma. Gastroenterology, *88*:1–7, 1985.

43. Harmon, C. et al.: Pulmonary involvement in mixed connective tissue disease (MCTD). Arthritis Rheum., *19*:801, 1976.
44. Germain, M.J., and Davidman, M.: Pulmonary hemorrhage and acute renal failure in a patient with mixed connective tissue disease. Am. J. Kidney Dis., *3*:420–424, 1984.
45. Martens, J., and Demedts, M.: Diaphragm dysfunction in mixed connective tissue disease. Scand. J. Rheumatol., *11*:165–167, 1982.
46. Derderian, S.S. et al.: Pulmonary involvement in mixed connective tissue disease. Chest, *88*:45–48, 1985.
47. Alpert, M.A. et al.: Cardiovascular manifestations of mixed connective tissue disease in adults. Circulation, *68*:1182–1193, 1983.
48. Oetgen, W.J. et al.: Cardiac abnormalities in mixed connective tissue disease. Chest, *2*:185–188, 1983.
49. Comens, S.M. et al.: Frequency of mitral valve prolapse in systemic lupus erythematosus, progressive systemic sclerosis and mixed connective tissue disease. Am. J. Cardiol., *63*:369–370, 1989.
50. Bennett, R.M., and Spargo, B.H.: Immune complex nephropathy in mixed connective tissue disease. Am. J. Med., *63*:534–541, 1977.
51. Bresnihan, B. et al.: Antiribonucleoprotein antibodies in connective tissue diseases: Estimation by counter-immunoelectrophoresis. Br. Med. J., *1*:610–611, 1977.
52. Rao, K.V. et al.: Immune complex nephritis in mixed connective tissue disease. Ann. Intern. Med., *84*:174–176, 1976.
53. Baldassare, A. et al.: Mixed connective tissue disease (MCTD) in children. Arthritis Rheum., *19*:788, 1976.
54. Fuller, T.J. et al.: Immune-complex glomerulonephritis in a patient with mixed connective tissue disease. Am. J. Med., *62*:761–764, 1977.
55. Halla, J.T. et al.: Circulating immune complexes in mixed connective tissue disease (MCTD). Arthritis Rheum., *21*:562–563, 1978.
56. Bennett, R.M., Bong, D.M., and Spargo, B.H.: Neuropsychiatric problems in mixed connective tissue disease. Am. J. Med., *65*:955–962, 1978.
57. Bernstein, R.F.: Ibuprofen-related meningitis in mixed connective tissue disease. Ann. Intern. Med., *92*:206–207, 1980.
58. Cryer, P.F., and Kissane, J.M. (Eds.): Clinicopathologic Conference. Mixed connective tissue disease. Am. J. Med., *65*:833–842, 1978.
59. de Rooij, D.J.R.A.M., van de Putte, L.B.A., and van Beusekom, H.J.: Severe thrombocytopenia in mixed connective tissue disease. Scand. J. Rheumatol., *11*:184–186, 1982.
60. Hyslop, D.L., Singsen, B.H., and Sharp, G.C.: Leukocyte function, infection, and mortality in mixed connective tissue disease (MCTD). Arthritis Rheum., *29*:S64, 1986.
61. Fraga, A. et al.: Mixed connective tissue disease in childhood. Relationship with Sjögren's syndrome. Am. J. Dis. Child., *132*:263–265, 1978.
62. Cooke, C.L., and Lurie, H.I.: Case report: Fatal gastrointestinal hemorrhage in mixed connective tissue disease. Arthritis Rheum., *20*:1421–1427, 1977.
63. Davis, J.D., Parker, M.D., and Turner, R.A.: Exacerbation of mixed connective tissue disease during salmonella gastroenteritis—Serial immunological findings. J. Rheumatol., *5*:96–98, 1978.
64. Samach, M., Brandt, L.J., and Bernstein, L.H.: Spontaneous pneumoperitoneum with pneumatosis cystoides intestinalis in a patient with mixed connective tissue disease. Am. J. Gastroenterol., *69*:494–500, 1978.
65. Thiele, D.L., and Krejs, G.J.: Secretory diarrhea in mixed connective tissue disease. Am. J. Gastroenterol., *80*:107–110, 1985.
66. Norman, D.A., and Fleischmann, R.M.: Gastrointestinal systemic sclerosis in serologic mixed connective tissue disease. Arthritis Rheum., *21*:811–819, 1978.
67. Eberhardt, K., Svantesson, H., and Svensson, B.: Follow-up study of 6 children presenting with a MCTD-like syndrome. Scand. J. Rheumatol., *10*:62–64, 1981.
68. Sanders, D.Y., Huntley, C.C., and Sharp, G.C.: Mixed connective tissue disease. J. Pediatr., *83*:642–645, 1973.
69. deRooij, D.J. et al.: Juvenile-onset mixed connective tissue disease: Clinical, serological and follow-up data. Scand. J. Rheumatol., *18*:157–160, 1989.
70. Hepburn, B.: Multiple antinuclear antibodies in mixed connective tissue disease: report of a patient with an unusual antibody profile. J. Rheumatol., *8*:635–638, 1981.
71. Peskett, S.A. et al.: Mixed connective tissue disease in children. Rheumatol. Rehabil., *17*:245–248, 1978.
72. Singsen, B.H.: Mixed connective tissue disease, scleroderma and morphea in childhood. *In* Brenneman's Textbook of Pediatrics. Edited by R. Wedgwood. New York, Harper & Row Publishers, 1981.
73. Jones, M.B. et al.: Fatal pulmonary hypertension and resolving immune-complex glomerulonephritis in mixed connective tissue disease. A case report and review of the literature. Am. J. Med. *65*:855–863, 1978.
74. Silver, T.M. et al.: Radiological features of mixed connective tissue disease and scleroderma-systemic lupus erythematosus overlap. Radiology, *120*:269–275, 1976.
75. Oetgen, W.J., Boice, J.A., and Lawless, O.J.: Mixed connective tissue disease in children and adolescents. Pediatrics, *67*:333–337, 1981.
76. Rosenberg, A.M. et al.: Pulmonary hypertension in a child with mixed connective tissue disease. J. Rheumatol., *6*:700–704, 1979.
77. Hosoda, Y. et al.: Mixed connective tissue disease with pulmonary hypertension: A clinical and pathological study. J. Rheumatol., *14*:826–830, 1987.
78. Whitlow, P.L., Gilliam, J.N., Chubick, A. and Ziff, M.: Myocarditis in mixed connective tissue disease. Arthritis Rheum., *23*:808–815, 1980.
79. Takeda, Y. et al.: Antigenic domains on the U1 small nuclear ribonucleoprotein-associated 70K polypeptide: A comparison of regions selectively recognized by human and mouse autoantibodies and by monoclonal antibodies. Clin. Immunol. Immunopathol., (in press), 1991.
80. Cram, D.S. et al.: Mapping of multiple B cell epitopes on the 70-kilodalton autoantigen of the U1 ribonucleoprotein complex. J. Immunol., *145*:630–635, 1990.
81. Query, C.C., Bentley, R.C., and Keene, J.D.: A specific 31-nucleotide domain of U1 RNA directly interacts with the 70K small nuclear ribonucleoprotein component. Mol. Cell. Biol., *9*:4872–4881, 1989.
82. Query, C.C., Bentley, R.C., and Keene, J.D.: A common RNA recognition motif identified within a defined U1 RANA binding domain of the 70K U1 snRNP protein. Cell, *57*:89–101, 1989.
83. Sunderrajan, E.V. et al.: Pulmonary inflammation in autoimmune MRL/MP-lpr/lpr mice. Am. J. Pathol., *124*:353–362, 1986.
84. Chen, J. et al.: Human autoantibody secreted by immortalized lymphocyte cell line against the 68K polypeptide of the U1 small nuclear ribonucleoprotein. Arthritis Rheum., *31*:1265–1271, 1988.
85. Billings, P.B., Allen, R.W., Jensen, F.C., and Hoch, S.O.: Anti-RNP monoclonal antibodies derived from a mouse strain with lupus-like autoimmunity. J. Immunol., *128*:1176–1180, 1982.
86. Alarcon-Segovia, D.: Immunological abnormalities in mixed connective tissue disease. *In* Mixed Connective Tissue Disease and Anti-nuclear Antibodies. Edited by R. Kasukawa and G.C. Sharp. Amsterdam, Elsevier Science Publishers B.V., 1987.

87. Fishbein, E., Alarcon-Segovia, D., and Ramos-Niembro, F.: Free serum ribonucleoprotein (RNP) in mixed connective tissue disease (MCTD). *In* Proceedings of the Fourteenth International Congress on Rheumatology, San Francisco, 1977.
88. Negoro, N. et al.: A solid-phase radioimmunoassay for the detection of nRNP immune complexes. J. Immunol. Methods, *91*:83–89, 1986.
89. Negoro, N. et al.: Nuclear ribonucleoprotein immune complexes in pericardial fluid of a patient with mixed connective tissue disease. Arthritis Rheum., *30*:97–101, 1987.
90. Genth, E. et al.: HLA-DR and Gm (1,3; 5,21) are associated with U1-nRNP antibody positive connective tissues disease. Ann. Rheum. Dis., *46*:189–196, 1987.
91. Black, C.M. et al.: HLA and immunoglobulin allotypes in mixed connective tissue disease. Arthritis Rheum., *31*:131–134, 1988.
92. Kaneoka, H. et al.: Molecular genetic analysis of HLA-DR and HLA-DQ genes among anti-U1 70kD autoantibody-positive connective tissue disease patients. Arthritis Rheum., (in press), 1991.
93. Wolff-Vorbeck, G. et al.: A human T cell clone recognizing small nuclear ribonucleoproteins (UsnRNP). *In* Molecular and Cell Biology of Autoantibodies and Autoimmunity. Edited by E.K.F. Bautz, J.R. Kalden, M. Homma, and E.M. Tan. Heidelberg, Springer-Verlag, 1989.
94. Hoffman, R.W. et al.: Association of immunoglobulin Km and Gm allotypes with specific antinuclear antibodies and disease susceptibility among connective tissue disease patients. Arthritis Rheum., *34*:453–458, 1991.
95. Ramos-Niembro, F., Alarcon-Segovia, D., and Hernandez-Ortiz, J.: Articular manifestations of mixed connective tissue disease. Arthritis Rheum., *22*:43–51, 1979.
96. Alarcon-Segovia, D.A., and Shiokawa, Y.: Chairmen's summary. *In* Mixed Connective Tissue Disease and Anti-nuclear Antibodies. Edited by R. Kasukawa and G.C. Sharp. Amsterdam, Elsevier Science Publishers B.V., 1987.
97. Lerner, M.R. et al.: Are snRNP's involved in splicing? Nature, *283*:220–224, 1980.
98. Nyman, U. et al.: Intranuclear localization of snRNP antigens. J. Cell Biol., *102*:137–144, 1986.

72

Polymyositis/Dermatomyositis

LAWRENCE J. KAGEN

Polymyositis and dermatomyositis are acquired, chronic, inflammatory muscle disorders of unknown cause. They occur in children and adults and are manifested by disability resulting from muscle weakness. A characteristic rash distinguishes dermatomyositis from polymyositis.

Although inflammation of muscle may develop in the course of other connective tissue disorders such as progressive systemic sclerosis, systemic lupus erythematosus, and Sjögren's syndrome, the terms polymyositis and dermatomyositis are reserved for the clinical situations in which chronic inflammatory myopathy is the dominant element in the absence of features diagnostic of other illness.

Symmetric proximal muscle weakness and histologic findings of inflammation and myofiber damage of muscle tissue, accompanied by evidence of increased amounts of certain sarcoplasmic constituents in the circulation and electrophysiologic signs of myopathy, are the chief clinical manifestations, along with characteristic changes of the skin in patients with dermatomyositis. In severe cases, impairment of deglutition and cardiorespiratory complications contribute to morbidity. Malignant neoplasms may be found in patients with myositis and may further complicate the outcome.

CLASSIFICATION

Several schemes for the classification of patients with inflammatory myopathy have been devised for the purpose of segregating patients into groups to study cause, prognosis, and response to therapy more efficiently.[1,2] Patients with polymyositis are usually grouped separately from those with dermatomyositis, malignant diseases, and other connective tissue disorders. Because of factors discussed later in this chapter, dermatomyositis of childhood also has its own category. Attempts to classify a disease without knowledge of its cause and with incomplete knowledge of its pathogenesis may be flawed and are subject to revision, however. In this light, Table 72–1 presents a grouping of patients with polymyositis, for purposes of discussion and further study.

In general, a female preponderance exists in myositis, especially in patients with features of other connective tissue disorders. This preponderance is also present in the dermatomyositis and polymyositis groups, however (Table 72–2). No female preponderance is found in childhood dermatomyositis or in adults with myositis associated with neoplasia.

Although inflammatory muscle disease may occur at any age, most cases are noted in the fifth and sixth decades of life. In a survey of 380 reported cases, 17% of the patients were age 15 or younger, 14% were from 15 to 30 years of age and 60% were between the ages of 30 and 60. An additional 9% of patients were over the age of 60.[3]

Although rare, inflammatory myopathy has been reported in infants less than a year old.[4] In this situation, recognition of myositis and its distinction from congenital myopathies are important because corticosteroid therapy is valuable in the treatment of infants with myositis.

These disorders generally occur less frequently than certain other connective tissue syndromes. The incidence of dermatomyositis and polymyositis has been estimated at 0.5 cases per 100,000 population in a racially mixed area of Tennessee over a 22-year period. Ethnic or racial factors are important, and the highest frequency is noted in black women.[5] An English survey over a 20-year period indicated an incidence of 8 cases per 100,000. The application of these figures to all populations is not precise; however, it is now estimated that

TABLE 72–1. CLASSIFICATION OF INFLAMMATORY MUSCLE DISEASE

1. Dermatomyositis
   childhood
   adult
2. Polymyositis
3. Myositis associated with other connective tissue disorders (e.g., systemic lupus erythematosus, rheumatoid arthritis, scleroderma, sarcoidosis)
4. Myositis with malignant neoplasm
5. Inclusion-body myositis
6. Myositis secondary to infectious agents
   viral (e.g., influenza, coxsackievirus, HIV)
   toxoplasmosis
   bacterial pyomyositis
   Lyme myositis
7. Drug- and toxin-induced myositis (e.g., penicillamine-related, eosinophilia-myalgia syndrome)

TABLE 72–3. SCHEME FOR TESTING MANUAL MUSCLE STRENGTH

GRADE	
0	No evident contraction
1	Trace of contraction
2	Poor—movement with gravity eliminated
3	Fair—movement against gravity
4	Good—movement against resistance
5	Normal

(Modified from Gardner-Medwin, D., and Walton, J.N.[10])

TABLE 72–2. DISTRIBUTION OF PATIENTS BY GROUP AND SEX

GROUP	NO. OF PATIENTS	PERCENTAGE OF TOTAL (%)	PERCENTAGE OF FEMALE PATIENTS (%)
Polymyositis	52	34	69
Dermatomyositis	45	29	58
Dermatomyositis of childhood	11	7	36
Myositis with neoplasm	13	8.5	57
Myositis with overlap features of other connective tissue disorders	32	21	90

(Based on 153 patients reviewed by Bohan, A., et al.[8])

one to five new cases per million people occur each year in the United States, with a frequency perhaps four times greater among black women.[5–7] As suggested in Table 72–2, the incidence in adults is greater than in children.

CLINICAL FEATURES

MUSCLE WEAKNESS

Muscular weakness is the dominant feature of myositis syndromes, with symmetric involvement of proximal muscles of the extremities, trunk, and neck. Difficulty with the lower extremities is often first characterized by an inability to climb stairs, to arise from a low seat or a squat, and to cross the legs. Walking may be limited, and gait may become poorly coordinated and waddling. Weakness of the upper extremities limits lifting, hanging up clothes, and combing the hair. Weakness of the anterior neck flexor muscles interferes with lifting the head from the supine position, and arising from bed becomes difficult. Severely affected patients may have difficulty in swallowing, and liquids may be regurgitated through the nose. Along with weakness and muscle pain, soreness with tenderness may be noted, particularly in patients whose disease progresses rapidly. Although weakness may be marked, little atrophy occurs initially. With time, affected muscles lose volume, and involvement may become more generalized and include distal muscles. Speech may be altered and may assume a nasal quality. Whereas virtually all patients have proximal muscle weakness, few progress to distal involvement or have impaired swallowing or speech. Dysphagia occurs in approximately 10 to 15% of patients.[8] Facial involvement is rare.[9]

Because weakness is the central cause of morbidity in patients with myositis, ongoing assessment of muscle strength is of prime importance in clinical evaluation. One must therefore combine careful questioning, to record changes in functional capabilities, with muscle strength testing. The most common muscle testing schemes employ a semiquantitative grading system (Table 72–3). The ability to assess muscle strength accurately is limited by several factors. First, one must be certain that the patient's effort is his best. Pain, fatigue, and malaise may interfere with full cooperation and invalidate the results of assessment. In addition, variables related to the observer also can be a factor. Joint position in which the test is done affects muscle length, mechanical advantage, and the resultant tension. For example, knee extensor muscles tested at a 60° angle of knee flexion (full extension is 0°) have greater force than at a 30° position. The differences between grades 4 and 5 of muscle strength are significant, but they are difficult to quantify precisely. Finally, tests of this nature are most useful for muscle groups of the extremities. For other muscles, such as those of the torso, additional testing methods must be used.

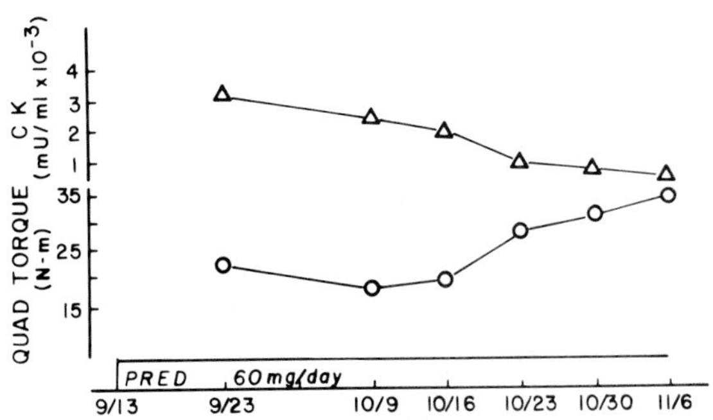

FIGURE 72–1. The use of biomechanical measurement of muscle strength during the course of polymyositis. Strength is recorded as the torque (force × lever arm) produced by the knee extensors (quadriceps femoris). This patient demonstrates an increase in strength concomitant with a fall in serum creatine kinase (CK) level after treatment with prednisone (pred). (Data from Dr. J. Otis and Mr. M. Kroll.)

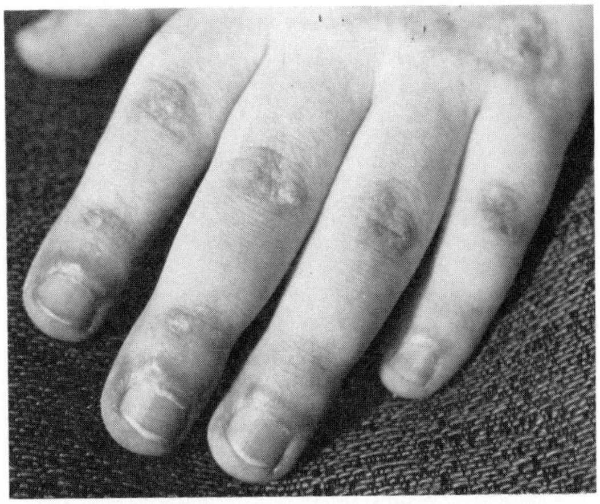

FIGURE 72–2. The rash of dermatomyositis over the hand of a child. Patches of erythematous, scaly plaques over knuckles, as well as periungual changes, are evident.

To approach some of the observer-related variables, as well as to standardize and increase reproducibility and sensitivity, several attempts have been made to introduce biomechanical methods and instruments into the clinical setting. The importance of such measurements has been stressed by Edwards and colleagues, who have reported that muscle strength correlates with metabolic studies of net losses and gains in total muscle mass and may be a better guide to progress than other laboratory measures.[11,12] Figure 72–1 demonstrates the use of biomechanical strength testing in a patient with polymyositis during initial therapy with prednisone. Torque production, an indicator of muscle strength of the quadriceps mechanism, rose after 6 to 7 weeks of prednisone therapy and was associated with a fall in serum creatine kinase activity, as well as with gains in functional ability. Not all muscle groups are affected equally in polymyositis and dermatomyositis. In the lower extremities, the quadriceps may manifest selective weakness compared to the hamstrings group, and significant lowering of the quadriceps/hamstrings ratio of strength occurs in severely ill patients.[13]

A study of polymyositis and dermatomyositis indicated a significant correlation between muscle strength and laboratory indices (serum enzymes and myoglobin) during the course of illness of some, but not all, patients.[14] Because laboratory guides are *not* correlated to disease activity in *all* patients, the need for *quantitative serial assessment of muscle strength* was emphasized.

A rapid method for evaluation of lower extremity strength has been standardized for men and women of various ages.[15]

RASH

The rash of dermatomyositis appears on the face, neck, chest, and extremities (Figs. 72–2 to 72–5). It is most common over the extensor surfaces of the extremities, particularly over the dorsum of the hands and the fingers. The rash is deep red and is slightly raised in small plaques over the wrists and knuckles. A whitish scale may be seen superficially. Similar patches occur over the elbows, the knees, and the medial malleoli of the ankles. Involvement of the scalp, upper arms, and outer thighs also occurs. At the nail beds, one sees hyperemia, telangiectasia and, with more marked involvement, destruction of the architecture of the nail bed. Dilated capillary loops at the nail fold, as well as over the knuckles and other areas of the fingers, may be seen.[16] In one study, abnormalities of nail fold capillaries were noted in 56% of patients with dermatomyositis and 21% of those with polymyositis. The severity of the capillary disturbance appeared to lessen with disease remission, but a clear correlation with activity of muscle inflammation was not demonstrable.[17] Cutaneous vasculitis, evidenced clinically by tender nodules, periungual infarctions, and digital ulcerations, has been noted in both adult and childhood dermatomyositis. In the adult, these lesions are less common and may be associated with an underlying malignant process. In a group of 76 adults studied, 7 had lesions of this nature, and 2 of these had an underlying malignant disease (28%). Of the total number of patients with malignant disease, 2 of 6 had these lesions.[18] A deep violet-red rash may be present on the face, particularly in the periorbital areas, which may also be edematous. Involvement is most prominent over the upper eyelids, and scaling may also occur here. Lilac suffusion or *heliotrope rash* over the upper eyelids is characteristic of dermatomyositis. A similar deep red-to-violaceous rash may appear on the forehead, neck, shoulders, and chest.

Although the heliotrope rash is characteristic, it is not absolutely diagnostic. Similar changes may occur in patients with allergic manifestations and during the course of trichinosis. A characteristic rash of this type has also been described in a patient with sarcoidosis and myopathy.[19]

Rash may appear before other signs of myopathy be-

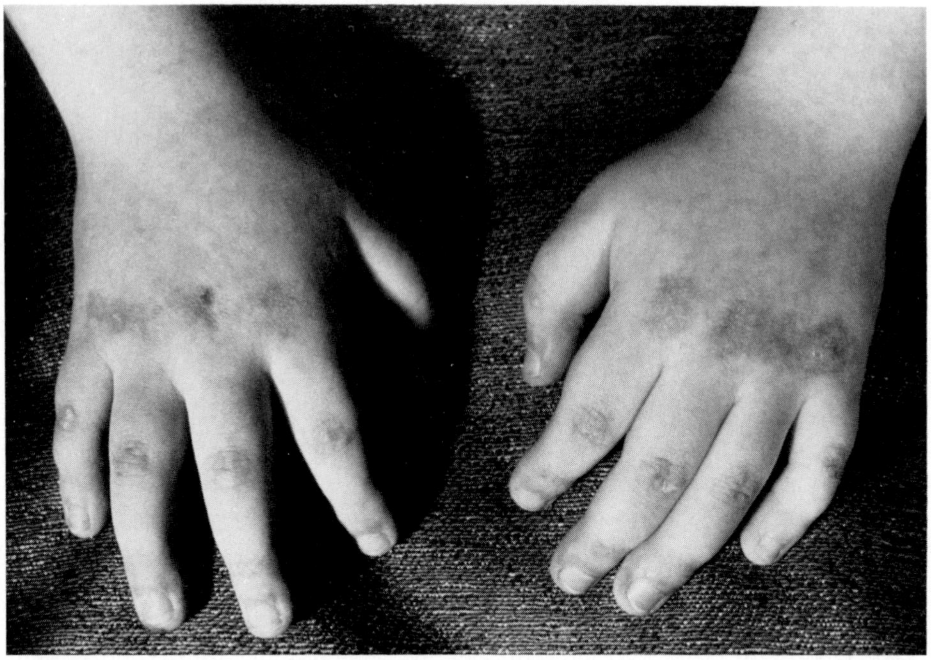

FIGURE 72–3. Dermatomyositis, showing a raised, reddened rash over the dorsum of the hands.

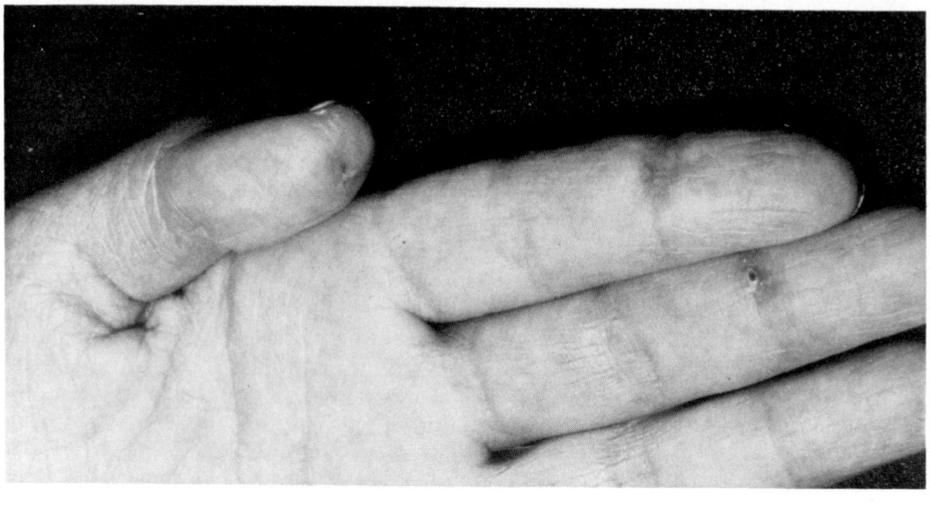

FIGURE 72–4. Punched-out ulcerated skin lesions over the volar surface of the hands (at the tip of the thumb and at the terminal creases of the second and third fingers) in a patient with dermatomyositis and adenocarcinoma of the large intestine.

come manifest. As extreme examples, 6 patients with classic heliotrope discoloration of the periorbital area with edema and a maculopapular violaceous rash over the interphalangeal joints with periungual telangiectasia did not develop clinical evidence of muscle involvement until months to years later.[20]

Histologic evaluation of skin biopsies in dermatomyositis reveals poikiloderma, that is, epidermal atrophy with liquefaction, degeneration of the basal cell layer, and vascular dilatation. Inflammatory infiltrates, composed of perivascular accumulations of lymphocytes and histiocytes in the upper dermis, are found along with few polymorphonuclear cells and occasional infiltrates around the pilosebaceous apparatus. Hyperkeratosis, dermal edema with increased deposits of mucin, and evidence of subcutaneous panniculitis may also be found.[21] Vascular endothelial changes characteristic of childhood dermatomyositis may be present in the skin (see the discussion on histology later in this chapter).

DYSPHAGIA

Difficulty in swallowing may result from several factors in patients with myositis. Decreased strength of pharyngeal contractions, disordered peristalsis, vallecular pooling, and weakness of the tongue may all interfere with normal swallowing. Patients with severe weakness of this type also have difficulties in elevating the palate and may have nasal speech. In addition, dysfunction of the cricopharyngeus muscle with spasm and improperly timed closure may occur in some patients and accentuate symptoms.[22] The importance of recognizing crico-

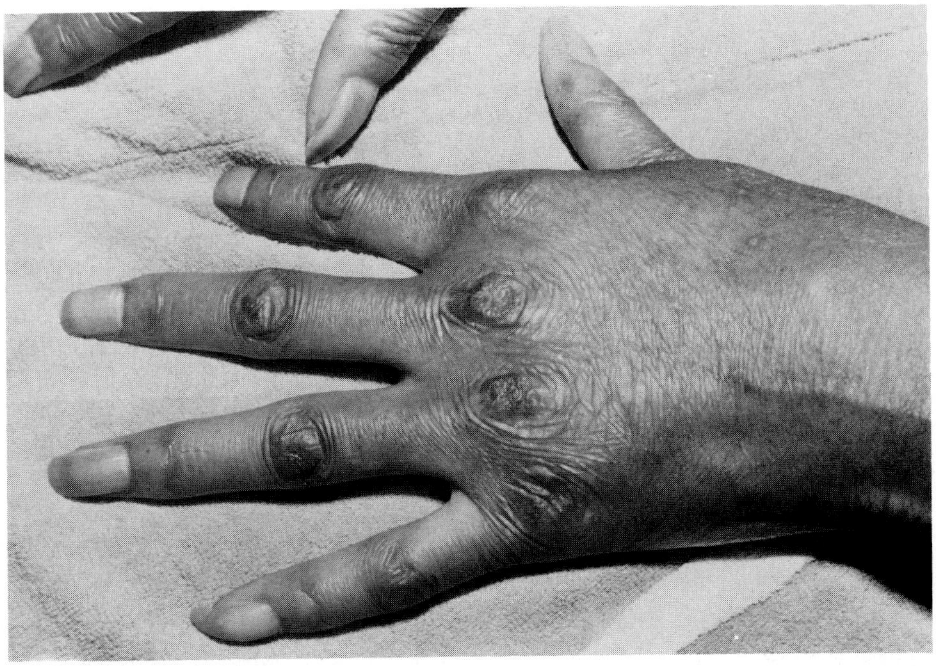

FIGURE 72–5. Papular, raised rash of the knuckle above the metacarpophalangeal and proximal interphalangeal joints in a patient with chronic dermatomyositis.

pharyngeal dysfunction resulting from constriction, fibrosis, or abnormal contraction lies in the possibility of surgical relief of obstruction. The occurrence of dysphagia among older patients with inclusion body myositis and its relief by myotomy have been noted. In these patients, weakness of the pharyngeal wall precludes timely emptying before the cricopharyngeal sphincter closes resulting in repetitive swallowing of the bolus and choking.[23] Appropriate investigation should be conducted in patients with dysphagia to determine to what extent cricopharyngeal dysfunction may be a complicating factor.[24]

Abnormalities of distal, as well as proximal, esophageal function and disturbances in gastric emptying have also been documented.[25,26]

Although found in only 10 to 15% of patients,[8] dysphagia is usually associated with severe disease and a poor prognosis.

PULMONARY MANIFESTATIONS

Several factors, including hypoventilation secondary to muscular weakness, infectious agents, aspiration in association with abnormalities in swallowing and, rarely, drug hypersensitivity, such as related to methotrexate,[27] may play a role in the association of pulmonary disease and myositis. In addition to these factors, interstitial pulmonary fibrosis or fibrosing alveolitis may be a significant feature of myositis syndromes.

Pulmonary fibrosis has been noted in 5 to 10% of patients, generally by roentgenography. The frequency of this disorder seems unrelated to a previous history of cigarette smoking and does not have the female preponderance seen in adults with myositis. Pulmonary function tests indicate restriction of ventilation with reduction of total lung capacity and vital capacity. Hypoxemia may be characterized by a moderate reduction in diffusing capacity. Dyspnea and cough are the major symptoms, and physical examination may reveal the presence of fine, crepitant, basilar rales. In approximately half the affected patients, pulmonary abnormalities are noted prior to the appearance of myopathy. In patients with severe myopathy, pulmonary involvement, including pulmonary hypertension, may be present, but its symptoms may be masked by the presence of peripheral muscle weakness.[28]

Alveolar septal fibrosis, interstitial mononuclear cell infiltrates containing mainly lymphocytes with smaller numbers of large mononuclear cells and plasma cells, hyperplasia of the type I alveolar epithelial cells, and increased numbers of free alveolar macrophages are seen histologically. These findings may be irregularly distributed and intermixed with areas of apparently uninvolved lung. Interstitial edema and vascular change marked by intimal and medial thickening of arteries and arterioles may also be evident. Three pathologic patterns of pulmonary involvement have been described. The first, that of bronchiolitis obliterans and organizing pneumonia, appears to have a better prognosis than that of interstitial pneumonia or that of diffuse alveolar damage.[29] Chest roentgenograms may show diffuse, linear, interstitial thickening, with an alveolar pattern of fibrosis. Patchy consolidation and "honeycomb" changes indicate more chronic and severe involvement. These changes may be associated with right-ventricular enlargement and with prominent hilar markings. Corticosteroid therapy may be followed by relief of dyspnea and by improvements in radiographic changes and abnormalities of pulmonary function, but some patients show no improvement. Therapeutic response may be better in patients with acute illness and lung biopsies showing inflammation of the alveolar wall, whereas fibrosis in the absence of inflammation is a sign of a poorer prognosis. Rapidly progressive fatal pulmonary insufficiency may occur, despite the early introduction of corticosteroid treatment. Carefully monitored therapy with these drugs is advisable, although generally applicable, statistically validated prognostic guides are still lacking. The progression of pulmonary dysfunction resulting from fibrosing alveolitis does stop in some patients.[30–34]

Ventilatory insufficiency as a result of weakness of muscles of respiration (e.g., the diaphragm and intercostal muscles) also contributes to defects in gas exchange. Loss of respiratory muscle strength, as assessed by inspiratory and expiratory pressures at the mouth, may be associated with a tendency toward hypercapnia.[35]

As indicated, pulmonary toxicity may occur in the course of therapy with certain agents, such as methotrexate and perhaps cyclophosphamide; such toxicity may play a role in the development of interstitial lung disease.[36]

CARDIAC MANIFESTATIONS

Cardiac abnormalities in patients with polymyositis and dermatomyositis occur frequently, but are rarely clinically symptomatic. First-, second-, and third-degree heart block, left bundle branch block, left axis deviation, and atrial and ventricular dysrhythmias have been noted. Myocarditis and congestive heart failure occur less often. At least half of patients have electrocardiographic abnormalities, with an increased frequency of mitral valve prolapse noted in one report.[37] Uncommonly, conduction abnormalities are so severe that an artificial cardiac pacemaker is required.[38] It is not certain whether the tendency to cardiac abnormalities is greater in more severely or chronically ill patients.

Postmortem evaluations have demonstrated myocarditis, as well as myocardial fibrosis.[39,40] Myocarditis is associated with congestive heart failure. One patient with bundle branch block had inflammation and necrosis involving the conduction system. Overall, arrhythmia is estimated to occur in 6%, congestive heart failure in 3%, bundle branch block in 5%, and high-grade heart block in 2% of patients.[8] Cardiac involvement may occur in both polymyositis and dermatomyositis, but it may go unnoticed unless electrocardiographic examinations are performed. Improvement in electrocardiographic abnormality in adults rarely occurs, although this has been noted in children.[41]

CALCINOSIS

Soft-tissue calcification can be a disabling complication of inflammatory muscle disease (Figs. 72–6 to 72–8). Most commonly, it occurs during the course of chronic childhood dermatomyositis. Calcification may invest the fascia surrounding muscle groups of the proximal

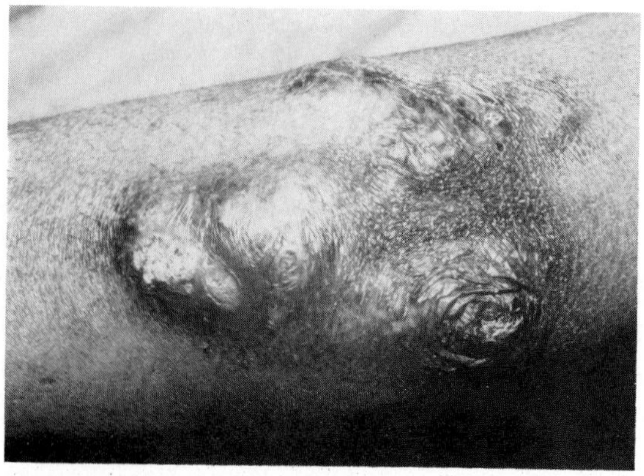

FIGURE 72–6. Subcutaneous calcific masses nearing the skin surface at the elbow of a patient with dermatomyositis.

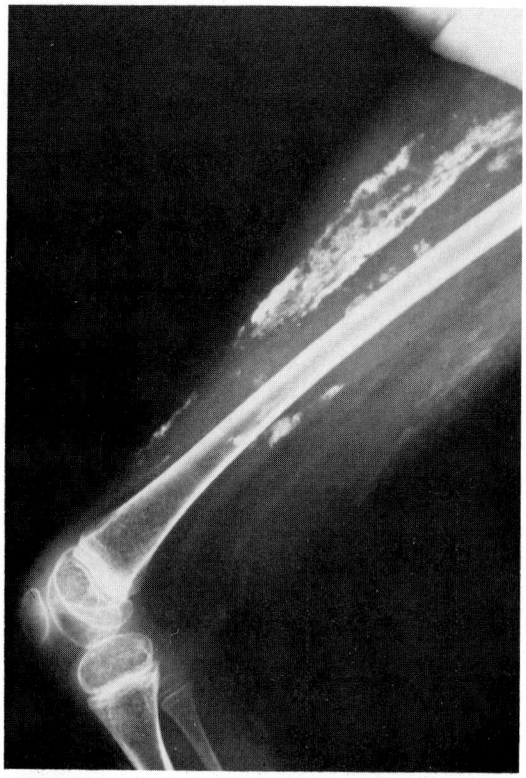

FIGURE 72–7. Subcutaneous and perimuscular calcific masses in the thigh of a child with dermatomyositis in remission.

extremities and may lead to diffuse "woody" induration that severely limits motion. Calcified masses may also appear under the skin and may open to the surface, draining calcareous material. A review of radiographs of 40 children with dermatomyositis has suggested the occurrence of four patterns of soft-tissue calcification. Deep linear and deep calcareal deposits were most common; superficial calcareal deposits were less common. The fourth pattern, characterized by lacy, reticular, subcutaneous calcification that could be widespread, was

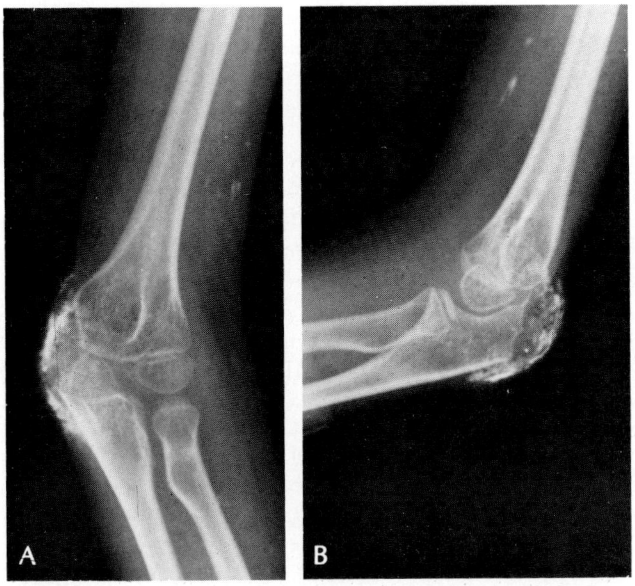

FIGURE 72–8. *A* and *B*, Subcutaneous calcification at the elbow and other areas of calcification in the upper arm of a child with dermatomyositis in remission.

associated with children with severe, unremitting illness.[42] Diagnostic sensitivity in detecting this abnormality, prior to accumulation of masses large enough to be seen radiographically, may be increased by bone-scanning techniques with ^{99m}technetium diphosphonate.[43] Treatment methods for calcinosis are generally unsatisfactory. Localized masses may be removed surgically, but extensive or more generalized involvement is a distressing problem. A number of therapies, including corticosteroids, diphosphonates, ethylenediaminotetraacetate, aluminum hydroxide gel, low-dose sodium warfarin (Coumadin), and probenecid, have been tried. The calcific deposits are sometimes resorbed spontaneously (see Chapter 97).

RENAL INVOLVEMENT

Renal disease is rare in patients with inflammatory myopathy. Renal insufficiency in patients with severe persistent myoglobinuria has been observed.[44] This complication may occur in both polymyositis and dermatomyositis. Although rare, glomerulonephritis of the focal-mesangial type or of the progressive-crescentic type has been recorded.[45,46]

FOCAL OR NODULAR MUSCLE INVOLVEMENT

Polymyositis may begin with a single, localized, nodular swelling in muscle. This swelling may then progress over months to generalized inflammatory myopathy. This unusual variant has been described as focal or nodular myositis.[47,48] In some patients, focal myositis of the gastrocnemius muscle has simulated thrombophlebitis.[49]

CHILDHOOD DERMATOMYOSITIS

Although a female preponderance exists among adults with myositis, such is not the case in children.[50]

The signs of rash and myopathy are similar to those previously described. In addition, evidence of vascular involvement may be prominent. Abnormalities of nail fold capillaries, including dilatation, avascular areas, and tortuosity, are present in over half the affected children, especially in those with severe disease.[51] Early changes are associated with thrombosis and hemorrhage, with later development of giant capillary loops and "bushy" formations representing areas of neovascularization. Although not all observers have noted a parallel course between the severity of systemic illness and these findings, this development may occur in certain patients. Moreover nail fold appearance may return to normal with disease remission.[52] Ulcerations of the gastrointestinal tract and hemorrhage related to vascular involvement of the digestive system are serious, life-threatening complications.[53] Perforations secondary to vasculopathy, ischemia, and necrosis may occur in several areas including the esophagus, duodenum, and colon. Individual patients may have multiple perforations.[54] This manifestation was described prior to the use of corticosteroid agents and represents a result of dermatomyositis rather than a complication of therapy.[2] Although vascular involvement of the gastrointestinal tract is the most prominent visceral complication of dermatomyositis, other areas may also be involved, including, rarely, the retina in which exudates, macular edema, and visual impairment have been described.[55]

Histologic evaluation of dermatomyositis reveals distinctive abnormalities related to pathologic changes of the vessel walls, as discussed later in this chapter.

RISK OF PREGNANCY

There are few reports of the effects of myositis on the risk of pregnancy; thus, predictive data are incomplete. The majority of these reports deal with dermatomyositis. Decreased fertility and increased fetal loss probably occur in some women with dermatomyositis. Exacerbations of disease during pregnancy have also been observed. No neonatal effects of dermatomyositis in surviving infants have been reported as yet.[56,57]

In the management of pregnant patients, it has been recommended that steroids be used as needed. Placental enzymes inactivate cortisol, prednisolone and, likely, prednisone and methylprednisolone. Dexamethasone and betamethasone, which are not inactivated, however, may have effects upon the fetus after crossing the placenta. If possible, cytotoxic therapy should be discontinued during pregnancy, and nonsteroidal anti-inflammatory medications avoided, particularly in the last 2 months, since they may induce premature closure of the ductus arteriosus resulting in pulmonary hypertension.[58]

LABORATORY AND OTHER DIAGNOSTIC STUDIES

The laboratory studies most used during the course of inflammatory muscle disease involve measurement of sarcoplasmic constituents, enzymes, and myoglobin released into the circulation as a consequence of muscle damage.

ENZYMES

Measurements of serum activities of creatine kinase, lactate dehydrogenase, aldolase, and aspartate aminotransferase (glutamic-oxaloacetic transaminase) are the most common enzyme tests. Elevations occur during periods of disease activity, and values return toward normal during remission or inactive disease.

An increase in serum creatine kinase activity is the most sensitive enzyme index of active muscle disease.[59] High creatine kinase activity is found in active disease, and the level falls during remission, sometimes weeks before clinically evident improvement. The level may then rise again if the therapeutic drug dosage is reduced too quickly or if a relapse is impending. Because aldolase, transaminase, and lactate dehydrogenase may be less consistently elevated in patients with myositis, estimation of creatine kinase levels is the most reliable enzyme test.[60]

In some situations, evaluations of serum enzyme activity are of limited use. From the technical point of view, the amount of enzyme is inferred from its activity, and factors that inhibit or promote activity influence the interpretation of test results. Inhibitors of creatine kinase activity have been described in serum. Dilution of serum samples with elevated creatine kinase levels may produce artifactual increases in creatine kinase activity,[61] and certain pharmacologic agents such as barbiturates, diazepam, and morphine may alter the removal rate of creatine kinase from the circulation and may increase its activity.[62] In addition, the question whether enzyme increases are due to tissue destruction, or whether cell membranes become leaky due to disease or pharmacologic agents, is difficult to answer. For example, following exercise, elevations of creatine kinase levels may be observed in the absence of histologically demonstrable evidence of tissue necrosis. In neuromuscular disorders other than myositis, falls in creatine kinase activity may occur without clinical change,[63] so this index may not always correlate with disease activity.

Rarely, in 1 to 5% of patients with polymyositis and dermatomyositis, the serum creatine kinase level alone may be normal, and in other patients, all serum enzyme levels tested are normal throughout the course of illness.[8] On the other hand, a series of 7 patients without creatine kinase elevation had a poor prognosis, with 5 patients having had either cancer or interstitial lung disease.[64] Taken together, therefore, the evidence suggests that serum enzyme evaluation is an important adjunct to the diagnosis and assessment of patients with myositis, but absolute correlations of strength and prognosis with the enzyme levels, particularly in patients with chronic illness, are often imprecise.

Creatine kinase exists as a dimer with three major isoenzymic forms: MM, MB, and BB. Creatine kinase-MM is the predominant form in skeletal muscle, where it represents approximately 95 to 98% of the total creatine kinase activity. The BB isoenzyme is the major component of brain and smooth muscle. The MB form is present in cardiac muscle to the extent of 20 to 30%, with the remainder as MM. The MB form may be present in skeletal muscle as well, in levels of 5% or less.[65–67] Creatine kinase-MB has been demonstrated in the circulation of patients with myositis in the absence of detectable, concomitant cardiac disease or dysfunction.[68–71] In these patients, creatine kinase-MB is probably synthesized in and released from skeletal muscle. Myofibers during embryologic development produce the B subunit and elaborate creatine kinase-MB, and skeletal muscle tissue in cell culture also produces this MB form.[72–74] These observations, combined with clinical information, suggest that regenerating myofibers within damaged skeletal muscle may be the source of the increased production of creatine kinase-MB.

MYOGLOBIN

Myoglobin, the respiratory heme protein of the muscle cell, is found in both skeletal and cardiac muscle, but not in other tissues. During the course of muscle disease or disorder, myoglobin may enter the circulation and, following renal clearance, may appear in the urine.[75] Hypermyoglobinemia is seen in most patients with dermatomyositis and polymyositis. Myoglobinuria is less prevalent.[44,76] From 70 to 80% of patients with active, untreated myositis have hypermyoglobinemia, with levels falling during periods of remission. Sequential determinations of serum myoglobin levels suggest rapid reductions with response to therapy, often before the activities of serum enzymes such as creatine kinase, lactic dehydrogenase, and glutamic-oxaloacetic transaminase return to normal. It is likely that the combined use of serum myoglobin determinations with the enzymes will offer advantages for the detection and assessment of myopathic states. In a study of patients with myositis,[77] 19% had hypermyoglobinemia in the absence of elevated creatine kinase levels. Myoglobinuria, although less frequent, also occurs in patients with inflammatory muscle disease, and persistent myoglobinuria has been associated with renal failure in these patients.[44] Because levels of myoglobin may undergo circadian variation, it is best to compare results from a standard time of day.[78]

ERYTHROCYTE SEDIMENTATION RATE

The erythrocyte sedimentation rate is often elevated in patients with active myositis in the range of 30 to 50 mm/hour as measured by the Westergren method. This value is normal, however, in many patients, and no correlation exists between the erythrocyte sedimentation rate and the grade of disability or degree of weakness.[6] During remission of the disease, this value generally approaches normal.

AUTOANTIBODIES

Patients with dermatomyositis may have circulating antibodies to certain nuclear and cellular constituents. These are discussed later, in the section on serologic factors.

ELECTROMYOGRAPHY

Patients with inflammatory muscle disease have evidence of myopathy on electromyographic examination; volitional contraction produces a pattern of activity characterized by short duration, low amplitude, and polyphasic potentials.[79] At rest, fibrillation potentials may be observed, presumably the result of involvement of terminal neural elements in the inflammatory process. Overall, 70 to 90% of patients studied have these findings; however, a few patients may have no demonstrable abnormalities. Generally, little or no correlation exists between the grade of disability at presentation and the electromyographic findings.[6,8]

Studies of patients with standard as well as single-fiber electromyography indicate an increase in the number of muscle fibers in individual motor units, along with abnormal jitter and blocking. These findings also suggest changes in the pattern of terminal innervation of the muscle, perhaps related to involvement of intramuscular nerves by inflammation, anoxia, or other factors coincident with inflammation, degeneration, and regeneration. In this connection, these changes may relate to the finding of fibrillation activity or to the occasional occurrence of fiber type grouping seen in affected tissues by histochemical techniques; these changes also suggest neural involvement.[80]

MUSCLE BIOPSY

Muscle biopsy is indicated in nearly all patients with suspected myositis before proceeding with what may be a long course of potentially hazardous therapy. Demonstration of inflammation confirms the diagnosis.

The optimal procedure for obtaining and processing muscle tissue requires coordination among clinician, surgeon, pathologist, and technologists. The site selected should be one of active involvement, but not one marked by advanced atrophic or end-stage disease. In addition, sites previously traumatized by electromyography needles, intramuscular injections, or surgical procedures should be avoided. In most cases, proximal muscle tissue of the extremity is usually selected. Cases of myositis with only spinal muscle involvement have been reported. Biopsy of the erector spinae muscles may be performed. Muscle is obtained at resting length for histologic processing.

In many cases, particularly when the clinician feels histologic evaluation is all that is desired, needle muscle biopsy may be employed. Its major advantages are ease of performance and low morbidity rate. A major drawback is the small size of the sample. If needed, however, multiple samples may be obtained. Expert handling of the small bits of tissue removed is critical to ensure their proper orientation for microtome sectioning. Contraction artifacts also may be encountered in needle biopsy samples. In a series of 30 patients, the overall diagnostic yield from needle biopsy was comparable to that expected with the open surgical procedure. Inflammation, necrosis, and degeneration were noted in most specimens studied. Two had only myofiber atrophy, and one had no abnormality. In addition, sequential needle biopsies have been employed to demonstrate response to therapy. Definite correlation in this regard may be difficult, however, because of uneven involvement of muscle tissue and because of persistent abnormalities in otherwise stable patients. In one group of patients examined by needle biopsy, failure to respond to corticosteroid therapy was associated with an increased number of myofiber internal nuclei.[81,82]

Open surgical biopsy, the present standard, is more time-consuming and is attended with more discomfort and morbidity than needle biopsy, but it obtains larger specimens with fewer chances for artifact, and it allows biochemical or electron-microscopic studies.

HISTOLOGIC EXAMINATION

The major findings in muscle tissue of patients with inflammatory myopathy are necrosis, phagocytosis of necrotic muscle tissue, perivascular and interstitial inflammation, and myofiber regeneration (Figs. 72–9 to 72–12). Signs of regeneration include the presence of myoblasts, seen as crescentic cells with basophilic cytoplasm within the sarcolemmal sheath. Myoblasts of this type may contain one or two nuclei and either few coarse myofibrils or none. Syncytial masses of such presumed progenitor cells with basophilic cytoplasm and immature myofibrils, as well as myotubes characterized by central nuclei, and large myofibers with peripheral basophilia may all be part of the regenerative process. Increased content of RNA and of certain enzymes such as lactate dehydrogenase and succinate dehydrogenase are noted in regenerating myofibers by histochemical techniques. The inflammatory infiltrate, the hallmark of myositis, consists of small and large lymphocytes, macrophages and, occasionally, plasma cells. Associated with the infiltrate of inflammatory cells, particularly in chronic cases, is an increase in collagen and connective tissue, which may separate bundles of myofibers as well as isolate and replace individual necrotic myofibers. Immunohistologic study has indicated that this connective tissue is rich in collagen types I to IV, and that concentrations of the amino terminal propeptides of procollagen III, the precursor of type III collagen, are increased in blood serum of patients with polymyositis and dermatomyositis.[83–86]

Anastomoses between the terminal cisternae of the

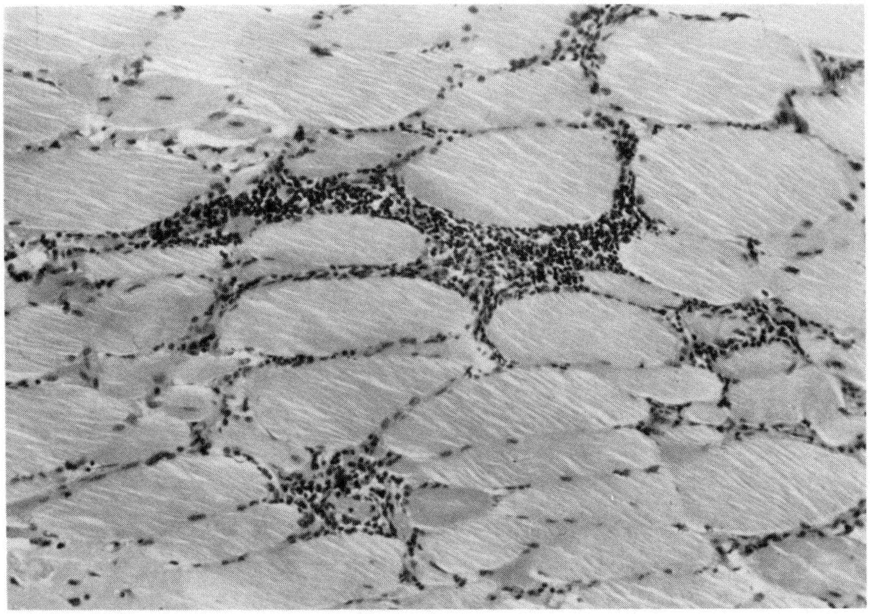

FIGURE 72–9. Infiltration of inflammatory cells between fibers with necrosis and areas of loss of fibers seen on microscopic examination of a muscle biopsy specimen.

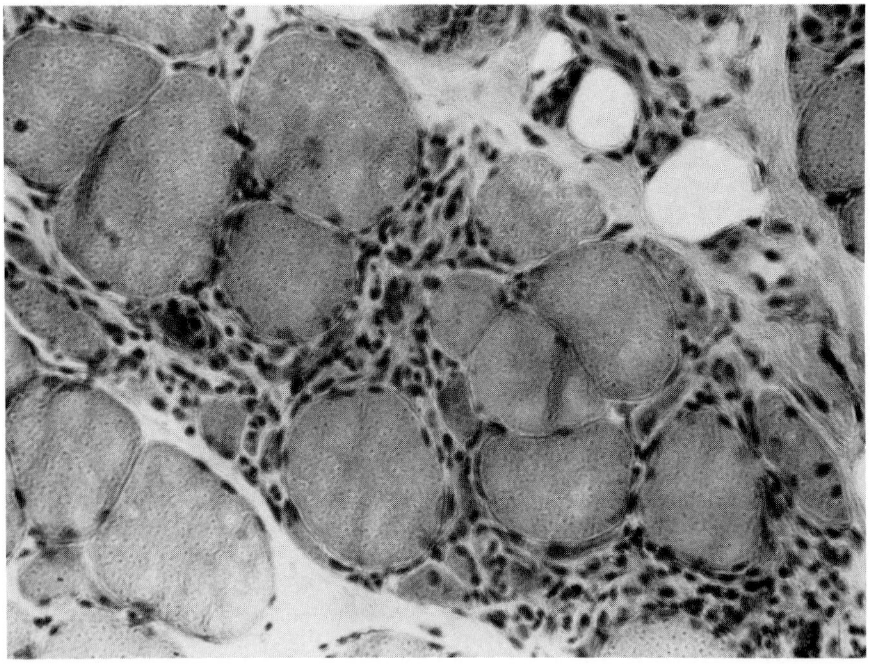

FIGURE 72–10. Inflammatory cell infiltrate with areas of necrosis and an increase in connective tissue and lipid (upper right).

sarcoplasmic reticulum and the transverse tubules have been observed by electron-microscopic examination in myositis. These abnormal anastomoses may furnish pathways for the leakage of intracellular constituents such as enzymes to the extracellular space.[87]

In patients with chronic disease, inflammatory changes may be less marked, and the histologic picture may be characterized by myofiber atrophy, fibrosis, and increased deposits or accumulations of lipid.

Table 72–4 indicates the results of muscle biopsy of 103 patients, all of whom had clinical findings of polymyositis.[6] Sixty-five percent of specimens showed sufficient inflammation for the diagnosis of myositis (groups 1 and 2); however, 17% of patients had no demonstrable abnormalities. The data suggest that muscle biopsy is strong diagnostic evidence in most patients with active disease, but a negative or nonspecific biopsy does not of itself exclude the diagnosis of polymyositis.

Another review indicated an overall frequency of 5% of patients with clinically evident myositis, but normal tissue on biopsy. Interestingly, this phenomenon was more frequent in patients with associated malignant tumors.[88]

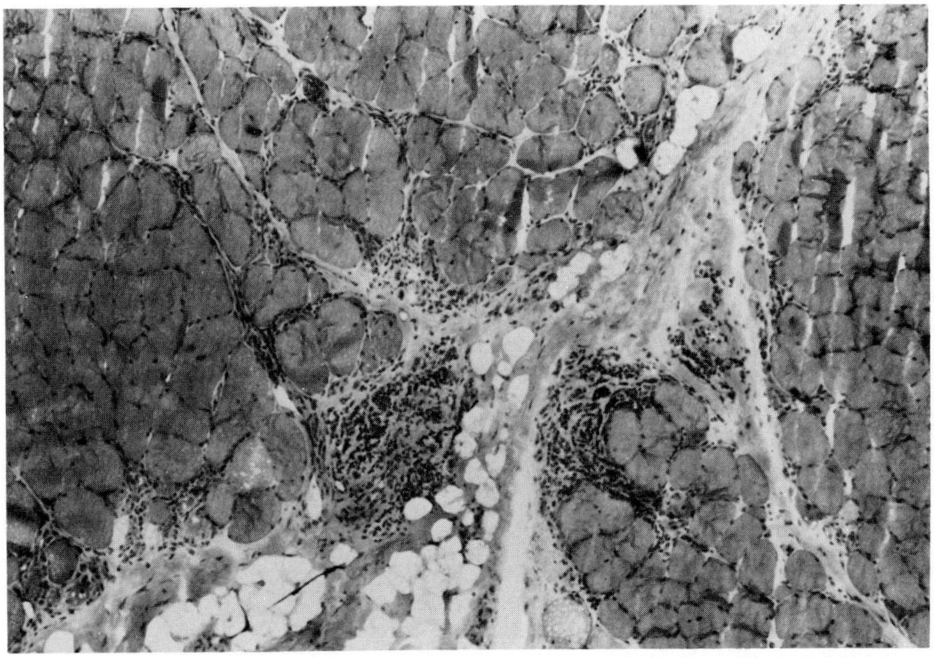

FIGURE 72–11. Low-power microscopic view demonstrating zones of inflammation and an increase in connective tissue and lipid in a patient with chronic polymyositis.

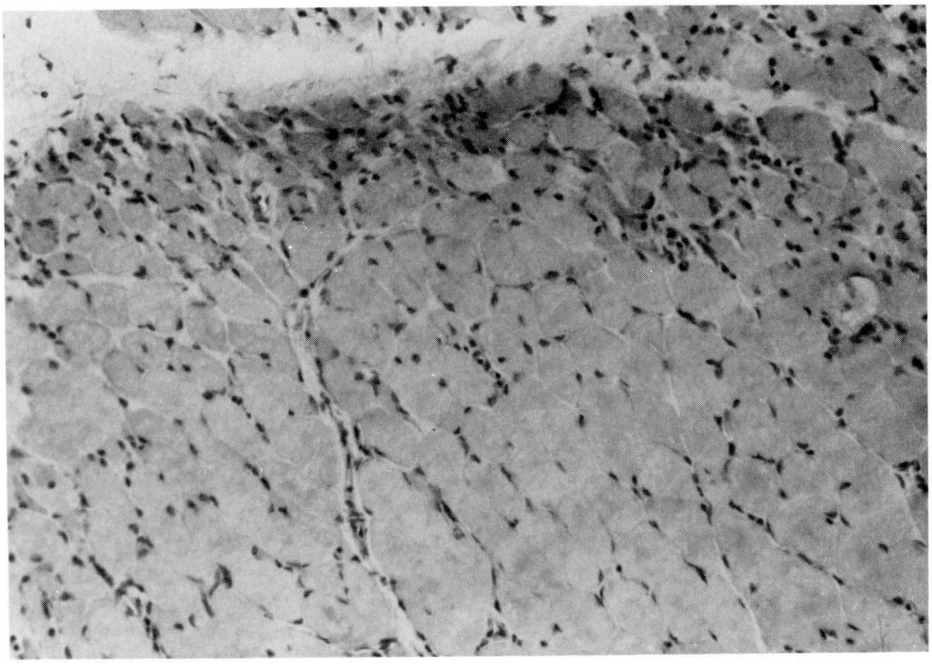

FIGURE 72–12. Perifascicular atrophy in a biopsy from a child with dermatomyositis.

Childhood Dermatomyositis

The histologic findings of childhood dermatomyositis, characterized by zonal loss of capillaries, muscle infarction, vasculopathy, and lymphocytic infiltration of blood vessels, set this entity apart from other types of inflammatory myopathy. Vasculopathy is the striking feature. In addition to an inflammatory component, swelling, necrosis, and obliteration of vessels also occur in the absence of nearby inflammatory cells. The endothelium of small vessels may appear prominent and hyperplastic. Biopsies from adults with dermatomyositis have also demonstrated reduced capillary density with focal depletion of capillaries and evidence of the presence of the complement membrane attack complex on clusters of capillaries. These observations suggest that capillaries may be a particular target site in both the childhood and adult forms of dermatomyositis.[89,90] These findings are supported by observations of muscle biopsy samples that generally appeared only minimally

TABLE 72–4. MUSCLE BIOPSY FINDINGS IN A GROUP OF 103 PATIENTS WITH MYOSITIS

FINDINGS	PERCENTAGE OF TOTAL (%)	
1. Fiber destruction, regeneration, perivascular and interstitial inflammation	46	65
2. Perivascular and interstitial inflammatory infiltrate with minimal fiber destruction	19	
3. Myofiber destruction and regeneration without inflammatory cell infiltrates	8	
4. Fiber atrophy and other nonspecific changes	11	
5. Normal tissue	17	

(Data adapted from DeVere, R., and Bradley, W.G.[6])

changed but nonetheless had abnormalities of the microvasculature including endothelial inclusions, microvacuoles, and capillary necrosis.[91] Elevated levels of C3d, fibrinopeptide A, and factor VIII-related antigen present in patients with juvenile dermatomyositis have also provided evidence of activation of complement and the coagulation system in this disorder.[92]

Electron-microscopic evaluation of endothelial cells reveals degeneration and areas of regeneration. Affected endothelial cells appear pleomorphic and contain cytoplasmic inclusions made up of aggregates of tubular structures, both free and circumscribed by endoplasmic reticulum. The tubular structures are 250 to 280 Å in diameter, and the aggregate masses are 0.4 to 2.7 μ across. These inclusion aggregates appear to distort the endothelial cells. Gaps are present between endothelial cells. Changes in the endothelium and the loss of the normal covering of underlying collagen may be factors in the formation of thrombi in such affected vessels. It has been suggested that there are two types of inclusions: the tubuloreticular type commonly found, and a cylindric type associated with cisternae present in more acute cases.[93]

Thrombosis may be seen in capillaries, small arteries, and veins in muscle tissue obtained from children with dermatomyositis. Associated with these findings of small-vessel damage and occlusion are ischemic changes in muscle. Myofiber atrophy occurs, as does infarction, particularly at the periphery of the muscle fasciculus. In addition to the changes in the blood vessels and the muscle ischemia, changes in sarcolemmal nuclei and cytoplasmic inclusions of the muscle cells are present. Signs of muscle regeneration with enlarged satellite cells are present. Immunoglobulin, fibrin, and complement components have also been identified in or near blood-vessel walls, but these constituents have not been directly related to the presence of inflammation or to the degree of vascular damage. Vasculopathy may also occur in tissue other than skeletal muscle. Endarteropathy, marked by endothelial cell abnormalities with tubuloreticular inclusions, has been found in the superficial dermis, along with dermal infiltrates of mononuclear cells. Endarteropathy and vascular damage in the gastrointestinal tract are believed to be factors in perforation of the small intestine, a grave complication of childhood dermatomyositis.[94,95] Vascular lesions affecting the retina and skin may occur. In the skin, the dermal microvasculature may show changes of endothelial swelling and damage, as well as concentric thickening of the basement membrane. Dropout of vessels and linear deposition of collagen also may be evident. It has been suggested that children with pronounced ulcerating cutaneous vasculitis may follow a more disabling course.[96]

THEORIES OF PATHOGENESIS

The cause or causes of dermatomyositis and polymyositis are not known. Several areas, however, have served as foci for study and discussion in speculating on possible pathogenetic mechanisms. In the context, the following topics are discussed: (1) the relation of the immune system to myositis; (2) the relation of infectious disease to myositis; and (3) the association of malignant disease with myositis.

IMMUNE SYSTEM

This discussion includes aspects of humoral and cellular immunity, and genetics.

Muscle Components

Early studies demonstrated the presence of antibody with specificity for muscle tissue and its components, but such autoantibodies are not specific for patients with clinically evident myositis. Antibodies and immune reactions to myoglobin,[97] myosin,[98] filamin and vinculin,[100] and troponin and tropomyosin components[99] have been found in higher titer in patients with inflammatory muscle disease compared to controls. Immunoglobulin and complement components have been observed deposited in muscle during the course of myositis. The presence of immunoglobulin deposits is not always correlated with the presence of inflammation in the areas in which it is found, however, nor are these deposits found only in patients with myositis.[101] Further, not all investigators have found immunoglobulins or complement components in affected muscle.[102] This topic is controversial. One study concluded that immunoglobulin associated with blood vessels, connective tissue, and necrotic fibers may be nonspecifically deposited. Using the immunoperoxidase method, researchers found the mononuclear cells of the inflammatory infiltrate to contain IgG and IgM in most biopsies studied.[103] Antigens of the terminal C5b-9 membrane-attack complex of the complement system were localized to the intramuscular arterioles and capillaries in muscle biopsy specimens of most patients with childhood dermatomyositis. Such vasculopathy may be of pathogenetic significance.[90]

In experimental myositis in animals, muscle-binding antibody may appear, but its presence is not correlated with the onset of illness, and no relationship exists between the titers of such antibody and the presence or severity of myositis. In this situation, muscle-binding antibody has not been demonstrated to be injurious to muscle,[104] although under other circumstances, antibody may be pathogenic.[105]

Little or no evidence exists for abnormalities in the humoral immune capabilities of most patients with inflammatory muscle disease, although the occurrence of myositis in certain patients with immunoglobulin or complement deficiency raises this issue. Hypogammaglobulinemic disorders of both the congenital and acquired types have been observed in association with dermatomyositis and polymyositis, and a patient with inflammatory myopathy associated with a deficiency of the second component of complement has been encountered.[106–108] Whether these associations suggest a relationship of myositis with a defective immune response against an unknown provoking agent is unknown at this time. The relationship of hypogammaglobulinemia and Echovirus infection is discussed below.

Nuclear and Cytoplasmic Antigens (see Chapters 67, 68, and 70)

Using tissue-cultured cells as substrate for immunocytologic studies has shown that many patients with polymyositis have serologic reactivity. The pattern of this reactivity is nuclear in over half the tested sera, with homogeneous cytoplasmic or nucleolar staining occurring less frequently. In addition, other patterns, including centromeric and cytoplasmic filamentous, have been observed rarely.[109] In childhood dermatomyositis, 86% of one group of patients demonstrated antinuclear antibodies, with anticytoplasmic antibodies also commonly seen.[110]

Progress toward identifying the nature of the antigens involved and the relationships of serologic reactivity to the type of disease has been great, although much remains to be done. The clearest relationships between antibody and clinical pattern are antinuclear RNP and PM-SLE overlap, anti-Jo-1 with polymyositis, and anti-Mi with dermatomyositis.[109] Several additional antibody-antigen systems have also been observed, but each specificity occurs in only a fraction of patients.

The Jo-1 antibody system is found in 20 to 30% of patients with polymyositis, but much less frequently in those with dermatomyositis. Antibody to Jo-1 was found in 47% of tested patients with polymyositis, but in none with dermatomyositis or myositis associated with malignancy. Fifty percent of the Jo-1-positive patients had pulmonary involvement.[88] There may be an association between its occurrence and the presence of HLA-DR3.[111] An association has become apparent between the presence of antibody and interstitial lung disease in patients with myositis. Nine of 14 patients (64%) reported from Japan had this antibody,[112] and similar findings have been reported from England and the United States. In the American series, 8 of 17 patients with polymyositis (47%), but none with dermatomyositis, had the Jo-1 antibody. An additional 2 of 13 patients with overlap syndromes also had Jo-1. Of these 10 patients, 5 had pulmonary involvement as defined by chest roentgenographs and/or diffusing capacity tests, whereas only 14.7% of the patients without the Jo-1 antibody had such involvement.[113] In the English experience, anti-Jo-1 was found in 25% of patients with myositis, but its prevalence in patients with both myositis and fibrosing alveolitis was 68% (13 of 19).[114] The Jo-1 antigen has been characterized as histidyl-tRNA synthetase.[115] Other antibodies have been detected in sera of patients with myositis against other RNA charging enzymes. Antithreonyl-tRNA synthetase was found in sera from patients with polymyositis, and one with an SLE-like syndrome.[116,117] This specificity, estimated to be present in 5% of cases, is much less common than Jo-1. Still less common is antialanyl-tRNA synthetase, estimated to occur in approximately 3% of patients with myositis.[118] Moreover, antibodies to the tRNA synthetases for isoleucine and glycine, as well as to other cell components important in translation, have been found in patients with polymyositis.[119–121] The presence of these antisynthetases too may be correlated with interstitial lung disease, although data in this regard are still preliminary. Table 72–5 lists antibodies with specificity for translation factors discovered thus far in patients with polymyositis. Their occurrence and specificity remain an intriguing mystery in this disorder.

Because the antibodies of this type are present in only some patients with myositis, their pathogenic role is uncertain. Such antibodies may have been stimulated by other etiologically important molecules, and theories of molecular mimicry and viral causation have been proposed. Immunochemical analysis has demonstrated that anti Jo-1 antibodies recognize multiple-conformation dependent and independent epitopes that vary

TABLE 72–5. ANTIBODIES WITH SPECIFICITY FOR TRANSLATION FACTORS IN POLYMYOSITIS

TYPE	APPROXIMATE % OF PATIENTS
1. Antisynthetases	
Antihistidyl t-RNA synthetase (Jo-1)	20
Antithreonyl t-RNA synthetase (PI-7)	4
Antialanyl t-RNA synthetase (PI-12)	3
Antiisoleucyl t-RNA synthetase (OJ)	1
Antiglycyl t-RNA synthetase (EJ)	1
2. Antibodies to other cytoplasmic factors	
AntiSRP (signal recognition particle)	3
AntiKJ (translation factor)	1
AntiFer (elongation factor 10γ)	<1
AntiMas (small RNA)	<1

Based on Targoff, I.N.[260]

among different patients with myositis. The anti Jo-1 response is polyclonal, although mainly of the IgG1 type. These observations suggest that the antibodies may be "antigen-driven." This means they arise, or their production may be stimulated, by exposure to antigen, rather than as the result of nonspecific B-cell activation. This finding generates the intriguing questions of why patients with idiopathic inflammatory muscle disease react in a specific manner with cell components critical to protein translation, and whether these components are involved in disease expression.[122,123]

The Mi-antibody system consists of two components. The Mi-1 antibody cross-reacts with bovine immunoglobulin and is present in a small proportion of patients with myositis, as well as in sera from patients with other disorders.[124] The Mi-2 antibody correlates strongly with dermatomyositis, but occurs in only a minority of patients. In one study, 11 of 52 adult and pediatric patients with dermatomyositis had Mi-2 antibody demonstrated by an enzyme-linked immunosorbent assay, but it was rare or absent in other disorders or in normal individuals. The nature of the Mi antigen is not yet known.[125]

The PM-1 or PM-Scl antibody is found in about 10% of patients with myositis, approximately one half of whom also have scleroderma features, and occurs in patients with scleroderma without discernible myositis. The PM-Scl antigen is most likely a protein associated with the cell nucleus and nucleolus.[126,127]

Patients with myositis in association with other connective tissue disorders or overlap syndromes may evince a number of other antigen-antibody systems, such as anti-Ku, seen with progressive systemic sclerosis (PSS) and systemic lupus erythematosus (SLE), as well as antibodies to nRNP, Ro, Scl-70, Sm, DNA, La, cytoskeletal components, nuclear pore, and ribonucleoprotein.

Cell-Mediated Immunity

Analysis of the inflammatory cell infiltrate in biopsy samples from patients with polymyositis suggests a role of cellular immunity in disease pathogenesis.

Immunohistochemical studies reveal that cytotoxic T8 cells and macrophages invade, and may destroy, muscle fibers in polymyositis and inclusion body myositis, but not in dermatomyositis. In dermatomyositis, the inflammatory exudate is predominantly perivascular and perimysial, consisting chiefly of B-lymphocytes at perivascular sites and of T-lymphocytes (mostly T8) at endomysial sites. In polymyositis, the inflammatory exudate is predominantly endomysial and focal, although perimysial and perivascular infiltrates are also conspicuous. B cells again are most prominent perivascularly, whereas T cells are most abundant at the endomysium with a particular increase of T8 cells at these sites. In both dermatomyositis and polymyositis, the relative proportions of T cells, T8 cells, and Ia-bearing T cells increase from the perivascular areas to the endomysium. Conversely, the relative proportion of B cells and T4 cells decreases in this direction. It has been suggested in dermatomyositis that the high percentage of B cells and the high T4/T8 ratios reflect helper T-cell stimulation of B cells to secrete immunoglobulin, and that humoral immune mechanisms may therefore be of importance in this disorder. In polymyositis, the close apposition of lymphocytes and macrophages to membranes of myofibers and the invasion of non-necrotic muscle fibers of mononuclear cells suggest a more central role for cell-mediated immune mechanisms in pathogenesis.[128] T-cell cytotoxicity may be enhanced by the presence of MHC class I antigens on the surface of myofibers, in polymyositis and dermatomyositis, which permit muscle cells to function as targets in these disorders.[129] In addition, lymphocytes and monocytes may display activation markers and IL2 receptors. Soluble IL2 receptors released from activated lymphocytes and IL1 receptors from activated monocytes may be detected in the circulation of patients with active polymyositis.[130–132]

Mononuclear cells from patients with either polymyositis or dermatomyositis, after incubation with autologous muscle, release factors suppressing the ATP-dependent calcium binding of the sarcoplasmic reticulum membrane. This process may play a role in the dysfunction of the sarcoplasmic reticulum of patients with myositis and, in turn, may contribute to inefficiency of the contraction-relaxation mechanism.[133,134] Peripheral blood mononuclear cells from patients with dermatomyositis also attach to and inhibit the proliferation of cultured skin fibroblasts implicating a potential mechanism for interstitial cell damage in this disease.[135]

Genetics

The possibility of a genetic influence in dermatomyositis and polymyositis has been suggested on the basis of studies of HLA associations, but this influence is not yet understood. HLA-B8/DR3 has been noted with increased frequency in many white children with dermatomyositis,[136,137] as well as in adults with polymyositis.[138,139] In addition, a strong association exists between DR3 and the presence of Jo-1 antibodies, as well as the presence of the haplotype HLA-DRW 52 with the translation-related antibodies (antisynthetases and antisignal recognition particle).[111,140] Associations of disease with HLA-B14 and B40 have also been noted.[141] A strong association has been found in juvenile dermatomyositis with the C4 null genes. C4A null is in linkage disequilibrium with DR3 and B8.[142]

INFECTIOUS AGENTS

Skeletal muscle may be the site of inflammation in a number of infectious disorders caused by diverse agents including bacteria, protozoa, viruses, and parasites. None of these disorders has been linked to the development of chronic polymyositis; however, the possible role of infectious agents is considered in this section, particularly in relation to viruses and to toxoplasmosis.

Viruses

Several viruses may produce muscle damage and inflammation, usually of a transient nature. Among the best characterized of these are Coxsackie, echo- and influenza viruses. One such postviral syndrome of childhood is termed *benign acute myositis*. In this disorder, children develop severe lower extremity pain, usually in the calves with soreness and cramps, 24 to 72 hours after an upper respiratory infection or apparent gastroenteritis. Boys are affected more frequently than girls. The average age is approximately 9 years. The prodromal illness is marked by fever, occasionally headache, and gastrointestinal or respiratory symptoms. During the period of severe myalgia, muscles may swell. Biopsy is rarely performed; however, inflammation of muscle was observed in one girl, and in another child, no abnormalities were noted. Results of virologic studies in this syndrome are consistent with recent infection, usually with influenza virus of either type A or type B. On occasion, adenovirus and parainfluenza viruses are also implicated. Most children recover completely within a week. Creatine kinase activity of serum is elevated and returns to normal in 2 weeks.[143]

This disease has an epidemic form. In one such outbreak, 17 children developed acute myositis, chiefly involving the gastrocnemius and soleus muscles. Influenza B virus was isolated from 11 of the 17 patients. Complete recovery occurred in 4 to 5 days.[144]

Adults also have been affected with myositis following influenza virus infection. In some cases, myositis was transient; in others, severe and prolonged disease occurred with myonecrosis, myoglobinuria, and renal failure. Although documentation of viral infection is most commonly serologic, virus has been isolated from respiratory secretions, and in a 65-year-old man with inflammatory myopathy following an influenza-like syndrome, influenza B virus was recovered from affected muscle and was seen in muscle by electron microscopy.[145]

Coxsackie virus has been seen by electron microscopy and has been isolated from muscle in children with inflammatory myopathy. Elevation of antibody titers to Coxsackie B viruses has been found in some adults and children with polymyositis and dermatomyositis.[146,147] Coxsackie B virus-specific probes prepared using molecular cloning techniques were used to detect viral RNA in skeletal-muscle biopsy samples; 5 of 9 patients with clinical myositis tested positive, whereas no viral sequences were detected in muscle from 4 patients with muscular dystrophy or from 6 normal children.[148]

Another study utilizing in situ hybridization with CDNA probes found evidence of enterovirus RNA in some patients with polymyositis as well as dermatomyositis.[149] Recently, hybridization studies with RNA probes have suggested that a virus related to Theiler's murine encephalomyelitis virus may be implicated in some patients with adult dermatomyositis.[150]

Hepatitis B virus also has been implicated in the pathogenesis of inflammatory muscle disease. Several instances of hepatitis B infection followed by myositis have been observed, with deposition of immunoglobulin, complement and, in one case, hepatitis surface antigen in muscle.[151]

Echovirus infection also has been associated with myositis, including patients with X-linked hypogammaglobulinemia. Recovery of this virus has been reported from several sites. In one patient with weakness, elevated serum enzyme levels, a myopathic electromyographic pattern, and biopsy evidence of inflamed muscle and fascia, echovirus 11 was recovered from muscle and cerebrospinal fluid. Treatment with immunoglobulin preparations containing specific antibody was followed by dramatic clinical recovery in this patient.[152] Not all patients have responded well in this manner, however. Accurate diagnosis is important in this viral syndrome because usual treatment for polymyositis with immunosuppressive agents may be detrimental.[153]

Other viruses, including herpes and Epstein-Barr viruses, have been implicated in myopathy and myositis. Particles seen by electron microscopy, possibly related to picorna-type virus, have been noted in muscle in several patients with myositis, as well as in patients with Reye's syndrome. In such instances, viral identification has not been definite, and questions have been raised regarding other origins for these structures, such as degeneration of cellular components.

Polymyositis has also been reported in patients infected with the human immunodeficiency viruses. Evidence of both necrotizing as well as inflammatory myopathy has been found in patients with AIDS.[154,155] In addition, HTLV-1 may also be found in muscle and may lead to a polymyositis-like illness.[156,157]

On the basis of available information, it is possible to conclude that viruses of several types may lodge in muscle and may lead to inflammation and myonecrosis. In some cases, as in patients with hypogammaglobulinemia, host factors may be important in viral infection and in disease severity.

Toxoplasma Gondii

This protozoan organism commonly infects individuals in the United States, and asymptomatic cysts may persist in muscle.[158,159] During the early invasion of muscle in man, it is not known whether an accompanying inflammatory response occurs; however, experimental murine infections are associated with mild focal myositis.[160] In certain cases, *Toxoplasma gondii* infection of muscle has been linked to severe myopathy. In some such patients, the diagnosis of toxoplasmosis was suggested by serologic tests, as well as by response to therapy. In others, in addition to serologic evidence, *Toxoplasma* organisms were seen in muscle biopsies. Of three patients with these organisms identified in muscle, polymyositis was the diagnosis in two, and dermatomyositis in one. Central nervous system disease and fever are common in such patients.[161–163]

Serologic evidence of toxoplasmosis has also been obtained in studies of patients with polymyositis. In an age-, sex-, and race-matched controlled study, 60% of patients with polymyositis had positive Sabin-Feldman tests with titers higher than in control subjects. In addition, complement-fixing antibody, usually suggestive of recent infection, was present in greater frequency (35%) and at higher titers than in control subjects. Responses of this type were not found in the polymyositis patients tested for antibody against rubella, measles, parainfluenza, and Epstein-Barr viruses. Patients with serologic evidence of recent toxoplasmosis generally had polymyositis of less than 2 years' duration.[164] Declines in antibody titers over time and an improvement coincident with sulfa-pyrimethamine therapy have also been reported.[165] In addition, a high frequency of specific IgM anti-*Toxoplasma* antibody, suggestive of recent infection, is also found. In one study, 48% of patients with inflammatory muscle disease and positive Sabin-Feldman tests had IgM antibody.[166] Current evidence suggests high frequency of recent toxoplasmosis among certain patients with polymyositis of recent onset. It is not known, however, whether *Toxoplasma gondii* in such patients is the causative agent of polymyositis or whether dormant, persistent forms may be reactivated or reintroduced to the immune system concurrent with inflammation in muscle.

Lyme Myositis

A necrotizing myopathy may occur during the course of Lyme disease with certain features such as proximal muscle weakness, dysphagia, and elevated serum enzyme activities overlapping those of polymyositis. Biopsies of muscle reveal myofiber necrosis as well as inflammatory cell infiltrates characterized predominantly by lymphocytes of the B and CD4 T types. Spirochetes have also been observed, indicating the possibility that Lyme myositis may be the result of direct invasion of the microorganism in such patients.[167–169]

MALIGNANT DISEASE

The association of malignant disease with inflammatory myopathy may offer an important clue to the pathogenesis of myositis. The basis for this association, initially noted over 100 years ago, is still poorly understood and remains controversial. The reported frequency of malignant disease in patients with dermatomyositis varies widely; however, several series reported a rate of approximately 15 to 20% of adults. Malignant disease in children with myositis is rare, although neoplasia and coincident dermatomyositis-like syndromes have been described. One review of this aspect listed two children with leukemia, one with agammaglobulinemia followed by lymphoma, and one with pituitary adenoma.

A retrospective survey of the literature to 1976 noted 258 cases of malignant disease concurrent with myositis. Most such cases were observed in the fifth and sixth decades of life, with a mean age of 52.6 years. The most frequent tumors were cancers of the breast and lung; malignant tumors of the ovary and stomach were also common. In this group, the temporal relation of the onset of the two disorders was reported in 167 patients. In 99 of these patients, myopathy was observed first, and the malignant process was discovered later, usually within a year. In 17 patients, both diseases were noted at the same time, and in 51, the tumor appeared first, and the myopathy was recognized later, usually within a year. The frequency of malignant disease in patients with myositis was 5 to 7 times that expected in the general population. Similar results have been noted in other retrospective surveys. One study over a 20-year period noted 7 of 27 patients with both dermatomyositis and malignant disease. This frequency, 26%, was not only greater than that expected in the general population, but also was greater than that reported in patients with RA or systemic lupus erythematosus. Of this group of 7 patients, 2 had breast cancer, 2 had cancer of the colon, and 3 had cancer of an unknown primary site. In most patients, the diagnosis of malignant disease was made at the same time as the diagnosis of dermatomyositis. Adding to the general impression of the significance of this relationship are case reports of patients with multiple neoplasms in whom recurrence of dermatomyositis-like signs was observed with the recurrence of the tumor or with the appearance of a new tumor.

In another group of 35 patients with dermatomyositis seen over a 20-year period, 12 had malignant disease. Of these, 6 of 9 showed improvement in the manifestations of dermatomyositis after treatment directed toward the neoplasm, and 3 had exacerbations of dermatomyositis with progression of the neoplasm. The course of the two disorders is not always parallel, however. Although the course may not be predictable, the coexistence of these disorders generally bespeaks a grave prognosis. The types of associated malignant diseases vary, as previously indicated; most neoplasms are carcinomas originating in the lung, breast, gastrointestinal tract, nasopharynx, ovary, and uterus. Lymphomas, sarcomas, and other malignant diseases are also observed.

The reason for this concurrence is unknown. The retrospective method of enumerating published case reports may place undue emphasis on this association, and the lack of prospective study leaves unanswered the question of the precise frequency of this association. Nonetheless, on the basis of available information, it is prudent to look for this coincidence, particularly in adults with dermatomyositis.

Because of the many kinds of malignant disorders noted, the varied times of the appearance of one disease relative to the other, and the lack of a predictable direct relationship in the short-term course of the illnesses, it seems unlikely that one illness is the direct cause of the other. It is possible that an alteration in host responsiveness, perhaps involving the immune apparatus, may underlie the mechanism of the expression of both illnesses. The frequency of malignant disease among adult patients with polymyositis/dermatomyositis, therefore, is in the range of 7 to 24%. If patients are excluded from analysis because the association of these disorders (e.g., neoplasms and myositis) was widely separated in time, the frequency is reduced by approximately one half. If host factors predispose to this association, however, there may be no reason to suppose a priori that the disorders would necessarily be coincident.[5,88,170–174]

With this knowledge in mind, the clinician may face the problem of whether and how to search for an occult malignant tumor in adults with dermatomyositis. At present there is no precise answer. Several studies have questioned the advisability of extensive "nondirected" testing; others have cited cases where extensive searches have discovered potentially treatable neoplasms.[175]

OTHER DISORDERS MARKED BY MYOSITIS

DRUG-RELATED STATES

Drugs are not usually the cause of myositis, although toxic and myopathic effects of medications are known. Myositis-like states are reported rarely in patients receiving sulfonamides, penicillin, isoniazid, azathioprine, and propylthiouracil. One agent that may produce inflammatory myopathy, however, is D-penicillamine. Most patients with this complication have received this agent for the treatment of RA. In one reported case, a patient had two muscle biopsies; myositis was not present prior to therapy and was seen after treatment with D-penicillamine.[176–180]

OTHER CONNECTIVE TISSUE DISORDERS

Myositis may be a prominent feature of other connective tissue disorders. Progressive systemic sclerosis, in particular, may begin in a manner indistinguishable from polymyositis and may later develop its own characteristic features. In undifferentiated or mixed connective tissue disorders, inflammatory myopathy is often a prominent element. Myositis also may complicate the course of systemic lupus erythematosus and of sarcoidosis. Although patients with RA do not generally have clinical signs of inflammatory myopathy, histologic examination may reveal the presence of inflammation in skeletal muscle, particularly in severely affected patients.[181] Myalgia and muscle weakness are noted in approximately one third of patients with Sjögren's syndrome. Severe myositis with profound weakness and marked elevation of serum enzyme levels is less common.[182,183]

INCLUSION BODY MYOSITIS

This disorder is marked by chronic progressive wasting and weakness with microscopic inclusions seen in both nuclei and cytoplasm of skeletal muscle cells. In contrast to dermatomyositis and polymyositis, this rare disorder occurs most frequently in middle-aged or elderly men. No skin rash is present. Most cases have occurred in elderly men. The disorder is usually slowly progressive and painless. Involvement of distal, as well as proximal, musculature may be marked. This feature, combined with loss of tendon reflexes and occasional asymmetric involvement at the outset, may suggest a neuropathy. Electromyographic testing, however, has revealed both myopathic signs with polyphasic potentials of brief duration and neuropathic features, such as fibrillation and long-lasting large amplitude potentials. EMG patterns may be varied. A pattern of fibrillation potentials, positive sharp waves, and short-duration small-amplitude motor unit potentials was found in over 50% of a series of 30 patients. Fibrillation potentials and positive sharp waves with a mixed pattern of short duration, small amplitude, and long-duration high-amplitude potentials were found in over 33%; fibrillations with positive sharp waves and long-duration high-amplitude potentials were found in approximately 7%.[184] Dysphagia occurs and creatine kinase elevation of a moderate degree is present in most, but not all, patients.

The distinguishing features of this disorder are seen on histologic examination of affected muscle. In addition to evidence of myonecrosis and inflammation, eosinophilic inclusions occur in the sarcoplasm, the nucleus, or both. Rimmed or lined vacuoles filled with basophilic granules are seen on cryostat sections stained with hematoxylin and eosin. These appear purplish with the Gomori trichrome stain. Paraffin sections usually do not reveal these granules, which are likely to be removed by solvents, but they do demonstrate the empty vacuoles. The inflammatory infiltrate of inclusion body myositis resembles that of polymyositis, with concentration of CD8 T-lymphocytes at endomysial areas. Nearby myofibers express class I MHC antigens.[129]

By electron microscopy, the nuclear and/or cytoplasmic inclusions are masses of filamentous material, often in crystalline arrays. The diameters of the filaments range from 10 to 25 nm and are greater in the cytoplasm. The pathogenesis of the inclusions is uncertain. Mumps virus antigen has been demonstrated by immunohistochemical techniques in both intranuclear and cytoplasmic inclusions in 8 cases. In 5 of these, frozen sections also showed mumps antigen-positive cytoplasmic inclusions without rimmed vacuoles.[185] These observations suggest that inclusion body myositis may be the result of chronic persistent mumps virus infection; however, serum mumps antibody titers in a few patients studied have not been elevated.[186–190] In situ hybridization with cDNA probes specific for mumps virus nucleocapsid gene and immunochemical probes for mumps antigens have failed to confirm the presence of mumps virus in studied patients.[191] Adenovirus type 2 was isolated from muscle tissue in one case.[192]

Inclusion body myositis is probably underrecognized.[193] It was documented in 17% of two large series of patients with inflammatory myopathy.[187,194] It is important to differentiate it from polymyositis because its natural history and treatment are different.

The natural history of this disease in most patients is generally slowly progressive. Corticosteroids, immunosuppressive drugs, or total body irradiation[195] are ineffective in isolated inclusion body myositis. An occasional case is followed by,[196] or associated with,[197–199] a diffuse connective tissue disease (e.g., SLE, Sjögren's syndrome, or immune thrombocytopenia). Some patients do, however, respond to corticosteroid therapy, and good responses have been reported.

It has been suggested that essential pathologic features of the muscle biopsy for diagnosis are at least one rimmed vacuole per low-power field, at least one group of atrophic fibers per low-power field, as well as endomysial inflammatory exudate and demonstration of typical filamentous inclusions by electron microscopy.[200]

TROPICAL PYOMYOSITIS

This disorder is marked by abscesses, apparently spontaneously occurring in skeletal muscle. Children and young adults chiefly in tropical areas are affected. One or more skeletal muscles such as biceps, pectoral, gluteal, or quadriceps become painful and tender. An accompanying fever is usually present. The involved area may resolve spontaneously or may swell and suppurate, yielding large numbers of microorganisms, most often *Staphylococcus aureus*. The presence of multiple abscesses suggests hematogenous spread. Occasionally, clinically involved areas may be bacteriologically sterile, and this observation has led to speculation that skeletal muscle may first be damaged by an unknown agent, and then colonized by *Staphylococcus*. Among candidates for such initiating agents have been tissue parasites, other bacteria and viruses, antecedent trauma, the presence of genetically variant hemoglobin, and nutritional deficiencies. The morbidity and mortality rates for tropical pyomyositis relate to the occurrence of staphylococcal septicemia and metastatic suppurative complications, such as osteomyelitis.[201,202]

This condition is becoming recognized with increasing frequency in temperate climates: 32 cases had been recorded in the United States as of 1984.[203] Some but not all patients had traveled to the tropics before disease onset. Staphylococci predominated in these patients also, but cases resulting from *Yersinia*[204] and streptococci[205,206] have been reported. Early recognition is important because 85% of the cases associated with the latter organism have proved fatal. Computerized tomography[207] and gray-scale ultrasonography[208] have been useful diagnostic methods. One case occurred in association with diabetes mellitus and rheumatoid arthritis.

EOSINOPHILIC MYOSITIS AND HYPEREOSINOPHILIC SYNDROMES

Myositis with eosinophilic infiltration may be part of hypereosinophilic syndromes, along with involvement of other organs and the central nervous system. In some patients, anemia, hypergammaglobulinemia, petechiae, Raynaud's phenomenon, and pulmonary and cardiac manifestations have been observed. Cardiac complications include endocardial and myocardial fibrosis, congestive heart failure, and arrhythmias. Peripheral neuropathy may be present. Circulating eosinophilia, which may not be constant in all cases, can be marked, with relative proportions of 20 to 60% of the circulating leukocytes. Leukocytosis is common. Response to corticosteroid therapy is inconsistent or poor. One patient responded after leukapheresis.[209,210] Myositis also may occur during the course of eosinophilic fasciitis.[211–214] Eosinophilic myositis may have a relapsing course with a benign prognosis.[213,214]

EOSINOPHILIA MYALGIA SYNDROME (EMS)

In the fall of 1989, public health authorities were alerted to a newly recognized epidemic illness that rapidly spread across the country. Astute observation, as well as epidemiologic follow-up investigation, revealed the cause to be associated with the ingestion of certain lots of commercial L-tryptophan usually taken to promote sleep. At present, it is believed that a contaminant was responsible for this vivid and unusual illness. Its manifestations included severe disabling myalgia and cramps, fatigue, weight loss, fever, skin changes, leukocytosis, and striking eosinophilia, as well as cardiopulmonary disease with pneumonia and pleural effusions. With time, evidence of fasciitis, skin thickening, edema, and scleroderma-like features developed in about one half the patients, usually with sparing of the hands, and without overt Raynaud's phenomena. Peripheral neuropathy manifested by hyperesthesia and paresthesia appeared in approximately two thirds of affected individuals (Table 72–6). Biopsies demonstrated the presence of inflammatory infiltrates within muscle as well as in the perimysium. Predominant cells were macrophages and T-lymphocytes of the CD4 type. Eosinophils were also noted, but in smaller numbers than in the

TABLE 72–6. EOSINOPHILIA MYALGIA SYNDROME

	%
Clinical Symptoms	
Myalgia	100
Arthralgia	73
Rash	60
Peripheral edema	59
Scleroderma-like skin changes	32
Alopecia	28
Neuropathy	27
Pulmonary infiltrates	17
Pulmonary effusions	12
Laboratory Findings	
Leukocytosis	100
Eosinophilia	100
Elevated aldolase	46
Elevated erythrocyte sedimentation rate (ESR)	33
Epidemiology	
Female	84
White race	97
Over age 45	87
Tryptophan use	97

Based on data of Swygert, L.A., et al.[215]

peripheral circulation. Similar infiltrates were also seen in epineural tissues. EMG studies revealed changes of demyelination and fibrillation potentials.

By July of 1990, over 1500 cases had been reported, with 27 fatalities. Eighty-four percent of the patients were women, 97% were white, and 97% had used tryptophan. Most patients were older than 45. Laboratory studies, in addition to the marked leukocytosis and eosinophilia, demonstrated elevated aldolase in approximately one half of patients, whereas creatine kinase was elevated in only 10%. The precise course of illness is still incompletely known. Some patients have improved after discontinuing L-tryptophan; others required medications generally including corticosteroids. Most treated patients have demonstrated improvement in clinical findings. The eosinophilia resolved soon after initiation of corticosteroids. However, the neuromuscular manifestations have often been slow to change, or resistant to therapy.

Chemical analysis of implicated lots of tryptophan has focused on the presence of a contaminant that appears to be a chemical derivative of tryptophan. A recent study performed in rats has noted EMS-like changes in animals to which lots containing this contaminant have been administered.

Over 90% of cases of this epidemic were observed after May of 1989. The epidemic ended abruptly after November when the U.S. Food and Drug Administration issued a recall of L-tryptophan products. The eosinophilia myalgia syndrome has brought to mind a previous epidemic that occurred in Spain from 1981 to 1982. This disease, caused by ingestion of denatured rapeseed oil sold as cooking oil, also produced eosinophilia, myalgia, myositis, scleroderma-like changes, and a progressive neuromuscular disorder. The precise pathogenesis of these disorders remains unknown; however, further investigation may shed light on their mechanisms as well as on other inflammatory disorders and eosinophilia.[215–222]

GRANULOMATOUS MYOPATHY

This entity may be associated with other disorders such as sarcoidosis or Crohn's disease of the bowel, or it may appear without the signs of other disease. Granulomatous myopathy occurring alone is generally observed in middle-aged women who have a chronically progressive, predominantly proximal pattern of muscle weakness, occasionally complicated by dysphagia. Histologic examination reveals groups of granulomas made up of loosely packed epithelioid cells and histiocytes, often in association with lymphocytes and a surrounding rim of collagenous fibers. Reticular fibers are present in the granuloma, as well as Langerhans-type giant cells.

Myositis may occur during the course of sarcoidosis, and granulomas have been observed in muscle tissue of patients with sarcoid myopathy, as well as in patients with sarcoidosis who have no muscular symptoms.[223–225]

Myositis may also accompany *chronic enteroviral meningoencephalitis* in children with X-linked (Bruton's) agammaglobulinemia.[226]

Metabolic muscle disorders are discussed in Chapter 112.

TREATMENT

In considering the approach to therapy, one should emphasize two features: the first is accuracy of diagnosis, and the second is precision of assessment of disease activity.

It is important to secure as accurate a diagnosis as possible before initiating a treatment program that may be lengthy and possibly hazardous. In this connection, the presence of an associated malignant disease or of another connective tissue disorder may affect the patient's prognosis and response to treatment.

The assessment of disease activity and of response to therapy depends on evaluating elements of the patient's medical history, physical examination, and laboratory findings. Exacerbations of disease may have manifestations similar to those present at the onset of the disease. Return of rash, arthralgia, and the spread of areas of telangiectasia may be early warnings of exacerbation and increased disease activity. Renewed weakness may be difficult to evaluate, and other factors, including therapy and the possibility of altered electrolyte balance, should be considered in the ongoing assessment of the patient's muscle strength and function. Laboratory findings, particularly increases in creatine kinase, lactate dehydrogenase, and serum myoglobin levels and, to a lesser extent, erythrocyte sedimentation rate, may accompany or may precede an exacerbation of inflammatory muscle disease. These laboratory findings may be less reliable in the chronically ill patient than at the onset of disease. Active inflammation in muscle, as well as vasculitis, may be present and may continue in the absence of chemical evidence of active disease.[227] In addition, other factors such as trauma, injections, the performance of electromyographic studies, and exertion may lead to transient elevations of serum enzymes unrelated to the progression of the disease. Patients returning to fuller schedules of activities after a period of bed rest, or those undertaking exercise programs too taxing for their clinical status, may experience muscle aching accompanied by serum enzyme elevations. All these considerations stress the need for careful analysis of changes in the patient's condition before adjusting the program of therapy.

The major approach to treatment involves the use of medications and physical measures, with a spirit of understanding and cooperation between physician and patient. The course of illness may be protracted, and periods of depression and frustration should be anticipated.

PHYSICAL THERAPY

Rest during periods of active inflammation and physical therapy to rebuild muscle strength during periods of remission are indicated. Passive range-of-motion exercises are important to prevent the development of contractures. Despite daily therapy, however, contractures may occur and may progress in severely affected patients.

PHARMACOLOGIC THERAPY

This form of treatment includes corticosteroids and immunosuppressive agents.

Corticosteroids

Corticosteroids are the mainstay of drug treatment for most patients. Although adequately controlled data are still insufficient to indicate the degree of effectiveness of agents of this class, corticosteroid therapy is generally considered beneficial and is recommended for both adults and children. One should be aware of spontaneous remissions of disease. Retrospective examinations of overall survival have not demonstrated the absolute value of corticosteroids; however, this information may be difficult to evaluate because of the lack of simultaneous comparison groups adequately matched for diagnostic classification, time of institution of therapy in relation to disease onset, variation of doses and types of treatment, and age and sex.

The usual practice is to begin oral corticosteroid therapy in the range of 40 to 80 mg/day prednisone for approximately 4 to 6 weeks or until the maximum benefit or remission of the disease is achieved. The dose may then be gradually reduced, with careful monitoring of symptoms, physical findings, and laboratory test results. For children, doses of 1 to 2 mg/kg body weight/day are used initially. Other approaches are possible; alternate-day therapy, as well as parenteral pulse therapy, has been used.[228,229] In general, corticosteroid dosage is reduced as clinical improvement is noted.[230,231] Maintenance dosage and the need to increase therapy are decided by the patient's response and the ensuing course. The suggestion, based upon a retrospective review, has been made to give an adequately large loading dose that is continued until the creatine kinase becomes normal, and is then followed by a slow rate of reduction or taper. Recent reviews have provided algorithms for this approach to therapy.[232,233]

In both children and adults, one sees the usual potentially serious complications of corticosteroid therapy. Hypertension, cardiovascular decompensation, exacerbation of diabetes mellitus, gastrointestinal ulceration, sepsis, and osteoporosis, as well as changes in physical appearance and psychologic state, have been problems. Questions regarding corticosteroid-induced myopathy are sometimes difficult to analyze, although in many patients treated on a long-term basis, corticosteroid-induced weakness may cause protracted disability.

Most patients with myositis unassociated with malignant disease can be treated with corticosteroids alone; however, this treatment may not always be optimal. Two such situations are as follows: (1) life-threatening progressive illness without response to adequate corticosteroid therapy; and (2) partially responsive illness requiring doses of corticosteroids that have side effects difficult or impossible to tolerate. Under these circumstances, one should consider adding other forms of therapy, such as immunosuppressive agents.

The response of patients who received prednisone (40 mg or more daily) for at least 4 weeks was studied in a review of 81 patients. Over 60% achieved normal or near normal muscle strength after 3 to 4 months. Morbidity among these patients included 8 with osteoporotic vertebral compression fractures, 7 with avascular necrosis of the femoral head, 7 with complicated peptic ulcer, 7 with posterior subcapsular cataracts, and 4 with diabetes mellitus.[174]

Immunosuppressive Agents

With regard to immunosuppressive agents, two general cautions should be observed. First, adequate and complete information about the effect of these drugs in myositis is lacking. The same problems mentioned in regard to corticosteroid therapy apply here, but because these agents have been less extensively used than corticosteroids, the amount of organized, controlled data on which to base judgments is even smaller. Second, although a number of different agents are classified together by virtue of immunosuppressive activity, current evidence is insufficient to relate this factor to therapeutic effectiveness. In addition, it is not known whether any two of these agents operate in a similar manner through similar mechanisms.

A number of agents have been used, including 6-mercaptopurine and chlorambucil, but most experience has been gained with methotrexate, azathioprine, and cyclophosphamide.

Methotrexate was first employed in the treatment of dermatomyositis many years ago;[234] since then, several reports have noted its usefulness, including its corticosteroid-sparing effects that allow reduction in corticosteroid dosage.[235] Methotrexate in conjunction with corticosteroid therapy may be given intravenously, initially at doses of 10 to 15 mg at intervals of 5 to 7 days, then with gradually increasing doses up to 50 mg or higher. The frequency of administration is then reduced from weekly to biweekly, and finally to monthly. Stomatitis is the most common side effect. Hepatotoxicity, bone-marrow suppression (usually evident as leukopenia), gastrointestinal hemorrhage, skin effects, nephropathy, and reduction of normal host defense against infection may be other complications of therapy. Drug-induced pneumonitis has been reported in patients receiving oral therapy.[27] Methotrexate, in biweekly injections of 2 to 3 mg/kg body weight or 7 mg/kg body weight with citrovorum factor, has been used in conjunction with corticosteroid therapy in children.[236] Oral methotrexate in weekly doses of approximately 7.5 to 30 mg has been used successfully also, and is currently becoming a popular method of administration.

Azathioprine has been added to corticosteroid treatment. A controlled study indicated that patients treated with azathioprine and corticosteroids showed improvements in functional ability and required less prednisone for maintenance than patients treated with prednisone alone.[237] The dosage was 2 mg/kg/day until the concurrent prednisone dosage could be reduced to less than 15 mg/day; then the azathioprine dose was reduced as tolerated. In general, dosages for active disease in most studies are in the range of 100 to 150 mg/day orally, with a decrease to 50 to 75 mg/day for maintenance therapy after remission of the disease. Dosages of 50 to 125 mg/day are prescribed for children.[236] Major areas of toxicity include bone-marrow suppression, chiefly leukopenia, gastrointestinal intolerance, hepatotoxicity, and increased susceptibility to infections.

Cyclophosphamide has probably been used in fewer patients than either methotrexate or azathioprine. The dosage has not been completely evaluated, but a range of 100 to 200 mg/day has been used. Toxicity includes bone-marrow suppression, increased susceptibility to infection, alopecia, and hemorrhage from the urinary bladder. Improvement in pulmonary function tests has been noted in a small group of patients with interstitial lung disease and myositis.[238] Conflicting results, however, have been reported. One group of 11 treated patients had poor results with only 6 being able to complete the full course of therapy and only 1 having a favorable response.[239]

Cyclosporine has also been used with improvement in small groups of patients. Dosages have ranged from 2.5 to 3.5 mg/kg/day. In one case, improvement was noted in a child treated with cyclosporine alone. Not all observers have reported success with this agent, however. Nephrotoxicity and the development of hypertension represent possible untoward reactions.[240,241]

Other concerns relative to the use of these agents, except methotrexate, relate to possible genetic damage and the risk of malignant disease. These associations have not been completely evaluated in patients with myositis, but they should be considered, particularly in young patients. Overall, substantial corticosteroid-sparing effects have been noted in approximately 40 to 50% of patients treated with immunosuppressive agents.[3]

Combined Immunosuppressive Drug Therapy

Two small, uncontrolled studies have documented successful treatment of steroid-resistant dermatomyositis/polymyositis[242,243] using combined immunosuppressive agents.*

Plasmapheresis

Plasmapheresis is a newly developed mode of treatment in patients judged to have a poor response to corticosteroids and immunosuppressive agents. Patients undergoing plasmapheresis have continued to receive corticosteroids and immunosuppressive agents during the period of pheresis therapy, which has sometimes lasted for several months or more. Most of a group of 35 patients treated in this manner were judged to be improved. Herpes zoster developed in 7 of 35 patients subjected to plasmapheresis.[244,245]

OTHER THERAPEUTIC CONSIDERATIONS

Other areas of treatment include management of calcinosis, for which medical therapy has, as of yet, not been very effective. Surgical removal of troublesome deposits may be helpful.

Several patients with evidence of recent *Toxoplasma gondii* infection have received therapy directed against this organism with sulfonamides, pyrimethamine, and folinic acid.

Hydroxychloroquine, 2 to 5 mg/kg, has been used in conjunction with steroids in childhood dermatomyositis with improvement in rash and strength as well as decrease of needed prednisone therapy. However, in one series, 2 of 9 treated patients also required cytotoxic agents, and retinal changes developed in 3 patients after 1 to 2 years.[246–247] Whole-body irradiation has been used with partial success in 2 patients with refractory dermatomyositis.[248]

PROGNOSIS

CHILDREN

The outlook for complete remission is good in at least 50% of children, and results are best with early diagnosis and treatment. Although severe, unresponsive disease is less common, the course of such patients may be complicated by respiratory infection, cardiac failure, and gastrointestinal hemorrhage, all of which unfavorably influence prognosis. Fatalities have occurred. Approximately 30 to 40% of children have chronic active disease and need protracted therapy. Calcinosis and joint contractures are sources of disability that, along with residual weakness, limit return to normal function when remission has occurred. Physical therapy, although not always effective, should be an early part of the therapeutic program to maximize chances for mobility and to decrease the likelihood of disabling contractures. The duration of disease activity in most children is generally 2 to 4 years.[227,231,249]

In one retrospective study, a monocyclic disease pattern was present in 25% of children, with full recovery in 2 years. The remainder had either a chronic, continuous, persistent pattern of disease or a polycyclic course with periods not requiring therapy and periods of relapses.[250] Rarely, late relapses in apparently well children may occur.[251]

ADULTS

The outlook in adult patients does not appear to be as good as in children. In general, patients with malignant disease have a poor outcome. Patients under 20 years

* *Editor's note:* I have relied on intravenous methotrexate combined with low-dose (50 to 100 mg/day) azathioprine for many years with gratifying results.[15]

of age have better chances for survival than those over age 55. Intercurrent infections, particularly pneumonia, severe muscle weakness, chronically active disease, and dysphagia all unfavorably influence prognosis. The overall survival rate has varied in several studied groups. One retrospective survey, which did not include patients with malignant disease, indicated a mortality rate of 39% in the first year.[252] A cumulative survival rate of 53% after 7 years was observed in a group of over 100 patients,[253] whereas a lower mortality rate of 28% was noted in another group of similar size after 6 years.[6] Taken together, the experience indicates a substantial mortality rate in adults with inflammatory muscle disease, even in groups from which patients with cancer have been excluded. In addition, most surviving patients have long-term disability and need medication. Relapses are common, and many, perhaps 20 to 30% of patients, demonstrate disease activity with deterioration of strength or elevation of serum enzyme levels and erythrocyte sedimentation rate for over 10 years. Many patients have a static clinical state with elevated serum enzyme levels for long periods.

Histologic estimate of the severity of abnormalities demonstrated by muscle biopsy is not a generally reliable indicator of outcome.

The outlook in the future, however, may not necessarily be as gloomy as these figures suggest. In one large series of patients, the mortality rate was 13.7% after a mean follow-up period of 4.3 years; 25% of the deaths were due to malignant disease, and 20% were due to sepsis. Recognition and prompt treatment of infections as well as careful monitoring and adjustment of medications may reduce the severity of complications and may improve the overall prognosis.[8]

A retrospective review of 27 patients indicated a more favorable outcome, with 52% of patients able to discontinue steroid therapy within an average 4½-year period of follow up.[254] A similar result was obtained in a Canadian series in which 42% of patients, by life-table analysis, terminated corticosteroids within 3 years of diagnosis. Thirty-two percent of these patients died, however, and functional disability was common.[255] Mortality rates over a 10-year period studied by review of death records indicated greatest overall mortality for nonwhite women.[256]

Factors that affect prognosis include age, cardiopulmonary disease, and dysphagia. A positive correlation has been found between age at diagnosis and duration of therapy, implying that older patients require longer treatment and do less well. In addition, delay in diagnosis has been associated with a poorer outcome, particularly in patients whose initiation of treatment was later than 24 months after the onset of muscular weakness.[257,258] Cutaneous necrotic lesions, especially on the trunk, in patients with dermatomyositis also were associated with a higher mortality.[259]

Of 39 patients aged 45 and older in another series, 30.8% died, compared to 2.7% of younger patients. Cardiac involvement also indicates a poor prognosis. Dysphagia occurred in the more severely ill patients, with a shortened life expectancy. The cumulative survival of all patients in this study was 73% after 8 years, which probably reflects a trend toward better outcomes in recent years.[88]

REFERENCES

1. Bohan, A., and Peter, J.B.: Polymyositis and dermatomyositis. N. Engl. J. Med., *292*:344–347, 403–407, 1975.
2. Walton, J.N., and Adams, R.D.: Polymyositis. Edinburgh, E.S. Livingstone, 1958.
3. Pearson, C.M., and Bohan, A.: The spectrum of polymyositis and dermatomyositis. Med. Clin. North Am., *61*:439–457, 1977.
4. Thompson, C.E.: Infantile myositis. Dev. Med. Child. Neurol., *24*:307–313, 1982.
5. Medsger, T.A., Dawson, W.N., and Masi, A.T.: The epidemiology of polymyositis. Am. J. Med. *48*:715–723, 1970.
6. DeVere, R., and Bradley, W.G.: Polymyositis: Its presentation, morbidity and mortality. Brain, *98*:637–666, 1975.
7. Pearson, C.M.: Polymyositis. Annu. Rev. Med., *17*:63–82, 1966.
8. Bohan, A., Peter, J.B., Bousman, R.L., et al.: A computer-assisted analysis of 153 patients with polymyositis and dermatomyositis. Medicine, *56*:255–286, 1977.
9. Pearson, C.M.: Polymyositis and dermatomyositis. *In* Arthritis and Allied Conditions, 9th Ed. Edited by D.J. McCarty. Philadelphia, Lea & Febiger, 1979, pp. 742–761.
10. Gardner-Medwin, D., and Walton, J.N.: The clinical examination of the voluntary muscles. *In* Disorders of Voluntary Muscle. Edited by J.N. Walton. Edinburgh, Churchill Livingstone, 1974, pp. 517–560.
11. Edwards, R.H.T., Wiles, C.M., and Round, J.M.: et al.: Muscle breakdown and repair in polymyositis. A case study. Muscle Nerve, *2*:223–229, 1979.
12. Young, A., and Edwards, R.H.T.: Dynamometry and muscle disease. Arch. Phys. Med. Rehabil., *62*:295–296, 1981.
13. Kroll, M.A., Otis, J.C., and Kagen, L.J.: Abnormalities in quadriceps-hamstring strength relationships in polymyositis and dermatomyositis. J. Rheum., *15*:1782–1788, 1988.
14. Kroll, M., Otis, J., and Kagen, L.: Serum enzyme, myoglobin and muscle strength relationships in polymyositis and dermatomyositis. J. Rheumatol., *13*:349–355, 1986.
15. Csuka, M.E., and McCarty, D.J.: A rapid method for measurement of lower extremity muscle strength. Am. J. Med., *78*:77–81, 1985.
16. Maricq, H.R., and LeRoy, E.C.: Patterns of finger capillary abnormalities in connective tissue diseases by "wide-field" microscopy. Arthritis Rheum., *16*:619–628, 1973.
17. Ganczarczyk, M.L., Lee, P., and Armstrong, S.K.: Nailfold capillary microscopy in polymyositis and dermatomyositis. Arthritis Rheum., *31*:116–119, 1988.
18. Feldman, D., Hochberg, M.C., Zizic, T., et al: Cutaneous vasculitis in adult polymyositis/dermatomyositis. J. Rheumatol., *10*:85–89, 1983.
19. Itoh, J., Akiquohi, I., Miderikena, R., et al.: Sarcoid myopathy with typical rash of dermatomyositis. Neurology, *30*:1118–1121, 1980.
20. Krain, L.S.: Dermatomyositis in 6 pateints without initial muscle involvement. Arch. Dermatol., *111*:241–245, 1975.
21. Janis, J.F., and Winkelmann, R.K.: Histopathology of the skin in dermatomyositis. Arch. Dermatol., 97:640–650, 1968.
22. Kagen, L.J., Hochman, R.B., and Strong, E.W.: Cricopharyngeal obstruction in inflammatory myopathy (polymyositis/dermatomyositis). Arthritis Rheum., *28*:630–636, 1985.

23. Wintzen, A.R., Bots, G.T.A.M., deBakker, H.M., et al.: Dysphagia in inclusion body myositis. J. Neurol. Neurosurg. Psychiatry, *51*:1542–1545, 1988.
24. Dietz, F., Logeman, J.A., Sahgal, V., et al.: Cricopharyngeal muscle dysfunction in the differential diagnosis of dysphagia in polymyositis. Arthritis Rheum., *23*:491–495, 1980.
25. De Merieux, P., Verity, M.A., Clements, R.J., and Paulus, H.E.: Esophageal abnormalities and dysphagia in polymyositis and dermatomyositis. Arthritis Rheum., *26*:961–968, 1983.
26. Horowitz, M., McNeil, J.D., Maddern, G.J., et al.: Abnormalities of gastric and esophageal emptying in polymyositis and dermatomyositis. Gastroenterology, *90*:434–439, 1986.
27. Arnett, F.C., Welton, J.C., Zizic, T.M., et al.: Methotrexate therapy in polymyositis. Ann. Rheum. Dis., *32*:536–546, 1973.
28. Hebert, C.A., Byrnes, T.J., Baethqe, B.A., et al.: Exercise limitation in patients with polymyositis. Chest, *98*:352–357, 1990.
29. Tazelaar, H.D., Viggiano, R.W., Pickersgill, J., and Colby, T.V.: Interstitial lung disease in polymyositis and dermatomyositis. Am. Rev. Respir. Dis., *141*:727–733, 1990.
30. Duncan, P.E., Griffin, J. P., Garcia, A., et al.: Fibrosing alveolitis in polymyositis. Am. J. Med., *57*:621–626, 1974.
31. Fergusson, R.J., Davidson, N., Nuki, G., et al.: Dermatomyositis and rapidly progressive fibrosing alveolitis. Thorax, *38*:71–72, 1983.
32. Frazier, A.R., and Miller, R.D.: Interstitial pneumonitis in association with polymyositis and dermatomyositis. Chest, *65*: 403–407, 1974.
33. Salmeron, G., Greenberg, D., and Lidsky, M.D.: Polymyositis and diffuse interstitial lung disease. Arch. Intern. Med., *141*:1005–1010, 1981.
34. Schwarz, M.I., Matthay, R.A., Sahn, S.A., et al.: Interstitial lung disease in polymyositis and dermatomyositis: analysis of six cases and review of the literature. Medicine, 55:89–104, 1976.
35. Braun, N.M.T., Arora, N.S., and Rochester, D.F.: Respiratory muscle and pulmonary function in polymyositis and other proximal myopathies. Thorax, *38*:616–623, 1983.
36. Dickey, B.F., and Myers, A.R.: Pulmonary disease in polymyositis/dermatomyositis. Semin. Arthritis Rheum., *14*:60–76, 1984.
37. Gottdiener, J.S., Sherbes, H.S., Hawley, R.J., et al.: Cardiac manifestations in polymyositis. Am. J. Cardiol., *41*:1141–1149, 1978.
38. Henderson, A., Cummings, W.J., Williams, D.O., et al.: Cardiac complications of polymyositis. J. Neurol. Sci., *47*:425–429, 1980.
39. Denbow, C.E., Lie, J.T., Tancredi, R., et al.: Cardiac involvement in polymyositis. Arthritis Rheum., *22*:1088–1092, 1979.
40. Haupt, H.M., and Hutchins, G.M.: The heart and cardiac conducting system in polymyositis-dermatomyositis. Am. J. Cardiol., *50*:998–1006, 1982.
41. Stern, R., Goodbold, J.H., Chess, Q., and Kagen, L.J.: ECG abnormalities in polymyositis. Arch. Intern. Med., *44*:2185–2189, 1984.
42. Blane, C.E., White, S.J., Braunstein, E.M., et al.: Patterns of calcification in childhood dermatomyositis. Am. J. Rad., *142*:397–400, 1984.
43. Sarmiento, A.H., Alba, J., Lanaro, A.E., et al.: Evaluation of soft-tissue calcifications in dermatomyositis with ^{99m}Tc-phosphate compounds: Case report. J. Nucl. Med., *16*:467–468, 1975.
44. Kagen, L.J.: Myoglobinemia and myoglobinuria in patients with myositis. Arthritis Rheum., *14*:457–464, 1971.
45. Dyck, R.F., Katz, A., Gordon, D.A., et al.: Glomerulonephritis associated with polymyositis. J. Rheumatol., *6*:336–344, 1979.
46. Kamata, K., Kobayashi, Y., Shigematsu, H., et al.: Childhood type polymyositis and rapidly progressive glomerulonephritis. Acta Pathol. Jpn., *32*:801–806, 1982.
47. Cumming, W.J.K., Weiser, R., Tech, R., et al.: Localized nodular myositis: A clinical and pathological variant of polymyositis. Q. J. Med., *46*:531–546, 1977.
48. Heffner, R.R., and Barron, S.A.: Polymyositis beginning as a focal process. Arch. Neurol., *38*:439–442, 1981.
49. Kalyanaraman, K., and Kalyanaraman, U.P.: Localized myositis presenting as pseudothrombophlebitis. Arthritis Rheum., *25*:1374–1377, 1982.
50. Pachman, L.M., and Cooke, N.: Juvenile dermatomyositis. A clinical and immunological study. J. Pediatr., *96*:226–234, 1980.
51. Spencer-Green, G., Crowe, W.E., and Levinson, J.E.: Nailfold capillary abnormalities and clinical outcome in childhood dermatomyositis. Arthritis Rheum., *25*:954–958, 1982.
52. Silver, R.M., and Maricq, H.R.: Childhood dermatomyositis: Serial microvascular studies. Pediatrics, *83*:278–283, 1989.
53. Banker, B.Q., and Victor, M.: Dermatomyositis (systemic angiopathy) of childhood. Medicine, *45*:261–289, 1966.
54. Downey, E.C., Jr., Woolley, M.M., and Hanson, V.: Required surgical therapy in the pediatric patient with dermatomyositis. Arch. Surg., *123*:1117–1120, 1988.
55. Winfield, J.: Juvenile dermatomyositis with complications. Proc. R. Soc. Med., *70*:548–551, 1977.
56. Guttierez, G., Dagnino, R., and Mintz, G.: Polymyositis/dermatomyositis and pregnancy. Arthritis Rheum., *27*:291–294, 1986.
57. King, C.R., and Chow, S.: Dermatomyositis and pregnancy. Obstet. Gynecol., *66*:589–592, 1985.
58. Kitridou, R.C.: Pregnancy in mixed connective disease, poly/dermatomyositis and scleroderma. Clin. Exp. Rheumatol., *6*:173–178, 1988.
59. Pennington, R.T.: Biochemical aspects of muscle disease. *In* Disorders of Voluntary Muscle. Edited by J.N. Walton. New York, Churchill Livingstone, 1981, pp. 415–447.
60. Vignos, P.J., and Goldwin, J.: Evaluation of laboratory tests in diagnosis and management of polymyositis. Am. J. Med., *263*:291–308, 1972.
61. Farrington, C., and Chalmers, A.H.: The effect of dilution on creatine kinase activity. Clin. Chim. Acta., *73*:217–219, 1976.
62. Roberts, R., and Sobel, B.E.: Effect of selected drugs and myocardial infarction on the disappearance of creatine kinase from the circulation in conscious dogs. Cardiovasc. Res., *11*:103–112, 1977.
63. Munsat, T.L., and Bradley, W.G.: Serum creatine phosphokinase levels and prednisone treated muscle weakness. Neurology, *27*:96–97, 1977.
64. Fudman, E.J., and Schnitzer, T.J.: Dermatomyositis without creatine kinase elevation. A poor prognostic sign. Am. J. Med., *80*:329–332, 1986.
65. Dawson, D.M., and Fine, I.H.: Creatine kinase in human tissues. Arch. Neurol., *16*:175–180, 1967.
66. Jockers-Wretou, E., and Pfleiderer, G.: Quantitation of creatine kinase isoenzymes in human tissues by an immunological method. Clin. Chim. Acta, *58*:223–232, 1975.
67. Mercer, D.W.: Separation of tissue and serum creatine kinase in human tissues. Arch. Neurol., *16*:175–180, 1967.
68. Brownlow, K., and Elevitch, F.R.: Serum creatine phosphokinase iso-enzyme (CPK_2) in myositis. J.A.M.A., *230*:1141–1144, 1974.
69. Goto, I.: Creatine phosphokinase isoenzymes in neuromuscular disorders. Arch. Neurol., *31*:116–119, 1974.
70. Larca, L.J., Coppola, J.T., and Honig, S.: Creatine kinase MB isoenzyme in dermatomyositis: A noncardiac source. Ann. Intern. Med., *94*:341–343, 1981.

71. Morton, B.D., III, and Statland, B.E.: Serum enzyme alterations in polymyositis. Am. J. Clin. Pathol., *73*:556–557, 1980.
72. Eppenberger, H.M., Richterich, R., and Aebi, H.: The ontogeny of creatine kinase isoenzymes. Dev. Biol., *10*:1–16, 1964.
73. Lough, J., and Bischoff, R.: Differentiation of creatine phosphokinase during myogenesis. Quantitative fractionation of isoenzymes. Dev. Biol., *57*:330–334, 1977.
74. Turner, D.C., Maier, V., and Eppenberger, H.M.: Creatine kinase and aldolase isoenzyme transitions in cultures of chick skeletal muscle cells. Dev. Biol., *37*:63–89, 1974.
75. Kagen, L.J.: Myoglobin: Methods and diagnostic uses. CRC Crit. Rev. Clin. Lab. Sci., *9*:273–320, 1978.
76. Kagen, L.J.: Myoglobinemia in inflammatory myopathies. J.A.M.A., *237*:1448–1452, 1977.
77. Nishikai, M., and Reichlin, M.: Radioimmunoassay of serum myoglobin in polymyositis and other conditions. Arthritis Rheum., *20*:1514–1518, 1977.
78. Bombardieri, S., Clerics, A., Riente, L., et al.: Circadian variations of serum myoglobin levels in normal subjects and patients with polymyositis. Arthritis Rheum., *25*:1419–1424, 1982.
79. Daube, J.R.: The description of motor unit potentials in electromyography. Neurology, *28*:623–625, 1978.
80. Henricksson, K.-G., and Stalberg, E.: The terminal innervation pattern in polymyositis; a histochemical and SFEMG study. Muscle Nerve, *1*:3–13, 1978.
81. Edwards, R.H.T., Isenberg, D.A., Wiles, C.H., et al.: The investigation of inflammatory myopathy. J. R. Coll. Physicians Lond., *15*:19–24, 1981.
82. Schwarz, H.A., Slavin, G., Ward, P., et al.: Muscle biopsy in polymyositis and dermatomyositis. A clinicopathological study. Ann. Rheum. Dis., *39*:500–507, 1980.
83. Duance, V.C., Black, C.H., Dubowitz, V., et al.: Polymyositis—an immunofluorescence study on the distribution of collagen types. Muscle Nerve, *3*:487–490, 1980.
84. Mastaglia, F.L., and Kakulas, B.A.: A histological and histochemical study of skeletal muscle regeneration of polymyositis. J. Neurol. Sci., *10*:471–487, 1970.
85. Myllyla, R., Myllyla, V.V., Tolonen, U., et al.: Changes in collagen metabolism in diseased muscle. I. Biochemical studies. Arch. Neurol., *39*:752–755, 1982.
86. Peltonen, L., Myllyla, R., Tolonen, U., et al.: Changes in collagen metabolism in diseased muscle. II. Immunohistochemical studies. Arch. Neurol., *39*:756–759, 1982.
87. Chou, S.-M., Nonaka, I., and Voice, G.F.: Anastomoses of transverse tubules with terminal cisternae in polymyositis. Arch. Neurol., *37*:257–266, 1980.
88. Hochberg, M.C., Feldman, D., and Stevens, M.B.: Adult onset polymyositis/dermatomyositis: An analysis of clinical and laboratory features and survival in 76 patients with a review of the literature. Semin. Arthritis Rheum., *15*:168–178, 1986.
89. Emslie-Smith, A.M., and Engel, A.G.: Microvascular changes in early and advanced dermatomyositis: A quantitative study. Ann. Neurol., *27*:343–356, 1990.
90. Kissel, J.T., Mendell, J.R., and Rommohan, K.W.: Microvascular deposition of complement membrane attack complex in dermatomyositis. N. Engl. J. Med., *314*:329–334, 1986.
91. Devisser, M., Emslie-Smith, A.M., and Engel, A.G.: Early ultrastructural alterations in adult dermatomyositis: Capillary abnormalities precede other structural changes in muscle. J. Neurol. Sci., *94*:181–192, 1989.
92. Scott, J.P., and Arroyave, C.: Activation of complement and coagulation in juvenile dermatomyositis. Arthritis Rheum., *30*:572–576, 1987.
93. Fidzianska, A., and Goebel, H.H.: Tubuloreticular structures (TRS) and cylindric confronting cisternae (CCC) in childhood dermatomyositis. Acta Neuropathol., *79*:310–316, 1989.
94. Banker, B.Q.: Dermatomyositis of childhood. J. Neuropathol. Exp. Neurol., *34*:46–75, 1975.
95. Crowe, W.E., Bove, K.E., Levinson, J.E., et al.: Clinical and pathogenetic implications of histopathology in childhood polydermatomyositis. Arthritis Rheum., *25*:126–139, 1982.
96. Bowyer, S.L., Clark, R.A.F., Ragsdale, C.G., et al.: Juvenile dermatomyositis: Histological findings and pathogenetic hypothesis for the associated skin changes. J. Rheumatol., *13*:753–759, 1986.
97. Herrera-Esparza, R., Magana, L., Moreno, J., et al.: Cell-mediated immunity to myoglobin in polymyositis. Ann. Rheum. Dis., *42*:182–186, 1983.
98. Wada, K., Ueno, S., Hazawa, T., et al.: Radioimmunoassay for antibodies to human skeletal muscle myosin in serum from patients with polymyositis. Clin. Exp. Immunol., *52*:297–304, 1983.
99. Koga, K., Abe, S., Hashimoto, H., and Yamaguchi, M.: Western-blotting method for detecting antibodies against human muscle contractile proteins in myositis. J. Immunol. Methods, *105*:15–21, 1987.
100. Yamamoto, T., Furukawa, S., Nojima, M., et al.: Anti-filamin and -vinculin antibodies in sera from patients with myasthenia gravis and polymyositis. Proc. Jpn. Acad. Ser. B., *62*:113–116, 1986.
101. Whitaker, J.N., and Engel, W.K.: Vascular deposits of immunoglobulin and complement in idiopathic inflammatory myopathy. N. Engl. J. Med., *286*:333–338, 1972.
102. Fessel, W.J., and Raas, M.C.: Autoimmunity in the pathogenesis of muscle disease. Neurology, *18*:1137–1139, 1968.
103. Fulthorpe, J.J., and Hudgson, P.I.: Immunocytochemical localization of immunoglobulins in the inflammatory lesions of polymyositis. J. Neuroimmunol., *2*:145–154, 1982.
104. Dawkins, R.L., Eghtedari, A., and Holborow, E.J.: Antibodies to skeletal muscle demonstrated by immunofluorescence in experimental autoallergic myositis. Clin. Exp. Immunol., *9*:329–337, 1971.
105. Korenyi-Both, A., and Kelemen, G.: Damage of skeletal muscle in rats by immunoglobulins. Acta Neuropathol., *34*:199–206, 1976.
106. Giuliano, V.J.: Polymyositis in a patient with acquired hypogammaglobulinemia. Am. J. Med. Sci., *268*:53–56, 1974.
107. Janeway, C.A., Gitlin, D., Craig, J.H., et al.: "Collagen disease" in patients with congenital agammaglobulinemia. Trans. Assoc. Am. Physicians, *69*:93–97, 1956.
108. Leddy, J.P., Griggs, R.C., Klemperer, M.R., et al.: Hereditary complement (C2) deficiency with dermatomyositis. Am. J. Med., *58*:83–91, 1975.
109. Reichlin, M., and Arnett, F.C.: Multiplicity of antibodies in myositis sera. Arthritis Rheum., *27*:1150–1156, 1984.
110. Montecucco, G., Revelli, A., Caporali, R., et al.: Autoantibodies in juvenile dermatomyositis. Clin. Exp. Rheumatol., *8*:193–196, 1990.
111. Arnett, F.C., Hirsch, T.J., Bias, W.B., et al.: The Jo-1 antibody system in myositis. Relationships to clinical features and HLA. J. Rheumatol., *8*:925–930, 1981.
112. Yoshida, S., Akizuki, M., Mimori, T., et al.: The precipitating antibody to an acidic nuclear antigen, the Jo-1, in connective tissue diseases, a marker for a subset of polymyositis with interstitial pulmonary fibrosis. Arthritis Rheum., *26*:606–611, 1983.
113. Hochberg, M.C., Feldman, D., Stevens, M.B., et al.: Antibody to Jo-1 in polymyositis/dermatomyositis: association with interstitial pulmonary disease. J. Rheumatol., *11*:663–665, 1984.
114. Bernstein, R.M., Morgan, S.H., Chapman, J., et al.: Anti-Jo-1 antibody: A marker for myositis with interstitial lung disease. Br. Med. J., *289*:151–152, 1984.
115. Mathews, M.B., and Bernstein, R.M.: Myositis autoantibody

inhibits histidyl-tRNA synthetase: A model for autoimmunity. Nature, *304*:177–179, 1983.

116. Mathews, M.B., Reichlin, M., Hughes, G.R.V., and Bernstein, R.M.: Anti-threonyl—tRNA synthetase, a second myositis-related autoantibody. J. Exp. Med., *160*:420–434. 1984.
117. Okada, N., Mukai, R., Harada, F., et al.: Isolation of a novel antibody, which precipitates ribonucleoprotein complex containing threonine tRNA from a patient with polymyositis. Eur. J. Biochem., *139*:425–429, 1984.
118. Bunn, C.C., Bernstein, R.M., and Mathews, M.B.: Autoantibodies against alanyl-tRNA synthetase and tRNA ala coexist and are associated with myositis. J. Exp. Med., *163*:1281–1291, 1986.
119. Targoff, I.N., Arnett, F.C., Berman, L., et al.: Anti KJ: A new antibody associated with the syndrome of polymyositis and interstitial lung disease. J. Clin. Invest., *84*:162–172, 1989.
120. Targoff, I.N.: Autoantibodies to aminoacyl-transfer RNA synthetases for isoleucine and glycine. J. Immunol., *144*:1737–1743, 1990.
121. Targoff, I.N., Johnson, A.E., and Miller, E.W.: Antibody to signal recognition particle in polymyositis. Arthritis Rheum., *33*:1361–1370, 1990.
122. Ramsden, D.A., Chen, J., Miller, F.W., et al.: Epitope mapping of the cloned human autoantigen histidyl-tRNA synthetase. J. Immunol., *143*:2267–2272, 1989.
123. Miller, F.W., Twitty, S.A., Biswas, T., and Plotz, P.H.: Origin and regulation of a disease-specific autoantibody response. J. Clin. Invest., *85*:468–475, 1990.
124. Targoff, I.M., Raghi, G., and Reichlin, M.: Antibodies to Mi-1 in SLE; relationship to other precipitins and reaction with bovine immunoglobulin. Clin. Exp. Immunol., *53*:76–82, 1983.
125. Targoff, I.N., and Reichlin, M.: The association between Mi-2 antibodies and dermatomyositis. Arthritis Rheum., *28*:796–803, 1985.
126. Treadwell, E.L., Alspaugh, M.A., Wolfe, J.F., and Sharp, G.C.: Clinical relevance of PM-1 antibody and physiochemical characterization of PM-1 antigen. J. Rheumatol., *11*:658–662, 1984.
127. Wolfe, J.F., Adelstein, E., and Sharp, G.C.: Antinuclear antibody with distinct specificity for polymyositis. J. Clin. Invest., *59*:176–178, 1977.
128. Engel, A.H., and Arahata, K.: Mononuclear cells in myopathies. Hum. Pathol., *17*:704–721, 1986.
129. Figarella-Branger, D., Pellissier, J.E., Bianco, N., et al.: Inflammatory and non-inflammatory inclusion body myositis. Acta Neuropathol., *79*:528–536, 1990.
130. Giorno, R., and Ringel, S.P.: Analysis of macrophages, activated cells and T cell subsets in inflammatory myopathies using monoclonal antibodies. Pathol. Immunopathol. Res., *5*:491–499, 1986.
131. Miller, F.W., Love, L.A., Barbieri, S.A., et al.: Lymphocyte activation markers in idiopathic myositis: Changes with disease activity and differences among clinical and autoantibody groups. Clin. Exp. Immunol., *81*:373–379, 1990.
132. Wolf, R.E., and Baethge, B.A.: Interleukin-1γ, interleukin-2, and soluble interleukin-2· receptors in polymyositis. Arthritis Rheum., *33*:1007–1014, 1990.
133. Kalovidouris, A.: Mononuclear cells from patients with polymyositis inhibit calcium binding by sarcoplasmic reticulum. J. Lab. Clin. Med., *107*:23–28, 1986.
134. Kalovidouris, A.E.: Dysfunction of the sarcoplasmic reticulum in polymyositis. Arthritis Rheum., *27*:299–304, 1984.
135. Saito, E., Kinoshita, M., Oshima, H., et al.: Damaging effect of peripheral mononuclear cells of dermatomyositis on cultured human skin fibroblasts. J. Rheumatol., *14*:936–941, 1987.
136. Friedman, J.M., Pachman, L.M., Maryjowski, M.L., et al.: Immunogenetic studies of juvenile dermatomyositis. Tissue Antigens, *21*:45–49, 1983.
137. Pachman, L.M., Jonasson, O., Cannon, R.A., and Friedman, J.M.: HLA-B8 in juvenile dermatomyositis. Lancet, *2*:567–568, 1977.
138. Behan, W.M.H., Behan, P.O., and Dick, H.A.: HLA-B8 in polymyositis. N. Engl. J. Med., *298*:1260–1261, 1978.
139. Hirsch, T.J., Enlow, R.W., Bias, W.B., et al.: HLA-D related (DR) antigens in various kinds of myositis. Hum. Immunol., *3*:181–186, 1981.
140. Goldstein, R., Duvic, M., Targoff, I.N., et al.: HLA-D region genes associated with autoantibody responses to histidyl-transfer RNA synthetase (Jo-1) and other translation-related factors in myositis. Arthritis Rheum., *33*:1240–1248, 1990.
141. Cumming, W.J.K., Hudgson, P., Lattimer, D., et al.: HLA and serum complement in polymyositis. Lancet, *2*:978–979, 1977.
142. Robb, S.A., Fielder, A.H.L., Saunders, C.E., et al.: C4 complement allotypes in juvenile dermatomyositis. Hum. Immunol., *22*:31–38, 1988.
143. Antony, J.H., Procopis, P.C., and Ouvrier, R.A.: Benign acute childhood myositis. Neurology, *29*:1068–1071, 1979.
144. Dietzman, D.E., Schaller, J.G., Ray, G., et al.: Acute myositis associated with influenza B infection. Pediatrics, *57*:255–258, 1976.
145. Gamboa, E.T., Eastwood, A.B., Hays, A.P., et al.: Isolation of influenza virus in myoglobinuric polymyositis. Neurology, *29*:1323–1335, 1979.
146. Christensen, M.L., Pachman, L.M., Schneiderman, R., et al.: Prevalence of Coxsackie B virus antibodies in patients with juvenile dermatomyositis. Arthritis Rheum., *29*:1365–1370, 1986.
147. Travers, R.L., Hughes, G.R.V., Cambridge, G., et al.: Coxsackie B neutralisation titres in polymyositis/dermatomyositis. Lancet, *1*:1268, 1977.
148. Bowles, N.E., Sewry, C.A., Dubowitz, V., et al.: Dermatomyositis, polymyositis and Coxsackie B virus infection. Lancet, *1*:1004–1007, 1987.
149. Yousef, G.E., Isenberg, D.A., and Mowbray, J.F.: Detection of enterovirus specific RNA sequences in muscle biopsy specimens from patients with adult onset myositis. J. Rheum. Dis., *49*:310–315, 1990.
150. Rosenberg, N.L., Rotbart, H.A., Abzug, M.J., et al.: Evidence for a novel picorna virus in human dermatomyositis. Ann. Neurol., *26*:204–208, 1989.
151. Damjanov, I., Moser, R.L., Katz, S.M., et al.: Immune complex myositis associated with viral hepatitis. Hum. Pathol., *11*:478–481, 1980.
152. Mease, P.J., Ochs, H.D., and Wedgewood, R.J.: Successful treatment of ECHO virus meningoencephalitis and myositis-fasciitis with intravenous immune globulin therapy in a patient with X-linked agammaglobulinemia. N. Engl. J. Med., *304*:1278–1281, 1981.
153. Crennan, J.M., VanScoy, R.E., McKenna, C.H., and Smith, T.F.: Echovirus polymyositis in patients with hypogammaglobulinemia. Am. J. Med., *81*:35–42, 1986.
154. Gabbai, A.A., Schmidt, B., Castelo, A., et al.: Muscle biopsy in AIDS and ARC: Analysis of 50 patients. Muscle Nerve, *13*:541–544, 1990.
155. Wrzolek, M.A., Sher, J.H., Kozlowski, P.B., and Chandrakant, R.: Skeletal muscle pathology in AIDS: An autopsy study. Muscle Nerve, *13*:508–515, 1990.
156. Morgan, O. StC., Mora, C., Rodgers-Johnson, P., and Char, G.: HTLV-1 and polymyositis in Jamaica. Lancet, *2*:1184–1187, 1989.
157. Wiley, C.A., Nerenberg, M., Cros, D., and Soto-Aguilar, M.C.: HTLV-1 polymyositis in a patient also infected with the human immunodeficiency virus. N. Engl. J. Med., *320*:992–995, 1989.
158. Feldman, H.A., and Miller, L.T.: Serological study of toxoplasmosis prevalence. Am. J. Hyg., *64*:320–335, 1956.

159. Remington, J.S., and Cavanaugh, E.N.: Isolation of the encysted form of *Toxoplasma gondii* from human skeletal muscle and brain. N. Engl. J. Med., *273*:1308–1310, 1965.
160. Henry, L., and Beverley, J.K.A.: Experimental myocarditis and myositis in mice. Br. J. Exp. Pathol., *50*:230–238, 1969.
161. Fonseca, R.C., Mullner, F., Segura, J.J., et al.: Miositis toxoplasmica aguda en un adulto. Acta Med. Cost., *16*:75–78, 1973.
162. Greenlee, J.E., Johnson, W.D., Jr., Campa, J.F., et al.: Adult toxoplasmosis presenting as polymyositis and cerebellar ataxia. Ann. Intern. Med., *82*:367–371, 1973.
163. Hendrickx, G.G.M., Verhage, J., Jennekens, P.G.I., et al.: Dermatomyositis and toxoplasmosis. Ann. Neurol., *5*:393–395, 1979.
164. Phillips, P.E., Kassan, S.S., and Kagen, L.J.: Increased toxoplasma antibodies in idiopathic inflammatory muscle disease. Arthritis Rheum., *22*:209–214, 1979.
165. Kagen, L.J., Kimball, A.C., and Christian, C.L.: Serologic evidence of toxoplasmosis among patients with polymyositis. Am. J. Med., *56*:186–191, 1974.
166. Magid, S.K., and Kagen, L.J.: Serological evidence for acute toxoplasmosis in polymyositis-dermatomyositis. Increased frequency of specific anti-toxoplasma IgM antibodies. Am. J. Med., *75*:312–320, 1983.
167. Schoenen, J., Sianard-Gainko, J., Carpentier, M., and Reznik, M.: Myositis during *Borrelia burgdorferi* infection (Lyme disease). J. Neurol. Neurosurg., Psychiatry, *52*:1002–1005, 1989.
168. Reimers, C.D., Pongratz, D.E., Neubert, U., et al.: Myositis caused by *Borrelia burgdorferi*: Report of four cases. J. Neurol. Sci., *91*:215–226, 1989.
169. Atlas, E., Novak, S.N., Duray, P.H., and Steere, A.C.: Lyme myositis: Muscle invasion by *Borrelia burgdorferi*. Ann. Intern. Med., *109*:245–246, 1988.
170. Arundell, F.D., Wilkinson, R.D., and Haserick, J.R.: Dermatomyositis and malignant neoplasms in adults. Arch. Dermatol., *82*:772–775, 1960.
171. Barnes, B.E.: Dermatomyositis and malignancy. Ann. Intern. Med., *84*:68–76, 1976.
172. Callen, J.P., Hyla, J.F., Bole, G.G., Jr., et al.: The relationship of dermatomyositis and polymyositis to internal malignancy. Arch. Dermatol., *116*:295–298, 1980.
173. Singsen, B.H., Waters, K.Q., Siegel, S.E., et al.: Lymphocytic leukemia, atypical dermatomyositis and hyperlipidemia in a 4-year-old boy. J. Pediatr., *88*:602–604, 1976.
174. Tymms, K.E., and Webb, J.: Dermatopolymyositis and other connective tissue diseases: A review of 105 cases. J. Rheumatol., *12*:1140–1148, 1985.
175. Richardson, J.B., and Callen, J.P.: Dermatomyositis and malignancy. Med. Clin. North Am., *73*:1211–1220, 1989.
176. Fayolle, J., Vallon, C., Claudy, A., et al.: Dermatomyosite déclenchée par l'isoniazide, avec syndrome biologique d'auto-immunisation de type lupique. Lyon Med., *233*:135–138, 1975.
177. Goldenberg, D.L., and Stor, R.A.: Azathioprine hypersensitivity mimicking an acute exacerbation of dermatomyositis. J. Rheumatol., *2*:346–349, 1975.
178. Fernandes, L., Swinson, D.R., and Hamilton, E.B.D.: Dermatomyositis complicating penicillamine treatment. Ann. Rheum. Dis., *36*:94–95, 1977.
179. Morgan, G.L., McGuire, J.L., and Ochoa, J.: Penicillamine-induced myositis in rheumatoid arthritis. Muscle Nerve, *4*:137–140, 1981.
180. Petersen, J., Halberg, P., Hojgaard, K., et al.: Penicillamine-induced polymyositis-dermatomyositis. Scand. J. Rheumatol., *7*:113–117, 1978.
181. Halla, J.T., Koopman, W.J., Fallahi, S., et al.: Rheumatoid myositis: Clinical and histologic features and possible pathogenesis. Arthritis Rheum., *27*:737–743, 1984.
182. Martinez-Lavin, M., Vaughan, J.H., and Tan, E.M.: Autoantibodies and the spectrum of Sjögren's syndrome. Ann. Intern. Med., *91*:185–190, 1979.
183. Ringel, S.P., Forstot, J.Z., Tan, E.M., et al.: Sjögren's syndrome and polymyositis or dermatomyositis. Arch. Neurol., *39*:157–163, 1982.
184. Joy, J.L., Oh, S.J., and Baysal, A.I.: Electrophysiological spectrum of inclusion body myositis. Muscle Nerve, *13*:949–951, 1990.
185. Chou, S.-M.: Inclusion body myositis: A chronic persistent mumps myositis? Hum. Pathol., *17*:765–777, 1986.
186. Carpenter, S., Karpati, G., Heller, I., et al.: Inclusion body myositis: A distinct variety of idiopathic inflammatory myopathy. Neurology, *28*:8–17, 1978.
187. Danon, M.J., Reyes, M.G., Perurena, O.H., et al.: Inclusion body myositis: A corticosteroid-resistant inflammatory myopathy. Arch. Neurol., *39*:760–764, 1982.
188. Eisen, A., Berry, K., and Gibson, G.: Inclusion body myositis (IBM): Myopathy or neuropathy? Neurology, *33*:1109–1114, 1983.
189. Julien, J., Vital, C., Vallat, J.M., et al.: Inclusion body myositis. J. Neurol. Sci., *55*:15–24, 1982.
190. Yunis, E.J., and Samaha, F.J.: Inclusion body myositis. Lab. Invest., *25*:240–248, 1971.
191. Nishino, H., Engel, A.G., and Rima, B.K.: Inclusion body myositis: The mumps virus hypothesis. Ann. Neurol., *25*:260–264, 1989.
192. Mikol, J., Felten-Papaiconomou, A., Ferchal, F.: Inclusion body myositis: Clinicopathological studies and isolation of an adenovirus type 2 from muscle biopsy specimen. Ann. Neurol., *11*:576–581, 1982.
193. Lazaro, R.P., Barron, K.D., Dentinger, M.P., et al.: Inclusion body myositis: Case reports and a reappraisal of an under-recognized type of myopathy. Mt. Sinai J. Med. (NY), *53*:137–144, 1986.
194. Carpenter, S., and Karpati, G.: The major inflammatory myopathies of unknown cause. Pathol. Annu., *16*:205–237, 1981.
195. Kelly, J.J., Madoc-Jones, H., Adelman, L.S., et al.: Total body irradiation not effective in inclusion body myositis. Neurology, *36*:1264–1266, 1986.
196. Yood, R.A., and Smith, T.W.: Inclusion body myositis and systemic lupus erythematosus. J. Rheumatol., *12*:568–570, 1985.
197. Chad, D., Good, P., Adelman, L., et al.: Inclusion body myositis associated with Sjögren's syndrome. Arch. Neurol., *39*:186–188, 1982.
198. Riggs, J.E., Schochet, S.S., Jr., Gutmann, L., et al.: Inclusion body myositis and chronic immune thrombocytopenia. Arch. Neurol., *41*:93–95, 1984.
199. Lane, R.J.M., Fulthorpe, J.J., and Hudgson, P.: Inclusion body myositis: A case with associated collagen-vascular disease responding to treatment. J. Neurosurg. Psychiatry, *48*:270–273, 1985.
199a. Cohen, M.R., Sulaiman, A.R., Garancis, J.C., and Wortmann, R.L.: Clinical heterogeneity and treatment response in inclusion body myositis. Arthritis Rheum., *32*:734–740, 1989.
200. Lotz, B.P., Engel, A.G., Nishino, H., et al.: Inclusion body myositis. Brain, *112*:727–747, 1988.
201. Joseph, S.C.: Pyomyositis. Am. J. Dis. Child., *130*:775–776, 1975.
202. Taylor, J.F., Fluck, D., and Fluck, D.: Tropical myositis: Ultrastructural studies. J. Clin. Pathol., *29*:1081–1084, 1976.
203. Gibson, R.K., Rosenthal, S.J., and Lukert, B.P.: Pyomyositis: Increasing recognition in temperate climates. Am. J. Med., *77*:768–772, 1984.
204. Brennessell, D.J., Robbins, N., and Hindman, S.: Pyomyositis

caused by *Yersinia enterocolitica*. J. Clin. Microbiol., *20*:293–294, 1984.
205. Moore, D.L., Delage, G., Labelle, H., et al.: Per acute streptococcal pyomyositis, report of 2 cases and review of the literature. J. Pediatr. Orthop., *6*:232–235, 1986.
206. Adams, E.M., Gudmundsson, S., Yocum, D.E., et al.: Streptococcal myositis. Arch. Intern. Med., *145*:1020–1023, 1985.
207. Lachiewicz, P.F., and Hadler, N.M.: Spontaneous pyomyositis in a patient with Felty's syndrome; diagnosis using computerized tomography. South Med. J., *79*:1047–1048, 1986.
208. Weinberg, W.G., and Dembert, M.L.: Tropical pyomyositis: Delineation by gray scale ultrasound. Am. J. Trop. Med. Hyg., *33*:930–932, 1984.
209. Ellman, L., Miller, L., and Rappaport, J.: Leukopheresis therapy of a hypereosinophilic disorder. J.A.M.A., *230*:1004–1005, 1974.
210. Layzer, R.B., Shearn, M.A., and Satya-Murti, S.: Eosinophilic polymyositis. Ann. Neurol., *1*:65–71, 1977.
211. Bjelle, A., Henriksson, K.-G., and Hofer, P.-A.: Polymyositis in eosinophilic fasciitis. Eur. Neurol., *19*:128–137, 1980.
212. Schumacher, H.R.: A scleroderma-like syndrome with fasciitis, myositis and eosinophilia. Ann. Intern. Med., *84*:49–50, 1976.
213. Serratrice, G., Pellissier, J.F., Cros, D., et al.: Relapsing eosinophilic perimyositis. J. Rheumatol., 7:199–205, 1980.
214. Sladek, G.D., Vasey, F.B., Sieger, B., et al.: Relapsing eosinophilic myositis. J. Rheumatol., *10*:467–470, 1983.
215. Swygert, L.A., Maes, E.E., Sewell, L.E., et al.: Eosinophilia-myalgia syndrome. Results of a national surveillance. J.A.M.A., *264*:1698–1703, 1990.
216. Shulman, L.E.: The eosinophilia-myalgia syndrome associated with ingestion of L-tryptophan. Arthritis Rheum., *33*:913–917, 1990.
217. Slutsker, L., Hoesly, F.C., Miller, L., et al.: Eosinophilia-myalgia syndrome associated with exposure to tryptophan from a single manufacturer. J.A.M.A., *264*:213–217, 1990.
218. Hertzman, P.A., Blevins, W.L., Mayer, J., et al.: Association of the eosinophilia-myalgia syndrome with the ingestion of tryptophan. N. Engl. J. Med., *322*:869–873, 1990.
219. Kaufman, L.D., Seidman, R.J., and Gruber, B.L.: L-tryptophan-associated eosinophilic perimyositis, neuritis, and fasciitis. Medicine, *69*:187–199, 1990.
220. Eidson, M., Philen, R.M., Sewell, C.M., et al.: L-tryptophan and eosinophilia-myalgia syndrome in New Mexico. Lancet *335*:645–648, 1990.
221. Mayeno, A.N., Lin, F., Foote, C.S., et al.: Characterization of "Peak E" a novel amino acid associated with eosinophilia-myalgia syndrome. Science, *250*:1707–1708, 1990.
222. Crofford, L.L., Rader, J.I., Dalakas, M.C., et al.: L-tryptophan implicated in human eosinophilia-myalgia syndrome causes fasciitis and perimyositis in the Lewis rat. J. Clin. Invest., *86*:1757–1763, 1990.
223. Hewlett, R.H., and Brownell, B.: Granulomatous myopathy: Its relationship to sarcoidosis and polymyositis. J. Neurol. Neurosurg. Psychiatry, *38*:1090–1099, 1975.
224. Menard, D.B., Haddad, H., Blain, J.G., et al.: Granulomatous myositis and myopathy associated with Crohn's colitis. N. Engl. J. Med., *295*:818–819, 1976.
225. Schimrigk, K., and Uldall, B.: The diseases of Besnier-Boeck-Schaumann and granulomatous polymyositis. Eur. Neurol., *1*:137–157, 1968.
226. McKinney, R.E., Katz, S.L., and Wilfert, C.M.: Chronic enteroviral meningoencephalitis in agammaglobulinemic patients. Rev. Infect. Dis., *9*:334–356, 1987.
227. Miller, J.J.: Late progression in dermatomyositis in childhood. J. Pediatr., *83*:543–548, 1973.
228. Uchino, M., Araki, S., Yoshida, O., et al.: High single-dose alternate-day corticosteroid regimens in treatment of polymyositis. J. Neurol., *232*:175–178, 1985.
229. Yanagisawa, T., Sueishi, M., Nawata, Y., et al.: Methyl prednisolone pulse therapy in dermatomyositis. Dermatologica, *167*:47–51, 1983.
230. Dubowitz, V.: Treatment of dermatomyositis in childhood. Arch. Dis. Child., *51*:494–500, 1971.
231. Rose, A.L.: Childhood polymyositis. Am. J. Dis. Child., *127*:518–522, 1974.
232. Oddis, C.V., and Medsger, T.A., Jr.: Relationship between serum creatine kinase level and corticosteroid therapy in polymyositis-dermatomyositis. J. Rheumatol., *15*:807–811, 1988.
233. Oddis, C.V., and Medsger, T.A.: Current management of polymyositis and dermatomyositis. Drugs, *37*:382–390, 1989.
234. Malaviya, A.N., Many, A., and Schwartz, R.S.: Treatment of dermatomyositis with methotrexate. Lancet, *2*:485–488, 1968.
235. Metzger, A.L., Haddad, H., Blain, J.G., et al.: Polymyositis and dermatomyositis: Combined methotrexate and corticosteroid therapy. Ann. Intern. Med., *81*:182–189, 1974.
236. Jacobs, J.C.: Methotrexate and azathioprine treatment of childhood dermatomyositis. Pediatrics, *59*:212–218, 1977.
237. Bunch, T.W.: Prednisone and azathioprine for polymyositis. Long-term follow-up. Arthritis Rheum., *24*:45–48, 1981.
238. Al-Janadi, M., Smith, C.D. and Karsh, J.: Cyclophosphamide treatment of interstitial pulmonary fibrosis in polymyositis/dermatomyositis. J. Rheumatol., *16*:1592–1596, 1989.
239. Cronin, M.E. and Plotz, P.H.: Current concepts in idiopathic inflammatory myopathies: Polymyositis, dermatomyositis and related disorders. Ann. Intern. Med., *111*:143–157, 1989.
240. Dantzig, P.: Juvenile dermatomyositis treated with cyclosporine. J. Am. Acad. Dermatol., *22*:310–311, 1990.
241. Heckmatt, J., Hasson, N., Saunders, C., et al.: Cyclosporin in juvenile dermatomyositis. Lancet, *1*:1063–1066, 1989.
242. Tiliakos, N.A.: Low dose cytotoxic combination therapy in intractable dermatopolymyositis. Arthritis Rheum., *30*:S14, 1987.
243. Wallace, D.J., Metzger, A.L., and White, K.K.: Combination immunosuppressive treatment of steroid-resistant dermatomyositis/polymyositis. Arthritis Rheum., *28*:590–592, 1985.
244. Bennington, J.A., and Dau, P.C.: Patients with polymyositis and dermatomyositis who undergo plasmapheresis therapy. Pathologic findings. Arch. Neurol., *38*:553–560, 1981.
245. Dau, P.C.: Plasmapheresis in idiopathic inflammatory myopathy. Arch. Neurol., *38*:544–552, 1981.
246. Olson, N.Y., and Lindsley, C.B.: Adjunctive use of hydroxychloraquine in childhood dermatomyositis. J. Rheumatol., *16*:1545–1547, 1989.
247. Woo, T.Y., Callen, J.P., Voorhees, J.L., et al.: Cutaneous lesions of dermatomyositis are improved by hydroxychloraquine. J. Am. Acad. Dermatol., *10*:592–600, 1984.
248. Kelly, J.J., Madoc-Jones, H., Adelman, L.S., et al.: Response to total body irradiation in dermatomyositis. Muscle Nerve, *11*:120–123, 1988.
249. Hill, R.H., and Wood, W.S.: Juvenile dermatomyositis. Can. Med. Assoc. J., *103*:1152–1156, 1970.
250. Spencer, C.H., Hanson, V., Singsen, B.H., et al.: Course of treated juvenile dermatomyositis. J. Pediatr., *105*:399–408, 1984.
251. Lovell, H.B., and Lindsley, C.B.: Late recurrence of childhood dermatomyositis. J. Rheumatol., *13*:821–822, 1986.
252. Carpenter, J.R., Bunch, T.W., Engel, A.G., et al.: Survival in polymyositis: Corticosteroids and risk factors. J. Rheumatol., *4*:207–214, 1977.
253. Medsger, T.A., Jr., Robinson, H., and Masi, A.T.: Factors affecting survivorship in polymyositis. Arthritis Rheum., *14*:249–258, 1971.
254. Hoffman, G.S., Franck, W.A., Raddatz, D.A., et al.: Presenta-

tion, treatment, and prognosis of idiopathic inflammatory muscle disease in a rural hospital. Am. J. Med., *75*:433–438, 1983.

255. Baron, M., and Small, P.: Polymyositis/dermatomyositis: Clinical features and outcome in 22 patients. J. Rheumatol., *12*:283–286, 1985.

256. Hochberg, M.C., Lopez-Aeuna, D., and Gittelsohn, A.M.: Mortality from polymyositis and dermatomyositis in the United States, 1968–1978. Arthritis Rheum., *26*:1465–1471, 1983.

257. McKendry, R.J.R.: Influence of age at onset on the duration of treatment in idiopathic adult polymyositis and dermatomyositis. Arch. Intern. Med., *147*:1989–1991, 1987.

258. Henriksson, K.G., and Lindvall, B.: Polymyositis and dermatomyositis 1990. Diagnosis, treatment and prognosis. Prog. Neurobiol., *35*:181–193, 1990.

259. Basset-Seguin, N., Roujeau, J.C., Gherardi, R., et al.: Prognostic factors and predictive signs of malignancy in adult dermatomyositis. Arch. Dermatol., *126*:633–637, 1990.

260. Targoff, I.N.: Immunologic aspects of myositis. Curr. Opin. Rheumatol., *1*:432–442, 1989.

73

Systemic Sclerosis (Scleroderma), Localized Forms of Scleroderma, and Calcinosis

THOMAS A. MEDSGER, JR.

SYSTEMIC SCLEROSIS (SCLERODERMA)

Systemic sclerosis is a generalized disorder of connective tissue characterized by fibrosis and degenerative changes in the blood vessels, skin, synovium, skeletal muscle, and certain internal organs, notably the gastrointestinal tract, lung, heart, and kidney.[1] Although there is an early, often clinically unappreciated inflammatory component, the hallmark of the disease is skin thickening (scleroderma) caused by excessive accumulation of connective tissue. Proliferative vascular changes leading to Raynaud's phenomenon and obliterative arteriolar and capillary lesions are prominent.

The term *scleroderma* traditionally has been applied to the cutaneous changes of both systemic sclerosis and a heterogeneous group of conditions designated collectively as *localized scleroderma*. In the latter disorders, dermal fibrosis is more circumscribed both vascular and internal organ involvement are absent, and characteristic serologic abnormalities are not present. Coexistence of these entities or transition from localized to systemic disease is extremely rare.

CLASSIFICATION OF SYSTEMIC SCLEROSIS

Clinical Subsets

Systemic sclerosis is divided into two major clinical variants, diffuse cutaneous and limited cutaneous disease, dependent primarily on the degree and extent of cutaneous involvement.[2,3] The term *overlap syndrome* is used when features commonly encountered in other connective tissue diseases are also present (Table 73–1).[4] A similar spectrum of disease is recognized in the classification systems proposed by other authors, including acrosclerosis and CREST syndrome (an acronym referring to the findings of *c*alcinosis, *R*aynaud's phenomenon, *e*sophageal hypomotility, *s*clerodactyly, and *t*elangiectasia),[5] which are closely analogous to limited cutaneous scleroderma.

The diffuse cutaneous variant is characterized by distal and proximal extremity and truncal skin thickening, whereas in the limited cutaneous subtype, these skin changes are most often restricted to the fingers and distalmost portions of the extremities and face. In addition, there are many differentiating demographic, clinical, laboratory and natural history features (Table 73–2). These differences are particularly important to the patient and managing physician because they serve as orientation to the expected subsequent natural history of disease by identifying potential complications and indicating the time frame during which they are most likely to occur.

Diffuse cutaneous disease is associated with palpable tendon friction rubs, arthritis with joint contractures, serum antitopoisomerase I (anti-Scl 70) antibodies, and earlier, more frequent occurrence of visceral disease affecting the gastrointestinal tract, lung, heart, and kidney. In contrast, limited cutaneous disease is correlated with calcinosis, telangiectases, serum anticentromere antibodies, and the occasional late development of pulmonary arterial hypertension or small bowel malabsorption.

Systemic sclerosis in overlap includes patients in either of the preceding two categories who also have convincing evidence of another connective tissue dis-

TABLE 73–1. CLASSIFICATION OF SCLERODERMA

I. **SYSTEMIC** (systemic sclerosis)
With diffuse cutaneous scleroderma: symmetric widespread skin fibrosis, affecting the distal and proximal extremities and often the trunk and face; tendency to rapid progression of skin changes and early appearance of visceral involvement
With limited cutaneous scleroderma: symmetric restricted skin fibrosis affecting the distal extremities (often confined to the fingers) and face; prolonged delay in appearance of distinctive internal manifestations (e.g., pulmonary arterial hypertension); prominence of calcinosis and telangiectasia
With "overlap": having either diffuse or limited skin fibrosis and typical features of one or more of the other connective tissue diseases

II. **LOCALIZED**
Morphea: single or multiple plaques of skin fibrosis
Linear scleroderma: single or multiple bands of skin fibrosis; includes scleroderma en coup de sabre (with or without facial hemiatrophy)
Eosinophilic fasciitis: fascial and deep subcutaneous fibrosis
Eosinophilia myalgia syndrome
Toxic oil syndrome

TABLE 73–2. COMPARISON OF CLINICAL AND LABORATORY FEATURES FOUND AT ANY TIME DURING THE COURSE OF SYSTEMIC SCLEROSIS (UNIVERSITY OF PITTSBURGH, 1981 TO 1990)

	DIFFUSE SCLERODERMA (n = 391)	LIMITED SCLERODERMA (n = 354)	OVERLAP SYNDROME (n = 82)
Demographic features			
Age (<40 at onset)	42%	50%	66%
Race (nonwhite)	10%	5%	16%
Sex (female)	77%	86%	82%
Duration of symptoms (years)	3.4	12.1	6.9
Organ system involvement			
Skin thickening (total skin score)*	36.6	6.6	9.9
Telangiectases	63%	88%	62%
Calcinosis	15%	49%	25%
Raynaud's phenomenon	91%	96%	92%
Arthralgias or arthritis	69%	26%	65%
Tendon friction rubs	62%	5%	17%
Joint contractures	91%	51%	62%
Skeletal myopathy	11%	5%	57%
Esophageal hypomotility	67%	73%	71%
Pulmonary fibrosis	35%	35%	42%
Pulmonary hypertension	<1%	11%	2%
Cardiac involvement	13%	6%	16%
"Scleroderma renal crisis"	16%	3%	7%
Laboratory data			
ANA positive (1:16+)	95%	90%	96%
Anticentromere antibody positive (1:40+)	2%	45%	4%
Anti-Scl 70 antibody positive (any titer)	32%	14%	4%
Cumulative survival from first diagnosis			
5 years	79%	82%	87%
10 years	56%	69%	72%

* As described in Steen, V.D., et al.[32]
ANA = antinuclear antibody.

ease, such as active myositis and a dermatomyositis rash, or leukopenia, glomerulonephritis, pleuropericarditis, or typical rash of systemic lupus erythematosus (SLE). Other subsets of systemic sclerosis undoubtedly exist, but their distinctive features have not been so clearly delineated.

Serologic Subsets

Since the identification of anti-topoisomerase and anticentromere antibodies and their observed strong association with diffuse cutaneous and limited cutaneous disease, respectively, the concept of serologic subsets within the spectrum of systemic sclerosis has been popular. Other serum autoantibodies, relatively specific for scleroderma have also been described and have raised the proportion of patients having one or more of these autoantibodies to nearly 85% of the total (Fig. 73–1). The limited cutaneous category contains anticentromere and anti-Th[6] subsets. Diffuse cutaneous disease includes anti-Scl 70 and anti-RNA polymerase I and III.[7,8] Overlap syndromes are associated with anti-U1RNP,[9] anti-PM-Scl,[10,11] and anti-U3 RNP.[12] Clinical

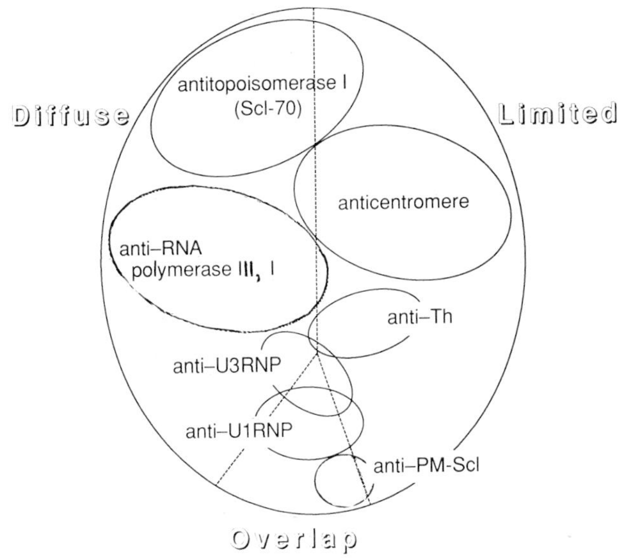

FIGURE 73–1. Classification of systemic sclerosis by clinical subjects and autoantibody types.

features associated with these autoantibodies are detailed later in the section on serum autoantibodies.

Criteria for Classification

These criteria are intended for description of large series of patients in research studies and not for diagnosis of an individual patient. A prospective multicenter study by the American College of Rheumatology (ACR) compared 264 systemic sclerosis patients with 413 persons having polymyositis-dermatomyositis, SLE, or isolated Raynaud's phenomenon for the purpose of developing such criteria.[13] Sclerodermatous skin change in any location proximal to the digits was found to be the major discriminating criterion for *definite* systemic sclerosis. Such thickening was present in 91% of systemic sclerosis cases and in fewer than 1% of comparison patients. With the addition of any two of three minor criteria these are specific sclerodactyly, digital pitting scars, bibasilar pulmonary interstitial fibrosis on chest roentgenogram, sensitivity rose to 97% and specificity was maintained at 98%.

In my experience, however, nearly 10% of individuals whom I believe to have definite systemic sclerosis do not satisfy these criteria.[14] They are patients with limited cutaneous disease and other convincing evidence of systemic sclerosis such as esophageal or small bowel hypomotility or pulmonary arterial hypertension. Modification of the ACR criteria to more adequately include patients with limited cutaneous involvement presents a challenge.

EPIDEMIOLOGY

Systemic sclerosis has been described in all races and is global in distribution. A U.S. community study detected nearly 20 new cases per million population at risk annually.[15] The disease is unusual in childhood. Overall, women are affected approximately three times as often as men, and this ratio is increased during the childbearing years. No significant racial differences have been found.

Several environmental factors have been implicated as predisposing to or precipitating systemic sclerosis.[16] The disease is more common among underground coal and gold miners and others occupationally exposed to silica dust, especially workers with intense exposure.[17] Systemic sclerosis has been reported to occur many years after the injection of paraffin or insertion of silicone breast implants.[18] Localized sclerodermatous changes, a Raynaud-like phenomenon, and osteolysis of the distal phalanges have been described in persons exposed to unfinished plastics in the manufacture of polyvinyl chloride, who also may develop a unusual form of hepatic and pulmonary fibrosis.[19] Another implicated substance is the antitumor drug bleomycin.[20] Use of chlorinated hydrocarbons closely related to vinyl chloride[21] and aromatic hydrocarbon solvents, such as benzene and toluene,[22] and exposure to the polymerization of epoxy resins[23] have also been associated with the development of sclerodermatous lesions, but the appearance of these skin changes is generally not typical.

Relatives of systemic sclerosis patients are often affected by other connective tissue diseases such as SLE, suggesting a heritable predisposition to this family of disorders. The number of reports of such familial disease has increased[24,25] and includes disease in consanguineous kindreds.[26,27] Serum antinuclear antibodies have been found in over 25% of blood relatives of patients but in only 5 to 8% of controls.[28,29] In one of these studies,[28] 21 of 58 family members with antinuclear antibodies had one or more clinical features of connective tissue disease. Similar findings in spouses of patients, however, raise the issue of environmental contributions.[28] Immunologic studies on identical twins discordant for systemic sclerosis showed striking abnormalities in the affected but not the normal twin, a point against a predominant genetic predisposition to disease.[30]

CLINICAL FEATURES

Initial Symptoms

Systemic sclerosis usually begins in persons between 30 and 50 years of age, but onset during childhood and among the elderly is reported. In most cases of limited cutaneous disease, the initial complaint is Raynaud's phenomenon. In contrast, patients with diffuse cutaneous disease most often have skin thickening or arthritis as the first manifestation. Rarely, the earliest clue is that of visceral involvement. Esophageal symptoms (dysphagia, heartburn) or pulmonary fibrosis may long antedate the development of cutaneous changes, and in fact, the latter may be entirely absent (systemic sclerosis sine scleroderma).[31]

FEATURES OF ORGAN SYSTEM INVOLVEMENT

Skin

Easily recognized phases are present in the evolution of scleroderma. Initially, patients complain about tight, puffy fingers, especially on arising in the morning (edematous phase). Pitting or nonpitting edema of the fingers ("sausaging") and hands may occur, which also frequently involves the forearms, legs, feet, and face. Edema may last indefinitely (e.g., fingers in limited cutaneous disease) or may be replaced gradually by thickening and tightening of the skin (indurative phase) after several weeks or months. In the limited cutaneous subset, changes are generally restricted to the fingers, hands, and face, whereas diffuse cutaneous disease first affects the distalmost extremities and then spreads at a variable rate to the forearms, upper arms, thighs, upper anterior chest, and abdomen. Affected skin becomes increasingly shiny, taut, thickened, and tightly adherent to underlying subcutis, thus impairing the mobility of muscles, tendons, and joints. During this phase, the dermis is markedly thickened but the epidermis is thinned, leading to loss of skin creases, hair, sweat, and oils. Facial changes may result in the development of a characteristic pinched, immobile, expressionless appearance, with thin, tightly pursed lips and reduced oral aperture (Fig. 73–2). Microstomia interferes with eating and with proper dental care. In limited cutaneous disease, skin thickening is much less prominent, and the most striking digital and facial finding consists of numerous telangiectases representing dilated capillary loops and venules (Fig. 73–3). After several years, the dermis tends to soften somewhat and in many cases reverts to normal thickness or actually becomes thinner than normal (atrophic phase) with many telangiectases.

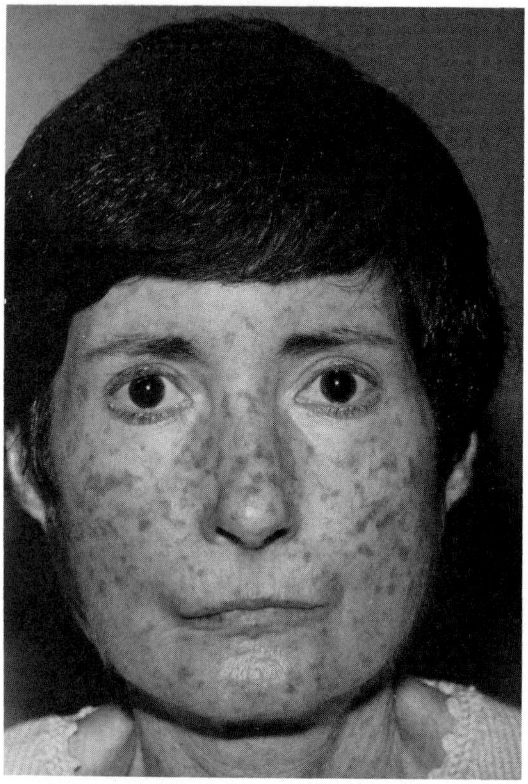

FIGURE 73–3. Face of a 45-year-old woman with limited cutaneous systemic sclerosis who had no skin thickening but had multiple telangiectases.

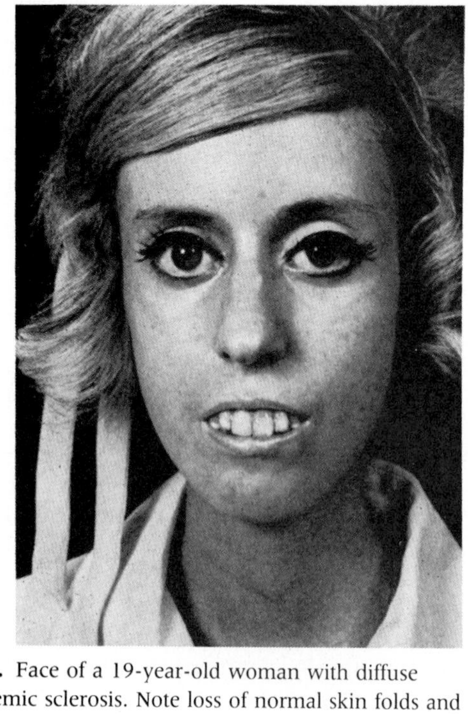

FIGURE 73–2. Face of a 19-year-old woman with diffuse cutaneous systemic sclerosis. Note loss of normal skin folds and retraction of lips.

The natural history of skin involvement in the two major variants of systemic sclerosis is notably different when one of several reported semiquantitative methods is used to measure the degree and extent of cutaneous thickening in multiple sites (Fig. 73–4).[32,33] In limited cutaneous disease, skin thickening remains minimal over many years and bears no relation to visceral sequelae. In contrast, in diffuse cutaneous scleroderma, early, accelerated increase in skin thickness occurs most often and reaches a peak after 1 to 3 years. Rapid progression of skin thickness is associated with the development of joint contractures and internal organ problems, including involvement of the gastrointestinal tract, lung, heart, and kidney. Thus, although extensive skin thickening per se does not influence prognosis, the associated visceral disease is clearly life threatening. After maximal skin thickening has developed most often slow but definite regression of this abnormality ensues and in some cases is remarkable.[34]

Skin thickening is frequently accompanied, and in some instances preceded, by impressive hyperpigmentation that spares the mucous membranes. This change is most prominent in the area of hair follicles, with surrounding hypopigmentation leading to a "salt-and-

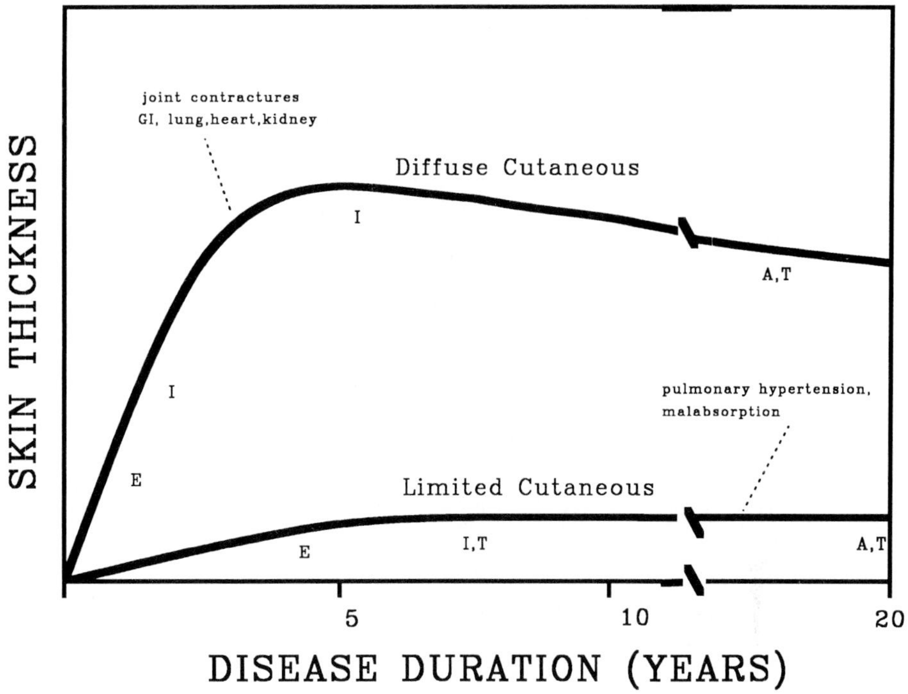

FIGURE 73–4. Schematic representation of the natural history of skin thickness and timing of some serious complications during the course of systemic sclerosis with the two major disease variants. E = edema; I = induration; A = atrophy; T = telangiectasia.

pepper" appearance. Hyperpigmentation is most striking over the course of superficial blood vessels[35] and tendons.[36]

In early disease, skin biopsy is less reliable for establishing a diagnosis than is physical examination. The weight and thickness of standard diameter full thickness skin-punch biopsy cores were found to be significantly increased and correlated closely with skin thickness score on physical examination.[37] Biopsy specimens obtained during the active indurative phase disclose a striking increase of compact collagen fibers in the reticular dermis and hyalinization and fibrosis of arterioles. Simultaneously, thinning of the epidermis occurs with loss of rete pegs and atrophy of dermal appendages. Variably large accumulations of mononuclear cells, chiefly T-lymphocytes, are encountered in the lower dermis and upper subcutis (Fig. 73–5).[38] Direct immunofluorescence is negative for immunoglobulins and complement components at the dermal–epidermal junction and in blood vessels.[39] Degranulated mast cells, which have been linked to fibrosis, are found in increased numbers and density in clinically involved skin from patients with early cutaneous disease (less than 3 years' duration).[40]

The skin overlying bony prominences, and especially over extensor surfaces of the proximal interphalangeal joints, becomes tightly stretched as a result of contractures and is extremely vulnerable to trauma. In such areas cutaneous thinning (atrophy) rather than induration occurs. Patients are often plagued by painful ulcerations at these sites and, less commonly, over the bony prominences of the olecranons and malleoli of the ankles. These ulcers heal extremely slowly and frequently

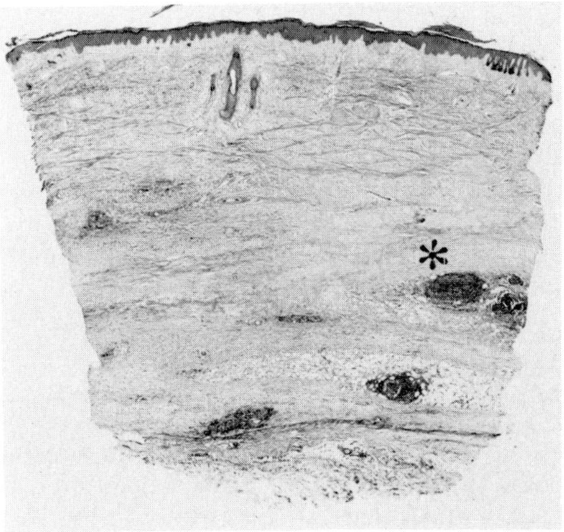

FIGURE 73–5. Photomicrograph of a skin-punch biopsy from the dorsum of the forearm of a 53-year-old woman with diffuse cutaneous systemic sclerosis. Skin appendages are atrophic, the dermis is thickened by deposition of dense collagenous connective tissue, and there are prominent collections of small round cells (*asterisk*) that were identified as T-lymphocytes.

become secondarily infected. Healing of skin in other locations, including surgical incisions, is normal.

Patients with limited scleroderma or late-stage diffuse disease commonly develop intracutaneous and subcutaneous calcifications. These deposits occur chiefly in the digital pads and periarticular tissues, along the extensor surfaces of the forearms, in the oleocranon bur-

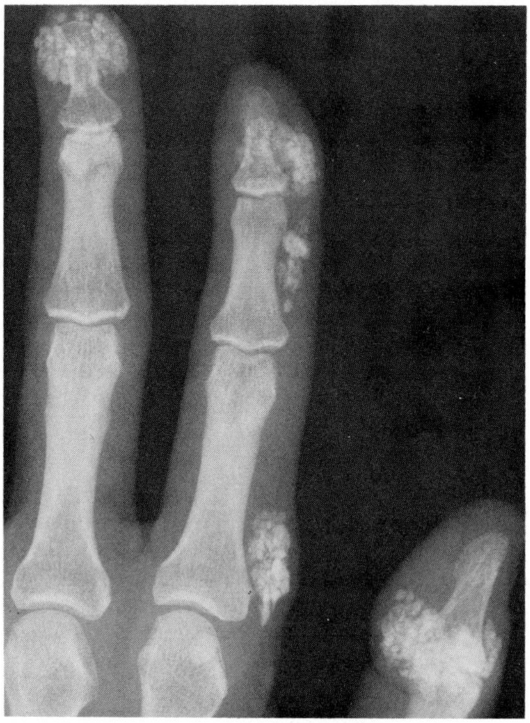

FIGURE 73–6. Close-up hand roentgenogram of a 46-year-old woman with limited cutaneous systemic sclerosis. Note extensive subcutaneous calcinosis.

sae, and in the prepatellar area. They vary in size from tiny punctate lesions of the fingers (Fig. 73–6) to large conglomerate masses in the forearms. Such calcinosis may be complicated by ulceration of overlying skin, intermittent extrusion of calcareous material, and secondary bacterial infection.

Peripheral Vascular System: Functional Abnormalities

Raynaud's phenomenon is defined as paroxysmal vasospasm of the fingers in response to cold exposure or emotional stress and occurs at some time during the disease in over 90% of persons with systemic sclerosis. Typically, the patient reports episodes of sudden pallor and/or cyanosis of the distal two thirds of the fingers, which become cold, numb, and painful. During rewarming, reactive hyperemia is common. The toes also may be affected, and rarely, the tip of the nose, earlobes, or tongue. Many patients with bilateral Raynaud's phenomenon but no obvious symptoms or signs of underlying connective tissue disease are referred to internists or rheumatologists for evaluation. Some of these individuals will develop a connective tissue disorder within the first 2 years after the onset of Raynaud's phenomenon.[41] After 2 years, few (less than 5%) will do so. The most frequent condition that evolves is limited cutaneous scleroderma.[42] Clinical clues antedating the later appearance of systemic sclerosis include sclerodactyly, puffy fingers, digital pitting scars, capillary microscopic abnormalities, and serum anticentromere or anti-Th antibodies.[6,43]

In most cases Raynaud's phenomenon begins contemporaneously with skin changes and/or rheumatic complaints or precedes these by a few months to a year. In patients with the limited cutaneous variant, Raynaud's phenomenon may antedate other evidence of disease by many years. In contrast, in up to 20% of patients with the diffuse cutaneous subtype, skin thickening precedes Raynaud's phenomenon. This latter order of events was correlated with subsequent diffuse skin thickening and an increased risk of renal involvement.[44] Because it is almost universal in systemic sclerosis, the presence or absence of Raynaud's phenomenon has little prognostic importance.

Patients with Raynaud's phenomenon, with or without scleroderma, have a persistently reduced digital pad temperature in the basal state and subnormal capillary blood flow in the fingers in both warm and cool environments.[45] Reduction in finger systolic blood pressure, unaltered by blockade of the sympathetic nervous system, has been observed.[46] Together with delay in rewarming of the fingers after cold exposure, these findings suggest structural as well as functional narrowing of blood vessels.

The plasma activity of a product of endothelial cells, factor VIII/von Willebrand factor antigen, was increased under basal conditions[47] and even more so after cold exposure.[48] Decreased platelet serotonin content, indicating its release;[49] increased serotonin-induced platelet aggregation;[50] and raised levels of circulating platelet aggregates and plasma β-thromboglobulin, presumed to reflect vascular injury and repair,[51,52] have been reported. Measurement of β-thromboglobulin may differentiate patients with systemic sclerosis from those with primary Raynaud's phenomenon.[52]

Structural Changes

Small areas of fingertip ischemic necrosis or ulceration are frequent, often leaving pitted scars. Gangrene of the terminal portions of the phalanges ensues in a few patients. Angiographic and autopsy studies have disclosed narrowing and obstruction of the digital arteries.[53] At necropsy, these showed prominent intimal and adventitial fibrosis without evidence of inflammation (Fig. 73–7). When severe, these changes led to considerable lumenal narrowing or occlusion. Recent or old thrombosis was frequently found, and 25% of vessels had a distinctive lesion, namely, telangiectases of the vasa vasorum.[53] Similar alterations of larger arteries, such as radial, ulnar, or popliteal changes, not due to atherosclerosis, have been noted.[53,54] These may be late complications of limited cutaneous scleroderma[54] and have been associated with anticardiolipin antibody.[55]

On microscopy the capillary circulation is altered by the appearance of "giant loops," and in diffuse scleroderma, by a paucity of nailfold vessels (Fig. 73–8).[56] Complete arrest of blood flow in these vessels has been observed after cold exposure.[57] Capillary microscopic

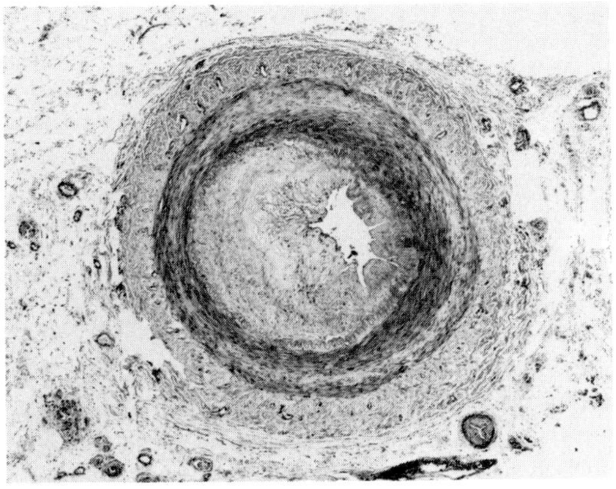

FIGURE 73–7. Photomicrograph of a digital artery obtained at autopsy from a 45-year-old woman with diffuse cutaneous systemic sclerosis who had Raynaud's phenomenon for over 20 years before her death. Near occlusion of the lumen is due to subintimal proliferation and striking periadventitial fibrosis.

patterns are interpreted from photographs,[58] and semiquantitative grading scales have been devised for both capillary size and extent of "avascularity."[59] These observations may be a useful permanent record of the state of the microvasculature. Nailfold biopsy has confirmed the accuracy of in vivo microscopy.[60] Such capillary changes are an early predictor of evolution to scleroderma in persons who clinically appear to have Raynaud's phenomenon alone,[61] and observed differences in patterns may discriminate patients with other diseases, such as SLE and rheumatoid arthritis (RA).[62] Although a relationship between reduced number and increased size of nailfold capillaries and visceral organ involvement in systemic sclerosis has been claimed,[63] not all authors agree.[64]

Joints, Tendons, and Bones

Symmetric polyarthralgias and joint stiffness of the fingers, wrists, knees, and ankles are frequent initial or early complaints. Generalized swelling of the fingers also occurs. It is difficult to ascertain the degree to which limitation of interphalangeal joint motion is caused by joint, periarticular, or tenosynovial disease, or by changes in the skin. Synovitis mimicking RA is uncommon but may be the first manifestation of diffuse cutaneous disease. Larger peripheral joints occasionally show evidence of inflammation, but contain scanty synovial fluid with predominantly mononuclear leukocytes numbering less than 2000/mm^3. Pathologic examination of synovium reveals variable numbers of chronic inflammatory cells, either in focal aggregates or scattered diffusely.[65] Fibrin deposition on the synovial surface is frequent. Patients with calcinosis may develop widespread calcification of the synovium and tendon sheaths.[66] The synovial fluid in such cases is milky or chalky and contains large numbers of basic calcium phosphate crystals.[67]

Some patients are aware of a "squeaking" sensation on movement of their extremities. A distinctive coarse, leathery crepitus (tendon friction rub) may be palpated over such areas during joint motion, particularly over the elbows, wrists, fingers, knees, and ankles. These rubs, which are due to fibrinous deposits on the surfaces of tendon sheaths and overlying fascia,[68] are relatively specific for diffuse cutaneous involvement, seldom occurring in the limited cutaneous variant or other inflam-

FIGURE 73–8. Nailfold capillary pattern of a patient with diffuse cutaneous systemic sclerosis (× 18). Note extensive avascular area along the edge of the nailfold and grossly enlarged capillary loops. (From Maricq, H.R.[59])

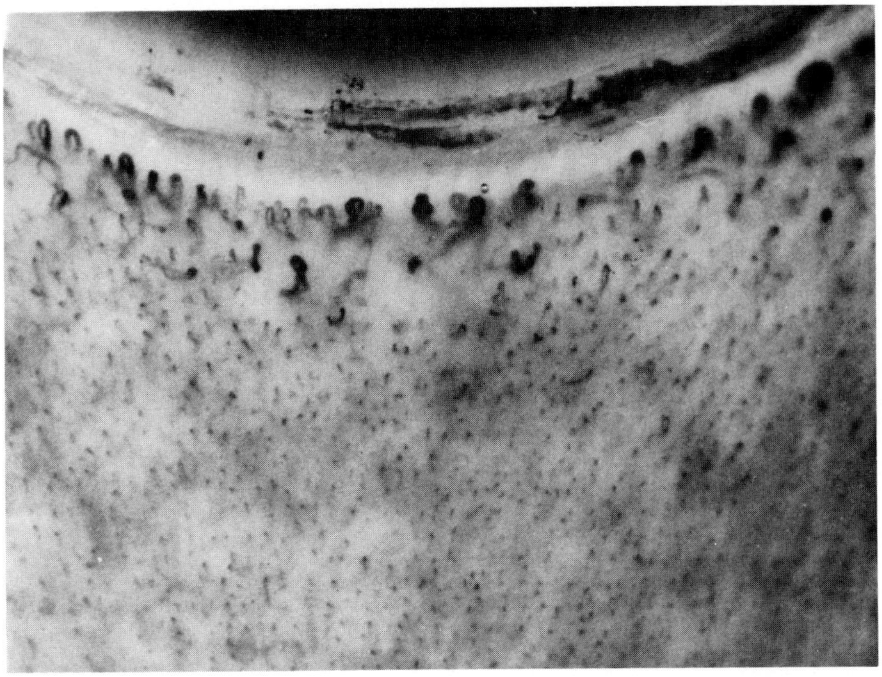

matory rheumatic conditions. Friction rubs often antedate an explosive increase in skin thickening. Carpal tunnel syndrome is caused by flexor tenosynovitis at the wrist. Flexion contractures ("bowed fingers") are attributed, at least in part, to tendinous and periarticular fibrosis and shortening.[69] These contractures, which occur commonly in the fingers, wrists, elbows, and ankles, usually become apparent within several months.

The most frequent bony radiographic abnormality is resorption of the tufts of the terminal phalanges of the fingers, rarely leading to complete dissolution of the terminal phalanx. The cause of tuft resorption is unknown but is presumed to be ischemic. A few patients develop severe erosive changes of the finger joints, which radiographically most closely resemble osteoarthritis (OA).[70] However, overlap with classic RA is also recognized.[71] Other examples of bone resorption include "notching" of the ribs[72] and dissolution of the condyle and ramus of the mandible,[73] both of which are reported only in patients with diffuse scleroderma.

Skeletal Muscle

In most instances, weakness and atrophy of skeletal muscle result from disuse secondary to joint contractures or chronic disease. However, approximately 20% of patients have a primary myopathy.[74] In most cases, this is a subtle process with weakness detected only by the examining physician, mild or no serum muscle enzyme elevation, and muscle biopsy showing focal replacement of myofibrils with collagenous connective tissue and perimysial and epimysial fibrosis without inflammatory changes. This bland myopathy is distinctive in that it does not occur in patients with other connective tissue diseases. It is nonprogressive and does not warrant intervention. A minority of patients exhibit more pronounced proximal muscle weakness and electrophysiologic, biochemical, and pathologic evidence of polymyositis.[74,75] These persons have been variably classified as having systemic sclerosis with myositis or systemic sclerosis in overlap with polymyositis.

Gastrointestinal Tract: Oral Cavity

Thinning of the lips (microcheilia) and reduced oral aperture (microstomia) are frequent. In the CREST variant, numerous lip and oral mucosa telangiectases are common. Atrophy of the mucous membrane and tongue papillae with impaired taste perception have been noted.[76] Thickening of the periodontal membrane occurs in up to 30% of patients and is due to fibrosis.[77] Loss of the lamina dura with gingivitis and subsequent loosening of the teeth also have been observed frequently. These events are compounded by the mechanical difficulty of maintaining good oral hygiene (finger contractures, limited oral opening) and by associated Sjögren's syndrome. Temporomandibular joint involvement may also be a factor in some patients.[73]

Esophagus and Stomach

Esophageal dysfunction eventually develops in nearly 80% of patients, thus constituting the most common visceral manifestation. No predilection for either the diffuse or limited subtype has been noted. In some cases, this abnormality occurs long before evidence of cutaneous disease.

As a result of incoordination of the normal propulsive peristalsis, solids (meat, bread) become "stuck" in the esophagus. Patients appreciate this problem in a retrosternal location and often need to ingest fluids in order to pass these foods. A second abnormality is incomplete closure of the lower esophageal sphincter, which leads to gastroesophageal reflux with peptic esophagitis. Although some patients are symptomatic, most complain about retrosternal burning pain, postprandial fullness, or acid regurgitation, especially on reclining at night, where the protective effect of gravity is eliminated. Despite the frequency of peptic esophagitis, and the presence of mucosal telangiectases in that area, esophageal hemorrhage is surprisingly unusual. After many years of inadequately treated reflux esophagitis, distal esophageal stricture is likely to develop, leading to reduced oral intake and, on occasion, loss of appreciable amounts of weight. Finally, pharyngoesophageal dysphagia, caused by dysfunction of striated rather than smooth muscle, may occur with or without associated polymyositis.[78]

All patients should have some assessment of esophageal function. Roentgenographic abnormalities are found in three fourths, including many who have no esophageal symptoms. Cinefluoroscopic examination, the standard method of evaluation, reveals diminished or absent peristaltic activity in the distal esophagus and gastroesophageal reflux. Esophageal pH monitoring may be useful in documenting the presence of reflux.[79] Chronic reflux predisposes to Barrett's metaplasia[80] and thus theoretically to adenocarcinoma of the esophagus, although there is no published support for this sequence of events in systemic sclerosis.[81] Incoordination and loss of contractile power and a reduction in the tone of the gastroesophageal sphincter are confirmed by manometric measurements, which are more sensitive but less well tolerated.[82] Radionuclide scintigraphy, both quantitative and patient accepted, gives very comparable results that correlate highly with abnormal distal esophageal pressure measurements.[83] Specificity for systemic sclerosis is lacking, however, because abnormal radionuclide studies have also been reported in other connective tissue diseases and in normal subjects.[84]

Gastric atony and dilatation may occur, but involvement of the stomach is remarkably uncommon when compared with other portions of the alimentary tract. Gastric acid secretion is unimpaired, but both hyperchlorhydria and increased basal and/or stimulated gastric acid output have been found.[85] In rare instances, telangiectases have been considered the source of serious bleeding from the distal esophagus, stomach, or other gastrointestinal tract sites, especially in persons with limited cutaneous disease.[86]

Histologic changes are most significant in the lower two thirds of the esophagus, where there is thinning of the mucosa and increased collagen in the lamina propria of the muscularis, which may be almost totally replaced by fibrous tissue. The walls of small arteries and arterioles are thickened and often surrounded by periadventitial deposits of collagen. Cellular infiltrates have been noted in the submucosa. The myenteric plexuses of Auerbach, which may be conspicuously lacking in ganglion cells, usually appear to be normal. Physiologic and pharmacologic studies of esophageal blood flow have not been performed.

Small Intestine

In a small proportion of patients, the illness is dominated by intestinal complaints consisting of severe bloating, abdominal cramps, and episodic diarrhea. These symptoms are due to striking hypomotility of the small intestine and may result in malabsorption, weight loss, and extreme wasting. Hypomotility favors the overgrowth of intestinal microorganisms that consume large amounts of vitamin B_{12} and interfere with normal fat absorption as a result of their deconjugation of bile salts. Radiographic findings include prolonged retention of barium in the atonic and widely dilated second and third portions of the duodenum (loop sign) and irregular flocculation or hypersegmentation of barium or localized areas of dilatation of the jejunum and/or ileum. The mucosal pattern of the distended jejunum contains prominent transverse folds (Fig. 73–9). The valvulae conniventes remain close to one another despite pronounced dilatation of the lumen (*''closed accordion'' sign*), presumably owing to excessive fibrosis of the submucosa. Similar changes are occasionally found in the ileum. Severe atony of the bowel produces a functional ileus (pseudo-obstruction) with symptoms simulating mechanical obstruction. Volvulus of a greatly dilated small intestine has been observed.[87]

Pneumatosis intestinalis is an occasional complication

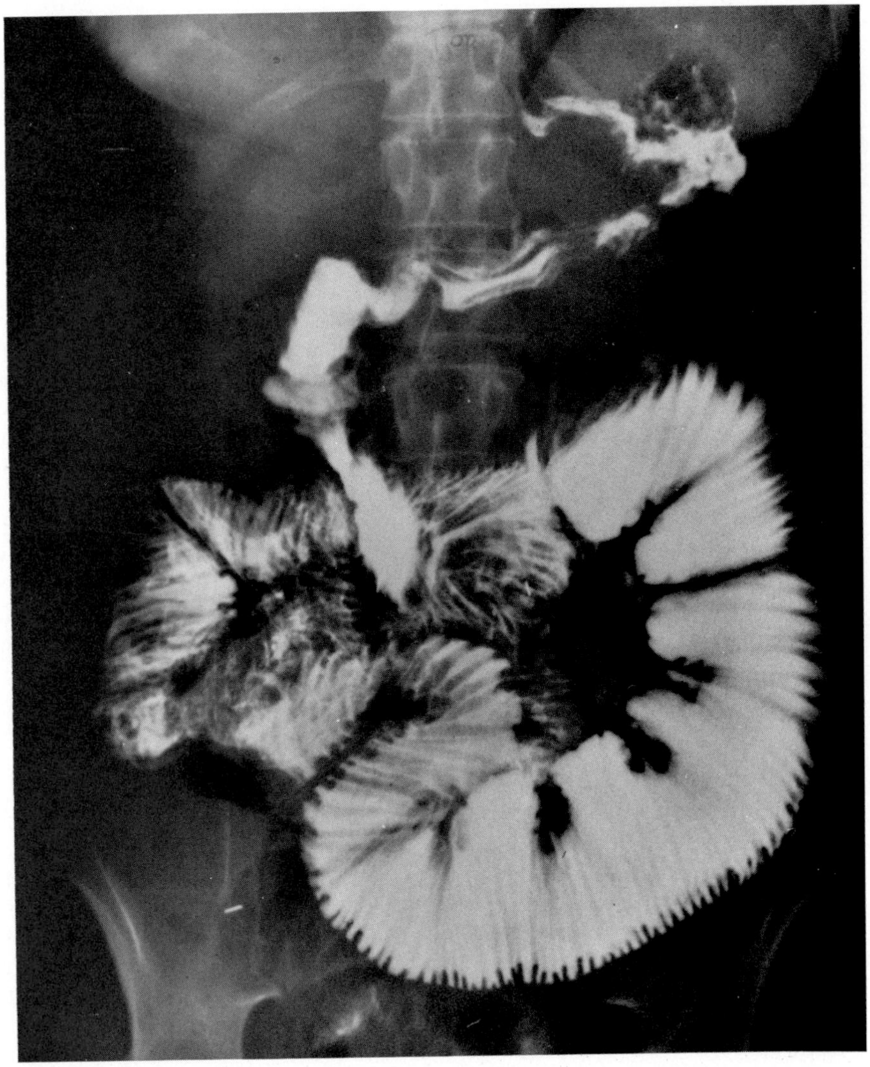

FIGURE 73–9. Upper gastrointestinal tract roentgenogram in a 46-year-old woman with diffuse cutaneous systemic sclerosis. Although dilatation of the jejunum is striking, its valvulae conniventes remain closely approximated (closed accordion sign).

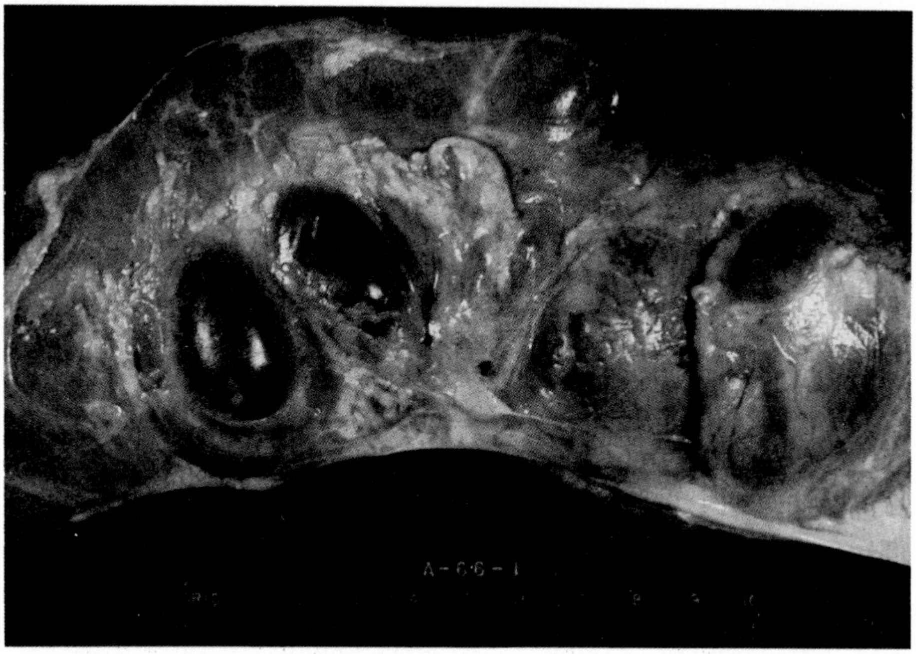

FIGURE 73–10. Gross appearance of the transverse colon from a patient with limited cutaneous scleroderma showing numerous wide-mouthed colonic diverticula, which had been demonstrated previously on barium enema.

of systemic sclerosis. Gas enters from the bowel lumen through small defects in the mucosa and muscularis mucosae and appears as numerous radiolucent cysts or linear streaks within the bowel wall. Rupture of these collections of air into the peritoneal space is occasionally accompanied by symptoms of partial bowel obstruction or by those mimicking a perforated viscus. Most often, however, this problem results in a benign pneumoperitoneum.

With the addition of serosal fibrosis, the pathologic changes in the small intestine are similar to those described for the esophagus, that is, normal mucosa or mild villous atrophy, infiltration of the lamina propria by lymphocytes and plasma cells, fibrous thickening of the submucosa, atrophy of smooth muscle with collagenous replacement, and thickening of the walls of small arteries and arterioles. Peroral biopsy specimens of the duodenum have revealed increased amounts of collagen surrounding and infiltrating Brunner's glands. Similar periglandular fibrosis is seen involving the esophageal, minor salivary, nasal mucosal, and thyroid glands.[88–90]

Colon

Constipation, either alone or alternating with diarrhea, may signal colonic involvement. Reduced motility of this organ has been reported,[91] and in one study the frequencies of anorectal and esophageal dysmotility were similar.[92] Patchy atrophy of the muscularis leads to the development of widemouthed diverticula, which usually occur along the antimesenteric border of the transverse and descending colon (Fig. 73–10). They are almost entirely unique to systemic sclerosis, having been described only in a single patient with amyloidosis.[93] Ordinarily, these outpouchings cause no difficulty, but rarely they may perforate or become impacted with fecal matter, producing obstruction.[94] Rectal incontinence and prolapse are rare but disabling problems.[95]

Lung

Lung involvement occurs in over 70% of patients[96] and during the past 10 years has emerged as the most common disease-related cause of death. The most prominent symptom is exertional dyspnea, which is present in nearly half of patients. Less often there is a chronic cough, which is nonproductive unless associated with superimposed infection, and rarely, one or more episodes of pleuritic chest pain. Many patients remain entirely asymptomatic, despite radiographic and functional evidence of pulmonary interstitial fibrosis, possibly because their physical activity is restricted. Physical examination sometimes reveals dry bibasilar "fibrotic" rales and rarely a pleural friction rub, but most commonly examination of the lungs proves unremarkable.

In over one third of patients with both diffuse and limited cutaneous scleroderma, the chest roentgenogram discloses a reticular pattern of linear, nodular, and lineonodular densities that are most pronounced in the lower lung fields. High-resolution computerized axial tomography is a more sensitive method for detecting these changes.[97] In some persons, the appearance is that of diffuse mottling or "honeycombing," indicative of cystic lesions. Large upper lobe cystic areas have been observed, most often associated with limited cutaneous involvement.[98]

Pulmonary function abnormalities occur in more

than two thirds of all patients, irrespective of disease variant.[72,99] A restrictive ventilatory defect, indicated by a reduction in forced vital capacity and decreased lung compliance, is most common. Impairment in gas exchange, evidenced by a reduced diffusing capacity for carbon monoxide, is usually present in patients with restrictive lung disease but is also common as an isolated defect without significant alteration in ventilation or roentgenographic evidence of fibrosis. A few patients have obstructive disease, but this finding is most often attributable to cigarette smoking.[100] In serial studies of pulmonary function, no excessive deterioration occurred in scleroderma patients compared with a normal population.[101,102] Some patients, however, do develop progressive, fatal respiratory failure; at highest risk are younger individuals, blacks, and males.[103]

The predominant histologic changes, present in nearly all cases at postmortem examination, consist of diffuse alveolar, interstitial, peribronchial, and pleural fibrosis (Fig. 73–11). A moderate degree of pulmonary hypertension, with a relatively slow progression, accompanies widespread pulmonary interstitial fibrosis, which very gradually obliterates more and more of the pulmonary vascular bed. Early in the disease, an inflammatory component is present. At this stage, gallium scanning is abnormal in many patients.[104,105] Alveolitis has been documented by bronchoalveolar lavage with large numbers of macrophages and lymphocytes and increased proportions of neutrophils and/or eosinophils in the lavage fluid,[106] especially in early disease.[106–109]

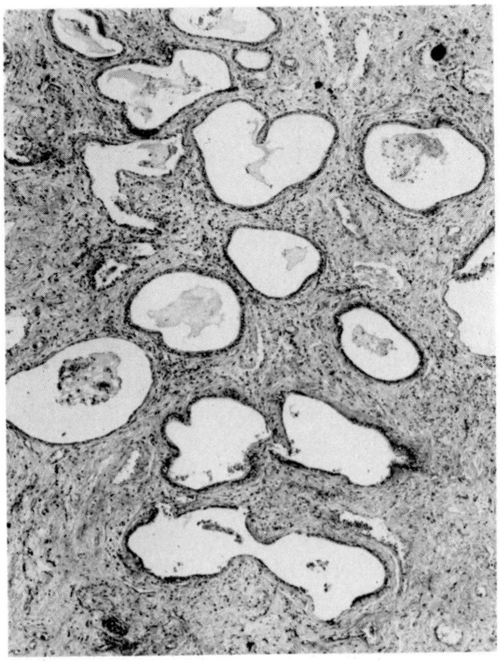

FIGURE 73–11. Photomicrograph of the lung of a 52-year-old woman with diffuse cutaneous systemic sclerosis who died as the result of respiratory insufficiency. Note the dramatic interstitial fibrosis and dilatation of air sacs (honeycomb lung).

It is believed that mononuclear cell products are important stimulants of the proliferation of lung fibroblasts.

A very different clinical entity, severe pulmonary arterial hypertension with cor pulmonale, and minimal or no pulmonary interstitial fibrosis, is encountered almost exclusively in patients with limited cutaneous involvement.[110] Less than 10% of patients in this subset develop pulmonary hypertension, which typically appears after 10 to 30 years of observation. This complication is heralded by rapid worsening of dyspnea, a markedly accentuated pulmonic component of the second heart sound, and ultimately, signs of right-sided cardiac failure. The diffusing capacity is extremely low, consistent with impaired gas exchange across thickened small pulmonary blood vessels. Diagnosis is confirmed by echocardiogram or by right-sided heart catheterization. The mean duration of survival from detection is 2 years, emphasizing the serious nature of this problem.[110] Pathologic findings include medial smooth muscle hypertrophy and uniform narrowing and/or occlusion of small pulmonary arteries caused by subintimal proliferative changes without evidence of vasculitis (Fig. 73–12).[110] The existence of "pulmonary Raynaud's phenomenon" is controversial.[111]

As expected, reduced diffusing capacity (40% or less of predicted normal) and an obstructive ventilatory defect were found to be associated with increased mortality.[112] Lung cancer occurs with increased frequency in late-stage systemic sclerosis, generally in the setting of long-standing pulmonary fibrosis with intense bronchiolar epithelial proliferation and cellular atypia and is independent of smoking.[113]

Heart

Cardiopulmonary and cardiovascular manifestations have been extensively reviewed.[96,114] Cardiac involvement may be classified as primary or secondary.[115,116] Primary disease consists of pericarditis with or without effusion, left ventricular or biventricular congestive failure, or a serious supraventricular or ventricular arrhythmia. Scleroderma patients develop atherosclerosis and hypertensive heart disease with frequencies similar to their occurrence in the general population. For this reason, one cannot assume that scleroderma is the cause of heart disease in these patients.

Acute symptomatic pericarditis is unusual. Small pericardial effusions and pericardial thickening are detected commonly by echocardiograpy, but cardiac tamponade is rare. Pericardial effusion may antedate renal involvement.[117] The few reported aspirates of pericardial fluid are exudates without evidence of immune complexes or complement activation.

Clinical evidence of congestive failure secondary to myocardial fibrosis occurs in fewer than 5% of patients, nearly all of whom have diffuse cutaneous scleroderma. New noninvasive radionuclide studies, however, show that more subtle abnormalities of ventricular function are frequent.[118] These changes are attributable to diffuse atrophy and fibrous replacement of functioning myo-

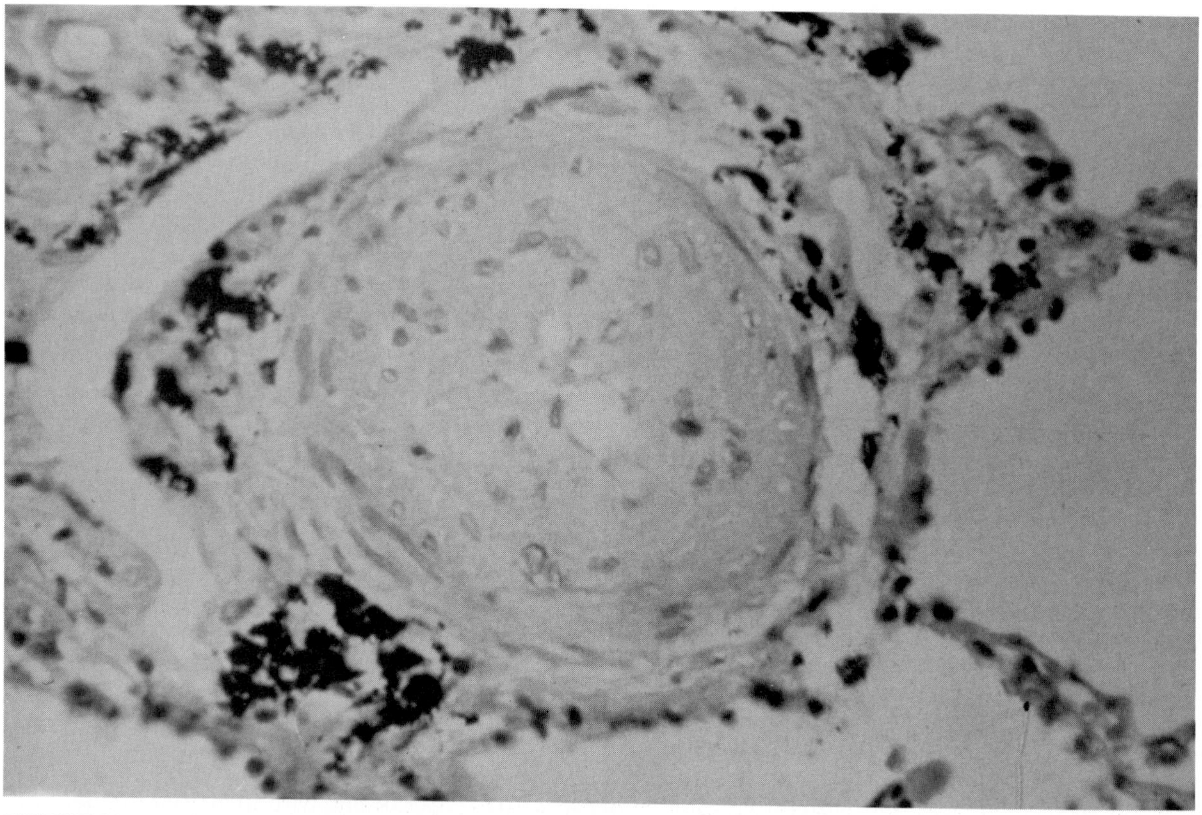

FIGURE 73–12. Photomicrograph of the lung of a 61-year-old woman with systemic sclerosis and limited scleroderma who died as the result of pulmonary arterial hypertension with cor pulmonale. There is significant intimal proliferation and medial hypertrophy of this small pulmonary artery and no interstitial fibrosis.

cardium. Myocarditis has been reported in four scleroderma patients who also had typical polymyositis.[119,120]

Although a few patients have exertional chest pain that mimics angina pectoris, coronary angiograms are most often normal. The autopsy findings of "contraction band necrosis" of the myocardium suggests that heart damage may be due to intermittent vascular spasm or "intramyocardial Raynaud's phenomenon."[121] Electrocardiographic evidence of myocardial ischemia and/or necrosis in the absence of the clinical syndrome of myocardial infarction has been noted.[122] Both resting and reversible exercise and cold-induced myocardial perfusion defects and left ventricular dysfunction have been detected,[123] especially in patients with diffuse disease,[118] raising the possibility that multiple vasospastic ischemic episodes led to myocardial fibrosis. These resting defects are reversible after administration of oral nifedipine[124] or intravenous dipyridamole.[125] The latter potent vasodilator was also used to determine coronary blood flow and resistance reserve, which were reduced in scleroderma cardiomyopathy patients compared with controls.[126]

Autopsies of patients with diffuse scleroderma may also show extensive degeneration of myocardial fibers with replacement by irregular patches of fibrosis that are prominent in, but not limited to, perivascular areas (Fig. 73–13). The large extramural coronary arteries are typically normal, but focal infiltrates of round cells and considerable thickening of smaller coronary vessels may occur.[127] Myocardial infarction is unusual.

Cardiac arrhythmias including complete heart block and other electrocardiographic abnormalities are encountered, as expected in cardiomyopathy regardless of cause. During 24-hour continuous electrocardiogram (Holter monitor), one fifth of scleroderma patients had conduction defects in a point-prevalence study.[128] Arrhythmias may exercise performance in up to one third of patients.[129] Careful dissection of the conduction system of several patients with rhythm disturbances, including complete heart block, has revealed fibrous replacement of the sinus node; atrioventricular node, particularly in its proximal segment;[130] and bundle branches.[131] In most cases, however, no specific morphologic changes have been identified in this tissue, and arrhythmias have been attributed to disturbances of the working myocardium.

Secondary causes of heart disease typically are due to the extracardiac stresses of pulmonary and systemic arterial hypertension. The former occurs chiefly in the limited cutaneous variant, as noted previously. Severe systemic arterial hypertension associated with renal in-

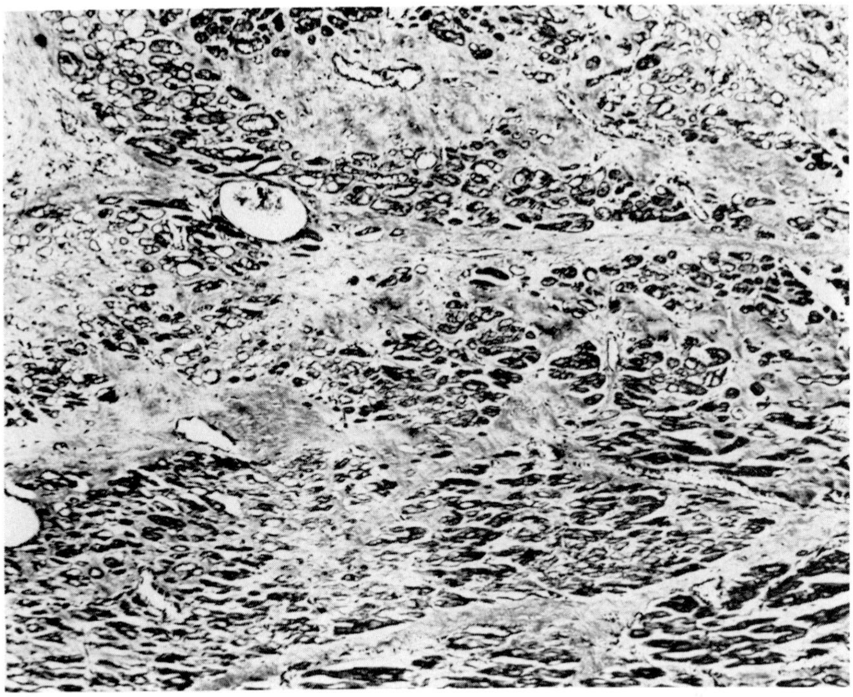

FIGURE 73–13. Photomicrograph of myocardium of a 52-year-old woman with diffuse cutaneous systemic sclerosis who died of congestive heart failure. Loss of normal myocardial fibers is extensive, and interstitial fibrosis is severe.

volvement (see following discussion) frequently leads to myocardial dysfunction.

Kidney

Renal disease is an important aspect of systemic sclerosis, and in previous decades, has been the major cause of death.[132] Clinically evident renal involvement is restricted almost exclusively to persons with diffuse cutaneous disease, especially those with rapidly progressive skin thickening of less than 3 years' duration.[133] Rarely is a person with the limited cutaneous variant affected unless misclassified during an early stage in the evolution of diffuse disease.

Twenty percent of diffuse cutaneous scleroderma patients develop a dramatic complication, termed *scleroderma renal crisis,* with the abrupt onset of highly malignant arterial hypertension, followed immediately by rapidly progressive oliguric renal insufficiency. In some populations, renal crisis is considerably less frequent for unknown reasons.[134] The appearance of hypertension is heralded by a variety of manifestations including severe headache, visual difficulties resulting from striking hypertensive retinopathy, seizures, or sudden left ventricular failure. Within several days or weeks, microscopic hematuria and proteinuria are noted, along with rapidly increasing azotemia, and finally oliguria or anuria. Proteinuria in the nephrotic range is unusual. Severe hypertension is typically associated with extremely high plasma renin levels.

On occasion, the blood pressure may remain within normal limits, and azotemia and severe microangiopathic hemolytic anemia become the dominant features.[135] Prior administration of adrenocorticotrophic hormone (ACTH) or a corticosteroid preparation has been reported as a precipitating factor in "scleroderma kidney," especially of the normotensive type,[135] but in most instances these drugs cannot be implicated. Sudden, severe volume depletion may also trigger renal crisis in the susceptible patient, who often has had clinically undetected reduced renal blood flow. Renal angiography during life and postmortem injection studies have demonstrated a striking constriction of interlobular arteries and afferent arterioles and a sharp decrease in glomerular filling (Fig. 73–14).[136]

Before the 1980s, survival for more than 3 to 6 months after the onset of this most dreaded complication was almost unknown; patients succumbed to renal or cardiac failure or to cerebral hemorrhage despite treatment with available antihypertensive agents. However, the aggressive use of potent new drugs that block the renin–angiotensin system appears to be uniformly successful in controlling hypertension, although renal insufficiency may nevertheless progress, requiring dialysis. In many instances, it has been possible to discontinue dialysis after several months.[137] Simultaneous remarkable reduction in skin thickness has been noted in some but not all patients who have survived renal crisis.[138]

Numerous small cortical infarcts are seen grossly in the affected kidneys with subintimal proliferative changes of the intralobular arteries. Focal microscopic alterations consist of intimal hyperplasia, with acid mucopolysaccharide deposition, and necrosis of the walls of these vessels, afferent arterioles, and glomerular tufts (Fig. 73–15). Only prominent fibrosis of the adventitia

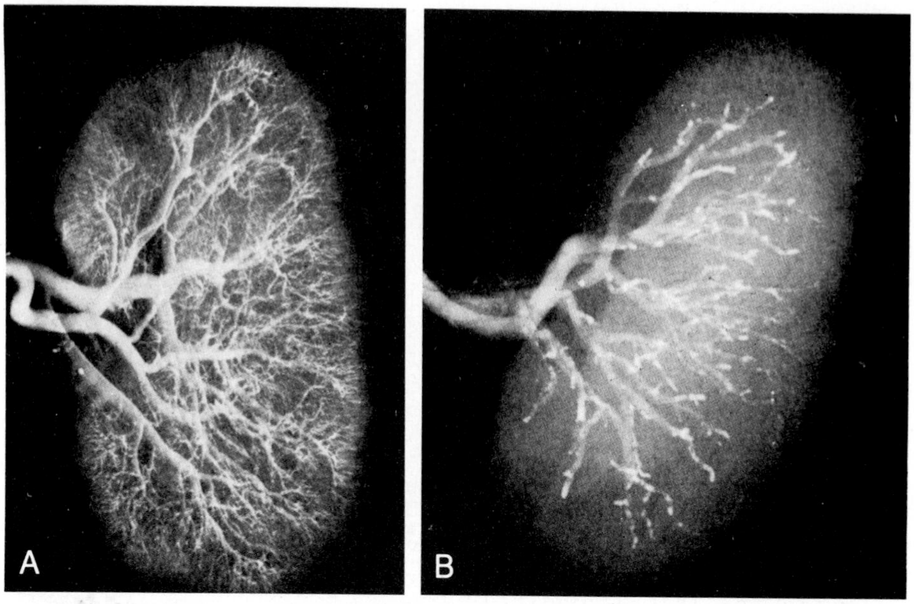

FIGURE 73–14. Roentgenograms of kidneys, injected postmortem, of two patients with diffuse cutaneous systemic sclerosis. *A*, Kidney of a man who died of cardiac disease without clinical evidence of renal involvement. Filling of the interlobular and smaller cortical vessels is normal. *B*, Kidney of a man who developed "scleroderma renal crisis" with malignant hypertension and renal failure. There is irregular narrowing of the interlobular vessels and little filling of smaller vessels supplying the renal cortex.

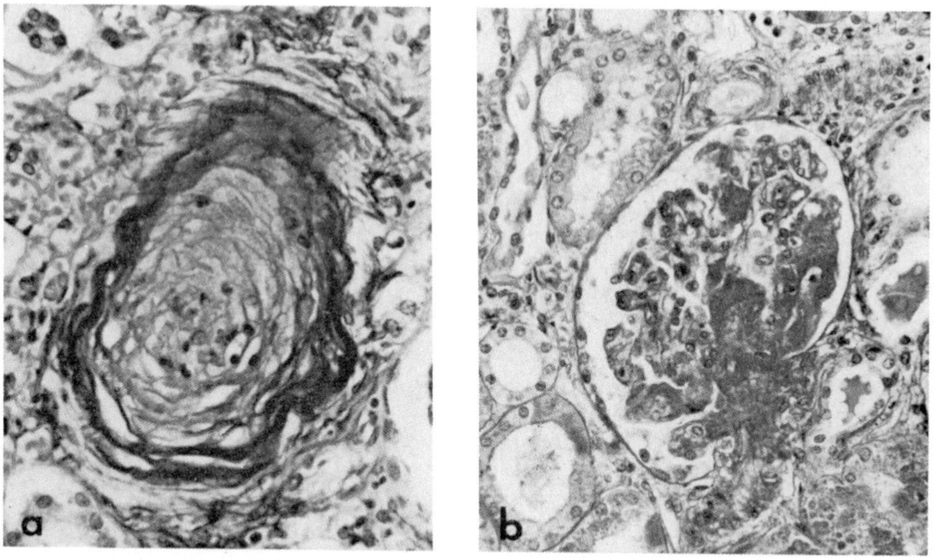

FIGURE 73–15. Photomicrographs of kidneys of two women who died of malignant arterial hypertension and renal insufficiency complicating diffuse cutaneous systemic sclerosis. *A*, Intimal hyperplasia with complete lumenal occlusion of an interlobular artery. Note reduplication and fraying of the internal elastic lamina (orcein stain). *B*, Fibrinoid necrosis of blood vessels in the glomerulus.

of the small vessels may distinguish this lesion from that of nonsclerodermatous malignant nephrosclerosis.[136] Identical histopathologic changes have been observed in the absence of hypertension.[139] These alterations are reminiscent of those encountered in the digital vessels, as discussed earlier.

Immunohistologic examination has revealed the regular presence of immunoglobulins (chiefly IgM); complement components (also reported in malignant hypertension not associated with systemic sclerosis); and fibrinogen in the walls of affected vessels.[140,141] Electron microscopic examination, however, has failed to reveal discrete electron-dense deposits or other features indicative of the presence of immune complexes.[140]

Symptomatic sclerodermatous involvement of the lower urinary tract is rare, although bladder wall connective tissue deposition and proliferative vascular lesions have been noted.[142]

Liver and Pancreas

Primary biliary cirrhosis occurs in some women with limited cutaneous scleroderma,[143] most frequently in association with Sjögren's syndrome.[144] These patients develop pruritus, jaundice, and hepatomegaly, with a pronounced elevation of serum alkaline phosphatase activity and antimitochondrial antibodies, most often directed against a 72,000-dalton M2 autoantigen.[145] Nodular regenerative hyperplasia of the liver has also been reported.[146] There is no convincing clinical evidence of pancreatic exocrine or endocrine dysfunction or increased pancreatic fibrosis at autopsy compared with controls.[147]

Blood

In typical systemic sclerosis, hematologic studies are normal, and abnormalities suggest either a specific complication or an associated illness.[148] Only a few patients have anemia classified as being due to chronic disease; blood loss (peptic esophagitis or telangiectases); excessive destruction (microangiopathic hemolysis); or metabolic causes (intestinal malabsorption). Their peripheral blood and bone marrow reflect these circumstances, and the marrow is not fibrotic. Autoimmune hemolytic anemia[149] and neutropenia[150] have been recorded. Leukopenia is often present when systemic sclerosis exists in overlap with SLE or with mixed connective tissue disease.[148] Impressive eosinophilia (over 500 cells per cubic millimeter) is unusual;[151] its presence should alert the physician to the possibility of one of the localized forms of scleroderma (discussed later in the chapter).

Nervous System

Primary disorders of the nervous system are seldom encountered. Most of the problems that occur are either purely coincidental or represent secondary compressive phenomena, for example, carpal tunnel syndrome.[152] Trigeminal sensory neuropathy, an occasional finding, is associated most closely with myositis and serum antiribonucleoprotein (anti-RNP) antibodies.[153] Cerebral arteritis has been reported[154] as well as vasculitis that is believed to be due to coexisting Sjögren's syndrome.[155] Impotence without other obvious cause has been described and is most likely due to reduced penile blood flow.[156] Autonomic neuropathy was observed in one patient and suspected in three others.[157]

Eyes and Ears

With the exception of keratoconjunctivitis sicca, most ocular disease in patients with systemic sclerosis is due to other conditions.[158] Hypertensive retinopathy found in persons with renal crisis has already been described. Patchy areas of nonperfusion have been noted in the choroidal capillary bed.[159] Sensorineural hearing loss was found in the majority of patients in one study and was not attributable to factors such as age, drugs, or noise.[160]

Sjögren's Syndrome

Dry eyes and dry mouth are frequent complaints. Lymphocytic infiltration of minor salivary glands on labial biopsy is present in approximately 15 to 20% of patients[90] In a similar proportion, periglandular and intraglandular fibrosis occur and are believed to be characteristic of scleroderma. Half of scleroderma patients with Sjögren's syndrome have serum anti-SSA/Ro and/or anti-SSB/La antibodies, but these autoantibodies occur almost exclusively in patients with glandular lymphocytic infiltration rather than fibrosis.[90] As in primary Sjögren's syndrome, vasculitis involving the skin (palpable purpura and leg ulcers) and peripheral nervous system (sensory neuropathy and mononeuritis multiplex) may occur.[155]

Thyroid Gland

Hypothyroidism, often clinically unrecognized, occurs in one fourth of patients with systemic sclerosis and is frequently accompanied by serum antithyroid antibodies.[161] As in the salivary glands, fibrosis is a prominent histologic finding,[89] whereas lymphocytic infiltration typical of Hashimoto's thyroiditis is unusual. Hyperthyroidism has also been noted.[162]

Serum Autoantibodies

Moderate hyper-γ-globulinemia (1.4 to 2.0 g/dL) occurs in over one third of patients and is most often countered in the setting of overlap conditions. Typically, IgG is increased, but IgM elevation has also been observed.[163] Monoclonal gammopathy has been described,[164] and a child with scleroderma, myositis, and IgA deficiency has been reported.[165] The level of serum complement is normal in all but a few patients. Mixed cryoglobulins and circulating immune complexes have been detected in small amounts[166,167] and were found to be present only in association with certain autoantibodies (Scl 70, nRNP, SSA/Ro, and SSB/La).[168] One third of patients have positive tests for rheumatoid factor, usually in low titer. Lupus erythematosus (LE) cells reactions and biologic false-positive serologic reactions for syphilis have been reported, most often in overlap syndromes, but are uncommon.

With the use of multiple substrates, antinuclear antibodies have been found in the sera of over 90% of pa-

TABLE 73–3. CLINICAL AND LABORATORY CHARACTERISTICS OF PATIENTS WITH SYSTEMIC SCLEROSIS ACCORDING TO SERUM AUTOANTIBODY TYPE

	AUTOANTIBODY SUBTYPE						
CHARACTERISTICS	ACA	Th	U1RNP	PM-Scl	U3RNP	RNA Pol I, III	Scl-70
ANA staining pattern	Centromere	Nucleolar	Speckled	Nucleolar	Nucleolar	Speckled/ nucleolar	Speckled
Proportion of all patients	25%	5%	10%	5%	5%	20%	15%
Clinical classification	Limited	Limited	Limited, overlap	Mixed, overlap	Mixed, overlap	Diffuse	Diffuse
Organ involvement	PHT	PHT, small bowel	Muscle	Muscle	Muscle, PHT	Skin, renal	Lung fibrosis
HLA association	None			DR3, w52			DR5

ANA = antinuclear antibody; HLA = human leukocyte antigen; PHT = "primary" pulmonary hypertension.

tients with systemic sclerosis.[169] The amounts are typically low as compared with those found in SLE, but titers of 1 : 1000 or greater are seen occasionally. In most instances, the pattern of nuclear fluorescence is that of fine or large speckles or threads, but nucleolar and occasionally diffuse (homogeneous) nuclear staining also occur. It is widely accepted that certain autoantibodies are highly specific for systemic sclerosis and also define clinically homogeneous patient subsets. In aggregate, seven autoantibodies account for nearly 85% of all patients with scleroderma. Their immunofluorescence patterns on routine antinuclear antibody testing and their clinical and immunogenetic associations are shown in Table 73–3.

Anti-topoisomerase I antibodies are found in 20% to over 50% of systemic sclerosis sera, but rarely in control specimens[170,171] and are associated with diffuse cutaneous scleroderma and pulmonary interstitial involvement.[171] Originally designated anti-Scl 70,[170] this antibody is now known to recognize the nuclear enzyme DNA topoisomerase I.[172]

Anticentromere antibodies appear morphologically as fine, discrete speckles directed against the centromeric portion of chromosomes observed in dividing cells.[173] They have remarkable specificity for limited cutaneous scleroderma, where they occur in over 50% of patients compared with fewer than 5% of patients with diffuse cutaneous disease.[174,175] These antibodies are found in a few persons with Raynaud's phenomenon alone, who may be at increased risk of developing limited scleroderma eventually.[176] Some patients with other diagnoses, including SLE and RA, have anticentromere antibodies,[177,177a,177b] although Raynaud's phenomenon is almost universally present in these cases. These predominantly IgG antibodies tend to persist in the serum for prolonged periods.[178] Immunoelectron microscopy has pinpointed the antigen as residing in the kinetochore region of chromosomes, but its precise identity is not yet known.[179] Three distinct antigens are recognized by nearly all anticentromere antibody-positive sera,[180] but their clinical relevance is unknown.

The coexistence of anti-topoisomerase I and anticentromere antibodies was reported in 2 of 121 patients,[181] but must be rare indeed because I have found no such occurrences in over 700 positive tests.

Some patients have high titers of antibody to nuclear ribonucleoprotein (anti-U1RNP); these persons tend to have myositis more frequently than those without high-titer anti-U1RNP.[182] Antibody directed against the nuclear antigen Ku, distinct from nRNP, has been found in a small proportion f Japanese patients, nearly all of whom had a scleroderma–polymyositis overlap syndrome.[183] Anti-Ku has been observed in both SLE and scleroderma patients in the United States.[183a] Both of the preceding are associated with speckled staining in routine antinuclear antibody testing. Antibodies to other components of dividing cells such as metaphase chromatin[184] and centrioles[185] have also been observed in sera of systemic sclerosis patients. The latter were reported in two patients with systemic sclerosis[186,187] and in one with Raynaud's phenomenon.[186]

Nucleolar immunofluorescence has been detected in 10 to 54% of scleroderma sera. These antibodies are relatively specific for systemic sclerosis, particularly in patients with associated Sjögren's syndrome. Several of the responsible nucleolar antigens have now been identified. A few patients with anti-topoisomerase I display nucleolar staining,[8] and antibody to RNA polymerase I has been detected.[188] The latter autoantibody appears to identify a group of women with otherwise typical diffuse cutaneous disease.[8] Anti-PM-Scl (previously termed *anti-PM-1*), which is also directed against a nucleolar antigen,[10] is associated with limited skin thickening and often with polymyositis.[11] Several newly described autoantibodies have helped to complete the picture of antinucleolar antibodies. Anti-Th accounts for approximately 10% of patients with limited cutaneous disease.[6] Anti-U3RNP identifies patients with both diffuse and limited skin disease, but two interesting subsets include black women with skeletal myopathy and a small group of individuals with diffuse disease and pulmonary arterial hypertension. New data have identified a large group of persons with diffuse disease who have anti-RNA polymerase III antibodies, some of whom also have anti-RNA polymerase I.[7] In contrast to the anti-RNA polymerase I sera, those with anti-RNA polymerase III activity display nuclear rather than nucleolar staining.

Anticardiolipin antibody has been detected in low concentration in 11 of 35 patients without vascular disease or other clinical associations.[189]

DISEASE COURSE

The course of systemic sclerosis is extremely variable. Early in the illness, it is difficult to judge prognosis with respect to either survival and disability. Many patients with diffuse cutaneous scleroderma experience steadily increasing sclerosis of the fingers and hands, leading to deforming flexion contractures. In others, mobility is maintained despite advancing skin changes. The most reliable early sign predicting subsequent severe diffuse skin involvement are the appearance of cutaneous thickening before the onset of Raynaud's phenomenon, rapid progression of scleroderma toward the more proximal parts of the extremities, tendon friction rubs, and serum anti-topoisomerase I or anti-RNA polymerase I or III antibodies. Often, later in the disease, spontaneous improvement in skin thickening occurs, and thus, the designation *"progressive"* is not uniformly applicable and should be abandoned.[34]

Clinical evidence of active disease consists of increase in the extent and severity of skin thickness as well as worsening of clinical or laboratory features of musculoskeletal or visceral involvement. Considering the pathophysiology of disease, several newly described laboratory studies may provide useful guides to disease activity. Microvascular damage is reflected by the release into plasma of factor VIII/von Willebrand factor antigen from injured endothelium,[48,190] lymphocyte activation by the serum level of interleukin-2 (IL-2)[191] and soluble IL-2 receptors,[192] and fibroblast activity by serum procollagen III peptide concentration.[193] Such tests also have the potential to be useful adjuncts in the performance of clinical trials.

Limited cutaneous scleroderma was initially considered to represent a benign variant associated with a relatively favorable prognosis. Raynaud's phenomenon, alone or in combination with swollen, puffy fingers, may be present for up to a decade or more before the diagnosis of systemic sclerosis is evident. The life span of patients with limited scleroderma is significantly longer than that of patients with diffuse scleroderma, in part because the former rarely, if ever, develop myocardial or renal involvement. Anticentromere antibody itself is often a clue to a good prognosis.[194] However, as noted previously, a small number of limited scleroderma patients acquire severe pulmonary arterial hypertension, which is independent of the presence of anticentromere antibody and is almost uniformly fatal.[110]

Several large survival studies have been reported and summarized.[195] The 5-year cumulative survival rate after either first physician diagnosis or entry to study has ranged from 34 to 73%, and researchers agree that male sex, older age, and involvement of the kidney, heart, and lung adversely affect outcome (Fig. 73–16). It is disturbing that long-term followup studies show continued excess mortality among patients with diffuse cutaneous disease.[195a,195b] To the extent that they are associated with the clinically defined subsets described previously, serum autoantibodies are also useful in predicting prognosis.[196]

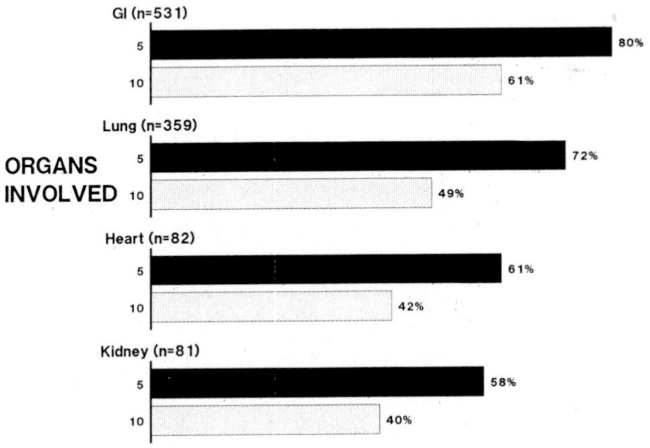

FIGURE 73–16. Cumulative survival rates in patients with systemic sclerosis 5 and 10 years after the first detection of certain types of visceral involvement (University of Pittsburgh, 1981 to 1990).

Childhood Disease

Systemic sclerosis is rare in childhood.[197] Most reported children have diffuse cutaneous disease[198] or overlap syndromes.[199] Clinical findings are similar to those in adults except for an increased frequency of myocardial involvement[198] and possibly a reduced frequency of "renal crisis."[198,200–202] Serum antinucleolar antibodies may be more commonly found in children than in adults.[203]

Pregnancy

There is controversy concerning both fertility and the frequency of spontaneous abortion.[204,205] Pregnancy appears to exert no consistent effect on the course of systemic sclerosis.[205–207] Conversely, the disease ordinarily does not interfere with pregnancy or parturition. Instances of hypertension alone,[205] serious and fatal third-trimester or postpartum renal involvement with severe hypertension,[207a,208] and nephrotic syndrome[209] have been reported but may be unrepresentative. In general, women with early diffuse disease should be advised not to become pregnant.

Malignancy

The published frequency of cancer in large clinical series has varied from 3 to 7%.[210–212] In the only studies in which population denominators and comparison groups have been used, several important associations have been detected. In two case series[210,213] and an epidemiologic study,[113] a subset of women developed breast cancer at or near the time of onset of scleroderma. Lung cancer is significantly more frequent than in the age- and sex-matched general population and occurs in the setting of long-standing scleroderma with pulmonary interstitial fibrosis and is independent of cigarette smoking.[113] Alveolar cell carcinoma, for many years believed to be a specific sequel of scleroderma, is only one of the lung tumors found and does not occur more often than expected.[113] Surprisingly few lymphoproliferative malignancies have been reported in systemic sclerosis patients. However, as might be expected, the use of immunosuppressive agents may be followed by an excessive number of late lymphoproliferative neoplasms.[214]

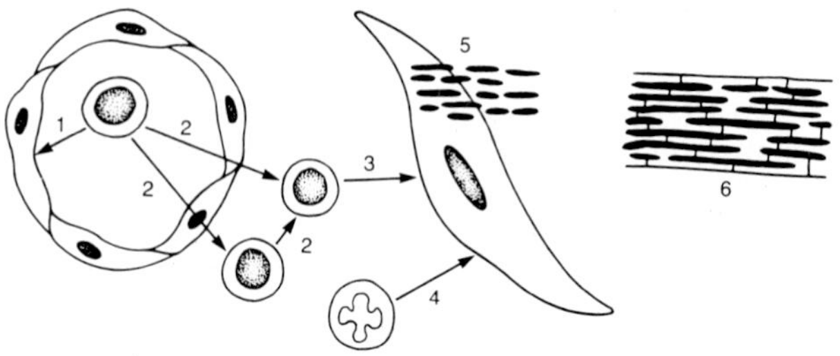

FIGURE 73–17. Schematic representation of pathophysiology of systemic sclerosis with possible sites for therapeutic intervention. Rational therapy would be designed (1) to prevent endothelial cell damage; (2) to alter communication between mononuclear cell subsets; (3) to prevent mononuclear cell stimulation of fibroblasts; (4) to prevent mast cell degranulation; (5) to block fibroblast production or extrusion of procollagen; or (6) to increase solubilization of preformed collagen.

TREATMENT

The first responsibility of the physician is to discuss the nature of the disease with the patient and family, who are often unreasonably pessimistic. Classification as diffuse cutaneous or limited cutaneous scleroderma is helpful in understanding the future risk of developing visceral complications and which ones they may be. Such discussion aids in establishing a good relationship between physician and patient, which is particularly important in this chronic, demanding disease. Diagrams of the blood vessels, skin, esophagus, and other appropriate illustrations are useful in instruction. Several excellent publications geared to patients and family members are available from arthritis and scleroderma support organizations, and these should be recommended.

Numerous vitamins, hormones, pharmaceuticals, and surgical procedures have been used to treat systemic sclerosis; nearly all of these therapies have been abandoned after initial enthusiasm and later critical evaluation. Improvement can hardly be expected in those manifestations that are the result of far-advanced tissue fibrosis. Too often, success has been claimed solely on the basis of a diminution in subjective complaints (e.g., a reduction in frequency of Raynaud's phenomenon, which occurs with virtually any new treatment) and poorly documented "softening" of the skin.

Evaluation of the effectiveness of treatment has proved difficult for several reasons.[215] Systemic sclerosis is variable in its severity and in its rate of progression; therefore, the classification of patients into subsets is important in interpreting the results of therapy. Because spontaneous improvement often occurs after several years, controlled trials are necessary. There are limitations in the availability and application of objective criteria for ascertaining improvement (or deterioration) in the condition, particularly with respect to visceral changes. Finally, the influence of psychologic factors on many of the symptoms is important.

Drugs

Fig. 73–17 summarizes some current concepts of the pathogenesis of systemic sclerosis and indicates those points at which therapeutic intervention might be considered.[216] *No drug or combination of drugs has been proved to be of value in adequately controlled prospective trials.* Anti-inflammatory agents and corticosteroids have been disappointing. Because of their potential toxicity, I restrict the use of corticosteroids to patients with inflammatory myopathy or symptomatic serositis. On occasion, refractory arthritis and the "edematous" phase of skin involvement respond favorably to relatively small doses of corticosteroids, such as prednisone 5 to 10 mg/day. Myositis, however, may require higher doses. There has been some concern that high-dose corticosteroid therapy may precipitate acute renal failure.[217]

In the past, attention has been focused on D-penicillamine, a compound that interferes with the intermolecular cross linking of collagen and also possesses immunosuppressive activity. Reports from England,[218] Denmark,[219] and the U.S.S.R.[220] have been optimistic. In two retrospective U.S. studies of early diffuse disease,[32,221] one with an untreated "comparison" group,[32] there was striking improvement in skin thickening, reduced frequency of subsequent renal involvement, and survival. D-penicillamine may also improve established interstitial lung disease when given for a prolonged period.[222,223] Its use may be accompanied by a variety of side effects, including some that are autoimmune in nature, such as nephrotic syndrome, glomerulonephritis,[224] pemphigus, and myasthenia gravis.[225] Up to one fourth of patients may be forced to discontinue the drug.[226] Adverse reactions occur with lower frequency when the D-penicillamine dose is increased slowly (over 6 to 8 months to a maximum of 1000 to 1500 mg/day). Careful monitoring of the white blood cell and platelet counts and of urine protein are recommended. Chemically related compounds such as N-acetylcysteine[227] and S-adenosylmethionine[228] have also been used with limited success.

Colchicine inhibits the accumulation of collagen by blocking the conversion of procollagen to collagen, probably through interference with microtubule-mediated transport or perhaps by stimulation of collagenase production. In one long-term open trial (mean followup 39 months), improvement in skin thickening occurred in 17 of 19 patients who received colchicine, 10 mg/week.[229] However, several other negative studies have been published and reviewed.[223,230] In none of these trials was colchicine toxicity a serious limiting factor.

A variety of potential beneficial effects can be hypothesized from the use of immunosuppressive drugs, including alterations in interactions between immunocompetent cells and inhibition of the effects of soluble mediators on fibroblast function. Azathioprine was considered beneficial in an uncontrolled study,[231] and 5-fluorouracil was reported to result in some cutaneous improvement but had unacceptable gastrointestinal toxicity.[232] Chlorambucil results have been mixed, but a recent 3-year double-blind controlled trial was negative.[233] As in RA,[234] late-developing malignancy may be a limiting feature of the use of alkylating agents.[214] Plasmapheresis has been advocated,[235–237] but its effect are not uniformly beneficial[238] and are difficult to evaluate because of confounding immunosuppressive and corticosteroid therapy. Cyclosporine A has been used in a limited number of patients,[239] but no trials are currently ongoing owing to an unacceptably high frequency of hypertension and renal insufficiency, which could be attributable either to the drug or to scleroderma. The effects of recombinant interferon-γ, an "immunomodulating" drug, are uncertain, but may be promising on the basis of an uncontrolled open trial.[240] Several abstracts have been published on the beneficial effects of methotrexate.[241,242] To date, there is no general agreement on the effectiveness of immunosuppressive drug therapy. Additional adequately controlled therapeutic trials are urgently needed.[215] The use of immunosuppressive measures seems justified in patients with rapidly progressive, life-threatening and/or disabling disease, provided there is informed consent and close surveillance for adverse effects.

Agents designed to protect injured endothelial cells and to prevent platelet aggregation and subsequent release of platelet-derived growth factors are a logical extension of the vascular hypothesis of scleroderma. Although increased circulating platelet aggregates and plasma β-thromboglobulin levels were reduced by treatment with dipyridamole and aspirin,[243] a randomized, double-blind 2-year trial of these agents versus placebo showed no significant improvement in the treatment group.[244] Lower doses of dipyridamole in the latter study could conceivably account for the ineffectiveness. This approach to systemic sclerosis should not be abandoned. A controlled trial of antihypertensive therapy did not result in any clinically meaningful improvement over a 24-month period.[245]

SUPPORTING MEASURES

Raynaud's Phenomenon

It must be recognized that in systemic sclerosis, preexisting structural damage underlies vasospastic episodes. Common sense self-management includes avoiding undue cold exposure, dressing warmly, and abstaining from tobacco use. Induced vasodilation[246] and biofeedback[247] may also be helpful. Various vasodilating drugs have been employed, including intra-arterial reserpine,[248] methyldopa,[249] adrenergic blocking agents, and α-receptor blocking and β-receptor stimulating drugs.[250] In general, these compounds have proved disappointing.

Several promising new pharmacologic agents have been effective in double-blind studies, including the calcium channel blocker nifedipine;[251,252] a direct vasodilator, prazosin;[253] an oral serotonin antagonist, ketanserin;[254] topical nitroglycerin;[255] PGE_1;[256] and prostacyclin.[257] Whether renin–angiotensin blockade benefits vascular disease in organs other than the kidney is unknown, although captopril did not ameliorate Raynaud's phenomenon or alter digital plethysmographic findings during cold challenge in one study.[258]

Thoracic sympathectomy may be followed by partial (usually transient) improvement in Raynaud's phenomenon but not by significant or sustained influence on the course of cutaneous changes or visceral sclerosis.[250] When large vessels are involved, such as radial or ulnar arteries, microvascular surgical reconstruction should be considered.[259] Digital tip amputation occasionally may be required, although the demarcation of tissue achieved by autoamputation is preferred.[259,260] Thus, if pain can be controlled with narcotic analgesics for the time necessary for such demarcation, tissue loss may be minimized. The development of "wet" gangrene of course would force amputation.

Calcinosis

Unfortunately, reliable treatment to eradicate calcinosis is not available. Surgical excision of large calcareous masses may be helpful in selected instances.[259] Soft tissue calcinotic deposits contain increased amounts of the amino acid 4-carboxyl-L-glutamic acid (Gla).[261] Thus, long-term inhibition of Gla with low-dose anticoagulant therapy may be useful,[262] but this form of therapy remains unproven. Suppression of local sterile inflammation surrounding these hydroxyapatite deposits has been achieved with colchicine.[263]

Skin

Special lotions, soaps, and bath oils should be used to relieve excessive skin dryness; taking unduly frequent baths and using household detergents may aggravate this symptom. Pruritus is a frequent and occasionally dominant problem in early diffuse cutaneous disease. There is no adequate therapy for pruritis, but fortunately it always disappears later in the course of the illness.

Digital tip ulcerations can be protected by plastic finger casts. Noninfected ulcers respond rapidly to the use of occlusive dressings, such as Duoderm, which are also protective. If these lesions become infected (almost always with staphylococci), half-strength hydrogen peroxide soaks and gentle local debridement are employed, and oral antibiotics are sometimes recommended. Deeper soft tissue infections, septic arthritis, and osteomyelitis must be treated vigorously with intravenous antibiotics, excision of infected and devitalized tissue, joint fusion, and rarely, amputation.

Joints and Muscles

Articular complaints may be treated with salicylates and other nonsteroidal anti-inflammatory drugs, with careful attention to their potential to aggravate gastroesophageal reflux. Corticosteroids are seldom necessary, but patients with true synovitis may benefit from prednisone, 5 to 7.5 mg/day, during the first 6 to 12 months of disease. Patients with diffuse cutaneous involvement often develop digital contractures with deformity. Dynamic splinting does not prevent the progression of this process,[264] but a vigorous daily exercise program to minimize loss of motion may be very beneficial. Proximal interphalangeal joint replacement arthroplasties have been performed later in disease, with improvement in hand function and appearance.[265] When severe finger contractures have occurred, and excessive flexion of the proximal interphalangeal (PIP) joints leaves them vulnerable to trauma with repeated skin breakdown and infection, including septic arthritis, joint replacement will not be effective; in this circumstance, PIP joint fusion is preferred.[259] After such fusions, hand function depends on the amount of motion present at the metacarpophalangeal joints. Surgical wound healing has been excellent.

Active polymyositis with proximal muscle weakness that is due to systemic sclerosis or attributable to an overlap syndrome should be treated with moderate doses of corticosteroids (prednisone, 20 to 30 mg/day), and methotrexate can be added in the event that response is incomplete. In contrast, bland myopathy with minimal elevation of serum creatine kinase and little or no progression of weakness is generally not treated pharmacologically.

Gastrointestinal Tract

Maintenance of the oral opening requires mouth-stretching exercises;[266] the patient must also maintain good oral hygiene and make regular visits to a dentist for prophylaxis. For edentulous individuals with microstomia, a flexible prosthesis has been designed to augment the exercise program.[267]

Patients who have difficulty in swallowing should learn to masticate carefully and to avoid foods likely to cause substernal dysphagia (e.g., meat, bread). Metoclopramide improves esophageal motility and is useful in some patients.[268] Cisapride stimulates both gastric and esophageal emptying.[269] Because nifedipine is capable of decreasing lower esophageal sphincter pressure and contraction amplitude in the body of the esophagus,[270] it may aggravate esophageal symptoms. In this respect, diltiazem may be a preferable agent.[271] Reflux esophagitis can be minimized by appropriate measures, such as assuming the upright position during and after eating, avoiding food before bedtime, raising the head of the bed on blocks to prevent nocturnal reflux, and taking an antacid 45 to 60 minutes after meals and at bedtime, histamine (H_2) receptor blockade[272] and cytoprotection with sucralfate. The latter should be given as a slurry to avoid development of a gastric bezoar, a complication observed in some patients with reduced gastric motility. Esophageal stricture may require periodic dilatation. Successful excision of strictures and correction of gastroesophageal reflux by gastroplasty combined with fundoplication have been reported.[273]

Transient improvement in steatorrhea and other signs of intestinal malabsorption may follow the administration of tetracycline or other broad-spectrum antibiotics, but the underlying hypomotility is unaffected. Metoclopramide significantly increases small bowel motility[274] but is not effective in patients with gross malabsorption. In advanced circumstances, one must replace calcium and fat-soluble vitamins, use medium-chain triglycerides and, often, resort to parenteral hyperalimentation.[275] In severe malabsorption, the likelihood of septicemia of catheter origin or other serious bacterial infection and premature death is high.

Lung

Patients with pulmonary fibrosis who have bacterial bronchitis or pneumonitis require prompt and vigorous antibiotic treatment. Prophylactic influenza and pneumococcal pneumonia vaccination should be given. In persons with documented inflammatory alveolitis which has been shown to predict subsequent decline in pulmonary function, high-dose corticosteroids (with or without immunosuppressive drugs) may be efficacious short-term therapy.[276,277] Evidence indicates that D-penicillamine is useful in the treatment of scleroderma interstitial lung disease.[278–280] When there is resting- or exercise-precipitated hypoxia, supplemental oxygen should be administered.

No effective therapy is available for "primary" pulmonary arterial hypertension unassociated with interstitial fibrosis. This complication typically comes to attention at an advanced stage. Numerous pharmacologic measures have been suggested, but only the serotonin antagonist, ketanserin,[281] calcium channel antagonists,[282] and captopril[283] are capable of lowering pulmonary artery pressure after their instillation into the artery. Unfortunately, the subsequent oral administration of these agents does not appear to alter the inexorably fatal course. Because those who develop right-sided cardiac failure often respond poorly to digitalis and easily become digitalis intoxicated, greater reliance is placed on the use of diuretics. Anticoagulation is often prescribed in this circumstance and should be used in individuals with high titer serum anticardiolipin antibody. Heart–lung or single-lung transplantation is an option that has not been adequately explored.

Heart

Symptomatic pericarditis is treated with nonsteroidal drugs or corticosteroids. Hemodynamically significant pericardial effusion should be managed with pericardiocentesis or, if recurrent, with an open pericardial window procedure. If myocarditis can be identified clinically or by endomyocardial biopsy, glucocorticoids should be tried. The typical progressive left ventricular failure caused by myocardial fibrosis is unaffected by any therapy and is uniformly fatal, unless some correctible nonsclerodermatous problem is also present. Serious arrhythmias complicate the former situation and respond inconsistently to antiarrhythmic drugs.

Kidney

The most important aspect of therapy for renal involvement is early detection. The high-risk patient is one with rapidly progressive diffuse cutaneous scleroderma. If such a person develops any one of a number of markers of renal disease, such as hypertension, proteinuria, azotemia, or microangiopathic hemolysis, it is recommended that stimulated plasma renin levels be obtained, and if they are elevated, treatment should begin immediately.[284] The availability of new and more potent antihypertensive agents and of improved dialysis procedures and care has dramatically improved survival.[137] The angiotensin-converting enzyme (ACE) inhibitors are the drugs of choice, but early aggressive therapy with other potent antihypertensive agents can be successful. Regardless, some individuals require dialysis.[285] Scleroderma patients may have inadequate vascular access and thus ineffective hemodialysis. Poor peritoneal clearance has been described,[286] but continuous ambulatory peritoneal dialysis has been successfully employed.[287]

Many renal failure patients receiving ACE inhibitors continuously have a slow reversal of renal vascular damage and can discontinue dialysis after several months.[137] A remarkable reduction in the degree of dermal thickening and induration has been observed in some but not all of these patients during dialysis.[138,288] Numerous successful renal transplantations have now been reported,[289] but typical scleroderma kidney histologic changes have been found in a transplanted organ[290] and in an allograft.[291]

LOCALIZED FORMS OF SCLERODERMA

The spectrum of localized scleroderma includes a variety of morphologic types of skin thickening, such as morphea (patches); generalized morphea (multiple confluent patches); subcutaneous morphea (patches with prominent subcutaneous involvement); linear scleroderma (bands); and eosinophilic fasciitis (confluent fascial and deep subcutaneous involvement). The clinical overlap between these disorders is considerable; for example, morphea coexists with both linear scleroderma and eosinophilic fasciitis. Other common features include peripheral blood eosinophilia; infiltration of affected tissues with mononuclear cells (especially lymphocytes and eosinophils); absence of the characteristic visceral and serologic changes of systemic sclerosis; and a tendency to be self-limited.[151] A summary of the clinical and laboratory findings in these conditions is found in Table 73–4. Other autoimmune disorders, such as Sjögren's syndrome, autoimmune hypothyroidism, and SLE, may be found in affected patients. Localized scleroderma is most often encountered during

TABLE 73–4. COMPARISON OF CLINICAL AND LABORATORY FINDINGS IN LOCALIZED FORMS OF SCLERODERMA

	MORPHEA, GENERALIZED; MORPHEA, LINEAR	EOSINOPHILIC FASCIITIS	EOSINOPHILIA MYALGIA SYNDROME	TOXIC OIL SYNDROME
Fever	0	0	+	+
Rash	0	0	+	+
Alopecia	0	0	+	+
Edema	0	+	+	+
Arthritis	±	+	+	+
Contractures	±	+	+	+
Myopathy	Rare	0	+	+
Pulmonary disease	0	0	+	+
Cardiac involvement	0	0	Rare	+
Neuropathy	0	0	+	+
Eosinophilia	+	+	+	+
Anemia	0	0	±	±
ANA	+	±	±	±
anti-ssDNA	+	0	0	0

0 = not reported; ± = unusual but reported; + = frequent (>10%); ANA = antinuclear antibody.

childhood. In some instances, the cutaneous changes appear soon after trauma and originate at the site of injury. Onset after mammoplasty has been reported,[292] and familial occurrence has been observed.[293]

MORPHEA, GENERALIZED MORPHEA, AND LINEAR SCLERODERMA

Discrete droplike patches (guttate morphea) or plaques may begin at any age or site. Most often, these patches are oval and are oriented in a dermatomal direction, that is, parallel to the course of sensory nerves and similar to the lesions of linear scleroderma. During their evolution, they become sclerotic and waxy or ivory-colored and may increase to a diameter of many centimeters. The surface is smooth, hairless, and ceases to sweat. During this active phase, a surrounding erythematous or violaceous border of inflammation is often visible. After several months or years, spontaneous softening of the skin occurs, with atrophy and hyperpigmentation or depigmentation; smaller patches may heal without trace. Lesions are confined entirely to the skin and adjacent superficial subcutis and are ordinarily of little consequence unless the face is involved or there is extensive dissemination (generalized morphea). Localized patches of morphea have been observed in a person with otherwise typical systemic sclerosis,[294] but it should be emphasized that this coincidence is extremely rare.

Early in morphea, the major histologic changes consist of new collagen deposition in the dermis and septae of the subcutaneous tissue and variable but often heavy infiltration of lymphocytes, plasma cells, and histiocytes. This inflammatory reaction is more intense than that usually encountered in systemic sclerosis. The coexistence of morphea and lichen sclerosis et atrophicus has been reported,[295] but some authors feel that these two conditions are unrelated and that confusion exists only because skin biopsies were not deep enough to show the diagnostic features of morphea in the reticular dermis and subcutis.[296] Inflammation and later fibrosis and atrophy of underlying subcutaneous tissue, fascia, and striated muscle may be present, suggesting an overlap with eosinophilic fasciitis.[297]

In linear scleroderma, which usually develops in childhood, a sclerotic band appears on the trunk, arm, or leg (Fig. 73–18) and may extend the entire length of the extremity. The location of these bands, even on the trunk, corresponds strikingly to established dermatomes. Frequently, multiple linear and morphea lesions are present in the same patient. The natural history of linear scleroderma is similar to that of morphea, with an active indurative phase followed in 1 or 2 years by softening and more normal pigmentation. Linear scleroderma in the frontoparietal area of the forehead and scalp (*en coupe de sabre*) may be associated with ipsilateral facial hemiatrophy[298] and rarely with neurologic abnormalities, such as seizures attributable to hemiatrophy of the brain.[299] Some patients develop a nonerosive arthropathy in a rheumatoid distribution, usually restricted to the small joints of the hands. The concurrence of linear scleroderma and other connective tissue diseases, especially SLE, has been reported.[300]

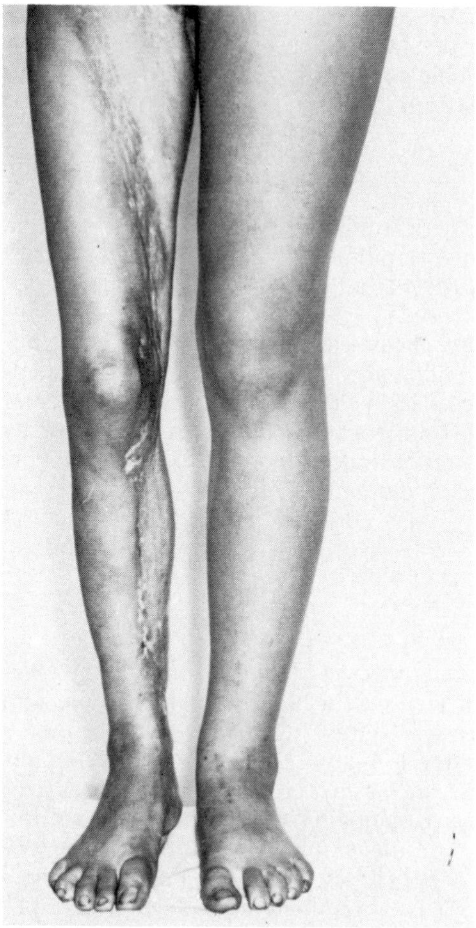

FIGURE 73–18. Localized scleroderma of the linear type in the thigh and leg of a 12-year-old girl. (Courtesy of Prof. Stephanie Jablonska.)

Inflammation and extensive fibrosis, similar to the findings in morphea, are present in the dermis, subcutis, and deep fascia in linear scleroderma. Extension into underlying muscle occasionally results in deforming fibrous contractures of the extremity joints, and neurovascular compromise has been reported rarely. A noninflammatory myopathy underlying areas of linear scleroderma has been described.[301] Linear scleroderma may coexist in the same extremity with melorheostosis, a peculiar linear fibrotic hyperostosis of bone[302]

Peripheral blood eosinophilia is often found in morphea, generalized morphea, and linear scleroderma.[151] Antinuclear antibodies, including high titers of antibodies to single-stranded DNA, have been noted in the serum of up to one third of patients with linear scleroderma, morphea, and generalized morphea.[303–305] Anti-single-stranded DNA antibodies accompany active disease, and titers decline during remission.[305] Two patients with linear scleroderma and one with morphea were found to have serum anticentromere antibodies.[306]

It is important to recognize that the majority of patients with these localized forms of scleroderma have a brief, self-limited disease. For active inflammation (extension of existing lesions and occurrence of new lesions), I recommend corticosteroids in low-to-moderate dose (prednisone, 7.5 to 20 mg/day) with reduction after several months. Often, depending on disease severity, I would also prescribe one of the following drugs: D-penicillamine,[307] etretinate,[308] or salazopyrin.[309]

EOSINOPHILIC FASCIITIS

This condition, which chiefly affects adults, is characterized by the rather abrupt onset of bilateral pain, swelling, and tenderness of the hands, forearms, feet, and legs, soon followed by induration of the skin and subcutaneous tissues of these parts.[310] In contrast to systemic sclerosis, the proximal extremities (forearms, arms, legs, thighs) are considerably more affected than are the distal areas such as hands, fingers, feet, and toes. Pronounced limitation of motion of the hands and feet and flexion contractures of the fingers may result. Carpal tunnel syndrome is an early feature in many patients. The induration often remains confined to the extremities but may spread to affect the trunk and rarely, the face. Although unilateral disease has been reported,[311] bilaterality is the rule and serves to distinguish this condition from linear scleroderma. Some cases have been thought to suggest a close relationship to systemic sclerosis,[312] but it in my opinion these diseases are entirely different, and distinguishing them from one another is seldom difficult.

Histologic diagnosis is best confirmed using a deep, wedge-shaped biopsy that includes "en bloc" the contiguous skin, subcutis, fascia, and muscle. Both inflammation and fibrosis are found in all layers, but they are most intense in the fascia and deeper layers of the subcutaneous tissue, which are often dramatically thickened (Fig. 73–19). Large numbers of lymphocytes, plasma cells, and histiocytes are present in the affected areas, and eosinophil infiltration may be striking, particularly early in the disease.[313] Immunoglobulin and complement component C3 have been identified in the inflamed tissues.[313]

Eosinophilic fasciitis is self-limited in most patients, with spontaneous improvement and occasionally complete remission after 2 to 5 years.[310] Some patients, however, have persistent or recurrent disease, while others are left with disabling joint contractures.[314] A variety of hematologic complications, including thrombocytopenia, aplastic anemia, and myelodysplastic syndromes, have developed in a small number of patients with eosinophilic fasciitis.[315–317] These conditions, suspected to be of autoimmune cause (both humoral and cell-mediated mechanisms have been described), may occur at any time in the course of the fasciitis and do not correlate with its severity.

Dramatic peripheral blood eosinophilia is the hallmark of this disease and is nearly universal.[313,314] The absolute number of eosinophils declines spontaneously later in the illness and parallels serum eosinophil chemotactic activity.[318] Hyper-γ-globulinemia (IgG)[313,319] and circulating immune complexes are found in nearly half of patients with eosinophilic fasciitis and tend to parallel disease activity.[320] Approximately one third have serum antinuclear antibodies, but no unique specificities have been identified.

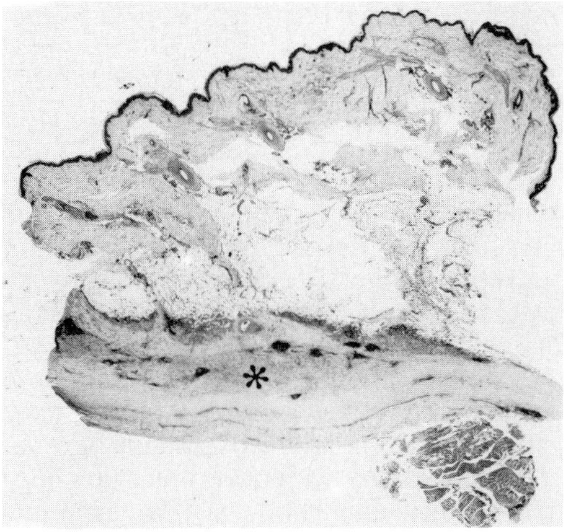

FIGURE 73–19. Photomicrograph of an en-bloc biopsy from the leg of a 35-year-old woman with eosinophilic fasciitis. Note thickening of the dermis, subcutaneous fibrous septa, and deep fascia (*asterisk*). The latter is infiltrated by large collections of cells that were identified as lymphocytes, plasma cells, histiocytes, and eosinophils.

Fasciitis has been preceded by unusually strenuous physical exertion, especially in younger men, and by allogeneic bone marrow transplantation.[321] The blood and tissue abnormalities described previously suggest an immune pathogenesis.[313,322] An association with autoimmune thyroiditis has been noted.[323]

Corticosteroids in moderate or small doses (prednisone, 10 to 20 mg/day) often result in prompt and substantial improvement in fasciitis and readily obliterate eosinophilia. Several reports have suggested that cimetidine treatment is effective.[324,325] Physical therapy may prove useful in the prevention or reduction of joint contractures. Treatment with antithymocyte globulin has been beneficial in two cases with associated aplastic anemia.[326,327]

EOSINOPHILIA MYALGIA SYNDROME

In the spring of 1989, an epidemic illness began in the United States that was characterized by the abrupt onset of constitutional features, severe myalgias, dyspnea and/or cough, and a variety of cutaneous lesions.[328] Prominent eosinophilia was noted, and the disorder was named the eosinophilia myalgia syndrome (EMS). A frequent later finding was diffuse fasciitis, which prompted classification as one of the systemic fibrosing diseases. The cause of this condition has not been precisely identified, but the disease is highly associated with ingestion of the amino acid L-tryptophan sold over the counter and produced by a single manufacturer in Japan.

Using a strict surveillance definition[329] established by the U.S. Communicable Disease Center to identify cases (severe incapacitating myalgias, total eosinophile count greater than 1000/mm^3, and absence of other recognized cause), over 2000 cases were reported, and more than 30 deaths have resulted. It is estimated that an equal number of unrecognized and/or unreported less severe instances of illness have occurred. A ban on the sale and distribution of L-tryptophan–containing products and an intense public awareness campaign ended this epidemic within 2 months. Several excellent reviews and the summary of a national conference on this disorder provide considerable detail about its clinical and laboratory features and natural history.[330–333]

The initial complaints include severe myalgias and muscle tenderness, often with cramps, followed by muscle weakness that is frequently asymmetrical and distal, consistent with a polyneuropathy. Cough and dyspnea are common. Most patients develop a rash, which is highly variable in its appearance, ranging from maculopapular to urticarial and always transient rather than persistent. Severe pruritus and alopecia are encountered. Later, edema of the extremities is found, followed by typical fasciitis of the extremities and/or trunk with prominent contractures. Morphea has also been described in these patients. True arthritis is unusual. After the acute illness, peripheral nervous system involvement may occur, with paresthesias, sensory loss, weakness, and/or paralysis. In such cases, physical examination frequently confirms a peripheral sensory neuropathy and/or mononeuritis multiplex. Clinically evident cardiac disease is rare but takes the form of a cardiomyopathy with congestive heart failure and arrhythmias.

The multisystem nature of EMS distinguishes it from classic eosinophilic fasciitis,[334] but it has been suggested that cases of the former long antedated the 1989 epidemic.[335] Peripheral blood eosinophilia is extremely common, often in excess of 50% of all white blood cells. Absolute eosinophil counts may exceed 5000/mm^3. Biopsies of deep subcutaneous tissue and fascia are identical histologically to those in eosinophilic fasciitis. Involved muscle shows chronic inflammatory cells located in perimysial and perivascular sites and microangiopathy but not true vasculitis or thrombosis. Myofibril degeneration is absent, but neurogenic atrophy may occur. Serum creatine kinase levels are normal. Serum aldolase and lactic dehydrogenase levels are often elevated, but the source and rationales for increased amounts of these enzymes are uncertain.

Nerve conduction studies and electromyography are often abnormal, and nerve biopsies have shown perineural and perivascular chronic inflammation, segmental demyelination, and axonal degeneration. Pulmonary interstitial mononuclear inflammatory changes are found, along with subintimal proliferation and medial hypertrophy of arterioles consistent with pulmonary arterial hypertension.[336] Pulmonary function test results, echocardiography, and right heart catheterization confirm pulmonary hypertension in some patients. An autopsy study has shown an unusual cardioneuropathy characterized by lymphocytic and fibrotic conduction system changes.[337]

The natural history of the EMS cannot yet be determined with certainty. Hospitalization was required in nearly 30% of cases. Death was rare (occurring in less than 2%), but almost always was attributed to ascending polyneuropathy with respiratory paralysis or myocardial and/or conduction system involvement. Although a few patients experienced disease progression, the majority improved spontaneously, but very slowly, after discontinuation of L-tryptophan. It is now clear that some chronic persistent damage to nerve and muscle may lead to irreversible neuropathy and joint contractures. Late subtle neuropsychiatric disturbances have been documented in a few patients.

Corticosteroids in moderate dosage (prednisone, 20 to 60 mg/day) are useful in reducing edema, rash, and pulmonary inflammation and in improving mobility and eliminating eosinophilia, but they appear to have little effect on neuropathy, fibrosis, and subsequent contractures. Repeat biopsies may continue to show mononuclear cell infiltration, and thus the prolonged use of moderate-to-high-dose corticosteroids does not appear to be beneficial. A variety of other anti-inflammatory and immunosuppressive agents has been used in small numbers of patients without uniform success. Some patients have become dependent on narcotics used for control of neuropathic pain.

Two state health departments mounted studies that unequivocally linked the development of the syndrome to the use of L-tryptophan.[338,339] The source, established by "trace-back" analysis, was a single Japanese manufacturer in virtually all cases.[340,341] The rate of disease was estimated to be as high as 80%, independent of age and sex, if large doses of implicated L-tryptophan (more than 4.0 g/day) were consumed.[342]

High-performance liquid chromatography analysis established that several distinctive "peaks" characterized the manufacturer's product.[340,343] The particular compound has now been identified as a dimer of L-tryptophan,[344] which may have been produced by one of several changes in the production process made shortly before the "hot lots" were distributed. Whether this contaminant is the causal agent or merely a marker for disease remains unknown. An animal model, the Lewis rat, develops mild fasciitis without eosinophilia after being fed the implicated material but does not after ingestion of unimplicated L-tryptophan.[345]

Although there is no clear-cut pathogenesis of EMS, it is certain that patients with active disease have elevated blood levels of the L-tryptophan metabolites kynurenine and quinolinic acid.[346] Increased peripheral metabolism resulting from induction of the enzyme indoleamine-2,3 dioxygenase is suspected, perhaps by products of activated mononuclear cells such as IL-2 and interferon-γ.

TOXIC OIL SYNDROME

A 1981 epidemic in Spain produced an illness remarkably similar to EMS. The cause was ingestion of adulterated industrial grade rapeseed oil, which had been illegally prepared and sold as cooking oil. Over 20,000 cases were reported, with several hundred deaths.[347–350] The initial symptoms were predominantly respiratory, with dyspnea, cough, pulmonary infiltrates, and noncardiac pulmonary edema. Intense peripheral blood eosinophilia was frequent. Subsequent stages of the disease were virtually identical to EMS, including severe myalgias, fasciitis, neuropathy, contractures, and the late development of pulmonary hypertension. Vascular, inflammatory, and fibrotic histologic findings were also similar. Despite more frequent early respiratory disease, elevated serum IgE levels, and thromboembolism in patients with toxic oil syndrome, the similarities between these two disorders are so striking that they should be considered very closely related in terms of pathogenesis. Comprehensive long-term followup has not been completed, but anecdotal information suggests that the majority of surviving toxic oil syndrome patients have made slow functional improvement over the past decade and have stable neurologic status and reduction in joint contractures.

DIFFERENTIAL DIAGNOSIS OF SCLERODERMA

Many other conditions with systemic features exhibit scleroderma-like, but often distinctive, skin changes and lack the typical visceral manifestations of systemic sclerosis (Table 73–5).[351,352]

Scleredema. Scleredema is characterized by symmetric, painless, edematous induration of the skin of the face, scalp, neck, trunk, and upper arms. In contrast to systemic sclerosis, the distal extremities are seldom affected. Recent streptococcal infection in childhood and diabetes mellitus[351] are its two most frequent associations. Other manifestations include hydrarthrosis, pleural and pericardial effusions, widespread involvement of skeletal or cardiac muscle, and macroglossia. Histochemical studies have revealed swollen collagen bundles and the accumulation of mucopolysaccharide (probably hyaluronic acid) in the dermis, subcutis, and skeletal muscle. This condition either resolves spontaneously after 6 to 12 months or persists for many years.

Porphyria Cutanea Tarda. In addition to bullae, hypopigmented plaque-like sclerodermatous induration of the skin and pigmentary changes occur in porphyria cutanea tarda, usually in sun-exposed areas.[353] Particularly on the face, long-standing lesions may ulcerate and contain dystrophic calcific deposits.[354] Bullae are

TABLE 73–5. DISORDERS ASSOCIATED WITH SKIN CHANGES THAT MAY RESEMBLE SCLERODERMA (PSEUDOSCLERODERMA)

PRIMARY CUTANEOUS DISEASES
Scleredema
Porphyria cutanea tarda; congenital porphyria
Scleromyxedema
Acrodermatitis chronica
Lichen sclerosus et atrophicus
Lipoatrophy
PRIMARY SYSTEMIC DISEASES IN WHICH CUTANEOUS FEATURES ARE ALSO PRESENT
Amyloidosis
Juvenile onset diabetes mellitus
Acromegaly
Carcinoid syndrome
Phenylketonuria
Werner's syndrome
Progeria
Rothmund's syndrome
Graft versus host disease
CHEMICAL AGENTS INDUCING SCLERODERMA-LIKE CONDITIONS
Vinyl chloride
Organic solvents, epoxy resins
Trichloroethylene
Bleomycin
Silicone or paraffin implantation
Contaminated L-tryptophan (eosinophilia myalgia syndrome)
Rapeseed oil (toxic oil syndrome)

rare in systemic sclerosis, and uroporphyrin excretion is normal.

Scleromyxedema. Scleromyxedema (lichen myxedematosus, papular mucinosis) is an unusual disorder in which a widespread lichenoid eruption of soft, pale red or yellowish papules is accompanied by diffuse thickening of the skin, especially involving the proximal extremities in a scleredema (neck, proximal upper extremity) distribution. Dense deposits of acid mucopolysaccharide, without glycosaminoglycan subunits on electron microscopy,[355] are found in the upper portion of the dermis. Proximal muscle weakness, dysphagia, and vacuolar myopathy have been reported.[356] Abnormal serum immunoglobulins (M components) have been detected in several patients, suggesting a relationship of this condition to myelomatosis.[357]

Acrodermatitis Chronica Atrophicans and Lichen Sclerosis et Atrophicus. These are uncommon disorders of unknown etiology in which cutaneous inflammation is followed by atrophy. The latter shows a high frequency of organ-specific serum antibodies, such as to thyroid and gastric parietal cells. Histologic overlap with localized scleroderma has been reported but is probably not justified (see preceding discussion).

Amyloidosis. Infiltration of the dermis may accompany amyloidosis of either the primary (multiple myeloma associated) or secondary type.[358] Firm, discrete hemispheric brown or yellow papules are described, but when the deposition of amyloid is diffuse and involves the fingers, hands, and face, the physical examination findings may mimic those of systemic sclerosis. Skin biopsies were positive for amyloid in involved skin in over half of amyloidosis cases and in clinically normal skin in over one third.[358]

Juvenile Onset Diabetes Mellitus. Digital sclerosis and mild finger contractures occur in one third of patients with insulin-dependent juvenile-onset diabetes mellitus.[359] These findings are correlated better with disease duration than with microvascular (retinal and renal) complications.[359]

Acromegaly. Considerable thickening of the skin and subcutaneous tissue may occur in acromegaly as a result of connective tissue hyperplasia.[37] Hypertrophy of the digital tufts is the rule, rather than the ischemic atrophy associated with systemic sclerosis.

Glycogen Storage Disease. Scleroderma-like skin induration has been observed in persons with glycogen storage disease of muscle.[360]

Carcinoid Syndrome. The occurrence of a peculiar localized cutaneous fibrosis in a few patients with the malignant carcinoid syndrome has suggested that 5-hydroxytryptamine (serotonin) metabolism might be deranged in systemic sclerosis.[361] Persons with scleroderma (and in one case an unaffected relative) have been reported to excrete excessive amounts of kynurenine and other intermediary metabolites of tryptophan.[362] The relationship of these metabolic alterations to those observed in EMS[356] are intriguing and perhaps indicate certain common pathogenetic mechanisms in the production of fibrosis.

Phenylketonuria. Atypical scleroderma of the trunk and extremities without visceral stigmata has been reported in children with phenylketonuria,[363] a disorder in which the absence of the enzyme phenylalanine hydroxylase ultimately leads to excessive urinary excretion of indolic compounds and decreased levels of plasma serotonin and urinary 5-hydroxyindoleacetic acid. Improvement follows conversion to a low-phenylalanine diet. Studies of nine children with scleroderma, aged 3 to 14 years, revealed normal urinary levels of both phenylalanine and D-hydroxyphenylacetic acid.[363]

Werner's Syndrome, Progeria, and Rothmund's Syndrome. The classic findings of Werner's syndrome, a rare hereditofamilial disorder, include growth retardation, premature graying of the hair and baldness, juvenile cataracts, and a high frequency of diabetes mellitus. Atrophy and hyperkeratosis of the skin with chronic ulcerations over pressure points in the feet may occur.[364] In progeria, a rare autosomal recessive syndrome, the corium and subcutis have been reported to be either thickened or atrophic,[365] and the thermal shrinkage and solubility of skin collagen resemble aged rather than normally growing connective tissue.[365] The nature of the primary defect in these conditions is unknown. Rothmund's syndrome is another heritable (recessive) disorder in which atrophy of the skin (poikiloderma), beginning in infancy, is associated with juvenile cataracts.

Vinyl Chloride- and Epoxy Resin-Associated Scleroderma. Workers who clean reactor vessels containing the polymerizing agent vinyl chloride (CH_2CHC1 may acquire a systemic illness with some features of systemic sclerosis.[366] These persons complain of soreness and tenderness of the fingertips and Raynaud's phenomenon. They develop patchy, nodular induration of skin on the dorsa of the hands and forearms, clubbing, synovial thickening of the PIP joints, hepatic portal fibrosis, splenomegaly, and pulmonary fibrosis. Roentgenograms reveal varying degrees of acro-osteolysis of the distal phalanges of the fingers, as well as erosive and sclerotic changes in the sacroiliac joints. Partial resorption of the mandible has been reported. Microvascular abnormalities distinct from those encountered in systemic sclerosis are observed on capillary microscopy,[367] and lumenal narrowing of the digital arteries has been seen on angiographic examination.[368] Occupational exposure to volatile compounds with similar chemical structures, including trichlorethylene, ethylenediamine, and benzene, has been reported to be associated with systemic sclerosis.[369] The vapor of epoxy resins is believed to lead to localized, primarily truncal cutaneous sclerosis and muscle weakness.[23] A biogenic amine is the suspected causative agent.

Bleomycin Toxicity. Administration of the tumoricidal drug bleomycin often leads to the development of nodules and/or plaques of thickened skin, the result of an increase of dense collagen deposition in the dermis.[370] More uniform induration of the skin, Raynaud's phenomenon,[371] and pulmonary fibrosis[372] mimic the findings in systemic sclerosis. The dermal fibrosis tends to recede following discontinuation of bleomycin. Cultured fibroblasts from affected skin demonstrate increased collagen synthesis.[20]

Silicone Injection. A variety of connective tissue disease syndromes has been reported to follow cosmetic surgery with injection of foreign substances (e.g., paraffin, silicone), chiefly for breast augmentation[18] The most common clinical entity recognized in this situation is systemic sclerosis. Atypical features include a reduced proportion of patients with esophageal hypomotility and serum antinuclear antibodies.

CALCINOSIS

Calcinosis, or pathologic calcification of the soft tissues, occurs in a variety of systemic and localized conditions (Table 73–6). Most of these disorders are considered in

TABLE 73–6. DISEASES ASSOCIATED WITH CALCIFICATION OF THE SOFT TISSUES IN THE EXTREMITIES

I. Metastatic calcification
Hypercalcemic conditions
Primary hyperparathyroidism
Hypervitaminosis D
Milk-alkali syndrome
Metastatic and other neoplasms of bone
Sarcoidosis
Hyperphosphatemic conditions
Chronic renal failure with secondary hyperparathyroidism
Hypoparathyroidism
Pseudohypoparathyroidism
Tumoral calcinosis (lipocalcinosis granulomatosis)
II. Dystrophic calcification
Connective tissue diseases
Systemic sclerosis, with both diffuse and limited scleroderma
Dermatomyositis-polymyositis
Ehlers-Danlos syndrome
Pseudoxanthoma elasticum
Metabolic disorders
Chondrocalcinosis articularis (pseudogout)
Gout
Diabetes mellitus
Alkaptonuria (ochronosis)
Porphyria cutanea tarda
Pseudopseudohypoparathyroidism
Werner's syndrome
Progeria
Myositis (or fibrodysplasia) ossificans progressiva
Vascular diseases
Medial sclerosis of arteries (Monckeberg's sclerosis)
Venous calcifications
Parasitic infestations
Other diseases
Neuropathic arthropathy
Calcific tendinitis
Para-articular limb joint ectopic calcification associated with paralysis and other neurologic disorders

detail in Chapters 108 to 110. Classifications of ectopic calcification generally separate these conditions into those that result from long-continued hypercalcemia and/or hyperphosphatemia (metastatic calcification) and those following some local abnormality in the affected tissue (dystrophic calcification).

METASTATIC CALCIFICATION

Calcareous deposits, which occur commonly in hypercalcemic states, are found in the kidney (nephrocalcinosis), stomach, lung, brain, eyes (band keratopathy), skin, subcutaneous and periarticular tissues, and arterial walls. The mild-alkali syndrome and vitamin D intoxication are two such conditions that may affect rheumatic disease patients who become hypercalcemic because of overzealous treatment to prevent duodenal ulcer or osteoporosis.[373] Calcification of the articular cartilage and menisci (chondrocalcinosis) and joint capsules is a well-recognized feature of hyperparathyroidism. For some persons, an attack of calcium pyrophosphate dihydrate (CPPD) crystal-induced synovitis (pseudogout) represents the first clinical manifestation of this disease. Accordingly, the possibility of primary hyperparathyroidism should be carefully considered in all patients with CPPD arthropathy. During the immediate postoperative period, patients whose parathyroid adenoma has been removed are at high risk to develop attacks of pseudogout.[374]

Soft-tissue calcification without ocular involvement and seldom affecting skin[375] is also found in normocalcemic-hyperphosphatemic hyperparathyroidism secondary to renal insufficiency, although renal calculus formation is less frequent than in the hypercalcemic states. Acute episodes of articular and periarticular inflammation, which appear to be related to the local deposition of microcrystalline calcium phosphate (and, at times, monosodium urate), have been described in patients undergoing hemodialysis for chronic renal failure.[376] The finding of subperiosteal juxta-articular bone erosions following calcinosis in the same location suggests that the calcification may induce erosions.[377] The removal of pyrophosphate, which appears to act as a physiologic inhibitor of calcification, may be responsible for this phenomenon.[378] Treatment with phosphate-binding agents has resulted in a significant reduction of serum phosphorus levels, disappearance of cutaneous calcinosis, and relief from the articular attacks,[376] although malabsorption of phosphate binders may be a problem.[379] Oxalosis secondary to end stage renal disease may be associated with chondrocalcinosis and highly inflammatory bursitis, tenosynovitis, and arthritis from calcium oxalate deposition.[380]

In hypoparathyroidism, pseudohypoparathyroidism, and pseudopseudohypoparathyroidism, calcification may occur in the brain, particularly in the basal ganglia, as well as in the subcutaneous tissue. Acute calcific periarthritis in hypoparathyroidism has been reported to occur in association with a fall in serum calcium,[381] similar to the same phenomenon in surgically treated primary hyperparathyroidism[374] and gout.

Radiographically obvious biopsy-proved metastatic calcification has been detected by bone scanning (Technetium 99 [^{99m}Tc]-labeled methylene diphosphonate) in numerous areas, including the lung, gastric wall, heart, and kidney.[382,383] Such uptake, caused by the affinity of the tracer for the surface of hydroxyapatite crystals, has now been shown in the subcutaneous tissues and skin.[384]

Tumoral Calcinosis

Although included in the category of metastatic calcification because of frequent elevation in serum phosphorus level and occasional increase in serum calcium values, tumoral calcinosis is separable from other forms of metastatic calcification because visceral involvement is absent. This rare entity, which has also been called *lipocalcinosis granulomatosis*, is characterized by the rapid development of large, multilobulated calcific masses in the subcutaneous tissue and muscles surrounding the hips, shoulders, elbows, hands, and chest wall in otherwise healthy young subjects. Smaller tumors occur adjacent to the spine, wrists, feet, lower ribs, sacrum, and ischium. There is no sex predilection, but there is a considerably increased prevalence among blacks and black Africans.[385] These firm, nontender deposits may increase to a diameter of 20 cm or larger over a period of months to years. Little or no articular limitation occurs unless masses become very large or are complicated by the development of fistulous tracts caused by either infection or attempts at surgical drainage. Nerve root impingement (especially sciatica) may result. Curiously, several patients have angioid streaks of the retina.

Most patients with tumoral calcinosis have normal serum calcium and alkaline phosphatase values, but hyperphosphatemia[386] and elevated levels of 1,25-dihydroxyvitamin D[387] have been noted in several cases. Rapid exchange of calcium between serum and calcific masses is evident, along with an increased intestinal absorption of dietary calcium, with no defect in the turnover of skeletal calcium.[386] An intrinsic renal proximal tubular defect allowing enhanced phosphate reabsorption has been postulated. Elevated 1,25-dihydroxyvitamin D levels are present after phosphate depletion, suggesting dysregulation of its synthesis or metabolism or an undiscovered stimulus for its production.[388] Approximately half of the patients with tumoral calcinosis reported to date have had affected siblings. This observation, together with the occurrence of hyperphosphatemia, has led to the suggestion that there is a heritable disturbance in the metabolism of phosphorus.[386] Although an autosomal recessive mechanism has been considered the report of this condition in four generations of one family, coupled with a unique dental lesion, suggests the possibility of an autosomal dominant heredity with variable expression.[389] Affected teeth have short, bulbous roots and nearly total obliteration of pulp cavities on panoramic radiographs.

On sectioning, calcific deposits are found to be composed of multilocular cysts enclosing pockets of milky fluid or pasty microcrystalline calcareous matter. The tissue lining the walls of these cysts contains mononuclear cells, which are rich in alkaline phosphatase and believed to be responsible for local accumulation of calcium phosphate. Foreign body giant cells are also present.[385] These mononuclear and multinucleated cells are structurally, and apparently functionally, similar to osteoblasts and osteoclasts, respectively.[386] The masses contain pure calcium carbonate and phosphate, a mixture of the two salts, or hydroxyapatite crystals.[390]

Treatment at present consists mainly of early surgical excision of the calcareous masses, which rarely occur at the same site. New deposits may appear in time around other joints. As a rule, the prognosis is good, although in some instances secondary infection of the deposits has led to multiple draining sinuses, cachexia, and amyloidosis. A low-calcium and low-phosphorus diet and large oral doses of antacids containing aluminum hydroxide have resulted in negative balances of both calcium and phosphorus with clinical improvement.[391] Intravenous calcitonin infusion has been reported to cause phosphaturia and a significant fall in serum phosphorus level.[392]

DYSTROPHIC CALCIFICATION

Many restrict the use of the term *calcinosis* to those patients in whom the deposition of calcium salts in the soft tissues occurs in the absence of any generalized disturbance in calcium or phosphorus metabolism.

Calcinosis Associated with Connective Tissue Disease

In systemic sclerosis, the calcareous deposits are generally confined to the extremities and are particularly frequent on the flexor surfaces of the terminal phalanges, around joints, and near other bony eminences (Fig. 73–20; see also Fig. 73–6). Most of these patients suffer from the limited cutaneous or CREST syndrome variant. In contrast, widespread encasing calcification of the skin, subcutaneous and periarticular tissues, as well as involvement of the deeper structures, occurs later in the course of polymyositis-dermatomyositis. This process includes tendons, tendon plaques, and nodules and is often associated with erosive arthropathy, serve joint contractures or ankylosis.[393] Calcinosis most often complicates childhood dermatomyositis (40 to 74% of cases) and is associated with late, suboptimal dosage of corticosteroids and severe myopathy unresponsive to steroids.[394] The latter type of patient more frequently demonstrates a linear, reticular pattern of calcification.[395] A case of vasculitis with destructive spinal discitis believed to be due to apatite has been described.[396]

The standard method of detection of dystrophic calcification has been the standard roentgenogram. However, a computed tomographic scanning has been reported to identify calcinosis in symptomatic but radiographically normal areas.[397] On microscopic examination, the precipitates of calcium in the skin are pleomorphic crystals, many in the shape of needles and large plates. They appear to develop in the elastic fibers of the connective tissue.[398,399] X-ray diffraction (Fig. 73–20) and electron microscopy identify these crystals as hydroxyapatite.[400]

As a rule, affected persons have normal concentrations of serum calcium, phosphorus, and alkaline phosphatase activity, but calcium balance studies have yielded conflicting data. In patients with cutaneous deposition (calcinosis cutis), increased absorption and retention of calcium have been evident, paradoxically with a more rapid disappearance rate of radiolabeled calcium injected intradermally.[401] When a woman with scleroderma and calcinosis was placed on a calcium-restricted diet, the bone resorption rate increased, and urinary excretion of calcium fell normally, but the net calcium accretion rate (which included extraosseous calcium deposition) remained constant.[402] Urinary excretion of a vitamin K-dependent calcium-binding protein γ-carboxyglutamic acid, or Gla, is increased in der-

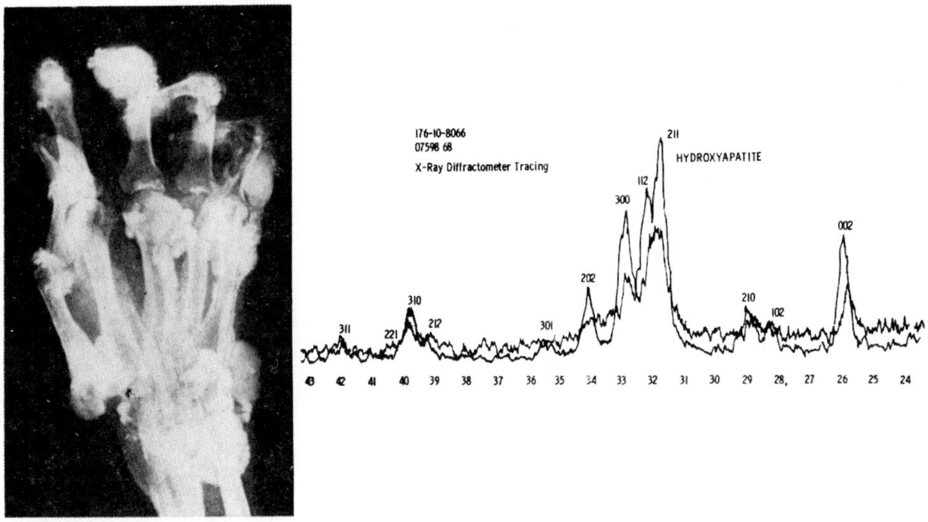

FIGURE 73–20. Dystrophic calcinosis. *Left,* Roentgenogram of the hand of a woman with polymyositis showing extensive calcinosis involving both subcutaneous tissues and tendon sheaths. *Right,* X-ray diffraction patterns. The labeled spectra are derived from a hydroxyapatite control, and the spectra with lower peak heights are from the patient. Correspondence of peak positions suggests the presence of hydroxyapatite. (See Chapter 109 for additional information on identification of calcium phosphate crystals).

matomyositis and scleroderma patients with calcinosis,[403,404] but it is premature to conclude that this substance plays a primary role in the pathogenesis of calcinosis.

The basis of the deposition of calcium salts in the dermis of patients with systemic connective tissue disorders is unclear. Several different forms of cutaneous, subcuticular, periarticular, and visceral calcification have been produced experimentally in the rat by calciphylaxis, but none serve as a model of human calcinosis. The initial precipitation of calcium salts in experimental cutaneous calcinosis in the rat occurs in areas rich in mucopolysaccharides or, in some instances, in collagen fibers, which appear to act as a matrix for this calcification. Calcification of porcine cardiac valve prostheses has been shown to occur on devitalized porcine connective tissue cells and collagen fibers, and abnormal collagen cross links have been implicated in this process.[405] Because polysaccharides may "shield" reactive sites on collagen fibrils and block mineral nucleation, calcinosis in scleroderma may be related to the diminution of mucopolysaccharides in the affected skin during later stages of the disease.

Numerous drugs, hormones, and a host of nonspecific measures have been used unsuccessfully in the treatment of calcinosis.[406,407] Oral low-dose anticoagulant therapy has been effective occasionally in preventing and reversing subcutaneous calcinosis.[262,404] Surgical excision of large calcareous masses may be helpful in selected instances.[408,409] Resolution of calcinosis in juvenile dermatomyositis was accompanied by serious hypercalcemia in one case.[410] Colchicine may be effective in reducing soft tissue inflammation surrounding such deposits.[263] Ectopic calcification following paraplegia or hip surgery in animals was prevented by indomethacin and prednisone plus low-dose radiation therapy.[411]

Myositis (or Fibrodysplasia) Ossificans Progressiva

Patients with this uncommon disorder have widespread ectopic calcification and ossification in fascia, aponeuroses, and other fibrous structures related to muscles. The initial symptoms usually appear in early childhood, often preceded by local trauma (Fig. 73–21). The disease occurs in families and appears to be transmitted as an autosomal dominant trait with irregular penetrance. Associated congenital anomalies of the digits include microdactyly or total absence of the thumbs and great toes.

The initial manifestation usually consists of a localized area of swelling, redness, and warmth in the neck or paravertebral area, often associated with extreme pain. After several days, the signs of inflammation subside, leaving an area of residual doughy firmness that appears fibromatous and gradually ossifies over the following weeks. Scanning with ^{99m}Tc pyrophosphate may be useful in the detection of areas of ossification before roentgenographic changes.[412] The replacement of the tendon and muscle by bone leads to characteristic contracture deformities. Once ossification occurs, further change is minimal. Recurring bouts of inflammation and ossification result in progressive damage to much of the striated musculature. Involvement of the muscles of the chest wall and back may lead to restrictive pulmonary disease.[413] Death usually ensues from respiratory failure and/or pulmonary infection resulting from ossification of the muscles of the thorax or from

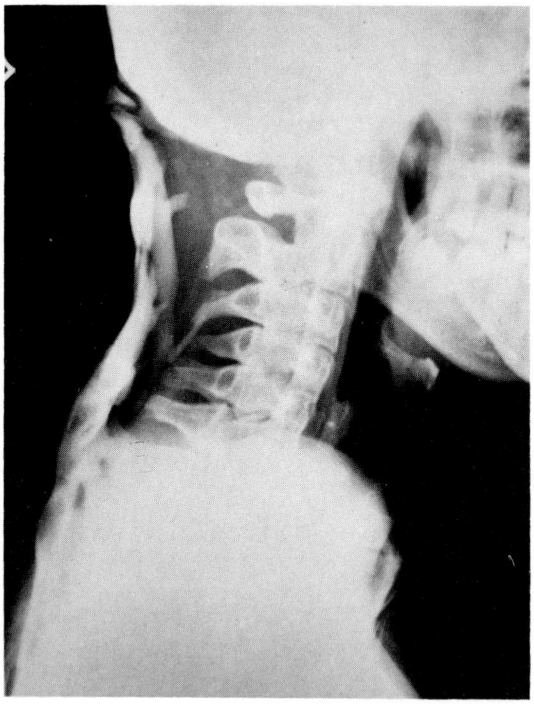

FIGURE 73–21. Roentgenogram illustrating new bone formation in the cervical area of a 17-year-old woman with myositis ossificans progressiva. She first noted pain, swelling, and limitation of motion in this area after trauma 10 years previously.

inanition as a result of damage to the muscles of mastication.

The administration of diphosphonates may suppress, at least temporarily, the development of new areas of mineralization following surgical excision of ectopic bone, but the ultimate value of these agents is as yet uncertain.[405,414] Corticosteroids may relieve the acute symptoms of inflammation and retard progression of the disease in some patients.[415]

Other Localized Calcific Syndromes

A variety of local and regional sites of calcification have been associated with rheumatic complaints. Intra-articular[416] and periarticular[417] calcification have followed intra-articular corticosteroid injections. In addition to the common syndromes of the shoulder and hip, idiopathic calcific tendinitis and tenosynovitis have produced instances of carpal tunnel syndrome[418] and wrist and finger flexor tenosynovitis,[419] all believed to be due to repeated minor trauma. A similar cause has been suggested for calcinosis cutis affecting the knee.[420] Synthetic retinoid therapy is associated with spinal hyperostosis, diffuse idiopathic skeletal hyperostosis (DISH), and extraspinal tendon and ligament calcification.[421] With DISH[422] and with ligamentum flavum calcification,[423] cervical myelopathy may result. Nontraumatic causes of neck pain now include calcific tendinitis of the longus colli muscle[424] and retropharyngeal calcific tendinitis.[425] Three siblings with multifocal calcific periarthritis and low levels of serum (hepatic) alkaline phosphatase have been reported.[426] It has been proposed that reduction of this enzyme may allow increased pyrophosphate levels, thus stimulating apatite growth.[427,428] A genetic predisposition to calcific periarthritis of the shoulder in diabetes mellitus patients with the HLA-B27 antigen has been suggested.[429]

REFERENCES

1. Medsger, T.A., Jr.: Systemic sclerosis (scleroderma), eosinophilic fasciitis, and calcinosis. *In* Arthritis and Allied Conditions. 11th Ed. Edited by D.J. McCarty. Philadelphia, Lea & Febiger, 1989, pp. 1118–1165.
2. LeRoy, E.C. et al.: Scleroderma (systemic sclerosis): Classification, subsets, and pathogenesis. J. Rheumatol., *152*:202–205, 1988.
3. Masi, A.T.: Classification of systemic sclerosis (scleroderma). *In* Systemic Sclerosis (Scleroderma). Edited by C.M. Black and A.R. Myers. New York, Gower Medical Publishing, 1985, pp. 7–15.
4. Sharp, G.C.: Association of progressive systemic sclerosis with other connective tissue diseases ("overlap syndromes"). *In* Systemic Sclerosis (Scleroderma). Edited by C.M. Black and A.R. Myers. New York, Gower Medical Publishing, 1985, pp. 33–35.
5. Winterbauer, R.H.: Multiple telangiectasia, Raynaud's phenomenon, sclerodactyly, and subcutaneous calcinosis: A syndrome mimicking hereditary hemorrhagic telangiectasia. Bull. Johns Hopkins Hosp., *114*:361–383, 1964.
6. Okano, Y., and Medsger, T.A., Jr.: Antibody to Th ribonucleoprotein (nucleolar 7-2 RNA protein particle) in patients with systemic sclerosis (scleroderma). Arthritis Rheum., *33*:1822–1828, 1990.
7. Okano, Y., and Medsger, T.A., Jr.: Unpublished observations, 1991.
8. Reimer, G. et al.: Correlates between autoantibodies to nucleolar antigens and clinical features in patients with systemic sclerosis (scleroderma). Arthritis Rheum., *31*:532–535, 1988.
9. Sharp, G.C. et al.: Mixed connective tissue disease. An apparently distinct rheumatic disease syndrome associated with a specific antibody to an extractable nuclear antigen (ENA). Am. J. Med., *52*:148–159, 1972.
10. Targoff, I.N., and Reichlin, M.: Nucleolar localization of the PM-Scl antigens. Arthritis Rheum., *28*:226–230, 1985.
11. Treadwell, E.L., Alspaugh, M.A., Wolfe, J.F., and Sharp, G.C.: Clinical relevance of PM-1 antibody and physiochemical characterization of PM-1 antigen. J. Rheumatol., *11*:658–662, 1984.
12. Okano, Y., Steen, V.D., and Medsger, T.A., Jr.: Clinical significance of autoantibody to nucleolar U3 ribonucleoprotein (RNP) in patients with systemic sclerosis (SSc). Arthritis Rheum., *34*:R29, 1991.
13. Masi, A.T. et al.: Clinical criteria for easly diagnosed systemic sclerosis: Preliminary results of the ARA Multicenter Cooperative Study. Arthritis Rheum., *21*:576–577, 1987.
14. Medsger, T.A., Jr.: Comment on Scleroderma Criteria Cooperative Study. *In* Current Topics in Rheumatology: Systemic Sclerosis. Edited by C.M. Black and A.R. Meyers. New York, Gower Medical Publishing, 1985, pp. 16–17.
15. Steen, V., Conte, C., Santoro, D. et al.: Twenty-year incidence survey of systemic sclerosis. (Abstract.) Arthritis Rheum., *31*:557, 1988.

16. Haustein, U.F., and Ziegler, V.: Environmentally induced systemic sclerosis-like disorders. Int. J. Dermatol., *24*:147–151, 1985.
17. Sluis-Cremer, G.K. et al.: Silica, silicosis, and progressive systemic sclerosis. Br. J. Ind. Med., *42*:838–843, 1985.
18. Kumagai, Y. et al.: Clinical spectrum of connective tissue disease after cosmetic surgery. Observations on eighteen patients and a review of the Japanese literature. Arthritis Rheum., *27*:1–12, 1984.
19. Veltman, G. et al.: Clinical manifestations and course of vinyl chloride disease. Ann. N.Y. Acad. Sci., *246*:6–17, 1975.
20. Finch, W.R. et al.: Bleomycin-induced scleroderma. J. Rheumatol., *7*:651–659, 1980.
21. Sparrow, G.P.: A connective tissue disorder similar to vinyl chloride disease in a patient exposed to perchlorethylene. Clin. Dermatol., *2*:17–22, 1977.
22. Walder, B.K.: Do solvents cause scleroderma? Int. J. Dermatol., *22*:157–158, 1983.
23. Yamakage, A., and Ishikawa, H.: Generalized morphea-like scleroderma occurring in people exposed to organic solvents. Dermatologica, *165*:186–193, 1982.
24. Jablonska, S., Chorzelski, T., and Blaszczyk, M.: Familial occurrence of scleroderma. *In* Scleroderma and Pseudoscleroderma. 2nd Ed. Edited by S. Jablonska. Warsaw, Polish Medical Publishers, 1975, pp. 35–55.
25. Sheldon, W.B. et al.: Three siblings with scleroderma (systemic sclerosis) and two with Raynaud's phenomenon from a single kindred. Arthritis Rheum., *24*:668–676, 1981.
26. Greger, R.E.: Familial progressive systemic scleroderma. Arch. Dermatol., *111*:81–85, 1975.
27. Muralidar, K. et al.: Familial scleroderma (case report). J. Assoc. Physicians India, *26*:307–309, 1978.
28. Maddison, P.J. et al.: Antinuclear antibodies in the relatives and spouses of patients with systemic sclerosis. Ann. Rheum. Dis., *45*:793–799, 1986.
29. Takehara, K., Moroi, Y., and Ishibashi, Y.: Antinuclear antibodies in the relatives of patients with systemic sclerosis. Br. J. Dermatol., *112*:23–33, 1985.
30. Dustoor, M.M., McInerney, M.M., Mazanec, D.J., and Cathcart, M.K.: Abnormal lymphocyte function in scleroderma: A study on identical twins. Clin. Immunol. Immunopathol., *44*:20–30, 1987.
31. Rodnan, G.P., and Fennell, R.H., Jr.: Progressive systemic sclerosis *sine* scleroderma. J. Am. Med. Assoc., *180*:665–670, 1962.
32. Steen, V.D., Medsger, T.A., Jr., and Rodnan, G.P.: D-penicillamine therapy in progressive systemic sclerosis (scleroderma). Ann. Intern. Med., *97*:652–658, 1982.
33. Kahaleh, M.B., Sultany, G.L., Smith, E.A., and Huffstutter, J.E.: A modified scleroderma skin scoring method. Clin. Exp. Rheumatol., *4*:367–369, 1986.
34. Black, C., Dieppe, P.K., Huskisson, T., and Hart, F.D.: Regressive systemic sclerosis. Ann. Rheum. Dis., *45*:384–388, 1986.
35. Jawitz, J.C., Albert, M.K., Nigra, T.P., and Bunning, R.D.: A new skin manifestation of progressive systemic sclerosis. J. Am. Acad. Dermatol., *2*:265–268, 1984.
36. Sukenik, S., Kleiner-Baumgarten, A., and Horowitz, J.: Hyperpigmentation along tendons in progressive systemic sclerosis. (Letter.) J. Rheumatol., *13*:474–475, 1986.
37. Rodnan, G.P., Lipinski, E., and Luksick, J.: Skin thickness and collagen content in progressive systemic sclerosis (scleroderma) and localized scleroderma. Arthritis Rheum., *22*:130–140, 1979.
38. Roumm, A.D. et al.: Lymphocytes in the skin of patients with progressive systemic sclerosis: Quantification, subtyping and clinical correlations. Arthritis Rheum., *27*:645–653, 1984.
39. Connolly, S.M., and Winkelmann, R.K.: Direct immunofluorescent findings in scleroderma syndromes. Acta Derm. Venereol. (Stockh.), *61*:29–36, 1981.
40. Hawkins, R.A., Claman, H.N., Clark, R.A.F., and Steigerwald, J.C.: Increased dermal mast cell populations in progressive systemic sclerosis: A link in chronic fibrosis? Ann. Intern. Med., *102*:182–186, 1985.
41. Sheiner, N.M., and Small, P.: Isolated Raynaud's phenomenon: A benign disorder. Ann. Allergy, *58*:114–117, 1987.
42. Gerbracht, D.D. et al.: Evolution of primary Raynaud's phenomenon (Raynaud's disease) to connective tissue disease. Arthritis Rheum., *28*:87–92, 1985.
43. Kallenberg, C.G.M., Wouda, A.A., Hoet, M.H., and vanVenrooij, W.J.: Development of connective tissue disease in patients presenting with Raynaud's phenomenon: A six year follow-up with emphasis on the predictive value of antinuclear antibodies as detected by immunoblotting. Ann. Rheum. Dis., *47*:634–641, 1988.
44. Young, E.A., Steen, V., and Medsger, T.A., Jr.: Systemic sclerosis without Raynaud's phenomenon. (Abstract.) Arthritis Rheum., *29*:S51, 1986.
45. Coffman, J.D., and Cohen, A.S.: Total and capillary fingertip blood flow in Raynaud's phenomenon. N. Engl. J. Med., *285*:259–263, 1971.
46. Hendriksen, O., and Kristensen, J.K.: Reduced systolic blood pressure in fingers of patients with generalized scleroderma (acrosclerosis). Acta Derm. Venereol. (Stockh.), *61*:531–534, 1981.
47. Belch, J.J.F. et al.: Vascular damage and factor-VIII-related antigen in the rheumatic diseases. Rheumatol. Int., *7*:107–111, 1987.
48. Kahaleh, M.B., Osborn, I., and LeRoy, E.C.: Increased factor VIII/von Willebrand factor antigen and von Willebrand factor activity in scleroderma and in Raynaud's phenomenon. Ann. Intern. Med., *94*:482–484, 1981.
49. Zeiler, J. et al.: Serotonin content of platelets in inflammatory rheumatic diseases. Correlation with clinical activity. Arthritis Rheum., *26*:532–540, 1983.
50. Friedhoff, L.T., Seibold, J.R. Kim, H.C., and Simester, K.S.: Serotonin induced platelet aggregation in systemic sclerosis. Clin. Exp. Rheumatol., *2*:119–123, 1984.
51. Kahaleh, M.B., Osborn, I., and LeRoy, E.C.: Elevated levels of circulating platelet aggregates and beta-thromboglobulin in scleroderma. Ann. Intern. Med., *96*:610–613, 1982.
52. Seibold, J.R., and Harris, J.N.: Plasma β-thromboglobulin in the differential diagnosis of Raynaud's phenomenon. J. Rheumatol., *12*:99–103, 1985.
53. Rodnan, G.P., Myerowitz, R.L., and Justh, G.O.: Morphologic changes in the digital arteries of patients with progressive systemic sclerosis (scleroderma) and Raynaud's phenomenon. Medicine, *59*:393–408, 1980.
54. Merino, J. et al.: Hemiplegia and peripheral gangrene secondary to large and medium size vessels involvement in CREST syndrome. Clin. Rheumatol., *1*:295–299, 1982.
55. Shapiro, L.S.: Large vessels, arterial thrombosis in systemic sclerosis associated with antiphospholipid antibodies. J. Rheumatol., *17*:685–688, 1990.
56. Maricq, H.R., Spencer-Green, G., and LeRoy, E.C.: Skin capillary abnormalities as indicators of organ involvement in scleroderma (systemic sclerosis). Am. J. Med., *61*:862–870, 1976.
57. Maricq, H.R., and LeRoy, E.C.: Capillary blood flow in scleroderma. Bibl. Anat., *11*:352–358, 1973.
58. Kenik, J.G., Maricq, H.R., and Bole, G.G.: Blind evaluation of the diagnostic specificity of nailfold capillary microscopy in the connective tissue diseases. Arthritis Rheum., *24*:885–891, 1981.
59. Maricq, H.R.: Comparison of quantitative and semiquantitative

estimates of nailfold capillary abnormalities in scleroderma spectrum disorders. Microvasc. Res., *32*:271–276, 1986.
60. Thompson, R.P. et al.: Nailfold biopsy in scleroderma and related disorders. Arthritis Rheum., *27*:97–103, 1984.
61. Harper, F.E. et al.: A prospective study of Raynaud's phenomenon and early connective tissue disease. A five-year report. Am. J. Med., *72*:883–888, 1982.
62. McGill, N.W., and Gow, P.J.: Nailfold capillaroscopy: A blinded study of its discriminatory value in scleroderma, systemic lupus erythematosus, and rheumatoid arthritis. Aust. N.Z. J. Med., *16*:457–460, 1986.
63. Houtman, P.M., Kallenberg, C.G.M., Wouda, A.A., and The, T.H.: Decreased nailfold capillary density in Raynaud's phenomenon: A reflection of immunologically mediated local and systemic vascular disease? Ann. Rheum. Dis., *44*:603–609, 1985.
64. Lovy, M., MacCarter, D., and Steigerwald, J.C.: Relationship between nailfold capillary abnormalities and organ involvement in systemic sclerosis. Arthritis Rheum., *28*:496–501, 1985.
65. Rodnan, G.P.: The nature of joint involvement in progressive systemic sclerosis (diffuse scleroderma). Clinical study and pathological examination of synovium in twenty-nine patients. Ann. Intern. Med., *56*:422–439, 1962.
66. Devogelaer, J.P. et al.: Intra-articular calcification in progressive systemic sclerosis. Clin. Rheumatol., *5*:262–267, 1986.
67. Brandt, K.D., and Krey, P.R.: Chalky joint effusion: The result of massive synovial deposition of calcium apatite in progressive systemic sclerosis. Arthritis Rheum., *20*:792–796, 1977.
68. Schumacher, H.R., Jr.: Joint involvement in progressive systemic sclerosis (scleroderma). A light and electron microscopic study of synovial membrane and fluid. Am. J. Clin. Pathol., *60*:593–600, 1973.
69. Palmer, D.G. et al.: Bowed fingers. A helpful sign in the early diagnosis of systemic sclerosis. J. Rheumatol., *8*:266–272, 1981.
70. Blocka, K.L.N. et al.: The arthropathy of advanced progressive systemic sclerosis: A radiographic survey. Arthritis Rheum., *24*:874–884, 1981.
71. Armstrong, R.D., and Gibson, T.: Scleroderma and erosive polyarthritis: A disease entity? Ann. Rheum. Dis., *41*:141–146, 1982.
72. Owens, G.R. et al.: Pulmonary function in progressive systemic sclerosis: Comparison of CREST syndrome variant with diffuse scleroderma. Chest, *84*:546–550, 1983.
73. Osial, T.A., Jr. et al.: Resorption of the mandibular condyles and coronoid processes in progressive systemic sclerosis (scleroderma). Arthritis Rheum., *24*:729–733, 1981.
74. Medsger, T.A., Jr.: Progressive systemic sclerosis: Skeletal muscle involvement. Clin. Rheum. Dis., *5*:103–113, 1979.
75. Clements, P.J. et al.: Muscle disease in progressive systemic sclerosis: Diagnostic and therapeutic considerations. Arthritis Rheum., *21*:62–71, 1978.
76. Foster, T.D., Fairburn, E.A.: Dental involvement in scleroderma. Br. Dent. J., *124*:353–356, 1968.
77. Rowell, N.R., and Hopper, F.E.: The periodontal membrane in systemic sclerosis. Br. J. Dermatol., *96*:15–20, 1977.
78. Rajapakse, C.N.A. et al.: Pharyngo-esophageal dysphagia in systemic sclerosis. Ann. Rheum. Dis., *40*:612–614, 1981.
79. Stentoft, P., Hendel, L., and Aggestrup, S.: Esophageal manometry and pH-probe monitoring in the evaluation of gastroesophageal reflux in patients with progressive systemic sclerosis. Scand. J. Gastroenterol., *22*:499–504, 1987.
80. Katzka, D.A. et al.: Barrett's metaplasia and adenocarcinoma of the esophagus in scleroderma. Am. J. Med., *82*:46–52, 1987.
81. Segel, M.C., Campbell, W.L., Medsger, T.A., and Roumm, A.D.: Systemic sclerosis (scleroderma) and esophageal adenocarcinoma: Is increased patient screening necessary? Gastroenterology, *89*:485–488, 1985.
82. Garrett, J.M. et al.: Esophageal deterioration in scleroderma. Mayo Clin. Proc., *46*:92–96, 1971.
83. Davidson, A., Russell, C., and Littlejohn, G.O.: Assessment of esophageal abnormalities in progressive systemic sclerosis using radionuclide transit. J. Rheumatol., *12*:472–477, 1985.
84. Tsianos, E.B. et al.: Esophageal manometric findings in autoimmune rheumatic disease: Is scleroderma esophagus a specific entity? Rheumatology Int., *7*:23–27, 1987.
85. Akesson, A,. Akesson, B., Gustafson, T., and Wollheim, F.: Gastrointestinal function in patients with progressive systemic sclerosis. Clin. Rheumatol., *4*:441–448, 1985.
86. Rosecrans, P.C.M. et al.: Gastrointestinal telangiectasia as a cause of severe blood loss in systemic sclerosis. Endoscopy, *12*:200–204, 1980.
87. Hendy, M.S., Torrance, H.B., and Warnes, T.W.: Small-bowel volvulus in association with progressive systemic sclerosis. Br. Med. J., *1*:1051–1052, 1979.
88. Elwany, S., Talaat, M., Kamel, N, and Stephanos, W.: Further observations on nasal mucosal changes in scleroderma. J. Laryngol. Otol., *98*:979–986, 1984.
89. Gordon, M.B. et al.: Thyroid disease in progressive systemic sclerosis (PSS): Increased frequency of glandular fibrosis and hypothyroidism. Ann. Intern. Med., *95*:431–435, 1981.
90. Osial, T.A., Jr. et al.: Clinical and serologic study of Sjögren's syndrome in patients with progressive systemic sclerosis. Arthritis Rheum., *26*:500–508, 1983.
91. Battle, W.M. et al.: Abnormal colonic motility in progressive systemic sclerosis. Ann. Intern. Med., *94*:749–752, 1981.
92. Hamel-Roy, J. et al.: Comparative esophageal and anorectal motility in scleroderma. Gastroenterology, *88*:1–7, 1985.
93. Kemp-Harper, R.A., and Jackson, D.C.: Progressive systemic sclerosis. Br. J. Radiol., *38*:825–834, 1965.
94. Robinson, J.C., and Teitelbaum, S.L.: Stercoral ulceration and perforation of the sclerodermatous colon: Report of two cases and review of the literature. Dis. Colon Rectum, *17*:622–632, 1974.
95. D'Angelo, G., Stern, H.S., and Myers, E.: Rectal prolapse in scleroderma: Case report and review of the colonic complications of scleroderma. Can. J. Surg., *28*:62–63, 1985.
96. Owens, G.R., and Follansbee, W.P.: Cardiopulmonary manifestations of systemic sclerosis. Chest, *91*:118–127, 1987.
97. Warrick, J.H., Bhalla, M., Schabel, S.I., and Silver, R.M.: High resolution computed tomography in early scleroderma lung disease. J. Rheumatol., *18*:1520–1528, 1991.
98. Kosaka, Y. et al.: Large cystic lesions of the upper lobes of the lungs in two patients with CREST syndrome. Arthritis Rheum., *27*:935–938, 1984.
99. Guttadauria, M. et al.: Pulmonary function in scleroderma. Arthritis Rheum., *20*:1071–1079, 1977.
100. Bjerke, R.D. et al.: Small airways in progressive systemic sclerosis (PSS). Am. J. Med., *66*:201–209, 1979.
101. Peters-Golden, M. et al.: Clinical and demographic predictors of loss of pulmonary function in systemic sclerosis. Medicine, *63*:221–231, 1984.
102. Greenwald, G.I. et al.: Longitudinal changes in lung function and respiratory symptoms in progressive systemic sclerosis. Am. J. Med., *83*:83–92, 1987.
103. Steen, V.D., Conte, C., Owens, G., and Medsger, T.A., Jr.: Natural history of severe pulmonary fibrosis in systemic sclerosis (SSc). (Abstract.) Arthritis Rheum., *33*:5157, 1990.
104. Baron, M. et al.: ^{67}Gallium lung scans in progressive systemic sclerosis. Arthritis Rheum., *261*:969–974, 1983.
105. Furst, D.E. et al.: Abnormalities of pulmonary vascular dynam-

ics and inflammation in early progressive systemic sclerosis. Arthritis Rheum., *24*:1403–1408, 1981.
106. Silver, R.M., Metcalf, J.F., Stanley, J.H., and LeRoy, E.C.: Interstitial lung disease in scleroderma analysis by bronchoalveolar lavage. Arthritis Rheum., *27*:1254–1261, 1984.
107. Konig, G. et al.: Lung involvement in scleroderma. Chest, *85*:318–324, 1984.
108. Rossi, G.A. et al.: Evidence for chronic inflammation as a component of the interstitial lung disease associated with progressive systemic sclerosis. Am. Rev. Respir. Dis., *131*:612–617, 1985.
109. Edelson, J.S. et al.: Lung inflammation in scleroderma: Clinical, radiographic, physiologic and cytopathological features. J. Rheumatol., *12*:957–963, 1985.
110. Stupi, A. et al.: Pulmonary hypertension (PHT) in the CREST syndrome variant of progressive systemic sclerosis (PSS). Arthritis Rheum., *29*:515–524, 1986.
111. Shuck, J.W., Oetgen, W.J., and Tesar, J.T.: Pulmonary vascular response during Raynaud's phenomenon in progressive systemic sclerosis. Am. J. Med., *78*:221–227, 1985.
112. Peters-Golden, M. et al.: Carbon monoxide diffusing capacity as predictor of outcome in systemic sclerosis. Am. J. Med., *77*:1027–1034, 1984.
113. Roumm, A.D. and Medsger, T.A., Jr.: Cancer and systemic sclerosis. Arthritis Rheum., *28*:1336–1340, 1985.
114. Follansbee, W.: The cardiovascular manifestations of systemic sclerosis (scleroderma). Curr. Probl. Cardiol., *11*:242–298, 1986.
115. Botstein, G.R., and LeRoy, E.C.: Primary heart disease in systemic sclerosis (scleroderma): Advances in clinical and pathologic features, pathogenesis and new therapeutic approaches. Am. Heart J., *102*:913–919, 1981.
116. Bulkley, B.H.: Progressive systemic sclerosis: Cardiac involvement. Clin. Rheum. Dis., *5*:131–149, 1979.
117. McWhorter, J.E., and LeRoy, E.C.: Pericardial disease in scleroderma (systemic sclerosis). Am. J. Med., *57*:566–574, 1974.
118. Follansbee, W.P. et al.: Physiologic abnormalities of cardiac function in progressive systemic sclerosis with diffuse scleroderma. N. Engl. J. Med., *310*:142–148, 1984.
119. West, S.G., Killian, P.J., and Lawless, D.J.: Association of myositis and myocarditis in progressive systemic sclerosis. Arthritis Rheum., *24*:662–667, 1981.
120. Carette, S., Turcotte, J., and Mathon, G.: Severe myositis and myocarditis in progressive systemic sclerosis. J. Rheumatol., *12*:997–999, 1985.
121. Smith, J.W. et al.: Echocardiographic features of progressive systemic sclerosis (PSS). Correlation with hemodynamic and postmortem studies. Am. J. Med., *66*:28–33, 1979.
122. Todesco, S. et al.: Cardiac involvement in progressive systemic sclerosis. Acta Cardiol., *5*:311–322, 1979.
123. Ellis, W.W. et al.: Left ventricular dysfunction induced by cold exposure in patients with systemic sclerosis. Am. J. Med., *80*:385–392, 1986.
124. Kahan, A. et al.: Nifedipine and thallium-201 myocardial perfusion in progressive systemic sclerosis. N. Engl. J. Med., *314*:1397–1402, 1986.
125. Kahan, A. et al.: Pharmacodynamic effect of dipyridamole on thallium-201 myocardial perfusion in progressive systemic sclerosis with diffuse scleroderma. Ann. Rheum. Dis., *45*:718–725, 1986.
126. Nitenberg, A. et al.: Reduced coronary flow and resistance reserve in primary scleroderma myocardial disease. Am. Heart J., *112*:309–315, 1986.
127. James, T.N.: De subitaneis mortibus: VIII. Coronary arteries and conduction system in scleroderma heart disease. Circulation, *50*:844–956, 1974.
128. Clements, P.J. et al.: The relationship of arrhythmias and conduction disturbances to other manifestations of cardiopulmonary disease in progressive systemic sclerosis (PSS). Am. J. Med., *71*:38–46, 1981.
129. Blom-Bulow, B., Jonson, B., and Bauer, K.: Factors limiting exercise performance in progressive systemic sclerosis. Semin. Arthritis Rheum., *13*:174–181, 1983.
130. Roberts, N.K., and Cabeen, W.R.: Atrioventricular nodal function in progressive systemic sclerosis. Electrophysiological and morphological findings. Br. Heart J., *44*:529–533, 1980.
131. Ridolfi, R.L., Bulkley, B.H., and Hutchins, G.M.: The cardiac conduction system in progressive systemic sclerosis. Clinical and pathologic features of 35 patients. Am. J. Med., *61*:361–366, 1976.
132. Traub, Y.M. et al.: Hypertension and renal failure (scleroderma renal crisis) in progressive systemic sclerosis. Report of a 25-year experience with 68 cases. Medicine, *62*:335–352, 1984.
133. Steen, V.D.: Factors predicting the development of renal involvement in progressive systemic sclerosis. Am. J. Med., *76*:779–786, 1984.
134. Sundar, A.S. et al.: Kidney in progressive systemic sclerosis. Indian J. Med. Res., *82*:534–539, 1985.
135. Salyer, W.R., Salyer, D.C., and Heptinstall, R.H.: Scleroderma and microangiopathic hemolytic anemia. Ann. Intern. Med., *78*:895–897, 1973.
136. Cannon, P.J. et al.: The relationship of hypertension and renal failure on scleroderma (progressive systemic sclerosis) to structural and functional abnormalities of the renal cortical circulation. Medicine, *53*:1–46, 1974.
137. Steen, V.D., Costantino, J.P., Shapiro, A.P., and Medsger, T.A., Jr.: Outcome of renal crisis in systemic sclerosis: relation to availability to angiotensin converting enzyme (ACE) inhibitors. Am. Intern. Med., *113*:352–357, 1990.
138. Beckett, V.L. et al.: Use of captopril as early therapy for renal scleroderma: A prospective study. Mayo Clin. Proc., *60*:763–771, 1985.
139. Moore, H.C., and Sheehan, H.L.: The kidney of scleroderma. Lancet, *1*:68–70, 1952.
140. Lapenas, D., Rodnan, G.P., and Cavallo, T.: Immunopathology of the renal vascular lesion of progressive systemic sclerosis (scleroderma). Am. J. Pathol., *91*:243–258, 1978.
141. McGiven, A.R., deBoer, W.G.R.M., and Barnett, A.J.: Renal immune deposits in scleroderma. Pathology, *3*:145–150, 1971.
142. Lally, E.V. et al.: Pathologic involvement of the urinary bladder in progressive systemic sclerosis. J. Rheumatol., *12*:778–781, 1985.
143. Culp, K.S. et al.: Autoimmune association of primary biliary cirrhosis. Mayo Clin. Proc., *57*:365–370, 1982.
144. Clarke, A.K., Galbraith, R.M., Hamilton, E.D.B., and Williams, R.: Rheumatic disorders in primary biliary cirrhosis. Ann. Rheum. Dis., *37*:42–47, 1978.
145. Alderuccio, F., Toh, B-H., Barnett, A.J., and Pedersen, J.S.: Identification and characterization of mitochondria autoantigens in progressive systemic sclerosis: Identity with the 74,000 dalton autoantigen in primary biliary cirrhosis. J. Immunol., *137*:1855–1859, 1986.
146. Russell, M.L., and Kahn, J.J.: Nodular regenerative hyperplasia of the liver associated with progressive systemic sclerosis: A case report with ultrastructural observation. J. Rheumatol., *10*:748:752, 1983.
147. D'Angelo, W.A. et al.: Pathologic observations in systemic sclerosis (scleroderma). Study of 58 autopsy cases and 58 matched controls. Am. J. Med., *46*:428–440, 1969.
148. Frayha, R.A., Shulman, L.E., and Stevens, M.B.: Hematological abnormalities in scleroderma. A study of 180 cases. Acta Haematol., *64*:25–30, 1980.

149. Sumithran, E.: Progressive systemic sclerosis and autoimmune haemolytic anemia. Postgrad. Med. J., *52*:173–176, 1976.
150. Waugh, D., and Ibels, L.: Malignant scleroderma associated with autoimmune neutropenia. Br. Med. J., *280*:1577–1578, 1980.
151. Falanga, V., and Medsger, T.A., Jr.: Frequency, levels and significance of blood eosinophilia in systemic sclerosis, localized scleroderma and eosinophilic fasciitis. J. Am. Acad. Dermatol., *17*:648–656, 1987.
152. Lee, P., Bruni, J., and Sukenik, S.: Neurological manifestations in systemic sclerosis (scleroderma). J. Rheumatol., *11*:480–483, 1984.
153. Farrell, D.A., and Medsger, T.A., Jr.: Trigeminal neuropathy in progressive systemic sclerosis. Am. J. Med., *73*:57–62, 1982.
154. Estey, E. et al.: Cerebral arteritis in scleroderma. Stroke, *10*:595–597, 1979.
155. Oddis, C.V. et al.: Vasculitis in systemic sclerosis: Association with Sjögren's syndrome and the CREST syndrome variant. J. Rheumatol., *14*:942–948, 1987.
156. Nowlin, N.S. et al.: Impotence in scleroderma. Ann. Intern. Med., *104*:794–798, 1986.
157. Sonnex, C., Paice, E., and White, A.G.: Autonomic neuropathy in systemic sclerosis: A case report and elevation of six patients. Ann. Rheum. Dis., *45*:957–960, 1986.
158. West, R.H., and Barnett, A.J.: Ocular involvement in scleroderma. Br. J. Ophthalmol., *63*:845–847, 1979.
159. Grennan, D.M., and Forrester, J.A.: Involvement of the eye in SLE and scleroderma. Ann. Rheum. Dis., *36*:152–156, 1977.
160. Tosti, A., Patrizi, A., and Veronesi, S.: Audiologic involvement in systemic sclerosis. Dermatologica, *168*:206, 1984.
161. Kahl, L.E. et al.: Prospective evaluation of thyroid function in patients with systemic sclerosis (scleroderma). J. Rheumatol., *12*:103–107, 1986.
162. Nicholson, D. et al.: Progressive systemic sclerosis and Graves' disease. Report of 3 cases. Arch. Intern. Med., *146*:2350–2352, 1986.
163. Barnett, A.J.: Some observations on the immunological status in scleroderma (progressive systemic sclerosis). Aust. N.Z. J. Med., *8*:622–627, 1978.
164. Kogo, Y. et al.: A case of the progressive systemic sclerosis (PSS) with high serum concentration of M protein. Jpn. Soc. Intern. Med., *64*:1167–1173, 1975.
165. Ja, S., Helm, S., and Wary, B.B.: progressive systemic scleroderma with IgA deficiency in a child. Am. J. Dis. Child., *135*:965–966, 1981.
166. Husson, J.M. et al.: Systemic sclerosis and cryoglobulinemia. Clin. Immunol. Immunopathol., *6*:77–82, 1976.
167. Chen, Z. et al.: Immune complexes and antinuclear, antinucleolar and anticentromere antibodies in scleroderma. J. Am. Acad. Dermatol., *11*:461–467, 1984.
168. French, M.A.H. et al.: Serum immune complexes in systemic sclerosis: Relationship with precipitating nuclear antibodies. Ann. Rheum. Dis., *44*:89–92, 1985.
169. Bernstein, R.M., Steigerwald, J.C., and Tan, E.M.: Association of antinuclear and antinucleolar antibodies in progressive systemic sclerosis. Clin. Exp. Immunol., *48*:43–51, 1982.
170. Douvas, A.S., Achten, M., and Tan, E.M.: Identification of a nuclear protein (Scl-70) as a unique target of human antinuclear antibodies in scleroderma. J. Biol. Chem., *254*:10514–10522, 1979.
171. Catoggio, L.J. et al.: Serological markers in progressive systemic sclerosis: Clinical correlations. Ann. Rheum. Dis., *42*:23–27, 1983.
172. Shero, J.H., Bordwell, B., Rothfield, N.F., and Earnshaw, W.C.: High titers of autoantibodies to topoisomerase I (Scl-70) in sera from scleroderma patients. Science, *231*:737–740, 1986.
173. Burnham, T.K., and Kleinsmith, D'A.M.: The "true speckled" antinuclear antibody (ANA) pattern: Its tumultuous history. Semin. Arthritis Rheum., *13*:155–159, 1983.
174. Catoggio, L.J. et al.: Autoantibodies in Argentine patients with systemic sclerosis (scleroderma). Arthritis Rheum., *28*:715–717, 1985.
175. Steen, V.D. et al.: Clinical and laboratory associations of anticentromere antibody (ACA) in patients with progressive systemic sclerosis (scleroderma). Arthritis Rheum., *27*:125–131, 1984.
176. Kallenberg, C.G.M. et al.: Antinuclear antibodies in patients with Raynaud's phenomenon. Clinical significance of anticentromere antibodies. Ann. Rheum. Dis., *41*:382–387, 1982.
177. Migliaresi, S.: Infrequency of anticentromere antibody in patients without systemic sclerosis and without Raynaud's phenomenon. Arthritis Rheum., *30*:358–359, 1987.
177a. Goldman, J.A.: Anticentromere antibody in patients without CREST and scleroderma: Association with active digital vasculitis, rheumatic and connective tissue disease. Ann. Rheum. Dis., *48*:771–775, 1989.
177b. Genth, E., Mierau, R., Genetzky, P. et al.: Immunogenetic associations of scleroderma-related antinuclear antibodies. Arthritis Rheum., *33*:657–665, 1990.
178. McCarty, G.A. et al.: Anticentromere antibody. Clinical correlations and association with favorable prognosis in patients with scleroderma variants. Arthritis Rheum., *26*:1–7, 1983.
179. Brenner, S. et al.: Kinetochore structure, duplication, and distribution in mammalian cells: Analysis by human autoantibodies from scleroderma patients. J. Cell Biol., *91*:95–102, 1981.
180. Earnshaw, W., Bordwell, B., Marino, C., and Rothfield, N.: Three human chromosomal autoantigens are recognized by sera from patients with anti-centromere antibodies. J. Clin. Invest., *77*:426–430, 1986.
181. Ruffatti, A. et al.: Association of anti-centromere and anti-Scl 70 antibodies in scleroderma. Report of two cases. J. Clin. Lab. Immunol., *16*:227–229, 1985.
182. Furst, D.E. et al.: Case control study of antibodies to ENA in progressive systemic sclerosis patients. J. Rheumatol., *11*:298–305, 1984.
183. Mimori, T. et al.: Characterization of a high molecular weight acidic nuclear protein recognized by autoantibodies in sera from patients with polymyositis-scleroderma overlap. J. Clin. Invest., *68*:611–620, 1981.
183a. Yaneva, M., and Arnett, F.C.: Antibodies against Ku protein in sera from patients with autoimmune diseases. Clin. Exp. Immunol., *76*:366–372, 1989.
184. Fritzler, M.J. et al.: An antigen in metaphase chromatin and the midbody of mammalian cells binds to scleroderma sera. J. Rheumatol., *14*:291–294, 1987.
185. Osborn, T.G. et al.: Anticentriole antibody in a patient with progressive systemic sclerosis. Arthritis Rheum., *29*:142–146, 1986.
186. Moroi, Y. et al.: Human anticentriole autoantibody in patients with scleroderma and Raynaud's phenomenon. Clin. Immunol. Immunopathol., *29*:381–390, 1983.
187. Osborn, T.G. et al.: Antinuclear antibody staining only centrioles in a patient with scleroderma. N. Engl. J. Med., *307*:253–254, 1982.
188. Reimer, G., Rose, K.M., Scheer, U., and Tan, E.M.: Autoantibody to RNA polymerase I in scleroderma sera. J. Clin. Invest., *79*:65–72, 1987.
189. Seibold, J.R., Knight, P.J., and Peter, J.B.: Anticardiolipin antibodies in systemic sclerosis (Letter.) Arthritis Rheum., *29*:1052–1053, 1986.
190. Greaves, M. et al.: Elevated von Willebrand factor antigen in

systemic sclerosis: relationship to visceral disease. Br. J. Rheumatol., *27*:281–285, 1988.
191. Kahaleh, M.B., and LeRoy, E.C.: Interleukin-2 in scleroderma: Correlation of serum level with extent of skin involvement and disease duration. Ann. Intern. Med., *110*:446–450, 1989.
192. Degiannis, D., Seibold, J.R., Czarnecki, M. et al.: Soluble interleukin-2 receptors in patients with systemic sclerosis. Arthritis Rheum., *33*:375–380, 1990.
193. Black, C.M. et al.: Serum type III procollagen peptide concentrations in systemic sclerosis and Raynaud's phenomenon: Relationship to disease activity and duration. Br. J. Rheumatol., *28*:98–103, 1989.
194. Miller, M.H. et al.: The clinical significance of the anticentromere antibody. Br. J. Rheumatol., *26*:17–21, 1987.
195. Medsger, T.A., Jr., and Masi, A.T.: Epidemiology of progressive systemic sclerosis. Clin. Rheum. Dis., *5*:15–25, 1979.
195a. Spooner, M.S., and LeRoy, E.C.: The changing face of severe scleroderma in five patients. Clin. Exp. Rheumatol., *8*:101–105, 1990.
195b. Altman, R.D., Medsger, T.A., Jr., Bloch, D.A., and Michel, B.A.: Predictors of survival in systemic sclerosis (scleroderma). Arthritis Rheum., *34*:403–413, 1991.
196. Giordano, M. et al.: Different antibody patterns and different prognoses in patients with scleroderma with various extent of skin sclerosis. J. Rheumatol., *13*:911–916, 1986.
197. Medsger, T.A., Jr., and Masi, A.T.: Epidemiology of systemic sclerosis (scleroderma). Ann. Intern. Med., *74*:714–721, 1971.
198. Suarez-Almazor, M.E. et al.: Juvenile progressive systemic sclerosis: Clinical and serologic findings. Arthritis Rheum., *28*:699–702, 1985.
199. Blaszczyk, M. et al.: Childhood scleromyositis: An overlap syndrome associated with PM-Scl antibody. Pediatr. Dermatol., *8*:1–8, 1991.
200. Singsen, B.H.: Scleroderma in childhood. Pediatr. Clin. North Am., *33*:1119–1139, 1986.
201. Hanson, V.: Dermatomyositis, scleroderma and polyarteritis nodosa. Clin. Rheum. Dis., *2*:455–464, 1976.
202. Cassidy J.T., Sullivan, D.B., Dabich, L., and Petty, R.E.: Scleroderma in children. Arthritis Rheum., *20*(Suppl.):351–354, 1977.
203. Bernstein, R.M., et al.: Autoantibodies in childhood scleroderma. Ann. Rheum. Dis., *44*:503–506, 1985.
204. Giordano, M., Valentini, G., Lupoli, S., and Giordano, A.: Pregnancy and systemic sclerosis. Arthritis Rheum., *28*:237–238, 1985.
205. Ballou, S.P., Morley, J.J., and Kushner, I.: Pregnancy and systemic sclerosis. Arthritis Rheum., *27*:295–298, 1984.
206. Mor-Yosef, S. et al.: Collagen diseases in pregnancy. Obstet. Gynecol. Surg., *39*:67–84, 1984.
207. Steen, V.D. et al.: Pregnancy in systemic sclerosis (Abstract.) Arthritis Rheum., *32*:151–157, 1989.
207a. Scarpinato, L., and MacKenzie, A.H.: Pregnancy and progressive systemic sclerosis: Case report and review of the literature. Cleve. Clin. Q., *52*:207–211, 1985.
208. Sood, S.V., and Kohler, H.G.: Maternal death from systemic sclerosis. (Report of a case of renal scleroderma masquerading as pre-eclamptic toxaemia.) J. Obstet. Gynecol. Br. Commw., *77*:1109–1112, 1970.
209. Palma, A. et al.: Progressive systemic sclerosis and nephrotic syndrome. Arch. Intern. Med., *141*:520–521, 1981.
210. Duncan, S.C., and Winkelmann, R.K.: Cancer and scleroderma. Arch. Dermatol., *115*:950–955, 1979.
211. Medsger, T.A., and Masi, A.T.: The epidemiology of systemic sclerosis (scleroderma) among male U.S. veterans. J. Chronic Dis., *31*:73–85, 1978.
212. Black, K.A. et al.: Cancer in connective tissue disease. Arthritis Rheum., *25*:1130–1133, 1982.
213. Lee, P. et al.: Malignancy in progressive systemic sclerosis. Association with breast carcinoma. J. Rheumatol., *10*:665–666, 1983.
214. Medsger, T.A., Jr.: Systemic sclerosis and malignancy—Are they related? J. Rheumatol., *12*:1041–1043, 1985.
215. Medsger, T.A., Jr.: Progressive systemic sclerosis. Clin. Rheum. Dis., *9*:655–670, 1983.
216. Medsger, T.A., Jr.: Treatment of systemic sclerosis. Rheum. Dis. Clin. North Am., *15*:513–531, 1989.
217. Helfrich, DJ., Banner, B., Steen, V.D., and Medsger, T.A., Jr.: Normotensive renal failure in systemic sclerosis. Arthritis Rheum., *32*:1128–1134, 1989.
218. Jayson, M.I.V., Lovell, C., and Black, C.M.: Penicillamine therapy in systemic sclerosis. Proc. R. Soc. Med., *70*:82–88, 1977.
219. Asboe-Hansen, G.: Treatment of generalized scleroderma: Updated results. Acta Derm. Venereol., *59*:465–467, 1979.
220. Ivanova, M.M. et al.: Treatment of systemic sclerosis with D-penicillamine. Ther. Arch., 7:91–99, 1977.
221. Jimenez, S.A., Andrews, R.P., and Myers, A.R.: Treatment of rapidly progressive scleroderma (PSS) with D-penicillamine: A prospective study. *In* Systemic Sclerosis (Scleroderma) Current Topics in Rheumatology. Edited by C.M. Black and A.R. Myers. New York, Gower Medical Publishing, 1985, pp. 387–393.
222. Steen, V.D. et al.: The effect of D-penicillamine on pulmonary findings in systemic sclerosis. Arthritis Rheum., *28*:882–888, 1985.
223. deClerck, L.S. et al.: D-Penicillamine therapy and interstitial lung disease in scleroderma. A long-term followup study. Arthritis Rheum., *30*:643–650, 1987.
224. Ntoso, K.A. et al.: Penicillamine-induced rapidly progressive glomerulonephritis in patients with progressive systemic sclerosis: Successful treatment of two patients and a review of the literature. Am J. Kidney Dis., *8*:159–163, 1986.
225. Tordres, C.F. et al.: Penicillamine-induced myasthenia gravis in progressive systemic sclerosis. Arthritis Rheum., *23*:900–908, 1980.
226. Steen, V.D., Blair, S., and Medsger, T.A., Jr.: The toxicity of D-penicillamine in systemic sclerosis. Ann. Intern. Med., *104*:699–705, 1986.
227. Furst, D.E. et al.: Measurement of clinical change in progressive systemic sclerosis: A 1 year double-blind placebo-controlled trial of N-acetylcysteine. Ann. Rheum. Dis., *38*:356–361, 1979.
228. Oriente, P. et al.: Progressive systemic sclerosis and S-adenosylmethionine. Clin. Rheum., *4*:360–361, 1985.
229. Alarcon-Segovia, D.: Progressive systemic sclerosis: Management. Part IV. Colchicine. Clin. Rheum. Dis., *5*:294–302, 1979.
230. Guttadauria, M., Diamond, H., and Kaplan, D.: Colchicine in the treatment of scleroderma. J. Rheumatol., *4*:272–275, 1977.
231. Jansen, G.T. et al.: Generalized scleroderma. Treatment with an immunosuppressive agent. Arch. Dermatol., *97*:690–698, 1968.
232. Casas, J. et al.: 5-Fluorouracil in the treatment of scleroderma: A randomised, double-blind, placebo controlled international collaborative study. Am. Rheum. Dis., *49*:926–928, 1990.
233. Furst, D.E. et al.: Preliminary results of a double-blind parallel, randomized trial of chlorambucil vs. placebo in progressive systemic sclerosis (PSS). (Abstract.) Arthritis Rheum., *29*:S29, 1986.
234. Baker, G.L. et al.: Malignancy following treatment of rheumatoid arthritis with cyclosphophamide. Am. J. Med., *83*:1–9, 1987.
235. Dau, P.C., Kahalen, M.D., and Sagebiel, R.W.: Plasmapheresis and immunosuppressive drug therapy in scleroderma. Arthritis Rheum., *24*:1128–1136, 1981.

236. Schmidt, C., Schooneman, F., Siebert, P., et al.: Traitement de la sclerodermie generalisee par echanges plasmatiques. Ann. Med. Interne (Paris), *139*:(Suppl. 1):20–22, 1988.
237. Capodicasa, G. et al.: Clinical effectiveness of apheresis in the treatment of progressive systemic sclerosis. Int. J. Artif. Organs, *6*:81–86, 1983.
238. Guillevin, L. et al.: Treatment of progressive systemic sclerosis with plasma exchange. Seven cases. Int. J. Artif. Organs, *6*:315–318, 1983.
239. Zachariae, H., and Zachariae, E.: Cyclosporin A in systemic sclerosis. Br. J. Dermatol., *116*:741–742, 1987.
240. Kahan, A., Amor, B., Menkes, C.J., and Straveh, G.: Recombinant interferon-gamma in the treatment of systemic sclerosis. Am. J. Med., *87*:237–277, 1989.
241. van den Hoogen, F.M.J., Boerbooms, A., Rasker, J., et al.: Treatment of systemic sclerosis with methotrexate: Results of a one-year open study. (Abstract.) Arthritis Rheum., *33*:566, 1990.
242. Bode, B.Y., Yocum, D.E., Gall, E.P., et al.: Methotrexate (MTX) in scleroderma: Experience in 10 patients. (Abstract.) Arthritis Rheum., *33*:566, 1990.
243. Kahaleh, M.D., Sherer, D.L., and LeRoy, E.C.: Endothelial injury in scleroderma. J. Exp. Med., *149*:1326–1335, 1979.
244. Beckett, V.L. et al.: Trial of platelet-inhibiting drug in scleroderma. Double-blind study with dipyridamole and aspirin. Arthritis Rheum., *27*:1137–1143, 1984.
245. Fries, J.F. et al.: A controlled trial of antihypertensive therapy in systemic sclerosis (scleroderma). Ann. Rheum. Dis., *43*:407–410, 1984.
246. Jobe, J.B. et al.: Induced vasodilation as treatment for Raynaud's disease. Ann. Intern. Med., *97*:706–709, 1982.
247. Yocum, D.E., Hodes, R., Sundstrom, W.R., and Cleeland, C.S.: Use of biofeedback training in treatment of Raynaud's disease and phenomenon. J. Rheumatol., *12*:90–93, 1985.
248. McFayden, I.J., Housley, E., and MacPherson, A.I.S.: Intra-arterial reserpine administration in Raynaud's syndrome. Arch. Intern. Med., *132*:526–528, 1973.
249. Varadi, D.P., and Lawrence, A.M.: Suppression of Raynaud's phenomenon by methyldopa. Arch. Intern. Med., *124*:13–18, 1969.
250. Blunt, R.J., and Porter, J.M.: Raynaud's syndrome. Semin. Arthritis Rheum., *10*:282–308, 1981.
251. Rodeheffer, R.J. et al.: Controlled double-blind trial of nifedipine in the treatment of Raynaud's phenomenon. N. Engl. J. Med., *308*:880–883, 1983.
252. Finch, M.B., Dawson, J., and Johnston, G.D.: The peripheral vascular effects of nifedipine in Raynaud's syndrome associated with scleroderma: A double-blind crossover study. Clin. Rheumatol., *5*:493–498, 1986.
253. Surwit, R.S., Gilgor, R.S., Allen, L.M., and Duvic, M.: A double-blind study of prazosin in the treatment of Raynaud's phenomenon in scleroderma. Arch. Dermatol., *120*:329–331, 1984.
254. Seibold, J.R., and Jageneau, A.H.M.: Treatment of Raynaud's phenomenon with ketanserin, a selective antagonist of the serotonin 2 (5-HT2) receptor. Arthritis Rheum., *27*:139–146, 1984.
255. Franks, A.: Topical glyceryl trinitrate as adjunctive treatment in Raynaud's disease. Lancet, *1*:76, 1982.
256. Mizushima, Y. et al.: A multicenter double blind controlled study of lipo-PGE_1, PGE_1 incorporated in lipid microspheres, in peripheral vascular disease secondary to connective tissue disorders. J. Rheumatol., *14*:97–101, 1987.
257. Keller, J. et al.: Inhibition of platelet aggregation by a new stable prostacyclin introduced in therapy of patients with progressive scleroderma. Arch. Dermatol. Res., *277*:323–325, 1985.
258. Tosi, S. et al.: Treatment of Raynaud's phenomenon with captopril. Drugs Exp. Clin. Res., *13*:37–42, 1987.
259. Jones, N.F., Raynor, S.C., and Medsger, T.A.: Microsurgical revascularisation of the hand in scleroderma. Br. J. Plast. Surg., *40*:264–269, 1987.
260. Gahhos, F., Ariyan, S., Frazier, W.H., and Cuono, C.B.: Management of sclerodermal finger ulcers. J. Hand Surg., *9A*:320–327, 1984.
261. Lian, J.B., Skinner, M., Glimcher, M.J., and Gallop, P.M.: The presence of γ-carboxyglutamic acid in the proteins associated with ectopic calcification. Biochem. Biophys. Res. Commun., *73*:349–355, 1976.
262. Berger, R.G. et al.: Treatment of calcinosis universalis with low-dose warfarin. Am. J. Med., *83*:72–76, 1987.
263. Fuchs, D. et al.: Colchicine suppression of local inflammation due to calcinosis in dermatomyositis and progressive systemic sclerosis. Clin. Rheumatol., *5*:527–530, 1986.
264. Seeger, M.W., and Furst, D.E.: Effects of splinting in the treatment of hand contractures in progressive systemic sclerosis. Am. J. Occup. Ther., *41*:118–121, 1987.
265. Norris, R.W., and Brown, H.G.: The proximal interphalangeal joint in systemic sclerosis and its surgical management. Br. J. Plast. Surg., *38*:526–531, 1985.
266. Naylor, W.P.: Oral management of the scleroderma patient. J. Am. Dent. Assoc., *105*:814, 1982.
267. Naylor, W.P., and Manor, R.C.: Fabrication of a flexible prosthesis for the edentulous scleroderma patient with microstomia. J. Prosthet. Dent., *50*:536–538, 1983.
268. Ramirez-Mata, M., Ibanez, G., and Alarcon-Segovia, D.: Stimulatory effect of metaclopramide on the esophagus and lower esophageal sphincter of patients with PSS. Arthritis Rheum., *20*:30–34, 1977.
269. Horowitz, M. et al.: Effects of cisapride on gastric and esophageal emptying in progressive systemic sclerosis. Gastroenterology, *93*:311–315, 1987.
270. Kahan, A. et al.: Nifedipine and esophageal dysfunction in progressive systemic sclerosis. A controlled manometric study. Arthritis Rheum., *28*:490–495, 1985.
271. Jean, F. et al.: Effects of diltiazem versus nifedipine on lower esophageal sphincter pressure in patients with progressive systemic sclerosis. Arthritis Rheum., *29*:1054–1055, 1986.
272. Hendel, L., Aggestrup, S., and Stentoft, P.: Long-term ranitidine in progressive systemic sclerosis (scleroderma) with gastroesophageal reflux. Scand. J. Gastroenterol., *21*:799–805, 1986.
273. Orringer, M.B. et al.: Combined collis gastroplasty-fundoplication operations for scleroderma reflux esophagitis. Surgery, *90*:624–630, 1981.
274. Rees, W.D.W. et al.: Interdigestive motor activity in patients with systemic sclerosis. Gastroenterology, *83*:575–580, 1982.
275. Levien, D.H., Fiallos, F., Barone, R., and Taffet, S.: The use of cyclic home hyperalimentation for malabsorption in patients with scleroderma involving the small intestines. J. Parenter. Enter. Nutr., *9*:623–625, 1985.
276. Kallenberg, C.G.M., Jansen, H.M., Elema, J.D., and The, T.H.: Steroid-responsive interstitial pulmonary disease in systemic sclerosis. Monitoring by bronchoalveolar lavage. Chest, *86*:489–492, 1984.
277. Silver, R.M., Miller, K.S., Kinsella, M.B., et al.: Evaluation and management of scleroderma lung disease using bronchoalveolar lavage. Am. J. Med., *88*:470–476, 1990.
278. Medsger, T.A., Jr.: D-Penicillamine treatment of lung involvement in patients with systemic sclerosis (scleroderma). Arthritis Rheum., *30*:832–834, 1987.
279. Steen, V.D. et al.: The effect of D-penicillamine on pulmonary findings in systemic sclerosis. Arthritis Rheum., *28*:882–888, 1985.
280. deClerck, L.S., Dequeker, J., Franc, L., and Demedts, M.: D-penicillamine therapy and interstitial lung disease in sclero-

derma: A long-term followup study. Arthritis Rheum., *30*:643–650, 1987.
281. Seibold, J.R. et al.: Acute hemodynamic effects of ketanserin in pulmonary hypertension secondary to systemic sclerosis. J. Rheumatol., *14*:519–524, 1987.
282. O'Brien, J.T., Hill, J.A., and Pepine, C.J.: Sustained benefit of verapamil in pulmonary hypertension with progressive systemic sclerosis. Am. Heart J., *109*:380–382, 1985.
283. Rouse, P.J., Lahiri, A., and Gumpel, J.M.: The CREST syndrome—Successful reduction of pulmonary hypertension by captopril. Postgrad. Med. J., *60*:672–674, 1984.
284. LeRoy, E.C.: Systemic sclerosis (scleroderma). *In* Textbook of Rheumatology. Edited by W.N. Kelley, E.D. Harris, Jr., S. Ruddy, and C.B. Sledge. Philadelphia, W.B. Saunders Co., 1985, pp. 1183–1205.
285. Brown, E.A., MacGregor, G.A., and Maini, R.N.: Failure of captopril to reverse the renal crisis of scleroderma. Ann. Rheum. Dis., *42*:52–53, 1983.
286. Nolph, K.D., Stolz, M.L., and Maher, J.L.: Altered peritoneal permeability in patients with systemic vasculitis. Ann. Intern. Med., *75*:753–755, 1971.
287. Copley, J.B., and Smith, B.J.: Continuous ambulatory peritoneal dialysis and scleroderma. Nephron, *40*:353–356, 1985.
288. Barker, D.J., and Farr, M.J.: Resolution of cutaneous manifestations of systemic sclerosis after hemodialysis. Br. Med. J., *1*:501, 1976.
289. LeRoy, E.C., and Fleischmann, R.M.: The management of renal scleroderma. Experience with dialysis, nephrectomy and transplantation. Am. J. Med., *64*:974–978, 1978.
290. Merino, G.E. et al.: Renal transplantation for progressive systemic sclerosis with renal failure. Am. J. Surg., *133*:745–749, 1977.
291. Woodhall, P.B. et al.: Apparent recurrence of progressive systemic sclerosis in a renal allograft. JAMA, *236*:1032–1034, 1976.
292. Byron, M.A., Venning, V.A., and Mowat, A.G.: Post-mammoplasty human adjuvant disease. Br. J. Rheumatol., *23*:227–229, 1984.
293. Taj, M., and Ahmad, A.: Familial localized scleroderma (morphoea). Arch. Dermatol., *113*:1132–1133, 1977.
294. Ikai, K. et al.: Morphea-like cutaneous changes in a patient with systemic scleroderma. Dermatologica, *158*:438–442, 1979.
295. Connelly, M.G., and Winkelmann, R.K.: Coexistence of lichen sclerosus, morphea, and lichen planus. J. Am. Acad. Dermatol., *12*:844–851, 1985.
296. Patterson, J.A.K., and Ackerman, B.: Lichen sclerosus et atrophicus is not related to morphea. A clinical and histologic study of 24 patients in whom both conditions were reputed to be present simultaneously. Am. J. Dermatol., *6*:323–335, 1984.
297. Mensing, H., and Schmidt, K.-U.: Diffuse fasciitis with eosinophilia associated with morphea and lichen sclerosus et atrophicus. Acta Derm. Venereol. (Stockh.), *65*:80–83, 1985.
298. Jablonska, S.: Scleroderma and Pseudoscleroderma. 2nd Ed. Warsaw, Polish Medical Publishers, 1975.
299. Rogers, B.O.: Transactions of the 3rd International Congress of Plastic Surgery (International Congress Series No. 66). Edited by T.R. Broadbent. Amsterdam, Excerpta Medica, 1963, pp. 681–689.
300. Dubois, E.L. et al.: Progressive systemic sclerosis (PSS) and localized scleroderma (morphea) with positive LE cell test and unusual systemic manifestations compatible with systemic lupus erythematosus (SLE): Presentation of 14 cases including one set of identical twins, one with scleroderma and the other with SLE. Review of the literature. Medicine, *50*:199–222, 1971.
301. Stern, L.Z. et al.: Myopathy associated with linear scleroderma. Neurology, *25*:114–119, 1975.
302. Soffa, D.J., Sire, D.J., and Dodson, J.H.: Melorheostosis with linear sclerodermatous skin changes. Radiology, *114*:577–578, 1975.
303. Falanga, V., Medsger, T.A., Jr., and Reichlin, M.: High titers of antibodies to single-stranded DNA in linear scleroderma. Arch. Dermatol., *121*:345–347, 1985.
304. Takehara, K. et al.: Antinuclear antibodies in localized scleroderma. Arthritis Rheum., *26*:612–616, 1983.
305. Falanga, V., Medsger, T.A., Jr., and Reichlin, M.: Antinuclear and anti-single-stranded DNA antibodies in morphea and generalized morphea. Arch. Dermatol., *123*:350–353, 1987.
306. Ruffatti, A. et al.: Anticentromere antibody in localized scleroderma. J. Am. Acad. Dermatol., *15*:637–642, 1986.
307. Moynahan, E.J.: Morphoea (localized cutaneous scleroderma) treated with low-dosage penicillamine (4 cases, including coup de sabre). Proc. R. Soc. Med., *66*:1083–1085, 1973.
308. Neuhofer, J., and Fritsch, P.: Treatment of localized scleroderma and lichen sclerosus with etretinate. Acta Derm. Venereol. (Stockh.), *64*:171–174, 1984.
309. Czarbecki, D.B., and Taft, E.H.: Generalized morphoea successfully treated with salazopyrine. Acta Derm. Venereol. (Stockh.), *62*:81–82, 1982.
310. Lakhanpal, S. et al.: Eosinophilic fasciitis: Clinical spectrum and therapeutic response in 52 cases. Semin. Arthritis Rheum., *17*:221–231, 1988.
311. Williams, H.J., Ziter, F.A.,, and Banta, C.A.: Childhood eosinophilic fasciitis—progression to linear scleroderma. J. Rheumatol., *13*:961–962, 1986.
312. Drosos, A.A., Papadimitriou, C.S., and Moutsopoulos, H.M.: An overlap of diffuse fasciitis with eosinophilia and scleroderma. Rheumatology, *4*:187–189, 1984.
313. Barnes, L. et al.: Eosinophilic fasciitis. A pathologic study of twenty cases. Am. J. Pathol., *96*:493–507, 1979.
314. Shulman, L.E.: Diffuse fasciitis with eosinophilia. A new syndrome? Trans. Assoc. Am. Physicians, *88*:70–86, 1975.
315. Hoffman, R. et al.: Diffuse fasciitis and aplastic anemia: A report of four cases revealing an unusual association between rheumatologic and hematologic disorders. Medicine, *61*:373–382, 1982.
316. Michet, C.J., Jr., Doyle, J.A., and Ginsburg, W.W.: Eosinophilic fasciitis. Report of 15 cases. Mayo Clin. Proc., *56*:27–34, 1981.
317. Doyle, J.A.: Eosinophilic fasciitis: Extracutaneous manifestations and associations. Cutis, *34*:259–261, 1984.
318. Wasserman, S.I. et al.: Serum eosinophilotactic activity in eosinophilic fasciitis. Arthritis Rheum., *25*:1352–1356, 1982.
319. Moore, T.L., and Zuckner, J.: Eosinophilic fasciitis. Semin. Arthritis Rheum., *9*:228–235, 1980.
320. Seibold, J.R. et al.: Circulating immune complexes in eosinophilic fasciitis. Arthritis Rheum., *25*:1180–1185, 1982.
321. Van Den Bergh, V. et al.: Diffuse fasciitis after bone marrow transplantation. Am. J. Med., *83*:139–143, 1987.
322. Kent, L.T., Cramer, S.F., and Moskowitz, R.W.: Eosinophilic fasciitis: Clinical, laboratory and microscopic considerations. Arthritis Rheum., *24*:677–683, 1981.
323. Smiley, A.M., Husain, M., and Indebaum, S.: Eosinophilic fasciitis in association with thyroid disease: A report of three cases. J. Rheumatol., *7*:871–876, 1980.
324. Laso, F.J., Pastor, I., and deCastro, S.: Cimetidine and eosinophilic fasciitis. Ann. Intern. Med., *98*:1026, 1983.
325. Solomon, G., Barland, P., and Rifkin, H.; Eosinophilic fasciitis responsive to cimetidine. Ann. Intern. Med., *97*:547–549, 1982.
326. Balaban, E.P. et al.: Treatment of cutaneous sclerosis and aplastic anemia with antithymocyte globulin. Ann. Intern. Med., *106*:56–58, 1987.

327. Joyce, R.A., Kahl, L.E., and Rodnan, G.P.: Aplastic anemia and eosinophilic fasciitis: Demonstration of T cell inhibition of colony formation and response to antithymocyte globulin. Arthritis Rheum., *27*:S74, 1984.
328. Hertzman, P.A., Blevins, W.L., Mayer, J., et al.; Association of the eosinophilia-myalgia syndrome with the ingestion of tryptophan. N. Engl. J. Med., *322*:869–873, 1990.
329. Centers for Disease Control: Eosinophilia-myalgia syndrome and L-tryptophan-containing products—New Mexico, Minnesota, Oregon, and New York, 1989. MMWR, *38*:785–788, 1989.
330. Kaufman, L.D., Seidman, R.J., and Gruber, B.L.: L-tryptophan associated eosinophilic perimyositis, neuritis, and fasciitis: A clinicopathologic and laboratory study of 25 patients. Medicin, *69*:187–199, 1990.
331. Varga, J., Heiman-Patterson, T.D., Emery, D.L., et al.: Clinical spectrum of the systemic manifestations of eosinophilia-myalgia syndrome. Semin. Arthritis Rheum., *19*:313–328, 1990.
332. Martin, R.W., Duffy, J., Engel, A., et al.: The clinical spectrum of the eosinophilia-myalgia syndrome associated with L-tryptophan ingestion. Ann. Intern. Med., *113*:124–134, 1990.
333. Hertzman, P.A., Falk, H., Kilbourne, E.M., et al.: The eosinophilia-myalgia syndrome: The Los Alamos Conference. J. Rheumatol., *18*:867–873, 1991.
334. Shulman, L.E.: The eosinophilia-myalgia syndrome associated with ingestion of L-tryptophan. (Editorial.) Arthritis Rheum., *33*:913–917, 1990.
335. Freundlich, B., Werth, V.P., Rook, A.H., et al.: L-tryptophan ingestion is associated with eosinophilic fasciitis but not progressive systemic sclerosis. Ann. Intern. Med., *112*:758–762, 1990.
336. Tazelaar, H.D., Myers, J.L., Drage, C.W., et al.: Pulmonary disease associated with L-tryptophan-induced eosinophilia-myalgia syndrome. Chest, *97*:1032–1036, 1990.
337. James, T.N.: Cardiac pathology in EMS. Presentation at the International eosinophilia-myalgia syndrome conference. Los Alamos National Laboratory, Los Alamos, NM, June 12–13, 1990.
338. Centers for Disease Control: Eosinophilia-myalgia syndrome and L-tryptophan containing products—New Mexico, Minnesota, Oregon, and New York, 1989. MMWR, *38*:785–788, 1989.
339. Eidsen, M., Philen, R., Sewell, C.M., et al.: L-tryptophan and eosinophilia-myalgia syndrome in New Mexico. Lancet, *335*:645–648, 1990.
340. Belongia, E.A., Hedberg, C.W., Gleich, G.J., et al.: An investigation of the cause of the eosinophilia-myalgia syndrome associated with tryptophan use. N. Engl. J. Med., *323*:357–365, 1990.
341. Slutsker, L., Hoelsly, F.C., Miller, L., et al.: Eosinophilia-myalgia syndrome associated with exposure to tryptophan from a single manufacturer. JAMA, *264*:213–217, 1990.
342. Kamb, M.L., Murphy, J.J., Jones, J.L., et al.: Eosinophilia-myalgia syndrome in L-tryptophan exposed patients in a South Carolina psychiatric practice. JAMA, *267*:77–82, 1992.
343. Centers for Disease Control: Analysis of L-tryptophan for the etiology of eosinophilia-myalgia syndrome. MMWR, *39*:589–591, 1990.
344. Mayeno, A.N., Lin, F., Foote, C.S., et al.: Characterization of "Peak E," a novel amino acid associated with eosinophilia-myalgia syndrome. Science, *250*:1707–1708, 1990.
345. Crofford, L.J., Rader, J.I., Dalakas, M.C., et al.: L-tryptophan implicated in human eosinophilia-myalgia syndrome causes fasciitis and perimyositis in the Lewis rat. J. Clin. Invest., *86*:1757–1763, 1990.
346. Silver, R.M., Heyes, M.P., Maize, J.C., et al.: Scleroderma, fasciitis, and eosinophilia associated with the ingestion of tryptophan. N. Engl. J. Med., *322*:874–881, 1990.
347. Kilbourne, E.M., Rigau-Perez, J.G., Heath, C.W., Jr. et al.: Clinical epidemiology of toxic-oil syndrome. Manifestations of a new illness. N. Engl. J. Med., *309*:1408–1414, 1983.
348. Toxic Epidemic Syndrome Study Group: Toxic epidemic: Spain 1981. Lancet, *2*:697–702, 1982.
349. Martinez Tello, F.J., Navas Palacios, J.J., Ricoy, J.R. et al.: Pathology of a new toxic syndrome caused by ingestion of adulterated oil in Spain. Virchows Arch. (Pathol. Anat.), *397*:261–285, 1982.
350. Ricoy, J.R., Cabello, A., Rodriguez, J., and Tellez, I.: Neuropathological studies on the toxic syndrome related to adulterated oil in Spain. Virchows Arch. (Pathol. Anat.), *397*:261–285, 1982.
351. Fleischmajer, R., and Pollock, J.L.: Progressive systemic sclerosis: Pseudoscleroderma. Clin. Rheum. Dis., *5*:243–261, 1979.
352. Rocco, V.K., and Hurd, E.R.: Scleroderma and scleroderma-liked disorders. Semin. Arthritis Rheum., *16*:22:69, 1986.
353. Ramsey, C.A. et al.: The treatment of porphyria cutanea tarda by venesection. Q. J. Med., *43*:1–24, 1974.
354. Grossman, M.E. et al.: Porphyria cutanea tarda. Clinical features and laboratory findings in 40 patients. Am. J. Med., *67*:277–286, 1977.
355. Maeda, H., Ishikaw, H., and Onta, S.: Circumscribed myxedema of lichen myxedematosus as a sign of faulty formation of the proteoglycan macromolecule. Br. J. Dermatol., *105*:239–245, 1981.
356. Helfrich, D.J., Walker, E.R., Martinez, A.J., and Medsger, T.A., Jr.: Scleromyxedema myopathy: Case report and literature review. Arthritis Rheum., *31*:1437–1441, 1988.
357. Lawrence, L.A., Tye, M.J., and Liss, M.: Immunochemical analysis of the basic immunoglobulin in papular mucinosis. Immunochemistry, *9*:41–49, 1972.
358. Rubinow, A., and Cohen, A.S.: Skin involvement in generalized amyloidosis. A study of clinically involved and uninvolved skin in 50 patients with primary and secondary amyloidosis. Ann. Intern. Med., *88*:781–785, 1978.
359. Siebold, J.R.: Digital sclerosis in children. Skin changes in insulin-dependent diabetes mellitus. Arthritis Rheum., *25*:1357–1361, 1982.
360. Jablonska, S., and Stachow, A.: Pseudoscleroderma concomitant with a muscular glycogenosis of unknown enzymatic defect. Acta Derm. Venereol., *52*:379–385, 1972.
361. Fries, J.F., Lindgren, J.A., and Bull, J.M.: Scleroderma-like lesions and the carcinoid syndrome. Arch. Intern. Med., *131*:550–553, 1973.
362. Houpt, J.B., Ogryzlo, M.A., and Hunt, M.: Tryptophan metabolism in man (with special reference to rheumatoid arthritis and scleroderma). Semin. Arthritis Rheum., *2*:333–353, 1973.
363. Kornreich, H.K. et al.: Phenylketonuria and scleroderma. J. Pediatr., *73*:571–575, 1968.
364. Epstein, C.J. et al.: Werner's syndrome. A review of its symptomatology, natural history, pathologic features, genetics and relationship to the natural aging process. Medicine, *45*:177–221, 1966.
365. Vilee, D.B., Nichols, G., and Talbot, N.B.; Metabolic studies in two boys with classical progeria. Pediatrics, *43*:207–216, 1969.
366. Sucio, I. et al.: Clinical manifestations in vinyl chloride poisoning. Ann. N.Y. Acad. Sci., *246*:53–69, 1975.
367. Maricq, H.R. et al.: Capillary abnormalities in polyvinyl chloride production workers. Examination by in vivo microscopy. J. Am. Med. Assoc., *236*:1368–1371, 1976.
368. Selikoff, I.J., and Hammond, E.C.: Editors and Conference Chairman: Toxicity of vinyl chloride-polyvinyl chloride. Ann. N.Y. Acad. Sci., *246*:1–337, 1975.
369. Owens, G.R., and Medsger, T.A., Jr.: Systemic sclerosis secondary to occupational exposure. Am. J. Med., *85*:114–116, 1988.

370. Cohen, I.S. et al.: Cutaneous toxicity of bleomycin therapy. Arch. Dermatol., *107*:553–555, 1973.
371. Vogelzang, N.J. et al.: Raynaud's phenomenon: A common toxicity after combination chemotherapy for testicular cancer. Ann. Intern. Med., *95*:288–292, 1981.
372. Yagoda, A. et al.: Bleomycin, an antitumor antibiotic. Clinical experience in 274 patients. Ann. Intern. Med., *77*:861–870, 1972.
373. Butler, R.C., Dieppe, P.A., and Keat, A.C.S.: Calcinosis of joints and periarticular tissues associated with vitamin D intoxication. Ann. Rheum. Dis., *44*:494–498, 1985.
374. Bilezikian, J.P., Auerbach, G.D., and Connor, T.B.: Pseudogout after parathyroidectomy. Lancet, *1*;445–446, 1973.
375. deGraaf, P. et al.: Metastatic skin calcifications: A rare phenomenon in dialysis patients. Dermatologica, *161*:28–32, 1980.
376. Moskowitz, R.W. et al.: Crystal-induced inflammation associated with chronic renal failure treated with periodic hemodialysis. Am. J. Med., *47*:450–460, 1969.
377. Andresen, J., and Nielsen, H.E.: Juxta-articular erosions and calcifications in patients with chronic renal failure. Acta Radiol. [Diagn.] (Stockh.), *22*:709–713, 1981.
378. Russell, R.G.G., Bisaz, S., and Fleisch, H.: Pyrophosphate and disphosphonates in calcium metabolism and their possible role in renal failure. Arch. Intern. Med., *124*:571–577, 1969.
379. Kovarik, J. et al.: Tumorous paraarticular calcifications due to undigested phosphate-binders in a patient undergoing regular hemodialysis. (Letter.) Clin. Nephrol., *21*:141–142, 1984.
380. Reginato, A.J. et al.: Arthropathy and cutaneous calcinosis in hemodialysis oxalosis. Arthritis Rheum., *29*:1387–1396, 1986.
381. Walton, K., and Swinson, D.R.: Acute calcific periarthritis associated with transient hypocalcaemia secondary to hypoparathyroidism. Br. J. Rheumatol., *22*:179–180, 1983.
382. Reference deleted.
383. Kim, E.E. et al.: Accumulation of Tc-99m-phosphonate complexes in metastatic lesions from colon and lung carcinomas. Eur. J. Nucl. Med., *5*:299–301, 1980.
384. Kantarjian, H.M. et al.: Uptake of ^{99m}Tc-methylene disphosphonate in calcinosis cutis. J. Am. Acad. Dermatol., 7:804–806, 1982.
385. McKee, P.H., Liomba, N.G., and Hutt, M.S.R.: Tumoral calcinosis: A pathological study of fifty-six cases. Br. J. Dermatol., *107*:669–674, 1982.
386. Lafferty, F.W., Raynolds, E.S., and Pearson, O.H.: Tumoral calcinosis: A metabolic disease of obscure etiology. Am. J. Med., *38*:105–118, 1965.
387. Zerwekh, J.E. et al.: Tumoral calcinosis: Evidence for concurrent defects in renal tubular phosphorus transport and in 1α,25-dihydrocholecalciferol synthesis. Calcif. Tissue Int., *32*:1–6, 1980.
388. Lufkin, E.G., Kumar, R., and Heath, H., III: Hyperphosphatemic tumoral calcinosis: Effects of phosphate depletion on vitamin D metabolism, and of acute hypocalcemia on parathyroid hormone secretion and action. J. Clin. Endocrinol. Metab., *56*:1319–1322, 1983.
389. Lyles, K.W. et al.: Genetic transmission of tumoral calcinosis: Autosomal dominant with variable clinical expressivity. J. Clin. Endocrinol. Metab., *60*:1093–1096, 1985.
390. Boskey, A.L. et al.: Chemical, microscopic, and ultrastructural characterization of the mineral deposits in tumoral calcinosis. Clin. Orthop. Rel. Res., *178*:258–269, 1983.
391. Mozartarian, G., Lafferty, F.W., and Pearson, O.H.: Treatment of tumoral calcinosis with phosphorus deprivation. Ann. Intern. Med., *77*:741–745, 1972.
392. Salvi, A. et al.: Phosphaturic action of calcitonin in pseudotumoral calcinosis. Horm. Metab. Res., *15*:260, 1983.
393. Kazmers, I.S., Scoville, C.D., and Schumacher, H.R.: Polymyositis associated apatite arthritis. J. Rheumatol., *15*:1019–1021, 1988.
394. Bowyer, S.L., Blane, C.E., Sullivan, D.B., and Cassidy, J.T.: Childhood dermatomyositis: Factors predicting functional outcome and development of dystrophic calcification. J. Pediatr., *103*:882–888, 1983.
395. Blane, C.E. et al.: Patterns of calcification in childhood dermatomyositis. Am. J. Radiol., *142*:397–400, 1984.
396. Zwillich, S.H., Schumacher, H.R., Jr., Hoyt, T.S. et al.: Universal spondylodiscitis in a patient with erosive peripheral arthritis and apatite crystal deposition. J. Rheumatol., *15*:123–218, 1988.
397. Randle, H.W., Sander, H.M., and Howard, K.: Early diagnosis of calcinosis cutis in childhood dermatomyositis using computed tomography. JAMA, *256*:1137–1138, 1986.
398. Leroux, J-L. et al.: Ultrastructural and crystallographic study of calcifications from a patient with CREST syndrome. J. Rheumatol., *10*:242–246, 1983.
399. Reference deleted.
400. Kawakami, T. et al.: Ultrastructural study of calcinosis universalis with dermatomyositis. J. Cutan. Pathol., *13*:135–143, 1986.
401. Marks, J.: Studies with ^{47}Ca in patients with calcinosis cutis. Br. J. Dermatol., *82*:1–9, 1970.
402. Kales, A.N., and Phang, J.M.: Dietary calcium perturbation in patients with abnormal calcium deposition. J. Clin. Endocrinol. Metab., *31*:204–212, 1970.
403. Lian, J.B. et al.: Gamma-carboxyglutamate excretion and calcinosis in juvenile dermatomyositis. Arthritis Rheum., *25*:1094–1100, 1982.
404. Moore, S.E., Jump, A.A., and Smiley, J.D.: Effect of warfarin sodium therapy on excretion of 4-carboxy-L-glutamic acid in scleroderma, dermatomyositis, and myositis ossificans progressiva. Arthritis Rheum., *29*:344–351, 1986.
405. Sherman, F.S., et al.: Collagen crosslinks: A critical determinant of bioprosthetic heart valve calcification. Trans. Am. Soc. Artif. Intern. Organs, *30*:577–581, 1984.
406. Russell, R.G.G., and Smith, R.: Diphosphonates: Experimental and clinical aspects. J. Bone Joint Surg., *55B*:66–86, 1973.
407. Dent, C.E., and Stamp, T.C.G.: Treatment of calcinosis circumscripta with probenecid. Br. Med. J., *1*:216–218, 1972.
408. Jones, N.F., Imbriglia, J.E., Steen, V.D., and Medsger, T.A., Jr.: Surgery for scleroderma of the hand. J. Hand Surg., *12A*:391–400, 1987.
409. Mendelson, B.C. et al.: Surgical treatment of calcinosis cutis in the upper extremity. J. Hand Surg., *2*:318–324, 1977.
410. Wilsher, M.L., Holdaway, I.M., and North, J.D.K.: Hypercalcaemia during resolution of calcinosis in juvenile dermatomyositis. Br. Med. J., *288*:1345, 1984.
411. Ahrengart, L., Lindgren, V., and Reinholt, E.P.: Comparative study of the effects of radiation, indomethacin, prednisolone and ethane-1-hydroxy-1′, 1-diphosphonate (EHDP) in the prevention of ectopic bone formation. Clin. Orthop. Res., *229*:265–273, 1988.
412. Suzuki, Y., Bisada, K., and Takeda, M.: Demonstration of myositis ossificans by ^{99m}Tc pyrophosphate bone scanning. Radiology, *111*:663–664, 1974.
413. Buhain, W.J., Rammohan, G., and Berger, H.W.: Pulmonary function in myositis ossificans progressiva. Am. Rev. Respir. Dis., *110*:333–337, 1974.
414. Smith, R.: Myositis ossificans progressiva. A review of current problems. Semin. Arthritis Rheum., *4*:369–380, 1975.
415. Illingworth, R.S.: Myositis ossificans progressiva (Munchmeyer's disease). Brief review with report of two cases treated with corticosteroids and observed for 16 years. Arch. Dis. Child., *46*:264–268, 1971.
416. Gilsanz, V., and Bernstein, B.H.: Joint calcification following

intraarticular corticosteroid therapy. Radiology, *151*:647–649, 1984.

417. Dalinka, M.K. et al.: Periarticular calcifications in association with intra-articular corticosteroid injections. Radiology, *153*:615–618, 1984.
418. Edwards, A.J., Sill, B.J., and Macfarlane, I.: Carpal tunnel syndrome due to dystrophic calcification. Aust, N.Z. J. Surg., *54*:491–492, 1984.
419. Selby, C.L.: Acute calcific tendinitis of the hand: An infrequently recognized and frequently misdiagnosed form of periarthritis. Arthritis Rheum., *27*:337–340, 1984.
420. Ellis, I.O., Foster, M.C., and Womack, C.: Plumber's knee: Calcinosis cutis after repeated minor trauma in a plumber. Br. Med. J., *288*:1723, 1984.
421. DiGiovanna, J.J., Helfgott, R.K., Gerber, L.H., and Peck, G.L.: Extraspinal tendon and ligament calcification associated with long-term therapy eith etretinate. N. Engl. J. Med., *315*:1177–1182, 1986.
422. Sakkas, L. et al.: Cervical myelopathy with ankylosing hyperostosis of the spine. Surg. Neurol., *24*:43–46, 1985.
423. Miyasaka, K. et al.: Myelopathy due to ossification or calcification of the ligamentum flavum: Radiologic and histologic evaluations. Am. J. Neurol. Radiol., *4*:629–632, 1983.
424. Widlus, D.M.: Calcific tendonitis of the longus colli muscle: A cause of atraumatic neck pain. Ann. Emerg. Med., *14*:1014–1017, 1985.
425. Benanti, J.C., Gramling, P., Bulat, P.I., and Chen, P.: Retropharyngeal calcific tendinitis: Report of five cases and review of the literature. J. Emerg. Med., *4*:15–24, 1986.
426. Caspi, D., Rosenbach, T.O., Yaron, M. et al.: Periarthritis associated with basic calcium phosphate crystal deposition and low levels of serum alkaline phosphatase—Report of three cases from one family. J. Rheumatol., *15*:823–827, 1988.
427. Chuck, A.J., Pattnick, M.G., Hamilton, E. et al.: Crystal deposition in hypophosphatasia: A reappraisal. Ann. Rheum. Dis., *48*:571–576, 1989.
428. Siegel, S.A., Hummel, C.F., and Carty, R.P.: The role of nucleoside triphosphate pyrophosphohydrolase in *in vitro* nucleoside triphosphate-dependent matrix vesicle calcification. J. Biol. Chem., *258*:8601–8607, 1983.
429. Zervas, J. et al.: HLA antigens in diabetics with calcified shouder periarthritis (CSP). Clin. Exp. Rheumatol., *4*:351–353, 1986.

74

Pathogenesis of Systemic Sclerosis

E. CARWILE LeROY

Despite our ability to identify the population at risk (capillary-positive, serology-positive patients with Raynaud's phenomenon) to develop the potentially lethal form of scleroderma (termed *generalized scleroderma*, or *systemic sclerosis*, SSc), our understanding of its pathogenesis is so meager that, except for the treatment and prevention of renal failure by inhibitors of angiotensin-converting enzymes, our patients continue to succumb to vascular insufficiency and fibrosis of the lung, gastrointestinal track, heart, and peripheral vasculature. One path to logical, effective therapeutic intervention seems to be increased understanding of the pathogenetic steps leading to fibrosis rather than continued futile attempts to dissolve mature scar tissue, a largely unsuccessful venture now for several centuries. This chapter includes a definition, selected comments regarding etiology, a pathophysiologic hypothesis, and a discussion of what is known regarding the pathogenesis of SSc. Pathogenesis is divided into extracellular matrix, fibroblast, endothelial cell, and immune cell sections, keeping in mind that autoimmune and inflammatory events, to be relevant to SSc, should be linked directly to the exuberant fibrosis that is its hallmark.

DEFINITION

Systemic sclerosis is operationally defined here as a disorder in which autoimmune events trigger widespread vascular and microvascular lesions characterized by endothelial cell activation/injury, which initiates proliferative, fibrotic interstitial reactions associated with vascular insufficiency and scarring of the skin, lungs, gastrointestinal system, heart, and kidneys. In skin, the dermis, subcutis, or deep fascia (eosinophilic fasciitis) may be involved. The epidermis, otherwise normal, is thinned in the late atrophic phase of the disease. This working definition is diagrammed in Fig. 74–1.

ETIOLOGY

The cause of SSc is not known.[1] Many exogenous–environmental triggers have been associated with SSc-like syndromes (Table 74–1). Whether they occur de novo or in hosts genetically predisposed to fibrosis is unknown. The large proportion of persons who develop fibrosis after exposure to bleomycin[2] and silica,[3] for example, suggests that either a fibrotic phenotype is common or that a sufficient stimulus can induce fibrosis in nearly anyone, as it does following radiation exposure, a consistent and predictable fibrotic stimulus. A pattern of inheritance for autoimmunity in general is more apparent than the inheritance of SSc per se.[4] Multiple triggers appear to be at least additive and possibly synergistic. As an example, when persons with limited SSc have a limb immobilized after bone fracture, diffuse skin involvement may occur in only the immobilized area. This does not occur in healthy casted subjects (except in the setting of reflex sympathetic dystrophy, which is usually reversible), suggesting that both the susceptibility (possibly autoimmune) and the immobilization trigger were needed for the development of taut skin.[5]

HYPOTHESIS

The hypothesis of an autoimmune attack on the endothelium,[6] in which fibrosis results from fibroblast activation after endothelial activation and/or injury, has led to renewed interest in HLA associations, in mechanisms of T-cell activation, and in the wide array of changes dependent on altered endothelial cell function. Here, cause and effect have not been sorted out. A selected activation of T cells, of endothelial cells, monocytes, or of fibroblasts which then direct a cycle of interactions (Fig. 74–1) seems plausible, inviting further study of what comes first.

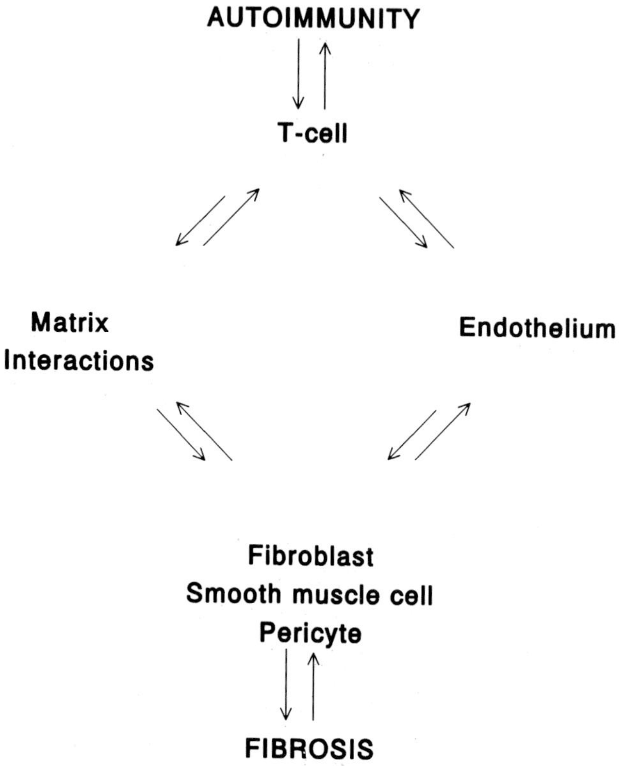

FIG. 74–1. Systemic sclerosis activation cycle.

TABLE 74–1. ENVIRONMENTAL TRIGGERS OF SYSTEMIC SCLEROSIS

OCCUPATIONAL
Silicosis
Vibration exposure (from sewing machines to bulldozers)
Solvents
Vinyl chloride (monochloroethylene)
Other halogenated, unsaturated hydrocarbons (dichloroethylene, trichloroethylene, etc.)
Other solvents (benzene and phenylenediamines)
Epoxy resins (electronics manufacturing)
THERAPEUTIC OR DIAGNOSTIC AGENTS
L-tryptophan (eosinophilia myalgia syndrome)
Practolol
Bleomycin, cis-platinum
x-Irradiation
FOODSTUFFS
Adulterated rapeseed oil (toxic oil syndrome)
COSMETICS
Breast implants (silicone mammoplasty)
Hair dyes
IATROGENIC
Chronic graft-versus-host disease (bone marrow transplants)
Carbidopa and hydroxytryptophan

THE EXTRACELLULAR MATRIX

Collagen deposition replacing subcutaneous fat was the first histologic feature of SSc to draw attention in the early days of microscopic pathology.[7] SSc fibroblasts propagated in vitro secreted increased quantities of total collagen.[8,9] Now that 14 collagen types (more than 20 genes) have been recognized and techniques are available to measure mRNA as well as secreted protein, it has been shown that SSc fibroblasts demonstrate a phenotype of activation of matrix gene expression that includes types I, III, and VI collagens, fibronectin, and proteoglycan; in addition, each of these matrix genes has been shown to be expressed in increased quantity at the transcriptional level, that is, increased levels of steady-state message (mRNA) constitutively in vitro and also for selected genes by in situ hybridization ex vivo.[1] Taken together, these findings are consistent with the activation of one or several DNA responsive elements by one or more protein complexes transactivating gene expression. To what degree message stability plays a role in SSc is unknown. In the well-studied example of ascorbate stimulation of collagen synthesis, both increased transcription and decreased decay of mRNA are operative in vitro.[10] Also, translational control of matrix synthesis has been shown at least for type I collagen; the best studied translational point of control is a feedback mechanism whereby both a fragment of the nonhelical aminoterminal region of α1(I) procollagen and a 22 amino acid peptide of the carboxyterminal region of α2(I) procollagen inhibit not only their own protein synthetic rates but also have an inhibitory influence on other collagens, other matrix gene products, and general protein synthetic rates, all without changes in mRNA levels.[11] Because mRNA levels from genes coding for matrix macromolecules are elevated and general protein synthetic rates are normal in SSc fibroblasts, a post-translational site for control of matrix deposition cannot explain the SSc fibroblast phenotype. Nonetheless, post-translational mechanisms to reduce matrix synthesis in vivo could be developed therapeutically. Along these lines it has been shown that SSc fibroblast overproduction of collagen is reduced by exposure in vitro to fragments of the aminoterminal region of α2(I) procollagen.[11] Proline analogues preventing collagen helix formation and enhancing nascent collagen chain degradation also have been proposed as therapeutic agents.[12]

Coordinate regulation of multiple genes coding for matrix macromolecules makes biologic sense and provides an investigative focus to define such regulation precisely. This could lead to a therapeutic strategy reducing the expression of all genes coding for matrix macromolecules simultaneously. When one examines the responsive elements of collagen genes, differences are more apparent than similarities; moreover, the results of elegant studies by de Crombrugghe et al. in mice were not applicable to human genes.[13,14] Each 5′ regulatory region of each gene coding for matrix macromolecules is characterized by multiple responsive elements that are not identical between species or between the genes coding for different matrix proteins. Two areas of the α2(I) procollagen gene seem promising for further study to understand SSc: these are a 5′ region between −324 and −224 (i.e., 224 bases 5′ from the initiation point of the transcriptional start site) and a region

(+418 to +1524) in the first intron. In the first site a specific regulatory element (−315 to −295 and composed of TCGN$_5$–GCCA) increases α2(I) collagen mRNA by binding to the transactivating protein NF1 and, most interestingly, is involved in the stimulation of mouse α2(I) collagen mRNA by transforming growth factor beta (TGF-β), a potent fibrokine (fibrogenic cytokine).[15] Whether a similar responsive element is present in the human α2(I) collagen gene is an important question. The intron story may be even more interesting. In the mouse α2(I) collagen gene, a tissue-specific enhancer element between +418 and +1524 has a strong homology to several viral enhancers. In contrast, although the study of the human gene is incomplete, there appears to be a negative responsive element in this region of the human α2(I) gene.[16,17] This and other examples of negative control of collagen gene regulation (repression) may occur by the methylation of cytosine/guanosine bases, a mechanism well studied in development since it was realized that virtually all genes are methylated and thereby inactivated in sperm. The regulation of methylation itself is incompletely understood, but if it controls human fibroblast collagen gene regulation and plays a role in the overexpression of collagen genes in the SSc fibroblast (i.e., overexpression representing a failure of methylation), then selective methylation could represent another potential therapeutic strategy in human fibrotic diseases. Therapeutic control of connective tissue matrix formation and breakdown remains a long-term goal of studies of SSc.

Among the matrix elements known to be elevated at the transcriptional level in SSc fibroblasts, fibronectin warrants further comment. It is a reasonable hypothesis, amenable to experimental testing, that increased amounts of fibronectin are deposited in the edematous, immune, inflammatory phase of SSc by activated cells (monocytes, endothelial cells, pericytes, or fibroblasts) with subsequent fibronectin matrix assembly generating a scaffolding on which future scar tissue is deposited. Alveolar macrophages and fibroblasts from involved SSc tissue both have been shown to produce increased amounts of fibronectin; and in both, fibronectin mRNA levels are increased, and TGF-β induced greater levels of fibronectin secretion in SSc fibroblasts than in control skin fibroblasts.[18] Fibronectin enhances fibroblast chemotaxis and proliferation and serves as a co-stimulatory signal for T cells already activated by an antigen-specific major histocompatibility complex-dependent (CD3) stimulus. Members of the B1 subfamily of integrins (termed very late antigens or VLA 3, 4, 5) bind fibronectin and provide co-stimulation to human CD4-positive T cells.[19] Fibronectin enhances platelet adhesion and activation by similar mechanisms. The pro-inflammatory and pro-immune features of fibronectin make it a potentially pivotal molecule in the fibrotic reaction.

FIBROBLAST STUDIES

Fibroblasts have been the major cell of tissue culture studies since Alexis Carrel (and his technician) propagated the same strain of cells for decades in the 1920s.[20] Hayflick used fibroblasts to define the concept of in vitro cell senescence in the 1960s. Currently, many metabolic and gene regulation studies, including those involving transfection and transgenic manipulation, use fibroblasts as the cell of choice. These cells are the major producers of extracellular matrix and display anchorage-dependent growth and density-dependent inhibition of proliferation (confluence). Although monotonously similar by morphologic criteria, fibroblasts are surprisingly heterogeneous in their capacity to proliferate and to produce collagen, tissue coagulation factor, and prostaglandins.[21,22] Thus, fibroblast studies in mass culture likely represent the average of a spectrum of cellular responses that require studies of cloned cells for precise definition. In studies using human diploid, nonimmortalized, nontransformed fibroblasts, clonal propagation is difficult because it requires most of the proliferative capacity of the cell, leaving only a brief life span for experiments. Unfortunately, immortalization of a patient's fibroblasts may alter the phenotypic characteristics under study. For example, immortalization of human skin fibroblasts by the large T antigen of the SV40 virus changes both their matrix gene expression and their growth characteristics, rendering them inappropriate as experimental controls. Immortalized cells from other species, such as mouse NIH 3T3 or baby hamster kidney (BHK), are not relevant to human disease. Likewise, tumor cells are not relevant to the study of human fibrotic disease because they differ in exactly the crucial phenotype characteristics, that is, matrix gene expression and cell growth behavior, which are abnormal in the disease phenotype. Thus, for the study of SSc fibroblast behavior, there seems to be little alternative to the labor-intensive propagation of cells from lesional skin obtained by biopsy as compared to skin fibroblasts from age, sex, biopsy site, and skin color-matched healthy subjects. Differences in both growth and matrix characteristics between adult skin, infant foreskin, and NIH 3T3 fibroblasts are great enough to disqualify the latter two cell lines for use as controls for SSc fibroblasts. Adult skin fibroblasts are the only control cells with reproducible growth and matrix characteristics.

Fibroblast proliferation is abnormal in SSc, occurring in the same cells showing abnormal matrix gene expression. In early studies of SSc fibroblast collagen synthesis, we realized that control skin fibroblasts showed increased collagen production when serum-supplemented media was replaced daily but that SSc fibroblasts were unresponsive to such frequent feeding schedules. Because platelet-derived growth factor (PDGF) is the major fibroblast mitogen of serum, we next noted that SSc fibroblasts were *selectively* unresponsive to added PDGF but not to other growth factors such as epidermal growth factor (EGF) or fibroblast growth factor (FGF),[24] suggesting that SSc fibroblasts might possess an active autocrine growth cycle involving PDGF.

Such autocrine activity was demonstrated when SSc fibroblasts continued to express the early mitogenic response proto-oncogene c-*myc* and continued to incorporate radioactively labeled thymidine into their nuclei (nuclear grain counts indicating continuing DNA synthesis) for several days when serum was reduced to submitogenic concentrations (<1%). Control adult skin fibroblasts ceased to express *myc* or take up thymidine within hours of serum removal.[25] TGF-β, a potent fibrokine, up-regulates cell responses to PDGF. We examined the capacity of TGF-β to enhance responses to PDGF by measuring the binding of labeled PDGF isoforms (AA,AB,BB) to SSc, adult skin, and infant foreskin fibroblasts before and after an 8-hour exposure to TGF-β in serum-free conditions. PDGF binding occurred through the dimerization of PDGF receptors α and β, to form homodimers (αα and ββ). All ligand isoforms bound to α-receptors, and AA ligand homodimers bound only to αα-homodimer–receptor complexes. Distinct differences between the three cell types were found. Foreskin cells showed decreased PDGF AA binding to half of their constitutive level after exposure to TGF-β; adult skin binding remained unchanged or increased slightly, while SSc fibroblast binding doubled after TGF-β exposure. The data show that SSc fibroblasts are hypersensitive to picomolar quantities of TGF-β as compared to control adult or foreskin fibroblasts.[23] The simplest way to increase the sensitivity of a cell to TGF-β with regard to PDGF binding is to expose it to TGF-β itself. Thus, TGF-β up-regulates its own expression as well as up-regulating expression and responsiveness to PDGF. The A-ligand–α-receptor system of PDGF may be more important for fibrogenesis than the B-ligand–β-receptor system, which is known to be important in oncogenesis and cell transformation. Perhaps resting adult fibroblasts express relatively low levels of PDGF-α receptors until they are exposed to TGF-β (or IL-1β, which also has this effect), at which time they increase α-receptor expression for several population doublings. This renders them exquisitely sensitive to autocrine or paracrine PDGF coming from an inflammatory and/or immune stimulus. (Cells other than platelets secrete PDGF, e.g., macrophages.) The regulation of the expression of the α-receptor of PDGF is a key area for future study. This fibroblast-proliferative pathway may be involved in not only SSc but also wound healing, keloid formation, atherosclerosis, and cirrhosis.

Other evidence of fibroblast activation has been described beyond the well-known enhanced transcriptional expression of several matrix genes and the autocrine up-regulation of PDGF A-ligand–α-receptor expression; lesional fibroblasts express the intercellular adhesion molecule (ICAM-1) in vitro.[26] And in situ studies demonstrate fibroblast and adjacent mononuclear cell expression of α1(I) collagen mRNA, TGF-β2, PDGF, and FGF—either separately or together—suggesting multiple cytokine effects in the fibroblast activation of SSc.[27–29]

ENDOTHELIAL CELLS

The vascular involvement in the spectrum of SSc disorders [limited and diffuse SSc, dermatomyositis, polymyositis, diffuse fasciitis with eosinophilia, and early, undifferentiated or mixed connective tissue disease (CTD)] is both similar to and distinctive from that seen in rheumatoid arthritis (RA), systemic lupus erythematosus (SLE), or systemic vasculitis, such as polyarteritis nodosa (PAN). Early in all of these disorders there is often an *arteriolar-capillary perivasculitis* with mononuclear cell collections containing T cells, B cells, and monocytes. Here the similarities end; SSc vascular lesions progress in two distinctive ways: (1) *arterial intimal proliferation* (the only vessels with a morphologically defined intima, internal to the internal elastic lamina) appears and progresses relentlessly, even while cutaneous involvement seems to be improving, and (2) in the *obliteration of arterioles and capillaries* with attrition of endothelial cells and basal lamina, which also proceeds inexorably.[30] Another difference is that in rare patients with RA, SLE, or in PAN, a true arteritis occurs, with mononuclear cells infiltrating all layers of arteries with disruption of arterial architecture and resulting in aneurysm formation; such arteritis does not occur in SSc. In SSc, both the intimal proliferation and microvascular obliteration are consistent with a recurring pattern of injury to endothelial cells or basal lamina or both, which the endothelium cannot effectively repair to return to its healthy state of regulating nonthrombogenicity, vasomotion, and vascular permeability.[6]

Four different but not necessarily exclusive possibilities could explain the mechanism of endothelial activation and/or injury in SSc: (1) a soluble molecule (cytokine and/or protease); (2) an endothelial or basal lamina (type IV collagen or laminin) specific antibody; (3) soluble immune complexes; or (4) an activated immune cell (most likely a T cell or monocyte). Some evidence exists for each of these possibilities.

In 1979 a soluble, 50-kDa activity was identified in SSc sera; this activity was directly and selectively cytotoxic to human umbilical vein endothelial cells.[31] Such SSc cytotoxic activity was inversely proportional to the deficient protease inhibitory activity found in SSc sera.[32] More than a decade later (failing to implicate TGF-β, tumor necrosis factor-α (TNF-α) or -β, an interferon, or an interleukin directly), the best candidate for this serum cytotoxic activity is a product of activated T cells, termed *granzyme one* for its localization in cytolytic T-cell granules.[33] Free granzyme one is present in SSc sera. Its blockade by specific antisera abrogates the endothelial cytotoxicity, of SSc sera, unifying possibilities one and four. Because granzyme one is a type IV collagenase, endothelial injury could occur via disruption of basal lamina, generating fragments to elicit autoimmune reactions and preventing full repair. Thus, fragments of type IV collagen and laminin released by granzyme one could explain the autoimmunity to these basal lamina components observed in SSc.[34,35] More study is needed to sort out how granzyme one influences endothelial function in vivo (its highest binding natural inhibitor is antithrombin III); at present it seems to fulfill the criteria proposed in 1979 for the SSc endothelial cell cytotoxic factor; parenthetically, microvascular endothelial cells are also affected adversely by SSc sera. If these observations are confirmed, attempts to understand the well-documented failure of SSc endothelial integrity in vivo, with disruption of its key nonthrombogenic and vasomotor roles, will turn to T-cell activation as discussed in the following paragraphs.

In vivo, endothelial cell function can be assessed in several reliable ways. The single best test seems to be the plasma level of factor VIII/von Willebrand factor; levels of factor VIII were elevated in SSc patients who, on biopsy, showed disruption of endothelial integrity.[36] Such elevated levels correlated inversely with levels of angiotensin-converting enzyme in the same patients. To guard against tissue injury or platelet release artifacts ex vivo, a normal platelet factor four level is an essential control, because the ex vivo platelet contribution to the levels detected in the assay can be substantial. Most SSc patients show elevations of factor VIII/von Willebrand factor, and the standard therapies for SSc (calcium channel blockers, antiplatelet regimens with aspirin and dipyridamole, d-penicillamine, and colchicine) do not consistently normalize them. Potential pathogenic roles for serotonin, epinephrine, platelet-activation factor, or thromboxane A_2 have not been studied sufficiently to permit comment. A therapeutic regimen that consistently normalizes serum levels of molecules reflecting endothelial cell perturbation and keeps them normal would become an important investigational tool to further decipher the prominent endothelial and vascular injury pattern as these lead directly to organ failure and determine prognosis in SSc patients. More emphasis on vascular therapies in SSc is needed before organ failure ensues. The success of angiotensin-converting enzyme inhibitors in preventing scleroderma renal crisis *before* the serum creatinine reaches 4 mg/dL is fitting testimony to the potential for effective vascular-oriented therapy in earlier stages of SSc.[37]

Anti-endothelial antibodies, functioning via an antibody-dependent cell cytotoxicity mechanism, have been found in about 25% of SSc patients;[36] circulating immune complexes are commonly detected in low titer but immunofluorescent studies of immunoglobulin and complement components in biopsy material have not been positive in most cases. Thus, direct antibody and immune complex mechanisms of vascular injury are viewed as either secondary or rare in SSc, in contrast to other rheumatic syndromes where they are often much more frequent and present in higher titer.

IMMUNE CELLS IN SYSTEMIC SCLEROSIS

Immune abnormalities in SSc have had a checkered history. In the early days of antinuclear antibody (ANA) serology, when substrates were nonhuman and nondividing cell nuclei (such as rat liver, mouse thymus, confluent 3T3 fibroblasts), the proportion of positive ANAs in SSc patients was below 30%, and patterns, usually speckled, were considered nonspecific. With the introduction of the human, rapidly dividing laryngeal carcinoma (HEp-2) cell line, positive serology in SSc jumped to >95% and includes antibodies to a group of very interesting biologic molecules (e.g., the rare Ku protein has been shown to be a leucine zipper nuclear protein, which serves as a trans-acting regulator of gene expression). The variety of serologies seen in the spectrum of SSc patients is shown in Table 74–2. Anti-centromere antibody has been the most helpful clinically because it is present early in patients with isolated Raynaud's phenomenon and it predicts the development of the limited cutaneous subset of SSc. Also, its absence predicts the diffuse SSc subset. Still, the revolution in SSc serology using the HEp-2 substrate has not made a major impact on our understanding of the pathogenesis of the disease. What it has done is to focus investigation on the contribution of the immune response to the vascular–microvascular injury pattern and the resultant fibrosis.[39] Here, too, there is progress.

Many avenues of inquiry lead to the notion that T-cell hyperactivity occurs in SSc. Absolute levels of circulating CD4 antigen, circulating CD4-positive cells, and ratios of CD4-positive/CD8-positive circulating cells are elevated. Serum levels of interleukin-2 (IL-2) and IL-2 receptors are also increased. IL-2 levels correlated positively with increases in skin tautness scores, the initial indication that these T-cell abnormalities may be relevant to the edema–inflammation–fibrosis cycle in the skin.[40,41]

The stimulus for T-cell hyperactivity is unknown. Self- or cross-reactive bacterial epitopes, to which each of the autoantibodies listed in Table 74–2 are reactive, are candidates for T-cell reactivity in SSc. Among these is laminin, a vascular scaffolding structural protein now shown to have major co-stimulatory activity when the T-cell receptor is engaged. Co-stimulation of T cells is a relatively new concept in human autoimmunity that can now be pursued in SSc. Autoimmunity to laminin is seen not only in SSc but also in other human fibrotic

TABLE 74–2. AUTOIMMUNE SEROLOGY IN SYSTEMIC SCLEROSIS

Anticentromere antibodies
Antinuclear antibodies (speckled, nucleolar, other)
Antinucleolar antibodies
RNA polymerase I
Fibrillarin (U3 RNA protein complex)
Nucleolar 4-65 RNA
U2 RNA protein complex
Polymyositis–systemic sclerosis overlap (Pm/Scl)
Antitopoisomerase I (formerly Scl-70)
Anticollagen type IV (basement membrane structure)
Antilaminin (basement membrane attachment protein)
Antiribonucleoprotein (RNP)
JO-1
SS-A (Ro), SS-B (La)
Ku

diseases such as trypanosomiasis (Chagas' disease) and leishmaniasis.[42] Reactivity seems to be to the galactosyl side chains on laminin.[43] It will be interesting to see if laminin's co-stimulatory action, probably via very late activation T-cell receptors (B_1 integrins), is also mediated by carbohydrate side chains.

The endothelial cell (EC) membrane could be the stimulus for T-cell hyperreactivity in SSc.[44] Antibodies to EC have been demonstrated in some SSc patients; moreover, SSc lymphocytes show increased adherence to human umbilical vein EC;[43] and, as already discussed, T-cell granzyme one, present in SSc sera, is cytotoxic to human EC, and antisera specific for human granzyme one abrogate the EC cytotoxicity of SSc sera.

Recent results have expanded the possibilities for T-cell–EC cooperation; a membrane-dependent component of EC induced healthy T cells to produce IL-2.[46] Because IL-2 may play a role in driving the T-cell contribution to fibrosis, a role for EC membrane components in normal T-cell IL-2 production could be relevant to SSc. In this system, using human peripheral blood mononuclear cells prestimulated by phorbol esters, human EC and formaldehyde-fixed EC exerted a co-stimulatory effect on IL-2 production not noted by EC-conditioned medium or relevant EC cytokines, including IL-1, IL-6, TNF, or gamma-interferon (IFN-γ). This co-stimulation seems to engage CD2 on the T-cell and lymphocyte function-related antigen (LFA-3) on the EC for full effect. Reagents blocking LFA-1 have a more modest blocking effect. The relevance of these findings to SSc may be that EC injury could precede IL-2–dependent T-cell hyperactivity and be a major stimulus to continued T-cell effects.[46] This raises the possibility that an external stimulus, such as bleomycin or L-trytophan, first disrupts EC, which sets off the T-cell responses, which include autoimmune (via CD3) and co-stimulatory effects of type IV collagen, fibronectin, and laminin. These findings raise a number of interesting experimental possibilities for the study of SSc and for our general understanding of T-cell–EC interactions.

We should not slight the monocyte in these considerations. It shares the same cellular lineage as EC, and along with dendritic cells (including subcutaneous papillary perivascular dendritic cells and epidermal Langerhans dendritic cells) and B cells, monocytes are major participants in antigen presentation and in cytokine activation and release. Interestingly, monocytes can also be stimulated by IL-2 to secrete active TGF-β. Monocyte activation can be demonstrated in SSc, but where this fits in cell activation leading to fibrosis is unclear.

The possibilities for T-cell, monocyte, EC, and fibroblast interactions are numerous. Cell–cell and cell–matrix interactions are being defined on a regular basis with integrins, adressins, adherins and selectins appearing in profusion. In addition, both membrane and soluble cytokines [including interleukins, interferons, lymphokines, monokines, and fibrokines (fibrogenic cytokines)] can change the microenvironment of microvascular and interstitial tissue in minutes. Brief cytokine exposure (e.g., 8 hours, TGF-β, 10 pM) induces persistent cellular activation, which continues for days after the ligand is removed and persists through several cell divisions to affect the gene expression of several generations of progeny. Perhaps this is because many cytokines (IL-1, TGF-β) induce the expression of their own mRNAs (autocrine transcriptional up-regulation), which perpetuate the biologic phenotype. Many of these stimuli also up-regulate the expression of their own receptors, rendering the cell exquisitely sensitive to future cytokine exposure. Such up-regulation may be a feature of cytokine cross talk, by which one cytokine up-regulates another (e.g., TGF-β stimulates PDGF-AA–ligand expression and PDGF-α–receptor activity). Thus, the signal transduction mechanisms of the original ligand–receptor interaction sets in motion a cascade of phosphorylation, G-protein–dependent, or ion-flux–dependent mechanisms, which continue to activate the nuclear and/or cytoplasmic apparatus essential for cellular activation. Whatever the precise mechanisms involved, all of these possibilities are immediately approachable experimentally, and each could lead to a novel form of therapeutic intervention in the fibrotic cycle of SSc and related fibrotic disorders.[47]

REFERENCES

1. LeRoy E.C., Smith, E.A., Kahaleh, M.B. et al.: A strategy for determining the pathogenesis of systemic sclerosis: Is transforming growth factor β the answer? Arthritis Rheum., *32*:817–825, 1989.
2. Thrall, R.S., McCormick, J.R., Jack, R.M. et al.: Bleomycin-induced pulmonary fibrosis in the rat. Am. J. Pathol., *95*:117–130, 1979.
3. Haustein, U.F., Herrmann, K., and Bohme, H.J.: Pathogenesis of progressive systemic sclerosis. Int. J. Dermatol., *25*:258–293, 1986.
4. Briggs, D., Black, C., and Welsh, K.: Genetic factors in scleroderma. Rheum. Dis. Clin. North Am., *16*:31–51, 1990.
5. Varga, J., and Jimenez, S.A.: Cutaneous sclerosis localized to one limb after immobilization in a patient with CREST syndrome. J. Rheum., *14*:637–638, 1987.
6. Kahaleh, M.B.: Vascular disease in scleroderma. Endothelial T lymphocyte-fibroblast interactions. Rheum. Dis. Clin. North Am., *16*:53–73, 1990.
7. Fleischmajer, R., Perlish, J.S., and Reeves, J.R.T.: Cellular infiltrates in scleroderma skin. Arthritis Rheum., *20*:975–984, 1977.
8. LeRoy, E.C.: Connective tissue synthesis by scleroderma skin fibroblasts in cell culture. J. Exp. Med., *135*:1351–1362, 1972.
9. LeRoy, E.C.: Increased collagen synthesis by scleroderma skin fibroblasts *in vitro*. J. Clin. Invest., *54*:880–889, 1974.
10. Chojkier, M., Houglum, K., Solis-Herruzo, J., and Brenner, D.A.: Stimulation of collagen gene expression by ascorbic acid in cultured human fibroblasts. A role for lipid peroxidation? J. Biol. Chem., *264*:16957–16962, 1989.
11. Wiestner, M., Krieg, T., and Horlein, D. et al.: Inhibiting effect of procollagen peptides on collagen biosynthesis in fibroblast cultures. J. Biol. Chem., *254*:7016–7023, 1979.
12. Uitto, J., Tan, E., and Ryhanen, L.: Inhibition of collagen accumulation in fibrotic processes: Review of pharmacologic agents and new approaches with amino acids and their analogues. J. Invest. Dermatol., *79*:113S–120S, 1982.

13. Schmidt, A., Rossi, P., and de Crombrugghe, B.: Transcriptional control of the mouse α_2(I) collagen gene: Functional deletion analysis of the promoter and evidence for cell-specific expression. Mol. Cell. Biol., *6*:347–354, 1986.
14. Hatanochi, A., Golumbek, P., and de Crombrugghe, B.: A CCAAT DNA binding factor consisting of two different components that are both required for DNA binding. J. Biol. Chem., *263*:5940–5947, 1988.
15. Ramirez, F., and Di Liberto, M.: Complex and diversified regulatory programs control the expression of vertebrate collagen genes. FASEB J., *4*:1616–1623, 1990.
16. Rossi, P., and de Crombrugghe, B.: Identification of a cell-specific transcriptional enhancer in the first intron of the mouse α_2 (type I) collagen gene. Proc. Natl. Acad. Sci. U.S.A., *84*:5590–5594, 1987.
17. Raghow, R., and Thompson, J.P.: Molecular mechanisms of collagen gene expression. Mol. Cell. Biochem., *86*:5–18, 1989.
18. Xu, W., LeRoy, E.C., and Smith, E.A.: Fibronectin release by systemic sclerosis and normal dermal fibroblasts in response to TGF-β. J. Rheumatol., *18*:241–246, 1991.
19. Shimizu, Y., Van Seventer, G.A., Horgan, K.J., and Shaw, S.: Costimulation of proliferative responses of resting CD4[4] T cells by the interaction of VLA-4 and VLA-5 with fibronectin or VLA-6 with laminin. J. Immunol., *145*:59–67, 1990.
20. Carrel, A., and Ebeling, A.H.: Age and multiplication of fibroblasts. J. Exp. Med., *34*:599, 1921.
21. Botstein, G.R., Sherer, G.K., and LeRoy, E.C.: Fibroblast selection in scleroderma. Arthritis Rheum., *25*:189–195, 1982.
22. Korn, J.H., and Downie, E.: Clonal interactions in fibroblast proliferation: Recognition of self vs non-self. J. Cell. Physiol., *141*:437–440, 1989.
23. Ishikawa, O., LeRoy, E.C., and Trojanowska, M.: Mitogenic effects of transforming growth factor β_1 on human fibroblasts involves the induction of platelet-derived growth factor α receptors. J. Cell. Physiol., *145*:181–186, 1990.
24. LeRoy, E.C., Mercurio, S., and Sherer, G.K.: Replication and phenotypic expression of control and scleroderma human fibroblasts: Responses to growth factors. Proc. Natl. Acad. Sci. U.S.A., *79*:1286–1290, 1982.
25. Trojanowska, M., Wu, L., and LeRoy, E.C.: Elevated expression of c-myc proto-oncogene in scleroderma fibroblasts. Oncogene, *3*:477–481, 1988.
26. Needleman, B.W.: Increased expression of intracellular adhesion molecule 1 on the fibroblasts of scleroderma patients. Arthritis Rheum., *33*:1847–1851, 1990.
27. Gay, S., Jones, R.E., Huang, G.-Q., and Gay, R.E.: Immunohistologic demonstration of platelet-derived growth factor (PDGF) and sis-oncogene expression in scleroderma. J. Invest. Dermatol., *92*:301–303, 1989.
28. Kulozik, M., Hogg, A., Lankat-Buttgereit, B., and Krieg, T.: Colocalization of transforming growth factor β_2 with α_1(I) procollagen mRNA in tissue sections of patients with systemic sclerosis. J. Clin. Invest., *86*:917–922, 1990.
29. Gruschwitz, M., Muller, P.U., Sepp, N. et al.: Transcription and expression of transforming growth factor type beta in the skin of progressive systemic sclerosis: A mediator of fibrosis? J. Invest. Dermatol., *94*:197–203, 1990.
30. Norton, W.L.: Comparison of microangiopathy of systemic lupus erythematosus, dermatomyositis, scleroderma, and diabetes mellitus. Lab. Invest., *22*:301–308, 1970.
31. Kahaleh, M.B., Sherer, G.K., and LeRoy, E.C.: Endothelial injury in scleroderma. J. Exp. Med., *149*:1326–1335, 1979.
32. Kahaleh, M.B., and LeRoy, E.C.: Endothelial injury in scleroderma. A protease mechanism. J. Lab. Clin. Med., *101*:553–560, 1983.
33. Kahaleh, M.B., Yin, T.: The molecular mechanism of endothelial cell (EC) injury in scleroderma (SSc): Identification of granzyme 1 (a product of cytolytic T cell) in SSc sera. (Abstract.) Arthritis Rheum., *33*(Suppl.):67, 1990.
34. Mackel, A.M., DeLustro, F., Harper, F.E., and LeRoy, E.C.: Antibodies to collagen in scleroderma. Arthritis Rheum., *25*:522–531, 1982.
35. Huffstutter, J.E., DeLustro, F.A., and LeRoy, E.C.: Cellular immunity to collagen and laminin in scleroderma. Arthritis Rheum., *28*:775–780, 1985.
36. Kahaleh, M.B., Osborn, I., and LeRoy, E.C.: Increased factor VIII/von Willebrand factor antigen and von Willebrand factor activity in scleroderma and Raynaud's phenomenon. Ann. Intern. Med., *94*:482–484, 1981.
37. Helfrich, D.J., Banner, B., Steen, V.D., and Medsger, T.A., Jr.: Normotensive renal failure in systemic sclerosis. Arthritis Rheum., *32*:1128–1134, 1989.
38. Marks, R.M., Czerniecki, M., Andrews, B.S., and Penny, R.: The effects of scleroderma serum on human microvascular endothelial cells. Arthritis Rheum., *31*:1524–1534, 1988.
39. Silver, R.M., and LeRoy, E.C.: Systemic sclerosis (scleroderma). *In* Immunological Disease. 4th Ed. Edited by M. Samter. Boston, Little, Brown. 1988, pp. 1459–1500.
40. Umehara, H., Kumagai, S., Ishida, H. et al.: Enhanced production of interleukin-2 in patients with progressive systemic sclerosis. Hyperactivity of CD4-positive T cells? Arthritis Rheum., *31*:401–407, 1988.
41. Kahaleh, M.B., and LeRoy, E.C.: Interleukin-2 in scleroderma: Correlation of serum level with extent of skin involvement and disease duration. Ann. Intern. Med., *110*:446–450, 1989.
42. Towbin, H., Rosenfelder, G., Wieslander, J. et al.: Circulating antibodies to mouse laminin in Chaqas disease. American cutaneous leishmaniasis, and normal individuals recognize terminal galactosyl (alpha 1-3-galactose epitopes. J. Exp. Med., *166*:419–432, 1987.
43. Gabrielli, A., Leoni, P., Danieli, G. et al.: Antibodies against galactosyl (α_{1-3}) galactose in connective tissue diseases. Arthritis Rheum., *34*:375–376, 1991.
44. Antibodies to endothelial cells. (Editorial.) Lancet, *337*:649–650, 1991.
45. Kahaleh, M.B., and Yin, T.: Enhanced lymphocyte-endothelial cell (EC) interaction in scleroderma (SSc). (Abstract.) Arthritis Rheum., *33*(Suppl.):A129, 1990.
46. Hughes, C.C.W., Savage, C.O.S., and Pober, J.S.: The endothelial cell as a regulator of T-cell function. Immunol. Rev., *117*:85–102, 1990.
47. Kovacs, E.J.: Fibrogenic cytokines: The role of immune mediators in the development of scar tissue. Immunol. Today, *12*:17–23, 1991.

75

Vasculitis

ANTHONY S. FAUCI
RANDI Y. LEAVITT

Vasculitis is a clinicopathologic process characterized by inflammation and damage to blood vessels. This process is usually associated with compromise of the vessel lumen and ischemic changes in the tissues supplied by the involved vessels.[1,2] Vasculitis might be the only manifestation of a disease. Alternatively, vasculitis can be a secondary component of another primary disease. For example, Wegener's granulomatosis and classic polyarteritis nodosa are *primary* vasculitic syndromes, whereas the vasculitides associated with underlying connective tissue diseases such as rheumatoid arthritis (RA) or systemic lupus erythematosus (SLE) are classified as *secondary* vasculitic syndromes.[1–3]

PATHOGENESIS

Most of the vasculitic syndromes are mediated, at least in part, by immunopathogenic mechanisms.[1,2] Foremost among these mechanisms is the immune complex model whereby antigen-antibody complexes either circulate and deposit in the vessel walls or are formed in situ at the area of tissue damage.[4,5] Although *circulating immune complexes* can be demonstrated in many of the vasculitic syndromes,[1,2,5] and evidence suggests deposition of complexes in various tissues, the causal role of these mechanisms in the inflammatory response of involved vessels remains unclear. In a few instances a causative antigen has been demonstrated in putative immune-complex–mediated disease. Hepatitis B antigen–associated systemic vasculitis is the prototype of immune-complex–mediated vasculitis in which an exogenous antigen is implicated.[6] In addition to the classic immune-complex–mediated vasculitis, other types of immunopathogenic mechanisms can damage vascular tissue. One of these is cell-mediated immune reactivity, a poorly documented form of damage to vascular tissue. Nonetheless, the histopathologic features of certain types of vasculitis suggest at least a component of *cell-mediated immune injury*. Granulomatous vasculitis might indeed represent a component of classic cell-mediated immune mechanisms in certain vasculitic syndromes,[1,2] and immune complexes themselves could trigger granulomatous responses.[7] Therefore, the presence of granulomas in or near vessels can indicate immune-complex mechanisms, cell-mediated immune responses, or both. Other mechanisms, such as tissue injury mediated directly by antibodies with specificity against the vessel itself or by cytotoxic effector cells in *antibody-dependent cellular cytotoxicity*, can play a role in vascular damage, but little evidence supports their contribution to the pathogenesis of any of the recognized vasculitic syndromes, with the exception of Kawasaki disease. The production of cytotoxic antibodies directed against mediator-induced endothelial cell antigens might play a role in the vascular damage seen in this condition.[8,9] It has been proposed that cytokine-mediated endothelial cell activation may play a role in the pathogenesis of other vasculitic syndromes.[10] Finally, it has been suggested that anti-neutrophil cytoplasmic antibodies (ANCAs) which are associated with Wegener's granulomatosis (see below) and have been shown to induce neutrophil activation are directly responsible for the vascular injury associated with the disorder.[11,12]

CLASSIFICATION

The clinical spectrum of the vasculitides is characterized by heterogeneity as well as overlap among the various syndromes. Considerable confusion and difficulty have hindered the categorization of these diseases. Any categorization scheme is empiric, but we have found an approach that is helpful in prognosis and in the design of therapeutic regimens.[1,2,13] This approach emphasizes the conceptual differences between disease that is predominantly systemic, almost invariably causing irreversible organ system dysfunction and even death if untreated, and those syndromes with primarily cutaneous manifestations, rarely resulting in irreversible dysfunction of vital organs. Some syndromes overlap these categories. A classification scheme of the clinical spectrum of vasculitis is shown in Table 75–1.

The first group, systemic necrotizing vasculitis, has been the most difficult to categorize. The original *classic polyarteritis nodosa* in contained within this group.[14] Lung involvement, granulomas, eosinophilia, and a history of allergy are not characteristic of this syndrome. Another syndrome, however, called *allergic angiitis and granulomatosis* or *Churg-Strauss syndrome,*[15] resembles classic polyarteritis nodosa in many respects, except lung involvement is the rule, and eosinophilia, granulomas, and allergy are common. The histopathologic features of these two syndromes differ in that the vasculitic lesions of classic polyarteritis nodosa are confined to the small and medium-sized muscular arteries, whereas those of classic allergic angiitis and granulomatosis involve blood vessels of various types and sizes, including small and medium-sized muscular arteries as well as veins and venules.[1,2]

A form of systemic necrotizing vasculitis that is probably more common than classic polyarteritis nodosa or allergic angiitis and granulomatosis has been recognized. This syndrome can have features that overlap several distinct vasculitic syndromes. We call this group the *polyangiitis overlap syndrome* (Table 75–2).[1,2,13,16] This group of systemic necrotizing vasculitides has a common denominator of involvement of multiple organ systems with the overriding tendency for irreversible organ-system dysfunction. In general, the prognosis for patients with this group of disorders is poor without appropriate and aggressive therapy.

TABLE 75–1. CLASSIFICATION OF THE VASCULITIS SYNDROMES

Systemic necrotizing vasculitis
- Classic polyarteritis nodosa
- Allergic angiitis and granulomatosis of Churg-Strauss
- Polyangiitis overlap syndrome

Hypersensitivity vasculitis
- Exogenous stimuli proved or suspected
  - Henoch-Schönlein purpura
  - Serum sickness and serum sickness-like reactions
  - Other drug-related vasculitides
  - Vasculitis associated with infectious diseases
- Endogenous antigens likely involved; vasculitis associated with
  - Neoplasms
  - Systemic connective tissue diseases
  - Other underlying diseases
  - Congenital deficiencies of the complement system

Wegener's granulomatosis

Giant cell arteritis
- Temporal arteritis
- Takayasu's arteritis

Other vasculitis syndromes
- Mucocutaneous lymph node syndrome (Kawasaki's disease)
- Isolated central nervous system vasculitis
- Thromboangiitis obliterans (Buerger's disease)
- Miscellaneous vasculitides

From Fauci, A.S.[13].

TABLE 75–2. TYPICAL CLINICOPATHOLOGIC FEATURES OF DISTINCT VASCULITIS SYNDROMES

VASCULITIC SYNDROME	VESSELS INVOLVED	PATHOLOGY	DISTINCTIVE FEATURES
Polyarteritis nodosa	Small and medium-sized arteries	Necrotizing vasculitis	Angiogram showing aneurysms in renal, hepatic, and visceral vasculature
Allergic angiitis and granulomatosis (Churg-Strauss syndrome)	Small and medium-sized arteries	Granulomatous vasculitis	Allergic history, eosinophilia, pulmonary involvement
Hypersensitivity vasculitis	Arterioles, capillaries, venules, rarely small muscular arteries	Leukocytoclastic vasculitis	Skin most commonly involved, usually single type of vessel involved
Henoch-Schönlein purpura	Venules, capillaries, arterioles	Leukocytoclastic vasculitis	Usually skin, gastrointestinal, renal involvement, IgA in immune complexes
Takayasu's arteritis	Medium and large arteries	Giant cell arteritis	Predilection for aortic arch
Temporal arteritis	Medium and large arteries	Giant cell arteritis	Predilection for branches of carotid
Wegener's granulomatosis	Small arteries and veins, medium arteries	Necrotizing granulomatous vasculitis	Involves upper and lower respiratory tracts, glomerulonephritis commonly seen, varying degrees of small vessel vasculitis

From Leavitt, R.Y., and Fauci, A.S.[16]

In contrast, the second broad category consists of predominantly cutaneous vasculitides and is called *hypersensitivity* vasculitis. Although these disorders can also be systemic, they most frequently remain cutaneous and do not consistently pose a threat of irreversible dysfunction of vital organs.[17–19] If the disease does remain confined to the skin and does not become systemic, aggressive therapy with high doses of corticosteroids or long-term administration of cytotoxic agents is indicated only in unusual circumstances.

The broad category of "hypersensitivity vasculitis" has been applied to a heterogeneous group of disorders thought to represent a hypersensitivity reaction to an identifiable antigenic stimulus such as drug or as infectious agent—hence the term "hypersensitivity."[2,5,13,18] The term is often confusing because many, if not most, of the vasculitic syndromes represent hypersensitivity reactions of one form or another. As discussed later, although the proved or suspected antigenic stimuli associated with this group are heterogeneous, these disorders generally share the characteristic involvement of small vessels and a predominant, often exclusive, involvement of the vessels of the skin. Confusion has resulted from the inclusion of this group with the more serious systemic conditions. This confusion is probably related to the variable degrees of organ system involvement other than cutaneous that can occur in the hypersensitivity vasculitides. Such involvement, however, is usually much less severe than in the systemic vasculitis of classic polyarteritis nodosa or Wegener's granulomatosis. The skin is exclusively involved, or if other organ systems are involved, the cutaneous disease dominates the clinical picture.[2,5,13,17–19] Finally, a syndrome indistinguishable from hypersensitivity vasculitis can appear as a secondary component of another underlying disease, such as a systemic connective tissue disease or neoplasm, and can thus lead to additional confusion.

Most of the remainder of the vasculitic syndromes such as Wegener's granulomatosis, temporal arteritis, or Takayasu's arteritis have distinctive enough clinical and pathologic features to permit them to be readily grouped into separate categories (Tables 75–1 and 75–2). Several of these distinctive syndromes are clearly systemic, but are not listed in the systemic necrotizing vasculitis group because they warrant separate classification.

SYSTEMIC NECROTIZING VASCULITIS (POLYARTERITIS NODOSA GROUP)

The systemic necrotizing vasculitis group includes (1) classic polyarteritis nodosa, (2) allergic angiitis and granulomatosis, and (3) the polyangiitis overlap syndrome.

CLASSIC POLYARTERITIS NODOSA

The first complete description of a vasculitic syndrome was made in 1866 by Kussmaul and Maier in an elegant clinicopathologic case report.[14] Classic peri-arteritis nodosa, as it was originally described[14] and further studied,[17,20] is a necrotizing vasculitis of small and medium-sized muscular arteries. The lesions are segmental, with a predilection for bifurcations of arteries with distal spread involving arterioles and, in some cases, circumferentially involving adjacent veins. This disorder is not primarily a venulitis. Histopathologically, in the acute states, polymorphonuclear leukocytes infiltrate all layers of the vessel wall and perivascular areas (Fig. 75–1). Subsequently, mononuclear cell infiltration occurs as the lesions become subacute and chronic. Intimal proliferation, vessel wall degeneration with fibrinoid necrosis, thrombosis, ischemia, and infarction are seen in

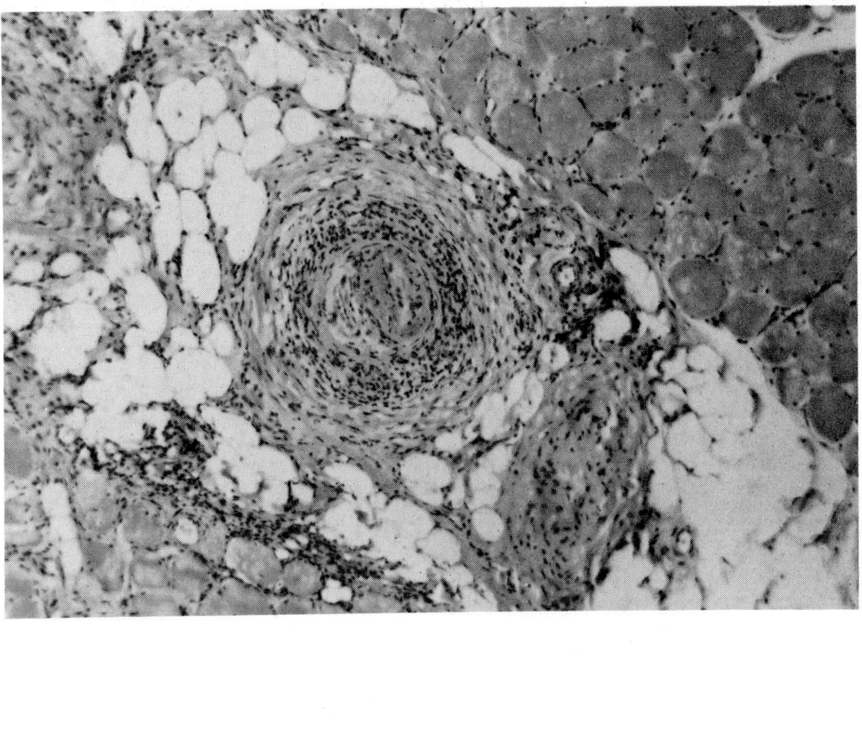

FIGURE 75–1. Muscle biopsy in a 36-year-old patient with classic polyarteritis nodosa. A small muscular artery is involved, with fibrinoid necrosis and inflammatory cell infiltrate. (Hematoxylin and eosin stain; magnification ×130.)

varying degrees. Generally, vascular lesions in various stages of development are found simultaneously. This finding might reflect the continuous deposition of immune complexes, such as one might expect in the vasculitis associated with persistent hepatitis B antigenemia.[6] Multiple organ systems are involved, and the clinicopathologic findings are consistent with the degree and location of vessel involvement and the resulting ischemic changes.[1,2]

Clinical Manifestations

The nature of the presenting problems may be nonspecific. *Vague symptoms* such as weakness, malaise, abdominal pain, extremity pain, headache, fever, and myalgias are frequent.[1,2] Less commonly, patients have signs and symptoms of neurologic and joint involvement. The nonspecific nature of the presentation and the uncommon occurrence of classic polyarteritis nodosa can contribute to the difficulty in establishing the diagnosis. The signs or symptoms and actual involvement might not correlate with those of documented vasculitis.

The clinical profile and manifestations in patients with classic polyarteritis nodosa are outlined in Table 75–3. These manifestations, together with the findings at autopsy summarized from several large series (Table 75–4), provide a striking witness to the scope and severity of the organ system involvement in this disease.

Variable degrees of renal involvement are seen in most patients, and this complication is a major cause of death. The renal disease can be primarily vascular with secondary ischemic changes in the glomeruli, it can be a primary glomerulitis, or it can be a combination of both. Hypertension, usually associated with elevated renin levels, can compound the severity of the renal disease or might itself be the predominant cause of renal dysfunction in the form of nephrosclerosis.[2,21,22] It was once thought that the hypertension of polyarteritis nodosa was almost exclusively associated with the healing stages of the renal polyarteritis nodosa or glomerulonephritis,[20] but it is now clear that hypertension can occur as an independent early finding before clinically apparent functional renal disease. Hypertension can dominate the clinical picture and can be directly responsible for certain of the associated cerebrovascular, cardiovascular, or renal manifestations.

Besides hypertensive cardiovascular disease, primary involvement of the coronary arteries is common, and cardiac involvement is a major cause of death.[23] Areas of myocardial infarction are frequently found at autopsy in the absence of a suggestive clear-cut history.[24] Polyarteritis nodosa in children is associated with a high incidence of coronary artery involvement,[21,25] but most of the cases in the United States formerly reported as polyarteritis nodosa of children, with its characteristic and unusual selective involvement of the coronary arteries, were in fact the arteritis of unrecognized mucocutaneous lymph node syndrome (Kawasaki disease).[26]

Gastrointestinal involvement is seen in over 50% of

TABLE 75–3. CLINICAL PROFILE AND MANIFESTATIONS IN PATIENTS WITH CLASSIC POLYARTERITIS NODOSA

CLINICAL PARAMETER	VALUE
General considerations	
Age (mean)	45 years
Sex ratio (male to female)	2.5 to 1
	Percentage (%)
Fever	71
Weight loss	54
Organ involvement	
Kidney	70
Musculoskeletal system	64
Arthritis or arthralgia	53
Myalgias	31
Circulatory system (hypertension)	54
Peripheral nerves	51
Gastrointestinal tract	44
Abdominal pain	43
Nausea or vomiting	40
Cholecystitis	17
Bleeding	6
Bowel perforation	5
Bowel infarction	1.4
Skin	43
Rash or purpura	30
Livedo reticularis	4
Heart	36
Congestive failure	12
Myocardial infarction	6
Pericarditis	4
Central nervous system	23
Cerebral vascular accident	11
Altered mental status	10
Seizure	4

From Cupps, T.R., and Fauci, A.S.[2]

TABLE 75–4. ORGAN INVOLVEMENT AT AUTOPSY IN CLASSIC POLYARTERITIS NODOSA

ORGAN SYSTEM	PERCENTAGE (%)
Kidney	85
Heart	76
Liver	62
Gastrointestinal tract	51
Jejunum	37
Ileum	27
Mesentery	24
Colon	20
Rectosigmoid	10
Duodenum	10
Gallbladder	10
Appendix	7
Muscle	39
Pancreas	35
Testes	33
Peripheral nerves	32
Central nervous system	27
Skin	20

From Cupps, T.R., and Fauci, A.S.[2]

patients and usually relates to involvement of the visceral arteries.[2] Symptoms and signs include nausea, vomiting, diarrhea, ileus, abdominal pain, ulceration with bleeding, infarction, or perforation of intra-abdominal organs. Depending on the severity of involvement, manifestations range from abdominal angina or steatorrhea, associated with partial obstruction of the superior mesenteric artery or its branches, to massive bowel infarction, resulting from acute involvement of the superior mesenteric artery.[21] Bowel perforation carries a high mortality rate. Significant abdominal involvement is often masked partially or completely in patients receiving daily corticosteroids, and an ischemic segment of bowel can go undetected until actual perforation has occurred.

Liver disease varies in classic polyarteritis nodosa. When hepatitis B antigenemia accounts for the vasculitis, hepatic involvement can relate to the underlying hepatitis and ranges from subclinical diseases to chronic active hepatitis.[6] Liver disease related directly to the vasculitis can lead to massive hepatic infarction.[27]

Neurologic manifestations are common. Mononeuritis multiplex resulting from vasculitis of the vasa nervorum is the most frequent finding. In a review of the neurologic manifestations of systemic necrotizing vasculitis (Table 75–1) including polyarteritis nodosa, 80% of patients had some form of nervous system disease.[28] The periperal nervous system was involved in 60% of this subset. Four patterns of neuropathy were seen: mononeuritis multiplex, extensive mononeuritis, cutaneous neuropathy, and polyneuropathy. The central nervous system was involved in the remaining 40%, and these patients predominantly had diffuse and focal disturbance of cerebral, cerebellar, and brain stem function.

Cutaneous Involvement. The question of the precise type of cutaneous involvement in classic polyarteritis nodosa is controversial because many cases of small-vessel hypersensitivity vasculitis have been included in reports of groups of patients said to have polyarteritis nodosa. Furthermore, skin involvement in the polyangiitis overlap syndrome can have features of both classic polyarteritis nodosa and hypersensitivity venulitis.[2,13,16] Skin involvement in classic polyarteritis occurs in approximately 20 to 30% of patients and is usually confined to the small muscular arteries of the subcutaneous tissues.[29] The lesions are generally manifested as painful erythematosus subcutaneous nodules, which can appear in crops and can range from a few millimeters to several centimeters in size. Another characteristic of skin involvement is *livedo reticularis* (Fig. 75–2). *Cutaneous polyarteritis nodosa* is characterized by a necrotizing vasculitis of small arteries of subcutaneous tissue.[30] The disease is a localized process with sparing of visceral arteries, and therefore is not a true systemic vasculitic syndrome. Cutaneous polyarteritis usually runs a chronic course and has a favorable long-term prognosis. Although the histologic lesion resembles that of classic polyarteritis nodosa, this disease is clinically similar to the hypersensitivity vasculitides.

Arthralgias are common in classic polyarteritis nodosa, but frank arthritis is rare. When small and medium-sized muscular arteries in skeletal muscle are involved, the muscles are almost invariably symptomatic (see Fig. 75–1). In addition, testicular or epididymal pain is characteristic, and testicular involvement is seen in approximately 30% of autopsies in classic polyarteritis nodosa (Table 75–4). Thus, when muscular or testicular pain is present, biopsy is likely to be helpful in

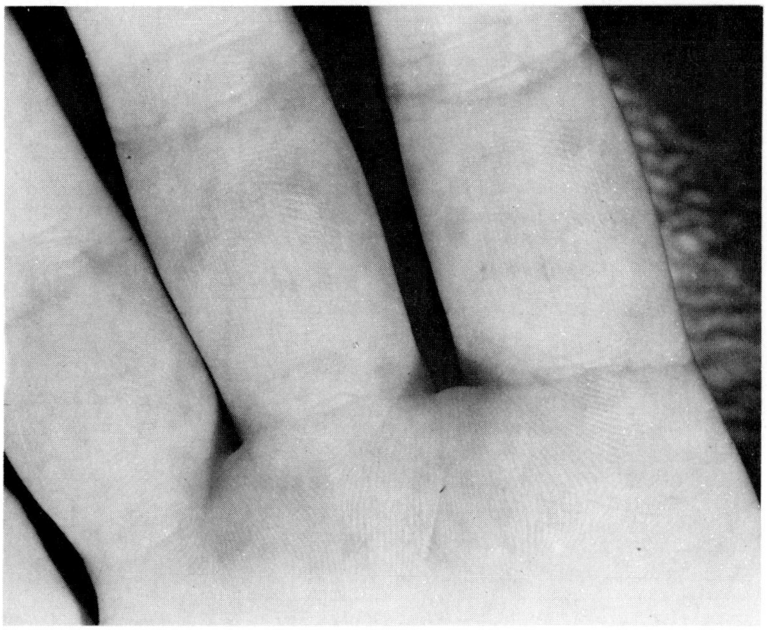

FIGURE 75–2. Livedo reticularis of the volar aspect of the proximal phalanges and distal palm in a patient with systemic lupus erythematosus. The lesions are nonpalpable and may be seen in a variety of vasculitic syndromes.

making the diagnosis, whereas blind biopsies of asymptomatic organs have a low diagnostic yield.

Diagnosis

No diagnostic laboratory findings are indicative of classic polyarteritis nodosa, and the many abnormalities are outlined in Table 75–5. The finding of hepatitis B antigenemia has been reported in up to 30% of patients with systemic vasculitis of the polyarteritis nodosa type,[6,31–33] but this finding in itself does not establish the diagnosis, which depends on characteristic clinical and pathologic manifestations.[34]

The mainstay of the diagnosis of classic polyarteritis nodosa is the *histopathologic demonstration of necrotizing vasculitis of small and medium-sized arteries in patients with compatible clinical manifestations.* It is preferable to perform a biopsy on accessible organs such as the skin, muscle, or testis, but these structures are not invariably involved, and "blind" biopsy has only limited value.

A characteristic feature of the polyarteritis nodosa type of necrotizing vasculitis is the finding of aneurysmal dilatations up to 1 cm in size in medium-sized arteries seen by angiogram in the renal, hepatic, and visceral vasculature (Fig. 75–3). It was formerly believed that this finding was virtually pathognomic of classic polyarteritis nodosa,[35,36] although multiple aneurysms of this type are seen in overlap syndromes in which vessels of various sizes are involved,[16,37] as well as in other disorders such as SLE[38] and fibromuscular dysplasia.[39] Demonstration of involved vessels on a visceral angiogram, however, is helpful in establishing the presence of systemic vascular disease and is valuable in clinical situations in which no involved organ is easily accessible for biopsy. *If a patient has signs and symptoms suggestive of polyarteritis nodosa without readily accessible tissue for biopsy, the diagnosis can be made on the basis of a positive visceral angiogram.*

TABLE 75–5. LABORATORY ABNORMALITIES IN PATIENTS WITH CLASSIC POLYARTERITIS NODOSA

LABORATORY ABNORMALITY	PERCENTAGE (%)
Erythrocyte sedimentation rate >10 mm/hr	94
Leukocytosis (WBC >10,000/mm³)	74
Anemia (hematocrit <35%)	66
Thrombocytosis (>400,000/mm³)	53
Renal function abnormality	70
Proteinuria	64
Hematuria	45
Casts	34
Complement abnormality	
Depressed CH_{50}	21
Depressed C3	70
Depressed C4	30
Rheumatoid factor ≥1:160	40
Immune complexes present	62.5
Cryoglobulins present	25

From Cupps, T.R., and Fauci, A.S.[2]

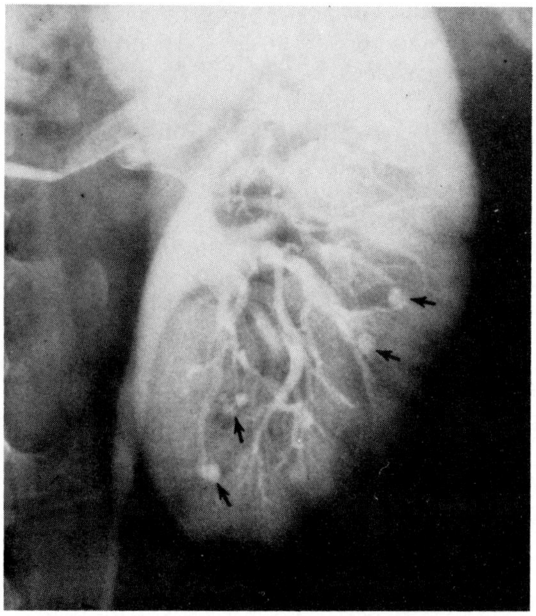

FIGURE 75–3. Renal angiogram in a patient with classic polyarteritis nodosa. Note the multiple intraparenchymal aneurysms (arrows).

Prognosis

The prognosis of untreated classic polyarteritis nodosa is poor. Although some cases have resolved spontaneously, the usual course of the disease is a relentless progression with intermittent acute flares.[1,2,33] The grave prognosis is reflected in the 5-year-survival rate of 13% reported for untreated patients improved to 48% with corticosteroid treatment, and to 90% in patients treated with combined cyclophosphamide and corticosteroids.[32,33,40] Survival rates are lower in patients with hypertension or renal disease initially. Death usually results from renal failure or from cardiovascular or gastrointestinal involvement. Persistent and uncontrolled hypertension often contributes to the late morbidity and mortality of this disease by compounding the renal disease and by leading to late cardiovascular and cerebrovascular disorders. Treatment is considered later in this chapter. However, patients with polyarteritis nodosa associated with hepatitis B virus antigenemia have been successfully treated with the antiviral agent vidarabine in combination with plasma exchange with and without corticosteroids.[41,42]

ALLERGIC ANGIITIS AND GRANULOMATOSIS (CHURG-STRAUSS SYNDROME)

The combination of allergic angiitis and granulomatosis is a disease characterized by granulomatous vasculitis of multiple organ systems.[15,43,44] Although the vascular lesions can be identical to those of classic polyarteritis nodosa, this disease is unique for the following reasons: (1) frequency of involvement of *pulmonary vessels,* (2) vasculitis of blood vessels of various types and sizes such as small and medium-sized muscular arteries, veins, arterioles, and venules, (3) intravascular and extravascular *granuloma* formation, (4) *eosinophilic tissue infiltrates*, and (5) association with severe *asthma* and *peripheral eosinophilia*. This disease can be thought of as a polyarteritis nodosa–like syndrome with strong allergic components and with pulmonary involvement as an essential element of the disease instead of a rarity.[1,43]

The clinical features of allergic angiitis and granulomatosis are listed in Table 75–6. Laboratory findings are similar to those in classic polyarteritis nodosa. An elevated erythrocyte sedimentation rate and leukocytosis are found in the majority of patients. An elevated total eosinophil count (greater than 1000/mm^3) is noted at some point in approximately 85% of patients. This peripheral eosinophilia is not seen in classic polyarteritis nodosa, but can be seen in the overlap syndromes described later. Elevated serum IgE levels have also been described, and circulating immune complexes containing IgE have been identified in some patients.[45] Unlike classic polyarteritis nodosa, no association exists with hepatitis B antigenemia.

The degree of severity of allergic angiitis and granulomatosis varies from patients to patient, and so prognosis is also variable. The overall prognosis remains poor, however, and in untreated patients, it is similar to that of classic polyarteritis nodosa. Treatment is discussed below.

TABLE 75–6. CLINICAL PROFILE AND MANIFESTATIONS IN ALLERGIC ANGIITIS AND GRANULOMATOSIS

CLINICAL PARAMETER	VALUE
General considerations	
Age (mean)	44 years
Sex ratio (male to female)	1.3 to 1
Duration (mean) of pulmonary symptoms prior to systemic symptoms	2 years
Fever	Majority of patients
Organ involvement	Percentage (%)
Lungs	96
Infiltrate on chest roentgenogram	93
Wheezing	82
Skin	67
Purpura	37
Nodules	35
Peripheral nerves	63
Circulatory system (hypertension)	54
Gastrointestinal tract	42
Heart	38
Kidney	38
Lower urinary tract	10
Musculoskeletal system	10
Arthritis or arthralgia	21

From Cupps, T.R., and Fauci, A.S.[2]

TABLE 75–7. CHARACTERISTICS OF THE POLYANGIITIS OVERLAP SYNDROME

PATIENT	OVERLAPPING SYNDROMES
1	SNV, not classified
2	PAN and Churg-Strauss
3	PAN and Churg-Strauss
4	TA and PAN
5	PAN and Churg-Strauss
6	Takayasu's arteritis and PAN
7	SNV, not classified
8	PAN and cutaneous vasculitis
9	HSP and PAN
10	Giant cell arteritis and Churg-Strauss or Wegener's granulomatosis
11	PAN and Wegener's granulomatosis
12	PAN and cutaneous vasculitis

SNV = systemic necrotizing vasculitis, PAN = polyarteritis nodosa, TA = temporal arteritis, HSP = Henoch-Schönlein purpura.
Adapted from Leavitt, R.Y., and Fauci, A.S.[16]

POLYANGIITIS OVERLAP SYNDROME

Many systemic necrotizing vasculitides manifest clinicopathologic characteristics that overlap classic polyarteritis nodosa and allergic angiitis and granulomatosis, as well as the hypersensitivity small-vessel group of vasculitides, and it is now clear that overlap can exist among any of the well-defined vasculitic syndromes (Tables 75–2 and 75–7).[16] This subgroup of systemic necrotizing vasculitis has been referred to as the *polyangiitis overlap syndrome*.[1,2,13,16,46] This syndrome has caused the most difficulty in classification and has appeared under different designations and categories. A typical, perplexing case is that of a young person with a multisystem necrotizing vasculitis with renal involvement and mononeuritis multiplex. The patient might or might not have hypertension, and visceral and renal angiograms might or might not demonstrate multiple aneurysms. By most generally accepted criteria, this patient would be diagnosed as having classic polyarteritis nodosa.[14,17] This same patient, however, could also have significant lung involvement, a small-vessel cutaneous venulitis, or history of allergy with or without eosinophilia and granulomas, none of which occur in classic polyarteritis nodosa. Recognition of the overlap syndrome avoids confusion as to appropriate diagnosis and therapy. This subgroup is indeed a "systemic" vasculitis with the same potential for irreversible organ system dysfunction. For this reason, we categorized all three of these subgroups under the major category of *systemic necrotizing vasculitis*.

TREATMENT

Corticosteroids are still the initial treatment of choice for the systemic necrotizing vasculitides, but the addition of a cytotoxic agent, such as cyclophosphamide, to the therapeutic regimen has resulted in striking remissions in a high percentage of patients within this category.[1,32]

Early reports showed an increase in survival rates from 13% in untreated patients to 48% in corticosteroid-treated patients.[40] Unlike in Wegener's granulomatosis, in which corticosteroids alone are inadequate therapy and a cytotoxic drug such as cyclophosphamide is essential for the induction of remission, treatment should be tailored to the degree, severity, and stage of the disease.[3,32] *Most patients require a combination of a cytotoxic agent and corticosteroids for maximal induction of remission,* but some treated with corticosteroids alone have a complete remission. On the other hand a few patients have such fulminant systemic vasculitis that they succumb to a devastating complication such as bowel perforation or infarction of other vital organs before any therapy has a chance to be effective. Patients with less-severe forms of systemic vasculitis in whom irreversible organ system dysfunction does not appear to be imminent may be treated initially with corticosteroids alone. Initial therapy with prednisone is 1 mg/kg per day in divided doses, followed by consolidation in a few weeks to a single daily dose. Depending on the clinical response, the patient should be treated with daily prednisone for approximately 1 to 2 months, with an attempt to convert to alternate-day therapy over the next month. If conversion is accomplished without relapse, an alternate-day regimen is maintained for several months to a year. The dose is then gradually tapered until the drug is discontinued or until a maintenance dose is reached.

If patients do not improve objectively after a month of corticosteroid therapy or if they initially have fulminant disease and deteriorating organ system function, a cytotoxic regimen should be started. We have had excellent results with oral cyclophosphamide at a dose of 2 mg/kg per day. A patient who cannot tolerate oral medication or a patient with bowel vasculitis in whom intestinal absorption is questionable should receive *cyclophosphamide intravenously* at the same dose. An aggressive surgical approach to the complications of ischemic bowel with early exploratory laparotomy, appropriate removal of necrotic bowel segments, and repeated operations for observation of the retained bowel can reduce the mortality rates associated with this most serious complication of systemic vasculitis. *Prednisone should always be given together with cyclophosphamide* during the induction phase of the therapeutic protocol because it usually takes 2 to 3 weeks to achieve an immunosuppressive effect from cyclophosphamide given at these doses. The combined regimen, which we use to treat the severe corticosteroid-resistant systemic vasculitides,[47] was originally developed for the treatment of Wegener's granulomatosis,[48] and is outlined in Table 75–8. *We have induced long-term clinical remission in most patients with systemic necrotizing vasculitis using this therapeutic protocol.*[32]

Although malignant diseases, chiefly leukemia and non-Hodgkin's lymphoma, have been noted in patients with polycythemia vera, Hodgkins' disease, or organ transplants treated with immunosuppressive drugs, only one instance of malignant lymphoma has occurred in over 200 patients treated by our group. This occurred in a patient with smoldering Wegener's granulomatosis treated for several years with cyclophosphamide. The patient developed an undifferentiated lymphoma and died.[49] In addition, bladder carcinoma has been reported to be associated with cyclophosphamide therapy, and seven of our patients (approximately 3%) have developed this complication.[50] Cyclophosphamide therapy is also rarely associated with bladder fibrosis, pulmonary fibrosis, and hypogammaglobulinemia.[46,47,51,52] More common side effects of cyclophosphamide include bone marrow suppression, gonadal dysfunction, and hemorrhagic cystitis (see Chapter 38).[46,47,51,52]

TABLE 75–8. COMBINED CYCLOPHOSPHAMIDE-PREDNISONE THERAPY FOR SEVERE SYSTEMIC VASCULITIS

Cyclophosphamide: Initial dose of 2 mg/kg/day orally; adjust so that white blood cell count remains above 3,000 to 3,500/mm³ (neutrophil count 1,000 to 1,500/mm³); continue therapy with frequent downward adjustments of dosage, to prevent severe neutropenia; continue therapy for a year following induction of complete remission, and then taper dose by 25-mg decrements every 2 months until discontinued.
Prednisone: Initial dose of 1 mg/kg/day in 3 to 4 divided doses for 7 to 10 days; consolidate to single morning dose by 2 to 3 weeks; continue single morning daily dose until patient has had 1 month's total corticosteroid treatment; convert to alternate-day regimen for the second month; maintain alternate-day regimen for the third month, followed by gradual tapering of alternate-day dose for the next 3 to 6 months.

From Fauci, A.S. and Leavitt, R.Y.[47]

Other cytotoxic agents such as azathioprine, chlorambucil, and methotrexate have been used in vasculitic syndromes with variable success,[47] but cyclophosphamide is the most effective agent in the induction of long-term remission. Large, single-bolus doses of corticosteroids or cyclophosphamide, or plasmapheresis,[53,54] have been administered to certain patients with vasculitic syndromes.[47] The efficacy of these regimens is not well established, however. (See Wegener's Granulomatosis, Treatment and Prognosis.)

HYPERSENSITIVITY VASCULITIDES

This heterogeneous group is characterized by inflammation of small vessels such as venules, capillaries, and arterioles.[17–19,29,55] The postcapillary venule is most commonly involved. Although hypersensitivity vasculitis can affect any organ system, cutaneous disease usually predominates, and life-threatening organ system dysfunction is rare.

This type of vasculitis was first described in association with a recognized antigenic stimulus such as a microbe or a drug, accounting for the term "hypersensitivity."[5,18,19] The vasculitic component of serum sickness and similar reactions falls within the category of the hypersensitivity vasculitides.[2] *The term is unfortunate be-*

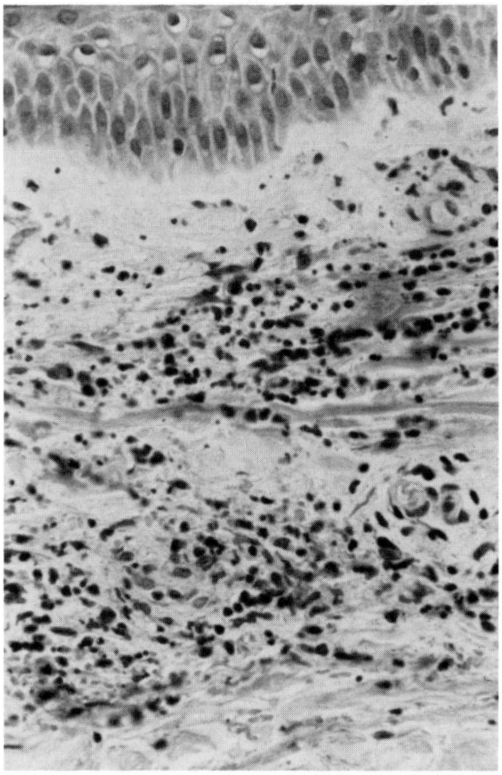

FIGURE 75–4. Skin biopsy in a patient with hypersensitivity vasculitis. Note the involvement of postcapillary venules with leukocytoclasis, as manifested by nuclear debris.

cause no inciting antigen can be identified or even suspected in most cases. Moreover, virtually all the recognized vasculitic syndromes have clinical and pathologic features that suggest underlying hypersensitivity or immunologic phenomena.

Other terms used synonymously with hypersensitivity vasculitis include *allergic vasculitis*[56] and *leukocytoclastic vasculitis*. The most common histopathologic pattern is the characteristic leukocytoclastic vasculitis involving the postcapillary venules (Fig. 75–4).[18,55] Mononuclear, predominantly lymphocytic infiltrates have been described also, however.[57] The typical macroscopic appearance of the lesion is that of *palpable purpura* caused by a combination of endothelial swelling, infiltration by leukocytes, and extravasation of erythrocytes.[1] The lesions range in size from pinpoint to several centimeters and can take the form of *papules, nodules, vesicles, bullae, ulcers,* or *recurrent urticaria.*

Although vasculitic skin lesions are the major features, the syndrome can be accompanied by systemic signs and symptoms such as fever, malaise, myalgia, and anorexia, as with the systemic vasculitides. The disease can consist of a single acute episode lasting only a few weeks, or it can be recurrent or, less commonly, chronic, lasting for months or years. Weight loss and the anemia of chronic disease can be seen in chronic hypersensitivity vasculitis. The skin lesions can be pruritic or painful, with a stinging or burning sensation. Lesions are most common in dependent areas such as the lower extremities in ambulatory patients and over the sacrum in bedridden patients, most likely as a result of hydrostatic pressure. As the lesions resolve or become chronic or recurrent, skin hyperpigmentation can result.

The hypersensitivity vasculitides comprise a number of subgroups (see Table 75–1), within which the extent of extracutaneous involvement varies. The approximate figures for extracutaneous involvement in the whole group include arthritis or arthralgias in 40%, renal involvement in 37%, gastrointestinal involvement in 15%, and peripheral neuropathy in 12% of patients.[2] Although pulmonary involvement is seen in up to 19% of patients with nonspecific patterns of infiltrates or effusion or both on chest radiographs, the significance of these findings is unclear because pulmonary vasculitis has rarely been demonstrated in these patients.[46,55] Those patients formerly diagnosed as having hypersensitivity vasculitis with significant extracutaneous involvement are now categorized within the "polyangiitis overlap" group, within the broader category of systemic vasculitis.

HENOCH-SCHÖNLEIN PURPURA

Henoch-Schönlein purpura, a distinctive subgroup of the hypersensitivity vasculitides, requires special mention not only because of its unique complex of manifestations, but also because *it typifies vasculitis that is usually confined to the skin but that might have significant extracutaneous manifestations.* This disorder is characterized by the clinicopathologic complex of nonthrombocytopenic purpura, skin lesions, joint involvement, and colicky abdominal pain, sometimes associated with gastrointestinal hemorrhage and renal disease.[19,58–62] The disease usually occurs in children, but adults of any age can be affected.[63] The male/female ratio is 1.5:1. This disease usually remits spontaneously within a week, but can recur a number of times for some weeks to months before remission is complete. Rarely, patients have recurrent disease for years. The characteristic skin lesions are manifested as palpable purpura and represent leukocytoclastic venulitis (Fig. 75–5). Fever is seen in 75% of patients. Glomerulitis usually consists of microscopic hematuria without clinically significant functional renal impairment; rarely, renal failure occurs.[59] Hypertension is seen in 13% of patients. The organ system involvement and clinical manifestations in children with Henoch-Schönlein purpura are listed in Table 75–9.

Because of the excellent prognosis, immunosuppressive therapy is rarely indicated. Treatment usually consists of supportive, symptomatic therapy. In patients with recurrent disease, corticosteroids in daily doses of 1 mg/kg for limited periods are recommended; the dose is then tapered to an alternate-day regimen and is ultimately discontinued.[2,64,65] It has been difficult to evaluate the efficacy of corticosteroid therapy because of spontaneous remissions and recurrences. The few patients who develop significant renal disease might re-

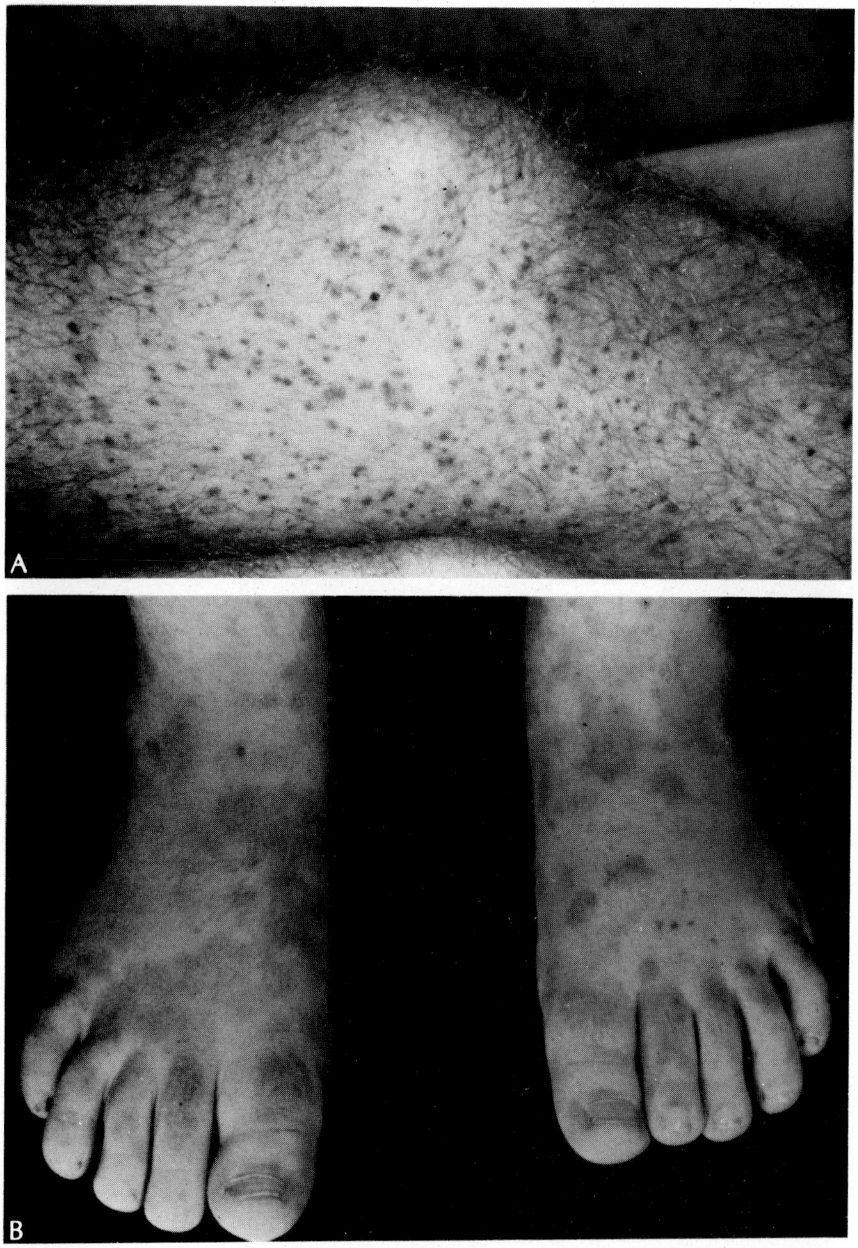

FIGURE 75–5. *A,* Palpable purpura and flexion contracture of the knee in a patient with Henoch-Schönlein purpura. The flexion contracture is due to the periarthritis frequently seen with this disease. *B,* The larger, deeper, and more ecchymotic-appearing lesions seen in the dependent extremities in a patient with Henoch-Schönlein purpura. Also note the three more superficial palpable purpuric lesions over the dorsum of the distal left forefoot and the anterior aspect of the right ankle.

quire cytotoxic therapy, according to the protocol already given for the systemic necrotizing vasculitides.

VASCULITIS ASSOCIATED WITH CONNECTIVE TISSUE DISEASE

Vasculitis can be associated with the entire spectrum of connective tissue disorders,[1,17,19,29,46,66] as discussed in other chapters devoted to the individual connective tissue diseases. Vasculitis is most common in RA, SLE, and Sjögrens syndrome.[66] Although we include vasculitis associated with other systemic connective tissue diseases under the category of hypersensitivity vasculitis, implying small-vessel disease of the skin, vasculitis in these diseases can be indistinguishable from the fulminant multisystem disorder of the systemic necrotizing vasculitis group. Cutaneous small-vessel disease is the most common associated vasculitis.[57]

TABLE 75–9. ORGAN INVOLVEMENT AND CLINICAL MANIFESTATIONS IN PEDIATRIC PATIENTS WITH HENOCH-SCHÖNLEIN PURPURA

INVOLVEMENT	PERCENTAGE (%)
Skin	100
Purpura	100
Ulceration	4
Joints	71
Gastrointestinal tract	68
Pain	57
Nausea or vomiting	50
Occult blood	42
Hematemesis or melena	35
Major bleeding	5
Intussusception	3
Kidney	
Hematuria	45
Microscopic	45
Macroscopic	26
Proteinuria	35
Functional impairment	9
Localized edema	32

From Cupps, T.R., and Fauci, A.S.[2]

The vasculitis associated with RA usually consists of typical leukocytoclastic vasculitis of the postcapillary venules of the skin resulting in palpable purpura and cutaneous ulceration.[57] In addition, the synovium and early rheumatoid nodules can manifest vasculitis.[67] Less commonly, patients with RA, particularly those with severely erosive and nodular disease and high-titer seropositivity for rheumatoid factor (RF),[68] develop a fulminant systemic vasculitis involving arterioles and medium-sized muscular arteries similar to that seen in the polyarteritis nodosa group of systemic necrotizing vasculitis.[69,70] Previously, it was believed that corticosteroid therapy either precipitated the development of or worsened the systemic vasculitis associated with RA,[71,72] although it is now thought that systemic vasculitis merely reflects severe RA, a condition that might require corticosteroid therapy.[66] For whatever reason, vasculitis associated with RA is much less common than it was in the 1950s and 1960s.

Cutaneous vasculitis develops in approximately 20% of patients with SLE,[73] typically small-vessel vasculitis resulting in palpable purpura, although patients can develop cutaneous infarction and chronic ulceration. A serious, much less common vasculitic complication of SLE is diffuse central nervous system vasculitis and visceral involvement similar to that seen in the polyarteritis nodosa group of systemic vasculitis.[73–75]

The mechanism is most likely immune complex deposition. The evidence for immune complex–mediated tissue damage is ample.[29,76] Treatment of most vasculitides in the diffuse connective tissue diseases is that of the primary underlying disease. If the vasculitis threatens vital organs, the treatment is as described for systemic vasculitis.

ESSENTIAL MIXED CRYOGLOBULINEMIA

Cryoglobulinemia can be present in a variety of disorders, with or without vasculitis. Indeed, cryoglobulinemia is present to a variable degree in many of the vasculitic syndromes under discussion. Several categories of cryoglobulinopathies exist, and vasculitides can be found in a number of them.[70,77,78] In the distinct syndrome called essential mixed cryoglobulinemia, identifiable underlying disease is not usually present.[78,80] In this syndrome, the vasculitis is generally confined to the skin, although some patients develop fulminant multisystem disease, particularly involving the kidney, with severe glomerulonephritis. Histopathologic examination of the purpuric skin lesions typically shows leukocytoclastic venulitis due to deposition of immune complexes, principally immunoglobulin M (IgM) RF directed against an IgG molecule—hence the term "mixed" cryoglobulinemia. Results of treatment are variable. When the disease remains confined to the skin, the prognosis is good. Patients with severe glomerulonephritis have a poor prognosis, however, because the disease has been reported to progress despite therapy with corticosteroids or even cytotoxic agents.[80,81] Plasmapheresis can be useful in this syndrome, but firm conclusions must await more extensive clinical trials.[82]

VASCULITIS ASSOCIATED WITH NEOPLASMS AND OTHER PRIMARY DISORDERS

The association between small-vessel cutaneous vasculitis and certain malignant diseases is a well-recognized but rare phenomenon.[83] Associated neoplasms usually are lymphoid or reticuloendothelial disorders such as Hodgkin's disease, other lymphomas, and multiple myeloma.[83–86] Although the vasculitis is usually a leukocytoclastic venulitis limited to the skin, systemic vasculitis in association with neoplasms also occurs rarely. Hairy cell leukemia has been associated with systemic vasculitis of the polyarteritis nodosa type.[87,88] An interesting syndrome of granulomatous vasculitis of the central nervous system (CNS) is associated with lymphoproliferative disorders, usually Hodgkin's disease, in which the vasculitis is found in areas not invaded by tumor.[89] Although the cause of vasculitis associated with neoplasms is not known, it could reflect a hypersensitivity reaction to tumor or tumor-related antigen with or without the formation and deposition of immune complexes. Treatment of the vasculitis should be directed at the underlying neoplasm.

An association exists between *atrial myxoma* and systemic vasculopathy.[90] Strictly speaking, this syndrome is not a true vasculitis, because the arterial lesions result from embolization of myxomatous tissue and secondary inflammation of the arterial wall (see Chapter 78).[91–93]

Leukocytoclastic vasculitis can be a minor component of many other primary diseases.[29] Such diseases include subacute bacterial endocarditis, chronic active hepatitis, ulcerative colitis, retroperitoneal fibrosis, primary biliary cirrhosis, and Goodpasture's syndrome. As

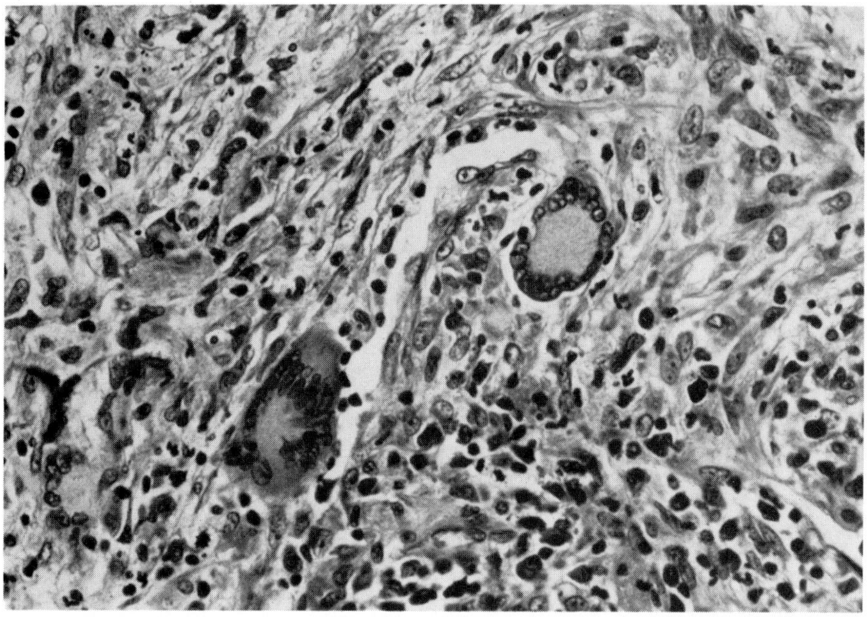

FIGURE 75–6. Lung biopsy in a patient with Wegener's granulomatosis. Histopathologic study reveals granulomatous vasculitis with multinucleated giant cells infiltrating the vessel wall. (Hematoxylin and eosin stain; magnification ×200.)

with other secondary vasculitides, therapy is directed at the underlying primary cause.

WEGENER'S GRANULOMATOSIS

Wegener's granulomatosis, a distinct clinicopathologic entity, is characterized by granulomatous vasculitis of the upper and lower respiratory tracts together with glomerulonephritis (Fig. 75–6). Variable degrees of disseminated vasculitis involving both small arteries and veins also can occur.[3,48] This disorder probably represents an aberrant hypersensitivity reaction to an unknown antigen, perhaps one that enters through the upper respiratory tract. No association with allergic diatheses, geographic location, travel, or domestic or occupational exposure are known, however. The male/female ratio is 1.3:1, and the mean age of onset is 40.6 years.[3]

CLINICAL MANIFESTATIONS

The presenting signs and symptoms of 85 cases of Wegener's granulomatosis are listed in Table 75–10.[3] Clinical presentations varied widely, but the typical findings related to the upper respiratory tract and included rhinorrhea, severe sinusitis, nasal mucosal ulcerations, and otitis media, usually secondary to blockage of the eustachian tube resulting from upper airway disease. Hearing loss was the initial complaint of several patients. A few patients had pulmonary disease without any evidence of upper airway disease. Symptoms included cough, hemoptysis, and less frequently, chest discomfort. Chest radiograph usually demonstrated pulmonary infiltrates. Other organ systems affected by Wegener's granulomatosis were occasionally the focus of initial complaints,

TABLE 75–10. PRESENTING SIGNS AND SYMPTOMS IN 85 PATIENTS WITH WEGENER'S GRANULOMATOSIS

	PATIENTS	
SIGN OR SYMPTOM*	Number	Percentage (%)
Pulmonary infiltrates	60	71
Sinusitis	57	67
Arthralgia or arthritis	37	44
Fever	29	34
Otitis	21	25
Cough	29	34
Rhinitis or nasal symptoms	19	22
Hemoptysis	15	18
Ocular inflammation (conjunctivitis, uveitis, episcleritis, or scleritis)	14	16
Weight loss	14	16
Skin rash	11	13
Epistaxis	9	11
Renal failure	9	11
Chest discomfort	7	8
Anorexia or malaise	7	8
Proptosis	6	7
Shortness of breath or dyspnea	6	7
Oral ulcers	5	6
Hearing loss	5	6
Pleuritis or effusion	5	6
Headache	5	6

* Miscellaneous: hoarseness or stridor, saddle nose deformity, and mastoiditis, three patients each; cranial nerve dysfunction, and mastoiditis, three patients each; cranial nerve dysfunction, three patients; parotid mass or pain, two patients each; nasolacrimal duct obstruction, thyroiditis, liver function test abnormality, blindness, peripheral neuropathy, ear pinna mass, pedal edema, adenopathy, anosmia, pericarditis, asthma, diabetes insipidus, and Raynaud's phenomenon, one patient each.

From Fauci, A.S., et al.[3]

often associated with the foregoing respiratory tract findings. Rarely, patients had renal failure in the absence of significant and easily detectable disease in other organ systems. Arthralgias were often present initially, as were other generalized manifestation of systemic inflammatory disease such as fatigue, malaise, anorexia, and weight loss. Fever often occurred, perhaps from the underlying inflammatory disease, although it was more commonly associated with secondary bacterial infection of the involved paranasal sinuses.

Although Wegener's granulomatosis is a generalized systemic disease with certain cardinal and characteristic features reflected in multiple organ system involvement (Table 75–11), it is essentially a true pulmonary-renal syndrome, and these two organ systems are largely responsible for the clinical course of the disease.

The characteristic and typical lung findings consist of multiple, *bilateral nodular infiltrates that usually cavitate* (Fig. 75–7). Pleural effusions occur in approximately 20% of patients, but hilar adenopathy is not seen, and pulmonary calcifications are rare.[48,94,95] Pulmonary function abnormalities are common and include obstruction to airflow as well as reduced lung volumes and diffusing capacity abnormalities.[96] Small areas of *atelectasis* frequently occur adjacent to parenchymal infiltrates during active pulmonary disease. Patients with documented endobronchial disease can develop atelectasis related to scarred endobronchial tissue or smoldering endobronchial disease accompanying quiescent disease in other organs.

TABLE 75–11. ORGAN OR SYSTEM INVOLVEMENT IN WEGENER'S GRANULOMATOSIS

	PATIENTS	
ORGAN OR SYSTEM	Number	Percentage (%)
Lung	80	94
Paranasal sinuses	77	91
Kidney	72	85
Joints	57	67
Nose or nasopharynx	54	64
Ear	52	61
Eye	49	58
Skin	38	45
Nervous system	19	22
Heart	10	12

From Fauci, A.S., et al.[3]

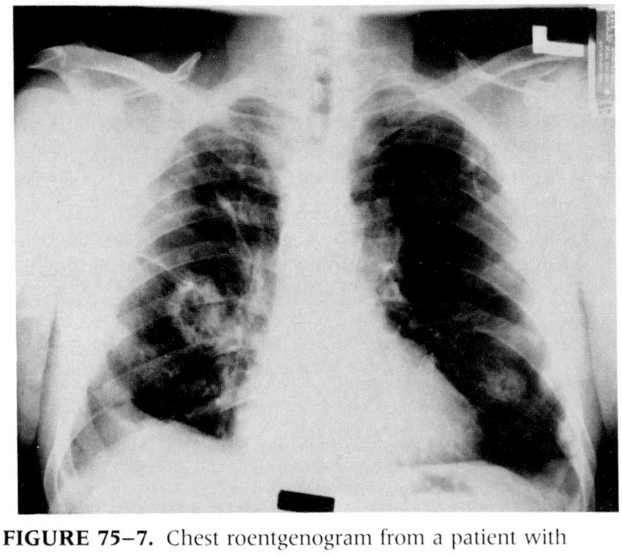

FIGURE 75–7. Chest roentgenogram from a patient with Wegener's granulomatosis showing multiple nodules and cavity formation.

Renal lesions range from mild focal and *segmental glomerulonephritis* with minimal urinary findings and little, if any renal functional impairment to *fulminant diffuse necrotizing glomerulonephritis* with proliferative and crescentic changes (Fig. 75–8).[48,94,97] Granulomas and true arteritis are rarely found on renal biopsy. Once present, glomerulonephritis can rapidly progress from mild to severe and can lead to fulminant renal failure within weeks and even days of its inception. Because extrarenal manifestations usually precede functional renal disease, often by months, it is critical to establish the diagnosis early with appropriate treatment to prevent irreversible renal failure.[3]

Most patients with Wegener's granulomatosis and serious sinus or nasal disease develop *secondary infection* of these tissues, almost surely because of mucosal damage and the subsequent impairment of host defenses.[3] Staphylococcus aureus is the predominant organism cultured from the nose or sinus of infected patients. Treated patients in complete remission often have an apparent relapse because of increased sinus symptoms together with an elevation of the erythrocyte sedimentation rate. Careful evaluation shows, however, that the symptoms and the erythrocyte sedimentation rate elevation are usually related to smoldering upper airway infection, and both respond promptly to antibiotics with or without drainage procedures. *This observation is important because increasing or reinstituting immunosuppressive therapy under these circumstances is obviously contraindicated.*

Anti-neutrophil cytoplasmic antibodies (ANCAs) have been shown to be a sensitive and specific marker for Wegener's granulomatosis.[11,12,98,99] ANCAs are an important adjunct in understanding and managing Wegener's granulomatosis; however, their precise role in the management of the disease is not well defined.[100] ANCAs can suggest a diagnosis of Wegener's granulomatosis in patients with atypical presentations, but a clinicopathologic diagnosis must be established and therapy should not be initiated on the basis of positive serology alone. ANCAs can be helpful in following patients during therapy, especially in distinguishing an infectious process from active disease.[98]

TREATMENT AND PROGNOSIS

Before the use of immunosuppressive therapy, the prognosis for patients with this disease was grave. Untreated, the disease usually ran a rapidly fatal course, particu-

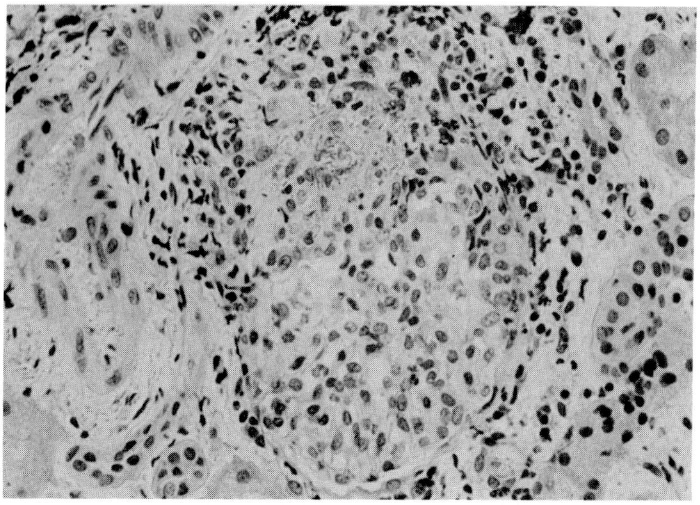

FIGURE 75–8. Photomicrograph of a kidney biopsy from a patient with Wegener's granulomatosis showing extensive involvement of the glomerulus with marked increase in cellularity (hematoxylin and eosin stain; original magnification; ×400). From Leavitt, R.Y., and Fauci, A.S.[46]

larly after the recognition of functional renal impairment. The mean survival rate of patients with untreated Wegener's granulomatosis was 5 months; 82% of patients died within a year, and more than 90% died within 2 years.[101] Wegener's granulomatosis was the first vasculitic syndrome in which the use of long-term, low-dose (2 mg/kg/per day) cytotoxic agents, in this case cyclophosphamide, together with alternate-day corticosteroid administration, was effective in inducing remissions in most patients.[48] We recorded complete remissions in 79 of 85 patients (93%) using this protocol.[3] The mean duration of remission for survivors was over 4 years, and some patients maintained remission without therapy for more than 10 years. This striking response of a formerly fatal non-neoplastic disease to a combination of low-dose cyclophosphamide and alternate-day corticosteroids has led to its use in other severe systemic vasculitic syndromes, as previously discussed.

Cyclophosphamide pulse therapy (monthly intravenous bolus) has been suggested in the therapy of systemic vasculitis because it is effective in the therapy of systemic lupus erythematosus.[102] Also, it is less toxic than daily cyclophosphamide therapy. However, we found that cyclophosphamide pulse therapy was not as effective as daily low-dose cyclophosphamide in the treatment of Wegener's granulomatosis.[103]

Trimethoprim/sulfamethoxazole has been reported to be effective therapy in some patients with Wegener's granulomatosis.[104–106] These observations are interestingly but largely anecdotal; more data are needed before definite conclusions regarding the role of trimethoprim/sulfamethoxazole in the therapy of Wegener's granulomatosis can be drawn.[105,107]

LYMPHOMATOID GRANULOMATOSIS

Lymphomatoid granulomatosis is characterized by infiltration of various organs with a polymorphic cellular infiltrate consisting of atypical lymphocytoid and plasmacytoid cells together with granulomatous inflammation in an angiocentric and angiodestructive pattern.[108–111] Strictly speaking, lymphomatoid granulomatosis is not a vasculitis, because it is not a true inflammation of blood vessels, but is rather an infiltration and invasion of blood vessel walls with atypical lymphoid cells in association with an intramuscular or extravascular granulomatous response. The disease probably represents one end of the spectrum of malignant lymphoma.[46,111–114] The term angiocentric immunoproliferative lesion has been proposed as an alternative to lymphomatoid granulomatosis.[111] The disease is included because it is often confused with certain vasculitic syndromes such as Wegener's granulomatosis.[115] The disease primarily involves the lungs, but skin, renal, and CNS disease have occurred in various patients.

Patients generally have nonspecific signs and symptoms such as fever, malaise, weight loss, and fatigue. Chest radiographs reveal bilateral nodular infiltrates resembling metastatic cancer.[108–110] The spectrum or organ system involvement in lymphomatoid granulomatosis is outlined in Table 75–12.[116]

Untreated disease is almost uniformly fatal.[108,109,117] We have treated 15 patients with lymphomatoid granulomatosis with a regimen of cyclophosphamide and alternate-day prednisone administration.[116] Approximately half the patients had a complete remission, and therapy was ultimately discontinued. Patients who did not have a remission developed the lymphoproliferative phase of the disease and ultimately died. Thus, the prognosis remains poor.

GIANT CELL ARTERITIDES

The giant cell arteritides include temporal or cranial arteritis and Takayasu's arteritis (see also Chapter 83). Both are panarteritides characterized by inflammation of medium-sized and large arteries. They are separable by the clear-cut difference in age range, the distribution of involved vessels, the associated syndromes, and the response to therapy. The characteristics of these diseases are outlined in Table 75–13.

TEMPORAL ARTERITIS

Temporal arteritis (see also Chapter 81) is well recognized by its classic clinical picture of fever, anemia, high erythrocyte sedimentation rate, and associated symptoms in a person more than 55 years old.[118–120] The diagnosis can often be made clinically and confirmed by biopsy of the temporal arteries. Because vessel involvement can be segmental and might be missed on routine biopsy, some authors have recommended local arteriography[121] and examination of multiple sections of bilateral biopsies.[122]

Polymyalgia rheumatica syndrome, closely associated with temporal arteritis, is characterized by stiffness, aching, and pain in the muscles of the neck, shoulder, lower back, hips, and thighs.[118,123,124] This syndrome is discussed in Chapter 81.

A well-recognized and serious complication of temporal arteritis, particularly in untreated patients, is ocular involvement, sometimes leading to sudden blindness.[125] The aorta and other large arteries can also be involved in patients with temporal arteritis.[126] Although the dramatic eye manifestations can appear suddenly, most patients have complaints relating to the head or eyes for months, and so one needs to pay careful attention to symptoms and rapid use of appropriate therapy. Temporal arteritis is generally exquisitely sensitive to corticosteroid therapy.[118,123,127] Treatment should begin with 40 to 60 mg prednisone daily, followed by gradual tapering to a daily maintenance dose of 7.5 to 10 mg, with upward readjustment of dosage if symptoms recur. Therapy should be continued for at least 1 to 2 years.[118,123,127,128] Although one should not attempt to induce initial remission of temporal arteritis with alternate-day therapy, many patients can be given alternate-day therapy in preparation for discontinuing the drug after induction of remission.[128] The prognosis of this disorder is good with corticosteroid therapy, and remissions usually are maintained after withdrawal of therapy, although relapse can occur.

TABLE 75–12. ORGAN OR SYSTEM INVOLVEMENT IN 15 PATIENTS WITH LYMPHOMATOID GRANULOMATOSIS

ORGAN OR SYSTEM	NO. OF PATIENTS (%)
Lung	15 (100)
Skin	8 (53)
Kidney	6 (40)
Lymph nodes	6 (40)
Central nervous system	5 (33)
Bone marrow	5 (33)
Liver	4 (27)
Peripheral nervous system	3 (20)
Eyes	3 (20)
Muscle	2 (13)
Paranasal sinuses	1 (7)
Thyroid gland	1 (7)
Epididymis	1 (7)

From Fauci, A.S., et al.[116]

TABLE 75–13. CHARACTERISTICS OF THE GIANT CELL ARTERITIDES

	TEMPORAL ARTERITIS	TAKAYASU'S ARTERITIS
Patients	Disease of the elderly; women more than men	More prevalent in young women; more common in the Orient, but neither racially nor geographically restricted
Blood vessels	Characteristically involves branches of carotid (temporal artery), but is a systemic arteritis and may involve any medium-sized or large artery	Large and medium-sized arteries with predilection for aortic arch and its branches; may involve pulmonary artery
Histopathologic features	Panarteritis; inflammatory mononuclear cell infiltrates; frequent giant cell formation within vessel wall; fragmentation of internal elastic lamina; proliferation of tunica intima	Panarteritis; inflammatory mononuclear cell infiltrates; intimal proliferation and fibrosis; scarring and vascularization of tunica media; disruption and degeneration of elastic lamina
Clinical manifestations	Classic complex of fever, anemia, high erythrocyte sedimentation rate, muscle aches in an elderly person; possible headache; strong association with polymyalgia rheumatica syndrome	Generalized systemic symptoms; local signs and symptoms related to involved vessels; occlusive phase
Complications	Ocular (sudden blindness)	Related to distribution of involved vessels; death usually occurs from congestive heart failure or cerebrovascular accidents
Diagnosis	Temporal artery biopsy; lesions may be segmental; multiple sections, arteriography, and bilateral biopsy may aid in diagnosis	Arteriography; biopsy of involved vessel
Treatment	Corticosteroids effective	Corticosteroids not of proved efficacy; cytotoxic agents currently being tested

From Fauci, A.S., Haynes, B.F., and Katz, P.[1]

TAKAYASU'S ARTERITIS

Usually seen in women in the second or third decade in life, Takayasu's arteritis is characterized by inflammation and stenosis of large and intermediate-sized arteries with frequent involvement of the aortic arch and its branches.[129–135] Diagnosis is usually made angiographically. Takayasu's arteritis is often referred to as "pulseless disease" because of the frequent involvement of the subclavian artery (Fig. 75–9A). Nonetheless, it has complex manifestations ranging from generalized, often vague, symptoms characteristic of a systemic inflammatory disease to local signs and symptoms relating to the involved vessels themselves, to the characteristic manifestation of compromised blood flow to the organs perfused by the involved vessels (Fig. 75–9B). Some patients experience no apparent inflammatory symptoms and signs but have initial ischemic findings and changes related to the involved organ systems. The most common and obvious findings are absent pulses in the

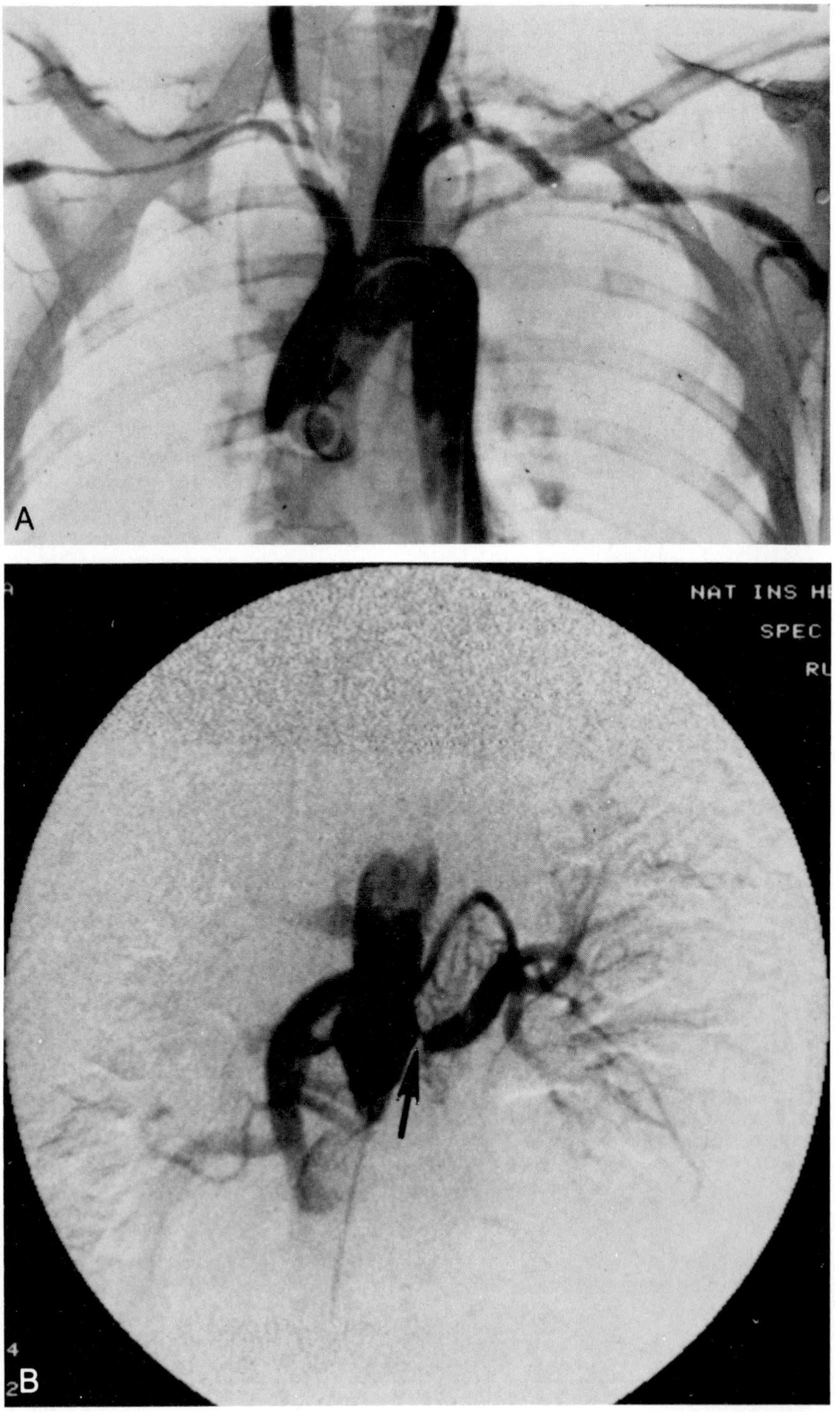

FIGURE 75–9. Subtraction angiograms from two patients with Takayasu's arteritis. *A,* Angiogram demonstrates severe involvement along a large segment of the right subclavian artery, as well as involvement of the right common carotid artery. *B,* Angiogram demonstrates marked narrowing of the left renal artery (arrow) and narrowing of the infrarenal aorta.

affected vessels. Bruits are common. The clinical course of the disease varies. Gradual deterioration is the rule, but the process can spontaneously remit, stabilize temporarily, insidiously progress, or abruptly decompensate. This variability has made it difficult to evaluate therapy. Despite reports of spontaneous remissions in untreated patients, the course is generally progressive and fatal within a few years. Death usually occurs from congestive heart failure or cerebrovascular accidents.[130] Corticosteroid therapy usually results in symptomatic improvement and angiographic stabilization.[134,135] We use cytotoxic agents in patients who have persistent or progressive disease while on corticosteroid therapy.[135,136] In addition to medical treatment, we take an aggressive approach to vascular reconstructive surgery aimed at preventing ischemic damage to organs with compromised vascular flow; necessary surgery can and should be performed on patients with active arteritis.[134–137] This approach to the therapy of Takayasu's arteritis appears to improve survival and decreased ischemic complication, but longer follow-up is necessary.[134–137]

MUCOCUTANEOUS LYMPH NODE SYNDROME (KAWASAKI DISEASE)

The mucocutaneous lymph node syndrome is an acute febrile illness of infants and young children originally described in Japan.[138,139] The cause is completely unknown, and although an infectious agent has been suspected, no etiologic agent has been identified.[138–140] Several causative agents such as *Propionibacterium acnes*, rickettsia, Epstein-Barr virus, and retroviruses have been implicated but not confirmed as etiologic agents.[138–141] Evidence suggests that Kawasaki disease could be associated with an antecedent respiratory illness.[141] In addition, some studies have shown an exposure to freshly shampooed rugs prior to the onset of Kawasaki disease.[142,143] The Centers for Disease Control (CDC) have established diagnostic criteria for Kawasaki disease. These include fever lasting 5 days or more without other explanation and four of the following manifestations of mucocutaneous inflammation: bilateral nonpurulent conjunctival injection, one or more changes in the lips or oral cavity (injected or fissured lips, injected pharynx, "strawberry tongue"), changes of peripheral extremities (desquamation of the skin of the fingertips, reddened palms or soles, edema of hands or feet), polymorphous exanthem, and nonsuppurative cervical adenitis.[144] The disease has been recognized with increasing frequency in the United States.[139] Its clinical manifestations are listed in Table 75–14. The condition is usually self-limited, and most patients recover uneventfully. Approximately 1 to 2% of patients, however, develop severe and often fatal complications, resulting from vasculitic involvement of the coronary arteries. In addition, atypical Kawasaki disease has been described, and includes patients with the typical coronary artery lesions who do not fulfill the CDC diagnostic criteria.[145] Many cases in the United States were formerly reported as polyarteritis nodosa of children, with its characteristic and unusual selective involvement of the coronary arteries, but actually were the arteritis of unrecognized Kawasaki disease.[26,146] Myocarditis, pericarditis, myocardial infarction, and cardiomegaly are also seen. Involvement of other vessels such as the aorta and the celiac, carotid, subclavian, and pulmonary arteries occurs much less frequently. Treatment with aspirin (30 mg/kg/per day) can lessen the incidence of cardiac complications. Corticosteroids can actually increase the incidence of cardiac complications.[138,139,147,148] High doses of intravenous gammaglobulin appear to decrease the incidence of cardiac abnormalities if administered early in the course of the disease.[149–151] It is now recommended that all patients with acute Kawasaki disease receive intravenous gammaglobulin.[152]

TABLE 75–14. CLINICAL MANIFESTATIONS OF MUCOCUTANEOUS LYMPH NODE SYNDROME (KAWASAKI'S DISEASE)

MANIFESTATIONS	PERCENTAGE (%)
Fever	95
Changes of the extremity	
Desquamation from finger tips	94
Erythematous palms and soles	88
Indurated edema	76
Polymorphous exanthem of body and trunk	92
Changes in lips and oral cavity	
Dry, red lips	90
Erythematous oral mucosa	90
Prominent tongue papillae	77
Congested conjunctivae	88
Swelling of cervical lymph nodes	75

From Cupps, T.R., and Fauci, A.S.[2]

VASCULITIS ISOLATED TO THE CENTRAL NERVOUS SYSTEM

In addition to the granulomatous vasculitis of the CNS already discussed in association with certain lymphoproliferative malignant disease, a syndrome of *isolated vasculitis of the CNS* exists (see also Chapter 79). This uncommon entity is characterized by vasculitis restricted to the vessels of the CNS in the apparent absence of systemic vasculitis or other systemic disease.[153–155] Presenting manifestations include severe headaches, altered mental function, and focal neurologic defects. Systemic symptoms such as fever, myalgia, arthralgia, and arthritis, common in the systemic vasculitides, are usually not present. Diagnosis is made by the clinical presentation together with angiographic studies or biopsy of the brain parenchyma and leptomeninges, when feasible.[155,156] Prognosis is generally poor, but corticosteroid therapy alone or together with cyclophosphamide in corticosteroid-resistant patients used in the regimen already described for systemic vasculitis can induce long-term remission.[13,47,153,155]

BEHÇET'S DISEASE

Behçet's disease (see also Chapter 64) of unknown origin is characterized by recurrent episodes of oral ulcers, eye lesions, genital ulcers, and other cutaneous lesions.[157] The underlying pathologic lesion is a vasculitis predominantly involving venules, although vessels of any size in any organ system can be affected. No therapy for Behçet's disease is uniformly acceptable.[158] Cyclosporin has been effective in treating patients with refractory disease but its use is limited by side effects such as renal dysfunction.[159] In addition, azathioprine proved useful in a controlled study of treatment of Behçet's disease.[160]

THROMBOANGIITIS OBLITERANS (BUERGER'S DISEASE)

This rare inflammatory occlusive peripheral vascular disease involves the arteries and veins. The disease is seen predominantly in men, usually between the ages of 20 to 40, but it can affect women.[161–163] It primarily involves medium-sized and small arteries as well as veins in a segmental fashion. The inflammatory process is associated with a thrombus and evolves through several stages. In the acute stage, the vessel wall and thrombus are infiltrated by polymorphonuclear leukocytes. Microabscess can be found within the thrombi.[164] A subacute stage follows, when mononuclear cells and giant cells can be seen, and ultimately a chronic stage develops, characterized by chronic inflammatory infiltrates, fibrosis, and recanalization of the vessel lumen. The entire process can be associated with migratory superficial thrombophlebitis.

Although the cause is unknown, the use of tobacco makes the disease much worse. Almost without exception, thromboangiitis obliterans occurs in heavy smokers.[161] No sufficient evidence suggests an immunologic pathogenesis.

The clinical presentation is variable and can be insidious or abrupt. Coldness of the distal extremities, color changes, dysesthesias, intense hyperemia, excruciating pain, ulceration, gangrene, and pulp atrophy are common.[161,164,165] Usually, acute attacks last 1 to 4 weeks, and the disease runs an indolent and recurrent course. Ultimately, the collateral circulation can no longer compensate for the progressive ischemia, and amputation of the involved distal extremities might be required. Various techniques such as anticoagulation, thromboendarterectomy, bypass operations, and sympathectomy have not improved the prognosis for the involved extremity.[165,166] The most effective approach to this disease seem to be meticulous local care of the involved area, together with complete abstinence from tobacco.

MISCELLANEOUS VASCULITIDES

A number of other syndromes show vasculitis as either a primary disease process or a secondary component of an underlying entity. *Erythema nodosum* is a common syndrome well recognized as a hypersensitivity manifestation of underlying disorders.[167] It is manifested as a painful, nodular, inflammatory process of the dermis and subcutaneous tissues. Vasculitis, predominantly of small venules, is a major component of its histopathologic picture.[168]

Other less common vasculitides that deserve mention are *erythema elevatum diutinum*,[169] *Cogan's syndrome*,[170] and *Eale's disease*.[171] Finally, some rare syndromes appear to be confined to single organs such as the vermiform appendix and the female breast.[172]

GENERAL APPROACH TO THE PATIENT

The vasculitides comprise a broad spectrum of clinicopathologic syndromes. In certain disorders, vasculitis is the predominant and most obvious manifestation in the absence of an underlying disease process. Other disorders are characterized by a vasculitic syndrome secondary to an underlying disease. Most vasculitic syndromes are associated directly or indirectly with immunopathologic mechanisms. Using various clinical, pathologic, and immunologic criteria, certain vasculitic syndromes can be clearly recognized and categorized as distinct entities, whereas others overlap different diseases within a broader category. It is important to categorize the vasculitis syndrome in a given patient, and particu-

TABLE 75–15. GENERAL APPROACH TO THE PATIENT WITH VASCULITIS

1. Categorize the syndrome correctly (specific syndrome; primary versus secondary; localized versus systemic).
2. Determine extent of disease activity.
3. Remove offending antigen if possible.
4. If associated with underlying disease, treat underlying disease when possible.
5. Use appropriate therapeutic agents immediately in diseases in which efficacy is clearly demonstrated, such as corticosteroids in temporal arteritis and cyclophosphamide and corticosteroids in Wegener's granulomatosis.
6. Avoid immunosuppressive therapy (corticosteroids or cytotoxic agents) in diseases that: (1) do not disseminate; (2) do not usually result in irreversible organ system damage; and (3) rarely respond to such agents.
7. Institute corticosteroids immediately in patients with systemic vasculitis; add a cytotoxic agent such as cyclophosphamide if response is not prompt or if disease is known to respond only to cytotoxic agents.
8. Continually attempt to taper corticosteroids to alternate-day regimens, and discontinue when possible.
9. Have a clear-cut understanding of goals and mechanisms of the long-term use of cytotoxic agents in the treatment of non-neoplastic diseases.
10. Use other agents if clinical situation dictates (e.g., nonsteroidal anti-inflammatory agents or plasmapheresis) based on results from therapeutic trials.

larly to identify disseminated systemic disease leading to irreversible organ system dysfunction if untreated or if inadequately treated. Such patients need prompt and aggressive treatment with corticosteroids and, in some cases, cytotoxic agents, such as cyclophosphamide. In contrast, patients with predominantly cutaneous disease without a high risk of systemic involvement can be treated much less aggressively. Appreciation of the scope of the vasculitic syndromes is essential for an appropriate diagnostic and therapeutic approach to individual patients (Table 75–15).

REFERENCES

1. Fauci, A.S., Haynes, B.F., and Katz, P.: The spectrum of vasculitis: Clinical, pathologic, immunologic, and therapeutic considerations. Ann. Intern. Med., *89*:660–676, 1978.
2. Cupps, T.R., and Fauci, A.S.: The Vasculitides. Philadelphia, W.B., Saunders, 1981.
3. Fauci, A.S., et al.: Wegener's granulomatosis: Prospective clinical and therapeutic experience with 85 patients for 21 years. Ann. Intern. Med., *98*:76–85, 1983.
4. Cochrane, C.G., and Dixon, F.J.: Antigen-antibody complex induced disease. *In* Textbook of Immunopathology. 2nd Ed. Vol. 1. Edited by P.A. Mesicher and H.F. Muller-Eberhard. New York, Grune & Stratton, 1976.
5. Sams, W.M. Jr.: Human hypersensitivity angiitis, an immune complex disease. J. Invest. Dermatol., *85*(Suppl.):144–148, 1985.
6. Sergent, J.S., et al.: Vasculitis with hepatitis B antigenemia: Long-term observation in nine patients. Medicine (Baltimore), *67*:354–359, 1976.
7. Spector, W.G., and Heesom, N.: The production of granulomata by antigen-antibody complexes. J. Pathol., *98*:31–39, 1969.
8. Leung, D.Y.M., Collins, T., Lapierre, L.A., and Geha, R.S.: IgM Antibodies present in the acute phase of Kawasaki syndrome lyse cultured vascular endothelial cell stimulated by gamma interferon. J. Clin. Invest., *77*:1428, 1986.
9. Leung, D.Y.M., et al.: Two monokines, interleukin-1 and tumor necrosis factor, render cultured vascular endothelial cells susceptible to lysis by antibodies circulating during Kawasaki syndrome. J. Exp. Med., *164*:1958, 1986.
10. Pober, J.S., and Cotran, R.S.: Cytokines and endothelial cell biology. Physiol. Rev., *70*:427–451, 1990.
11. Van der Woude, F.J., Daha, M.R., and Van Es, L.A.: The current status of neutrophil cytoplasmic antibodies. Clin. Exp. Immunol., *78*:143, 1989.
12. Jennette, J.C., and Falk, R.J.: Antineutrophil cytoplasmic autoantibodies and associated diseases: A review. Am. J. Kidney Dis., *15*:517, 1990.
13. Fauci, A.S.: The vasculitis syndromes. *In* Harrison's Principles of Internal Medicine. 12th Ed. Edited by E. Braunwald, et al. New York, McGraw-Hill, 1991.
14. Kussmaul, A., and Maier, K.: Uber eine bischer nicht beschreibene eigenthumliche Arterienekrankung (Periarteritis nodosa), die mit Morbus Brightii und rapid fortschreitender allgemeiner Muskellähmung einhergeht. Dtsch. Arch. Klin., *1*:484–517, 1966.
15. Churg, J., and Strauss, L.: Allergic granulomatosis, allergic angiitis and periarteritis nodosa. Am. J. Pathol., *27*:277–301, 1951.
16. Leavitt, R.Y., and Fauci, A.S.: Polyangiitis overlap syndrome: Classification and prospective clinical experience. Am. J. Med., *81*:79, 1986.
17. Zeek, P.M.: Periarteritis nodosa: Critical review. Am. J. Clin. Pathol., *22*:777–790, 1952.
18. Price, N., and Sams, W.M. Jr.: Vasculitis. Dermatol. Clin., *1*:475–491, 1983.
19. Alarcón-Segovia, D.: The necrotizing vasculitides. A new pathogenetic classification. Med. Clin. North Am., *61*:241–260, 1977.
20. Rose, G.A., and Spencer, H.: Polyarteritis nodosa. Q. J. Med., *26*:43–81, 1957.
21. Fauci, A.S.: Vasculitis. *In* Clinical Immunology. Edited by E.W. Parker. Philadelphia, W.B. Saunders, 1980.
22. White, R.H., and Schambelan, M.: Hypertension, hyperreninemia, and secondary hyperaldosteronism in systemic necrotizing vasculitis. Ann. Intern. Med., *92*:199, 1980.
23. Holsinger, D.R., Osmundson, P.J., and Edwards, J.E.: The heart in periarteritis nodosa. Circulation, *25*:610–618, 1962.
24. Sheps, S.G.: Vasculitis. *In* Peripheral Vascular Diseases. 4th Ed. Edited by J.F. Fairburn, J.L. Juergens, and J.A. Spittel. Philadelphia, W.B. Saunders, 1972, pp. 351–385.
25. Roberts, F.B., and Fetterman, G.H.: Polyarteritis nodosa in infancy. J. Pediatr., *63*:519–529, 1963.
26. Landing, B.H., and Larson, E.J.: Are infantile periarteritis nodosa with coronary artery involvement and fatal mucocutaneous lymph node syndrome the same? Comparison of 20 patients from North American with patients from Hawaii and Japan. Pediatrics, *59*:651–662, 1977.
27. Mowrey, F.H., and Lundberg, E.A.: The clinical manifestations of essential polyangiitis (periarteritis nodosa) with emphasis on the hepatic manifestations. Ann. Intern. Med., *40*:1141–1155, 1967.
28. Moore, P.M., and Fauci, A.S.: Neurologic manifestations of systemic vasculitis. A retrospective and prospective study of the clinicopathologic features and responses to therapy in 25 patients. Am. J. Med., *71*:517–524, 1981.
29. Gilliam, J.N., and Smiley, J.D.: Cutaneous necrotizing vasculitis and related disorders. Ann. Allergy, *37*:328–339, 1976.
30. Diaz-Perez, J.L., and Winkelmann, R.K.: Cutaneous periarteritis nodosa. Arch. Dermatol., *110*:407–414, 1974.
31. Duffy, J., et al.: Polyarthritis, polyarteritis and hepatitis B. Medicine, *55*:19–37, 1976.
32. Fauci, A.S., et al.: Cyclophosphamide therapy of severe systemic necrotizing vasculitis. N. Engl. J. Med., *301*:235–238, 1979.
33. McMahon, B.J., Heyward, W.L., Templin, D.W., et al.: Hepatitis B–associated polyarteritis nodosa in Alaskan eskimos: Clinical and epidemiologic features and long-term follow-up. Hepatology, 97–101, 1989.
34. Lightfoot, R.W. Jr., et al.: The American College of Rheumatology 1990 criteria for the classification of polyarteritis nodosa. Arthritis Rheum., *33*:1088–1093, 1990.
35. Bron, K.M., Stroot, C.A., and Shapiro, A.P.: The diagnostic value of angiographic observations in polyarteritis nodosa. Arch. Intern. Med., *116*:450–453, 1965.
36. Dornfeld, L., Lecky, L.W., and Peter, J.B.: Polyarteritis and intrarenal artery aneurysms. JAMA, *215*:1950–1952, 1971.
37. Fauci, A.S., Doppman, J.L., and Wolff, S.M.: Cyclophosphamide-induced remissions in advanced polyarteritis nodosa. Am. J. Med., *64*:890–894, 1978.
38. Longstreth, P.L., Lorobkin, M., and Palubinskas, A.J.: Renal microaneurysms in a patient with systemic lupus erythematosus. Radiology, *113*:65–66, 1974.
39. Meyers, D.S., Grim, C.E., and Kertzer, W.F.: Fibromuscular dysplasia of the renal artery with medial dissection. A case simulating polyarteritis nodosa. Am. J. Med., *56*:412–416, 1974.
40. Frohnert, P.P., and Sheps, S.G.: Long-term follow-up study of periarteritis nodosa. Am. J. Med., *43*:8–14, 1967.
41. Guillevin, L., Merrouche, Y., Gayraud, M., et al.: Periarteritis nodosa associated with hepatitis B virus. Determination of a

new therapeutic strategy: 13 cases [in French]. Press Med., *17*:1522–1526, 1988.
42. Trepo, C., Ouzan, D., Delmont, J., Tremisi, J.: Superiority of a new curative etiopathogenic treatment of hepatitis B-related polyarteritis, using a short corticosteroid course, vidarabine, and plasma exchanges. Presse Med., *17*:1527, 1988.
43. Lanham, J.C., Elkon, K.B., Pusey, C.D., and Hughes, G.R.: Systemic vasculitis with asthma and eosinophilia: A clinical approach to the Churg-Strauss syndrome. Medicine (Baltimore), *63*:65–81, 1984.
44. Masi, A.T., et al.: The American College of Rheumatology 1990 criteria for the classification of the Churg-Strauss syndrome (allergic granulomatosis and angiitis). Arthritis Rheum., *33*:1094–1100, 1990.
45. Manger, B.J., Krapf, F.E., Gramatzki, M., et al.: IgE-containing circulating immune complexes in Churg-Strauss vasculitis. Scand. J. Immunol., *21*:369–373, 1985.
46. Leavitt, R.Y., and Fauci, A.S.: Pulmonary vasculitis. Am. Rev. Respir. Dis., *134*:149–166, 1986.
47. Fauci, A.S., and Leavitt, R.Y.: Systemic vasculitis. *In* Current Therapy in Allergy, Immunology, and Rheumatology-3, Edited by L.M. Lichtenstein and A.S. Fauci. Philadelphia, B.C. Decker, 1988.
48. Fauci, A.S., and Wolff, S.M.: Wegener's granulomatosis: Studies in eighteen patients and a review of the literature. Medicine (Baltimore), *52*:535–561, 1973.
49. Ambrus, J.L., and Fauci, A.S.: Diffuse histiocytic lymphoma in a patient treated with cyclophosphamide for Wegener's granulomatosis. Am. J. Med., *76*:745–747, 1984.
50. Pedersen-Bjergaard, J., et al.: Carcinoma of the urinary bladder after treatment with cyclophosphamide for non-hodgkin's lymphoma. N. Engl. J. Med., *318*:1028–1032, 1988.
51. Ahmed, A.R., and Hombal, S.M.: Cyclophosphamide (Cytoxan): A review on relevant pharmacology and clinical uses. J. Am. Acad. Dermatol., *11*:1115–1126, 1984.
52. Young, K.R., and Fauci, A.S.: Cytotoxic and other immunoregulatory agents. *In* Textbook on Rheumatology. Edited by W.N. Kelley, E.D., Harris Jr., S. Ruddy, and C.B. Sledge. Philadelphia, W.B. Saunders, 1989.
53. Lockwood, C.M., et al.: Reversal of impaired splenic function in patients with nephritis or vasculitis (or both) by plasma exchange. N. Engl. J. Med., *300*:524–530, 1979.
54. Kauffmann, R.H., and Houwert, D.A.: Plasmapheresis in rapidly progressive Henoch-Schönlein glomerulonephritis and the effect on circulating IgA immune complexes. Clin. Nephrol., *16*:155–160, 1981.
55. Winkelmann, R.K., and Ditto, W.B.: Cutaneous and visceral syndromes of necrotizing or "allergic" angiitis: A study of 38 cases. Medicine (Baltimore), *43*:59–89, 1964.
56. Ackroyd, J.F.: Allergic purpura, including purpura due to foods, drugs, and infections. Am. J. Med., *14*:605–632, 1953.
57. Soter, N.A.: Clinical presentations and mechanisms of necrotizing angiitis of the skin. J. Invest. Dermatol., *67*:354–359, 1976.
58. Lindenauer, S.M., and Tank, E.S.: Surgical aspects of Henoch-Schönlein purpura. Surgery, *59*:982–987, 1966.
59. Ansell, B.M.: Henoch-Schönlein purpura with particular reference to the prognosis of the renal lesion. Br. J. Dermatol., *82*:211–215, 1970.
60. Ballard, H.S., Eisinger, R.P., and Gallo, G.: Renal manifestations of the Henoch-Schönlein syndrome in adults. Am. J. Med., *49*:328–335, 1970.
61. Cream, J.J., Gumpel, J.M., and Peachy, R.D.G.: Schönlein-Henoch purpura in the adult. Q. J. Med., *39*:461–484, 1970.
62. Heng, M.C.: Henoch-Schönlein purpura. Br. J. Dermatol., *112*:235–240, 1985.
63. Roth, D.A., Wilz, D.R., and Theil, G.B.: Schönlein-Henoch syndrome in adults. Q. J. Med., *55*:145–152, 1985.
64. Cupps, T.R., and Fauci, A.S.: Cutaneous vasculitis. *In* Current Therapy in Allergy and Immunology 1983–1984. Edited by L.M. Lichenstein and A.S. Fauci. Philadelphia. B.C. Decker, 1983.
65. Swerlick, R.A., and Lawley, T.J.: Cutaneous vasculitis: its relationship to systemic disease. Med. Clin. North Am., *73*:1221–1235, 1989.
66. Christian, C.L., and Sergent, J.S.: Vasculitis syndromes: Clinical and experimental models. Am. J. Med., *61*:385–392, 1976.
67. Glass, D., Soter, N.A., and Schur, P.H.: Rheumatoid vasculitis. Arthritis Rheum., *19*:950–952, 1976.
68. Mongan, E.S., et al.: A study of the relation of seronegative and seropositive rheumatoid arthritis to each other and to necrotizing vasculitis. Am. J. Med., *47*:23–35, 1969.
69. Sokoloff, L., and Bunim, J.J.: Vascular lesions in rheumatoid arthritis. J. Chronic Dis., *5*:668–687, 1957.
70. Brouet, J.C., et al.: The occurrence and nature of precipitating antibodies in anti-DNA sera. Clin. Immunol. Immunopathol., *2*:310–324, 1974.
71. Kemper, J.W., Baggenstoss, A.H., and Slocumb, C.H.: The relationship of therapy with cortisone to the incidence of vascular lesions in rheumatoid arthritis. Ann. Intern. Med., *46*:831–851, 1957.
72. Schmid, F.R., et al.: Arteritis in rheumatoid arteritis. Am. J. Med., *30*:56–83, 1961.
73. Estes, D., and Christian, C.L.: The natural history of systemic lupus erythematosus by prospective analysis. Medicine, *50*:85–95, 1971.
74. Klemperer, P., Pollack, A.D., and Baehr, G.: Pathology of disseminated lupus erythematosus. Arch. Pathol., *32*:569–631, 1941.
75. Mintz, G., and Fraga, A.: Arteritis in systemic lupus erythematosus. Arch. Intern. Med., *116*:55–66, 1965.
76. Conn, D.L., McDuffie, F.C., and Dyck, P.J.: Immunopathologic study of sural nerves in rheumatoid arthritis. Arthritis Rheum., *15*:135–143, 1972.
77. Grey, H.M., and Kohler, P.F.: Cryoimmunoglobulins. Semin. Hematol., *10*:87–112, 1973.
78. Gorevic, P.D., Kassab, H.J., Levo, Y., et al.: Mixed cryoglobulinemia: Clinical aspects and long-term follow-up of 40 patients. Am. J. Med., *69*:287–308, 1980.
79. LoSpalluto, J., et al.: Cryoglobulinemia based on interaction between a gamma macroglobulin and 7S gamma globulin. Am. J. Med., *32*:142–147, 1962.
80. Meltzer, M., et al.: Cryoglobulinemia—A clinical and laboratory study. II. Cryoglobulin with rheumatoid factor activity. Am. J. Med., *40*:837–856, 1966.
81. Golde, D., and Epstein, W.: Mixed cryoglobulins and glomerulonephritis. Ann. Intern. Med., *69*:1221–1227, 1968.
82. Shumak, K.H., and Rock, G.A.: Therapeutic plasma exchange. N. Engl. J. Med., *310*:762–771, 1984.
83. Greer, J.M., Longley, S., Edwards, N.L., et al.: Vasculitis associated with malignancy: Experience with 13 patients and literature review. Medicine, *67*:220–230, 1988.
84. McCombs, R.P.: Systemic "allergic" vasculitis. Clinical and pathological relationships. JAMA, *194*:157–567, 1965.
85. Sams, W.M., Harville, D.D., and Winkelmann, R.K.: Necrotizing vasculitis associated with lethal reticuloendothelial diseases. Br. J. Dermatol., *80*:555–567, 1968.
86. Copeman, P.W.M., and Ryan, T.J.: The problems of classification of cutaneous angiitis with reference to histopathology and pathogenesis. Br. J. Dermatol., *81*:2–14, 1970.
87. Hughes, G.R.V., et al.: Polyarteritis nodosa, hairy cell leukemia. Lancet, *1*:678–681, 1978.

88. Goedert, J.J., et al.: Polyarteritis nodosa, hairy cell leukemia and splenosis. JAMA, *71*:323–326, 1981.
89. Rewcastle, N.B., and Tom, M.I.: Non-infectious granulomatous angiitis of the nervous system associated with Hodgkin's disease. J. Neurol. Neurosurg. Psychiatry, *25*:52–58, 1962.
90. Leonhardt, E.T.G., and Kullenberg, K.P.G.: Bilateral atrial myxomas with multiple arterial aneurysms—A syndrome mimicking polyarteritis nodosa. Am. J. Med., *62*:792–794, 1977.
91. Burton, C., and Johnston, J.: Multiple cerebral aneurysms and cardiac myxoma. N. Engl. J. Med., *282*:35–37, 1970.
92. Price, D.L., et al.: Cardiac myxoma. A clinicopathologic and angiographic study. Arch. Neurol., *23*:558–567, 1970.
93. Huston, K.A., et al.: Left atrial myxoma simulating peripheral vasculitis. Mayo Clin. Proc., *53*:752–756, 1978.
94. Wolff, S.M., et al.: Wegener's granulomatosis. Ann. Intern. Med., *81*:523–525, 1974.
95. Maquire, R., et al.: Unusual radiographic findings of Wegener's granulomatosis. AJR, *130*:133–138, 1978.
96. Rosenberg, D.M., et al.: Functional correlates of lung involvement in Wegener's granulomatosis. Am. J. Med., *69*:387–394, 1980.
97. Fauci, A.S., Balow, J.E., and Wolff, S.M.: Effect of cytotoxic therapy on the renal lesions of Wegener's granulomatosis. *In* Proceedings of the Sixth International Congress of Nephrology. Edited by S. Giovannetti, V. Bonomini, and G.D'Amico. Basel, S. Karger, 1976.
98. Nölle, B., Specks, U., Lüdermann, J., et al.: Anticytoplasmic autoantibodies: Their immunodiagnostic value in Wegener's granulomatosis. Ann. Intern. Med., *111*:28–40, 1989.
99. Specks, U., Wheatley, C.L., McDonald, T.J., et al.: Anticytoplasmic autoantibodies in the diagnosis and follow-up of Wegener's granulomatosis. Mayo Clin. Proc. *64*:28–36, 1989.
100. Van der Woude, F.J., Daha, M.R., and Van Es, L.A.: Review: The current status of neutrophil cytoplasmic antibodies. Clin. Exp. Immunol., *78*:143–148, 1989.
101. Walton, E.W.: Giant-cell granuloma of the respiratory tract (Wegener's granulomatosis). Br. Med. J., *2*:265–270, 1958.
102. Balow, J.E., Austin, H.A., Tsokos, G.C., et al.: Lupus nephritis. Ann. Intern. Med., *106*:79–94, 1987.
103. Hoffman, G.S., Leavitt, R.Y., Fleisher, T.A., et al.: Treatment of Wegener's granulomatosis with intermittent high-dose intravenous cyclophosphamide. Am. J. Med., *89*:403–410, 1990.
104. DeRemee, R.A., McDonald, T.J., and Weiland, L.H.: Wegener's granulomatosis: Observation on treatment with antimicrobial agents. Mayo Clin. Proc., *60*:27–32, 1985.
105. DeRemee, R.A.: The treatment of Wegener's granulomatosis with trimethoprim/sulfamethoxazole: Illusion or vision? Arthritis Rheum., *31*:1068–1072, 1988.
106. Israel, H.L.: Sulfamethoxazole-tremethoprim therapy for Wegener's granulomatosis. Arch. Intern. Med., *148*:2293–2295, 1988.
107. Leavitt, R.Y., Hoffman, G.S., and Fauci, A.S.: Response: The Role of trimethoprim/sulfamethoxazole in the treatment of Wegener's granulomatosis. Arthritis Rheum., *31*:1073–1074, 1988.
108. Liebow, A.A., Carrington, C.R.B., and Friedman, P.J.: Lymphomatoid granulomatosis. Hum. Pathol., *3*:457–458, 1972.
109. Katzenstein, A.-L.A., Carrington, C.B., and Liebow, A.A.: Lymphomatoid granulomatosis: A clinico-pathologic study of 152 cases. Cancer, *43*:360–373, 1979..
110. Patton, W.F., and Lynch, J.P. III: Lymphomatoid granulomatosis: Clinicopathologic study of four cases and literature review. Medicine (Baltimore), *51*:1–12, 1982.
111. Lipford, E.H. Jr., Margolick, J.B., Longo, D.L., et al.: Angiocentric immunoproliferative lesions: A clinicopathologic spectrum of post-thymic T cells proliferations. Blood, *72*:1674–1681, 1988.
112. Colby, T.V., and Carrington, C.B.: Lymphoreticular tumors and infiltrates of the lung. Pathol. Annu., *18*:27–70, 1983.
113. Colby, T.V., and Carrington, C.B.: Pulmonary lymphomas: Current concepts. Hum. Pathol., *14*:884–887, 1983.
114. Colby, T.V., and Carrington, C.B.: Pulmonary lymphomas simulating lymphomatoid granulomatosis. Am. J. Surg. Pathol., *6*:19–32, 1982.
115. Fauci, A.S.: Granulomatous vasculitides: Distinct but related. Ann. Intern. Med., *87*:782–783, 1977.
116. Fauci, A.S., et al.: Lymphomatoid granulomatosis: Prospective clinical and therapeutic experience over 10 years. N. Engl. J. Med., *306*:68–74, 1982.
117. Israel, H.L., Patchefsky, A.S., and Saldana, M.J.: Wegener's granulomatosis, lymphomatoid granulomatosis, and benign lymphocytic angiitis and granulomatosis of lung: Recognition and treatment. Ann. Intern. Med., *87*:691–699, 1977.
118. Hamilton, C.R. Jr., Shelley, W.M., and Tumulty, P.A.: Giant cell arteritis: Including temporal arteritis and polymyalgia rheumatic. Medicine (Baltimore), *50*:1–27, 1971.
119. Goodman, B.W.: Temporal arteritis. Am. J. Med., *67*:839–852, 1979.
120. Huston, K.A., and Hunder, G.G.: Temporal arteritis: a 25-year epidemiologic, clinical, and pathologic study. Ann. Intern. Med., *88*:162–167, 1978.
121. Hunder, G.G., et al.: Superficial temporal arteriography in patients suspected of having temporal arteritis. Arthritis Rheum., *15*:561–570, 1972.
122. Klein, R.G., et al.: Skip lesions in temporal arteritis. Mayo Clin. Proc., *51*:504–510, 1976.
123. Healey, L.A., Parker, F., and Wilske, K.R.: Polymyalgia rheumatic and giant cell arteritis. Arthritis Rheum., *14*:138–141, 1971.
124. Chuang, T.-Y., et al.: Polymyalgia rheumatic. A 10-year epidemiologic and clinical study. Ann. Intern. Med., *97*:672–680, 1982.
125. Wagener, H.P., and Hollenhorst, R.W.: The ocular lesions of temporal arteritis. Am. J. Opthalmol., *45*:617–630, 1958.
126. Ninet, J.P., Bachet, P., Dumontet, C.M., et al.: Subclavian and axillary involvement in temporal arteritis and polymyalgia rheumatic. Am. J. Med., *88*:13–20, 1990.
127. Beever, D.G., Harper, J.E., and Turk, K.A.D.: Giant cell arteritis—The need for prolonged treatment. J. Chronic Dis., *26*:561–570, 1973.
128. Cupps, T.R.: Temporal arteritis. *In* Current Therapy in Allergy Immunology and Rheumatology-3. Edited by L.M. Lichtenstein and A.S. Fauci. Philadelphia, B.C. Decker, 1988.
129. McKusick, V.A.: A form of vascular disease relatively frequent in the Orient. Am. Heart J., *63*:57–64, 1962.
130. Nakao, K., et al.: Takayasu's arteritis. Clinical report of eight-four case and immunological studies of severe cases. Circulation, *35*:1141–1151, 1967.
131. Vinijchaikul, L.: Primary arteritis of the aorta and its main branches (Takayasu's arteriopathy). Am. J. Med., *43*:15–27, 1967.
132. Fraga, A., et al.: Takayasu's arteritis: frequency of systemic manifestations (study of 22 patients) and favorable response to maintenance steroid therapy and adrenocorticosteroids (12 patients). Arthritis Rheum., *15*:617–624, 1972.
133. Ishikawa, K.: Natural history and classification of occlusive thromboaortopathy (Takayasu's disease). Circulation, *57*: 617–624, 1978.
134. Hall, S., et al.: Takayasu arteritis: A study of 32 North American patients. Medicine (Baltimore), *64*:89–99, 1985.

135. Schelhamer, J.H., et al.: Takayasu's arteritis and its therapy. Ann. Intern. Med., *103*:121–126, 1985.
136. Leavitt, R.Y., and Fauci, A.S.: Takayasu's arteritis. *In* Current Therapy and Allergy, Immunology, and Rheumatology-4. Edited by L.M. Lichtenstein and A.S. Fauci. Philadelphia, B.C. Decker, in press.
137. Giordano, J.M., Leavitt, R.Y., Hoffman, G.S., and Fauci, A.S.: Experience with surgical treatment for Takayasu's disease. J. Vasc. Surg., *109*:252–258, 1991.
138. Rowley, A.H., Gonzalex-Crussi, F., and Shulman, S.T.: Kawasaki syndrome. Rev. Infect. Dis., *10*:1–15, 1988.
139. Melish, M.E., and Hicks, R.V.: Kawasaki's syndrome: Clinical features, pathophysiology, etiology, and therapy. J. Rheumatol., *17*(Suppl. 24):2–10, 1990.
140. Melish, M.E.: Kawasaki syndrome: A new infectious disease? J. Infect. Dis., *143*:317, 1981.
141. Rauch, A.M.: Kawasaki syndrome: Issues in etiology and treatment. Adv. Pediatr. Infect. Dis., *4*:163–182, 1989.
142. Ichida, F., et al.: Epidemiologic aspects of Kawasaki disease in a Manhattan hospital. Pediatrics, *84*:235–241, 1989.
143. Patriarca, P., Rogers, M., Morens, D., et al.: Kawasaki syndrome: Association with the application of rug shampoo. Lancet, *3*:578–580, 1982.
144. Rauch, A., and Hurwitz, E.: Centers for Disease Control case definition for Kawasaki syndrome. Pediatr. Infect. Dis., *4*:702–703, 1985.
145. Levy, M., and Koren G.: Atypical Kawasaki disease. Pediatr. Infect. Dis. J., *9*:122–126, 1990.
146. Tanaka, N., Sekimoto, K., and Naoe, S.: Kawasaki disease. Relationship with infantile periarteritis nodosa. Arch. Pathol., *100*:81–86, 1976.
147. Kato, H., Koike, S., and Yokoyama, T.: Kawasaki disease: Effect of treatment on coronary artery involvement. Pediatrics, *63*:175–179, 1979.
148. Shulman, S.T., et al.: Management of Kawasaki syndrome. Pediatr. Infect. Dis. J., *8*:663–665, 1989.
149. Newburger, J.W., et al.: Treatment of Kawasaki syndrome with intravenous gammaglobulin. N. Engl. J. Med., *315*:341–346, 1986.
150. Nagashima, M., Matsushima, M., Matsuoka, H., et al.: High-dose gammaglobulin therapy for Kawasaki disease. J. Pediatr., *110*:710–712, 1987.
151. Furusho, K., et al.: High dose intravenous gammaglobulin for Kawasaki disease. Lancet, *2*:1055–1057, 1984.
152. American Academy of Pediatrics: Intravenous γ-globulin use in children with Kawasaki disease. Pediatrics, *82*:122–123, 1988.
153. Cupps, T.R., Moore, P.M., and Fauci, A.S.: Isolated angiitis of the central nervous system. Prospective diagnostic and therapeutic considerations. Am. J. Med., *74*:97–105, 1983.
154. Calabrese, L.H., and Mallek, J.A.: Primary angiitis of the central nervous system: Report of 8 new cases, review of the literature, and proposal for diagnostic criteria. Medicine, *67*:20–39, 1988.
155. Moore, P.M.: Diagnosis and management of isolated angiitis of the central nervous system. Neurology, *39*:167–173, 1989.
156. Stein, R.L., et al.: Cerebral angiography as a guide for therapy in isolated central nervous system vasculitis. JAMA, *257*:2193–2195, 1987.
157. O'Duffy, J.D., Carney, J.A., and Deodhar, S.: Behçet's disease. Report of 10 cases, 3 with new manifestations. Ann. Intern. Med., *75*:561–570, 1971.
158. O'Duffy, J.D.: Behçet's syndrome. *In* Current Therapy in Allergy, Immunology and Rheumatology-3. Edited by L.M. Licthenstein and A.S. Fauci. Philadelphia, B.C. Decker, 1988.
159. Masuda, K., Nakajima, A., Urayama, A., et al.: Double-masked trial of cyclosporine versus colchicine and long-term open study of cyclosporin in Behçet's disease. Lancet, *1, 8647*:1093–1096, 1989.
160. Yazici, H., et al.: A controlled trial of azathioprine in Behçet's disease. N. Engl. J. Med., *322*:281–285, 1990.
161. Lie, J.T.: The rise and fall and resurgence of thromboangiitis obliterans (Buerger's disease). Acta Pathol. Jpn., *39*:153–158, 1989.
162. Leavitt, R.Y., Bressler, P.R., and Fauci, A.S.: Buerger's disease in a young women. Am. J. Med., *80*:1003–1005, 1986.
163. Lie, J.T.: Thromboangiitis obliterans (Buerger's disease) in women. Medicine (Baltimore), *66*:65–72, 1987.
164. Williams, G.: Recent views on Buerger's disease. J. Clin. Pathol., *22*:573–578, 1969.
165. Hill, G.L.: A rational basis for management of patients with the Buerger syndrome. Br. J. Surg., *61*:476–481, 1974.
166. Shionoya, S., et al.: Diagnosis, pathology, and treatment of Buerger's disease. Surgery, *75*:195–199, 1974.
167. Blomgren, S.E.: Erythema nodosum. Semin. Arthritis. Rheum., *4*:1–24, 1974.
168. Winkelman, R.K., and Förstrom, L.: New observations in the histopathology of erythema nodosum. J. Invest. Dermatol., *65*:441–446, 1975.
169. Katz, P., et al.: Erythema elevatum diutinum: Skin and systemic manifestations, immunologic studies, and successful treatment with dapsone. Medicine (Baltimore), *56*:443–455, 1977.
170. Cheson, B.D., Bluming, A.Z., and Alroy, J.: Cogan's syndrome: A systemic vasculitis. Am. J. Med., *60*:549–555, 1976.
171. Miller, S.J.H.: Clinical Ophthalmology. Bristol, Wright, 1987.
172. Thaell, J.F., and Save, G.L.: Giant cell arteritis involving the breasts. J. Rheumatol., *10*:329–331, 1983.

76

Pseudovasculitis Syndromes

LEONARD H. SIGAL

Vasculitis must be considered in the differential diagnosis of any patient with a multisystem illness. Conversely, some syndromes may present features compatible with vasculitis but are ultimately related to specific underlying diseases with known pathophysiology. The embolic phenomena of subacute bacterial endocarditis[1] or other infectious diseases[2] may present in such a fashion. Atrial myxoma and multiple cholesterol embolization syndrome (MCES) are less frequently encountered mimics of systemic necrotizing vasculitis.

ATRIAL MYXOMA

Patients with cardiac myxomas typically present with and are treated for cardiac disease. These patients, however, often have significant extracardiac manifestations, sometimes in the absence of findings referable to the heart. Uniformly fatal and usually undiagnosed ante mortem until the last three decades, myxoma is now a curable entity because of early diagnosis (by echocardiography and angiography) and effective treatment (open heart surgery).

Cardiac myxoma has been reported in stillborn infants and in individuals 95 years old, but its peak incidence is in the third to sixth decade, and mean age at occurrence is about 45 years.[3] A female predominance has been described. Familial cardiac myxoma has been reported,[3] including a description of a family with myxoma associated with lentigines and endocrine overactivity.[4]

The incidence of primary cardiac neoplasms in unselected autopsies is between 0.0017 and 0.33%; about 80% are benign. Myxomas account for about half of these, typically arising as solitary pedunculated tumors near the fossa ovalis. Approximately 70% are left atrial and 18% right atrial in origin.[3] Systemic manifestations of both left and right atrial myxomas are well described. Only about 12% of myxomas arise in the ventricles. Ventricular myxomas are more often sessile and therefore less likely to cause obstruction to blood flow.[3] Extracardiac manifestations of ventricular myxomas have not been documented.

The signs and symptoms of atrial myxomas include obstructive, embolic, and systemic or constitutional manifestations.[5] Congestive heart failure, systolic or diastolic murmurs (usually suggestive of atrioventricular valve dysfunction), chest pain, and dyspnea may be caused by tumoral obstruction of blood flow. Embolic disease occurs in about half of patients with left atrial myxomas, and the brain is affected in about half of these[6] (Fig. 76–1A and B). Neurologic manifestations include peripheral and cranial neuropathy, hemiparesis, seizures, syncope,[7] and progressive intellectual impairment.[8] Peripheral and visceral embolization also occurs.[6] Constitutional symptoms such as fever, weight loss, malaise, and fatigue are present in 90% of cases.[3] Isolated fever may result in evaluation of a fever of unknown origin.

In the absence of cardiac manifestations, diagnosis is often missed. Isolated fever may result in evaluation of a fever of unknown origin. Myxoma presenting with extracardiac manifestations may mimic rheumatologic or vasculitic syndromes (Table 76–1). Patients with myxoma can experience Raynaud's phenomenon, arthralgia or true arthritis, petechial and erythematous maculopapular skin rashes,[6,9] and finger pulp lesions.[6] The combination of embolic and constitutional findings may mimic endocarditis or the Libman-Sacks lesion of systemic lupus erythematosus.[6] Tender calf muscles and elevated serum levels of muscle enzymes may suggest polymyositis or dermatomyositis.[6]

Systemic necrotizing vasculitis was the initial diagnosis in 10 reported cases of myxoma;[6] findings in these

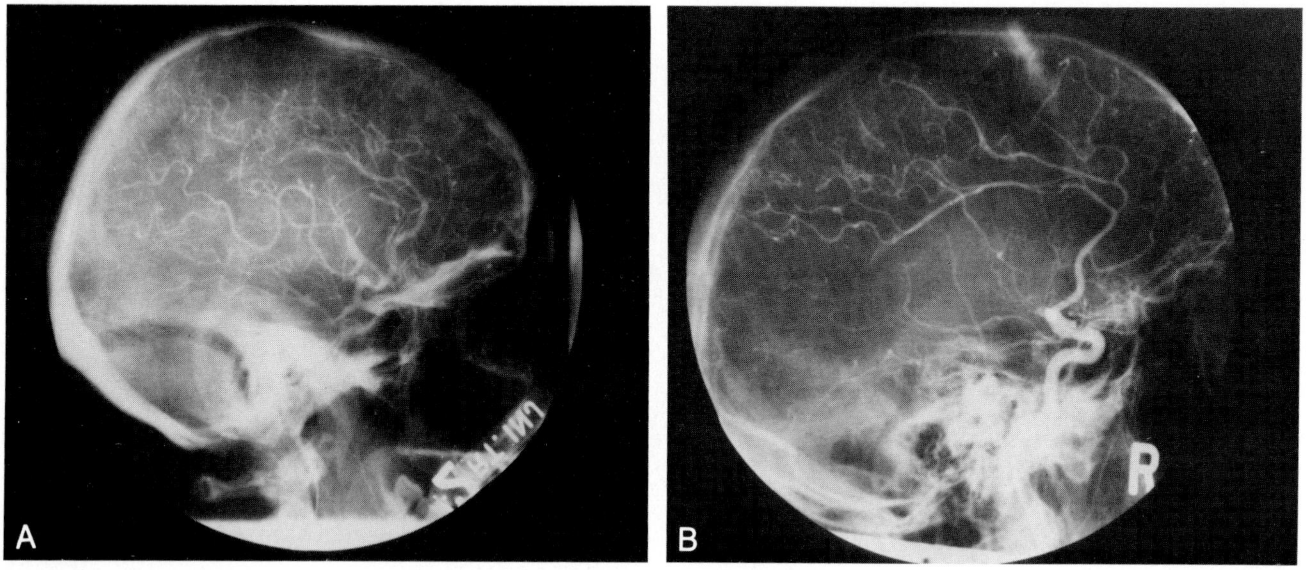

FIGURE 76–1. *A,* Right internal carotid angiogram showing occlusion of the middle cerebral and pericallosal arteries; left carotid angiogram (not shown) in the same patient showed occlusion of the posterior angular branch of the left middle cerebral artery. Echocardiogram was normal, but cardiac angiography showed a filling defect in the left atrium. A left atrial myxoma was surgically removed. *B,* Right internal carotid angiogram of a second patient showing a fusiform aneurysm at the bifurcation of the right middle cerebral artery (From Roeltgen, D.P., Weimer, G.R., and Patterson, L.F.: Delayed neurologic complications of left atrial myxoma. Neurology (NY), *31*:8–13, 1981. By permission of authors and editor.

patients included fever, weight loss, Raynaud's phenomenon, myalgia, arthritis, central and peripheral nervous system lesions, and pleural effusions. The systemic findings may suggest polymyalgia rheumatica or giant cell arteritis, and the importance of considering myxoma in the elderly has been stressed. The isolated central nervous presentation of myxoma[6,9,10] may simulate isolated central nervous system vasculitis (granulomatous angiitis of the nervous system[11] (see Chapter 77). There has been a report of the antiphospholipid antibody syndrome presenting with an intracardiac mass, thus mimicking a myxoma, itself a mimic of vasculitis.[12]

Laboratory abnormalities (Table 76–2) are nonspecific and include elevated sedimentation rate and C-reactive protein, leukocytosis (usually granulocytic), anemia (microcytic–hypochromic, or normocytic–normochromic), and abnormal urinalysis (microhematuria and proteinuria). Elevated levels of α-2- and γ-globulins are nearly universal. Polycythemia has been associated with both left and right atrial myxomas. Antibodies to double-stranded DNA[13] and antibodies capable of binding to heart muscle (but not to myxoma) have been identified. Hypocomplementemia, thrombocytopenia, consumption coagulopathy, and microangiopathic, hemolytic anemia have been described.[6] Liver function abnormalities, including frank jaundice, may occur more frequently than has been appreciated.[6] Angiography of the celiac, renal, and cerebral circulation may reveal aneurysms similar to those seen in polyarteritis nodosa[6] (Fig. 76–1A and B).

Cardiac angiography has been replaced by transthoracic echocardiography as the best diagnostic tool, although the latter may be falsely negative.[10] A recent report suggests that transesophageal echocardiography may be an even more sensitive test for myxoma.[14] The diagnosis also has been made by pathologic examination of muscle biopsy and embolectomy samples, retrospectively in three instances.[6]

The immunopathogenesis of the constitutional and laboratory findings in myxoma is unclear. Tumor necrosis or tissue death that was due to embolism is thought to cause fever and systemic symptoms. The hyperglobulinemia has been attributed to an immune response to polysaccharide antigens released from the tumor, which may continue even after its surgical removal;[6] liver dysfunction is said to be "on an immune basis."[6] Systemic autoimmune reactivity and circulating immune complexes have been suggested, but neither has been demonstrated. Myxoma cells have been shown to produce B-cell stimulatory factor-2 (BSF-2) or B-cell differentiation factor (BCDF).[15] It seems likely that the BSF-2–BCDF molecule is identical to interferon β-2;[16] thus, myxoma tumor cells may produce an immunologic mediator of its systemic manifestations.

Therapy consists of excision. Steroid therapy of cases mistakenly diagnosed as vasculitis has produced little or no clinical response[6] and does not substitute for surgery. Clinical and laboratory abnormalities usually resolve after tumor removal, but Raynaud's phenomenon may persist long after curative surgery.[6] Progression of cere-

TABLE 76–1. VARIOUS PRESENTATIONS OF CARDIAC MYXOMA

CONDITION MIMICKED	CLINICAL FINDINGS	LABORATORY FINDINGS
RHEUMATOLOGIC		
Connective tissue disease	Fever, weight loss, fatigue Arthralgia/arthritis Myalgia Raynaud's phenomenon Pleuritis Pericarditis Central and peripheral nervous system abnormalities Petechial skin rash	Elevated ESR, CRP Anemia Thrombocytopenia Coagulopathy Urinalysis: proteinuria, hematuria, hypocomplementemia Antibodies to double-stranded DNA
Polymyositis/dermatomyositis	Tender muscles Weakness Elevated CPK, SGOT	Elevated CPK, SGOT Biopsy revealing muscle necrosis and vasculitis
Systemic necrotizing vasculitis	Fever, weight loss, fatigue Arthralgia/arthritis Myalgia Central and peripheral nervous system abnormalities Petechial skin rash Elevated ESR, CRP	Elevated ESR, CRP Urinalysis: proteinuria, hematuria, anemia, microangiopathy Coagulopathy Liver function test Abnormalities Hypocomplementemia
NONRHEUMATOLOGIC		
Subacute bacterial endocarditis	Fever, weight loss, fatigue Peripheral emboli Petechial rash Arthralgia Myalgia Heart murmur	Elevated ESR, CRP Urinalysis: proteinuria, hematuria, anemia, microangiopathy Thrombocytopenia Coagulopathy
Thrombotic, thrombocytopenic purpura	Fever Peripheral emboli Petechial skin rash Central and peripheral nervous system abnormalities Urinalysis: proteinuria, hematuria, anemia, microangiopathy Coagulopathy	Urinalysis: proteinuria, hematuria, anemia, microangiopathy Coagulopathy

CPK = creatine phosphokinase; CRP = C-reactive protein; ESR = erythrocyte sedimentation rate; SGOT = serum glutamate oxaloacetate transaminase.

TABLE 76–2. LABORATORY ABNORMALITIES REPORTED IN CARDIAC MYXOMA

Elevated erythrocyte sedimentation rate
Elevated C-reactive protein
Elevated α-2- and γ-globulins
Anemia: normocytic–normochromic, microcytic–hypochromic, microangiopathic hemolytic
Polycythemia (with cyanosis and decreased arterial oxygen tension)
Thrombocytopenia
Leukocytosis (rarely eosinophilia)
Elevated liver function tests: SGOT, LDH, alkaline phosphatase, bilirubin
Elevated muscle enzymes: SGOT, CPK, aldolase
Hypocomplementemia
Antibodies to double-stranded DNA
Urinalysis: proteinuria, hematuria

CPK = creatine phosphokinase; LDH = lactic dehydrogenase; SGOT = serum glutamate oxaloacetate transaminase.

bral aneurysmal changes may occur after tumor removal,[10] suggesting that the aneurysms are due to metastatic myxoma rather than to an organizing thrombus.[6] Tumor recurrences may be associated with recrudescence of symptoms and new abnormalities of previously normalized laboratory tests.[6]

MULTIPLE CHOLESTEROL EMBOLIZATION SYNDROME

Ulcerating plaques found in an atherosclerotic aorta may release atheromatous emboli containing cholesterol crystals.[17] Larger emboli can occlude major arteries,[18] with loss of pulse, pallor, ischemia, and ultimate tissue death. MCES is due to the occlusion of smaller vessels (usually less than 200 μm) by showers of cholesterol crystals from plaques. MCES is therefore typically seen in patients with severe atherosclerosis, generally men in the sixth to eighth decade, but one report documents MCES in a 26-year-old.[19] Embolization may occur after a known event, such as abdominal trauma, aortic surgery, angiography, or Valsalva maneuver.[6,20] A "purple toe" syndrome has been described following the initiation of warfarin therapy.[18,21,22] As described by Feder and Auerbach, this includes (1) purple discoloration of the plantar surfaces of toes, 3 to 8 weeks after the start of therapy; (2) complete blanching on moderate pressure; (3) fading of the color after elevation of the affected leg, (4) pain and tenderness in the toes on palpation, and (5) waxing and waning of color over time without complete resolution.[18] A similar or identical syndrome can follow streptokinase[23] or tissue plasminogen activator[24] therapy. MCES may also occur spontaneously,[25] in which case it may present with the multisystem manifestations and laboratory abnormalities suggestive of systemic necrotizing vasculitis, giant cell arteritis, or polymyositis.[6] Transesophageal echocardiography may provide a more sensitive means of detecting protruding atheromatous plaques of the aortic arch, which may be an occult source of such emboli.[26]

Although the lower aorta is the most common source of the crystals that cause MCES, embolization occurs throughout the body. The most obvious lesions are cutaneous (Fig. 76–2A and B). Autopsy studies have demonstrated evidence of cholesterol crystals embolizing to the kidney, pancreas, spleen, thyroid, adrenal, liver, gastrointestinal tract, gallbladder, brain, spinal cord, bone marrow, and heart.[27] These emboli are capable of causing clinically significant damage to many of these organs (Table 76–3). Peripheral pulses are typically intact.

It may be difficult to distinguish the clinical manifestations of necrotizing vasculitis from those of MCES. Fever, weight loss, and fatigue are common in both. Livedo reticularis is seen in about 50% of patients with MCES[28] attributed to incomplete blockage of the arteries supplying the skin[29] and may be preceded by intense myalgia.[29] Petechial and purpuric lesions and localized skin necrosis are well described in both syndromes[6] (Fig. 76–2A and B). Peripheral neuropathy has been described rarely in MCES,[6] and mononeuritis is frequent in vasculitis. Retinal involvement in systemic vasculitis includes hypertensive changes, retinal artery occlusion, and vasculitis, while in MCES bright orange-yellow lesions, consisting of embolic cholesterol crystals and known as *Hollenhorst plaques* may be seen at retinal arteriolar bifurcations.[19] With the exception of true arthritis, which is very rare in MCES, all of the clinical manifestations of polyarteritis frequently accompany MCES.

Central nervous system deficits, including cranial nerve palsies, hemiparesis, dysphasia, blindness, cerebrovascular accidents, and declining mental function[6] may occur in MCES.

Sneddon's syndrome is a progressive, noninflammatory arteriopathy affecting medium-sized vessels. Intimal hyperplasia, adventitial fibrosis, irregularities of the internal elastic lamella, and thrombosis are seen in biopsies of affected vessels, not atherosclerosis.[30,31] Its pathogenesis is obscure and treatment unsuccessful,[31] but the syndrome may mimic MCES or vasculitis. Some of these patients have circulating anticardiolipin antibodies, and a pathogenetic relationship between these antibodies and the vasculopathy has been suggested.[32,33]

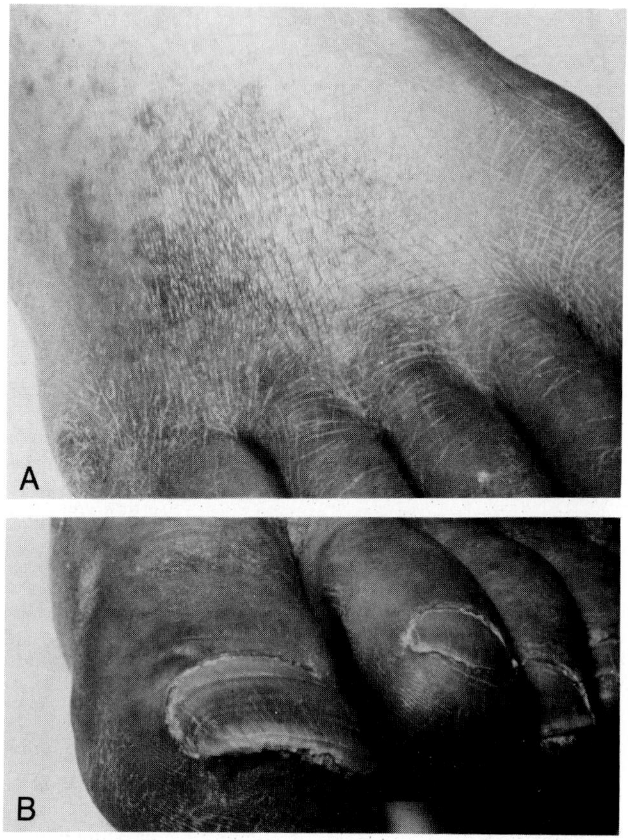

FIGURE 76–2. *A,* Purpuric rash over dorsum of affected foot. *B,* Purplish discoloration is seen at the tips of the first and second toes. (From Young, D.K., Burton, M.F., and Herman, J.F.: Multiple cholesterol emboli syndrome simulating systemic necrotizing vasculitis. J. Rheumatol., *13*:423–426, 1986. By permission of authors and editor.

Elevated serum glutamic oxaloacetic transaminase, creatinine phosphokinase, and aldolase in the presence of painful muscles have led to the erroneous diagnosis of polymyositis. In this case, biopsy of a gastrocnemius muscle proved diagnostic of MCES.[6]

Leukocytosis, eosinophilia, and eosinophiluria have been reported in MCES.[6] Elevated erythrocyte sedimentation rate, frequently over 100 mm/hour, is the rule. Hypocomplementemia and thrombocytopenia have been reported,[34] although the former has been disputed.[35] In one report, three of four patients had antinuclear antibodies and hypocomplementemia, while three had a positive test for rheumatoid factor.[36] Cryoglobulins were weakly positive in the only two cases tested.[36,37] Consumption coagulopathy has also been reported.[38,39] Elevated serum amylase is often found, occasionally in the presence of clinical pancreatitis.[6]

TABLE 76–3. MANIFESTATIONS OF MULTIPLE CHOLESTEROL EMBOLIZATION SYNDROME

NEURAL
Amaurosis fugax
Myelopathy
Stroke
Peripheral neuropathy
CARDIOVASCULAR
Myocardial infarction—with or without preceding history of angina
GASTROINTESTINAL
Abdominal pain with gastrointestinal bleeding
Bowel infarction
Pancreatitis
RENAL
Progressive renal failure—with or without proteinuria
Hypertension
Necrotizing glomerulonephritis
DERMAL
Isolated "purple toes" or "purple toes" with abdominal aortic aneurysm
Gangrene
Skin
Penis and scrotum
Petechial and purpuric lesions; livedo reticularis
MUSCULAR
Tender myalgia
SYSTEMIC
Giant cell arteritis
Systemic necrotizing vasculitis

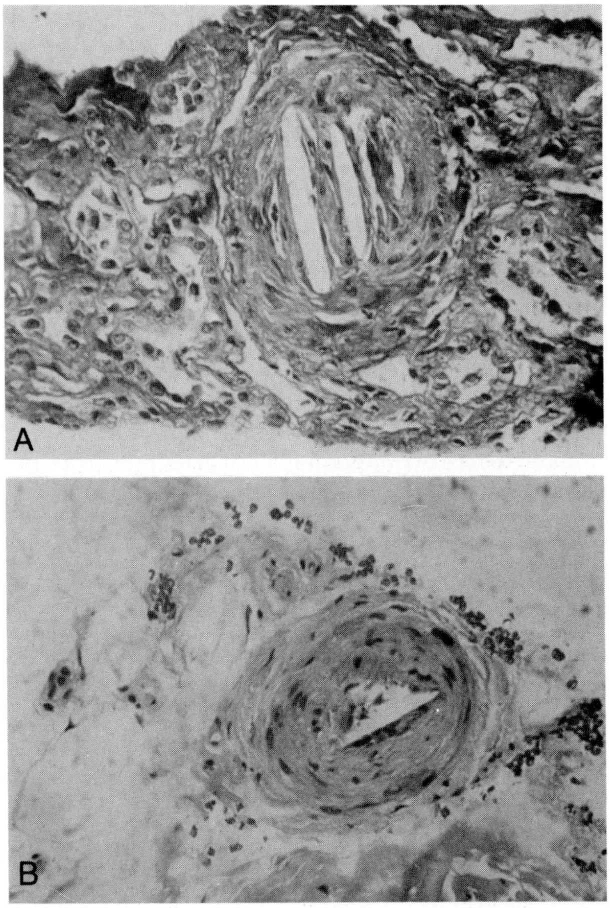

FIGURE 76–3. *A*, Histologic section of a skin biopsy from affected foot showing recent hemorrhage and a subcutaneous arteriole with medial thickening containing a cholesterol cleft (hematoxylin and eosin stained, magnification 320×). *B*, Histologic section of a renal biopsy showing luminal obstruction of an interlobular artery with intimal fibroblastic proliferation surrounding cholesterol clefts (trichrome stained, magnification 320×). (From Young, D.K., Burton, M.F., and Herman, J.F.: Multiple cholesterol emboli syndrome simulating systemic necrotizing vasculitis. J. Rheumatol., *13*:423–426, 1986. By permission of authors and editor.

Proteinuria is common, but hematuria and red blood cells casts have not been reported.[6] Rapidly progressive renal failure is the exception in MCES, but slow deterioration of renal function occurring approximately 2 weeks after embolization is common.[17] Renal failure is often severe and irreversible, but it may be mild and can resolve spontaneously.[6,17,33] The renal failure of MCES must be differentiated from possible renal failure that is due to the contrast dyes.[40]

Diagnosis is usually made by muscle (quadriceps or gastrocnemius), kidney, or skin biopsy[6] (Fig. 76–3A). Biopsy of other affected tissues, such as bone marrow and jejunum, have also been diagnostic. Routine tissue fixation dissolves the cholesterol crystals, leaving "clefts" in the tissue as evidence of the presence of crystal emboli[19,25] (Fig. 76–3B). Early lesions may have eosinophils as part of the cellular infiltrate. In properly fixed biopsy specimens, crystals, or collections of crystals, are surrounded by macrophages and foreign body giant cells.[6] Biopsies of older lesions may reveal only intimal fibrosis without damage to the rest of the arterial wall.[6] In experimental models of MCES using human atheroma extract, the cholesterol crystals or "clefts" disappear after 1 month so that their absence in pathologic specimens probably does not rule out the diagnosis of MCES.[6] Within 1 day of embolization, a panarteritis develops; fibroblastic reaction of the intima and occasional giant cell formation effectively block the lumen within 3 days.[6] Vascular spasm may be a factor in diminished tissue perfusion, although one study suggested that spasm does not contribute to decreased renal perfusion in MCES.[41]

Bone marrow[37] and prostatic[42] samples have also demonstrated cholesterol clefts in affected individuals. Two renal biopsies in MCES revealed necrotizing glomerulonephritis;[43,44] in one case the linear distribution of IgG suggested the presence of anti-glomerular basement membrane antibodies.[44]

MCES has occurred coincident with heparin and/or coumadin therapy of between 3 weeks' and 3 months' duration[6,21,22] and after the start of streptokinase[23] or tissue plasminogen activator[24] therapy. The resolution of MCES after discontinuation of anticoagulants suggests that anticoagulant-induced thrombolysis may allow cholesterol crystals to be released from atherosclerotic plaques, causing MCES.

Cholesterol, atheroma lipids, and nonlipid atheroma

components have thrombogenic activity.[39,45] Atheroma contents are capable of activating complement[34,35] in the presence of immunoglobulin and an intact classic complement pathway.[46] Atheroma-activated complement (probably C5a) can cause aggregation of neutrophils, perhaps contributing to local endothelial damage.[46]

Therapy should be directed at removal of the atherosclerotic source of emboli.[6,17] Anti-platelet therapy, vasodilators, and low molecular weight dextran have proved ineffective.[6] Discontinuation of anticoagulant therapy seems well advised, as already noted. Corticosteroid therapy has been reported as being moderately effective or of no value, but exacerbation of MCES accompanied the discontinuation of such therapy in a case initially treated for presumed vasculitis, suggesting that corticosteroid withdrawal may be hazardous.[6] Aggressive diagnostic workup of suspected vasculitis with MCES in mind is suggested, especially in the elderly. The long-term prognosis of patients with MCES is unclear, but in one series with retinal atheroembolic plaques, 15% were dead within 1 year and 54% were dead by 7 years of followup.[47]

REFERENCES

1. Churchill, M.A. Jr., Geraci, J.E., and Hunder, G.G.: Musculoskeletal manifestations of bacterial endocarditis. Ann. Intern. Med., *87*:754–759, 1977.
2. Weber, D.J., Gammon, W.R., and Cohen, M.S.: The acutely ill patient with fever and rash. *In* Principles and Practice of Infectious Diseases. 3rd edition. Edited by G.L. Mandell, R.G. Douglas Jr., and J.E. Bennett. New York, Churchill Livingstone, 1990.
3. Wold, L.E., and Lie, J.T.: Cardiac myxomas. A clinicopathologic profile. Am. J. Pathol., *101*:219–240, 1980.
4. Carney, J.A. et al.: The complex of myxomas, spotty pigmentation, and endocrine overactivity. Medicine (Baltimore), *64*:270–283, 1985.
5. Markel, M.L., Waller, B.F., and Armstrong, W.F.: Cardiac myxomas: A review. Medicine, *66*:114–125, 1987.
6. Sigal, L.H.: Pseudovasculitis syndromes. *In* Arthritis and Allied Conditions. 11th Ed. Edited by D.J. McCarty. Philadelphia, Lea & Febiger, 1989, p. 2045.
7. Knepper, L.E., Biller, J., Adams, H.P. Jr., and Bruno, A.: Neurologic manifestations of atrial myxoma: A 12-year experience and review. Stroke, *19*:1435–1440, 1988.
8. Frank, R.A., Shalen, P.R., Harvey, D.G. et al.: Atrial myxoma with intellectual decline and cerebral growths on CT scan. Ann. Neurol., *5*:396–400, 1979.
9. Feldman, A.R., and Koeling, J.H., III: Cutaneous manifestations of atrial myxoma. J. Am. Acad. Dermatol., *21*:1080–1084, 1989.
10. Roeltgen, D.P., Weimer, G.R., and Patterson, L.F.: Delayed neurologic complications of left atrial myxoma. Neurology, *31*:8–13, 1981.
11. Sigal, L.H.: The isolated neurologic presentation of vasculitic and rheumatologic syndromes. A review. Medicine (Baltimore), *66*:157–180, 1987.
12. Leventhal, L.J., Borofsky, M.A., Bergey, P.D., and Schumacher, H.R., Jr.: Antiphospholipid antibody syndrome with right atrial thrombosis mimicking an atrial myxoma. Am. J. Med., *87*:111–113, 1989.
13. Byrd, W.E., Matthews, O.P., and Hunt, R.E.: Left atrial myxoma presenting as a systemic vasculitis. Arthritis Rheum., *23*:240–243, 1980.
14. Obeid, A.I., Marvasti, M., Parker, F., and Rosenberg, J.: Comparison of transthoracic and transesophageal echocardiography in diagnosis of left atrial myxoma. Am. J. Cardiol., *63*:1006–1008, 1989.
15. Hirano, T., Taga, T., Yasukawa, K. et al.: Human B-cell differentiation factor defined by an anti-peptide antibody and its possible role in autoantibody production. Proc. Natl. Acad. Sci. USA, *84*:228–231, 1987.
16. Sehgal, P.B., May, L.T., Tamm, I., and Vilcek, J.: Human β_2 interferon and B-cell differentiation factor BSF-2 are identical. Science, *235*:731–732, 1987.
17. Smith, M.C., Ghose, M.K., and Henry, A.R.: The clinical spectrum of renal cholesterol embolization. Am. J. Med. *71*:174–180, 1981.
18. Kempczinski, R.F.: Lower-extremity arterial emboli from ulcerating atherosclerotic plaques. JAMA, *241*:807–810, 1979.
19. Kalter, D.C., Rudolph, A., and McGarran, M.: Livedo reticularis due to multiple cholesterol emboli. J. Am. Acad. Dermatol., *13*:235–242, 1985.
20. Colt, H.G., Begg, R.J., Saporito, J.J. et al.: Cholesterol emboli after cardiac catheterization: Eight cases and a review of the literature. Medicine, *67*:389–400, 1988.
21. Feder, W., and Auerbach, R.: "Purple toes": An uncommon sequela of oral coumadin drug therapy. Ann. Intern. Med., *59*:911–917, 1961.
22. Hyman, B.T., Landas, S.K., Ashman, R.F. et al.: Warfarin-related purple toes syndrome and cholesterol microembolization. Am. J. Med., *82*:1233–1237, 1987.
23. Schwartz, M.W., and McDonald, G.B.: Cholesterol embolization syndrome—Occurrence after intravenous streptokinase therapy for myocardial infarction. JAMA, *258*:1934–1935, 1987.
24. Shapiro, L.S.: Cholesterol embolization after treatment with tissue plasminogen activator. N. Engl. J. Med., *321*:1270, 1989.
25. Darsee, J.: Cholesterol embolism: The great masquerader. South. Med. J., *72*:174–180, 1979.
26. Tunick, P.A., and Kronzon, I.: Protruding atherosclerotic plaque in the aortic arch of patients with systemic embolization: A new finding seen by transesophageal echocardiography. Am. Heart J., *120*:658–660, 1990.
27. Hendel, R.C., Cuenoud, H.F., Giansiracusa, D.F., and Alpert, J.S.: Multiple cholesterol emboli syndrome—Bowel infarction after retrograde angiography. Arch. Int. Med., *149*:2371–2374, 1989.
28. Deschamps, P., Leroy, D., and Mandard, J.C.: Cutaneous crystal cholesterol emboli. Acta Derm. Venereol., *60*:266–269, 1980.
29. Ho, S.W.-C., Thatcher, G.N., and Matz, L.R.: Reversible renal failure due to renal cholesterol embolism. Aust. N.Z. J. Med., *12*:531–533, 1982.
30. Rebollo, M., Val, J.F., Garijo, F. et al.: Livedo reticularis and cerebrovascular lesions (Sneddon's syndrome). Brain, *106*:965–979, 1983.
31. Rumpl, E., Neuhofer, J., Pallua, A. et al.: Cerebrovascular lesions and livedo reticularis (Sneddon's syndrome)—A progressive cerebrovascular disorder? J. Neurol., *231*:324–330, 1985.
32. Gratan, C.E.H., Burton, J.L., and Boon, A.P.: Sneddon's syndrome (livedo reticularis and cerebral thrombosis) with livedo vascultitis and anticardiolipin antibodies. Br. J. Dermatol., *120*:441–447, 1989.
33. Burton, J.L.: Livedo reticularis, porcelain-white scars, and cerebral thrombosis. Lancet, *1*:1263–1264, 1988.
34. Cosio, F.G., Zager, R.A., and Sharma, H.M.: Atheroembolic renal disease causes hypocomplementemia. Lancet, *2*:118–121, 1985.
35. Firth, J.D., North, J.P.: Does atheroembolic renal disease cause hypocomplementemia? (Letter.) Lancet, *2*:1133, 1985.

36. Leroy, D., Michel, M., and Mandard, J.: Association of disseminated intravascular coagulation and cutaneous crystal cholesterol emboli. Ann. Dermatol. Venereol. (Stockh.), *108*:665–681, 1981.
37. Cappiello, R.A., Espinoza, L.R., Adelman, H. et al.: Cholesterol embolism: A pseudovasculitis syndrome. Semin. Arthritis Rheum., *18*:240–246, 1989.
38. Lyford, C.L., Connor, W.E., Hoak, J.C., and Warner, E.D.: The coagulant and thrombogenic properties of human atheroma. Circulation, *36*:284–293, 1967.
39. Thurlbeck, W.M., and Castleman, B.: Atheromatous emboli to the kidneys after aortic surgery. N. Engl. J. Med., *257*:442–447, 1957.
40. Cronin, R.E.: Southwestern Internal Medicine Conference: Renal failure following radiologic procedures. Am. J. Med. Sci., *298*:342–356, 1989.
41. Zdon, M.J., Crawford, B., and Hermreck, A.: Renal function, microcirculation, and the role of PGI_2 following atheromatous embolization. Curr. Surg., *40*:209–211, 1983.
42. Knechtges, T.C., and Defever, B.A.: Cholesterol emboli in transurethral curettings: Report of 4 cases. J. Urol., *114*:102–106, 1975.
43. Goldman, M., Thoua, Y., Dhaene, M., and Toussaint C.: Necrotizing glomerulonephritis associated with cholesterol microemboli. Br. Med. J., *290*:205–206, 1985.
44. Hannedouche, T., Godin, M. Courtois, H. et al.: Necrotizing glomerulonephritis and renal cholesterol embolization. Nephron, *42*:271–272, 1986.
45. Jeynes, B.J., and Warren, B.A.: Thrombogenicity of components of atheromatous material. An animal and in vitro model of cerebral atheroembolism. Arch. Pathol. Lab. Med., *105*:353–357, 1981.
46. Hammerschmidt, D.E., Greenberg, C.S., Yamada, O. et al.: Cholesterol and atheroma lipids activate complement and stimulate granulocytes. A possible mechanism for amplification of ischemic injury in atherosclerotic states. J. Lab. Clin. Med., *98*:68–77, 1981.
47. Pfaffenbach, D.D., and Hollenhorst, R.W.: Morbidity and survivorship of patients with embolic cholesterol crystals in the ocular fundus. Am. J. Opthalmol., *75*:66–72, 1973.

77

Cerebral Vasculitis

LEONARD H. SIGAL

Central nervous system abnormalities are common in vasculitic and rheumatic syndromes. The underlying diagnosis can usually be made on the basis of the associated clinical and laboratory findings. Occasionally, however, the underlying disease is otherwise silent in a patient with only neurologic complaints. In this circumstance, the clinician must differentiate between a neurologic presentation of a systemic inflammatory disease and an isolated central nervous system (CNS) process. The systemic necrotizing vasculitides[1,2] and their CNS manifestations[3–5] have been reviewed. The purpose of this chapter is to discuss the clinical, laboratory, and pathologic findings of *isolated CNS vasculitis* (ICNSV, also known as *granulomatous angiitis of the nervous system*—GANS—or *primary angiitis of the central nervous system*—PACNS) and to compare it with herpes zoster ophthalmicus (HZO) with delayed contralateral hemiplegia, more properly known as *herpes zoster–associated cerebral angiitis* (HZO-CA). Other primary CNS vasculitides, the systemic vasculitides, and other rheumatic diseases that can produce CNS symptoms are also discussed briefly. These subjects have been reviewed previously.[6]

ICNSV is an angiitis, frequently granulomatous (thus GANS, the older name for this syndrome), affecting cerebral and spinal cord leptomeningeal and parenchymal small arteries and occurring in the absence of symptomatic systemic necrotizing vasculitis. In the past HZO-CA has often been considered a form of ICNSV/GANS. Post-herpetic angiitis superficially resembles the latter, but it is less severe, more limited in extent, related to a known pathogenic agent, and more likely to resolve. The differences in severity and extent of involvement help differentiate these two conditions.

CENTRAL NERVOUS SYSTEM VASCULITIS ASSOCIATED WITH SYSTEMIC VASCULITIS

Until recently, the diagnosis of CNS vasculitis in patients with known systemic vasculitis was often made clinically, without proof that vasculitis was actually the cause of CNS dysfunction. Because CNS dysfunction is often due to damage to other organs such as the lung or kidney in systemic lupus erythematosus, progressive systemic sclerosis, or rheumatoid arthritis rather than to vasculitis,[7–9] it is imperative that a more precise evaluation be completed. Angiography and biopsy are now considered essential for diagnosis and proper management.[9–11] The angiographic findings of cerebral arteritis include narrowing and dilatation of vessels, changes in blood flow, and associated masses.[10] "Vasculitic" angiographic changes can be seen in a variety of inflammatory,[10,11] infectious,[12] and noninflammatory diseases.[13,14] Angiographically diagnosed CNS "vasculitis" has occasionally spontaneously resolved in days.[15–17] Thus, biopsy is necessary to differentiate true vasculitis from vasospasm or other causes of angiographic changes.

ISOLATED CNS VASCULITIS (ICNSV)

ICNSV was first described as a separate entity by Cravioto and Feigin in 1959. Two cases described by Harbitz in 1922 in his review of cerebral arteritis are compatible with the diagnosis of its synonym, GANS. A review of the English literature in 1987 summarized 61 cases of GANS,[6] and 30 cases have been collected since then.[15,18–30] In 1987, 39 cases of HZO-CA were reviewed,[6] and 8 cases have been collected since then.[31–35]

The presenting signs and symptoms of these cerebral angiitides are usually nonspecific, often suggesting global CNS dysfunction. Confusion, headache, change in personality, paresis, cranial neuropathy, or loss of consciousness can suggest a variety of diagnoses at first evaluation; patients with ICNSV have been mistakenly diagnosed as having viral encephalitis, primary or metastatic tumor, syphilis, tuberculosis, sarcoidosis, or multiple sclerosis.

Reported cases of ICNSV are summarized in Table 77–1. Men outnumbered women by 4 to 3. The mean age was 43 years, with a range from 3 to 78 years. Presenting symptoms included headache (65%), weakness (45%), and confusion or "possible psychiatric disorder" (45%). Aphasia or dysphasia, nausea or vomiting, disorders of memory, lethargy, seizure disorder, or frank loss of consciousness were seen in approximately 15 to 30% of cases. Associated or antecedent disorders included hypertension, renal failure, diabetes mellitus, ileitis, upper respiratory infection, Hodgkin's or non-Hodgkin's lymphoma, and other malignancies in a small proportion of cases.

TABLE 77–1. COMPARISON OF THE CLINICAL FEATURES OF ISOLATED CENTRAL NERVOUS SYSTEM (ICNSV) AND HERPES ZOSTER–ASSOCIATED CEREBRAL ANGIITIS (HZO-CA)

	ICNSV	HZO-CA
Demographic Data		
Number of cases	91	47
Average age	43.1	60.3
Sex (male/female)	55/36	30/17
Clinical Features (%)		
Headache	65	11
Weakness	45	70
Confusion/psychiatric disorder	45	40
Nausea/vomiting	23	5
Aphasia/dysphasia	27	8
Seizure	20	6
Lethargy	18	14
Memory disturbance	17	4
Loss of consciousness	14	2
Incoordination	18	6
Numbness	9	6
Stiff neck	9	0
Physical Findings (%)		
Fever	20	6
Hypertension	16	4
Maculopapular rash	3	0
Hemiplegia/single limb paresis	48	72
Pathologic lower extremity reflexes	30	18
Funduscopic abnormalities	16	0
Ataxia	6	10
Tremor	2	2
Myelopathy	8	0
Cranial nerve disorder	29	45
II	2	8
III	5	15
IV	1	0
V	1	11
VI	8	11
VII	18	44
VIII	3	2
IX	1	0
X	1	2
XI	0	4
XII	0	8
Horner's syndrome	0	4

TABLE 77–2. COMPARISON OF THE LABORATORY FEATURES OF ISOLATED CENTRAL NERVOUS SYSTEM (ICNSV) AND HERPES ZOSTER–ASSOCIATED CEREBRAL ANGIITIS (HZO-CA)

LABORATORY TEST (% ABNORMAL)	ICNSV	HZO-CA
Increased erythrocyte sedimentation rate	62	30
Cerebrospinal fluid		
Normal	5	2
Increased pressure	65	33
Lymphocytic pleocytosis	75	95
Increased protein	65	63
Decreased glucose	28	7
Electroencephalogram		
Normal	33	14
Diffuse slowing	43	32
Diffuse slowing, unilateral predominance	14	2
Unilateral slowing	6	37
Diffuse slowing, plus focal abnormality	12	10
Focal abnormality	5	17
Other		
Brain scan abnormal	54	50
Brain computerized tomography abnormal	67	68
Cerebral angiography abnormal	82	95

Fever and elevated blood pressure were noted in about one fifth of patients; dermatologic abnormalities were described in only two cases. Neurologic evaluation was remarkable for muscle weakness in about one half of patients; pathologic lower extremity reflexes were elicited in most patients with lower extremity motor findings. Funduscopy revealed papilledema or vascular changes in 16% of patients. Cranial neuropathy, usually facial or abducens, occurred in 29%.

The erythrocyte sedimentation rate (ESR) was usually accelerated (Table 77–2). Serologies for syphilis were uniformly negative, an important finding because meningovascular syphilis can be clinically indistinguishable from ICNSV.[6,12] Cerebrospinal fluid analysis was abnormal in 95% of patients tested, usually revealing increased pressure and total protein, lymphocytic pleocytosis, and normal glucose levels (Table 77–2). Electroencephalograms were abnormal in 74% of the patients tested, usually diffusely slow, often with superimposed lateral or focal findings. Cerebral angiography, computerized axial tomography (CAT), and radionuclide brain scan were valuable, in that order, in identifying disease.

The angiographic images of the internal carotid artery and its branches are numbered, the lowest number

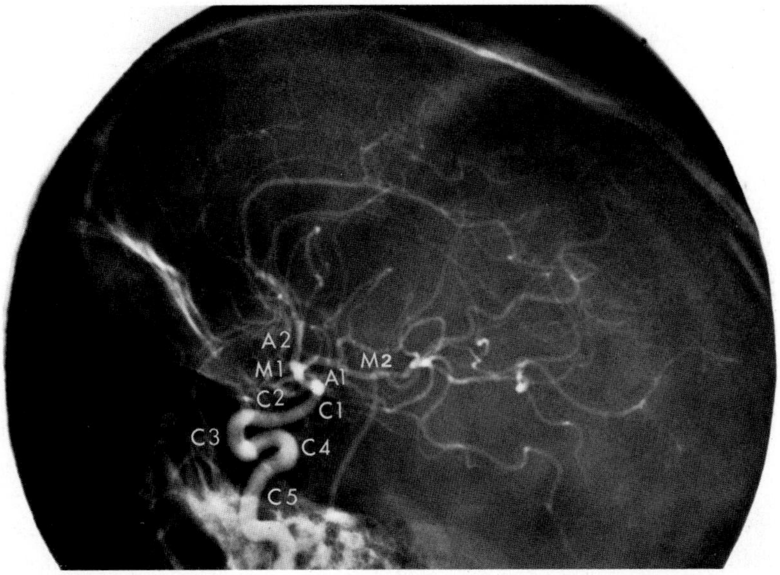

FIGURE 77–1. Angiogram of the internal carotid artery and its branches. The omega-shaped loop consisting of C2, C3, and C4 is called the carotid siphon. The internal carotid enters the skull at the carotid foramen, passes anteromedially, and then rises vertically (C5) to pass forward opposite the sella turcica (C4). The artery then passes upward within the dura (C3) and emerges below and medial to the anterior clinoid (C2) and gives rise to the ophthalmic artery. The Gasserian nucleus lies immediately adjacent to the siphon and to the initial branches of the anterior and middle cerebral arteries. The carotid then bifurcates (C1) to form the anterior and middle cerebral arteries. The anterior cerebral artery is directed anteromedially (A1) till it reaches the midline, where it turns upward (A2) to be joined by the anterior communicating artery. Thereafter, the frontopolar and pericallosal arteries arise. The medial portions of the frontal and parietal lobes and the corpus callosum are supplied by these vessels. The middle cerebral artery extends laterally (M1) and gives off three branches, which supply the basal ganglia, internal capsule, and lateral aspects of the frontal, parietal, and temporal lobes.

being assigned to the regions nearest the bifurcation of the internal carotid artery, the origin of the anterior and middle cerebral arteries (Fig. 77–1). Cerebral angiography in ICNSV reveals diffuse or localized abnormalities of large, intermediate, and small arteries in the distribution of several of the cerebral arteries (Fig. 77–2). These changes include beading, aneurysms, circumferential or eccentric vessel irregularities, and avascular mass effect. Magnetic resonance imaging (MRI) can be more sensitive than computerized tomography in identifying foci of infarction or edema, but there is still insufficient experience to identify the role of MRI in the work-up of a patient with ICNSV. None of the abnormalities seen with any of these tests is specific. Biopsy is the *only* absolutely diagnostic procedure.

Postmortem and biopsy examination with ICNSV reveals an inflammatory process of small arteries and arterioles (typically 200 to 500 μm in diameter) affecting parenchymal and leptomeningeal more than subcortical vessels (Fig. 77–3; Table 77–3). Multinucleate giant cells of the Langhans and foreign body type, granulomata, macrophages, and lymphocytes are present, often adjacent to a disrupted elastic lamella. Intimal proliferation and fibrosis are frequent. Relative sparing of the media compared to the other vessel wall layers is often cited in descriptions of GANS, in contradistinction to giant cell arteritis, which GANS resembles histologically.[6] Veins are affected about half the time, but usually far less severely than the arteries.

Significant vasculitis is rarely seen outside of the cranium, although spinal cord, temporal arteries, and cranial nerves are affected rarely. Eleven of the postmortem examinations showed pathology outside the nervous system, most notably in lung and kidney. In none of these cases were the lesions of any clinical significance (Table 77–3).

The early reports of cerebral vasculitis suggested a uniformly dismal prognosis, with death inexorably following diagnosis by 1 day to 9½ months (mean, 45 days; median 16.5 days). In more recent experience, the diagnosis of ICNSV has been made antemortem and there have been successes using high-dose corticoste-

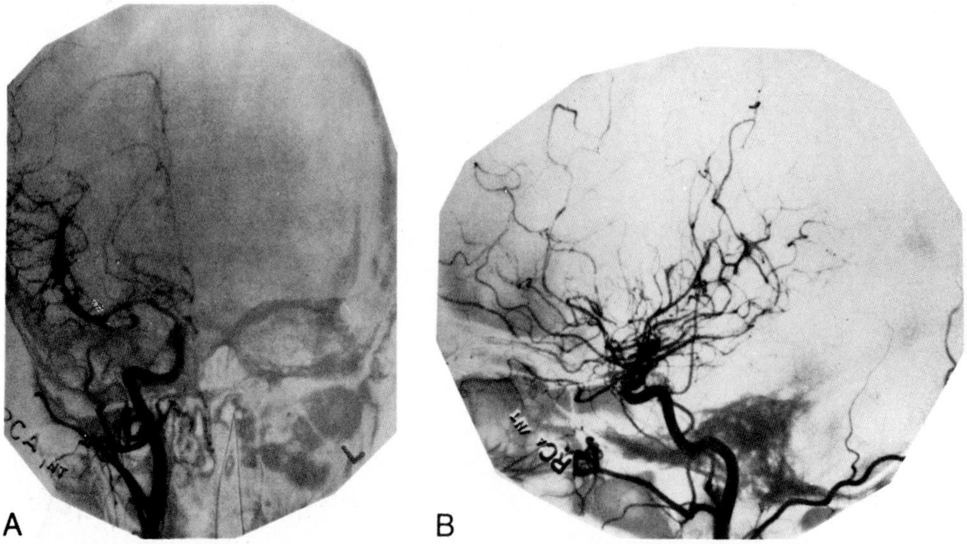

FIGURE 77–2. *A*, Right carotid angiogram (anteroposterior view) in a patient with isolated central nervous system vasculitis (ICNSV). Focal narrowing of multiple vessels in both the anterior and posterior cerebral arterial systems. *B*, Right carotid angiogram (lateral view) in a patient with ICNSV. Beading and multiple irregularities are seen both proximally and distally. From Sigal, L.H.[6]

TABLE 77–3. HISTOPATHOLOGY OF ISOLATED CENTRAL NERVOUS SYSTEM VASCULITIS (ICNSV) COMPARED WITH HERPES ZOSTER-ASSOCIATED CEREBRAL ANGIITIS (HZO-CA)

	ICNSV		HZO-CA	
	Biopsy (19)[1]	Autopsy (41)	Biopsy (5)	Autopsy (11)
Type of Cellular Infiltrate in Vessels				
Granulomata	5[2]	30		4
Epithelial cells	5	11	1	0
Multinucleate giant cells	13	40	3	4
Lymphocytes	14	39	3	7
Histiocytes	6	14		6
Type of Vessels Affected				
Arterioles	8	14	1	1
Small arteries	9	17	1	3
Medium arteries	1	9		2
Large arteries	0	6		2
Disrupted elastic lamella	5	15	1	5
Veins	3	20	1	0
Arteries more affected than veins		13/19		
Veins more affected than arteries		1/19		
Peripheral nerves affected		0		0
Spinal cord affected		7		
Cranial nerves affected		3		1
Non-nervous system foci of vasculitis noted at autopsy		11		0
Lung		7		
Kidney		7		
Coronary vessels		5		
Liver		3		
Lymph nodes		2		
Spleen, stomach, prostate, testis, uterus		1		

[1] Number of cases reported in each category

[2] Number of cases where each feature has been reported.

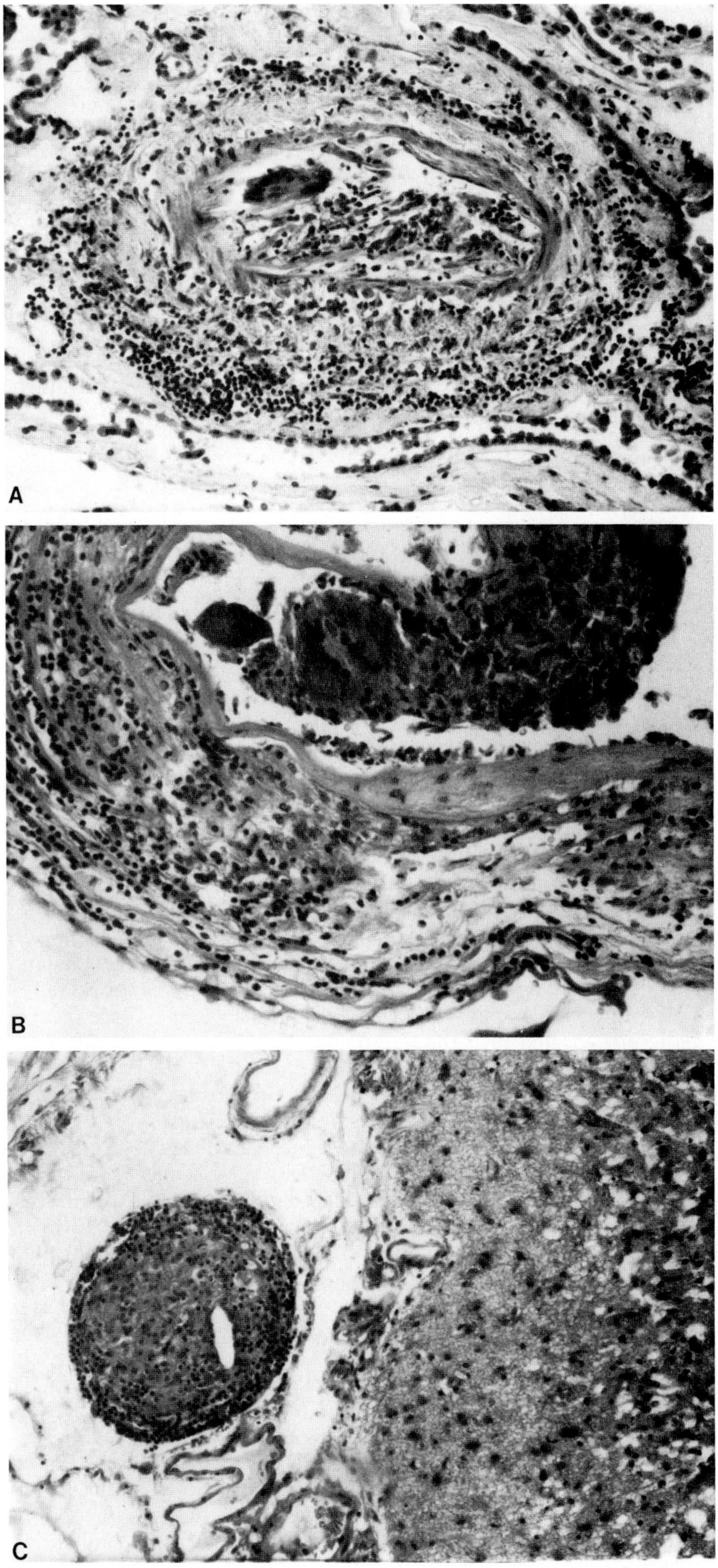

FIGURE 77–3. *A,* Photomicrograph of a postmortem specimen from the choroid plexus of a patient with ICNSV. Near occlusion of the vessel is secondary to subintimal reaction. Inflammatory infiltrate in the media and adventitia with lymphocytes and giant cell is seen (magnification ×205). *B,* Photomicrograph of a postmortem specimen from the subarachnoid space of a patient with ICNSV. A more fully developed mononuclear cell reaction is seen with a giant cell and more vessel wall damage than in *A*. Damage to the internal elastic lamella is seen (magnification ×256). *C,* Photomicrograph of a postmortem specimen from the cerebral cortex of a patient with ICNSV. A vessel with severe wall damage and near total loss of the lumen is seen. Damage of the external granular layer is seen with necrosis and reactive gliosis in the molecular layer of the cortex (magnification ×160). From Sigal, L.H.[6]

TABLE 77–4. OUTCOME OF PATIENTS WITH ISOLATED CENTRAL NERVOUS SYSTEM VASCULITIS (ICNSV) OR HERPES ZOSTER–ASSOCIATED CEREBRAL ANGIITIS (HZO-CA), IN NUMBERS OF PATIENTS

TREATMENT AND OUTCOME	ICNSV	HZO-CA
No treatment		
Fatal or progressive	38	14
No progression	1	8
Improved	2	18
Corticosteroids		
Fatal or progressive	4	0
Temporary response	4	1
No progression	4	0
Improved	13	2
Corticosteroids + cytotoxic agent		
Fatal or progressive	2	
No progression	3	
Improved	19	
No follow-up available	1	4
Total	91	47

roids (dexamethasone or prednisone) and cytotoxic agents (cyclophosphamide or azathioprine) (Table 77–4). In one case, radiotherapy and corticosteroid treatment of underlying Hodgkin's disease was associated with resolution of cerebral vasculitis.[6]

The cause of ICNSV is unknown. The relative sparring of media and intima suggests that the causative agent might reach the vessel from without, rather than hematogenously. Intracranial spread of an agent is compatible with the nonsystemic nature of ICNSV. The disrupted elastica might be the focus of inflammation, as has been suggested in giant-cell arteries.[6] An angiitis similar to GANS can be produced in turkeys inoculated intravenously with *Mycoplasma gallisepticum*, with *Mycoplasma* found attached to or in the cerebral arterial wall at the lesions.[6] Two patients with GANS had *Mycoplasma*-like inclusion bodies within giant cells in the vasculitis lesion, located near the internal elastica, but cultures for *Mycoplasma* were negative.[6]

Alternatively, a preceding viral infection could be the culprit. In one case of GANS, electron microscopic studies of glial cells revealed intranuclear virus-like particles in an aggregate of about 100 nm in diameter. A few appeared to be budding from the nuclear membrane, and some had electron-dense cores. No cytoplasmic particles were found (6). Complement consumption in the intrathecal space suggested a role for local immune reactivity in ICNSV.[20] Human immunodeficiency virus can produce CNS vasculitis histologically similar to ICNSV (see Chapter 122).[6,36]

There is certainly clinical (and likely etiologic) heterogeneity of the syndrome known as ICNSV.[6,25] As noted earlier, angiographic evaluation is a mainstay of the diagnostic work-up. In a review of 125 cerebral angiograms, Roubenoff and colleagues found it to be a very safe procedure, although there was a higher incidence of complications and death in patients whose angiograms were abnormal. The diagnoses in the 16 cases with abnormal angiograms were as follows: SLE (in 4), Sjögren's syndrome (1), giant cell arteritis (1), Takayasu's arteritis (1), cutaneous vasculitis (1), and ICNSV (8). Using a logistic model, the predictors of complications due to angiography were the presence of a previous stroke and an abnormal cerebrospinal fluid. Using similar analysis, predictors of an abnormality on angiogram were an abnormal fluid analysis and a history of a previous rheumatic disease.[37]

As noted above, angiography by itself is not sufficient to make a specific diagnosis. Angiograms have been described as normal in biopsy-proven cases of ICNSV.[15,19] On the other hand, biopsies of angiographically abnormal vessels have been reported as normal,[15–17] perhaps a testament to the patchy distribution of ICNSV, or an example of "benign cerebral vasculitis" or perhaps reversible vasospasm.[16] Thus, biopsy is a crucial part of the evaluation of an individual with isolated CNS disease due to presumed "vasculitis." Many reports suggest that the leptomeningeal vessels are often affected, so that *a combined cortical* and *leptomeningeal biopsy* offers the best chance of diagnosis. The diagnostic yield can be increased by using an angiogram to guide the biopsy to the affected area.[6] Temporal artery biopsy is not indicated in the diagnostic evaluation of likely ICNSV. An abnormal angiogram followed by a normal biopsy raises the possibility of vasospasm. In this circumstance therapeutic decisions should be dictated by the overall clinical status of the patient and the progression of the neurologic abnormalities.

HERPES ZOSTER OPHTHALMICUS–ASSOCIATED CEREBRAL ANGIITIS (HZO-CA)

In this entity a 4:3 male predominance is seen as in ICNSV, but the patients are somewhat older (average age, 60 years; range 7 to 96 years), probably because zoster infections are more common in an older population. Neurologic sequelae follow the HZO by 1 week to 2 years. There were five patients in whom the delays were 117 days, 4, 5, and 6 months, and 2 years; if these are excluded, the mean and median delay were both about 31 days.

The clinical presentation of HZO-CA differs from that of ICNSV, however. With the exception of more frequent and severe weakness, HZO-CA is usually a milder illness (Table 77–1). Only 3 of the 10 ESRs reported (30%) were accelerated. The CSF findings were also usually abnormal. Focal or unilateral electroencephalographic abnormalities were more common in HZO-CA than in ICNSV. The angiographic findings in HZO-CA are characteristic,[6] with segmental, unilateral involvement of vessels in the distribution of the middle cerebral artery, and occasionally of the internal carotid artery (Fig. 77–4). The results of tissue examination in 16 patients (5 biopsy specimens and 11 autopsies) revealed similarities with results of examinations of patients with ICNSV (Fig. 77–5).

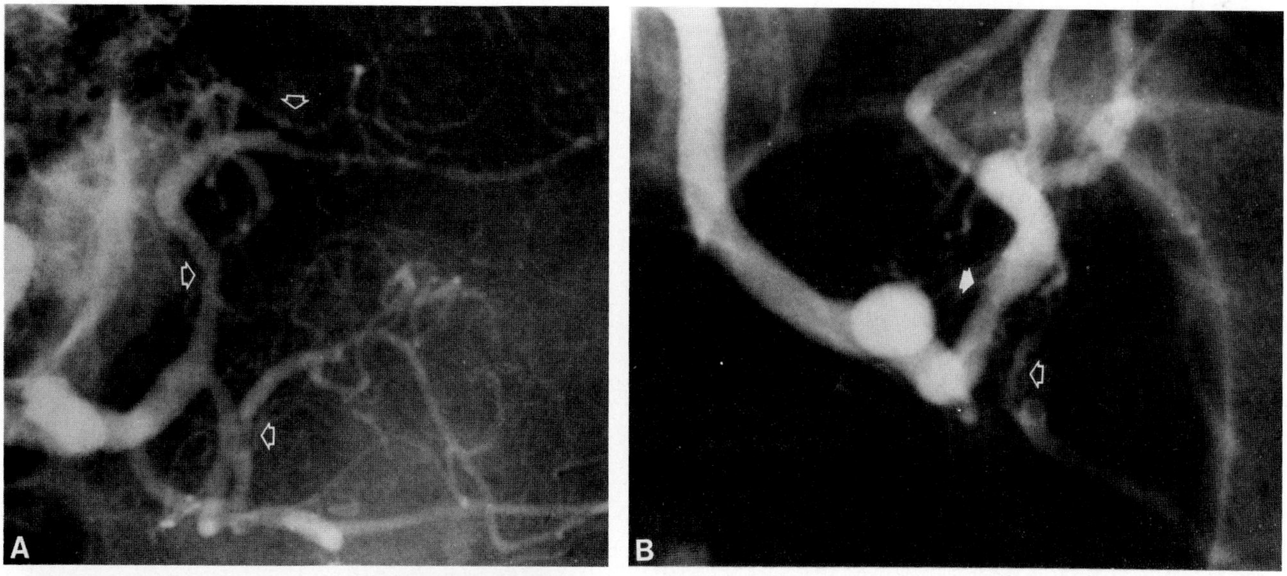

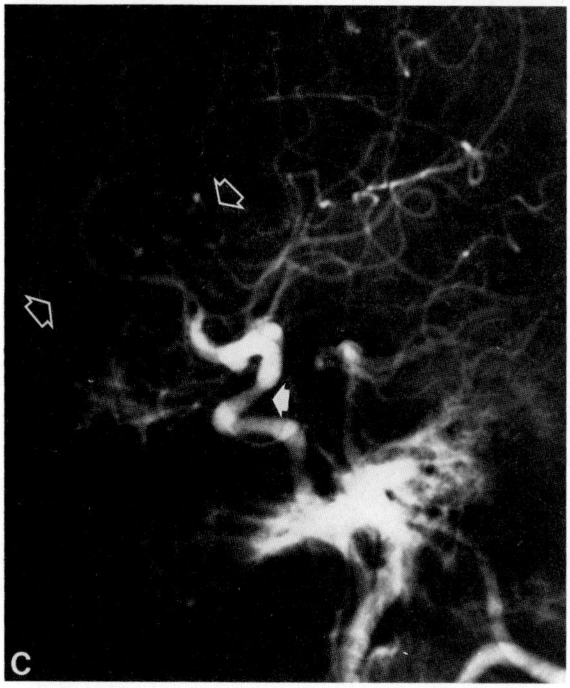

FIGURE 77–4. *A*, Left internal carotid angiogram (anteroposterior view) in a patient with contralateral hemiplegia following herpes zoster ophthalmicus. Note narrowing of the M1 portion of the left middle cerebral artery and the A1 portion of the left anterior cerebral artery (open arrow). Segmental beading is seen more distally. *B*, Right internal carotid angiogram (oblique view) in a patient with contralateral hemiplegia following herpes zoster ophthalmicus. Note narrowing of the right intracranial carotid artery (filled arrow) and irregularity of the A1 portion of the right anterior cerebral artery (open arrow). *C*, Right retrograde brachial cerebral angiogram (lateral view) in a patient with contralateral hemiplegia following herpes zoster ophthalmicus. Of note is narrowing of the right intracranial carotid artery in the region of the carotid siphon (filled arrow) and irregularities of the distal anterior and middle cerebral arteries (open arrow). From Sigal, L.H.[6]

In contrast to ICNSV, the prognosis in HZO-CA is encouraging (Table 77–4). Only two reported cases were treated with corticosteroids. Corticosteroids and acyclovir therapy was associated with improvement in one case. Corticosteroid therapy was thought to be beneficial in a second case, but death due to intracranial hemorrhage from a vasculitic aneurysm supervened. An additional patient was treated with aspirin, 500 mg daily, and dipyridamole, 75 mg t.i.d., with no disease progression.[6]

Herpes zoster–associated neurologic system disease includes the following entities: zoster radiculopathy, zoster myelitis, cranial neuropathy (including Ramsay-Hunt syndrome), zoster meningoencephalitis, and remote leukoencephalitis. The pathogenesis of HZO-CA is still unclear, and theories relating to this syndrome have been summarized elsewhere.[6] Virus can spread from the eye by intra-axonal or neuroglial pathways to the Gasserian nucleus, where it causes inflammation. Contiguous spread of inflammation can then engulf the overlying vessels, causing tissue damage downstream.[6] Virus-like particles have been described in smooth muscle cells in the walls of affected vessels (Fig. 77–6).

Although histologically similar, ICNSV and HZO-CA are clearly distinct clinical entities. ICNSV is diffuse, as seen both by angiography and in its clinical manifesta-

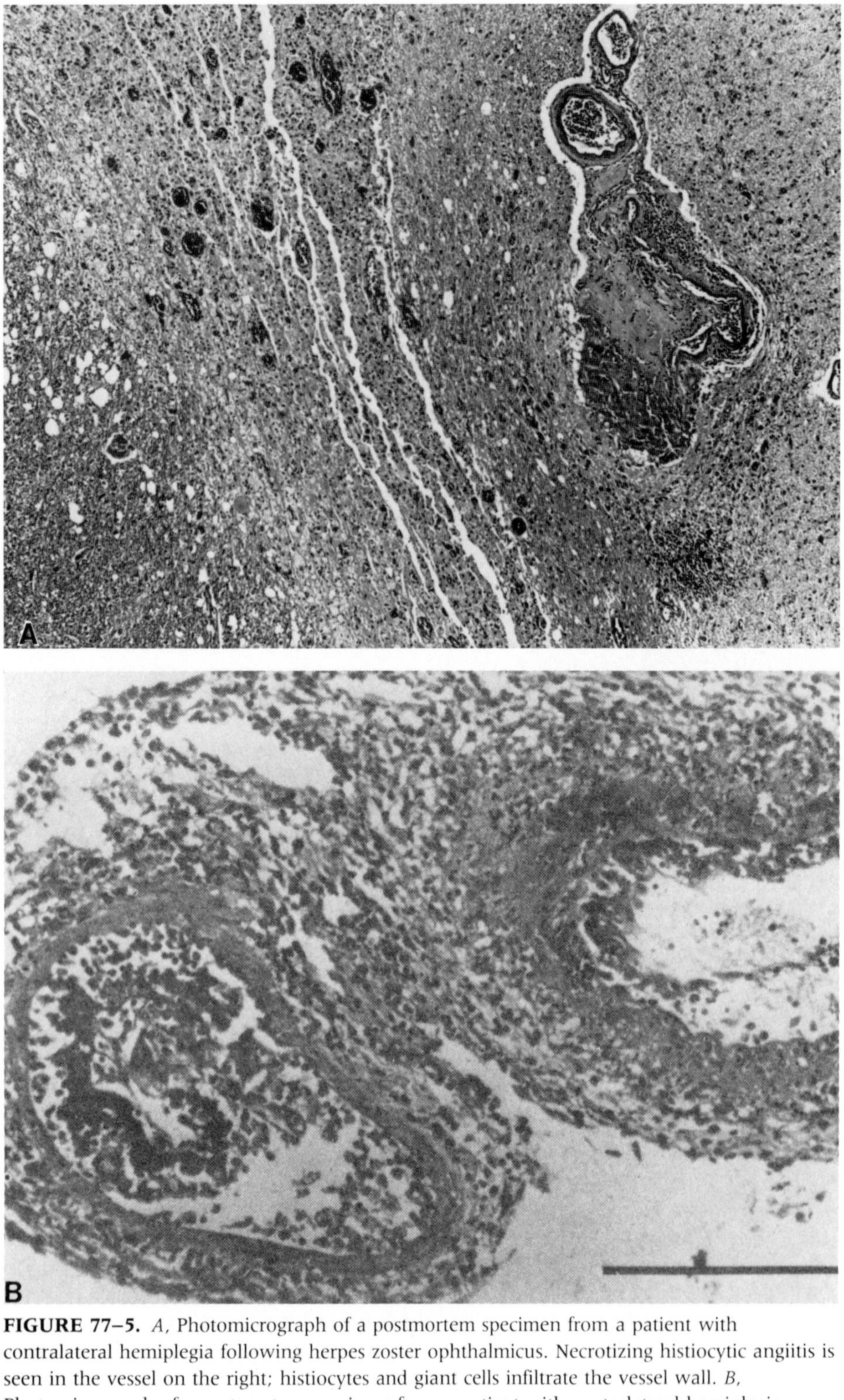

FIGURE 77–5. *A*, Photomicrograph of a postmortem specimen from a patient with contralateral hemiplegia following herpes zoster ophthalmicus. Necrotizing histiocytic angiitis is seen in the vessel on the right; histiocytes and giant cells infiltrate the vessel wall. *B*, Photomicrograph of a postmortem specimen from a patient with contralateral hemiplegia following herpes zoster ophthalmicus. Two small basilar arteries with heavy mononuclear and histocytic infiltrate. Granulomatous inflammatory process is segmental; fibrinoid necrosis is also seen involving the wall of one artery. From Sigal, L.H.[6]

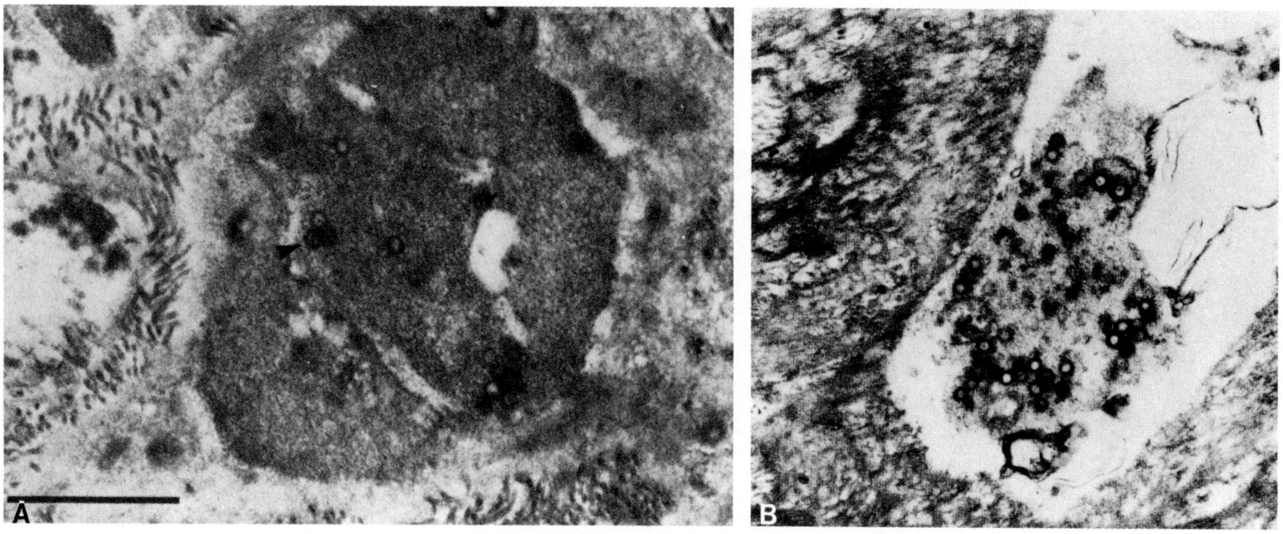

FIGURE 77–6. *A*, Electron micrograph of a postmortem specimen from a patient with contralateral hemiplegia following herpes zoster ophthalmicus. This area of granulomatous angiitis reveals intranuclear particles characteristic of herpes virus nucleocapsids, which are found in smooth muscle cells but not in endothelial cells. *B*, Electron micrograph of a postmortem specimen from a patient with contralateral hemiplegia following herpes zoster ophthalmicus. The nucleus of a smooth muscle is seen as a clear space, with darker cytoplasm around it. Hexagonal virions measuring 115 nm in diameter, consistent with herpes virus, are seen within an inclusion body composed of debris. From Sigal, L.H.[6]

tions, with a poor prognosis. Angiitis after herpes zoster ophthalmicus is localized, less severe, and has a somewhat better prognosis even in the absence of therapy. Also, the known antecedent infection with herpes zoster suggests the pathogenesis of HZO-CA, whereas the etiology of ICNSV remains completely unknown.

Many rheumatic diseases can damage the nervous system, usually in the setting of systemic disease; Table 77–5 lists these as three separate classes. The four primary CNS vasculitides are usually not associated with systemic disease (Table 77–6).

Cogan's syndrome is defined by episodes of acute interstitial keratitis or scleritis/episcleritis with vestibuloauditory dysfunction, usually in young adults.[38–40] Interstitial keratitis and vestibuloauditory abnormalities are found in other diseases including polyarteritis nodosa, Wegener's granulomatosis, and rheumatoid arthritis. Interstitial keratitis can be caused by congenital syphilis, tuberculosis, and viral infections, each of which must be excluded. A syndrome of subacute encephalopathy, sensorineural hearing loss, and retinal arteriolar occlusions in young adults due to occlusive nonvasculitic vasculopathy has also been described.[41–43] The presence of retinal and neuropsychiatric findings and the absence of interstitial keratitis or other inflammation of the anterior segment of the eye differentiates this syndrome from Cogan's syndrome.

Eales' disease is an isolated peripheral retinal vasculitis in young adults, often leading to visual loss.[44,45] It must be distinguished from the retinal vasculitis of other syndromes such as Wegener's granulomatosis, systemic lupus erythematosus, Behçet's syndrome, sickle cell disease, sarcoidosis, and tuberculosis. Retinal vasculitis

TABLE 77–5. VASCULITIS AND OTHER RHEUMATIC SYNDROMES MIMICKING ICNSV

Other primary CNS vasculitides
Cogan's syndrome
Eales disease
Isolated spinal cord arteritis
Systemic vasculitides that often affect the CNS
Polyarteritis nodosa group
Classic polyarteritis nodosa
Churg-Strauss vasculitis
Drug abuse–associated vasculitis
Hepatitis B virus–associated vasculitis
Giant cell arteritis
Takayasu's aortitis
Wegener's granulomatosis
Lymphomatoid granulomatosis
Henoch-Schönlein purpura
Cryoglobulinemia
Rheumatic syndromes associated with CNS disease due to vasculitis or other mechanisms
Systemic lupus erythematosis
Progressive systemic sclerosis
Mixed connective tissue disease
Sjögren's syndrome
Rheumatoid disease
Juvenile rheumatoid arthritis
Polymyositis/dermatomyositis
Behçet's syndrome
Lyme disease
Ankylosing spondylitis
Reiter syndrome

TABLE 77–6. THE PRIMARY CENTRAL NERVOUS SYSTEM VASCULITIDES

DISEASE	AGE AT ONSET (YRS)	SEX (M/F)	WITH CNS DISEASE (%)	ISOLATED OR PREDOMINANT CNS PRESENTATION	OTHER REPORTED CNS MANIFES-TATIONS	OTHER FEATURES OF THE SYNDROME	TESTS OF DIAGNOSTIC VALUE
ICNSV	30–50	4/3	100	Headache Cererovascular syndromes Confusion/psychiatric disorders Aphasia/dysphasia Seizures Ataxia Cranial neuropathy Transverse myelopathy		—	Angiography Leptomeningeal and cortical biopsy
Cogan's syndrome	15–30	1/1.2	2–5	Meningoen-cephalitis Seizures Ataxia Cerebrovascular syndromes Cranial neuropathy Organic mental syndromes	Inferior cerebellar artery occlusion Headache	Nonsyphilitic interstitial keratitis (90–100%) or scleritis/episcleritis Vestibuloauditory abnormalities (100%) Systemic necrotizing vasculitis in "atypical cases" (30%) Aortic insufficiency	Ophthalmologic examination Auditory evaluation
Eales disease	25–45	1.5/1	Rare	Optic disc vasculitis		—	Ophthalmologic examination Fluorescein-angiography
Isolated spinal cord arteritis	25–60			Myelopathy		Heroin addiction	Myelography Angiography Biopsy

rarely accompanies anterior uveitis.[46] Spinal cord arteritis, presenting with myelopathy, can be the first manifestation of systemic diseases, or can occur as isolated cord arteritis.[47–49]

The use of intravenous *methamphetamine*[49–51] or *cocaine*[52,53] can also cause CNS vasculitis in the absence of any systemic vascular abnormality. CNS vasculitis has also accompanied *ephedrine* abuse[54] and the use of *phenylpropanolamine*, a major ingredient in many over-the-counter diet pills, decongestants, and stimulants. Most of these patients took the drug at the recommended dose and had no systemic manifestation of vascular damage.[55,56] This syndrome could represent spasm rather than true vasculitis.[56]

CNS vasculitis associated with other rheumatic syndromes can occur with or without systemic vasculitis. A description of the primary CNS presentation of these syndromes can be found elsewhere.[6] There is usually evidence of systemic rheumatic disease or of systemic vasculitis to suggest the proper diagnosis. In few circumstances will there be no systemic extracranial manifestations, but cases of systemic lupus erythematosus, progressive systemic sclerosis, Sjögren's syndrome, Behçet's syndrome, cryoglobulinemia, and lymphomatoid granulomatosis have been reported without extracerebral manifestations. The diagnosis was sometimes delayed up to 5 years before the extracranial disease became manifest. In most circumstances, however, a complete clinical evaluation will reveal the underlying disease.

According to the data summarized here, a patient with suspected ICNSV should be evaluated quickly. If the diagnosis is confirmed by biopsy, treatment with high doses of corticosteroids is indicated. Cyclophosphamide also has been used in 24 patients, only two of whom deteriorated. The addition of a cytotoxic agent might be warranted, but further experience is needed before a definitive opinion can be rendered. The usually less severe, self-limited, neurologic sequelae in HZO-CA and its better outcome suggest that in most cases therapy is not necessary. In severe cases corticosteroid therapy might be indicated. Whether acyclovir should also be given remains to be investigated.

REFERENCES

1. Cupps, T.R., and Fauci, A.S.: The vasculitides. Major problems in internal medicine, vol. 21. Philadelphia, W.B. Saunders, 1981.
2. Fan, P.T., Davis, J.A., Somer, T., et al.: A clinical approach to systemic vasculitis. Semin. Arthritis Rheum., 9:248–304, 1980.
3. Cohen, S.B., and Hurd, E.R.: Neurological complications of con-

nective tissue and other "collagen-vascular" diseases. Semin. Arthritis Rheum., *11*:190–212, 1981.

4. Moore, P.M., and Cupps, T.R.: Neurological complications of vasculitis. Ann. Neurol., *14*:155–167, 1983.
5. Moore, P.M., and Fauci, A.S.: Neurologic manifestations of systemic vasculitis: A retrospective and prospective study of the clinicopathologic features and responses to therapy in 25 patients. Am. J. Med., *71*:517–524, 1981.
6. Sigal, L.H.: The neurologic presentation of vasculitic and rheumatologic syndromes: A review. Medicine, *66*:157–180, 1987.
7. Feinglass, E.J., Arnett, F.C., Dorsch, C.A., et al.: Neuropsychiatric manifestations of systemic lupus erythematosus: Diagnosis, clinical spectrum, and relationship to other features of the disease. Medicine, *55*:323–339, 1976.
8. Estey, E., Lieberman, A., Pinto, R., et al.: Cerebral arteritis in scleroderma. Stroke, *5*:595–597, 1979.
9. Bryant, G., Weinblatt, M., Rumbaugh, C., and Coblyn, J.S.: Angiographically proven central nervous system vasculitis: A review of fourteen cases. Arthritis Rheum., *25*:S15, 1982.
10. Ferris, E.J., and Levine, H.L.: Cerebral arteritis: Classification. Radiology, *109*:327–341, 1973.
11. Sole-Llenas, J., and Pons-Tortella, E.: Cerebral angiitis. Neuroradiology, *15*:1–11, 1978.
12. Vatz, K., Scheibel, R., Keiffer, S., and Ansari, K.: Neurosyphilis and diffuse cerebral angiography: A case report. Neurology, *24*:472–476, 1974.
13. Ferris, E.J., Rudikoff, J.C., and Shapiro, J.H.: Cerebral angiography of bacterial infection. Radiology, *90*:727–734, 1968.
14. Leeds, N.E., and Rosenblatt, R.: Arterial wall irregularities in intracranial neoplasms: The shaggy vessel brought into focus. Radiology, *103*:121–124, 1972.
15. Koo, E.H., and Massey, E.W.: Granulomatous angiitis of the central nervous system: Protean manifestations and response to treatment. J. Neurol. Neurosurg. Psychiatry, *51*:1126–1133, 1988.
16. Serdaru, M., Chiras, J., Cujas, M., and Lhermitte, F.: Isolated benign cerebral vasculitis or migrainous vasospasm? J. Neurol. Neurosurg. Psychiatry, *47*:73–76, 1984.
17. Beresford, H.R., Hyman, R.A., and Sharer, L.: Self-limited granulomatous angiitis of the cerebellum. Ann. Neurol., *5*:490–492, 1979.
18. Younger, D.S., Hays, A.P., Brusi, J.C.M., and Rowland, L.P.: Granulomatous angiitis of the brain: An inflammatory reaction of diverse etiology. Arch. Neurol., *45*:514–518, 1988.
19. Vanderzant, C., Bromberg, M., MacGuire, A., and McCune, W.J.: Isolated small-vessel angiitis of the central nervous system. Arch. Neurol., *45*:683–687, 1988.
20. Langlois, P.F., Sharon, G.E., and Gawryl, M.S.: Plasma concentrations of complement-activation complexes correlate with disease activity in patients diagnosed with isolated central nervous system vasculitis. J. Allergy Clin. Immunol., *83*:11–16, 1989.
21. Clinicopathologic conference. Am. J. Med., *85*:407–413, 1988.
22. Ibrahim, W.N., and Paroski, M.W.: Communicating hydrocephalus as a complication of isolated CNS angiitis—A case report. Angiology, *38*:635–641, 1987.
23. Cupps, T.R., Moore, P.M., and Fauci, A.S.: Isolated angiitis of the central nervous system: Prospective diagnostic and therapeutic experience. Am. J. Med., *74*:97–105, 1983.
24. DeReuck, J., Crevits, L., Sieben, G., et al.: Granulomatous angiitis of the nervous system: A clinicopathologic study of one case. J. Neurol., *227*:49–53, 1982.
25. Calabrese, L.H., and Mallek, J.A.: Primary angiitis of the central nervous system: Report of 8 new cases, review of the literature, and proposal for diagnostic criteria. Medicine, *67*:20–39, 1987.
26. Moore, P.M.: Diagnosis and management of isolated angiitis of the central nervous system. Neurology, *39*:167–173, 1989.
27. Matsell, D.G., Keene, D.L., Jimenez, C., and Humphreys, P.: Isolated angiitis of the central nervous system in childhood. J. Can. Sci. Neurol., *17*:151–154, 1990.
28. Zimmerman, R.S., Young, H.F., and Hadfield, M.G.: Granulomatous angiitis of the nervous system: A case report of long-term survival. Surg. Neurol., *33*:206–212, 1990.
29. Biller, J., Loftus, C.M., Moore, S.A., et al.: Isolated central nervous system angiitis first presenting as spontaneous intracranial hemorrhage. Neurosurgery, *20*:315–320, 1987.
30. Brown, D.G., Greer, J.M., Webster, E.M., et al.: Central nervous system vasculitis. Ann. Allergy, *58*:162–163, 209–212, 1987.
31. Tabbaa, M., and Selhorst, J.B.: Angiography in herpes zoster ophthalmicus and delayed contralateral hemiparesis. Neurology, *35*:442–443, 1985.
32. Blue, M.C., and Rosenblum, W.I.: Granulomatous angiitis of the brain with herpes zoster and varicella encephalitis. Arch. Pathol. Lab. Med., *107*:126–128, 1983.
33. Mackenzie, R.A., Ryan, P., Karnes, W.E., and Okazaki, H.: Herpes zoster arteritis: Pathological findings. Clin. Exp. Neurol., *23*:219–224, 1987.
34. Gasperetti, C., and Song, S.K.: Contralateral hemiparesis following herpes zoster ophthalmicus. J. Neurol. Neurosurg. Psychiatry, *48*:338–341, 1985.
35. O'Donohue, J.M., and Enzmann, D.R.: Mycotic aneurysm in angiitis associated with herpes zoster ophthalmicus. AJNR, *8*:615–619, 1987.
36. Scaravilli, F., Daniel, S.E., Harcourt-Webster, N., and Guiloff, R.J.: Chronic basal meningitis and vasculitis in acquired immunodeficiency syndrome—A possible role for human immunodeficiency virus. Arch. Pathol. Lab. Med., *113*:192–195, 1989.
37. Roubenoff, R., Healy, R.A., Wang, H., and Hellmann, D.: Central nervous system angiography: Safety and predictors of a positive result in 110 consecutive patients. Arthritis Rheum., *33*:S132, 1990.
38. Bicknell, J.M., and Holland, J.V.: Neurologic manifestations of Cogan syndrome. Neurology, *28*:278–281, 1978.
39. Cogan, D.G.: Syndrome of nonsyphilitic interstitial keratitis and vestibulo-auditory symptoms. Arch. Ophthalmol., *33*:144–149, 1945.
40. Haynes, B.F., Kaiser-Kupfer, M.I., Mason, P., and Fauci, A.S.: Cogan syndrome: Studies in thirteen patients, long-term follow-up, and a review of the literature. Medicine, *59*:426–441, 1980.
41. Coppeto, J.R., Currie, J.D., Monteiro, M.L.R., and Lessell, S.: A syndrome of arterial-occlusive retinopathy and encephalopathy. Am. J. Ophthalmol., *98*:189–203, 1983.
42. Monteiro, M.L.R., Swanson, R.A., Coppeto, J.R., et al.: A microangiopathic syndrome of encephalopathy, hearing loss, and retinal arteriolar occlusions. Neurology, *35*:1113–1121, 1985.
43. Susac, J.O., Hardman, J.M., and Selhorst, J.B.: Microangiography of the brain and retina. Neurology, *29*:313–316, 1979.
44. Hayreh, S.S.: Optic disc vasculitis. Br. J. Ophthalmol., *56*:652–670, 1972.
45. Scheie, H.G., and Albert, D.M.: Textbook of Ophthalmology. 9th Ed. Philadelphia, W.B. Saunders, 1977, pp. 32, 37, 204–207, 366.
46. Nolan, J., and Cullen, J.F.: Retinal vasculitis associated with anterior uveitis. Br. J. Ophthalmol., *51*:361–364, 1967.
47. Feasby, T.E., Ferguson, G.G., and Kaufman, J.C.E.: Isolated spinal cord arteritis. Can. J. Neurol. Sci., *2*:143–146, 1975.
48. Jellinger, K.: Spinal cord arteriosclerosis and progressive vascular myelopathy. J. Neurol. Neurosurg. Psychiatry, *30*:195–206, 1967.
49. Judice, D.J., LeBlanc, J.H., and McGarry, P.A.: Spinal cord vasculitis presenting as a spinal cord tumor in a heroin addict: Case report. J. Neurosurg., *48*:131–134, 1978.

50. Halpern, M., and Citron, B.P.: Necrotizing angiitis associated with drug abuse. AJR, *111*:663–671, 1971.
51. Citron, B.P., Halpern, M., McCarron, M., et al.: Necrotizing angiitis associated with drug abuse. N. Engl. J. Med., *283*:1003–1011, 1970.
52. Kaye, B.R., and Fainstat, M.: Cerebral vasculitis associated with cocaine abuse. JAMA, *258*:2104–2106, 1987.
53. Cregler, L.L., and Mark, H.: Medical complications of cocaine abuse. N. Engl. J. Med., *315*:1495–1500, 1986.
54. Wooten, M.R., Khangure, M.S., and Murphy, M.J.: Intracerebral hemorrhage and vasculitis related to ephedrine abuse. Ann. Neurol., *13*:337–340, 1981.
55. Glick, R., Hoying, J., Cerullo, L., and Perlman, S.: Phenylpropanolamine: An over-the-counter drug causing central nervous system vasculitis and intracerebral hemorrhage: Case report and review. Neurosurgery, *20*:969–974, 1987.
56. Forman, H.P., Levin, S., Stewart, B., et al.: Cerebral vasulitis and hemorrhage in an adolescent taking diet pills containing phenylpropanolamine: Case report and review of literature. Pediatrics, *83*:737–741, 1989.

78

Sjögren's Syndrome and Connective Tissue Diseases Associated With Other Immunologic Disorders

NORMAN TALAL

SJÖGREN'S SYNDROME

Sjögren's syndrome is a chronic inflammatory disease characterized by diminished lacrimal and salivary gland secretion (the sicca complex) resulting in keratoconjunctivitis sicca (KCS) and xerostomia.[1] The glandular insufficiency is secondary to lymphocytic and plasma cell infiltrations. The term *autoimmune exocrinopathy* has been introduced for Sjögren's syndrome.[2] Both a primary and a secondary form of this disease are recognized. Approximately 25% of patients with an associated rheumatoid arthritis (RA) are considered to have *secondary* Sjögren's syndrome; a small percentage may have another associated connective tissue disease. *Primary* Sjögren's syndrome is diagnosed in the absence of another connective tissue disease.

Sjögren's syndrome is particularly important among the autoimmune diseases for two reasons. First, perhaps 2 to 3 million individuals are affected in the United States, the majority undiagnosed. Second, in Sjögren's syndrome a benign autoimmune process can terminate in a malignant lymphoid disorder. Thus, it is a "crossroads" disease that offers potential insight into the mechanisms whereby immunologic dysregulation may predispose a person to a malignant transformation of B cells already involved in an autoimmune process.[3]

HISTORICAL BACKGROUND

A number of patients with various combinations of dry mouth, dry eyes, and chronic arthritis were described by European clinicians between the years 1882 and 1925. In 1892, Mikulicz[4] reported a man with bilateral parotid and lacrimal gland enlargement associated with massive round cell infiltration. In 1925, Gougerot described three patients with salivary and mucous gland atrophy and insufficiency progressing to dryness. Two years later, Houwer emphasized the association of filamentary keratitis, the major ocular manifestation of the syndrome, with chronic arthritis. In 1933, Henrik Sjögren[4] reported detailed clinical and histologic findings in 19 women with xerostomia and keratoconjunctivitis sicca, of whom 13 had chronic arthritis. In 1953, Morgan and Castleman[4] concluded that Sjögren's syndrome and Mikulicz's disease were the same entity.

ETIOLOGIC FACTORS

Autoimmune disorders have a multifactorial origin with elements of (1) genetic control related to the activity of specific immune response genes; (2) immunologic control exerted by regulatory T-dependent lymphocytes (suppressor and helper T cells); (3) possible viral influences, although such influences are not yet clearly established; and (4) sex hormone modulation of immune regulation in which estrogens enhance and androgens suppress autoimmunity.[5]

Sjögren's syndrome is one of several autoimmune diseases associated with the histocompatibility antigens HLA-B8 and HLA-DR3. This genetic predisposition is seen in several other organ-specific autoimmune conditions such as celiac disease, dermatitis herpetiformis, myasthenia gravis, Graves' disease, chronic active hepatitis, idiopathic Addison's disease, and insulin-dependent diabetes mellitus. Recent attention has focused on the HLA-D region, with the suggestion that gene interaction at the HLA-DQ locus is related to high-titered autoantibody responses and a more severe autoimmune disease.[6] There is also an association with HLA-DRw52 (previously known as MT2), which is a supertypic specificity encoded by an HLA-DRβ2 gene in linkage disequilibrium with HLA-DR3, -DR5, -DRw6, and -DRw8.[4] Primary Sjögren's syndrome in males is associated with HLA-DRw52 but not with HLA-B8 or HLA-DR3.[7] A familial relationship has been observed that focuses on immunogenetic and autoantibody factors.[8] Several spontaneously autoimmune mouse strains, particularly the MRL mice, have features of Sjögren's syndrome.

The presence of multiple serum autoantibodies is a characteristic feature of Sjögren's syndrome. Some of these reactions are organ-specific (e.g., against salivary duct epithelium), whereas others, such as antinuclear and rheumatoid factor (RF), are not. Two autoantibody systems, designated Ro/SSA and La/SSB, occur in the vast majority of primary Sjögren's syndrome patients and to a lesser extent in patients with systemic lupus erythematosus (SLE). A true Sjögren's syndrome/SLE overlap syndrome exists.[9] The antigens are RNA protein complexes. La/SSB binds to terminal uridine-rich regions of RNA polymerase III transcripts. Antibodies to gag proteins of human immunodeficiency virus-1 (HIV-1) have been reported in 30% of patients with primary Sjögren's syndrome[10] and also in patients with SLE in association with a particular idiotype.[11] A human intracisternal A-type retroviral particle has been seen when Sjögren's syndrome salivary gland homogenates are cocultured with a human T-cell line.[12] Transgenic mice containing the HTLV-1 tax gene develop salivary gland lesions resembling Sjögren's syndrome.[13]

The mechanisms responsible for the glandular destruction are beginning to be understood. There are numerous HLA-DR-positive glandular epithelial cells in the Sjögren's syndrome salivary glands[14,15] (Table 78–1). In close proximity to these HLA-Dr–positive epithelial cells are the lymphoid infiltrates in which activated T-helper cells are the most prominent population represented.[15,16] Activated T cells are also prominent in the pseudolymphoma lesions of Sjögren's syndrome patients with generalized lymphoproliferation.[17] There are fewer B cells, but these too are in an activated state and produce large amounts of immunoglobulin.[4] This seems particularly important in light of the subsequent development of B-cell lymphomas in 5 to 10% of Sjögren's syndrome patients, and the production of monoclonal immunoglobulins in the Sjögren's syndrome salivary glands.

TABLE 78–1. IMMUNOLOGIC FINDINGS IN THE SALIVARY GLANDS IN SJÖGREN'S SYNDROME

Many HLA-DR + glandular epithelial cells
Many T-helper cells expressing activation markers
Fewer activated B cells
Production of monoclonal immunoglobulins
Absence of natural killer cells

Natural killer cells carry the cell surface marker Leu-11b and are important for several immunoregulatory functions including natural host defense against malignancy. There is defective natural killer cell function in the blood of Sjögren's syndrome patients[18] and absent Leu-11b natural killer cells in the salivary gland lesions.[19] These results suggest that the salivary gland in Sjögren's syndrome may serve as an initial nidus for lymphoma development. This hypothesis is supported by an immunohistologic study suggesting that the myoepithelial sialadenitis of Sjögren's syndrome may contain areas of confluent lymphoid proliferation producing mostly monoclonal IgM/κ.[20] These lesions were considered "early lymphomas," analogous to carcinoma in situ, which after a variable latent period transform into true lymphomas. β-2-Microglobulin, a component of lymphocyte membranes that may play an immunologic role, is increased in serum and saliva of patients with Sjögren's syndrome.[4]

PATHOLOGIC FEATURES

The classic lesion is a lymphocytic and plasma cell infiltrate of salivary, lacrimal, and other exocrine glands in the respiratory tract, gastrointestinal tract, and vagina. Both major (parotid, submaxillary) and minor (gingival, palatine) salivary glands are affected. The term *benign lymphoepithelial lesion* has been used to describe the characteristic histologic appearance in the salivary glands. These lesions may be present without xerostomia and other features of Sjögren's syndrome. The earliest infiltrates may be scattered around small intralobular ducts. The histologic picture is varied and includes acinar atrophy, generally in proportion to the extent of lymphoid infiltration, occasional germinal center formation, and proliferative or metaplastic changes in the duct lining cells. The proliferation may progress to form the characteristic epimyoepithelial islets (Fig. 78–1), which are seen in about 40% of parotid

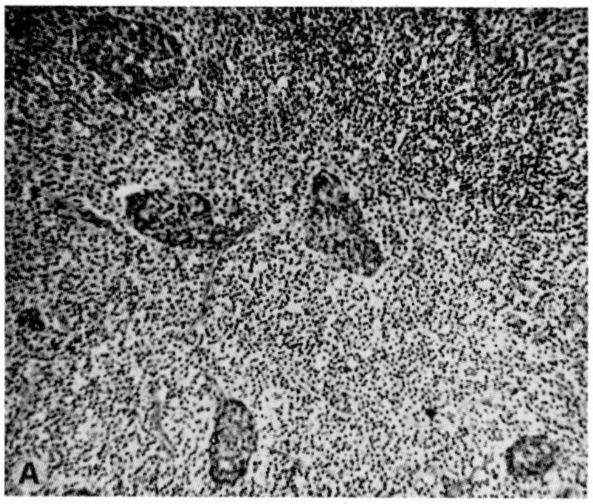

FIGURE 78–1. Extensive lymphoid proliferation and formation of epimyoepithelial islets in the parotid gland of a patient with Sjögren's syndrome. (From Bloch, K.J., Buchanan, W.W., Wohl, M.J., and Bunim, J.J.: Sjögren's syndrome. A clinical, pathological, and serological study of sixty-two cases. Medicine, *44*:187–236, 1965.)

biopsy specimens. In some patients, adipose replacement may be more prominent than lymphoid infiltration. Typically, the lobular architecture is preserved; some lobules may be spared, while others are virtually destroyed.

When mucosal glands in the trachea and bronchi are involved, benign-appearing lymphoid infiltrates are again a prominent feature. More extensive lymphoid infiltrates may involve the lung, kidney, or skeletal muscle, resulting in functional abnormalities of these organs.

In some patients, the lymphoid infiltrates in salivary glands, lymph nodes, or parenchymal organs will be more pleomorphic, more primitive, or more invasive than in others, suggesting the possibility of a malignant disorder. Lymph node architecture can be destroyed, and malignant lymphoma may be diagnosed if such abnormal cells predominate. When it is not possible to distinguish a benign from a malignant process, the term *pseudolymphoma* is used.[4]

The immunophenotyping technique and the immunogenotyping technique[21] now permit the diagnosis of monoclonal B-cell proliferations in tissue lymphoid infiltrates that are difficult to diagnose by conventional microscopy. Such molecular approaches may well increase diagnostic accuracy to the point where the imprecise term *pseudolymphoma* can be abandoned.

CLINICAL FEATURES[1]

More than 90% of patients are women; the mean age is 50 years. The disease occurs in all races and in children.[22] The two most common presentations are (1) the insidious and slowly progressive development of the sicca complex in a patient with chronic RA and (2) the more rapid development of a severe oral and ocular dryness, often accompanied by episodic parotitis, in an otherwise well patient.

About 50% of patients with keratoconjunctivitis sicca have additional features of Sjögren's syndrome. The most common ocular complaint is a sensation, described as "gritty" or "sandy," of a foreign body in the eye. Other symptoms include burning, accumulation of thick, ropy strands at the inner canthus, particularly on awakening, decreased tearing, redness, photosensitivity, eye fatigue, itching, and a "filmy" sensation that interferes with vision. Patients complain of eye discomfort and difficulty in reading or in watching television. Inability to cry is *not* a common complaint. Lacrimal gland enlargement occurs infrequently. Ocular complications include corneal ulceration, vascularization, or opacification, followed rarely by perforation.

The distressing manifestations of salivary insufficiency include the following: (1) difficulty with chewing, swallowing, and phonation; (2) adherence of food to buccal surfaces; (3) abnormalities of taste or smell; (4) fissures of the tongue, buccal membranes, and lips, particularly at the corners of the mouth; (5) frequent ingestion of liquids, especially at meal times; and (6) rampant dental caries. Patients are unable to swallow a dry cracker or toast without ingesting fluids and express displeasure at the suggestion. They may carry bottles of water or other fluids with them and may awaken at night for sips of water. The dentist may notice that fillings are loosening.

Dryness may also involve the nose, the posterior pharynx, the larynx, and the tracheobronchial tree and may lead to epistaxis, hoarseness, recurrent otitis media, bronchitis, or pneumonia.

Half these patients have parotid gland enlargement (Fig. 78–2), often recurrent and symmetric and sometimes accompanied by fever, tenderness, or erythema. Superimposed infection is rare. Rapid fluctuations in gland size are not unusual. A particularly hard or nodular gland may suggest a neoplasm.

The arteritis of Sjögren's syndrome resembles classic RA in its clinical, pathologic, and roentgenographic features. Keratoconjunctivitis sicca develops in about 10 to 15% of patients with RA. Arthralgias and morning stiffness without joint deformity may occur in patients with the sicca complex. Fluctuations in the course of the arthritis are not accompanied by parallel alterations in the symptoms of the sicca complex. Splenomegaly and leukopenia suggestive of Felty's syndrome, and vasculitis with leg ulcers and peripheral neuropathy, may appear even in the absence of RA. Raynaud's phenomenon occurs in 20% of patients.

Skin or vaginal dryness and allergic drug eruptions are frequent. Episodic lower extremity purpura, sometimes preceded by itching or other prodromal signs, may

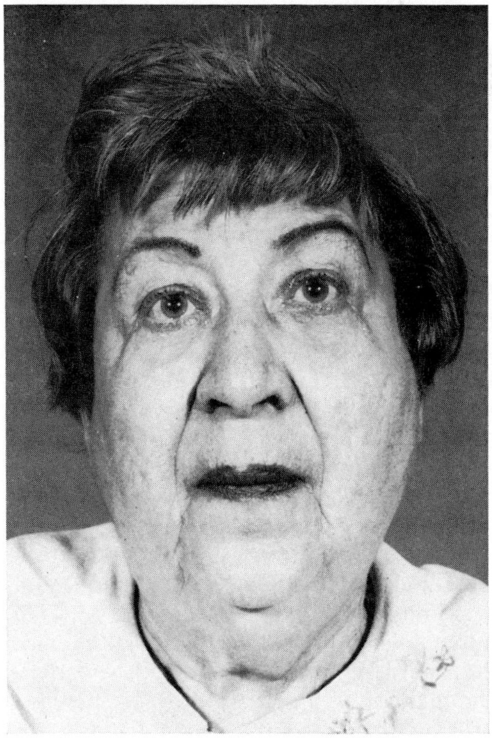

FIGURE 78–2. Bilateral parotid gland enlargement in a patient with severe xerostomia and Sjögren's syndrome.

be the presenting complaint.[23] Glomerulonephritis develops rarely and should suggest either coexisting SLE or cryoglobulinemia. Cryoglobulins occur in up to a third of patients and may contain monoclonal immunoglobulin (IgM).[24] Overt or latent abnormalities of the renal tubular function, such as occurs in diabetes insipidus, renal tubular acidosis, and Fanconi syndrome, occur with greater frequency.[4] A variety of pulmonary disorders may be present.[25–28]

Severe proximal muscle weakness and, rarely, tenderness may be early symptoms leading to a diagnosis of polymyositis. Weakness may also be associated with electrolyte imbalance, nephrocalcinosis, and the clinical findings of renal tubular acidosis. Peripheral or cranial neuropathy may cause symptoms of dysesthesia or paraesthesia. Facial pain and numbness can accompany trigeminal neuropathy and may contribute to the oral discomfort caused by the dryness. Focal and diffuse central nervous system (CNS) disease may include cognitive disorders,[29] may mimic multiple sclerosis,[30] and has been associated with vasculitis and CNS synthesis of immunoglobulins.

Although chronic thyroiditis of the Hashimoto type is present in 5% of patients, clinical hypothyroidism is rare. Sjögren's syndrome was found in 52% of patients with primary biliary cirrhosis and in 35% of patients with active chronic hepatitis.[4] Gastric achlorhydria, acute pancreatitis, and adult celiac disease have been reported in Sjögren's syndrome. Cervical or other lymph node enlargement may be the first indication of malignant lymphoma or pseudolymphoma (Fig. 78–3).

PHYSICAL FINDINGS

An elderly woman presenting with joint deformities, reddened eyes, and parotid gland enlargement should immediately suggest the diagnosis. In many patients, however, the findings are less obvious. The parotid glands may have any consistency but are usually firm and nontender. Persistent bilateral parotid swelling may give rise to the so-called "chipmunk faces."

Gross inspection of the eyes may reveal nothing abnormal, a mucous thread, or conjunctival congestion. Lacrimal enlargement may not be apparent even when these glands are involved. The *Schirmer test*, in which a strip of Whatman No. 41 filter paper is folded and placed in the lower conjunctival sac, is a simple but crude measure of tear formation. Five minutes later, the moistened portion normally measures 15 mm or more. Most patients with Sjögren's syndrome moisten less than 5 mm of the test paper. More reliable diagnostic signs are obtained with rose bengal or fluorescein dye and biomicroscopic examination. Normally, no stain is visible a few minutes after dye instillation. Grossly visible or microscopic staining of the bulbar conjunctiva or cornea indicates the presence of small, superficial erosions. Biomicroscopy may also reveal increased amounts of corneal debris and attached filaments of corneal epithelium (filamentary keratitis).

The tongue and mucous membranes are characteristi-

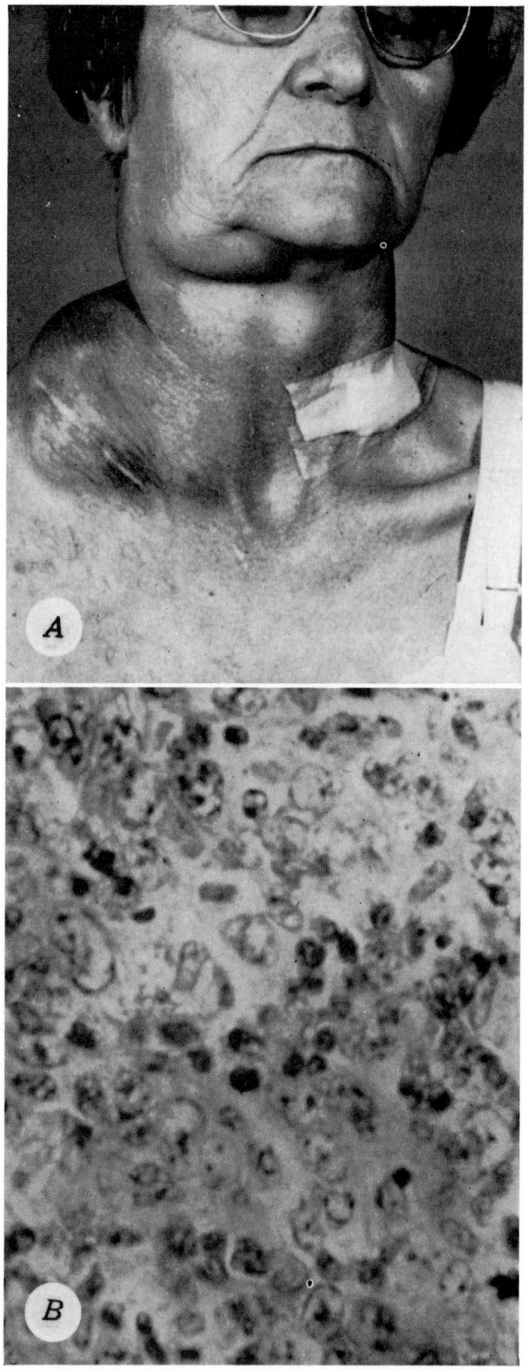

FIGURE 78–3. *A*, Several hard, matted lymph nodes are present in the neck and submandibular region in this patient with Sjögren's syndrome of 20 years' duration. She has had intermittent, cervical lymphadenopathy for the last 6 years, with histologic diagnosis of pseudolymphoma made on four occasions. *B*, On biopsy, many abnormal reticulum cells with large nuclei and prominent nucleoli are found. The diagnosis is reticulum cell sarcoma. (Courtesy of Pediatric Clinics of North America.)

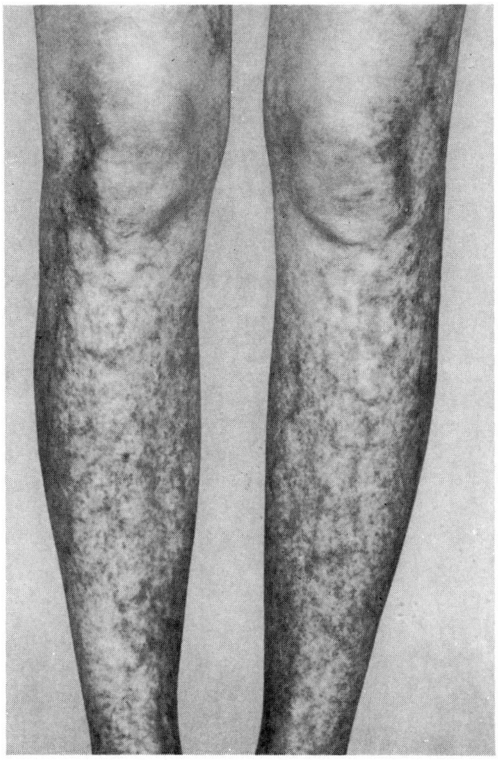

FIGURE 78–4. Characteristic appearance of the legs of a patient with Sjögren's syndrome and intermittent, dependent, nonthrombocytopenic purpura.

cally dry, red, and "parchment-like." The lips may be dry and cracked. A tongue depressor adheres to oral surfaces, and the normal pool of saliva in the sublingual vestibule, visible when the tongue is elevated, is not present. A residual brownish pigmentation over the shins suggests past episodes of purpura (Fig. 78–4). Cervical or other lymph node enlargement may be the first indication of malignant lymphoma or pseudolymphoma. Splenomegaly occurs in 25% of patients.

LABORATORY FINDINGS

Parotid salivary flow rates can be measured by means of Carlson-Crittenden cups placed over the orifices of the parotid ducts and secured by suction. Flow is then stimulated by placing lemon juice on the tongue. Parotid secretion depends on age, sex, and other factors. Normal stimulated parotid flow rate should be about 0.5 to 1.0 mL/min/gland. Flow rates are reduced or unobtainable in Sjögren's syndrome.

Two techniques can be employed for visualizing the salivary glands. Secretory sialography is performed by introducing a radiopaque contrast medium through a small polyethylene catheter inserted into the orifice of the parotid duct.[31] After injection of 0.5 to 1.0 mL contrast material, the catheter is plugged, and radiographs are made (injection phase). The catheter is then removed, and emptying is encouraged by stimulation with lemon juice. Films are taken again 5 minutes later (secretory phase). A normal sialogram shows fine arborization of parotid ductules with little retention of contrast medium. In patients with Sjögren's syndrome, one sees gross distortion of the normal pattern with marked retention. The sialectasis may appear punctate, globular, or cavitary (Fig. 78–5). This procedure is performed much less frequently now than in the past.

The second method depends on the uptake, concentration, and excretion of the radionuclide ^{99m}Tc (pertechnetate) by the salivary gland. Patients are studied by sequential salivary scintigraphy in which the gland image is recorded visually on a γ-scintillation camera over 60 to 80 minutes. Both uptake and release of radionuclide are measured. Most patients show decreased function.[4] The scintigraphic findings parallel the degree of xerostomia, the salivary flow rate determinations, and the results of secretory sialography (Fig. 78–6).

Involvement of minor salivary glands in the lower lip has led to the use of lower lip biopsies and histologic confirmation of the diagnosis. The procedure is performed under local anesthesia with the patient seated in a dental chair. An elliptic incision is made with a scalpel in the labial mucosa parallel to the vermillion border. Patients generally experience discomfort for 24 to 48 hours; approximately 1% complain of more persistent localized numbness. Lymphocytic infiltration can be measured by means of the focus scoring method, in which the number of foci, defined as 50 or more round cells per 4 mm^2 of sectioned tissue, is determined on the biopsy specimen. Although various authorities still disagree somewhat about precise diagnostic criteria for Sjögren's syndrome, a focus score greater than 1 is probably the best criterion for the oral component and far superior to the subjective evaluation of xerostomia.[32]

A mild normocytic, normochromic *anemia* occurs in about 25% of patients, *leukopenia* in 30%, *eosinophilia* (about 6% eosinophils) in 25%, and an elevated *erythrocyte sedimentation rate* (greater than 30 mm/hour by the Westergren method), in over 90%.

About half the patients have hyper-γ-globulinemia, which is generally a diffuse elevation of all immunoglobulin classes. The most hyperglobulinemic patients may not have RA, but rather polymyopathy, purpura, vasculitis, or renal tubular acidosis. Monoclonal IgM may be seen. Cryoglobulinemia, often of the mixed IgM–IgG type, may be present, particularly in patients with glomerulonephritis or pseudolymphoma. Hyperviscosity associated with IgG rheumatoid factor (RF) and intermediate complexes has been reported. Some patients with lymphoma have hypo-γ-globulinemia. A mild hypoalbuminemia is common. Levels of circulating immune complexes are increased, and reticuloendothelial clearance is defective in Sjögren's syndrome.

RF is detected in over 90% of sera when pooled human F II γ-globulin is used as antigen and in 75% when rabbit γ-globulin is employed. Thus, many patients who do not have RA have RF. RF may disappear,

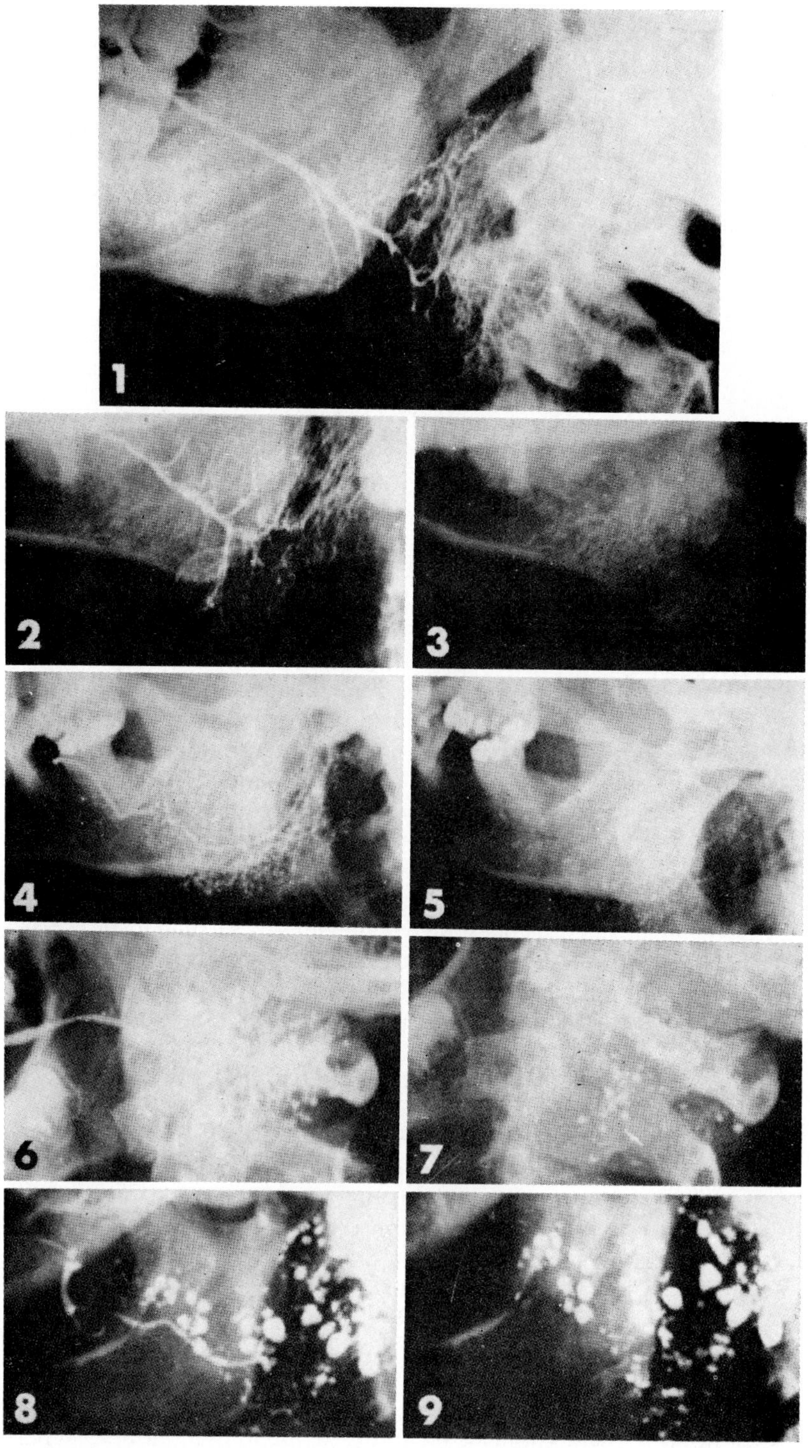

FIGURE 78–5. Appearance of secretory sialography in normal individuals and in patients with Sjögren's syndrome. *1*, Injection phase, normal pattern. *2*, Injection phase, punctate sialectasis. *3*, Secretory phase, punctate sialectasis. *4*, Injection phase, punctate sialectasis with intermediate duct involvement. *5*, Secretory phase, punctate sialectasis with intermediate duct involvement. *6*, Injection phase, globular sialectasis. *7*, Secretory phase, globular sialectasis. *8*, Injection phase, cavitary and destructive sialectasis. *9*, Secretory phase, cavitary and destructive sialectasis. (From Bloch, K.J., Buchanan, W.W., Wohl, M.J., and Bunim, J.J.: Sjögren's syndrome. A clinical, pathological, and serological study of sixty-two cases. Medicine, *44*:187–231, 1965.)

or diminish markedly in titer when lymphoma develops.[4]

The LE cell phenomenon occurs in 20% of patients who also have RA. This phenomenon is otherwise rare, unless SLE is also present.

Antinuclear factors, giving a homogenous or speckled pattern of immunofluorescence, are seen in about 70% of patients. Antibodies to native DNA are occasionally present in low titer. Thyroglobulin antibodies, detected by hemagglutination, are present in about 35% of patients.

The presence of multiple serum autoantibodies is a characteristic feature of Sjögren's syndrome as it is in SLE. Antibodies to Ro/SSA occur in the vast majority of primary Sjögren's syndrome patients (as determined by sensitive solid-phase assays) and are associated with RF,

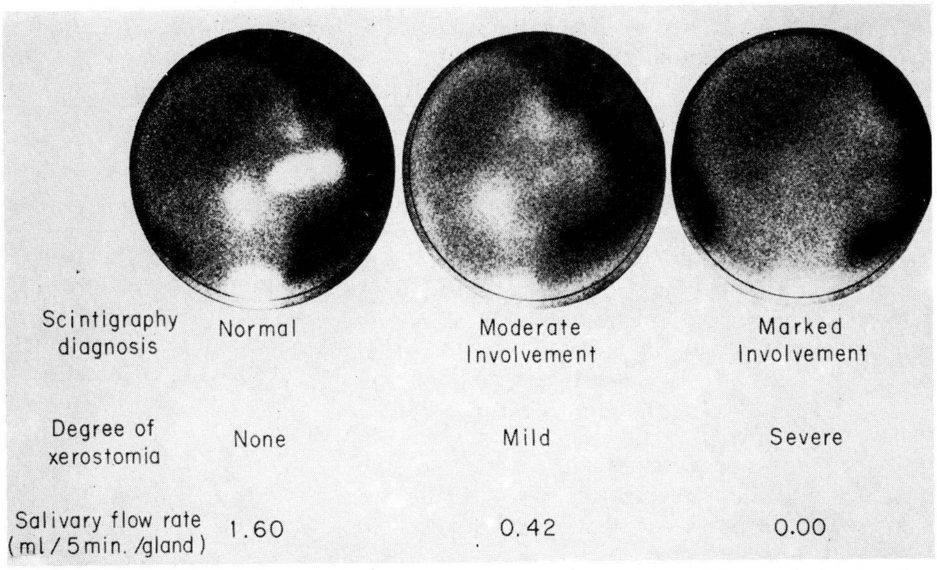

FIGURE 78–6. Comparative studies of salivary function in Sjögren's syndrome illustrating the results achieved with scintigraphy employing ^{99m}Tc (pertechnetate).

TABLE 78–2. IMMUNOLOGIC FINDINGS IN THE PERIPHERAL BLOOD IN SJÖGREN'S SYNDROME

Polyclonal hyper-γ-globulinemia
Autoantibodies (ANA+ and RF+)
Anti-Ro (SS-A) and anti-La (SS-B)
Monoclonal immunoglobulins
Deficient IL-2 production
Impaired T-cell function
Decreased natural killer cell function
Increased CD5+ B cells[36]

ANA+ = antinuclear antibody positive; IL-2 = interleukin 2; RF+ = rheumatoid factor positive; CD5+ = CD5 positive.

hyper-γ-globulinemia, vasculitis, the neonatal lupus syndrome, and DQ heterozygosity (DQ1, DQ2). This autoantibody is often accompanied by anti-La/SSB. Both autoantibodies also occur in SLE but to a lesser extent than in Sjögren's syndrome. The relationship between Sjögren's syndrome and SLE can be confusing, not only for the sharing of these autoantibodies but also because, rarely, patients may change disease expression during the course of their illness and therefore present a true Sjögren's syndrome–SLE overlap syndrome.[1]

The immunologic findings in the peripheral blood of patient with Sjögren's syndrome are summarized in Table 78–2. There is a marked polyclonal hyper-γ-globulinemia with the presence of RF, antinuclear antibodies (ANAs), and in particular anti-Ro (SS-A) and anti-La (SS-B). Monoclonal immunoglobulins including homogenous light-chain bands are frequently found in the blood as well as in the urine by sensitive electrophoretic techniques.[33] Studies using peripheral blood lymphocytes demonstrate that many Sjögren's syndrome patients have deficient interleukin-2 (IL-2) production.[34] There is a decrease in peripheral blood T cells in about one third of patients. Abnormalities in T-cell function may be present, particularly in patients with systemic features. These patients often have alterations in T-cell subsets and decreased intracellular signaling demonstrated by various T-cell activators.[35] Natural killer cell activity is also diminished as a consequence of immunoregulatory abnormalities rather than intrinsic deficits. CD5-positive B cells, the cells that circulate in chronic lymphocytic leukemia, are increased in the peripheral blood of patients with primary Sjögren's syndrome. These cells are thought to have immunoregulatory functions and are also increased in the blood of RA patients.

An increase in salivary β_2-microglobulin concentration correlates with the degree of lymphocytic infiltration found on labial biopsy. Serum β_2-microglobulin levels can be increased, particularly in patients with associated renal or lymphoproliferative complications.[4]

LYMPHOMA AND MACROGLOBULINEMIA

An increased incidence of non-Hodgkin's lymphoma in patients with Sjögren's syndrome was first reported in the 1960s. The chronic antigenic stimulation was suggested as a possible trigger for a malignant transformation event. There are now about 200 reported examples of this association. Indeed, the risk of lymphoma development is 44 times greater in Sjögren's syndrome than in the normal population. The autoimmune disorder may precede the development of lymphoma by intervals ranging from 0.5 to 29 years. Certain extraglandular disease features (e.g., splenomegaly) as well as parotid swelling are more likely to occur in patients predisposed to lymphoma.

In most patients, significant lymphoproliferation remains confined to salivary and lacrimal tissue and has a chronic, benign course of stable or progressive xerostomia and xerophthalmia. Even after 15 years or more of benign disease, however, some patients develop an extension of lymphoproliferation to extraglandular sites such as lung, kidney, lymph nodes, skin, gastrointestinal tract, and bone marrow. Persistent or massive parotid gland enlargement may also suggest lymphoma.

When such "extraglandular" lymphoproliferation occurs, diagnosis is often difficult, and clinically and histologically the disease may simulate frankly malignant lymphoproliferative disorders such as Waldenström's macroglobulinemia or non-Hodgkin's lymphoma. Because the subsequent clinical course is frequently that of lymphoma, ending fatally, the early recognition of extraglandular lymphoproliferation in Sjögren's syndrome and the prompt institution of appropriate therapy are important.

The extraglandular lymphoid infiltrates are of two general types. They may be highly pleomorphic and include small and large lymphocytes, plasma cells, and large reticulum cells. In a lymph node the cells may distort the normal architecture and may extend beyond the capsule; the distinction between benign and malignant lesions is thereby made difficult. The term "pseudolymphoma" has been applied[4] when the lesions show tumor-like aggregates of lymphoid cells but do not meet the usual histologic criteria for malignancy (Fig. 78–7).

In pseudolymphoma, the site of extraglandular lymphoproliferation determines the clinical presentation. Striking regional lymphadenopathy may be the predominant clinical feature. On the other hand, lymphoid infiltration may be selectively excessive in a distant organ such as kidney or lung. These organs may become functionally impaired, giving rise to renal abnormalities or pulmonary insufficiency. Renal tubular acidosis may develop through such a mechanism.

Features that should alert the clinician to the possibility of extraglandular lymphoproliferation in a patient with Sjögren's syndrome are regional or generalized lymphadenopathy, hepatosplenomegaly, pulmonary infiltrates, renal insufficiency, purpura, leukopenia, hyper-γ-globulinemia, and elevated serum β_2-microglobulin. Vasculitis may be present, but arthritis is rare in such patients. The entity of pseudolymphoma cannot be clearly defined, but it occupies the middle portion of a spectrum ranging from benign disease to frankly malignant disease, such as Waldenström's macroglobulinemia.

The second type of extraglandular lymphoid infiltrate is histologically malignant and enables one to make the specific diagnosis of lymphoproliferative neoplasm. These lesions may also appear after several years of apparently benign disease; they may or may not be preceded by pseudolymphoma, and they are often resistant to therapy. Although the histologic diagnosis may vary, the lymphoma generally belongs to the B-cell lineage and often contains intracellular immunoglobulin. Some patients may also have serum immunoglobulin spikes, which tend to be IgMκ in Western countries but non-IgM in Japan.

A low IgM level may herald the presence or development of malignant lymphoproliferation and can be a sign of a poor prognosis. A fall in the serum IgM level is often accompanied by a reduction in the RF titer and may precede the onset of generalized hypo-γ-globulinemia.

DIAGNOSIS

Clinically, a "sicca-like" syndrome may be caused by a number of other disease processes including acquired immune deficiency syndrome (AIDS), hyperlipoproteinemias IV and V, hemochromatosis, sarcoidosis, and amyloidosis. The use of anticholinergic or antidepressive drugs as well as numerous other medications may cause xerostomia. Thus, it is essential to establish the presence of focal lymphoid infiltrates and autoimmunity in a patient suspected of having Sjögren's syndrome.

A viral cause for the autoimmune rheumatic diseases has long been suspected but never proven. This possibility has become even more likely because of reports that salivary gland infiltrates and parotid swelling resembling Sjögren's syndrome develop in patients infected with HIV.

HIV-associated salivary gland disease can occur in adults or children or after transfusion and may be seen with either AIDS-related complex or AIDS itself. HIV-related disease must now be added to the differential diagnosis of any patient presenting with parotid swelling. Xerostomia is present in almost all of these patients. Salivary flow rates may be reduced. Dry eyes and arthralgias may also be present. Generalized lymphadenopathy, lymphocytic pulmonary infiltrates, and CNS symptoms can occur as well as antinuclear or rheumatoid factor. Anti-Ro/SSA or anti-La/SSB antibodies do not occur. The proper diagnosis can be made by screening for antibodies to HIV with Western blot analysis.

The diagnosis of secondary Sjögren's syndrome, which should be suspected in any patient with RA, can be made when either keratoconjunctivitis sicca or a positive labial salivary gland biopsy are present. Generally, the arthritis precedes or is concurrent with the sicca complex. Other connective tissue diseases, such as scleroderma, SLE, or polymyositis, may substitute for RA in this definition.

Many patients have symptoms of oral or ocular dryness without an underlying connective tissue disease and appear to have primary Sjögren's syndrome. If arthritis does not develop within the first 12 months of the sicca complex, the chances are only 10% that it will appear later.

As with most diseases, obtaining the patient's medical history is the important first step in making the diagnosis. Many patients, on casual questioning, reply that their mouths feel dry. More significant is the requirement for frequent fluids during the course of the day or the admission that they awaken at night because of oral dryness. The dramatic negative response to the thought of ingesting a dry cracker is a helpful clue. Patients should be asked to describe their ocular complaints.

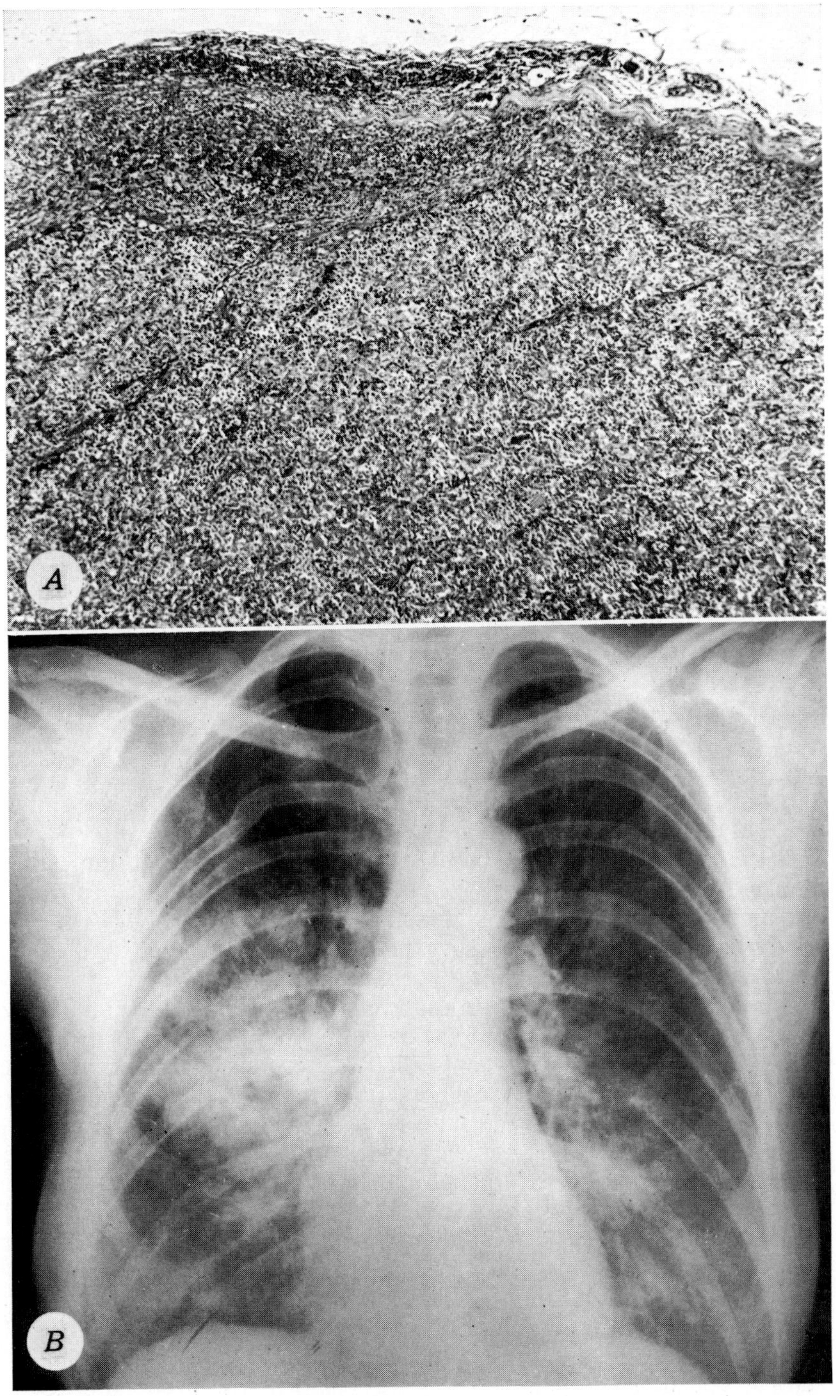

FIGURE 78–7. Pseudolymphoma can distort the normal lymph node architecture with penetration of cells through *(A)* the capsule, or *(B)* it may appear as pulmonary infiltrates in chest radiogram. (From Bloch, K.J., Buchanan, W.W., Wohl, M.J., and Bunim, J.J.: Sjögren's syndrome. A clinical, pathological, and serological study of sixty-two cases. Medicine, *44*:187–236, 1965.)

They often use the expression "gritty" or "sandy" to characterize the discomfort of xerophthalmia.

Objective evidence of salivary or lacrimal glands insufficiency should be sought in any patient with a suggestive history. Such evidence includes a careful ophthalmologic examination with biomicroscopic examination, measurement of salivary flow, and a labial salivary gland biopsy.

The varied clinical presentation and the multisystemic nature of Sjögren's syndrome may make the diagnosis obscure. As indicated in Table 78–3, the disease may become manifest in several different ways. Unilateral or asymmetric glandular enlargement may suggest a possible tumor. Hyperglobulinemic purpura or other features of cutaneous vasculitis may be prominent. The initial symptoms may be related to a renal tubular disorder such as renal gravel or calculi, or they may suggest a severe degenerative or inflammatory muscle disease. Peripheral neuropathy may be a prominent feature, and trigeminal nerve involvement can cause facial discom-

TABLE 78–3. CLINICAL PRESENTATION OF SJÖGREN'S SYNDROME

1. Sicca complex—dry eyes and dry mouth
2. Rheumatoid arthritis—or other connective tissue disease
3. Salivary gland enlargement
4. Purpura—nonthrombocytopenic; hyperglobulinemic
5. Renal tubular acidosis—or other tubular disorder
6. Polymyopathy
7. Neurologic-peripheral or CNS
8. Chronic liver disease
9. Chronic pulmonary disease
10. Lymphoma—local or generalized
11. Immunoglobulin disorder—cryoglobulinemia; macroglobulinemia

fort. CNS symptoms have recently been emphasized. The disease may appear initially as a chronic active hepatitis or biliary cirrhosis. Pulmonary disease may be related to dryness and infection or to lymphoid infiltration of the lung. Malignant lymphoma or an immunoglobulin disorder may first attract medical attention.

TREATMENT

Most often, Sjögren's syndrome is a relatively benign disease. Conservative management is therefore the best guide to therapy.

The sicca complex is treated with fluid replacement as often as necessary. Several readily available ophthalmic preparations, such as Tearisol, Liquifilm, and 0.5% methylcellulose, adequately replace the deficient tears. In severe situations, patients instill these drops as often as every half hour to hour. If corneal ulceration is present, patching of the eye and application of boric ointment may be necessary. Soft contact lenses are sometimes used to protect the cornea. Plastic-wrap occlusion or diving goggles may prevent tear evaporation at night. Topical corticosteroids are generally avoided unless specifically indicated because corneal thinning and subsequent perforation may occur. The use of diuretics, some antihypertensive drugs, and antidepressants may further diminish lacrimal and salivary gland function.

It is more difficult to compensate for the salivary insufficiency. Various saliva substitutes have not proved useful. Bromhexine, a mucolytic agent, has been used abroad. The frequent ingestion of fluids, particularly with meals, is often the best solution. Patients should see their dentists every 4 months and should pay scrupulous attention to proper oral hygiene. The careful use of a mouth-rinsing apparatus after eating may reduce the incidence of caries. Patients should avoid a high sucrose intake or the frequent use of sugar-containing candies to decrease oral dryness. Vigorous dental plaque control and topical application of fluoride should be routine. Oral candidiasis may be treated with nystatin tablets for a prolonged course, with separate treatment of dentures.

Proper humidification of the home environment is helpful in reducing respiratory infections and other complications of the sicca complex. Patients should be encouraged to live with their disability. They require sympathetic understanding.

The management of RA or other associated disorders is not altered by the presence of Sjögren's syndrome. No controlled studies evaluating the efficacy of corticosteroids or immunosuppressive drugs in the treatment of the sicca complex have been reported. In view of the benign nature of this problem and the potential hazards of these agents, such therapy does not seem justified.

On the other hand, corticosteroids or immunosuppressive drugs are indicated in the treatment of pseudolymphoma, particularly when the patient has renal or pulmonary involvement. Cyclophosphamide, 75 to 100 mg daily, has diminished extraglandular lymphoid infiltrates and restored salivary gland function in some patients.

Malignant lymphoma should be treated with intensive chemotherapy, surgery, or radiotherapy as indicated by the location and extent of disease. These malignant and often fatal lesions require rapid and skilled intervention.

CONNECTIVE TISSUE DISEASE ASSOCIATED WITH OTHER IMMUNOLOGIC DISORDERS

HYPO-γ-GLOBULINEMIA

The functions of the immune system can be divided between those dependent on the secretion of antibody by plasma cells and those dependent on an intact thymus and specifically sensitized lymphocytes. One or both of these two functional systems, humoral and cellular immunity, respectively, may be defective in a variety of different immunodeficiency syndromes described in recent years.

A deficiency of humoral immunity results in a failure to produce specific antibody, a severe depression of serum γ-globulin concentration, and the absence of germinal center formation in lymph nodes and spleen. Five immunologically and structurally distinct classes of γ-globulin are known: IgG, IgM, IgA, IgD, and IgE. All immunoglobulin classes may be depressed simultaneously, or selective deficiencies may be present with normal or elevated levels of the remaining classes. The term *dys-γ-globulinemia* has been applied to describe the latter condition.

Hypo-γ-globulinemia may be congenital or acquired. Congenital hypo-γ-globulinemia is a sex-linked recessive disease usually heralded by recurrent pyogenic infections after the age of 6 months. Cellular immunity is generally intact, the level of IgG is usually less than 0.2 g/dL, and the other immunoglobulin classes are absent. These patients lack circulating B cells and tissue plasma cells.

Acquired hypo-γ-globulinemia, also termed the common, variable-onset form, occurs in both sexes, often becomes symptomatic between the ages of 15 and 35 years, and is frequently associated with autoimmunity, as well as with pyogenic infection. Cellular immunity can be defective, and thymomas may occur. Circulating B-lymphocytes are generally normal in number but have a diminished ability to synthesize and to secrete immunoglobulin. Suppressor T-cell function may be present.

Selective IgA deficiency, the most common immunodeficiency disorder, appears to predispose persons to a variety of diseases. The incidence of IgA deficiency in the normal population varies between 1:800 and 1:600. The cause is unknown, but an arrest in B-cell maturation has been suggested. The other immunoglobulins are either normal or increased.

In addition to an enhanced susceptibility to bacterial and other infections, both congenital and acquired hypo-γ-globulinemia may be accompanied by watery diarrhea and malabsorption producing a sprue-like syndrome, a chronic polyarthritis resembling RA, or other connective tissue or lymphoproliferative disease. Frequently, the malabsorption is associated with infestation by Giardia lamblia.

CLINICAL AND DIAGNOSTIC FEATURES

The chronic polyarthritis associated with hypo-γ-globulinemia often starts in the knees and then involves the ankles, wrists, and fingers.[4] Pain is infrequent, but joint effusion is common. Subcutaneous nodules are rare. The incidence of arthritis in patients with hypo-γ-globulinemia varies between 8 and 29%.[37,38]

Many characteristic features of RA, such as morning stiffness and symmetric joint swelling, are present. Radiograms show demineralization of the bones and narrowing of the joint spaces. Erosions are rare, and extensive joint destruction has not been reported. RF is absent from the serum.

Synovial biopsies may show lymphocytic infiltration, but no B-lymphocytes or plasma cells are found.[39] An excessive suppressor T-cell activity has been reported in the synovium.[40] Other patients, however, may have chronic synovitis without these features. A suggestion that relatives of patients had a high incidence of RA and hyper-γ-globulinemia has not been substantiated.

In addition to polyarthritis, other disorders that may be associated with hypo-γ-globulinemia include scleroderma, SLE, dermatomyositis, idiopathic thrombocytopenic purpura, Sjögren's syndrome, hemolytic anemia, and pernicious anemia. Patients with the acquired form may have marked lymphadenopathy and splenomegaly, and, occasionally, autoantibodies associated with SLE or hemolytic anemia. Intestinal lymphoid nodular hyperplasia may accompany the malabsorption. Lymphoreticular malignant tumors and thymomas have been reported. Three patients developed panhypo-γ-globulinemia during the course of SLE.[41,42]

Some patients have a selective IgA deficiency associated with autoimmune disease or with serologic abnormalities suggestive of autoimmunity. Recurrent sinopulmonary infections are common in these patients. Allergies, ataxia telangiectasia, gastrointestinal tract disease, and malignant tumor may be present. Immunologic abnormalities include increased serum IgA and IgM concentrations, serum 7S IgM, abnormal κ/λ ratios, and antibodies reacting with IgG, IgA, milk, bovine proteins, and human tissue antigens.[4] The clinical presentations associated with selective IgA deficiency include RA, SLE, Sjögren's syndrome, dermatomyositis, pernicious anemia, chronic active hepatitis, Coombs'-positive hemolytic anemia, and thyroiditis.[4] Cellular immunity is generally normal. Selective IgA deficiency occurs in approximately 4% of patients with SLE or juvenile RA (JRA).

Quantitative immunoglobulin determinations are essential for diagnosis. Immunoglobulin concentrations may be slightly higher in the acquired form but are still depressed. Isohemagglutinins either are absent or are present in low titers (1:10). A failure to develop an antibody response to a specific antigenic challenge may help to establish the diagnosis if immunoglobulin levels are borderline. *Live attenuated vaccines should not be used for immunization.*

Abnormalities of cellular immunity may be seen, including absent delayed hypersensitivity skin test reactions, depressed responses to mitogenic stimulation, and decreased numbers of rosette-forming T-lymphocytes.

Serum and secretory IgA may be selectively absent in IgA-deficient patients. Some subjects may have normal secretory IgA or have increased amounts of serum and secretory 7S IgM.

TREATMENT

Commercial γ-globulin is given at regular intervals, starting at doses of 0.2 mL/kg and increasing progressively. The arthritis associated with hypo-γ-globulinemia usually responds promptly to this treatment. Anaphylactoid reactions to γ-globulin have been noted. Fresh-frozen plasma may also be used. Patients with selective IgA deficiency should not be given γ-globulin, because they may react to the foreign IgA and may develop anaphylactoid transfusion reactions.

ETIOLOGIC FACTORS

The immunologic events occurring locally in the synovium and joint space in these patients may be similar to those in typical RA, despite the hypo-γ-globulinemia and impaired ability to produce specific antibody or RF.

The pathogenesis of the autoimmune and connective tissue diseases probably depends on genetic, immunologic, and viral factors. The immunologic deficiency present in these patients predisposes them to pyogenic respiratory tract infections and to unexplained diarrhea and malabsorption, as well as to autoimmunity. Perhaps their altered immune status renders them more susceptible to disorders induced by unusual pathogens such as latent viruses. The peculiar susceptibility of patients with selective IgA deficiency supports this concept. IgA, the major secretory immunoglobulin, may play an important host defense role in the respiratory and gastrointestinal tract. Deficiency of IgA in these critical areas may permit the entry and establishment of foreign pathogens that induce antigenic alterations and contribute to the development of autoimmunity.

The use of intravenous γ-globulin as treatment for several autoimmune diseases may shed new light on the mechanisms involved in pathogenesis.

HYPERGLOBULINEMIC PURPURA

Clinical Features

Hyperglobulinemic purpura affects women predominantly and is characterized by hyper-γ-globulinemia and episodes of purpura of the lower extremities. Described originally by Waldenström, this disorder is not to be confused with another entity, Waldenström's macroglobulinemia. Patients often have no other associated illness, although myeloma, arthritis, and Sjögren's syndrome may develop.[4] Prodromal symptoms such as burning or itching of the legs may precede by several hours and announce the onset of another episode of purpura. A chronic brownish pigmentation of the skin often appears as the residue of these attacks.

Laboratory Findings

The erythrocyte sedimentation rate and γ-globulin concentration are elevated. RF and antinuclear factor are frequently present in the serum.

Anti-γ-globulins of the IgG type are a feature of this disease and result in immune complexes with sedimentation properties intermediate between 7S and 19S immunoglobulins. These "intermediate complexes" are formed by interactions of the IgG anti-IgG with itself and with other normal IgG molecules. The resulting pattern on serum paper electrophoresis is generally polydispersed, that is, polyclonal, but it may appear monoclonal. IgA complexes may also be involved, and the complexes may increase when the ambient temperature falls.

Etiologic Factors

This disorder seems to occupy a middle ground between autoimmune and lymphoproliferative diseases. It is distinguished immunologically from RA by the frequent presence of IgG rather than IgM RF, that is, anti-IgG antibody.

The exact relation of the hyper-γ-globulinemia to the purpura is not understood. The circulating immune complexes become deposited in small blood vessels and give rise to vascular injury and extravasation of blood. The cooler skin temperature and orthostatic pressure changes may play a role in this process.

CRYOGLOBULINEMIA

Cryoglobulins are immunoglobulins with the physiochemical characteristic of precipitation in the cold followed by resolution on warming. Three types of cryoglobulins have been defined[4] as follows: (1) isolated monoclonal immunoglobulins produced by proliferating cells in Waldenström's macroglobulinemia or multiple myeloma; (2) mixed cryoglobulins in which a monoclonal component, usually IgM, has antibody activity against polyclonal IgC; and (3) mixed polyclonal cryoglobulins, which are usually anti-immunoglobulin immune complexes, but may also contain other molecules such as β1C or lipoprotein.

Cryoglobulins also occur in rheumatoid vasculitis, cutaneous vasculitis,[4] and SLE.[4] They appear to represent circulating immune complexes and, in SLE, may contain antibodies to nucleoproteins and to lymphocyte antigens.

Clinical and Diagnostic Features

Cryoglobulins of either monoclonal or immune complex (mixed) nature may produce Raynaud's phenomenon, numbness, urticaria, vascular occlusions, tissue infarction, and digital ulcerations. Cutaneous and vasomotor symptoms are more severe in types 1 and 2 cryoglobulinemia. Types 2 and 3 are more often associated with renal and neurologic involvement, chronic vascular purpura, and Raynaud's phenomenon. Immunoproliferative disorders are associated with types 1 and 2, and autoimmunity with type 3.

Mixed cryoglobulins may also be associated with a symptom complex, occurring predominantly in women, that includes arthralgias, purpura, especially involving the lower extremities, weakness, vasculitis, and diffuse glomerulonephritis. RF is present, and Sjögren's syndrome or thyroiditis may occur.

Forty patients with essential mixed cryoglobulins represented 32% of all cryoglobulinemic patients seen in an 18-year period.[43] Seventy percent had evidence of hepatic dysfunction, and 60% had serologic evidence of prior infection with hepatitis B virus. Many patients had severe renal disease with glomerular deposits of IgA, IgM, and complement. All cryoglobulins had RF activity. Renal involvement indicated a poor prognosis, and widespread vasculitis was found frequently during postmortem examination.

The laboratory finding that confirms the diagnosis is the cryoglobulin in the serum. From 24 to 48 hours in the cold may be required to precipitate the cryoglobulin from serum. Anywhere from 20 to 60% of the mixed cryoprecipitate is IgM. The presence of IgG is required to precipitate IgM, and IgM behaves like an antibody to IgG. Cryoprecipitation occurs in the absence of complement, although complement may be associated with the complex, and serum complement levels are generally depressed. The IgM is a fairly typical RF binding to the Fc portion of IgG. The IgM may be a monoclonal (Waldenström-type) paraprotein; mixed IgA-IgG cryoglobulinemia has also been reported.

One patient had mixed cryoglobulinemia, Sjögren's syndrome, and pulmonary lymphoid infiltrates, with an associated hypo-γ-globulinemia and increased susceptibility to bacterial infection.[4] The IgM was monoclonal and reacted specifically with IgG subclasses 1, 2, and 4 but not with subclass 3. Serum concentrations of IgG 1, 2, and 4 were 10% of normal. These three subclasses also showed reduced synthesis and shortened survival times, whereas IgG-3 had a normal synthetic rate and survival time. The hypo-γ-globulinemia was due in part to a rapid elimination of IgG through its interaction with the IgG-reactive monoclonal IgM.

Hyperviscosity due to an IgM-IgG interaction has been reported in association with RA.

Treatment

Corticosteroids, immunosuppressive drugs, plasmapheresis, penicillamine, and splenectomy have been used with limited success.

Etiologic Factors

The "mixed cryoglobulins" probably represent a special example of an immune complex phenomenon that has highly unusual physicochemical properties, both in vitro and in vivo. The cold precipitability in vitro makes it possible to identify, to isolate, and to characterize the individual components of the complex. The in vivo properties of the complex probably contribute in a major way to the findings of vascular insufficiency. The purpuric lesions may be caused by cryoprecipitation in the small skin capillaries, which reach a temperature (30°C) at which these aggregates are known to precipitate. The complexes may also induce glomerulonephritis and may be responsible for hypo-γ-globulinemia with increased susceptibility to infection.

These cryoglobulins illustrate in an impressive way the dramatic pathologic consequences of immune complex formation and deposition. They shed no light on the mechanism leading to their production, although their ready availability in serum may contribute to further investigation. If viral or tissue antigens are involved in the initial stages of their production, then the specificity of antibodies in the cryocomplex may conceivably be directed against such antigens.

MALIGNANT LYMPHOMA

Enough published reports of the association of connective tissue disease and malignant lymphoma, two rare conditions, now exist that a mere coincidental relationship may not be the best explanation. There is an increased risk of lymphoma, leukemia, and multiple myeloma in patients with RA. The association of Sjögren's syndrome with lymphoproliferation was discussed earlier in this chapter.

Patients with coexisting SLE and malignant lymphoma have been reported.[4] Four patients had Hodgkin's disease, two had lymphosarcoma, and one each had mixed cell lymphoma, reticulum cell sarcoma, and chronic lymphocytic leukemia. All but two died of the malignant disease. Two had hypo-γ-globulinemia. One patient had hematoxylin bodies, onion-skin lesions in the spleen, and hypo-γ-globulinemia with an increase in IgM. The IgM showed cryoprecipitability, was an antinuclear factor, and contained only λ light chains.

The association of RA with monoclonal gammopathies is noteworthy. In a series of 16 patients with arthritis, 6 had multiple myeloma, 8 had asymptomatic monoclonal immunoglobulin "spike" on serum protein electrophoresis, and 1 each had Waldenström's macroglobulinemia or heavy-chain disease. These patients had RF, and their arthritis antedated the development of the paraprotein by as much as 26 years. Such patients should be distinguished from those with multiple myeloma or Waldenström's macroglobulinemia in whom amyloid deposition or the bony lesions themselves can mimic RA.

The connective tissue diseases may predispose patients to the subsequent development of lymphoid or plasma cell malignant disorders, possibly as a consequence of chronic viral infection or prolonged antigenic stimulation, perhaps coupled with impaired cellular immunity and immunologic surveillance.

REFERENCES

1. Talal, N., Moutsopoulos, H.M., and Kassan, S.S. (eds.): Sjögren's Syndrome: Clinical and Immunologic Aspects. New York, Springer-Verlag, 1987.
2. Strand, V., and Talal, N.: Advances in the diagnosis and concept of Sjögren's syndrome (autoimmune exocrinopathy). Bull. Rheum. Dis., *30*:1046–1052, 1980.
3. Talal, N. (ed.): Second International Symposium on Sjögren's Syndrome: A Model for Understanding Autoimmunity. London, Academic Press, 1989.
4. Talal, N.: Sjögren's Syndrome and Connective Tissue Disease Associated with Other Immunologic Disorders. *In* Arthritis and Allied Conditions. 11th Ed. Edited by D.J. McCarty. Philadelphia, Lea & Febiger, 1989, pp. 1197–1213.
5. Ansar Ahmed, S., Penhale, W.J., and Talal, N.: Sex hormones, immune responses, and autoimmune diseases: Mechanisms of sex hormone action. Am. J. Pathol., *121*:531–551, 1985.
6. Harley, J.B., Reichlin, M., Arnett, F.C., et al.: Gene interaction at HLA-DQ enhances autoantibody production in primary Sjögren's syndrome. Science, *232*:1145–1147, 1986.
7. Molina, R., Provost, T.T., Arnett, F.C., et al.: Primary Sjögren's syndrome in men. Clinical, serologic, and immunogenetic features. Am. J. Med., *80*:23–31, 1986.
8. Arnett, F., Hamilton, R.G., Reveille, J.D., et al.: Genetic studies of Ro(SS-A) and La(SS-B) autoantibodies in families with systemic lupus erythematosus and primary Sjögren's syndrome. Arthritis *32*:413–419, 1989.
9. Provost, T., Talal, N., Bias, W., et al.: Ro(Ss-A) positive Sjögren's/lupus erythematosus (SC/LE) overlap patients are associated with the HLA-DR3 and/or DRw6 phenotypes. J. Invest. Dermatol., *91*:369–371, 1988.
10. Talal, N., Dauphinee, M., Dang, H., et al.: Detection of serum antibodies to retroviral proteins inpatients with primary Sjögren's syndrome (autoimmune exocrinopathy). Arthritis Rheum., *33*:774–781, 1990.
11. Talal, N., Garry, R., Alexander, S.S., et al.: A conserved idiotype and antibodies to retroviral proteins in systemic lupus erythematosus. J. Clin. Invest., *85*:1866–1871, 1990.
12. Garry, R.F., Fermin, C.D., Hart, D.J., et al.: Detection of a human

intracisternal A-type retroviral particle antigenically related to HIV. Science (Reports), 1127–1129, 1990.
13. Green, J.E., Hinrichs, S.H., Vogel, J., and Jay, G.: Exocrinopathy resembling Sjögren's syndrome in HTLV-1 tax transgenic mice. Nature (Letters), *341*:72–74, 1989.
14. Fox, R.I., Bumol, T., Fantozzi, R., et al.: Expression of histocompatibility antigen HLA-DR by salivary gland epithelial cells in Sjögren's syndrome. Arthritis Rheum., *29*:1105–1111, 1986.
15. Lindahl, G., Hedfors, E., Klareskog, L., and Forsum, U.: Epithelial HLA-DR expression and T lymphocyte subsets in salivary glands in Sjögren's syndrome. Clin. Exp. Immunol., *61*:475–482, 1985.
16. Adamson, T.C., III, Fox, R.I., Frisman, D.M., and Howell, F.V.: Immunohistologic analysis of lymphoid infiltrates in primary Sjögren's syndrome using monoclonal antibodies. J. Immunol., *130*:203–208, 1983.
17. Fox, R.I., Adamson, R.C., Fong, S., et al.: Lymphocyte phenotype and function in pseudolymphoma associated with Sjögren's syndrome. J. Clin. Invest., *72*:52, 1983.
18. Miyasaka, N., Seaman, W., Bakshi, A., et al.: Natural killing activity in Sjögren's syndrome: An analysis of defective mechanisms. Arthritis Rheum., *26*:954–960, 1983.
19. Fox, R.I., Hugli, T.E., Lanier, L.L., et al.: Salivary gland lymphocytes in primary Sjögren's syndrome lack lymphocyte subsets defined by Leu-7 and Leu-11 antigens. J. Immunol., *135*:207, 1985.
20. Schmid, U., Helbron, D., and Lennert, K.: Development of malignant lymphoma in myoepithelial sialoadenities (Sjögren's syndrome). Pathol. Anat., *395*:11, 1982.
21. Fishleder, A., Tubbs, R., Hesse, B., and Levine, H.: Uniform detection of immunoglobulin-gene rearrangement in benign lymphoepithelial lesions. N. Engl. J. Med., *316*:1118–1122, 1987.
22. Chudwin, D.S., Daniels, T.E., Wara, D.W., et al.: Spectrum of Sjögren's syndrome in children. J. Pediatr., *98*:213–217, 1981.
23. Ferreiro, J.E., Pasarin, G., Quesada, R., and Gould, E.: Benign hypergammaglobulinemic purpura of Waldenstrom associated with Sjögren's syndrome. Case report and review of immunologic aspects. Am. J. Med., *81*:734–740, 1986.
24. Tzioufas, A.G., Manoussakis, M.N., Costello, R., et al.: Cryoglobulinemia in autoimmune rheumatic diseases. Evidence of circulating monoclonal cryoglobulins in patients with primary Sjögren's syndrome. Arthritis Rheum., *29*:1098–1104, 1986.
25. Constantopoulos, S.H., Papadimitriou, C.S., and Moutsopoulos, H.M.: Respiratory manifestations in primary Sjögren's syndrome. A clinical, functional, and histologic study. Chest, *88*:226–229, 1985.
26. Fairfax, A.J., Haslam, P.L., Pavia, D., et al.: Pulmonary disorders associated with Sjögren's syndrome. Am. J. Med., *199*:279–295, 1981.
27. Segal, I., Fink, G., Machtey, I., et al.: Pulmonary function abnormalities in Sjögren's syndrome and the sicca complex. Thorax, *36*:286–289, 1981.
28. Vitali, C., Tavoni, A., Viegi, G., et al.: Lung involvement in Sjögren's syndrome: A comparison between patients with primary and with secondary syndrome. Ann. Rheum. Dis., *44*:455–461, 1985.
29. Alexander, E.L., Lijewski, J.E., Jerdan, M.S., and Alexander, G.E.: Evidence of an immunopathologic basis for central nervous system disease in primary Sjögren's syndrome. Arthritis Rheum., *29*:1223–1231, 1986.
30. Alexander, E.L.: Primary Sjögren's syndrome with central nervous system disease mimicking multiple sclerosis. Ann. Intern. Med., *104*:323–330, 1986.
31. Dijkstra, P.F.: Classification and differential diagnosis of sialographic characteristics in Sjögren's syndrome. Semin. Arthritis Rheum., *10*:10–17, 1980.
32. Daniels, T.E.: Labial salivary gland biopsy in Sjögren's syndrome. Arthritis Rheum., *27*:147–156, 1984.
33. Moutsopoulos, H.M., Costello, R., Drosos, A.A., et al.: Demonstration and identification of monoclonal proteins in the urine of patients with Sjögren's syndrome. Ann. Rheum. Dis., *44*:109, 1985.
34. Miyasaka, N., Murota, N., Yamaoka, K., et al.: Interleukin 2 defect in the peripheral blood and the lung in patients with Sjögren's syndrome. Clin. Exp. Immunol., *65*:497–505, 1986.
35. Dauphinee, M., Tovar, Z., Ballester, A., and Talal, N.: The expression and function of CD3 and CD5 in patients with primary Sjögren's syndrome. Arthritis Rheum., *32*:420–429, 1989.
36. Dauphinee, M., Tovar, Z., and Talal, N.: B cells expressing CD5 are increased in Sjögren's syndrome. Arthritis Rheum., *31*:642–647, 1988.
37. Lederman, H.M., and Winkelstein, J.A.: X-linked agammaglobulinemia: An analysis of 96 patients. Medicine, *63*(3):145–156, 1985.
38. Preston, S.J., and Buchanan, W.W.: Rheumatic manifestations of immune deficiency. Clin. Exp. Rheumatol., *7*(5):547–555, 1989.
39. Abrahamsen, T.G., Froland, S.S., Kass, E., et al.: Lymphocytes from synovial tissue of a boy with X-linked hypogammaglobulinemia and chronic polyarthritis. Arthritis Rheum., *22*:71–78, 1979.
40. Chattopadhyay, J., Natvig, B., and Chattopadhyay, H.: Excessive suppressor T-cell activity of the rheumatoid synovial tissue in X-linked hypogammaglobulinemia. Scand. J. Immunol., *11*:455–459, 1980.
41. Ashman, R.F., et al.: Panhypogammaglobulinemia in systemic lupus erythematosus: In vitro demonstration of multiple cellular defects. J. Allergy Clin. Immunol., *70*:465–473, 1982.
42. Tsokos, G.C., Smith, P.L., and Balow, J.E.: Development of hypogammaglobulinemia in a patient with systemic lupus erythematosus. Am. J. Med., *81*:1081–1084, 1986.
43. Gorevic, P.D., et al.: Mixed cryoglobulinemia: Clinical aspects and long-term follow-up of 40 patients. Am. J. Med., *69*:287–308, 1980.

79

Rheumatic Fever

ANGELO TARANTA

Once the most common cause of acute polyarthritis, rheumatic fever has become a rarity in the West, and many physicians have completed their training without seeing a single case.[1] Since the mid-1980s, however, the disease may be staging a comeback.[2]

HISTORY AND GEOGRAPHY

The description of rheumatic fever as a syndrome resulted from the integration of manifestations originally described independently and thought to be unrelated, that is, *acute articular rheumatism, valvular heart disease,* and *chorea* (Fig. 79–1), to which were then added *subcutaneous nodules* and *erythema marginatum.*[1,3] Later, a number of entities were recognized as mimics of rheumatic fever or of rheumatic heart disease and were identified separately as viral carditis, Yersinia arthritis, and mitral valve prolapse, among others.[4]

While these conceptual changes occurred, the incidence of the disease also changed. Although records from the past are poor and details are lacking, the incidence of rheumatic fever seems to have increased with industrialization and urbanization and then decreased with the consequent affluence, a process completed in the postindustrial West and still ongoing in the developing countries.[4,5]

Availability of penicillin[5a] and improvement in the standard of living (especially a decrease of crowding in the home) have been credited with contributing to the decrease of rheumatic fever in this century; yet the most striking decline may have occurred during the 1970s, when our standard of living did not improve and our use of penicillin did not increase. The strep seems to outsmart us.

PATHOLOGY AND IMMUNOPATHOLOGY

In patients dying of acute rheumatic fever, pancarditis is usually present. Tiny translucent nodules or verrucae, form on the edge of the valves, which can no longer close properly; the valves are "regurgitant" or "incompetent." The myocardium is pale, flabby, edematous, and mildly hypertrophic; the heart chambers are dilated. Fibrin and serosanguineous fluid may be present in the pericardial cavity.

Microscopically, diffuse degeneration and swelling of muscle fibers may be apparent, along with fibrinoid degeneration of collagen. Perivascular foci of degeneration or necrosis may be surrounded by clusters of large mononuclear and giant multinuclear cells,[6] largely of monocyte or macrophage lineage.[7] These clusters, known as *Aschoff bodies*, or nodules, are considered specific for *acute* rheumatic fever, but they may persist long after any other evidence of active disease. Immunofluorescent study reveals immunoglobulins and complement in cardiac myofibers, vessel walls,[8] and pericardium.[9] Valvular lymphoid infiltrates contain a predominance of T cells.[10]

In the joints, a sterile exudate may be found that is deficient in complement components with respect to simultaneously determined serum levels;[11] there is no synovial hypertrophy, no bony erosion, and no cartilage loss.

Chorea affects the basal ganglia, as one would expect from the symptoms, but also, diffusely, other parts of the brain. *Subcutaneous nodules* resemble recently formed rheumatoid nodules; both consist of a central area of necrosis surrounded by parallel rows of elongated fibroblasts, as in a palisade ("palisading" fibroblasts), surrounded by loose connective tissue.[12]

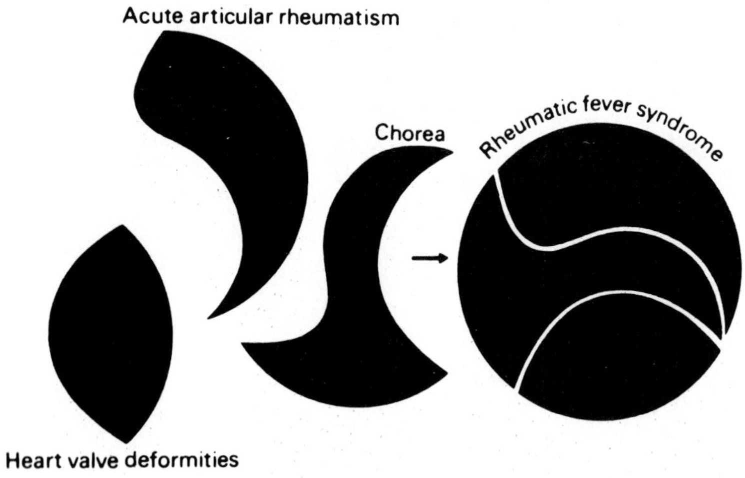

FIGURE 79–1. Historical development of the concept of rheumatic fever syndrome from the integration of disease manifestations previously described independently of each other. (From Taranta, A., and Markowitiz, M.[5])

INCIDENCE AND CAUSE

Like the infections that lead to it, rheumatic fever affects mostly children of 5 to 15 years of age but also is seen in young adults. In the early 1980s, its incidence in various locales in the United States was reported to be as low as 0.23 to 1.88/100,000/year among children and adolescents, but incidence rates 10 times as high have been reported since the mid-1980s in several locales.[2]

Sore throats accompanied by scarlatiniform rash, that is, scarlet fever, have long been known to precede some attacks of rheumatic fever. In the remainder of patients, rheumatic fever is preceded by a sore throat without rash or by a pharyngitis without soreness of the throat, recognizable as a streptococcal infection only by antibody tests.

If streptococcal pharyngitis is treated and the organisms eradicated from the throat, rheumatic fever fails to appear;[13] if patients who have had previous attacks of rheumatic fever receive continual antistreptococcal prophylaxis, the disease does not recur.[14] The few failures to prevent rheumatic fever can be traced to failures to achieve the aims of prophylaxis, which are to eradicate the streptococci from the throat in the case of initial attacks and to prevent streptococci from initiating infections in the case of recurrences.

In 1941, Kuttner and Krumwiede[15] reported that an epidemic of type 4 streptococcal pharyngitis among children convalescing from rheumatic fever failed, surprisingly, to cause recurrences. Conversely, a number of serologic types have been associated with rheumatic fever outbreaks, notably 5, 18, 24, 3, and 14.[16] The mucoid colony type is frequent among streptococci associated with rheumatic fever and so is the absence of "serum opacity factor."[16a] Fischetti has classified M proteins into class I, which share a surface-exposed antigenic domain associated with rheumatic fever, and class II, which produce the serum opacity factor and are associated with skin infections.[16b] The observation that rheumatic fever seems to be coming back in some parts of the country without a concomitant increase of streptococcal infections could be explained by a shift to "rheumatogenic" streptococcal types or strains.[2]

The well-known correlation of rheumatic fever with poverty seems to be mediated mainly by crowding: the larger the number of persons per room, the higher the prevalence of rheumatic heart disease.[17] Crowding leads to multiple close contact,[5] which facilitate streptococcal contagion and seems to favor the selection of more virulent strains. In the 1979 edition of this book, I called attention to the shrinking of family living space in this country and wondered whether it would affect rheumatic fever incidence. In the recent epidemic of rheumatic fever in Utah, the patients were not poor, but the patients' family size was double that of the average family in Utah as a whole, and the majority of patients share bedrooms with other family members.[2]

Although all attacks of rheumatic fever follow a streptococcal infection, only a few streptococcal infections are followed by rheumatic fever, and the reason remains elusive. The severity of the infection may be a factor; although rheumatic fever follows 3% of severe infections (i.e., those accompanied by fever, exudate, swollen and tender cervical lymph nodes, persistence of positive streptococcal throat cultures, and subsequent antistreptolysin O response),[18] only 0.3 to 0.1%, or even fewer, of the less severe infections lead to rheumatic fever.[19] Host factors may be important, as the concordance rate for rheumatic fever is seven times higher in monozygotic (18.7%) than dizygotic twin pairs (2.5%).[20] HLA type I antigens seem to have no reproducible relationship to susceptibility to rheumatic fever, but among type II antigens, HLA-DR4 may be associated with the disease among whites.[21] Moreover, certain B-cell alloantigens have been reported in the majority of rheumatic patients and in the minority of controls.[22] Recently defined by monoclonal antibodies, they are much more prevalent among rheumatic fever patients than among controls in disparate parts of the world. But whether these markers are determined genetically, or are amplified by the rheumatic fever attack, or both, remains uncertain.[22]

PATHOGENESIS

Little is known about the chain of events that links streptococcal infections in the throat to the manifestations, distant in space and subsequent in time, of rheumatic fever. The streptococci do not migrate from the throat to the joints or to the heart, which are demonstrably sterile, but their products diffuse. Some of them are cardiotoxic in experimental animals and could be the mediators of tissue damage in rheumatic fever, but an indirect or immune pathogenesis is considered more likely.[23]

Several streptococcal antigens cross-react immunologically with human tissue antigens. As a result, the immune response to streptococci may be blunted because their antigens may be erroneously recognized as "self" by the lymphocytes, and whatever response is elicited may boomerang, in part, on the host because the host's antigens may be mistaken as foreign. The latter "mistake," which is called autoimmunity, may be the mechanism of tissue damage in rheumatic fever, especially in rheumatic carditis, as the well-studied cross-reactions of streptococcal antigens with heart antigens suggests.[23] Circulating immune complexes may also play a role.[24]

Considering the variety of manifestations of the rheumatic fever syndrome, some fleeting, others chronic, some exudative, other proliferative, it would not be surprising if more than one pathogenetic mechanism were at work.

CLINICAL FINDINGS

The natural history of rheumatic fever may be said to start with the streptococcal pharyngitis that precedes it by an interval ("latent period") of 2 to 3 weeks (mean 18.6 days). The latent period of rheumatic fever is a little longer than that of poststreptococcal glomerulonephritis and is of the same length in first attacks and in recurrences.[25]

The onset of the attack is acute when the presenting manifestation is arthritis but usually gradual when the presenting manifestation is carditis alone, and the symptom is heart failure. The onset of chorea may be acute but is often preceded by subtle behavioral changes that can be interpreted as a manifestation of chorea only in retrospect. Subcutaneous nodules and erythema marginatum are seldom, if ever, the presenting manifestations of rheumatic fever.

JOINT INVOLVEMENT

In the classic, untreated case, the arthritis of rheumatic fever affects several joints in quick succession, each for a short time (Fig. 79–2). The arthritis predilects large joints and often affects the lower limbs at first and later spreads to the arms.[26]

Joint involvement is more common, and also more severe, in young adults (nearly 100% in first attacks)[26] than in teenagers (82%) and in children (66%).[27] Rheumatic polyarthritis may be excruciatingly painful, but it is always transient. The arthritis is characteristically acute, almost like in gout, reaching its maximum intensity within a day or two in any given joint. The *pain* is usually more prominent than the objective signs of inflammation. Conversely, joints seldom are very swollen and only slightly tender.

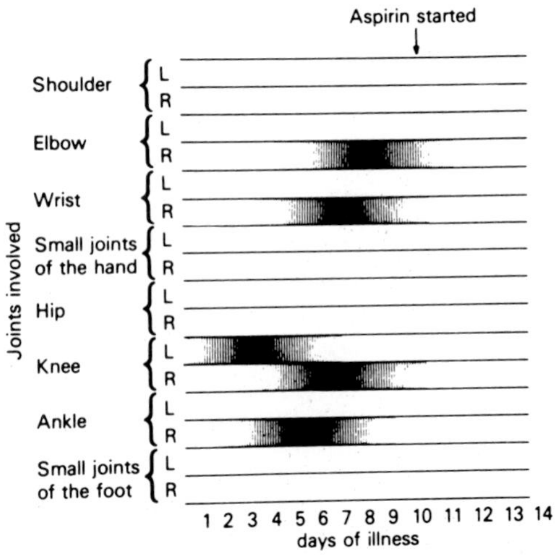

FIGURE 79–2. Time course of the migratory polyarthritis of rheumatic fever. Notice that even in the absence of treatment, the involvement of each joint is short-lived, but the cumulative involvement of all joints is less so. Note also that arthritis rapidly responds to aspirin.

When the disease is allowed to express itself fully, unchecked by anti-inflammatory treatment, the number of affected joints may be as high as 16, and about half of these patients develop arthritis in more than 6 joints.[28] Each joint is maximally inflamed for only a few days, or a week at the most, after which the inflammation decreases, usually to appear in another joint (migratory polyarthritis). Because the arthritis in the first joint(s) is often still present when other joints start to be inflamed, the arthritis of rheumatic fever has also been called additive. Tenosynovitis is often seen in adults.[28a] Considering all joints, the polyarthritis may be severe for a week in two thirds of the patients, and for 2 or at the most 3 weeks in the others, and may then persist in a mild form for another week or two.[28] Radiologic examination shows only effusion.

Under the usual circumstances of medical practice, however, many patients with joint complaints are treated empirically and prematurely with aspirin or other anti-inflammatory drugs; "migration" of the arthritis is then stopped, or the arthralgia is prevented from blooming into arthritis, depriving the clinician of useful data and the patient of a firm diagnosis. Conversely, administration of aspirin just a few days later, after the disease has declared itself, may further confirm the diagnosis of rheumatic fever by a characteristically rapid and complete therapeutic response.

Some patients may have only the subjective manifestations of joint involvement, such as arthralgia or polyarthralgia, which are very nonspecific. More often, objective evidence is present but not detected, hence the quip, "Arthralgia is arthritis without a good physical examination."

CARDITIS

Rheumatic carditis is the most important manifestation of acute rheumatic fever, because it may lead to chronic rheumatic heart disease and even to death from heart failure during the acute attack. More commonly, however, carditis causes no symptoms, only signs, and is diagnosed by auscultation when a patient is examined because of arthritis or chorea.

Criteria for the clinical diagnosis of rheumatic carditis include organic heart murmur(s) not previously present, enlargement of the heart, congestive heart failure, and pericardial friction rubs or signs of effusion, but significant murmurs are almost always present. In some patients, Doppler echocardiography may detect a valvular lesion that cannot be picked up by auscultation.[2] Patients whose rheumatic fever consists only of asymptomatic carditis may later develop chronic rheumatic heart disease, despite the absence of a medical history of recognized rheumatic fever.

The incidence of carditis in rheumatic fever varies with age, but in a direction opposite to that of arthritis; it is present in 90 to 92% of children under the age of 3 years,[29] in 50% of children aged 3 to 6 years, in 32% of teenagers aged 14 to 17,[27] but in only 15% of adults with a first attack of rheumatic fever.[26] In addition to being less frequent, carditis is less severe in adults than in children. The mitral valve is the most common site of involvement; a high-pitched, usually loud, long, blowing apical systolic murmur indicates *mitral regurgitation*. Functional or innocent systolic murmurs may be mistaken for it, especially when their loudness is increased by fever or anemia. Unlike the murmur of mitral regurgitation, however, most functional systolic murmurs are heard best along the left sternal border, in the third to second interspace or at the lower left sternal border. The functional systolic murmurs are limited to the first two thirds of systole and usually have a midsystolic accentuation. Their pitch is generally low, and they lack the "blowing" or "steam-jet" quality of mitral regurgitation murmurs. Some functional murmurs have a "groaning" or "twanging-string" quality; they are often heard best along the lower left sternal margin or between it and the apex. Depending on its loudness, the murmur of mitral regurgitation may persist after the acute rheumatic episodes, or it may disappear.

A mid-diastolic or Carey-Coombs murmur, usually following a third heart sound, is common in patients with rheumatic fever and acute mitral regurgitation. This murmur does not indicate mitral stenosis and disappears after the edema of the leaflets subsides. Physiologic third heart sounds may be mistaken for mid-diastolic murmurs. Differentiation of the two rests mainly on the perceptible duration of the latter.

The second most common valvular lesion during acute rheumatic fever is *aortic regurgitation*. This disorder produces a high-pitched decrescendo diastolic murmur that begins immediately after the second heart sound; it may be short and faint and therefore difficult to hear.[30]

Pericarditis can be detected clinically in up to 10% of patients with acute rheumatic fever. Pericardial effusion is occasionally striking, but cardiac tamponade is rare.

Congestive failure is the most serious manifestation of rheumatic carditis. Usually, it develops in patients with severe involvement of more than one valve. It occurs in 5 to 10% of first episodes of rheumatic carditis and is more frequent during recurrences. The diagnosis is established by careful physical examination, history taking, and review of chest roentgenograms.

ELECTROCARDIOGRAPHIC FINDINGS

Prolongation of the PR interval occurs in 28 to 40% of patients with rheumatic fever, much more frequently than in other febrile illnesses,[31] and therefore is useful in diagnosis. This prolongation does not correlate with residual heart disease,[32] however, and is not useful in prognosis.

CHOREA

Sydenham's chorea, chorea minor, or "St. Vitus' dance" is a neurologic disorder consisting of involuntary movements, muscular weakness, and emotional liability. The movements are abrupt and purposeless, not rhythmic or repetitive. They disappear during sleep but may occur at rest and may interfere with voluntary activity. The movements can be suppressed by the will of the patient, for a while. They may affect all voluntary muscles, but the involvement of the hands and face is usually the most obvious. Grimaces and inappropriate smiles are common (Fig. 79–3). Handwriting usually becomes clumsy and provides a convenient way of following the patient's course. Speech is often slurred. The movements are commonly more marked on one side and occasionally are completely unilateral (hemichorea).

The muscular weakness is best revealed by asking the patient to squeeze the examiner's hands. The examiner feels that the pressure of the patient's grip increases and decreases continually and capriciously—the relapsing grip, or "milking" sign.

The emotional changes manifest themselves in outbursts of inappropriate behavior, crying, and restlessness. There are no sensory losses or pyramidal tract involvement. In doubtful cases the choreic movements can be elicited by asking patients to stretch their hands in front of them, to stretch their fingers out, to close their eyes, and to stick their tongues out, one movement added to the other. By the time patients stick out their tongues, their fingers wiggle and their eyelids flutter. When the arms are projected straight forward, one sees flexion of the wrist, hyperextension of the metacarpophalangeal (MCP) joints, straightening of the fingers,

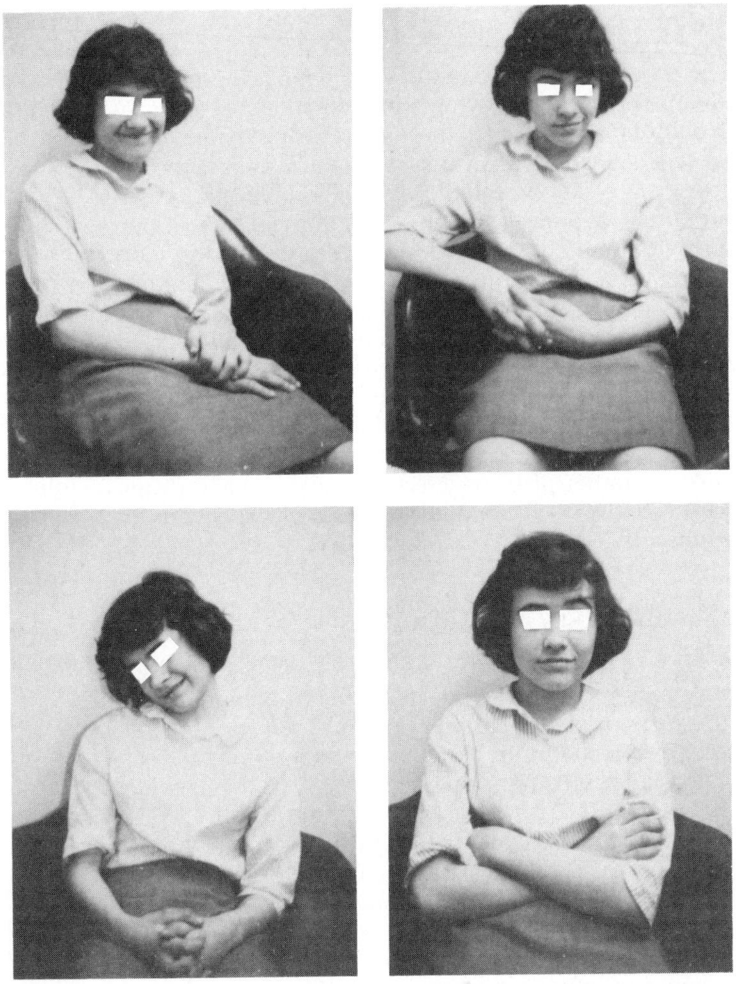

FIGURE 79–3. Grimaces and inappropriate smiles in a patient with chorea.

and abduction of the thumb ("spooning" or "dishing" of the hands). When patients are asked to raise their arms above their heads, they also pronate one or both hands (pronator sign).

Chorea may follow streptococcal infections after a longer latent period than that of other rheumatic manifestations. Some patients with chorea never develop other rheumatic symptoms, but other patients develop chorea weeks or months after arthritis[33] (Fig. 79–4). In either case, examination of the heart may reveal organic murmurs.

Patients who have had Sydenham's chorea have a marked tendency to develop it again. In most such patients intercurrent strep infections can be demonstrated serologically, but in a minority they cannot.[33a]

The incidence of chorea among rheumatic attacks has varied widely and seemed to be decreasing, but in the recent Utah epidemic, it was 31%.[2] Chorea is rare after puberty, and does not occur in adults, with the exception of rare cases during pregnancy ("chorea gravidarum"). Finally, it is the only manifestation with a marked sex predilection. Chorea is twice as frequent in girls as in boys; after puberty, this sex predilection increases.[34]

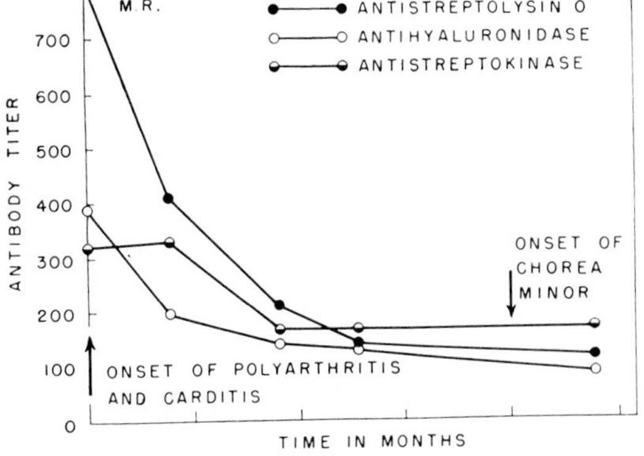

FIGURE 79–4. Chorea appearing 4 months after the onset of polyarthritis and carditis. Intercurrent streptococcal infections were ruled out by the falling titers of three streptococcal antibodies. (From Taranta, A., and Stollerman, G.H.[33])

SUBCUTANEOUS NODULES

The subcutaneous nodules of rheumatic fever are firm and painless. The overlying skin is not inflamed and can usually be moved over the nodules. The diameter of these roundish lesions varies from a few millimeters to 1 or even 2 cm. They are located over bony surfaces or prominences or near tendons; their number varies from a single nodule to a few dozen and averages three or four; when numerous, they are usually symmetric. These nodules are present for 1 or more weeks, rarely for more than a month. They are smaller and shorter lived than the nodules of rheumatoid arthritis (RA). Rheumatic subcutaneous nodules generally appear only after the first few weeks of illness, usually *only* in patients with carditis.[35] The frequency of their appearance, or rather of their detection, varies widely (from 34%[36] to 1%[27]). Rheumatic nodules are very rare in adults.

ERYTHEMA MARGINATUM

Erythema marginatum is an evanescent, nonpruritic, pink skin rash, which appears on the trunk and sometimes the proximal parts of the limbs, but not on the face. It is made up of a variable number of individual skin lesions, starting as erythematous spots that may be slightly raised. Each lesion extends centrifugally, while the skin in the center gradually returns to normal; hence the name *erythema marginatum.* The outer edge of the lesion is sharp, whereas the inner edge is soft[37] (Fig. 79–5).

The individual lesions may appear and disappear in a matter of hours, usually to return. They may change in shape and size almost as fast as smoke rings, which they resemble both in shape and in the centrifugal manner in which they expand and dissolve. A hot shower may make them more evident. Erythema marginatum, like nodules, occurs *only* in patients with carditis[35] and has been reported from 13%[38] to 2%[39] of patients with rheumatic fever. Erythema marginatum is very rare in adults.

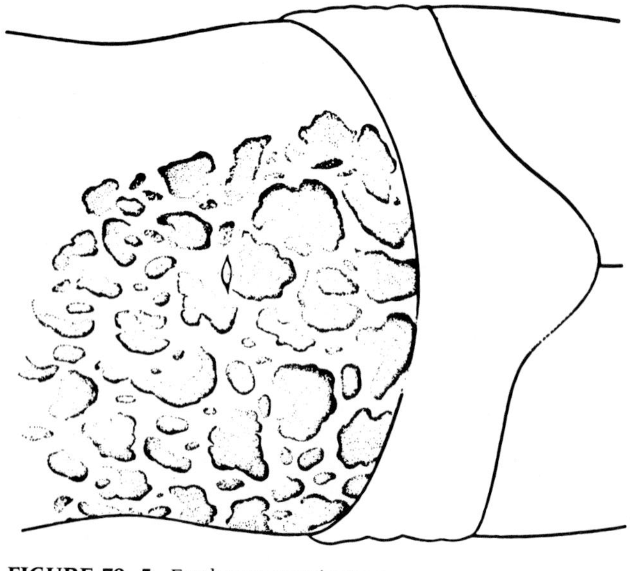

FIGURE 79–5. Erythema marginatum.

OTHER MANIFESTATIONS

Fever is regularly present in rheumatic fever with arthritis; it is often present in isolated carditis but seldom in isolated chorea. It is a remittent type of fever (unlike the wide swings of juvenile rheumatoid arthritis) that usually does not exceed 104°F and returns to normal in 2 to 3 weeks even without treatment.[40]

Anorexia, nausea, and vomiting may occur, mostly as manifestations of congestive heart failure or salicylate intoxication. Epistaxis seems to have been frequent once but is not common now.

DURATION OF THE ATTACK AND SEQUELAE

An episode of rheumatic fever is customarily considered to end when the patient's erythrocyte sedimentation rate returns to normal, usually several weeks after the subsidence of arthritis. By this criterion, the duration of the episode is 109 ± 57 days,[27] less than 12 weeks in 80% of cases and less than 15 weeks in 90%.[35] A few patients develop chronic rheumatic activity.[41]

Sequelae involve primarily the heart and depend on the occurrence and on the severity of carditis during the acute attack. In addition, patients who have had rheumatic fever develop it again after streptococcal infections with an attack rate much higher than in the general population (see following discussion). This propensity can also be considered a sequela.

JACCOUD'S ARTHRITIS (OR ARTHROPATHY OR SYNDROME) (see also Chapter 43)

Jaccoud's arthritis is also called, more descriptively, *chronic postrheumatic fever arthropathy.* It is a rare, indolent, slowly progressive process that deforms the fingers and sometimes the toes.[42–46] The deformity consists of ulnar deviation of the fingers, flexion of the MCP joints, and hyperextension of the proximal interphalangeal joints, just as in RA, but without the joint pains, heat, and swelling of the latter. The ulnar deviation occurs mostly in the fourth and fifth digits and is at first correctable, but later may become fixed. The toes may be affected similarly. Although no true erosions are present, notches or "hooks," thought to be due to the mechanical effect of ulnar deviation, are sometimes seen in roentgenograms on the ulnar side of each metacarpal head ("Bywater's hooks"). Rheumatoid factor (RF) is absent; the erythrocyte sedimentation rate is normal.

In classic cases, Jaccoud's arthropathy appears after multiple, prolonged, and severe attacks of rheumatic fever. It is thought to be the end result of the repeated inflammation of the fibrous articular capsules in the small joints of the hand, perhaps depending on individual predisposition. Patients with systemic lupus erythematosus (SLE) may develop a similar arthropathy,[47,48] and some patients develop it without having either SLE or rheumatic fever.[49,50] The prognosis of Jaccoud's arthropathy is good. Patients, alarmed by the deformity, may fear that it will extend to joints in other parts of the body, but this does not happen.

RECURRENCES

The attack rates of rheumatic fever after streptococcal pharyngitis are much higher in patients who have already had a previous attack than in those who have not. The recurrence rate per infection is highest in the first year after the rheumatic attack. The rate decreases sharply in the following 2 years, and then seems to level off[51] (Fig. 79–6).

Rheumatic fever recurs only among patients who develop a streptococcal antibody response, and the recurrence rate per infection increases with the magnitude of the antibody rise. At each level of antibody response, streptococcal infections are more likely to lead to recurrences of rheumatic fever in patients with pre-existing rheumatic heart disease than in patients with previous rheumatic fever attacks but without heart disease (Table 79–1).

The same clinical manifestations present in the initial episode of rheumatic fever tend to reappear in recurrences[53] (Table 79–2). Conversely, manifestations absent in the first episodes are usually absent in recurrent attacks. This is especially important in the case of the most serious manifestation, carditis.[54]

MORTALITY RATE

Of the many deaths ultimately caused by rheumatic fever, only a minority occur during an acute episode, and even fewer occur during the initial attack. Case-fatality rates of 0.36%,[27] 0.6%,[38] and 1.6%[35] have been reported in first episodes and rates of 2.3%[38] and 3%[27] in recurrences. None died among the 74 patients of the recent Utah epidemic.[2]

LABORATORY FINDINGS

EVIDENCE OF RECENT STREPTOCOCCAL INFECTION

Eighty percent of patients with acute rheumatic fever observed early in their course have elevated antistreptolysin O titers. The remaining 20% have elevation of one or more of the other streptococcal antibodies tested, such as antistreptokinase, antihyaluronidase, antideoxyribonuclease B, and antinicotinamide-adenine dinucleotidase.[56,57] All these antibody tests are based on the principle of inhibition of a specific toxic or enzymatic activity of streptococcal culture filtrate.

A simple, rapid test based on a different principle, the agglutination of sheep red blood cells coated with a mixture of streptococcal antigens, is commercially avail-

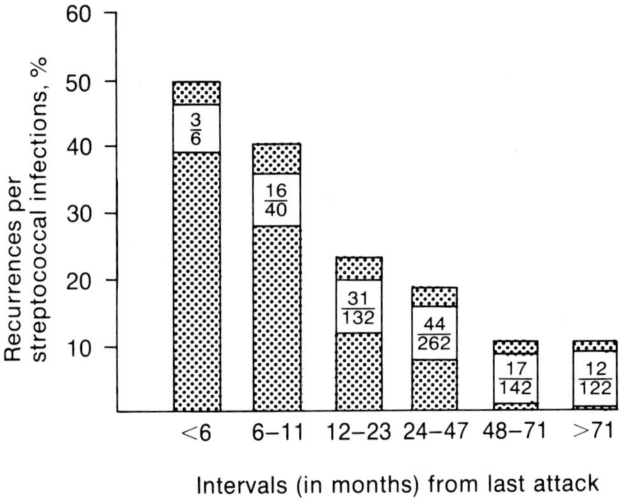

FIGURE 79–6. Decrease of the rheumatic fever recurrence rate per infection with time lapsed since the latest rheumatic episode. (From Spagnuolo, M., et al.[51])

TABLE 79–1. RATIO OF RHEUMATIC FEVER RECURRENCES TO STREPTOCOCCAL INFECTIONS IN PATIENTS STRATIFIED FOR PRE-EXISTING RHEUMATIC HEART DISEASE AND FOR RISE IN ANTISTREPTOLYSIN O (ASO)

ASO RISE IN NUMBER OF TUBE DILUTIONS	PRE-EXISTING HEART DISEASE (%)	NO PRE-EXISTING HEART DISEASE (%)
0–1	3:24 (13)	1:79 (1)
2	10:38 (26)	3:50 (6)
3	6:16 (38)	5:34 (15)
4+	9:16 (56)	9:26 (35)

(Data from Taranta, A. et al.[52])

TABLE 79–2. MAJOR CLINICAL MANIFESTATIONS OF RHEUMATIC FEVER RECURRENCES ACCORDING TO MANIFESTATIONS OF THE FIRST EPISODE

INITIAL MANIFESTATIONS (ISOLATED OR COMBINED WITH OTHERS)	MANIFESTATIONS OF RECURRENCES (ISOLATED OR COMBINED WITH OTHERS)		
	Polyarthritis No. (%)	Carditis No. (%)	Chorea No. (%)
Polyarthritis (N = 149)	110 (74)	51 (34)	18 (12)
Carditis (N = 89)	44 (49)	62 (70)	2 (2)
Chorea (N = 68)	11 (16)	10 (15)	54 (79)

(Data from Roth, I.R., Lingg, C., and Whittemore, A.[53])

able (Streptozyme). It is more sensitive than any other single streptococcal antibody test, simpler, and it takes only a few minutes to perform. In small series, it was positive at a dilution of 1:200 in 100% of rheumatic fever cases,[58] but there have been problems with its reproducibility.

NONSPECIFIC LABORATORY MANIFESTATIONS

Nonspecific laboratory manifestations include an elevated erythrocyte sedimentation rate, positive tests for C-reactive protein, moderate leukocytosis, and anemia. With the exception of "pure" or isolated chorea, untreated rheumatic fever is consistently accompanied by an elevated erythrocyte sedimentation rate and an elevated serum C-reactive protein.

OTHER LABORATORY ABNORMALITIES

Synovial fluid examination is useful to exclude other processes, especially septic arthritis. Synovial leukocyte counts vary (from 600 to 80,000/mL, with a mean of 16,000,[26] from 2,600 to 96,000/mL, with a mean of 29,000),[11] and polymorphonuclear leukocytes predominate (73 to 100%, with a mean of 90%,[26] 56 to 95%, with a mean of 83%).[11] The levels of C3, C4, and C1q are decreased with respect to simultaneously determined serum levels.[11] Interestingly, the viscosity of the fluid is high and gives a good mucin clot on addition of acetic acid.

Heart antibodies are demonstrable by a variety of techniques in the serum of patients with rheumatic fever, but they are also found in serum of patients with uncomplicated streptococcal infections or with acute glomerulonephritis, although usually at a lower titer.[23]

Subclinical liver involvement, manifested by transient enzyme elevations, has long been known to occur in rheumatic fever patients treated with aspirin,[59] but it may also occur without therapy.[26]

DIAGNOSIS

No single manifestation is so characteristic as to be diagnostic; the greater the number of clearly recognized manifestations, the firmer the diagnosis. The most common presentation, but also the least specific, is *arthritis without carditis*. There is no diagnostic laboratory test.

Because the prognosis varies according to the manifestations of the acute attack, the diagnosis of rheumatic fever should be qualified by mention of the manifestations diagnosed, such as "rheumatic fever with polyarthritis only."

JONES CRITERIA

T.D. Jones divided the manifestations of rheumatic fever into "major" and "minor" according to their diagnostic usefulness (Table 79–3) and proposed that the presence of two major or of one major and two minor manifestations indicates a high probability of rheumatic fever. These criteria have been widely accepted and have proved useful, especially in preventing overdiagnosis.[60]

DIFFERENTIAL DIAGNOSIS

The differential diagnosis varies according to the presenting manifestations. It is always prudent to exclude bacteremia by blood cultures; polyarthralgia and polyarthritis, as well as heart murmurs, are frequent manifestations of infective endocarditis.[61] Disseminated gonococcal infection is a frequent cause of acute, often migratory polyarthralgia and polyarthritis in adolescents and adults. Polyarthralgia and polyarthritis occur in preicteric and anicteric viral hepatitis, which can be recognized by a high serum glutamic-oxaloacetic transaminase level, positive tests for hepatitis B surface antigen, and sometimes an accompanying urticarial rash and low serum complement.[62] RA of acute onset does not respond to aspirin as readily as does rheumatic fever; in its juvenile form, RA is not infrequently accom-

TABLE 79–3. JONES CRITERIA (REVISED) FOR GUIDANCE IN THE DIAGNOSIS OF RHEUMATIC FEVER

Major Manifestations	Minor Manifestations
Carditis	Clinical
Polyarthritis	Fever
Chorea	Arthralgia
Erythema marginatum	Previous rheumatic fever or rheumatic heart disease
Subcutaneous nodules	Laboratory
	Erythrocyte sedimentation rate, C-reactive protein, leukocytosis
	Prolonged P-R interval

PLUS

Supporting evidence of preceding streptococcal infection such as increased antistreptolysin O or other streptococcal antibodies; positive throat culture for group A streptococci; or recent scarlet fever.

The presence of two major criteria, or of one major and two minor criteria, indicates the probable presence of rheumatic fever if supported by evidence of a preceding streptococcal infection. The absence of the latter should make the diagnosis suspect, except when rheumatic fever is first discovered after a long latent period from the antecedent infection, as in Sydenham's chorea or low-grade carditis.

(Courtesy of the American Heart Association.)

panied by high antistreptolysin O titers, which increase diagnostic confusion,[63] and RF tests are usually negative. The arthritis is persistent, however, and prolonged observation yields the diagnosis. Antinuclear antibody (ANA) tests, regularly positive in patients with SLE, are negative in patients with rheumatic fever, and the clinical pictures usually differ. Particularly troublesome may be the differentiation from a serum-sickness type of reaction, with fever and polyarthritis, which may occur after administration of penicillin for pharyngitis; urticaria or angioneurotic edema, if present, may help in the diagnosis. Polyarthritis may follow a number of viral infections, especially rubella, as well as rubella vaccination.[64]

Isolated rheumatic carditis may be difficult to distinguish from viral carditis, with which it has many features in common, such as pericarditis, cardiomegaly, heart failure, and even heart murmurs.[65] In dubious cases, one should attempt viral isolation from stools and pharyngeal washings and look for an appropriate antibody response, which may help at least in a retrospective diagnosis. Left atrial myxoma may also mimic isolated rheumatic carditis.[66]

Chorea must be differentiated from tics, which are repetitive, stereotyped, localized movements, and from benign familial chorea, a rare disorder transmitted as an autosomal dominant trait and beginning in childhood.[67]

Subcutaneous nodules must sometimes be differentiated from enlarged lymph nodes, especially in rubella. Rarely, nodules clinically and histologically indistinguishable from rheumatic or rheumatoid nodules occur in an isolated fashion and are benign.[68] Erythema marginatum must sometimes be differentiated from cutis marmorata, a fixed, reticular, bluish discoloration of the skin. An evanescent rash resembling erythema marginatum has been reported in Lyme arthritis.

In Scandinavian countries, infections with Yersinia enterocolitica have been associated with acute polyarthritis, carditis, and abdominal pains, all of which may cause diagnostic confusion.[69] Febrile diarrhea, frequent in Yersinia infections, may help in the differentiation.

In doubtful cases, and maybe in all cases of acute polyarthritis in Scandinavia, the agglutination test for Yersinia should be performed.

Among blacks, another cause of diagnostic confusion is sickle cell anemia, which may mimic rheumatic fever because of heart murmurs and arthralgias but may also coexist with it.[70]

TREATMENT

GENERAL MEASURES AND BED REST

All patients with rheumatic fever should be examined daily for the first 2 weeks of the illness, primarily to watch for the development of carditis and to start treatment promptly should heart failure occur. Patients should be kept comfortable, and rest generally helps, but strict and prolonged bed rest, once the rule, appears useless.

ANALGESICS OR ANTI-INFLAMMATORY AGENTS

Patients with arthralgia alone or with mild arthritis and no carditis may be given analgesics only. This is particularly wise when the diagnosis is not definite. Patients with moderate or severe arthritis but no carditis, or with carditis but no cardiomegaly or fever, are treated with aspirin, 40 mg/lb/day for the first 2 weeks and 20 mg/lb/day for the following 4 to 6 weeks. Larger doses may be necessary to control arthritis. In patients with carditis and cardiomegaly but without congestive failure, with or without polyarthritis, treatment should be started with aspirin. In patients with marked cardiomegaly, aspirin is often insufficient to control fever, discomfort, and tachycardia, or it does so only at toxic or near-toxic doses. These patients may then be treated with corticosteroids.

Patients with carditis and heart failure, with or without polyarthritis, should receive corticosteroids, starting with a dose of prednisone, 40 to 60 mg/day, to be increased if heart failure is not controlled. In cases of extreme acuteness and severity, therapy should be started by intravenous administration of methylprednisolone, 10 to 40 mg, followed by oral prednisone. In 2 to 3 weeks, prednisone may be slowly withdrawn; one should decrease the daily dose at the rate of 5 mg every 2 to 3 days. When the dose is tapered, aspirin at standard doses may be added and continued for 3 to 4 weeks after prednisone is discontinued. This "overlap" therapy reduces the incidence of post-therapeutic clinical rebounds.

The termination of anti-inflammatory treatment may be followed in all patients with rheumatic fever by transient reappearance, within 2 to 3 weeks, of laboratory or clinical abnormalities.[71]

Unfortunately, most well-controlled studies have failed to prove that treatment with corticosteroids decreases the incidence of residual rheumatic heart disease.[72,73] Nevertheless, such treatment is indicated in patients with severe carditis and heart failure because in many clinicians' experience corticosteroids help avert death during the acute attack. Patients with refractory cardiac failure may benefit from the insertion of a prosthetic valve.[2]

PREVENTION OF RECURRENCES (SECONDARY PREVENTION)

For all its simplicity, secondary prevention is the finest achievement of medicine in this disease. Its importance is out of proportion to the reduction in the number of rheumatic fever attacks because recurrences are more dangerous than first attacks.

Best results are obtained with 1.2 million U benzathine penicillin G given intramuscularly every 4 weeks. This treatment is especially useful in high-risk patients, that is, those with rheumatic heart disease, a previous rheumatic attack within the past 3 years, or multiple attacks, or in those unlikely to take daily medication. Additional risk factors are youth (childhood and adolescence), exposure to young people, and crowding in the home. In countries where rheumatic fever is rife, injections every 3 weeks have been advocated.[74]

Second best is continual oral medication. It success depends on the compliance of the patient. Sulfadiazine, at a dose of 0.5 g once daily in children weighing less than 60 pounds and 1 g in others, and oral penicillin, at a dose of 200,000 to 250,000 U twice a day, are about equally effective.

For maximum protection, continual prophylaxis may be maintained for the lifetime of the patient, particularly if rheumatic heart disease is present.[75]

PREVENTION OF INFECTIVE ENDOCARDITIS

Rheumatic heart disease predisposes patients to infective endocarditis. *It is advisable to administer appropriate antibiotics prophylactically to patients with rheumatic heart disease before they are exposed to a procedure that causes bacteremia.*[76]

PREVENTION OF INITIAL EPISODE (PRIMARY PREVENTION)

Although prevention of recurrences is both important and attainable, rheumatic fever can be eradicated only by preventing initial episodes, that is, by accurate diagnosis and appropriate treatment of streptococcal pharyngitis.[75] A relaxation of our vigilance had been suggested by the "virtual disappearance" of rheumatic fever,[1] but its return suggests otherwise.[2] Penicillin, or in the patient who is hypersensitive to it, another antibiotic, must be given *for at least 10 days* to eradicate the streptococci from the pharynx. Family members and other close contacts of the patient should have throat cultures, and if these are positive, should be treated similarly and simultaneously.

REFERENCES

1. Bland, E.F.: Rheumatic fever: The way it was. Circulation, *76*:1190–1195, 1987.
2. Bisno, A.L.: The resurgence of acute rheumatic fever in the U.S. Annu. Rev. Med., *41*:391–329, 1990.
3. Murphy, G.E.: Evolution of our knowledge of rheumatic fever: Historical survey with particular emphasis on rheumatic heart disease. Bull. Hist. Med., *14*:123–147, 1943.
4. El-Sadr, W., and Taranta, A.: The spectrum and the specter of rheumatic fever in the 1980's. Clin. Immunol. Update, 1979. Edited by E.C. Franklin. Elsevier, New York, 1979, pp 183–209.
5. Taranta, A., and Markowitz, M.: Rheumatic Fever. 2nd Ed. Boston, Kluwer Academic Publishers, 1989.

5a. Massell, B.F., Chute, C., Walker, A., Kurland, G.: Penicillin and the marked decrease in morbidity from rheumatic fever in the U.S. N. Engl. J. Med., *318*:280–285, 1988.

6. Murphy, G.E.: The characteristic rheumatic lesions of striated and of non-striated or smooth muscle cells of the heart. Genesis of the lesions known as Aschoff bodies and those myogenic components known as Aschoff cells or as Antischkow cells or myocytes. Medicine, *42*:73–117, 1963.
7. Husby, G., Arora, R., Williams, R., et al.: Immunofluorescence studies of florid rheumatic Aschoff lesions. Arthritis Rheum., *2*:207–211, 1986.
8. Kaplan, M., Bolande, R., Rakita, L., and Blair, J.: Presence of bound immunoglobulins and complement in myocardium in acute rheumatic fever. J. Clin. Invest., *56*:111–117, 1975.
9. Persellin, S.T., Ramirez, G., and Moatamed, F.: Immunopathology of rheumatic pericarditis. Arthritis Rheum., *25*:1054–1058, 1982.
10. Raisada, V., Williams, R., Chopra, P., et al.: Tissue distribution of lymphocytes in rheumatic heart valves as defined by monoclonal anti-T cell antibodies. Am. J. Med., *74*:90–96, 1983.
11. Svartman, M., Potter, E.V., Poon-King, T., and Earle, D.P.: Immunoglobulins and complement components in synovial fluid of patients with acute rheumatic fever. J. Clin. Invest., *56*:111–117, 1975.
12. Benedek, T.G.: Subcutaneous nodules and the differentiation of rheumatoid arthritis from rheumatic fever. Semin. Arthritis Rheum., *4*:305–321, 1984.
13. Wannamaker, L.W., et al.: Prophylaxis of acute rheumatic fever by treatment of the preceding streptococcal infection with various amounts of depot penicillin. Am. J. Med., *10*:673–695, 1951.
14. Taranta, A., and Gordis, L.: The prevention of rheumatic fever: Opportunities, frustrations, and challenges. Cardiovasc. Clin., *4*:1–10, 1972.
15. Kuttner, A.G., and Krumwiede, E.: Observations on the effect of streptococcal upper respiratory infections on rheumatic children: A three-year study. J. Clin. Invest., *20*:273–287, 1941.
16. Stollerman, G.H.: Rheumatogenic group A streptococci and the return of rheumatic fever. Adv. Intern. Med., *35*:1–26, 1990.

16a. Kaplan, E.L., Johnston, D.R., and Cleary, P.P.: Group A streptococcal serotypes isolated from patients and sibling contacts during the resurgence of rheumatic fever in the US. in the mid-1980's. J. Infect. Dis., *159*:101, 1989.

16b. Bessen, D., Jones, K.F., and Fischetti, V.A.: Evidence for two distinct classes of streptococcal M-protein and their relation to rheumatic fever. J. Exp. Med., *169*:269, 1989.

17. Perry, B.C., and Roberts, M.A.F.: A study on the variability in the incidence of rheumatic heart disease within the city of Bristol. Br. Med. J., *22*(Suppl.):154–158, 1937.
18. Rammelkamp, C.H., Jr.: Epidemiology of streptococcal infections. Harvey Lect., *15*:113–142, 1955–1956.
19. Stollerman, G.H., Siegel, A.C., and Johnson, E.E.: Variable epidemiology of streptococcal disease and the changing pattern of rheumatic fever. Mod. Concepts Cardiovasc. Dis., *34*:45–48, 1965.
20. Taranta, A. et al.: Rheumatic fever in monozygotic and dizygotic twins. *In* Proceedings of the Tenth International Congress of Rheumatology. Minerva Med., *2*:96–98, 1961.
21. Ayoub, E.M., Barrett, D.J., Maclaren, N.K., and Krischer, J.P.: Association of class II human histocompatibility leukocyte antigens with rheumatic fever. J. Clin. Invest., *6*:2019–2026, 1986.
22. Froude, J., Gibofsky, A., Buskizk, D.R., et al.: Cross-reactivity between streptococcus and human tissue: A model of molecular mimicry and autoimmunity. Curr. Top. Microbiol. Immunol., *145*:5–26, 1989.
23. Zabriskie, J.B.: Rheumatic fever: The interplay between host, genetics, and microbe. Lewis A. Conner memorial lecture. Circulation, *6*:1077–1086, 1985.
24. Friedman, J., van de Rign, I., Ohkuni, H., et al.: Immunological studies of post-streptococcal sequelae. Evidence for presence of

streptococcal antigens in circulating immune complexes. J. Clin. Invest., *76*:1027–1034, 1986.

25. Rammelkamp, C.H., Jr., and Stolzer, B.L.: The latent period before the onset of acute rheumatic fever. Yale J. Biol. Med., *34*:386–398, 1961–1962.
26. Barnert, A.L., Jerry, E.E., and Persellin, R.H.: Acute rheumatic fever in adults. JAMA, *232*:925–928, 1975.
27. Feinstein, A.R., and Spagnuolo, M.: The clinical patterns of acute rheumatic fever: A reappraisal. Medicine, *41*:279–305, 1962.
28. Graef, I., Parent, S., Zitron, W., Wyckoff, J: Studies in rheumatic fever. The natural course of acute manifestations of rheumatic fever uninfluenced by "specific" therapy. Am. J. Med. Sci., *185*:197–210, 1933.

28a. Wallace, M.R., Garst, P.D., Papadimos, T.J., et al.: The return of acute rheumatic fever in young adults. JAMA, *262*:2557–2561, 1989.

29. Rosenthal, A., Czoniczer, G., and Messell, B.F.: Rheumatic fever under three years of age. A report of 10 cases. Pediatrics, *41*:612–619, 1968.
30. Feinstein, A.R., and Di Masa, R.: The unheard diastolic murmur in acute rheumatic fever. N. Engl. J. Med., *260*:1331–1333, 1959.
31. Mirowski, M., Rosenstein, B.J., and Markowitz, M.: A comparison of atrioventricular conduction in normal children and in patients with rheumatic fever, glomerulonephritis, and acute febrile illnesses. A quantitative study with determination of the P-R index. Pediatrics, *33*:334–340, 1964.
32. Feinstein, A.R., and Spagnuolo, M.: Prognostic significance of valvular involvement in acute rheumatic fever. N. Engl. J. Med., *260*:1001–1007, 1959.
33. Taranta, A., and Stollerman, G.H.: The relationship of Sydenham's chorea to infection with group A streptococci. Am. J. Med., *20*:170–175, 1956.

33a. Berrios, X., Quesney, F., Morales, A., et al.: Are all recurrences of "pure" Sydenham chorea true recurrences of acute rheumatic fever? J. Pediatr., *107*:867–872, 1985.

34. Aron, A.M., Freeman, J.M., and Carter, S.: The natural history of Sydenham's chorea. Review of the literature and long-term evaluation with emphasis on cardiac sequelae. Am. J. Med., *38*:83–95, 1965.
35. Massell, B.F., Fyler, D.C., and Rey, S.B.: The clinical picture of rheumatic fever: Diagnosis, immediate prognosis, course and therapeutic implications. Am. J. Cardiol., *1*:436–449, 1958.
36. Bywaters, E.G.L., and Thomas, G.T.: Bed rest, salicylates, and steroid in rheumatic fever. Br. Med. J., *1*:1628, 1962.
37. Perry, B.C.: Erythema marginatum (rheumaticum). Arch. Dis. Child., *12*:233–238, 1937.
38. United Kingdom and United States Joint Report: The treatment of acute rheumatic fever in children: A cooperative clinical trial of ACTH, cortisone and aspirin. Circulation, *11*:343–377, 1955.
39. Sanyal, S.K., Thapar, M.K., Ahmed, S.H., et al.: The initial attack of acute rheumatic fever during childhood in North India: A prospective study of the clinical profile. Circulation, *49*:7–12, 1974.
40. McMinn, F.J., and Bywaters, E.G.L.: Differences between the fever of Still's disease and that of rheumatic fever. Ann. Rheum. Dis., *18*:293–297, 1959.
41. Taranta, A., Spagnuolo, M., and Feinstein, A.R.: Chronic rheumatic fever. Ann. Intern. Med., *56*:367–388, 1962.
42. Bittl, J.A., and Perloff, J.K.: Chronic postrheumatic fever arthropathy of Jaccoud. Am. Heart. J., *105*:515–517, 1983.
43. Bywaters, E.G.L.: The relation between heart and joint disease including "rheumatoid heart disease" and chronic post-rheumatic arthritis (type Jaccoud). Br. Heart J., *12*:101, 1950.
44. Girigis, F.L., Popple, A.W., Bruckner, F.E.: Jaccoud's arthropathy. A case report and necropsy study. Ann. Rheum. Dis., *37*:561–565, 1978.
45. Ruderman, J.E., and Abruzzo, J.L.: Chronic postrheumatic fever arthritis (Jaccoud's): Report of a case with subcutaneous nodules. Arthritis Rheum., *9*:640–647, 1966.
46. Zvaifler, N.J.: Chronic postrheumatic-fever (Jaccoud's) arthritis. N. Engl. J. Med., *267*:10–14, 1962.
47. Bywaters, E.G.L.: Jaccoud's syndrome: A sequel to the joint involvement of systemic lupus erythematosus. Clin. Rheum. Dis., *1*:125–148, 1975.
48. Esdaile, J.M., Danoff, D., Rosenthall, L., Gutkowski, A.: Deforming arthritis in systemic lupus erythematosus. Ann. Rheum. Dis., *40*:124–126, 1981.
49. Ignaczak, T., Espinoza, L.R., Kantor, O.S., Osterland, C.K.: Jaccoud arthritis. Arch. Intern. Med., *35*:557–579, 1975.
50. Murphy, W.A., and Staple, T.W.: Jaccoud's arthropathy viewed. AJR, *118*:300–307, 1973.
51. Spagnuolo, M., Pasternak, B., and Taranta, A.: Risk of rheumatic fever recurrences after streptococcal infections. Prospective study of clinical and social factors. N. Engl. J. Med., *285*:641–647, 1971.
52. Taranta, A., Kleinberg, E., Feinstein, A.R., et al.: Rheumatic fever in children and adolescents. A long-term epidemiologic study of subsequent prophylaxis, streptococcal infections, and clinical sequelae. V. Relation of the rheumatic fever recurrence rate per streptococcal infection to pre-existing clinical features of the patients. Ann. Intern. Med., *60*:58–67, 1964.
53. Roth, I.R., Lingg, C., and Whittemore, A.: Heart disease in children. A. Rheumatic Group. I. Certain aspects of the age at onset and of recurrences in 488 cases of juvenile rheumatism ushered in by major clinical manifestations. Am. Heart J., *13*:36–60, 1937.
54. Feinstein, A.R., and Spagnuolo, M.: Mimetic features of rheumatic fever recurrences. N. Engl. J. Med., *262*:533–540, 1960.
55. Taranta, A.: Rheumatic fever made difficult: Critical review of pathogenetic theories. Pediatrician, *5*:74–95, 1976.
56. Stollerman, G.H., Lewis, A.J., Schultz, I., Taranta, A.: Relationship of immune response to group A streptococci to course of acute, chronic and recurrent rheumatic fever. Am. J. Med., *20*:163–169, 1956.
57. Taranta, A., Wood, H.F., Feinstein, A.R., et al.: Rheumatic fever in children and adolescents. A long-term epidemiologic study of subsequent prophylaxis, streptococcal infections, and clinical sequelae. IV. Relation of the rheumatic fever recurrence rate per streptococcal infection to the titers of streptococcal antibodies. Ann. Intern. Med., *60*:(Suppl. 5):47–57, 1964.
58. Bisno, A.L., and Ofek, I.: Serologic diagnosis of streptococcal infection. Comparison of a rapid hemagglutination technique with conventional antibody tests. Am. J. Dis. Child., *127*:676–681, 1974.
59. Manso, C., Taranta, A., and Nydick, S.: Effect of aspirin administration on serum glutamic oxaloacetic and glutamic pyruvic transaminase in children. Proc. Soc. Exp. Biol. Med., *93*:84–88, 1956.
60. American Heart Association: Jones Criteria (revised) for guidance in the diagnosis of rheumatic fever. Circulation, *69*:204A–208A, 1984.
61. Doyle, E.F., Spagnuolo, M., Taranta, A., et al.: The risk of bacterial endocarditis during antirheumatic prophylaxis. JAMA, *201*:807–812, 1967.
62. Fernandez, R., and McCarty, D.L.: The arthritis of viral hepatitis. Ann. Intern. Med., *74*:207–211, 1971.
63. Roy, S.B., Sturges, G.P., and Massell, B.F.: Application of the antistreptolysin-O titer in the evaluation of joint pain and in the diagnosis of rheumatic fever. N. Engl. J. Med., *254*:95–102, 1956.
64. Cooper, L.Z., Ziring, P.R., Weiss, H.J., et al.: Transient arthritis after rubella vaccination. Am. J. Dis. Child., *118*:218–225, 1969.
65. Ward, C.: Observations of the diagnosis of isolated rheumatic carditis. Am. Heart J., *91*:545–550, 1976.

66. Lortscher, R.H., Toews, W.H., Nora, J.J., et al.: Left atrial myxoma presenting as rheumatic fever. Chest. *66*:302–303, 1974.
67. Chun, R.W.M., Daly, R.F., Mansheim, B.J., Wolcott, G.J.: Benign familial chorea with onset in childhood. JAMA, *225*:1603, 1973.
68. Taranta, A.: Occurrence of rheumatic-like subcutaneous nodules without evidence of joint or heart disease. N. Engl. J. Med, *266*:13–16, 1962.
69. Laitinen, O., Leirisalo, M., and Allander, E.: Rheumatic fever and *Yersinia* arthritis; Criteria and diagnostic problems in a changing disease pattern. Scand. J. Rheumatol., *4*:145–157, 1975.
70. Mazzara, J.T., Burns, G.C., Mueller, H.S., Ayres, S.M.: Coexistence of sickle-cell anemia and rheumatic heart disease. N.Y. State J. Med., *71*:2426–2430, 1971.
71. Feinstein, A.R., Spagnuolo, M., and Gill, F.A.: The rebound phenomenon in acute rheumatic fever 1. Incidence and significance. Yale J. Biol. Med., *33*:259–278, 1961.
72. Combined Rheumatic Fever Study Group: A comparison of short-term, intensive prednisone and acetylsalicylic acid therapy in the treatment of acute rheumatic fever. N. Engl. J. Med., *272*:63–70, 1965.
73. United Kingdom and United States Joint Report: The evolution of rheumatic heart disease in children: Five-year report of a cooperative clinical trial of ACTH, cortisone and aspirin. Circulation, *22*:1503, 1960.
74. Ayoub, E.M.: Prophylaxis in patients with rheumatic fever: Every three or every four weeks? J. Pediatr., *115*:89–91, 1989.
75. American Heart Association: Prevention of rheumatic fever. Circulation, *70*:1118A–1122A, 1984.
76. Shulman, S.T., Amzen, D.P., Bisno, A.L., et al.: Prevention of bacterial endocarditis. Circulation, *70*:1122A–1123A, 1984.

80

Relapsing Polychondritis

DAVID E. TRENTHAM

Relapsing polychondritis is an uncommon entity whose manifestations are frequently widespread and dramatic. The essential features are inflammation with progressive loss of structural integrity of some cartilaginous tissues and involvement of organs of special sense such as the eye, the middle and inner ears, and the vestibular apparatus. Aortic insufficiency can also occur.

Before 1958, the medical literature contained only 10 single case reports, but since that time the condition has become widely recognized as a distinct clinical entity.[1–6] Many of the earlier authors did not realize that similar patients had been described before, and each invented his own descriptive terms for the disease. Thus, some of the terms used for relapsing polychondritis were "systemic chondromalacia," "panchondritis," and "chronic atrophic polychondritis." "Relapsing polychondritis" best describes the undulating clinical course that this syndrome follows, although admittedly it does not take into account the frequent involvement of some noncartilaginous structures.

CLINICAL FEATURES

The earliest identifiable report of relapsing polychondritis, published in 1923 by Jaksch-Wartenhorst,[7] still provides a clear picture of the disease. His patient, a 32-year-old brewer, first became ill with arthritic swellings and pain in several finger joints and then in the wrists, left hand, right knee, and toes of the right foot. There was also a febrile response. One-and-a-half months later, burning pain developed in both external ears, which slowly swelled and, within the next 3 months, receded and shrank, leaving a flabby deformity of both auricles. Two or three months later, without pain, the midsegment of the nose slowly collapsed, leaving a saddle-nose deformity. At that time, there was nearly complete stenosis of both auditory canals and some diminution of hearing, even when the canals were held open. Associated dizziness and tinnitus also occurred. Somewhat later, crepitation developed in both knees and in the spine.

The disease occurs equally in both sexes. It is most common in the middle decades of life, but cases have been reported in children and the elderly. Although it is often fatal, the clinical course is highly variable and may be self-limited. One study reported a 7-year average life span in 11 patients from the time of appearance of symptoms of death, but the spectrum of survival ranged widely, from 10 months to over 20 years.[3] The causes of death were usually respiratory failure that was due to airway stenosis (or collapse) and complicating pulmonary infection and cardiovascular failure that were due to intractable aortic insufficiency.[1,3] Table 80–1 summarizes many of the clinical manifestations and their incidence.

Inflammation of isolated or multiple cartilages predominates, often with an initial febrile response and involvement of one or several structures of the eye. Onset is usually acute in the first and subsequent attacks unless the latter are modified by glucocorticoid therapy. Typically, the pinnas, or cartilaginous portions of the ears, swell and become purplish-red and exquisitely tender, so that it is impossible to rest them on a pillow. The soft earlobes are always spared. The external auditory canals, especially the meatus, also swell and may close almost completely; hearing is thereby reduced. Inflammation of the inner ear producing serous otitis media and obstruction of the eustachian tube from cartilage involvement in its nasopharyngeal portion can further impair hearing.[8] A labyrinthine type of vertigo may develop. Often, the episclerae are inflamed. Joint inflammation or simple arthralgias occasionally occur during these attacks. Sometimes, the cartilaginous por-

TABLE 80–1. INCIDENCE OF VARIOUS CLINICAL FEATURES IN RELAPSING POLYCHONDRITIS*

MANIFESTATION	NO. AFFECTED/NO. REPORTED	FREQUENCY (%)
Ear cartilage involvement	45/51	88
Nasal cartilage involvement	40/49	82
Fever	21/26	81
Arthropathy	40/51	78
Laryngotracheal involvement	33/47	70
Episcleritis or conjunctivitis	29/48	60
Defective hearing	21/44	48
Costochondral cartilage involvement	21/45	47
Iritis	11/41	27
Labyrinthine vertigo†	—	25
Aortic valve lesion with insufficiency‡	10/74	14

* Modified from Dolan, D.L. et al.[3]
† Rough approximation of incidence. These organ systems were not always clearly described.
‡ Data from Arkin, C.R., and Masi, A.T.,[1] and others.

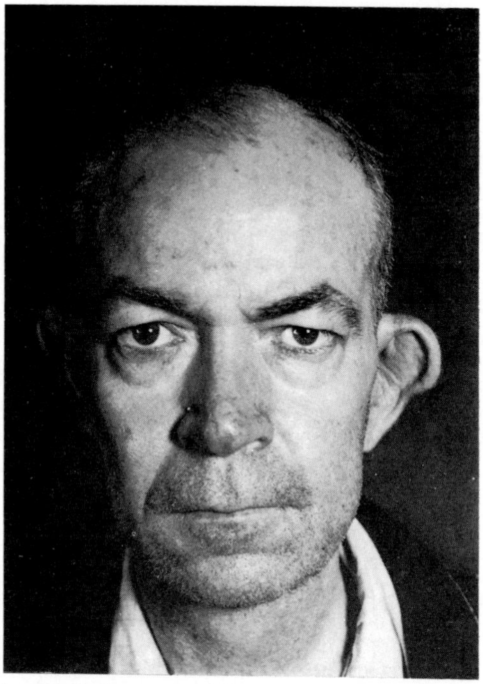

FIGURE 80–1. Classic drooping of the left external ear in a man with recurrent episodes of polychondritis.

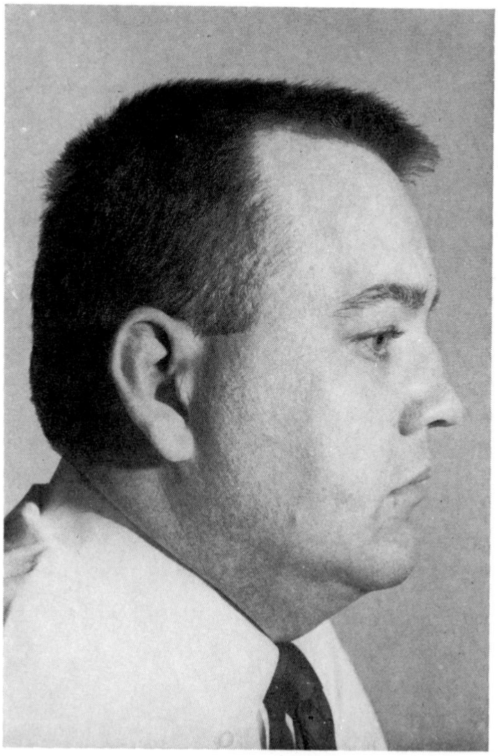

FIGURE 80–2. The characteristic saddle-nose deformity had developed painlessly 3 months earlier.

tion of the bridge of the nose becomes inflamed during the first or later episodes.

An attack lasts from a few days to many weeks, and may, if left untreated, progress in a subacute or smoldering fashion to involve additional cartilaginous structures and special sense organs. As the inflammatory phase subsides, the external ear may shrink, owing to the thinning of the cartilage or the loss of its structural integrity, so that the pinna droops forward from lack of support (Fig. 80–1). This condition may occur during the first episode or not until after several attacks. Similarly, the cartilaginous nasal septum may erode (Fig. 80–2), leaving a step-shaped or saddle nose, which is also characteristic for this condition.

The two most serious complications of relapsing polychondritis are: (1) an involvement of the cartilaginous structures of the respiratory tract and (2) progressive aortic insufficiency. In the mildest forms of the disease, the respiratory tract involvement consists of hoarseness, slight cough, and minimal tenderness of the larynx and trachea. In more severe instances, there may be extensive inflammation and edema of the laryngeal and epiglottal cartilages, necessitating emergency tracheostomy. A similar process may also involve the tracheal and bronchial rings so that diffuse narrowing of the airways may ensue. This complication may be fatal, owing to asphyxia and/or superimposed respiratory infection. Moreover, in such circumstances, tracheostomy may be inadequate to maintain adequate pulmonary ventilation. If the patient survives one or more chondrolytic attacks on the air passages, the cartilages may be left with some loss of structural support in the involved regions. The trachea and bronchi may then become diffusely or focally narrowed because of varying degrees of stenosis, or the cartilages may lose all or nearly all of their architectural support. They then appear at autopsy as floppy collapsible tubes. In such patients, intubation is useless because of the collapse throughout even the smallest bronchi.[9] As if such serious involvement of the respiratory apparatus is not enough, further embarrassment to breathing may, on occasion, be caused by tenderness and swelling of one or several costosternal cartilages. In rare instances, partial or complete dissolution may result, leaving a flail anterior chest plate.

Aortic insufficiency, the other life-threatening complication, has been described in approximately 10 to 15% of cases.[1,2] The aortic regurgitation is due to progressive dilatation of the aortic ring and, often, the ascending aorta, rather than to inflammation of the valve leaflets. This pattern of involvement helps to differentiate the aortic insufficiency of relapsing polychondritis from the regurgitation that occurs in ankylosing spondylitis, Reiter's syndrome, and certain other rheumatic diseases (Table 80–2). Rarely, polychondritis can be associated with dilatation of the annulus of the mitral and tricuspid valves.[2] Prosthetic valves have been inserted successfully in some patients.[1]

Eye lesions are common and include episcleritis, conjunctivitis and, less frequently, iritis. Usually, the inflammation smolders at a low level or resolves as an attack subsides. Rarely have serious sequelae resulted, but proptosis, cataracts, severe keratitis, and even blindness have occurred in isolated instances.[2]

TABLE 80–2. AORTIC INSUFFICIENCY

CONDITION	DISEASE CAUSING
Valvulitis	Rheumatic fever Rheumatoid arthritis Ankylosing spondylitis* Endocarditis Reiter's syndrome* Behçet's syndrome*
Congenital	Bicuspid aortic valve
Dilatation of valve ring	Marfan's syndrome Syphilis Relapsing polychondritis Secondary to dissecting aneurysm Idiopathic

* Also dilatation of valve ring

Articular involvement is variable, usually consisting of subacute swelling and pain in one or several large joints of the extremities. The articulations of the spine, either the true apophyseal cartilages or the intervertebral discs, are rarely involved. Serious peripheral joint damage has not been a common occurrence. However, it may resemble low-grade rheumatoid arthritis (RA) or, conversely, may culminate in osteophyte formation that even limits joint mobility. In a series of 23 patients, arthritis was the presenting symptom in 35% and was a significant clinical feature during the course of relapsing polychondritis in 85% of patients.[10]

Minor hematopoietic, hepatic, and renal involvement has been described,[3] but in some cases, this may have represented another associated disease process.

The most curious clinical feature is the selectivity of the chondritic process. Not only are some cartilages and cartilaginous structures spared while others are extensively involved, but there exists in some patients a remarkable unilaterality so that only one ear or one eye may be affected, even after multiple attacks. Other disorders to be considered in the differential diagnosis of relapsing polychondritis, such as a bacterial perichondritis, trauma or frostbite, Wegener's granulomatosis, lethal midline granuloma, or Cogan's syndrome,[2] do not produce multifocal chondritic lesions. However, polychondritis may develop in patients with a variety of connective tissue diseases, including systemic lupus erythematosus, vasculitis, adult or juvenile rheumatoid arthritis, and Sjögren's syndrome.[1,2]

In a large single-institution analysis,[6] the 5- and 10-year probabilities for survival after the diagnosis of relapsing polychondritis were 74 and 55%, respectively. Infection, systemic vasculitis, and malignancy were the most frequent causes of death. Surprisingly, only 10% of the fatalities were attributable to airway involvement. Anemia at the time of diagnosis was a marker for shortened survival; a saddle-nose deformity or systemic vasculitis were additional unfavorable prognostic signs in younger patients.

LABORATORY OBSERVATIONS

As may be anticipated, aside from diagnostic biopsy findings, the laboratory features are nonspecific.[3] The most common findings are noted during the active disease process. They consist of an increased erythrocyte sedimentation rate, some degree of leukocytosis and anemia, occasional low titer positivity for rheumatoid factor or antinuclear antibody, and modest serum protein alterations, such as a decreased albumin and increased α- and γ-globulins.

The roentgenographic finding that is of the greatest value, diagnostically, is tracheal stenosis. After multiple inflammation attacks, the external ears may show calcific deposits. This finding is not specific for relapsing polychondritis, however, because it may result from other inflammatory conditions such as frostbite. The joints may show moderate destructive changes, often spotty and asymmetric, but sometimes suggestive of RA. On a chest film, major airways may be narrowed. The closure may be focal or diffuse and is most clearly visualized by tracheal tomography (Fig. 80–3). In the presence of aortic insufficiency, cardiomegaly is commonly found.

PATHOLOGY

The histopathology of relapsing polychondritis is highly characteristic[5,9,11–13] Acidophilic (pink) coloration of the cartilage matrix, in contrast to the usual basophilic (blue) hue, is seen by routine hematoxylin and eosin staining (Fig. 80–4). Focal or diffuse infiltration by predominantly mononuclear inflammatory cells, with occasional polymorphonuclear leukocytes and plasma cells in the perichondrial tissues, is associated with the dissolution of cartilage from its periphery inward (Fig. 80–5). Fibroblastic granulation tissue frequently coexists and leads to partial sequestration of the cartilage matrix (see Fig. 80–4). This vigorous reparative response may culminate in the production of new cartilage.[12] Evidence of necrotizing angiitis or thrombosis is lacking. Rarely, calcium salts are found in the cartilage. Examination of the ocular globe in one patient revealed mononuclear inflammatory cells and plasma cells scattered about the episcleral vessels.

In involved cardiac and aortic structures, the aortic valve leaflets are normal, whereas the ascending aorta, especially the aortic ring, is dilated, with a loss of basophilia and degeneration, necrosis, and fibrosis. The primary pathologic change in the aortic ring and ascending aorta is in the media, with a loss of elastic tissue, a

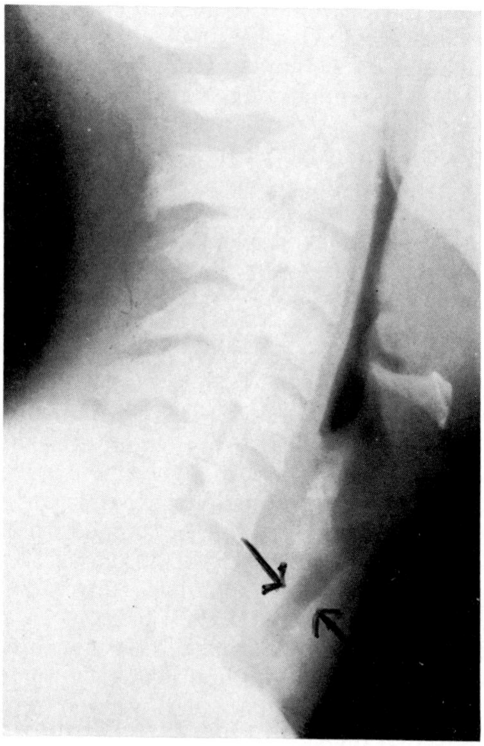

FIGURE 80–3. Significant stenosis of the tracheal airway as demonstrated by air tomography in a 50-year-old woman with relapsing polychondritis.

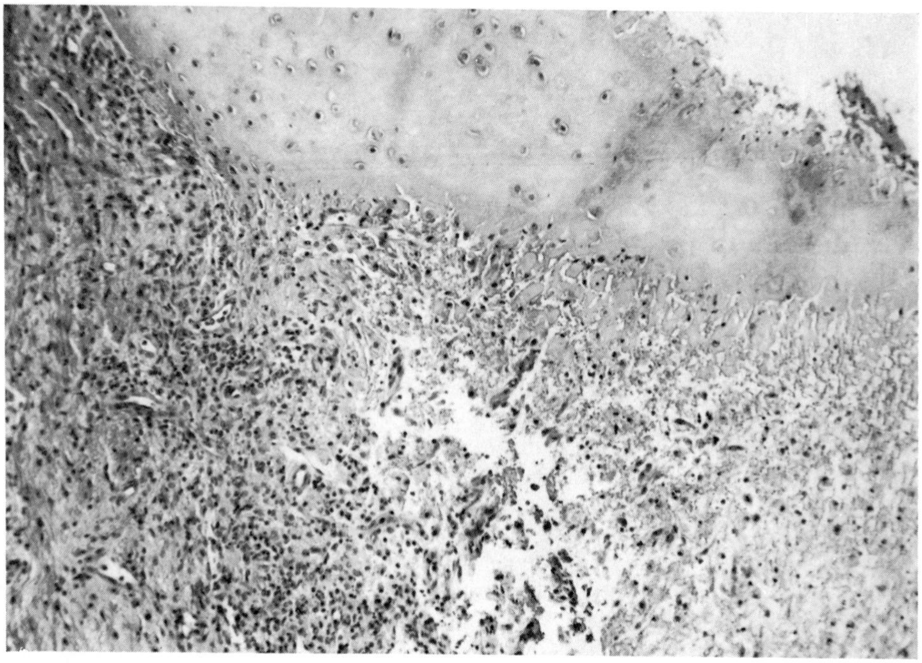

FIGURE 80–4. Chondrocyte necrosis, destruction of the matrix, and loss of basophilia in the elastic cartilage of the ear, sequestration of segments of cartilage by contiguous granulation tissue, and infiltration by inflammatory cells. These histopathologic features are characteristic of the cartilage lesion in relapsing polychondritis.

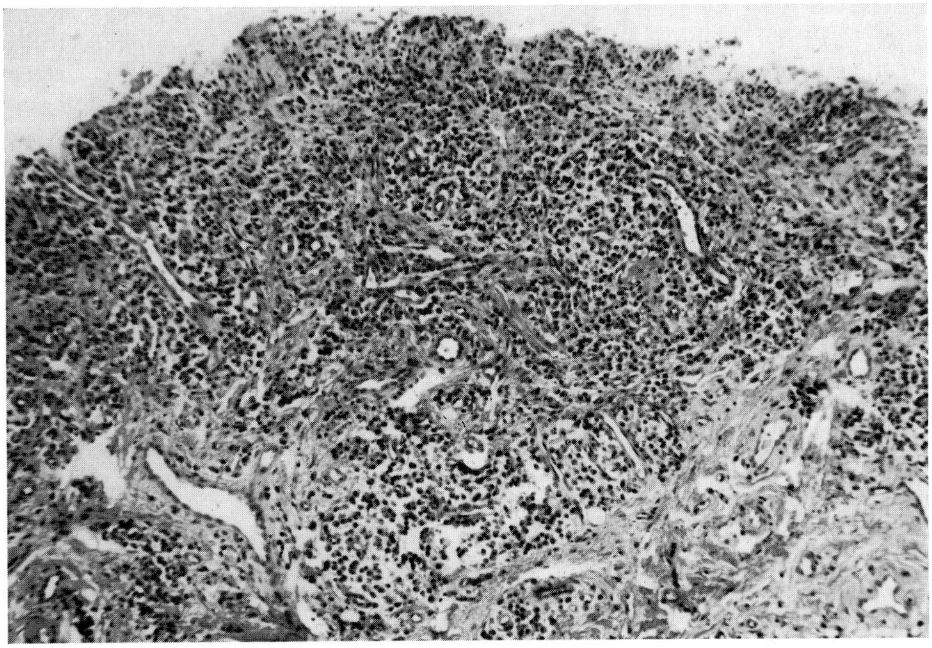

FIGURE 80–5. Marked cellular infiltration composed of mononuclear inflammatory cells, plasma cells, and histiocytes in the perichondrial tissues in relapsing polychondritis. Connective tissue and blood vessel elements have proliferated, but no vasculitis is present in this exuberant granulation tissue.

decrease in basophilia, and fibrosis. Associated focal acute and chronic inflammation occurs in these areas as well as in the adventitial blood vessels and in the vasa vasorum.

Histochemical studies have confirmed these findings and have revealed a loss of metachromasia in the residual cartilage matrix, with some preservation of metachromasia in the cytoplasm and in the immediate perilacunar zones around chondrocytes.[9] In the aorta, there was a moderate loss in neutral or acidic polysaccharides by the toluidine blue, azure A (pH 2.0), or PAS-alcian blue methods. Hale's method for sulfated mucopolysaccharides showed marked depletion of these components in the abnormal aortas and aortic rings.

By electron microscopy, cartilage from patients with active relapsing polychondritis contains greatly increased numbers of "matrix granules."[14] These are small (less than 10 nm in diameter) stellate granules of medium electron density and are compatible with particles of cartilage matrix composed primarily of proteoglycan. These granules are usually not membrane limited and are seen in normal cartilage in small numbers. "Matrix vesicles," also present in these specimens, are larger than the matrix granule, measure about 1000 nm, and are located extracellularly. Ultrastructurally, the vesicles and dense granules found in the lesions are more compatible with lysosomes than typical matrix vesicles or granules, because they are usually larger and more irregular in shape, and because they often contain multiple myelin-like laminated structures. The matrix vesicles possess a significant amount of alkaline phosphatase and adenosine triphosphatase activities, but a low acid phosphatase activity, which is usually a marker for lysosomes. The origin of these cartilage matrix vesicles is uncertain. Because they are extracellular, it is likely that they are budding from cellular membranes containing cytoplasmic debris. Other investigators have recognized a few dense bodies, which they interpreted as lysosomes, in the chondrocytes of the lesion.[14] Furthermore, they observed a large number of extracellular dense bodies containing multiple vesicles. The significance of this observation is unknown.

Immunofluorescence studies of specimens from patients with relapsing polychondritis have identified granular deposits of immunoglobulin G (IgG), IgA, IgM, and C3 at the lesional junction of fibrous and cartilaginous tissue, suggesting the presence of immune complexes.[2,12,13,15]

PATHOGENESIS

The cause of relapsing polychondritis is unknown. The loss of acid mucopolysaccharides and many of the other cartilage changes that may be secondary events could be caused by release of lysosomal enzymes, especially proteases, either from chondrocytes or from other cellular elements. Thus, it is of potential interest that intravenously administered crude papain, a proteolytic enzyme, induced a noninflammatory dissolution of the ear cartilages of rabbits within 4 hours.[16] This reaction also involved a rapid loss of cartilage metachromasia. In addition, 3 to 6 weeks after a single intravenous injection of crude papain into rabbits, focal plaque lesions that were due to alterations of connective tissue of the media occurred in the ascending aorta and arch. Some of these lesions progressed by metaplasia into partially developed cartilage and bone.[17] It has been postulated that these lesions resulted from the release, by papain, of large amounts of sulfated mucopolysaccharides, which are then deposited in various organs and especially in the aortic wall. A similar mechanism may be operative in relapsing polychondritis, with an endogenous proteolytic enzyme, perhaps lysosomal, being responsible for the chondrolysis.

The identification of immunoglobulins in the lesions and the occasional coexistence of another systemic connective tissue disease are consistent with the possibility that autoimmune mechanisms cause the cartilage damage.[1,2,12,13,15,18–21] The ability of an autoimmune response to produce inflammation in both cartilage and ocular tissue could be explained by the reactivity being directed to a constituent shared by both structures. Type II collagen fulfills this requirement. Type II collagen is a brisk immunogen in rodents, and immunization with this protein can induce an inflammatory arthritis in rats or mice that resembles RA morphologically.[22] Recently, it has been observed that auricular chondritis, with immunoglobulin and complement deposits at the site of the lesion, occurred on occasion in rats with type II collagen-induced arthritis.[12,20] Because antibodies to type II collagen have been detected in the serum of patients during the acute stage of polychondritis, there is increasing, although indirect, evidence that immunologic responses to cartilage and ocular collagen participate in the pathogenesis of relapsing polychondritis.[18,19,21]

Based on these findings, a hypothetical scheme can be proposed to partially explain the pathogenesis of relapsing polychondritis. Clones of autoreactive T and/or B cells emerge, by as yet undefined mechanisms, that are sensitized to type II collagen. Autoantibodies and perhaps lymphokines induce inflammation in cartilage (and the eye), which leads to chondrocyte death and matrix dissolution. Fibroblasts and chondroblasts then attempt to repair the lesion. Occasionally, the cycle of injury and repair is repeated, accounting for the relapsing nature of the disease. Substances released into the blood during the destruction of cartilage are injurious to the structural integrity of major blood vessels and trigger the characteristic aortic lesion. Much remains to be learned about the pathogenesis of relapsing polychondritis.

THERAPY

Aside from prosthetic valve replacement for aortic insufficiency, therapy has consisted primarily of supportive measures and the use of glucocorticoids. An acute inflammatory attack of affected cartilages may be moderated or brought under complete control with prednisone, 20 to 60 mg/day.[1,2] As the attack subsides, the dosage may be reduced to a maintenance level of 10 to 15 mg daily. In some patients, the anti-inflammatory and abortive effects of prednisone diminish over months or years so that the maintenance dosage must be raised gradually in an effort to prevent further severe attacks. On occasion, it is necessary to eventually administer doses approximating 30 mg of prednisone daily to provide satisfactory suppression of inflammation of cartilages and episcleritis. Glucocorticoids have no obvious effect on inhibiting the development of the aortic lesions. In patients who are truly refractory to prednisone, other types of immunosuppressive drugs may be attempted.[1] Cyclosporin has been used successfully.[21] Short courses of low-dose methotrexate or cyclosporin can be helpful adjunctive therapy in patients with severe or life-threatening disease. The efficacy of dapsone has been overstated. Because the attacks are frequently self-limited and the response to prednisone is delayed, however, attempts to curtail the inflammation with glucocorticoids should not be abandoned prematurely.

REFERENCES

1. Arkin, C.R., and Masi, A.T.: Relapsing polychondritis: Review of current status and case report. Semin. Arthritis Rheum., *5*:41–62, 1975.
2. Case Records of the Massachusetts General Hospital (Case 51-1982). N. Engl. J. Med., *307*:1631–1639, 1982.
3. Dolan, D.L., Lemmon, G.B., and Teitelbaum, S.L.: Relapsing polychondritis: Analytical review and studies on pathogenesis. Am. J. Med., *41*:285–299, 1966.
4. Hughes, R.A.C. et al.: Relapsing polychondritis: Three cases with a clinico-pathological study and literature review. Q. J. Med., *41*:363–380, 1972.
5. Kaye, R.L., and Sones, D.A.: Relapsing polychondritis: Clinical and pathologic features in fourteen cases. Ann. Intern. Med., *60*:653–664, 1964.
6. Michet, C.J., Jr., McKenna, C.H., Luthra, H.S., and O'Fallon, W.M.: Relapsing polychondritis: Survival and predictive role of early disease manifestations. Ann. Intern. Med., *104*:74–78, 1986.
7. Jacksch-Wartenhorst, R.: Polychondropathia. Weiner Archive Innere Med., *6*:93–100, 1923.
8. Moloney, J.R.: Relapsing polychondritis—Its otolaryngological manifestations. J. Laryngol. Otol., *92*:9–15, 1978.
9. Verity, M.A., Larson, W.M., and Madden, S.C.: Relapsing polychondritis: Report of two necropsied cases with histochemical investigation of the cartilage lesion. Am. J. Pathol., *42*:251–269, 1963.
10. O'Hanlan, M. et al.: The arthropathy of relapsing polychondritis. Arthritis Rheum., *19*:191–194, 1976.
11. Kindblom, L.-G. et al.: Relapsing polychondritis: A clinical, pathologic-anatomic and histochemical study of two cases. Acta Pathol. Microbiol. Scand. (A), *85*:656–664, 1977.
12. McCune, W.J. et al.: Type II collagen-induced auricular chondritis. Arthritis Rheum., *25*:266–273, 1982.
13. Valenzuela, R. et al.: Relapsing polychondritis: Immunomicroscopic findings in cartilage of ear biopsy specimens. Hum. Pathol., *11*:19–22, 1980.
14. Hashimoto, K., Arkin, C.R., and Kang, A.H.: Relapsing polychondritis: An ultrastructural study. Arthritis Rheum., *20*:91–99, 1977.
15. Rogers, P.H., Boden, G., and Tourtellotte, C.D.: Relapsing polychondritis with insulin resistance and antibodies to cartilage. Am. J. Med., *55*:243–248, 1973.
16. McCluskey, R.T., and Thomas, L.: The removal of cartilage matrix, in vivo, by papain: The identification of crystalline papain protease as the cause of the phenomenon. J. Exp. Med., *108*:371–384, 1958.
17. Tsaltas, T.T.: Metaplasia of aortic connective tissue to cartilage

and bone induced by the intravenous injection of papain. Nature, *196*:1006–1007, 1962.
18. Foidart, J.M. et al.: Antibodies to type II collagen in relapsing polychondritis. N. Engl. J. Med., *299*:1203–1207, 1978.
19. Ebringer, R. et al.: Autoantibodies to cartilage and type II collagen in relapsing polychondritis and other rheumatic diseases. Ann. Rheum. Dis., *40*:473–479, 1981.
20. Cremer, M.A. et al.: Auricular chondritis in rats: An experimental model of relapsing polychondritis induced with type II collagen. J. Exp. Med., *154*:535–540, 1981.
21. Svenson, K.L.G. et al.: Cyclosporin A treatment in a case of relapsing polychondritis. Scand. J. Rheumatol., *13*:329–333, 1984.
22. Trentham, D.E.: Collagen arthritis as a relevant model for rheumatoid arthritis: Evidence pro and con. Arthritis Rheum., *25*:911–916, 1982.

81

Polymyalgia Rheumatica and Giant Cell Arteritis

LOUIS A. HEALEY

Polymyalgia rheumatica (PMR) is a syndrome of older patients characterized by pain and stiffness in the neck, shoulders, and pelvic girdle persisting for at least a month, often accompanied by a rapid erythrocyte sedimentation rate (ESR) and dramatically relieved by prednisone in low dose.

Scattered reports of patients with this syndrome appeared in the British and European literature in the latter half of this century under various names including anarthritic rheumatoid disease. In 1957, Barber introduced the name polymyalgia rheumatica, which has been generally accepted. In 1932, Horton described the first patients with temporal arteritis, which he predicted was "a focal localization of an unknown systemic disease."[1] In 1951, Porsman pointed out the similarity of PMR to the prodrome of temporal arteritis, and this relation was confirmed in 1963 by Alestig and Barr when they demonstrated giant cell arteritis on biopsy of asymptomatic temporal arteries in patients with PMR. The first case report of this syndrome in the United States appeared in 1966, and since then the disease has been widely recognized and reported. The annual incidence has been estimated at 53 per 100,000 for persons over the age of 50. Giant cell arteritis is about one fourth as common and seems to be increasing in frequency in recent years, but this may reflect a greater awareness of the diagnosis rather than a true increase.[2]

The cause of PMR and of giant cell arteritis is unknown. The histologic appearance of the arteritis suggests a cell-mediated immune response, but no evidence confirms this. Both conditions are rare in patients less than 50 years of age and become more common with increasing age. Despite the strong predilection of PMR for whites, immunogenetic studies have not been revealing. Epidemiologic investigations indicate that PMR and particularly giant cell arteritis are very common in Scandinavia, nearly as common in Olmstead County, Minnesota, and less common in the southern United States. (See also Chapter 3.)

RELATION OF POLYMYALGIA TO GIANT CELL ARTERITIS

The relationship between PMR and giant cell arteritis was recognized because of the frequency with which the two conditions appeared in the same patients as well as the biopsy study of Alestig and Barr. In Scandinavian studies, the coincidence is so high (almost 50% of PMR patients also have temporal arteritis) that the two are considered manifestations of the same disease.[3] This is not true in the rest of Europe or in North America, where the corresponding figure is between 15 and 20%. The two syndromes often appear coincidentally or within months of one another, but in one third of patients, the interval between their onsets may be as long as 10 years. PMR is not necessarily the prodrome; arteritis may appear first. Many patients appear to have PMR alone; they respond well to low-dose prednisone and never develop clinical evidence of arteritis.

Because of this experience, temporal artery biopsy and high-dose steroid treatment are not recommended for the patient who only has PMR symptoms. If no symptoms suggest cranial arteritis, or if a temporal artery biopsy is negative, the risk of blindness is slight. These patients are best treated with low-dose prednisone but should be informed that they have a 15% chance of developing arteritis in the future. They should be instructed in the significance of headache, diplopia, blurred vision, or jaw claudication and told to call their physician promptly if these symptoms appear.

CLINICAL PICTURE

Polymyalgia rheumatica occurs twice as often in women as men. The typical patient is a white woman over age 60, previously in excellent health. Patients complain of pain in the neck, shoulders, upper arms, lower back, and thighs. At times, the onset is abrupt; patients go to bed feeling well and awaken as stiff and sore as if they had chopped a cord of wood. Gelling and morning stiffness are marked. Patients describe graphically how difficult it is to get out of bed in the morning or to get out of a car after a trip. Symptoms may be widespread, or a single area such as pectoral or pelvic girdle may predominate. At times the onset is gradual, starting in one shoulder much like bursitis but soon spreading and becoming symmetric.

Despite the severity of the complaints, little is to be found on physical examination other than tenderness and limited motion in the shoulders. Radiographs are unrevealing. The ESR which may be very elevated, often provides a clue to the diagnosis. Other acute-phase reactants such as C-reactive protein and fibrinogen are also increased but are not more specific than the ESR. Rheumatoid factor and antinuclear antibodies are not present. Despite the perception of patients that their symptoms are in the muscles, serum creatine kinase levels, electromyograms, and muscle histology are all normal.

By contrast, in polymyositis, for which these tests do demonstrate inflammation of muscle, the main symptom is weakness. Patients with PMR are not weak; although pain and stiffness make motion difficult, muscle strength is normal.

Arthroscopy and biopsy have shown nonspecific inflammation of synovial tissue in the shoulders.[4] This synovitis is consistent with the marked morning stiffness and gelling that are so typical of PMR and help differentiate if from other pain syndromes such as osteoarthritis, fibrositis, or malignancy. The demonstration of synovitis also explains why the most difficult differential is to separate PMR from the onset of rheumatoid arthritis (RA) when rheumatoid factor is not present. In RA, the small joints of the hands and feet tend to be involved as opposed to the proximal distribution of joints in PMR. Some PMR patients, however, have synovitis of the wrists with swelling and carpal tunnel syndrome or synovitis of the knees with effusions, and it is not possible to make a definite diagnosis until later in their course.

TREATMENT

The response of PMR to prednisone is truly dramatic. Some patients are almost well the next day. The improvement is so invariable that if the response is not seen within a week the diagnosis should be doubted. The usual dose is 10 to 20 mg/day, which, following the clinical response, is tapered to a daily maintenance dose of 5 to 7.5 mg after several weeks. Aspirin and other anti-inflammatory drugs are less effective. For the rare patient who requires a higher dose of prednisone, methotrexate is also effective. PMR was initially considered to be a self-limited condition that lasted for 1 to 2 years, but experience has shown that this is not always the case. Some patients require prednisone for longer periods, sometimes for as long as 10 years. Despite such prolonged treatment, patients remain free of symptoms of 5 mg a day and develop no joint destruction.

Recurrence has proven to be frequent, appearing in 30% of patients who were able to stop prednisone after a year or 2 of initial treatment. The symptom-free interval has varied from months to 8 years. The sedimentation rate is often normal when pain and stiffness reappear. The recurrence may be similar to the initial episode, or the synovitis may involve wrist and metacarpophalangeal (MCP) joints, presenting the picture known as seronegative RA. In either case, the recurrence responds to low-dose prednisone without joint destruction. Involvement of the metatarsophalangeal (MTP) joints helps to distinguish true RA from this benign synovitis.[5]

Long-term observations have also shown no increased association of PMR with seropositive RA, malignancy, or other diseases except for giant cell arteritis.

GIANT CELL ARTERITIS

Giant cell arteritis (also called *temporal* or *cranial arteritis*) may involve any medium or large artery, but there is a predilection for the aortic branches to the head and neck. As the most superficial and accessible, temporal arteritis was the first manifestation recognized (Fig. 81–1). In contrast to polyarteritis, the small arterioles are spared, and thus pulmonary and renal manifestations are not seen in this syndrome. Stroke or myocardial infarction are rare, and their frequency is not increased for this age group. The clinical manifestations can readily be divided into localized or systemic (Table 81–1).

The local manifestations (Table 81–2) depend on the

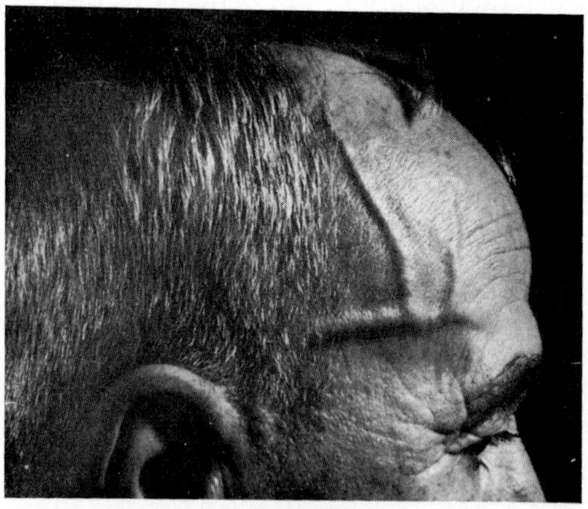

FIGURE 81–1. Temporal arteritis. The swollen temporal artery is tender and painful.

TABLE 81–1. MANIFESTATIONS OF GIANT CELL ARTERITIS

Systemic	
	Fever
	Anemia
	Anorexia
	Malaise
	Weight loss
	Abnormal liver function tests
Local	
	Headache
	Blindness
	Scalp necrosis
	Tongue gangrene
	Jaw claudication
	Diplopia, brachial paralysis, peripheral neuropathy
	Aortic arch syndrome

TABLE 81–2. SYMPTOMS SUGGESTIVE OF CRANIAL ARTERITIS

Temporal or occipital headache
Scalp tenderness
Amaurosis fugax
Diplopia
Jaw claudication
Cough
Unexplained fever, anemia, weight loss

artery involved and may include the typical headache (temporal); posterior headache (occipital); sudden unilateral blindness (ophthalmic); transient diplopia that is due to paralysis of an extraocular muscle; pain in the jaw on chewing (facial). This last is also pathognomonic of cranial arteritis. Aortic involvement also may occur, producing symptoms of an aortic arch syndrome as well as aneurysm and possibly rupture. Unexplained cough is an intriguing symptom that may reflect involvement of an arterial branch in the neck. The systemic manifestations may include fever, hypoproliferative anemia, weight loss, malaise, and abnormal liver function tests, particularly the serum alkaline phosphatase. At times systemic symptoms may predominate, posing a diagnostic problem such as fever of unknown origin, unexplained anemia, or a picture simulating an occult cancer. In such patients, the rapid ESR often provides the clue that leads to biopsy of an asymptomatic temporal artery and establishes the diagnosis.

PATHOLOGY

Inflammation is located on either side of the internal elastic lamina, which is markedly fragmented. The infiltrate consists of histiocytes, lymphocytes, and the giant cells for which the lesion is named. The lumen is narrowed by the thickened edematous intima and may at times be occluded (Fig. 81–2). Electron microscopic examination reveals histiocytes and giant cells in close proximity to fragments of elastic lamina whose ground substance is altered and looks dense and granular. The inflammation is distributed in skip fashion interspersed with normal-appearing artery, so that biopsy of a sizable

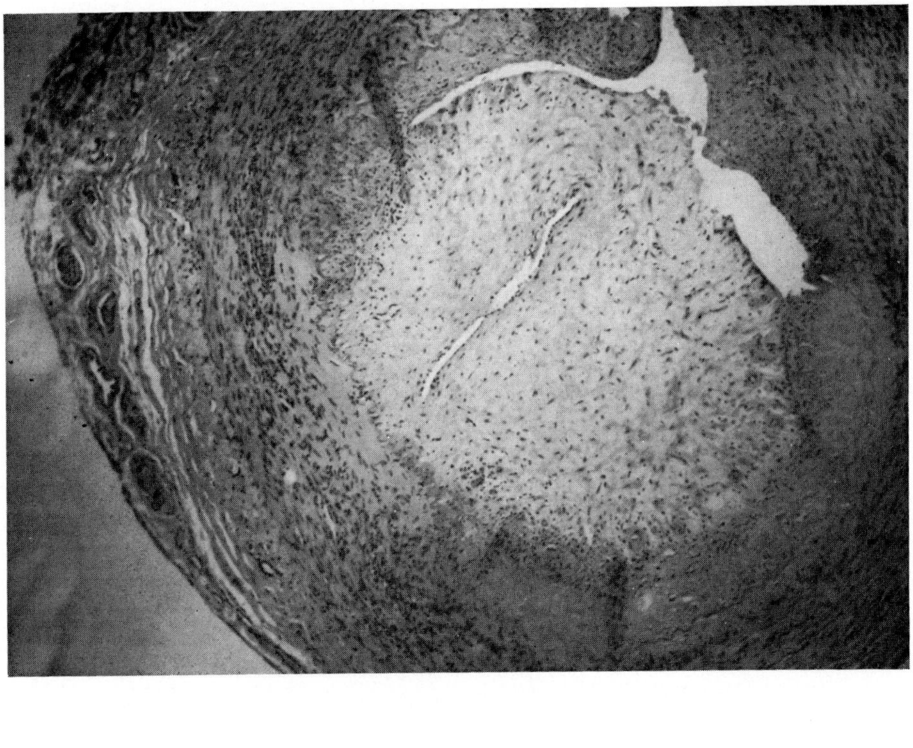

FIGURE 81–2. Giant cell arteritis. Cross section of temporal artery showing inflammatory infiltrate, giant cells, fragmentation of elastic lamina, and intimal thickening; the lumen is almost occluded by thrombus. Separation at upper right is artifact.

segment is more likely to yield the diagnosis. Despite this distribution, adequate biopsy specimens, bilateral if necessary, correctly predicted the subsequent outcome with 90% accuracy.[6]

TREATMENT

Giant cell arteritis responds to prednisone, but the dose required for control of inflammation is higher than that needed for the treatment of PMR. Because of the risk of blindness, it is customary to treat with at least 50 mg of prednisone a day for 1 month. Alternate-day steroid has not been effective initial therapy. It has not yet been proven that a large pulse dose of 1000 mg of methylprednisolone intravenously will more reliably protect vision than the standard recommended oral dose. Symptoms respond rapidly to prednisone. An occasional patient may experience some loss of vision within the first few days of starting treatment, but for the most part, this schedule has prevented blindness.

Treatment with high-dose prednisone for 1 month effectively suppresses the inflammation, and late recurrences of arteritis are rare (less than 1%). The dose is then gradually tapered over the next 6 months. While the ESR is initially a good indicator of inflammation, it does not accurately reflect the activity of the arteritis in its subsequent course. Attempting to treat to maintain an normal ESR will almost invariably result in steroid toxicity with osteoporosis and vertebral collapse. Unlike PMR, for which late recurrences are frequent, giant cell arteritis usually occurs as a single episode. Most instances of what may appear as resistant disease represent patients with a persistently elevated ESR and nonspecific symptoms.

REFERENCES

1. Horton, B.T., Magath, B.T., and Brown, G.E.: An undescribed form of arteritis of the temporal vessels. Proc. Staff Meet. Mayo Clin., 7:700–701, 1932.
2. Machado, E.B.V. et al.: Trends in incidence and clinical presentation of temporal arteritis in Olmstead County, Minnesota, 1950–1985. Arthritis Rheum., *31*:745–749, 1988.
3. Chou, C.-T., and Schumacher, H.R.: Clinical and pathologic studies of synovitis in polymyalgia rheumatica. Arthritis Rheum., *27*:1107–1118, 1984.
4. Bengtsson, B.-A.: Giant cell arteritis. Curr. Opin. Rheum., *2*:60–65, 1990.
5. Healey, L.A., and Sheets, P.K.: The relation of polymyalgia rheumatica to rheumatoid arthritis. J. Rheumatol., *15*:750–752, 1988.
6. Hall, S., and Hunder, G.G.: Is temporal artery biopsy prudent? Mayo Clin. Proc., *59*:793–796, 1984.

SECTION VII

Miscellaneous Rheumatic Diseases

82

Fibromyalgia, Restless Legs Syndrome, Periodic Limb Movement Disorder, and Psychogenic Pain

MUHAMMAD B. YUNUS
ALFONSE T. MASI

FIBROMYALGIA SYNDROME

Rheumatologists, like other physicians, are trained to diagnose and treat diseases that have clear-cut objective findings and abnormal laboratory tests. If they encountered a patient who complained of pain in muscles and joints and yet found little on physical examination or laboratory tests, then the conclusion was often "all psychologic" or worse, malingering. Although such thinking is changing, many physicians still do not accept such patient's problem as being real and find it even harder to offer any help to these suffering individuals. Although some of these patients may have serious psychopathology as a cause of their pain, it is more likely that a majority have a definable rheumatic pain syndrome with objective findings of tenderness on palpation at characteristic spots and that their consistent symptoms and signs over time have a physiologic basis. This syndrome, fibromyalgia, will be discussed here along with other related conditions and psychogenic pain.

HISTORICAL ASPECTS

By the eighteenth century, European physicians were able to distinguish "articular rheumatism" from soft tissue pain; the latter category was generally called muscular rheumatism.[1] In 1904, Sir William Gowers hypothesized that back pain of muscular origin and muscular rheumatism in general were due to an inflammation of the fibrous tissue.[2] This concept found legitimacy by Stockman's purported findings of "increased and edematous fibrous tissue" in the nodules apparently observed in muscular rheumatism.[3] Thus, the term "fibrositis" coined by Gowers[2] became established on an apparent pathologic basis. Several muscle biopsy reports later claimed to have shown inflammatory or degenerative changes,[4] but these were found to be invalid by critical review because of a lack of defined criteria of case selection and an absence of control specimens.[5] Fibromyalgia is clearly not an inflammatory or degenerative condition.

Until the 1960s, description of "fibrositis" did not clearly distinguish between the localized form, such as "fibrositis of the neck," and a syndrome of generalized aching. In 1968, Trout described "fibrositis" as a syndrome of generalized musculoskeletal pain, fatigue, poor sleep, and tenderness on palpation of certain muscles and tendon insertion sites.[6] Smythe's description of fibromyalgia with a set of empirically suggested criteria for diagnosis and published in the eighth edition of this textbook in 1972 drew attention of rheumatologists to this ubiquitous syndrome.[7] Moldofsky in 1975 demonstrated that an abnormal sleep pattern (alpha intrusion into the non-REM delta sleep by sleep electroencephalogram) is of etiologic importance in "fibrositis."[8] In 1977, Smythe further refined his suggested criteria.[9]

"Fibrositis," however, remained unrecognized by a majority of physicians. The major issue was: does "fibrositis" exist as a clinical entity separate from the normal population? Are poor sleep, fatigue, and those intriguing tender points significantly more common in "fibrositis" than matched normal controls? Such questions led to the first controlled and quantitative study of the clinical characteristics of fibromyalgia by Yunus et al.[10] It confirmed the astute descriptions of "fibrositis" by Trout[6] and by Smythe.[7,9] Yunus et al. also argued in favor of the term "fibromyalgia," which was earlier suggested by Hench,[11] and proposed a set of criteria for diagnosis based on data employing normal controls. Additionally, several associated features (e.g., irritable bowel syndrome, headaches, subjective swelling of soft tissues, and paresthesia) were shown to be significantly more common in fibromyalgia than normal controls, raising the syndrome concept.[10] These observations were subsequently confirmed by other studies.[12–14] Thus, an era of controlled investigations in fibromyalgia began in the early 1980s, generating further research interest in this neglected area. The classification of fibromyalgia was later validated by the multicenter criteria study based on appropriate pain controls and blinded observations.[14]

DEFINITION, TERMINOLOGY, AND CLASSIFICATION

Fibromyalgia is a form of nonarticular rheumatism characterized by musculoskeletal aching and tenderness on palpation of tendinomusculoskeletal sites, called *tender points*.[9,10,12–14] We emphasized using the term fibromyalgia (Latin *fibra* = fiber, Greek *mys* = muscle, Greek *algos* = pain + *ia* = condition) rather than "fibrositis" was because the latter term implied inflammation, which is absent in this condition, and because fibrositis meant different things to different people.[10,15,16] Fibromyalgia was subclassified as *primary, secondary, concomitant*, and *localized*.[16] Patients with *primary fibromyalgia* have diffuse, widespread musculoskeletal pain and multiple tender points in the absence of an underlying, causative, or significant concomitant condition. A condition such as osteoarthritis may partly explain a patient's localized pain, but does not account for her diffuse, widespread pain or tenderness on palpation. These patients have *concomitant fibromyalgia*. Studies have shown that the characteristics of fibromyalgia in these patients are not significantly different from those of primary fibromyalgia.[14,17] Thus, primary and concomitant fibromyalgia may both be grouped as fibromyalgia. We, however disagree with the assertion that the distinction between primary and secondary fibromyalgia should be abandoned.[14] One can not abandon a concept without proper study. "Secondary fibromyalgia" in the multicenter criteria study was, in fact, concomitant fibromyalgia. We have documented cases of polymyalgia rheumatica and active polymyositis that fulfilled criteria for fibromyalgia and that subsequently remitted with appropriate treatment; these cases are examples of *secondary fibromyalgia*, which needs further studies. *Localized fibromyalgia* is characterized by pain in a few (usually 1 to 4) contiguous anatomic sites, and is often due to a strain or trauma factor, such as neck pain following an automobile accident. Such patients generally do not have tender points below the waist. Many patients with localized pain with or without a history of trauma, however, subsequently develop widespread pain and tender points, fulfilling the standard criteria for fibromyalgia. Localized fibromyalgia, however, should not be called fibromyalgia without proper qualification. The relationship between localized fibromyalgia and myofascial pain syndrome is not clear; these conditions will be discussed later in this chapter.

PREVALENCE AND DEMOGRAPHIC FEATURES

Fibromyalgia is common. Its prevalence in rheumatology clinics has varied from 6 to 20%.[15] The prevalence of fibromyalgia was found to be 5.7% and 2.1% in a nonreferral general internal medicine clinic[18] and family practice clinic,[19] respectively. Among the inhabitants of a southern Swedish city who were aged 50 to 70 years, the prevalence of fibromyalgia was found to be 1.0% (by the criteria of Yunus et al.)[10], as compared with a rheumatoid arthritis prevalence of 0.7%.[20] Considering methodologic issues, it is likely that these studies have underestimated the true prevalence of fibromyalgia.

The most common age of fibromyalgia patients seen in a rheumatology clinic is between 40 and 50 years, and most are women (80 to 90%);[13] such female preponderance (88%) has also been noted in a family practice setting,[19] as well as in a population study.[20] Fibromyalgia has also been well described among children[21] and in persons aged 60 years or older.[17] It is a chronic condition. The mean duration of symptoms on presentation in a rheumatology clinic was 5 to 10 years (Table 82–1). The preponderance of caucasians in most studies might simply reflect the selective patient population seen in the private clinics, although a racial predisposition cannot be ruled out. Fibromyalgia has been well described in many European countries.[22–24]

TABLE 82–1. AGE, SEX, AND SYMPTOM DURATION AMONG FIBROMYALGIA PATIENTS SEEN IN RHEUMATOLOGY CLINICS IN SEVERAL SELECTED SERIES

	YUNUS ET AL.[13] n = 113	GOLDENBERG[12] n = 118	WOLFE ET AL.[25] n = 293	COMBINED* n = 524
Mean age (yrs.)	40	43	49	44
% Females	94	87	89	90
% Caucasian	98	92	93	94
Duration of symptoms (yrs.)	7	5	NR†	6

* Results are based on the mean values of the 3 series[12,13,25]
† NR = Not reported

TABLE 82–2. SYMPTOMS IN FIBROMYALGIA BASED ON RELATIVELY LARGE SERIES OF WELL DEFINED PATIENTS SEEN IN RHEUMATOLOGY CLINICS*

SYMPTOMS	% FREQUENCY (MEAN)*	% FREQUENCY (RANGE)
Musculoskeletal		
Pain at multiple sites[10,12–14,25]	100	100–100
Stiffness[10,12–14,22,25]	78	76–84
"Hurt all over"[13,14,25]	64	60–69
Swollen feeling in soft tissues[10,12,13,22]	47	32–64
Non-musculoskeletal		
Fatigue (most times of the day)[10,12–14,22,25]	86	75–92
Morning fatigue[12–14,22,25]	78	75–80
Poor sleep†[10,13,22,25]	65	56–72
Paresthesia[10–14,22]	54	26–74
Associated symptoms		
Self-assessed anxiety[10,13,14,22]	62	48–72
Headaches[10–14,22]	53	44–56
Dysmenorrhea[13,14]	43	40–45
Irritable bowel symptoms[10–14,22]	40	30–53
Self-assessed depression[13,14]	34	31–37
Sicca symptoms[30,32]	15	12–18
Raynaud's phenomenon‡[14,30]	13	9–17
Female urethral syndrome[31]	12	

* Mean values derived from percentage figures reported in the referred studies.
† Based on the question "Do you sleep well?" or a similar question.
‡ Definition specified as "dead white pallor on exposure to cold."

SYMPTOMS

Symptoms are listed in Table 82–2. It is worth emphasizing that these symptoms are based on studies done in rheumatology clinics, and their frequencies are subject to several biases, including referral bias. The most common and characteristic symptoms in primary fibromyalgia syndrome (PFS) or fibromyalgia are pain, fatigue and sleep disturbance.[10,12–14,22,25]

Pain is the primary reason for a rheumatology consultation. Fibromyalgia patients express more kinds of words for pain than do patients with rheumatoid arthritis (RA), including aching, shooting, throbbing, and penetrating.[26] Among our sample of 64 fibromyalgia patients, the two most spontaneously used words were aching (53%) and burning (38%). Most fibromyalgia patients have widespread pain involving the spine and all the limbs; the mean number of sites of the pain complaints was 19 in one study.[13] Common sites of pain (as a symptom) (Table 82–3) have varied in several reports,[13,26–28] probably because of methodologic differences. Pain in the spine and muscles is significantly more common in fibromyalgia than in RA.[13] Cervical, thoracic, and lumbar pain were present in 85%, 72%, and 79% of patients, respectively, in the multicenter study.[14] We agree with Wolfe's observation that pain is predominantly articular in some patients and muscular in others.[27]

Pain in fibromyalgia is commonly aggravated by cold or humid weather, mental anxiety or stress, and poor sleep, similar to pain in RA patients.[13] Pain or stiffness is particularly present in the morning or the evening, but 30% of patients described no consistent pattern.[17]

Stiffness is present in most patients (Table 82–2). The mean standard deviation (± SD) of duration of morning stiffness was 110 ± 234 minutes in our study.[13] No significant correlation between duration of morning stiffness and any important fibromyalgia feature, including pain severity, number of tender points, or poor sleep was found.[13]

Fatigue, a common symptom in fibromyalgia,[12–14,22,25] is usually present throughout the day and can be severe. It is the presenting feature in some patients. The expression from a typical patient is "I am always tired"; other common descriptions of this symptom are "total exhaustion" and "lack of energy." Fatigue is accentuated by physical activities, and many patients state that they are too weak to do anything. In one of our studies employing univariate statistics, general fatigue correlated with morning fatigue, mental stress, and poor sleep.[13] *Poor sleep* is also common in fibromyalgia. Patients' perception of poor sleep when asked "do you sleep well?" correlated with morning fatigue,[13] which is present in about 75 to 80% of patients. Many patients described their sleep to be "light." Morning fatigue, present in 75 to 80%,[13] may be a better indication of sleep quality than other clinical sleep parameters.

Subjective soft tissue swelling is present in about half of the patients.[10,12,13,22] It is usually present in the extremities, both in articular and nonarticular locations.[17] Objective joint swelling is absent in primary fibromyalgia.[10] *Paresthesias,* also common in fibromyalgia,[10,12–14,22] are described as tingling, numbness, or pins and needles, and are more commonly present in the upper extremity than the lower extremity or the

TABLE 82–3. COMMON SITES OF PAIN COMPLAINTS REPORTED IN SEVERAL SERIES (% OF PATIENTS)

SITE	LEAVITT ET AL.[26] n = 50	McCAIN[28] n = 50	WOLFE[27] n = 81	YUNUS ET AL.[13] n = 113	COMBINED* n = 294
Hands	62	76	62	52	63
Wrists	52	—†	51	—	(52)
Elbows	48	—	43	42	(44)
Arms	58	80	—	47	(62)
Shoulders	62	92	90	46	73
Neck	70	68	93	74	76
Chest wall	30	20	71	—	(40)
Upper back	48	—	—	—	(48)
Lower back	78	88	94	55	79
Hips	68		63	41	(57)
Thighs	66	64	—	—	(65)
Knees	70	76	75	51	68
Legs	76	60	—	—	(68)
Ankles	54	20	54	34	41
Feet	46	48	70	36	50

* Average of percentage figures of the four cited studies; parenthesis used if a site is reported in less than four studies.
† Percentage not reported.

trunk in a nonsegmental distribution.[17,29] The whole extremity can be involved (either diffusely or in a radiating pattern) in some patients.[17] These symptoms occasionally are the presenting complaint.[29]

Associated features have been reported to be significantly more common in fibromyalgia than in controls (Table 82–2).[10,12–14,22,30,31] *Irritable bowel syndrome, tension headache,* and *primary dysmenorrhea* are present in about 40 to 50% of patients. *Female urethral syndrome,* defined as urinary frequency, dysuria, and suprapubic discomfort in the presence of sterile urine, was present in 12% of fibromyalgia patients, as compared with none of 50 patients with other rheumatic conditions.[31] Twenty-six percent of fibromyalgia patients in the multicenter study had urinary urgency, as compared with 15% of other pain controls, but urinary tract infection was not specifically ruled out among these patients.[14] Müller reported dysuria in 32% of fibromyalgia patients as compared with 4% in normal controls.[23]

Self-assessed global anxiety and mental stress evaluated by simple questions are present in about 50 to 70%, and *depression* by similar evaluation in about 30% of patients.[10,13,14,22] Psychologic status thus assessed may be useful, because it correlates with pain severity[33] and perhaps prognosis.

Several "connective tissue disease (CTD) features", such as *Raynaud's phenomenon* when defined as "dead white discoloration" of the extremities on exposure to cold temperature, and *dry mouth* not due to any medication, are present in about 10% of patients.[20] In our study of 153 fibromyalgia patients and 80 normal controls, 9% of patients and 3% of controls had Raynaud's phenomenon ($p < 0.06$), whereas dry mouth was present in 12% of patients and in none of the controls ($p < 0.005$).[30] Dinerman et al. have described a subgroup of patients with these CTD features along with a positive Schirmer's test in those with dry mouth, positive antinuclear antibodies, and low serum C3. None of these patients fulfilled accepted diagnostic criteria for systemic lupus or another connective tissue disease on follow-up.[32] Bennett et al. reported cold-induced vasospasm in 12 (41%), elevated levels of platelet α_2-adrenergic receptors in 11 (38%), and Raynaud's phenomenon in 3 (10%) of 29 fibromyalgia patients.[34] The significance of these observations, including their relevance to possible pathophysiologic mechanisms, is not clear. It seems likely that unrelated and concomitant CTD features prompted patient referral. None of our patients with dry mouth had a positive Schirmer's test, and the frequency of positive antinuclear antibody (ANA) among our referred fibromyalgia patients was not significantly different from a matched control population (see laboratory tests).[30] Vaerøy et al. reported a *decreased* vasoconstrictory response to cold pressor test without objective demonstration of Raynaud's phenomenon among 27 fibromyalgia patients as compared with 29 nonpain controls.[35] A true association between Raynaud's phenomenon and fibromyalgia remains unproven.

SIGNS

Examination of the joints, muscle strength, sensory system, and reflexes is normal in primary fibromyalgia,[10] but patients with another concomitant rheumatic or nonrheumatic condition will have signs of that condition (e.g., osteoarthritis). The most characteristic physical sign in fibromyalgia is the presence of *multiple tender points* on firm digital palpation.[9,10,12–14] A pressure dolorimeter has also been used to "quantitate" such tenderness,[18] but it is impractical for daily clinical use.[14] The validity of tender points in fibromyalgia is established by the fact that they are significantly more common than in normal controls[10] as well as in patients with other types of rheumatic conditions having chronic pain by blinded observation.[14] Tender points provide high sensitivity and specificity for fibromyalgia. Controlled studies have also shown a high inter- and intraobserver reliability,[36] as well as their consistency over time.[37] A set of nine pairs of tender points were most discriminating in the multicenter criteria study,[14] but fibromyalgia patients are tender at many more sites.[6,10,38] In fact, a subgroup of these patients are tender all over on palpation; psychologic or other characteristics of these patients are currently unknown.

Campbell et al. found that fibromyalgia patients are not different from controls in their tenderness in certain control points (e.g., forehead, nail of the thumb, and midfoot),[18] but this finding has been disputed.[14,39] We use the forehead as a control site during routine examination. A steady and firm force of about 4 kg using the pulp of the finger produces a sensation of mere pressure on the forehead in a large majority of fibromyalgia patients. A patient is then asked to differentiate between pressure and pain, which is further graded as mild (with no physical signs of grimace or withdrawal of a body part), moderate, and severe, the latter two grades being accompanied by a visible physical sign. The above described technique of palpation should be applied to all examination sites (Fig. 82–1). However, it should be noted that the exact site of maximal tenderness on palpation can vary somewhat from patient to patient, and a physician should palpate for such an area of tenderness within a centimeter or so of the sites shown in Figure 82–1. Although a "typical" patient has many sites of pain complaint and many tender points, we found that fibromyalgia patients may be classified into four groups based on a varying number of sites of pain complaint and of tender points (Fig. 82–2).[13]

Other signs found in fibromyalgia are *skin-fold tenderness* (elicited by grasping a fold of cutaneous and subcutaneous tissue) and *cutaneous hyperemia* following examination of a tender point or skin-fold tenderness.[13,14,40] The strong correlation between skin-fold tenderness and tender points[40] limits diagnostic usefulness of the former.[14,40] Cutaneous hyperemia at tender point sites is significantly more common in patients with fibromyalgia than in normal controls,[13] but not other "pain" controls, such as patients with RA.[13,14] *Reticular skin discoloration* of moderate or severe degree in the extremities was found to be present in 24% of patients in one study,[41] and in 15% in another.[14]

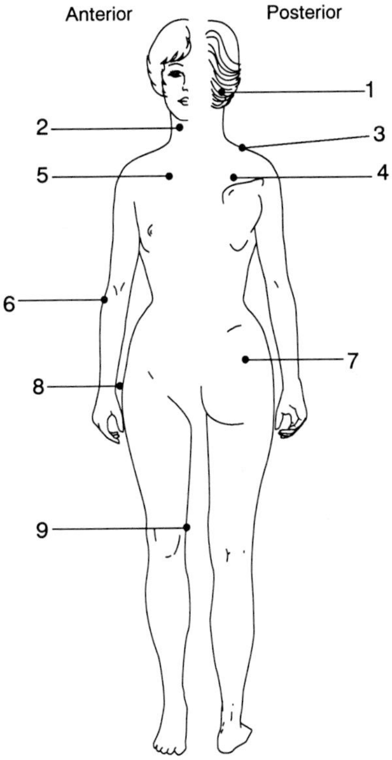

FIGURE 82–1. Locations of nine bilateral tender point sites for the American College of Rheumatology classification criteria for fibromyalgia. *1*, Suboccipital muscle insertions; *2*, cervical, at the anterior aspects of the intertransverse spaces at C5–C7; *3*, trapezius, at the midpoint of the upper border; *4*, supraspinatus, at the origin, above the scapular spine near the medial border; *5*, second rib, at the costochondral junction; *6*, lateral epicondyle, 2 cm distal to the epicondyle; *7*, gluteal, in upper outer quadrant of the buttock; *8*, greater trochanter, just posterior to the trochanteric prominence; *9*, knee, at the medial fat pad proximal to the joint line.

LABORATORY TESTS

Routine laboratory tests, including complete blood count, erythrocyte sedimentation rate, chemistry profile including muscle enzymes, and radiographs of the involved joints are normal in primary fibromyalgia.[10] However, fibromyalgia might coexist with other conditions, as stated earlier. ANA test results are not significantly different in fibromyalgia patients than in controlled populations.[30,42] Eleven percent of our 153 fibromyalgia patients and 10% of age- and sex-matched pain-free healthy controls had a positive ANA test in a titer of 1:20 or greater; the figures were 7% and 5% for patients and controls, respectively, for a titer of 1:80 or greater.[30] None of these patients had antibodies to native DNA or low complement levels, and none satisfied criteria for a connective tissue disease. Results of radionuclide, scintigraphic[43] and electromyographic[44] studies are normal in fibromyalgia. Immunoreactant deposits of IgG type at the dermal-epidermal junctions in skin biopsy specimens of fibromyalgia patients have been reported in 12 to 76% of patients.[45] A controlled and blinded study showed that 19 (53%) of 36 patients and 2 (17%) of only 12 controls had these deposits ($p < 0.05$).[46] The significance of these deposits in some patients is not clear, but they are thought to represent an increased vascular permeability, and not a true immunologic phenomenon.[45,46]

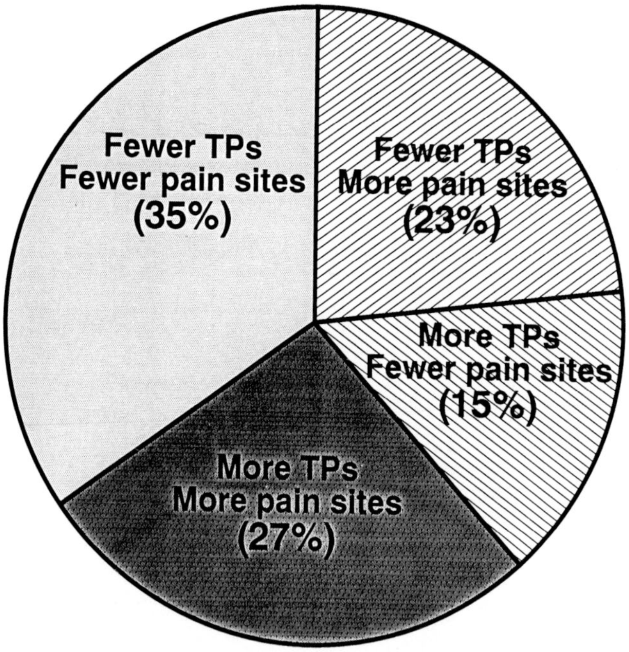

FIGURE 82–2. The number of tender points (TPs) and of sites of the pain complaint may be present in varying combinations of fibromyalgia, as shown in this chart. Fewer TPs = fewer than 6 TPs (defined as severe pain on palpation); more pain sites = more than 14 sites of pain. From Yunus, M.B., Masi, A.T., and Aldag, J.C.[13]

DIAGNOSIS

A diagnosis of fibromyalgia should be made in the presence of characteristic features (Table 82–2; Fig. 82–1), and not by an exclusion of other conditions alone. The multicenter criteria for the classification of fibromyalgia[14] require (1) widespread musculoskeletal aching (i.e., axial pain—pain in the cervical or thoracic or lumbosacral or anterior chest region) plus pain in the right side of the body, the left side of the body, above the waist, and below the waist, and (2) presence of mild or greater tenderness (as defined under physical signs) in 11 of the 18 sites (Fig. 82–1). The definition of widespread pain will thus be met if a patient has this symptoms in as few as three separate areas (e.g., neck, right shoulder, and left knee), although most patients have pain in many more sites.[14] Widespread pain should be present for at least 3 months. These criteria provided a sensitivity of 88% and specificity of 81% against other rheumatic conditions, with an accuracy of 85%.

A lower required number of tender points (i.e., four of five) in the previously published criteria of Yunus et al.[10,40] is explained by the fact that the definition of tender points used in those criteria involved *severe* tenderness, as opposed to *mild* or greater tenderness in the multicenter criteria study.[14] Our criteria of 1981[10] and of 1989,[40] which were frequently used by other investigators, provided an accuracy of 80% and 84%, respectively, in the multicenter data set when 'tender point'' was appropriately defined.[14]

In clinical practice, not all patients will have an adequate number of tender points (particularly in the hands of inexperienced physicians) or widespread aching as defined above. However, for practical management purpose, these patients may be diagnosed as having fibromyalgia if they otherwise have the characteristic clinical picture described above.

CONCOMITANT AND SECONDARY FIBROMYALGIA

These conditions, defined earlier, are important to recognize. A patient with severe widespread pain, pronounced fatigue, and multiple tender points, but having only mild, concomitant RA, might receive inappropriate therapy (e.g., a large dose of corticosteroids or an immunosuppressive agent), if concomitant fibromyalgia is not diagnosed.

For a diagnosis of *secondary* (as opposed to concomitant) fibromyalgia, we suggest that at least 80% of fibromyalgia features (e.g., pain, fatigue, and number of tender points) should remit following appropriate therapy of a causative condition (e.g., polymyalgia rheumatica). Hypothyroidism with aching, stiffness, and fatigue is often cited as an example of secondary fibromyalgia. However, most cases of hypothyroidism in a fibromyalgia patient are concomitantly present, because fibromyalgia features, including tender points, rarely remit satisfactorily with full replacement dose of thyroxine.[47]

DIFFERENTIAL DIAGNOSIS

Various conditions can be confused with fibromyalgia; these and the key differentiating points are shown in Table 82–4. Chest pain may be a prominent feature in some fibromyalgia patients, leading to hospitalization and expensive cardiac work-up.[48] Localized chest-wall tenderness on palpation often reproduces the patient's chest pain, but in our opinion, this sign alone should not be used to rule out intrathoracic pathology. These patients with fibromyalgia usually have other features of the syndrome, including musculoskeletal aching and multiple tender points at other sites. Depression and somatization disorder may mimic fibromyalgia and will be discussed under Pain in Psychiatric Conditions and Psychogenic Pain. It is important to appreciate that the conditions listed in Table 82–4 (e.g., polymyalgia rheumatica) can coexist with fibromyalgia. In this example, fibromyalgia should be suspected if a patient's pain continues despite an adequate treatment of polymyalgia rheumatica with corticosteroids and the patient has other features of fibromyalgia including multiple tender points. Regional or localized fibromyalgia is described below.

THE CONCEPT OF FIBROMYALGIA FORMING A SPECTRUM OF DYSFUNCTIONAL DISORDERS

In 1981, Yunus et al. observed that irritable bowel syndrome (IBS) and tension headaches are significantly more common in patients with fibromyalgia than in

TABLE 82–4. PRESENTING FEATURES OF FIBROMYALGIA WITH CONFOUNDING DIAGNOSES AND KEY POINTS OF DIFFERENTIATION

PRESENTING FEATURES	CONFOUNDING DIAGNOSIS	ABSENT IN FIBROMYALGIA
Joint pain and subjective swelling	Arthritis	Objective joint swelling
Diffuse muscular aching and stiffness	Polymyalgia rheumatica	↑ ESR, ↓ Hb, weight loss
Muscle fatigue, weakness	Myopathy	Objective weakness, ↑ muscle enzymes
Fatigue, sensitivity to cold, muscle pain	Hypothyroidism	↓ T4, ↑ TSH
Back pain/stiffness	Ankylosing spondylitis	Sacroiliitis
Sciatica-type pain	Disc herniation	Neurologic and radiologic findings
Chest pain	Cardiac or pleural pain	Typical history of cardiac pain, pleural rub, EKG, chest radiograph or other laboratory findings of an intrathoracic disease

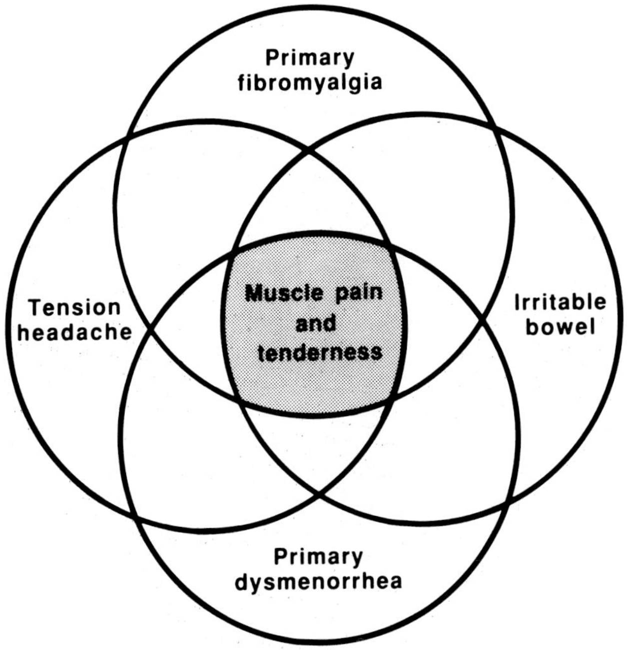

FIGURE 82–3. Fibromyalgia, irritable bowel, tension headache, and primary dysmenorrhea are overlapping syndromes that share many common features, including muscle pain and tenderness. From Yunus, M.B., Masi, A.T., and Aldag, J.C.[13]

matched normal controls.[10] Subsequently, Yunus in 1984 suggested the concept that fibromyalgia, IBS, tension headache, and primary dysmenorrhea form a spectrum of similar conditions with several features in common (e.g., preponderance or exclusiveness of female sex, muscle pain and tenderness, and lack of a specific diagnostic test) (Fig. 82–3).[16] These conditions can also share other findings (e.g., poor sleep, fatigue, and psychologic distress) in a subgroup of patients. Subsequent studies have confirmed a significantly increased frequency of IBS, headaches, dysmenorrhea,[13] and female urethral syndrome[31] in fibromyalgia patients as compared with controls with other causes of pain. The concept of a spectrum of common dysfunctional disorders is important, because they might share pathophysiologic mechanism (e.g., aberration of neuroendocrine factors—see Hypothesis of Pathophysiologic Mechanisms below) and demonstration of a contributory mechanism in one of them may provide a clue in another. These syndromes may result from a dysfunction of normal physiologic homeostasis provided by restorative sleep and good mental and physical health (hence the use of the term "dysfunctional" rather than "functional"). Additionally, their known overlapping features in a given patient are often useful in diagnostic and management considerations, helping one to avoid unnecessary investigations. As a group, these conditions probably constitute the most common chronic disorder in medicine causing significant pain and disability, and yet they receive few research dollars for scientific studies. Besides those mentioned above, other conditions can also form the spectrum with overlapping features. These include temporomandibular dysfunctional pain syndrome,[49,50] hearing/vestibular dysfunction,[51] and chronic fatigue syndrome.[52]

PATHOPHYSIOLOGIC STUDIES IN FIBROMYALGIA

Muscle Studies

An uncontrolled study of muscle biopsy from a tender point in the trapezius muscle had shown no inflammatory changes by light microscopy, type 2 fiber atrophy and motheaten appearance of type 1 fibers by histochemistry, and several changes by electron microscopy (EM), including myofibrillar lysis with glycogen and mitochondrial deposition and papillary projections of sarcolemmal membrane.[53] Controlled studies by Bengtsson and her colleagues showed no significant differences in light microscopic and histochemical findings between patients and controls, with the possible exception of ragged red fibers, which were found in 29% of patients and 17% of controls.[54] Our controlled and blinded EM study of muscle biopsy showed no significant differences between patients and pain-free healthy controls grossly matched for physical activities.[55] An interesting observation in a controlled study was the significant presence of "rubber band–like" structures in the glycerinated biopsies of the quadriceps muscle in fibromyalgia patients.[56,57] It was suggested that these bands cause a cascade of muscle pull, causing pain.[56,57] The same group of investigators reported a decrease in the dynamic strength of the quadriceps muscles in fibromyalgia.[57] Adenosine triphosphate, adenosine diphosphate, and phosphoryl creatine were decreased in the biopsy of trapezius muscle tender points in fibromyalgia patients as compared with normal controls.[58] Lund et al. have also reported decreased microcirculation in the tender points of fibromyalgia-affected muscles when compared with muscles of normal controls, as determined by multipoint oxygen electrode.[59] These findings[58,59] may indicate relative ischemia in the tender muscles of fibromyalgia, but may also be secondary to deconditioning in this condition.[60] Another controlled study, in which level of physical fitness as estimated by V_{O_2} max was similar between patients and controls, found that exercising muscle blood flow as determined by xenon-133 clearance was significantly decreased among fibromyalgia patients; this study also showed that over 80% of fibromyalgia patients were below the average level of fitness seen in the age- and sex-matched population controls.[60] Ischemia of muscles, however, was not reflected in the oxygen uptake (V_{O_2}) relative to work rate in the preliminary report of Sietsema et al., the results being within the predicted normal range.[61] The presence of significant ischemia in tender muscles in fibromyalgia remains questionable.

Immunologic Parameters

These have been reviewed by Caro.[45] Elevated numbers of T helper cells and decreased natural killer cells have been reported in preliminary investigations. Lymphocyte subsets and cytokine levels have also been investigated in fibromyalgia, with generally negative results.[62] Circulating immune complexes are normal.[45] Considering the small sample size and inadequate information on study methodology, further studies are warranted in this area.

Psychologic Studies

Important findings in several psychologic studies of fibromyalgia are summarized in Table 82–5.[63–71,73] Taken together, these findings might lead one to conclude that a subgroup of fibromyalgia patients (about 30 to 40%) seen in a referral rheumatology clinic have significant psychologic problems, including anxiety, depression, and stress. The only study of nonreferred patients seen in an internal medicine outpatient clinic found no significant differences between patients with fibromyalgia and other patients in their psychologic status as measured by the Beck Depression Inventory, the Spielberger State and Trait Anxiety Inventory, and the Symptom Check List of 90 items (SCL-90-R).[66] Primarily because of an earlier study by structured interview wherein depression was found to be significantly more common in fibromyalgia than in RA,[67] Hudson and Pope suggested that fibromyalgia is an "affective spectrum disorder."[72] But however, only 14 RA patients were studied, permitting no such firm conclusion.[67]

A causal relationship between depression and fibromyalgia in general appears unlikely for the following reasons: (1) Several studies indicate that depression was no more common in fibromyalgia than in RA.[66,68,69,73] We had blindly assessed 35 fibromyalgia and 33 RA patients as well as 31 pain-free normal controls by Psychiatric Diagnostic Interview, or PDI (all subjects wore special gloves so that RA patients could not be identified during the interview), and found no significant differences between the groups in any lifetime diagnoses of psychiatric disorders; depression was present in 34% of fibromyalgia, 39% of RA, and 26% of normal control subjects.[73] (2) The dose of an antidepressant drug that is effective in fibromyalgia[74,75] is subtherapeutic in depression. (3) Cortisol nonsuppression in fibromyalgia does not correlate with depression in fibromyalgia[76] (see Neurohormonal Dysfunction, below). (4) Platelet binding of ^{3}H-imipramine was reported to be increased in fibromyalgia is a preliminary report,[77] whereas it is decreased in depression.[78]

A subgroup of patients seen in a rheumatology clinic do show more psychologic distress compared with RA patients by the Minnesota multiphasic personality inventory (MMPI), even after adjustment of data for pain or pain-related questions.[79] Three studies have shown a significantly greater level of mental stresses in patients with fibromyalgia than in RA controls;[64,70,71] stress, in fact, accounted for most of the abnormal findings of psychologic distress measured by the SCL-90-R (Symptom Checklist of 90 items of various psychological categories, such as somatization, anxiety, and depression).[71] It is now clear that an abnormal psychologic status is not required for clinical manifestations of fibromyalgia.[33,63–72] In our study of the relationship between clinical features of fibromyalgia and psychologic status, we found that the central features of fibromyalgia (e.g., number of sites of pain complaints and of tender points on palpation) were independent of the psychologic status, but pain severity was correlated with psychologic factors.[33] Finally, our above-mentioned data gathered by PDI,[73] as well as other studies,[67,69] indicate that a small number of fibromyalgia patients have a pattern of expressing excessive somatic symptoms. Whether fibromyalgia in these patients is secondary to a somatization disorder or somatization is concomitantly present is unknown. Finally, the psychologic status of fibromyalgia patients seen in a primary care setting needs to be evaluated, because the degree of psychologic abnormality seen in a rheumatology clinic is likely to be influenced by referral bias.

Sleep Studies

Clinically, 70 to 80% of fibromyalgia patients complain of nonrestorative sleep (Table 82–2) and aggravation of pain by poor sleep.[13] Several sleep electroencephalogram (EEG) studies have been reported (Table 82–6).[8,80–85] Moldofsky and associates first docu-

TABLE 82–5. SUMMARY OF PSYCHOLOGIC STUDIES IN FIBROMYALGIA

PRIMARY AUTHOR	MAJOR TESTS USED	NO. OF SUBJECTS (SITE OF STUDY)	MAIN FINDINGS	OTHER FINDINGS/ COMMENTS
Payne[63]	MMPI	30 FM,* 30 RA,† 30 other arthritides (hospitalized patients)	FM patients more psychologically disturbed with greater variability than controls	Hospitalized FM patients are likely to have greater psychopathology
Ahles[64]	MMPI, Life Events Inventory (LEI)	45 FM, 30 RA and 32 NC‡ (rheumatology clinic)	Among FM patients, 36% were normal, 33% had chronic pain profile, and 31% were psychologically disturbed by MMPI; LEI scores were higher in FM than controls	Overall greater psychologic abnormalities in FM than controls
Wolfe[65]	MMPI, Family Inventory of Life Events, Self-motivation questionnaire	46 FM and 43 RA (rheumatology clinic)	In FM group, 28% were normal, 34% had somatic concern, and 37% were psychologically disturbed by MMPI; stress and motivation normal	MMPI overall more abnormal in FM than RA, but 65% of FM patients were similar to RA
Clark[66]	Beck Depression Inventory, Spielburger State and Trait Anxiety Inventory, SCL-90-R	22 FM and 22 clinic controls (general internal medicine outpatient)	Findings in fibromyalgia not significantly different from controls	Only study not including patients seen by referral; small sample size
Hudson[67]	Diagnostic Interview Schedule	31 FM and 14 RA (rheumatology clinic)	26% FM (vs. 0% RA) patients had current depression and 71% had current or past depression (vs. 13% in RA)	Number of RA patients were too small for a valid comparison
Ahles[68]	Zung Depression Scale	45 FM and 29 RA (rheumatology clinic)	29% of FM and 31% of RA patients were depressed	Essentially no difference in depression scores between FM and RA
Kirmayer[69]	Diagnostic Interview Schedule	20 FM and 23 RA (rheumatology clinic)	Psychiatric diagnoses, including depression, not significantly different between FM and RA groups	Rather small study sample
Dailey[70]	Hassles Scale, (daily stress) Social Support Inventory	28 FM and 20 RA (rheumatology clinic)	FM patients scored higher in daily stresses than RA, with no difference in social support	Rather small study sample
Uveges[71]	Hassles Scale (daily stress), SCL-90-R	25 FM and 22 RA (rheumatology clinic)	Greater psychologic distress by SCL-90-R and daily stresses in FM than RA; abnormal findings in SCL-90-R in FM were mostly explained by daily stress scores	Rather small study sample
Ahles[73]	Psychiatric Diagnostic Interview	35 FM, 33 RA, and 31 NC (rheumatology clinic)	Psychiatric disorders, including depression, not significantly different between the FM, RA, and NC groups	Only diagnostic interview study with blinded assessment

* FM = Fibromyalgia
† RA = Rheumatoid arthritis
‡ NC = Normal, healthy pain-free controls

mented an objective sleep abnormality in fibromyalgia by demonstrating an alpha anomaly in the restorative, non-REM (NREM) sleep pattern.[8] In the first part of that sleep EEG study, 7 of the 10 patients had this anomaly and another three had no stage 3 or 4 sleep at all (the stages providing NREM restful sleep). In the second part, alpha anomaly was induced in the NREM sleep of six healthy volunteers by a variety of auditory stimuli (Fig. 82–4). Following this sleep deprivation, the volunteers developed significantly increased musculoskeletal tenderness by dolorimetry as compared with baseline values. Two other blinded and controlled studies from the same center reaffirmed the above sleep EEG abnormalities in fibromyalgia (Table 82–6).[80,81] A definite confirmation of the abnormal finding of alpha anomaly in NREM sleep by independent centers em-

TABLE 82–6. SUMMARY OF CONTROLLED SLEEP ELECTROENCEPHALOGRAPHIC STUDIES IN FIBROMYALGIA

PRIMARY AUTHOR	TYPE OF PUBLICATION; NO. OF SUBJECTS; STUDY DESIGN	MAJOR FINDINGS	COMMENTS
Moldofsky*[8]	Full length; 10 FM† (7 females, 3 males) and 6 NC‡ (all males); open design	7 of 10 patients had alpha anomaly in NREM sleep and 3 had no stage 3 or 4 sleep. NCs developed pain and mood symptoms of FM following stage 4 sleep deprivation	Patients and controls not matched by age or sex; however, FM features might have been greater if controls were females
Ware[82]	Abstract; 15 FM and 12 depressed patients; blinded study	60% FM and 40% of depressed patients showed alpha anomaly of NREM sleep (p not significant)	An addition of normal controls would have been desirable. Study details not known
Molony[83]	Full length; 7 FM and 6 NC; blinded study	Significantly increased miniarousal/h and increased % of transitional sleep in FM compared to NC	Small study sample. Results consistent with those of Moldofsky et al.[8] and Gupta et al.[80]
Gupta*[80]	Full length; 6 FM and 6 with dysthymic disorder; blinded study	FM patients had more alpha anomaly in NREM than those with dysthymic disorder ($p < 0.01$)	Small study sample
Moldofsky*[81]	Full length; 9 FM, 9 FM secondary to febrile illness, and 10 NC; blinded study	Greater alpha anomaly of NREM sleep in FM patients than normal controls	
Herisson[84]	Abstract; 12 FM and NC (n = ?); blindedness not stated	Significantly decreased stage 4 NREM sleep and alpha anomaly in NREM sleep in FM compared to NC	Details of study not known
Doherty[85]	Abstract; 10 FM and 10 OA§ patients; ? open study	Alpha anomaly of NREM sleep was not noted in any patient	Details of the study not stated, hence difficult to interpret

* Studies from the same center.
† FM = Fibromyalgia
‡ NC = Normal controls
§ OA = Osteoarthritis

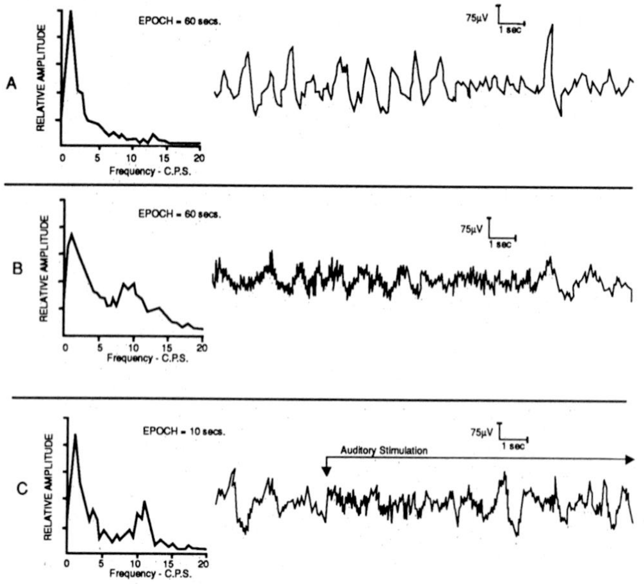

FIGURE 82–4. Frequency spectra and raw EEGs from *A*, non-REM (stage 4) sleep in a healthy subject showing that most amplitude is concentrated at 1 cps (delta); *B*, non-REM sleep in a fibromyalgia patient showing amplitude at both 1 cps (delta) and 8 to 10 cps (alpha); and *C*, non-REM sleep of a healthy subject during stage 4 sleep deprivation, showing a clear association between an auditory stimulus and alpha onset. From Moldofsky, H., Scarisbrick, P., England, R., and Smythe, H.[8]

ploying a satisfactory sample size in a detailed paper is eagerly awaited. It is clear that an NREM sleep anomaly is not specific for fibromyalgia,[86] and it is not known whether the putative sleep anomaly is due to a unique endogenous abnormality secondary to anxiety or depression, or if it simply results from the nocturnal pain of fibromyalgia.

Neurohormonal Dysfunction

Based on observations in animal studies that pain and sleep are mediated by serotonin,[87] it has been suggested that fibromyalgia is due to a deficiency of this neurotransmitter.[88] Several studies have focused on the amino acid tryptophan,[88–90] a precursor of serotonin. Available data support the notion that serum or plasma tryptophan and its transport ratio (calculated by the plasma concentration of tryptophan divided by the sum concentrations of other large neutral amino acids, and presumably a better indicator of the brain entry of tryptophan) reflect the brain concentration of this amino acid.[91] The following findings support the serotonin deficiency hypothesis in fibromyalgia: (1) there is an inverse relationship between plasma tryptophan and morning pain;[88] (2) serum or plasma tryptophan levels are decreased in fibromyalgia patients as compared with normal controls;[89,90] (3) the transport ratio of plasma tryptophan is significantly decreased when compared with normal controls;[90] (4) cerebrospinal fluid (CSF) levels of 5-hydroxy indole acetic acid, a metabolite of serotinin, is lower in patients than in controls;[92] (5) administration of parachlorophenylalanine, a selective inhibitor of serotonin synthesis, in migraine sufferers produced a fibromyalgia-like syndrome with diffuse musculoskeletal pain and hyperalgesia to touch;[93] and (6) serotonergic drugs have been effective in fibromyalgia in controlled studies.[74,75] An aberrance of serotonin metabolism in fibromyalgia is further suggested by increased platelet binding of ^{3}H-imipramine compared with healthy controls.[77] Although a consensus is emerging in support of the serotonin deficiency hypothesis in fibromyalgia, it should be noted that the above-mentioned studies are mostly preliminary, involving small numbers of patients, and that free plasma tryptophan has been found to be normal in another preliminary report involving 20 patients and 20 controls.[94] Moreover, it appears that serotonin deficiency is present in only a minority subgroup of patients, and the role of other neurohormonal factors would seem important.

Both serum[94,95] and CSF[96] levels of β-endorphin have been reported to be normal. Although plasma substance P is normal,[97] the CSF level of substance P has been reported to be elevated compared with a group of patients who had a spinal tap for neurologic symptoms but who subsequently were found not to have a neurologic disease.[98] This study would have been more meaningful if appropriately age- and sex-matched normal controls were used. Plasma[99] and urinary[99,100] catecholamine levels were normal, but significantly lower levels of 3-methoxy 4-hydroxy phenylglycol (MHPG), a metabolite of norepinephrine, and of homovanillic acid (a metabolite of dopamine) were reported in a preliminary study.[101] Some of these findings might be relevant to fibromyalgia, once the physiology of pain is examined.[98,101]

Some hormonal abnormalities have been described in fibromyalgia. Two preliminary studies described cortisol nonsuppression to dexamethasone in 25 to 35% of patients, as compared with 0 to 5% of patients with RA.[76,102] Ferraccioli et al. found no correlation between nonsuppression of cortisol and depression (as assessed by Zung Depression Inventory), but there was a strong correlation of this endocrine abnormality with stress as measured by the stress symptom questionnaire of Aro and Hassan.[76] These investigators also found a hyperprolactinemic response to TRH in 33% of 24 fibromyalgia patients, as compared with 9% of 11 RA patients.[76] These interesting findings may provide a biologic marker for psychologic or other features in fibromyalgia, and need to be confirmed in a larger series of patients.

PHYSIOLOGY OF PAIN

An overview of the physiology of pain, described elsewhere,[103,104] is useful for an understanding of the possible pathophysiologic mechanisms in fibromyalgia. Nociception is the sensation of pain associated with tissue injury. Pain sensation is initiated by activation of pain receptors at the nerve endings in peripheral tissues. Relevant to pain are three classes of afferent sensory fibers: myelinated, large diameter (5 to 15 μm) A-β fibers that transmit touch and pressure; thinly myelinated, smaller diameter (1 to 5 μm) A-δ fibers that carry precise, sharp, and fast pain, as well as temperature; and unmyelinated thin (diameter 0.25 to 1.5 μm) C fibers that transmit dull, diffuse, nonprecise, and burning pain, as well as touch and temperature. Nociception served by A-δ fibers depends on stimulation of high-threshold mechanoreceptors (e.g., those activated by strong, tissue-damaging pressure). By contrast, a majority of the C fibers are polymodal (i.e., they are stimulated by noxious mechanical, thermal, and chemical stimuli). Substance P (SP) is the neurotransmitter for C fibers at both peripheral receptors and dorsal horn synapses. Several chemical substances released from damaged tissues can activate nociceptors; these include bradykinin, serotonin, prostaglandin, and histamine. Prolonged ischemia can also stimulate high-threshold mechanoreceptors.

Afferent sensory fibers synapse in the spinal cord before ascending to supraspinal structures (Fig. 82–5A, B). A-δ fibers end mostly in lamina I of the dorsal horn, but some fibers synapse at lamina V (Fig. 82–5B). Different C fibers synapse in lamina II and III, that is, substansia gelatinosa (not shown in Fig. 5B), as well as lamina V. Both A-δ and C fibers then cross to the opposite side, forming the spinothalamic tract, which is divided into two distinct tracts. The neospinothalamic tract, which relays mostly from the A-δ fibers,[104] stays laterally as it ascends, sending branches to the periacqueductal gray (PAG) of the midbrain, before synapsing in the posterior thalamus, where third-order neurons arise to terminate in the somatosensory cortex. The neospinothalamic system serves to pinpoint the precise location of a noxious stimulus. The paleospinothalamic tract, which transmits pain carried mostly by peripheral C fibers and which is implicated in chronic pain,[104] swings medially to send synapsing fibers to the reticular formation of the brain stem, with further connections to the intralaminar nuclei (ILN) of the thalamus, which also receive fibers directly from the spinal cord (Fig. 82–5A). The fibers from the ILN project diffusely to the cortex, including the limbic structures, with prefrontal predominance. The paleospinothalamic tract is responsive to noxious stimuli, but also serves the autonomic and motor functions that sometimes accompany such stimuli. The emotional component of pain is supposedly served by the limbic connections of this tract.

It appears likely that pain impulses entering thalamus and reticular formation can produce conscious perception of pain.[104] The function of the cerebral cortex is to integrate the cognitive and behavioral aspects of pain.[103,104] It seems likely that the cortex modulates pain inhibition, although the main fibers for this function arise at the PAG in the midbrain.[103]

A most significant discovery in pain physiology was the identification of the inhibitory pathways mediated by the enkephalin and similar neurotransmitter sys-

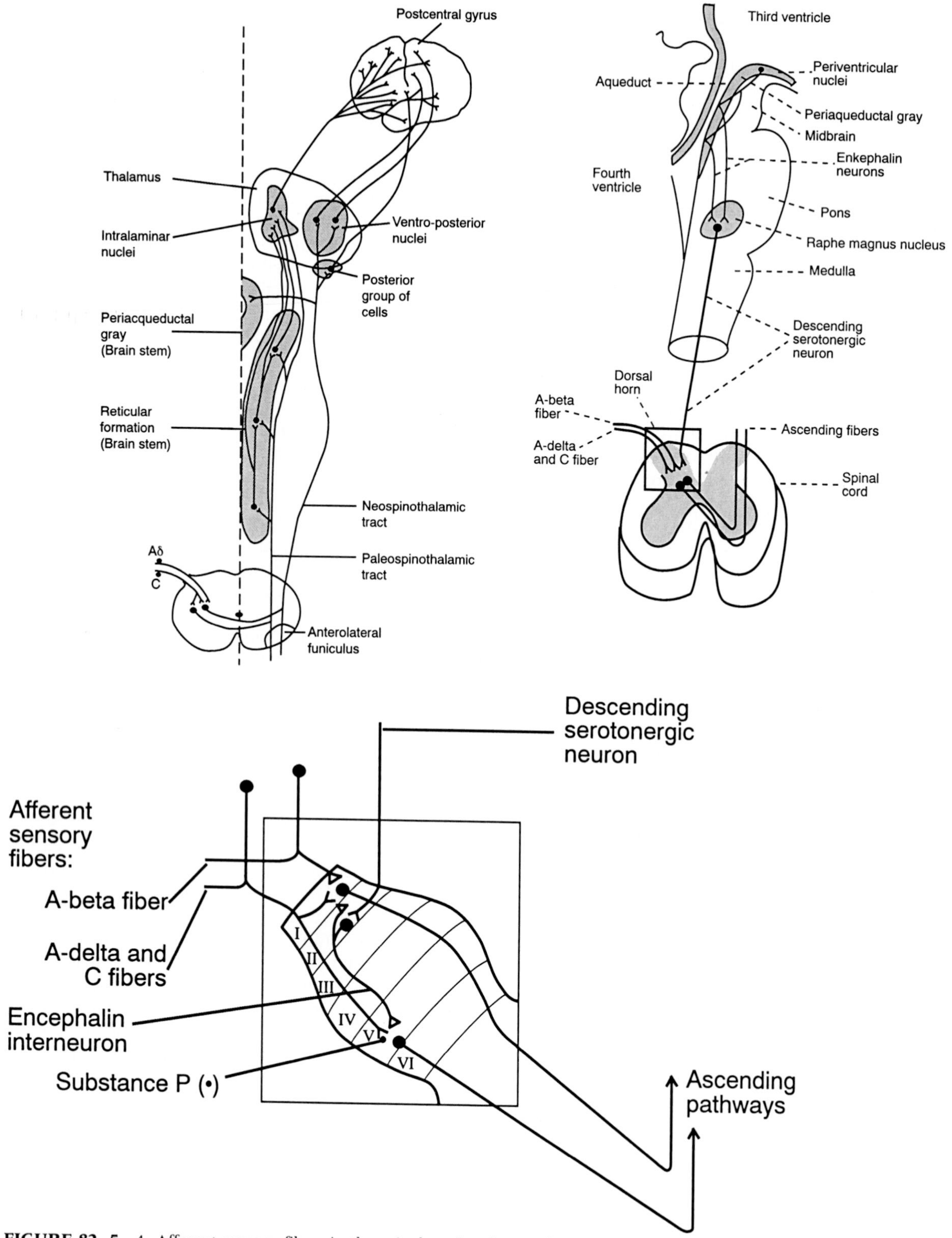

FIGURE 82–5. *A*, Afferent sensory fibers in the spinal cord and ascending pathways. From Bowsher, D.: Medical Times, *114*:83, 1986. *B*, Details of the dorsal horn showing laminae I–VI and approximate sites of interactions between afferent sensory fibers, descending pathways, and enkephalin interneurons (see text); open terminals indicate stimulation and closed ones inhibition. From McCain, G.A.[102] *C*, Descending inhibitory pathway of pain showing enkephalinergic and serotonergic neurons and their interaction with afferent sensory fibers at the dorsal horn. Adapted from Guyton, A.C.[104]

tems. Such a system at least partly explains great variability in individual response to a similarly intense noxious stimulus. The inhibitory system, operative mostly at the dorsal horn of the spinal cord level, originates in the brain stem as well as in the peripheral tissues. The descending inhibitory pathways have three major components (Fig. 82–5C): (1) the PAG area of midbrain, (2) the raphe magnus nucleus (RMN) in the upper medulla and pons, and (3) local pain inhibitory fibers at the dorsal horn. The enkephalinergic fibers arise from the PAG (as well as the periventricular area of the hypothalamus), synapsing with serotonergic fibers at the RMN,[103,104] which then presynaptically inhibit the incoming A-δ and C fibers at the dorsal horn through activation of the local enkephalinergic interneurons (Fig. 82–5B). However, serotinergic neurons can also cause direct postsynaptic inhibition.[104] The peripheral component of the inhibitory system is activated by the myelinated A-β fibers (Fig. 82–5B) by such non-nociceptive stimuli as rubbing, massaging, and transcutaneous nerve stimulation (TENS), which inhibit nociceptive A-δ and C fibers at the dorsal horn. The dorsal horn thus acts as a "gate" that controls pain by regulating the excitatory and the inhibitory stimuli before pain transmission ascends to the supraspinal level.

Apart from the above-mentioned enkephalinergic and serotonergic inhibitory systems, there is evidence that inhibitory noradrenergic neurons, originating in the locus coeruleus in the pons, also descend to the dorsal horn laminae and contribute to the "gate control."[103] Thus, the preliminary findings of an increased level of substance P[98] (an excitatory neurotransmitter) and a decreased level of MHPG in the CSF of fibromyalgia patients[101] may partly explain the increased pain sensitivity in these patients.

HYPOTHESES OF PATHOPHYSIOLOGIC MECHANISMS IN FIBROMYALGIA

Based on available information from several studies and normal mechanisms of pain described above, the following tentative hypotheses on mechanisms of fibromyalgia pain may be described.

Peripheral mechanisms. The presence of pathologic changes in muscles has been suggested,[105] but such a mechanism is unlikely to be the primary defect in fibromyalgia. Muscle damage, causing elaboration of such algogenic substances as prostaglandins, histamines, or potassium ions and activating the peripheral nociceptors, has not been demonstrated in fibromyalgia. Moreover, the pain and tenderness in fibromyalgia is global with widespread involvement of not only muscles, but also skin, ligaments, and the bone (such as the shin of the leg). Nonsteroidal anti-inflammatory drugs (NSAIDs) with their predominant peripheral action are not effective.[37,74] Tricyclic agents with their predominantly central mode of action, on the other hand, are the only drugs that have been beneficial in fibromyalgia in controlled studies.[74,75,106] Several peripheral factors, if present, may provide *additional* stimuli for pain, however. These factors include microtrauma from physical deconditioning, overactivity, hyperlaxity, and mechanical stress from the spine. The deconditioning present in many fibromyalgia patients is probably a *secondary* phenomenon due to pain and fatigue.

Central Mechanisms. Neurohormonal factors may be the primary aberration in fibromyalgia, perhaps in genetically predisposed individuals (Fig. 82–6). Limited data suggest genetic factors in fibromyalgia.[107] Serotonin deficiency is an attractive candidate for explaining pain and sleep disturbance,[87] two important features in fibromyalgia. However, available data do not suggest serotonin deficiency in all patients,[89,90,94] and aberrations of other neurotransmitters, such as norepinephrine[101] and substance P,[98] are likely to be present. These neurohormonal dysfunctions would decrease the normal pain threshold generally, so that tissue damage with production of algogenic substances would not be necessary to cause peripheral activation of nociception.

Ischemia. Although ischemia may be present in some muscle fibers more than others,[59] it appears that generalized ischemia significant enough to cause an abnormal oxygen uptake following exercise is absent.[61] Moreover, decreased microcirculation in muscles[59] may well be secondary to physical deconditioning.[60]

Local Stresses. Based on the work of Kellgren and Lewis, who demonstrated that an injection of hypertonic saline solutions deep in the structures of the cervical spine not only causes local tenderness but also distant and diffuse aching, Smythe suggested that the peripheral pain of fibromyalgia originates in the cervical and lumbar spinal structures.[108] Whether fibromyalgia patients have *abnormal* biomechanical stresses in these spinal segments is not known, however. Poor posture may also cause abnormal stress on muscles and spine.

Autonomic Dysfunction. Sympathetic blockade regionally and by stellate ganglion blockade decreased pain and the number of tender points in one controlled study.[109] Although the mechanisms of pain relief often sympathectomy is unknown, improvement of muscle hypoxia has been suggested to be one of them. However, the mechanism for such pain relief may also be central, because sympathectomy improves pain of reflex sympathetic dystrophy (RSD) due to a central cause.[110] An undefined autonomic dysfunction may also explain the subjective swollen feeling in fibromyalgia. Alternatively, this symptom, as well as paresthesia, may be related to pain itself. Total sites of "swollen feeling/paresthesia" correlated with total sites of pain, but not with the psychologic status in fibromyalgia.

Psychologic Abnormality. Anxiety, depression, and emotional stress are likely to aggravate pain,[33] although they are not essential for expression of fibromyalgia features.[66] This is not unique for fibromyalgia, however, because the pain of other conditions, such as RA,[111] is also known to be correlated with these psychologic factors. *Nonspecific stressful stimulus*, such as an infection, may also precipitate onset of fibromyalgia in a patient who is otherwise genetically or neurohormonally predisposed. The exact mechanism of such a stimulus is unknown, however.

Fatigue. Utilizing a twitch interpolation technique, Stokes et al. concluded that the fatigue of the chronic fatigue syndrome, a condition with overlapping features of fibromyalgia (see below), is central in origin.[112] The chemical neurotransmitter for fatigue is unknown, but it is interesting that an increased opioid activity has been postulated in chronic fatigue syndrome.[113] Additional factors leading to fatigue in fibromyalgia include depression, stress, and poor sleep; the latter two factors were correlated with fatigue in one of our studies.[13]

In summary, it appears likely that the major features of fibromyalgia—pain, tender points, fatigue, and poor sleep—are all predominantly due to central neurohormonal factors that may be further amplified by several other interrelated or independent factors, as depicted in Figure 82–6. A vicious cycle of pain leads to poor sleep, inactivity, stress, and depression, which in turn accentuate pain and ensure the chronicity of this painful syndrome.

MANAGEMENT OF FIBROMYALGIA

Management of fibromyalgia is more art than science at this time, because the pathophysiologic basis of therapy is incompletely understood and few controlled data exist regarding efficacy of several measures employed by practicing physicians (Table 82–7). Details of fibromyalgia management have been published elsewhere.[16,114]

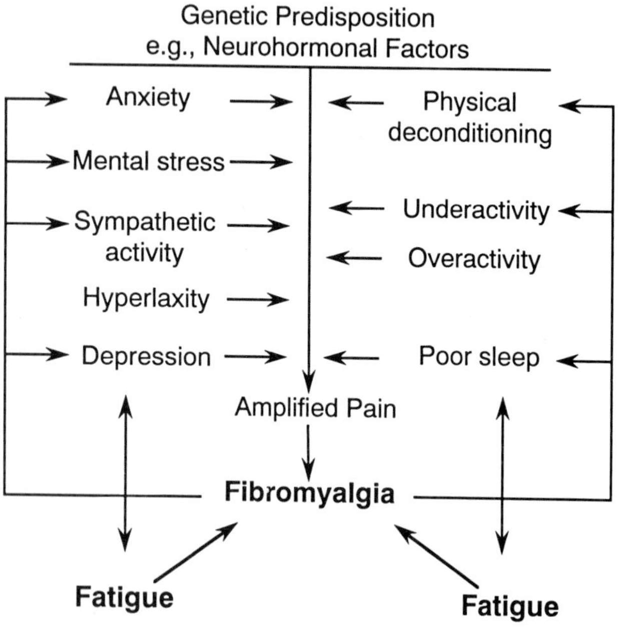

FIGURE 82–6. Postulated pathophysiologic mechanisms in fibromyalgia, showing a probable interaction between central (e.g., neurohormonal) and peripheral mechanisms.

TABLE 82–7. MANAGEMENT OF FIBROMYALGIA

Firm diagnosis and assurance regarding benign nature of fibromyalgia
Patient education; avoidance of aggravating factors
Management of psychologic factors
Behavioral changes
Physical exercises and physical fitness
Physical therapy
Use of simple analgesics (e.g., acetaminophen) and psychotropic drugs (e.g., amitriptyline and cyclobenzaprine—(see text for others)
Injection of tender points with local anesthetics
Referral to psychiatrists; pain clinic

Management begins with the initial patient contact. These patients are often apprehensive, possibly because of previous negative experiences with other physicians. An attitude of caring and understanding by the physician of the patient's suffering is essential for successful management, as is psychologic support on an ongoing basis with patience and empathy.

Firm Diagnosis and Assurance. Fibromyalgia can be diagnosed in a large majority of cases by its positive clinical features. Routine blood tests (such as CBC, ESR, and chemistry profile) may be ordered, but "one more test" on successive visits creates anxiety in a patient and should be avoided. Once a diagnosis is made, the physician should assure the patient that no underlying serious condition such as crippling arthritis, life-threatening cancer, or systemic lupus is present. The fundamentally benign nature of fibromyalgia without tissue damage should be emphasized. Such reassurance alone is helpful in most patients.

Patient Education Including Avoidance of Aggravating Factors and Utilization of Beneficial Modalities. This is an integral part of management. Explanation of probable or possible physiologic mechanisms is helpful. The interacting factors as shown in Figure 82–6 should be explained in clear and simple language. A brief handout including this information is useful. Important contributing or aggravating factors include poor sleep, overwork, trauma, anxiety, stress, depression, lack of physical conditioning, poor posture, and obesity.[13] The relative importance of these factors varies a great deal from patient to patient, and should be stressed for remedial action accordingly. Patients should be encouraged to utilize relieving factors (e.g., local heat and stretching exercises).[13]

Addressing Psychologic Factors. Many patients are apprehensive about being told that their pain is "all psychologic." They should be reassured that although their pain is not *caused* by psychologic factors, it may be *aggravated* by anxiety, stress, and depression.[13,33] These factors are not present in all patients, but are prominent in some. An underlying cause for anxiety, depression, or stress, such as marital disharmony, stress at work, or problems with growing or grown-up children, should be discretely discussed with an empathetic attitude during multiple visits. Excessive dependence on a physician should, however, be discouraged, and patients should always be guided to assume major responsibility in the management of their stress and pain. Appropriate psychologic counseling from a psychologist or a psychiatrist may be needed in some patients. Despite some questions about methodology, biofeedback was reported to be beneficial in a controlled study,[24] as was hypnotherapy in another controlled report of 40 refractory fibromyalgia patients with psychologic distress.[115] Rest, relaxation, and recreation are particularly important in an overworked and tense individual.

Behavioral Changes. These are crucial to successful therapy in fibromyalgia. Behavioral changes begin with the patient's acceptance of the fact that he or she has chronic pain, and that the improvement really lies in his or her own hands. Success is enhanced by having a definite goal in mind, particularly in daily life. The overall goal may be defined as being a happy and functional person. Daily goals should focus on physical exercises and getting usual chores done, as well as rest and recreation. It is helpful to write down these goals at the beginning of a day and keep a diary or graph of progress. The initial goals need to be modest for a patient with "severe pain." For example, the patient might be asked to begin with cleaning half a room or walking only a block. Two aspects of behavior are important: operant behavior and pacing one's activities.

Patients with chronic pain, irrespective of cause, often develop *operant behavior*, which can simply be defined as an unconscious but voluntary behavior of an individual that is influenced by the consequences of that behavior.[116] For example, readily available help for a patient who cannot do any house work at all because of pain will reinforce the negative pain behavior in that patient, whereas an expectation by the family members that this patient looks after such necessary work reasonably well discourages such unproductive behavior. Pacing one's activities, however, is important to avoid pain and subsequent operant behavior of shunning responsibilities. Operant behavior should not be confused with malingering.

Increasing Physical Fitness and Exercise Tolerance. Most fibromyalgia patients have flabby muscles and poor physical conditioning because of inactivity and a lack of regular exercise.[60] Such deconditioning may perpetuate pain (Fig. 82–6). Well-defined physical activities keep a patient busy, increase physical fitness, and generally encourage a healthy mental attitude. Doing group exercises at a medical or health center works better than individual efforts in many patients. A blinded, controlled study of cardiovascular fitness training three times a week for 20 weeks demonstrated significantly decreased pain and tender points and improvement of global health and psychologic status.[117] Such vigorous exercises might work by increasing endogenous endorphins in the central nervous system. Restorative sleep is also promoted by regular exercises. Brisk walking and swimming exercises in warm water can help patients attain cardiovascular fitness. The keys to success in achieving such fitness are motivation and starting at a low level with cautiously graded increments.

Physical Therapy. Various modes of physical therapy, including stretching and muscle-strengthening exercises, local heat, massage, and electric stimulation, have been used in chronic pain, but their efficacy in fibromyalgia has not been determined by controlled studies. In a controlled study of 145 patients with chronic low back pain, many of whom had "chronic lumbar sprain" and "myofascial pain," transcutaneous electric nerve stimulation (TENS) was found to be ineffective, although 52% of patients in the stretching exercise group improved, as compared with 37% in the nonexercise group ($p < 0.02$).[118] However, most patients discontinued their exercises after 2 months. We emphasize good posture and weight loss, as well as graduated muscle strengthening for ligamentous laxity, if present.

Analgesics. Relatively safe analgesics, such as acetaminophen, may be tried, although their true efficacy in controlled studies is unknown. Nonsteroidal anti-inflammatory drugs have not been found to be more effective than placebo in two controlled studies.[37,74] They should be particularly avoided in elderly patients who are at a greater risk of developing gastrointestinal and other serious side effects. Addictive and narcotic drugs should not be prescribed for chronic use in fibromyalgia.

Use of Psychotropic Agents. Two double-blind, placebo-controlled studies have established the beneficial effects of the tricyclic agent amitriptyline in the treatment of fibromyalgia with improvement in pain, sleep disturbance, and tender points.[74,75] Such a drug may be prescribed if the previously described measures do not significantly help a patient, or if the patient has severe symptoms during initial periods of consultation. The dose used in the two studies mentioned above was too small (25 mg and 50 mg at bedtime, respectively), and the response occurred too early to be attributed to the antidepressant effects of this drug. Cyclobenzaprine, a tricyclic compound, was also shown to have beneficial effects in fibromyalgia in a double-blind, placebo-controlled study, although a one-tail test of significance was used.[106] These tricyclic drugs can improve sleep, and it has been suggested that they also increase synaptic levels of serotonin, dopamine, and noradrenaline.[119] Although no specific studies are available for fibromyalgia, we have empirically used imipramine, nortriptyline, doxepin, and trazodone in small doses (10 to 50 mg) at bedtime. We have also used fluoxetine, a serotonergic drug, at a dose of 20 mg in the morning along with a tricyclic agent in the evening in some cases. S-adenosylmethionine, an antidepressant with an anti-inflammatory property (not available in the United States) was found useful in a placebo-controlled trial.[120] Some patients with fibromyalgia do have significant depression and will require larger, adequate doses of an antidepressant drug. Tricyclic agents should not be referred to as "antidepressants" to a fibromyalgia patient, because most patients are not significantly depressed and might resent using a drug for depression. A tranquilizer (e.g., alprazolam) may be added in an overtly anxious patient. A combination of alprazolam and ibuprofen was thought to be beneficial in one study.[121]

Injection of Tender Points. This mode of therapy is practical only if a patient has most pain in a limited number of sites (one to four) with well-identifiable tender points (TPs). A combination of 1 ml of 1 or 2% lidocaine and a similar amount of a corticosteroid preparation, such as triamcinolone diacetate or methylprednisolone acetate,* is injected after an injection of 2 to 3 ml of lidocaine alone in a precisely located TP. The initial injection of the local anesthetic should be gently and slowly carried out with a fine-gauge needle (e.g., size 27) of appropriate length (e.g., 1 to 1½ in.) in a "spoke wheel" radial fashion. Dizziness, usually transient, can be avoided by using a 1% solution of lidocaine and injecting slowly, particularly in an elderly patient. Although no controlled data are available, our experience shows that the effect of local injections lasts between 2 weeks and 2 to 3 months, depending on such factors as underlying psychopathology. Systemic corticosteroids were not useful in a controlled fashion in fibromyalgia[122] and should not be used.

Referral to a Psychiatrist, Psychologist, and Pain Clinic. Such consultations should not generally be considered at an early phase of management. Some patients do require a consultation for significant psychologic disturbance (e.g., severe anxiety, stress, depression, and somatization disorder). Referral to a pain clinic is sometimes helpful. Our pain clinic physicians have occasionally used stellate ganglion block for severe upper extremity pain in some patients with apparent success.

Management of fibromyalgia is challenging and not always satisfactory, and will remain so until its pathophysiologic mechanisms are better known. In the meantime, the nonspecific, supportive measures as described above might help many suffering individuals.

PROGNOSIS

Limited data exist regarding the course or prognosis of fibromyalgia patients seen in a rheumatology clinic. Felson and Goldenberg interviewed 39 fibromyalgia patients by telephone on a yearly basis and reported that 67% had moderate or severe symptoms over a period of 3 years, and that those with initially severe symptoms did poorly.[123] Similar results were reported by Ongchi et al.[124] Hawley et al. assessed 75 patients by a monthly questionnaire and found that their symptoms remained relatively stable over 1 year, and that psychologic status, pain, and functional disability were independent determinants of disease severity.[125] Further studies are needed to evaluate the prognosis and prognostic factors in fibromyalgia.

FUNCTIONAL DISABILITY AND WORK STATUS

The performance of 28 fibromyalgia and 26 RA patients, during five standardized work tasks showed that the former performed 59% and the latter 62% of the work accomplished by matched sedentary normal control subjects.[126] About 10% of patients considered themselves disabled, but only 6% actually received disability benefits—none specifically for fibromyalgia.[126] At this time most government agencies do not recognize fibromyalgia as a legitimate cause for disability payments. We have sometimes recommended disability for a severely symptomatic patient who (1) has documented consistent symptoms and TPs over time, (2) does not seem to have a predominant psychiatric cause for her or his disability as evaluated by a psychiatrist, (3) is unable to perform even a physically nondemanding job on a part-time basis, and (4) has significant functional impairment by a standardized questionnaire (e.g., Health Assessment Questionnaire) as well as on standardized tasks of work as determined by a specially equipped disability determination center. Fibromyalgia becomes and remains a disabling condition in a significant number of cases.

CONDITIONS SIMILAR OR RELATED TO FIBROMYALGIA

REGIONAL OR LOCALIZED FIBROMYALGIA (MYOFASCIAL PAIN SYNDROME)

Many patients with generalized fibromyalgia first experience symptoms of a localized nature (e.g., in the neck, trapezei, or the back, with or without a history of trauma).[22] However, when a patient presents with such localized symptoms, it is difficult to predict if their symptoms are going to spread to other areas. Host predisposition, mental stress and other psychologic factors, poor sleep, and trauma are possible determinants of subsequent progression to generalized fibromyalgia. Although the total number of sites involved can be as many as seven (e.g., neck, two trapezei, both shoulder joints, and two arms),[40] these areas are contiguous and do not fulfill the criteria of widespread pain of fibromyalgia. The number of TPs in these patients is smaller than in fibromyalgia,[14,40] but some patients do have widespread TPs, suggesting that they represent forme fruste cases of fibromyalgia and may well develop widespread pain symptoms at a later date. Undoubtedly

* *Editor's note*: Flourinated corticosteroids may cause significant soft tissue atrophy. I reserve them for intrasynovial use only.

there is an overlap with several fibromyalgia features, such as poor sleep and fatigue (which are, however, less common than fibromyalgia).[14,40] We had termed this regional pain syndrome localized fibromyalgia,[15,16] but there is no general agreement regarding terminology at this time. Such a syndrome may have a varied cause, including obvious or repetitive trauma, postural imbalance, and a referred pain from the disease in the cervical region, or it may simply reflect an initial stage of generalized fibromyalgia. The term myofascial pain syndrome (MPS) is commonly used in the physical medicine literature to characterize such patients with localized pain and tenderness, with added requirements that they also have, on palpation, referred pain (trigger points), taut band, and a local twitch response.[127] Unfortunately, these added features have not been validated in controlled and blinded studies. The only such study, in fact, demonstrated that taut bands and twitch response were equally frequent among MPS, fibromyalgia, and normal control subjects when assessed blindly by four MPS experts who also differed significantly between themselves in identifying TPs.[128] Patients with localized fibromyalgia seem to respond fairly well to local injections of their TPs with a local anesthetic.[127]

REPETITIVE STRAIN INJURY SYNDROME

An epidemic of upper-extremity pain and tenderness has recently been described in Australia among workers whose occupation involves repetitive use of their upper extremities.[129] The syndrome, abbreviated as RSI, is similar to the regional fibromyalgia syndrome described above, but seems to be clouded by emotional, social, and medicolegal (related to compensation) factors with an exaggerated response of chronic pain and dysfunction. Often the soft tissue tenderness is diffuse, including tenderness over tendons. There are many overlapping features of fibromyalgia in these patients, including multiple (sometimes generalized) TPs, irritable bowel syndrome, headaches, poor sleep, and paresthesias.

CHRONIC FATIGUE SYNDROME

Patients with chronic fatigue syndrome (CFS) present with severe and debilitating fatigue in the absence of an organic cause.[130,131] Initially a chronic Epstein-Barr virus (EBV) infection was implicated, but it soon became clear that there was no causative relationship between EBV and (CFS), although many viruses may nonspecifically trigger it.[130,131] Although this condition has been variously called postviral fatigue syndrome, epidemic neuromyasthenia, and chronic EBV syndrome, CFS is commonly used in the United States.

Empirical criteria proposed by the Centers for Disease Control (CDC) are listed in Table 82–8.[130] It is now clear that the CDC criteria are too restrictive. Manu et al. found that only 6 of their 135 patients with debilitating fatigue in the absence of an organic cause fulfilled the CDC criteria.[132] No satisfactory criteria based on appropriate data are available at this time. Several immunologic abnormalities have been described, including lymphocytosis, decreased cytolytic activity of natural killer cells, and an elevated ratio of CD4 to CD8 in a subgroup of patients.[131] Whether these findings reflect an initial triggering viral infection with a defect in immunologic

TABLE 82–8. CRITERIA FOR CASE DEFINITION OF CHRONIC FATIGUE SYNDROME AS PROPOSED BY CENTERS FOR DISEASE CONTROL (CDC)*

A. *Major Criteria*
New onset debilitating fatigue for at least 6 months, in the absence of an organic or chronic psychiatric disease.

B. *Symptom Criteria*
1. Mild fever (oral temp. 37.5° C–38.6° C)
2. Sore throat
3. Painful lymph nodes
4. Generalized muscle weakness
5. Myalgia
6. Unusually prolonged fatigue after exercise
7. Generalized headaches (if severity or pattern is different from headache prior to onset of current fatigue)
8. Migratory arthralgia without joint swelling
9. Neuropsychologic symptoms (one or more of the following: photophobia, transient scotoma, forgetfulness, irritability, confusion, difficulty thinking, inability to concentrate, depression)
10. Hypersomnia or insomnia
11. Main symptoms developing over a few days

C. *Physical Criteria*
1. Low grade oral temp. (37.6° C–38.6° C)
2. Nonexudative pharyngitis
3. Palpable or tender cervical/axillary lymph nodes (<2 cm in diameter)

To fulfill the criteria, a patient must satisfy the major criteria plus 8 of 11 symptom criteria (or 6 of 11 symptom criteria and 2 of 3 physical criteria).

* Adapted from Holmes, G.P., Kaplan, J.E., Gentz, N.M., et al.[130]

containment or if they are of any pathophysiologic significance is unclear.[131]

CFS and fibromyalgia are similar, overlapping syndromes.[133] A significant number of 50 fibromyalgia patients had such common CFS symptoms as recurrent pharyngitis (54%), recurrent adenopathy (33%), low-grade fever (28%) and acute onset with flu-like symptoms (55%).[134] Conversely, among 27 patients with CFS, TPs were found to be significantly more common than in 10 healthy controls, and two thirds of them had chronic myalgia.[133] Other striking similarities between the two syndromes include a female preponderance with a similar age distribution, arthralgia, myalgia, headache, paresthesia, irritable bowel syndrome, and depression.[133] Thus, patients with CFS may represent a subgroup of fibromyalgia patients with severe fatigue, and present to physicians predominantly for this problem.

RESTLESS LEGS SYNDROME

Restless legs syndrome (RLS) is characterized by an unpleasant, difficult-to-describe sensation usually in the calf of the legs, but sometimes in the feet and the thighs that occurs during rest or before sleep.[135,136] The sensation is variously described as "crawling of insects," "full of writhing worms," and "funny numbness." Unlike paresthesia of peripheral neuritis, which is constantly present irrespective of activities, the discomfort of RLS is present during inactivity, typically in the evening while resting in a sitting position and before sleep. The symptoms are usually improved or relieved by movements of the legs and the feet as well as by walking. Men and women are equally affected, the common age being between 50 and 60 years. A wide variety of conditions have been described to be associated with RLS; however, true association is probably limited to iron deficiency, pregnancy, and uremia.[135] About one third of patients with RA had RLS, according to one report.[137] In our preliminary analysis, 30% of 134 female fibromyalgia patients had RLS, as compared with 2% of 88 female normal controls of similar age ($p < 0.001$) and 18% of 57 female RA patients ($P < 0.05$). The difference between RA patients and normal conrols was significant ($P < 0.005$). RLS has shown a consistent association with nocturnal myoclonus (see below). Pathophysiologic mechanisms of RLS are unknown, but a central mechanism, including decreased dopamine activity, has been suggested.[138] No pathologic changes have been demonstrated in leg muscles. Laboratory tests are normal, with the exception of iron deficiency in some patients.

A large number of drugs are said to be effective in RLS, but only clonazepam (0.5 to 2 mg), carbamazepine (100 to 300 mg), and levodopa (100 to 200 mg) taken at bedtime have been found to be useful in double-blind placebo controlled studies.[135] RLS is a benign condition, but the symptoms are severe enough to significantly interfere with social life, such as going to movies, in some patients.

PERIODIC LIMB MOVEMENT DISORDER (NOCTURNAL MYOCLONUS)

Periodic limb movement disorder (PLMD) is the new term recommended in the International Classification of Sleep Disorders, replacing the older term *nocturnal myoclonus*.[139] PLMD is known to be significantly associated with restless leg syndrome; both conditions frequently occur in the same patient.[136] PLMD is characterized by repetitive, stereotyped brief movements of one or both lower extremities that occur primarily during non-REM sleep.[136,139,140] The sudden movement involves dorsiflexion of the ankle and the toes, with or without flexion of the leg at the knee and of the hip at the trunk. The muscle contraction complex usually lasts between 0.5 and 4.0 seconds, recurring approximately every 20 to 40 seconds, over a period of several minutes to hours, with predictable and remarkable regularity. Coleman et al. suggested that 40 or more such movements are required by electromyography for a diagnosis of PLMD.[140] Clinically, patients describe themselves as restless sleepers and find their bed sheets in disarray in the morning. Often the sleep partners complain of being kicked, although patients themselves may not be aware of such activities. The mean age of onset is between 47 to 56 years, with no significant gender differences; older patients have been reported to have more-severe symptoms.[136] PLMD should be distinguished from "sleep starts" (hypnic jerks), which occur at the onset of sleep, usually involving all the extremities as well as the trunk simultaneously.

Patients with PLMD complain of excessive daytime sleepiness and insomnia,[140] but a causal relationship has not been established.[139] Moldofsky et al. described nine fibromyalgia patients with nocturnal myoclonus, eight of whom also had an alpha anomaly in NREM sleep called alpha-delta sleep.[141] Nocturnal myoclonus occurred in 16% of 44 fibromyalgia patients by polysomnographic evaluation.[142] PLMD may also occur in patients with Parkinson's disease treated with levodopa and in obstructive and central sleep apnea, which should be ruled out appropriately.[136] Clonazepam at a bedtime dose of 0.5 to 2 mg is considered the first choice of treatment; this drug was effective in a placebo-controlled trial.[136] Other drugs often used include baclofen (20 to 40 mg at bedtime), temazepam, and imipramine.[136] Tricyclic drugs in general are believed to aggravate PLMD.[136]

PAIN IN PSYCHIATRIC CONDITIONS, INCLUDING PSYCHOGENIC PAIN

Regional or widespread pain may be a manifestation of several psychiatric disorders, including anxiety, depression, hypochondriasis, somatization disorder, and somatoform pain disorder.[143] These conditions should be diagnosed by other criteria besides musculoskeletal pain. The criteria published in Diagnostic and Statistical Manual of Mental Disorders (DSM-III-R) offer helpful guidelines,[143] but should not be used exclusively for the purpose of definite diagnosis.

Generalized anxiety disorder is characterized by unrealistic or excessive anxiety about several life circumstances (e.g., financial difficulties and misfortunes happening to children). A logical assessment or explanation of the situation fails to allay the persistent anxiety state. DSM-III criteria for a *major depressive syndrome* require the presence of five or more of the following: depressed mood, much-diminished interest in the pleasures of life, significant weight loss, sleep disturbance, fatigue, diminished ability to think or concentrate nearly everyday, feeling of worthlessness, and recurrent suicidal thoughts. Because fatigue and sleep problems are related to fibromyalgia per se irrespective of psychologic status, the focus for diagnosis of depression in a patient with musculoskeletal pain should be on the mood and related symptoms. As stated earlier, most fibromyalgia patients are not depressed. Depression, if present, is more likely to be concomitant or secondary to pain in fibromyalgia.

The essential feature of *hypochondriasis* is the patient's preoccupation that she or he may have a serious disease that is not supported by clinical or laboratory evidence. The preoccupation involves bodily functions (e.g., sweating, heartbeat, and body odor) or a minor cough or pain, which persist despite reassurances by a physician. *Somatization disorder* is characterized by many physical complaints that begin before the age of 30 years. Major symptoms for screening purposes include vomiting, difficulty in swallowing, pain in extremities, breathlessness at rest, amnesia, burning sensation in sexual organs, and painful menstruation. It has been suggested that two or more of these seven symptoms might indicate the diagnosis, but formal diagnosis requires the presence of at least 13 of the 35 symptoms listed in DSM-III-R.[143] Despite multiple complaints, less than 10% of fibromyalgia patients satisfy the criteria for somatization disorder by structured interview studies.[143]

In *somatoform pain disorder* (older terminology: *psychogenic pain*), a patient is preoccupied with pain, but in contrast with such dysfunctional disorders as tension headache or fibromyalgia, there is an absence of known pathophysiologic mechanism or of consistent physical findings (e.g., TPs). Unlike the psychiatric conditions mentioned above, pain dominates the picture.

The distinction between fibromyalgia and various psychiatric conditions described above may be difficult in some patients. Part of the problem arises from the fact that no data exist comparing an adequate number of patients with fibromyalgia and those with psychiatric diseases with regards to fibromyalgia and psychiatric features. For example, the proportion of patients in a psychiatric population who fulfill criteria for fibromyalgia is unknown. No criteria studies have included such a population as a control group; hence, the specificity of reported fibromyalgia criteria against psychiatric conditions with pain is not known.

General clinical experience suggests that patients with a predominant psychiatric or psychologic problem have an obsession with pain that is always severe, described with many bizarre or unusual words, resistant to any form of therapy, and sometimes involving unusual sites such as the sexual organs. Symptoms and TPs lack consistency among these patients. Patients suspected of having a significant psychiatric problem should be evaluated by a psychiatrist. Data do not suggest that the number of sites of pain complaints, the "hurt all over" symptom, and the number of TPs in are helpful in distinguishing fibromyalgia patients with or without psychologic disturbance.[33] Patients who are sore literally everywhere when touched are likely to have a significant or predominant psychiatric condition, but no data exist to support this notion.

Finally, the problem of distinguishing fibromyalgia from a psychiatric condition is compounded by the fact that a patient may have both conditions, in which case the pain is accentuated by the psychologic factor.[33] Occasionally a patient may also have an additional concomitant organic pathology such as thoracic outlet syndrome, spinal stenosis, or malignancy. A careful history-taking and examination are needed to sort out comorbidities in such patients.

REFERENCES

1. Reynolds, M.D.: The development of the concept of fibrositis. J. Hist. Med. Allied Sci., *38*:5–35, 1983.
2. Gowers, W.R.: Lumbago: Its lessons and analogues. Br. Med. J., *1*:117–121, 1904.
3. Stockman, R.: The causes, pathology and treatment of chronic rheumatism. Edinburgh Med. J., *15*:107–116, 223–235, 1904.
4. Simons, D.G.: Muscle pain syndromes—Part II. Am. J. Phys. Med., *55*:15–42, 1976
5. Yunus, M.B., and Kalyan-Raman, U.P.: Muscle biopsy findings in primary fibromyalgia and other forms of nonarticular rheumatism. Rheum. Dis. Clin. North Am., *15*:115–134, 1989.
6. Traut, E.F.: Fibrositis. J. Am. Geriatr. Soc., *16*:531–538, 1968.
7. Smythe, H.A.: Non-articular rheumatism and the fibrositis. *In* Arthritis and Allied Conditions: A Textbook of Rheumatology. ed 8, Edited by J.L. Hollander and D.J. McCarty, Jr. Philadelphia, Lea & Febiger, 1972, pp. 874–884.
8. Moldofsky, H., Scarisbrick, P., England, R., and Smythe, H.: Musculoskeletal symptoms and non-REM sleep disturbance in patients with "fibrositis" syndrome and healthy subjects. Psychosom. Med., *37*:341–351, 1975.
9. Smythe, H.A., and Moldofsky, H.: Two contributions to understanding of the "fibrositis" syndrome. Bull. Rheum. Dis., *28*:928–931, 1977.
10. Yunus, M.B., Masi, A.T., Calabro, J.J., et al.: Primary fibromyalgia (fibrositis): Clinical study of 50 patients with matched normal controls. Semin. Arthritis Rheum., *11*:151–171, 1981.
11. Hench, P.K.: Nonarticular Rheumatism, 22nd rheumatism review: Review of the American and English literature for the years 1973 and 1974. Arthritis Rheum. Suppl., *19*:1081–1089, 1976.
12. Goldenberg, D.L.: Fibromyalgia syndrome: An emerging but controversial condition. JAMA, *257*:2782–2787, 1987.
13. Yunus, M.B., Masi, A.T., and Aldag, J.C.: A controlled study of

primary fibromyalgia syndrome: Clinical features and association with other functional syndromes. J. Rheumatol., *16*(Suppl. 19):62–71, 1989.
14. Wolfe, F., Smythe, H.A., Yunus, M.B., et al.: The American College of Rheumatology 1990 criteria for classification of fibromyalgia: Report of the multicenter criteria committee. Arthritis Rheum., *33*:160–172, 1990.
15. Yunus, M.B.: Fibromyalgia syndrome: A need for uniform classification. J. Rheumatol., *10*:841–844, 1983.
16. Yunus, M.B.: Diagnosis, etiology, and management of fibromyalgia syndrome: An update. Compr. Ther., *14*:8–20, 1988.
17. Yunus, M.B., Holt, G.S., Masi, A.T., and Aldag, J.C.: Fibromyalgia syndrome among the elderly: Comparison with younger patients. J. Am. Geriatr. Soc., *35*:987–995, 1988.
18. Campbell, S.M., Clark, S., Tindall, E.A., et al.: Clinical characteristics of fibrositis: I. A 'blinded', controlled study of symptoms and tender points. Arthritis Rheum., *26*:817–824, 1983.
19. Hartz, A., and Kirchdoerfer, E.: Undetected fibrositis in primary care practice. J. Fam. Practice, *25*:365–369, 1987.
20. Jacobsson, L., Lindgärde, F., and Manthorpe, R.: The commonest rheumatic complaints of over six weeks' duration in a twelve-month period in a defined Swedish population. Scand. J. Rheumatol., *18*:353–360, 1989.
21. Yunus, M.B., and Masi, A.T.: Juvenile primary fibromyalgia syndrome. Arthritis Rheum., *28*:138–144, 1985.
22. Bengtsson, A., Henriksson, K.G., and Jrfeldt, L., et al.: Primary fibromyalgia: A clinical and laboratory study of 55 patients. Scand. J. Rheumatol., *15*:340–347, 1986.
23. Müller, W.: The fibrositis syndrome: Diagnosis, differential diagnosis and pathogenesis. Scand. J. Rheumatol., *65*(Suppl.): 40–53, 1987.
24. Ferraccioli, G., Ghirelli, L., Scita, F., et al.: EMG-biofeedback training in fibromyalgia syndrome. J. Rheumatol., *14*:820–825, 1987.
25. Wolfe, F., Hawley, D.J., Cathey, M.A., et al.: Fibrositis: Symptom frequency and criteria for diagnosis. J. Rheumatol., *12*:1159–1163, 1985.
26. Leavitt, F., Katz, R.S., Golden, H.E., et al.: Comparison of pain properties in fibromyalgia patients and rheumatoid arthritis patients. Arthritis Rheum., *29*:775–781, 1986.
27. Wolfe, F.: The clinical syndrome of fibrositis. Am. J. Med., *81*:7–14, 1986.
28. McCain, G.A., and Scudds, R.A.: The concept of primary fibromyalgia (fibrositis): Clinical value, relation and significance to other chronic musculoskeletal pain syndromes. Pain, *33*:273–287, 1988.
29. Simms, R.W., and Goldenberg, D.L.: Symptoms mimicking neurologic disorders in fibromyalgia syndrome. J. Rheumatol., *15*:1271–1273, 1988.
30. Yunus, M.B., Hussey, F.X., Aldag, J.C., and Masi, A.T.: Antinuclear antibodies and connective tissue disease features in primary fibromyalgia (abstract). Arthritis Rheum., *34*:R12, 1991.
31. Wallace, D.J.: Genitourinary manifestations of fibrositis: An increased association with the female urethral syndrome. J. Rheumatol., *17*:238–239, 1990.
32. Dinerman, H., Goldenberg, D.L., Felson, D.T., et al.: A prospective evaluation of 118 patients with fibromyalgia syndrome: Prevalence of Raynaud's phenomenon, sicca syndrome, ANAs, low complement and IG deposition at the dermal epidermal junction. J. Rheumatol., *13*:368–373, 1986.
33. Yunus, M.B., Ahles, T.A., Aldag, J.C., and Masi, A.T.: Relationship of clinical features with psychological status in primary fibromyalgia. Arthritis Rheum., *34*:15–21, 1991.
34. Bennett, R.M., Clark, S.R., Campbell, S.M., et al.: Symptoms of Raynaud's syndrome in patients with fibromyalgia. Arthritis Rheum., *34*:264–269, 1991.
35. Vaerøy, H., Qiao, Z.G., Morkrid, L., and Forre, O.: Altered sympathetic nervous system response in patients with fibromyalgia (fibrositis syndrome). J. Rheumatol., *16*:1460–1465, 1989.
36. Tunks, E., Crook, J., Norman, G., and Kalaher, S.: Tender points in fibromyalgia. Pain, *34*:11–19, 1988.
37. Yunus, M.B., Masi, A.T., and Aldag, J.C.: Short-term effects of ibuprofen in primary fibromyalgia syndrome: A double blind, placebo controlled trial. J. Rheumatol., *16*:527–532, 1989.
38. Simms, R.W., Goldenberg, D.L., Felson, D.T., and Mason, J.H.: Tenderness in 75 anatomic sites: Distinguishing fibromyalgia patients from controls. Arthritis Rheum., *31*:182–187, 1988.
39. Quimby, L.G., Block, S.R., and Gratwick, G.M.: Fibromyalgia: Generalized pain intolerance and manifold symptom reporting. J. Rheumatol., *15*:1264–1270, 1988.
40. Yunus, M.B., Masi, A.T., and Aldag, J.C.: Preliminary criteria for primary fibromyalgia syndrome (PFS): Multivariate analysis of a consecutive series of PFS, other pain patients, and normal subjects. Clin. Exp. Rheumatol., *7*:63–69, 1989.
41. Caro, X.J.: Immunofluorescent detection of IgG at the dermal-epidermal junction in patients with apparent primary fibrositis syndrome. Arthritis Rheum., *27*:1174–1179, 1984.
42. Bengtsson, A., Ernerudh, J., Vrethem, M., and Skogh, T.: Absence of autoantibodies in primary fibromyalgia. J. Rheumatol., *17*:1682–1683, 1990.
43. Yunus, M.B., Berg, B.C., and Masi, A.T.: Multiphase skeletal scintigraphy in primary fibromyalgia syndrome: A blinded study. J. Rheumatol., *16*:1466–1468, 1989.
44. Zidar, J., Bäckman, E., Bengtsson, A., and Henriksson, K.G.: Quantitative EMG and muscle tension in painful muscles in fibromyalgia. Pain, *40*:249–254, 1990.
45. Caro, X.J.: Is there an immunologic component to the fibrositis syndrome? Rheum. Dis. Clin. North Am., *15*:169–186, 1989.
46. Caro, X.J., Wolfe, R., Johnston, W.H., et al.: A controlled and blinded study of immunoreactant deposition at the dermal-epidermal juntion of patients with primary fibrositis syndrome. J. Rheumatol., *13*:1086–1092, 1986.
47. Carette, S., and Lefrancois, L.: Fibrositis and primary hypothyroidism. J. Rheumatol., *15*:1418–1421, 1988.
48. Pellegrino, M.J.: Atypical chest pain as an initial presentation of primary fibromyalgia. Arch. Phys. Med. Rehabil., *71*:526–528, 1990.
49. Erickson, P.-P., Lindman, R., Stal, P., and Bengtsson, A.: Symptoms and signs of mandibular dysfunction in primary fibromyalgia syndrome. Swed. Dent. J., *12*:141–149, 1988.
50. Blasberg, B., and Chalmers, A.: Temporomandibular pain and dysfunction syndrome associated with generalized musculoskeletal pain: A retrospective study. J. Rheumatol., *16*(Suppl. 19):87–90, 1989.
51. Gester, J.C., and Hadj-Dijilani, A.: Hearing and vestibular abnormalities in primary fibrosis syndrome. J. Rheumatol., *11*:679–680, 1984.
52. Goldenberg, D.L.: Fibromyalgia and its relation to chronic fatigue syndrome, viral illness and immune abnormalities. J. Rheumatol., *16*(Suppl. 19):91–93, 1989.
53. Kalyan-Raman, U.P., Kalyan-Raman, K., Yunus, M.B., et al.: Muscle pathology in primary fibromyalgia syndrome: Light microscopic, histochemical and ultrastructural study. J. Rheumatol., *11*:808–813, 1984.
54. Bengtsson, A., Henriksson, K.G., and Larsson, J.: Muscle biopsy in primary fibromyalgia: Light microscopical and histochemical findings. Scand. J. Rheumatol., *15*:1–6, 1986.
55. Yunus, M.B., Kalyan-Raman, U.P., Masi, A.T., et al.: Electron microscopic studies of muscle biopsy in primary fibromyalgia syndrome: A controlled and blinded study. J. Rheumatol., *16*:97–101, 1989.

56. Bartels, E.M., Danneskiold-Samsøe, B.: Histological abnormalities in muscle from patients with certain types of fibrositis. Lancet, *1*:755–757, 1986.
57. Bach-Andersen, R., Jacobsen, S., Danneskiold-Samsøe, B., et al.: New diagnostic tools in primary fibromyalgia. *In* Advances in Pain Research and Therapy, Vol. 17. Edited by J.R. Fricton and E.A. Awad. New York, Raven Press, 1990, pp. 269–276.
58. Bengtsson, A., Henriksson, K.G., and Larsson, J.: Reduced high-energy phosphate levels in the painful muscles of patients with primary fibromyalgia. Arthritis Rheum., *29*:817–821, 1986.
59. Lund, N., Bengtsson, A., and Thorborg, P.: Muscle tissue oxygen pressure in primary fibromyalgia. Scand. J. Rheumatol., *15*:165–173, 1986.
60. Bennett, R.M., Clark, S., Goldberg, L., et al.: Aerobic fitness in patients with fibrositis: A controlled study of respiratory gas exchange and xenon^{133} clearance from exercising muscle. Arthritis Rheum., *32*:454–460, 1989.
61. Sietsema, K.E., Cooper, D.M., and Caro, X.J.: Oxygen utilization during muscular exercise in patients with primary fibromyalgia patients (abstract). Arthritis Rheum., *33*(Suppl.):5137, 1990.
62. Wallace, D.J., Peter, J.B., Bowman, R.L., et al.: Fibromyalgia, cytokines, fatigue syndromes and immune regulation. *In* Advances in Pain Research and Therapy, Vol. 17. Edited by J.R. Fricton and E.A. Awad. New York, Raven Press, pp. 277–287.
63. Payne, T.C., Leavitt, F., Garron, D.C., et al.: Fibrositis and psychological disturbance. Arthritis Rheum., *25*:213–217, 1982.
64. Ahles, T.A., Yunus, M.B., Railey, S.D., et al.: Psychological factors associated with primary fibromyalgia syndrome. Arthritis Rheum., *27*:1101–1106, 1984.
65. Wolfe, F., Cathey, M.A., Kleinheksel, S.M., et al.: Psychological status in primary fibrositis and fibrositis associated with rheumatoid arthritis. J. Rheumatol., *11*:500–506, 1984.
66. Clark, S., Campbell, S.M., Forehand, M.E., et al.: Clinical characteristics of fibrositis. II. A "blinded" controlled study using standard psychological tests. Arthritis Rheum., *28*:132–137, 1985.
67. Hudson, J.I., Hudson, M.S., Plinter, L.F., et al.: Fibromyalgia and major affective disorders: A controlled phenomenology and family history study. Am. J. Psychiatry, *142*:441–446, 1985.
68. Ahles, T.A., Yunus, M.B., and Masi, A.T.: Is chronic pain a variant of depressive disease? The case of primary fibromyalgia syndrome. Pain, *29*:105–111, 1987.
69. Kirmayer, L.J., Robbins, J.M., and Kapusta, M.A.: Somatization and depression in fibromyalgia syndrome. Am. J. Psychiatry, *145*:950–954, 1988.
70. Dailey, P.A., Bishop, G.D., Russell, I.J., and Fletcher, E.M.: Psychological stress and the fibrositis/fibromyalgia syndrome. J. Rheumatol., *17*:1380–1385, 1990.
71. Uveges, J.M., Parker, J.C., Smarr, K.L., et al.: Psychological symptoms in primary fibromyalgia syndrome: Relationship to pain, life stress and sleep disturbance. Arthritis Rheum., *33*:1279–1283, 1990.
72. Hudson, J.I., and Pope, H.G.: Fibromyalgia and psychopathology: Is fibromyalgia a form of "affective spectrum disorder?" J. Rheumatol., *15*:1551–1556, 1988.
73. Ahles, T.A., Khan, S.A., Yunus, M.B., et al.: Psychiatric status of primary fibromyalgia and rheumatoid arthritis patients and nonpain controls: A blinded comparison of DSM-III diagnoses. Am. J. Psychiat., *148*:1721–1726, 1991.
74. Goldenberg, D.L., Felson, D.T., and Dinerman, H.: A randomized controlled trial of amitriptyline and naproxen in the treatment of patients with fibromyalgia. Arthritis Rheum., *29*:1371–1377, 1986.
75. Carette, S., McCain, G.A., Bell, D.A., and Fam, A.G.: Evaluation of amitriptyline in primary fibrositis: A double-blind, placebo-controlled study. Arthritis Rheum., *29*:655–659, 1986.
76. Ferraccioli, G., Cavalieri, F., Salaffi, F., et al.: Neuroendocrine findings in primary fibromyalgia and in other chronic rheumatic conditions (rheumatoid arthritis, low back pain). J. Rheumatol., *17*;869–873, 1990.
77. Russell, I.J., Bowden, C.L., Michalek, J., et al.: Imipramine receptor density on platelets of patients with fibrositis syndrome: Correlation with disease severity and response to therapy (abstract). Arthritis Rheum., *30*:S63, 1987.
78. Briley, M.S., Raisman, R., and Langer, S.Z.: Human platelets possess high affinity binding sites for H-imipramine. Eur. J. Pharmacol., *58*:347–348, 1979.
79. Leavitt, F., and Katz, R.S.: Is the MMPI invalid for assessing psychological disturbance in pain related organic conditions? J. Rheumatol., *16*:521–526, 1989.
80. Gupta, M.A., and Moldofsky, H.: Dysthymic disorders and rheumatic pain modulation disorder (fibrositis syndrome): A comparison of symptoms and sleep physiology. Can. J. Psychiatry, *31*:608–616, 1986.
81. Moldofsky, H., Saskin, P., and Lue, F.A.: Sleep and symptoms in fibrositis syndrome after a febrile illness. J. Rheumatol., *15*:1701–1704, 1988.
82. Ware, J.C., Russell, I.J., and Campas, E.: Alpha intrusions into the sleep of depressed and fibromyalgia syndrome patients (abstract). Sleep Res., *15*:286, 1986.
83. Molony, R.L., MacPeek, D.M., Schiffman, P.L., et al.: Sleep, sleep apnea and the fibromyalgia syndrome. J. Rheumatol., *13*:797–800, 1986.
84. Herisson, C., Simon, L., Touchon, J., and Billiard, M.: Sleeping disorders, fibrositis and mianserin treatment (abstract). Arthritis Rheum., *32*(Suppl.):S70, 1989.
85. Doherty, M., Patrick, M., and Smith, J.: Sleeping electroencephalograms in patients with primary fibromyalgia syndrome and osteoarthritis (abstract). Arthritis Rheum., *33*(Suppl.):S22, 1990.
86. Moldofsky, H., Lue, F.A., and Smythe, H.A.: Alpha EEG sleep and morning symptoms in rheumatoid arthritis. J. Rheumatol., *10*:373–379, 1983.
87. Chase, T.N., and Murphy, D.J.: Serotonin and central nervous systems function. Annu. Rev. Pharmacol., *13*:181–197, 1973.
88. Moldofsky, H., and Warsh, J.J.: Plasma tryptophan and musculoskeletal pain in nonarticular rheumatism ("fibrositis syndrome"). Pain, *5*:65–71, 1978.
89. Russell, I.J., Michalek, J.E., Vipraio, G.A., et al.: Serum amino acids in fibrositis/fibromyalgia concentration. J. Rheumatol., *16*(Suppl. 19):158–163, 1989.
90. Yunus, M.B., Dailey, J.W., Aldag, J.C., et al.: Plasma tryptophan and other amino acids in primary fibromyalgia: A controlled study. J. Rheumatol., *19*:90–94, 1992.
91. Gibson, C.J.: Control of monoamine synthesis by precursor availability. *In* Handbook of Neurochemistry. Edited by A. Lajtha. New York, Plenum Press, 1985, pp. 309–324.
92. Houvenagel, E., Forzy, G., Cortet, B., and Vincent, G.: 5-Hydroxy indole acetic acid in cerebrospinal fluid in fibromyalgia. Arthritis Rheum., *33*(Suppl.):S55, 1990.
93. Sicuteri, F.: Headache as a possible expression of deficiency of brain 5-hydroxytryptamine (central denervation supersensitivity). Headache, *12*:69–72, 1972.
94. Simon, L., Aboukrat, P., Herisson, C., and Bressot, N.: Free plasmatic tryptophan and plasma beta-endorphins in primary fibromyalgia syndrome (abstract). Arthritis Rheum., *33* (Suppl.):S56, 1990.
95. Yunus, M.B., Denko, C.W., and Masi, A.T.: Serum beta endorphin in primary fibromyalgia syndrome: A controlled study. J. Rheumatol., *13*:183–186, 1986.

96. Vaerøy, H., Helle, R., Forre, O., et al.: CSF levels of beta-endorphin in patients with fibromyalgia. J. Rheumatol., *15*: 1804–1806, 1988.
97. Reynolds, W.J., Chiu, B., and Inman, R.D.: Plasma substance P in fibrositis. J. Rheumatol., *15*:1802–1803, 1989.
98. Vaerøy, H., Helle, R., Forre, Ø., et al.: Elevated CSF levels of substance P and high incidence of Raynaud's phenomenon in patients with fibromyalgia: New features for diagnosis. Pain, *32*:21–26, 1988.
99. Yunus, M.B., Dailey, J.W., Aldag, J.C., et al.: Plasma and urinary catecholamines in primary fibromyalgia. J. Rheumatol., *19*:95–97, 1992.
100. Russell, I.J.: Neurohormonal aspects of fibromyalgia syndrome. Rheum. Dis. Clin. North Am., *15*:149–168, 1989.
101. Russell, I.J., Vaerøy, H., Javors, M., and Nyberg, F.: Cerebrospinal fluid biogenic amines in fibrositis/fibromyalgia syndrome. Arthritis Rheum., *33*(Suppl.):S55, 1990.
102. McCain, G.A.: Nonmedicinal treatments in primary fibromyalgia. Rheum. Clin. North Am., *15*:73–90, 1989.
103. Bonica, J.J.: Biochemistry and modulation of nociception and pain. *In* The Management of Pain. 2nd Ed. Edited by J.J. Bonica. Philadelphia, Lea & Febiger, 1990, pp. 95–121.
104. Guyton, A.C. (ed.): Textbook of Medical Physiology. Philadelphia, W.B. Saunders, 1991, pp. 520–531.
105. Bennett, R.M.: Beyond fibromyalgia: Ideas on etiology and treatment. J. Rheumatol., *16*(Suppl. 19):185–191, 1989.
106. Bennett, R.M., Gatter, R.A., Campbell, S.M., et al.: A comparison of cyclobenzaprine and placebo in the management of fibrositis. Arthritis Rheumatol., *31*:1535–1542, 1988.
107. Pellegrino, M.J., Waylonis, G.W., and Sommer, A.: Familial occurrence of primary fibromyalgia. Arch. Phys. Med. Rehab., *70*:61–63, 1989.
108. Smythe, H.A.: Nonarticular rheumatism and psychogenic musculoskeletal syndromes. *In* Arthritis and Allied Conditions: A Textbook of Rheumatology, 11th ed. Edited by D.J. McCarty. Philadelphia, Lea & Febiger, 1989, pp. 1241–1254.
109. Bengtsson, A., and Bengtsson, M.: Regional sympathetic blockade in primary fibromyalgia. Pain, *33*:161–167, 1988.
110. Schott, G.D.: Mechanisms of causalgia and related clinical conditions. Brain, *109*:717–738, 1986.
111. Creed, F.: Psychological disorders in rheumatoid arthritis: A growing consensus? Ann. Rheum. Dis., *49*:808–812, 1990.
112. Stokes, M.J., Cooper, R.G., and Edwards, R.H.T.: Normal muscle strength and fatigability in patients with effort syndromes. Br. Med. J., *297*:1014–1017, 1988.
113. Prieto, J., Subira, M.L., and Serrano, M.: Naloxone-reversible monocyte dysfunction in patients with chronic fatigue syndrome. Scand. J. Immunol., *30*:13–20, 1989.
114. Masi, A.T., and Yunus, M.B.: Fibromyalgia—Which is the best treatment? A personalized, comprehensive, ambulatory, patient-involved management programme. Baillieres Clin. Rheumatol., *4*:333–370, 1990.
115. Haanen, H.C.M., Hoenderdos, H.T.W., vanRomunde, L.K.J., et al.: Controlled trial of hypnotherapy in the treatment of refractory fibromyalgia. J. Rheumatol., *18*:72–75, 1990.
116. Fordyce, W.E.: Behavioral Methods for Chronic Pain and Illness. St. Louis, C.V. Mosby, 1976.
117. McCain, G.A., Bell, D.A., Mai, F.M., and Holliday, P.D.: A controlled study of the effects of a supervised cardiovascular fitness training program on the manifestations of primary fibromyalgia. Arthritis Rheum., *31*:1135–1141, 1989.
118. Deyo, R.A., Walsh, N.E., Martin, D.C., et al.: A controlled trial of transcutatneous electrical nerve stimulation (TENS) and exercise for chronic low back pain. N. Engl. J. Med., *322*: 1627–1634, 1990.
119. Willner, P.: Antidepressants and serotonergic neurotransmission: An integrative review. Psychopharmacology, *85*:387–404, 1985.
120. Jacobsen, S., Danneskiold-Samsøe, B., and Andersen, R.B.: Oral S-adenosylmethionine in primary fibromyalgia: Double-blind placebo controlled evaluation. Scand. J. Rheumatol., in press.
121. Russell, I.J., Fletcher, E.M., Michalek, J.E., et al.: Treatment of primary fibromyalgia syndrome with ibuprofen and alprazolam: A double blind, placebo-controlled study. Arthritis Rheum., *34*:552–560, 1991.
122. Clark, S., Tindall, E., and Bennett, R.M.: A double blind crossover trial of prednisone versus placebo in the treatment of fibrositis. J. Rheumatol., *12*:980–983, 1985.
123. Felson, D.T., and Goldenberg, D.L.: The natural history of fibromyalgia. Arthritis Rheum., *29*:1522–1526, 1986.
124. Ongchi, D.R., Dill, E.R., and Katz, R.S.: How often do fibromyalgia patients improve? (abstract). Arthritis Rheum., *33* (Suppl.):S136, 1990.
125. Hawley, D.J., Wolfe, F., and Cathey, M.A.: Pain, functional disability, and psychological status: A 12-month study of severity in fibromyalgia. J. Rheumatol., *15*:1551–1556, 1988.
126. Cathey, M.A., Wolfe, F., and Kleinheksel, S.M.: Functional ability and work status in patients with fibromyalgia. Arthritis Care Res., *1*:85–98, 1988.
127. Travell, J.G., and Simons, D.G.: Myofascial Pain and Dysfunction: The Trigger Point Manual. Baltimore, Williams & Wilkins, 1983.
128. Wolfe, F., Simons, D., Friction, J., et al.: The fibromyalgia and myofascial pain syndromes: A study of tender points and trigger points in persons with fibromyalgia, myofascial pain syndrome and no disease (abstract). Arthritis Rheum., *33*(Suppl.):S137, 1990.
129. Littlejohn, G.O.: Fibrositis/fibromyalgia syndrome in the workplace. Rheum. Dis. Clin. North Am., *15*:45–60, 1989.
130. Holmes, G.P., Kaplan, J.E., Gantz, N.M., et al.: Chronic fatigue syndrome: A working case definition. Ann. Intern. Med., *108*:387–389, 1988.
131. Komaroff, A.L., Goldenberg, D.: The chronic fatigue syndrome: Definition, current studies and lessions for fibromyalgia research. J. Rheumatol., *16*(Suppl. 19):23–27, 1989.
132. Manu, P., Lane, T.J., and Mathews, D.A.: The frequency of the chronic fatigue syndrome in patients with symptoms of persistent fatigue. Ann. Intern. Med., *109*:554–556, 1989.
133. Goldenberg, D.L.: Fibromyalgia and its relation to chronic fatigue syndrome, viral illness and immune abnormalities. J. Rheumatol., *16*(Suppl. 19):91–93, 1989.
134. Buchwald, D., Goldenberg, D.L., Sullivan, J.L., and Komaroff, A.L.: The "chronic, active Epstein-Barr virus infection" syndrome and primary fibromyalgia. Arthritis Rheum., *30*:1132–1136, 1987.
135. Clough, C.: Restless legs syndrome. Br. Med. J., *294*:262–263, 1987.
136. Krueger, B.R.: Restless legs syndrome and periodic movements of sleep. Mayo Clin. Proc., *65*:999–1006, 1990.
137. Reynolds, G., Blake, D.R., Hall, H.S., and Williams, A.: Restless legs syndrome and rheumatoid arthritis. Br. Med. J., *292*:659–660, 1986.
138. Montplaisir, J., Godbout, R., Poirier, G., and Bédard, M.A.: Restless legs syndrome and periodic movements in sleep: Physiopathology and treatment with L-dopa. Clin. Neuropharmacol., *9*:456–463, 1986.
139. Thorpy, M.J., and McGregor, P.A.: The use of sleep studies in neurologic practice. Semin. Neurol., *10*:111–122, 1990.
140. Coleman, R.M., Pollak, C.P., and Weitzman, E.D.: Periodic

movements in sleep (nocturnal myoclonus): Relation to sleep disorders. Ann. Neurol., *8*:416–421, 1980.

141. Moldofsky, H., Tullis, C., Lue, F.A., et al.: Sleep-related myoclonus in rheumatic pain modulation disorder (fibrositis syndrome) and in excessive daytime somnolence. Psychosom. Med., *46*:145–151, 1984.

142. Hamm, C., Derman, S., and Russell, I.J.: Sleep parameters in fibromyalgia syndrome (abstract). Arthritis Rheum., *32*(Suppl.):S70, 1989.

143. Diagnostic and Statistical Manual of Mental Disorders, DSM-IIIR, 3rd Ed. revised. Washington, D.C., American Psychiatric Association, 1987, pp. 218, 233, 251–253, 257–267.

83

Neuropathic Joint Disease (Charcot Joints)

MICHAEL H. ELLMAN

Neuropathic joint disease is a progressive degenerative arthritis with characteristic clinical and roentgenologic features. Described by J.M. Charcot in 1868[1] in patients with "l'ataxie locomotrice progressive," or tabes dorsalis, it is now most commonly seen in the mid- and forefoot of patients with diabetes mellitus (Fig. 83–1). The arthritis develops after sensory loss to a joint and continued weight bearing; for unknown reasons, however, not all patients who meet these criteria develop neuroarthropathy.

It seems fitting that the eponym *Charcot joint* be retained as synonymous with neuropathic joint disease. Jean-Martin Charcot (1825 to 1893) was a master of medicine with virtuoso contributions in neurology, psychiatry, and rheumatology.[2] He is considered a "father" of neurology, and his interest in arthritis was keen and included a thesis, written in 1853, entitled *Primary Progressive Chronic Articular Rheumatism.*[3] His progressive attitude toward medicine was revealed in a lecture at the Hospital of the Salpetriere in Paris in 1867, when he stated that the essential difference between ancient and modern medicine was that in the latter, "physicians could profit by the errors of their predecessors, which roads ought to remain closed to speculation and which, on the contrary, they may traverse without fear of losing themselves."[2]

Charcot's description of neuropathic joint disease has remained the best. He emphasized the *suddenness* of the arthritis, "most commonly without any pain whatever, or any febrile reaction." Charcot described the *swelling* of the joint and the presence of a *hydrarthrosis.* "On puncture being made, a transparent lemon-colored liquid has been frequently drawn from the joint." He also mentioned *cracking sounds* at the articular surfaces, *luxations* developing, rapid *wasting* of the muscles, the presence of *foreign bodies,* and to the etiology of this arthritis, "produced . . . by the more or less energetic movements to which the patient sometimes continues to subject the affected members. . . ." Charcot felt that the joint changes were subordinate to sclerotic changes in the spinal cord, a concept of a "trophic" injury to nerves that became known as the "French theory" of neuropathic joint disease.[1,4,5] This view was violently disputed by Volkmann and Virchow, who espoused the "German theory," that neuropathic arthritis had a mechanical origin produced by insensitive joints and repeated subclinical trauma.[4–6] Charcot also described a hyperacute variant of the disease with swelling and other signs of inflammation of such severity that joint sepsis is suspected.

Schultze and Kahler described the relationship between syringomyelia and neuropathic joint disease in 1888.[7] Dearborn,[8] in 1932, described the disease in congenital insensitivity to pain in a patient who billed himself as the "human pin cushion." Jordan,[9] in 1936, chronicled neuropathic joint disease in diabetic neuropathy. By 1964, Robillard et al.[10] reviewed 100 cases of diabetic neuropathic joint disease in the medical literature, and in 1974, Clouse and co-workers[11] reported 90 cases of neuropathic joint disease and diabetes mellitus seen at a single institution over a 13-year span. "Neuropathic-like" joint disease without neurologic deficits was described in patients receiving intra-articular corticosteroids[12–16] and in some individuals with calcium pyrophosphate dihydrate (CPPD) crystal deposition disease.[17–28]

Neuropathic joint disease has been described in a host of other diseases as disparate as yaws[29] and meningomyelocele.[30] It is now most frequently seen by diabetologists, podiatrists, and rheumatologists in patients with

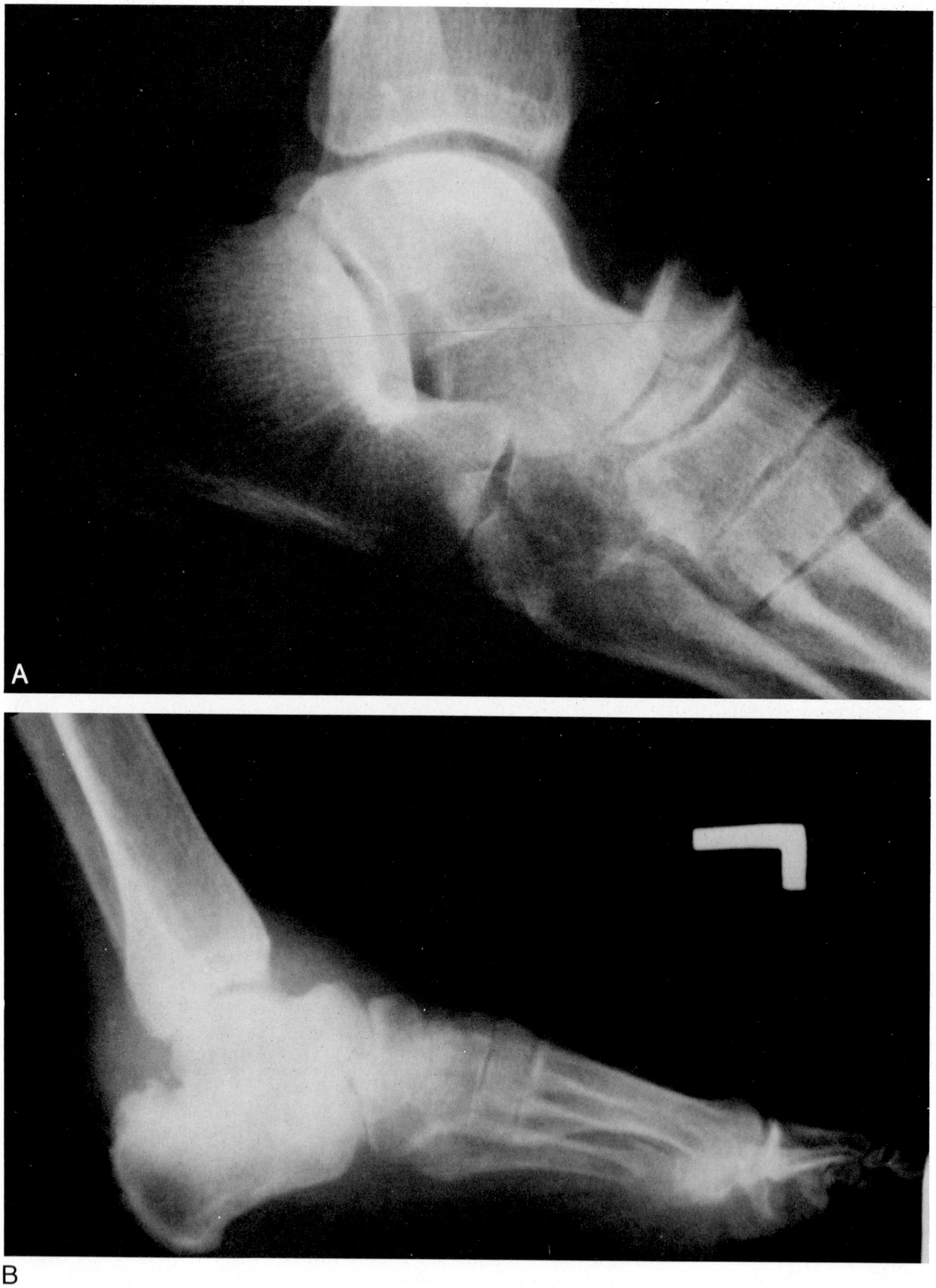

FIGURE 83–1. The roentgenographic appearance of neuropathic joint disease of the foot and ankle has great variety. The foot is now the most common site of neuroarthropathy. *A*, This patient with diabetes mellitus had only moderate discomfort with the dislocation of the navicular bone, which was the first indication of neuropathic joint disease. *B*, Massive soft tissue swelling surrounding the joint is common in the neuropathic ankle and is frequently seen in neuroarthropathy accompanying diabetes mellitus, tabes dorsalis, congenital insensitivity to pain, or meningomyelocele.

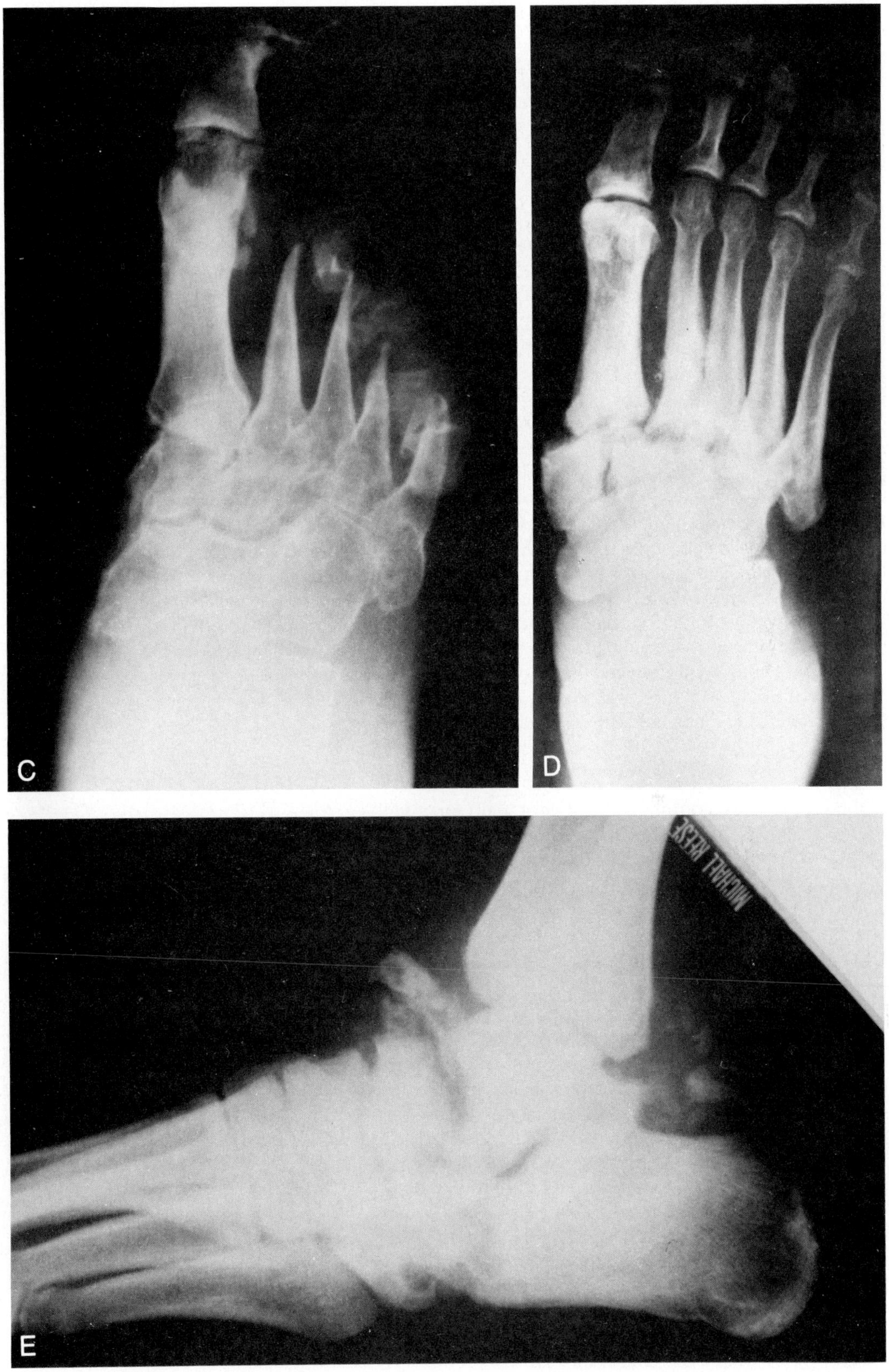

FIGURE 83–1. (*Continued*) *C,* There is striking osteolysis of the metatarsals ("sucked candy" appearance) and the phalanges in this patient with chronic diabetes mellitus. *D,* This patient with diabetes mellitus exhibits destruction, fragmentation, and displacement of the tarsometatarsal joints, which are sometimes described as "Lisfranc's fracture-dislocation" (Lisfranc actually described amputation at that site).[36,93] *E,* Another patient with diabetes mellitus with typical soft tissue swelling and fragmentation of the navicular bone has sharply defined osseous debris at the dorsum and posterior foot and ankle.

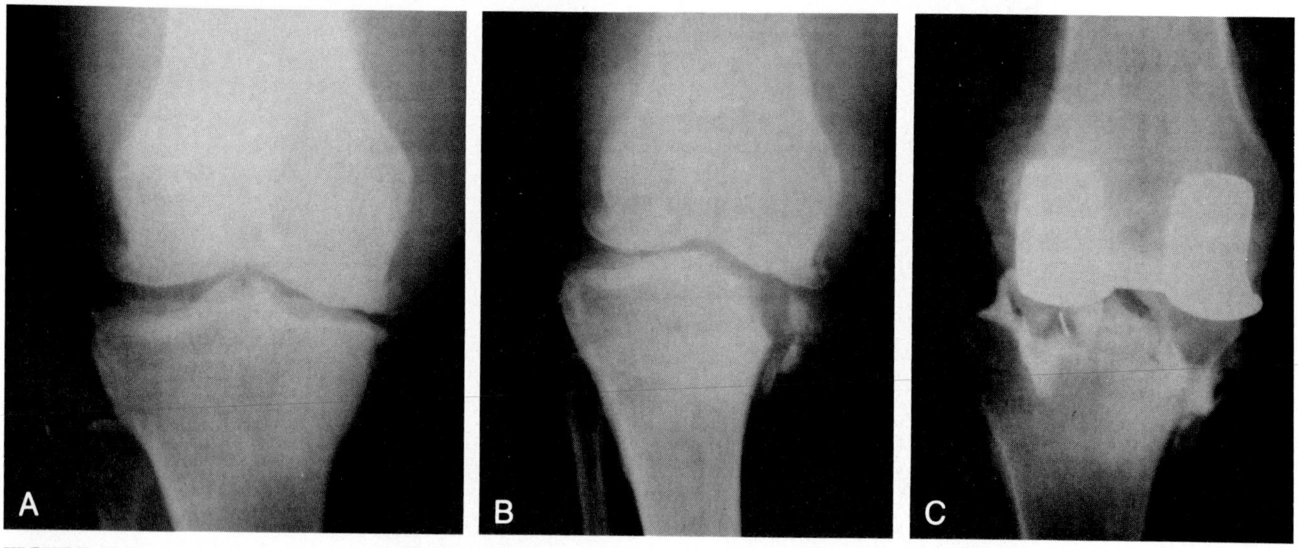

FIGURE 83–2. Neuroarthropathy of the knee joint in tabes dorsalis. *A*, This patient with tabes dorsalis was initially thought to have osteoarthritis and had been scheduled for total knee surgery, although there was minimal pain, and the large joint effusion was atypical for primary osteoarthritis. *B*, A preoperative knee roentgenogram showed sharply defined fragmentation of bone at the medial tibial joint margin and a massive joint effusion, clues to the diagnosis of neuropathic joint disease that were, unfortunately, ignored by the surgeons. *C*, Two weeks after total knee surgery, the prosthesis had subluxed, and the knee was unstable. The patient had minimal knee pain but was not able to bear weight. Total joint replacement surgery is generally contraindicated in neuropathic joints (see text).

diabetes mellitus complaining of foot pain or swelling.[10,11,31–39] If the disease is diagnosed early and treatment instituted promptly, the outcome is often surprisingly successful.[10,31,33–37,39–42]

CLINICAL FEATURES

The diseases giving rise to neuropathic joint disease have changed over the last several decades, as has the clinical picture. The decline in new cases of syphilis and the success of antibiotic treatment in curing existing cases has made tabetic neuropathic joint disease uncommon. These patients typically had monoarticular involvement, usually of the knee, with the hip, ankle, and lower axial skeleton less frequently involved.[5,33,43–47] A "painless" lower extremity monoarticular arthritis in a patient with a neurologic deficit was usually ascribed to neurosyphilis.[5,33,44–48] Synovitis, progressive joint instability, bony overgrowth, and fragmentation led to the characteristic "bag of bones" sensation noted when the involved joint was palpated[5,33,45,49] (Figs. 83–2 and 83–3).

Pain is often the presenting symptom, although some patients have none, even after gross joint disintegration. *Absent deep pain sensation*, tested by squeezing the achilles tendon, is the neurologic sine qua non.

Most patients with neuropathic joint disease now have diabetes mellitus with peripheral neuropathy as the underlying cause. These patients usually present to

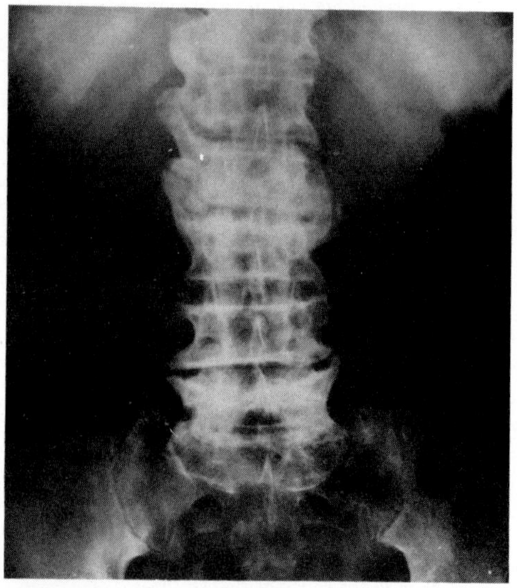

FIGURE 83–3. Neuropathic joint disease of the axial skeleton may mimic osteoarthritis or ankylosing hyperostosis. Irregular narrowing of the disc spaces, a vertebral fracture, subchondral sclerosis, and bulky-headed osteophytes resembling *"les becs des parroquets"* have developed in this 78-year-old man. (From Rodnan, G.P.[107])

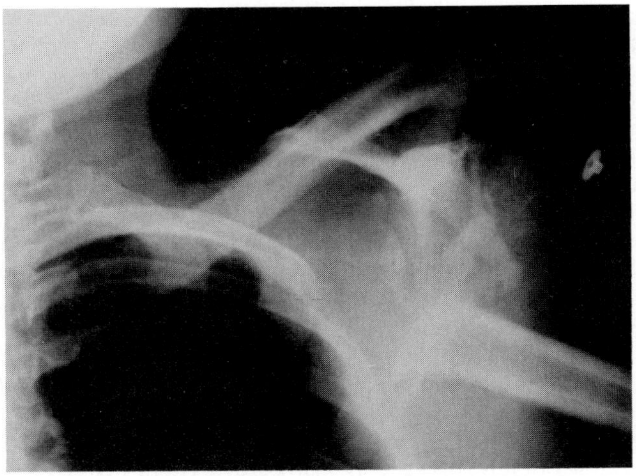

FIGURE 83–4. Shoulder neuroarthropathy is usually due to syringomyelia. Sterile inflammatory joint fluid was observed, and this patient experienced constant pain. The osteolysis of the proximal humerus and cloudy calcification of soft tissue are typical. Some patients have painless swelling; the progression of osteolysis may be exceedingly rapid (see text).

the rheumatologist with a painful and swollen mid- or forefoot or ankle with roentgenographic abnormalities demonstrating soft tissue swelling and demineralization suggestive of early infection[11,31,32,35,39,50,51] (See Fig. 83–1).

Upper extremity neuropathic joint disease is usually caused by syringomyelia.[33,52–55] Proximal joints are most often involved, especially the shoulder (Fig. 83–4). The joints are swollen, warm, and often painful; subluxations may be seen early. In some patients, rapid dissolution of bone occurs.[56,57]

Noninflammatory (Group 1) joint fluid is frequently present when large joints are involved, although about half of the fluids obtained are grossly bloody or markedly zanthochromic.[58] Inflammatory joint fluid containing CPPD crystals has been observed in some patients.[17,20] Such fluid without the presence of CPPD crystals should raise the possibility of sepsis. Although uncommon, infection poses diagnostic difficulties because patients may complain of only mild increases in joint pain or swelling.[59–62] Most of the reported cases of septic arthritis in large joint neuropathic disease have been caused by staphylococci, although tuberculous arthritis has been described.[59–62] Perforating ulcerations of the foot in patients with neuropathic joint disease is distressingly common and often associated with infection. This was described in 1818 as *"plantaire mal perforant."*[39,63,64]

The relative lack of pain makes a diagnosis of other complicating disorders difficult. For example, a traumatic false aneurysm developed after a hip fracture in a patient with tabes dorsalis and neuropathic joint disease. No pain was noted by the patient despite a large expanding hematoma, and the diagnosis was made only by presence of ecchymosis in the flank accompanied by a falling hemoglobin.[65]

Spontaneous fractures and dislocations are both very common in tabes dorsalis, diabetic neuropathy, congenital indifference to pain, and spinal dysraphism, and often call attention to the underlying disorder.[43,50,66–74] Untreated fractures or dislocations may hasten the development and progression of the neuroarthropathy.[69–74a]

The diagnosis of neuropathic joint disease is usually considered in a patient with arthritis accompanying a neurologic disorder. Most patients experience relatively less pain than expected, allowing continued use of the joint.[5,45,75] The progression of the disease process varies widely.[4,33] Many patients have sudden and dramatic symptoms with collapse of the joint because of intra- or juxta-articular fractures.[69,72] The radiologic appearance is typical and nearly specific for the disease, although early in the course it may closely mimic the changes seen in osteoarthritis.[3,11,25] Joint disease may progress so slowly that review of serial roentgenograms correlated with the clinical features may be needed to confirm the diagnosis.[25,49] In other patients, acute fractures, dislocations, subluxations, and gross disruption of the joint confirm the diagnosis on a single roentgenogram.[25,27]

RADIOLOGIC FEATURES

The roentgenographic appearance may be the first clue to the presence of neuroarthropathy. Joint effusion, soft tissue swelling, and osteophytes difficult to distinguish from primary osteoarthritis are early changes that are not diagnostic.[25,48,49] Subluxation, para-articular debris, and bony fragmentation strongly suggest the diagnosis of neuropathic joint disease.[5,25,49]

More advanced roentgenographic changes include massive soft tissue enlargement, marked joint effusion, fractures, depression, and absorption of subchondral bone, and bony proliferation seen as osteophytes and sclerosis.[25,33,48] Fragments of bone may accumulate in tissue distant from the joint. The focal disruption of bone and cartilage with collection of debris into the synovial and para-articular tissues may produce roentgenographic clues to the diagnosis before gross fragmentation becomes evident.[25,48]

Malalignment with angular deformity and subluxation of the joint contribute to the fracturing. Pseudarthroses form at some joint surfaces as a result of fractures and deformities leading to new bone approximations.[11,25,48,49,74]

Hodgson et al., in 1948,[76] directed attention to the difficulty in separating the roentgenographic picture of neuroarthropathy from that of local infection. These authors found infection in the contiguous soft tissue in most of their patients with "neurotrophic" bone lesions and postulated that osteomyelitis contributed to the roentgenographic picture of neuropathic joint disease.[76] Resnick and Niwayama[25] emphasized that the bony margins produced by osseous fragmentation in neuropathic joint disease are well defined and sharp; "fuzzy" bony contours are atypical for neuroarthropathy and suggest infection or the presence of other inflammatory processes.

Bone scintigraphy with ^{99m}Tc-labeled diphosphonate revealed markedly abnormal uptake, even early in the disease.[77,78] Radiopharmaceutical uptake was increased within 2 minutes after injection, indicating increased local blood flow.[77] Gallium-67 (radiogallium) is an indicator of inflammation, and its accumulation in neuroarthropathy may be intense. Its distribution is less dependent on blood flow than is localization of ^{99m}Tc-labeled diphosphonate.[79,80] Of historical interest, six cases of neuropathic joint disease have been studied with angiography and three by lymphangiography.[81,82] All showed increased local vascularity by angiography, whereas lymphangiography was normal. Computed tomography (CT) has been helpful in evaluating neuroarthropathy in the axial skeleton.[83–87]

The diagnosis of infection in a Charcot joint remains difficult. The superimposition of the sometimes subtle clinical and radiographic findings of osteomyelitis on top of the neuroarthropathy is often diagnostically challenging. The sudden worsening of a previously stable neuropathic foot, increasing erythema without trauma, and systemic symptoms are clues to the possibility of infection. Osteomyelitis in the absence of chronic skin ulcers has been unusual in our experience. Positive blood or tissue or bone cultures for a micro-organism will clarify the situation.

Indium-111 neutrophil imaging has been studied in several series of patients with suspected osteomyelitis (see Fig. 83–5). Maurer et al.[88] reported 13 patients with diabetic neuroarthropathy, 4 of whom had osteomyelitis. Three of the four patients with infection had a positive scintigram, but the negative results in eight of the nine patients without osteomyelitis were even more helpful. Seabold et al.[89] compared ^{111}In-leukocyte imaging with that obtained with ^{99m}Tc-diphosphonate and magnetic resonance imaging (MRI) in patients with neuroarthropathy and suspected osteomyelitis. A negative ^{111}In-WBC study indicated that osteomyelitis was unlikely, but positive imaging with any of the preceding techniques was compatible with infected neuroarthropathy alone. Splittgerber et al.[90] and Kalen et al.[91]—the latter studying spinal neuroarthropathy—had similar findings. Leukocyte imaging has the disadvantages of a long preparation time and low radionuclide count rates with poor spatial resolution. There may also be difficulty separating soft tissue from bony infection.

MRI has the ability to delineate soft tissue inflammation from bony structures[80] and is very helpful in diagnosing osteomyelitis.[92] It gives abnormal results in almost all patients with Charcot joints and is a sensitive tool for diagnosing the arthritis at the earliest stage and for quantifying the extent of the abnormalities. Seabold et al.[89] found MRI abnormalities in all seven of the Charcot patients they studied, finding decreased signal intensity on T1 images and increased signal on T2 and short TI inversion recovery (STIR) images in joints and adjacent bone marrow (see Fig. 83–6).

Resnick and Niwayama[25] stated, "The radiographic picture is that of a disorganized joint, characterized by simultaneously occurring bone resorption and formation. The degree of sclerosis, osteophytosis and fragmentation in this articular disorder is greater than that in any other process."

See Figures 83–5 and 83–6.

DIABETIC NEUROARTHROPATHY

The roentgenographic picture in diabetes mellitus has been divided into a *destructive* type affecting tarsal bones and an *absorptive or mutilating* type confined to the forefoot, with gradual disappearance of the epiphyseal ends with "pencil point" or "sucked candy" narrowing (see

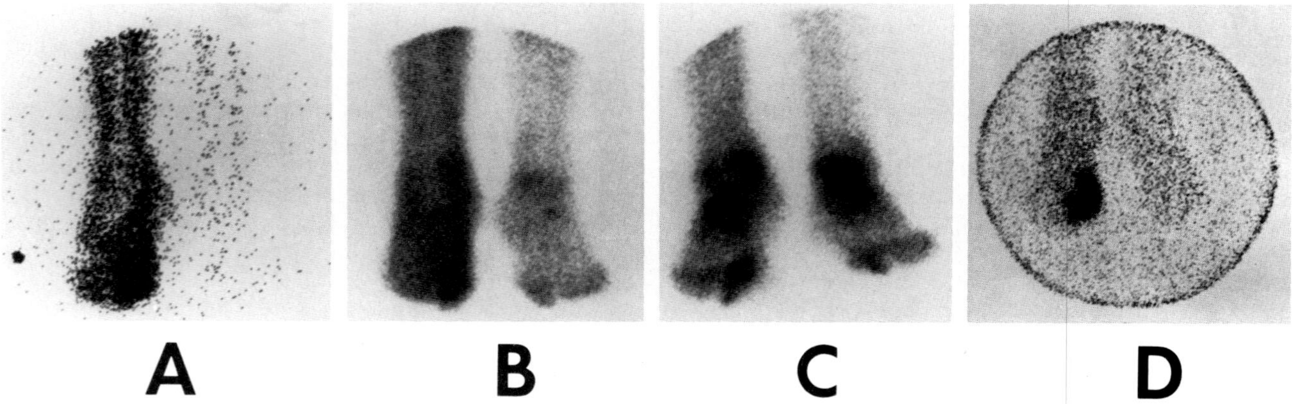

FIGURE 83–5. Selections from the three phases of a triple-phase ^{99m}Tc-labeled diphosphonate bone scintigram are shown. *A*, radionuclide angiogram; *B*, blood pool image; and *C*, delayed bone image in a patient with arthritis of the foot and ankle with suspected infection. *D*, The ^{111}Indium-labeled WBC scan demonstrates accumulation at the first toe. This site proved to be the only site of osteomyelitis.

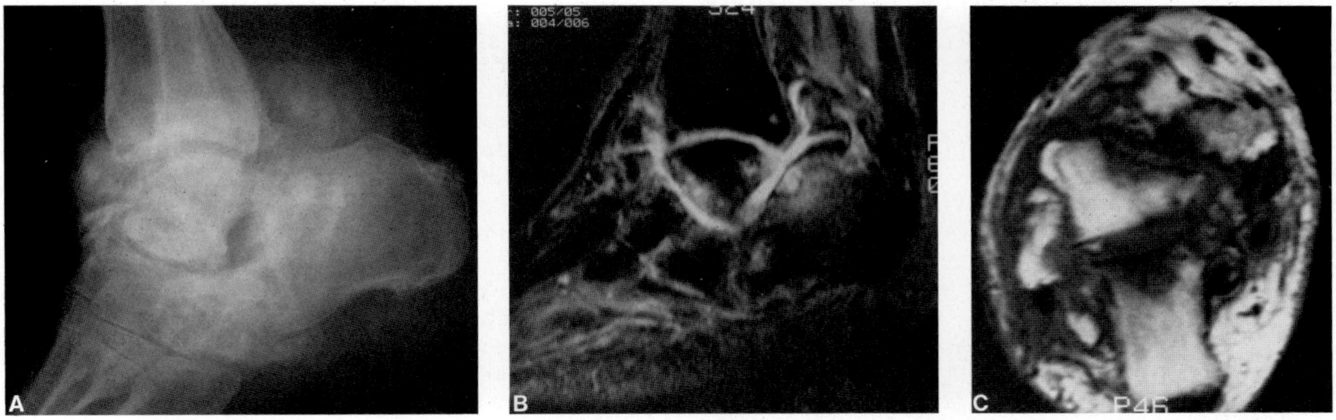

FIGURE 83–6. *A,* A lateral radiograph demonstrating neuroarthropathy involving the ankle with bony fragmentation, sclerosis, and soft tissue swelling. The appearance of this hypertrophic type of Charcot arthropathy has been described as "osteoarthritis with a vengeance." *B,* Sagittal view of the same ankle as in *A* with short TI inversion recovery [STIR] (STIR-fat suppression technique) demonstrating foci (areas of high intensity) of bone marrow edema within the talus, which could represent either infection or fracture. *C,* Coronal view MRI of the same ankle (SE 600/20) picturing the bony fragmentation medial to the talus and calcaneous, soft tissue edema, tenosynovitis surrounding the peroneous longus and brevis tendons, and low signal focus in the calcaneous, probably representing sclerotic bone. (All photographs courtesy of Dr. Tom Grant.)

Fig. 83–1C).[10,25,32,38,39,41,51] These types are not mutually exclusive. Destructive changes at the tarsometatarsal area are sometimes referred to as a "Lisfranc fracture-dislocation"[4,93] (see Fig. 83–1D).

Forgacs[94] described the three roentgenographic stages of diabetic neuropathic joint disease, with stage I (initial findings) demonstrating only osteoporosis and cortical defects leading to stage II (progression) with osteolysis and fragmentation. In stage III (healing), there is deformity, ankylosis, refilling of cortical defects, and restitution.[94]

TABES DORSALIS

The location of the joint involved may be the only differentiation between tabetic and diabetic neuropathic joint disease. Although nearly every joint has been involved in tabes dorsalis, the knee is most commonly affected, followed by the hip[5,33,47,48,66] (see Fig. 83–2). Steindler[46] found genu varum deformity in 26 of 42 tabetic Charcot knees and free joint bodies in 24. Flattening of the tibial condyles was an early sign.[44] In some cases intramuscular and ligamentous ossifications formed a sheath of bone around the knee joint.[46]

Axial neuroarthropathy is common in tabes dorsalis; 6 to 21% of tabetic neuropathic joints occur in the spine[40,43,84,86,95–103] (see Fig. 83–3). Syringomyelia, paraplegia, and diabetes mellitus may also be associated with axial neuropathic joint disease, and rapid destruction of bone may occur.[85,91,96,100,104,105] The axial neuroarthropathy of tabes dorsalis occurs most often in men in the sixth and seventh decades of life. Bone atrophy and hypertrophy often co-exist, analogous to the peripheral arthropathy.[101] Local bony outgrowths have been described as *"les becs de parroquets."*[100,101] Resnick and Niwayama[25] compared the roentgenographic features of axial arthropathy in tabes dorsalis with disorders that may mimic it such as infection, degenerative disc disease and CPPD crystal deposition disease.

SYRINGOMYELIA

The neuroarthropathy in syringomyelia usually occurs in the shoulders, elbows, and cervical spine. The latter may be indistinguishable from ordinary cervical spondylosis.[25,96,106,107] Large effusions and the loss of bone, especially the proximal humerus, are characteristic[55–57,106,108] (see Fig. 83–4).

CALCIUM PYROPHOSPHATE DIHYDRATE CRYSTAL DEPOSITION DISEASE

A destructive arthropathy resembling Charcot joints has been described in CPPD crystal deposition disease per se.[17–19,21–28] Jacobelli et al. have suggested synergism between it and tabes dorsalis.[20] Typical chondrocalcinosis with subsequent joint collapse and fragmentation, especially in the knee or hip, may suggest underlying CPPD crystal deposition[22–26] (Fig. 83–7).

PATHOPHYSIOLOGY

Charcot postulated a role for spinal cord lesions in the pathogenesis of neuropathic joint disease. Volkmann and Virchow felt that the spectacular joint destruction

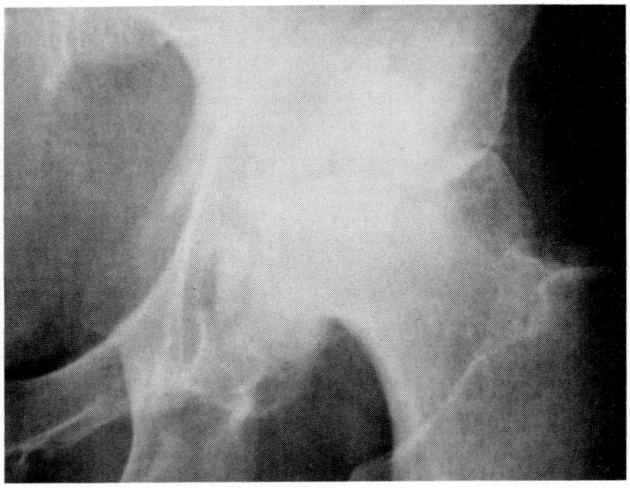

FIGURE 83–7. This elderly patient with no neurologic disease has calcium pyrophosphate dihydrate deposition disease with rapid, painful destruction of the hips, referred to as *neuropathic-like* or *pseudoneuropathic joint*. Joint replacement is not contraindicated if the patient is otherwise well.

was primarily mechanical, caused by multiple episodes of trauma not perceived by the patient because of insensitivity of the affected joints.[4–6,109]

Eloesser[110] followed a series of cats with posterior nerve root rhizotomy on one side; the contralateral side served as a control. Charcot joints developed only on the denervated side. Cats with posterior nerve root rhizotomy followed by induction of deforming arthritis with thermocautery developed accelerated neuropathic joint disease. Bone composition and strength under a given stress load was the same on both the rhizotomy side or the control side. Neuropathic joint disease resulting from nerve resection produced in healthy cats obviously could not be ascribed to syphilis or other infectious causes; trauma and lack of pain and proprioception could be the only cause of neuropathic joint disease. There was no osseous atrophy produced by disturbance in the nerve roots, making Charcot's trophic theory untenable.[110]

Corbin and Hinsey[111] followed 13 cats with one hind limb completely denervated (lumbar sympathectomy and resection of L4-S3 dorsal roots) from 2 weeks to >3 years. No changes in the bones or joints were found as long as ambulation was restricted. In cats allowed to run free, hip arthritis developed. The authors concluded that activity was crucial to the development of arthritis and that nerves had no specific "trophic" function to joints.

Unilateral dorsal root ganglionectomy followed by transection of the ipsilateral anterior cruciate ligament in dogs produced remarkable gross and histologic lesions that resembled early neuroarthropathy.[112] Dogs with transection of the anterior cruciate ligament only (no ganglionectomy) had more pain, as evidenced by limping, than did those with both cruciate ligament transection and ganglionectomy. Dogs subjected only to unilateral ganglionectomy, but no joint damage, developed no evidence of degenerative joint lesions.

Finsterbush and Friedman,[113] however, found that sensory denervation of the hind limb in rabbits produced chondrocyte degeneration even in rabbits with the affected limb immobilized by a plaster cast. These cellular changes progressed over time in both rhizotomized immobilized and active rabbits. The authors postulated that the effects were mediated through altered nutrition produced by the nerve injury, not trauma, thus supporting Charcot's theory of nerve injury-mediated "trophic" changes in the joint.

Brower and Allman[114] also championed the Charcot "trophic" theory and nervous system control of bone and joint metabolism. They studied 91 roentgenograms of neuropathic joints. Approximately one half of the patients had tabes dorsalis, syringomyelia, or diabetes mellitus, but fully a third of their patients had no known underlying neurologic disease. Four of their patients were bedridden when the neuropathic joint disease developed, and the arthritis sometimes occurred with such rapidity that trauma could not be causal. They also noted striking bone resorption that also could not be adequately explained by trauma and suggested that increased bone blood flow with active bone resorption initiated by neurally controlled vascular reflex changes best explained their radiographic findings.

Evidence indicates that blood flow to Charcot joints is increased. Increased vascularity with increased venous draining and filling was shown by Kiss et al.[80] and Rabaiotti et al.[81] The latter authors commented that in some respects neuropathic joint vascularity was similar to that found in certain malignancies. Bone scintigraphy in neuropathic joint disease reveals diffuse and focal increases in joint uptake both at 2 minutes and 4 hours after injection.[77,78] Scintigraphy demonstrated more extensive abnormalities than did conventional radiographs, and these sometimes preceded roentgenographic changes.[77,78] Although the increased blood flow to the neuropathic joints could be secondary to the arthritis, the disparity between the scintigrams and the roentgenograms was marked.[78] A primary autonomic nerve defect resulting in increased blood flow and increased osteoclastic activity allowing bone damage after minor trauma was postulated.[77] Three diabetic patients developed neuroarthropathy of the ankle or foot after revascularization procedures restored blood flow to a neuropathic lower extremity, emphasizing that *adequate blood flow* plus neuropathy and trauma are necessary for the development of Charcot joints.[115,116]

The role of local anesthesia as a prerequisite for developing neuropathic joint disease remains controversial. The frequent development of neuropathic joints in patients insensitive to pain attest to the role of sensory nerves, yet many patients with neuropathic joint disease experience significant pain and near normal sensation.[5,33] The majority of these patients have neurologic disease with diminished proprioception or diminished protective reflexes.

The underlying neuropathy may be subtle. Dyck et al.[68] studied patients with neuropathic joint disease without overt neurologic signs; subclinical neuropathy and other factors such as trauma, obesity, and excessive activity were found. Sophisticated computer-assisted sensory examinations, nerve conduction velocities, and periosteal nociception testing were needed to detect the presence of the neurologic disorder in some of these patients.

The role of fractures was thoroughly studied by Johnson,[70] when he reviewed 188 cases of neuropathic joint disease, 84 of which were tabetic. Fractures were of major importance in initiating or worsening the arthritis in the majority of patients.[70,74A] The serious prognostic results of fractures were further reported on by Clohisy and Thompson[117] in 18 juvenile-onset diabetes mellitus patients who had neuroarthropathy and fracture that were followed for a minimum of 1 year. Four of the patients became nonambulatory, and 14 depended on orthoses. Charcot, in his original article, called attention to the frequency of spontaneous fractures in tabes dorsalis.[1] El-Khoury and Kathol[69] described unusual fractures in six diabetic patients, followed by the development of neuropathic joint disease. Even minor fractures may cause joint instability and increased susceptibility to abnormal stresses.[67,70,74] When stress fractures or sprains occur in normal persons, pain stops further injurious activities. Such warning may not happen in patients with neurologic deficits. Trauma was identified as a precipitating cause in 13 of 55 cases of neuropathic joint disease.[42] Newman[74] described spontaneous fractures of the foot and ankle in a patient with diabetic neuropathy that led to neuropathic joint disease. Neuropathic ankle joint disease developed in one patient after traumatic severance of the sciatic nerve.[118] However, in another patient, denervation of the ankle joint as treatment for unrelenting pain did not cause neuropathic joint disease.[119]

PATHOLOGY

The histologic findings in neuropathic joint disease are similar to those of osteoarthritis, with differences mainly of degree.[5,48,75,120,121] Floyd et al.[122] stated that the essential pathologic difference between the two conditions is the presence of an active pannus in neuroarthropathy. Microscopic bone and cartilage fragments in the synovium are almost universal[48,120–123] (Fig. 83–8). Horwitz[121] stressed the importance of synovial debris in the early stages of neuropathic joint disease; in three of five patients, the finding of cartilage and bone detritus "ground" into the synovium first suggested the diagnosis. Few studies have been conducted of tissues from early neuropathic joints or the underlying nerve lesions.

In contrast, many authors have provided detailed descriptions of chronic neuropathic joints.[5,45,46,48,75,114] There is degeneration and disappearance of joint cartilage followed by eburnation of the bone ends that have been denuded of cartilage. In some areas, there is proliferation of cartilage resulting in new bone formation. The coincidental occurrence of massive bony disintegration and production of exuberant quantities of new bone is striking.[5,42,46] Extra-articular bony fragments and periosteal bone production co-exist with erosions and fractures and the devitalized bone. Intra- and extra-articular osteophytes and exostosis are found on gross examination.[75]

Several authors describe a hypertrophic and atrophic form of neuropathic joint disease.[46,48,124] Extra- and intra-articular exostosis, osteocytosis, and ossification of soft tissue are predominant in the former, whereas joint displacement and bone resorption characterize the latter. King[75] postulated that the hypertrophic changes are due to the stimulation of cellular proliferation by products of bone dissolution.

The microscopic changes defend on the stage and se-

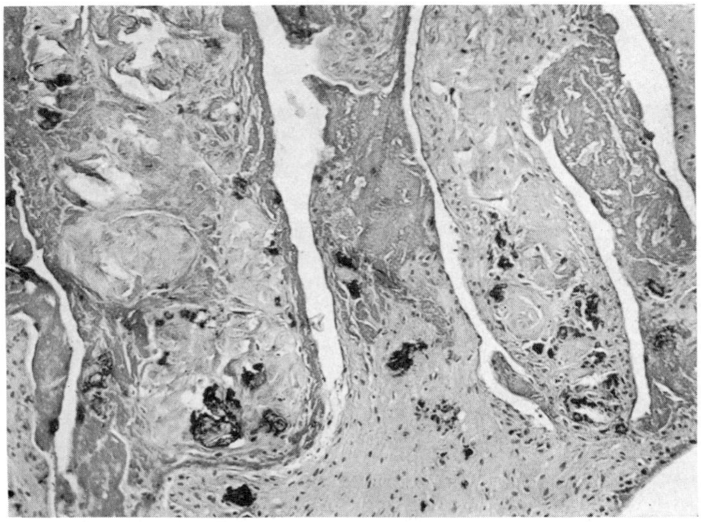

FIGURE 83–8. Photomicrograph of synovium from a neuropathic hip secondary to syphilitic tabes dorsalis. Note the surface hyalinization, dense fibrosis, and scattered areas of calcification. The presence of synovial proliferation and bone and cartilage detritus is very typical of neuropathic joint disease (hematoxylin and eosin stain). (From Rodnan, G.P.[107])

verity of the disease and the area of tissue examined. King[75] commented on the great variety of appearances presented by the diseased bone and cartilage, and Steindler[46] described cartilage hyperplasia. Some cartilage is invaded by pannus, leading to its destruction.[46] A synovial cyst measuring 5 cm in diameter that presented as a slowly enlarging mass has been described.[125] O'Connor et al.[112] found a variety of cartilage abnormalities in dogs subjected to anterior cruciate ligament transection after dorsal root ganglionectomy. Diminution of cartilage thickness, decreased cellularity, and staining with safranin O was common, although in other areas, hypercellularity and brood capsules were present.[112]

DIABETIC NEUROPATHIC JOINT DISEASE

It is not surprising that diabetes mellitus is the most common underlying condition in neuropathic joint disease. Perhaps 10 million Americans have diabetes mellitus, approximately 6% of the middle-aged population, and most diabetics have clinical or electromyographic evidence of neuropathy.[64,126–129] Deaths from diabetes mellitus are declining, and diabetic patients are living longer, increasing their risk of developing neuropathic joint disease.[64]

Jordan[9] reviewed the neurologic manifestations of 226 diabetic patients at the Joslin Diabetic Center in 1936. The incidence of arthropathy was estimated to be between 0.1 and 0.5%, with an approximately equal sex ratio.[64,94] The mean age at diagnosis of neuropathic joint disease is 55 years, and the mean duration of diabetes mellitus before the diagnosis of neuroarthropathy is 18 years, with a range of 8 months to 43 years.[11,39] Esses et al.[60] described neuropathic arthritis in a 21-year-old diabetic patient. In one study of 90 diabetic patients with neuropathic joint disease, all had peripheral neuropathy.[11]

The preponderance of neuropathic joint disease occurring in diabetic rather than tabetic patients is a recent phenomenon. As late as 1964, tabes dorsalis accounted for 37 of a series of 52 cases with diabetes mellitus only accounting for four.[130]

The most common sites of neuropathic joints in diabetes are the tarsal and metatarsal joints with ankle involvement slightly less frequent.[10,11,31,32,34,35,124] The ankles were affected in 12% of 101 patients with neuropathic joint disease, while 24% had bilateral foot disease.[39] Frykberg[35] found approximately 20% bilateral foot disease in his patients. Sinha et al.[39] reported that bony deformity was most common at the tarsometatarsal joints, skin ulceration at the metatarsophalangeal joints, and soft tissue swelling at the ankle. Metatarsophalangeal joint involvement may be more common than expected, found in 15 of 21 patients with diabetic neuroarthropathy.[131] Antecedent trauma was recalled most commonly in patients with tarsometatarsal joint disease. Neuropathic joint disease developing after fractures or dislocations in diabetic patients is common.[37,50,67,69,74a,116] Diabetic neuroarthropathy uncommonly occurs in joints above the ankle, but knee, spinal, and even upper extremity joint involvement have been reported.[104,132,133] Cauda equina syndrome has complicated diabetic neuropathic joint disease.[85]

Diabetic neuropathy has been described since 1798.[64,127] Distal, bilaterally symmetric polyneuropathy, predominantly sensory, is the most common finding. The distal portions of the longest nerves are affected first, explaining the inordinate degree of foot involvement.[64,127] There is diminution of the nocifensive reflex, which is due to loss of small fibers responsible for pain sensation.[64,127,129] The sensory loss and recurrent everyday trauma combined with normal motor function and blood flow allow the occurrence of abnormal joint hypermobility with development of external rotation and eversion of the foot. The stress of weight bearing leads to gradual, or at times sudden, breakdown of the foot.[10,109,127]

The patient presents because of foot pain, although it is generally accepted that the pain in diabetic neuropathic joint disease is less than expected for the degree of deformity.[34,35,39,52,134–137] Swelling almost always precedes pain and may be the only manifestation of early disease.[36] Soft tissue ankle swelling is especially typical with ankle neuropathic joint disease.[11,39] (see Fig. 83–1B). Deep tendon reflexes of the ankle are diminished, with absent or diminished pain and vibration sensation and proprioception in most patients.[64,127,129] The foot is erythematous, and the pulses are usually bounding.[34,35] Increased mobility of the toes, especially in extension with crepitation on palpation, may be present.[39] Tarsometatarsal joint involvement may produce bony deformities with dorsal prominence or plantar protrusions. Downward collapse of the tarsal bones may produce convexity of the volar surface, forming a "rocker" foot or sole.[11,34,35,39] Callus formation occurs over weight-bearing areas, especially the metatarsophalangeal joints, and are frequent sites of infection. This combined surgical and medical problem of perforating ulcers in the foot with a neurologic deficit and arthritis is difficult to manage.[63,137–140]

TABES DORSALIS

The joint disorder that accompanied lesions of the central nervous system (CNS) described by Charcot was caused by tabes dorsalis; he emphasized the suddenness of the swelling and the lack of pain or fever. Swelling and hydroarthrosis would occur after a few days; and a week or 2 later "cracking sounds" developed, leaving a hypermobile joint with wearing away of the articular bones. "Besides the wearing down of the articular surfaces—you may notice the presence of foreign bodies, of bony stalactites, and in a word, of all the customary accompaniments of arthritis deformans. . . ."[1]

Late tertiary syphilis includes cardiovascular, neurologic, and gummatous lesions. The neurologic lesions may be asymptomatic (abnormal cerebral spinal fluid only) or symptomatic, including tabes dorsalis.[141] The posterior spinal column at the fasciculus gracilis is principally involved, but the fasciculus cuneatus may be affected, accounting for the loss of proprioception.[53,103] The proprioceptive loss is generally compensated by intact visual pathways.[53,103]

The VDRL or other nonspecific tests for syphilis such as the RPR (rapid reagen) test are often negative in neurosyphilis because of prior treatment or the passage of time, but the specific tests, FTA-abs and TPHA-tp, are positive in greater than 95% of patients with neurosyphilis. Testing of cerebrospinal fluid may be helpful; a positive cerebrospinal fluid VDRL usually indicates active syphilis, whereas a positive cerebrospinal fluid FTA usually indicates neurosyphilis.[141]

The best single clinical criterion for diagnosing tabetic neuropathy is the absence of deep pain sensation.[107] The Argyll Robertson pupil may be absent or the irregularity in pupil size slight.[45,46,103,122] A careful sensory examination is required. Absent knee reflexes are common.[45,46,103,122] Neuropathic joint disease may be the first sign of tabes dorsalis. The classic picture of a large, firm, painless, unstable joint is not always present, and the arthritis may remain undiagnosed for some time.[44,122,130]

Neuropathic joint disease occurs in 4 to 10% of tabetics. Key[44] considered it rare in persons less than 40 years of age. A history of syphilis is obtained in less than half the patients.[44,122] The mean interval between the onset of the syphilis and the development of the neuropathic joint is 19 years. In Key's series of 69 cases, a total of 92 joints were involved; 18 patients had two joints and 5 had three joints affected. The knee was affected in 39, the foot and ankle, 29; the hip, 15; the spine, 5; the elbow, 2; and the shoulder and wrist joint, 1 each.[44] In another series,[47] the knee was involved in 66% of the tabetic neuropathic joints and the ankle in 26%; 28% of their patients had polyarticular involvement. Women comprised one third of these cases,[47] but in most series, men outnumbered women to a greater extent.[4,45,46,66] Beetham et al.[66] also described a patient with extensive polyarticular involvement.

The onset of joint disease in neurosyphilis is not always acute, the joint swelling may continue for months or years before disintegration occurs.[44,47,66] Swelling is the prominent sign of disease onset in the knee, ankle, and foot, but in the hip, a pathologic fracture is usually the presenting finding. In the spine, deformity is frequently the first finding.[5,9,46,130]

Spinal neuroarthropathy is common.[84,95–97,99,100,102,103] As late as 1980, Wirth et al.[103] described 18 tabetic neuropathic spinal arthropathies culled from two institutions, and Campbell and Doyle[97] found eight cases within a 2-year period. The lesions are usually in the lumbar or lower dorsal vertebra with vertebral body destruction leading to posterior or lateral displacement, resulting in kyphotic and scoliotic deformity. Usually no bone tenderness occurs, but considerable discomfort may be caused by compression of nerve roots.[95,97,103] A "thud" on flexion–extension movement of the spine is said to be characteristic.[99]

The incidence of tabes dorsalis is decreasing, but the disorder has not disappeared.

SYRINGOMYELIA

Syringomyelia has been frequently associated with neuropathic joint disease,[4,52,54,56,106,108] since the original description by Schultze and Kahler in 1888[7] (see Fig. 83–9). Approximately 25% of syringomyelia patients have neuropathic arthritis, predominantly in the shoulders, elbows, and cervical spine, followed by the wrist, carpal, and small hand joints[25,106,108] (Fig. 83–10). Sternoclavicular joint involvement with massive swelling and destruction has been reported.[142]

Syringomyelia (from the Greek *syrinx*—pipe or tube) is a chronic progressive, degenerative disorder of the spinal canal characterized clinically by weakness and atrophy of the hands and arms and segmental anesthesia of the dissociated type (loss of pain and temperature sensation but preservation of touch) especially at the neck, shoulders, and arms.[53,108] There is cavitation of the central portion of the spinal canal, usually in the cervical region.[53] The very high incidence of neuropathic joint disease in syringomyelia as compared to tabes dorsalis and diabetes mellitus is probably ex-

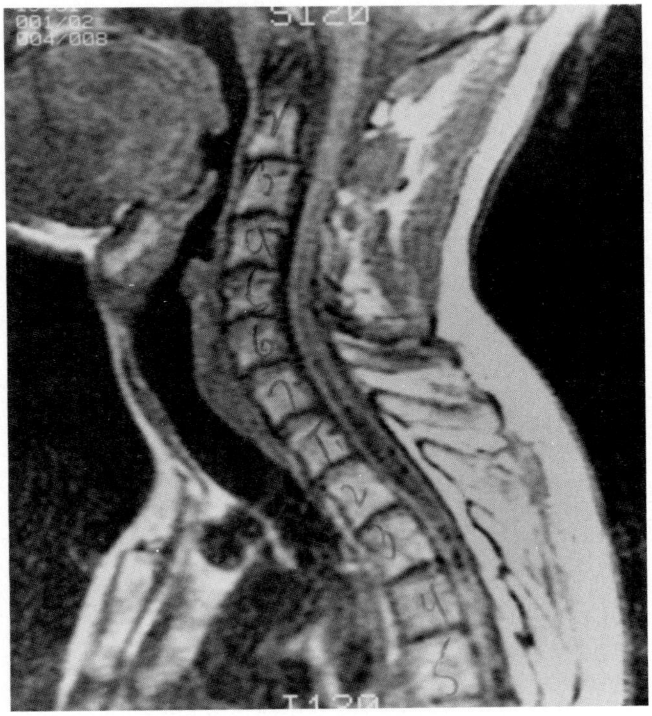

FIGURE 83–9. Sagittal section from a magnetic resonance imaging study of the cervical spine in a patient with syringomyelia demonstrating a fluid-filled cavity within the spinal canal.

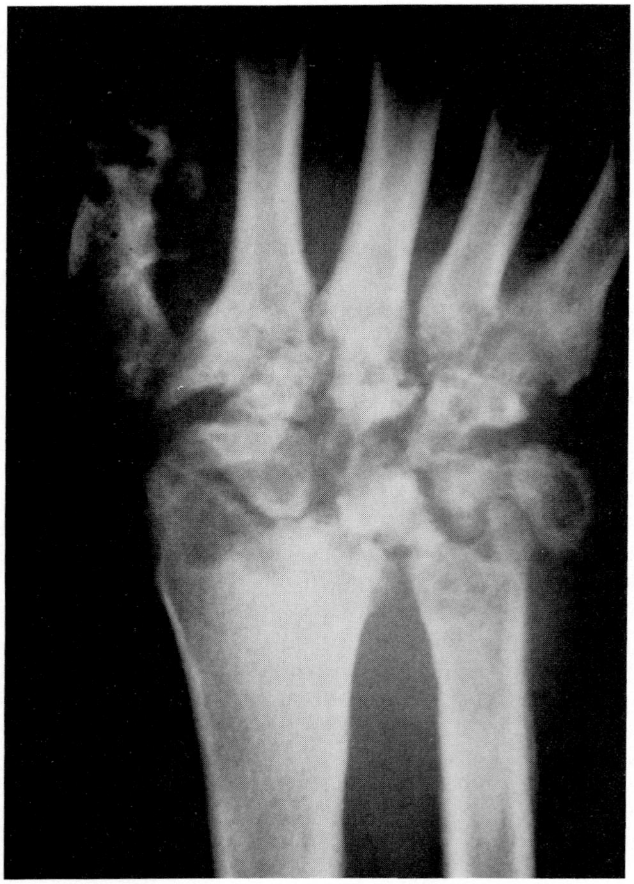

FIGURE 83–10. The wrist involvement in this patient with syringomyelia resembles the tarsometatarsal changes of the foot in diabetic neuroarthropathy. The combination of bony destruction and repair is frequently seen in neuropathic joint disease.

plained by the more profound sensory loss that occurs in syringomyelia.[4,53] Amyotrophy and upper extremity areflexia are common in syringomyelia. Deep aching or boring pain is frequent.[53]

Neuropathic joint disease may occur early or late in the course of syringomyelia.[53,55,101,106] Painful shoulder involvement was found in two patients as the first manifestation of syringomyelia,[54] and rapid bone dissolution may occur.[56] Multiple joints may be involved, even mimicking rheumatoid arthritis (RA).[143] In one series, three patients complained of pain, while in three others, the condition was painless.[55] Swelling was so pronounced that it limited arm motion in all.[55] In two patients, no bony roentgenographic changes were found at the onset of the swelling, but gradually, extensive joint destruction and calcification in the soft tissue developed, followed by slow resorption of bone.[54] Cervical spine involvement is common in syringomyelia; early roentgenographic changes may be indistinguishable from cervical spondylosis.[25,108]

When neuropathic joint disease occurs in the upper extremity, syringomyelia should be considered the most likely cause. The loss of deep tendon reflexes in the upper extremities, analgesia, and thermal anesthesia support the diagnosis.[53] The diagnosis is confirmed by MRI of the syrinx (see Fig. 83–9). Unfortunately, even with early diagnosis, treatment is unsatisfactory. Decompression of the distended syrinx may temporarily alleviate the symptoms.[53]

CALCIUM PYROPHOSPHATE DIHYDRATE CRYSTAL DEPOSITION DISEASE

Jacobelli et al.[20] described the occurrence of CPPD crystal deposition and neuropathic joint disease in four patients, three with tabes dorsalis, and one with no neurologic abnormalities but with a history of syphilis and positive VDRL and FTA-abs tests. All four patients had severe arthropathy of the knees, originally considered to be only neuropathic joint disease, until careful search revealed generalized CPPD crystal deposition. The patient without neurologic deficit developed an *acute* Charcot joint with collapse of the medial tibial plateau 24 hours after his first attack of pseudogout.[17] As only 5 to 10% of tabetic patients develop neuropathic joints and the prevalence of CPPD deposition at age 70 years is about 5%, crystal deposition and neuropathic joint disease were postulated as analogous to the experimental findings of Eloesser already discussed.[20] Bennett et al.[17] suggested that the presence of CPPD crystals in joint fluid may explain some of the episodes of acute inflammation seen in some neuropathic joints.

CPPD crystal deposition and neuropathic joint disease were described in two patients without neurologic abnormalities or laboratory evidence of syphilis;[19] the destructive arthropathy was described as neuropathic-like because of the presence of pain and lack of neurologic deficit.

Menkes et al.[24] described 15 cases of neuropathic-like destructive arthropathy in 125 patients with CPPD crystal deposition collected over a 3-year period. Knees, shoulders, hips, and wrists were most commonly involved.

Resnick et al.[26] also described severe destructive arthropathy occurring frequently in his series of patients with CPPD crystal deposition. This variant has been called *pseudoneuropathic joint disease*.[21]

There is little doubt that CPPD crystal deposition alone can be associated with a destructive arthropathy,[21] but it is important to separate neuropathic-like joint disease from true neuropathic joint disease because the former patients may be candidates for prosthetic joint surgery while the latter are not.

INTRA-ARTICULAR CORTICOSTEROIDS

The possibility of iatrogenic neuropathic-like joint disease with intra-articular corticosteroids remains a concern.[12–16,144] This form of local treatment of arthritis was popularized by Hollander et al. in 1951.[145] By 1961, Hollander and associates[146] reported on more than 100,000 injections (articular and soft tissue) with careful observations on results and adverse effects. Instability of joints was noted in 0.7% of repeatedly injected weight-bearing joints. Proprioception or sensation loss was exhibited in the unstable joints, but in only four joints was "the absorption of bone extensive." Kendall[147] had even a lower incidence of untoward events in a series of 6700 injections in 2256 patients.

Chandler et al.[13] reported the rapid deterioration and development of a neuropathic-like hip joint in a patient with osteoarthritis injected at approximately monthly intervals (approximately 18 injections). Sweetnam et al.[16] described "steroid arthropathy" in four patients with rapid painless destruction of the hips; two had received intra-articular steroids and two had been treated with oral corticosteroids. Steinberg et al.[15] described neuropathic-like changes in a knee of a patient with rheumatoid arthritis (RA) treated locally with 22 corticosteroid injections over a period of 2 years. Alarcon-Segovia and Ward[12] described a similar case that developed after the patient received four to six yearly injections over a 6-year period.

Such neuropathic-like changes after local intra-articular steroid use is believed to result from the temporary suppression of pain induced by the medication, encouraging overuse of the damaged joint.[14] Hollander et al.[146] advised protection from trauma and rest of weight-bearing joints after intra-articular corticosteroid therapy.

Although reported cases of neuropathic-like joint disease with intra-articular corticosteroid use may only represent a small fraction of the actual number of cases, it still must be uncommon. It is certainly not true neuropathic joint disease, although the corticosteroids may well interfere with normal protective sensory processes.

The early reports of neuropathic-like joint disease were associated with short-lived, relatively soluble corticosteroid preparations used repeatedly in weight-bearing joints. The deleterious effects of the newer, now more commonly used, much less soluble intra-articular corticosteroids are unclear. Benefits from judicious intra-articular corticosteroids seem to greatly outweigh the risk of inducing joint instability and destruction (see also Chapter 39).

CONGENITAL INSENSITIVITY TO PAIN

Congenital insensitivity to pain, although rare, is so frequently associated with neuropathic joints that the diagnosis should be considered in children or young adults with atypical arthritis[8,12,148–157] Insensitivity to pain was first described in a sideshow participant advertised as the "human pin cushion."[8] "The patient cannot recall any pain except headache—and his memory is good." The diagnostic criteria are (1) pain sensation is absent from birth, (2) the entire body is affected, and (3) all other sensory modalities should be intact or only minimally impaired, with preservation of the deep tendon reflexes.[156] Subtle varieties of the condition include *congenital insensitivity to pain with anhidrosis*[158] and *congenital sensory neuropathy* with neuropathic joint disease where all modalities of patients with congenital insensitivity to pain report an intact peripheral nervous system,[160] although neuropathologic changes have been described.[149,158]

Fractures of the metaphysis and diaphysis of long bones with epiphyseal separation and soft-tissue ulcerations occur frequently and are often unrecognized.[155] The roentgenographic appearance of injury (destruction) and repair (proliferation) of bone, occasionally complicated by infection, is similar to that seen in other causes of neuropathic joint disease.[155] The ankle is most frequently involved, with joints of the feet, elbows, spine, and hip joints less commonly involved.[161] In a patient with bilateral leg amputation because of congenital insensitivity to pain, hand and wrist arthropathy developed after use of the upper extremities for weight bearing.[162] *Pain asymbolia*, an acquired equivalent of congenital insensitivity to pain, has not been reported in association with neuroarthropathy.

SPINAL DYSRAPHISM

The disorders of fusion of the dorsal midline structures at the primitive neural tube (especially meningomyelocele) are the most frequent cause of neuropathic joint disease in children.[30,107,155,163] Evident at birth, the neurologic findings depend on the level of the lesion.[30,53] The neuropathic joint disease most commonly affects the tarsal articulations and the ankle.[30,155,163] Lower extremity long bone fractures are common in meningomyelocele because of osteoporosis that is due to immobility and sensory neuropathy.[71,155,163,164] Children with myelomeningocele had less neuropathic joint disease and their fractures healed quicker than in children with congenital insensitivity to pain because children with the former walked less.[155] The joints of children with meningomyelocele often are protected by braces at an early age, which apparently decreases the incidence of neuropathic joint disease.[155]

MISCELLANEOUS

Children with thalidomide disease also may develop neuropathic joint disease.[165] Because some adults treated with thalidomide also develop severe sensory peripheral neuropathy, McCredie[165] hypothesized that the embryo developed neuropathy at the time of thalidomide exposure, which later led to the neuropathic joint disease in childhood.

Neuropathic joint disease has been reported in familial amyloid neuropathy,[166] nonfamilial amyloid neuropathy in a dialysis patient,[167] amyloidosis associated with Waldenstrom's macroglobulinemia,[168] the myelopathy of pernicious anemia,[169] spinal cord trauma,[130,170–172] familial dysautonomia,[173] multiple sclerosis,[4] paraplegia,[91,171] idiopathic,[174–176] arachnoiditis secondary to tuberculosis,[177] adhesive arachnoiditis,[178] and neuropathy associated with leprosy.[4,179] It has also been reported in acromegaly,[180] yaws,[29] juvenile RA,[181] scleroderma (with cervical osteolysis),[83] and in patients undergoing chronic hemodialysis.[182]

Neuropathic joint disease of the forefoot was described in 59 severe alcoholic patients with polyneuropathy who were hospitalized at a single institution during a 3-year period.[183] Patients were excluded if diseases usually associated with neuropathic joint disease such as diabetes mellitus, amyloidosis, or syphilis were present. The patients were chronic heavy drinkers, mean age 46.7 years; painless foot ulcers, infections, chronic venous insufficiency and repeated bouts of cellulitis or lymphangitis were frequent. The association of alcohol and neuropathic joint disease had been described infrequently before this report.[4,33,63]

A variety of other neurologic disorders may be associated with neuropathic joint disease. Because the common denominator of this arthritis is sensory loss and continued weight bearing, any disease with those features may be complicated by neuropathic joint disease. Hereditary sensory neuropathy,[184–186] progressive hypertrophic polyneuritis,[187] and peroneal muscular atrophy (Charcot-Marie-Tooth disease)[188] have all been associated with neuropathic joint disease. Bruckner and Kendall[188] described seven cases of neuropathic joint disease associated with the latter. These patients had more severe muscle wasting and sensory loss than did Charcot-Marie-Tooth patients without neuropathic joint disease.[188] Neuroarthropathy of the shoulder developed in two patients with no underlying sensory abnormalities.[189] Charcot arthropathy may develop before signs of an underlying neurologic disease become apparent. The patients described were followed for 14 and 2 years, respectively. In another patient, Charcot shoulder was an initial manifestation of Arnold-Chiari malformation.[190]

MANAGEMENT

Most patients with neuropathic joint disease seen by rheumatologist will have foot involvement resulting from diabetic neuropathy. Either painful or painless swelling in a diabetic foot should be considered possible neuropathic joint disease. An aggressive approach to diagnosis and treatment may help the patient. Molded or contour shoes, bracing, patient education, and foot elevation bring relief to most patients when treated early.[34,35,37,41,75,109,150,191] Several authors state that control of the diabetes mellitus improves the arthropathy.[31,78]

Infection has to be excluded or treated before conservative treatment can begin. The intense inflammation of untreated, acute Charcot arthropathy with its frequent exacerbations can make differential diagnosis difficult. Help from radiologic study has been described (see preceding section entitled, "Radiologic Features"). Osteomyelitis always must be considered in a worsening neuroarthropathy.

A team approach provides optimal treatment. The ideal team may consist of the attending physician, who treats the diabetes mellitus and other medical disorders if present and guides the patient through the slow recovery process; the rheumatologist; orthopedist; and orthotist, who patiently and skillfully reworks and redesigns the orthotics so that the patient is always comfortable. Podiatric consultation has been invaluable to us on many occasions for advice about the underlying arthropathy and ongoing treatment of the other foot disorders that diabetic patients so frequently experience.

Treatable conditions that cause neurologic disorders such as syphilis, yaws, and leprosy should always be kept in mind, but even when the underlying neurologic disease may be untreatable, prompt joint immobilization, cessation of weight bearing, accommodative foot wear, and patient education often stabilize the neuropathic joint.[37,72,109] Fractures heal with immobilization.[70] Sprains should be treated with immobilization.[36,70] Reduction of edema and treatment of infection and ulcerations are required for successful therapy of the diabetic foot.[34,35,37] Refractory plantar ulcers can be successfully treated with a wide plantar exposure, excision of the ulcer, and a generous saucerization of the convexity of the rocker bottom bony prominence.[140] Immobilization or arthrodesis of the spine often provides successful treatment in axial skeleton neuroarthropathy.[40,98,102,172] Crutch walking is usually needed for hip joint neuropathic involvement. A patellar tendon-bearing orthosis has successfully reduced weight bearing in patients with neuropathic joint disease of the ankle or foot.[32,192]

Arthrodesis of a neuropathic joint may fail because of nonunion or pin fracture,[193,194] but successful fusion is possible and is often required for treatment of the neuropathic knee.[42,148,193,195–197] Drennan et al.,[195] in 1971, described successful knee arthrodesis in eight patients. The high rate of fusion was attributed to adequate bone resection and debridement, complete synovectomy, and firm interval fixation (bleeding bone to bleeding bone). Samilson et al.[42] emphasized the need for early arthrodesis. Arthrodesis of the spine is successful in achieving stability and relieving pain in most instances.[40,98,103] Shibata et al.[198] successfully fused 19 of 26 ankles after intramedullary nailing with a follow-up of an average of 9 years.

Total joint replacement is generally contraindicated in neuropathic joint disease, although pain has been relieved with hip arthroplasty even through the joints have later subluxed or loosened.[33,199–201] Charnley,[202] the innovator of total hip joint surgery, warned against total joint replacement in neuropathic joint disease. Total glenohumeral joint replacement is contraindicated.[203] The rapidity of loosening and subluxation of total joint prosthesis in neuropathic joint disease attest to the need for proprioception and deep pain sensation to stabilize even carefully reconstructed joints.

Sprenger and Foley[204] reviewed hip replacement surgery in neuropathic joint disease and described successful hip surgery in a patient with neurosyphilis. At 7-year followup, the patient was well and the hip prosthesis was stable. The authors ascribed the excellent result, contrary to the experience of other surgeons, to the lack of ataxia in their patient.

Soudry et al.[205] reported nine total knee arthroplasties in seven patients with neuropathic joint disease. Excellent results were obtained in eight and good results in one with an average followup of 3 years. The histologic and radiologic findings were diagnostic of neuropathic joint disease, but four patients with clinically apparent neurologic abnormalities had no definable neurologic disease. Posterior stabilized components, ligamentous balancing, resection of adequate bone, bone grafting if required, or the use of a custom, augmented prosthesis were considered the reasons for this unusual rate of success.[205]

Lumbar sympathectomy was helpful in the diabetic foot with neuropathic joint disease in two patients with impaired circulation.[206] Clinical healing occurred in three patients treated with nonweight bearing and the use of a pulsed electromagnetic field, inducing a weak electrical current in bone.[207] Amputation of the foot is occasionally required. Exostectomies, when indicated, also have been reported to be helpful.[191]

REFERENCES

1. Charcot, J.M.: Du Cerveau ou de la moelle epiniere. Arch. Physiol. Nom. Pathol., *1*:161–178, 379–399, 1868.
2. Owen, A.R.G.: Hysteria, hypnosis and healing: the work of J-M. Charcot. New York, Ganett Publications, 1971.
3. Pemberton, R., and Osgood, R.B. (eds.): The Medical and Orthopaedic Management of Chronic Arthritis. New York, Macmillan, 1934.
4. Bruckner, F.E., and Howell, A.: Neuropathic joints. Semin. Arthritis Rheum., *2*:47–69, 1972.
5. Delano, P.J.: The pathogenesis of Charcot's joints. AJR, *56*:189–200, 1946.
6. Volkmann, R., and Virchow, R. cited by Delano, P.J.: The pathogenesis of Charcot's joints. AJR, *56*:189–200, 1946.
7. Schultze, F., and Kahler, O. cited by Bruckner, F.E., and Howell, A.: Neuropathic joints. Semin. Arthritis Rheum., *2*:47–69, 1972.
8. Dearborn, G.V.N.: A case of congenital general pure analgesia. J. Nerv. Med. Dis., *75*:612–615, 1932.
9. Jordan, W.R.: Neuritic manifestations in diabetes mellitus. Arch. Intern. Med., *57*:307–366, 1936.
10. Robillard, R., Gagnon, P.A., and Alarie, R.: Diabetic neuroarthropathy: Report of four cases. Can. Med. Assoc. J., *91*:795–804, 1964.
11. Clouse, M.E., Gramm, H.F., Legg, M., and Flood, T.: Diabetic osteoarthropathy: Clinical and roentgenographic observations in 90 cases. AJR, *121*:22–34, 1974.
12. Alarcon-Segovia, D., and Ward, L.E.: Charcot-like arthropathy in rheumatoid arthritis: Consequence of overuse of a joint repeatedly injected with hydrocortisone. JAMA, *193*:136–138, 1965.
13. Chandler, G.N., Jones, P.T., Wright, V., and Hartfall, S.J.: Charcot's arthropathy following intra-articular hydrocortisone. Br. Med. J., *1*:952–953, 1959.
14. Chandler, G.N., and Wright, V.: Deleterious effect of intra-articular hydrocortisone. Lancet, *2*:661–663, 1958.
15. Steinberg, C.L., Duthie, R.B., and Piva, A.E.: Charcot-like arthropathy following intra-articular hydrocortisone. JAMA, *181*:851–854, 1962.
16. Sweetnam, D.R., Mason, R.M., and Murray, R.O.: Steroid arthropathy of the hip. Br. Med. J., *1*:1392–1394, 1960.
17. Bennett, R.M., Mall, J.C., and McCarty, D.J.: Pseudogout in acute neuropathic arthropathy. A clue to pathogenesis? Ann. Rheum. Dis., *33*:563–567, 1974.
18. Genant, H.K.: Roentgenographic aspects of calcium pyrophosphate dihydrate crystal deposition disease (pseudogout). Arthritis Rheum., *3*:307–328, 1976.
19. Helms, C.A., Chapman, G.S., and Wild, J.H.: Charcot-like joints in calcium pyrophosphate dihydrate deposition disease. Skeletal Radiol., *7*:55–58, 1981.
20. Jacobelli, S., McCarty, D.J., Silcox, D.C., and Mall, J.C.: Calcium pyrophosphate dihydrate crystal deposition in neuropathic joints: Four cases of polyarticular involvement. Ann. Intern. Med., *79*:340–347, 1973.
21. McCarty, D.J., Jr.: Arthritis and Allied Conditions. 10th Ed. Philadelphia, Lea & Febiger, 1985.
22. McCarty, D.J., Jr., and Haskin, M.E.: The roentgenographic aspects of pseudogout (articular chondrocalcinosis): An analysis of 20 cases. Am. J. Roentgenol. Radium Ther. Nucl. Med., *90*:1248–1257, 1963.
23. Martel, W. et al.: Further observations on the arthropathy of calcium pyrophosphate crystal deposition disease. Radiology, *141*:1–15, 1981.
24. Menkes, C.J. et al.: Destructive arthropathy in chondrocalcinosis articularis. Arthritis Rheum., *19*:329–348, 1976.
25. Resnick, D., and Niwayama, G.: Diagnosis of bone and joint disorders with emphasis on articular abnormalities. Philadelphia, W.B. Saunders, 1981.
26. Resnick, D. et al.: Clinical radiographic and pathologic abnormalities in calcium pyrophosphate dihydrate deposition disease (CPPD): Pseudogout. Radiology, *122*:1–15, 1977.
27. Richards, A.J., and Hamilton, E.B.D.: Spinal changes in idiopathic chondrocalcinosis articularis. Rheumatol. Rehabil., *15*:138–142, 1976.
28. Richardson, B.C., and Genant, H.K.: Destructive arthropathy in chondrocalcinosis: A case report. Orthopedics, *5*:1482–1486, 1982.
29. Smith, F.H.: Charcot-like joints in yaws. U.S. Naval Med. Bull. *46*:1832–1843, 1946.
30. Nellhaus, G.: Neurogenic arthropathies (Charcot's joints) in children. Clin. Pediatr., *14*:647–653, 1975.
31. Antes, E.H.: Charcot joint in diabetes mellitus. JAMA, *156*:602–603, 1954.
32. Bailey, C.C., and Root, H.F.: Neuropathic foot lesions in diabetes mellitus. N. Engl. J. Med., *236*:397–401, 1947.
33. Eichenholtz, S.N.: Charcot joints. Springfield, IL Charles C Thomas, 1966.
34. Frykberg, R.G.: Neuropathic arthropathy: The diabetic Charcot foot. Diabetes Educator, *9*:17–20, 1984.
35. Frykberg, R.G. and Kozak, G.P.: Neuropathic arthropathy in the diabetic foot. Am. Fam. Physician, *5*:105–113, 1978.
36. Herzwurm, P.J., and Barja, R.H.: Charcot joints of the foot. Contemp. Orthoped., *14*:17–22, 1987.
37. Jackson, W.P.U., and Louw, J.H.: The diabetic foot. S. Afr. Med. J., *56*:87–92, 1979.
38. Pogonowska, M.J., Collins, L.C., and Dobson, H.L.: Diabetic osteopathy. Radiology, *89*:265–271, 1967.

39. Sinha, S., Munichoodappa, C.S. and Kozak, G.P.: Neuroarthropathy (Charcot joints) in diabetes mellitus. Medicine, *51*:191–210, 1972.
40. Briggs, J.R., and Freehafer, A.A.: Fusion of the Charcot spine. Clin. Orthop., *53*:83–93, 1967.
41. Calabro, J.J., and Garg, S.L.: Neuropathic joint disease. Am. Fam. Physician, *2*:90–95, 1973.
42. Samilson, R.L., Sankaran, B., Bersani, F.A., and Smith, A.D.: Orthopedic management of neuropathic joints. Arch. Surg., *78*:115–121, 1959.
43. Charcot, J.M.: Arthropathies, inxations et fractures spontanees chez une ataxique. Bull. Mem. Soc. Anat. Paris, *48*:744–747, 1873.
44. Key, J.A.: Clinical observations on tabetic arthropathies (Charcot joints). Am. J. Syphilis, *16*:429–447, 1932.
45. Soto-Hall, R., and Haldeman, K.O.: The diagnosis of neuropathic joint disease (Charcot joint). An analysis of 40 cases. JAMA, *114*:2076–2078, 1940.
46. Steindler, A.: The tabetic arthropathies. JAMA, *96*:250–256, 1931.
47. Wile, U.J., and Butler, M.G.: A critical survey of Charcot's arthropathy. Analysis of eighty-eight cases. JAMA, *94*:1053–1055, 1930.
48. Potts, W.J.: The pathology of Charcot joints. Ann. Surg., *86*:596–606, 1927.
49. Katz, I., Rabinowitz, J.G., and Dziadiw, R.: Early changes in Charcot's joints. AJR, *86*:965–974, 1961.
50. Esses, S., Langer, F., and Gross, A.: Charcot's joints: A case report in a young patient with diabetes. Clin. Orthop., *156*:183–186, 1981.
51. Kraft, E., Spyropoulos, E., and Finby, N.: Neurogenic disorders of the foot in diabetes mellitus. AJR, *124*:17–24, 1975.
52. Bhaskaran, R., Suresh, K., and Iyer, G.V.: Charcot's elbow—A case report. J. Postgrad. Med., *27*:194–196, 1981.
53. Rowland, L.P. (ed.): Merritt's Textbook of Neurology. Philadelphia, Lea & Febiger, 1984.
54. Sackellares, J.C., and Swift, T.R.: Shoulder enlargement as the presenting sign of syringomyelia: Report of two cases and review of the literature. JAMA, *236*:2878–2879, 1976.
55. Skall-Jensen, J.: Osteoarthropathy in syringomyelia: Analysis of seven cases. Acta Radiol., *38*:382–388, 1952.
56. Meyer, G.A., Stein, J., and Poppel, M.H.: Rapid osseous changes in syringomyelia. Radiology, *69*:415–418, 1957.
57. Norman, A., Robbins, H., and Milgram, J.E.: The acute neuropathic arthropathy—A rapid, severely disorganizing form of arthritis. Radiology, *90*:1159–1164, 1968.
58. Ropes, M.W., and Bauer, W.: Synovial fluid changes in joint disease. Cambridge, MA, Harvard University Press, 1953.
59. Bennet, K., and Hinricson, H.: A case of tuberculous infection of the knee with clinical and roentgenographic appearance of Charcot's disease. J. Bone Joint Surg., *16*:463–466, 1934.
60. Goodman, M.A., and Swartz, W.: Infection in a Charcot joint: A case report. J. Bone Joint Surg., *67A*:642–643, 1985.
61. Martin, J.R., Root, H.S., Kim, S.O., and Johnson, L.G.: Staphylococcus suppurative arthritis occurring in neuropathic knee joints: A report of four cases with a discussion of the mechanisms involved. Arthritis Rheum., *8*:389–402, 1965.
62. Rubinow, A., Spark, E.C., and Canoso, J.J.: Septic arthritis in a Charcot joint. Clin. Orthop., *147*:203–206, 1980.
63. Classen, J.N.: Neurotrophic arthropathy with ulceration. Ann. Surg., *6*:891–894, 1964.
64. Marble, A. et al. (eds.): Joslin's Diabetes Mellitus. 12th Ed. Philadelphia, Lea & Febiger, 1985.
65. Boynton, E.L. et al.: False aneurysm in a Charcot hip. J. Bone Joint Surg., *68A*:462–464, 1986.
66. Beetham, W.P., Jr., Kaye, R.L., and Polley, H.F.: Charcot's joints: A case of extensive polyarticular involvement, and discussion of certain clinical and pathologic features. Ann. Intern. Med., *58*:1002–1012, 1963.
67. Coventry, M.B., and Rothacker, G.W., Jr.: Bilateral calcaneal fracture in a diabetic patient. J. Bone Joint Surg., *61A*:462–464, 1979.
68. Dyck, P.J. et al.: Neurogenic arthropathy and recurring fractures with subclinical inherited neuropathy. Neurology, *33*:357–367, 1983.
69. El-Khoury, G.Y., and Kathol, M.H.: Neuropathic fractures in patients with diabetes mellitus. Radiology, *134*:313–316, 1980.
70. Johnson, J.T.H.: Neuropathic fractures and joint injuries: Pathogenesis and rationale of prevention and treatment. J. Bone Joint Surg., *49A*:1–30, 1967.
71. Korhonen, B.J.: Fractures in myelodysplasia. Clin. Orthop., *79*:145–155, 1971.
72. Kristiansen, B.: Ankle and foot fractures in diabetics provoking neuropathic joint changes. Acta Orthop. Scand., *51*:975–979, 1980.
73. Muggia, F.M.: Neuropathic fracture: Unusual complication in a patient with advanced diabetic neuropathy. JAMA, *191*:336–338, 1965.
74. Newman, J.H.: Spontaneous dislocation in diabetic neuropathy. A report of six cases. J. Bone Joint Surg., *61B*:484–488, 1979.
74a. Slowman-Kovacs, S.D., Braunstein, E.M., and Brandt, K.D.: Rapidly progressive charcot arthropathy following minor joint trauma in patients with diabetic neuropathy. Arthritis Rheum., *33*:412–417, 1990.
75. King, E.J.S.: On some aspects of the pathology of hypertrophic Charcot's joints. Br. J. Surg., *18*:113–124, 1930.
76. Hodgson, J.R., Pugh, D.G., and Young, H.H.: Roentgenologic aspects of certain lesions of bone: Neurotrophic or infectious? Radiology, *50*:65–71, 1948.
77. Edmonds, M.E. et al.: Increased uptake of bone radiopharmaceutical in diabetic neuropathy. Q. J. Med., *224*:843–855, 1985.
78. Eymontt, M.J., Alavi, A., Dalinka, M.K., and Kyle, G.C.: Bone scintigraphy in diabetic osteoarthropathy. Radiology, *140*:475–477, 1981.
79. Glynn, T.P., Jr.: Marked gallium accumulation in neurogenic arthropathy. J. Nucl. Med., *22*:1016–1017, 1981.
80. Mack, J.M., and Spencer, R.P.: Role of radiopharmaceuticals in detection of osteomyelitis. *In* Nuclear Medicine—Annual 1990. Edited by L.M. Freeman. New York, Raven Press, 1990.
81. Kiss, J., Martin, J.R., McConnell, F., and Wlodek, G.: Angiographic and lymphoangiographic examination of neuropathic knee joints. J. Can. Assoc. Radiol. *19*:19–24, 1968.
82. Rabaiotti, A., Rossi, L., Schittone, N., and Gandini, G.E.: Vascular changes in tabetic arthropathy. Ann. Radiol. Diag., *3*:115–121, 1960.
83. Clement, G.B. et al.: Neuropathic arthropathy (Charcot joints) due to cervical osteolysis: A complication of progressive systemic sclerosis. J. Rheumatol., *11*:545–548, 1984.
84. Moran, S.M., and Mohr, J.A.: Syphilis and axial arthropathy. South Med. J., *76*:1032–1035, 1983.
85. Race, M.C., Keppler, J.P., and Grant, A.E.: Diabetic Charcot Spine as cauda equina syndrome: An unusual presentation. Arch. Phys. Med. Rehabil. *66*:463–465, 1985.
86. Raynor, R.B.: Charcot's spine with neurological deficit: Computed tomography as an aid to treatment. Neurosurgery, *19*:108–110, 1986.
87. Kapila, A., and Lines, M.: Neuropathic spinal arthropathy: CT and MR findings. J. Comput. Assist. Tomogr., *11*:736–739, 1987.
88. Maurer, V. et al.: Infection in diabetic osteoarthropathy: Use of Indium-labelled leukocytes for diagnosis. Radiology, *161*:221–225, 1986.

89. Seabold, J.E. et al.: Indium-111-leukocyte/technetium-99m-MDP bone and magnetic resonance imaging: Difficulty of diagnosing osteomyelitis in patients with neuropathic osteoarthropathy. J. Nucl. Med., *31*:569–556, 1990.
90. Splittgerber, G.F. et al.: Combined leukocyte and bone imaging used to evaluate diabetic osteoarthropathy and osteomyelitis. Clin. Nucl. Med., *14*:156–159, 1989.
91. Kalen, V. et al.: Charcot arthropathy of the spine in longstanding paraplegia. Spine, *12*:42–47, 1987.
92. Meyers, S.P., and Wiener, S.N.: Diagnosis of hematogenous pyogenic vertebral osteomyelitis by magnetic resonance imaging. Arch. Intern. Med., *151*:683–687, 1991.
93. Giesecke, S.B., Dalinka, M.K., and Kyle, G.C.: Lisfranc's fracture–dislocation: A manifestation of peripheral neuropathy. AJR, *131*:139–141, 1978.
94. Forgacs, S.: Stages and roentgenological picture of diabetic osteoarthropathy. Fortschr. Rontgenstr., *126*:36–42, 1977.
95. Alergant, C.D.: Tabetic spinal arthropathy: Two cases with motor symptoms due to root compression. Br. J. Vener. Dis., *36*:261–265, 1960.
96. Brain, R., and Wilkinson, M.: Cervical arthropathy in syringomyelia, tabes dorsalis and diabetes. Brain, *81*:275–289, 1958.
97. Campbell, D.J., and Doyle, J.O.: Tabetic Charcot's spine. Report of eight cases. Br. Med. J., *1*:1018–1020, 1954.
98. Cleveland, M., and Wilson, H.J., Jr.: Charcot disease of the spine: A report of two cases treated by spine fusion. J. Bone Joint Surg., *41A*:336–340, 1959.
99. Culling, J.: Charcot's disease of the spine. Proc. R. Soc. Med., *67*:1026–1027, 1974.
100. Feldman, F., Johnson, A.M., and Walter, J.F.: Acute axial neuropathy. Radiology, *111*:1–16, 1974.
101. Holland, H.W.: Tabetic spinal arthropathy. Proc. R. Soc. Med., *46*:747–752, 1953.
102. Thomas, D.F.: Vertebral osteoarthropathy of Charcot's disease of the spine. Review of the literature and report of two cases. J. Bone Joint Surg., *34B*:248–255, 1952.
103. Wirth, C.R., Jacobs, R.L., and Rolander, S.D.: Neuropathic spinal arthropathy: A review of the Charcot spine. Spine, *5*:558–567, 1980.
104. Zucker, G., and Marder, M.J.: Charcot spine due to diabetic neuropathy. Am. J. Med., *12*:118–124, 1952.
105. Crim, J.R. et al.: Spinal neuroarthropathy after traumatic paraplegia. AJNR, *9*:359–362, 1988.
106. Rataj, R.: Artropatic w jamistorci rdzenia. Neurol. Neurochir. Pol., *14*:439–445, 1964.
107. Rodnan, G.P.: Neuropathic joint disease (Charcot joints.) *In* Arthritis and Allied Conditions. 10th Ed. Edited by D.J. McCarty. Philadelphia, Lea & Febiger, 1985.
108. Williams, B.: Orthopaedic features in the presentation of syringomyelia. J. Bone Joint Surg., *61B*:314–323, 1979.
109. Lippmann, H.I., Perotto, A., and Farrar, R.: The neuropathic foot of the diabetic. Bull. N.Y. Acad. Med., *52*:1159–1178, 1976.
110. Eloesser, L.: On the nature of neuropathic affections of the joints. Ann. Surg., *66*:201–207, 1917.
111. Corbin, K.B., and Hinsey, J.C.: Influence of the nervous system on bone and joints. Anat. Rec., *75*:307–317, 1939.
112. O'Connor, B.L., Palmoski, M.J., and Brandt, K.D.: Neurogenic acceleration of degenerative joint lesions. J. Bone Joint Surg., *67A*:562–572, 1985.
113. Finsterbush, A., and Friedman, B.: The effect of sensory denervation on rabbits' knee joints. J. Bone Joint Surg., *57A*:949–956, 1975.
114. Brower, A.C., and Allman, R.M.: Pathogenesis of the neurotropic joint: Neurotraumatic vs neurovascular. Radiology, *139*:349–354, 1981.
115. Edelman, S.V. et al.: Neuro-osteopathy (Charcot's joint) in diabetes mellitus following revascularization surgery. Three case reports and a review of the literature. Arch. Intern. Med., *147*:1504–1508, 1987.
116. Frykberg, R.G.: Osteoarthropathy. Clin. Podiatr. Med. Surg., *4*:351–359, 1987.
117. Clohisy, D.R., and Thompson, R.C., Jr.: Fractures associated with neuropathic arthropathy in adults who have juvenile onset diabetes. J. Bone Joint Surg., *70A*:1192–1200, 1988.
118. Kernwein, G., and Lyon, W.F.: Neuropathic arthropathy of the ankle joint resulting from complete severance of the sciatic nerve. Ann. Surg., *115*:267–279, 1942.
119. Casagrande, P.A., Austin, B.P., and Indeck, W.: Denervation of the ankle joint. J. Bone Joint Surg., *33A*:723–730, 1951.
120. Collins, D.H.: The Pathology of Articular and Spinal Diseases. Baltimore, Williams & Wilkins, 1949.
121. Horwitz, T.: Bone and cartilage debris in the synovial membrane: Its significance in the early diagnosis of neuroarthropathy. J. Bone Joint Surg., *30A*:579–588, 1948.
122. Floyd, W., Lovell, W., and King, R.E.: The neuropathic joint. South. Med. J., *52*:563–569, 1959.
123. Rodnan, G.P., Yunis, E.J., and Totten, R.S.: Experience with punch biopsy of synovium in the study of joint disease. Ann. Intern. Med., *53*:319–331, 1960.
124. Raju, U.B., Fine, G., and Partamian, J.O.: Neuropathic neuroarthropathy (Charcot's joints). Arch. Pathol. Lab. Med., *106*:349–351, 1982.
125. Brenner, M.A. et al.: The diabetic foot with synovial cyst. Cutis, *46*:142–144, 1990.
126. Barrett-Connor, E.: The prevalence of diabetes mellitus in an adult community as determined by history or fasting hyperglycemia. Am. J. Epidemiol. *111*:705–712, 1980.
127. Martin, M.M.: Diabetic neuropathy: A clinical study of 150 cases. Brain, *76*:594–624, 1953.
128. Ostrander, L.D., Jr., Lamphiear, D.E., and Block, W.D.: Diabetes among men in a general population: Prevalence and associated physiological findings. Arch. Intern. Med., *136*:415–420, 1976.
129. Mulder, D.W., Lambert, E.H., Bastron, J.A., and Sprague, R.G.: The neuropathies associated with diabetes mellitus: A clinical and electromyographic study of 103 unselected diabetic patients. Neurology, *11*:275–284, 1961.
130. Storey, G.: Charcot joint. Br. J. Vener. Dis., *40*:109–117, 1964.
131. Scartozzi, G., and Kanat, I.O.: Diabetic neuropathy of the foot and ankle. J. Am. Podiatr. Med. Assoc., *80*:298–303, 1990.
132. Campbell, W.L., and Feldman, F.: Bone and soft tissue abnormalities of the upper extremity in diabetes mellitus. AJR, *24*:7–16, 1975.
133. Feldman, M.J., Becker, K.L., Reefe, W.E., and Longo, A.: Multiple neuropathic joints, including wrist, in a patient with diabetes mellitus. JAMA, *209*:1690–1692, 1969.
134. Reiner, M. et al.: The neuropathic joint in diabetes mellitus. Clin. Podiatr. Med. Surg., *5*:421–437, 1988.
135. Brooks, A.P.: The neuropathic foot in diabetes: Part II. Charcot's neuropathy. Diabetic Med., *3*:116–118, 1986.
136. Harrelson, J.M.: Management of the diabetic foot. Orthop. Clin. North Am., *20*:605–619, 1989.
137. Mizel, M.S.: Diabetic foot infections. Orthop. Rev., *18*:572–577, 1989.
138. Hart, T.J., and Healey, K.: Diabetic osteoarthropathy versus diabetic osteomyelitis. J. Foot Surg., *25*:464–468, 1986.
139. Subbarao, J. et al.: Diabetic neuro-osteoarthropathy. Rehabilitation of a patient with both ankle joints involved and associated skin problems. Orthop. Rev., *15*:85–92, 1986.
140. Leventen, E.O.: Charcot foot—A technique for treatment of chronic plantar ulcer by saucerization and primary closure. Foot Ankle, *6*:295–299, 1986.

141. Mandell, G.L., Douglas, R.G., Jr., and Bennett, J.E.: Principles and Practice of Infectious Diseases. 2nd Ed. New York, John Wiley & Sons, 1985.
142. Chidgey, L.K.: Neuropathic sternoclavicular joint secondary to syringomyelia. A case report. Orthopedics, *11*:1571–1573, 1988.
143. Steinberg, V.L.: Clinical reports: Syringomyelia with multiple neuropathic joints. Ann. Phys. Med., *3*:103–104, 1956.
144. Mankin, H.J., and Congler, K.A.: The acute effects of intra-articular hydrocortisone on articular cartilage in rabbits. J. Bone Joint Surg., *48A*:1383–1388, 1966.
145. Hollander, J.L., Brown, E.M., Jr., Jessar, R.A., and Brown, C.Y.: Hydrocortisone and cortisone injected into arthritis joints. Comparative effects of and use of hydrocortisone as a local antiarthritic agent. JAMA, *147*:1629–1635, 1951.
146. Hollander, J.L., Jessar, R.A., and Brown, E.M., Jr.: Intra-synovial corticosteroid therapy: A decade of use. Bull. Rheum. Dis., *11*:239–240, 1961.
147. Kendall, P.H.: Untoward effects following local hydrocortisone injection. Ann. Physical Med., *4*:170–175, 1958.
148. Abell, J.M., Jr., and Hayes, J.T.: Charcot knee due to congenital insensitivity to pain. J. Bone Joint Surg., *46A*:1287–1291, 1964.
149. Drummond, R.P., and Rose, G.K.: A twenty-one year review of a case of congenital indifference to pain. J. Bone Joint Surg., *57B*:241–243, 1975.
150. van der Houwen, H.: A case of neuropathic arthritis caused by indifference to pain. J. Bone Joint Surg., *43B*:314–317, 1961.
151. Mooney, V., and Mankin, H.J.: A case of congenital insensitivity to pain with neuropathic arthropathy. Arthritis Rheum., *9*:820–829, 1966.
152. Murray, R.O.: Congenital indifference to pain with special reference to skeletal changes. Br. J. Radiol., *30*:2–6, 1957.
153. Petrie, J.G.: A case of progressive joint disorders caused by insensitivity to pain. J. Bone Joint Surg., *35B*:399–401, 1953.
154. Sandell, L.L.: Congenital indifference to pain. J. Fac. Radiol., *9*:50–56, 1958.
155. Schneider, R., Goldman, A.B., and Bohne, W.H.O.: Neuropathic injuries to the lower extremities in children. Radiology, *128*:713–718, 1978.
156. Silverman, F.N., and Gilden, J.J.: Congenital insensitivity to pain: A neurologic syndrome with bizarre skeletal lesions. Radiology, *72*:176–189, 1959.
157. Thrush, D.C.: Congenital insensitivity to pain: A clinical genetic and neurophysiological study of four children from the same family. Brain, *96*:369–386, 1973.
158. Swanson, A.G., Buchan, G.C., Alvord, E.C., Jr.: Anatomic changes in congenital insensitivity to pain. Arch. Neurol., *12*:12–18, 1965.
159. Johnson, R.H., and Spalding, M.K.: Progressive sensory neuropathy in children. J. Neurol. Neurosurg. Psychiatry, *27*:125–130, 1964.
160. Feindel, W.: Note on the nerve endings in a subject with arthropathy and congenital absence of pain. J. Bone Joint Surg., *35B*:402–407, 1953.
161. Piazza, M.R. et al.: Neuropathic spinal arthropathy in congenital insensitivity to pain. Clin. Orthop., *236*:175–179, 1988.
162. Parker, R.D., and Froimson, A.I.: Neurogenic arthropathy of the hand and wrist. J. Hand Surg., *11A*:709–710, 1986.
163. Gyepes, M.T., Newbern, D.H., and Neuhauser, E.B.D.: Metaphyseal and physeal injuries in children with spina bifida and meningomyelocele. AJR, *95*:168–177, 1965.
164. Handelsman, J.E.: Spontaneous fractures in spina bifida. J. Bone Joint Surg., *54B*:381, 1972.
165. McCredie, J.: Thalidomide and congenital Charcot's joints. Lancet, *2*:1058–1061, 1973.
166. Pruzanski, W., Baron, M., and Shupak, R.: Neuroarthropathy (Charcot joints) in familial amyloid polyneuropathy. J. Rheumatol., *8*:477–481, 1981.
167. Peitzman., S.J. et al.: Charcot arthropathy secondary to amyloid neuropathy. JAMA, *235*:1345–1347, 1976.
168. Scott, R.B., et al.: Neuropathic joint disease (Charcot joints) in Waldenstrom's macroglobulinemia with amyloidosis. Am. J. Med., *54*:535–538, 1973.
169. Halonen, P.I., and Jarvinen, K.A.J.: On the occurrence of neuropathic arthropathies in pericious anemia. Ann. Rheum. Dis., *7*:151–155, 1948.
170. Kettunen, K.O.: Neuropathic arthropathy caused by spinal cord trauma. Ann. Chir. Gynaecol., *46*:95–100, 1957.
171. Slabaugh, P.B., and Smith, T.K.: Neuropathic spine after spinal cord injury. J. Bone Joint Surg., *60A*:1005–1006, 1978.
172. Sobel, J.W., Bohlman, H.H., and Freehafer, A.A.: Charcot's arthropathy of the spine following spinal cord injury. J. Bone Joint Surg., *67A*:771–776, 1985.
173. Brunt, P.W.: Unusual cause of Charcot joints in early adolescence (Riley-Day Syndrome). Br. Med. J., *4*:277–278, 1967.
174. Blanford, A.T., Keane, S.P., McCarty, D.J., and Albers, J.W.: Idiopathic Charcot joint of the elbow. Arthritis Rheum., *21*:723–726, 1978.
175. Chillag, K.J., and Stevens, D.B.: Idiopathic neurogenic arthropathy. J. Pediatar. Orthop. 5:597–600, 1985.
176. Meyn, M., Jr., and Yablon, I.G.: Idiopathic arthropathy of the elbow. Clin. Orthop., *97*:90–93, 1973.
177. Nissenbaum, M.: Neurothrophic arthropathy of the shoulder secondary to tuberculous arachnoiditis. A case report. Clin. Orthop., *118*:169–172, 1976.
178. Wolfgang, G.L.: Neurotrophic arthropathy of the shoulder. A complication of progressive adhesive arachnoiditis. Clin. Orthop., *87*:217–221, 1972.
179. Horibe, S. et al.: Neuroarthropathy of the foot in leprosy. J. Bone Joint Surg., *70B*:481–485, 1988.
180. Daughaday, W.H.: Extreme gigantism: Analysis of growth velocity and occurrence of severe peripheral neuropathy and neuropathic arthropathy (Charcot joints). N. Eng. J. Med., *23*:1267–1270, 1977.
181. Rothschild, B.M., and Hanissian, A.S.: Severe generalized (Charcot-like) joint destruction in juvenile rheumatoid arthritis. Clin. Orthop., *155*:75–80, 1981.
182. Meneghello, A., and Bertoli, M.: Neuropathic (Charcot's) joints in dialysis patients. Fortschr. Rontgenstr., *141*:180–184, 1984.
183. Thornhill, H.L., Richter, R.W., Shelton, M.L., and Johnson, C.A.: Neuropathic arthropathic (Charcot forefoot) in alcoholics. Orthop. Clin. North Am., *4*:7–20, 1973.
184. Heller, I.H., and Robb, P.: Hereditary sensory neuropathy. Neurology, *5*:15–29, 1955.
185. Murray, T.J.: Congenital sensory neuropathy. Brain, *96*:387–394, 1973.
186. Pallis, C., and Schneeweiss, J.: Hereditary sensory radicular neuropathy. Am. J. Med., *32*:110–118, 1962.
187. Russell, W.R., and Garland, H.G.: Progressive hypertrophic polyneuritis with case reports. Brain, *53*:376–384, 1930.
188. Bruckner, F.E., and Kendall, B.E.: Neuroarthropathy in Charcot-Marie-Tooth disease. Ann. Rheum. Dis., *28*:577–583, 1969.
189. Kuur, E.: Two cases of Charcot's shoulder arthropathy. Acta Orthop. Scand., *58*:581–583, 1987.
190. David, R.P. et al.: Charcot shoulder as the initial symptom in Arnold-Chiari malformation with hydromyelia: Case report. Mt. Sinai J. Med. (NY), *55*:406–408, 1988.
191. Goldman, F.: Identification, treatment, and prognosis of Charcot joint in diabetes mellitus. J. Am. Podiatry Assoc., *10*:485–490, 1982.
192. Gristina, A.G., Nicastro, J.F., Clippinger, F., and Rovere, G.D.: Neuropathic foot and ankle patellar-tendon-bearing orthosis.

As an adjunct to patient management. Orthop. Rev., *6*:53–59, 1977.
193. Brashear, H.R.: The value of the intramedullary nail for knee fusion particularly for the Charcot joint. Am. J. Surg., *87*:63–65, 1954.
194. Stack, J.K.: Experiences with intramedullary fixation in knee fusion. Am. J. Surg., *83*:291–299, 1952.
195. Drennan, D.B., Fahey, J.J., and Maylahn, R.J.: Important factors in achieving arthrodesis of the Charcot knee. J. Bone Joint Surg., *53A*:1180–1193, 1971.
196. Frymoyer, J.W., and Hoaglund, F.T.: The role of arthrodesis in reconstruction of the knee. Clin. Orthop., *101*:82–92, 1974.
197. Wiseman, L.W.: Neurogenic arthritis and the problems of arthrodesis of the neurogenic knee. Clin. Orthop., *8*:218–226, 1956.
198. Shibata, T. et al.: The results of arthrodesis of the ankle for leprotic neuroarthropathy. J. Bone Joint Surg., *72A*:749–756, 1990.
199. Coventry, M.B. et al.: Geometric total knee arthroplasty. II. Patient date and complications. Clin. Orthop., *94*:177–184, 1973.
200. Ritter, M.A., and DeRosa, G.P.: Total hip arthroplasty in a Charcot joint: A case with a six-year follow-up. Orthop. Rev., *6*:51–53, 1977.
201. Robb, J.E. et al.: Total hip replacement in a Charcot joint: Brief report. J. Bone Joint Surg., *70B*:489, 1988.
202. Charnley, J.: Present status of total hip replacement. Ann. Rheum. Dis., *30*:560–564, 1971.
203. Fenlin, J.M., Jr.: Total glenohumeral joint replacement. Orthop. Clin. North Am., *6*:565–583, 1975.
204. Sprenger, T.R., and Foley, C.J.: Hip replacement in a Charcot joint: A case report and historical review. Clin. Orthop., *165*:191–194, 1982.
205. Soudry, M. et al.: Total knee arthroplasty in Charcot and Charcot-like joints. Clin. Orthop., *208*:199–204, 1986.
206. Parsons, H., and Norton, W.S., II: The management of diabetic neuropathic joints. N. Engl. J. Med., *244*:935–938, 1951.
207. Bier, R.R., and Estersohn, H.S.: A new treatment for Charcot joint in a diabetic foot. J. Am. Podiatry Med. Assoc., *77*:63–69, 1987.

84

Amyloidosis

ALAN S. COHEN

Although amyloid was probably described by several physicians in the 17th century,[1] Rokitansky, in 1842, observed a unique disorder causing a waxy, enlarged liver and, occasionally, similar changes in the spleen.[2] Virchow noted the more widespread recurrence of this waxy material in other organs and subsequently observed that the "lardaceous" liver and spleen stained with iodine and sulfuric acid. Because he believed that it had a certain similarity to cellulose, Virchow named the material "amyloid."[3,4] This substance was studied for many years at the autopsy table or in experimental animals, usually with amyloid induced by infection, until direct biopsy procedures and the Congo red test and stain were introduced in the 1920s.[5–7] In the subsequent 30 years, many clinical and experimental studies were done on what was then considered to be a rare "degenerative" condition. It has become apparent, however, that amyloidosis is not as rare as was thought; it is often of great clinical significance, it is associated with many diseases, and as discovered in the past several decades, it is sometimes genetically determined.[8]

Amyloidosis may be defined as the extracellular deposition of the fibrous protein amyloid in one or more sites of the body. This protein has unique ultrastructural properties, x-ray diffraction, and biochemical characteristics. The substance may be local and isolated with no clinical consequences, it may grossly involve any organ system of the body and may thus lead to severe pathophysiologic changes, or the disorder may fall between these two extremes. The natural history is poorly understood, and the clinical diagnosis may not be made until the disease is far advanced.

CLASSIFICATION

Until recently, the diagnosis of amyloidosis was rarely made during the lifetime of the patient. It is therefore not surprising that most of the older systems of classification depended on the distribution of amyloid in the various organs and on the staining properties of the deposit. Patients with heart, gastrointestinal tract, skin, nerve, and tongue involvement were considered to have "primary" amyloidosis, and those with liver, spleen, kidney, and adrenal involvement, "secondary" amyloidosis. Amyloidosis of any type can involve any organ, however, with variable severity. Furthermore, routine stains do not enable one to distinguish "types" of amyloidosis.

The following clinical classification has been accepted by most authors: (1) *primary amyloidosis,* in which one sees no evidence of pre-existing or coexisting disease; (2) *amyloidosis associated with multiple myeloma;* (3) *secondary,* or reactive or acquired, amyloidosis, with evidence of chronic infection, such as osteomyelitis, tuberculosis, or leprosy, or chronic inflammatory disease, such as rheumatoid arthritis (RA) or ankylosing spondylitis; (4) *heredofamilial amyloidosis,* which is the amyloidosis associated with familial Mediterranean fever and a variety of neuropathic, renal, cardiovascular, and other syndromes; (5) *local amyloidosis,* in which local deposits, often resembling tumors, are seen in isolated organs without evidence of systemic involvement; and (6) amyloidosis involving the brain, including the amyloid of Alzheimer's disease and of Down's syndrome as well as that of Creutzfeldt-Jakob syndrome and related spongioform disorders; and (7) amyloidosis of the endocrine system, especially that of the pancreas in adult-onset diabetes.

With the recent progress in delineating the chemical composition of various amyloid proteins, a more exact clinicoimmunochemical classification is now possible. Each of several amyloid proteins has a serum protein precursor, as follows: (1) *the light chains of immunoglobulins* in AL (primary or myeloma associated) amyloidosis, (2) *the acute-phase reactant, serum amyloid A, (SAA)* in

TABLE 84–1. THE 1990 GUIDELINES FOR NOMENCLATURE AND CLASSIFICATION OF AMYLOID AND AMYLOIDOSIS

AMYLOID PROTEIN*	PROTEIN PRECURSOR	PROTEIN TYPE OF VARIANT	CLINICAL SYNDROMES
AA	apo SAA		Reactive (secondary) Familial Mediterranean fever Familial amyloid nephropathy with urticaria and deafness (Muckle-Wells syndrome)
AL	κ, λ, e.g., κIII	Aκ, A, e.g., A κIII	Idiopathic (primary), myelomar, or macroglobulinemia-associated
AH	IgG 1 (1)	A1	
ATTR	Transthyretin	met-30 met-111 TTR or Ile-122	FAP Portuguese Familial amyloid cardiomyopathy, Danish Systemic senile amyloidosis
AApo A-1	apo A-1	Arg-26	FAP, Iowa
AGel	Gelsolin	Asn-187†, (15)	Familial amyloidosis, Finnish
ACys	Cystatin C	Gln-68	Hereditary cerebral hemorrhage with amyloidosis, Icelandic
AB	B protein precursor, e.g., BPP_{695}‡	Gln-618 (22)†	Alzheimer's disease Down syndrome Hereditary cerebral hemorrhage with amyloidosis, Dutch
$A\beta_2M$	β-Microglobulin		Associated with chronic dialysis
AScr	Scrapie protein precursor 33–35^{kD} cellular form	Scrapie protein 27–30, e.g., Leu-102	Creutzfield-Jakob disease, and so forth Gerstmann-Straussler-Scheinker syndrome
ACal	(Pro)calcitonin	(Pro)calcitonin	Medullary carcinomas of the thyroid
AANF	Atrial natriuretic factor		Isolated atrial amyloid
AIAPP	Islet amyloid		In islets of Langerhans, diabetes type II, insulinoma

AA = amyloid A protein; apo = apolipoprotein; L = immunoglobulin light chain; H = immunoglobulin heavy chain.
(Modified from Husby et al.[9])
* Nonfibrillar proteins, e.g., amyloid P protein, excluded.
† Amino acid positions in the mature precursor proteins. The position in the amyloid fibril protein is given in parentheses.
‡ Number of amino acid residues.

AA (secondary or acquired) amyloidosis; and (3) transthyretin in heredofamilial amyloidosis and many others (Table 84–1).[9] Several forms of localized amyloidosis, especially those associated with endocrine organs and with the aged heart or brain, have also been identified.

PRIMARY AMYLOIDOSIS AND THAT RELATED TO MULTIPLE MYELOMA (AL)

Although the term *primary amyloidosis* delineates disease in which no predisposing cause is found, it should not be misconstrued as a peculiar clinical type of amyloidosis easily distinguishable from the others. The classic distinctions between primary and secondary amyloidosis based solely on organ distribution are not completely valid. Routine staining cannot distinguish the primary from the secondary type, and under the electron microscope, all types of amyloidosis have an identical fibrillar nature. Only in the early 1970s was the biochemical composition of the amyloid fibril in this form found to be unique and to consist of fragments of or whole immunoglobulin light chains (κ or λ) in both primary amyloidosis and that associated with multiple myeloma.[10,11] Since then it has been shown that treatment with the potassium permanganate stain, followed by Congo red staining, allows gross differentiation, because secondary amyloid deposits lose their Congo red reactivity, whereas primary, myeloma, and heredofamilial deposits do not. Recently a case of heavy chain–related amyloid has been described.[12]

Certain features that alert the clinician to the diagnosis of primary amyloidosis are unexplained proteinuria, peripheral neuropathy, progressive numbness and tingling of the feet, enlarged tongue, increased heart size, unexplained electrocardiographic abnormalities, malabsorption, hepatomegaly, and orthostatic hypotension. Laboratory abnormalities are nonspecific and may or may not include proteinuria, an elevated erythrocyte sedimentation rate, and Bence Jones protein or M component in the patient's serum or urine. The patient frequently has symptoms for several years before the correct diagnosis is made. A biopsy of an involved organ is necessary to confirm the diagnosis. All patients said to have primary amyloidosis should be thoroughly investigated for evidence of other disease, to rule out unsuspected inflammatory disorders and malignant tumors.

Multiple myeloma is a malignant condition with an increased prevalence of amyloid disease. From 6 to 15% of such patients have amyloidosis, the features of which are often indistinguishable from the primary type.

Whereas organ involvement in the various types of amyloidosis usually overlaps, involvement of the synovial membrane is found almost exclusively in patients with multiple myeloma.[13] This joint disease may mimic the features of RA.

SECONDARY OR REACTIVE (AA) AMYLOIDOSIS

The frequency of amyloidosis in the general population is not known. Most available data are based on postmortem studies, which are unreliable because they are performed on a selected group of patients and special staining for amyloidosis is not routine. The prevalence of amyloid at autopsy in many general hospitals around the world is about 0.5%. In Japan, it is low (0.1%), whereas in countries such as Portugal and Israel, where hereditary amyloid syndromes are known, the prevalence is much greater. Moreover, studies in patients with chronic infectious disease who have an increased risk of developing amyloidosis, such as patients with chronic tuberculosis or leprosy, have shown a high prevalence on postmortem examination, up to 50% in some series.

Patients with chronic inflammatory conditions treated by the rheumatologist may develop amyloidosis. These rheumatic conditions include RA, ankylosing spondylitis, juvenile RA (JRA), Reiter's syndrome, the arthritis associated with psoriasis, and other miscellaneous disorders. Tuberculosis, leprosy, paraplegia, and RA have a high incidence. The development of secondary amyloidosis in a patient with one of the aforementioned diseases is often heralded by proteinuria, hepatomegaly, or splenomegaly. The interval between the onset of the rheumatic disease and the appearance of amyloid is unpredictable. Secondary amyloid deposits are composed of a protein moiety termed *protein AA*, which has a unique amino acid sequence and is distinct from immunoglobulin light chains.

HEREDOFAMILIAL (AF) AMYLOIDOSIS

Hereditary amyloid syndromes have been described in many geographic locations; each family and each type described are associated with characteristic organ involvement and clinical manifestations. Generally, the mode of transmission is autosomal dominant, with the exception of familial Mediterranean fever, a condition common in the Near East and affecting Sephardic Jews, Armenians, Turks, and Arabs, for which autosomal recessive transmission has been described. Classification by organ involvement is occasionally helpful because distinct clinical syndromes occur. The biochemical nature and specific point mutations of many of these syndromes have been elucidated.[8–12] Multiple kinships with hereditary amyloidosis of the peripheral nervous system are especially prevalent. Reports of such hereditary syndromes have been appearing in the literature at a rate of about one new syndrome or kinship per year. The amyloid of familial Mediterranean fever is composed of AA protein, whereas the amyloid of most other familial syndromes studied to date is composed of transthyretin.

LOCALIZED AMYLOIDOSIS

In addition to systemic deposition, amyloid may be present in small, focal amounts, sometimes resembling tumors, in any area of the body. Common locations are the lung, skin, larynx, eye, and bladder. In these patients, one rarely sees evidence of systemic disease. Blood vessel involvement is common in primary and secondary amyloidosis. If such involvement is found in a local form, one should investigate further for more widespread disease. Amyloid also may occur in approximation to endocrine organs. Islet amyloid polypeptide (IAPP) has been described in the pancreatic islets of patients with type 2 diabetes mellitus.[14]

AMYLOIDOSIS IN AGED PERSONS

For reasons not completely understood, amyloidosis occurs more frequently with aging.[15,16] In one series, virtually all consecutive autopsies in individuals over 65 years of age demonstrated small deposits of amyloid.[17] Although usually clinically inapparent, small deposits are often found in the heart, brain, pancreas, and spleen of elderly patients. Occasionally, by virtue of its specific location, such as in the conducting system of the heart, symptoms are severe. Although the pathogenesis of amyloidosis in the process of aging is not clear, the staining properties and the ultrastructure of the amyloid found in the elderly are identical to those of the other types. The major form was originally called *senile cardiac amyloid* and has subsequently been termed *senile systemic amyloid* (SSA) and *isolated atrial amyloid*. The latter amyloid consists of atrial natiuretic factor (ANF), and the former, of transthyretin, usually the normal molecule.[18] Occasionally, mutated transthyretin (MET-111) appears to be responsible.

β-Protein has been identified as the major constituent of the amyloid of Alzheimer's syndrome. This material can be isolated from the senile plaques and angiopathic lesions.

AMYLOIDOSIS AND CHRONIC HEMODIALYSIS

Amyloidosis has been identified as a major complication of long-term hemodialysis. Its manifestations include the carpal tunnel syndrome, osteoarthropathy, spondyloarthropathy, and lytic bone lesions made up of amyloid. Synovial deposits occur as well. This amyloid is made up of intact β_2-microglobulin, leading to studies demonstrating extensive and progressive amyloid deposition after 5 to 10 years of hemodialysis.

HISTOPATHOLOGIC FEATURES AND STRUCTURE

GROSS APPEARANCE

Amyloid is an amorphous, eosinophilic, glassy, hyaline extracellular substance ubiquitous in distribution. It may be identified by the classic iodine and dilute sulfuric acid stain first used by Virchow. When successful, this stain imparts a blue-purple color to the amyloid, but it is inconsistent and currently only of historical interest. Small amounts of amyloid do not produce gross organ abnormalities. With larger amounts, the involved organs take on a rubbery, firm consistency. They may have a waxy, pink or gray appearance. Organ enlargement, especially of the liver, kidney, spleen, and heart, may be prominent when the deposits are large. In patients with long-standing renal involvement, however, the kidneys may become small and pale. The heart, in addition to being enlarged by the interstitial myocardial involvement, may have nodular elevations on its pericardial and endocardial surfaces, as well as lesions in the valves. Nerves are often normal, even when involved, but they may become thickened and nodular. Other gross findings are variable and depend on the presence or absence of local nodular deposits.

TINCTORIAL PROPERTIES

Microscopically, amyloid is pink when stained with hematoxylin and eosin and shows crystal violet or methyl violet metachromasia, although it is orthochromatic when stained with toluidine blue.

Congo red remains one of the most widely used stains. When formalin fixed, Congo-red–stained sections are viewed in the polarizing microscope; a unique green birefringence is present.[19,20] *This is the single most useful procedure for establishing the presence of amyloid.* Amyloid has also been stained with fluorochromes to produce a secondary fluorescence, and thioflavine dyes in particular are sensitive indicators of amyloid. The lack of specificity of these dyes, however, makes it mandatory to employ them primarily for screening.

A histochemical method that is useful in differentiating AA from AL amyloid has been described.[21] After incubation with potassium permanganate, AA amyloid, the amyloid of the secondary disorder, loses its affinity for Congo red, whereas AL amyloid, that of primary or myeloma-related amyloidosis, does not. In addition, immunocytochemical methods, using specific anti-AA, anti-AL, and antiprealbumin antisera, allow for even more precise delineation of the type of amyloid in a tissue section.[22]

LIGHT-MICROSCOPIC APPEARANCE

By light microscopy, amyloid is almost invariably extracellular in connective tissue. The deposits may be focal in almost any area of the body, but perivascular amyloid is most often present. The amyloid may involve bone marrow, spleen, capillaries, venules, veins, arterioles, or arteries. The heart may have focal or diffuse interstitial deposits in the myocardium, endocardium, or pericardium. In the kidney, the glomerulus is primarily affected, although interstitial, peritubular, and vascular amyloid may be prominent. In early lesions, small nodular or diffuse deposits appear near the basement membrane; as the disease progresses, the glomerulus may be massively laden, with apparent occlusion of the capillary bed. Atrophic glomeruli laden with amyloid may show marked thickening in the area of Bowman's capsule. Rarely, the glomerulus is replaced almost entirely by connective tissue. Tubular dilation, casts, and interstitial amyloid deposits may be found in the medulla.

In the gastrointestinal tract, one may see perivascular deposits alone, or irregular or diffuse deposits may be found in the submucosa, in the muscularis mucosa, or in the subserosa. The amyloid may appear at any level or portion of the gastrointestinal tract, including the gallbladder and pancreas. Hepatic deposits again may be perivascular only, but more commonly, diffuse amyloid is found between the Kupffer and parenchymal cells. Primary amyloid involves the liver at least as significantly as does secondary and possibly more so.[23] In the nervous system, amyloid has been described along peripheral nerves, in autonomic ganglia, in senile plaques, and in vessels of the central nervous system (CNS). It may be found in any portion of the orbit including the vitreous humor and the cornea.

The bronchopulmonary tract may be involved focally or extensively. The unique aspect of pulmonary or pleural involvement is that although amyloid in virtually all areas of the body remains without evidence of resorption or foreign body reaction, pulmonary amyloid deposits may be accompanied by large numbers of macrophages about and within the lesions. These deposits may also contain islets of cartilage and of ossification. No area of the body is spared, and this ubiquitous distribution produces varying clinical symptoms and signs.

ULTRASTRUCTURE

On direct examination under the electron microscope, amyloid consists of fine fibrils[24] (Fig. 84–1). All types of human amyloid, whether primary, secondary, or heredofamilial, no matter how classified, consist of these fine, nonbranching rigid fibrils that in tissue sections measure approximately 100 Å in diameter.[25] When distant from the cell, these fibrils are usually arranged in random array, but close to cells; they may be parallel

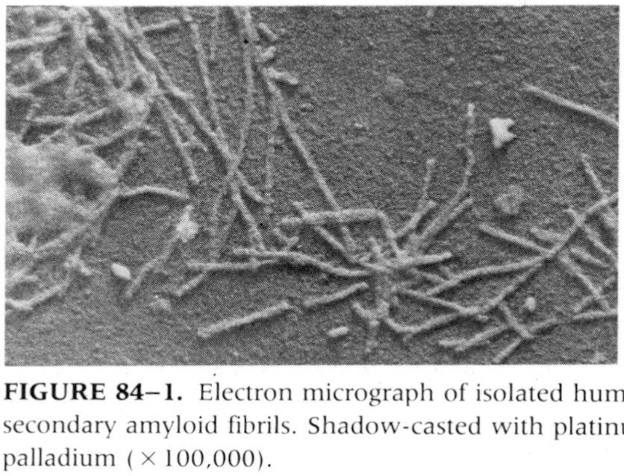

FIGURE 84–1. Electron micrograph of isolated human secondary amyloid fibrils. Shadow-casted with platinum-palladium (× 100,000).

or perpendicular to the plasmalemma with which they occasionally appear to merge. Intracellular fibrils of dimensions comparable to those outside the cell are sometimes observed. Their precise nature has not yet been established.

The amyloid fibrils are usually seen in earliest and closest relationship to the mesangial cell in the kidney,[26] although as deposits enlarge, they appear in comparable relationship to the endothelial and finally epithelial cell. In the liver, these fibrils first border the Kupffer cell, but they finally fill the space of Disse and are seen about the hepatic cell as well. In many other locations, amyloid fibrils have been found close to blood vessels, pericytes, and endothelial cells. Thus, although the cell processing amyloid fibrils may appear to be in the reticuloendothelial or macrophage family, this complex process involves, in AA amyloid, the macrophage, the hepatocyte, and probably the reticuloendothelial system or macrophage again.

The amyloid fibrils thus visualized can be extracted from amyloid-laden tissues for more definitive ultrastructural, chemical, and immunologic study. When isolated, these fibrils can be specially stained, either positively or negatively with phosphotungstic acid, and their delicate, thin, nonbranching fibrous character can thereby be illustrated. The individual fibril has a diameter of about 70 Å, and the fibrils aggregate laterally. Each fibril is made up of filaments, and subunit protofibrils about 30 to 35 Å in diameter have also been defined.[25] X-ray diffraction of isolated amyloid fibrils reveals a cross-β pattern, the "pleated sheet" of Pauling and Corey, indicating that the polypeptide chain runs transversely to the fiber axis of the specimen.[27,28]

A second substance, P-component (plasma component or pentagonal unit) with different ultrastructure, x-ray diffraction pattern, and chemical characteristics, has also been isolated from amyloid and is identical to a circulating α-globulin present in minute amounts. This substance is not responsible for the characteristic tinctorial properties or ultrastructure of amyloid.[29] Amyloid P-component (AP) is distinct on electron microscopy and consists of a pair of pentagonally structured subunits (i.e., each of the pair has five units of 22,000 daltons each, with a total molecular weight [MW] 220,000). C-reactive protein and hamster female protein have similar ultrastructural appearances, and the three belong to a family of proteins now termed *pentraxins*. The physiologic role of AP and its serum counterpart, SAP, is not known, although it has had a stable evolutionary conservation.[30]

BIOCHEMISTRY OF AMYLOID FIBRILS

Amyloid deposits are mainly composed of insoluble fibrillar material that contains a protein backbone. A more precise biochemical identification of constituent amyloid fibril proteins has been made possible with the development of appropriate isolation and purification techniques since the early 1970s. Amino acid analyses have indicated that the amyloid proteins contain all of the common amino acids, with no reports of hydroxyproline, hydroxylysine, desmosine, or isodesmosine (uncommon residues present in collagen and elastin). There is a preponderance of aspartic and glutamic acid residues, which can constitute up to 20% of the total amino acid content. This tends to create a highly polyanionic environment, which is characteristic of amyloid fibrils. Identification of the major protein component of the fibril has become the basis for defining the clinical type of amyloid with certainty. Mucopolysaccharide and glycosaminoglycan residues may be present in some types of amyloid.[31–33]

AL AMYLOID

The first systemic form of amyloid to be defined biochemically was the immunoglobulin or primary type, identified in 1970,[11,34] by N-terminal sequence analysis as the variable (V_L) segment of a κ I light chain in two amyloid fibril preparations.

The protein associated with idiopathic (primary) amyloid and that associated with multiple myeloma consist of a portion of the variable region of either κ- or λ-light chains, or the whole molecule. These proteins have an MW of 5 to 25 kd and begin at the amino terminus of the variable region of the light chain. In AL amyloid, however, λ-chain is more common than κ in a 2:1 ratio,[35] while in multiple myeloma and in the monoclonal gammopathies, there is a κ chain predominance. Almost all subgroups of κ- and λ-light chains have been found in amyloid, but some such as λ VI are particularly amyloidogenic.[36,37]

Because the primary proteins consist of the variable fragments of light chains, they also have idiotypic antigenic determinants. As a rule, little cross-reactivity has been noted between the amyloid proteins belonging to the different subgroups.[38] This lack of common antibody contributes to the diagnostic dilemma in identifying the type of amyloid in the patient with systemic disease. Tissue biopsy specimens are now analyzed for AA amyloid by immunocytochemistry to rule out the secondary form of amyloid. If the test results are negative, the specimens can be examined for transthyretin by the same methods to exclude hereditary amyloidosis. If test results are still negative, one may not be able to define precisely the amyloid, although the potassium permanganate stain noted earlier is of assistance.

AA AMYLOID

Amyloid A protein (AA) was among the first to be clearly defined.[39] It is associated with chronic inflammatory (e.g., RA) and chronic infectious diseases (e.g., osteomyelitis, tuberculosis) and with familial Mediterranean fever. AA is a 76 amino acid 85-kd molecule, heterogeneous at the amino terminus and found in many species. As opposed to AL proteins where individual variations are the norm, AA proteins all have the same amino acid sequence. The 12.5-kd serum protein

SAA[40] that circulates with high-density lipoproteins and is itself an apolipoprotein[41] is its putative precursor.[42] SAA synthesis takes place in the liver, and interleukin-1 (IL-1) mediates its production. It is a sensitive acute-phase serum protein whose level can increase many hundred times in inflammation. That SAA, a nonspecific and widespread acute-phase phenomenon,[43,44] is elevated in the serum does not by itself indicate the presence of AA amyloid. SAA is polymorphic,[45,46] consisting of a family of six proteins of which $SAA_{1\alpha}$ (occasionally a mixture of $SAA_{1\alpha}$ and $SAA_{1\beta}$) is the form identified in the AA deposit. The genes for SAA are reportedly in the short arm of chromosome 11. Extensive studies in the mouse model of AA amyloid have further defined the product–precursor relationship of SAA to AA, the polymorphism of SAA, and the possible pathogenesis of the deposits.[42,47,48]

HEREDITARY AMYLOID PROTEINS

A Transthyretin Prealbumin

The literature on new and distinct hereditary amyloid proteins has expanded enormously. A major constituent especially in familial amyloid polyneuropathies (FAP) has been found to be transthyretin (prealbumin).[49] Amino acid sequencing has shown (in type I FAP in Portuguese, Japanese, Swedish, Greek, and Italian patients) single amino acid substitutions, that is, methionine for valine at position 30 in the 127 amino acid molecule (ATTR met 30).[50–54]

Many other single amino acid variants of transthyretin have been reported in patients of various ethnic backgrounds.[55] All are inherited as autosomal dominant traits. (These mutations and major associated clinical features are listed in Table 84–4, shown later in the section entitled "Hereditary Amyloidosis.") Transthyretin is a 127 amino acid single polypeptide chain that is expressed in hepatocytes, encoded on chromosome 1; its cDNA has been cloned and genomic structure reported. Its secondary, tertiary, and quarternary crystallographic structure is also known.[56,57] It circulates as a tetranomer composed of monomers that have an extensive β-structure and have eight strands organized into two, four-stranded units.

Nontransthyretin Molecules

Other proteins have been reported in hereditary amyloid deposits. These include apolipoprotein AI in patients of Scottish-Irish-English background[58] and gelsolin (with an Asn 15 substitution) in the hereditary cranial nerve neuropathy and vitreous opacity amyloid syndrome reported from Finland.[59]

In the Icelandic syndrome of hereditary cerebral amyloid with hemorrhage, cystatin C with a Gln 68 substitution has been reported. In the clinically similar syndrome of the Dutch, β-protein has been found.[60] Finally, in familial Mediterranean fever and in Muckle-Wells syndrome associated amyloid, AA protein has been identified.

CHRONIC HEMODIALYSIS-ASSOCIATED AMYLOID (Aβ2M)

One of the first neuropathies recognized as having an association with amyloid was the carpal tunnel syndrome. Indeed, in AL amyloid an incidence of about 20% has been reported. The syndrome has also been described in certain FAP syndromes. Carpal tunnel syndrome has been increasingly associated with chronic hemodialysis (5 to 10+ years' duration) and is caused by amyloid deposits.[61] More prominent musculoskeletal lesions, including juxta-articular radiolucent bone cysts, isolated bone cysts, destructive arthropathies of large joints, and spondyloarthropathies, may also complicate long-term hemodialysis. These lesions are also caused largely by amyloid deposits.[62] Such deposits are composed of β_2-microglobulin, an 11,800-dalton molecule, whose normal level of 1 to 2 mg/L increases to 50 to 100 mg/L in patients with renal failure treated with hemodialysis.[63–65] Changes in the standard hemodialysis membranes to allow the elimination of β_2-microglobulin could potentially reduce or eliminate this complication.

A β-PROTEIN (ALZHEIMER'S DISEASE-RELATED AMYLOID)

The lesions in the brains of patients with Alzheimer's disease consist of plaques, neurofibrillary tangles (intraneuronal), and variable blood vessel changes (congophilic angiopathy). All of these lesions stain positively with Congo red, and this reaction has been variously attributed to different proteins. These changes are also seen in the brains of individuals with Down's syndrome. A specific amyloidogenic protein termed β-protein,[66,67] or A_4, which has a unique amino acid sequence, has been identified in these lesions.

The precursor protein of Aβ is APP or (ABPP) (amyloid precursor protein), a large polypeptide that, inserted into the cell membrane, has a large extracellular and small or intracellular component. Aβ insists of approximately 40 amino acids, 28 or which are extracellular.[68] The serine protease inhibitor α_1-antichymotrypsin has also been found in close association with β-protein (Aβ).[69] The latter is also the protein of the amyloid of the Dutch form of hereditary cerebral amyloidosis with bleeding.

The unusual spongioform encephalopathies in animals (scrapie; bovine spongioform encephalopathy) and in man (kuru, Creutzfeldt-Jakob disease; Gerstmann-Straussler-Scheinker syndrome) are all associated with amyloid plaques in the brain from which the amyloid protein AScr (prion protein) (PrP) (scrapie-associated protein) (SAF protein) (proteinase-resistant protein) can be isolated. These diseases are most unusual as a result of their transmissible nature and have led to the concept of a distinctive infectious amyloidosis.[70]

AMYLOID OF ENDOCRINE ORGANS

The amyloid of medullary carcinoma of the thyroid is related to thyrocalcitonin.[71]

Local amyloid deposits in the atria of the heart have been found to consist of a hormone called atrial natiuretic factor (AANF).[72] The extensive deposits of amyloid in systemic senile amyloidosis, however, are made up of normal transthyretin in most cases.

The association of adult-onset diabetes mellitus and local pancreatic islet amyloid is well-known. This protein has been identified as islet amyloid polypeptide (IAPP). It has been found in insulinomas also.[73] AIAPP is a 37 amino acid molecule derived from the large preproIAPP.[74]

P-COMPONENT OF AMYLOID

In addition to the characteristic fibrils described, a minor second component, the P-component, has been noted in most amyloid deposits.[29] P-component (AP) has been recognized by electron microscopy as a pentagonal unit measuring about 90 Å in diameter on the outside and 40 Å on the inside. It appears to consist of five globular subunits of 25 to 30 Å, which may aggregate laterally to form short rods. On immunoelectrophoresis, this component migrates as an α-globulin, and it possesses antigenic identity with a constituent of normal human plasma. The amino acid sequence is distinct from that of the amyloid fibrils. The MW, that of a doublet, is about 230,000 daltons. AP is associated with all types of amyloid.

Human AP has been isolated from plasma by affinity chromatography. Characterization and comparison of the isolated P-component proteins from tissue and plasma demonstrate immunologic and sequence identity.[75] Its complete gene sequence has been determined.[76]

AP also has substantial homology in amino acid sequence, molecular appearance, and subunit composition to C-reactive protein, but differences in MW (C-reactive protein has about half the MW of SAP) and in other parameters suggest that although these substances are analogous and may have evolutionary relationships to one another, they are indeed distinct.[75,77,78] SAP in humans does not usually behave as an acute-phase reactant, although it does become elevated in patients with malignant disease.[79] The unique relationship between SAP and amyloid fibrils, both AA and AL, is at least partly due to a calcium-dependent binding of SAP in vitro to isolated fibrils.[80,81]

IMMUNOBIOLOGY OF AMYLOID

The origin and pathogenesis of amyloidosis are unknown. Advances in characterization of the chemical structure of amyloid may provide insight into these complex mechanisms. Ultrastructural studies of amyloid-laden tissues in an animal model have led to the concept that cytoplasmic invaginations, containing tufts of amyloid fibers, cell–amyloid interface, were the sites of amyloid formation.[82] Electron-microscopic autoradiographic studies have revealed high concentrations of fibrils adjacent to reticuloendothelial cells; this finding suggests their involvement.

The availability of animal models for acquired (secondary) systemic amyloidosis has advanced our understanding of this disease.[83] With these models, some important concepts regarding the pathogenesis of amyloid, such as the two-phase concept of amyloid induction,[84] transfer of amyloid,[85,86] and involvement of the reticuloendothelial system in amyloid fibril formation,[87,88] were developed.

The mechanism of acute-phase SAA elevation has also been studied. The origin of SAA as an acute-phase reactant has become a prototype for the study of the regulation of acute-phase reactant synthesis. It is believed that acute-phase proteins are produced as part of the systemic host response to localized injury, and numerous studies suggest that circulating mediators are released at the site of injury. One of the functions of these mediators is to stimulate hepatic synthesis of acute-phase reactants. This mediator of SAA synthesis is IL-1, a soluble monokine elicited by inflammation and antigenic stimulation, with many target cells including T cells, hepatocytes, synovial cell fibroblasts, brain cells, and B cells.[89,90]

It is now recognized that all amyloid proteins (with one exception) derive from a larger precursor molecule (i.e., SAA and AA; whole light chains and AL; precalcitonin and calcitonin) or from a specific point mutation (varieties of ATTR). The exception is β_2-microglobulin (B2M), which consists of intact molecules. In all instances, there are two phases of amyloidogenesis: (1) the period of elevated SAA or B2M or mutated ATTR for prolonged periods without the occurrence of amyloid, then, (2) the phase of actual amyloid formation.

AP has been regarded as a potential scaffold for the accumulation of amyloid fibrils, but no direct evidence proves this notion. Glycosaminoglycans (GAGs) have long been known to be associated with amyloid deposits. Although highly sulfated GAGs predominate, no precise studies have proven that they play more than an incidental role.

This two-phase aspect of amyloid deposition, first described by Teilum,[84] has been invoked many times. It is attractive because of the apparent proteolysis that takes place. In this model, some investigators feel that a substance known as amyloid-enhancing factor (AEF)—identified by its biologic activity in sharply decreasing the lag phase (induction time) of experimental amyloidosis—plays a critical pathogenetic role.[91] This hypothesis can be tested when AEF is isolated and clearly identified.

Among many treatments purported to influence the course of amyloidosis, colchicine has played an important role in studies of the acquired systemic variety that can occur in situations of chronic and recurrent acute inflammation. Since the observation that colchicine treatment of patients with familial Mediterranean fever lessens or prevents amyloid deposition, this drug has been used to treat all types of systemic amyloidosis. Colchicine has blocked or delayed the development of AA amyloidosis in the mouse model of the disease.[92,93] The therapeutic value of dimethyl sulfoxide in amyloidosis was first reported in a mouse model in 1976, and clinical trials have since been undertaken.[94]

Animal models for other than the AA type of amyloidosis are scarce.[95] Spontaneous amyloidosis has been reported in a few strains of mice and other species; however, in most cases, the models have been poorly defined with regard to reproducibility and the biochemical and immunologic characteristics of the amyloid. A mouse model for spontaneous aging amyloidosis seems valuable because of the high predictable incidence of amyloidosis, the absence of apparent predisposing conditions for acquired amyloidosis, and the preliminary biochemical and immunologic findings for the uniqueness of its amyloid protein.[96]

Thus, amyloidosis the disease and amyloid the substance have been more precisely defined in modern biochemical terms. Further categorization will doubtless be possible, with clinicopathologic implications concerning pathogenesis and diagnosis. A clearer delineation of the relation of animal models of acquired amyloidosis to the other systemic and localized forms of the disease in terms of mediators and amyloid-enhancing factor will also contribute to a better understanding of the origin and pathogenesis of this complex disorder.

CLINICAL ASPECTS

DIAGNOSIS

Although the specific diagnosis of amyloidosis depends on tissue examination with appropriate stains,[19] the disease must first be suspected on clinical grounds. When a patient who has a disorder predisposing him to amyloid formation develops hepatomegaly, splenomegaly, malabsorption, or, most important, proteinuria, amyloidosis should be suspected. Moreover, in heredofamilial syndromes,[8] especially those with an autosomal dominant mode of transmission and characterized by peripheral neuropathy, particularly that starting in the lower limb, carpal tunnel syndrome, vitreous opacities, macroglossia, nephropathy, or cardiopathy, the diagnosis of amyloidosis should be considered. Finally, primary systemic AL amyloidosis should be suspected in patients with a diffuse, noninflammatory, infiltrative disease involving blood vessels, heart, or gastrointestinal tract or tissues such as kidney or liver. (See Table 84-2).

For screening purposes, a subcutaneous abdominal fat-pad aspiration may be the simplest and most useful procedure[97,98] (Fig. 84–2). Complications are almost nonexistent; no absolute contraindications exist, and with appropriate staining and interpretation, the overall sensitivity is in the range of 90%. Until this procedure is more generally used, however, it is good practice to perform a rectal biopsy for diagnosis (Fig. 84–3). If this procedure is contraindicated or if the patient refuses, gingival biopsy is recommended. Skin biopsy, of both involved and uninvolved skin, is also useful in all types of amyloidosis.[99] If results of the aforementioned procedures are negative in patients who have renal disease, hepatic disease, or other organ involvement, biopsy of the appropriate site is undertaken with the standard precautions against bleeding. All tissue obtained must be stained with Congo red and examined under a polarizing microscope for green birefringence. If a polarizing microscope is not available, a light microscope may be adapted.[19] Electron-microscopic examination of tissue sections when biopsies are negative is not helpful.

Amyloid deposits can be further classified immunohistochemically by the use of specific antisera to AA,

TABLE 84–2. CLINICAL DIAGNOSIS OF AMYLOIDOSIS

SUSPECT AMYLOID IN PATIENTS WITH		
AA (Secondary)	AL (Primary)	Hereditary Amyloidosis
Chronic infection (Osteomyelitis, tuberculosis) or	Monoclonal immunoglobulin in urine or serum	Family history of neuropathy
Chronic inflammation (Rheumatoid arthritis) (Granulomatous ileitis) Who develop any of the following	And any of the following	And any of the following
Proteinuria	Unexplained nephrotic syndrome	Early sensorimotor disassociation
Hepatomegaly	Hepatomegaly	Vitreous opacities
Splenomegaly	Carpal tunnel syndrome	Renal disease
Unexplained gastrointestinal disease	Macroglossia	Autonomic nervous system symptoms
	Malabsorption or unexplained diarrhea or constipation	Cardiovascular disease
	Peripheral neuropathy	Gastrointestinal disease
	Cardiomyopathy	

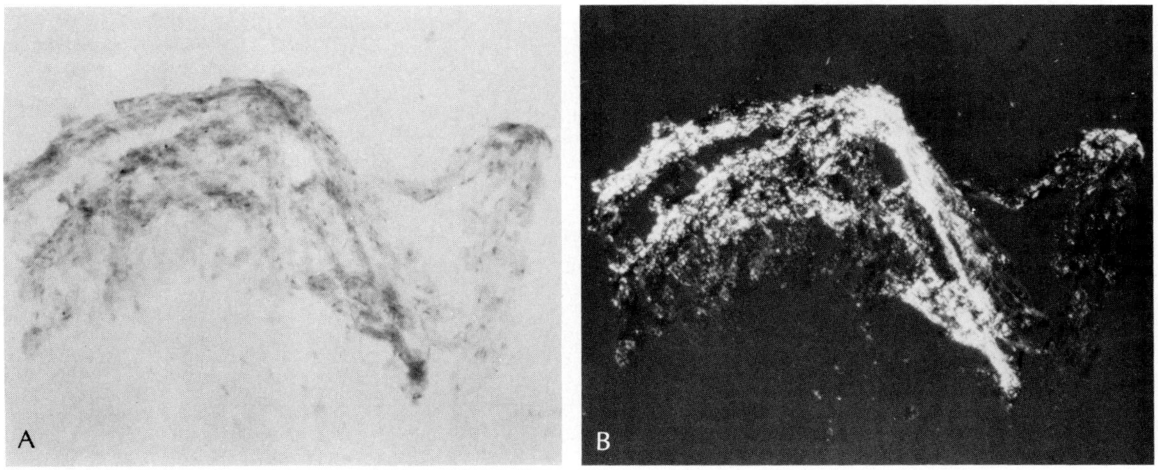

FIGURE 84–2. Light micrographs of an abdominal fat biopsy stained with Congo red and hematoxylin nonpolarized (A) and polarized (B), the latter demonstrating green birefringence (×90).

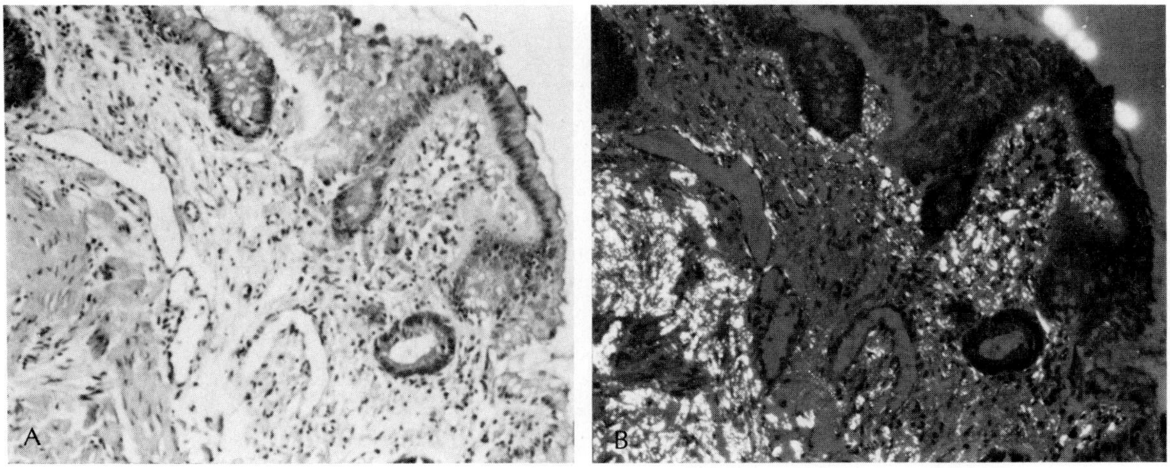

FIGURE 84–3. Light micrographs of a rectal biopsy stained with Congo red and hematoxylin nonpolarized (A) and polarized (B), the latter demonstrating green birefringence (×90).

transthyretin, and other amyloid proteins.[22] A less precise delineation can be made with potassium permanganate treatment of an unstained slide. This will render AA protein unreactive with Congo red, while AL proteins retain their positive reaction (Table 84–3).

AMYLOIDOSIS AS A RHEUMATIC DISEASE

Amyloid can directly involve articular structures and may be present in the synovial membrane (Figs. 84–4, 84–5), as well as in the synovial fluid.[100] It may also occur in the articular cartilage.[101] Amyloid arthritis can mimic many rheumatic diseases because it can become manifest as a symmetric, small-joint arthritis associated with nodules, morning stiffness, and fatigue.[13] The diagnosis of RA can be made in error, and differentiation is imperative because of the great difference in prognosis. When diagnostic arthrocentesis is done and amorphous material is seen in the fluid, a Congo red stain should be used and the material viewed under a polarizing microscope. Individuals with nodules and no erosive disease, as well as patients whose nodules enlarge precipitously, should be looked at more critically. When excessive soft tissue boggy thickening is present, the patient may also have amyloid disease. Amyloidosis should be suspected in those patients with multiple myeloma with articular manifestations. Indeed, most, but not all, patients with amyloid arthropathy (excluding those on chronic hemodialysis) do eventually seem to have multiple myeloma.[13,102]

One might expect that amyloidosis of the joints would not be limited to multiple myeloma and would be present in patients with systemic or generalized primary amyloidosis and with generalized secondary amy-

TABLE 84–3. DIAGNOSIS OF AMYLOIDOSIS

BIOPSY		
Common Sites	Occasional Sites	Rare Sites
Subcutaneous abdominal fat aspirate	Small intestine	Kidney
Rectum	Muscle	Liver
Skin	Nerve	Bone marrow
Gingiva		Synovium
		Spleen
APPROPRIATE STAIN		
Congo red, viewed in polarizing microscope	Potassium permanganate pretreatment then Congo red stain	
Other	Immunofluorescent or immunoperoxidase stains with specific antisera	
Cotton dyes (comparable to Congo red)		
Thioflavin (less specific)		
Crystal violet (less sensitive)		

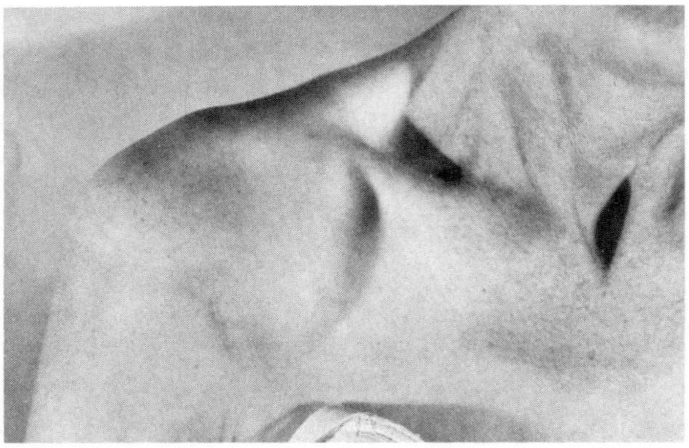

FIGURE 84–4. "Shoulder pad" sign in a 52-year-old woman with primary amyloidosis and widespread amyloid arthropathy simulating arthritis.

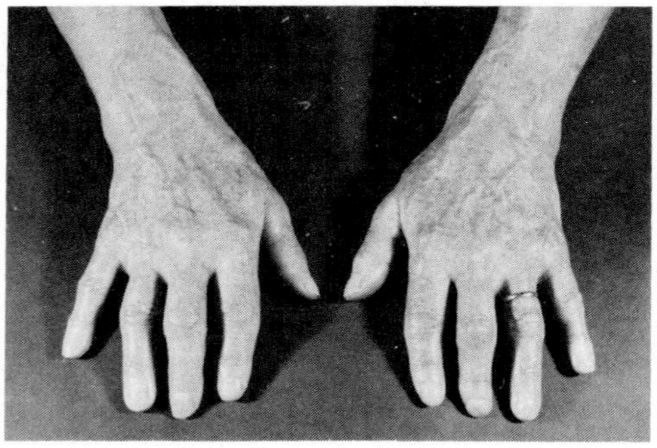

FIGURE 84–5. The hands of the patient in Figure 84–4 showing flexion contractures of the fingers from synovial thickening of the metacarpophalangeal and proximal interphalangeal joints and flexor tendons.

loidosis. Clinical arthropathy that is due to amyloid in generalized secondary amyloidosis is unusual, however. Few data are available from systemic analysis of joint disease for the presence of amyloid. In a report of 289 joint biopsies,[103] some suggestion of amyloid was found in 83 (28.7%). In most other autopsy series of patients with RA, either no mention is made of amyloid in joints or, in the few joints appropriately examined, none is found. Because of the widespread involvement of small blood vessels throughout the body in both primary and secondary disease, small amounts of perivascular amyloid may be found.

Amyloid has been found in association with degenerative joint disease,[104,105] as well as chondrocalcinosis.[106] Egan and associates found amyloid in 6 of 13 cartilage specimens, 4 of 18 articular capsules, and 2 of 16 synovial membranes from patients with osteoarthritis of the hip.[107] The clinical significance of such deposits is not known.

In summary, clinically significant amyloid arthritis can be characterized as follows. The joints most frequently involved are shoulders, wrist, knees, and fingers. The period of morning stiffness associated with the early lesions is shorter than in RA. The joints are often swollen and firm, and occasionally tender, but redness and severe tenderness have not been noted. Swelling of the shoulders may resemble shoulder pads (see Fig. 84–4). Subcutaneous nodules are present in almost 70% of cases, whereas rheumatoid factor is uncommon. Roentgenograms show soft tissue swelling. Erosions about the joints were noted only once among 20 patients studied. Generalized osteoporosis, with or without osteolytic lesions, however, is common and is seen in 80% of patients.

The synovial fluid is usually benign and appears to have the characteristics of a traumatic effusion or a low-grade inflammation. It is generally described as viscous, yellow, or xanthochromic; mucin clot is good to poor. The leukocyte count is usually low, with a median of about 1000 cells/mm^3 but counts as high as 10,000 cells/mm^3 have been reported. Usually, one sees a predominance of mononuclear cells. Free-amyloid-containing bodies, presumably synovial villi, were found in the sediment of three fluids extensively studied, and possible free amyloid itself.[100] The synovial membrane may have lining-cell amyloid, subsynovial amyloid, or perivascular deposits. Multiple myeloma predominates.

The observation in 1985 that B2M was the amyloid protein causing carpal tunnel syndrome in patients treated with chronic hemodialysis led to a clearer appreciation of the extent and nature of the osteoarticular complications of that procedure.[107a] Dialysis arthritis can be disabling and commonly affects the shoulders, hips, hands, knees, and cervical and lumbar spine.[108] Morning stiffness, pain, swelling, limited motion, and tenderness are common signs and symptoms. Although other types of arthritis may occur in chronic dialysis (i.e., crystal synovitis, septic arthritis, osteoarthritis, parathyroid-associated articular symptoms), amyloid arthritis predominates. Synovial fluid aspiration and the usual differential diagnostic procedures are indicated. The amyloid itself can be in synovial fluid, can line the synovium, can cause small or large subsynovial or isolated bone cysts, or can cause a destructive spondylarthropathy, especially at C4–C6. Occasionally, it appears in nonarticular sites and has caused intestinal pseudo-obstruction[109] and subcutaneous tumors of the skin.[110] The multiple bone and joint manifestations have been extensively reviewed.[62,111]

GENERAL MANIFESTATIONS

The clinical manifestations of amyloidosis vary and depend entirely on the affected structures.[3,112,113]

Renal Involvement

Renal involvement may consist of mild proteinuria or frank nephrosis, or in some cases, the urinary sediment may show only a few red blood cells.[114] The renal lesion is usually irreversible and in time leads to progressive azotemia and death. The prognosis does not appear to be related to the degree of the proteinuria. When azotemia finally develops, if it is due to the amyloid process and not to a reversible superimposed condition, the prognosis is grave. In a group of patients with secondary amyloidosis, those with some residual function remained comfortable for long periods, but once the patient's serum creatinine level was over 3 mg/dL, or the creatinine clearance was under 20 mg/mL, the prognosis was poor.[115] In another series, the mean survival after the time of biopsy was 29 months,[116] but in five cases, evidence showed regression of the disease. Hypertension is rare, except in long-standing amyloidosis. Serial films of the kidneys may or may not show a diminution in size. Renal tubular acidosis or renal vein thrombosis may occur. Localized accumulation of amyloid may be noted in the ureter, bladder, or other genitourinary tract tissue. In recent years the prognosis has improved considerably, which is due to successful dialysis or renal transplantation.

Hepatic Involvement

Although hepatomegaly is common, liver function abnormalities are minimal and occur late in the disease. The most useful older tests of hepatic involvement with amyloid are the Bromsulphalein (BSP) extraction and the serum alkaline phosphatase level. Liver scans have variable, nonspecific results, but bone-seeking radionuclides, such as ^{99m}Tc diphosphonate, have recently shown increased liver uptake because of the high calcium content of amyloid.[117] Signs of intrahepatic cholestasis are uncommon.[118] In our series in which liver tissue from 54 patients was examined, whether the disorder was primary or secondary, all had some amyloid present, either in the parenchyma or in blood vessels.[119] The remarkable degree to which liver parenchyma can be replaced by amyloid was seen in a patient whose liver was palpable below the iliac crest and weighed 7200 g; BSP extraction during life in this patient had been 17%, with only a modest elevation of the serum alkaline phosphatase level. Splenomegaly may be massive, although usually it does not cause symptoms unless traumatic rupture occurs. Amyloidosis of the spleen is not usually associated with leukopenia and anemia.

Cardiac Involvement

Cardiac manifestations consist primarily of enlargement and congestive heart failure, either with or without murmurs and arrhythmias.[120] Although these manifestations reflect predominantly diffuse myocardial amyloid deposition, the endocardium, valves, and pericardium may be involved. Pericarditis with effusion is rare, although one must frequently distinguish between constrictive pericarditis and restrictive myocardiopathy. The clinical features and the demonstration of a left ventricular end-diastolic pressure exceeding that of the right are useful in distinguishing restrictive myocardiopathy from constrictive pericarditis, but even left heart catheterization and quantitative left ventriculography are not always enough to make the differential diagnosis.[121] Echocardiographic study has demonstrated symmetric thickening of the left ventricular wall, hypokinesia, decreased systolic thickening of the interventricular septum and left ventricular posterior wall, and the small-to-normal size of the left ventricular cavities.[122]

Hearts heavily infiltrated with amyloid may or may not exhibit an enlarged silhouette. Fluoroscopic study shows decreased mobility of the ventricular wall; angiographic studies usually show a thickened ventricular wall, decreased ventricular mobility, and the absence of rapid ventricular filling in early diastole.

The first signs of cardiac amyloid are often those of intractable heart failure. Electrocardiographic abnormalities include a low-voltage QRS complex and abnormalities in atrioventricular and intraventricular conduction, often resulting in varying degrees of heart block. Electrocardiographic abnormalities are frequent, often without previous infarct.[123] Because of their propensity to conduction defects and arrhythmias, patients with cardiac amyloidosis appear to be especially sensitive to digitalis, and this drug should be used in small doses and with caution. Binding of digoxin by isolated amyloid fibrils may play a role in such sensitivity.[124]

More recent noninvasive techniques have added to our understanding of the extent of cardiac amyloid and the associated functional abnormalities. For example, ^{99m}Tc pyrophosphate or diphosphonate scintigraphy is a sensitive and specific test for amyloid in patients with congestive heart failure of obscure origin. It is not useful, however, as an indicator of early cardiac amyloid in patients without electrocardiographic or other abnormalities.[125] Although M-mode echocardiography can, by the presence of thickened ventricular walls with a small or normal left ventricle, suggest amyloid, two-dimensional echocardiography adds substantial new information. It demonstrates thickened ventricles with a normal left ventricular cavity and a unique diffuse hyperrefractile "granular" sparkling appearance.[126] Thirty-one patients with documented cardiac amyloidosis were compared to 39 control subjects with left ventricular hypertrophy to determine specific two-dimensional echocardiographic features of amyloid. In 16 patients, increased myocardial echogenicity was present when a single short-axis view was examined, and these patients had a sensitivity of 63% and a specificity of 74% for the diagnosis of amyloidosis. When complete echocardiograms were reviewed, an improved sensitivity of 87% and specificity of 81% based on increased echogenicity was seen. Increased atrial septal thickness was present in 60% of amyloid patients and in no controls. The combination of increased myocardial echogenicity and increased atrial thickness was 60% sensitive and 100% specific for the diagnosis of amyloidosis. Detailed 24-hour electrocardiographic monitoring of patients with amyloid heart disease has revealed a significant number of high-grade ventricular arrhythmias and a lesser incidence of clinically significant bradycardia.[123]

Skin Lesions

Involvement of the skin is one of the most characteristic manifestations of AL (primary) amyloidosis. The lesions may consist of raised, waxy, often translucent papules or plaques, usually clustered in the folds about the axillae, the anal or inguinal regions, the face and neck, or mucosal areas such as the ear or tongue. The patient may also have purpuric areas, nodules or tumefactions, alopecia, a yellowish waxy discoloration, glossitis, and xerostomia. The lesions are seldom pruritic. Involvement of the skin or mucosa may be inapparent, even on close inspection, yet may be disclosed at biopsy. Gentle rubbing of the skin with one's finger may induce bleeding (purpura). Skin involvement can also occur in secondary amyloidosis. Amyloid was demonstrated in biopsy of the skin, with or without clinical lesions, in 42% of a group of 12 patients with secondary disease and in 55% of a group of 38 patients with primary disease.[99] All of a group of 8 patients with hereditary amyloid neuropathy studied by us had positive skin biopsies.

Gastrointestinal Involvement

Gastrointestinal findings in amyloidosis are common and may result from direct infiltration at any level or from infiltration of the autonomic nervous system. Symptoms and signs include those of obstruction, ulceration, malabsorption, hemorrhage, protein loss, and diarrhea. Infiltration of the tongue may lead to macroglossia, which may become incapacitating; alternatively, the tongue, although not enlarged, may become stiffened and firm to palpation. Infiltration of the tongue is especially characteristic of primary amyloidosis or amyloidosis accompanying multiple myeloma, but it may also occur in secondary amyloidosis.

Gastrointestinal bleeding may initiate from a number of sites, notably the esophagus, stomach, or large intestine, and may be severe or even fatal. Amyloid infiltration of the esophagus or small bowel may lead to clinical and radiologic changes of obstruction. A variable pattern has been observed in esophageal motility studies.[127] Malabsorption is sometimes seen. Amyloidosis may develop in association with other entities involving the gastrointestinal tract, especially tuberculosis, granulomatous enteritis, lymphoma, and Whipple's disease. Differentiation of these conditions from diffuse amyloidosis of the small bowel may be difficult. Similarly, amyloidosis of the stomach may mimic gastric carcinoma, with obstruction, achlorhydria, and the radiologic appearance of tumor masses. Patients may also have alternating constipation and diarrhea.

Neurologic Involvement

Neurologic manifestations are common and include peripheral neuropathy, postural hypotension, inability to sweat, Adie's pupil, hoarseness, and sphincter involvement.[128] These manifestations are especially prominent in the heredofamilial amyloidoses.[8] Cranial nerves are generally spared, except for those involving the pupillary reflexes and in the Finnish form of hereditary amyloid. The protein concentration of the cerebrospinal fluid may be increased. Infiltrates of the cornea or vitreous body may be present in hereditary amyloid syndromes. Amyloid may infiltrate the thyroid or other endocrine glands, but it rarely causes endocrine dysfunction. Local amyloid deposits almost invariably accompany medullary carcinoma of the thyroid. Amyloid infiltration of muscle may lead to pseudomyopathy.

Respiratory Tract Involvement

The nasal sinuses, larynx, and trachea may be involved by accumulations of amyloid that block the ducts, in the case of the sinuses, or the air passages. Amyloidosis of the lung may include diffuse involvement of the bronchi or alveolar septa. The lower respiratory tract is frequently involved in primary amyloidosis and in that associated with dysproteinemia.[129] Pulmonary symptoms attributable to amyloid are present in about 30% of patients, and in some individuals, these are the most serious disease manifestations. In secondary amyloidosis, pulmonary disease is a frequent histopathologic complication, but seldom gives rise to clinically significant symptoms. Amyloid may form a localized mass in the bronchi or alveolar tissue and may resemble a neoplasm. In such cases, local excision should be attempted; if successful, this procedure may be followed by a prolonged remission.

Hematologic Manifestations

Hematologic changes may include fibrinogenopenia, increased fibrinolysis, and selective deficiency of clotting factors, especially factor X.[130] Minor bleeding most often occurs in the absence of clotting abnormalities, however, and is due to local vessel amyloid infiltrates.[131]

PROGNOSIS

The course of amyloidosis is difficult to document because it is rarely possible to date its time of onset. Amyloidosis seldom develops in patients with RA of less than 2 years' duration. The mean duration of arthritis in one series at the time of recognition of amyloidosis was 16 years.[132]

When amyloidosis develops in patients with multiple myeloma, manifestations leading to the initial hospitalization are more apt to be related to the amyloid than to the myeloma.[112] Life expectancy is less than a year in such cases.

In amyloidosis accompanying sepsis such as osteomyelitis, at least partial remission has been reported after treatment of the primary disease.

Established, generalized amyloidosis in man, although usually progressive, may have a better prognosis than was once thought. Primary amyloid progresses less rapidly in women, who may also show a better response to treatment than men.[133] The chief cause of death in secondary (AA) amyloidosis is renal failure, whereas in primary amyloid, cardiac disease heads the list.[134] Sudden death may occur from arrhythmias. Occasionally, gastrointestinal hemorrhage, sepsis, respiratory failure, or intractable heart failure may cause death.

AMYLOIDOSIS AND RHEUMATOLOGIC DISEASE

The type of amyloid that complicates the inflammatory rheumatic diseases is AA (secondary or reactive) amyloid. This is true of the amyloid of RA, ankylosing spondylitis (AS), JRA, and other diffuse connective diseases.

Rheumatoid Arthritis

A variety of studies between the 1950s and 1970s reported a varying incidence of amyloid in RA of 2%, 5%, 12½%, 24%, 26%, 43%, and 60%.[135–141]

The earlier literature was affected by the method in which amyloid was diagnosed in the tissue. Crystal violet metachromasia and other histochemical and fluorescent stains as well as Congo red were used. The current standard is the demonstration of green birefrigence on polarization microscopy after Congo red staining and has been generally accepted since 1980.

In 1986 Laakso, Matru, Isomaki, and Koota reported a 10-year observation of 500 men and 500 women with RA together with a control population. Thirty-one RA patients and one control subject died of amyloidosis.[142] Boers, Croonen, Kijkmans, et al. in 1987 studied the renal abnormalities in 132 autopsied patients with RA and found amyloidosis in 11%.[143] Those with amyloid generally had arthritis of longer duration. Other investigators in the older[144] as well as more recent literature[145,146] have confirmed the 5 to 15% overall incidence of amyloid in RA. In our review of 19 RA patients who died of amyloid, the mean duration of arthritis before the onset of amyloid was 16 years (range, 1 to 40 years).[147]

The level of apoSAA, the precursor of AA amyloid, in diseases such as RA and JRA is extremely high, whereas in osteoarthritis, where systemic amyloidosis is rare, the level is virtually normal. In systemic lupus erythematosus (SLE) also, AA is a rare complication and the SAA level is only modestly elevated.[148]

In RA, the earliest clinical manifestation of amyloidosis is proteinuria. Indeed, the appearance of proteinuria in an RA patient should suggest the possibility of amyloidosis and trigger the appropriate diagnostic tests. Patients may also present with gastrointestinal symptoms, less often with hepatomegaly or splenomegaly. Amyloid may be diffusely present throughout the gastrointestinal tract; that may be the reason for positive gingival and rectal biopsies, and for the gastrointestinal bleeding that can occur. Such patients, however, rarely have clinically significant cardiovascular amyloid. In a patient with known amyloidosis and significant cardiovascular disease, one must think either of another cause or the possibility that the patient has AL or heredofamilial, rather than AA, amyloid. The mean duration of life of patients with secondary amyloid is relatively long. Patients have been reported with survivals of over 20 years. In such individuals, the most important predictor of improvement is the effective treatment of their primary disorder, the rheumatoid disease.

Juvenile Rheumatoid Arthritis

JRA is also known to be complicated by amyloidosis. In one large series of 1272 patients, 51 cases of amyloidosis (4%) were found. When the 243 who were followed for 15 years were evaluated, 7.4% had amyloid.[149] There is, however, a clear difference in the frequency of secondary amyloidosis in JRA in European countries as compared to the United States. One of the highest frequencies is in Poland, where 10.6% of patients had secondary amyloidosis. In the United States, the frequency was approximately 0.14%.[150] The reasons for these remarkable differences are obscure. In a study from Germany in 1981, a total incidence of 3.1% was found.[151] An overall incidence of 10% was believed to be the general European incidence.[152]

Ankylosing Spondylitis

Ankylosing spondylitis has been said not to have a very high association with secondary amyloidosis although sporadic cases have been reported. Ennevaara and Oka in 1963 reported three cases,[153] and in 1970 Pasternack, Ahonen, and Kuhlback reported amyloid in 3 out of 14 renal biopsies in patients with AS.[154] In 1980 Lehtinen reviewed the causes of death in 79 patients with AS between 1952 and 1959. Death was due to renal amyloid in 18% and was related to the cause of death in another 3.8%.[155] In our referral group of amyloid patients, we saw 49 patients with proven AA (secondary) amyloidosis between 1962 and 1987. Thirty had rheumatic diseases, with AS in 6, RA in 11, and JRA in 13.[156]

Psoriatic Arthritis

Although amyloidosis is said to be rare in this condition, David, Abraham, Weinberger, and Feurman reported 13 cases in 1982,[157] and Lofberg, Thysell, Westman, et al. noted that, of 42 AA cases, 2 had psoriatic arthritis and 1, psoriasis with AS.[158]

Reiter's Syndrome

Until recently, amyloid was almost never reported in Reiter's syndrome. In 1979, however, Miller, Brown, and Arnett found widespread bowel amyloid in a patient with Reiter's, which led to death.[159] Several similar cases have been reported since then, but clearly, this is a rare complication.

Behçet's Syndrome

Dilsen, Konic, Aral, et al. in 1988 noted 24 cases of amyloidosis in patients with Behçet's syndrome; 12 of those were Turkish.[160] A year later Tasdemir, Sivri, Turgan, et al. reported six new cases from Turkey.[161] However, only 5 of 1130 patients registered in a Behçet's clinic had amyloidosis.[162]

Sjögren's Syndrome

Amyloidosis has been reported in Sjögren's syndrome. However, in some cases investigated more extensively, it became clear that amyloidosis involving various glandular tissue, leading to dry eyes and dry mouth, actually mimicked Sjögren's syndrome. This occurred in what appeared to be AL amyloid and in AA amyloid found in various glandular tissues of patients with RA as well. It is possible that patients with widespread nodular squamous amyloid may be more prone to develop amyloid in glandular tissue and mimic Sjögren's syndrome.[163,164]

Vasculitis Syndromes

Amyloidosis has been reported in polymyalgia rheumatica, in temporal arteritis, in the Churg-Strauss syndrome, in nodular nonsuppurative panniculitis, in cerebral amyloid angiopathy with giant cell arthritis, and in Takayasu's syndrome. Some of this may be related to vessel injury and to tissue aging where there is an increased incidence of amyloid in vessel walls, particularly along the internal elastic lamina.[165]

Muscle Disease

Patients with amyloid (particularly primary) may develop extensive deposits in the muscle and subsequent stiffness and weakness. Although it was thought that the weakness caused muscle atrophy, more extensive electromyographic studies have suggested that this may be due as much to sarcolemmal conduction as well as to fibril atrophy.[166] In some studies, muscle amyloid was remarkably outlined by ^{99}Tc pyrophosphate.[167] These cases are very difficult to separate clinically from myositis, so muscle biopsies and special amyloid stains must be obtained.

Scleroderma

Many of the symptoms and signs of diffuse AL amyloidosis mimic those of scleroderma. Patients can have esophageal abnormalities with dysphagia.[168] They may have small and large bowel problems including alternating diarrhea and constipation. Smooth shiny skin may be due to either scleroderma or amyloidosis. Therefore, biopsies are absolutely vital. There are reported cases for which there is clear-cut evidence of scleroderma and amyloidosis occurring together.[169,170]

Systemic Lupus Erythematosus

One of the earliest cases of amyloid in SLE was reported in 1956 by Wegelius.[171] It is a very rare association. Only a few cases (12 to 20) have been reported.[172–175] Three patients with mixed connective tissue disease and amyloid have been recorded.[176]

Osteoarthritis and Amyloid

Because amyloidosis is essentially associated with inflammatory rheumatic diseases, it has been surprising to find that some authors reported it in association with osteoarthritis (OA), in particular, in areas in which calcium pyrophosphate dihydrate crystals also appear. Perhaps the earliest report was that of Bywaters and Dorling in 1970, when they noted amyloid in articular cartilage and along synovial lining cells.[177] It has also occurred in the fibrous capsules of joints, in the periarticular tissue, and in the intervertebral discs. In a necropsy study in 1981 of 91 unselected individuals (medium age 70), Goffin, Thoua, and Potvliege reported an overall incidence of 56% of amyloid microdeposits in hips and sternoclavicular joints.[178] Their presence correlated significantly only with age. The deposition began earliest in the sternoclavicular joint, where the fibrocartilage disc was almost exclusively involved. Ryan, Liang, and Kozin found articular or periarticular amyloid associated with chrondrocalcinosis.[179] Egan et al. reported that 10 of 18 consecutive patients who underwent knee or hip arthropathy for OA had amyloid present in surgically removed articular tissues.[107] It was found in 6 of 13 cartilage specimens, 4 of 18 articular capsules, and 2 of 16 synovial membranes. In three of the cartilage specimens, it was adjacent to focal deposits of calcium pyrophosphate dihydrate crystals. In a study of 100 consecutive operations on herniated disc, Ladefoged searched for intervertebral amyloid in 30 nonselective autopsies.[180] He found that 28 of the 30 specimens (93%) contained amyloid deposits and that amyloid was extensive throughout other surgically removed articular tissue as well.[181]

HEREDITARY AMYLOIDOSIS

The seminal work of Andrade in 1952 established hereditary amyloidosis as an important and well-defined clinical entity.[182] For many years, these diseases were defined according to whether they were inherited as autosomal dominants (most were), or recessives (familial Mediterranean fever), and by their clinical characteristics and ethnic distribution. Most hereditary amyloidoses were characterized by lower limb neuropathy and were defined as *familial amyloid polyneuropathies,* a term popularized since the mid-1960s. They were reported in persons of Portuguese, Japanese, and Swedish extraction and had similar clinical manifestations. These included peripheral neuropathy with early sensorimotor dissociation; autonomic neuropathy (with constipation, diarrhea, impotence); cardiomyopathy with arrhythmias and congestive failure; renal disease; severe wasting; and a life span of 10 to 15 years from mean onset of disease at age 25 to 40. The amyloid protein was identified as transthyretin (prealbumin),[49] and a single amino acid variant transthyretin was found.[51–53] There has been an explosion of new genetic data in recent years. In addition to the classic FAPs, syndromes with more marked cardiovascular, CNS, or other involvement have been identified. The original substitution of methionine for valine at position 30 has been shown to be accompanied by an increasing number of point mutations involving position 30, 33, 36, 42, 50, 58, 60, 77, 84, 90, 111, and 114 of transthyretin. Transthyretin is not the only protein responsible for hereditary amyloid. Apolipoprotein A-I, gelsolin, and cystatin C, each with their unique point mutations, have also been identified (Table 84–4).

The protein usually involved, however, is transthyretin, a well-identified 127 amino acid polypeptide whose structure was elucidated by x-ray diffraction in 1974.[183] The molecule circulates as a tetramer, is made up of four identical monomers, and binds thyroxin and retinol-binding protein. In many forms of FAP, circulating transthyretin levels are depressed, even in some asymptomatic carriers.[184,185]

The overview of the classification of hereditary amyloid in Table 84–1 is expanded in Table 84–4 to include all the proteins that have been identified and point mutations in the hereditary amyloidoses through 1990.

The most recently described transthyretin variants include Asn-90 in a Sicilian-Italian family whose clinical manifestations included the usual neuropathy plus vitreous opacities,[186] several Japanese families from Osaka, one with a Cys-114,[187] one with Gly-42, and another kinship with an Arg-50 substitution.[188] The amyloid of most cases of senile systemic amyloid has been attributed to normal transthyretin.[189] However, an Ile-122 variant[190] was found in an elderly black man with severe senile systemic amyloid and was further characterized as a homogeneous transthyretin mutation consistent with an autosomal recessive inheritance.[191]

That amyloid might consist of totally unexpected molecules was further illustrated when the Finnish hereditary amyloid with its cranial neuropathy and vitreous opacities was found to consist of gelsolin, the actin-modulating protein.[192,193] The hereditary recessive disorder familial Mediterranean fever, attributed to amyloid A protein, was found to occur in a presumably autosomal dominant fashion in a family of German background.[194]

In Iceland, the curious hereditary cerebral amyloid disease characterized by intracranial bleeding has been shown to be caused by the cysteine proteinase inhibitor, cystatin C.[195] A hereditary cerebral amyloid has also been found in the Dutch. This amyloid, however, is the β-protein (seen in Alzheimer's disease) and has been shown to be associated with a point mutation at position Gln-22 in the amyloid protein.[196]

TREATMENT

No specific therapy exists for any variety of amyloidosis. Rational therapy should be directed at the following: (1) decrease of chronic antigenic stimuli producing amyloid; (2) inhibition of the synthesis of the amyloid fibril; (3) inhibition of its extracellular deposition; (4) promotion of lysis or mobilization of existing deposits; and (5) genetic counseling for patients with the hereditary forms.

The progression of secondary amyloidosis is apparently retarded by eradication of the predisposing disease, although many such reports are not substantiated by biopsy proof of resorption. Although the average survival in most large series is 1 to 4 years, I have been treating some patients with amyloidosis for 5 to more than 10 years.

Among the many agents used to treat amyloidosis has been whole liver extract, but most clinicians have noted little effect on the course of the disease. Similarly, corticosteroids have little if any effect on amyloidosis. Ascorbic acid in large doses has been used, but proof of efficacy is lacking. The findings that immunoglobulin light-chain fragments are incorporated into primary amyloid and its presumed synthesis from plasma cells have led to the use of alkylating agents. These agents cause bone marrow depression, however, and acute leukemia has developed in some patients receiving melphalan.[197] Moreover, immunosuppressive agents used experimentally actually enhance amyloid deposition. Despite this, recent melphalan/prednisone regimens

TABLE 84–4. HEREDITARY AMYLOID SYNDROMES—1990

CLINICAL ASPECTS	GEOGRAPHIC OR ETHNIC ASSOCIATION	PROTEIN AND MUTATION
FAP—Distal limb peripheral neuropathy (sensory/motor); autonomic neuropathy with alternate constipation and diarrhea; nephropathy; cardiopathy with congestive failure (CHF) and arrhythmias; pupillary abnormalities in late disease (scalloped pupil); occasional vitreous opacities	Portuguese, Japanese, Swedish, Greek, Italian, Turkish	Transthyretin Met 30 (ATTR Met 30)
FAP—Peripheral neuropathy; autonomic neuropathy; cardiopathy, no renal (yet)	USA/German	ATTR Ala 30
FAP—Similar; few details known (neuropathy, diarrhea, vitreous opacities)	Israeli (Polish extraction)	ATTR Ile 33
FAP—Cardiomyopathy, vitreous opacities, mild neuropathy, renal (early report)	USA/Greek	ATTR Pro 36
FAP—Peripheral neuropathy; gastrointestinal (early report)	Japanese (Osaka)	ATTR Gly 42
FAP—Peripheral neuropathy; liver (early report)	Japanese	ATTR Arg 50
FAP—Cardiopathy; vitreous opacities	USA/Maryland/German extraction	ATTR His 58
FAP—Severe cardiopathy (often late in life); less peripheral neuropathy; occasional carpal tunnel syndrome	USA/West Virginia/ Appalachia (English-Irish-German extraction)	ATTR Ala 60
FAP—Neuropathy, diarrhea, nephropathy, cardiomyopathy	USA/Illinois/Texas (German extraction)	ATTR Tyr 77
FAP—Marked carpal tunnel syndrome; marked vitreous opacities, gastrointestinal symptoms	USA/Indiana (Swiss extraction)	ATTR Ser 84
FAC—Late onset cardiopathy; vitreous opacities; no neuropathy as yet (early report)	USA/Italian	ATTR Asn 84
FAP—Severe cardiomyopathy; mild sensory neuropathy; vitreous opacities	USA/Italian	ATTR Asn 90
FAC—Primarily heart disease with congestive failure and arrhythmias	Danish	ATTR Met 111
FAP—Peripheral neuropathy; vitreous opacities; gastrointestinal; kidney; (heart probable, early report)	Japanese (Osaka)	ATTR Cys 114
FAP—Lower limb neuropathy; nephropathy	USA/Iowa (Scottish-Irish-English)	Apolipoprotein AI Arg 26 (AApoAI Arg 26)
FAP—Cranial nerve neuropathy; skin changes; lattice corneal dystrophy; nephropathy	Finnish	Gelsolin Asn 187 (15) (AGel Asn 187 (15))
Hereditary cerebral hemorrhage with amyloidosis; cerebral angiopathy with spontaneous bleeds	A) Icelandic B) Dutch	A) Cystatin C Glu 68 (ACys Gln 68) B) β-Protein
Familial(?) amyloid (senile systemic) cardiopathy; heart disease in elderly patients; diagnosis at autopsy	Black	ATTR Ile 122
Familial Mediterranean fever—fever; joint pain; polyserositis; skin rash; mostly autosomal recessive	Sephardic Jews, Armenians, Kurds	AA
Familial nephropathy with urticaria and deafness (Muckle-Wells syndrome)		AA

FAC = familial amyloid cardiomyopathy; FAP = familial amyloid polyneuropathy.
(From Cohen, A.S.: Amyloidosis. Bull. Rheum. Dis. *40*:3, 1991.)

have suggested that this program significantly improves life expectancy in AL amyloid. In a prospective randomized study of melphalan/prednisone and of colchicine, no difference in survival was found when the groups were analyzed in aggregate. Significant differences favoring melphalan/prednisone were found when only one regimen was analyzed or when survival from the time of entry to the study to the time of death was studied.[198]

Amyloid deposition in the mouse model is inhibited by colchicine.[92,93] Colchicine prevents both acute attacks in patients with familial Mediterranean fever and deposition of the associated AA amyloid.[199] In our series of patients with AL amyloidosis, using historical controls and prospective treatment with colchicine, the mean duration of life was significantly longer in the colchicine-treated individuals (approximately doubled).[200] Because neither immunosuppressive therapy nor colchicine is a specific form of treatment, further studies of other agents are needed. At the moment, one or the other of these therapies, and possibly the combination (depending on the clinical circumstances) represent optimal therapy. Conservative, supportive measures, attention to organ involvement, and avoidance of overtreatment with agents that have increased hazard in amyloidosis remain vital aspects of management.

Surgery also has a role in the management of amyloid disease.[201] This may vary from the excision of local deposits and the removal of chronic infectious lesions to kidney transplantation. Two patients with severe renal amyloidosis and azotemia had bilateral nephrectomy and renal transplantation, followed by immunotherapy.[202] One patient died of infection 5 months later, and the donor kidney showed no evidence of amyloidosis. The second patient lived 10 years after receiving a transplanted kidney. Biopsies of her kidney after 2 and 4 years showed no amyloid. Notwithstanding the hazards of operating on patients with systemic amyloidosis who may have cardiac involvement, carefully selected patients would probably benefit from kidney transplantation.

REFERENCES

1. Cohen, A.S.: General introduction and a brief history of amyloidosis. *In* Amyloidosis. Edited by J. Marrink and M.H. Van Rijswijk. Dordrecht, The Netherlands, Martin Nijhoff, 1986.
2. Rokitansky, C.: Handbuch der Pathologischen Anatomie Vol. 3. Vienna, Braumuller and Seidel, 1842.
3. Cohen, A.S.: Amyloidosis. N. Engl. J. Med., *277*:522–530, 574–583, 628–638, 1967.
4. Cohen, A.S.: The constitution and genesis of amyloid. *In* International Review of Experimental Pathology, Vol. 4. Edited by G.W. Richter and M.A. Epstein. New York, Academic Press, 1965.
5. Bennhold, H.: Eine spezifische Amyloidfarbung mit Kongorot. Munchen. Med. Wochenschr., *69*:1537–1538, 1922.
6. Bennhold, H.: Ueber die Ausscheidung intravenos einverleibter Farbstoffe bei Amyloidkranken. Verh. Dtsch. Ges. Inn. Med., *34*:313, 1922.
7. Waldenstrom, H.: On the formation and disappearance of amyloid in man. Acta Chir. Scand., *63*:479–507, 1928.
8. Cohen, A.S.: Inherited systemic amyloidosis. *In* The Metabolic Basis of Inherited Disease. Edited by J.B. Standbury, J.B. Wyngaarden, and D.S. Fredrickson. New York, McGraw-Hill, 1972.
9. Husby, G., Araki, S., Benditt, E., et al.: The 1990 Guidelines for nomenclature and classification of amyloid and amyloidosis. *In* Amyloid and Amyloidosis—1990. Edited by J.B. Natvig et al. Dordrecht, The Netherlands, Kluwer, 1990, pp. 7–11.
10. Glenner, G.G. et al.: Amyloid fibril proteins: Proof of homology with immunoglobulin light chains by sequence analyses. Science, *172*:1150–1151, 1971.
11. Glenner, G.G. et al.: Creation of "amyloid" fibrils from Bence Jones proteins in vitro. Science, *174*:712–714, 1971.
12. Eulitz, M., Weiss, D.T., and Solomon, A.: Immunoglobulin heavy-chain associated amyloidosis. Proc. Natl. Acad. Sci. U.S.A., *87*:6542–6546, 1990.
13. Cohen, A.S., and Canoso, J.J.: Rheumatological aspects of amyloid disease. Clin. Rheum. Dis., *1*:149–161, 1975.
14. Westermark, P., Wernstedt, C., Wilander, E., et al.: Islet cell amyloid in type 2 human diabetes mellitus and adult diabetic cats contain a novel putative polypeptide hormone. Am. J. Pathol., *127*:414–417, 1987.
15. Cohen, A.S., and Kneapler, D.: Senile amyloidosis. *In* Handbook of Diseases of Aging. Edited by H.T. Blumenthal. New York VanNostrand Reinhold, 1983.
16. Schwartz, P.: Senile cerebral, pancreatic insular and cardiac amyloidosis. Trans. N.Y. Acad. Sci., *27*:393–413, 1965.
17. Wright, J.R. et al.: Relationship of amyloid to aging. Medicine, *48*:39–60, 1969.
18. Westermark, P., Natvig, J.B., and Johansson, B.: Characterization of an amyloid fibril protein from senile cardiac amyloid. J. Exp. Med., *146*:631–636, 1977.
19. Cohen, A.S.: Diagnosis of amyloidosis. *In* Laboratory Diagnostic Methods in the Rheumatic Diseases. 2nd Ed. Edited by A.S. Cohen, Boston, Little, Brown, 1975.
20. Cooper, J.H.: An evaluation of current methods for the diagnostic histochemistry of amyloid. J. Clin. Pathol., *22*:410–413, 1969.
21. Wright, J.R., Calkins, E., and Humphrey, R.L.: Potassium permangantate reaction in amyloidosis: A histologic method to assist in differentiating forms of the disease. Lab. Invest., *36*:274–281, 1977.
22. Shirahama, T., Skinner, M., and Cohen, A.S.: Immunocytochemical identification of amyloid in formalin fixed paraffin sections. Histochemistry, *72*:161–171, 1981.
23. Chopra, S., Rubinow, A., Koff, R.S., and Cohen, A.S.: Hepatic amyloidosis. Histopathologic analysis of primary (AL) and secondary (AA) forms. Am. J. Pathol., *115*:186–193, 1984.
24. Cohen, A.S., and Calkins, E.: Electron microscopic observations on a fibrous component in amyloid of diverse origins. Nature [Lond.], *183*:1202–1203, 1959.
25. Shirahama, T., and Cohen, A.S.: High resolution electron microscopic analysis of the amyloid fibril. J. Cell Biol., *33*:679–708, 1967.
26. Shirahama, T., and Cohen, A.S.: Fine structure of the glomerulus in human and experimental renal amyloidosis. Am. J. Pathol., *51*:869–911, 1967.
27. Eanes, E.D., and Glenner, G.G.: X-ray studies on amyloid filaments. J. Histochem. Chem., *16*:673–677, 1968.
28. Bonar, L., Cohen, A.S., and Skinner, M.M.: Characterization of the amyloid fibril as a cross-B protein. Proc. Soc. Exp. Biol. Med., *131*:1373–1375, 1969.
29. Sinner, M. et al.: P-component (pentagonal unit) of amyloid: Isolation, characterization and sequence analysis. J. Lab. Clin. Med., *84*:604–614, 1974.
30. Skinner, M., and Cohen, A.S.: Amyloid P-component. *In* Methods in Enzymology. Edited by G. DiSabato. Orlando, FL, Academic Press, 1988.
31. Cohen, A.S.: Preliminary chemical analyses of partially purified amyloid fibrils, Lab. Invest., *15*:66–83, 1966.
32. Newcombe, D.S., and Cohen, A.S.: Solubility characteristics of isolated amyloid fibrils. Biochim. Biophys. Acta, *104*:480–486, 1965.
33. Pras, M. et al.: The characterization of soluble amyloid prepared in water. J. Clin. Invest., *47*:924–933, 1968.
34. Glenner, G.G. et al.: An amyloid protein: The amino terminal variable fragment of an immunoglobulin light chain. Biochem. Biophys. Res. Commun., *41*:1287–1289, 1970.
35. Kyle, R.A., and Gertz, M.A.: Systemic amyloidosis. Crit. Rev. Oncol./Hematol., *10*:49–87, 1990.
36. Skinner, M., Benson, M.D., and Cohen, A.S.: Amyloid fibril protein related to immunoglobulin lambda-chains. J. Immunol., *114*:1433–1435, 1975.
37. Sletten, K., Husby, G., and Natvig, J.B.: N-terminal amino acid sequence of amyloid fibril protein AP. Prototype of a new lambda-variable subgroup, V lambda V. Scand. J. Immunol., *3*:833–836, 1974.
38. Isersky, C. et al.: Immunochemical cross reaction of human immunoglobulin light chains. J. Immunol., *8*:486–493, 1972.
39. Benditt, E.P., Erikssen, N., Hermondson, N.A., and Ericsson, L.H.: The major proteins of human and amyloid substance: common properties including unusual N-terminal amino acid sequences. FEBS Lett., *19*:169–173, 1971.
40. Levin, M., Pras, M., and Franklin, E.C.: Immunologic studies of the major nonimmunoglobulin protein of amyloid. Identification and partial characterization of a related serum component. J. Exp. Med., *138*:373–381, 1973.
41. Benditt, E.P., and Eriksen, N.: Amyloid protein SAA is associ-

ated with high density lipoprotein from human serum. Proc. Natl. Acad. Sci. U.S.A., *74*:4025–4028, 1977.
42. Miura, K., Ju, S.T., Cohen, A.S., and Shirahama, T.: Generation and use of site-specific antibodies to serum amyloid A for probing amyloid A development. J. Immunol., *144*:610–613, 1990.
43. Benson, M.D. et al.: Kinetics of serum amyloid protein A in casein-induced murine amyloidosis. J. Clin. Invest., *59*:412–417, 1977.
44. Sipe, J.D. et al.: The role of interleukin I on acute phase serum amyloid A (SAA) and serum amyloid P (SAP) biosynthesis. Ann. N.Y. Acad. Sci., *389*:137–150, 1982.
45. Moyner, K., Sletten, K., Husby, G., and Natvig, J.B.: An unusually large (83 amino acid residues) amyloid fibril protein AA from a patient with Waldenstrom's macroglobulinaemia and amyloidosis. Scand. J. Immunol., *11*:549–554, 1980.
46. Strachan, A., Shephard, E.G., Bellstedt, D.U., et al.: Human serum amyloid A protein: Behavior in aqueous and urea-containing solutions and antibody production. Biochem. J., *263*:365–370, 1989.
47. Rienhoff, H.Y., Jr., Huang, J.H., Xioxia, L., and Liao, W.S.L.: Molecular and cellular biology of serum amyloid A. Mol. Biol. Med., *7*:287–298, 1990.
48. Meek, R.L., Eriksen, N., and Benditt, E.P.: Serum amyloid A in the mouse: Sites of uptake and mRNA expression. Am. J. Pathol., *135*:411–419, 1989.
49. Costa, P.P., Figueira, A.S., and Bravo, F.R.: Amyloid fibril protein related to prealbumin in familial amyloidotic polyneuropathy. Proc. Natl. Acad. Sci. U.S.A., *75*:499–503, 1978.
50. Saraiva, M.J.M., Costa, P.P., Birken, S., and Goodman, D.S.: Presence of an abnormal transthyretin (prealbumin) in Portuguese patients with familial amyloidotic polyneuropathy. Trans. Assoc. Am. Physicians, *96*:261–270, 1983.
51. Tawara, S. et al.: Amyloid fibril protein in type I familial amyloidotic polyneuropathy in Japanese. J. Lab. Clin. Med., *98*:811–822, 1981.
52. Benson, M.D.: Partial amino acid sequence homology between an heredofamilial amyloid protein and human plasma prealbumin. J. Clin. Invest., *67*:1035–1041, 1981.
53. Skinner, M., and Cohen, A.S.: The prealbumin nature of the amyloid protein in familial amyloid polyneuropathy (FAP)—Swedish variety. Biochem. Biophys. Res. Commun., *99*:1326–1332, 1981.
54. Saraiva, M.J.M., Sherman, W., and Goodman, D.S.: Presence of a plasma transthyretin (prealbumin) variant in familial amyloidotic polyneuropathy in a kindred of Greek origin. J. Lab. Clin. Med., *108*:17–22, 1986.
55. Benson, M.D.: Inherited amyloidosis. J. Mol. Genet., *28*:73–78, 1991.
56. Blake, C.C.F., Geisow, M.J., and Oatley, S.I.: Structure of prealbumin: Secondary, tertiary and quarternary interactions determined by Fourier refinement at 1.8A. J. Mol. Biol., *121*:339–356, 1978.
57. Blake, C.C.F.: Structural and functional aspects of the transthyretin (TTR) molecule. *In* Familial Amyloid Polyneuropathy. Edited by P.P. Costa, A.F. Frietas, and M.J.M. Saraiva. Portugal, Archivos de Medicina, 1990, pp. 41–47.
58. Nichols, W.C., Dwulet, F.E., Leipnieks, J., and Benson, M.D.: Variant apolipoprotein A1 as a major constitutent of a human hereditary amyloid. Biochem. Biophys. Res. Commun., *156*:762–768, 1988.
59. Maury, C.P.J., Alli, K., and Baumann, M.: Finnish hereditary amyloidosis. Amino acid sequence homology between the amyloid fibril protein and human plasma gelsoline. FEBS Lett., *260*:85–87, 1990.
60. Levy, E., Carman, M.D., Fernandez-Madred, I.J., et al.: Mutation of the Alzheimer's disease amyloid gene in hereditary cerebral hemorrhage, Dutch type. Science, *248*:1124–1126, 1990.
61. Bardin, T. et al.: Synovial amyloidosis in patients undergoing long term hemodialysis. Arthritis Rheum., *28*:1052–1058, 1985.
62. Bardin, T. et al.: Hemodialysis associated amyloidosis and beta 2 microglobulin: A clinical and immunohistochemical study. Am. J. Med., *83*:419–424, 1987.
63. Gejyo, F. et al.: A new form of amyloid protein associated with chronic hemodialysis identified as β_2-microglobulin. Biochem. Biophys. Res. Commun., *129*:701–706, 1985.
64. Connors, L.H. et al.: In vitro formation of amyloid fibrils from intact β_2-microglobulin. Biochem. Biophys. Res. Commun., *131*:1063–1068, 1985.
65. Shirahama, T. et al.: Histochemical and immunohistochemical characterization of amyloid associated with chronic hemodialysis as β_2-microglobulin. Lab. Invest., *53*:705–709, 1985.
66. Glenner, G.G., and Wong, C.W.: Alzheimer's disease: Initial report of the purification and characterization of a novel cerebrovascular amyloid protein. Biochem. Biophys. Res. Commun., *120*:885–890, 1984.
67. Masters, C.L. et al.: Neuronal origin of a cerebral amyloid: Neurofibrillary tangles of Alzheimer's disease contain the same protein as the amyloid of plaque cores and blood vessels. EMBO J., *4*:2757–2763, 1985.
68. Selkoe, D.J.: Deciphering Alzheimer's disease: The amyloid precursor protein yields new clues. Science, *248*:1058–1060, 1990.
69. Abraham, C.R., Selkoe, J., and Potter, H.: Immunochemical identification of the serine protease inhibitor alpha-1 antichymotrypsin in the brain of amyloid deposits of Alzheimer's disease. Cell, *52*:487–501, 1988.
70. Brown, P., Goldfarb, L.G., and Gajdusek, D.C.: The new biology of spongioform encephalopathy: infectious amyloidosis with a genetic twist. Lancet, *337*:1019–1022, 1991.
71. Westermark, P.: Amyloid of medullary carcinoma of the thyroid: partial characterization. Uppsala J. Med. Sci., *80*:88–92, 1975.
72. Johanson, B., Wernstedt, C., and Westermark, P.: Atrial natriuretic peptide deposited as atrial amyloid fibrils. Biochem. Biophys. Res. Commun., *148*:1087–1092, 1987.
73. Westermark, P., Wernstedt, C., Wilander, E., et al.: Islet cell amyloid in type 2 human diabetes mellitus and adult diabetic cats contain a novel putative polypeptide hormone. Am. J. Pathol., *127*:414–417, 1987.
74. Johnson, B., Wernstedt, C., and Westermark, P.: Islet amyloid, islet-amyloid polypeptide and diabetes mellitus. N. Engl. J. Med., *321*:513–518, 1989.
75. Skinner, M. et al.: Studies on amyloid protein AP. *In* Amyloid and Amyloidosis. Edited by G.G. Glenner, P.P. Costa, and A.F. Freitas. Amsterdam, Excerpta Medica, 1980.
76. Mantzouranis, E.C. et al.: Human serum amyloid P component. J. Biol. Chem., *260*:7752–7756, 1985.
77. Oliveira, E.B., Gotschlich, E.C., and Liu, L.: Primary structure of human C-reactive protein. J. Biochem. Chem., *254*:489–502, 1979.
78. Skinner, M. et al.: Characterization of P-component (AP) isolated from amyloidotic tissue: Half-life studies human and murine AP. Ann. N.Y. Acad. Sci., *389*:190–198, 1982.
79. Skinner, M. et al.: Serum amyloid P-component levels in amyloidosis. Connective tissue diseases, infection and malignancy as compared to normal serum. J. Lab. Clin. Med., *94*:633–638, 1979.
80. Pepys, M.B. et al.: Binding of serum amyloid P-component (SAP) by amyloid fibrils. Clin. Exp. Immunol., *38*:284–293, 1979.
81. Pepys, M.B. et al.: Isolation of amyloid P component (Protein

AP) from normal serum as a calcium-dependent binding protein. Lancet, *1*:1029–1032, 1977.

82. Cohen, A.S., Shirahama, T., and Skinner, M.: Electron-microscopy of amyloid. *In* Electron Microscopy of Proteins. Vol. 3. Edited by J.R. Harris. London, Academic Press, 1982.
83. Skinner, M. et al.: Murine amyloid protein AA in casein-induced experimental amyloidosis. Lab. Invest., *36*:420–427, 1977.
84. Teilum, G.: Pathogenesis of amyloidosis: The two phase cellular theory of local secretion. Acta Pathol. Microbiol. Scand., *61*:21–45, 1964.
85. Hardt, F., and Kanlov, P.: Transfer amyloidosis. Int. Rev. Exp. Pathol., *16*:273, 1964.
86. Kisilevsky, R., Boudreau, L., and Foster, D.: Kinetics of amyloid deposition. The effects of dimethylsulfoxide and colchicine therapy. Lab. Invest., *48*:60–67, 1983.
87. Shirahama, T., and Cohen, A.S.: Intralysosomal formation of amyloid fibrils. Am. J. Pathol., *81*:101–116, 1975.
88. Cohen, A.S., Gross, E., and Shirahama, T.: The light and electron microscopic authoradiographic demonstration of local amyloid formation in spleen explants. Am. J. Pathol., *47*:1079–1111, 1965.
89. Sipe, J.D. et al.: The role of interleukin 1 in acute phase serum amyloid A (AA) and serum amyloid P (SAP) biosynthesis. Ann. N.Y. Acad. Sci., *389*:137–150, 1982.
90. Sipe, J.D. et al.: Detection of a mediator derived from endotoxin-stimulated macrophages that induces the acute phase serum amyloid A response in mice. J. Exp. Med., *150*:597–606, 1979.
91. Axelrad, M.A., and Kisilevsky, R.: Biological characterization of amyloid enhancing factor. *In* Amyloid and Amyloidosis. Edited by G.G. Glenner, P.P. Costa, and A.F. Freitas. Amsterdam, Excerpta Medica, 1980.
92. Kedar, I. et al.: Colchicine inhibition of casein-induced amyloidosis in mice. Isr. J. Med. Sci., *10*:787–789, 1974.
93. Shirahama, T., and Cohen, A.S.: Blockage of amyloid induction by colchicine in an animal model. J. Exp. Med., *140*:1102–1107, 1974.
94. Osserman, E.F., Sherman, W.H., and Kyle, R.A.: Further studies of therapy of amyloidosis with dimethyl sulfoxide (DMSO). *In* Amyloid and Amyloidosis. Edited by G.G. Glenner, P.P. Costa, and A.F. Freitas. Amsterdam, Excerpta Medica, 1980.
95. Cohen, A.S., and Shirahama, T.: Amyloidosis, model no. 17, supplemental update. *In* Handbook: Animal Models of Human Disease. Edited by C.C. Capen et al. Washington, D.C. Registry of Comparative Pathology, Armed Forces Institute of Pathology, 1980, fascicle 2.
96. Takeda T. et al.: A new murine model of accelerated senescence. Mech. Ageing Dev., *17*:183–194, 1981.
97. Libbey, C.A. et al.: Diagnosis of amyloidosis and differentiation of secondary amyloid by analysis of abdominal fat tissue aspirate. Arthritis Rheum., *24*:5,125, 1981.
98. Libbey, C.A., Skinner, M., and Cohen, A.S.: The abdominal fat tissue aspirate for the diagnosis of systemic amyloidosis. Arch. Intern. Med., *143*:1549–1552, 1983.
99. Rubinow, A., and Cohen, A.S.: Skin involvement in generalized amyloidosis. A study of clinically involved and uninvolved skin in 50 patients with primary and secondary amyloidosis. Ann. Intern. Med., *88*:781–785, 1978.
100. Gordon, D.A., Pruzanski, W., and Ogryzlo, M.A.: Synovial fluid examination for the diagnosis of amyloidosis. Ann. Rheum. Dis., *32*:428–430, 1973.
101. Bywaters, E.G.L., and Dorling, J.: Amyloid deposits in articular cartilage. Ann. Rheum. Dis., *29*:294–306, 1970.
102. Gordon, D.A. et al.: Amyloid arthritis simulating rheumatoid disease in five patients with multiple myeloma. Am. J. Med., *55*:142–154, 1973.
103. Laine, V., Vaino, K., and Ritama, V.V.: Occurrence of amyloid in rheumatoid arthritis. Acta Rheumatol. Scand., *1*:43–46, 1955.
104. Christensen, H.E., and Sorenson, K.L.: Local amyloid formation of capsule fibrosa in arthritis coxae. Acta Pathol. Microbiol. Scand. [A], *233*:128–131, 1972.
105. Goffin, Y.A., Thoua, Y., and Potvliege, P.R.: Microdeposition of amyloid in the joints. Ann. Rheum. Dis., *40*:27–33, 1981.
106. Ryan, L.M. et al.: Amyloid arthropathy in the absence of dysproteinemia: A possible association with chondrocalcinosis. Arthritis Rheum., *21*:587–588, 1978.
107. Egan, M.S. et al.: The association of amyloid deposits and osteoarthritis. Arthritis Rheum., *25*:204–208, 1982.
107a. Gejyo, F., Yamada, T., Odani, S., et al.: A new form of amyloid protein associated with chronic hemodialysis was identified as B2-microglobulin. Biochem. Biophys. Res. Commun., *129*:701–706, 1985.
108. Sethi, D., Naunton-Morgan, T.C., Brown, E.A., et al.: Dialysis arthropathy: A clinical biochemical radiological and histological study of 36 patients. Q. J. Med., *77*:1061–1082, 1990.
109. Shinoda, T., Komatsu, M., Aizawa, T., et al.: Intestinal pseudo-obstruction due to dialysis amyloidosis. Clin. Nephrol., *32*:284–289, 1989.
110. Campistol, J.M., Sole, M., Munoz-Gomez, J., et al.: Systemic involvement of dialysis amyloidosis. Am. J. Nephrol., *10*:389–396, 1990.
111. Munoz-Gomez, J., and Sole, M.: Dialysis arthropathy of amyloid orgin. J. Rheumatol., 17:723–724, 1990.
112. Cathcart, E.S., and Cohen, A.S.: A clinical analysis of the course and prognosis of 42 patients with amyloidosis. Am. J. Med., *44*:955–969, 1968.
113. Kyle, R., and Bayrd, E.: Amyloidosis: Review of 236 cases. Medicine, *54*:271–299, 1975.
114. Cohen, A.S.: Renal amyloidosis. *In* Textbook of Nephrology. Edited by S.G. Massry and R.J. Glassock. Baltimore, Williams & Wilkins, 1983.
115. Tribe, C.R.: Amyloidosis in chronic paraplegia. *In* Renal Failure in Paraplegia. London, Pitman Medical Publishing, 1969.
116. Triger, D.R., and Joekes, A.M.: Renal amyloidosis—A fourteen-year follow-up. Q. J. Med., *42*:15–40, 1973.
117. Yood, R.A. et al.: Soft tissue uptake of bone seeking radionuclide in amyloidosis. J. Rheumatol., *8*:760–766, 1981.
118. Rubinow, A., Koff, R.S., and Cohen, A.S.: Severe intrahepatic cholestasis in primary amyloidosis. A report of 4 cases and a review of the literature. Am. J. Med., *64*:937–946, 1978.
119. Cohen, A.S., and Skinner, M.: Amyloidosis of the liver. *In* Diseases of the Liver. 7th Ed. Edited by L. Schiff and E.R. Schiff. Philadelphia, J.B. Lippincott (in press), 1991.
120. Buja, L.M., Khoi, N.B., and Roberts, W.C.: Clinically significant cardiac amyloidosis. Am. J. Cardiol., *26*:394–405, 1970.
121. Meaney, E. et al.: Cardiac amyloidosis, constrictive pericarditis and restrictive cardiomyopathy. Am. J. Cardiol., *38*:547–556, 1976.
122. Child, J.S. et al.: Echocardiographic manifestations of infiltrative cardiomyopathy. A report of seven cases due to amyloid. Chest, *70*:726–731, 1979.
123. Falk, R.: Cardiac involvement in amyloidosis. *In* Amyloidosis. Edited by J. Marrink and M.H. van Rijswijk. Dordrecht, The Netherlands, Martin Nijhoff, 1986.
124. Rubinow, A., Skinner, M., and Cohen, A.S.: Digoxin sensitivity in amyloid cardiomyopathy. Circulation, *63*:1285–1288, 1981.
125. Falk, R.H. et al.: Sensitivity of technetium-99m-pryophosphate scintigraphy for the diagnosis of cardiac amyloidosis. Am. J. Cardiol., *51*:826–830, 1983.
126. Siqueira-Filho, A.G. et al.: M-mode and two-dimensional echo-

cardiographic features in cardiac amyloidosis. Circulation, *63*:188–196, 1981.
127. Rubinow, A., Burakoff, R.B., Cohen, A.S., and Harris, L.D.: Esophageal manometry in systemic amyloidosis. Am. J. Med., *75*:951–956, 1983.
128. Cohen, A.S., and Rubinow, A.: Amyloid neuropathy. *In* Peripheral Neuropathy. 2nd Ed., Vol. 2. Edited by P.J. Dyck, P.K. Thomas, and E.H. Lambert. Philadelphia, W.B. Saunders, 1983.
129. Celli, B.R. et al.: Patterns of pulmonary involvement in systemic amyloidosis. Chest, *74*:543–547, 1978.
130. Furie, B., Greene, E., and Furie, B.C.: Syndrome of acquired factor X deficiency and systemic amyloidosis in vivo studies of the fate of factor X. N. Engl. J. Med., *297*:81–85, 1977.
131. Yood, R.A. et al.: Bleeding and impaired hemostasis in 100 patients with amyloidosis. JAMA, *49*:1322–1324, 1983.
132. Cohen, A.S.: Amyloidosis associatd with rheumatoid arthritis. Med. Clin. North Am., *52*:643–653, 1968.
133. Anderson, J.J., Mason, J.H., Skinner, M., and Cohen, A.S.: Sex differences in survival with primary amyloidosis. Arthritis Rheum. *30*:S9, 1987.
134. Cohen, A.S. et al.: The life span of patients with primary (AL) amyloidosis and the effect of colchicine treatment. *In* Amyloidosis. Edited by G.G. Glenner et al. New York, Plenum Publishing, 1986.
135. Ozdemir, A.L., Wright, J.R., and Calkins, E.: Influence of rheumatoid arthritis on amyloidosis of aging. N. Engl. J. Med., *285*:534–538, 1971.
136. Bland, J.H.: Clinical incidence of renal amyloidosis in rheumatoid arthritis. J. Maine Med. Assoc., *56*:251–254, 1965.
137. Brun, C., Olsen, T.S., Raaschou, F., and Sorensen, A.W.S.: Renal biopsy in rheumatoid arthritis. Nephron, *2*:65–81, 1965.
138. Gedda, P.O.: On amyloidosis and other causes of death in rheumatoid arthritis. Acta Med. Scand., *150*:443–452, 1955.
139. Calkins, E., and Cohen, A.S.: The diagnosis of amyloidosis. Bull. Rheum. Dis., *10*:215–218, 1960.
140. Siegmeth, W., and Eberl, R.: Amyloidosis. *In* Rheumatoid Arthritis Organ Manifestations and Complications. Basel, Documenta Geigy, 1977, pp. 30–36.
141. Teilum, G., and Lindahl, A.: Frequency and significance of amyloid changes in rheumatoid arthritis. Acta Med. Scand., *149*:449–455, 1954.
142. Laakso, M., Mutru, O., Isomaki, H., and Koota, K.: Mortality from amyloidosis and renal disease in patients with rheumatoid arthritis. Ann. Rheum. Dis., *45*:663–667, 1986.
143. Boers, M., Croonen, A.M., Kijkmans, B.A.C., et al.: Renal findings in rheumatoid arthritis: Clinicial aspects of necropsies. Ann. Rheum. Dis., *46*:658–663, 1987.
144. Missen, G.A.K., and Taylor, J.D.: Amyloidosis in rheumatoid arthritis. J. Pathol. Bacteriol., *71*:179–192, 1956.
145. Husby, G.: Amyloidosis and rheumatoid arthritis. Clin. Exp. Rheumatol., *3*:173–180, 1985.
146. Mutru, O., Laakso, M., Isomaki, H., and Koota, K.: Ten year mortality and causes of death in patients with rheumatoid arthritis. Br. Med. J., *290*:1811–1813, 1985.
147. Cohen, A.S.: Amyloidosis associated with rheumatoid arthritis. Med. Clin. North Am., *52*:643–653, 1968.
148. Benson, M.D., and Cohen, A.S.: Serum amyloid A protein in amyloidosis, rheumatic and neoplastic diseases. Arthritis Rheum., *22*:36–42, 1979.
149. Schnitzer, T.J., and Ansell, B.M.: Amyloidosis in juvenile chronic polyarthritis. Arthritis Rheum., *20*(Suppl.):245–252, 1977.
150. Baum, J., and Gutowska, G.: Death in juvenile rheumatoid arthritis. Arthritis Rheum., *20*(Suppl.):253–255, 1977.
151. Stoeber, E.: Prognosis in juvenile chronic arthritis: Follow-up of 433 chronic rheumatic children. Eur. J. Pediatr., *135*:225–228, 1981.
152. Dhillon, V., Woo, P., and Isenberg, D.: Amyloidosis in the rheumatic diseases. Ann. Rheum. Dis., *48*:696–701, 1989.
153. Ennevaara, K., and Oka, M.: Amyloidosis in ankylosing spondylitis. Ann. Rheum. Dis., *22*:336–341, 1963.
154. Pasternack, A., Ahonen, H., Kuhlback, B.: Renal vascular changes in ankylosing spondylitis. Acta Med. Scand., *187*:519–523, 1970.
155. Lehtinen, K.: Cause of death in 79 patients with ankylosing spondylitis. Scand. J. Rheumatol., *9*:145–147, 1980.
156. Gridley, J., Skinner, M., Anderson, J., and Cohen, A.S.: Rheumatic disease resulting in secondary (AA) amyloidosis. Arthritis Rheum., *31*(Suppl.):124, 1988.
157. David, M., Abraham, D., Weinberger, A., and Feurman, E.J.: Generalized pustular psoriasis, psoriatic arthritis and nephrotic syndrome associated with systemic amyloidosis. Dermatologica, *165*:168–171, 1982.
158. Lofberg, H., Thysell, H., Westman, K., et al.: Demonstration and classification of amyloidosis in needle biopsies of the kidneys with special reference to amyloidosis of the AA-type. Acta Pathol. Microbiol. Immunol. Scand., *95*:357–363, 1987.
159. Miller, L.D., Brown, E.C., and Arnett, F.C.: Amyloidosis in Reiter's syndrome. J. Rheumatol., *6*:225–231, 1979.
160. Dilsen, N., Konic, M., Aral, O., et al.: Behcet's disease associated with amyloidosis in Turkey and in the world. Ann. Rheum. Dis., *47*:157–163, 1988.
161. Tasdemir, I., Sivri, B., Turgan, C., et al.: The expanding spectrum of a disease. Behcet's disease associated with amyloidosis. Nephron, *52*:154–157, 1989.
162. Yurdakul, Y., Tuzuner, N., Yurdakul, I., et al.: Amyloidosis in Behcet's syndrome. Arthritis Rheum., *33*:1586–1589, 1990.
163. Clinicopathological Conference: Subcutaneous masses and adenopathy in a 77 year old man with Sjogren's syndrome and amyloidosis. Am. J. Med., *86*:585–590, 1989.
164. Bonner, H., Ennis, R.S., Geelhoed, G.W., and Tarpley, T.M.: Lymphoid infiltration and amyloidosis of lung in Sjogren's syndrome. Arch. Pathol., *95*:42–44, 1973.
165. Meretoja, J., and Tarkkanen, A.: Amyloid deposits of internal elastic lamina in temporal arteritis. Ophthalmologica, *170*:337–344, 1975.
166. Doriguzi, C., Mongini, T., Troni, W., and Monga, G.: Early sarcolemmal dysfunction in skeletal muscle amyloidosis. J. Neurol., *234*:52–54, 1987.
167. Johnston, J.B., Raynor, H.L., Trevenen, C., and Greenberg, D.: Skeletal muscle uptake of Tc 99m pyrophosphate in amyloidosis. Am. J. Hematol., *93*:13–20, 1982.
168. Rubinow, A., Burakoff, R.B., and Cohen, A.S.: Esophageal manometry in systemic amyloidosis. A study of 30 patients. Am. J. Med., *75*:951–956, 1983.
169. Horwitz, H.M., DiBeneditte, J.D., Allegra, S.R., and Baumann, H.M.: Scleroderma, amyloidosis and extensor tendon rupture. Arthritis Rheum., *25*:1141–1143, 1982.
170. Holzmann, H., Horting, G.W., and Missmahl, H.P.: Pericollagenous amyloid in the skin and interal organs in scleroderma. Klin. Wochenschr., *47*:390–391, 1969.
171. Wegelius, O.: Amyloidosis of the kidneys, adrenals and spleen as a complication of acute disseminated lupus erythematosus treated with ACTH and cortisone. Acta Med. Scand., *156*:91–95, 1956.
172. Pettersson, T., Tornroth, T., Totterman, K.J., et al.: AA amyloidosis in systemic lupus erythematosus. J. Rheumatol., *14*:835–838, 1987.
173. ter Borg, E.J., Janssen, S., van Rijswijk, M.H., et al.: AA amyloidosis associated with systemic lupus erythematosus. Rheumatol. Int., *8*:141–143, 1988.

174. Carstein, P.H.B., Ogden, L.L., and Peak, W.P.: Renal amyloidosis associated with systemic lupus erythematosus. Am. J. Clin. Pathol., *74*:835–838.
175. Sweet, J., Bear, R.A., and Lang, A.P.: Amyloidosis and systemic lupus erythematosus. Hum. Pathol., *12*:853–856, 1981.
176. Phrainen, H.I., Helve, A.T., Tornroth, T., and Pettersson, T.E.: Amyloidosis in mixed connective tissue disease. Scand. J. Rheumatol., *18*:165–168, 1989.
177. Bywaters, E.G.L., and Dorling, J.: Amyloid deposits in articular cartilage. Ann. Rheum. Dis., *29*:294–306, 1970.
178. Goffin, Y.A., Thoua, Y., and Potvliege, P.R.: Microdeposition of amyloid in the joints. Ann. Rheum. Dis., *40*:27–33, 1981.
179. Ryan, L.M., Liang, G., and Kozin, F.: Amyloid arthropathy: Possible association with chrondrocalcinosis. J. Rheumatol., *9*:273–278, 1982.
180. Ladefoged, C.: Amyloid in intervertebral discs: A histopathological investigation of intervertebral discs from 30 randomly selected autopsies. Appl. Pathol., *3*:96–104, 1985.
181. Ladefoged, C., Merrild, U., and Jorgensen, B.: Amyloid deposits in surgically removed articular and periarticular tissue. Histopathology, *15*:289–296, 1989.
182. Andrade, C.: A peculiar form of peripheral neuropathy: Familial atypical generalized amyloidosis with special involvement of peripheral nerve. Brain, *75*:408–426, 1952.
183. Blake, C.C.F., Geisow, M.F., Swan, I.D.A., et al.: Structure of human plasma prealbumin at 2.5 A resolution. J. Mol. Biol., *80*:1–12, 1974.
184. Skinner, M., Connors, L.H., Rubinow, A., and Libbey, C.A.: Lowered prealbumin in patients with familial amyloid polyneuropathy (FAP) and their non-affected but at risk relatives. Am. J. Med. Sci., *289*:17–21, 1985.
185. Benson, M.D., and Dwulet, F.E.: Prealbumin and retinol binding protein serum concentrations in Indiana type hereditary amyloidosis. Arthritis Rheum., *26*:1493–1498, 1983.
186. Skare, J.C., Saraiva, M.J., Alves, I.L., et al.: A new mutation causing familial amyloidotic polyneuropathy. Biochem. Biophys. Res. Commun., *164*:1240–1246, 1989.
187. Ueno, S., Uemichi, T., Yorifuji, S., and Tarvi, S.: A novel variant of transthyretin (Tyr^{114} to Cys) deduced from the nucleotide sequence of gene fragments from familial amyloidotic polyneuropathy in Japanese sibling cases. Biochem. Biophys. Res. Commun., *169*:143–147, 1990.
188. Ueno, S., Uemichi, T., Takahashi, N., et al.: Two novel variants of transthyretin identified in Japanese cases with familial amyloidotic polyneuropathy: Transthyretin (Glu^{42} to Gly) and transthyretin (Ser^{50} to Arg). Biochem. Biophys. Res. Commun., *169*:1117–1121, 1990.
189. Westermark, P., Sletten, K., Johansson, B., and Cornwell, G.G., III: Fibril in senile systemic amyloidosis is derived from normal transthyretin. Proc. Natl. Acad. Sci. U.S.A., *87*:2843–2845, 1990.
190. Gorevic, P.D., Prelli, F.C., Wright, J., et al.: Senile systemic amyloidosis identification of a new prealbumin (transthyretin) variant in cardiac tissue. J. Clin. Invest., *83*:836–843, 1989.
191. Jacobson, D.R., Gorevic, P.D., and Buxbaum, J.N.: A homogenous transthyretin variant associated with senile systemic amyloidosis: Evidence for a late-onset disease of genetic etiology. Am. J. Hum. Genet., *47*:127–136, 1990.
192. Maury, C.P.J.: Gelsolin-related amyloidosis. Identification of the amyloid protein in Finnish hereditary amyloidosis as a fragment of variant gelsolin. J. Clin. Invest., *87*:1195–1199, 1991.
193. Haltia, M., Ghiso, J., Prelli, F., et al.: Amyloid in familial amyloidosis, Finnish type, is antigenically and structurally related to gelsolin. Am. J. Pathol., *136*:1223–1228.
194. Gertz, M.A., Petitt, R.M., Perrault, J., and Kyle, R.A.: Autosomal dominant familial Mediterranean fever-like syndrome with amyloidosis. Mayo Clin. Proc., *62*:1095–1100, 1987.
195. Ghiso, J., Jensson, O., and Frangione, B.: Amyloid fibrils in hereditary cerebral hemorrhage with amyloidosis of Icelandic type is a variant of gamma-trace basic protein (cystatin C). Proc. Natl. Acad. Sci. U.S.A., *83*:2974–2978, 1986.
196. Timmers, W.F., Tagliavini, F., Haan, J., and Frangione, B.: Parenchymal preamyloid and amyloid deposits in the brains of patients with hereditary cerebral hemorrhage with amyloidosis-Dutch type. Neuroscience Lett., *118*:223–226, 1990.
197. Kyle, R.A., Pierre, R.V., and Bayrd, E.D.: Primary amyloidosis and acute leukemia associated with melphalan therapy. Blood, *44*:333–337, 1974.
198. Kyle, R.A., Griepp, P.R., Garton, J.P., and Gertz, M.A.: Primary systemic amyloidosis. Comparison of melphalan/prednisone versus colchicine. Am. J. Med., *79*:708–716, 1985.
199. Zemer, D. et al.: Colchicine in the prevention and treatment of the amyloidosis of familial Mediterranean fever. N. Engl. J. Med., *314*:1001–1005, 1986.
200. Cohen, A.S. et al.: Survival of patients with primary (AL) amyloidosis: Colchicine treated cases from 1976–1983 compared with cases seen in previous years (1961–1973). Am. J. Med., *82*:1182–1190, 1987.
201. O'Doherty, D.P., Neoptolemos, J.P., and Wood, V.F.: Place of surgery in the management of amyloid disease. Br. J. Surg., *74*:83–88, 1987.
202. Cohen, A.S. et al.: Renal transplantation in two cases of amyloidosis. Lancet, *2*:513–516, 1971.

85

Sarcoidosis

H. RALPH SCHUMACHER, JR.

Sarcoidosis is a systemic disease characterized by a noncaseating granulomatous reaction of unknown origin. Our present concept of this syndrome has evolved from the early descriptions by Hutchinson, Besnier, and Boeck,[1] as well as by Schaumann.[2] Symptoms and signs depend on the organs affected, most frequently the lymph nodes, lungs, liver, skin, and eyes. Muscle, spleen, bones, parotid glands, central nervous system, blood vessels, endocrine glands, and almost any other tissue, including the joints, may also be involved. Although generally a chronic disease, its onset can be acute, with hilar adenopathy, erythema nodosum, fever, and articular manifestations. This acute form is often termed *Lofgren's syndrome.*[3]

PATHOLOGIC FEATURES

The characteristic histopathologic features of epithelioid tubercles with minimal necrosis and no true caseation, in contrast to the lesions of tuberculosis, are the hallmark of sarcoidosis (Figs. 85–1, 85–2).[4] Studies on skin (Kveim reactions) and pulmonary lesions have identified large numbers of T-lymphocytes around the epithelioid cells. At least in the lung lesions, these are enriched with T4 "helper" cells and activated cells.[5,6] Sarcoid granulomas often contain Langhans-type giant cells with three frequent types of cytoplasmic inclusions: (1) asteroid bodies, which appear to consist of criss-crossing bundles of collagen; (2) Schaumann bodies, which are round or oval, laminated calcifications containing hydroxyapatite (Fig. 85–3); and (3) irregular, poorly stained, anisotropic, glasslike fragments.[7] Such granulomas, even with the typical inclusions, are not pathognomonic for sarcoidosis. Similar granulomatous tissue reactions can be seen in histoplasmosis, coccidioidomycosis, tuberculosis, lymphoma, Hodgkin's disease, bronchogenic carcinoma, other tumors, foreign body granuloma, drug reactions, beryllium poisoning, syphilis, and leprosy. Functional impairment in sarcoidosis appears to result from both the active granulomatous disease and the secondary fibrosis.

CAUSE AND PREVALENCE

Many have speculated on the possible causes of sarcoidosis. The incidence of tuberculosis in sarcoidosis is 4%, and an unusual reaction to Mycobacterium tuberculosis or to atypical mycobacteria is one suggested mechanism. High titers of antibody to a number of viruses and other organisms have been reported in sarcoidosis. Clustering of cases has raised suspicion of infectious factors.[8] Circulating immune complexes can be identified in up to 50% of cases, but their pathogenetic role is not clear. Alveolar macrophages may show increased receptor-mediated phagocytosis and express increased complement receptors.[9] Despite cutaneous anergy and decreased circulating T-lymphocytes, there is considerable evidence of cell-mediated immune reactivity in the pulmonary lesions.[10] Patients who have HLA antigen B8 may be more likely to express their sarcoidosis as erythema nodosum and acute arthritis.[11] HLA-DR3 may predispose individuals to sarcoid arthritis.[12] Several series in this country show a higher incidence of sarcoidosis in black females than in the general population. The disease may begin at any age, including infancy, but it is most commonly diagnosed in the third and fourth decades. Females predominate slightly over males. Sarcoidosis has a worldwide distribution, with the estimated incidence of the disease reaching as high as 64/100,000 in Sweden. American veterans after World War II had an incidence of 11/100,000.

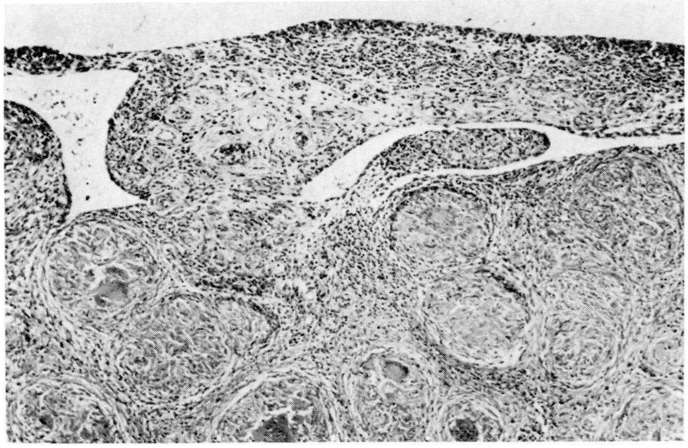

FIGURE 85–1. Granulomatous synovitis of the elbow in chronic sarcoid arthritis. (Hematoxylin and eosin stain, ×60.) The synovial tissue is crowded with discrete, noncaseating miliary tubercles. At the surface, the villi are hypertrophied and infiltrated with leukocytes and fibroblasts. The articular cartilage of this joint is intact, and the subchondral bone (olecranon and lateral condyle of humerus) is free of tubercles. (From Sokoloff, L., and Bunim, J.J.[4])

TABLE 85–1. DIAGNOSTIC FEATURES OF SARCOIDOSIS

1. Noncaseating granulomas on biopsy; one must exclude other causes of granulomas.
2. Hilar and right paratracheal adenopathy in 90%.
3. Skin lesions, uveitis, or involvement of almost any tissue.
4. Onset most often in third and fourth decades, but cases reported at all ages.
5. Impaired delayed hypersensitivity in 85%.
6. Frequent hyperglobulinemia.
7. Increased angiotensin-converting enzyme levels in about 80%.
8. Hypercalciuria in most; hypercalcemia in some.

GENERAL MANIFESTATIONS AND PROGNOSIS

The severity of manifestations can vary from an asymptomatic chest roentgenogram to death in approximately 4%. The most common symptoms and signs are fatigue (27%), malaise (15%), cough (30%), shortness of breath (28%), and chest pain (15%). Ninety-two percent of patients have abnormal chest roentgenograms. Pulmonary parenchymal involvement is more ominous than the more frequent hilar adenopathy. Restrictive lung disease and cor pulmonale can develop. Granulomatous uveitis is the most frequent visual problem. Skin lesions occur in 30% of cases. They may be nondescript, but commonly are papular or nodular, erythematous or violaceous lesions, which show the typical granulomas on histologic examination. Erythema nodosum is common in sarcoidosis of acute onset. Liver involvement is almost always asymptomatic and is evidenced mainly by hepatomegaly. An elevated alkaline phosphatase level may suggest the presence of liver granulomas.

The acute sarcoidosis, accompanied by erythema nodosum, hilar adenopathy, and arthralgia, generally has the best prognosis. Despite the similar sarcoid tissue reaction, Truelove has urged physicians to distinguish this syndrome from sarcoidosis.[13] Certainly, most patients with this acute syndrome have a full remission within 2 years, but up to 16% may have some chronic disease.[14]

DIAGNOSIS

The diagnosis of sarcoidosis is established by the demonstration of typical noncaseating granulomas in the absence of other identifiable causes of such granulomas (Table 85–1). Impaired delayed hypersensitivity on skin testing is characteristic but not invariable. Impaired tuberculin sensitivity after bacille Calmette Guérin vaccination may persist even after apparent recovery from sarcoidosis. Antibody production is normal. The elevated immunoglobulins are of little help in the differential diagnosis. Leukopenia, anemia, eosinophilia, hypercalcemia, and elevated erythrocyte sedimentation rates may be seen. Hypercalciuria is found in most cases. The serum level of angiotensin-converting enzyme (ACE) is typically elevated in active pulmonary or articular sarcoidosis.[15] ACE is produced by the granulomas, which also secrete 1,25 dihydrocholecalciferol, responsible for the absorptive hypercalciuria. Although increased ACE levels are seen in about 80% of patients, they are not unique to sarcoidosis and may also occur in inflammatory diseases of the liver,[16] Gaucher's disease, leprosy, silicosis, asbestosis, hyperthyroidism, and diabetes. ACE levels fall with successful therapy and may be useful in following treatment.[17] These levels can also be followed along with other findings in patients with mild disease who are not treated, to look for early clues to exacerbation.

Tissue diagnosis is most expeditiously established by biopsy of a skin lesion or an accessible superficial lymph node. With such superficial material, additional evidence of generalized disease is also needed because foreign body reactions can be difficult to distinguish from sarcoidosis. Liver samples also can show granulomas, especially if the liver is palpably enlarged, but a granulomatous liver reaction is common in other liver diseases,[18] and such granulomas are not as helpful in diagnosis as lymph node lesions. Mediastinoscopy in experienced hands is a safe and reliable method of obtaining lymph node tissue for diagnosis if hilar adenopathy is present. Transbronchial lung biopsy, using the fiberoptic bronchoscope, is an attractive initial biopsy procedure yielding diagnoses in about 60% of cases in one series.[19] In typical Lofgren's syndrome with asymptomatic hilar and right paratracheal adenopathy, one can sometimes observe the patient without performing a biopsy.[20] Biopsies with serial sections often show granulomas in asymptomatic muscles.[21] Israel and Sones found muscle tissue positive in 89% of patients with erythema nodosum or arthralgia.[22]

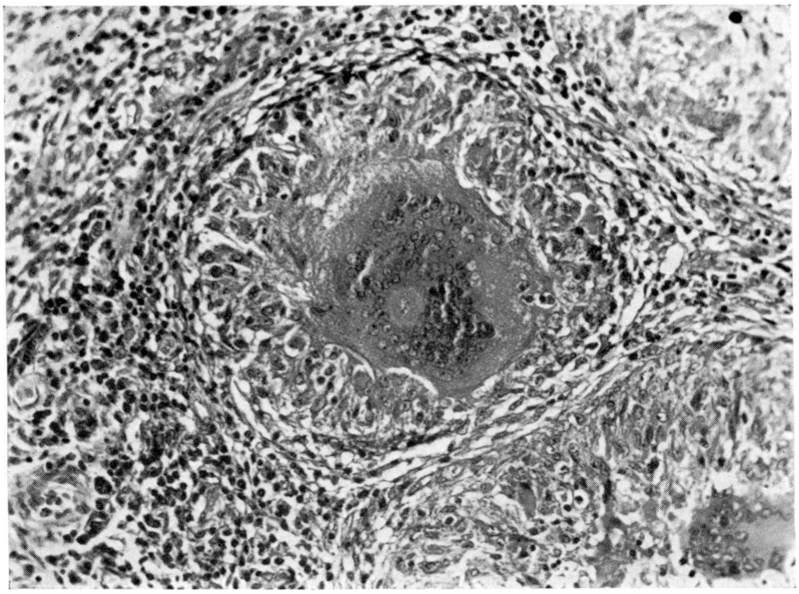

FIGURE 85–2. Multinucleated giant cell in the center of a tubercle of epithelioid cells. Surrounding the tubercle is a layer of fibroblasts and a cuff of lymphocytes, plasma cells, and mononuclear cells. This figure is an area from Figure 85–1 under higher magnification. (×175.) (From Sokoloff, L., and Bunim, J.J.[4])

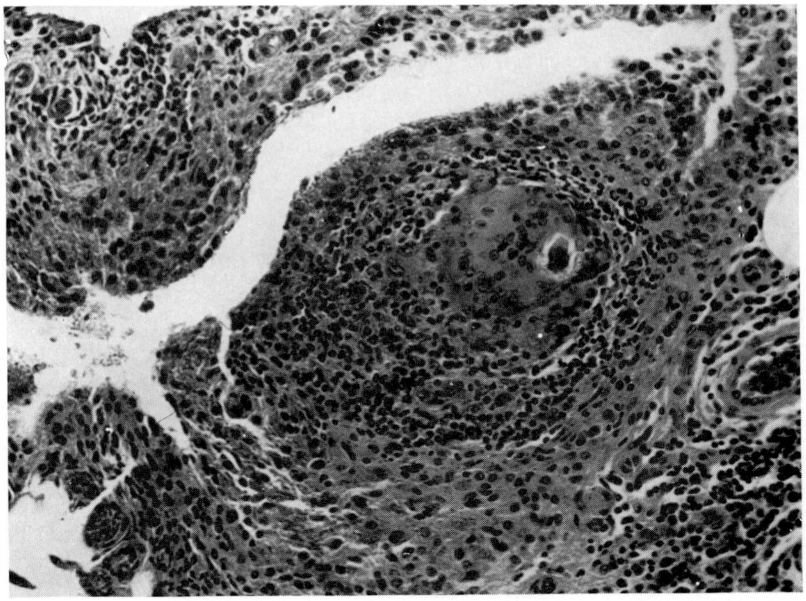

FIGURE 85–3. Section of synovial tissue from the knee of a 33-year-old black woman with sarcoid polyarthritis of about 6 weeks' duration showing granulomatous synovitis and a Schaumann body. This Schaumann body appears in the cytoplasm of a giant cell as a circular clear space and consists of a colorless, crystalloid material that is doubly refractive. No bacteria or fungi are found with Brown-Brenn, Ziehl-Neelsen, or periodic acid-Schiff stains. (From Sokoloff, L., and Bunim, J.J.[4])

An intradermal injection of 0.2 mL of a 10% saline suspension of sarcoid tissue (the Kveim test) has been used for diagnosis. A positive reaction consists of the development of a local sarcoid granuloma at the injection site. Positive test results can be obtained in 80% of patients with sarcoidosis, most often in those with prominent adenopathy, but standardization of preparations has been difficult, and reliable material is not generally available.[23]

^{67}Gallium scintigrams can assist in evaluating activity in alveolitis,[17] and they may be abnormal even in patients with normal chest roentgenograms.[24] Bronchoalveolar lavage showing more than 35 to 45% T-lymphocytes also suggests active alveolitis. Some patients without elevated numbers of lymphocytes in lavages have also responded to corticosteroid therapy, however.[17]

SPECIFIC MUSCULOSKELETAL MANIFESTATIONS

MUSCLE

Sarcoid granulomas in muscle are often asymptomatic, but they may be accompanied by local pain and tenderness, cramps, pseudohypertrophy, palpable nodules, and occasionally associated fasciitis. A symmetric proximal myopathy with weakness has also been described and has been reported to occur without evident sarcoidosis in other tissues.[25,26] Involved muscles often show noncaseating granulomas as well as lymphocytic infiltration, muscle necrosis, and regeneration. Creatine kinase levels may be elevated. Calcification of muscles and other soft tissues occasionally occurs in hypercalcemic patients. Neurosarcoidosis can produce a variety of musculoskeletal symptoms,[27] as can vascular sarcoid.

BONE

Phalangeal cysts, often considered a helpful diagnostic clue in sarcoidosis (Fig. 85–4), were described in 14% of patients in one series.[12] Although some of these cysts are due to sarcoid granulomas, others may be unrelated to the sarcoidosis. Other bones, including the skull and vertebrae, may also develop cysts from sarcoid granulomas. Large lytic or sclerotic vertebral lesions can be seen.[28] Bone sarcoidosis is usually asymptomatic. The overlying cortex is typically intact, although cortical dissolution with scalloping or acro-osteolysis and fractures through large cysts have been described.[29] The phalangeal lesions of sarcoidosis can also be associated with osteosclerosis.[30] Cystic bone lesions only occasionally extend into the joint, in which they may cause arthritis.[4] Some destructive bony lesions are associated with overlying purplish red, nodular cutaneous masses, termed *lupus pernio*,[7] or with a diffuse dactylitis.[31]

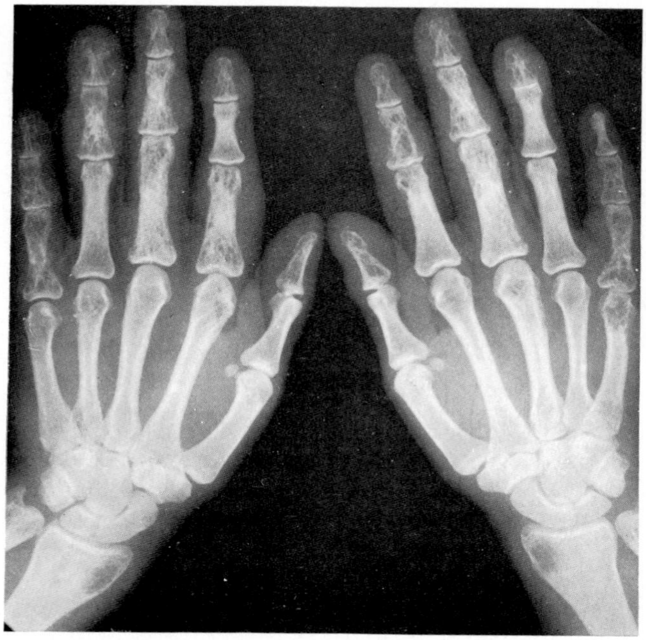

FIGURE 85–4. Roentgenograms of the hands showing unusually severe bone lesions of sarcoidosis. The bone cysts have not broken through the articular cortex. The hands shown in Figure 85–5 have similar bone changes, but with extension into the distal interphalangeal joints.

JOINTS

Arthritis was first described with sarcoidosis in 1936, and since then, arthritis, periarthritis, or arthralgia has been reported in 2 to 38% of patients in various series.[12,32–34] Chronic sarcoidosis is associated with fewer joint complaints than the acute form. Table 85–2 outlines the features of sarcoid arthropathy.

In acute sarcoidosis with hilar adenopathy, fever, and erythema nodosum, up to 89% of patients have articular symptoms, and 69 and 63% had articular or periarticular swelling in the series of Lofgren[3] and James et al.,[35] respectively. Ankles and knee joints are most frequently involved in acute sarcoidosis. Most other joints are occasionally involved. Heel pad pain is common; monoarthritis is unusual.[32] The patient generally has a dramatic, tender, warm, erythematous swelling that often is clearly periarticular rather than synovial. Such changes are occasionally difficult to separate from adjacent cutaneous erythema nodosum, and the histologic appearance of the lesions is identical. Joint motion is often painless; pain is much less than one would expect, considering the inflammatory signs. The frequency of a severe, localized tenderness has been emphasized.[36]

Roentgenograms show only soft-tissue swelling. Such articular findings may antedate erythema nodosum by as much as 2 weeks and suggest careful watch for the skin lesions. Both skin and joint lesions may antedate hilar adenopathy for up to several weeks. Ankle and knee involvement is often symmetric; joint involvement can be progressive. The acute inflammation often raises a suspicion of rheumatic fever, gonococcal or other infectious arthritis, and gout. Joint aspiration often yields no synovial fluid. When an effusion is aspirated, leukocyte counts can be as high as 42,500/mm^3, with 90% neutrophils.[37] Most effusions are only mildly inflammatory, however, with leukocyte counts of less than 1000/mm^3, predominantly lymphocytes and large mononuclear cells.

TABLE 85–2. SARCOID ARTHROPATHY

ACUTE SARCOIDOSIS (LOFGREN'S SYNDROME)

1. Often periarticular and tender, erythematous, warm swelling.
2. Ankles and knees almost invariably involved.
3. Joint involvement possibly the initial manifestation (chest film normal).
4. Joint motion possibly normal and pain absent or minimal
5. Synovial effusions infrequent and generally only mildly inflammatory
6. Usually nonspecific mild synovitis on synovial biopsy.
7. Self-limited in weeks to 4 months.

CHRONIC SARCOIDOSIS

1. Arthritis possibly acute and evanescent, recurrent, or chronic.
2. Noncaseating granulomas often demonstrable in synovium.
3. Usually nondestructive, despite chronic or recurrent disease.

Cultures are negative, and crystals cannot be identified by compensated, polarized light. Several patients with this syndrome, including an early case described by Hutchinson, had been thought to have gout before synovial fluid crystal identification was available to confirm the presence of gouty arthritis.[38] That sarcoid arthritis may respond dramatically to colchicine further confuses the issue. Elevated uric acid levels have been noted in a small percentage of patients with sarcoidosis,[34] but recent studies suggest that hyperuricemia should not be anticipated unless it is a result of drugs or renal failure. Needle synovial biopsy specimens in acute sarcoidosis most often show only mild nonspecific synovitis and some lining cell proliferation. Although much of the inflammation in acute sarcoidosis may be periarticular, synovial granulomas are occasionally found during open surgical biopsy.[4] Caplan et al. have described an identical periarthritis in 19 patients with hilar adenopathy, none of whom had erythema nodosum.[39] These workers found sarcoid granulomas in the subcutaneous tissue over three of seven inflamed ankles, but no granulomas in an open joint biopsy. Angiotensin-converting enzyme levels need not be elevated in patients with acute sarcoidosis without pulmonary parenchymal involvement.[11]

The joint manifestations of acute sarcoidosis subside in 2 weeks to 4 months, although rare patients may develop chronic sarcoid arthritis. Erythema nodosum and a similar arthropathy can also be seen in lepromatous leprosy, ulcerative colitis, regional enteritis, tuberculosis, coccidioidomycosis, histoplasmosis, oral contraceptive and possibly other drug use, pregnancy, and psittacosis and other infections. Other cases are idiopathic.

In sarcoidosis of more insidious onset, joint manifestations are less common. In such cases, even with widespread systemic granulomatous disease, the arthritis may still be mild and evanescent, as in acute sarcoidosis. Arthritis can also be recurring or protracted with polysynovitis, however. Even in patients with chronic synovitis, joint destruction is infrequent, and most roentgenograms show only soft-tissue swelling. The destructive joint disease occasionally seen in sarcoidosis is illustrated in Fig. 85–5. Such severe arthritis is most common in patients with multisystemic granulomatous disease. Arthritis may occur as an initial manifestation, or after years of systemic disease. Thus, such a variety of patterns can be seen that a high index of suspicion is needed to lead to biopsy and other diagnostic studies to differentiate this disorder from rheumatoid or other types of arthritis.

Reports of synovial fluid analysis are infrequent. We recently found joint-fluid leukocyte counts of 250 to 6250/mm^3 with predominantly mononuclear cells in six patients with arthritis associated with chronic sarcoidosis.[40] Sokoloff and Bunim found noncaseating granulomas in three of five surgical synovial biopsy specimens from patients with chronic arthritis.[4] In addition, the synovium showed diffuse chronic inflammation including plasma cells. None of their patients, and only 3.3% of those studied by Owen et al.,[37] had any elevation of rheumatoid factor, but others have found rheumatoid factor in as many as 38% of patients with sarcoidosis.[41] The presence of rheumatoid factor does not correlate with the presence or severity of joint disease. Tenosynovitis at the wrists and elsewhere can also be seen. Finger clubbing and hypertrophic osteoarthropathy[42] are occasional complications of pulmonary sarcoidosis.

Arthritis in early-childhood sarcoidosis has been described, with especially large, painless, boggy synovial and tendon sheath effusions.[43] The course of the disease is indolent, and constitutional symptoms are few. Despite prolonged synovitis, no erosive radiographic changes are seen. Synovial biopsy samples may show granulomas. Interestingly, the sarcoidosis reported in young children is associated with potentially devastating uveitis, but not with hilar adenopathy, so the relation of the syndrome to adult sarcoidosis is not clear.

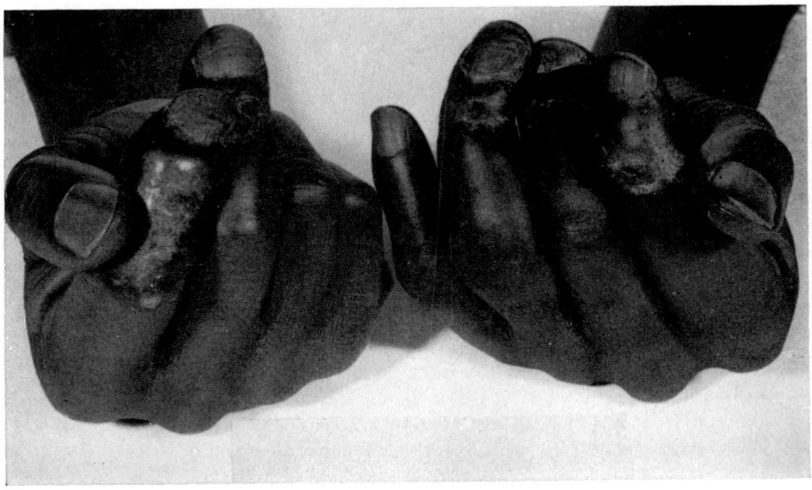

FIGURE 85–5. The hands of a 33-year-old black man with sarcoidosis of 5 years' duration. Depigmented skin lesions are present on the dorsum of fingers, and the distal phalanx of the left fourth finger is displaced. Note the fusiform swelling of the proximal interphalangeal joint of the fourth and fifth fingers of left hand (asymmetric). This patient does not have psoriasis. (From Sokoloff, L., and Bunim, J.J.[4])

TREATMENT

Many patients with minimal symptoms require no treatment. No curative agent exists. Adrenal corticosteroids are commonly used to try to suppress potentially serious active inflammatory reactions, such as ocular disease, pulmonary parenchymal disease, and central nervous system involvement, and are often effective. Corticosteroids can also lower persistently elevated serum calcium levels. Initial doses of 20 to 60 mg prednisone are tapered to the lowest effective maintenance dose. Alternate-day dosage seems effective for maintenance therapy. Objective long-term benefits from corticosteroids have often been difficult to demonstrate,[44] but improved vital capacity even in severe disease has been shown in one series.[45] Spontaneous remission can occur. Active articular disease almost always shows at least temporary improvement with corticosteroid therapy. When these agents are used, isoniazid coverage may be needed. Because joint disease is often self-limited, however, rest, salicylates, and other analgesics are often all that is required. Salicylates are not as dramatically effective as in rheumatic fever. Colchicine shortens attacks of acute arthritis in some patients,[36] but it is by no means invariably effective. Chloroquine or hydroxychloroquine have been reported to help cutaneous sarcoidosis[46] and may help some bone sarcoidosis.[47] Uncontrolled reports of methotrexate[48] and azathioprine[49] use in sarcoidosis have suggested benefit in these patients.

REFERENCES

1. Boeck, C.: Multiple benign sarkoid of the skin. J. Cutan. Genitourin. Dis., *17*:543–550, 1899.
2. Schaumann, J.N.: Etude sur le lupus pernio et ses rapports avec les sarcoides et la tuberculose. Ann. Dermatol. Syph., *6*:357–373, 1916–1917.
3. Lofgren, S.: Primary pulmonary sarcoidosis. I. Early signs and symptoms. Acta Med. Scand., *145*:424–431, 1953.
4. Sokoloff, L., and Bunim, J.J.: Clinical and pathological studies of joint involvement in sarcoidosis. N. Engl. J. Med., *260*:842–847, 1959.
5. Hunninghake, G.W., and Crystal, R.G.: Pulmonary sarcoidosis: a disorder mediated by excess helper T-lymphocyte activity at sites of disease activity. N. Engl. J. Med., *305*:429–434, 1981.
6. Konttinen, Y.T. et al.: Inflammatory cells of sarcoid granulomas detected by monoclonal antibodies and an esterase technique. Clin. Immunol. Immunopathol., *26*:380–389, 1983.
7. Longcope, W.T., and Freiman, D.G.: A study of sarcoidosis. Medicine, *31*:1–32, 1952.
8. Veale, D., and Fitzgerald, O.: Acute sarcoid arthropathy—An infective cause? Br. J. Rheum., *29*:158–159, 1990.
9. Petterson, H.B., Johnson, E., and Osen, S.S.: Phagocytosis of agarose beads by receptors for C3b (CRI) and iC3b (CR3) on alveolar macrophages from patients with sarcoidosis. Scand. J. Immunol., *32*:669–677, 1990.
10. Van Maarsseven, A.C.M., Mullink, H., Alons, C.L., and Stam, J.: Distribution of T cell subsets in different portions of sarcoid granulomas. Hum. Pathol., *17*:493–500, 1986.
11. Fitzgerald, A.A., and Davis, P.: Arthritis, hilar adenopathy, erythema nodosum complex. J. Rheumatol., *9*:935–938, 1982.
12. Krause, A., and Goebel, K.M.: Class II MHC antigen (HLA DR3) predisposes to sarcoid arthritis. J. Clin. Lab. Immunol., *24*:25–27, 1987.
13. Truelove, L.H.: Articular manifestations of erythema nodosum. Ann. Rheum. Dis., *19*:174–180, 1960.
14. Neville, E., Walker, A.N., and James, D.G.: Prognostic factors predicting the outcome of sarcoidosis: an analysis of 818 patients. Q. J. Med., *LII*:525–533, 1983.
15. Sequeira, W., and Stinar, D.: Serum angiotensin converting enzyme levels in sarcoid arthritis. Arch Int. Med., *146*:125, 1986.
16. Matsuki, K., and Sakata, T.: Angiotensin-converting enzyme in disease of the liver. Am. J. Med., *73*:549–551, 1982.
17. Lawrence, E.C. et al.: Serial changes in markers of disease activity with corticosteroid treatment in sarcoidosis. Am. J. Med., *74*:747–756, 1983.
18. Fagan, E.A., Moore-Gillon, J.C., and Turner-Warwick, M.: Multiorgan granulomas and mitochondral antibodies. N. Engl. J. Med., *308*:572–575, 1983.
19. Koontz, C.H., Joyner, L.R., and Nelson, R.A.: Transbronchial lung biopsy via the fiberoptic bronchoscope in sarcoidosis. Ann. Intern. Med., *85*:64–66, 1976.
20. Winterbauer, R.H., Belic, N., and Moores, K.D.: A clinical interpretation of bilateral hilar adenopathy. Ann. Intern. Med., *78*:65–71, 1973.
21. Stjernberg, N. et al.: Muscle involvement in sarcoidosis. Acta Med. Scand., *209*:213–216, 1981.
22. Israel, H.L., and Sones, M.: Selection of biopsy procedures for sarcoidosis diagnosis. Arch. Intern. Med., *113*:255–260, 1964.
23. James, D.G.: Editorial: Kveim revisited, reassesed. N. Engl. J. Med., *292*:859–860, 1975.
24. Nosal, A. et al.: Angiotensin-1-converting enzyme and gallium scan in non-invasive evaluation of sarcoidosis. Ann. Intern. Med., *90*:328–331, 1979.
25. Wolfe, S.M., Pinals, R.S., Aelion, J.A., et al.: Myopathy in sarcoidosis. Semin. Arthritis Rheum., *16*:300–306, 1987.
26. Janssen, M., Dijkmans, A.C., and Fulderink, F.: Muscle cramps in the calf as presenting symptom of sarcoidosis. Ann. Rheum. Dis., *50*:51–52, 1991.
27. Chapelon, C., Ziza, J.M., Piette, J.C., et al.: Neurosarcoidosis: Signs course and treatment in 35 confirmed cases. Medicine, *69*:261–276, 1990.
28. Perlman, S.G. et al.: Vertebral sarcoidosis with paravertebral ossification. Arthritis Rheum., *21*:271–277, 1978.
29. Sartoris, D.J., Resnick, D., Resnick, C., Yaghmai, I.: Musculoskeletal manifestations of sarcoidosis. Semin. Roentgenol., *20*:376–386, 1985.
30. McBrine, C.S., and Fisher, M.S.: Acrosclerosis in sarcoidosis. Radiology, *115*:279–281, 1975.
31. Liebowitz, M.R. et al.: Sarcoid dactylitis in black South African patients. Semin. Arthritis Rheum., *14*:232–237, 1985.
32. Gumpel, J.M., Johns, C.J., and Shulman, L.E.: The joint disease of sarcoidosis. Ann. Rheum. Dis., *26*:194–205, 1967.
33. Siltzbach, L.E., and Duberstein, J.L.: Arthritis in sarcoidosis. Clin. Orthop., *57*:31–50, 1968.
34. Spilberg, I., Siltzbach, L.E., and McEwen, C.: The arthritis of sarcoidosis. Arthritis Rheum., *12*:126–137, 1969.
35. James, D.G., Thomson, A.D., and Wilcox, A.: Erythema nodosum as a manifestation of sarcoidosis. Lancet, *2*:218–221, 1956.
36. Kaplan, H.: Sarcoid arthritis with a response to colchicine. N. Engl. J. Med., *268*:778–781, 1960.
37. Owen, D.S. et al.: Musculoskeletal sarcoidosis and rheumatoid factor. Med. Coll. VA Q., *8*:217–220, 1972.
38. Kaplan, H., and Klatskin, G.: Sarcoidosis, psoriasis, and gout: Syndrome or coincidence? Yale J. Biol. Med., *32*:335–352, 1960.
39. Caplan, H.I., Katz, W.A., and Rubenstein, M.: Periarticular in-

flammation, bilateral hilar adenopathy and a sarcoid reaction. Arthritis Rheum., *13*:101–111, 1970.
40. Palmer, D.G., and Schumacher, H.R.: Synovitis with non-specific histologic changes in synovium in chronic sarcoidosis. Ann. Rheum. Dis., *43*:778–782, 1984.
41. Oreskes, I., and Siltzbach, L.E.: Changes in rheumatoid factor activity during the course of sarcoidosis. Am. J. Med., *55*:60–67, 1968.
42. Rahbar, M., and Sharma, O.P.: Hypertrophic osteoarthropathy in sarcoidosis. Sarcoidosis, *7*:125–127, 1990.
43. North, A.F. et al.: Sarcoid arthritis in children. Am. J. Med., *48*:449–455, 1970.
44. Young, R.J. et al.: Pulmonary sarcoidosis: a prospective evaluation of glucocorticoid therapy. Ann. Intern. Med., *73*:207–212, 1970.
45. Emirgil, C., Sobol, B.J., and Williams, M.H.: Long-term study of pulmonary sarcoidosis. The effect of steroid therapy as evaluated by pulmonary function studies. J. Chronic Dis., *22*:69–86, 1969.
46. Jones, E., and Callen, J.P.: Hydroxychloroquine is effective therapy for control of cutaneous sarcoidal granulomas. J. Am. Acad. Dermatol., *23*:487–489, 1990.
47. De Simone, D.P., Brillant, H.L., Basile, J., et al.: Granulomatous infiltration of the talus and abnormal vitamin D metabolism in a patient with sarcoidosis; successful treatment with hydroxychloroquine. Am. J. Med., *87*:694–696, 1989.
48. Lacher, M.J.: Spontaneous remission or response to methotrexate in sarcoidosis. Ann. Intern. Med., *69*:1247–1248, 1968.
49. Krebs, P., Abel, H., and Schonberger, W.: Behandling der boeckschan sarkoidose mit immunosuppressiven substanzen. Erfahrungen mit Azatioprin (Imurel). Munchen. Med. Wochenschr., *111*:2307–2311, 1969.

86

Arthritis Associated with Hematologic Disorders, Storage Diseases, Disorders of Lipid Metabolism, and Dysproteinemias

MICHAEL H. WEISMAN

The significance of recognizing rheumatic manifestations originating from chronic systemic illness cannot be overemphasized. If a complaint or a physical finding is a presenting manifestation, then a delay in recognition can be avoided. Conversely, once a chronic illness is established, certain osteoarticular complications may dominate the clinical picture, as in hemophilia.[1,2] On occasion, therapy for a chronic illness produces an important clinical problem, hemodialysis-related arthropathy, for example.[3] Rheumatic signs and symptoms have been described in a diverse collection of hematologic conditions, storage diseases, disorders of lipoprotein metabolism, and in diseases related to immunoglobulin production and elimination.[4] Their clinical and pathophysiologic aspects are summarized here. Many of the older references are provided in the preceding version of this chapter.[4]

LEUKEMIAS AND HEMATOLOGIC SYNDROMES

The earliest manifestations of *leukemia* often include rheumatic signs and symptoms.[5–7] Children with leukemia are frequently misdiagnosed as having septic arthritis, acute rheumatic fever, juvenile rheumatoid arthritis (JRA), or Still's disease. The clinical picture may be confused further by the presence of a nondiagnostic or preleukemic (cytopenic) peripheral smear or the absence of radiographic evidence of the skeletal changes of leukemia despite severe bone pain. Most patients with leukemia show a combination of arthritis and periarthritis in a polyarticular distribution with knee and ankle joint predominance. In very young children, a diffuse dactylitis resembling sickle cell disease may occur;[8] in others the findings may be monoarticular or oligoarticular.[6,7,9] Synovial fluid analysis is almost always nondiagnostic, with leukocyte cell counts ranging from noninflammatory (50 cells/mm^3) to very inflammatory (45,000 cells per cubic millimeter).[10]

Unfortunately, delay in diagnosis often occurs. In children, bone pain out of proportion to objective evidence of arthritis, lymph node enlargement, and hematologic abnormalities have been stressed as distinguishing features.[9] Marked anemia, leukopenia, or thrombocytopenia in the setting of bone or joint pain in a child should alert the clinician to search for leukemia. Bone pain is most likely a consequence of leukemic involvement of the periarticular periosteum; however, leukemic infiltration into synovium or juxta-articular bone, as well as hemorrhage, may play a role.[7] Other, still unknown, mechanisms must be involved, because several studies have shown no synovial, periosteal, or periarticular bony leukemic infiltration.[10,11] Blast cells were seen in synovial fluid by light microscopy in a patient with acute lymphoblastic leukemia,[12] and immunologic evidence of B lymphocyte synovial infiltration was found in another patient with chronic B-cell leukemia-associated arthritis of the knees.[13]

Less dramatic articular involvement may also occur in the *chronic leukemias,* appearing late in the disease course, heralding disease exacerbation or blast crisis.[4,7,14] Patients with acute as well as chronic leukemias have a higher than expected frequency of positive tests for antinuclear antibodies and rheumatoid factor;[4,7,9] the significance of this finding is unknown. Chronic lymphocytic leukemia of T-cell origin has produced a picture of nonerosive polyarthritis resembling seronegative RA with skin nodules and T-cell infiltration of skin, synovial tissues, and bone marrow.[14] (See Chapter 122 for HTLV-1-associated rheumatic syndromes described by Nishioka and his colleagues.) Polymyositis has been reported in association with leukemias.[15]

Bone scintigraphy may show increased juxta-articular uptake as an important clue to the diagnosis of leukemic arthropathy.[16] Conventional roentgenograms reveal a multiplicity of abnormalities in acute leukemia[4,17–19] including osteopenia, lytic lesions, cortical and periosteal defects, distortion of trabecular patterns, pathologic fractures, osteosclerosis, and periosteal new bone. Children may display juxta-epiphyseal radiolucent bands in actively growing metaphyseal cortices at the ends of long bones. This particular abnormality, however, is nonspecific and is associated with other disturbances of osteogenesis.[19] Similar radiographic abnormalities occur in the chronic leukemias with the proximal portions of the femora and humeri, the pelvic bones, and the vertebrae most often affected.[19] Osteolytic and sclerotic changes in these areas may represent foci of a blastic crisis.[16]

False-positive or false-negative studies plague the diagnostician in many of these cases. A 9-year-old child with chronic myelogenous leukemia presented with aseptic necrosis of the femoral head, documented by biopsy with a normal radiograph.[20] Bone scintigraphy performed in another case with in vivo labeled granulocytes, revealed abnormal intravascular persistence of the labeled cells. Acute leukemia, restricted to the bone marrow, was discovered.[21] Typical "cold" lesions on bone scanning, thought to be infection, later turned out to be acute leukemia in two children.[22] Such scanning may localize pathologic changes, but diagnosis requires tissue.

Hairy cell leukemia (*HCL*), felt to be B cell in origin and presenting in middle-aged men with associated splenomegaly and cytopenias, may be accompanied by vasculitis and/or arthritis.[4] Systemic vasculitis follows usually within 2 years of the onset of HCL.[23,24] Most cases resemble polyarteritis nodosa (PAN), but a few display cutaneous small vessel vasculitis alone; mononuclear cells in the vessel walls are the predominant histologic feature.[24] A substantial number of patients with HCL have been reported to manifest arthritis or arthralgia. Oligoarthritis, dermal vasculitis, or erythema nodosum was found in 10 of 37 HCL patients in one series, suggesting an autoimmune mechanism for these rheumatic findings.[25] The link between HCL and vasculitis has not been explained; studies have failed to reveal signs of immune complex mechanisms.[26] Hairy cell infiltration of vessel walls has been demonstrated in a few cases.[24] The absence of correlation between the activity of HCL and its nonleukemic manifestations such as vasculitis or other "autoimmune" features remains a mystery.[25] Finally, destructive bone involvement, a direct manifestation of HCL, has been reported in 11 cases and may be favorably affected by radiation therapy.[27]

A review of 162 cases of *myelodysplastic syndromes* (insidious onset, usually in the elderly, ineffective hematopoiesis, normo- or hypercellular bone marrow, cytopenias, possible transformation to acute leukemias) revealed 10% with several rheumatic manifestations including cutaneous vasculitis, "lupus-like" syndrome, neuropathy, and concomitant rheumatic disease.[28] The majority of those with rheumatic features came from a subgroup called "refractory anemia with excess blasts." The potential immunologic imbalance created by the neoplastic transformation of the pluripotent stem cell was postulated as predisposing toward vasculitis. Because the rheumatic manifestations may precede the onset of ineffective hematopoiesis, the combination of clinical features of vasculitis and/or connective tissue disease, one or more cytopenias, and antinuclear antibody (ANA) negativity suggest a workup for a myelodysplastic syndrome.[28]

Neuroblastoma, known to mimic many of the clinical manifestations of childhood leukemia, may display a variety of musculoskeletal complaints. In a series of 109 children, 20 presented with complaints of hip pain, back pain, limp, or leg weakness.[29] Many were misclassified and initially treated as having septic arthritis. Compared to 74 children with hip sepsis, however, the anemia was more pronounced and should have suggested correct diagnosis earlier.[29]

Two rarer hematologic conditions may also be associated with osteoarticular signs and symptoms. *Sinus histiocytosis with massive lymphadenopathy* (SHML)—a benign childhood entity presenting with cervical adenopathy, leukocytosis, and hyper-γ-globulinemia—has produced osseous abnormalities in large joints resembling leukemia or metastatic neuroblastoma.[30] *Extramedullary hematopoiesis* of the deep synovium was found in a patient with myelofibrosis.[31] An elbow effusion was accompanied by a superficial synovitis.

Treatment of articular signs and symptoms in general should be subsumed by the management of the underlying malignancy. But joint symptoms in some patients with acute leukemia, however, have been suppressed by salicylates or other anti-inflammatory agents, a response that further confused the diagnosis.[4] The disappearance of bone and joint pain is often one of the first indications of response to antileukemic therapy.

LYMPHOMA

MALIGNANT LYMPHOMAS

Skeletal involvement is commonly seen in the *lymphomas*.[4,17,18,32] Bone defects, roentgenographically evident in as many as 15% of patients with *Hodgkin's disease*, have been found at postmortem examination in up to 50% of such patients.[4,32] Sites of involvement include the spine, pelvis, ribs, femur, skull, and shoulder. Symptoms referable to these lesions include deep pain, unremitting and worse at night, as well as pain caused by pathologic fracture, particularly in vertebrae. Diagnostic difficulty, however, may arise when articular signs or symptoms occur in the absence of radiographically evident bone lysis or lymph node enlargement. The diagnosis of reticulum cell sarcoma was established by the demonstration of malignant cells in synovial fluid from a symptomatic joint at a time when such cells were absent from the peripheral blood and bone marrow.[33] Such direct involvement of joint tissues is unusual.[34] One patient with a poorly differentiated, diffuse lymphoma initially had sternoclavicular joint arthritis.[35]

Six cases of *non-Hodgkin's lymphoma* primarily in joint tissues (capsule and/or synovium) have been reported.[36] Patients may present with either polyarticular disease or with monoarthritis. Lymphadenopathy and splenomegaly may not be apparent, and conventional radiographs typically do not reveal bone destruction in the vicinity of the involved joint. A synovial and/or bone biopsy was required for diagnosis.[36]

Primary *non-Hodgkin's lymphoma of bone* or *reticulum cell sarcoma of bone* without involvement of regional lymph nodes or distant viscera is a morphologically diverse condition affecting primarily young men. Involvement is usually localized to the ends of long bones.[37–39] A middle-aged woman presenting clinically with a monoarthritis showed a fine periosteal reaction along the distal femoral metaphysis radiographically; the synovial fluid was bloody and noninflammatory.[39] Malignant cells infiltrated the medullary canals and hyperplastic synovial villi. This lymphoma arose in bone, expanded to the contiguous synovium but did not extend into the joint space. Conventional synovial fluid analyses as well as cytologic examinations are nondiagnostic in such cases, reflecting the periarticular nature of the process. Computerized tomography (CT) and/or bone scintigraphy may suggest a periarticular focus. Tissue examination, of either synovium or bone, is critical to establishing a diagnosis.

Angioimmunoblastic lymphadenopathy with dysproteinemia (AILD) is a lymphoproliferative disease with unique histopathologic features and a fatal prognosis.[40–42] A 70-year-old man with sicca syndrome displayed extranodal histologic features of AILD on lip and kidney biopsies.[42] In another case the generalized manifestations of a nodular, poorly differentiated lymphocytic lymphoma (*follicular small cleaved cell lymphoma*) produced polymyalgia rheumatica symptoms and an extensive perivascular lymphomatous infiltrate of the temporal arteries without frank vasculitis.[43] This patient displayed prominent features of temporal or giant cell arteritis at the time the lymphoma was disseminating. A seronegative rheumatoid-like arthritis can be seen in AILD, and in one case the synovium was infiltrated with AILD.[44] The arthritis disappeared with chemotherapy-induced remission.

The underlying reasons for the occurrence of rheumatic manifestations in the lymphoproliferative disorders are not known; multiple mechanisms may play a role. The prevalence of "autoimmune perturbations" from 637 cases were noted to be 8%, compared to 1.7% in a comparison population of myeloproliferative disorders.[45] As prognosis improved in the lymphoproliferative disorders, the proportion of patients with autoimmune disorders increased. Tumor infiltration, by itself, is not sufficient to cause these secondary syndromes. A biopsy of synovium in a patient with arthritis associated with cutaneous T-cell lymphoma revealed nonspecific findings, suggesting a "reactive" arthritis.[46] Erythema nodosum was observed to occur in a patient with non-Hodgkin's lymphoma; its time course suggested a relationship to chemotherapy with cellular breakdown and release of neoantigens.[47]

MULTIPLE MYELOMA AND AMYLOID ARTHROPATHY

In most cases, pain in the back or proximal extremities, frequently the earliest symptom of *multiple myeloma*, is attributable to disease of the bone, and roentgenograms often reveal osteoporosis and osteolytic defects.[17,18,48] Persons with multiple myeloma may develop amyloid arthropathy. Pain and swelling of the joints, most commonly the shoulders, wrists, knees, and fingers, is the hallmark of the disease (see also Chapter 84). One may note prominent enlargement of the shoulders (shoulder-pad sign) and a rubbery, hard consistency of the periarticular connective tissue resulting from deposition of amyloid protein.[4] Amyloid deposits can be identified by histochemical and electron-microscopic techniques in articular cartilage, in perichondrocytic lacunae, in synovium, and in synovial fluid debris including fragments of synovial villi[49,50] (Fig. 86–1).

The presence of morning stiffness, fatigue, polyarticular involvement, periosteal nodular deposits of amyloid, and occasional bony erosion and destruction may closely simulate the clinical features of RA[4,49–51] (see also Chapter 84). However, the duration of morning stiffness is shorter and fatigue is more prominent than in RA, and the synovial fluid findings are completely inconsistent with RA. In amyloid arthropathy, synovial fluid viscosity is preserved, and it contains fewer leukocytes (200 to 4500/mm^3), predominantly mononuclear cells.[4,49–51] Synovial fluid pellets, stained with Congo red and viewed under polarized light, demonstrate yellow-green intracellular and extracellular amyloid.[49] Although the radiographic findings of amyloid arthropathy may be superficially reminiscent of RA, extensive soft tissue nodular masses, well-defined cystic lesions with or without surrounding sclerosis, and preservation of joint space are more characteristic of amyloid joint disease.[48,52] Many of these lesions resemble gouty arthritis. Lucencies, cysts, and osteolytic defects are often present but do not directly abut the articular surface. An exceptional case has been reported with multiple myeloma and typical findings of amyloid joint disease; radiographs, however, revealed typical rheumatoid erosions of the carpus and ulnar styloid as well as joint space narrowing of the metacarpophalangeal and proximal interphalangeal joints.[52] Biopsy revealed amyloid deposits without evidence of synovial inflammation.

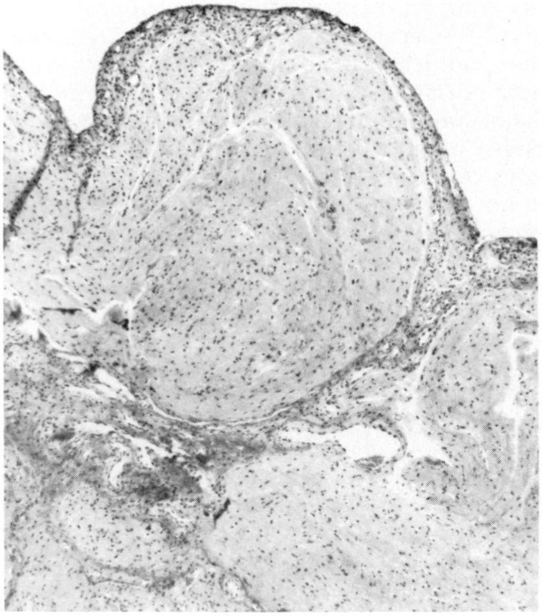

FIGURE 86–1. Photomicrograph of synovium obtained from the right shoulder of a 56-year-old woman with multiple myeloma who had developed pain in this shoulder and inability to use her arm 10 days earlier, following a fall. The humerus was dislocated. At the time of open reduction of this dislocation, large deposits of amyloid were found in the glenoid fossa. Note the mass of amyloid covered by a thin rim of synovium. The material in this nodule stained metachromatically with crystal violet.

Amyloidosis occurs in association with all forms of myeloma, including the IgD and pure Bence Jones varieties, but it is found most frequently in patients with pure light chain disease or with monoclonal IgA myelomas[4,53] (see also Chapter 84). Although typical amyloid arthropathy is found most frequently in association with multiple myeloma, it has been reported with primary amyloidosis.[4] In contrast, it is rare and indeed may not occur in those with generalized secondary amyloidosis. The incidence of typical amyloid arthropathy in multiple myeloma is estimated to be about 5%.[50] Amyloid deposits may be seen in small quantities from synovial biopsy specimens in some patients with secondary amyloidosis.[4]

Amyloid is frequently deposited in the carpal tunnel and may compress the median nerve, causing carpal tunnel syndrome.[4] Prevalence figures range from 20% of all cases of amyloid itself[51] to 45% of all patients with amyloid arthropathy reported in a review of the literature from 1931 to 1975[4] (see also Chapter 84). The concurrence of multiple myeloma, symmetric polyarthropathy, and carpal tunnel syndrome strongly suggests amyloidosis. Amyloidogenic proteins, the chemical structure of the fibrils, and information about the molecular biology of the amyloidoses are discussed in Chapter 84.

Skeletal involvement in multiple myeloma may be limited to diffuse osteoporosis, but one may also see circumscribed lytic areas, expansile lesions, or ill-defined diffuse areas of bone destruction ("moth-eaten" bone).[54] Scintigraphic or magnetic resonance examination may be helpful by demonstrating osseous lesions not detected by conventional radiography (see Chapter 6). Patients with Waldenstrom's macroglobulinemia may also exhibit bony changes including osteoporosis, isolated or multiple osteolytic defects resembling those seen in multiple myeloma, and multilocular cyst-like lesions found in the supra-acetabular portions of the iliac bones.[4,55] Typical amyloid arthropathy has been described in one patient with Waldestrom's macroglobulinemia,[4] and neuropathic joint disease secondary to amyloid neuropathy in another.[55]

POEMS syndrome is an acronym suggested for the combination in a single patient of plasma cell dyscrasia with polyneuropathy, organomegaly, endocrinopathy, M protein, and skin changes.[56] Other findings include hyperhidrosis, skin thickening, hyperpigmentation, gynecomastia or amenorrhea, and hirsutism. In addition to the radiographic presence of sclerotic plasmacytomas in the spine and pelvis, bony proliferation is apparent at sites of tendon and ligament attachment to bone, often with associated irregular bony excrescences involving the posterior elements of the spine.[57] The significance of paraproteins in the pathogenesis of this disorder, including its endocrine manifestations, is unknown.

An acquired form of amyloidosis is now recognized as a frequent accompaniment of long-term hemodialysis, and several reviews have addressed the important issues of etiopathogenesis, clinical characteristics, and management.[3,58] Amyloid in this syndrome has thus far been demonstrated primarily in articular and periarticular structures with generally negative results obtained from abdominal fat aspirations.[59] However, positive fat aspirates were found in in 3 of 12 patients treated with dialysis for nearly 11 years. Amyloid was found deposited in colon mucus and in rectal biopsy specimens as well, suggesting that, with time, dialysis patients may develop systemic amyloidosis.[60]

Arthralgias, knee swelling, painful stiff shoulders, and carpal tunnel syndrome are prominent and frequent features.[58,60,61] Studies of synovial fluid are not extensive; available data suggest that the fluid is generally noninflammatory or grossly bloody.[58,60,62,63] Synovial fragments staining with Congo red are common and helpful diagnostically.[62] The overall frequency of dialysis-related amyloid relates to the length of time on dialysis. Many of the pathologic features are similar to those observed in the amyloid arthropathy of myeloma, including erosions and radiolucent cysts in the hand and wrist, a destructive arthropathy needing surgery, or femoral neck cysts leading to pathologic fractures.[64,65] Subchondral bone cysts and/or erosions may be present for years, followed by relatively rapid narrowing of cartilage and collapse of subchondral bone.[58]

Hemodialysis-related amyloid is composed of β_2-microglobulin.[66,67] In renal failure, the serum level of this protein increases in conjunction with serum creatinine; its gradual accumulation in the tissues is felt to be responsible for the syndrome.[58] Use of the standard cuprophane dialysis membrane appears to have been important for the amyloid accumulations.[68] Hemofiltration with more highly permeable membranes reduces serum levels of this molecule and attendant amyloidosis.[68,69] The factors responsible for the largely articular and osseous accumulation, and the molecular mechanisms responsible for its deposition, remain to be elucidated.

Synovial amyloid obtained at the time of knee arthroscopy has been shown to contain β_2-microglobulin,[63] confirming other studies of amyloid from tissues obtained from the carpal tunnel or from bone.[66,70,71] The clinical spectrum of osteoarticular manifestations has broadened to include a destructive spondyloarthropathy.[72,73] Of 80 patients undergoing long-term hemodialysis, 9% developed an erosive spondylarthropathy with intervertebral disc space narrowing and major erosions at the vertebral end plates.[74,75] The prevalence of lesions attributable to renal osteodystrophy was almost identical to the prevalence of amyloid-related osteoarthropathy.[74]

The cervical vertebrae are most often affected radiologically, although many patients remain asymptomatic.[76] Further, it is clear that spinal destructive lesions have a multifactorial pathogenesis. From a series of 100 dialyzed cases, two groups were identified.[77] Those patients in whom arthropathy occurred early were older, had chondrocalcinosis, and had no carpal tunnel syndrome or osteoarticular bone defects. The second group of patients experienced later-onset disease, shoulder pain, juxta-articular bone cysts, and no chondrocalcinosis. Amyloidosis was identified in the second group.[77]

The generic term *dialysis-related arthropathy* has been suggested because of the complex and multiple mechanisms operating in these patients.[78] Among the factors deemed to be important are age, pre-existing joint disease, length of dialysis, synovial iron deposits, deposition of amyloid in cysts, and hyperparathyroidism.[78] When two different dialysis membranes, cellulose and polyacrylonitrile, were examined for their influence on the prevalence of signs and symptoms of amyloidosis, no differences were noted.[79] In a study of 56 peritoneal dialysis patients, similar findings to hemodialysis patients (carpal tunnel, shoulder pain, subchondral cysts, destructive arthropathies) were noted.[80] Finally, the relationship between inflammatory synovitis, amyloid deposition, and cystic radiolucent lesions in carpal bones has not been fully clarified.[81] There is no question that great concern is being raised about this newly recognized syndrome that is unique to the dialytic patient.[82,83] Potential modifications of dialysis techniques need to be explored, but it is also quite evident that diagnostic studies have advanced faster than have effective management strategies.

SICKLE CELL DISEASE AND OTHER HEMOGLOBINOPATHIES

The rheumatic manifestations of *sickle cell disease* are felt to be major contributing factors to its long-term morbidity.[84] Sickle cell crisis is frequently associated with severe periarticular pain and objective signs of arthritis manifested by warmth, swelling, and tenderness.[4] Joint involvement is almost always monarticular or pauciarticular, and the knees and elbows are most commonly involved. Synovial fluid is usually not inflammatory and is often clear, with a normal viscosity and a leukocyte count of fewer than 1000 cells per cubic millimeter, containing a low percentage of polymorphonuclear leukocytes. Sickled erythrocytes can be seen in these effusions. A few reports note sterile inflammatory effusions with high cell counts and no crystals.[4] Crystal-induced synovitis has been documented in a few reports,[85,86] the mechanism of hyperuricemia and secondary gout in sickle cell disease is discussed in Chapter 105.

Synovial biopsies obtained at the time of acute joint disease show little cellular infiltrate, prominent congestion of small blood vessels, and in a few cases, definite microvascular thrombosis.[4] Microvascular obstruction probably leads to infarction of synovium and adjacent bone and may account for joint effusions and inflammation. The painful crisis very likely results from ischemia of bone marrow in an intermediate zone of blood supply between the main nutrient artery and the perforating synovial vessels. Maximal intensity of bone pain in juxta-articular areas supports this hypothesis.[87]

Bone marrow scans using Technetium (^{99m}Tc) sulfur colloid and other isotopes reveal diminished uptake in the bone marrow adjacent to painful joints, suggesting infarction.[4] Scintigraphic defects occur in the absence of roentgenographic evidence of marrow or bone infarction and may precede these findings by many months. A normal scan in a symptomatic area may suggest another process, such as infection. On occasion, however, joint inflammation is followed by a rapid destruction of the articular cartilage. The presence of prominent lymphocytic and plasma cell infiltrates in these patients suggests a possible immune-mediated mechanism. Cryoprecipitable immune complexes have been implicated in sickle cell nephropathy,[88] and an abnormality of the alternate pathway of complement activation has been demonstrated in the serum of patients with sickle cell disease.[89] No evidence for immune mechanisms in sickle cell arthropathy has yet been uncovered, however.

The skeletal lesions characteristic of this hemoglobinopathy may be separated into those related to hyperplasia of bone marrow and those resulting from local thrombosis and infarction.[4] Bone marrow proliferation is associated with widening of medullary cavities, thinning of cortices, coarsening and irregularity of trabecular markings, and cupping of vertebral bodies. Lesions believed to result from sickle cell thrombosis and infarction include cortical bone infarcts with periostitis and periosteal elevation, bone marrow lysis, sclerosis and fibrosis, and most notably, avascular necrosis (AVN) of the femoral and humeral heads. Less commonly, one sees infarction in the distal portion of the femur, the radius, patella, and the vertebrae.[4]

The radiographic features vary with the age of the patient, presumably related to the different areas of the skeleton vulnerable to ischemia at specific times of maturity.[90] Subchondral and intraosseous hemorrhages contribute to the destruction of articular cartilage in the hip. Avascular necrosis of the femoral head has been reported in patients with S-S (sickle cell) disease and sickle cell trait, as well as in those with hemoglobin S-C disease, sickle cell thalassemia, and hemoglobin S-F disease.[4] Avascular necrosis occurs in 20 to 68% of patients with S-C disease but in only 4 to 12% of those with S-S disease.[4] In one study, the incidence of AVN was not increased in patients with sickle cell trait, when compared with age-matched control subjects with A-A hemoglobin.[91] Total hip replacement has been successful in some patients with these hemoglobinopathies.[92]

Although it has generally been assumed that infarction of the femoral head is caused by sickle cell thrombosis of the fine leakage of plasma proteins.

Young children with sickle cell disease may have transient swelling and tenderness of their hands and feet as a result of periostitis of the metacarpal, metatarsal, and proximal phalangeal bones, a condition known as sickle cell dactylitis.[4,93] Dactylitis may occur even before the diagnosis of sickle cell disease is established. In addition to periosteal elevation and subperiosteal new bone formation, roentgenograms reveal radiolucent areas intermingled with areas of increased density, giving a moth-eaten appearance. These changes have been interpreted as representing infarction.[4] In most cases, the integrity of the affected bones is restored to normal in several months without residual deformity or alteration in growth. The rarity of this "hand-and-foot" syndrome after the fourth year of life is explained by the recession of red marrow from the cooler distal bones and its replacement by fibrous tissue.[4]

Another striking skeletal complication of sickle cell disease is salmonella osteomyelitis, which may be multifocal.[4] The first radiographic signs of this infection, which usually starts in the medullary cavity of the long tubular bones, is periosteal proliferation. Bony destruction extending throughout the shaft then follows. Septic arthritis, although less common than osteomyelitis, has been reported to be due to many organisms, including salmonellae,[4] staphylococci, Escherichia coli, Fusobacterium varium,[94] and Serratia liquefaciens.[95] Staphylococci and Serratia organisms have also been responsible for osteomyelitis in these patients.[4] After successful treatment with antibiotics, the bones usually heal with minimal deformity. The serum of many patients with sickle cell anemia is deficient in opsonin for salmonellae and pneumococci, and their leukocytes are therefore limited in their ability to phagocytose these microorganisms.[96] This impairment has been attributed to a defective alternative complement pathway.[97] Local vascular insufficiency associated with sickling may also adversely affect the host response to infection and the efficacy of antibiotic treatment.[98] A clear distinction between acute osteomyelitis and vaso-occlusive bone crises was not possible because the typical radiographic and clinical aspects of osteomyelitis also were noted in many cases of aseptic bone infarction.[99]

In a comparative review and characterization of 14 osteoarticular infections in 13 children, however, fever was present in all cases, immature neutrophil forms (bands) were commonly seen in the peripheral blood, and the erythrocyte sedimentation rate (ESR) was elevated in 80% of cases. Bone infections were almost exclusively gram-negative, and septic arthritis alone was almost always gram-positive.[100] In 14 patients with septic arthritis associated with sickle cell disease, a staphylococcus was identified in 11 and salmonella in only 2.[101] Although proof from the literature is lacking, the epiphyseal vessels, occlusion may be the result of fat emboli. Systemic fat embolization, apparently originating in infarcted necrotic bone marrow, has been reported in hemoglobin S-C disease, as well as in sickle cell anemia.[4]

Although the pathogenesis of sickle cell arthropathy is thought to be ischemic in origin, it remains unclear of the associated noninflammatory synovial effusions represent "sympathetic effusions" or occur as a result of synovial ischemia. The incidence and pattern of articular disease was studied prospectively for 2½ years in 37 consecutive patients attending a sickle cell clinic in Jamaica.[87] Gout and ischemic bone necrosis were excluded. Twelve patients developed arthritis during a painful crisis; 13 patients had miscellaneous causes of arthritis, and 12 others displayed noninflammatory ankle effusions associated with the spontaneous development or deterioration of leg ulcers. Painful crises were associated with arthritis 20% of the time. The leg ulcers were felt to be vaso-occlusive in origin, and the chronic ankle joint effusions resolved with ulcer healing. It was hypothesized that synovial ischemia occurs in parallel with the ischemic leg ulcer, supporting the concept of primary synovial involvement.[87] If small synovial vessels participate in this process, as has been demonstrated during crises, the resultant ischemia could conceivably cause permeability changes in synovial capillary endothelium with choice of drainage technique (needle vs. open) in the initial management of sickle cell joint sepsis should be no different from the approach taken toward a patient with septic arthritis in the setting of any chronic underlying illness.

Although the pattern and prognosis of septic arthritis in sickle cell disease varies in different parts of the world, a large Nigerian experience emphasises several important points.[102] In 50 septic joints in 31 patients, the following observations were made: The hip was the most common site; polyarticular involvement occurred in 39% of cases; and contiguous osteomyelitis was present in 84%. Severe complications occurred in 76% of cases, mostly relating to delayed diagnosis and to the high frequency of hip joint infection. In contrast to most American studies, septic arthritis was not uncommon. This complication represented 12% of a total of 266 skeletal events seen in 207 consecutive patients over 5 years. In contrast, an American series of 600 children followed for 10 years reported only three cases of septic arthritis, all of whom had contiguous osteomyelitis of adjacent bone.[103] Two of these involved the hip or shoulder, a rare site for sickle cell arthropathy accompanying hemolytic crises.

A specific osteoarthropathy has been described in patients with β-*thalassemia* major, as well as in those with thalassemia minor.[104,105] Twenty-five of 50 patients between the ages of 5 and 33 years with β-thalassemia major had evidence of periarticular disease marked by pain and swelling of the ankles and pain on compression of the malleoli, calcaneus, and forefoot.[104] Synovial fluid obtained from the ankle joint in two of these patients was noninflammatory. Hyperplasia of the synovial lining cells and a heavy deposition of hemosiderin were found. Radiographic changes included osteopenia, widened medullary spaces, thin cortices with coarse trabeculations, and evidence of microfractures. The presence of microfractures was confirmed histologically; increased osteoblastic and resorptive (osteoclastic) surfaces, with iron deposits at the calcification front and cement lines, were noted. The arthropathy in these persons appears to be related to the underlying bone disease, although the role of iron overload in the pathogenesis remains to be fully evaluated. A similar form of pauciarticular, nonerosive, seronegative arthropathy was observed in persons with thalassemia minor.[105] Bilateral AVN of the femoral heads has been reported in a patient with this condition.[106]

Recurrent episodes of arthritis in thalassemia minor have been described as gout-like, lasting less than 10 days, and self-limited.[107] The ESR is always normal, and the synovial fluid from four cases showed 1500 and 8000 leukocytes per cubic millimeter, mostly mononuclear cells, and no crystals. Synovial biopsy revealed nonspecific, mildly inflammatory synovitis with local infiltration by lymphocytes and plasma cells and lining cells one to three layers thick. The authors speculated that the synovial inflammation followed primary compromise of the microvasculature. No evidence of bone disease was uncovered in contrast to thalassemia major, in which arthropathy is related to juxta-articular bone disease.

The rare, but reported, convergence of two chronic joint diseases (sickle cell, RA) in the same patient poses diagnostic and treatment confusion, although the radiographic features of each are distinctive.[108] Intra-articular corticosteroids may precipitate sickle cell crisis.[109]

STORAGE DISEASES

The *lysosomal storage diseases* are uncommon inborn errors of metabolism resulting from the deficiency or absence of specific lysosomal hydrolases.[110,111] Because the lysosome breaks down aging macromolecules, the enzyme deficiencies result in accumulation and storage of large amounts of substrate in multiple organ systems and connective tissue, including the skeleton. The target tissues are related to the sites of normal degradation of the specific macromolecule. Most cases represent inherited autosomal recessive traits, with the notable exception of Fabry's disease, an X-linked disorder with manifestations in females. The lysosomal storage diseases include most of the lipid storage disorders, the mucopolysaccaridoses, the mucolipidoses, glycoprotein storage diseases, and others. Skeletal features of the most common gangliosidoses and certain other storage diseases are discussed here.

GAUCHER'S DISEASE

Gaucher's disease is a heritable lysosomal sphingolipid storage disease characterized by the accumulation of the glycolipid glucocerebroside, or glucosylceramide, in reticuloendothelial cells in the bone marrow, spleen, liver, lymph nodes, and other internal organs.[4,112] Three clinical forms of Gaucher's disease are recognized. Type 1, by far the most common, is the chronic, non-neuronopathic, "adult" form of the disease; type 2 is the infantile or acute neuronopathic form, with an average survival rate of less than 1 year; and type 3 is the juvenile or subacute neuronopathic form. All are transmitted as autosomal recessive disorders. In type 1 the patient is deficient in lysosomal glucocerebrosidase, whereas in type 2, both this enzyme and a soluble β-glucosidase are lacking.[112] The adult form is 30 times more frequent among Ashkenazic Jews; this form may be diagnosed at any age, but it is one of the lysosomal storage diseases most likely to present to an internist.

Osteoarticular complaints are an important feature in both type 1 and type 3 Gaucher's disease. Symptoms result from infiltration of the bone marrow by lipid-laden histiocytes (Gaucher's cells) and are often the earliest disease manifestation.[4,112] The most common rheumatic complaint is acute, severe pain in the extremities, particularly in a hip, knee, or shoulder. Such painful bone crises are more common in children, but they occur in both juvenile and adult forms of the disease. When accompanied by signs of inflammation and fever, such episodes may mimic pyogenic osteomyelitis and have been called "pseudo-osteomyelitis."[4,113] In many ways, these crises resemble those of sickle cell anemia. Their exact cause is unknown, but vasospasm or vascular occlusion of end arteries within bone may result from deposition of Gaucher's cells and may increase the intramedullary pressure, leading to ischemia, necrosis, and local hemorrhage. Symptoms may last from days to weeks, but they eventually resolve.

The patient may also have pathologic fractures of long bones, as well as compression deformity of vertebrae causing low back pain.[4] In rare cases, the patient has migratory polyarthritis, the nature of which is poorly understood. Joint disease is usually monarticular or pauciarticular and involves the large points, in which it appears to be related to changes in adjacent bone.[4] Small joint involvement, including the proximal inter-

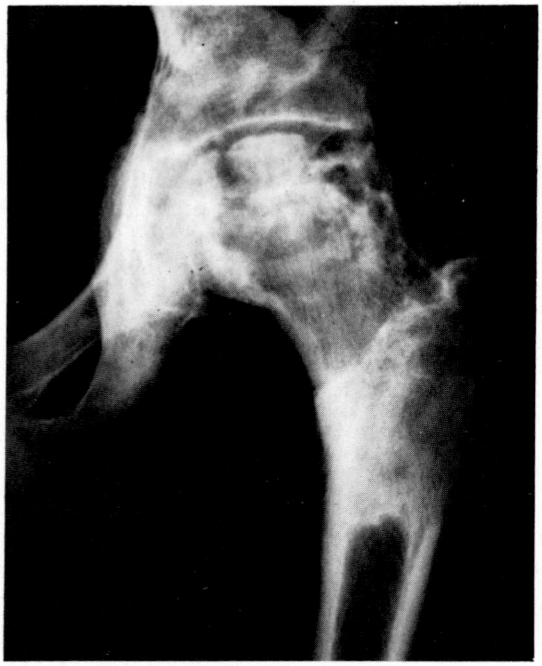

FIGURE 86–2. Roentgenogram of the left hip joint of a 22-year-old man with Gaucher's disease illustrating avascular necrosis of the head of the femur. This roentgenogram was obtained 2 years after the onset of pain in the hip.

phalangeal joints, is most uncommon.[114] Several reports cite severe degenerative hip disease as a result of AVN and collapse of the head of the femur[4,115] (Fig. 86–2). Total hip arthroplasty has been successful in such patients, but it is associated with increased intraoperative blood loss; the likelihood of loosening of the prosthesis may also be greater, perhaps because infiltration of the medullary cavity by Gaucher's cells prevents adequate cement fixation.[115] Recurrent AVN of the capital femoral epiphysis has been observed.[4]

Changes in the femoral neck may lead to pathologic fracture or to coxa vara deformity. On occasion, invasion of the head of the humerus gives rise to degenerative arthropathy of the shoulder.[4] Discovertebral changes have been described.[116]

Splenectomy, performed on some persons with thrombocytopenia, with hypersplenism, or with mechanical problems resulting from an enlarged spleen, may be followed by accelerated skeletal manifestations,[117] although this latter point is controversial. Following splenectomy, cerebroside storage may occur at an increased rate in liver and bone and may lead more rapidly to OA, aseptic necrosis, and pathologic fractures.[118] Many patients with long-standing disease have elevated serum immunoglobulin levels, often monoclonal.[4] Some patients with Gaucher's disease appear to progress from monoclonal dysproteinemia to overt multiple myeloma.[119]

One of the most consistent roentgenographic features of Gaucher's disease is widening of the femur just superior to the femoral condyles, creating the well-known "Erlenmeyer flask" appearance.[4] Similar flaring is less common in the tibia and humerus, together with changes in the other long bones, pelvis, skull, vertebrae, and mandible.[4] Characteristically, areas of rarefaction are mingled with patchy sclerosis and cortical thickening, resulting from new bone formation. The diagnosis of Gaucher's disease can be established by demonstrating large kerasin-filled Gaucher's cells in the bone marrow, as well as by analyzing peripheral blood leukocytes for residual β-glucocerebrosidase and β-glucosidase activities.[120,121] Administration of purified glucocerebrosidase to patients with Gaucher's disease produces a significant reduction of glucocerebroside in the liver and a reduction to normal levels of this substance in the erythrocytes.[4,112] The gene for glucocerebrosidase has been cloned, and organ transplantation, enzyme replacement, and allogeneic bone marrow transplantation are under active investigation.[112]

FABRY'S DISEASE

Fabry's disease, or glycolipid lipidosis, is a hereditary, X-linked disorder of glycosphingolipid metabolism characterized by the progressive accumulation of birefringent deposits of trihexosylceramide in endothelial, perithelial, and smooth muscle cells of blood vessels; in ganglion and perineural cells of the autonomic nervous system; in epithelial cells of the cornea; and in kidney, bone marrow, and many other tissues.[122] Such pathologic storage is due to a defect in the activity or absence of the lysosomal enzyme L-galactosidase A (ceramide trihexosidase), required for the normal catabolism of trihexosylceramide, which is derived from kidney and the membranes of senescent erythrocytes. Death usually occurs in the fifth or sixth decade as a result of renal failure or from the cardiac and cerebral complications of arterial hypertension or vascular disease. Heterozygous women may exhibit the disease in an attenuated form.

The disorder is characterized by a typical rash, known as *angiokeratoma corporis diffusum universale,* consisting of widespread telangiectasia or angiokeratoma. These pinpoint lesions, which occupy the dermal papillae, are venules with multiple layers of basement membrane in the vascular walls and may represent the ectopic placement of small collecting veins. They are thought to arise by alteration of the existing microvasculature rather than as a result of newly proliferating microvessels (neovascularization).[123] Vasospasm similar to that seen in Raynaud's disease, induced by changes in temperature and associated with paresthesias and burning in the extremities, are seen in many patients and are caused by deposits in the cells of the autonomic nervous system.[124] A study of forearm hemodynamics in eight patients with Fabry's disease revealed increased vascular resistance, decreased venous capacitance, and decreased forearm blood flow.[124]

The patient may also have painful swelling of the fingers, elbows, and knees.[122] A characteristic deformity consisting of limitation in extension of the distal interphalangeal joints of the fingers has been described.[4] Avascular necrosis of the head of the femur or talus and multiple, small, infarct-like opacities in the femoral head may occur.[4] Involvement of the metacarpal and metatarsal bones and of the temporomandibular joint has been reported,[21] as well as osteoporosis of the dorsal vertebrae.[4] The diagnosis of Fabry's disease is established by demonstration of the characteristic birefringement lipid material in skin and demonstration of deficient α-galactosidase activity in plasma or leukocytes.[122] Efforts have been made to determine whether an allograft, in the form of a kidney transplant, might provide a sufficient amount of α-galactosidase A to correct the metabolic defect. This question, as well as that of the value of other forms of enzyme replacement therapy, remains controversial.[122,125]

FARBER'S DISEASE

Farber's disease, or disseminated lipogranulomatosis, was first described in 1952 by S. Farber. This rare, progressive sphingolipidosis of early childhood is characterized by painful and swollen joints, periarticular and subcutaneous nodules, dysphonia, pulmonary infiltrations, and retardation of mental and motor development.[4] The patient accumulates ceramide, a glycolipid, in the cytoplasm of neurons and certain other cells attributable to a heritable deficiency in the lysosomal enzyme acid ceramidase, which catalyzes the conversion of ceramide to sphingosine and fatty acids.[126] Ceramide may accumulate in lysosomes of cultured diploid fibroblasts from persons with Farber's disease who are deficient in acid ceramidase.[127]

Articular disease, usually appearing between 2 weeks and 4 months of age, has been the dominant initial manifestation in the handful of patients recognized to date. Typically, pain and swelling of the interphalangeal and metacarpophalangeal joints, the ankles, wrists, knees, and elbows occur. Nodular masses develop on tendon sheaths and in para-articular tissues, as well as at points of pressure such as the occiput and the lumbosacral region. Nodules have also been found in the conjunctiva, the external ear, and the external nares. These patients often develop flexion contractures of the fingers and other joints. Ankylosis may follow. Swelling and granuloma formation in the epiglottis and larynx are responsible for a disturbance in swallowing and episodes of lung infection. A hoarse voice may be a clue to the correct diagnosis.[128] Few children survive past the age of 2 years, and the usual cause of death is pulmonary disease. The data on familial occurrence of Farber's disease are compatible with autosomal recessive inheritance.[126]

Fibroblasts, histiocytes, and macrophages with foamy cytoplasm-containing material having the staining properties of glycolipid are found in granulomatous deposits in the larynx, pleura, myocardium, pericardium, synovium, bones, liver, spleen, lymph nodes, cerebral cortex, and lung. Abnormal lipid is also present in the cytoplasm or neurons of the central nervous system. Roentgenographic changes consist of generalized body demineralization, juxta-articular erosions of long bones, and irregular disruption of trabeculae in the metacarpal bones and phalanges.[4] Specific diagnosis consists of the demonstration of diminished acid ceramidase in cultural skin fibroblasts or leukocytes.[126]

LIPOCHROME HISTIOCYTOSIS

This rare, familiar disorder is marked by pulmonary infiltrates, splenomegaly, hyper-γ-globulinemia, increased susceptibility to infection, and lipochrome pigment granulation of the histiocytes. In the first report of this syndrome, one of three affected sisters had RA with typical nodules, and a second had transient episodes of joint inflammation; the serum of all three contained rheumatoid factor in high titer.[4] The peripheral blood leukocytes of these patients have impaired respiration and hexose monophosphate shunt activity after phagocytosis and are deficient in their capacity to kill staphylococci.[129]

MULTICENTRIC RETICULOHISTIOCYTOSIS

Multicentric reticulohistiocytosis, or *lipodermatoarthritis,* is a rare disorder seen in adults and is characterized by a profusion of histiocytic nodules in the skin and mucous membranes and by severe, often mutilating polyarthritis[4,130–145] (Fig. 86–3A, B).

To date just over 90 cases have been reported. The disease affects women three times as often as men and has a worldwide distribution. There is no evidence that the disorder is heritable. Isolated lesions can occur, so-called solitary reticulohistiocytoma.[4]

Although the disorder has been thought to represent a lipid storage disease,[4] definitive evidence has not been presented. It is most likely that the histiocytes and giant cells contain a variety of nonspecifically accumulated lipid; it is not known with certainty whether this event is primary or secondary. Most lipid studies in multicentric reticulohistiocytosis reveal a varied and inconsistent pattern, suggesting a secondary accumulation. This latter phenomenon is generally referred to as a storage histiocytosis, defined by an accumulation of a normal or abnormal substance secondary to an alteration or disturbance in its metabolism by the mononuclear-phagocytic system.[4] It has been suggested, based on observations of normal lipid turnover studies, that multicentric reticulohistiocytosis is considered to be one of the conditions referred to as normolipidemic xanthomatosis.[132]

The disease appears to be inflammatory in nature. The lesions in skin and synovium resemble experimentally produced granulomas, containing activated histiocytes that fuse to form cells of increasing size. These larger cells, or megalocytes, may eventually coalesce to

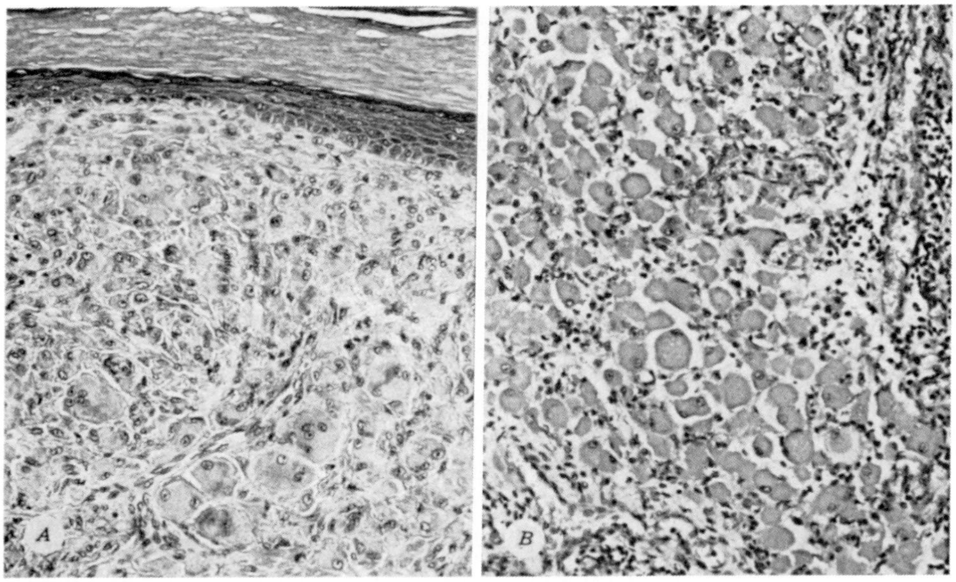

FIGURE 86–3. Photomicrograph of *A*, a skin nodule and *B*, synovium (knee) from a 54-year-old woman with multicentric reticulohistiocytosis. Numerous histiocytes and multinucleated giant cells contain large amounts of periodic-acid-Schiff-positive material ($\times$ 185).

form giant cells and may have granules that contain a variety of lipids, including triglycerides, cholesterol esters, and phospholipids.[4,138,139]

The role of lymphocyte–histiocyte interaction in the pathogenesis of multicentric reticulohistiocytosis is suggested by histochemical, immunochemical, and ultrastructural investigations. Staining techniques indicate that abundant lymphocytes are present in early nodules with reduction in their numbers as the nodule matures. The multicentric reticulohistiocytosis cell appears to be an activated macrophage.[130] Studies of interleukin-1 (IL-1) and PGE_2 secretion suggest that the mononuclear cell/macrophage may play a pathogenetic role in the disease.[133]

Severe bone and joint destruction is the hallmark of multicentric reticulohistiocytosis. This may occur without cartilage loss or with less cartilage loss than occurs in RA. Bony sites other than joints are destroyed, in addition to the typical areas of damage in the distal interphalangeal joints and the posterior facet joints of the lumbosacral spine. The severe bone and joint destruction is probably due to erosion of cartilage and bone by collagenase, elastase, and other degradative enzymes released by the proliferating, activated histiocytes, although direct evidence is still lacking.

The major difference between RA and multicentric reticulohistiocytosis is seen in the synovium. In multicentric reticulohistiocytosis, microscopic examination shows dense infiltrations of the dermis and synovium by a granulomatous proliferation of histiocytes and multinucleated giant cells containing large amounts of periodic acid-Schiff (PAS)–positive material. Similar cells have been observed in the bone marrow, lymph nodes, bone and periosteum, muscle, larynx, and endocardium.[4] There is no characteristic composition of the synovial fluid in multicentric reticulohistiocytosis; a wide range of cell counts are noted with protein content usually above 4 g/dL. In the few synovial fluid samples examined the cell count has varied from 700 to 93,000 cells per millimeter[4,140] with predominance of either mononuclear or polymorphonuclear cells.[4] Foamy giant cells have been found in the synovial fluid as well as in the synovium.[4,138] The presence of these large cells, known as megalocytes, may be a helpful early diagnostic clue.[138] Electron microscopic study of these unusual macrophages showed inclusions resembling the Golgi apparatus and seemingly developing from smooth endoplasmic reticulum.[4] Pericardial or pleural effusions may occur.[140] Gallium scanning has further suggested that pulmonary involvement may be part of the spectrum of MR.[135]

In approximately two thirds of patients, the first sign of the disease is polyarthritis, followed months to years later (average 3 years) by a nodular skin eruption. In the remaining patients, nodules appear first or are noted at the same time as the joint symptoms. The polyarthritis is usually symmetric, often simulates RA, and may involve all of the peripheral joints, including the distal interphalangeal (DIP) joints of the fingers, as well as the spinal and temporomandibular joints. Joint stiffness may be a prominent early complaint. The joints are swollen, tender, and may be inflamed. Large joint effusions may be present.[4] The most frequent joints affected are (in decreasing order): the interphalangeal joints, shoulders, knees, wrists, hips, feet, ankles, elbows, and spine. Marked DIP joint destruction is one of the distinguishing features of this disease.[4] In one half of cases, severely deforming arthritis mutilans appears. The degree of destruction may be inversely related to age of onset.[4]

Although the disease may remit spontaneously, chronic active disease is the rule. Many patients suffer severe destructive changes, particularly of the fingers (main en lorgnette) and less often of the hip and toe joints. The tendon sheaths on the flexor and extensor surfaces of the wrists may be involved, and Dupuytren's contracture or carpal tunnel syndrome has been described.[4]

The skin lesions consist of firm, reddish brown or yellow papulonodules, most commonly on the face and hands, ears, forearms, and elbows, scalp, neck, and chest.[4] Small tumefactions resembling coral beads are seen around the nailfold (Fig. 86–4). These lesions may remain discrete, or they may coalesce into diffuse plaques. They may be pruritic.[140] The nodules usually wax and wane and may disappear without a trace. Xanthelasma is noted in a third of these patients. About half of the patients develop mucosal papules on the lips, tongue, buccal membrane, nasal septum, and gingiva, as well as on the pharynx and larynx. Oral manifestations, including temporomandibular joint involvement, may dominant the clinical picture.[136]

Fever, weakness, and weight loss may occur during the disease course. Mild anemia, monoclonal gammopathy, or ESR elevation may occur.[140] Endocardial tissue (at post mortem) and pleural biopsy specimens as well as perirenal fat have shown involvement.[4]

Roentgenograms reveal rapidly progressive, symmetric joint destruction with loss of cartilage and absorption of subchondral bone, disproportionately severe when compared with the mildness of the symptoms. The radiologic features of multicentric reticulohistiocytosis are summarized in Table 86–1. The findings shown in Table 86–1 are in direct contrast to the typical radiographic feature of OA, in which erosions begin centrally or RA, in which prominent cartilage loss and periarticular osteopenia occur early, or the seronegative spondyloarthropathies, which show periostitis with ill-defined margins.[141]

Patients with multicentric reticulohistiocytosis have an increased incidence of coexistent malignant disease. Perhaps as many as 25% develop a neoplasm.[138,140] Twenty-eight cases of associated neoplasm were reported in 82 subjects with MR; the papulonodular skin involvement was the initial manifestation (alone or concurrent with the arthritis) in 90% of the reviewed cases, and a firm diagnosis of multicentric reticulohistiocytosis was made before the neoplasm was discovered in 73% of the subjects.[131] A wide spectrum of tumors appears to be associated with the disease. Multicentric reticulohistiocytosis has served as a marker for tumor recurrence, and therapy directed at the tumor caused regression of the disease.[131] The frequency of tumor association should sharply heighten the index of suspicion for neoplasm, especially during the first year after the diagnosis of multicentric reticulohistiocytosis.

As mentioned already, multicentric reticulohistiocytosis may become quiescent spontaneously. Although the mucocutaneous nodules may shrink or even disappear completely, the patient is often left with serious joint disability and, at times, a disfigured, leonine facies.[4] Treatment with anti-inflammatory corticosteroids may cause temporary regression of the cutaneous le-

TABLE 86–1. CHARACTERISTIC RADIOLOGIC FEATURES OF THE ARTHROPATHY OF MULTICENTRIC RETICULOHISTIOCYTOSIS

Well-circumscribed erosions spreading inward from the joint margins
Widened joint spaces
Predominance of changes in the interphalangeal, metacarpophalangeal, and metatarsophalangeal joints
Early and severe atlantoaxial joint involvement with erosion of the odontoid process, leading to subluxation
Erosion of the distal ends of the clavicles
Absent or minimal periosteal reaction
Absent or disproportionately mild osteopenia when compared with the severity of erosive changes
Prominent, uncalcified soft tissue nodules

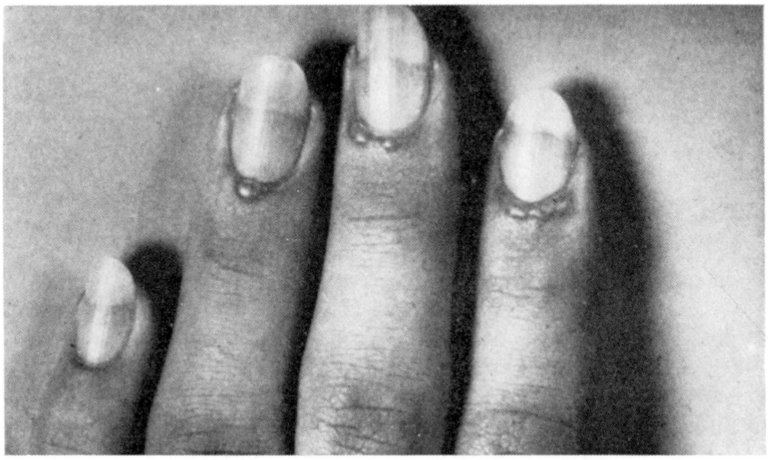

FIGURE 86–4. The fingers of a 16-year-old girl who had polyarthritis for 8 months and reddish brown "coral beads" around the nailfold for 5 months. Typical infiltrates of multicentric reticulohistiocytosis were found in biopsy specimens of both skin and synovium. (From Barrow and Holubar.)

sions, but these agents have little effect on the arthritis.[4] Dramatic clinical responses to cytotoxic drug therapy may occur. Both nodule formation and joint disease abated in one patient after treatment with cyclophosphamide.[4] The skin lesions were successfully treated with topical nitrogen mustard in another patient, whose skin and joint lesions later responded to cyclophosphamide.[4,142] Treatment with alkylating agents reportedly has been effective.[4] Two cases of coexisting multicentric reticulohistiocytosis and primary biliary cirrhosis were successfully treated with cyclophosphamide.[143] A patient with multicentric reticulohistiocytosis with salivary gland involvement and pericarditis responded to a regimen of prednisone, cyclophosphamide, and vincristine.[144] Azathioprine therapy controlled neither the arthritis nor the size and number of cutaneous nodules.[4,140]

The Mayo Clinic experience with alkylating agents (cyclophosphamide, 1.75 to 2.2 mg/kg; chlorambucil, 0.1 mg/kg for 6 to 24 months) appears quite favorable.[134] Complete remission occurred in 5 of 6 cases. It was suggested that remission might persist after the drug has been discontinued, but proof is lacking.

The presence of hypothyroidism, biopsy-proved Sjögren's syndrome, and anti-Ro (SS-A) in a patient with multicentric reticulohistiocytosis has led to speculation about its association with autoimmune diseases.[145]

In one report, four family members developed a reticulohistiocytosis-like disorder during childhood or adolescence.[146] The disease was characterized by a histiocytic papulonodular eruption on the face and hands; symmetric destructive polyarthritis, chiefly of the hands and wrists; and ocular involvement with cataract, uveitis, and glaucoma. The histologic changes in these patients differed from those of multicentric reticulohistiocytosis in several respects, however, including the absence of typical multinucleated giant cells and histiocytes with a "ground-glass" appearance of the cytoplasm.

HYPERLIPOPROTEINEMIAS

Articular and tendinous manifestations are important features of certain heritable disorders of lipid transport or lipoprotein metabolism.[147,148] The hyperlipoproteinemias are a result of a defect in either the synthesis or the degradation of lipoprotein particles. Often, dramatic articular signs and symptoms may be the first indication of the lipid disease and should alert the physician to an underlying disorder that may respond to dietary modification or drug therapy. Patients with type II hyperlipoproteinemia exhibit tendinous, tuberous, and periosteal xanthomas as well as xanthelasma, corneal ulcers, and early, rapidly progressive atherosclerosis. Tendinous xanthomas are located in Achilles and patellar tendons and in the extensor tendons of the hands and feet.[4,147] Tendon xanthomas have also been found in the plantar aponeurosis, in the fascia, and in periosteum overlying the lower tibia and the peroneal tendons. Xanthomas are situated within the tendon fibers and not on the tendon sheath, and they cannot be separated from the tendon on movement. They contain large, lipid-lined histiocytes within the collagenous connective tissue. Tendon xanthomas are composed of cholesterol and phospholipid.[4] Tuberous xanthomas are soft, subcutaneous masses occurring over extensor surfaces, especially of the elbows, knees, and hands, as well as on the buttocks. Persons homozygous for type II hyperlipoproteinemia develop extensive xanthomas in childhood, whereas those who are heterozygous develop tendinous xanthomas after age 30 and lack tuberous xanthomas.

Tendinous and tuberous xanthomas also occur in type III and type IV hyperlipoproteinemia.[148] A distinctive clinical feature of the type III disorder is lipid deposition, or plane xanthomas, in the palms of the hands.[148] Types I, IV, and V hyperlipoproteinemia are characterized by eruptive xanthomas over the knees, buttocks, shoulders, and back.[149]

Several studies have described individual rheumatic syndromes associated with type II hyperlipoproteinemia.[150] Recurrent episodes of migratory polyarthritis have been reported in about 50% of patients homozygous for type II hyperlipoproteinemia.[4] Arthritis occurs chiefly in large peripheral joints, and inflammation varies from mild to severe. Severely inflamed joints are swollen, warm, and red, and joint involvement is symmetric. Episodes of arthritis are self-limited, resembling acute attacks of gout, lasting several days to 2 weeks. In some patients, the illness resembles rheumatic fever because of the evanescent arthritis, the presence of (atherosclerotic) aortic valvular disease, an elevated ESR, and a false-positive increased titer of antistreptolysin O caused by hyperlipoproteinemia. The valvular disease and the elevated ESR may occur in persons without arthritis and are presumably direct results of the elevated lipoproteins.

In patients heterozygous for type II hyperlipoproteinemia, recurrent Achilles tendinitis is a common problem. This finding has been reported in adults, adolescents, and children.[4] In addition to Achilles tendinitis, monarticular arthritis involving the knee or great toe is seen,[4] and in some heterozygous type II patients, migratory "polyarthritis" involving up to six joints has been reported.[4] Affected joints include the knee, the proximal interphalangeal joints, the ankle, the wrist, the elbow, the shoulder, and the hip. The polyarthritis may represent an inflammatory periarthritis or peritendinitis.[4] Synovial fluid from these joints contained no crystals, and the cell counts were low (fewer than 200 neutrophils per cubic millimeter).

A review of 73 heterozygotes with familial hypercholesterolemia revealed a 40% prevalence of symptoms, including Achilles pain (18%), Achilles tendinitis (11%), oligoarticular arthritis (7%), and polyarticular or rheumatic fever-like arthritis (4%).[150] Symptoms appear quite diverse, recurrent, even incapacitating, yet they are short-lived, and no progression to joint damage is noted, unlike that observed in some homozygous patients. Attacks are "gout-like," with symptom-free intervals. Tendon xanthomas were present in many of these patients, but they may be absent before the onset of symptoms.[150] Because symptoms may occur long before appearance of xanthomata or coronary artery insufficiency, the recognition of the significance of these unique joint complaints may lead to an early diagnosis of familial hypercholesterolemia and primary prevention of its consequences. A patient with high concentrations of low-density lipoprotein (LDL) cholesterol (type IIa) and gout-like attacks of periarthritis was treated with a low-cholesterol diet and colestipol with resolution of the joint abnormality and lowering of cholesterol.[151]

The role of cholesterol crystals in the pathogenesis of this syndrome remains controversial, however. Cholesterol itself appears not locally toxic, and the individual contribution of inflammatory, mechanical, or as yet undiscovered factors remains to be established.[152–154]

An arthropathy resembling that seen in type II hyperlipoproteinemia occurs in patients with type IV hyperlipoproteinemia.[155,156] These persons have predominantly an asymmetric oligoarthritis involving both small and large joints, including the proximal interphalangeal and metacarpophalangeal joints in the hands, wrists, shoulders, knees, ankles, tarsus, and metatarsophalangeal joints. In some cases, the inflammatory disease is mild and persistent, and in others it is episodic and recurrent.

Morning stiffness and para-articular hyperesthesia have been described in these patients.[156] Synovial fluids were noninflammatory and free of crystals. Radiographs in many of these patients show prominent para-articular bone cysts (Fig. 86–5). One such cyst was grossly yellow and mucinous, and on microscopic examination it showed only fibrous tissue and fat cells (Fig. 86–6). No granulomata, no cholesterol deposits, and no lipid-laden histiocytes were observed. Synovial biopsy in one case revealed moderate hyperplasia of the synovial villi, prominent stromal vessels, and a moderate mononuclear infiltrate. Four patients experienced decreased severity of articular symptoms after reduction or normalization of serum lipid levels.[155]

Skeletal lesions associated with other hyperlipoproteinemias have also been reported. One patient with probable type V hyperlipoproteinemia had cystic lesions in both proximal femurs. Curettage yielded yellowish fragments that on microscopic examination showed foamy histiocytes and a granulomatous reaction around cholesterol clefts.[4] Secondary hyperlipoproteinemia can occur in association with the nephrotic syndrome, pancreatitis, alcoholism, hypothyroidism, and diabetes mellitus, and may be associated with musculoskeletal complaints. Joint changes secondary to infiltration of foam cells in subchondral bone in secondary hyperlipoproteinemia resemble those developing in patients with biliary cirrhosis.[4]

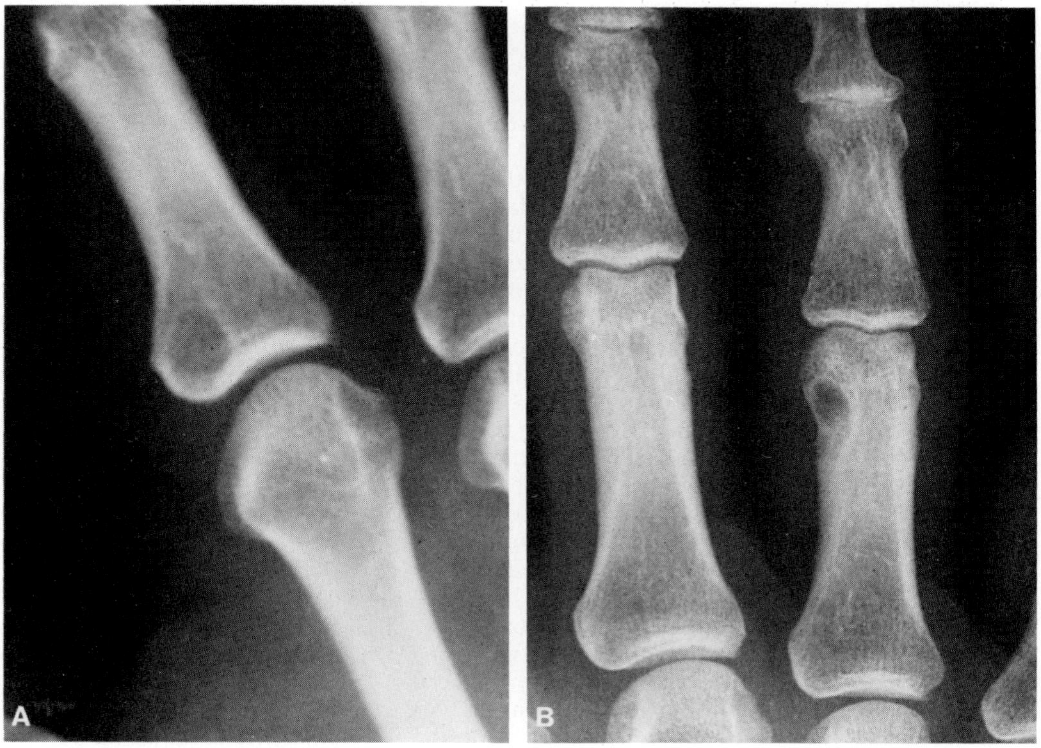

FIGURE 86–5. *A* and *B*, Roentgenograms showing prominent para-articular bone cysts in the fingers of two patients with arthritis associated with type IV hyperlipoproteinemia. Both patients had polyarticular inflammatory disease.

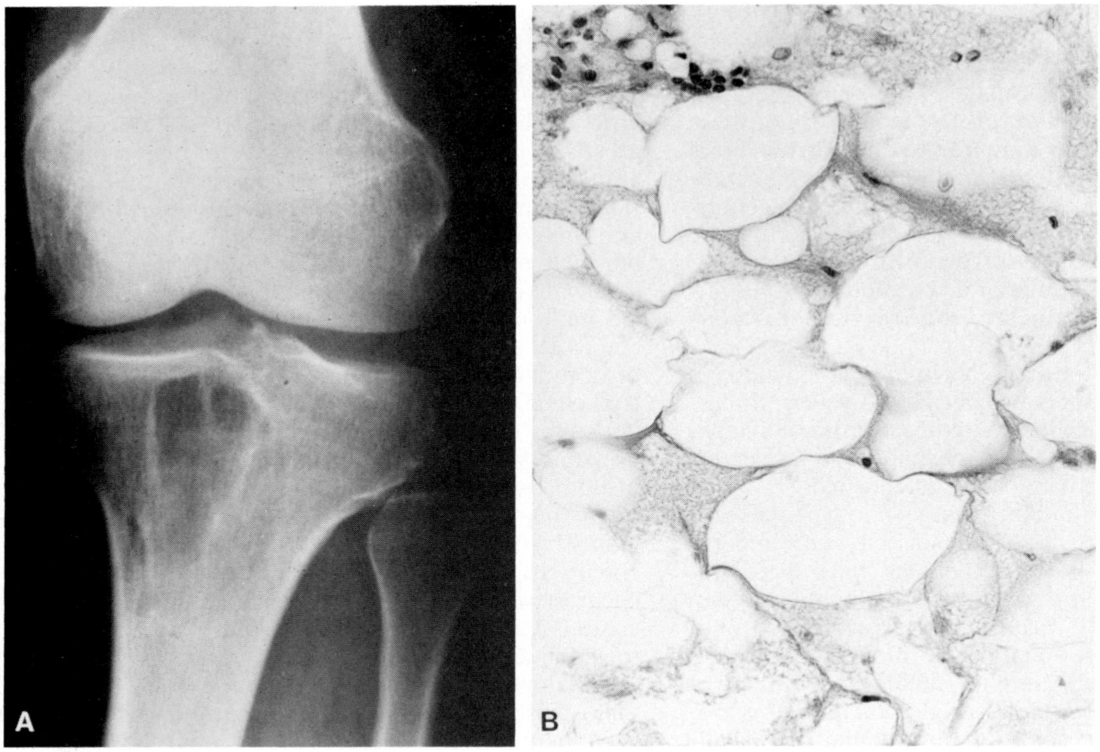

FIGURE 86–6. A patient with arthritis associated with type IV hyperlipoproteinemia and prominent knee symptoms had a large cyst in the proximal tibia, *A*. Tissue removed from the cyst at biopsy, *B*, was yellow and mucinous and on microscopic examination showed fibrous tissue and many fat cells (×400).

Cerebrotendinous xanthomatosis (CTX) is a rare autosomal recessive disorder characterized by progressive cerebellar ataxia, dementia, spinal cord paresis, subnormal intelligence, tendon xanthomas, and cataracts.[157] Cholestanol, or dihydrocholesterol, accumulates in the nervous tissue, tendons, and other tissues throughout the body. The underlying defect involves a deficiency of a hepatic mitochondrial 26-hydroxylase enzyme involved in bile acid synthesis; treatment with chenodeoxycholic acid inhibits the abnormal bile acid synthesis, reduces plasma cholestanol concentrations, and offers the promise of preventing progression of the disease.[157] Tendon xanthomas may appear as early as the second decade but usually not until the third or fourth decade. The Achilles tendons are the most common sites, but xanthomas may also occur in the triceps tendons, at the tibial tuberosities, and in the extensor tendons of the hands. Tuberous xanthomas and xanthelasma may also occur.

Tendon xanthomas constitute a feature of *sitosterolemia with xanthomatosis*, another rare, newly recognized familial lipid storage disease marked by the accumulation of plant sterols in the blood and tissues.[157,158] These persons have an increased intestinal absorption of dietary sitosterol coupled with decreased removal, but the underlying metabolic defect has not yet been defined. The patient's serum cholesterol level may be normal or moderately elevated.[158] Inheritance is autosomal recessive. Tendon xanthomas indistinguishable histologically from those found in hyperlipoproteinemia appear during childhood, initially in the extensor tendons of the hands and later in the patellar, plantar, and Achilles tendons. Sitosterolemia should be considered in the differential diagnosis of a patient who presents with xanthomas in childhood and who does not have familial hypercholesterolemia or the CTX syndrome. Because some of these persons may not have an elevated cholesterol level, measurement of plasma sterols is necessary to establish this diagnosis.[157]

BLEEDING DISORDERS

Hemophilia is the collective designation for a group of hereditary hemorrhagic diseases in which there is a qualitative or quantitative deficiency of plasma procoagulant proteins.[159] Hemophilia A is an X-linked recessive disorder secondary to decreased levels of properly functioning factor VIII (also known as antihemophilic factor, AHF). This disorder accounts for 80% of true hemophilias; hemophilia B is also X-linked and is not clinically distinguishable from hemophilia A.[159] For hemophilia B, the deficiency resides in factor IX (also known as plasma thromboplastin component, PTC, or Christmas factor). Von Willebrand's disease and factor

XI (plasma thromboplastin antecedent, PTA) deficiency account for a very small number of cases. Patients are subject to abnormal bleeding, the frequency and intensity varying with the level of the deficient factor. In addition to skin bruising, patients experience recurrent bleeding into the gastrointestinal and genitourinary tracts and hemorrhage into the musculoskeletal system.[4,160] Hemorrhage is the bleeding manifestation most commonly requiring treatment; it has been described in all of the hereditable coagulation disorders (except factor V deficiency) and as a complication of anticoagulant drugs.[161–163] Recurrent hemarthroses are painful, acute episodes that may lead ultimately to a self-sustaining synovitis and result in a deforming joint disease with permanent disability.[4,159,160]

Pathogenesis and Anatomic Findings

Hemophilic hemarthrosis usually but not always follows trauma. The injury is often trivial and is apparent neither to the young patient nor to his parents. The results of joint hemorrhage have been well studied in naturally hemophilic dogs, which develop an arthropathy comparable with that encountered in humans.[164] The initial lesion consists of synovial or subsynovial hemorrhage. Rupture of blood into the joint cavity provokes an inflammatory reaction characterized by effusion, villous hypertrophy, hyperplasia of the lining cells, and infiltration by lymphocytes and plasma cells.[4,165] This reaction gradually subsides several days to weeks after cessation of hemorrhage. Hemoglobin is released into the joint cavity and synovial tissues after lysis of erythrocytes has occurred. Hemosiderin remains in the synovium for an indefinite period, appearing as finely particulate matter within the phagocytic lining cells.[4] Additional coarser aggregates of this iron-containing pigment, lying free or within macrophages, are found in deeper portions of the synovium. The presence of large amounts of hemosiderin in this location distinguishes this variety of synovial siderosis from hemochromatosis.

Repeated hemorrhage is marked by hyperplasia of the synovial lining cells and by gradually increasing synovial fibrosis and hemosiderosis, leading to rigidity of the subsynovial tissue and joint capsule. Although these changes may account for some degree of limited joint motion, it is the damage to the cartilage and bone that is most harmful to joint function.[4] Marginal erosion of the cartilage owing to encroachment of the hyperplastic synovium and more central, irregular, "map-like" degeneration attributable to subchondral hemorrhage occur.[4] The demonstration of plasmin (fibrinolysin) in joint fluid during the course of acute hemarthrosis and the finding of numerous siderosomes suggest that the loss of cartilage may in part result from enzymatic degradation. Siderosomes are membrane-bound lysosomal bodies with aggregates of iron-containing particles believed to be lysosomal organelles in which hemoglobin and its derivatives are digested.

A marked increase in cathepsin-D and acid phosphatase activity in synovial tissue and a lesser increase in acid phosphatase activity in the joint fluid of patients with chronic hemophilic arthropathy occurs.[4] These enzymes are inactive at neutral pH and probably contribute little to extracellular connective tissue degradation. Nevertheless, such findings indicate that the synovial tissue is "activated" and may release other degradative enzymes or may form pannus and directly invade and destroy contiguous cartilage and bone. Supporting this concept are studies of proliferative synovium isolated from a hemophilic boy, which secreted latent collagenase and proteoglycanase in amounts equal to those produced by rheumatoid synovium.[165]

In tissue culture, hemophilic synovium generated PGE at rates similar to those of rheumatoid synovium, producing brisk breakdown of cartilage proteoglycans.[166] Immunopathologic mechanisms for perpetuation of the chronic synovitis in hemophilia have not been demonstrated; joint tissue from seven subjects showed no immune globulin deposits.[167] In summary, activated hemophilia synovium has the potential for considerable connective tissue destruction with a marked degradative effect on cartilage.

In experimental hemarthrosis in rabbits, the synthesis of both ribonucleic acid and protein by articular cartilage was initially unimpaired despite repeated daily intra-articular injection of autologous blood.[4] When such injections were continued for several weeks or months, however, definite alterations occurred in the cartilage matrix, consisting at first of altered metachromasia, followed by superficial and deep erosions, accompanied by a reduction in proteoglycan concentration and depressed chondrocyte synthetic activity.[4] The deposition of iron pigment in both synovium and cartilage plays a significant role in the pathogenesis of the degeneration of articular cartilage.[168] Degradation of ground substance surrounding chondrocytes containing iron suggests that local release of degradative enzymes may be prompted by the retained pigment.[4] Proteoglycan loss alerts the resilience and compressibility of normal cartilage and may accelerate its destruction.

Articular cartilage damage caused by repeated joint hemorrhage is accompanied by the development of cavities or "cysts" in the subchondral bone (Fig. 86–7). These lesions can become large and have been thought to be the results of intraosseous bleeding. In hemophilic dogs these cysts communicated with the synovial cavity at points of cartilage and subchondral bone erosion, at the margin of the articular cartilage, or at the site of ligamentous attachments.[164] These and similar observations in human hemophilic joint disease suggest that cyst development relates more to secondary degenerative changes in articular cartilage and subchondral bone than to intraosseous bleeding per se.[4] The final answer on the cause of the hemophiliac subchondral cyst is far from complete. Pathoanatomic evidence suggests that an expanding cyst is produced primarily through biomechanical forces. The initial event may be a subchondral hematoma beneath the load-bearing surface; centrifugal expansion of its developing fibrous wall might

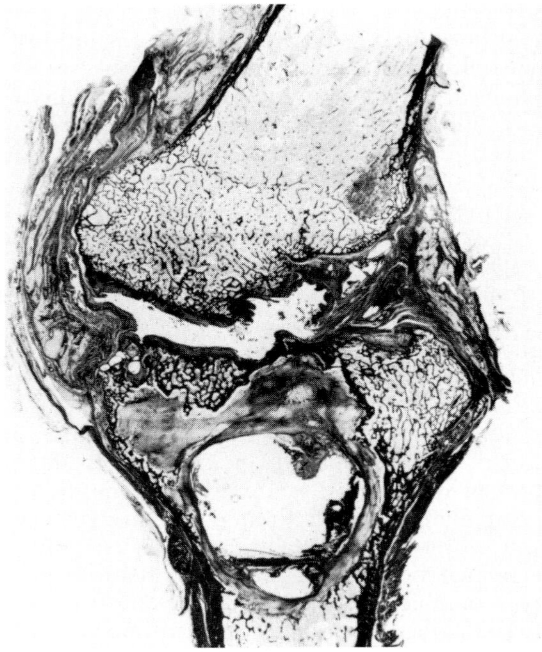

FIGURE 86–7. Sagittal section of the knee joint of a 49-year-old man with advanced hemophilic arthropathy. The femoral condyle appears flattened, and the patella has virtually disappeared. The head of the tibia has undergone massive cystic resorption. The articular cartilage has disappeared from most of the joint surfaces, which have undergone partial fibrous ankylosis on the popliteal aspect on the right and have been replaced by fibrous tissue. The cyst in the tibia is lined by loose-textured fibrous tissue. The synovial and capsular tissues are thickened and infiltrated with many hemosiderin-laden mononuclear cells. (From Sokoloff.)

destroy bone and cartilage, with the end result producing a large osteochondral defect displaying discrete vertical margins and a depressed sclerotic bony base. The process proceeds from within to without or toward the joint surface. Characteristic knee intercondylar widening noted radiologically is felt to be the evolution of these cysts in the load-bearing portion of the patellofemoral articulation.[169]

A striking but less specific finding in young patients is accelerated maturation and hypertrophy of the epiphyses adjacent to affected joints. Chronic hyperemia of the epiphyseal cartilage, induced by repeated hemarthrosis, may be responsible for this change.

In addition to hemarthrosis, bleeding into muscle and bone may occur. The terms *hemophilic pseudotumor* and *hemophilic cyst* have been applied to the destructive lesions that follow massive muscle, subperiosteal, or intraosseous hemorrhages. Such hematomas, if not optimally treated, subsequently organize, become vascularized, and are locally destructive to soft tissue and bone. In the adult, these hematomas occur most often in the pelvis, thigh, or leg,[4] whereas in children, they occur distal to the elbow or knee and are less destructive.

Soft tissue bleeding may be dangerous because of neurovascular compression, severe destruction and contracture of muscle, including Volkmann's contracture,[4] cyst rupture, sinus formation, or chronic infection. One of the most dramatic examples of hemophilic bleeding involves the iliopsoas muscle.[4] Hemorrhage into the closed fascial compartment that contains the iliopsoas muscle and the femoral nerve is marked by the development of sudden, severe pain in the groin and thigh, followed by the appearance of a tender mass, a hematoma, in the iliac fossa and the groin, flexion contracture of the hip, and signs of femoral nerve palsy. Bleeding into the gastrocnemius or soleus muscle, or both may lead to a talipes equinus deformity. Repeated bleeding in and around the joints and associated muscle atrophy inevitably lead to instability of the weight-bearing articulations.

Although hemarthrosis secondary to anticoagulant therapy is usually a self-limited process once the drug has been discontinued,[4,161–163] in one case the arthritis progressed after medication was withdrawn.[170]

Clinical Features

Hemarthrosis occurs in approximately 80 to 90% of patients with hemophilia[4,160] and constitutes the most common major hemorrhagic event in the disease. Bleeding into the joints is particularly frequent when the patient's level of antihemophilic globulin is less than 1 to 2% of normal.[4] Most patients first experience articular symptoms between the ages of 1 and 5 years, and they usually have repeated hemarthroses during the remainder of the first decade of life; thereafter, these episodes ordinarily become less and less frequent.[4] Patients with levels of antihemophilic globulin greater than 5% of normal generally experience fewer episodes of hemarthrosis, and these occur only after more severe trauma.

A clinical and radiologic survey of 139 hemophiliac patients provided unique observations on the prevalence of arthropathy because of the inclusion of many patients with mild-to-moderate disease (factor levels 6 to 60%). In contrast to earlier observations, a significant (one-third) prevalence of definite arthritis was seen in this mild-to-moderate group, although it was less severe, mostly affecting one or two joints.[160] Even subjects with factor levels up to 20% experienced arthropathy; those with factor levels of less than 5% were at risk for severe polyarthritis. And some patients without a history of bleeding demonstrated severe articular changes radiographically, an anomaly suggesting that subclinical bleeding occurs and may remain confined to the synovium.

Joint hemorrhage occurs most commonly in a knee, ankle, or elbow and less frequently in the shoulders, hips, wrists, fingers, and toes.[4,160] Generally, only a single joint is involved in each episode, but two joints may be affected simultaneously. The patient often has repeated hemorrhaging at the same site.[4]

The affected joint is swollen, warm, and often exquisitely painful and tender. Associated muscle spasm leads to flexion of the extremity. In instances of milder bleeding, the normal configuration and full motion of the joint may be restored within a matter of days, and the patient may experience little more than transient stiffness on reambulation. In the case of protracted bleeding, and particularly when repeated injury of the joint leads to renewed hemorrhage, symptoms may persist for weeks to months. Thermograms and radionuclide scanning have been used to assess the effects of acute hemarthrosis,[171] and it has been suggested that ^{99m}Tc scintigraphy may be useful to follow patients sequentially.[172] Ultrasonographic studies have proved useful in demonstrating deeper bleeding, such as retroperitoneal hemorrhage.[4]

After repeated severe hemarthrosis, the joint gradually fails to return to full normal form and function, and loss of muscle power and mass is progressive. Examination discloses thickening of the periarticular soft tissues, crepitation, atrophic muscle accentuating the bony enlargement of the joint, and various deformities, the most common of which are flexion contractures of the elbow and knee. Flexion contracture of the knee is frequently accompanied by posterior subluxation of the tibia. Occasionally, joints develop fibrous or (rarely) bony ankylosis.[4]

Bleeding into the hip joint during childhood may lead to dislocation,[4] as well as to flattening and destruction of the capital epiphysis and deformity of the femoral neck, with resultant shortening of the extremity. Synovial hyperemia may be accompanied by epiphyseal hyperemia and epiphyseal overgrowth. In growing children, this process may cause axial deviation including cubitus valgus, coxa valga, genu valgum, and pes valgus. Any one of these structural abnormalities may be asymmetric.

Bleeding episodes often necessitate long periods of bed rest, which, in turn, delay neuromotor maturation.[4] Approximately one half of all patients with hemophilia have some permanent changes in their peripheral articulations, and only the rare person with severe hemophilia (less than 2% of the normal level of antihemophilic globulin) escapes some residual deformity.[4,160] In many cases, only a few joints are involved in this chronic arthropathy, usually knees and elbows, and many other joints remain normal despite repeated bleeding episodes. Although hemarthroses were noted to be equally common in both factor VIII and IX deficiencies in a large referral hemophiliac clinic, arthritis was more frequently present in those with factor VIII deficiency. Hemarthroses and arthritis were exceptional in von Willebrand's disease.[160] An occasional patient with von Willebrand's disease, however, may display a progressive severe arthropathy.[173]

In addition to muscle atrophy as a result of joint inflammation and disuse, hemophiliacs have demonstrated other features of a neuromyopathy. Electromyographic assessments revealed reduced numbers of functioning motor units and a "myopathic" motor unit potential; serum creatine phosphokinase levels are frequently increased, and muscle biopsies show type 2 fiber atrophy.[174]

Although the presence of hemophilia is suspected readily in a person with a recognized bleeding tendency, the diagnosis may be much less obvious in the occasional child or adult in whom hemarthrosis is the initial symptom of the disease or in whom minor hemorrhagic episodes have been overlooked. It is especially important to recognize this condition, because unsuspecting surgical intervention often has disastrous consequences.[4]

Roentgenographic Findings

In acute intra-articular hemorrhage, one sees distention of the joint capsule and increased density of the soft tissues. An accompanying subperiosteal hemorrhage, followed by thickening or, in some cases, by atrophy of the underlying cortex may be evident. Subchondral hemorrhage may lead to defects in epiphyseal ossification centers.

Chronic hemophilic joint disease is characterized by irregular narrowing or obliteration of the joint space and later by marginal spurring and sclerosis of bone, which often contains one or more areas of cystic translucency[4,175] (Figs. 86–8 to 86–15). These cystic areas may be quite large. The periarticular soft tissues may be thickened and increased in density, and they occasionally contain fine opacities. These opacities were traditionally attributed to the deposition of hemosiderin in the synovium, a view that has been disputed. Certain roentgenographic features are characteristic but not pathognomonic of chronic hemophilic arthropathy. These findings include enlargement of the head of the radius in patients with elbow involvement;[4] flattening of the inferior portion of the ("squared-off") patella in advanced disease of the knee;[4] widening of the intercondylar notch of the femur; and flattening of the talus.[4,176] JRA and hemophilia may share morphologic characteristics and radiologic pattern of involvement. The isolated tibiotalar involvement noted of hemophilia and the high frequency of intertarsal disease found in JRA may be useful in differentiating these two conditions.[176] Aseptic necrosis of the femoral head, as well as of the talus, may also been seen.[4] In rare cases, chondrocalcinosis has been described in hemophiliacs.[4] An episode of acute pseudogout masqueraded as hemarthrosis in a patient with hemophilia.[177]

Management

Has modern treatment of hemophilia (e.g., demand therapy and home treatment programs) reduced the long-term morbidity of the associated arthropathy? A study using historical controls suggested a reduction in its prevalence as well as its severity.[160] A review of demand therapy in classic (factor VIII) disease patients

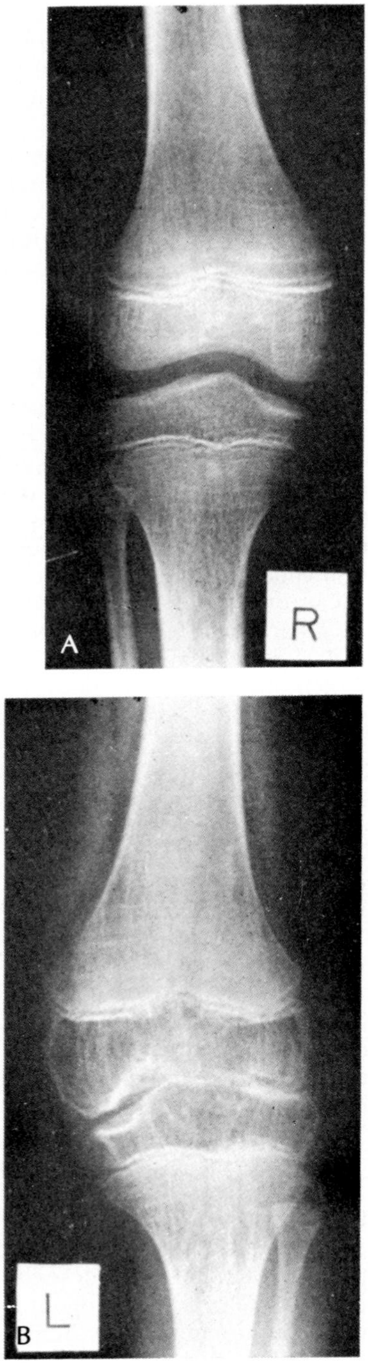

FIGURE 86–8. *A* and *B*, Roentgenograms of the knee of a 9-year-old boy with hemophilia and repeated hemarthroses involving the left knee, *B*. Note the loss of articular cartilage, the irregularity of bony surfaces, and the hypertrophy of the epiphyses of femur and tibia. The right knee, *A*, appears normal.

indicates that many of those with normal range of motion as well as those with marked or severe limitation maintained their range of motion for over 6 years. Nevertheless, some patients with mild disease showed progression in spite of demand therapy.[178] The unchecked use of factor VIII replacement from human sources is not without risk. There is a need to identify those patients who may have additional requirements or who may benefit from more aggressive therapy.

A recent review of hemophilia arthritis provides a basis for an improved prognosis in the modern era.[179] An international cooperative study to determine the role of clotting factor replacement on the outcome of arthritis is in progress. The interim report (at 4 years) suggested that progression related to the frequency of first bleeds. Early use of factor replacement delayed but did not prevent arthritis. Frequent, as well as prophylactic, use of factor replacement may have prevented joint disease in a small subset of patients.[179] It was speculated that, although several aspects of hemophilia arthritis are already treatable, the availability of purified monoclonal antibody and of recombinant factor concentrates free of infectious agents may make this type of arthritis ultimately preventable.[179]

Approximately 23 cases of septic arthritis complicating hemophilia have been reported, 15 patients without and 8 cases with human immunodeficiency concomitant human immunodeficiency virus (HIV) infection.[180–192] A review comparing pyogenic arthritis with spontaneous hemarthrosis in hemophiliac subjects has been published,[193] and although this complication is relatively uncommon, it carries serious morbidity. Key clinical features suggesting sepsis include monarticular involvement, most often the knee; association with an underlying arthropathy; presence of Staphylococcus aureus; invariable fever, leukocytosis (white blood cell count greater than 10,000/mm^3); and presence of factors predisposing to sepsis (intravenous drug use, hemodialysis, prior aspirations, or surgical procedures).[193] A case of pneumococcal septic arthritis, with multiple joint involvement, has been reported.[189] Based on a comparison with the findings in uncomplicated hemarthrosis, it was recommended that a patient with fever of 1°C (1.8°F) and an acute joint inflammation should have an aspiration to rule out infection.[193] Arthrocentesis in uncomplicated hemarthrosis does not modify its clinical course and may increase the risk of additional bleeding. The decision to perform the procedure should be made only when infection is suspected. In addition to the predisposing factors already discussed, infection should be considered when joint symptoms are prolonged despite standard factor replacement therapy. Hemophiliac patients traditionally have been thought not to be predisposed to joint infection, and it is a rare problem considering the degree of joint damage, frequent trauma, and bleeding that they experience.[185] The number of episodes of pyogenic arthritis in hemophilia, however, equaled the number of episodes of joint sepsis in RA in an admission survey from a Denver hospital.[193]

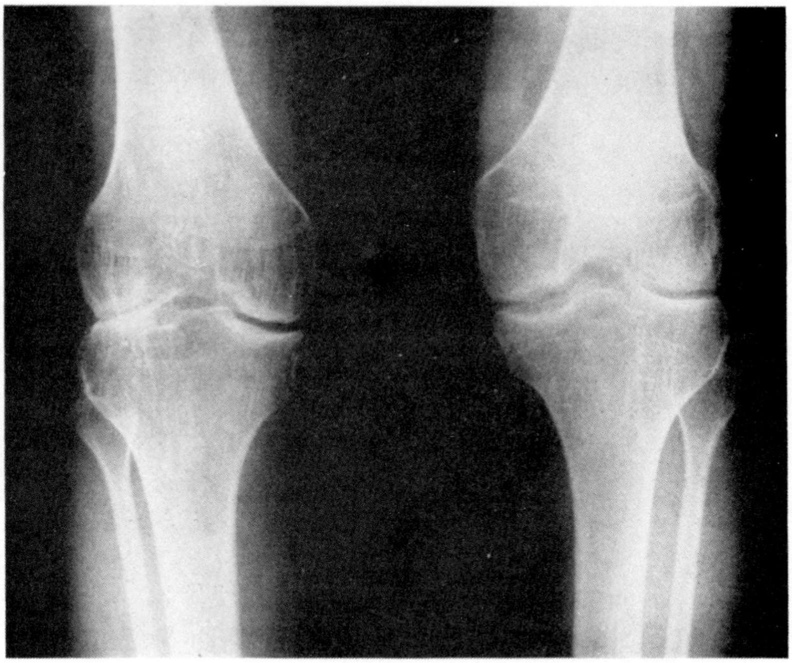

FIGURE 86–9. Roentgenograms of the knees of the patient in Fig. 86–8 at the age of 17 years. During the 8 years since the roentgenograms in Fig. 86–8 were obtained, the patient had many more episodes of joint hemorrhage involving both knees. Note the irregular narrowing of the joint space and early osteophyte formation.

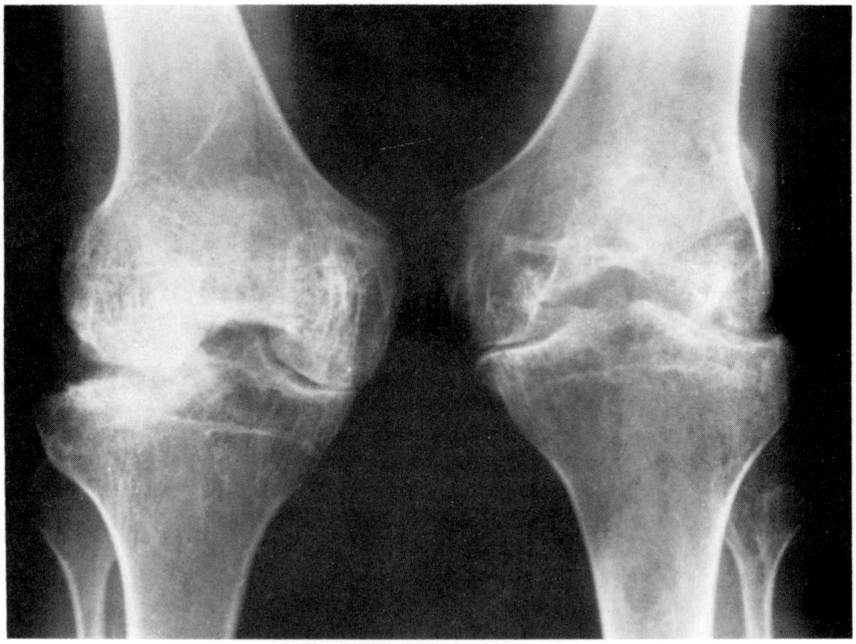

FIGURE 86–10. Roentgenogram of the knees of a 23-year-old man with hemophilia illustrating severe secondary degenerative joint disease.

It was further postulated that there is a greater frequency of septic arthritis in HIV-positive hemophiliac patients.[190,192]

Hemarthroses and chronic arthropathy are reported in factor XIII deficiency[194] and in von Willebrand's disease (VWD).[195] Bleeding does not appear to be rare in factor XIII deficiency, which is characterized by a qualitatively unstable clot. Articular hemorrhage in factor XIII deficiency occurs usually 12 to 36 hours after trauma; destructive joint sequelae, however, are uncommon.[194] Although earlier reports indicated that hemarthrosis occurred in only 5 to 10% of severe VWD patients, 4 out of 35 patients in a later study were affected; 3 of the 4 were girls. None had violent trauma, and bleeding into the ankle predominated.[195] Recurrent hemarthrosis in the shoulder of a 56-year-old man taking warfarin produced a destructive arthropathy in the absence of a pre-existing joint abnormality.[170]

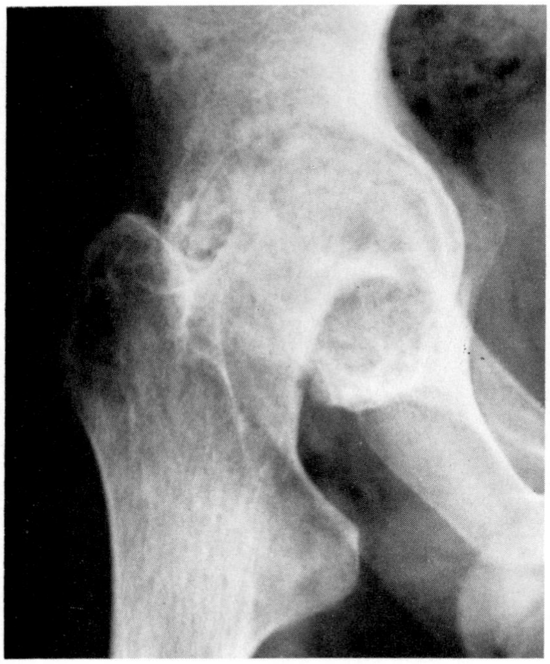

FIGURE 86–11. Roentgenogram of the right hip of the patient in Fig. 86–10 illustrating severe degenerative joint disease and protrusio acetabuli.

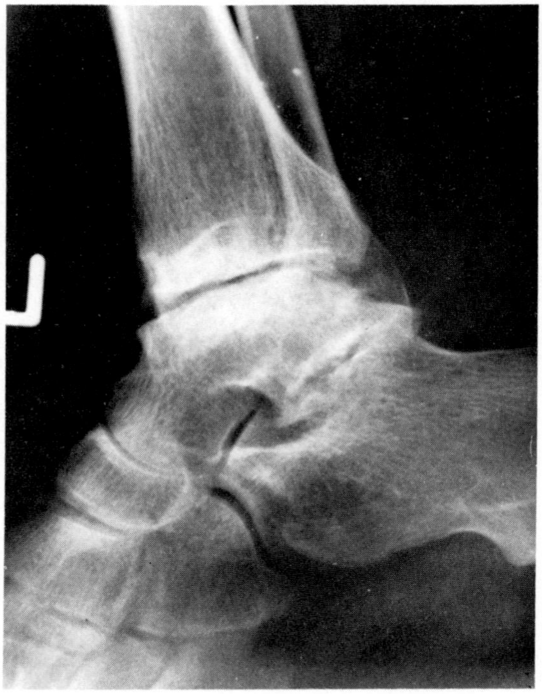

FIGURE 86–12. Roentgenogram of the ankle of a 26-year-old man with hemophilia. Note the loss of cartilage and subchondral sclerosis in both ankle and subtalar joints.

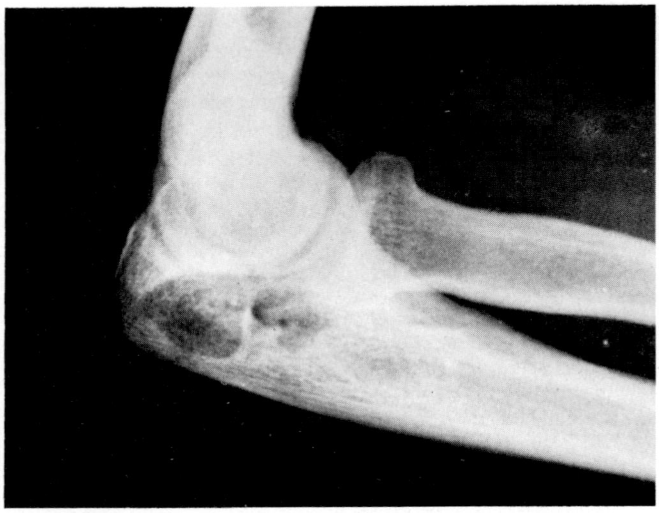

FIGURE 86–13. Roentgenogram of the elbow of a 27-year-old man with hemophilia illustrating large subchondral erosion in the ulna.

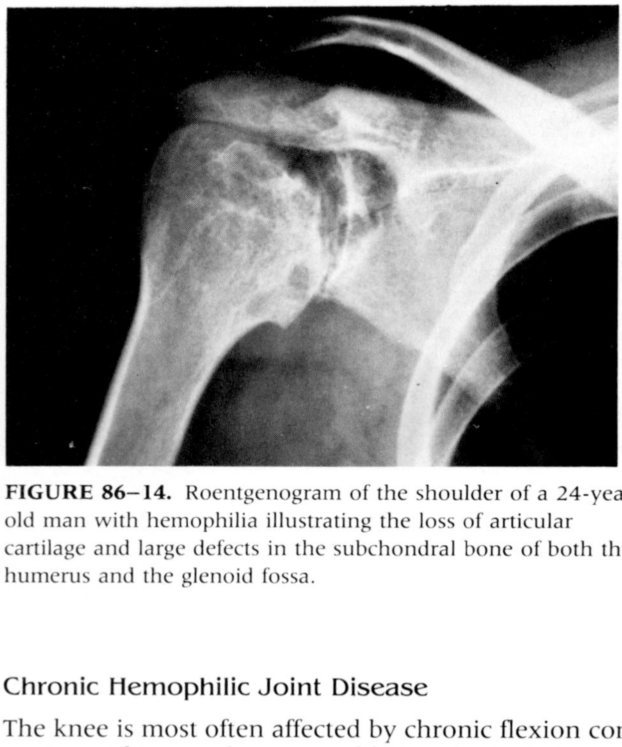

FIGURE 86–14. Roentgenogram of the shoulder of a 24-year-old man with hemophilia illustrating the loss of articular cartilage and large defects in the subchondral bone of both the humerus and the glenoid fossa.

Chronic Hemophilic Joint Disease

The knee is most often affected by chronic flexion contracture. This may be correctable by physical therapy. Stable weight bearing may be achieved by means of traction, wedging casts, quadriceps setting exercises, and later, active resistive exercises.[4] The use of a long leg-extension brace and crutches may be required for many months or years to prevent recurrence of the contracture.[4]

The use of surgical procedures for the correction of chronic joint deformities was once limited because of the risk of uncontrollable hemorrhage until potent fac-

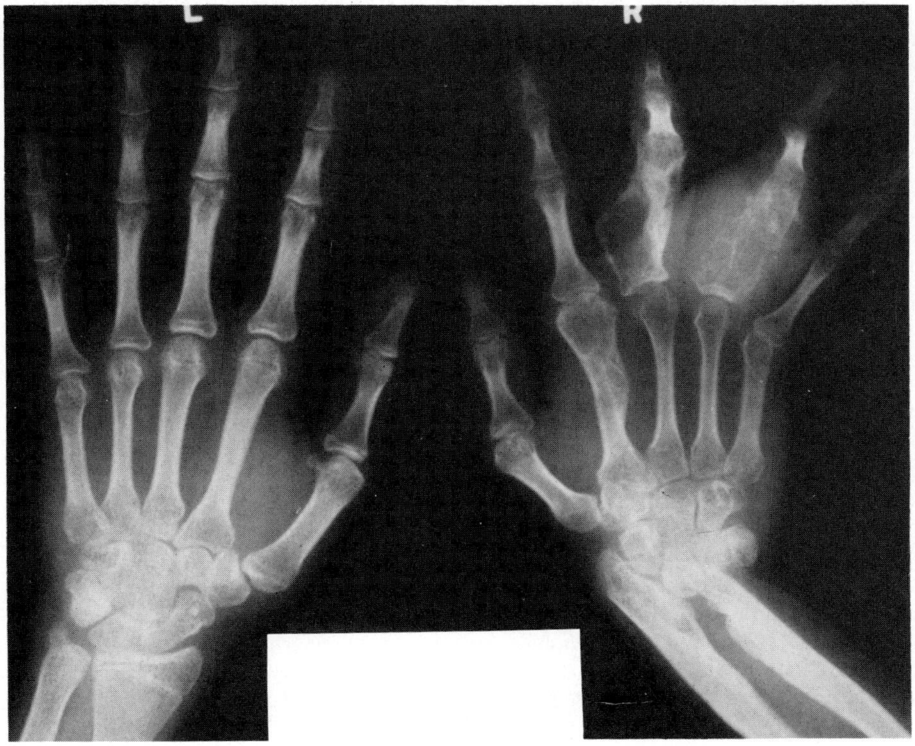

FIGURE 86–15. Roentgenogram of the right hand of a 16-year-old boy with hemophilia illustrating the destruction of bone of the proximal phalanges of the fourth and fifth fingers resulting from hemophilic pseudotumor (normal left hand for comparison).

tor concentrates became available.[196] The prospect of orthopedic rehabilitation is now excellent. Many procedures are now successful, including supracondylar wedge osteotomy or correction of valgus deformity of the knee;[4] wedge osteotomy of the tibia;[4] lengthening of the Achilles and other tendons of the feet for correction of equinus contracture;[4,160,196] compression arthrodesis of the knee, hip, and ankle;[4,196] and total knee and total hip replacement.[196,197] Heroic operations, such as drainage or radical excision of hematoma and pseudotumor and the amputation of an extremity in cases of uncontrollable, life-threatening bleeding, or infection are now also possible.[4] An analysis of 76 individual operative procedures revealed three that were particularly successful: (1) supracondylar correction of knock knee; (2) interochanteric correction of coxa valga; and (3) evacuation of iliacus hematoma in patients with femoral nerve paralysis.[4]

Synovectomy is a hemostatic procedure and should probably be limited to patients under the age of 20 years with radiographically less advanced arthropathy when conservative therapies are not successful.[198] The procedure has proved successful in control of repeated or intractable hemorrhage.[4] Synoviorthesis with osmic acid is less effective than synovectomy in preventing recurrent hemarthrosis, but because of its simplicity, it has been recommended for use in younger patients.[199] Intra-articular radioactive gold (^{198}Au) decreased bleeding frequency and halted the progression of the disease when used when the arthropathy was still reversible.[200]

In a study of 50 joints treated with radioactive gold (^{198}Au) or rhenium (^{186}Re), 60% of joints displayed no further bleeding, and 88% were improved overall.[201] The procedure reduced AHF requirements, was inexpensive, and could be repeated. The danger of extra-articular isotopic spread with chromosomal damage was thought to be minimal.[201]

Hemophilic pseudotumor has been treated successfully surgically, as well as with x-irradiation.[4,202] Many uncontrollable, destructive pseudotumors have been excised successfully.[4] In the management of fractures in the hemophilic patient, rigid immobilization has been essential. In addition to the maintenance of hemostasis during healing, internal stabilization may be required.[203]

The acquired immune deficiency syndrome (AIDS) has been reported in many patients with hemophilia, all of whom had been exposed to factor VIII or factor IX concentrates as well as other blood components. AIDS in hemophiliacs appears to be reaching epidemic proportions. Most of the patients with hemophilia and AIDS have died of opportunistic infections within a short time. Hemophiliacs are even more difficult to manage than other AIDS patients because diagnostic and therapeutic procedures may be complicated by bleeding diathesis.[204]

Purification methods (heat, lyophilization, pasteurization, organic solvent, and detergent) and donor screening have greatly reduced the risk of virus transmission in commercial factor preparations. A formulation of factor VIII purified by affinity chromatography has been approved for marketing by the U.S. Food and Drug Administration (FDA).[205] Nevertheless, until plasma-free factor VIII manufactured by recombinant DNA techniques becomes available, the risk of viral transmission is still present and must be considered when deciding to use factor concentrates.

Management

Detailed discussions of factor replacement therapy and the treatment of spontaneous hemarthroses are readily available.[206,207] Certain well-established principles deserve reiteration: acute hemarthrosis should be recognized early and treated with intensive factor infusion therapy. Both patient and parents must be instructed in this process to minimize joint damage and loss of schooling. Chronic joint disease should be managed with aggressive factor VIII or factor IX replacement as well as orthopedic and physical therapy measures for muscle building and increasing joint stability, intervals of non-weight bearing, and correction of flexion contractures.[206] However, the cornerstone of therapy in hemophilia is to immediately and adequately correct the hemostatic defect once bleeding is suspected.[208] The majority of patients with severe and moderately severe hemophilia can achieve that goal through a comprehensive multidisciplinary program of intensive self-education and a supervised self-therapy program at home.

The overriding principle is to achieve hemostasis quickly and with sufficient duration to allow wound healing. The amount of factor required depends on the location, severity, duration, and nature of the bleeding episode, as well as the long-term goals in the individual patient. The optimum or ideal dosage of factor VIII or IX varies.[206] Infusions should be given every 24 hours to achieve a minimal hemostatic level of 30% for mild hemorrhages (early hemarthrosis) and 50% for a major bleeding episode (advanced hemarthrosis) to be maintained for one or more days until resolution of the lesion occurs. Management includes repeated laboratory measurements of factor VIII or IX levels.[206,207]

Nonsteroidal anti-inflammatory drugs (NSAIDs) have been used in hemophiliac patients although the general principles of management include their avoidance.[207] No change in platelet function, bleeding time, or coagulation measures occurred with the nonacetylated salicylate salsalate. Ibuprofen did not affect the frequency of bleeding episodes or need for replacement concentrate while significantly reducing pain compared to placebo.[209] D-penicillamine reduced chronic inflammation in a rabbit model of hemarthrosis-induced arthritis and reduced the number of joint bleeding episodes in three of four hemophiliacs with chronic synovitis in uncontrolled observations.[210]

REFERENCES

1. Madhok, R., York, J., and Sturrock, R.D.: Haemophilic arthritis. Ann. Rheum. Dis., *50*:588–591, 1991.
2. Sturrock, R.D.: Hematologic disorders with rheumatic manifestations. Curr. Opin. Rheumatol., *1*:551–553, 1989.
3. Kleinman, K.S., and Coburn, J.R.: Amyloid syndromes associated with hemodialysis. Kidney Int., *35*:567–575, 1989.
4. Weisman, M.H.: Arthritis associated with hematologic disorders, storage diseases, disorders of lipid metabolism, and dysproteinemias. *In* Arthritis and Allied Conditions, Daniel J. McCarty, Philadelphia, Lea & Febiger, 1989.
5. Schwarzer, A.C., and Schreiber, L.: Rheumatic manifestations of neoplasia. Curr. Opin. Rheumatol., *1*:545–550, 1989.
6. Fink, C.W., Windmiller, J., and Sartain, P.: Arthritis as the presenting feature of childhood leukemia. Arthritis Rheum., *15*:347–349, 1972.
7. Spilberg, I., and Meyer, G.J.: The arthritis of leukemia. Arthritis Rheum., *15*:630–635, 1972.
8. Case Records of the Massachusetts General Hospital, N. Engl. J. Med. *314*:973–981, 1986.
9. Schaller, J.: Arthritis as a presenting manifestation of malignancy in children. J. Pediatr., *81*:793–797, 1972.
10. Weinberger, A., Schumacher, H.R., and Schimmer, B.M.: Arthritis in acute leukemia: Clinical and histopathological observations. Arch. Intern. Med., *141*:1183–1187, 1981.
11. Luzar, M.J., and Sharma, H.M.: Leukemia and arthritis: Including reports on light, immunofluorescent and electron microscopy of the synovium. J. Rheumatol., *10*:132–135, 1983.
12. Yoon, S.S. et al.: A case of leukemia-associated arthritis—Identification of leukemic cells in synovial fluid by light microscopy. J. Korean Med. Sci., *2*:255–258, 1987.
13. Gagnerle, F. et al.: Arthritis of the knees in B cell chronic lymphocytic leukemia: A patient with immunologic evidence of B lymphocytic synovial infiltration. Arthritis Rheum., *31*:815–816, 1988.
14. Soebergen, E.M. et al.: T cell leukemia presenting as chronic polyarthritis. Arthritis Rheum., *25*:87–91, 1982.
15. Evans, F.J., and Hilton, J.H.B.: Polymyositis associated with acute monocytic leukemia: Case report and review of the literature. Can. Med. Assoc. J., *91*:1272–1275, 1964.
16. Valimaki, M., Vuopio, P., and Luewendahl, K.: Bone lesions in chronic myelogenous leukemia. Acta Med. Scand., *210*:403–408, 1981.
17. Greenfield, G.B.: Radiology of Bone Diseases. 5th Ed. Philadelphia, J.B. Lippincott, 1990.
18. Hudson, T.L.: Radiologic-Pathologic Correlation of Musculoskeletal Lesions. Baltimore, Williams & Wilkins, 1987.
19. Resnick, D., and Haghighi, P.: Myeloproliferative disorders. *In* Diagnosis of Bone and Joint Disorders. 2nd Ed. Edited by D. Resnick and G. Niwayama. Philadelphia, W.B. Saunders, 1988, pp. 2459–2496.
20. Salimi, Z., Vas W., and Sundaram M.: Avascular bone necrosis in an untreated case of chronic myelogenous leukemia. Skeletal Radiol., *17*:353–355, 1988.
21. Holl, G. et al.: False-positive granulocyte scintigraphy in a patient with acute leukemia. Eur. J. Nucl. Med., *14*:628, 1988.
22. Caudle, R.J. et al.: Childhood acute lymphoblastic leukemia presenting as "cold" lesions on bone scan: A report of two cases. J. Pediatr. Orthop., *7*:93–95, 1987.
23. Elkton, R.B., Hughes, G.R.V., and Catovsky, D.: Hairy cell leukemia with polyarthritis nodosa. Lancet, *2*:280–282, 1979.
24. Gabriel, S.E. et al.: Vasculitis in hairy cell leukemia: Review of literature and consideration of possible pathogenetic mechanisms. J. Rheumatol., *13*:1167–1172, 1986.
25. Westbrook, C.A., and Golde, D.W.: Autoimmune disease in hairy cell leukemia: Clinical syndromes and treatment. Br. J. Haematol., *61*:349–356, 1985.
26. Weinstein, A.: Systemic vasculitis and hairy cell leukemia. J. Rheumatol., *9*:349–350, 1982.
27. Demames, D.J., Lane, N., and Beckstead, J.H.: Bone involvement in hairy-cell leukemia. Cancer, *49*:1697–1701, 1982.

28. Castro, M. et al.: Rheumatic manifestations in myelodysplastic syndrome. J. Rheumatol., *18*:721–727, 1991.
29. Aston, J.W., Jr.: Pediatric update #16. The orthopaedic presentation of neuroblastoma. Orthop. Rev., *19*:929–932, 1990.
30. Puczynski, M.S., Demos, T.C., and Suarez, C.R.: Sinus histiocytosis with massive lymphadenopathy: Skeletal involvement. Pediatr. Radiol, *15*:259–261, 1985.
31. Heinicke, M.H., Zarrabi, M.H., and Gorevic, P.D.: Arthritis due to synovial involvement by extramedullary haematopoiesis in myelofibrosis with myeloid metaplasia. Ann. Rheum. Dis., *42*:196–200, 1983.
32. Newcomer, L.N. et al.: Bone involvement in Hodgkin's disease. Cancer, *49*:338–342, 1982.
33. Emkey, R.D. et al.: A case of lymphoproliferative disease presenting as juvenile rheumatoid arthritis: Diagnosis by synovial fluid examination. Am. J. Med., *54*:825–828, 1977.
34. Martin, V.M. et al.: Lymphosarcomatous arthropathy. Ann. Rheum. Dis., *32*:162–166, 1973.
35. Adamsky, A., Varetzky, A., and Klajman, A.: Malignant lymphoma presenting as sternoclavicular joint arthritis. Arthritis Rheum., *23*:1330–1331, 1981.
36. Dorfman, H.D., Siegel, H.L., Perry, M.C., and Oxenhandler, R.: Non-Hodgkin's lymphoma of the synovium simulating rheumatoid symptoms. Arthritis Rheum., *30*:155–161, 1987.
37. Dosovetz, D.E. et al.: Primary lymphoma of bone. Cancer, *51*:44–46, 1983.
38. Dosovetz, D.E. et al.: Primary lymphoma of bone. Cancer, *50*:1009–1014, 1982.
39. Rice, D.M. et al.: Primary lymphoma of bone presenting as monarthritis. J. Rheumatol., *11*:851–854, 1984.
40. Frizzera, G., Moran, E.M., and Rappoport, H.: Angioimmunoblastic lymphadenopathy: Diagnostic and clinical course. Am. J. Med., *59*:803–818, 1975.
41. Pangalis, G.A. et al.: Angio-immunoblastic lymphadenopathy: Long-term follow-up study. Cancer, *52*:318–321, 1983.
42. Bignon, Y.I. et al.: Angioimmunoblastic lymphadenopathy with dysproteinaemia (AILD) and sicca syndrome. Ann. Rheum. Dis., *45*:519–522, 1986.
43. Webster, E., Corman, L.C., and Braylan, R.C.: Syndrome temporal arteritis with perivascular infiltration by malignant cells in a patient with follicular small cleaved cell lymphoma. J. Rheumatol., *13*:1163–1166, 1986.
44. Boumpas, D.T. et al.: Synovitis in angioimmunoblastic lymphadenopathy with dysproteinemia simulating rheumatoid arthritis. Arthritis Rheum., *33*:578–582, 1990.
45. D'uhrsen, U. et al.: Spectrum and frequency of autoimmune derangements in lymphoproliferative disorders: Analysis of 637 cases and comparison with myeloproliferative diseases. Br. J. Haematol., *67*:235–239, 1987.
46. Seleznick, M.J. et al.: Polyarthritis associated with cutaneous T cell lymphoma. J. Rheumatol., *16*:1379–1382, 1989.
47. Thomson, G.T. et al.: Erythema nodosum and non-Hodgkin's lymphoma. J. Rheumatol., *17*:383–385, 1990.
48. Resnick, D.: Plasma cell dyscrasias and dysgammaglobulinemias. *In* Diagnosis of Bone and Joint Disorders. 2nd Ed. Edited by D. Resnick. Philadelphia, W.B. Saunders, 1988, pp. 2358–2403.
49. Gordon, D.A., Pruzanski, W., and Ogryzlow, M.A.: Synovial fluid examination for the diagnosis of amyloidosis. Ann. Rheum. Dis., *32*:428–430, 1973.
50. Hickling, P., Wilkens, M., and Newman, G.R.: A study of arthropathy in multiple myeloma. Q. J. Med., *200*:417–433, 1981.
51. Hall, S., and Luthra, H.S.: Rheumatologic manifestations of amyloid disease. Minn. Med., *66*:631–632, 1983.
52. Leonard, P.A., Clegg, D.O., and Lee, R.G.: Erosive arthritis in a patient with amyloid arthropathy. Clin. Rheumatol., *4*:212–217, 1985.
53. Stone, M.J., and Frenkel, E.P.: The clinical spectrum of light chain myeloma: A study of 35 patients with special reference to the occurrence of amyloidosis. Am. J. Med., *58*:601–619, 1975.
54. Gompels, B.M., Votaw, M.L., and Martel, W.: Correlation of radiologic manifestations of multiple myeloma with immunoglobulin abnormalities and prognosis. Radiology, *104*:509–514, 1972.
55. Scott, R.B. et al.: Neuropathic joint disease (Charcot joints) in Waldenstrom's macroglobulinemia with amyloidosis. Am. J. Med., *54*:535–538, 1973.
56. Bardwick, P.A. et al.: Plasma cell dyscrasia with polyneuropathy, organomegaly, endocrinopathy, M Protein and skin changes: The POEMS syndrome. Medicine, *59*:311–322, 1980.
57. Resnick, D., Haghighi, P., and Guerra, J., Jr.: Bone sclerosis and proliferation in a man with multisystem disease. Invest. Radiol., *19*:1, 1984.
58. Bardin, T.: Dialysis related amyloidosis. J. Rheumatol., *14*:647–649, 1987.
59. Noel, L.H., et al.: Tissue distribution of dialysis amyloidosis. Clin. Nephrol., *27*:175–178, 1987.
60. Munoz-Gomez, J., Gomez-Perez, R., Llopart-Buisan, E., and Sole-Arques, M.: Clinical picture of the amyloid arthropathy in patients with chronic renal failure maintained on haemodialysis using cellulose membranes. Ann. Rheum. Dis., *46*:573–579, 1987.
61. Brown, E.A., Arnold, I.R., and Gower, P.E.: Dialysis arthropathy: Complication of long term haemodialysis. Br. Med. J., *292*:163–166, 1986.
62. Munoz-Gomez, J., Gomez-Perez, R., Sole-Arques, M., and Llopart-Buisan, E.: Synovial fluid examination for the diagnosis of synovial amyloidosis in patients with chronic renal failure undergoing haemodialysis. Ann. Rheum. Dis., *46*:324–326, 1987.
63. Bruckner, F.E. et al.: Synovial amyloid in chronic haemodialysis contains B2 microglobulin. Ann. Rheum. Dis., *46*:634–637, 1987.
64. Huaux, J.P. et al.: Erosive azotemic osteoarthropathy: Possible role of amyloidosis. Arthritis Rheum., *28*:1075–1076, 1985.
65. Bardin, T. et al.: Synovial amyloidosis in patients undergoing long term hemodialysis. Arthritis Rheum., *28*:1052–1058, 1985.
66. Gejyo, F. et al.: A new form of amyloid protein associated with hemodialysis was identified as B2 microglobulin. Biochem. Biophys. Res. Commun., *129*:701–706, 1985.
67. Gorevic, P.D. et al.: Polymerization of intact beta-2 microglobulin in tissue causes amyloidosis in patients on chronic hemodialysis. Proc. Natl. Acad. Sci. USA, *83*:7908–7912, 1986.
68. Vanderbroucke, J.M. et al.: Possible role of dialysis membrane characteristics in amyloid osteoarthropathy. Lancet, *1*:1210–1211, 1986.
69. Chanard, J. et al.: B-2 microglobulin associated amyloidosis in chronic haemodialysis patients. Lancet, *1*:1212, 1986.
70. Casey, T.T., Stone, W.J., and Di Raimondo, C.R.: Tumoral amyloidosis of bone of β2 microglobulin origin in association with long term hemodialysis. Hum. Pathol., *17*:731–738, 1986.
71. Gorevic, P.D. et al.: Beta-2 microglobulin is an amyloidogenic protein in man. J. Clin. Invest., *76*:2425–2429, 1985.
72. Sebert, J.L. et al.: Destructive spondylarthropathy in hemodialyzed patients: Possible role of amyloidosis. Arthritis Rheum., *29*:301–303, 1986.
73. Munoz-Gomez, J., and Estrada Laza, P.: Destructive spondyarthropathy in hemodialyzed patients. Arthritis Rheum., *29*:1171–1172, 1986.
74. Hardouin, P. et al.: Current aspects of osteoarticular pathology

in patients undergoing hemodialysis: Study of 80 patients: Part 1. Clinical and radiological analysis. J. Rheumatol., *14*:780–783, 1987.
75. Hardouin, P. et al.: Current aspects of osteoarticular pathology in patients undergoing hemodialysis: Study of 80 patients: Part 2. Laboratory and pathologic analysis. Discussion of the pathogenic mechanism. J. Rheumatol., *14*:784–787, 1987.
76. Fiocchi, O., Bedani, P.L., Orzincolo, C., et al.: Radiological features of dialysis amyloid spondylarthropathy. Int. J. Artif. Organs, *12*:216–222, 1989.
77. Bindi, P., Lavaud, S., Bernieh, B., et al.: Early and late occurrences of destructive spondylarthropathy in haemodialysed patients. Nephrol. Dial. Transplant, *5*:199–203, 1990.
78. Hurst, N.P., van den Berg, R., Disney, A., et al.: Dialysis related arthropathy: A survey of 95 patients receiving chronic haemodialysis with special reference to β 2 microglobulin related amyloidosis. Ann. Rheum. Dis., *48*:409–420, 1989.
79. Brunner, F.P., Brynger, H., Ehrich, J.H., et al.: Case control study of dialysis arthropathy: The influence of two different dialysis membranes: Data from the EDTA Registry. Nephrol. Dial. Transplant, *5*:432–436, 1990.
80. Cronelis, F., Bardin, T., Faller, B., et al.: Rheumatic syndromes and β_2-microglobulin amyloidosis in patients receiving long-term peritoneal dialysis. Arthritis Rheum., *32*:785–788, 1989.
81. Ogawa, H., Saito, A., and Ono, M.: Inflammation as the possible cause of cystic radiolucencies in carpal bones of patient on hemodialysis. ASAIO Trans., *35*:317–319, 1989.
82. Bardin, T., and Kuntz, D.: The arthropathy of chronic haemodialysis. Clin. Exp. Rheumatol., *5*:379–386, 1987.
83. Maury, C.P.: β_2-Microglobulin amyloidosis. A systemic amyloid disease affecting primarily synovium and bone in long-term dialysis patients. Rheumatol. Int., *10*:1–8, 1990.
84. Huo, M.H., Friedlaender, G.E., and Marsh, J.S.: Orthopaedic manifestations of sickle-cell disease. Yale J. Biol. Med., *63*:195–207, 1990.
85. Reynolds, M.D.: Gout and hyperuricemia associated with sickle-cell anemia. Semin. Arthritis Rheum., *12*:404–413, 1983.
86. Leff, R.D., Aldo-Benson, M.A., and Fife, R.S.: Tophaceous gout in patients with sickle cell-thalassemia: Case report and a review of the literature. Arthritis Rheum., *26*:928–929, 1983.
87. de Ceulaer, K. et al.: Non-gouty arthritis in sickle cell disease: Report of 37 consecutive cases. Ann. Rheum. Dis., *43*:599–603, 1984.
88. Strauss, J. et al.: Cryoprecipitable immune complex nephropathy and sickle cell disease. Ann. Intern. Med., *81*:114–115, 1974.
89. Johnston, R.B., Jr., Newman, S.L., and Struth, A.G.: An abnormality of the alternate pathway of complement activation in sickle cell disease. N. Engl. J. Med., *288*:803–808, 1973.
90. Ben Dridi, M.F. et al.: Radiological abnormalities of the skeleton in patients with sickle-cell anemia. A study of 222 cases in Tunisia. Pediatr. Radiol., *17*:296–302, 1987.
91. Dorwart, B.B. et al.: Absence of increased frequency of bone and joint disease with hemoglobin AS and AC. Ann. Intern. Med., *86*:66–67, 1977.
92. Gunderson, C., D'Ambrosia, R.D., and Shoij, H.: Total hip replacement in patients with sickle-cell disease. J. Bone Joint Surg., *59A*:760–762, 1977.
93. Worrall, V.T., and Butera, V.: Sickle-cell dactylitis. J. Bone Joint Surg., *58A*:1161–1163, 1976.
94. Moxley, G.F., Owne, D.S., and Irby, R.: Septic arthritis due to Fusobacterium varium in patient with sickle-cell anemia. J. Rheumatol., *10*:161–162, 1983.
95. Harden, W.B. et al.: Septic arthritis due to Serratia liquefaciens. Arthritis Rheum., *23*:946–947, 1980.
96. Hand, W.L., and King, N.L.: Serum opsonization of Salmonella in sickle cell anemia. Am. J. Med., *64*:388–395, 1978.
97. Wilson, W.A., Hughes, G.R., and Lachmann, P.J.: Deficiency of factor B of the complement system in sickle cell anaemia. Br. Med. J., *1*:367–369, 1976.
98. Palmer, D.W.: Septic arthritis in sickle-cell thalassemia: Pathophysiology of impaired response to infection. Arthritis Rheum., *18*:339–345, 1975.
99. Bennett, O.M., and Namnyak, S.S.: Bone and joint manifestations of sickle cell anaemia. J. Bone Joint Surg., *72B*:494–499, 1990.
100. Syrogiannopoulos, G.A., McCracken, G.H., Jr., and Nelson, J.D.: Osteoarticular infections in children with sickle cell disease. Pediatrics, *78*:1090–1096, 1986.
101. Sankaren-Kutty, M., Sadat-Ali, M., and Kutty, M.K.: Septic arthritis in sickle cell disease. Int. Orthop., *12*:255–257, 1988.
102. Ebong, W.W.: Septic arthritis in patients with sickle-cell disease. Br. J. Rheumatol., *26*:99–102, 1987.
103. Rao, S.P., Miller, S., and Solomon, N.: Acute bone and joint manifestations of sickle cell disease in children. N.Y. State J. Med., *86*:254–260, 1986.
104. Gratwick, G.M. et al.: Thalassemic osteoarthropathy. Ann. Intern. Med., *88*:494–501, 1978.
105. Schlumph, U. et al.: Arthritis in thalassemia minor. Schweiz. Med. Wochenschr., *107*:1156–1162, 1977.
106. Abou Rizk, N.A., Nasr, F.W., and Frayha, R.A.: Aseptic necrosis in thalassemia minor. Arthritis Rheum., *20*:1147–1148, 1977.
107. Gerster, J.C., Dardel, R., and Guggi, S.: Recurrent episodes of arthritis in thalassemia minor. J. Rheumatol., *11*:352–354, 1984.
108. Marino, C., and McDonald, E.: Rheumatoid arthritis in a patient with sickle cell disease. J. Rheumatol., *17*:970–972, 1990.
109. Gladman, D.D., and Bombardier, C.: Sickle cell crisis following intraarticular steroid therapy for rheumatoid arthritis. Arthritis Rheum., *30*:1065–1068, 1987.
110. Scriver, C.R. et al. (eds.): The Metabolic Basis of Inherited Disease. 6th Ed. New York, McGraw-Hill, 1989.
111. Beaudet, A.L.: Lysosomal storage diseases. *In* Harrison's Principles of Internal Medicine. 12th Ed. Edited by E. Braunwald et al. New York, McGraw-Hill, 1991, pp. 1845–1860.
112. Barranger, J.A., and Gerins, E.I.: Glucosylceramide lipidosis: Gaucher Disease. *In* The Metabolic Basics of Inherited Diseases. 6th Ed. Edited by C.R. Scriver et al. New York, McGraw-Hill, 1989, pp. 1677–1698.
113. Schubiner, H., Lefourdeau, M., and Murray, D.L.: Pyogenic osteomyelitis versus pseudo-osteomyelitis in Gaucher's disease. Clin. Pediatr., *20*:667–669, 1981.
114. Wrizman, Z., Tennenbaum, A., and Yatziv, S.: Interphalangeal joint involvement in Gaucher's disease, Type 1, resembling juvenile rheumatoid arthritis. Arthritis Rheum., *25*:706–707, 1982.
115. Lan, M.M. et al.: Hip arthroplasties in Gaucher's disease. J. Bone Joint Surg., *63A*:591–601, 1981.
116. Colhoun, E.N. et al.: Unusual disco-vertebral changes in Gaucher's disease. Br. J. Radiol., *60*:925–928, 1987.
117. Rose, J.S. et al.: Accelerated skeletal deterioration after splenectomy in Gaucher type I disease. AJR, *139*:1202–1204, 1982.
118. Shiloni, E. et al.: The role of splenectomy in Gaucher's disease. Arch. Surg., *118*:929–932, 1983.
119. Garfinkle, B. et al.: Coexistence of Gaucher's disease and multiple myeloma. Arch. Intern. Med., *142*:2229–2230, 1982.
120. Kudoh, T., and Wenger, D.A.: Diagnosis of metachromatic leukodystrophy, Krabbe's disease, and Farber's disease after uptake of fatty acid labeled cerebroside sulfate into cultured skin fibroblasts. J. Clin. Invest., *70*:89–97, 1982.

121. Pouard, A.C. et al.: Enzymological diagnosis of a group of lysosomal storage diseases. Med. J. Aust., *2*:549–553, 1980.
122. Desnick, R.J., and Bishop, D.F.: Fabry disease: α-Galactosedase deficiency. *In* The Metabolic Basis of Inherited Disease. 6th Ed. New York, McGraw-Hill, 1989, pp. 1751–1796.
123. Braverman, I.M., and Ken, Y.A.: Ultrastructure and three dimensional reconstruction of several macular and papular telangiectases. J. Invest. Dermatol., *81*:489–497, 1983.
124. Seino, I. et al.: Peripheral hemodynamics in patients with Fabry's disease. Am. Heart J., *105*:783–787, 1983.
125. Ahlmen, J. et al.: Clinical and diagnostic considerations in Fabry's disease. Acta Med. Scand., *211*:309–312, 1982.
126. Moser, H.W. et al.: Ceramidase deficiency: Farber liprogranulomatoses. *In* The Metabolic Basis of Inherited Disease. 6th Ed. New York, McGraw-Hill, 1989, pp. 1645–1654.
127. Chen, W.W., and Deeker, G.L.: Abnormalities of lysosomes in human diploid fibroblasts from patients with Farber's disease. Biochim. Biophys. Acta, *718*:185–192, 1982.
128. Jameson, R.A., Holt, P.J. and Keen, J.H.: Farber's disease (lysosomal acid ceramidase deficiency). Ann. Rheum. Dis., *46*:559–561, 1987.
129. Rodey, G.E. et al.: Defective bactericidal activity of peripheral blood leukocytes in lipochrome histiocytosis. Am. J. Med., *49*:327–332, 1970.
130. Heathcote, J.G., Buenther, L.G., and Wallace, A.C.: Multicentric reticulohistiocytosis: A report of a case and a review of the pathology. Pathology, *17*:601–608, 1985.
131. Nunnink, J.C., Krusinski, P.A., and Yates, J.W.: Multicentric reticulohistiocytosis and cancer: A case report and review of the literature. Med. Pediatr. Oncol., *13*:273–279, 1985.
132. Kes'anieml, Y.A., Ehnholm, C., and Miettinen, T.A.: Multicentric reticulohistiocytosis, another lipid disorder with normolipidemic xanthomatosis? Atherosclerosis, *68*:179–189, 1987.
133. Zagala, A., Guyot, A., Bensa, J.C., and Phelip, X.: Multicentric reticulohistiocytosis: A case with enhanced interleukin-1, prostaglandin E2 and interleukin-2 secretin. J. Rheumatol., *15*:136–138, 1988.
134. Ginsburg, W.W., O'Duffy, J.D., Morris, J.L., and Huston, K.A.: Multicentric reticulohistiocytosis: Response to alkylating agents in six patients. Ann. Intern. Med., *1*:384–388, 1989.
135. Widman, D., Swayne, L.C., and Rozan, S.: Multicentric reticulohistiocytosis: Assessment of pulmonary disease by gallium-67 scintigraphy. J. Rheumatol., *15*:132–135, 1988.
136. Yoshimura, Y., Sugihara, T., Kishimoto, H., and Nagaoka, S.: Multicentric reticulohistiocytosis accompanied by oral and temporomandibular joint manifestations. J. Oral Maxillofac. Surg., *45*:84–86, 1987.
137. Katz, R.W., and Anderson, K.F.: Multicentric reticulohistiocytois. Oral Surg. Oral Med. Oral Pathol., *65*:721–725, 1988.
138. Freemont, A.J., Jones, C.I.P., and Denton, J.: The synovium and synovial fluid in multicentric reticulohistiocytosis—A light microscopic, electron microscopic and cytochemical analysis of one case. J. Clin. Pathol., *3*:860–866, 1983.
139. Tani, M. et al.: Multicentric reticulohistiocytosis: Electromicroscopic and ultracytochemical studies. Arch. Dermatol., *117*:495–499, 1981.
140. Hall, S. et al.: Multicentric reticulohistiocytosis. Arthritis Rheum., *27*:S79, 1984.
141. Scutellari, P.N., Orzincolo, C., and Trotta, F.: Case report 375: Multicentric reticulohistiocytosis. Skeletal Radiol., *15*:394–397, 1986.
142. Brandt, F. et al.: Topical nitrogen mustard therapy in multicentric reticulohistiocytosis. J. Am. Acad. Dermatol., *6*:260–262, 1982.
143. Doherty, M., Martin, M.F.R., and Dieppe, P.A.: Multicentric reticulohistiocytosis associated with primary biliary cirrhosis: Successful treatment with cytotoxic agents. Arthritis Rheum., *27*:344–348, 1984.
144. Furey, N.D. et al.: Multicentric reticulohistiocytosis with salivary gland involvement and pericardial effusion. J. Am. Acad. Dermatol., *8*:679–685, 1983.
145. Carey, R.N. et al.: Multicentric reticulohistiocytosis and Sjögren's syndrome. J. Rheumatol., *12*:1193–1195, 1985.
146. Zayid, I., and Farraj, S.: Familial histiocytic dermatoarthritis: A new syndrome. Am. J. Med., *54*:793–800, 1973.
147. Goldstein, J.L., and Brown, M.S.: Familial hypercholesterolemia. *In* The Metabolic Basis of Inherited Disease. 6th Ed. New York, McGraw-Hill, 1989, pp. 1215–1250.
148. Mahley, R.W., and Rall, S.C.: Type 3 hyperlipoproteinemia (dysbetalipoproteinemia). *In* The Metabolic Basis of Inherited Disease. 5th Ed. New York, McGraw-Hill, 1989, pp. 1195–1213.
149. Brunzell, J.D.: Familial liproprotein lipase deficiency and other causes of the chylomicronemia syndrome. *In* The Metabolic Basis of Inherited Disease. 6th Ed. New York, McGraw-Hill, 1989, pp. 1165–1180.
150. Mathon, G. et al.: Articular manifestations of familial hypercholesterolaemia. Ann. Rheum. Dis., *44*:599–602, 1985.
151. Carroll, G.J., and Bayliss, C.E.: Treatment of the arthropathy of familial hypercholesterolaemia. Ann. Rheum. Dis., *42*: 206–209, 1983.
152. Rimon, D., and Cohen, L.: Hypercholesterolemic (type II hyperlipoproteinemic) arthritis. J. Rheumatol., *16*:703–705, 1989.
153. Rooney, P.J.: Atheroma, arthritis and all that. J. Rheumatol., *16*:570–571, 1989.
154. Wysenbeck, A.J., Shaui, E., and Beigel, Y.: Musculoskeletal manifestations in patients with hypercholesterolemia. J. Rheumatol., *16*:643–645, 1989.
155. Buckingham, R.B., Bole, G.G., and Bassett, D.R.: Polyarthritis associated with type IV hyperlipoproteinemia. Arch. Intern. Med., *135*:286–290, 1975.
156. Goldman, J.A. et al.: Musculoskeletal disorders associated with type-IV hyperlipoproteinaemia. Lancet, *2*:449–452, 1972.
157. Bjorken, I., and Skrede, S.: Familial diseases with storage of sterols other than cholesterol. *In* The Metabolic Basis of Inherited Disease. 6th Ed. New York, McGraw-Hill, 1989, pp. 1283–1302.
158. Shulman, R.S. et al.: Beta-sitosterolemia and xanthomatosis. N. Engl. J. Med., *294*:482–483, 1976.
159. Colman, R.W., Hirsh, J., Marder, V.J., and Salzman, E.W. (eds.): Hemostasis and Thrombosis: Basic Principles and Clinical Practice. 2nd Ed. Philadelphia, J.B. Lippincott, 1987.
160. Steven, M.M. et al.: Haemophilic arthritis. Q. J. Med., *58*:181–197, 1986.
161. Katz, A.L., and Alepa, F.P.: Hemarthrosis secondary to heparin therapy. (Letter.) Arthritis Rheum., *19*:996, 1976.
162. Wild, J.H., and Zvaifler, N.J. Hemarthrosis associated with sodium warfarin therapy. Arthritis Rheum., *19*:98–102, 1976.
163. Andes, W.A., and Edmunds, J.O.: Hemarthroses and warfarin: Joint destruction with anticoagulation. Thromb. Haemost., *28*:187–189, 1983.
164. Swanton, M.C., and Mepocki, G.P.: Pathology of joints in canine hemophilia A. *In* Handbook of Hemophilia. Edited by K.M. Brinkous and H.C. Hemker. Amsterdam, Excerpta Medica, 1975, pp. 313–332.
165. Mainardi, C.L. et al.: Proliferative synovitis in hemophilia: Biochemical and morphologic observations. Arthritis Rheum., *21*:137–144, 1978.
166. McLardy Smith, P.D., Ashton, I.K., and Duthie, R.B.: A tissue culture model of cartilage breakdown in haemophilic arthropathy. Scand. J. Haematol. [Suppl.], *40*:215–220, 1984.

167. Andes, W.A., Walker, P.D., Edmunds, J.O., and Wulff, K.M.: Hemophilic arthropathy–An immunologic study of the synovium. Scand. J. Haematol. [Suppl.], *40*:221–224, 1984.
168. Sokoloff, L.: Biochemical and physiological aspects of degenerative joint diseases with special reference to hemophilic arthropathy. Ann. N.Y. Acad. Sci., *240*:285–290, 1975.
169. Speer, O.P.: Early pathogenesis of hemophilic arthropathy: Evolution of the subchondral cyst. Clin. Orthop., *185*:250–265, 1984.
170. Riley, S.A., and Spencer, G.E., Jr.: Destructive monarticular arthritis secondary to anticoagulant therapy. Clin. Orthop., *223*:247–251, 1987.
171. Forbes, C.D. et al.: A comparison of thermography, radioisotope scanning and clinical assessment of the knee joints in haemophilia. Clin. Radiol., *26*:41–45, 1975.
172. Steven, M.M. et al.: Radio-isotopic joint scans in haemophilic arthritis. Br. J. Rheumatol., *24*:263–268, 1985.
173. Macfarlane, J.D., Kroon, H.M., and Caekebeke-Peerlinck, K.M.: Arthropathy in von Willebrand's disease. Clin. Rheumatol.,. *8*:98–102, 1989.
174. Defaria, C.R., Demelo-Souza, S.E., and Pinheiro, E.D.: Haemophilic neuromyopathy. J. Neurol. Neurosurg. Psychiatry, *42*:600–605, 1979.
175. Resnick, D.: Bleeding disorders. *In* Diagnosis of Bone and Joint Disorders. 2nd Ed. Edited by D. Resnick and G. Niwayama. Philadelphia, W.B. Saunders, 1988, pp. 2497–2522.
176. Morgante, D., Pathria, M., Sartoris, D.J., and Resnick, D.: Subtalar and intertarsal joint involvement in hemophilia and juvenile chronic arthritis: Frequency and diagnostic significance of radiographic abnormalities. Foot Ankle, *9*:45–48, 1988.
177. Leonello, P.P., Cleland, L.G., and Norman, J.E.: Acute pseudogout and chondrocalcinosis in a man with mild hemophilia. J. Rheumatol., *8*:841–844, 1981.
178. Brettler, D.B. et al.: A long-term study of hemophilic arthropathy of the knee joint on a program of factor VIII replacement given at time of each hemarthrosis. Am. J. Hematol., *18*:13–18, 1985.
179. Madhok, R., Vork, J., and Sturrock, R.D.: Haemophilic arthritis. Am. Rheum. Dis., *50*:588–591, 1991.
180. Houghton, G.R.: Septic arthritis of the hip in a hemophiliac. Clin. Orthop., *129*:223–244, 1977.
181. Moseley, P. et al.: Hemophilia, maintenance hemodialysis, and septic arthritis. Arch. Intern. Med., *141*:138–139, 1981.
182. Rosner, S.M., and Bhogal, R.S.: Infectious arthritis in a hemophiliac. J. Rheumatol., *8*:519–521, 1981.
183. Wilkins, R.M., and Wiedel, J.D.: Septic arthritis of the knee in a hemophiliac. A case report. J. Bone Joint Surg., *65*:267–268, 1983.
184. Goldsmith, J.C., Silberstein, P.T., Fromm, R.E., Jr., and Walker, D.Y.: Hemophilic arthropathy complicated by polyarticular septic arthritis. A case report. Acta Haematol. (Basel), *71*:121–123, 1984.
185. Cobb, W.B.: Septic polyarthritis in a hemophiliac. J. Rheumatol., *11*:87–891, 1984.
186. Scott, J.P., Maurer, H.S., and Dias, L.: Septic arthritis in two teenaged hemophiliacs. J. Pediatr., *107*:748–751, 1985.
187. Hofmann, A., Wyatt, R., and Bybee, B.: Septic arthritis of the knee in a 12-year-old hemophiliac. J. Pediatr. Orthop., *4*:498–499, 1984.
188. Ragni, M.V., and Hanley, E.N.: Septic arthritis in hemophilic patients and infection with human immunodeficiency virus (HIV). Ann. Intern. Med., *110*:168–169, 1989.
189. Mba, E.C., and Njoku, O.S.: Polyarticular pneumococcal pyarthrosis in a young haemophiliac. Acta Haematol. (Basel), *77*:62–63, 1987.
190. Bleasel, J.F., York, J.R., and Rickard, K.A.: Septic arthritis in human immunodeficiency virus infected haemophiliacs. Br. J. Rheumatol., *29*:494–496, 1990.
191. Hartmann, L.C., and Nauseef, W.M.: Group B streptococcal polyarthritis complicating hemophilia B. Acta Haematol. (Basel), *84*:95–97, 1990.
192. Pappo, A.S., Buchanan, G.R., and Johnson, A.: Septic arthritis in children with hemophilia. Am. J. Dis. Child., *143*:1226–1228, 1989.
193. Ellison, R.T., 3rd, and Reller, L.B.: Differentiating pyogenic arthritis from spontaneous hemarthrosis in patients with hemophilia. West J. Med., *144*:42–45, 198.
194. Thakker, S., McGehee, W., and Quismorio, F.P., Jr.: Arthropathy associated with factor XIII deficiency. Arthritis Rheum., *29*:808–811, 1986.
195. Sankarankutty, M., and Evans, D.I.: Chronic arthropathy in von Willebrand's disease. Clin. Lab. Haematol., *5*:149–156, 1983.
196. Mazza, J.J., et al.: Antihemophilic factor VIII in hemophilia: Use of concentrates to permit major surgery. JAMA, *211*:1818–1823, 1970.
197. Small, M. et al.: Total knee arthroplasty in hemophilic arthritis. J. Bone Joint Surg., 163–165, 1983.
198. Matsuda, Y., and Duthie, R.B.: Surgical synovectomy for haemophilic arthropathy of the knee joint: Long-term follow-up. Scand. J. Haematol. (Suppl.), *40*:237–247, 1984.
199. Gamba, G., Grignani, G., and Ascari, E.: Synoviorthesis versus synovectomy in the treatment of recurrent haemophilic haemarthrosis: Long term evaluation. Thromb. Haemost., *45*:127–129, 1981.
200. Ahlberg, A., and Pettersson, H.: Synoviorthesis with radioactive gold in hemophiliacs. Acta Orthop. Scand., *50*:513–517, 1979.
201. Fernandez-Palazzi, F., de Bosch, N.B., and de Vargas, A.F.: Radioactive synovectomy in haemophilic haemarthrosis: Follow-up on fifth cases. Scand. J. Haematol. [Suppl.], *40*:291–300, 1984.
202. Hilgartner, M.W., and Arnold, W.D.: Hemophilic pseudotumor treated with replacement therapy and radiation: Report of a case. J. Bone Joint Surg., *57A*:1145–1146, 1975.
203. Fell, E., Bentley, G., and Rizza, C.R.: Fracture management in patients with haemophilia. J. Bone Joint Surg., *56B*:643–649, 1974.
204. Evatt, B.L. et al.: The acquired immunodeficiency syndrome in patients with hemophilia. Ann. Intern. Med., *100*:499–504, 1984.
205. The Medical Letter, *29* (Jan. 1):1–4, 1988.
206. Rizza, C.R., and Matthews, J.M.: The management of patients with coagulation factor deficiencies. *In* Human Blood Coagulation, Hemostasis, and Thrombosis. 3rd Ed. Edited by R. Biggs and C.R. Rizza. Oxford, Blackwell Scientific Publications, 1984, pp. 273–318.
207. Roberts, H.R., and Jones, M.R.: Hemophilia and related conditions. *In* Hematology. 4th Ed. Edited by W.J. Williams, et al. New York, McGraw-Hill, 1990, pp. 1453–1473.
208. Levine, P.H.: Efficacy of self therapy in hemophilia: A study of 72 patients with hemophilia A and B. N. Engl. J. Med., *291*:1381–1384, 1974.
209. Steven, M.M. et al.: Non-steroidal anti-inflammatory drugs in haemophilic arthritis. A clinical and laboratory study. Haemostasis, *15*:204–209, 1985.
210. Corrigan, J.J., Jr., et al.: Treatment of hemophilic arthritis with DS-penicilliamine: A preliminary report. Am. J. Hematol., *19*:255–264, 1985.

87

Heritable and Developmental Disorders of Connective Tissue and Bone

REED E. PYERITZ

Theoretically, any disorder can be described or studied by two fundamental approaches: etiology and pathogenesis. Either can be useful, depending on the need. Understanding causes leads to reliable classification, diagnosis, and prevention; understanding mechanisms leads to effective prognosis and treatment. Unfortunately, the two approaches are often thought to be similar or even interchangeable—misconceptions that confuse nosology, management, and clinical investigation. Knowledge of etiology, no matter how refined, may shed no light on how the clinical manifestations (the phenotype) develop. For example, the "cause" of sickle cell disease is known at the highest level of resolution possible, the specific nucleotide mutation, whereas the mechanisms by which the diverse clinical features appear remain largely obscure. Conversely, the pathogenesis of acute gout is far better understood than is the etiology in most cases.

Consideration of the role of genetic factors in the disorders of a given system perforce focuses on etiology. The traditional approach has been to divide all disorders into nongenetic and genetic ones, and the latter into mendelian, chromosomal, and multifactorial categories. This scheme retains some didactic utility, provided it is recognized that no disorder is purely genetic or environmental in cause, and that all involve some interaction of genes and environment to produce the abnormal phenotype.

In *mendelian disorders*, a single mutant gene is of overriding importance, although its effect may be modulated by other genetic and environmental factors. These conditions occur in families in simple inheritance patterns, that is, autosomal dominant, autosomal recessive, or X-linked. Nearly all these disorders are individually rare (prevalences of $1/10^4$ to $1/10^6$ in the general population), but because so many are now known (over 5000 in one tabulation[1]), in the aggregate they represent a substantial category of disease. The heritable disorders of connective tissue are all examples.

Chromosomal disorders are those in which an abnormal phenotype is associated with a chromosome aberration visible with the light microscope. For example, the Down syndrome is caused by the presence of three copies of chromosome 21 (trisomy 21), or by the patient's having two normal chromosomes 21, and an additional copy of a short segment of the long arm of chromosome 21, usually attached to one of the other chromosomes. The number of syndromes associated with chromosome aberrations continues to grow as improved cytogenetic techniques enhance resolution,[2] resulting in blurring of the distinctions between mendelian and cytogenetic disorders. For example, susceptibility to retinoblastoma and the Wilms tumor–aniridia syndrome are inherited as autosomal dominant traits, but in some cases such susceptibility is due to deletions of chromosomes 13 and 11, respectively.[3] In one instructive family, the Greig cephalopolysyndactyly syndrome occurred only in relatives having an apparently balanced translocation between chromosomes 3 and 7.[4] Disruption of the gene responsible for this rare condition by the breakage and reunion of chromosome segments, without the visible loss of chromosomal material, is the most likely causal explanation.

The term *multifactorial* has a specific and a general meaning. Disorders such as pyloric stenosis, clubfoot, and idiopathic scoliosis, which conform to empiric predictions of recurrence, concordance in monozygotic twins, and differences in prevalence between sexes, are classified as multifactorial in the narrow sense.[5] On the other hand, any condition in which genes are a necessary, but insufficient, part of the cause and that is distributed in families in ways that do not fulfill any mendelian pattern can be described as multifactorial in the broad sense. Disorders in this latter category tend to be relatively common and include much of what is diagnosed as rheumatoid arthritis, osteoarthritis, and the "acquired" disorders of connective tissue (e.g., lupus and scleroderma).

Several excellent texts provide comprehensive coverage of genetic principles fundamental to an understanding of these concepts and those that will emerge from review of individual disorders.[6,7]

HERITABLE DISORDERS OF CONNECTIVE TISSUE AND BONE

This category of human disease was defined in 1955 by McKusick,[8] and in its first incarnation included only osteogenesis imperfecta, Marfan syndrome, Ehlers-Danlos syndrome, pseudoxanthoma elasticum, and gargoylism. Over more than three decades, upward of 200 distinct, mendelian disorders of connective tissue have been described and are now subject to periodic review by international committees, charged with consensus development of diagnostic criteria and nosologic boundaries (Table 87–1).[9,10] Although their classification remains rooted in phenotypic distinctions, study of the causes of these disorders at the biochemical and nucleic acid level is providing greatly increased understanding of their genesis.

The complexity of connective tissue is emphasized in Chapters 11–15 and in recent reviews.[11,12] Discovery of specific biochemical defects has only begun to be instructive about the pathogenesis of the heritable disorders of connective tissue and how the macromolecular components interact.[13–18] These disorders are as much inborn errors of metabolism as are the familial defects in amino acid and carbohydrate metabolism first investigated by Garrod at the turn of the century. With careful study, each of these disorders can serve as a window to normal structure and function of connective tissue.

TABLE 87–1. GENERAL CLASSIFICATION OF THE HERITABLE DISORDERS OF CONNECTIVE TISSUE AND BONE

CATEGORIES	BASIC DEFECT(S)
Marfan syndrome	Fibrillin and perhaps other components of microfibrils
Stickler syndrome	Type II collagen in some families
Ehlers-Danlos syndromes	Types I or III collagen in some patients
Familial articular hypermobility syndromes	?
Osteogenesis imperfecta	Various defects in type I collagen
Skeletal dysplasia with predominant joint laxity	?
Cutis laxa	?
Pseudoxanthoma elasticum	Calcification of elastic fibers
Osteochondrodysplasias	Most ? Type II collagen in spondylcepiphyseal dysplasias
Epidermolysis bullosa	Increased collagenase in one form
Disorders secondary to metabolic defects	
Alcaptonuria	Homogentisic acid oxidase deficiency
Homocystinuria	Cystathionine β-synthase deficiency
Disorders of copper transport	
Occipital horn syndrome	Decreased serum copper and ceruloplasmin
Menkes syndrome	Excess copper bound to metallothionein
Heteroglycanoses	
Mucopolysaccharidoses	Deficiencies of lysosomal hydrolases
Phosphotransferase deficiencies	Inability to modify lysosomal hydrolases
Fucosidosis	Deficiency of α-fucosidase
Mannosidosis	Deficiency of α-mannosidase
Aspartylglucosaminuria	Deficiency of aspartamido-N-Ac-glucos-amine-amidohydrolase
GM_1 gangliosidosis	Deficiency of β-galactosidase
Sialidoses	Deficiency of various neuraminidases
Sialuria	Intralysosomal neuraminic acid retention
Galactosialidosis	Deficiency of β-galactosidase and neuraminidase
Mucosulfatidosis	Deficiency of multiple suifatases
Geleophysic dysplasia	?
Miscellaneous disorders	
Buschke-Ollendorff syndrome	?
Familial cutaneous collagenoma	?
Wrinkly skin syndrome	?

The disorders chosen for description in this chapter are relatively common and important in clinical rheumatology, highly instructive as to general principles, or both.

MARFAN SYNDROME

Patients with the Marfan syndrome have diverse abnormalities, especially in the skeletal, ocular, cardiovascular, and pulmonary systems.[19,20] The diagnosis is based solely on the clinical features and the autosomal dominant inheritance pattern.[9] Although a variety of biochemical abnormalities have been described, none has proven to be the long-sought basic defect. Attention has been focused on elastic fibers because they are highly disorganized and even fragmented in the aortic media and dermis,[21–22] but if the defect were in elastin, the pathogenesis of increased length of long bones and dislocated lenses would be difficult to explain. A recently discovered, 350,000-dalton glycoprotein, fibrillin, is a constituent of both elastic fibers and the microfibrils that are so ubiquitous throughout the connective tissue.[23] Studies of Marfan patients and their relatives suggest that defects in synthesis of fibrillin account for some cases.[22,24] However, given the wide interfamilial variation in the phenotype of the Marfan syndrome and the precedent with other hereditary disorders, genetic heterogeneity is anticipated.[25]

Skeletal Features. Patients with the Marfan syndrome are excessively tall, or at least taller than unaffected relatives (Fig. 87–1). Body proportions are irregular (dolichostenomelia), with an abnormally low ratio of the upper segment to the lower segment (US/LS). In practice, two measurements are made with the patient standing: height and lower segment (top of the pubic symphisis to floor). In normal adult white persons, the mean ratio is about 0.92; in adult African-American persons, it is about 0.87. The excessive length of the lower extremities is primarily responsible for the abnormally low US/LS in the Marfan syndrome. The US/LS varies with age, race, sex, and degree of vertebral column deformity in all persons, so that an isolated determination in a suspected patient must be interpreted with caution. The arms also show excessive length, with the span of adult patients usually exceeding their height by more than 3%. The metacarpal index, based on the ratio of length to width of metacarpals, is said to be useful but requires a radiograph of the hands.

The ribs undergo excessive longitudinal growth as well. Depression of the sternum (pectus excavatum), protrusion (pectus carinatum; see Fig. 87–1), or their asymmetric combination often results.

The vertebral column is frequently deformed. Most often, the normal thoracic kyphos is lost, resulting in a "straight back" or an outright thoracic lordosis. Sco-

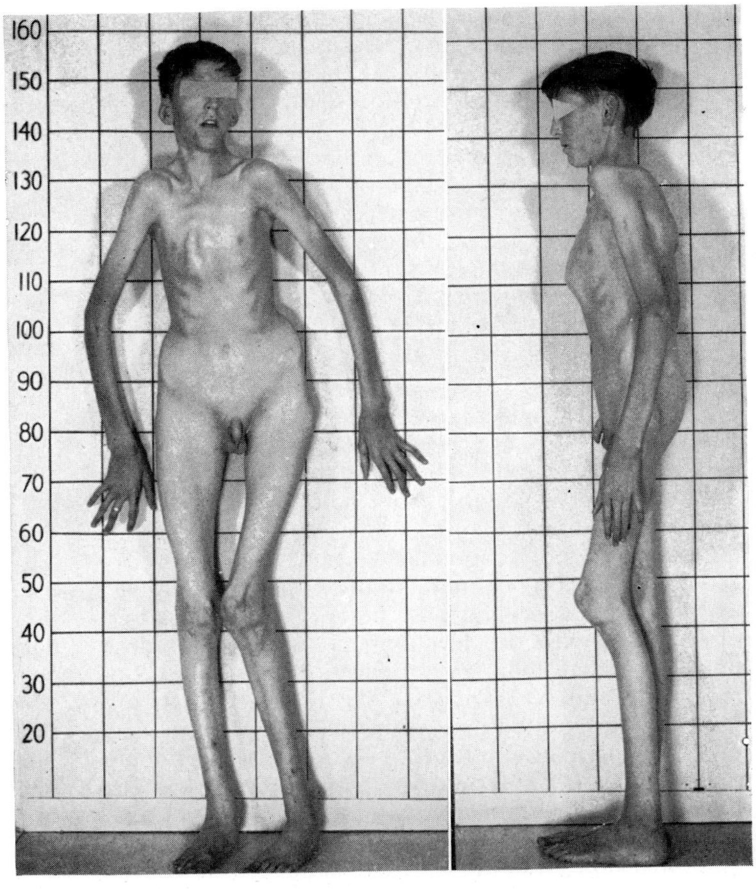

FIGURE 87–1. Marfan syndrome in a 14-year-old boy. Note arachnodactyly, relatively long limbs (dolichostenomelia), pectus carinatum, sparse subcutaneous fat, unilateral genu valgum, and pes planus. Ectopia lentis and scoliosis were also present. This patient died of aortic rupture at 15 years of age.

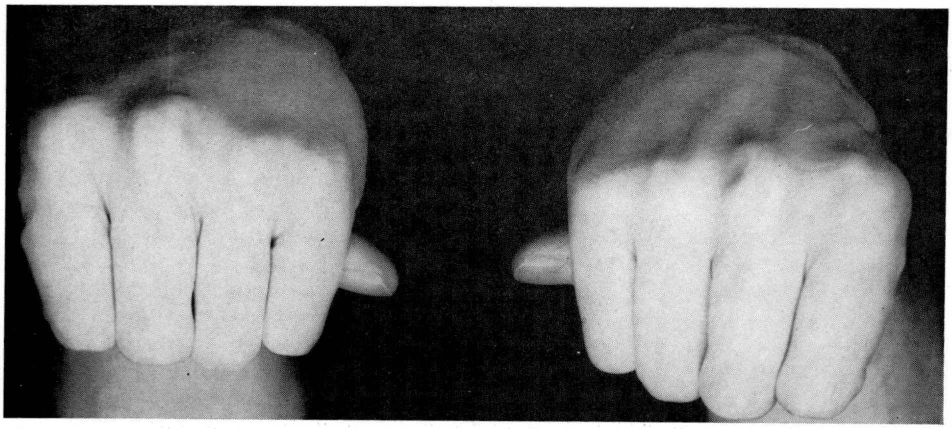

FIGURE 87–2. The Steinberg thumb sign in a patient with Marfan syndrome. A positive test, such as this, consists of the distal phalanx of the thumb protruding beyond the ulnar border of the clenched fist and reflects both longitudinal laxity of the hand and a long thumb.

liosis may involve multiple segments and may progress rapidly, particularly during the adolescent growth spurt.

Loose-jointedness is often striking in patients with the Marfan syndrome. Flat feet (pes planus), hyperextensibility at the knees (genu recurvatum), elbows, and fingers, congenital dislocation of the hip, and recurrent dislocation of the patellae are manifestations of the loose-jointedness. A relatively narrow palm of the hand, long thumb, and longitudinal laxity of the hand are the bases for the *Steinberg thumb sign* (Fig. 87–2): the thumb apposed across the palm extends well beyond the ulnar margin of the hand. Another simple, but nonspecific, test is the *wrist sign:* the first and fifth digits, when wrapped around the contralateral wrist, overlap appreciably in the Marfan syndrome (Fig. 87–3).

Joint laxity is so variable, even among relatives affected by the Marfan syndrome, that for a time distinct disorders were suspected. About 10% of patients have some restriction of extension at one or more joints, usually of congenital onset; although a separate congenital contractual arachnodactyly syndrome undoubtedly exists,[26] all patients with this signal feature should be evaluated as if they had the Marfan syndrome so that serious problems in other systems are not overlooked.[27] Similarly, the "marfanoid hypermobility syndrome"[28] is not worth distinguishing as a separate entity.

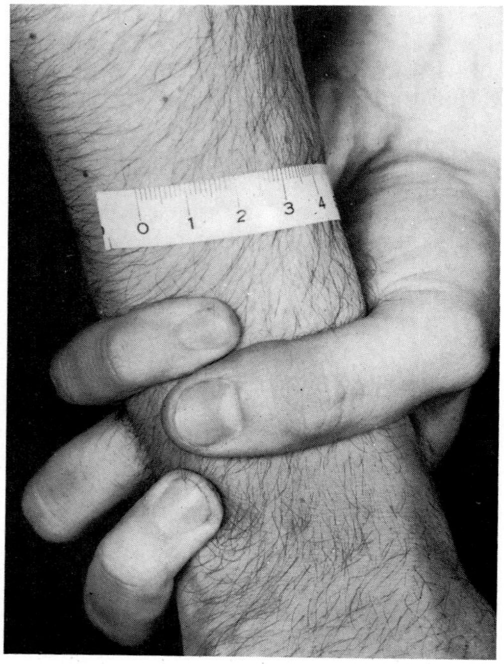

FIGURE 87–3. The wrist sign in a patient with Marfan syndrome. In a positive test, the first phalanges of the thumb and fifth digit substantially overlap when wrapped around the opposite wrist.

Other Features. Most patients with the Marfan syndrome have myopia, and about half have subluxation of the lenses (ectopia lentis). The ascending aorta bears the main stress of ventricular ejection, leading to progressive dilatation beginning in the sinuses of Valsalva. Aortic regurgitation and dissection are the main causes of death.[29] Before the development of reliable surgical procedures and their early application,[30,31] life expectancy was reduced, on average, by one-third in patients with the Marfan syndrome. Mitral valve prolapse occurs in 80% of patients and leads to severe mitral regurgitation in about 10%. Hernias are frequent, cystic changes in the lungs lead to pneumothorax,[32] and striae distensae over the pectoral and deltoid areas and thighs are often first noticed in adolescence. Dural ectasia is usually an incidental finding on plain radiographs, computed tomography, or magnetic resonance imaging of the vertebral column; occasional patients have problems with spinal fluid dynamics or spinal anesthesia as a consequence.

Management of the Skeletal Manifestations. Most Marfan patients can lead long and productive lives, especially now that the success of cardiovascular surgery in repairing the aorta has improved. Thus, all patients deserve aggressive and prophylactic management of all organ systems at risk. For the skeletal system, management must begin in childhood, because most problems are progressive during the years of growth.

Initial management of vertebral column deformity is by bracing. If abnormal curves can be stabilized, persistent bracing may be necessary until the skeleton matures. The presence of thoracic lordosis, rather common in the Marfan syndrome, unfortunately limits the effectiveness of most braces. Whenever scoliotic curves exceed 40 to 45°, surgical stabilization and fusion are required. Curves of moderate severity can progress after skeletal maturity is reached, and adults with vertebral column deformity evident on bedside examination should be monitored formally every year or two.

Tall stature per se is usually not a problem in males. Girls, on the other hand, often suffer much psychosocial turmoil as a result of their height. Analysis of growth shows that the average height for girls parallels the ninety-fifth percentile of the normal female growth curve; the average adult height is thus close to 6 feet.[34] Early induction of puberty by administration of ethinyl estradiol (0.05 mg/10 kg in a single oral dose daily) and medroxyprogesterone (2.5 mg/10 kg on days 25 to 28) results in accelerated skeletal maturation. If therapy is begun well before the age of physiologic menarche (I begin around 8 years of age) then adult height is clearly lessened.[34] Furthermore, by accelerating the "adolescent" growth spurt, there is less time for scoliosis to progress, and deformity is mitigated. Once the epiphyses are nearly fused or once the girl attains the age of physiologic menarche, hormonal therapy can be discontinued.

Deformity of the anterior chest also tends to worsen during adolescence as a result of rapid rib growth. Repair of either pectus excavatum or pectus carinatum for cosmetic indications should thus be delayed until midadolescence, when the defect is not likely to recur.[35]

Uncommonly disability can result from hyperextensibility at other joints. Dislocation of the patellae and the first metacarpal-phalangeal joints, severe pes planus, and metatarsus valgus are the most frequent problems. Physical therapy, muscular strengthening, and well-fitted shoes are useful. Surgery for these problems should be avoided if possible.

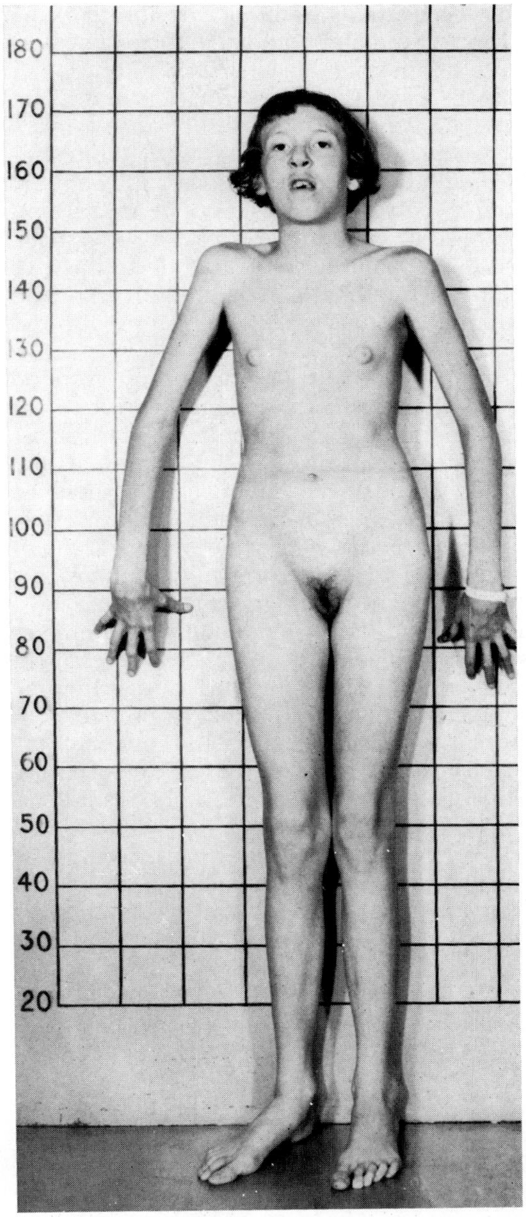

FIGURE 87–4. Homocystinuria in a 12-year-old girl. Note the excessive height, long, narrow feet, and mild anterior chest deformity. The teeth were crowded, ectopia lentis was present, and the joints showed moderate restriction of motion. Despite several episodes of pulmonary embolism and thrombophlebitis, she was active at 40 years of age.

HOMOCYSTINURIA

Homocystinuria is an inborn error in the metabolism of methionine in which activity of the enzyme cystathionine β-synthase is deficient. Clinical features are superficially similar to those of the Marfan syndrome and include ectopia lentis, dolichostenomelia, arachnodactyly, and chest and spinal deformity (Fig. 87–4).[36] Generalized osteoporosis, "tight" joints, arterial and venous thrombosis, malar flush, psychiatric disturbance, and mental retardation are features of homocystinuria usually not found in the Marfan syndrome.[36–39] Aortic aneurysm and mitral prolapse are not features of homocystinuria. Homocystinuria is an autosomal recessive disorder, unlike the Marfan syndrome, which is a dominant trait. The hand in homocystinuria has none of the longitudinal laxity present in the Marfan syndrome, and the appendicular joints tend to have reduced mobility. Back pain resulting from osteoporosis occurs in some patients.

The pathogenesis of the three cardinal groups of manifestations—mental retardation, connective tissue disorder (ectopia lentis, osteoporosis, reduced joint mobility), and thrombosis—is not understood. Perhaps the reduced sulfhydryl groups of homocysteine or other substances that accumulate proximal to the block interfere with cross linking of collagen, fibrillin, and other proteins of the extracellular matrix, thus accounting for the connective tissue manifestations. Such a mechanism occurs in the thiolism caused by prolonged administration of penicillamine, a compound structurally similar to homocysteine. An alternative, but not necessarily exclusive, hypothesis focuses on the deficiency of cysteine that results from the inability to join homocysteine with serine. Cysteine is one of the three amino acids that forms glutathione, the deficiency of which predisposes to damage from free radicals.

Over half the patients with homocystinuria respond to large doses of vitamin B_6 (pyridoxine) with clearing of homocystine from the urine, lowering of plasma methionine and cysteine, raising of cystine to normal, and reducing the likelihood of developing clinical manifestations.[37] Pre-existent mental retardation and ectopia lentis are not improved by pyridoxine treatment in patients who show biochemical correction, emphasizing the need for early diagnosis and therapy. Because most states include testing for elevated blood methionine as part of the newborn screening program, early treatment is possible. Newborns with B_6-responsive cystathionine β-synthase deficiency have sufficient pyridoxine from maternal sources to prevent hypermethioninemia during the first week of life, and thereby escape detection.[37] With supplementary folic acid (1 mg daily), as little as 20 mg of pyridoxine daily may be effective, although usually a dosage of 100 to 300 mg is required. In vitamin B_6-nonresponders, a low methionine diet is the mainstay of management,[38] although pyridoxine and folate should be included because of a tendency for unsupplemented patients to develop deficiency of these cofactors. Because the low-methionine diet is relatively unpalatable, especially for people who begin protein restriction after infancy, alternative forms of therapy are being explored. The methyl donor betaine, when taken in pharmacologic doses of several grams per day, results in a lowering of homocysteine plasma concentrations and a concomitant increase in methionine and cysteine.[37] Long-term clinical trials are needed. In addition, sulfinpyrazone, dipyridamole, or aspirin, singly or in combination, may be useful in preventing thrombotic episodes in all homocystinurics, even though platelet survival is normal in most patients.[40]

WEILL-MARCHESANI SYNDROME

The Weill-Marchesani syndrome is another systemic disorder with ectopia lentis as a conspicuous feature (Fig. 87–5). The skeletal features are the antithesis of those in the Marfan syndrome: the patients are short, with particularly short hands and feet, and have stiff joints, especially in the hands. The hands sometimes show atrophy of the abductor pollicis brevis muscle consistent with carpal tunnel compression. The Weill-Marchesani syndrome is autosomal recessive, but heterozygotes are shorter of stature than average.[41]

THE EHLERS-DANLOS SYNDROMES

The Ehlers-Danlos syndromes (EDSs) are a group of disorders of considerable diversity, largely caused by extensive genetic heterogeneity. The cardinal and unifying features relate to the joints and skin—hyperextensibility of skin, easy bruisability, dystrophic scarring, in-

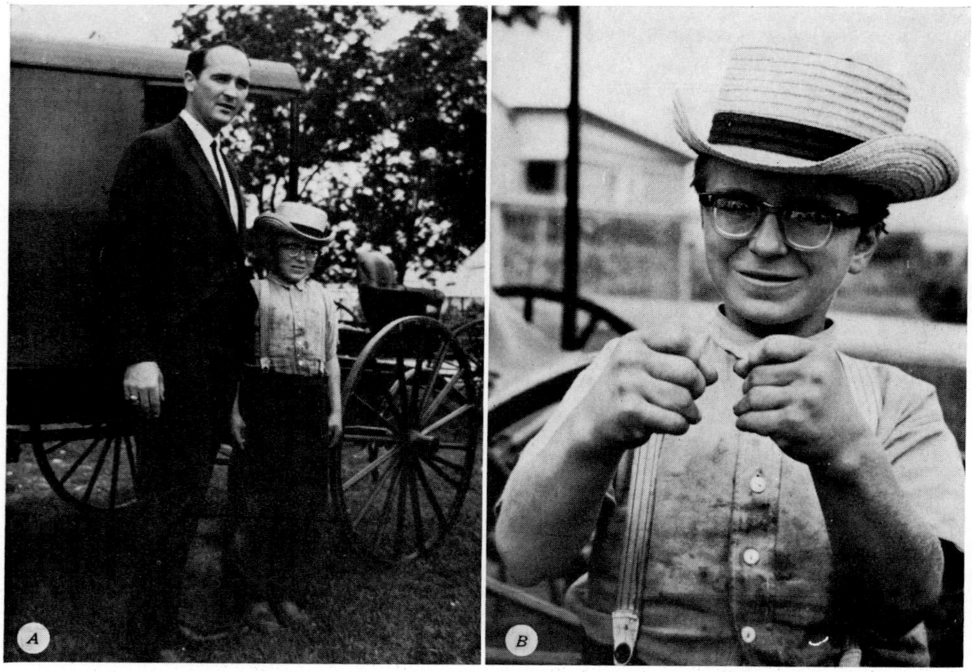

FIGURE 87–5. Weill-Marchesani syndrome in a 15-year-old Amish boy. *A*, Boy shown with normal adult male. Ectopia lentis was present, and attacks of acute glaucoma had occurred. *B*, The fingers were short with knobby joints and restricted flexion. Flattening of the thenar eminence was consistent with carpal tunnel compression.

creased joint mobility, and abnormal tissue fragility.[9] Internal manifestations, which include rupture of great vessels, hiatal hernia, diverticula of the gastrointestinal and genitourinary tracts, spontaneous rupture of the bowel, and spontaneous pneumothorax, tend to occur only in specific types of EDS.

The classification of EDS has been set at nine general types on the basis of phenotypic and inheritance characteristics (Table 87–2).[9] Biochemical studies have demonstrated considerable heterogeneity within individual types.[11,13,14,42] This extensive phenotypic and biochemical characterization nonetheless fails the clinician as often as it helps; nearly half of all patients who have at least one "cardinal" manifestation defy categorization.

EDS I (Gravis Form) and EDS II (Mitis Form). Generalized hyperextensibility of joints (Fig. 87–6), together with stretchability of skin, led in the past to characterization of the affected persons as "India rubber men." Other features are bruising and fragility of the skin, with gaping wounds caused by minor trauma and with poor retention of sutures.[43] Congenital dislocation of the hips in the newborn, habitual dislocation of selected joints in later life, joint effusions, clubfoot deformity of the feet, and spondylolisthesis are all consequences of the loose-jointedness. Hemarthroses and "hemarthritic disability" have been described and are analogous to bruising of the skin. Scoliosis is sometimes severe. Severe leg cramps occurring at rest and of unclear cause are troublesome to some patients.

Both of these types are inherited as autosomal dominant traits and tend to breed true within a family. They differ from one another only in severity; hence, the differentiation is somewhat subjective (Fig. 87–7).[9] The biochemical defects have not been characterized in either type, although abnormalities of the collagens most common in skin (types I and III) have long been suspected.[14,16,43,44]

Management of both EDS I and EDS II stresses prevention of trauma and great care in treating wounds. Some patients, particularly young boys, wear skin guards to protect their lower legs from the repeated minor injuries that lead to frequent hemorrhage, unsightly scars, and absence from school. Patients should be dissuaded from demonstrating their joint laxity as entertainment for their friends. Because the ligaments and joint capsules are lax, joint stability can be im-

TABLE 87–2. EHLERS-DANLOS SYNDROMES

TYPE	INHERITANCE	SKELETAL FEATURES	OTHER FEATHERS	BASIC DEFECT
I	AD	Marked joint hypermobility	Skin hyperextensibility and fragility	?
II	AD	Less severe than type I		?
III	AD	Marked joint hypermobility	None	?
IV	AD, AR	Hypermobile digits	Arterial and bowel rupture	Deficient type III collagen
V	X-L	Similar to type II		?
VI	AR	Marked joint hypermobility	Rupture of globe	Lysyl hydroxylase
VII	AD, AR	Marked joint hypermobility and dislocations; short stature	Minimal skin change	Defect in procollagen cleavage
VIII	AD	Variable joint hypermobility	Periodontitis	?
X	AD	Mild joint hypermobility	Mild skin changes; MVP	? Defect in fibronectin

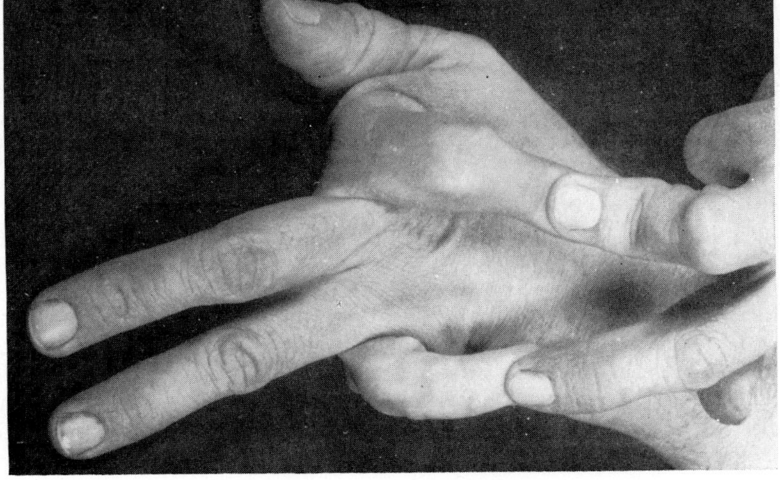

FIGURE 87–6. Joint hypermobility in the Ehlers-Danlos syndrome, type I.

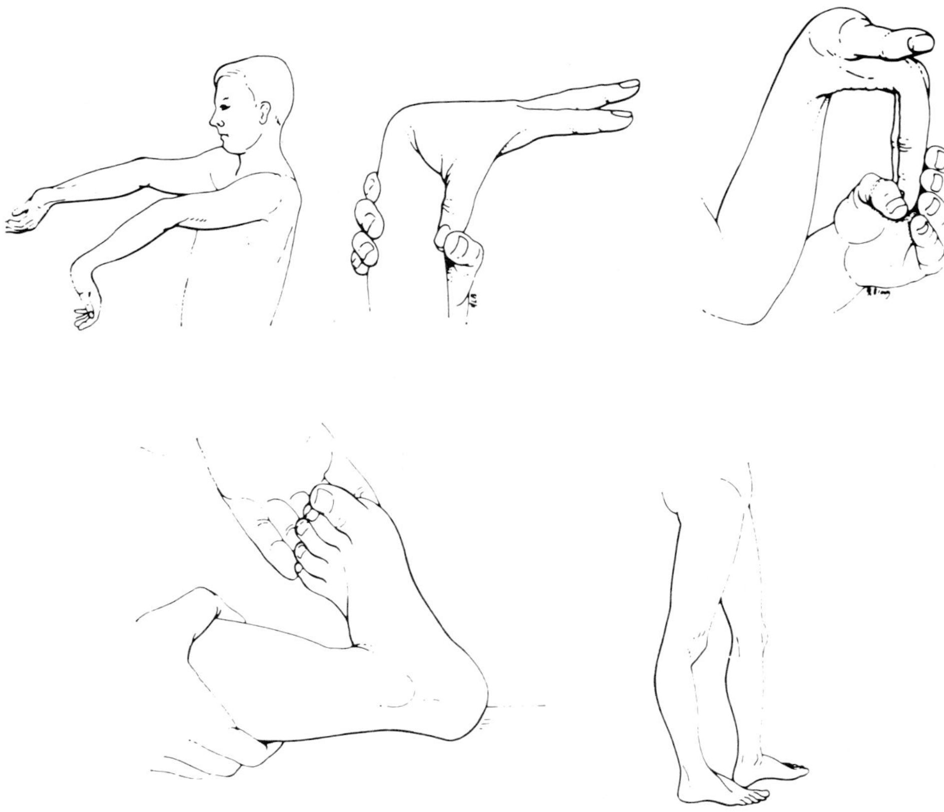

FIGURE 87–7. A method for evaluating joint mobility.[59] Excessive joint laxity is judged to exist when at least three of the following five conditions are present: (1) elbows and (2) knees extend beyond 180°; (3) thumb touches the forearm on flexing the wrist; (4) fingers are parallel to the forearm on extending the wrist and metacarpal joints; and (5) foot dorsiflexes to 45° or more.

proved only by developing the muscles. Care must be employed, however, in weight lifting and other forms of exercise because of fragility of tendons.

EDS III (Benign Hypermobility Form). This condition has moderate dermal hyperextensibility and minimal fragility. The joint hyperextensibility ranges from extreme to bordering on normal.[43] All too often, patients with mild joint laxity without joint instability or skin manifestations are labeled as EDS III, particularly if relatives show a similar manifestation. In some cases, such labeling causes more harm than good, unless one makes it clear that little if any disability is likely to result.

EDS IV (Arterial Form). This condition is by far the most serious type of EDS because of a propensity for spontaneous rupture of arteries and bowel.[44–46] This type is particularly heterogeneous genetically, the unifying theme being abnormal production of type III collagen.[11,46] Skin involvement is variable, with thin, nearly translucent skin present in some, and mildly hyperextensible skin the only feature in others. Joint laxity is also variable, but is generally limited to the digits. Affected women have a high risk of aortic rupture during pregnancy.[47] Inheritance is usually autosomal dominant.

EDS V. The phenotype of this rare, X-linked form resembles EDS II most closely.[48] Although a deficiency of lysyl oxidase was claimed in one pedigree, this has not been confirmed or found in any other family.

EDS VI (Ocular-Scoliotic Form). Fragility of the ocular globe and a propensity to severe scoliosis, in addition to the skin and joint involvement seen in EDS I, are the hallmarks of this autosomal recessive form of EDS.[44,49] This is the first of the heritable disorders of connective tissue to have its basic defect elucidated, by Krane and colleagues in 1972.[50] Collagen in this condition contains little hydroxylysine because of deficiency of the enzyme that hydroxylates selected lysyl residues in the nascent collagen chains. Because hydroxylysine is normally involved, along with lysine, in cross linking of collagen, the clinical features of EDS VI are readily explained. Vitamin C is a necessary cofactor of lysyl hydroxylase and, in high doses, may be beneficial in some cases of EDS VI[51] (comparable to the benefit of vitamin B_6 in some cases of homocystinuria).

EDS VII (Arthrochalasis Multiplex Congenita). Profound loose-jointedness with congenital dislocations dominates the clinical picture. The patients are moderately short of stature and the skin is variably, but usually mildly, involved.[44,52] An inability to convert type I procollagen to mature collagen, by cleavage of the N-propeptide, has been found in all patients who have been studied.[13,14,42,53,54] The genetic heterogeneity of EDS VII is instructive. Deficiency of procollagen N-peptidase, the enzyme that cleaves the propeptide from the amino-terminal end of type I procollagen, is deficient in fibroblasts from a minority of patients.[42] But most have had normal N-peptidase activity and an amino acid sequence alteration around the site of the procollagen molecule where cleavage occurs. Two general types of mutations have been seen thus far. At the cleavage site, amino acids in either the $\alpha1(I)$ or the $\alpha2(I)$ procollagen chain are mutated, disrupting the α-helix conformation requisite for peptidase activity. Alternatively, a deletion (or theoretically an insertion) of amino acids anywhere in either of the procollagen chains proximal to the N-peptidase cleavage site causes misregister of the three chains and disruption of the α-helix. Deficiency of peptidase activity would likely be an autosomal recessive trait. In distinction, the mutations causing amino acid alterations have all affected only one allele for either $\alpha1(I)$ or $\alpha2(I)$ procollagen. Because neither parent was affected in any of the cases examined biochemically so far, the mutation likely occurred in a parental gonad. The patients, however, should they choose to reproduce, will have a 50% chance of having an affected offspring, and their condition will readily be identified as an autosomal dominant trait.

EDS VIII (Periodontitis Form). This rare condition is characterized by severe periodontal disease, with early loss of both primary and permanent teeth. Presence of manifestations of EDS I and EDS IV has varied in the few reported kindreds.[44] The basic defect is unknown, and inheritance is autosomal dominant. The phenotypes of EDS IV and VIII overlap, and all such patients should be screened for deficiency of type III collagen.[55]

EDS IX. This disorder has been reclassified as a disorder of copper transport (see Table 87–1).

EDS X (Fibronectin Deficiency). One pedigree was reported with a phenotype inherited as an autosomal recessive, characterized by features of EDS II, and associated with abnormal platelet aggregation.[56] The platelet defect was corrected by exogenous plasma fibronectin.

FAMILIAL ARTICULAR HYPERMOBILITY SYNDROMES

This category of disorders includes generalized articular hypermobility with or without subluxation.[9] Specifically excluded are the skeletal dysplasias with joint hypermobility (e.g., the Larsen syndrome) and the EDS syndromes (which all have some degree of skin involvement).

Familial Articular Hypermobility, Uncomplicated Type. This is a relatively common, autosomal dominant condition of unknown biochemical defect. Joint hypermobility is generalized, but rarely causes dislocation or disability.[57,58] The incidence of congenital dislocation of the hip may be increased in families with this condition,[59] which is also known as familial simple joint laxity.

Familial Articular Hypermobility, Dislocating Type. The cardinal feature of this autosomal dominant condition is instability of multiple appendicular joints; recurrent dislocation is the usual clinical finding. Joint hyperextensibility is variable but usually mild, and skin involvement is uncommon.[60] This condition, which has been called both familial joint instability syndrome and Ehlers-Danlos type XI, may cause considerable disability. Clinical variability within a family is the rule, emphasizing the need for a comprehensive family history, including examination of close relatives if possible (Fig. 87–8).

This is an extremely difficult condition to manage successfully. For most patients, diagnosis is established only after multiple orthopedic surgical attempts (usually disappointing) to prevent recurrent dislocation of shoulders, knees, or elbows. As in EDS I and II, physical therapy of affected joints to increase periarticular muscle strength should be attempted first.

SKELETAL DYSPLASIAS WITH PREDOMINANT JOINT LAXITY

Many of the osteochondrodysplasias have variable degrees of joint laxity or instability as part of the overall phenotype. Several disorders, however, have such prominent joint hypermobility as to be the cardinal sign, and have been grouped in one category.

Larsen Syndrome. The Larsen syndrome is characterized by multiple congenital dislocations and characteristic facies: prominent forehead, depressed nasal bridge, and widely spaced eyes.[61] Dislocation occurs at the knees (characteristically anterior displacement of the tibia on the femur), hips, and elbows. The metacarpals are short, with cylindrical fingers lacking the usual tapering. Cleft palate, hydrocephalus, abnormalities of spinal segmentation, and moderate-to-severe short stature have occurred in some. Several instances of multiple affected siblings with normal parents are known, suggesting autosomal recessive inheritance, but parent-child involvement also occurs, consistent with dominant inheritance. Thus, at least two clinically indistinguishable forms of the Larsen syndrome exist.

Radiographic features that are helpful in diagnosis, in addition to congenital segmentation anomalies of the spine and congenital hip dislocation, are multiple ossification centers in the calcaneus and carpus.[62]

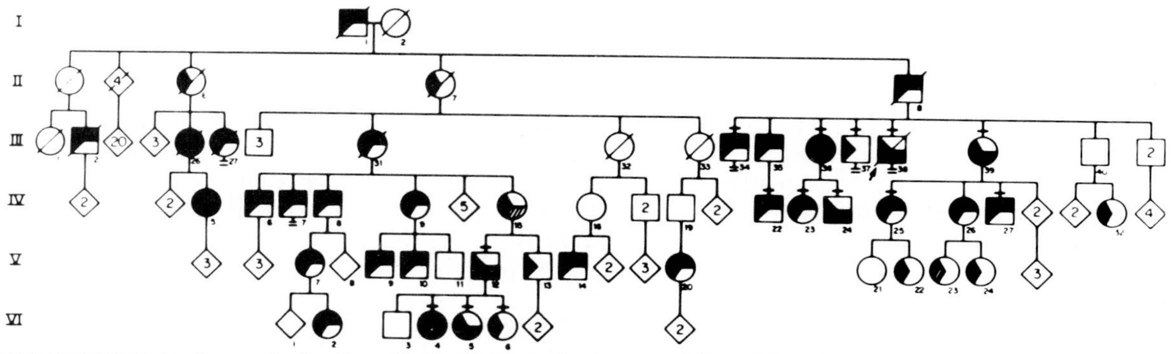

FIGURE 87–8. Pedigree of a family with familial articular hypermobility, dislocating type. The autosomal dominant transmission and variability of the phenotype are both well illustrated. Pedigree symbols: ◐ = joint hypermobility; ◔ = hip dislocation; ◒ = patella dislocation; ◍ = possibly affected; ♁ = examined by authors; ⌀ = deceased. From Horton, W.A., et al.[60]

TABLE 87–3. OSTEOGENESIS IMPERFECTA SYNDROMES

TYPE	INHERITANCE	SKELETAL FEATURES	OTHER FEATURES
IA	AD	Variable bone fragility and short stature, wormian bones	Blue sclerae, opalescent teeth, hearing loss
IB	AD	Variable bone fragility and short stature, wormian bones	Blue sclerae, normal teeth, hearing loss
II	Most sporadic, due to heterozygosity for a new mutation in type I collagen	In utero fractures, little calvarial calcium	Blue sclerae, pulmonary hypertension, neonatal death usual
III	Most sporadic; some AR	Moderately severe fragility, variable deformity, scoliosis, joint laxity	Variable sclerae, some with opalescent teeth
IVA	AD	Variable bone fragility and short stature, wormian bones	Normal sclerae, opalescent teeth, hearing loss
IVB	AD	Variable bone fragility and short stature, wormian bones	Normal sclerae and teeth, hearing loss

Desbuquois Syndrome. Desbuquois and colleagues described patients with short stature, joint laxity, prominent eyes, broad terminal phalanges, and supernumerary digits. The most characteristic radiographic features are extracarpal ossification centers and prominence of the lesser trochanter of the femur.[63] This rare condition can be inherited as an autosomal recessive trait, but may be genetically heterogeneous, so that sporadic cases should not be counseled that they have no risk of having an affected offspring.

OSTEOGENESIS IMPERFECTA SYNDROMES

Several phenotypically distinct osteogenesis imperfecta (OI) syndromes, and even more classification schemes, exist.[9,14] The disorders share osseous, ocular, dental, aural, and cardiovascular involvement. The classification enjoying current application is based on clinical and inheritance pattern criteria (Table 87–3).[9] At the current rapid pace of defining basic biochemical defects in collagen, a nosology grounded in objective data is a reasonable expectation.[11]

Type 1 OI is the most common form and is associated with wide intrafamilial variability.[67,68] One patient might be extremely short of stature, with frequent fractures and much disability, whereas an affected relative leads an unencumbered, vigorous life. Type II encompasses the classic "OI congenita" variants, most of which are lethal in infancy, if not in utero.[65,69,70] Molecular characterization of type II is progressing rapidly, at both the collagen and the DNA level.[66] Most cases arise as the result of a new mutation (the phenotype thus being transmissible as a dominant, if the patient could live and reproduce). A few patients have affected siblings and normal but sometimes consanguineous parents, consistent with autosomal recessive inheritance. Type III OI comprises miscellaneous phenotypes that cannot be classified better.[71] Most cases include severe skeletal deformity and short stature as distinguishing features. Most occur sporadically. Type IV OI is similar to type I, only rarer and not associated with blue sclerae.[72,73]

Skeletal Features. "Brittle bones" are a familiar and dramatic feature of all the OI variants. Sometimes fractures occur in utero, particularly in type II, and permit radiographic antenatal diagnosis. In such cases, the limbs are likely to be short and bent at birth. Multiple rib fractures give a characteristic "beaded" appearance on radiographs.[62,69] Other patients with types I or IV have few fractures or may escape them entirely, although blue sclerae or deafness indicates the presence of the mutant gene. Brittleness and deformability result from a defect in the collagenous matrix of bone. The skeletal aspect of OI is, therefore, a hereditary form of osteoporosis. "Codfish vertebrae" (scalloping of the superior and inferior vertebral bodies by pressure from the expansile intervertebral disc) or flat vertebrae are observed, particularly in older patients in whom senile or postmenopausal changes exaggerate the change, or young patients immobilized after fracture or orthopedic surgery. Usually the frequency of fractures decreases at puberty for patients with types I, III, and IV. Because of failure of union of fractures, pseudarthrosis (especially of humerus or femur) occurs in some. Hypertrophic callus occurs frequently in patients with OI and is often difficult to distinguish from osteosarcoma. Debate continues as to whether the risk of true osteosarcoma is increased in any form of OI; regardless, the risk is not great, but worthy of consideration whenever skeletal pain occurs in the absence of fracture, particularly in an older patient. Loose-jointedness is sometimes striking in type I OI; dislocation of joints can result from deformity secondary to repeated fracture, ligamentous laxity, or rupture of tendons (especially the Achilles and patellar).

Ocular Features. Blue sclerae are present in types I, II, and III OI and are a valuable clue to the diagnosis. The cornea, like the sclera, is abnormally thin. The ocular features are usually not of great functional importance.

Aural Features. Hearing loss becomes detectable in many patients by the second or third decade of life. It was long assumed that deafness in OI was the result of precocious otosclerosis; alternatively, otosclerosis is such a common disorder in the general population that many OI patients are likely to develop it. A variety of aural abnormalities occurs in OI, and symptomatic hearing loss is nearly always multifactorial.[74] The tympanic membrane may be thin, the pinna deformed, the ossicles disconnected, or the stapedial footplate thickened or degenerated. A surprisingly high percentage of patients have a sensorineural component, owing in part to cochlear deformity, cochlear hair loss, and tectorial membrane distortion.[74] Thus, each patient must be evaluated in considerable detail to determine whether hearing impairment is present and whether it is conductive, sensorineural, or mixed.

Dental Features. The characteristic dental manifestation of OI is opalescent teeth caused by a defect in dentin morphogenesis.[75] This finding is easily ascertained by direct observation of the blue or brown opalescent deciduous or permanent teeth or by the typical radiographic changes. This dental abnormality can be useful diagnostically because opalescent teeth, of all of the pleiotropic OI manifestations, tends to breed true in families. It thus forms the basis for subdividing types I and IV into disorders with and without opalescent teeth. Affected teeth wear poorly; enamel loss is secondary to fracture of the underlying dentin.

Other Features. Unusual bruising occurs in some patients, probably owing to a defect in the connective tissue in the walls of small blood vessels or in the supporting connective tissues. No consistent defect of the coagulation mechanism or of platelet function has been demonstrated.

Mitral valve prolapse occurs in about 15% of patients with OI type I, several times more frequently than in the general population, and occasionally may progress to mitral regurgitation. Aortic dilatation and regurgitation also occur but are infrequent.[29,76]

The differential diagnosis of osteogenesis imperfecta includes idiopathic juvenile osteoporosis,[77] juvenile osteoporosis with ocular pseudoglioma and mental retardation,[78] Cheney syndrome (osteoporosis, multiple wormian bones, acro-osteolysis),[79] pycnodysostosis (dwarfism, brittle bones, absent ramus of mandible, persistent cranial fontanelles, acro-osteolysis),[80] and hypophosphatasia.[81] When children with unrecognized OI are taken to the emergency room on account of a new fracture, and radiographs show multiple healed fractures, the possibility of child abuse may be raised and the parents unjustly accused. Conversely, we encountered a patient who was clearly abused and battered, but whose parents tried repeatedly and nearly successfully to have their child diagnosed as having a variant of OI.

STICKLER SYNDROME

The cardinal features of this relatively common (at least 1 per 10,000 in the population) autosomal dominant condition are severe, progressive myopia, vitreal degeneration, retinal detachment, progressive sensorineural hearing loss, cleft palate, mandibular hypoplasia, hypermobility and hypomobility of joints, epiphyseal dysplasia, and variable disability resulting from joint pain, dislocation, or degeneration.[82,83] In one large clinic for craniofacial anomalies, 6.6% of all patients with cleft palate but without cleft lip had Stickler syndrome.[84] This condition, also called progressive arthro-ophthalmopathy, is clearly underdiagnosed, in part because patients often do not have the full syndrome and in part because the physician fails to obtain a detailed family history that might suggest a hereditary condition. Some nosologic confusion persist as well. The ocular features, first described in 1938, have been called the Wagner syndrome by ophthalmologists, but this is clearly a distinct condition. Some patients with typical ocular and aural features have severe midfacial hypoplasia (not just flat malae), a thick calvarium, and abnormal frontal sinuses, findings termed the Marshall syndrome[85]; while this nosologic splitting is supported by some,[86] most ascribe the phenotypic differences to the variable expression of a single mutation.[87,88] Similarly the Weissenbacher-Zweymüller syndrome has been recognized as a severe, neonatal form of the Stickler syndrome.[88,89] The Stickler syndrome should be strongly considered in any infant with "swollen" wrists, knees, or ankles, the Robin sequence (hypognathia, cleft palate, and glossoptosis), or flared ("dumbbell"-shaped) femoral metaphyses; in any adult with precocious degenerative arthritis of the hip, especially if relatives are similarly affected; and in any person with spontaneous retinal detachment.

The Stickler syndrome in some families has been linked to the $\alpha 1$(II) procollagen locus.[91–93] Some families do not demonstrate linkage to the COL2A1 locus, however, and genetic heterogeneity is likely. Nonetheless, the Stickler syndrome became the first human disease shown to be due to a heritable defect in the principal collagenous component of cartilage. Subsequently, a number of chondrodysplasias[94,95] and a mild spondyloepiphyseal dysplasia, inherited as an autosomal dominant trait, that predisposed to generalized osteoarthritis[96] have proven to have mutations at the COL2A1 gene.

CUTIS LAXA

The cardinal feature of these conditions is dermatologic: the skin is lax and loose, with none of the hyperelasticity seen in the Ehlers-Danlos variants. Beyond childhood, the prominent skinfolds and excessive wrinkling give a prematurely aged appearance. Both congenital (usually autosomal recessive) and late-onset (autosomal dominant) forms occur, and the basic defects, which presumably affect elastic fibers, are unclear. The skeletal system is largely unaffected, but the condition is of importance to rheumatologists on account of the *phenocopy* that they may inadvertently cause in the offspring of their patients. A phenocopy is a disorder of nongenetic cause that mimics a hereditary disorder. Some fetuses exposed to D-penicillamine, as a result of maternal treatment of rheumatic disorders, Wilson's disease, or cystinuria, develop a congenital syndrome indistinguishable from the severe, autosomal recessive form of cutis laxa.[97] Neither the susceptible period of pregnancy nor the threshold dosage has been established.

PSEUDOXANTHOMA ELASTICUM

The characteristic features occur in the skin, retina, and arteries. In areas of flexural stress, yellowish papules develop over time, giving the skin the appearance of that of a plucked chicken. As Bruch's membrane fragments, angioid streaks develop in the retina; hemorrhages lead to progressive visual loss. An arteriolarsclerosis, similar histopathologically to that of Mönckeberg, develops and leads to loss of peripheral pulses, myocardial infarction, and gastrointestinal hemorrhage. The skeleton is not involved in any obvious way. Both autosomal recessive (the most common) and autosomal dominant forms occur. The basic defect is unclear, but the pathognomonic dermatopathologic finding is calcification of elastic fibers. Restriction of nutritional calcium intake in early life may retard progression of the disease.[98]

CONSTITUTIONAL DISEASES OF BONE

In addition to the disorders of connective tissue already discussed, a wide array of hereditary conditions affect the skeleton. According to a standard nomenclature,[10,62,99] they are classified broadly as osteochondrodysplasias, dysostoses, idiopathic osteolyses, and primary metabolic abnormalities. The most common or instructive examples will be presented here.

OSTEOCHONDRODYSPLASIAS

These disorders affect cartilage or bone growth and development. This category is divided into defects primarily of tubular bones, defects primarily of the spine, or defects of both the appendicular and axial skeleton. In some conditions, such as multiple epiphyseal dysplasia (MED), only the skeleton is involved. In others, such as spondyloepiphyseal dysplasia (SED) congenita, other organs are affected as well; the Stickler syndrome can be classified among this group. Achondroplasia merits special attention because it is the most common of the skeletal dysplasias.

Multiple Epiphyseal Dysplasia (MED). This group of disorders is defined by disordered growth of the epiphyses of one or more pairs of joints that leads to a strong predisposition to early degenerative arthritis. Because of diversity in clinical phenotype and inheritance pattern among affected families, MED is undoubtedly heterogeneous. The most common form is autosomal dominant and comes to attention when a child is evaluated for short stature, abnormalities of gait, or hip pain. Occasionally the diagnosis is not made until the third or fourth decade, when degenerative arthritis of the hips or occasionally of other joints occurs.

The most characteristic radiographic features occur in epiphyses of the limbs, with mild to no involvement of the spine and a normal skull. Joints are symmetrically involved. Appearance of ossification is delayed, and the centers then become irregular or even fragmented.[62] Cone-shaped epiphyses of the metacarpals and phalanges may lead to brachydactyly and deformity of the interphalangeal joints, but surprisingly little pain or disability. The hips are nearly always affected, with abnormal ossification of the capital femoral epiphyses leading to a flattened femoral head (Fig. 87–9). The acetabulum is usually affected, and protrusio acetabuli is often seen.

The differential diagnosis includes Legg-Perthes disease, which is distinguished by being asymmetric, involving the metaphysis, sparing the acetabulum, and usually improving spontaneously; the spondyloepiphyseal dysplasias (especially in males, the tarda form), in which the spine is more severely affected than the limbs; and untreated hypothyroidism.

Spondyloepiphyseal Dysplasia (SED) Congenita. As the name implies, short stature and gross skeletal deformity is obvious at birth.[99] Platyspondyly contributes more to reduced height than does dysplasia of the limbs, which tends to be more severe proximally. Associated clinical features are cleft palate, pectus carinatum, kyphoscoliosis, vitreoretinal degeneration, myopia, and retinal detachment. The cervical spinal cord is vulnerable to subluxation of C1 on C2. In some respects, SED congenita is a more severe phenotype of the Stickler syndrome. The two disorders have the same biochemical basis.[93,94] The phenotypes of patients with SED congenita comprise a clinical continuum, with severity positively correlated with how close the amino acid change is to the carboxyl end of the procollagen molecule, which determines the degree of post-translational overmodification that occurs.[100] Many cases of SED congenita are sporadic, with little likelihood that the affected women will reproduce because of the significant restriction in abdominal size. Pedigrees with autosomal dominant transmission and the direct analysis of mutations suggest that most mutations that cause this disorder are heterozygous.

The radiographic features include a normal skull; platyspondyly; delayed ossification of a dysplastic odontoid; severe disorganization and delay in limb ossification centers, more severe proximally and especially so at the femoral capital epiphyses; irregular, horizontal acetabula; mild involvement of the carpus; and minimal involvement of the digits.[62,99] Whether two clinical subgroups can be distinguished based on the severity of coxa vara is unconfirmed.[101]

Premature degenerative arthritis can be crippling; early, aggressive realignment of the legs may have a role, but long-term followup is still in progress.

Spondyloepiphyseal Dysplasia Tarda. Although several types of late-onset SED may occur, the vast majority of patients are male and occur in pedigrees consistent with X-linked recessive inheritance.[102] The condition is often not diagnosed until degenerative arthritis develops in the shoulders and hips in late childhood or early adulthood. The radiographic findings in the femoral capital epiphyses and proximal humeral epiphyses are difficult to distinguish from MED. The spine, however, is not only more severely affected, but characteristic (Fig. 87–10).

Pseudoachondroplastic Dysplasia. This disorder, which has both dominant and recessive forms, affects the epiphyses and the spine, and is therefore classified as a spondyloepiphyseal dysplasia.[62] The skeletal changes, which can be severe and debilitating, are distinct from achondroplasia, despite the name. Short stature is not evident at birth, but growth falls off the standard curves by a year or two of age.[103] Typically the head and the face are spared. Chondrocytes show accumulation of proteoglycan-like material in the endoplasmic reticulum. In the autosomal dominant form, however, pseudoachondroplasia is not linked with the gene for chondroitin sulfate core protein.[104]

Achondroplasia. This most common of the osteochondrodysplasias may occur as frequently as 1 per 50,000 births, and is the classic form of "short-limbed" dwarfism. In the medical literature before 1950, one has to view a diagnosis of "achondroplasia" with a healthy degree of skepticism because many conditions that affected the limbs more than the spine were so diagnosed. Achondroplasia is evident at birth,[62,106] is heritable as an autosomal dominant trait (but most cases arise through sporadic mutation in a parental gamete), and affects other organ systems only secondarily.[107] Midfacial hypoplasia produces a characteristic facies. General habitus and appearance are typified by rhizomelic (proximal) shortening of the limbs, flexion contractures of the elbows, bowed legs, hyperlordosis of the lumbosacral spine, and excessive body weight. Constriction on the craniocervical junction, particularly from a small foramen magnum,[108] can produce quadriparesis, sleep apnea, and sudden death in infants.[109] The entire vertebral canal is constricted, and many patients develop neurologic problems from impingement of the cord, roots, or cauda equina at ages ranging from early adolescence to late adulthood.[110–112] The entire range of neurologic complications is only partly understood.[113] Joint laxity of the shoulders and the knees can precipitate recurrent subluxation and predispose to degenerative arthritis.

The basic defect, which is not yet understood,[105] affects enchondral bone and produces diagnostic radiographic features. The skull base is short and the face small compared to the cranium; megalencephaly is part of the syndrome[106] but may be accentuated by hydrocephalus.[113] The posterior border of the vertebrae is scalloped and the pedicles are short. In the lumbar spine, the interpedicular distance narrows caudally. In infants, a thoracolumbar gibbus is common, and if it persists, anterior vertebral wedging results. The pelvis has square ilia with horizontal acetabular roofs and small sciatic notches. The metaphyses of the limbs are widened.[62]

Many patients benefit greatly from occupational and physical therapy, back braces, weight reduction, and various surgical procedures. Suboccipital craniectomy can be lifesaving in infancy. Straightening bowed legs can improve both gait and appearance.[114] By employing surgical techniques for lengthening limbs, pioneered

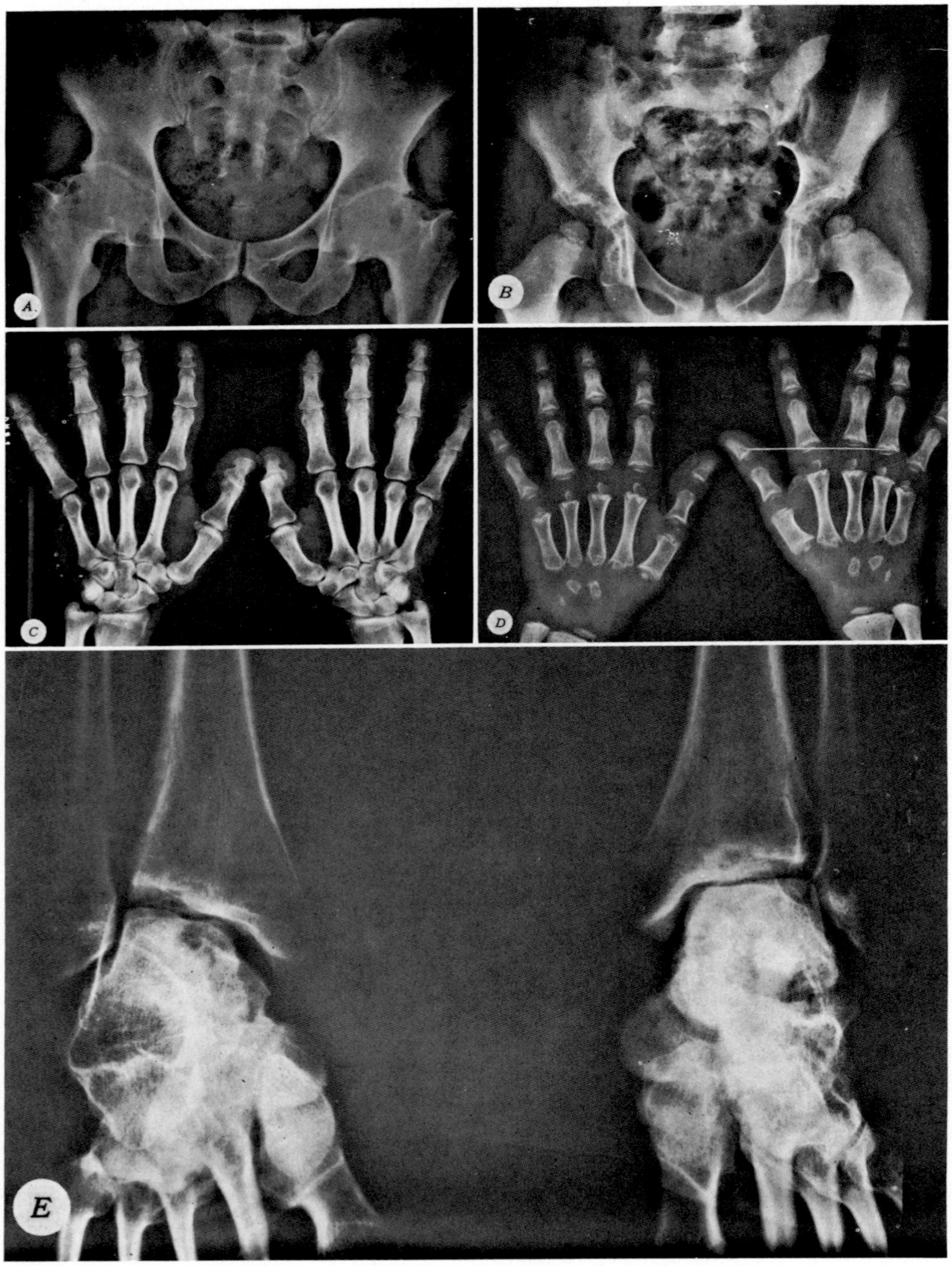

FIGURE 87–9. Multiple epiphyseal dysplasia (MED) in father and son. Both were short of stature, the father being 153.7 cm (61.5 inches) tall. *A*, Hips in the father at 44 years of age showing advanced degenerative changes. *B*, Hips in the son at 10 years of age showing small femoral capital epiphyses and irregularities of the acetabula. *C*, Hands of the father showing brachydactyly, a short carpus, and degenerative joint disease. *D*, Hands of the son at 10 years of age showing dysplastic epiphyses and delayed development of the carpal bones. *E*, Sloping of the distal tibia is a clue to the diagnosis of MED in the adult.

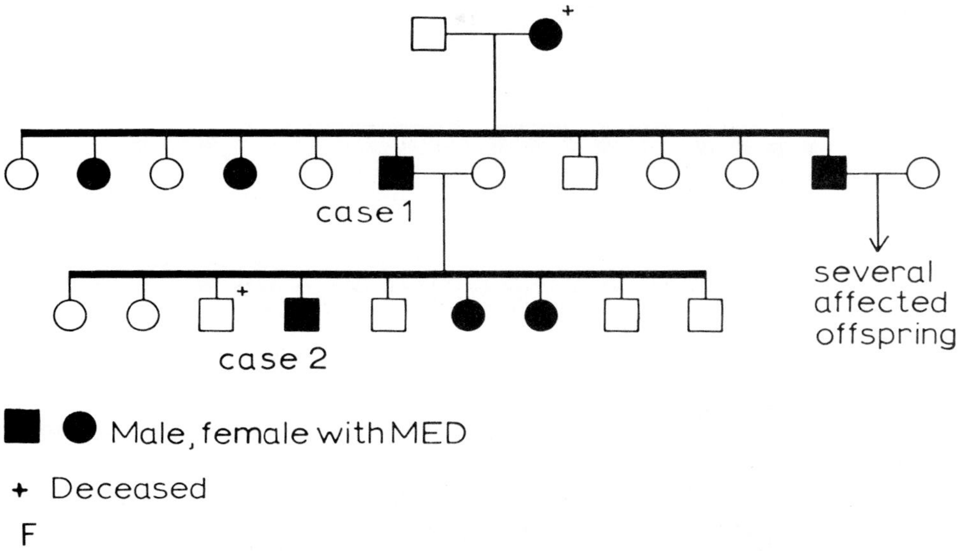

FIGURE 87–9. (*Continued*) *F*, Family pedigree, in which cases 1 and 2 are the father and son illustrated here, demonstrates typical autosomal dominant inheritance of MED.

by the Soviet orthopedist G. A. Ilizarov, it is possible to increase the stature and arm span of people with achondroplasia, or indeed with many skeletal dysplasias.[115] The incidences of vascular, neurologic, and infectious complications of the procedure have diminished with technical modifications and wider experience. Considerable debate continues, however, over whether the functional, cosmetic, and psychologic benefits are worth the protracted disability, potential morbidity, and psychosocial and economic costs.[116] Extended laminectomy for spinal stenosis, if performed early in the evolution of neurologic complications, can restore function.[112]

Craniodiaphyseal Dysplasia. This rare syndrome of uncertain cause and inheritance affects the skeleton generally and the craniofacies most severely. Hyperostosis and sclerosis of the skull and facial bones cause progressive nasal obstruction and cranial nerve impingement, ultimately producing deafness and blindness.[117] The long bones lack modelling, are more cylindrical then usual, and develop extensive diaphyseal and cortical thickening. Stature may be reduced considerably.

Hyperostosis Cranialis Interna. This autosomal dominant condition is limited to the calvaria and base of the skull.[118] Patients present with recurrent palsy of the facial nerve, and develop progressive impairment of balance, smell, taste, and vision.

DYSOSTOSES

This group of disorders involves malformations of individual bones, either singly or in combination. Some involve primarily the cranium and face (e.g., mandibulofacial dysostosis[119]), others the spine (e.g., Klippel-Feil deformities), and others the extremities (e.g., brachydactyly, symphalangism, polydactyly, and syndactyly[120]).

Symphalangism. Harvey Cushing applied this term to a condition of hereditary ankylosis of the proximal interphalangeal joints.[121] Fusion of carpal and tarsal bones also occurs in this autosomal dominant disorder.

Camptodactyly. Limited extension of the digits is a feature of over 25 syndromes, including the Marfan syndrome, but occasionally is an isolated abnormality inherited as an autosomal dominant trait.[122] Permanent flexion contractures are present at the proximal interphalangeal joints without limitation of flexion, typically accompanied by hyperextension at the metacarpophalangeal joints, and sometimes at the distal interphalangeal joints. Camptodactyly may be limited to the fifth finger, or other fingers. Rarely the thumb may be involved as well, with severity decreasing in the radial direction. A contracture band can often be felt on the volar surface of the affected proximal interphalangeal joint, and the transverse skin crease is invariably absent there. Camptodactyly is present from birth or early childhood and shows little tendency to progression. Because of compensatory hyperextension at the metacarpophalangeal joints, the contracture causes little disability. As was pointed out by Archibald Garrod, camptodactyly, when it involves multiple fingers, is often accompanied by "knuckle pads," thickened skin on the dorsal aspect of the proximal interphalangeal joints.[122] Camptodactyly is sometimes confused with Dupuytren's contracture, which is late in onset and has its primary site of contracture in the palm.

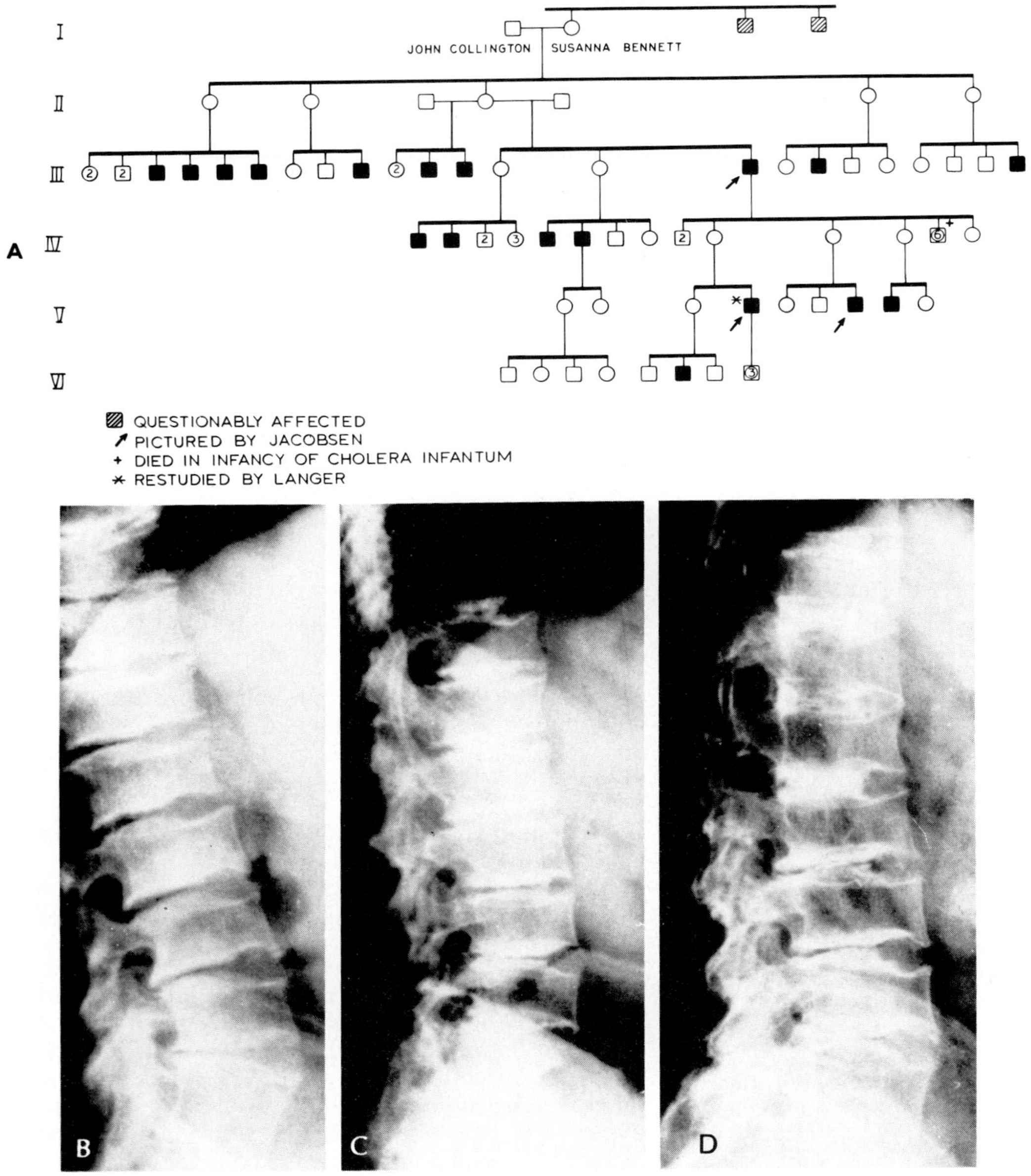

FIGURE 87–10. X-linked spondyloepiphyseal dysplasia tarda. *A*, Partially updated pedigree of family reported by Jacobsen.[105] *B* through *D*, Radiographic changes in the spine are progressive; the heaping up of the posterior portion of the superior vertebral plate (*B*) is particularly distinctive. At first glance, the late changes (*D*) suggest those of alkaptonuria.

IDIOPATHIC OSTEOLYSES

In the several rare heritable conditions that belong to this category,[123,124] progressive dissolution of bone occurs, with predictable debilitating and disfiguring consequences. In no case is either the cause or the pathogenesis understood.

PRIMARY METABOLIC ABNORMALITIES

In each of the disorders in this category, an inborn error disrupts metabolism of a constituent of cartilage or bone. In many cases, the constituent is also present in the connective tissue of other organs, and associated features of each syndrome may be either primary or secondary to skeletal involvement.

Mucopolysaccharidoses

The conditions in this subgroup of the heteroglycanoses are the result of inborn errors of mucopolysaccharide metabolism. Although phenotypically diverse, the individual disorders share mucopolysacchariduria and deposition of mucopolysaccharides in various tissues. Numerous distinct types of mucopolysaccharidoses (MPS)

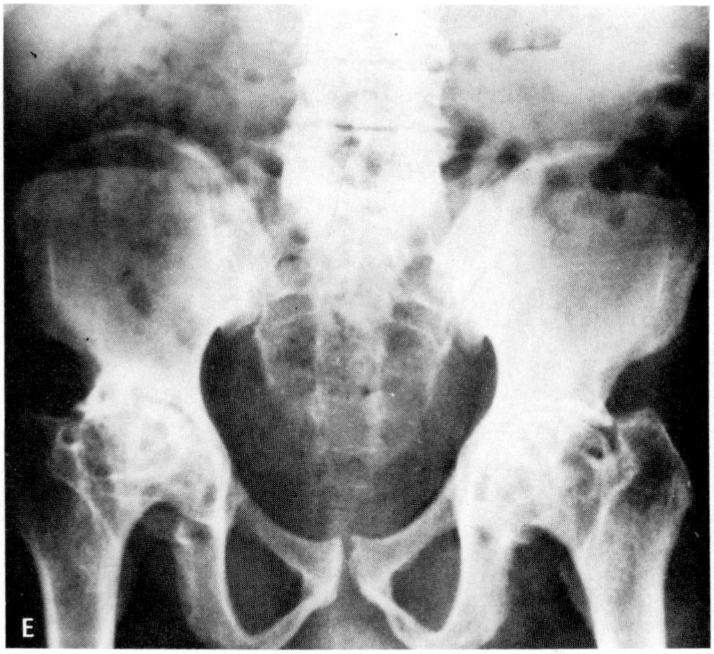

FIGURE 87–10. (*Continued*) *E*, Late changes in the hips. Note the deep acetabula. Radiographs courtesy of Dr. Leonard O. Langer, Jr., Minneapolis.

can be distinguished on the basis of combined phenotypic (i.e., clinical), genetic, and biochemical analysis.[125] Table 87–4 summarizes the distinctive features of each. Additional biochemical and clinical variants undoubtedly remain to be described. All these disorders are recessive, one being X-linked and the others autosomal.

Glycosaminoglycans (acid mucopolysaccharides) are the major constituents of the relatively amorphous part of the extracellular matrix that has been in the past referred to as "ground substance." The size, composition, and structure of proteoglycans vary widely in the human body (Chapter 12), but the hyaluronate backbone, core protein side chains, and link proteins that bind the glycosaminoglycan moieties are common to all. Proteoglycans, regardless of structural nuances and tissue distribution, share catabolic pathways; in particular, glycosaminoglycan degradation is largely catalyzed by lysosomal hydrolases. Thus, a deficiency of one enzyme will affect the metabolism of a variety of glycosaminoglycans in a variety of tissues and is largely responsible for the pleiotropism of the MPS disorders, that is, the diversity of phenotypic features associated with a single mutant gene. All the MPS disorders are characterized by abnormal urinary excretion of glycosaminoglycans—"mucopolysacchariduria" of dermatan sulfate, heparan sulfate, and keratan sulfate—which is useful in screening and specific diagnosis.

Mucopolysacchariduria can be identified by several standard screening tests, at least one of which is part of the standard battery performed when a "metabolic screen" is ordered. Fractionation and characterization of the urinary mucopolysaccharides are useful in separating the several types of MPS. For example, MPS III (Sanfilippo syndrome—the heparan sulfate excretors) and MPS IV (Morquio syndrome—the keratan sulfate excretors) in young subjects may be distinguished from the other types, especially MPS IH (Hurler syndrome—dermatan sulfate excretors), mainly by chemical analysis.

Studies with radioactive sulfate indicate accumulation of label in cultured fibroblasts and delayed washout, compatible with the conclusion that these disorders are due to a degradative defect. The specific lysosomal enzyme deficient in each is now known (see Table 87–4). Like other lysosomal disorders, MPS have six distinctive characteristics:

1. Intracellular storage of material occurs.
2. The storage material is heterogeneous because the degradative enzymes are not strictly specific, for example, in MPS IH, ganglioside is deposited in brain and predominantly mucopolysaccharide in the liver, and two glycosaminoglycans are excreted in the urine.
3. Deposition is vacuolar, that is, membrane-bound, when viewed with the electron microscope.
4. Many tissues are affected.
5. The disorder is clinically progressive.
6. Replacement therapy is at least theoretically possible, through replacing the missing enzyme by the process of endocytosis.

The possibility of replacement therapy in MPS is more than theoretic. Normal cells or the medium in which they have grown, when mixed with MPS fibroblasts, correct the metabolic defect. This finding indicates the production of a diffusible correction factor by normal cells, which is found also in normal urine. The correc-

TABLE 87–4. THE GENETIC MUCOPOLYSACCHARIDOSES

NUMBER	EPONYM	CLINICAL MANIFESTATIONS	GENETICS	URINARY MPS	ENZYME-DEFICIENCY
MPS I H (252800)*	Hurler	Clouding of cornea, grave manifestations, death usually before age 10	Homozygous for MPS IH gene	Dermatan sulfate heparan sulfate	α-L-iduronidase
MPS I S	Scheie	Stiff joints, cloudy cornea, aortic valve disease, normal intelligence and (?) lifespan	Homozygous for MPS IS gene	Dermatan sulfate, heparan sulfate	α-L-iduronidase
MPS I H/S	Hurler-Scheie	Intermediate phenotype	Genetic compound of MPS IH and MPS IS genes	Dermatan sulfate, heparan sulfate	α-L-iduronidase
MPS II-XR severe (309900)	Hunter, severe	No corneal clouding, milder course than in MPS IH, death before 15 years	Hemizygous for X-linked gene	Dermatan sulfate, heparan sulfate	Iduronate sulfatase
MPS II-XR, mild	Hunter, mild	Survival to 30s to 60s, fair intelligence	Hemizygous for X-linked allele	Dermatan sulfate, heparan sulfate	Iduronate sulfatase
MPS III A (252900)	Sanfilippo A	Indistinguishable phenotype: Mild somatic, severe central nervous system effects	Homozygous for Sanfilippo A gene	Heparan sulfate	Heparan N-sulfatase (sulfamidase)
MPS III B (252920)	Sanfilippo B		Homozygous for Sanfilippo B gene	Heparan sulfate	N-acetyl-α-D-glucosaminidase
MPS III C (252930)	Sanfilippo C		Homozygous for Sanfilippo C gene	Heparan sulfate	Acetyl-CoA: α-glucosaminide N-acetyltransferase
MPS III D (252940)	Sanfilippo D		Homozygous for Sanfilippo D gene	Heparan sulfate	N-acetylglucosamine-6-sulfate sulfatase
MPS IV A (253000)	Morquio A	Severe, distinctive bone changes, cloudy cornea, aortic regurgitation, thin enamel	Homozygous for Morquio A genes	Keratan sulfate	Galactosamine-6-sulfate sulfatase
MPS IV B (253010)	Morquio B (O'Brien-Arbisser)	Mild bone changes, cloudy cornea, hypoplastic odontoid, normal enamel	Homozygous for Morquio B gene	Keratan sulfate	β-galactosidase
MPS V	No longer used				
MPS VI, severe (253200)	Maroteaux-Lamy, classic severe	Severe osseous and corneal change; valvular heart disease, striking WBC inclusions; normal intellect; survival to 20s	Homozygous for Maroteaux-Lamy (M-L) gene	Dermatan sulfate	Arylsulfatase B (N-acetylgalactosamine 4-sulfatase)
MPS VI, intermediate	Maroteaux-Lamy, intermediate	Moderately severe changes	Homozygous for allele at M-L locus or genetic compound	Dermatan sulfate	Arylsulfatase B (N-acetylgalactosamine 4-sulfatase)
MPS VI, mild	Maroteaux-Lamy, mild	Mild osseous and corneal change, normal intellect; aortic stenosis	Homozygous for allele at M-L locus	Dermatan sulfate	Arylsulfatase B (N-acetylgalactosamine 4-sulfatase)
MPS VII (253230)	Sly	Hepatosplenomegaly dysostosis multiplex, mental retardation, WBC inclusions	Homozygous for mutant gene at β-glucuronidase locus	Dermatan sulfate, heparan sulfate	β-glucuronidase
MPS VIII (253230)	No longer used				

* Entry number in McKusick, V.A.[1]

tion factor is the enzyme specially deficient in the given disorder. Several trials of enzyme replacement therapy, by plasma exchange and fibroblast transplantation, have been attended by limited success, however, particularly in reversing established neurologic defects.[126]

Bone marrow transplantation has been used in patients with MPS disorders that do and do not affect the brain.[127,128] In either case, some improvement in somatic features (such as corneal clouding and joint stiffness) may occur, but mental retardation or other severe neurologic problems have been resistant to the presence of enzyme in the bloodstream. Also at this time, the complications of bone marrow transplantation limit early intervention with this method when prevention of somatic features, rather than their reversal, might be possible.[129]

The differential features of MPS are summarized in Table 87–4, and the clinical features of MPS IH, MPS IS, and MPS II are illustrated in Figures 87–11, 87–12, and 87–13, respectively. The nosologic validity of this classification is supported by the findings of cocultivation of fibroblasts. Mutual correction of their metabolic defects occurs when fibroblasts from MPS I and MPS II, MPS I and MPS III, and other combinations are mixed. Failure of cross-correction between cultured fibroblasts of two patients indicates that they have the same enzyme deficiency, and that the mutations underlying them at a minimum are allelic, if not identical.[125]

MPS V does not exist in the present classification. It was previously the numeric designation for the Scheie syndrome, a disorder distinct clinically from the other MPS (Fig. 87–12). In vitro studies, however, showed no cross-correction between Hurler and Scheie fibroblasts, and the same enzyme, α-L-iduronidase, was subsequently found deficient in the two disorders. One interpretation is that the Hurler and Scheie syndromes are due to homozygosity for two different mutations at the gene locus determining the structure of α-L-iduronidase. Thus, both are designated MPS I. The Hurler syndrome, MPS IH, is analogous to hemoglobin SS disease, a severe disorder, and the Scheie syndrome, MPS IS, to hemoglobin CC disease, a mild disorder. If the notion that MPS IH and MPS IS are due to allelic genes is correct, then a Hurler-Scheie genetic compound comparable to SC disease should exist. Indeed, patients with phenotypic features intermediate to MPS IH and MPS IS have been identified and are designated MPS IH/S. Some are likely true genetic compounds, whereas others are likely homozygotes (because of parental consanguinity) for other mutant alleles at the α-L-iduronidase

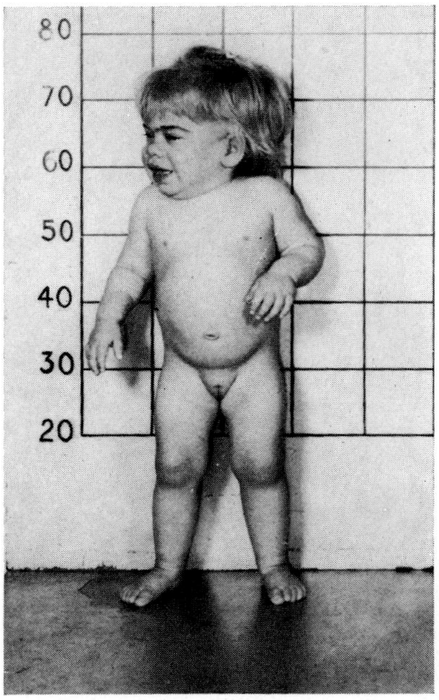

FIGURE 87–11. Mucopolysaccharidosis IH (Hurler syndrome) in a 2-year-old girl. Note the coarse facial features, prominent abdomen from hepatosplenomegaly, claw hands, and short stature. The joints generally had moderate restriction of motion. The patient died of congestive heart failure at 12 years of age.

locus.[130] Allelic variation at the loci responsible for MPS II and MPS VI presumably accounts for the severe and mild forms of those disorders.

Skeletal Features. Relative short stature is the rule in all patients with the MPS disorders, and can be profound in MPS IH, MPS II, MPS IV (the Morquio syndrome being the prototype "short trunk" form of dwarfism), and MPS VI. Radiographically, the skeletal dysplasia is similar in character in all but MPS IV, differing among the others largely in severity. The term dysostosis multiplex has been applied, but is not specific for MPS, similar changes occurring in a variety of storage disorders. The chief radiographic features are a thick calvaria, an enlarged J-shaped sella turcica, a short and wide mandible, biconvex vertebral bodies, hypoplasia of the odontoid, broad ribs, short and thick clavicles, coxa valga, metacarpals with widened diaphyses and pointed proximal ends, and short phalanges.[61]

For the disorders compatible with survival to adulthood without severe retardation (MPS IS, MPS II mild, MPS IV, MPS VI), progressive arthropathy and transverse myelopathy secondary to C1-C2 subluxation account for considerable disability. Cervical fusion should be considered whenever upper motor neuron signs appear. Joint replacement, particularly of the hips, has been beneficial in MPS IS.[124]

Stiff joints are a more or less striking feature of all forms except MPS IV. Like other somatic features, such as coarse facies, reduced joint mobility is less striking in MPS III. In the Scheie syndrome, stiff hands, together with clouding of the cornea, lead to the main disability. In that condition, as in the others, carpal tunnel syndrome contributes to the disability. Early decompression can be beneficial.

Regardless of the presence or severity of mental retardation or of the average life span, the major causes of death have as their pathogenesis the accumulation of glycosaminoglycan in soft tissues. The myocardium, cardiac valves, and coronary arteries are prime sites, and death from cardiac failure secondary to restrictive cardiopathy, severe valvular disease, or myocardial infarction is common (but often unrecognized) in MPS IH and MPS IIA.[29] Infiltration of the oropharynx and middle airways progresses to cause major clinical problems in most patients who survive cardiac disease.[131,132] When attempting any procedure that requires sedation or anesthesia in a patient with an MPS disorder, maximal precautions to protect the airway must be employed. If possible, procedures should be performed under local anesthetic. Intubation of the airway should be attempted only after careful assessment of the anatomy, and with full respect for the possibility of atlantoaxial instability.

Phosphotransferase Deficiencies

Mucolipidosis II (ML II) is also called I-cell disease (because of conspicuous inclusions in cultured cells). Mucolipidosis III (ML III) is also called pseudo-Hurler polydystrophy. Neither shows mucopolysacchariduria despite lysosomal storage of mucopolysaccharide and a demonstrable defect in degradation of mucopolysaccharides. Both are inherited as autosomal recessive conditions and some forms are likely allelic. The basic biochemical defect rests with an enzyme, UDP-*N*-acetylglucosamine:lysosomal enzyme, *N*-acetylglucosaminylphosphotransferase, responsible for post-translational modification of lysosomal enzymes.[133] This defect results in multiple enzyme deficiencies and accumulation in tissues of both mucopolysaccharides and mucolipids.

ML II is a severe Hurler-like disorder. ML III is a distinctive disorder with stiff joints, cloudy cornea, carpal tunnel syndrome, short stature, coarse facies, and sometimes mild mental retardation, compatible with survival to adulthood[134] (Fig. 87–14).

Mannosidosis

Deficiency of α-mannosidase, one of the many acid hydrolases found in lysosomes, causes phenotypic abnormalities of widely varying severity. Males and females are affected with equal frequency, and asymptomatic parents of patients have reduced levels of α-mannosidase, both features of autosomal recessive inheritance. Although the clinical conditions were initially thought to be limited to a severe and a mild form (designated types I and II), enough variation has been described to

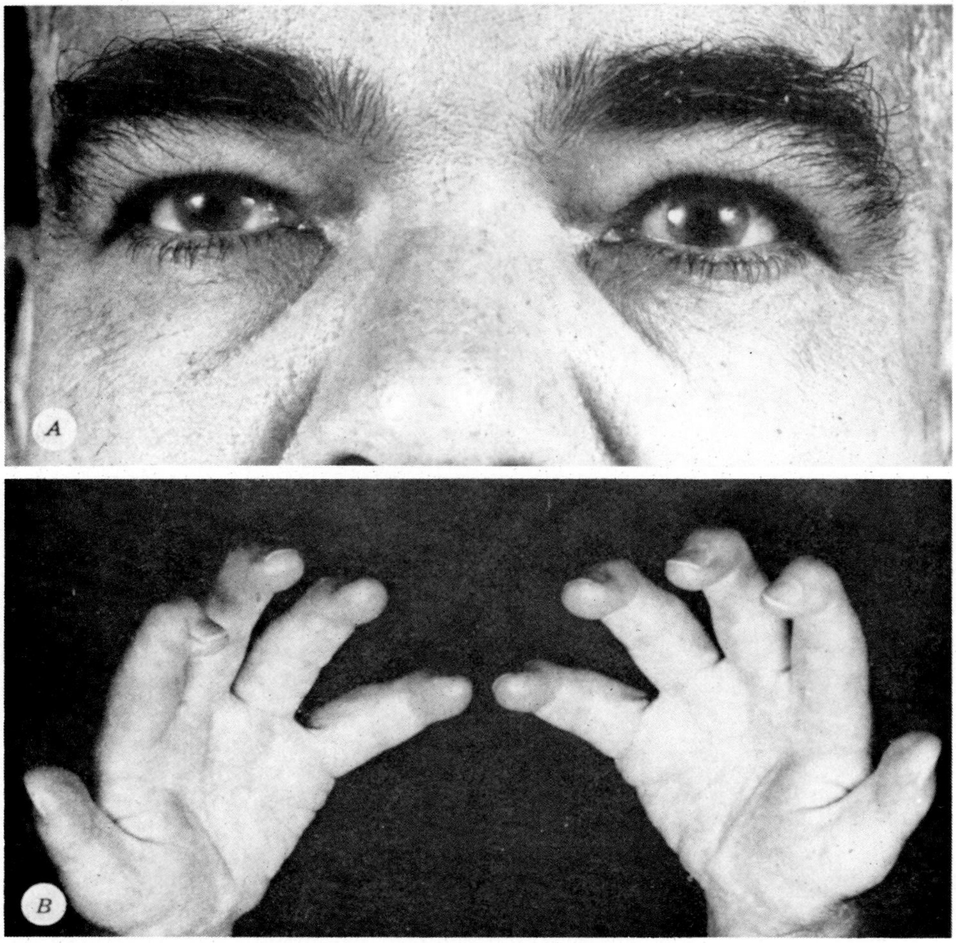

FIGURE 87–12. Mucopolysaccharidosis IS (Scheie syndrome) in a 54-year-old attorney. *A*, Clouding of the cornea was densest peripherally. *B*, The hands were clawed; atrophy of the lateral aspect of the thenar eminences indicated carpal tunnel compression.

suggest a spectrum of phenotypes, presumably caused by an allelic series of mutations.[135,136]

The most severe phenotype resembles the Hurler syndrome (MPS IH) in terms of coarse facial features, short stature, mental and motor retardation, hepatomegaly, and skeletal changes of dysostosis multiplex. Patients with severe mannosidosis have typical spoke-like posterior cataracts and lymphocytes with clear cytoplasmic vacuoles, however. Death in infancy from recurrent respiratory infections is common. At the other end of the phenotypic continuum, patients may not be diagnosed until adulthood, have mild coarsening of facies, clear corneas, IQs in the borderline normal range, and joint hypermobility; they come to medical attention because of degenerative arthritis of the hips or cardiac problems similar to those described in the mucopolysaccharidoses.

The diagnosis is suggested by screening urine for oligosaccharides and confirmed by documenting decreased activity of α-mannosidase in cultured fibroblasts.

The name of this autosomal recessive cause of short stature derives from the characteristic "happy-natured" facies. The skeletal dysplasia is more prominent in the hands and feet; bones are short and wide with relatively normal epiphyses.[137] Obstruction of the airway and cardiac valvular dysfunction cause early morbidity. Histologic examination of soft tissues shows cytoplasmic inclusions typical of lysosomal accumulation of incompletely catabolized macromolecules. A biochemical defect has not yet been defined.

OTHER DISORDERS THAT SIMULATE ARTHRITIDES

Hypophosphatemic Bone Disease. At least three distinct hereditary disorders have short stature, bowed legs, and reduced serum phosphate as cardinal features. The autosomal dominant and recessive forms are uncommon; the former responds to 1,25-$(OH)_2D_3$ (hydroxycholecalciferol) supplementation and the latter to oral phosphate.

Rickets has largely been eliminated as a medical con-

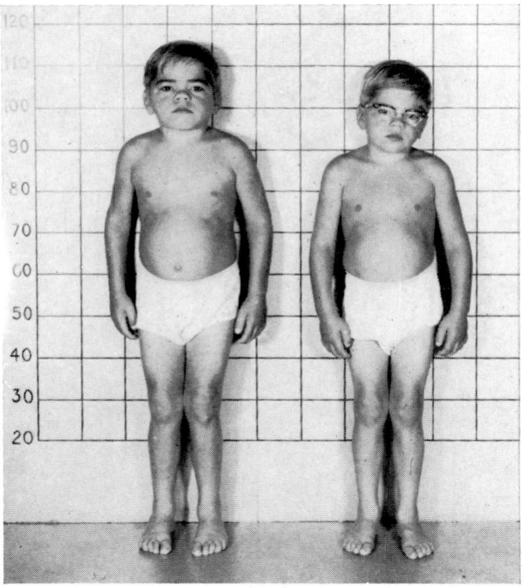

FIGURE 87–13. Mucopolysaccharidosis II, mild (the Hunter syndrome, mild variant) in brothers, 7 and 6 years of age. Note the short stature, coarse facies, prominent abdomen, and clawed hands. Intellect was normal.

cern because of supplementation of the diet with vitamin D and exposure to sunlight. As a result, the cases that are seen are highly likely to have a genetic basis. Fuller Albright and colleagues described the first instance of a patient with rickets who responded only to supraphysiologic doses of vitamin D.[138] This condition, now termed *familial hypophosphatemic rickets* or vitamin D–resistant rickets, is inherited as an X-linked dominant trait. Males and females both have reduced renal tubular reabsorption of phosphate that results in hypophosphatemia; however, serum calcium remains normal and patients do not develop muscle weakness or tetany. The skeletal features, which are more severe in males (Fig. 87–15), are those of rickets and osteomalacia. In infancy and childhood, the epiphyses are broad and the metaphyses cupped; the epiphyses fuse early, the limbs bow, and the endplates of the vertebrae become sclerotic; in adults, generalized bony sclerosis, scoliosis, protrusio acetabuli, and spinal stenosis from calcification of the ligamentum flavum are features. In adults, peripheral bone mass tends to be reduced, whereas axial bone mass is increased,[139] consistent with degenerative arthritis of the legs rather than vertebral fractures being the most frequent late complication.[140] The gene defect is expressed in teeth, resulting in abnormal secondary dentin, an effect apparently unrelated to

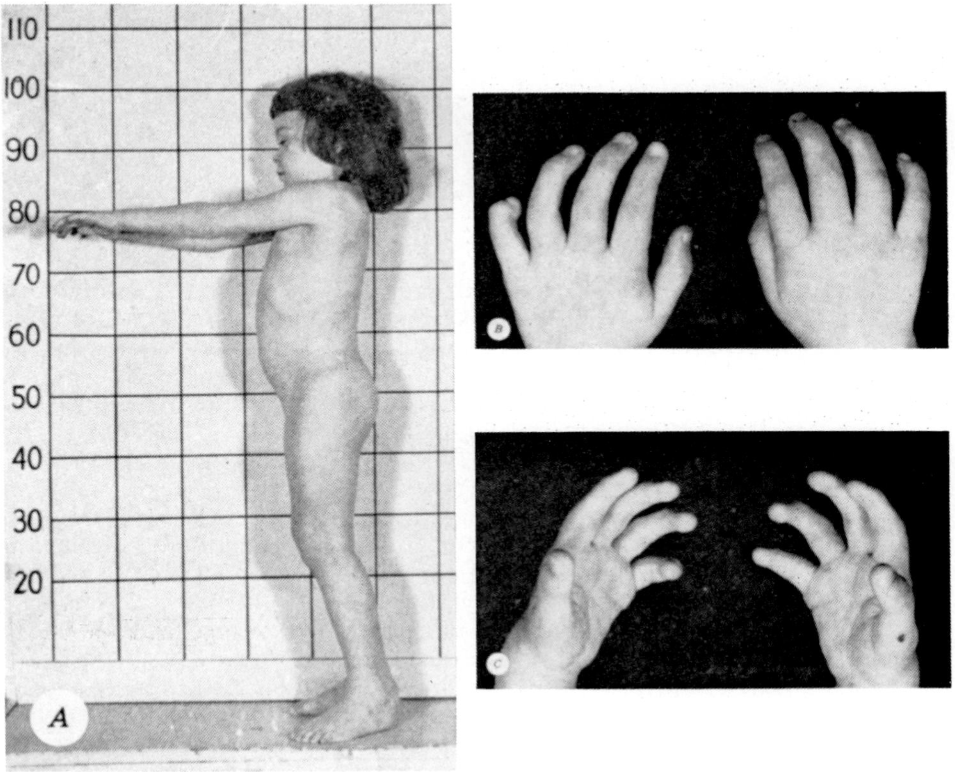

FIGURE 87–14. Mucolipidosis III (pseudo-Hurler polydystrophy) in a 6-year-old girl. *A*, Note the short stature and coarse facies. The corneas were clouded, motion of all joints was restricted, a murmur of aortic regurgitation was present, and intellect was mildly deficient. *B* and *C*, The hands were clawed, and atrophy of the thenar eminences indicated carpal tunnel compression, for which an operation was performed at 13 years of age, with some benefit.

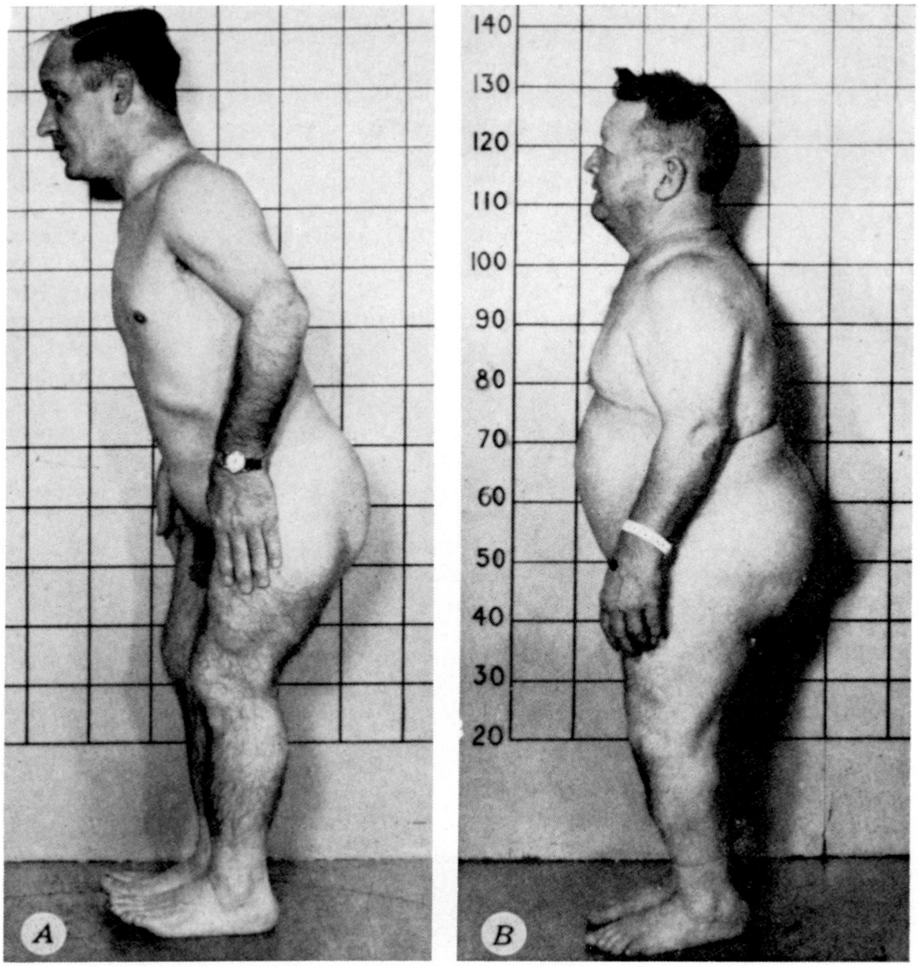

FIGURE 87–15. Ankylosing arthropathy in two men with vitamin D-resistant rickets. *A*, 41-year-old man. *B*, 61-year-old man. The younger man is the more severely affected, but both have almost complete ankylosis of the spine and similar changes in some peripheral joints. Note the short stature.

hypophosphatemia.[141] Therapy with both oral phosphate and vitamin D can prevent skeletal changes. 1α-hydroxyvitamin D_3 is preferable to vitamin D or calcidiol in producing optimal linear growth.[142]

In the hypocalcemic form of vitamin D–resistant rickets, an autosomal recessive disease, a defect in the cellular receptor for 1,25-dihydroxyvitamin D_3 has been found.[143]

Fibrodysplasia Ossificans Progressiva (FOP). This disorder, formerly called myositis ossificans progressiva, is uncommon and its biochemical defect is unknown.[144] Characterized by progressive ossification of ligaments, tendons, and aponeuroses, FOP begins an inexorable, progressive course in the first year or so of life, usually with a seemingly inflammatory process and nodule formation on the back of the thorax, neck, or scalp. Local heat, as well as leukocytosis and elevated sedimentation rate, is observed at this stage. Acute rheumatic fever is sometimes diagnosed. A valuable clue to the correct diagnosis is a short great toe with or without a short thumb; this is the leading cause of congenital hallux valgus.[145]

Most cases of this autosomal dominant disorder are the consequence of new mutation. Life expectancy is considerably reduced, with progressive restriction in lung capacity contributing to respiratory insufficiency and terminal pneumonia.[146]

Hypoparathyroidism. Hypocalcemia and its systemic consequences can be due to either inadequate or ineffective parathyroid hormone. Both classes of defects have multiple genetic causes. Aplasia of the parathyroid glands occurs as part of the DiGeorge sequence (3rd and 4th branchial arch syndrome), which is occasionally associated with an interstitial deletion of chromosome 22 (del22q11).[147]

Lack of effect of parathyroid hormone leads to elevated hormone levels in the face of hypocalcemia and hyperphosphatemia. The effect on the skeleton is historically termed Albright hereditary osteodystrophy; there are at least two forms of this condition, now called pseudohypoparathyroidism types IA and IB.[148] Patients with the autosomal dominant type IA have a syndrome of short stature, variable mental retardation, and ectopic calcification, especially of the basal ganglia and the paraspinal

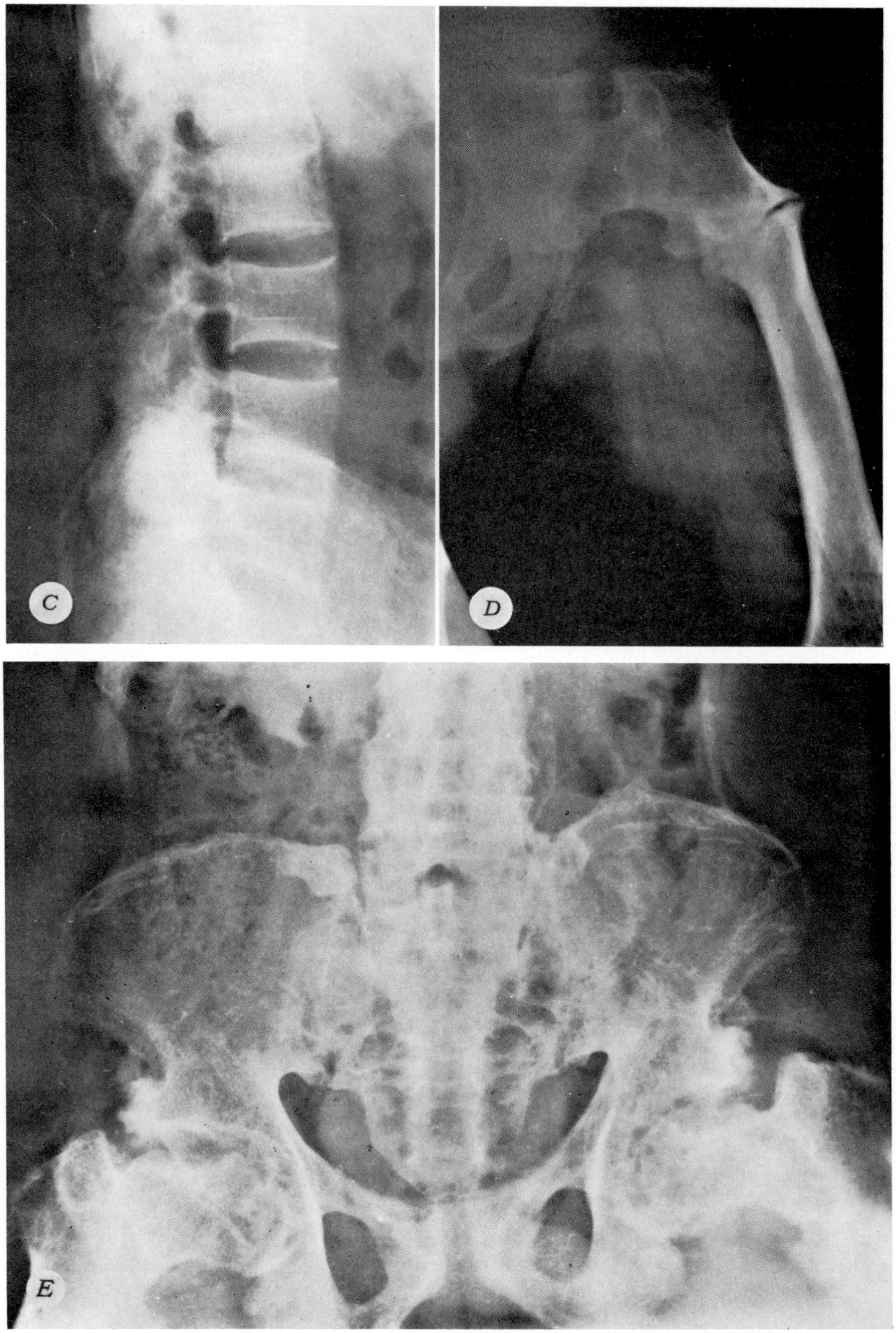

FIGURE 87–15. (*Continued*) *C*, Lateral radiograph of the lower spine in the older patient. *D*, Left femur of the younger patient. Pseudofractures were situated symmetrically in the subtrochanteric area of both femurs. *E*, Pelvis of the 41-year-old patient.

ligaments. A characteristic skeletal change is shortening of the metacarpals and metatarsals, especially the fourth. Most of these patients fail to increase urinary cAMP in response to parathyroid hormone, a phenomenon now recognized as due to the basic defect, reduced function or synthesis of the α subunit of the stimulatory G protein of adenylate cyclase.[149] The G proteins are normal in type IB, and patients with this form of parathyroid hormone resistance have normal appearance.

Arthrogryposis Multiplex Congenita (AMC). The phenotype of congenital rigidity of multiple joints is of complex etiology, pathogenesis, and clinical presentation.[150–153] In many instances, the disorder is a deformation of joints resulting from immobilization of the developing fetus, so that the proper stimulus for joint development is lacking. The cause of the immobilization may be a prenatal disorder of the brain, spinal cord, peripheral nerves, vasculature, or muscle. The affected baby is born with the arms and legs fixed in postures dictated by the position of the embryo and fetus in development. In addition to joint rigidity, dislocation of the hips and micrognathia are frequent findings. The Drachman theory of fetal immobilization as one cause of AMC was developed from studies of the effects of neuromuscular blocking agents on chick embryos. His theory is supported by observation of AMC in an infant born of a mother who received tubocurarine in early pregnancy for treatment of tetanus.[150] The hereditary syndromes that include AMC are exceedingly heterogeneous; at least 3 X-linked conditions affecting predominantly the distal joints have been described.[153]

REFERENCES

1. McKusick, V.A.: Mendelian Inheritance in Man. Catalogs of Autosomal Dominant, Autosomal Recessive and X-linked Phenotypes, 9th Ed. Baltimore, Johns Hopkins Press, 1990.
2. Gardner, R.J., and Sutherland, G.R.: Chromosome Abnormalities and Genetic Counseling. New York, Oxford University Press, 1989.
3. Emanuel, B.S.: Molecular cytogenetics: Toward dissection of the contiguous gene syndromes. Am. J. Hum. Genet., *43*:575–578, 1988.
4. Tommerup, N., and Nielsen, F.: A familial reciprocal translocation t(3:7)(p21.1;p13) associated with the Greig polysyndactyly-craniofacial anomalies syndrome. Am. J. Med. Genet., *16*:313–321, 1983.
5. Holmes, L.B.: Inborn errors of morphogenesis: A review of localized hereditary malformations. N. Engl. J. Med., *291*:763–773, 1974.
6. Emery, A., and Rimoin, D.L. (eds.): Principles and Practice of Medical Genetics, 2nd Ed. London, Churchill Livingstone, 1990.
7. Gelehrter, T.D., and Collins, F.S.: Principles of Medical Genetics. Baltimore, Williams & Wilkins, 1990.
8. McKusick, V.A.: The cardiovascular aspects of Marfan's syndrome: A heritable disorder of connective tissue. Circulation, *11*:321–342, 1955.
9. Beighton, P., et al.: International nosology of heritable disorders of connective tissue, Berlin, 1986. Am. J. Med. Genet., *29*:581–594, 1988.
10. Rimoin, D.L.: International nomenclature of constitutional diseases of bone with bibliography. Birth Defects, *15*(10):30, 1979.
11. Beighton, P., et al.: Molecular nosology of the heritable disorders of connective tissue. Am. J. Med. Genet., 1991, in press.
12. Fleishmajer, R., Olsen, B.R., and Kuch, K. (eds.): Biology, Chemistry, and Pathology of Collagen. New York, New York Academy of Sciences, 1985.
13. Royce, P.M., and Steinmann, B. (eds.): Extracellular Matrix and Inheritable Disorders of Connective Tissue. New York, Wiley-Liss, 1991.
14. Byers, P.H.: Disorders of collagen biosynthesis and structure. *In* The Metabolic Basis of Inherited Disease. Edited by C.R. Scriver, et al. New York, McGraw-Hill, 1989, pp. 2805–2842.
15. Pyeritz, R.E.: Heritable defects in connective tissue. Hosp. Pract., *22*:153–168, 1987.
16. Holbrook, K.A., and Byers, P.H.: Skin is a window on heritable disorders of connective tissue. Am. J. Med. Genet., *34*:105–121, 1989.
17. Solursh, M.: Extracellular matrix and cell surface as determinants of connective tissue differentiation. Am. J. Med. Genet., *34*:30–34, 1989.
18. Indik, Z., et al.: Structure of the elastin gene and alternative splicing of elastin mRNA: Implications for human disease. Am. J. Med. Genet., *34*:81–90, 1989.
19. Pyeritz, R.E., and McKusick, V.A.: The Marfan syndrome: Diagnosis and management. N. Engl. J. Med., *300*:772–777, 1979.
20. Pyeritz, R.E.: The Marfan syndrome. *In* Extracellular Matrix and Inheritable Disorders of Connective Tissue. Edited by P.M. Royce and B. Steinmann. New York, Wiley-Liss, 1991.
21. Perejda, A.J., et al.: Marfan's syndrome: Structural, biochemical, and mechanical studies of the aortic media. J. Lab. Clin. Med., *106*:376–383, 1985.
22. Hollister, D.W., et al.: Marfan syndrome: immunohistologic abnormalities of the elastin-associated microfibrillar fiber system. N. Engl. J. Med., *323*:152–159, 1990.
23. Sakai, L.Y., Keene, D.R., and Engvall, E.: Fibrillin, a new 350-kD glycoprotein, is a component of extracellular microfibrils. J. Cell Biol., *103*:2499–2509, 1986.
24. Dietz, H.C., et al.: Defects in the fibrillin gene cause the Marfan syndrome: linkage evidence and identification of a recurrent de novo missense mutation. Nature, 1991, in press.
25. Pyeritz, R.E.: Marfan syndrome (editorial). N. Engl. J. Med., *323*:987–989, 1990.
26. Beals, R.K., and Hecht, F.: Congenital contractural arachnodactyly: A heritable disorder of connective tissue. J. Bone Joint Surg., *53A*:987–993, 1971.
27. Morse, R.P., et al.: Diagnosis and management of Marfan syndrome in infants. Pediatrics, *86*:888–895.
28. Walker, B.A., Beighton, P.H., and Murdoch, J.L.: The marfanoid hypermobility syndrome. Ann. Intern. Med., *71*:349–352, 1969.
29. Pyeritz, R.E.: Cardiovascular manifestations of heritable disorders of connective tissue. Prog. Med. Genet., *5*:191–302, 1983.
30. Svensson, L.G., et al.: Impact of cardiovascular operation on survival in the Marfan patient. Circulation, *80*(Suppl. I):233–242, 1988.
31. Gott, V.L., et al.: Composite graft repair of Marfan aneurysm of the ascending aorta: Results in 100 patients. Ann. Thorac. Surg., 1991, in press.
32. Hall, J., Pyeritz, R.E., Dudgeon, D.L., and Haller, J.A., Jr.: Pneumothorax in the Marfan syndrome: Prevalence and therapy. Ann. Thorac. Surg., *37*:500–504, 1984.
33. Pyeritz, R.E., et al.: Dural ectasia is a common feature of the Marfan syndrome. Am. J. Hum. Genet., *43*:726–732, 1988.

33a. Francomano, C.A., et al.: The Stickler syndrome: Evidence for close linkage to the structural gene for type II collagen. Genomics, *1*:293–296, 1987.

34. Pyeritz, R.E., Murphy, E.A., Lin, S.J., and Rosell, E.M.: Growth and anthropometrics in the Marfan syndrome. *In* Endocrine Genetics and Genetics of Growth. Edited by C.J. Papadatos and C.S. Bartsocas. New York, A.R. Liss, 1985, pp. 355–366.

35. Arn, P.H., et al.: Clinical outcome of pectus excavatum in the Marfan syndrome and in the general population. J. Pediatr., *115*:954–958, 1989.

36. Pyeritz, R.E.: Homocystinuria. *In* McKusick's Heritable Disorders of Connective Tissue. Edited by P. Beighton. St. Louis, C.V. Mosby, 1991.

37. Mudd, S.H., Levy, H.L., and Skovby, F.: Disorders of transulfuration. *In* The Metabolic Basis of Inherited Disease. Edited by C.R. Scriver, et al. New York, McGraw-Hill Book Co., 1989, pp. 693–734.

38. Abbott, M.H., Folstein, S.E., Abbey, H., and Pyeritz, R.E.: Psychiatric manifestations of homocystinuria due to cystathionine beta-synthase deficiency. Am. J. Med. Genet., *26*:959–969, 1987.

39. Mudd, S.H., et al.: The natural history of homocystinuria due to cysthathionine beta-synthase deficiency. Am. J. Hum. Genet., *36*:1–31, 1985.

40. Hill-Zobel, R.L., et al.: Kinetics and biodistribution of ^{111}In-labeled platelets in homocystinuria. N. Engl. J. Med., *307*:781–786, 1982.

41. Maumenee, I.H.: The Weill-Marchesani syndrome. *In* McKusick's Heritable Disorders of Connective Tissue. Edited by P. Beighton. St. Louis, C.V. Mosby, 1991.

42. Minor, R.R., et al.: Defects in the processing of procollagen to collagen are demonstrable in cultured fibroblasts from patients with the Ehlers-Danlos and osteogenesis imperfecta syndromes. J. Biol. Chem., *261*:10006–10014, 1986.

43. Beighton, P.: The Ehlers-Danlos syndromes. *In* McKusick's Heritable Disorders of Connective Tissue. Edited by P. Beighton. St. Louis, C.V. Mosby, 1991.

44. Steinmann, B., Superti-Furga, S., and Royce, P.M.: The Ehlers-Danlos syndrome. *In* Extracellular Matrix and Inheritable Disorders of Connective Tissue. Edited by B. Steinmann and P.M. Royce. New York, Wiley-Liss, 1991.

45. Pyeritz, R.E., Stolle, C.A., Parfrey, N.A., and Myers, J.C.: Ehlers-Danlos syndrome IV due to a novel defect in type III procollagen. Am. J. Med. Genet., *19*:607–622, 1984.

46. Byers, P.H., et al.: Clinical and ultrastructural heterogeneity of type IV Ehlers-Danlos syndrome. Hum. Genet., *47*:141–150, 1979.

47. Rudd, N.L., et al.: Pregnancy complications in type IV Ehlers-Danlos syndrome. Lancet, *1*:50–53, 1983.

48. Beighton, P., and Curtis, D.: X-linked Ehlers-Danlos syndrome type V: The next generation. Clin. Genet., *27*:472–478, 1985.

49. Wenstrup, R.J., Murad, S., and Pinnell, S.R.: Ehlers-Danlos syndrome type VI: Clinical manifestations of collagen lysyl hydroxylase deficiency. J. Pediatr., *115*:405–409, 1989.

50. Krane, S.M., Pinnell, S.R., and Erbe, R.W.: Lyso-protocollagen hydroxylase deficiency in fibroblasts from siblings with hydroxylysine deficient collagen. Proc. Natl. Acad. Sci. U.S.A., *69*:2899–2903, 1972.

51. Elsas, L.J., II, Miller, R.L., and Pinnell, S.R.: Inherited human collagen lysyl hydroxylase deficiency: Ascorbic acid response. J. Pediatr., *92*:378–384, 1978.

52. Hass, J., and Hass, R.: Arthrochalasis multiplex congenita: Congenital flaccidity of the joints. J. Bone Joint Surg., *40A*:663–674, 1958.

53. Steinmann, B., et al.: Evidence for a structural mutation of procollagen type I in a patient with the Ehlers-Danlos syndrome type VII. J. Biol. Chem., *155*:8887–8893, 1980.

54. Weil, D., et al.: Temperature-dependent expression of a collagen splicing defect in the fibroblasts of a patient with Ehlers-Danlos syndrome type VII. J. Biol. Chem., *264*:16804–16809, 1989.

55. Hartsfield, J.K. Jr., and Kousseff, B.G.: Phenotypic overlap of Ehlers-Danlos syndrome types IV and VIII. Am. J. Med. Genet., *37*:465–470, 1990.

56. Arneson, M.A., et al.: A new form of Ehlers-Danlos syndrome: Fibronectin corrects defective platelet function. JAMA, *244*:144–147, 1980.

57. Kirk, J.A., Ansell, B.M., and Bywaters, F.G.L.: The hypermobility syndrome: Musculoskeletal complaints associated with generalized joint hypermobility. Ann. Rheum. Dis., *26*:419–425, 1967.

58. Beighton, P., Grahame, R., and Bird, H.: Hypermobility of Joints. 2nd Ed. New York, Springer-Verlag, 1989.

59. Wynne-Davies, R.: Acetabular dysplasia and familial joint laxity: Two etiologic factors in congenital dislocation of the hip. J. Bone Joint Surg., *52B*:704–716, 1970.

60. Horton, W.A., et al.: Familal joint instability syndrome. Am. J. Med. Genet., *6*:221–228, 1980.

61. Latta, R.J., et al.: Larsen's syndrome: A skeletal dysplasia with multiple joint dislocations and unusual facies. J. Pediatr., *78*:291, 1971.

62. Wynne-Davies, R., Hall, C.M., and Apley, A.G.: Atlas of Skeletal Dysplasias. Edinburgh, Churchill Livingstone, 1985.

63. Sconyers, S.M., et al.: A distinct chondrodysplasia resembling Kniest dysplasia: Clinical, roentgenographic, histologic, and ultrastructural findings. J. Pediatr., *103*:898–904, 1983.

64. Sillence, D.O.: Osteogenesis imperfecta: An expanding panorama of variants. Clin. Orthop., *159*:11–25, 1981.

65. Cole, W.G., et al.: The clinical features of three babies with osteogenesis imperfecta resulting from the substitution of glycine by arginine in the proα1(I) chain of type I procollagen. J. Med. Genet., *27*:228–235, 1990.

66. Byers, P.H.: Brittle bones—fragile molecules: Disorders of collagen gene structure and expression. Trends Genet., *6*:293–300, 1990.

67. Paterson, C.R., McAllion, S., and Miller, R.: Heterogeneity of osteogenesis imperfecta type I. J. Med. Genet., *20*:203–205, 1983.

68. Constantinou, C.D., et al.: Phenotypic heterogeneity in osteogenesis imperfecta: The mildly affected mother of a proband with a lethal variant has the same mutation substituting cysteine for α1-glycine 904 in a type I procollagen gene (COL1A1). Am. J. Hum. Genet., *47*:670–679, 1990.

69. Sillence, D.O., et al.: Osteogenesis imperfecta type II. Delineation of the phenotype with reference to genetic heterogeneity. Am. J. Med. Genet., *17*:407–423, 1984.

70. Cohn, D.H., et al.: Lethal osteogenesis imperfecta resulting from a single nucleotide change in one human pro alpha 1(I) collagen allele. Proc. Natl. Acad. Sci. U.S.A., *83*:6045–6057, 1986.

71. Sillence, D.O., et al.: Osteogenesis imperfecta type III. Delineation of the phenotype with reference to genetic heterogeneity. Am. J. Med. Genet., *23*:821–832, 1986.

72. Paterson, C.R., McAllion, S., and MIller, R.: Osteogenesis imperfecta with dominant inheritance and normal sclerae. J. Bone Joint Surg., *65B*:35–39, 1983.

73. Tsipouras, P., et al.: Molecular heterogeneity in the mild autosomal dominant forms of osteogenesis imperfecta. Am. J. Hum. Genet., *36*:1172–1179, 1984.

74. Bergstrom, L.V.: Fragile bones and fragile ears. Clin. Orthop., *159*:58–63, 1981.

75. Levin, L.S.: The dentition in the osteogenesis imperfecta syndromes. Clin. Orthop., *159*:64, 1981.

76. Hortop, J., et al.: Cardiovascular involvement in osteogenesis imperfecta. Circulation, *73*:54–61, 1986.
77. Dent, C.E., and Friedman, M.: Idiopathic juvenile osteoporosis. Q. J. Med., *34*:177–210, 1965.
78. Neuhauser, G., Kaveggia, E.G., and Opitz, J.M.: Autosomal recessive syndrome of pseudogliomatous blindness, osteoporosis, and mild mental retardation. Clin. Genet., *9*:324–332, 1976.
79. Weleber, R.G., and Beals, R.K.: The Hadju-Cheney syndrome. J. Pediatr., *88*:243–249, 1976.
80. Meredith, S.C., Simon, M.A., Laros, G.S., and Jackson, M.A.: Pycnodysostosis: A clinical pathological, and ultramicroscopic study of a case. J. Bone Joint Surg., *60A*:1122–1128, 1978.
81. Rasmussen, H.: Hypophosphatasia. *In* The Metabolic Basis of Inherited Disease. Edited by J.B. Stanbury, et al. New York, McGraw-Hill Book Co., 1983, pp. 1497–1507.
82. Herrmann, J., et al.: The Stickler syndrome (hereditary arthro-ophthalmopathy). Birth Defects, *11*:76–103, 1975.
83. Liberfarb, R.M., Hirose, T., and Holmes, L.B.: The Wagner-Stickler syndrome: A study of 22 families. J. Pediatr., *99*:394–399, 1981.
84. Shprintzen, R.J., Siegel-Sadewitz, V.L., Amato, J., and Goldberg, R.B.: Anomalies associated with cleft lip, cleft palate, or both. Am. J. Med. Genet., *20*:585–595, 1985.
85. Marshall, D.: Ectodermal dysplasia: Report of kindred with ocular abnormalities and hearing defect. Am. J. Ophthalmol., *45*:143–156, 1958.
86. Ayme, S., and Preus, M.: The Marshall and Stickler syndromes: Objective rejection of lumping. J. Med. Genet., *21*:34–38, 1984.
87. Baraitser, M.: Marshall/Stickler syndrome. J. Med. Genet., *19*:139–140, 1982.
88. Winter, R.M., et al.: The Weissenbacher-Zweymüller, Stickler, and Marshall syndromes: Further evidence for their identity. Am. J. Med. Genet., *16*:189–199, 1983.
89. Kelley, T.E., Wells, H.H., and Tuck, K.B.: The Weissenbacher-Zweymüller syndrome: Possible neonatal expression of the Stickler syndrome. Am. J. Med. Genet., *11*:113–119, 1982.
90. Francomano, C.A., et al.: The Stickler syndrome: Evidence for close linkage to the structural gene for type II collagen. Genomics, *1*:293–296, 1987.
91. Knowlton, R.G., et al.: Genetic linkage analysis of hereditary arthro-ophthalmopathy (Stickler syndrome) and the type II procollagen gene. Am. J. Hum. Genet., *45*:681–688, 1989.
92. Priestley, L., Kumar, D., and Sykes, B.: Amplification of the COL2A1 3-prime variable region used for segregation analysis in a family with the Stickler syndrome. Hum. Genet., *85*:525–526, 1990.
93. Ahmad, N.N., et al.: A stop codon in the gene for type II procollagen (COL2A1) causes one variant of arthro-ophthalmopathy (the Stickler syndrome). Am. J. Med. Genet., *47*:A206, 1990.
94. Lee, B., et al.: Identification of the molecular defect in a family with spondyloepiphyseal dysplasia. Science, *244*:978–980, 1989.
95. Vissing, H., et al.: Glycine to serine substitution in the triple helical domain of proalpha-1(II) collagen results in a lethal perinatal form of short-limbed dwarfism. J. Biol. Chem., *264*:18265–18267, 1989.
96. Ala-Kokko, L., et al.: Single base mutation in the type II procollagen gene (COL2A1) as a cause of primary osteoarthritis associated with a mild chondrodysplasia. Proc. Natl. Acad. Sci. U.S.A., *87*:6565–6568, 1990.
97. Solomon, I., Abrams, G., Dinner, M., and Berman, L.: Neonatal abnormalities associated with D-penicillamine treatment during pregnancy. N. Engl. J. Med., *296*:54–55, 1977.
98. Renie, W.A., Pyeritz, R.E., Combs, J., and Fine, S.L.: Pseudoxanthoma elasticum: High calcium intake in early life correlates with severity. Am. J. Med. Genet., *19*:235–244, 1984.
99. Spranger, J.: Radiologic nosology of bone dysplasias. Am. J. Med. Genet., *34*:96–104, 1989.
100. Murray, L.W., et al.: Type II collagen defects in the chondrodysplasias. I. Spondyloepiphyseal dysplasias. Am. J. Hum. Genet., *45*:5–15, 1989.
101. Wynne-Davies, R., and Hall, C.: Two clinical variants of spondyloepiphyseal dysplasia congenita. J. Bone Joint Surg., *64B*:435–441, 1982.
102. Bannerman, R.M., Ingall, G.B., and Mohn, J.F.: X-linked spondyloepiphyseal dysplasia tarda: Clinical and linkage data. J. Med. Genet., *8*:291–301, 1971.
103. Horton, W.A., et al.: Growth curves for height for diastrophic dysplasia, spondyloepiphyseal dysplasia congenita, and pseudoachondroplasia. Am. J. Dis. Child., *136*:316–319, 1982.
104. Finkelstein, J.E., et al.: Analysis of the chondroitin sulfate proteoglycan core protein (CSPGCP) gene in achondroplasia and pseudoachondroplasia. Am. J. Hum. Genet., *48*:97–102, 1990.
105. Jacobsen, A.W.: Hereditary osteochondro-dystrophia deformans. JAMA, *113*:121–124, 1939.
106. Horton, W.A., et al.: Standard growth curves for achondroplasia. J. Pediatr., *93*:435–438, 1978.
107. Nicoletti, B., Kopits, S.E., Ascani, E., and McKusick, V.A. (eds.): Human Achondroplasia. New York, Plenum, 1988.
108. Hecht, J.T., et al.: Computerized tomography of the foramen magnum: Achondroplastic values compared to normal standards. Am. J. Med. Genet., *20*:355–360, 1985.
109. Reid, C.S., et al.: Cervicomedullary compression in young patients with achondroplasia: Value of comprehensive neurologic and respiratory evaluation. J. Pediatr., *110*:522–530, 1987.
110. Lutter, I.D., and Langer, I.O.: Neurological symptoms in achondroplastic dwarfs—surgical treatment. J. Bone Joint Surg., *59A*:87–92, 1977.
111. Pyeritz, R.E., Sack, G.H., Jr., and Udvarhelyi, G.B.: Thoracolumbosacral laminectomy in achondroplasia: Long-term results in 22 patients. Am. J. Med. Genet., *28*:433–444, 1987.
112. Streeten, E.A., et al.: Extended laminectomy for spinal stenosis in achondroplasia. *In* Human Achondroplasia. Edited by B. Nicoletti, et al. New York, Plenum, 1988, pp. 261–274.
113. Hurko, O., Pyeritz, R.E., and Uematsu, S.: Neurologic considerations in achondroplasia. *In* Human Achondroplasia. Edited by B. Nicoletti, et al. New York, Plenum, 1988, pp. 153–162.
114. Kopits, S.E.: Correction of bowleg deformity in achondroplasia. Johns Hopkins Med. J., *146*:206–209, 1980.
115. Ascani, E., et al.: Round table: discussion on extensive leg lengthening. *In* Human Achondroplasia. Edited by B. Nicoletti, et al. New York, Plenum, 1988, pp. 415–442.
116. Weiss, J., et al.: Round table: social and psychological implications of extensive limb lengthening. *In* Human Achondroplasia. Edited by B. Nicoletti, et al. New York, Plenum, 1988, pp. 463–474.
117. Brueton, L.A., and Winter, R.M.: Craniodiaphyseal dysplasia. J. Med. Genet., *27*:701–706, 1990.
118. Manni, J.J., et al.: Hyperostosis cranialis interna: A new hereditary syndrome with cranial-nerve entrapment. N. Engl. J. Med., *322*:450–454, 1990.
119. Rovin, S., et al.: Mandibulofacial dysostosis, a familial study of five generations. J. Pediatr., *65*:215–221, 1964.
120. Temtamy, S., McKusick, V.A.: The Genetics of Hand Malformations. New York, AR Liss, 1978.
121. Strasburger, A.K., et al.: Symphalangism: Genetics and clinical aspects. Bull. Johns Hopkins Hosp., *117*:108–127, 1965.
122. Welch, J.P., and Temtamy, S.A.: Hereditary contractures of the fingers (camptodactyly). J. Med. Genet., *3*:104–113, 1966.
123. Renie, W.A., and Pyeritz, R.E.: Idiopathic multicentric osteolysis in a 78-year-old woman. Johns Hopkins Med. J., *148*:165–171, 1981.

124. Carnevale, A., Canun, S., Mendoza, L., and del Castillo, V.: Idiopathic multicentric osteolysis with facial anomalies and nephropathy. Am. J. Med. Genet., *26*:877–886, 1987.
125. Neufeld, E.F., and Meunzer, J.: The mucopolysaccharidoses. *In* The Metabolic Basis of Inherited Disease. 6th Ed. Edited by C.R. Scriver, et al. New York, McGraw-Hill, 1989, pp. 1565–1588.
126. Brown, F.R., III, et al.: Administration of iduronate sulfatase by plasma exchange to patients with the Hunter syndrome: A clinical study. Am. J. Med. Genet., *13*:309–318, 1982.
127. Hobbs, J.R., et al.: Reversal of clinical features of Hurler's disease and biochemical improvement after treatment by bone-marrow transplantation. Lancet, *2*:709–712, 1981.
128. Krivit, W., et al.: Bone-marrow transplantation in the Maroteaux-Lamy syndrome (mucopolysaccharidosis type VI): Biochemical and clinical status 24 months after transplantation. N. Engl. J. Med., *311*:1606–1611, 1984.
129. Lenarski, C., et al.: Bone marrow transplantation for genetic diseases. Hematol. Oncol. Clin. North Am., *4*:589–602, 1990.
130. Mueller, C.T., Shows, T.B., and Optiz, J.M.: Apparent allelism of the Hurler, Scheie, and Hurler/Scheie syndromes. Am. J. Med. Genet., *18*:547–556, 1984.
131. Young, I.D., and Harper, P.S.: Long-term complications in Hunter's syndrome. Clin. Genet., *16*:125–132, 1979.
132. Semenza, G.L., and Pyeritz, R.E.: Respiratory complications of the mucopolysaccharide storage disorders. Medicine, *67*:209–219, 1988.
133. Nolan, C.M., and Sly, W.S.: I-cell disease and pseudo-Hurler polydystrophy: Disorders of lysosomal enzyme phosphorylation and localization. *In* The Metabolic Basis of Inherited Disease. 6th Ed. Edited by C.R. Scriver, et al. New York, McGraw-Hill, 1989, pp. 1589–1602.
134. Kelly, T.E., et al.: Mucolipidosis III (pseudo-Hurler polydystrophy): Clinical and laboratory studies in a series of 12 patients. Johns Hopkins Med. J., *137*:156–175, 1975.
135. Yunis, J.J., et al.: Clinical manifestations of mannosidosis—a longitudinal study. Am. J. Med., *61*:841–848, 1976.
136. Desnick, R.J., et al.: Mannosidosis: Clinical, morphologic, immunologic, and biochemical studies. Pediatr. Res., *10*:985–996, 1976.
137. Shohat, M., et al.: Geleophysic dysplasia: A storage disorder affecting the skin, bone, liver, heart, and trachea. J. Pediatr., *117*:227–232, 1990.
138. Albright, F., Butler, A.M., and Bloomberg, E.: Rickets resistant to vitamin D therapy. Am. J. Dis. Child., *54*:529 1937.
139. Reid, I.R., et al.: X-linked hypophosphatemia: skeletal mass in adults assessed by histomorphometry, computed tomography, and absorptiometry. Am. J. Med., *90*:63–69, 1991.
140. Reid, I.R., et al.: X-linked hypophosphatemia: A clinical, biochemical, and histopathologic assessment of morbidity in adults. Medicine, *68*:336–352, 1989.
141. Shields, E.D., et al.: X-linked hypophosphatemia: the mutant gene is expressed in teeth as well as in kidney. Am. J. Hum. Genet., *46*:434–442, 1990.
142. Balsan, S., and Tieder, M.: Linear growth in patients with hypophosphatemic vitamin D-resistant rickets: Influence of treatment regimen and parental height. J. Pediatr., *116*:365–371, 1990.
143. Hughes, M.R., et al.: Point mutations in the human vitamin D receptor gene associated with hypocalcemic rickets. Science, *242*:1702–1705, 1988.
144. Rogers, J.G.: Fibrodysplasia ossificans progressiva. *In* Extracellular Matrix and Inheritable Disorders of Connective Tissue. Edited by B. Steinmann and P.M. Royce. New York, Wiley-Liss, 1991.
145. Schroeber, H.W., Jr., and Zasloff, M.: The hand and foot malformations in fibrodysplasia ossificans progressiva. Johns Hopkins Med. J., *147*:73–78, 1980.
146. Conner, J.M., and Evans, D.A.P.: Fibrodysplasia ossificans progressiva: The clinical features and natural history of 34 patients. J. Bone Joint Surg., *64B*:76–83, 1982.
147. Greenberg, F., et al.: Cytogenetic findings in a prospective series of patients with DiGeorge anomaly. Am. J. Hum. Genet., *43*:605–611, 1988.
148. Spiegel, A.M.: Albright's hereditary osteodystrophy and defective G proteins (editorial). N. Engl. J. Med., *322*:1461–1462, 1990.
149. Patten, J.L., et al.: Mutation in the gene encoding the stimulatory G protein of adenylate cyclase in Albright's hereditary osteodystrophy. N. Engl. J. Med., *322*:1412–1419.
150. Drachman, D.B.: The syndrome of arthrogryposis multiplex congenita. Birth Defects, 7:90–97, 1971.
151. Hall, J.G., Reed, S.D., and Greene, G.: The distal arthrogryposes: Delineation of new entities—review and nosologic discussion. Am. J. Med. Genet., *11*:185–239, 1982.
152. Smith, D.W.: Recognizable Patterns of Human Deformation. Philadelphia, W.B. Saunders Co., 1981.
153. Hall, J.G., et al.: Three distinct types of X-linked arthrogryposes seen in 6 families. Clin. Genet., *21*:81097, 1982.

88

Hypertrophic Osteoarthropathy

ROY D. ALTMAN

Clubbing was first recorded circa 400 B.C. by Hippocrates,[1,2] yet little is known of its etiopathogenesis. Von Bamberger and Marie noted the association of clubbing with bone and joint changes in 1890, describing the syndrome of hypertrophic osteoarthropathy (HPO).[2,3] HPO includes (1) clubbing of fingers and toes, (2) periostitis with new osseous formation of long bones, and (3) arthritis. HPO has also been called familial idiopathic hypertrophic osteoarthropathy, Marie-Bamberger syndrome, osteoarthropathic hypertrophiante and pneumique, and secondary hypertrophic osteoarthropathy.

HPO is classified as either primary or secondary. The primary (hereditary) form usually appears during childhood. The secondary form, often associated with neoplasms or infectious diseases, can appear at any age. Originally the associated diseases were intrathoracic, but HPO can be associated with numerous extrathoracic diseases. Insidious development of symptoms and signs with mild rheumatic complaints over a period of months or years characterizes HPO associated with suppurative disease. In contrast, rapidly progressing HPO with prominent joint pain and stiffness is often associated with malignant diseases.

CLINICAL FEATURES

CLUBBING

Rarely symptomatic, except for its unsightliness, clubbing is often observed by a physician rather than by the patient. Symptoms include clumsiness, stiffness, and burning or warmth of finger tips. Clubbing is the most constant feature of HPO and is not invariably accompanied by periostitis or synovitis.[4–6] It is unclear whether clubbing without the other features of HPO is a separate disease of a *forme fruste* of HPO.[4,7] Isolated clubbing does not distinguish primary from secondary disease except that clubbing without periostitis is more often idiopathic. Increased digital blood flow is a constant feature.

Softening of the nail bed causing a fluctuant, "rocking" sensation to palpation of the proximal nail is the first sign of clubbing. Subsequently, there is periungual erythema with telangiectasia, local warmth, and sweating. The nail shows increased convexity in the sagittal and cross-sectional planes with loss of the normal 15° angle between the proximal nail and dorsal surface of the phalanx (Fig. 88–1). Excessive distal phalangeal resorption can lead to acrolysis of fingers and toes.[8]

Frequently associated changes include excessive sweating or warmth of the fingertips, eponychia, paronychia, breaking or loosening of the nail, hangnails, and accelerated nail or cuticle growth. In advanced stages "drumstick" fingers (Fig. 88–2) and hyperextensibility of the distal interphalangeal joints develop (Fig. 88–1). Similar changes occur in the toes. Spade-like enlargement of the hands and feet can occur as clubbing evolves over months or years.

Clubbing can be recognized quantitatively by measuring the diameter of each thumb and finger at the base of the nail and at the distal interphalangeal joint. A sum of the 10 ratios (digital index) greater than 10 indicates clubbing.[9] This ratio is independent of age or sex. Another quantitative technique uses a "shadowgram" for measurement of the hyponychial angle.[10] A quick qualitative method involves placing the dorsal surfaces of the contralateral ring or fourth fingers together.[11] A gap normally appears between the fingers at the nailbed. With clubbing, as the nail bed becomes elevated, this gap disappears.

There are isolated reports of unilateral clubbing,[4] sometimes associated with aneurysms of the aorta or the subclavian or innominate artery, as well as with axillary tumors, subluxations of the shoulder, apical

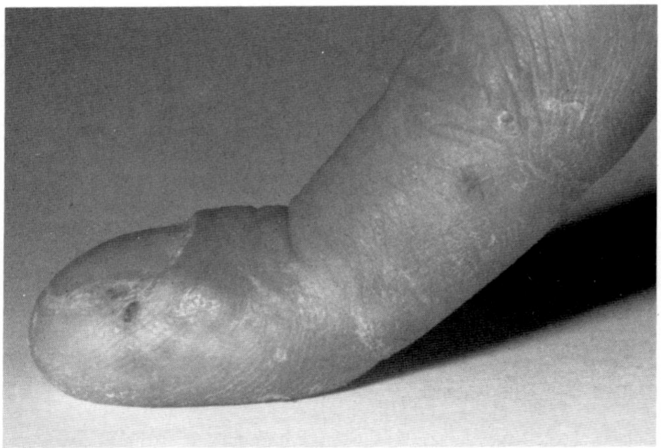

FIGURE 88–1. Lateral view of a distal digit with clubbing demonstrating loss of the normal 15° angle at the nail-nailbed junction and hyperextensibility of the distal interphalangeal joint.

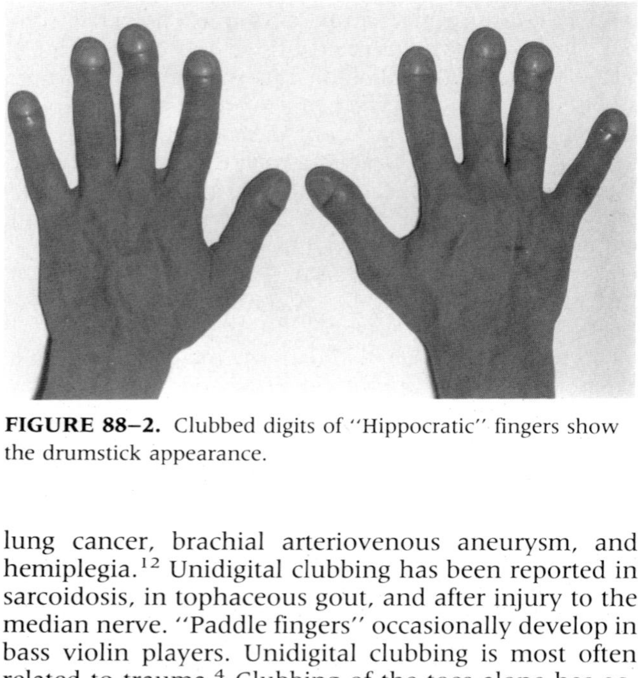

FIGURE 88–2. Clubbed digits of "Hippocratic" fingers show the drumstick appearance.

lung cancer, brachial arteriovenous aneurysm, and hemiplegia.[12] Unidigital clubbing has been reported in sarcoidosis, in tophaceous gout, and after injury to the median nerve. "Paddle fingers" occasionally develop in bass violin players. Unidigital clubbing is most often related to trauma.[4] Clubbing of the toes alone has accompanied an infected abdominal aortic aneurysm.

PERIOSTITIS

Periostitis can be asymptomatic. When present, symptoms include mild aching pain to deep-seated aching or burning pain, and tenderness over the long bones. A unique feature is aggravation of bone pain on dependency of the limbs often relieved by elevation, suggesting that local vascular stasis plays a role in production of pain. The extent of periostitis depends on its duration and not on whether the disease is primary or secondary. The patient might complain of heat and swelling over the feet and legs. The distal extremities often appear broadened with a palpable, firm, mildly pitting edema. Tenderness to pressure and warmth over the distal tibia, feet, radius, and ulna is usually present.

ARTHRITIS

The arthritis can affect few or many joints. Symptoms range from fleeting arthralgias to severe constant joint pain. Pain is usually symmetric and involves the knees, metacarpophalangeal joints, wrists, elbows, and ankles.[13] Local warmth and erythema of the overlying skin, restricted joint motion, and swelling accompany pain. Ingestion of alcohol might worsen joint pain and swelling.[14] Hypopigmentation of the skin and induration of the subcutaneous tissue around an affected joint suggest scleroderma. Effusions are usually mild but can be massive, particularly in HPO associated with cyanotic congenital heart disease.

ADDITIONAL FINDINGS

HPO can be accompanied by signs of autonomic dysfunction such as flushing, blanching, and profuse sweating, most severe in hands and feet. Coarsening of the facial features and thickened furrowed skin of the face (leonine facies) and scalp might develop. Occasionally, patients develop gynecomastia, often associated with elevated levels of urinary estrogens.[15,16]

Proposed diagnostic criteria of digital clubbing with periostitis show a sensitivity of 86%.[17]

CLINICAL SUBSETS

PACHYDERMOPERIOSTOSIS

Primary HPO is also referred to as pachydermoperiostosis or the Touraine-Solente-Golé syndrome. It has a bimodal onset with peaks at 1 and 15 years of age.[17] The disease occurs within families and appears to be transmitted by an autosomal dominant gene with variable expression.

Symptoms are usually limited to one or two decades of life.[14,18,19] The onset of clubbing is insidious with "spade-like" enlargement of hands and feet. Symptoms include cosmetic unsightliness, reduced dexterity, and awkwardness of the hands. There might be vague joint pain or bone pain or both,[18] which might be exacerbated by alcohol ingestion.[14]

Cylindric thickening of forearms and legs due to both bony and soft tissue proliferation accompanies clubbing.[18,20] Recurrent, mildly symptomatic joint effusions[19] and acrolysis involving the distal phalanges of hands and feet might occur.[21] There is often excessive sweating, particularly of the hands and feet. Thickening and furrowing of facial skin with deep nasolabial folds and a corrugated scalp produces the leonine features. The thickened skin is often "greasy." The facial features, greasy skin, and sweating are uncommon in secondary HPO. Gynecomastia, female hair distribution, striae, acne vulgaris, and cranial suture defects rarely occur.[6] Nailfold capillary microscopy might reveal dilated, irregular, serpiginous loops.[22]

SECONDARY HYPERTROPHIC OSTEOARTHROPATHY

HPO can accompany other illnesses, particularly pulmonary neoplasms or infection of the lungs, mediastinum, and pleura.

HPO has been observed in 5 to 10% of patients with intrathoracic neoplasms,[23–25] especially bronchogenic carcinoma[26] and pleural tumors.[27] HPO can also accompany lung abscess, bronchiectasis, chronic bronchitis, and empyema, and was associated with Pneumocystis carinii pneumonia in a patient with acquired immunodeficiency syndrome (AIDS).[28] With improved therapy of chronic infections, HPO is now most often associated with chronic pneumonitis, pneumoconiosis, pulmonary tuberculosis, mediastinal Hodgkin's disease, sarcoidosis, immunodeficient children with recurrent pneumonitis, and cystic fibrosis.[29–31] HPO presenting with arthralgias can be the initial manifestation of interstitial pulmonary fibrosis.[32] Numerous neoplasms have been reported with HPO, many in association with intrathoracic metastases.[33–38] Metastatic lesions per se are an uncommon cause of HPO, however.

Congenital heart malformations with cyanosis can cause clubbing.[39] HPO is seldom seen in uncomplicated congenital heart disease without cyanosis. Other cardiac diseases that can be associated with HPO include patent ductus arteriosis[40] and cardiac rhabdomyosarcoma.[41] Up to 31% of patients with cyanotic congenital heart disease develop HPO, a fact that relates to the degree of right to left shunt.[42] Clubbing in bacterial endocarditis might indicate embolization.

Gastrointestinal diseases associated with HPO include ulcerative colitis, regional enteritis, amebic colitis, subpherenic abscess, cirrhosis, idiopathic steatorrhea, sprue, neoplasms of the small intestine, multiple colonic polyposis, and carcinoma of the colon, esophagus, or liver.[43] HPO can also accompany rarer diseases such as primary cholangiolitic cirrhosis,[44,45] secondary hepatic amyloidosis (perhaps related to infection), and biliary atresia,[4,46] HPO confined to the lower extremities has been reported in association with an infected abdominal aneurysm.[47]

Less commonly HPO occurs after thyroidectomy for Graves' disease, and in hyperthyroidism, pregnancy, purgative abuse, connective tissue diseases, and hyperparathyroidism.[4,25,48–51]

THYROID ACROPACHY

This uncommon condition is characterized by clubbing of the fingers and asymptomatic periosteal proliferation of the bones of the hands and feet.[52,53] It is associated with prior or active hyperthyroidism (Graves' disease), and accompanies exophthalmos and localized nonpitting soft tissue swelling of the extremities or pretibial myxedema. Long-acting thyroid stimulator (LATS) has been found in these cases.[54]

LABORATORY AND ROENTGENOGRAPHIC FINDINGS

No tests are specific for HPO. Antinuclear antibody tests and tests for rheumatoid factor have been negative in most patients but the erythrocyte sedimentation rate is often elevated. Synovial fluids are group I (non-inflammatory), clear, and of high viscosity; they usually have total leukocyte counts below 2000/mm^3 with fewer than 50% polymorphonuclear leukocytes.[55,56] Serum and synovial fluid C3 and C4 levels have been normal in secondary HPO.[56]

Roentgenograms are diagnostically important. Subperiosteal new bone appears symmetrically in the distal diaphyseal regions of long bones, especially of the legs and forearms, and less commonly in the phalanges (Fig. 88–3). Rarely, patients have symptomatic disease in the absence of radiologic changes.[57] The subperiosteal new bone is often reduplicated in multiple layers, producing an "onion skin" appearance. In older patients digital tuft hypertrophy contrasts with acroosteolysis in younger patients.

Skeletal imaging using technetium-99m (^{99m}Tc) bisphosphonate produces an abnormal pattern.[59,60] A pericortical linear accumulation of radiotracer along the long bones (Fig. 88–4) and proximal phalanges along with increased periarticular uptake reflecting synovitis is characteristic. Involvement of the skull, scapulae, clavicles, and patellae is frequently noted. Asymmetric or irregular distribution (or both) is seen in fewer than 20% of patients. Differentiation from metastatic cancer is not difficult because this disease produces a diffuse pattern of radionuclide distribution.

PATHOLOGY

Histopathologic changes are similar in the primary (hereditary) and secondary forms of HPO. In clubbed phalanges, there is edema of the distal digital soft parts, thickening of the blood vessel walls, cellular infiltration, fibroblastic proliferation, and growth of new collagenous tissue resulting in the uniform enlargement of terminal segments. Nailbed and finger pulp mast cell counts have been found to be lower in clubbed fingers as compared to control fingers.[61]

Periostitis developing at the distal end of metacarpals, metatarsals, long bones of the forearms, and legs[62] and, in severe disease, in the ribs, clavicles, scapulae, pelvis, and malar bones is accompanied by round cell infiltration and edema of the periosteum, synovial membrane, articular capsule, and neighboring subcutaneous tissues. These changes are followed by periosteal elevation, deposition of subperiosteal osteoid, and subsequent mineralization. The distal long bones eventually become ensheathed with a cuff of new bone (Fig. 88–5).

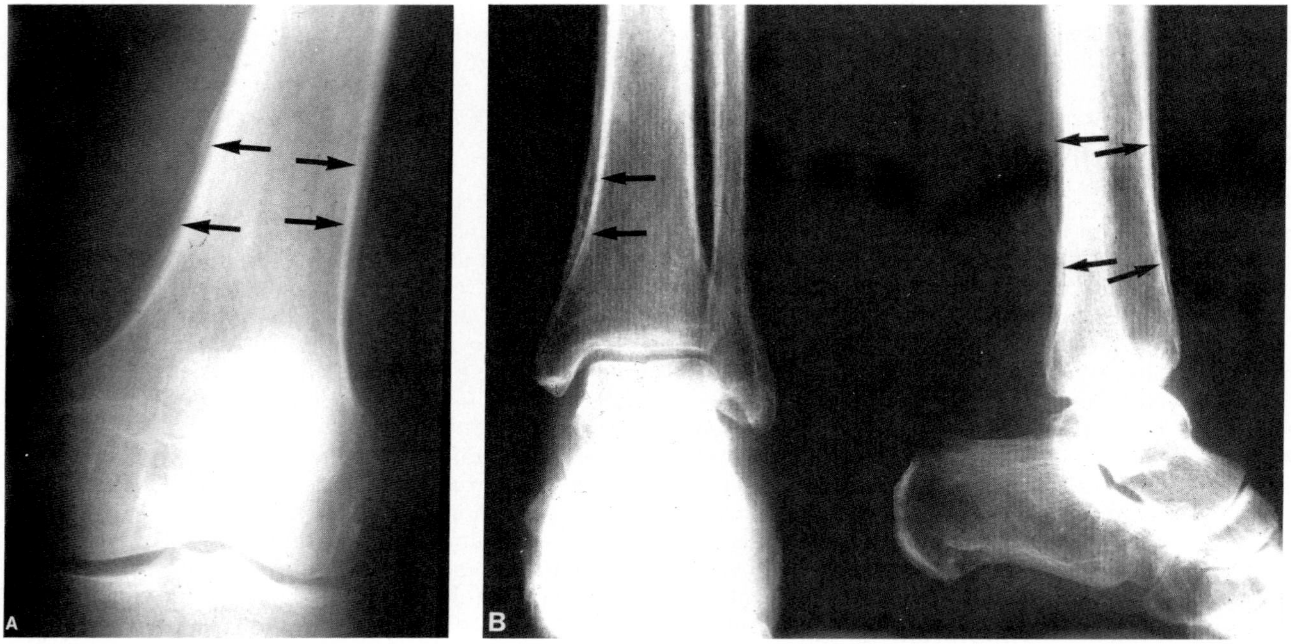

FIGURE 88–3. Hypertrophic osteoarthropathy. Radiodense bands along a margin of the shaft (arrows) indicate new osseous formation beneath the elevated periosteum. The appearance of these typical lesions is similar in the distal femur (*A*) to that of the distal tibia (*B*).

Concurrent with thickening, there is accelerated resorption of endosteal and haversian bone. The bony structure is weakened and pathologic fractures sometimes occur. With advancing disease, these pathologic alterations spread proximally along the bony shafts.

Synovial membranes adjoining the involved bones are often edematous and infiltrated with lymphocytes, plasma cells, and a few neutrophils. Advancing proliferative fibrous tissue at joint margins is sometimes associated with cartilage degeneration. Electron microscopic studies of the synovial membranes reveal alterations of the microcirculation, with dilatation of capillaries and venules, endothelial cell gaps, and multilamination of small vessel basement membranes.[55] The significance of subendothelial electron-dense deposits in the synovial membranes of patients with secondary HPO is unclear.[55] Negative immunofluorescent staining for γ-globulins and complement has been reported.[61]

ETIOLOGY AND PATHOGENESIS

The nature of the genetic factors operative in the hereditary form of HPO is unknown, although angiographic studies have demonstrated hypervascularization of the finger pads.[63] In secondary HPO, it has been postulated that the vascular proliferation and osteogenesis is produced by (1) obscure autonomic reflexes stimulated at the site of underlying disease, (2) a high arteriolar pulse pressure, possibly also involving autonomic reflexes, (3) toxins liberated by primary malignant lesions, or (4) osteoblastic-stimulating agents released at the site of malignant pulmonary lesions or by the pluripotential cells of pleural membranes.

Another theory implicates the development of pulmonary arteriovenous shunts that allows a hormone or toxin normally inactivated in the lungs to escape into the systemic circulation and cause the pathologic changes. One suspected vasoactive substance is reduced ferritin.

Factors conditioning an individual with intrathoracic disease to develop HPO are unknown, but there is evidence for a local circulatory disorder.[4,64] A locally acting circulating vasodilator has been demonstrated in some patients.[65] Increased vascularity of clubbed fingers in secondary HPO has been shown by measurement of skin temperature, infrared photography, nailfold capillarioscopy, and postmortem arteriography.[22,66,67] Elevated digital pulse pressure and blood flow has been shown to return to normal after removal of the pulmonary lesion.[4] Perhaps anomalous vascular control leads to such altered blood flow patterns.[68] Plasma growth hormone levels were elevated in patients with primary bronchial (especially small cell) neoplasms and clubbing.[69] Elevated excretion of urinary estrogens have been found in three patients with pulmonary lesions.[70] A polypeptide substance differing from immunoreactive growth hormone but related to somatotopins might be a mediator in HPO.[71] Striking resolution of symptoms and signs has been shown to follow simple denervation of the hilum or vagotomy on the same side as the le-

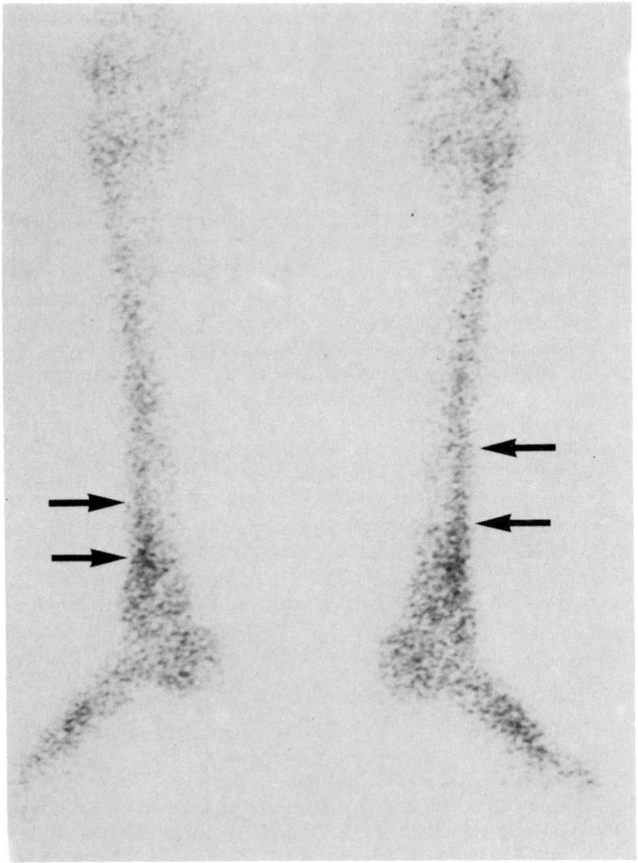

FIGURE 88–4. Bone scan utilizing technetium-99m labeled methylene bisphosphonate demonstrating periosteal localization of the nuclide to the anterior tibiae and radius (arrows).

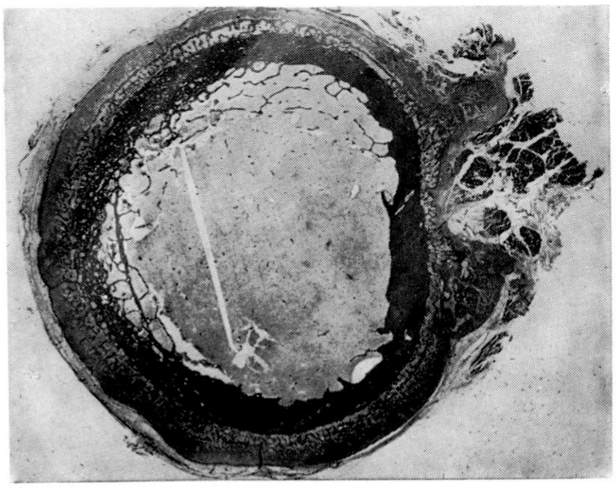

FIGURE 88–5. Cross section through a metatarsal of a patient with hypertrophic osteoarthropathy. The periosteum shows thickening with an irregular cuff of new bone deposited over the cortex. From Bartter, F.C., and Bauer, W.: *In* Textbook of Medicine. Edited by Cecil and Loeb. Philadelphia, W.B. Saunders.

sion.[23,25,72,23] Thoracotomy without denervation in these studies was ineffective.

Circulating tumor antigen-antibody complexes have been described in patients with a variety of tumors, including lung carcinomas. The electron microscopic findings seem equivocal but raise the possibility that the synovitis seen in HPO associated with bronchogenic carcinoma might be immune complex-mediated.

Prostaglandin-E_1 used in infants to maintain potency of the ductus arteriosus has been associated with widespread subperiosteal hyperostosis, implying a pathogenic role for this prostaglandin.[74]

DIFFERENTIAL DIAGNOSIS

The presence of clubbing, which is the most constant feature of HPO, simplifies diagnosis, and a primary disease must be sought. If acute polyarthritis precedes clubbing, the case might be mislabeled as rheumatoid arthritis.[75] In most instances, roentgenograms reveal subperiosteal new bone,[76] which must be differentiated from that resulting from local tumors, lymphangitis, syphilis, or the hemorrhages of trauma or scurvy. Swelling and tenderness of the lower legs might falsely suggest thrombophlebitis, and bony pains might be misinterpreted as peripheral neuritis. The spoon-shaped nails of hypochromic anemia are easily distinguishable. HPO sometimes superficially suggests scleroderma.

Associated diseases should be excluded before assigning a patient to the ill-defined hereditary or idiopathic group. This point is emphasized because of the danger of overlooking infection, a resectable tumor, or another treatable condition. Separation of primary and secondary HPO should not be difficult because the hereditary or idiopathic syndrome begins after puberty, follows a self-limited course of one to two decades, and occurs in other family members.[20]

Florid reactive periostitis occurs in young adults, is not associated with clubbing, and is more painful than the periostitis of HPO.[77]

TREATMENT

Clubbing is most often asymptomatic and usually requires no treatment. Disabling symptoms relating to periostitis, synovitis, or both often respond dramatically to removal of the primary pulmonary lesion or to intrathoracic vagotomy.[25,78]

Nonsteroidal anti-inflammatory drugs (NSAIDs) have been beneficial in reducing discomfort. Aspirin in modest doses or another NSAID is frequently effective.[38] Indomethacin[79] and perhaps flurbiprofen can be most effective. Chemical vagotomy by atropine[80,81] or propantheline bromide has reportly relieved symptoms.[82] Analgesics are appropriate. Adrenocortical steroid derivatives can be useful.[83] Radiotherapy to the primary tumor site[84] or to metastatic lesion[85] as well as chemotherapy[86] has relieved joint symptoms. Complete disappearance of HPO is described after appropriate therapy for empyema, lung abscess, bronchiectasis, pneumonia, and bacterial endocarditis.[87]

Treatment of idiopathic HPO is symptomatic.

REFERENCES

1. Hippocrates (c. 400 B.C.): The Genuine Works of Hippocrates. Vol I. Translated by F. Adams. London, Syndenham Society, 1849, p. 249.
2. Marie, P.: De l'osteoarthropathie hypertrophiante pneumique. Rev. Med., *10*:1–36, 1890.
3. von Bamberger, E.: Uber Knochen veranderungen bei chronishen Lungenund. Herzkran Kenheiten Klin. Med., *18*:193, 1890–1891.
4. Mendlowitz, M.: Clubbing and hypertrophic osteoarthropathy. Medicine, *21*:269–306, 1942.
5. Fischer, D.S., Singer, D.H., and Feldman, S.M.: Clubbing, a review, with emphasis on hereditary acropachy. Medicine, *43*:459, 1965.
6. Reginato, A.R., Schinpachasse, Y., and Guerrero, R.: Familial idiopathic hypertrophic osteoarthropathy and cranial suture defects in children. Skeletal Radiol., *8*:105–109, 1982.
7. Seaton, D.R.: Familial clubbing of fingers and toes. Br. Med. J., *1*:614, 1938.
8. Hedayati, H., Barmada, R., and Skosey, J.L.: Acrolysis in pachydermoperiostosis. Arch. Intern. Med., *140*:1087–1088, 1980.
9. Vazquez-Abad, D., Pineda, C., and Martinez-Lavin, M.: Digital clubbing: A numerical assessment of the deformity. J. Rheumatol., *16*:518–520, 1989.
10. Sinniah, D., and Omar, A.: Quantitation of digital clubbing by shadowgram technique. Arch. Dis. Child., *54*:145–146.
11. Schamroth, L.: Personal experience. S. Afr. Med. J., *50*:297–300, 1976.
12. Denham, M.J., Hodkinson, H.M., and Wright, B.M.: Unilateral clubbing in hemiplegia. Gerontol. Clin., *17*:7–12, 1975.
13. Shulman, L.E.: Hypertrophic osteoarthropathy. Bull. Rheum. Dis., *7*:135, 1957.
14. Mueller, M., and Trevarthen, D.: Pachydermoperiostosis: Arthropathy aggravated by episode alcohol abuse. J. Rheumatol., *8*:862–864, 1981.
15. Ginsburg, J.: Observations on the peripheral circulation in hypertrophic pulmonary osteoarthropathy. Q. J. Med., *27*:335–352, 1958.
16. Jao, J.Y., Barlow, J.J., and Krant, M.J.: Pulmonary hypertrophic osteoarthropathy, spider angiomata and estrogen hyperexcretion. Ann. Intern. Med., *70*:581–584, 1969.
17. Martinez-Lavin, et al.: Primary hypertrophic osteoarthropathy. Semin. Arthritis Rheum., *17*:156–162, 1988.
18. Vogl, A., and Goldfischer, S.: Pachydermoperiostosis. Primary or idiopathic hypertrophic osteoarthropathy. Am. J. Med., *33*:166–187, 1962.
19. Lauter, S.A., Vasey, F.B., Huttner, I., and Osterland, C.K.: Pachydermoperiostosis: Studies on the synovium. J. Rheumatol., *5*:85, 1978.
20. Touraine, A., Solente, A., and Golé, L.: Un syndrome osteodermo pathique. La pachydermie plicaturee avec pachyperiostose des extermites. Presse Med., *43*:1820–1824, 1935.
21. Fam, A.G., Chin-Sang, H., and Ramsay, C.A.: Pachydermoperiostosis: Scintographic, plethysmographic, and capillarscopic observations. Ann. Rheum. Dis., *42*:98–102, 1983.
22. Matucci-Cerinic, M., et al.: Pachydermoperiostosis (primary hypertrophic osteoarthropathy): Report of a case with evidence of endothelial and connective tissue involvement. Ann. Rheum. Dis., *48*:240–246, 1989.
23. Lansbury, J.: Connective tissue manifestations of neoplastic disease. Geriatics, *9*:319–324, 1954.
24. Wierman, W.J., Clagett, O.T., and McDonald, J.R.: Articular manifestations in pulmonary diseases: An analysis of their occurrence in 1,024 cases in which pulmonary resection was performed. JAMA, *155*:1459–1463, 1954.
25. Christian, C.L., Chairman Editorial Committee: 19th Rheumatism Review. Arthritis Rheum., *13*:615, 1970.
26. Freeman, M.H., and Tonkin, A.K.: Manifestations of hypertrophic pulmonary osteoarthropathy in patients with carcinoma of the lung. Demonstration by ^{99m}Tc-pyrophosphate bone scans. Radiology, *120*:363–365, 1976.
27. Briselli, M., Mark, J., and Dickersin, G.R.: Solitary fibrous tumors of the pleura: Eight new cases and review of 360 cases in the literature. Cancer, *1*:2678–2689, 1981.
28. Bhat, S., et al.: Hypertrophic osteoarthropathy associated with Pneumocystis carinii pneumonia in AIDS. Chest, *95*:1208–1209, 1989.
29. Beluffi, G., et al.: Secondary hypertrophic osteoarthropathy in two children with humoral immunodeficiencies. J. Belge Radiol., *71*:99–102, 1988.
30. Matthay, M.A., et al.: Hypertrophic osteoarthropathy in adults with cystic fibrosis. Thorax, *31*:572–575, 1976.
31. West, S.G., Gilbreath, R.E., and Lawless, O.J.: Painful clubbing and sarcoidosis. JAMA, *246*:1338–1339, 1981.
32. Kupfer, Y., Groopman, J.E., Aswini Lenora, R., and Tessler, S.: Pulmonary hypertrophic osteoarthropathy as the initial manifestation of interstitial fibrosis. N. Y. State J. Med., *89*:234–235, 1989.
33. Martin, C.L.: Complications produced by malignant tumors of the nasopharynx. Am. J. Roentgenol., *41*:377, 1939.
34. Trivedi, S.A.: Neurilemmoma of the diaphragm causing severe hypertrophic pulmonary osteoarthropathy. Br. J. Tuberc. Dis. Chest, *52*:214, 1958.
35. Lofters, W.S., and Walker, T.M.: Hodgkin's disease and hypertrophic pulmonary osteoarthropathy. West Indian Med. J., *28*:227, 1978.
36. McNeil, M.M., Sage, R.E., and Dale, B.M.: Hypertrophic osteoarthropathy complicating primary bone lymphoma—Association with invasive Phycomyosis and Aspergillus infections. Aust. N. Z. J. Med., *11*:71–75, 1981.
37. Solimbu, C., Marchetta, P., Firooznnia, H., and Rafu, M.: Hypertrophic osteoarthropathy in metastatic renal cell carcinoma. J. Urol., *22*:669–672, 1983.
38. Lokich, J.J.: Pulmonary osteoarthropathy: Association with mesenchymal tumor metastases to the lungs. JAMA, *238*:37, 1977.
39. McLaughlin, G.E., McCarty, D.J. Jr., and Downing, D.F.: Hypertrophic osteoarthropathy associated with cyanotic congenital heart disease. Ann. Intern. Med., *67*:579–587, 1967.
40. Williams, B., Ling, J., Leight, L., and McGaff, C.J.: Patent ductus arteriosus and osteoarthropathy. Arch. Intern. Med., *111*:346, 1963.
41. Pascuzzi, C.A., Parkin, T.W., Bruwer, A.J., and Edwards, J.E.: Hypertrophic osteoarthropathy associated with primary rhabdomyosarcoma of the heart. Mayo Clin. Proc., *32*:30, 1957.
42. Martinez-Lavin, M., et al.: Hypertrophic osteoarthropathy in cyanotic congenital heart disease. Arthritis Rheum., *25*:1186–1192, 1982.
43. Peirce, T.H., and Weir, D.G.: Hypertrophic osteoarthropathy associated with a non-metastasizing carcinoma of the oesophagus. J. Jr. Med. Assoc., *66*:160–162, 1973.
44. Buchan, D.J., and Mitchell, D.M.: Hypertrophic osteoarthropathy in portal cirrhosis. Ann. Intern. Med., *66*:130–135, 1967.
45. Kieff, E.D., and McCarty, D.J.: Hypertrophic osteoarthropathy

with arthritis and synovial calcification in a patient with alcoholic cirrhosis. Arhtritis Rheum., *12*:261–268, 1969.

46. Epstein, O., Dick, R., and Sherlock, S.: Prospective study of periostitis and finger clubbing in primary biliary cirrhosis and other forms of chronic liver disease. Gut, *22*:203–206, 1981.
47. Sorin, S.B., Askari, A., and Rhodes, R.S.: Hypertrophic osteoarthropathy of the lower extremities as a manifestation of arterial graft sepsis. Arthritis Rhuem., *23*:768–770, 1980.
48. Souders, C.R., and Manuell, J.L.: Skeletal deformities in hyperparathyroidism. N. Engl. J. Med., *250*:594–597, 1954.
49. Lovell, R.R.H., and Scott, G.B.D.: Hypertrophic osteoarthropathy in polyarteritis. Ann. Rheum., Dis., *15*:46, 1956.
50. Borden, E.C., and Holling, H.E.: Hypertrophic osteoarthropathy and pregnancy. Ann. Intern. Med., *71*:577, 1969.
51. Diamond, M.T.: The syndrome of exophthalmos, hypertrophic osteoarthropathy and localized myxedema: A review of the literature and report of a case. Ann. Intern. Med., *50*:206–213, 1959.
52. Kinsella, R.A. Jr., and Back, D.K.: Thyroid acropachy. Med. Clin. North Am., *52*:393–398, 1968.
53. Prabhu, R., Berger, H.W., Subietas, A., and Lee, M.: Lymphomatoid granulomatosis, report of a patient with severe anemia and clubbing. Chest, *78*:883–885, 1980.
54. Lynch, P.J., Maize, J.C., and Sisson, J.C.: Pretibial myxedema and nonthyrotoxic thyroid disease. Arch. Dermatol., *107*:107–111, 1973.
55. Schumacher, H.R.: Articular manifestations of HPO in bronchogenic carcinoma. A clinical and pathologic study. Arthritis Rheum., *19*:629–636, 1976.
56. Vidal, A.F., et al.: Structural and immunologic changes of synovium of hypertrophic osteoarthropathy (HPO). Arthritis Rheum., *20*:139, 1977.
57. Horn, C.R.: Hypertrophic pulmonary osteoarthropathy with radiographic evidence of new bone formation. Thorax, *35*:479, 1980.
58. Pineda, C., Fonseca, C., and Martinez-Lavin, M.: The spectrum of soft tissue and skeletal abnormalities of hypertrophic osteoarthropathy. J. Rheumatol., *17*:626–632, 1990.
59. Donnelly, B., and Johnson, P.M.: Detection of hypertrophic pulmonary osteoarthropathy of skeletal imaging with 99m Tc–labeled diphosphonate. Radiology, *114*:389–391, 1975.
60. Rosenthal, L., and Kirsh, J.: Observations on radionuclide imaging in hypertrophic pulmonary osteoarthropathy. Radiology. *120*:359–362, 1976.
61. Marshall, R.: Observations of the pathology of clubbed fingers with special reference to mast cells. Am. Rev. Respir. Dis., *113*:395–397, 1976.
62. Gall, E.A., Bennett, G.A., and Bauer, W.: Generalized hypertrophic osteoarthropathy. Am. J. Pathol., *27*:349–381, 1951.
63. Jajic, I., et al.: Primary hypertrophic osteoarthropathy (HPO) and changes in the joints. Scand. J. Rheumatol., *9*:89–96, 1980.
64. Mendlowitz, M., and Leslie, A.: Experimental simulation in dogs of cyanosis and hypertrophic osteoarthropathy which are associated with congenital heart disease. Am. Heart J., *24*:141–152, 1942.
65. Shneerson, J.M.: Digital clubbing and hypertrophic osteoarthropathy: The underlying mechanisms. Br. J. Dis. Chest, *75*:113–131, 1981.
66. Harter, J.S.: Joint manifestations (discussion). J. Thorac. Surg., *9*:505, 1939–1940.
67. Rominger, E.: Ein fall von morbus caeroleus mit demonstration der hautkapillaren am lebenden nach weibund elektro kardiographischen untersuchungen. Dtsch. Med. Wochenschr., *46*:168, 1920.
68. Doyle, L.: Pathogenesis of secondary hypertrophic osteoarthropathy: A hypothesis. Eur. Respir. J., *2*:105–106, 1989.
69. Goshney, M.A., Gosney, J.R., and Lye, M.: Plasma growth hormone and digital clubbing in carcinoma of the bronchus. Thorax, *45*:545–547, 1990.
70. Ginsburg, J., and Brown, J.B.: Increased estrogen excretion in hypertrophic pulmonary osteoarthropathy. Lancet, *2*:1274–1276, 1961.
71. Audebert, A.A., et al.: Osteoarthropathie hypertrophiante pneumique associee a une quadruple secretion hormonale paraneoplasique. Semin. Hop. Paris, *458*:529–530, 1982.
72. Semple, T., and McCluskie, R.A.: Generalized hypertrophic osteoarthropathy in association with bronchial carcinoma. Br. Med. J., *1*:754–759, 1955.
73. Haslock, I., and Vasanthakumar, V.: Case report. Disappearing hypertrophic osteoarthropathy. Br. J. Rheumatol., *27*:143–145, 1988.
74. Drvaric, D.M., et al.: Prostaglandin-induced hyperostosis. A case report. Clin. Orthop. Res., *246*:300–304, 1989.
75. Polley, H.F., et al.: Articular reactions with localized fibrous mesothelioma of the pleura. Ann. Rheum. Dis., *11*:314, 1952.
76. Greenfield, G.B., Schorsch, H.A., and Ahkoln, A.: The various roentgen appearances of pulmonary hypertrophic osteoarthropathy. Am. J. Roentgenol. Rad. Ther. Nucl. Surg., *101*:927–931, 1967.
77. Nance, K.V., Renner, J.B., Brashear, H.R., and Siegal, G.P.: Massive florid reactive periostitis. Pediatr. Radiol., *20*:186–189, 1990.
78. LeRoux, B.T.: Bronchial carcinoma with hypertrophic pulmonary osteoarthropathy. S. Afr. Med. J., *42*:1074–1075, 1968.
79. Altman, R.D.: Personal observation.
80. Day, W.H., and Hagelsten, J.O.: Blocking of the vagus nerve relieving osteoarthropathy in lung diseases. Dan. Med. Bull., *11*:131–133, 1964.
81. Lopez-Enriquez, E., Morales, A.R., and Robert, F.: Effect of atropine sulfate in pulmonary hypertrophic osteoarthropathy. Arthritis Rheum., *23*:822–824, 1980.
82. Schwartz, H.A.: Pro-Banthine for hypertrophic osteoarthropathy. Arthritis Rheum., *23*:1588, 1981.
83. Holling, H.E., and Brodey, R.S.: Pulmonary hypertrophic osteoarthropathy. JAMA, *178*:977–982, 1961.
84. Steinfeld, A.D., and Munzenrider, J.E.: The response of hypertrophic pulmonary osteoarthropathy to radiotherapy. Radiology, *113*:709–711, 1974.
85. Rao, G.M., et al.: Improvement in hypertrophic pulmonary osteoarthropathy after radiotherapy to metastases. Am. J. Radiol., *133*:944–946, 1979.
86. Evans, W.K.: Reversal of hypertrophic osteoarthropathy after chemotherapy for bonchogenic carcinoma. J. Rheumatol., *7*:93–97, 1980.
87. Shapiro, C.M., and Mackinnon, J.: The resolution of hypertrophic pulmonary osteoarthropathy following treatment of subacute bacterial endocarditis. Postgrad. Med. J., *56*:513–515, 1980.

SECTION **VIII**

Regional Disorders of Joints and Related Structures

89

Traumatic Arthritis and Allied Conditions

ROBERT S. PINALS

In its broadest sense, the term "traumatic arthritis" circumscribes a diverse collection of pathologic and clinical states that develop after single or repetitive episodes of trauma (Table 89–1). Although these conditions may be encountered frequently by the rheumatologist, interest in the area has been casual, and studies of basic mechanisms of disease have been few as compared with those in the other rheumatic diseases. Because surgeons are more likely to deal with the sequelae of trauma, it is not surprising that the most significant contributions are to be found in the orthopedic literature. The credulous assignment of etiologic roles to trauma in early writings stands in sharp contrast to modern attitudes on the subject. Rheumatoid arthritis, tuberculous arthritis, gout, and other rheumatic diseases were formerly attributed to trauma, which might alter the structural integrity of joints, predisposing them to inflammation. As other pathogenetic mechanisms have been revealed, it has become less necessary to invoke "unrecognized trauma," which was previously such a convenient explanation for poorly understood disorders. Even in osteoarthritis, once the bellwether of traumatic disorders, considered by some to be synonymous with traumatic arthritis, increasing emphasis is being placed on altered cartilage metabolism, leaving an even smaller role for "multiple microtraumata."

ACUTE TRAUMATIC SYNOVITIS

Following a direct blow or forced inappropriate motion to a joint, swelling and pain may develop. Because the knee is most commonly affected, the following discussion will be directed at that joint, but one might follow a similar approach for a traumatic synovitis in the elbow, shoulder, or ankle. On examination, an effusion is usually evident, which should be aspirated to determine whether hemarthrosis is present and to aid in further examination of the joint. Hemarthrosis is usually present if fluid appears within 2 hours after the injury. In about half the cases, swelling occurs within 15 minutes. On the other hand, nonbloody effusions generally appear 12 to 24 hours after injury. With hemarthrosis there is usually more pain, and at times a low-grade fever. Fractures, internal derangements, or major ligamentous tears must be ruled out by examination and radiographs, which suggest a cause for the bleeding in up to 75% of hemarthrosis. With arthroscopy and more sophisticated imaging techniques a broader range of pathology can be revealed.[1–3] In a prospective series of 100 traumatic hemarthrosis in nonathletes, magnetic resonance imaging (MRI) and arthroscopy, with ligament testing under anesthesia, demonstrated significant lesions in 99 even though routine roentgenograms were negative.[1] Anterior cruciate ligament tears were found most frequently (67%), particularly with recreational injuries. Other causes included collateral and posterior cruciate ligament tears, meniscal and capsular tears, and chondral fractures. Although not indicated routinely, MRI permits identification of occult fractures and "bone bruises" (multiple impaction fractures), which can result in hemarthrosis.[4] The presence of fat globules floating on the surface of bloody fluid usually indicates a fracture. At times, sufficient fat may be present to be detectable on a lateral knee radiograph as a radiolucent layer in the suprapatellar pouch[5] (Fig. 89–1). A similar appearance has been described in the elbow and hip. Among patients with hip trauma and negative roentgenograms, lipohemarthrosis on computed tomography is usually associated with an intra-articular fracture.[6] Hemorrhagic fluid usually does not clot; coagulation may indicate more profound tissue damage and a poorer prognosis. Rarely, a chylous effusion may occur, either with or without an intra-articular fracture or hemarthrosis.[7,8]

TABLE 89–1. CLASSIFICATION OF TRAUMATIC ARTHRITIS AND ALLIED CONDITIONS

I.	Articular trauma, single episode.
	A. Traumatic synovitis, without disturbance of articular cartilage or disruption of major supporting structures. This type includes acute synovitis, with or without hemarthrosis, and most sprains. Healing is expected within several weeks, without permanent tissue damage.
	B. Disruptive trauma, with infraction of the articular cartilage or complete rupture of major supporting structures. This type includes intra-articular fractures, meniscal tears, and severe sprains.
	C. Post-traumatic osteoarthritis. This type includes cases of disruptive trauma in which major residual damage is present. Patients may have deformity, limited motion, or instability of joints.
II.	Repetitive articular trauma. This type includes a variety of conditions related to occupation or sports and results in localized chronic arthritis.
III.	Induction or aggravation of another specific rheumatic disease by acute or repetitive trauma.
IV.	Conditions in which trauma may be one of several etiologic factors, or in which a relationship has been suggested but not established: osteochondritis dissecans, osteitis pubis, Tietze's syndrome, and hypermobility syndrome.
V.	Disorders of extra-articular structures, such as tendons, bursae, and muscles, in which trauma commonly plays an etiologic role.
VI.	Nonmechanical types of trauma, such as arthropathy following frostbite, radiation, and decompression.

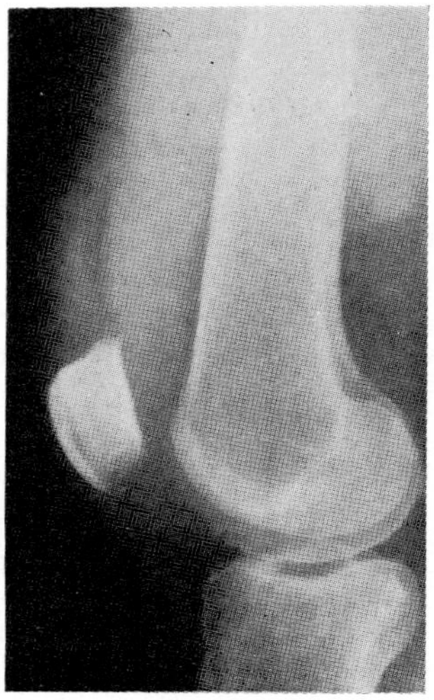

FIGURE 89–1. Traumatic hemarthrosis. Liquid fat and a fat-blood level are visible in the joint. (From Berk, R.N.[5])

In the absence of gross bleeding, examination of the fluid reveals a variable number of red blood cells and 50 to 2000 white blood cells, of which only a few are neutrophils. The protein content, mostly albumin, is two or three times that of normal fluid. Viscosity is slightly reduced, but the mucin clot is good. Synovial biopsy reveals some vasodilatation, edema, and an occasional small focus of synovial cell proliferation with mild lymphocytic infiltration.[9]

Rarely, a high leukocyte count in traumatic synovial effusions is accompanied by intra- and extracellular lipid globules, suggesting that lipid droplet phagocytosis might have provoked an inflammatory reaction.[10] This hypothesis was supported by studies of dog knees subjected to blunt trauma, which resulted in clear effusions containing fat globules. Intra-articular injection of autologous fat was shown to induce phagocytosis and mild inflammation[11] (see Chapter 112).

Treatment may include such measures as cold packs initially and heat later; compression dressings; splinting with a brace that permits limited motion; graded quadriceps exercises; repeated aspiration if significant volumes of fluid reaccumulate; and a period of bed rest or partial weight-bearing, depending on the severity of the injury. Early arthroscopic surgery is being advocated with increasing frequency, particularly in athletes with cruciate ligament or meniscal disruption.[3,12] Prognosis is excellent in the absence of improper treatment, such as cylinder cast immobilization, which may result in muscle atrophy and loss of motion, or premature weight-bearing, which may in turn lead to an extended duration of synovitis.

SPRAINS

A sprain may be defined as a stretching or tearing of a supporting ligament of a joint by forced movement beyond its normal range. In its simplest form, there is minimal disruption of fibers, swelling, pain, and dysfunction. Severe sprains may cause total rupture of ligaments, marked swelling and hemorrhage, and joint instability, which may be permanent if untreated. Sprains occur most frequently in the ankle, but are also common in the knee, low back, and neck.

ANKLE SPRAINS

Most ankle sprains result from unintentional weight-bearing on the inverted, plantar-flexed foot. There is partial or total disruption of one or more of the three main lateral supporting structures, which unite the fibula above with the calcaneus and talus below (Fig. 89–2). Rupture of the anterior talofibular ligament is most common; this structure prevents anterior displacement of the talus out of the ankle joint mortise. With additional force, the calcaneofibular ligament, which prevents excessive inversion, may also rupture. The third ligament, the posterior talofibular ligament, is seldom torn with the usual type of injury. If it also tears, a completely unstable ankle results. Stretching of the medial supporting structures usually results in fracture

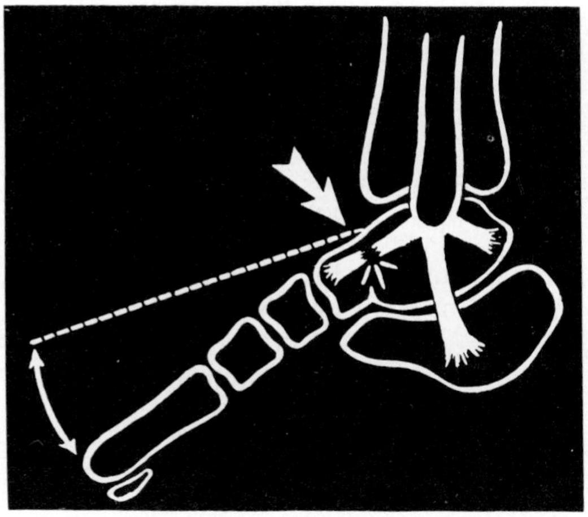

FIGURE 89–2. A severe ankle sprain, occurring in equinus and inversion, can result in rupture of the anterior talofibular ligament (arrow). (From Pipkin, G.: Clin. Orthop., 3:8, 1954.)

and avulsion of the medial malleolus rather than a sprain.

The patient presents with severe pain and swelling on the outer aspect of the foot and ankle. Much of the early swelling is due to hemorrhage, resulting in ecchymosis several hours later. A history of something snapping, giving away, or slipping out of place may suggest a complete ligament rupture. The nature of the treatment largely depends on assessment of the integrity of these ligaments. This is most easily accomplished soon after the injury, before swelling and pain make forced motion difficult. Local anesthesia may be required for proper examination. Some orthopedists insist upon stress roentgenograms after all severe sprains.[13]

Early treatment of simple sprains may include elevation, ice packs, and compression dressing to prevent swelling; injection of local anesthetics to permit early motion; and adhesive strapping. Full weight-bearing is permitted on the following day. A lift on the outer border of the heel will maintain eversion and prevent strain on the injured ligament. Strapping, or later an elastic support, is continued until healing is complete.[14]

Severe sprains may demand additional treatment, such as walking plaster for 4 to 6 weeks when the anterior talofibular ligament is ruptured, and early or late surgical repair for marked instability.[13,14] A followup study of patients with long-standing lateral ligament instability demonstrated a high incidence of degenerative changes in the articular cartilage of the medial joint surface.[15]

OTHER SPRAINS

Knee sprains are considered in Chapter 91, and low back sprains in Chapter 95. Shoulder "sprain" is actually a subluxation of the acromioclavicular joint, commonly seen in body contact sports. Wrist "sprain" is usually a fractured navicular bone, often missed on initial roentgenograms. Traumatic torticollis may be called a neck sprain. Following a sudden twist or wrenching of the neck, pain and muscle spasm may result in involuntary assumption of a "wry neck" position. Spontaneous remission occurs after 1 to 2 weeks. Measures such as a cervical collar, traction, and heat may be helpful. The actual structures involved in neck sprain have not been well defined.

PELLEGRINI-STIEDA SYNDROME; PERIARTICULAR OSSIFICATION

A linear calcific density may develop in the area of the medial collateral ligament after acute knee trauma. A hematoma may be the initial event. Calcification is noted on roentgenograms obtained as early as 3 or 4 weeks after the injury. Few biopsies have been obtained in the early stages; those performed later show bone rather than a calcific deposit. The initial injury may be minor or may produce a fracture, torn meniscus, or ligamentous rupture. Initial signs and symptoms, as well as subsequent disability, are related more to this associated trauma than to the Pellegrini-Stieda lesion itself. Periarticular heterotopic bone formation might occur after total hip replacement.[16–17] (See Chapter 54.) This does not cause pain but might limit motion. The ossification is usually well delineated on roentgenograms after 6 to 12 weeks.

ECTOPIC BONE FORMATION AFTER SPINAL CORD INJURY

Paraplegic and quadriplegic patients may develop ossification in soft tissues adjacent to joints that are located below the level of the neurologic lesion.[17,18] The hips and knees are most commonly involved. This complication occurs in about 20% of patients with spinal cord injury and occasionally in other neurologic conditions. Although some of the milder cases may not be detected by physical examination, many patients have swelling, warmth, and erythema in the affected area, suggesting alternative diagnoses, such as cellulitis and thrombophlebitis. These signs may appear as early as 3 weeks after the injury, when radiographic findings are minimal or absent. At this stage, serum alkaline phosphatase may be elevated, and soft tissue uptake of radionuclide may be increased on a bone scan. After about 2 months, a firm mass of trabeculated bone may be detected on physical examination and demonstrated radiologically. This finding is often accompanied by loss of joint motion and occasionally by complete ankylosis. Serious functional impairment may result; for instance, the patient may be unable to sit because hip flexion is lost.

There is some evidence to suggest that early treatment with indomethacin, diphosphonates, or radiotherapy delays the formation of ectopic bone. With conservative management, however, including range of motion exercises, functional outcomes can be acceptable. The osseous deposit may be excised when it reaches maturity, but it recurs in most patients.

The pathogenesis of this condition is unknown; participation of various systemic and local factors has been proposed.[17,18]

Patients with spinal cord injury may also develop hydrarthrosis or hemarthrosis of the knee, presumed to be of traumatic origin.[18,19] The effusion, which may precede the ossification, has a normal cell count but a discordantly high protein concentration.[19]

DISRUPTIVE ARTICULAR TRAUMA: POST-TRAUMATIC OSTEOARTHRITIS

Permanent joint damage may be the end result of various types of trauma, including fractures through the articular surface, dislocations, internal derangements, major ligamentous ruptures, and wounds, often with sepsis and foreign body implantation (Fig. 89–3). There may be permanent or progressive structural alterations, e.g., deterioration of articular cartilage, limitation of joint motion, instability, or angular deviation.[20] Arthritis is more likely to develop in the legs than in the arms because of greater weight-bearing loads. Pathologically and radiographically, the condition has most of the characteristics of osteoarthritis. However, a specific traumatic episode should not be definitely accepted as etiologically related to osteoarthritis unless there is evidence establishing the following points: (1) the joint was normal prior to injury; (2) records document either an effusion or structural damage shortly after the injury; and (3) similar disease has not occurred in nontraumatized joints. Other points favoring a traumatic origin are the occurrence of significant isolated osteoarthritis in a joint not usually involved by the idiopathic variety (such as ankle, wrist, elbow, or metacarpophalangeal joint) and radiologic demonstration of foreign bodies and healed fractures near the joint in question.

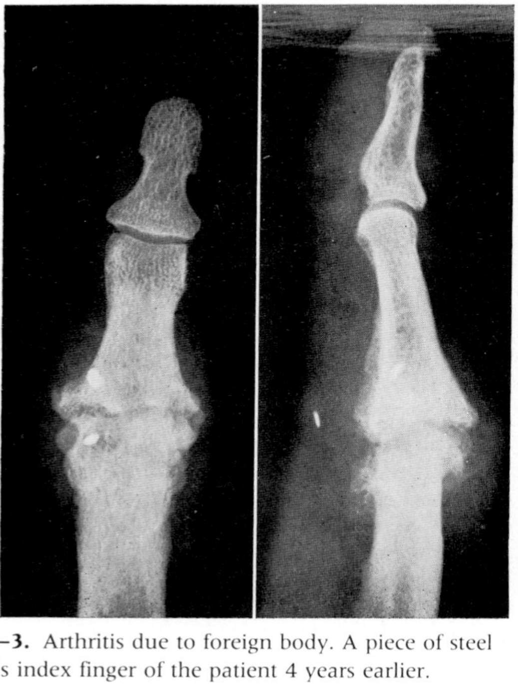

FIGURE 89–3. Arthritis due to foreign body. A piece of steel lodged in this index finger of the patient 4 years earlier. Swelling of the finger began about 2 years later and has continued to date. Roentgenograph shows marked deformity of the proximal interphalangeal joint of the right index finger. This consists of marked hypertrophic changes with possible ankylosis of the joint. There are two small opaque foreign bodies in relation to the palmar and radial aspects of the joint.

REPETITIVE ARTICULAR TRAUMA

Osteoarthritis may develop in joints that are repeatedly traumatized as a result of certain occupations and sports. Radiographic abnormalities, such as joint space narrowing, subcortical cysts, and marginal osteophytes, are common in some groups studied, but many of the affected individuals are asymptomatic. These changes occur in the hands and wrists of boxers and stone workers using pneumatic hammers, in the ankles of soccer players, in the first metatarsophalangeal joints of ballet dancers, and in the elbows of foundry workers.

ROLE OF TRAUMA IN OTHER TYPES OF ARTHRITIS

Trauma plays an important role in the development of neuropathic joint disease (see Chapter 84). Attacks of gouty arthritis and pseudogout often develop in recently injured joints. Rheumatoid arthritis occasionally begins in a joint that has been injured or subjected to a surgical procedure. In a followup study of patients who had sustained a serious fracture, the incidence of rheumatoid arthritis was found to be marginally greater than in control subjects.[21] Post-traumatic onsets of seronegative spondyloarthropathy,[22,23] as well as septic and tuberculous arthritis, have been described. A history of recent or old trauma to the affected joint is sometimes obtained from patients with septic or tuberculous arthritis. The evidence in these situations is anecdotal and difficult to evaluate. Data have not been gathered in an organized fashion, and the mechanisms involved are not well understood. In many instances, the trauma has been minimal, perhaps representing an unrelated antecedent to the joint disease.

In the absence of appropriate studies, the putative etiologic or precipitating role of trauma in chronic inflammatory arthritis remains speculative, but cannot be dismissed.

Pre-existing arthritis may certainly be aggravated by trauma, but the magnitude and duration of exacerbation reasonably attributable to trauma are unknown, and each case must be considered on its own merits. Only minor force would be required to cause rupture of a frayed wrist extensor tendon or collateral ligament in a patient with rheumatoid arthritis. Other acute episodes, such as abrupt increase in joint swelling or rupture of the posterior knee joint capsule, are commonly associated with unusual resistive exercise. Sanguineous joint fluid is sometimes aspirated from a knee or shoulder in patients with rheumatoid arthritis who report sudden increase in pain and swelling following relatively minor trauma. It is presumed that pinching or compressing the hypertrophied synovium may result in bleeding. In such cases, the synovial fluid hematocrit is fairly low, usually less than 10%.

BENIGN HYPERMOBILITY SYNDROME

Generalized joint hypermobility due to ligamentous laxity occurs in about 5% of the population. The condition is regarded by some as a familial disorder that predisposes the affected individual to articular injuries, leading to chronic or recurrent arthralgia. The term "hypermobility syndrome" refers to healthy subjects with joint laxity in the absence of major features of the Marfan or Ehlers-Danlos syndromes, and arthralgia for which no other explanation could be found. The syndrome has a marked female preponderance.[24] Symptoms first appear in children or young adults.[25,26] Hypermobile individuals are often able to hyperextend the knee and elbow beyond 10°, to achieve sufficient lumbar flexion to place both palms on the floor without bending the knees, and to passively oppose the thumb to the flexor aspect of the forearm. Lacking the stability afforded by normal ligaments, hypermobile subjects may be more vulnerable to the adverse effects of injury and overuse, including sprains, traumatic synovitis, recurrent dislocations, tendinitis, and temporomandibular joint dysfunction.[27] An associated systemic connective tissue abnormality is possible. A group of patients with mitral valve prolapse in one study had a higher frequency of joint hypermobility than controls.[29] A marfanoid habitus,[30] thin skin, and uterine prolapse[31] may also be associated with hypermobility. In a study of skin biopsies from selected patients with hypermobility, most of whom also had mitral valve prolapse, an increased content of type III collagen was demonstrated.[32] See also Chap 87.

ACUTE BONE ATROPHY (SUDECK'S ATROPHY; REFLEX DYSTROPHY)

After trauma to an extremity, a few patients develop severe pain, edema, vasomotor abnormalities, and atrophy of bone, muscle, and skin. Many labels have been applied to this syndrome, depending on the feature of particular interest to the describer: *Sudeck's atrophy, Leriche's post-traumatic osteoporosis, Weir Mitchell's causalgia, peripheral trophoneurosis, reflex dystrophy,* and *chronic traumatic edema*. The term "causalgia" should probably be reserved for cases in which there has been injury to a major nerve trunk, but the resulting intense burning pain is not confined to the distribution of the nerve and may not differ from that which occurs in reflex dystrophy without nerve injury.[33,34] Most patients are adults, but the condition can also occur in children.[35–37] Another variant, the "shoulder-hand syndrome," is usually not related to trauma and is described in detail in Chapter 100.

The antecedent injury may be a fracture, but it is often fairly trivial, such as a sprain or laceration, and it may occur with about equal frequency in an upper or lower extremity.[36] Pain, of a quality and degree inappropriate for the injury, may begin immediately or not until several weeks after the trauma.[34,36] Disinclination to move the extremity is also an early feature that is closely linked to the pain. The limb is painful on motion and may have striking cutaneous hyperalgesia and cold sensitivity. An early hyperemic stage may be noted in some cases, but a cold, moist, cyanotic, edematous hand or foot is more typical after 2 or 3 months. Roentgenograms, usually normal during the first month, later show patchy osteopenia, often periarticular in distribution initially, but diffuse later. Radionuclide bone scans show increased uptake in most adults, but normal or reduced uptake is more often characteristic in children.[36,37] With continued immobility, muscle and skin atrophy occur and joint motion is lost.

Pathogenesis and management are discussed in Chapter 99. It should be emphasized that early identification of patients and restoration of active motion are the keys to successful treatment. Early treatment with simple, conservative measures, including graded active exercises, heat, and elevation, may produce good results. Long-standing disease, with advanced atrophy of skin, muscle, and bone, may be largely irreversible. To obviate this irreversibility, more aggressive therapies have been proposed, but none has been studied in controlled trials. These measures include oral corticosteroids, sympathetic nerve blocks,[38] and regional intravenous injection of corticosteroids, analgesics, or sympatholytic agents, and transcutaneous nerve stimulation.[34,36a]

Another syndrome characterized by pain and osteopenia has been described in several reports since 1959 as *migratory osteolysis, regional migratory osteoporosis,* and *transient osteoporosis of the hip*. The condition was first described during pregnancy, but subsequently has been noticed most often in middle-aged men, who develop a painful swelling in one region of a lower extremity, rarely with preceding trauma.[39] Either the hip, knee, or foot may be involved. Pain is often severe, especially on motion and weight-bearing. Although radiographs may be normal during the first 2 or 3 weeks of symptoms, severe osteoporosis in the painful region is readily apparent thereafter. This condition is unlikely to be related to disuse because uptake of a bone-seeking radioisotope is increased in the affected area during the first week, prior to immobilization of the extremity. This disorder is self-limited, with resolution of signs and symptoms in several months and eventual return of bone density to normal. Subsequent attacks may occur in other areas but not in previously involved joints.

Nothing is known of the pathogenesis of this syndrome, but its resemblance to Sudeck's atrophy has been noted and a strong association with type IV hyperlipoproteinemia has been demonstrated.[40]

OSTEOCHONDRITIS DISSECANS

This local disorder of subchondral bone is most commonly found in the knees of adolescents and young adults. A devitalized fragment of bone, with its articular cartilage still present, demarcates from its original site, usually on the lateral portion of the medial femoral condyle. Partial or complete detachment may occur eventually, with resulting signs and symptoms of a "loose body" in the joint; less frequently, the fragment may lodge in the intercondylar notch and may remain clinically silent.

Antecedent trauma, though common, seems to be only one of several etiologic factors. Anomalous ossification centers, locally deficient blood supply, and genetic factors[41] are particularly important in the younger age group, whereas trauma plays a greater role in adults. The trauma involved may be "endogenous," such as repeated contact between an unusually prominent tibial spine or aberrantly situated cruciate ligament and the femoral condyle. Osteochondritis has a different arthroscopic appearance from osteochondral fracture, and only the latter results in hemarthrosis.[42]

The clinical picture in patients with knee involvement consists of mild discomfort rather than pain. This discomfort is aggravated by exercise, but there may also be some aching at rest. With separation of the fragment, the patient may complain of instability or "giving-way." Often an unusual stance, due to external rotation of the tibia, may be noted. This stance diminishes contact between the tibial spine and the usual site of osteochondritis on the medial condyle, near the intercondylar notch. A sign that correlates with this may be demonstrated by forcing the tibia into internal rotation while slowly extending the knee from 90° of flexion. At about 30°, the patient complains of pain, which is relieved immediately by external rotation of the tibia.

Roentgenograms may be normal for as long as 6 months after the injury; the typical picture is that of a bony sequestrum lodged in a sharply defined cavity (Fig. 89–4). The lesion has a similar appearance when it occurs in other locations, such as the elbow (capitellum), ankle (talus), hip, and metatarsal head.[43,44] Occasionally, multiple sites are involved particularly in individuals from predisposed families.[41]

Treatment is conservative if the fragment remains in place. Loose fragments may be treated surgically, with either removal or fixation.[44] The immediate prognosis is good, but some patients may develop osteoarthritis later in life.[45]

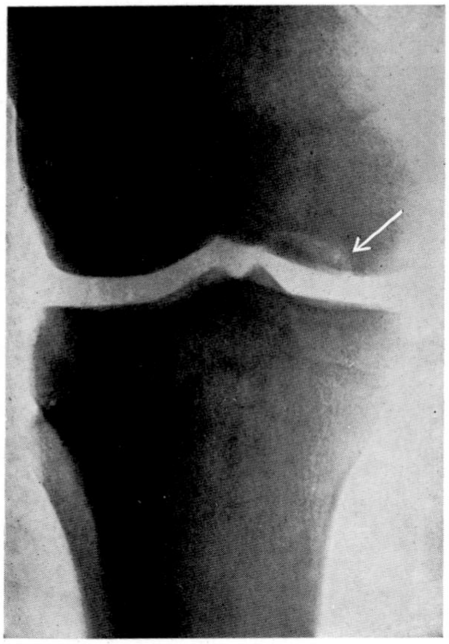

FIGURE 89–4. Osteochondritis dissecans. Arrow indicates osseous fragment.

EPIPHYSEAL OSTEOCHONDRITIS

Necrosis of an entire epiphysis is a common localized disorder in childhood. Vascular insufficiency is thought to be the most significant etiologic factor; trauma is often mentioned, but seldom established as a primary cause. Experimental evidence suggests that compression fractures may lead to disorderly epiphyseal ossification characteristic of osteochondritis.[46] In the hip *(Legg-Calvé-Perthes disease),* osteochondritis occurs in younger children (2 to 10 years of age), usually presenting with a limp rather than with pain. In the knee *(Osgood-Schlatter disease)*, older children (9 to 15 years of age) develop pain and swelling in the tibial tubercle; this condition may result from a traction injury.[46] Osteochondritis of the vertebrae *(Scheuermann's disease)* presents with kyphosis and is described in Chapter 95.

Generalized osteochondritis involving small joints in the hands and wrists, as well as the joints already mentioned, is a rare but definite entity. This condition must be differentiated from the polyarthritides.[47]

TIETZE'S SYNDROME; COSTOCHONDRITIS

Tietze's syndrome is a benign condition in which painful enlargement develops in the upper costal cartilages.[48] The syndrome occurs with the same frequency in both sexes and on both sides of the chest. Involvement of only a single costal cartilage is found in 80% of patients, the second and third costal cartilages being most affected. Onset of pain is either acute or insidious, usually without prior injury, with the exception of trauma, which may have occurred during vigorous coughing in a minority of cases. Pain is sometimes severe, is aggravated by motion of the rib cage, and may radiate to the shoulder and arm. Palpation of a firm tender fusiform swelling of the costal cartilage confirms the diagnosis. Biopsy usually shows normal cartilage, occasionally some edema of the perichondrium, and, rarely, nonspecific chronic inflammation in the surrounding tissues. The duration is variable, from a week to several years. Some patients have multiple episodes, but spontaneous remission is the rule. The swelling has been attributed to cartilaginous hypertrophy by some and to abnormal angulation by others, but nothing is known of the pathogenesis. Treatment may include analgesics, heat, local infiltration with corticosteroid, intercostal nerve block, and reassurance that symptoms are not due to heart disease.

Other disorders may produce pain, tenderness, or evidence of inflammation in the costochondral joints, but not a hard swelling as in Tietze's syndrome. They include rheumatoid arthritis, fibrositis, gout, pyogenic infection, and the anterior chest wall syndrome that may follow myocardial infarction.

The most common cause of chest wall pain in individuals who do not have a generalized rheumatic disease is an ill-defined condition usually called *costochondritis*[49] or *perichondritis*.[50] The pain may be severe, radiating widely, but is often worse on the left side. In some cases it is aggravated by coughing, deep respiration, and motion of the thorax. Anxiety and hyperventilation are common accompaniments. Some episodes are brief and self-limited, but others are chronic, recurrent, and disabling. Tenderness over the costal cartilages, simulating or accentuating the spontaneous pain, is the main physical finding. The xiphoid may be tender in patients with generalized costochondritis, but there is also a syndrome of *isolated xiphoidalgia*, which may result in epigastric pain suggestive of various intra-abdominal disorders. Reproduction of the pain by pressing over the xiphoid is the essential diagnostic maneuver. Little is known of the etiology and pathology of these conditions. In most cases there is no evidence for a traumatic cause, but emotional factors are frequently involved. Care must be taken to rule out coronary artery disease, which may occasionally be associated with chest wall hyperalgesia.

Sudden episodes of sharp pain at the costal margin may be caused by the *slipping rib* or *rib-tip syndrome*.[51] This condition is due to hypermobility of the anterior end of a costal cartilage, usually that of the tenth rib, as a result of past trauma. The patients, usually middle-aged of either sex, complain of upper abdominal pain, precipitated by movement and by certain postures. A snapping sensation and point tenderness at the rib tip, relieved by a local anesthetic injection, will confirm the diagnosis.

A rare inflammatory condition, sternoclavicular hyperostosis, can also cause widespread pain, tenderness, and swelling in the anterior chest wall. This can be associated with palmoplantar pustulosis, severe acne, and spondyloarthropathy.[52,53]

Painless enlargement of all the costochondral junctions (the acromegalic rosary) is a common clinical sign of previous or current growth hormone excess.[54]

OSTEITIS PUBIS

Surgical trauma in the retropubic area may occasionally provoke an inflammatory process in the pubic symphysis and adjacent bone.[61] Osteitis pubis may occur after prostate or bladder surgery and, more rarely, following herniorrhaphy or childbirth. Several weeks postoperatively, the patient develops pain over the symphysis radiating down the inner aspects of the thighs, often aggravated by coughing and straining. Physical findings include an antalgic gait, point tenderness over the symphysis, spasm in the abdominal and hip adductor muscle groups, and a low-grade fever. Radiographs may be normal initially, but rarefaction and osteolysis develop around the symphysis within 2 to 4 weeks. A sterile chronic inflammatory process is usually noted on biopsy, but a true osteomyelitis may be discovered in a minority of patients, generally those with more marked bone destruction and fever.[55] Tuberculosis and metastatic disease must also be considered in the differential diagnosis. Similar radiographic findings may be observed in ankylosing spondylitis and occasionally in chondrocalcinosis or in other types of polyarthritis, but pain is minimal or absent. Although spontaneous remission may be expected in osteitis pubis, disabling symptoms may persist for many months. The gamut of anti-inflammatory drugs has been used with varying success. Other measures, such as immobilization, wearing a tight pelvic belt, and surgical debridement have been advocated. The pathogenesis is uncertain, but there is general agreement that one or more factors, in addition to trauma, may contribute.

Traumatic osteitis pubis in athletes, particularly soccer players, may be a result of an avulsion stress fracture at the origin of the gracilis muscle near the symphysis.[56]

SYNOVIAL CYSTS OF THE POPLITEAL SPACE: "BAKER'S CYSTS"*

Six primary bursae are associated with muscles and tendons on the posteromedial aspect of the knee. Communications between two bursae and between a bursa and the knee joint are common. Popliteal cysts may arise in three ways: (1) accumulation of fluid in a noncommunicating bursa; (2) distention of a bursa by fluid originating as a result of a lesion in the knee joint; and (3) posterior herniation of the joint capsule in response to increased intra-articular pressure. The communication between joint and cyst is generally narrow and the anatomy such that a flap-valve mechanism may be operative, allowing free passage of fluid from knee to cyst, but not in the opposite direction.[57]

Popliteal cysts may be seen at all ages. Those in children are usually unassociated with joint disease and

* *Editors note*: Robert Adams, an Irish surgeon, described the popliteal cyst including the vohelike openings connecting it to the joint space of the knee in his textbook and illustrated it in his atlas in 1857. William Morant Baker was 18 years old at this time.

are often bilateral.[58] Most disappear spontaneously. In about half of all cases, some abnormality is evident in the knee joint, including osteoarthritis, rheumatoid arthritis, internal derangements, and a variety of other conditions. Only a few patients have a history of trauma. In most patients with knee joint disease, a connection between the cyst and joint can be demonstrated with arthrography. The cyst itself usually causes only mild discomfort; other symptoms may be related to the associated joint lesions. A fluctuant swelling is present in the popliteal area, occasionally extending well into the calf and presenting superficially at the medial border of the gastrocnemius. The differential diagnosis, which includes aneurysms, benign neoplasms, varicosities, and thrombophlebitis, is greatly facilitated by modern imaging techniques.[58–60] The histopathologic characteristics of the cysts are varied and do not particularly correspond to the presumed origin, bursal or hernial. Most have a thin fibrous wall, lined by a single layer of flat cells. Others have structural characteristics of a synovial membrane, particularly those occurring in patients with rheumatoid arthritis. A few have a thickened, inflamed wall coated with fibrin, but no villus formation.

Definitive treatment is essentially surgical. In some cases, correction of knee joint pathology (such as synovectomy in a patient with rheumatoid arthritis) may result in spontaneous disappearance. Aspiration of the cyst and corticosteroid injections are often palliative.

Synovial cysts in rheumatoid arthritis are seen in many other joints. Occasionally, a communicating cyst of traumatic or nonspecific origin may be seen elsewhere. For instance, a cyst connecting with the hip joint may present anteriorly as a mass in the groin or posteriorly with sciatic pain.

GANGLION

A ganglion is a cystic swelling that may be found near, and often attached to, a tendon sheath or joint capsule, and is believed to be derived from these structures.[61] A slender connection may be demonstrated histologically and radiographically.[62] The thick mucoid material within the ganglion contains hyaluronic acid, although no true synovial membrane lines the cavity. The most common location is on the dorsum of the wrist (Fig. 89–5), but ganglia are also frequently noted on the volar aspect of the wrist, the fingers, and the dorsum of the foot. Ganglia of the flexor tendon sheaths, at the base of the fingers, are common in typists. They have been reported near many other joints and also attached to the tibial periosteum. In most instances, there has been no definite relationship to trauma. Small ganglia are more likely to be painful than larger ones, probably because they are in the process of expanding. Most patients have few symptoms other than unsightly swelling and slight discomfort on motion.

Ganglia frequently disappear spontaneously.[63] Treatment is not necessarily required, but is often demanded by the patient for cosmetic reasons. Most cases may be treated successfully by puncturing the cyst wall with a large bone needle, aspiration of the contents, and injection of a corticosteroid preparation. If the ganglion recurs after this procedure, surgical excision may be performed.

TENOSYNOVITIS; STENOSING TENOVAGINITIS

Tenosynovitis is an inflammation of the cellular lining membrane of the fibrous tube (vagina) through which a tendon moves. It may be produced by various diseases (e.g., rheumatoid arthritis, gout, gonococcal arthritis), but even more commonly by trauma. Such trauma may occur from a direct blow, from abnormal pressure upon a tendon (such as from the stiff counter of a new shoe on the Achilles tendon) or, most often, from a short period of unusual activity involving a certain muscle-tendon unit. In industrial settings the wrist and thumb extensors are frequently involved, often related to a new type of repetitive work or to resumption of work after vacation. The condition is identified by tenderness,

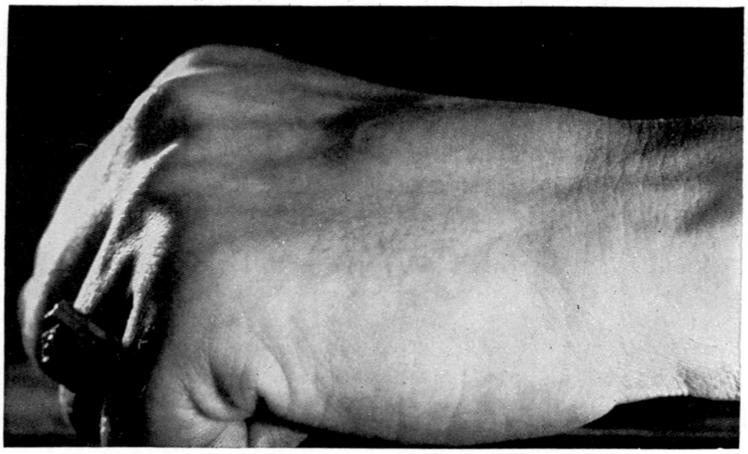

FIGURE 89–5. Ganglion arising from extensor tendon sheaths. An oval and flattened cystic mass is on the dorsum of the hand.

swelling, and palpable crepitus over the tendon as it is moved (peritendinitis crepitans). Remission usually occurs if the affected part is rested for a few days.

Stenosing tenovaginitis is primarily a disorder of the fibrous wall of the tendon sheath, particularly at locations where the tendon passes through a fibrous ring or pulley. Generally, an osseous groove comprises part of the ring, which is completed by a thickening of the tendon sheath. Such arrangements are found over bony prominences, such as the radial styloid and the flexor surfaces of the metacarpal and metatarsal heads. With prolonged mechanical stress from either tendon motion under an excessive load or external pressure, such as from the handles of pruning shears, abnormal proliferation of fibrous tissue in the ring constricts the lumen of the tendon sheath. Secondary changes may then occur in the tendon, usually with enlargement distal to the constriction. There may be a snapping sensation with movement of the enlarged segment of tendon through the narrowed ring ("trigger finger" and "snapping thumb"). Further progression may produce locking in flexion; the tendon may be pulled through the constriction by its own flexor muscle but not by its weaker extensor antagonist. When extension is forced, the bulbous portion suddenly pops back through the constriction, and the digit "unlocks." Tenosynovitis due to mechanical stress may also contribute to pain and loss of motion.

Stenosing tenovaginitis of the abductor pollicis longus and extensor pollicis brevis at the radial styloid is known as *de Quervain's disease*. It is a common disorder among individuals who perform repetitive manual tasks involving grasping with the thumb accompanied by movement of the hand in a radial direction (Fig. 89–6). Occurrence during pregnancy, followed by spontaneous resolution, has also been reported.[64] Symptoms include pain in the area of the radial styloid and weakness of grip. Examination reveals tenderness and thickening over the involved tendons and limited excursion of the thumb; locking and snapping seldom occur. The classic test is the demonstration of *Finkelstein's sign*. The thumb is placed in the palm of the hand and grasped by the fingers; ulnar deviation of the wrist elicits a sharp pain if inflammation of the tendon sheath is present.

The most common locations for stenosing tenovaginitis are the thumb flexor and extensor tendons and the finger flexors, but occasionally other sites are involved. These sites include the flexor carpi radialis tendon, resulting in pain at the base of the thenar eminence, the common peroneal sheath, causing pain on the lateral aspect of the ankle, and the tibialis posterior tendon, presenting with pain below and behind the medial malleolus after prolonged standing and walking.

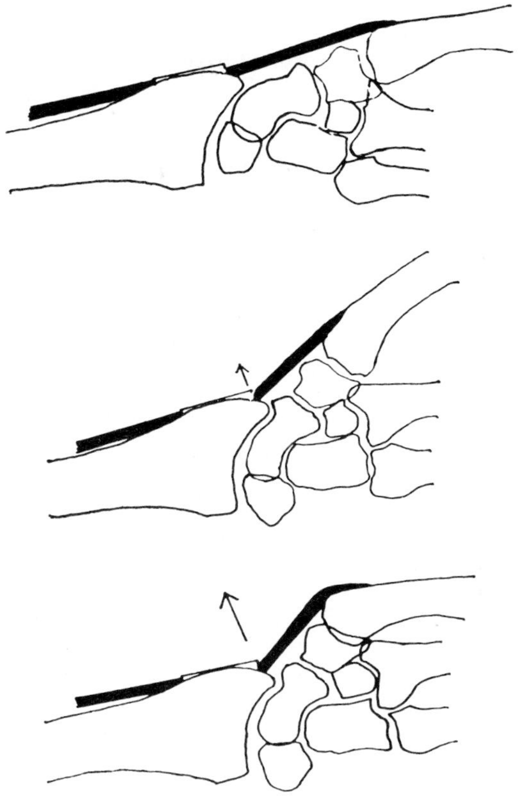

FIGURE 89–6. *Top*, Wrist and thumb in neutral position, tendons relaxed. *Center*, Radial deviation of wrist and thumb relaxed, minor tearing stress applied to retinaculum. *Bottom*, Radial deviation of wrist while gripping, strong tearing stress applied to retinaculum. (From Muckart, R.D.: Stenosing tendovaginitis of abductor pollicis longus and extensor pollicis brevis at the radial styloid (de Quervain's disease). Clin. Orthop., *33*:201–207, 1964.)

TREATMENT OF STENOSING TENOVAGINITIS

Conservative measures such as (1) cessation of the repetitive activity thought to have provoked the condition, (2) immobilization with splints, and (3) local corticosteroid injections often result in improvement, but recurrences are common. Tenosynovitis may subside, but the area of fibrous constriction is unlikely to be greatly altered by this approach, particularly when the duration of symptoms exceeds 4 months.[65] It is sometimes necessary to resort to surgical excision of this portion of the sheath. In all the locations, the operation is simple and results in permanent remission, even allowing resumption of full activity in most cases. Trigger finger and snapping thumb may be treated successfully without surgery, with resolution of symptoms in nearly 90% after one or two local corticosteroid injections.[66]

CARPAL AND TARSAL TUNNEL SYNDROMES

Tenosynovitis in the flexor compartment of the wrist, where the tendons are enclosed in a bony canal, roofed by a rigid transverse carpal ligament, may result in compression and degeneration of the medial nerve that shares this space.

An entrapment neuropathy of the posterior tibial nerve behind and below the medial malleolus may be caused by tenosynovitis of the tendons that accompany the nerve through an osseofibrous tunnel. These and other nerve entrapment syndromes are described in Chapter 98.

OTHER FORMS OF TENDINITIS AND BURSITIS

Painful conditions attributed to strain or injury of tendons and their attachments to bone are often loosely described by the term tendinitis. The supraspinatus and bicipital tendons of the shoulder, which are commonly affected, are discussed in Chapter 97. Frequently, tendinitis is related to a particular occupation or sport. For instance, a baseball pitcher, at the end of his delivery, stretches the attachment of the long head of the triceps to the inferior glenoid rim. This movement results in pain in the posterior axillary fold. It is presumed that inflammatory changes occur in the tendon attachment; treatment includes rest, local corticosteroid injections, and ultrasonography. Baseball pitchers and golfers may also develop a similar condition at the *medial* epicondyle of the elbow. Jumper's knee refers to tendinitis of the patellar tendon, at its attachment to the lower pole of the patella[67] or the quadriceps attachment to the upper pole.[68] Semimembranosus tendinitis can cause postero medial knee pain aggravated by weight-bearing exercise.[69]

TENNIS ELBOW (EPICONDYLITIS)

This is a common condition, most often found in middle-aged men, in which pain derives from the origin of the wrist and finger extensors at the lateral epicondyle. Although first described in tennis players, most cases are not related to that sport, but may be provoked by any exercise or occupation that involves repeated and forcible wrist extension or pronation-supination. The right elbow is involved more often than the left; the condition is seldom bilateral. Pain is usually gradual in onset, but is sometimes related to a specific traumatic incident. It often radiates to the forearm and dorsum of the hand. Physical examination reveals point tenderness at or near the lateral epicondyle, with little or no swelling. Elbow joint motion is unrestricted and painless, but resisted wrist extension results in accentuation of pain. Many possibilities have been expressed for the pathogenesis,[70] including tendon rupture, radiohumeral synovitis, periostitis, neuritis, aseptic necrosis, and displacement of the orbicular ligament. The majority of cases are believed to be due to an injury to the common extensor tendon at or near its attachment to the lateral epicondyle.

Management should be directed toward modifying the provocative activity. Many treatments have been proposed, including massage, ultrasonography, anti-inflammatory drugs, braces, and several surgical procedures. The most common approach, local corticosteroid injection, is usually successful.[70] In one study, 10% of patients continued to have symptoms after initial therapy with ultrasonography or corticosteroid injection.[71] The rate of response was greater with local injection, but recurrences were more common.

BURSITIS

Bursae are closed sacs, lined with a cellular membrane resembling synovium. They serve to facilitate motion of tendons and muscles over bony prominences. There are over 80 bursae on each side of the body. Many are nameless, and additional ones may form at almost any point subjected to frequent irritation. Excessive frictional forces or, at times, direct trauma may result in an inflammatory process in the bursal wall, with excessive vascularity, exudation of increased amounts of viscous bursal fluid, and fibrin-coating of the lining membrane. Only small numbers of inflammatory cells are found in bursal fluid in traumatic bursitis, but there may be a greater leukocyte response in bursitis secondary to other rheumatic diseases, such as rheumatoid arthritis or gout. Septic bursitis is usually caused by organisms introduced through punctures, wounds, or cellulitis in the overlying skin. Traumatic bursitis may be complicated by infection or hemorrhage.[73] "Beat knee" and "beat shoulder" in miners are examples of this condition. Continuous abrasion of the skin with stone dust results in cellulitis, and repeated scraping of the bursa against rough stone surfaces leads to hemorrhage. With modification of occupations and habits, many of the classic forms of bursitis are encountered less frequently, e.g., "housemaid's knee," "weaver's bottom," and "policeman's heel." Sports-related bursitis (e.g., "wrestler's knee," a prepatellar bursitis found in 10% of college wrestlers) is receiving greater emphasis.[74]

Subdeltoid bursitis, which is described in detail in Chapter 100, is a very common bursitis. The following other types are also frequently seen.

Trochanteric Bursitis. Trochanteric bursitis is an inflammation of one or more of the bursae about the gluteal insertion on the femoral trochanter. This condition is most common in females and usually has insidious onset, preceded by apparent trauma in only about a fourth of the cases.[75,76] Aching pain on the lateral aspect of the hip and thigh is aggravated by lying on the affected side. The patient experiences tenderness posterior to the trochanter and pain with external rotation of the hip and with active abduction against resistance, but not with flexion and extension.

Olecranon Bursitis. An inflammation with effusion at the point of the elbow occurs frequently with rheumatoid arthritis and gout as well as after trauma.[77] Pain is usually minimal, except when pressure is exerted on the swollen bursa. Elbow motion is unimpaired and usually painless. The swelling often subsides if additional trauma is prevented with a sponge ring. Fluid from the bursa is often serosanguineous with a low leukocyte concentration. Septic bursitis here is common.

Achilles Bursitis. In this condition, an inflammation of the bursa occurs just above the attachment of the Achilles tendon to the os calcis. Achilles bursitis is often related to trauma from tight shoes ("pump bumps") and perhaps to an unusual configuration of the posterior calcaneus (see Chapter 92).

Calcaneal Bursitis. An inflammation of a bursa occurs at the point of attachment of the plantar fascia to the os calcis (see Chapter 92).

Bunion. A painful bursitis occurs over the medial surface of the first metatarsophalangeal joint, usually with a hallux valgus (see Chapter 92).

Ischial Bursitis. An inflammation of the bursa separating the gluteus maximus from the underlying ischial tuberosity is usually produced by prolonged sitting on hard surfaces ("weaver's bottom").

Prepatellar Bursitis. This type of bursitis is a swelling between the skin and lower patella or patellar tendon, resulting from frequent kneeling (Fig. 89–7). Pain is usually slight unless there is direct pressure on the swollen area.

Anserine Bursitis. This inflammation of the sartorius bursa on the medial aspect of the tibia is said to occur in women whose legs are disproportionately large. The characteristic complaint is pain with stair climbing. In one series of bursitis in various locations, anserine bursitis was found to be the most common.[76] Inflammation in another, nameless bursa located at the anterior edge of the medial collateral ligament also gives pain on the inner aspect of the knee,[78] but with point tenderness in a different area.

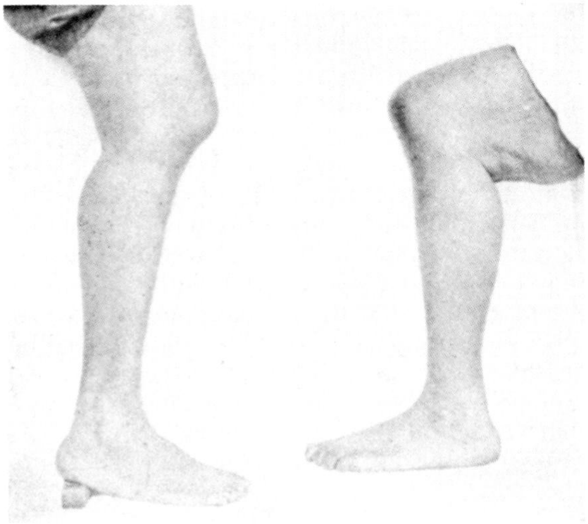

FIGURE 89–7. Bilateral prepatellar bursitis (housemaid's knee) in a scrubwoman. (From Lewin: Orthopedic Surgery for Nurses. Philadelphia, W.B. Saunders.)

Iliopectineal or Iliopsoas Bursitis. With this inflammation of a bursa between the iliopsoas and inguinal ligament, the patient complains of groin pain radiating to the knee. He often adopts a shortened stride to prevent hyperextension of the hip while walking. Examination reveals tenderness just below the inguinal ligament, lateral to the femoral pulse, and pain on hyperextension of the hip. Iliopsoas bursitis can also be a secondary manifestation of rheumatoid or osteoarthritis of the hip, presenting with an inguinal mass and leg swelling.[79,80]

Treatment. In general, therapy includes protection from irritation and trauma, either by modifying the patient's activities or by using appropriate padding. Anti-inflammatory drugs, heat, and ultrasound are also commonly employed. Local corticosteroid injections are usually successful, but there are occasional local complications such as infection and skin atrophy, particularly with olecranon bursitis.[77] Surgical excision is reserved for refractory cases.

CALCIFIC TENDINITIS AND PERIARTHRITIS

Some cases of tendinitis and bursitis are associated with calcific deposits, most commonly with subdeltoid bursitis and trochanteric bursitis, but occasionally with tendinitis, bursitis, or periarthritis around the wrist, knee, or elbow. In these instances, the attacks are less likely to be preceded by recognized trauma. The attacks tend to be abrupt in onset, with intense local inflammatory signs resembling an attack of gout. These episodes, which may be examples of crystal-induced inflammation, are described further in Chapters 100 and 111.

INJURIES TO MUSCLES AND TENDONS

The following clinical features are suggestive of rupture of muscles and tendons:

1. The patient has a history of sudden sharp pain or a snapping sensation that occurs during vigorous muscular effort.
2. The patient is unable to perform certain definite movements following this pain or snapping sensation.
3. The diagnosis is more certain if a defect is apparent in the belly of the muscle or in the tendon, with subsequent ecchymosis.
4. Soft tissue imaging often reveals a defect in the muscle.[81,82]
5. Electrical stimulation of the muscle causes it to contract and produce pain at the site of a tear in either the muscle or tendon.
6. Local anesthetic injection eliminates pain and permits testing of muscular function in those patients in whom the diagnosis is difficult.

The supraspinatus muscle or tendon is the most likely to be torn in the upper extremity. The calf muscles and the quadriceps are the most vulnerable in the lower extremity.

Because of their great tensile strength, rupture seldom occurs in the tendons, but rather at the muscle-tendon junction or at the bony insertion. Attrition of the musculotendinous cuff, secondary to local trauma by pulley systems and bony prominences, may lead to necrobiotic changes that predispose to rupture. Trauma is the immediate and direct cause of rupture; sudden application of a stretching force on a strongly contracting muscle results in tearing of muscle fibers, followed by hemorrhage, edema, and localized spasm ("charley horse"). In some cases, the primary mechanism is extreme passive stretching of a tendon attachment, such as the avulsion of the abductor insertion in the groin in a water skier falling with widely abducted hips. Muscle fatigue results in incomplete relaxation and predisposes to stretch injuries. Therefore, these injuries are more likely to occur in poorly conditioned athletes.

Tendon rupture, common in rheumatoid arthritis, is caused by the lytic effect of tenosynovial inflammation and, in addition, mechanical abrasion of tendons due to disruption of the contiguous bone. Injection of corticosteroids for tendinitis has also been said to predispose to tendon rupture, especially in the Achilles tendon.

Tears in the supraspinatus tendon occur in older individuals. It is presumed that attrition and trauma both contribute to the rupture (see Chapter 100).

Rupture of the long head of the biceps may be the final result of chronic frictional attrition of the tendon within the bicipital groove (see Chapter 100). The rupture may be accompanied by transient pain over the anterior aspect of the shoulder. The belly of the muscle assumes a spherical shape and lies closer to the elbow than normal. Surgical repair is often possible, but not mandatory, since disability is generally mild.

The greater or lesser rhomboid muscles may be strained by a sudden uncoordinated movement of the shoulder. This injury occurs frequently in industrial practice. These muscles arise from the ligamentum nuchae and the spinous process of the seventh cervical of the fifth dorsal vertebrae, and they insert into the vertebral border of the scapula. Contraction of these muscles draws this border of the scapula upward.

Following injury to the rhomboid muscles, there is a localized tenderness between the mid-dorsal spine and the scapula. Pain occurs at this point if the shoulder is passively flexed forward or if it is extended against resistance.

Other muscles arising from the spinous processes and inserting on the scapula or humerus include the levator scapulae, latissimus dorsi, and trapezius muscles. Strains of these muscles give a clinical picture somewhat similar to that for injury to the rhomboids.

Rupture of the pectoralis major muscle may occur in weight lifters during bench pressing,[83] or may be caused by an abrupt traction injury, with sudden sharp pain in the shoulder and a snapping sensation. A tender mass is felt in the muscle, and there is ecchymosis of the overlying skin. Evacuation of the hematoma and surgical repair are the treatments of choice.

Rupture of the rectus abdominus muscle may at times be mistaken for intraperitoneal disease (such as appendicitis). Rupture of this muscle may occur following a severe bout of coughing or sneezing, during pregnancy or labor, or following influenza or typhoid fever (with degeneration of the muscle fibers). A large hematoma may form as a result of tears of branches of the epigastric vessels. The hematoma may require evacuation surgically.

Rupture of the quadriceps muscle or tendon is relatively common. This injury occurs at the point of attachment of the tendon to the patella or at the musculotendinous junction; occasionally, a tear may occur through the purely tendinous or muscular portions. The usual cause of this condition is a violent contraction of the muscle, such as falling on a flexed knee. The patient is unable to actively extend the knee, and a hiatus is seen in the tendon or muscle.

When the patellar tendon is ruptured, the patella lies higher than usual, a gap is noted, active knee extension is lost, and joint effusion is usually present. A roentgenogram will confirm the diagnosis.

Partial rupture of one of the calf muscles, termed "tennis leg," usually involves a belly of the gastrocnemius muscle. Symptoms include a snap with sudden burning pain in the calf during a strong muscular contraction. The pain may extend to the popliteal space; it is aggravated by passive dorsiflexion of the ankle and may be confused with thrombophlebitis.[84] Treatment includes adhesive strapping to immobilize the ankle in plantar flexion for several weeks, followed by heat, massage, and exercises.

Spontaneous rupture of the posterior tibial tendon results in pain, tenderness, and swelling behind and below the medial malleolus, with loss of stability of the foot.[85,86] This injury is usually preceded by chronic symptoms suggestive of tenosynovitis and is often associated with planovalgus feet. Treatment is either surgical repair, in cases diagnosed early, or an arch support.

Injury to the Achilles tendon may occur in runners or in middle-aged men unaccustomed to exertion who indulge in weekend athletics involving jumping (such as basketball and volleyball). There may be rupture at the musculotendinous junction or avulsion at the attachment to the calcaneus. Examination reveals a depression over the tendon and inability to flex the ankle against resistance. In partial rupture, the pain may be mild. Swelling and ecchymosis may conceal the depression usually noted with complete tears. Partial rupture may be treated conservatively with immobilization of the foot in plantar flexion; complete tears usually require surgical intervention.[87] Sonography has been suggested as an inexpensive imaging technique that differentiates between conditions requiring surgery and those that will respond to conservative therapy.[88] Magnetic resonance imaging allows more precise preoperative assessment.[89]

The anterior tibial compartment syndrome is an ischemic necrosis of muscle caused by swelling after unaccustomed exercise. The muscles in this compartment are confined by a tight fascial sheath, resulting in a compromised blood supply when swelling occurs. Examination shows a marked weakness of the involved muscle and local swelling and erythema. Sensation in the first two toes is often lost because of compression of the deep peroneal nerve. Immediate fasciotomy must be performed to prevent irreversible destruction of the muscle. Less frequently, similar problems may arise from high pressure in other muscle compartments of the lower leg[90] and thigh.[91]

FIBROTIC INDURATION AND CONTRACTURE OWING TO REPEATED INTRAMUSCULAR INJECTIONS

Certain drugs may cause local destruction of muscle tissue at injection sites, leading to fibrosis and contracture. Self-administration of pentazocine (Talwin) by patients with chronic pain has resulted in the most striking examples of this condition.[92] The characteristic features are woody induration of the quadriceps, deltoids, and other muscles; needle marks and ulcerations in the overlying skin; and marked muscle shortening.

RUNNING INJURIES

The extraordinary popularity of running has engendered special interest in associated injuries and increased awareness of biomechanical aspects, including running techniques, conditioning, and equipment. These activities are often centered in special runners' clinics, in which the therapeutic goals may differ from those of conventional medicine. Emphasis is placed on continued participation and enhanced performance, in addition to the traditional aims of symptomatic relief and prevention of permanent tissue damage. The spectrum of running injuries encompasses virtually all the categories of musculoskeletal trauma (Table 89–2). About one third of running injuries involve the knee; heel pain is next in frequency. Certain pre-existing conditions may predispose the runner to injury. For instance, a high-arched foot (pes cavus) does not pronate sufficiently to absorb shock during running, leading to Achilles tendinitis or plantar fasciitis. Running on a hyperpronated or flat foot may result in lateral ankle pain. Incongruity, faulty tracking, or laxity in the patellofemoral joint may predispose to patellar pain or chondromalacia. Recrudescent symptoms from virtually any previous articular derangement may develop when the individual begins to run regularly. Ill-fitting or poorly constructed footwear, hard or irregular running surfaces, poor running posture or technique, and inadequate warmup or tendon stretching also increase the likelihood of injury. Detailed discussion of these matters is available elsewhere.[93–96]

Stress fractures, also called fatigue fractures, are partial, cortical fractures related to prolonged, repetitive mechanical loading. A complete fracture may eventually result if the activity is continued. Currently, running is probably the most common cause. The presenting symptom is pain, which is generally aggravated by weight-bearing and relieved by rest. In some areas, such as the tibia and fibula, tenderness, warmth, and swelling may occur over the fracture. The diagnosis is usually made radiographically, but typical findings of a linear cortical radiolucency or a localized area of periosteal new bone formation may not be present during the first week or two of symptoms. Therefore, negative radiographs should be repeated if a stress fracture is strongly suspected. A radionuclide scintigram shows increased uptake at the stress fracture site at this early stage,[97] but this expensive procedure is seldom justified in typical cases. The treatment of stress fractures depends on their location and severity. If the fibula is involved, continuation of running at a reduced level may be possible. At the other extreme, femoral fractures occasionally require surgical intervention.

Knee problems represent about a third of running injuries. They most frequently involve tracking abnormalities of the patella, often in relation to underlying anatomic and biomechanical factors (see Chapter 88). Internal derangements are seldom caused by running, but patients with pre-existing, asymptomatic lesions are likely to develop pain and swelling under the stress of running. *"Overuse" synovitis* in the apparent absence of intra-articular pathology is noted occasionally with rapid increases in mileage. This condition should be managed with temporary cessation until the effusion resolves, with gradual resumption of the running program later. Lateral knee pain may result from the *iliotibial band friction syndrome*. A thick strip of fascia lata, which inserts into the lateral tibial condyle, may im-

TABLE 89–2. COMMON DISORDERS IN RUNNERS

DISORDER	SITES OF INVOLVEMENT
Stress fracture	Tibia, fibula, metatarsus, femur
Compartmental syndromes	
Sprains	
Bursitis	Retrocalcaneus, anserine, ischium, trochanter
Fasciitis	Plantar area, iliotibial band
Tendinitis	Achilles, anterior and posterior tibial, peroneal, quadriceps, patella
Tendon and muscle rupture	Achilles, hamstrings
Intra-articular disorders	Chondromalacia, meniscal tears, plica, "overuse" synovitis, osteoarthritis
Cervical and lumbar disc degeneration	

pinge on the femoral condyle during repeated flexion and extension of the knee, particularly in individuals with tibia vara and hyperpronated feet.

Heel pain, the second most frequent complaint among runners, results from various conditions that can usually be distinguished by physical examination and radiographs. These conditions include plantar fasciitis, calcaneal bursitis, Achilles tendinitis and/or rupture, and calcaneal stress fractures. Treatment includes instruction in running technique to avoid excessive heel strike, heel pads and orthotic devices, stretching exercises, temporary cessation or reduction in running, and anti-inflammatory drugs.

Degenerative arthritis and disc disease may produce pain and limited activity among older runners, but there is little evidence that running causes osteoarthritis in previously normal hips and knees.[96] Substitution of an alternative exercise program with less impact loading, such as swimming or walking, may be recommended in such cases.

REPETITION STRAIN INJURY

Vague regional symptoms that are difficult to ascribe to a specific musculoskeletal injury may be encountered in patients whose occupations require fixed positions and repetitive movements, such as musicians,[98,99] assembly line workers, or accounting machine and computer operators.[100] The complaints include muscular fatigue, stiffness and aching, weakness, paresthesia, and incoordination. Mental stress, various environmental factors, and adverse working conditions may influence the symptoms. Multiple pathogenetic factors may be involved, including muscle fatigue, tenosynovitis, nerve entrapments, compartment syndromes, synovitis, ligamentous strain and referred pain from the cervical spine.[101] A muscle biopsy study has identified some differences in fiber type distribution and subtle ultrastructural changes compared with normal controls.[102] Treatment usually depends on careful analysis and modification of performing techniques and may include rest, anti-inflammatory drugs, and local injections.

RADIATION ARTHROPATHY FOLLOWING NONMECHANICAL TRAUMA

Because articular cartilage is relatively radioresistant, the effects of radiation on joints are usually secondary to destruction of osteoblasts. Vascular damage (endarteritis) may also contribute to osteonecrosis. Since the field of radiotherapy is more likely to include the axial skeleton than the extremities, radiation arthropathy is usually seen in the hips, shoulder, spine, and sacroiliac and temporomandibular joints. Radiation changes are dose-related; the threshold is 3000 rads, with cell death occurring at 5000 rads. Their occurrence depends not only on dosage, but on age, various technical factors, and superimposed trauma or infection. The time of onset of clinical manifestations is generally greater than 1 year, and is often several years after irradiation. Adults may present with aseptic necrosis, fracture, or protrusio acetabuli[103] (Fig. 89–8). Children may develop slipped capital femoral epiphysis,[104] and scoliosis or kyphosis[105] resulting from injury to the epiphyseal plates, leading subsequently to wedge deformities of the vertebral bodies.

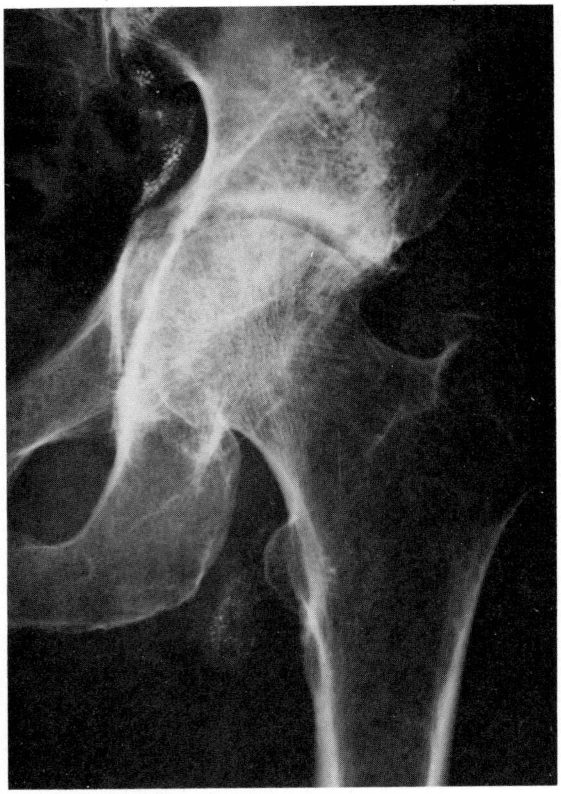

FIGURE 89–8. Radiation necrosis of acetabulum with protrusio acetabuli resulting from pathologic fractures.

Changes resembling degenerative arthritis are occasionally found only in joints that had been included in the field of radiation many years previously. Radiographic findings include narrowing of the joint space, marginal new bone formation, and periarticular osteoporosis. Occasionally, chondrocalcinosis and ankylosis may occur. A few examples of "rheumatoid-like" arthritis with soft tissue swelling have been noted. The spine may be involved, showing narrowing and calcification of intervertebral discs.

Irradiation of the rib cage may result in osteochondritis, with pain and swelling in the costal cartilages. These symptoms may suggest cancer of Tietze's syndrome, but, in contrast to these conditions, erythema exists in the tender area. High-dose ultrasound[106] and diathermy have been reported to cause exacerbations of synovitis in rheumatoid arthritis (see Chapter 49).

FROSTBITE ARTHROPATHY

Frostbite injury to the distal extremities may occasionally involve the joints, in addition to overlying soft tissues. Skeletal changes are not apparent until several months after frostbite, and include demineralization, juxta-articular cysts, and joint space narrowing. The late development of osteophytes results in a clinical picture closely resembling that of osteoarthritis, with Heberden's and Bouchard's nodes.[107] In children, destruction of the phalangeal epiphyses may lead to premature closure and digital growth impairment.[108] These changes may be the result of direct chondrocyte injury during cold exposure.

REFERENCES

1. Casteleyn, P.P., Handelberg, F., and Opdecam, P.: Traumatic haemarthrosis of the knee. J. Bone Joint Surg., *70B*:404–406, 1988.
2. Noyes, F.R., et al.: Arthroscopy in adult traumatic hemarthrosis of the knee; incidence of anterior cruciate tears and other injuries. J. Bone Joint Surg., *G2A*:687–695, 1980.
3. Zarins, B., and Adams, M.: Knee injuries in sports. N. Engl. J. Med., *318*:950–960, 1988.
4. Mink, J.H., and Deutsch, A.L.: Occult cartilage and bone injuries of the knee: Detection, classification, and assessment with MR imaging. Radiology, *170*:823–829, 1989.
5. Berk, R.N.: Liquid fat in the knee joint after trauma. N. Engl. J. Med., *277*:1411–1412, 1967.
6. Egund, N., Nilsson, C.T., Wingstrand, H., et al.: CT scans and lipohaemarthrosis in hip fractures. J. Bone Joint Surg., *72B*:379–382, 1990.
7. Reginato, A.J., Feldman, E., and Rabinowitz, J.L.: Traumatic chylous knee effusion. Ann. Rheum. Dis., *44*:793–797, 1985.
8. White, R.E., Wise, C.M., and Agudelo, C.A.: Post-traumatic chylous joint effusion. Arthritis Rheum., *28*:1303–1306, 1985.
9. Lindblad, S., and Wredmark, T.: Traumatic synovitis analysed by arthroscopy and immunohistopathology. Br. J. Rheumatol., *29*:422–425, 1990.
10. Graham, J., and Goldman, J.A.: Fat droplets and synovial fluid leukocytosis in traumatic arthritis. Arthritis Rheum., *21*:76–80, 1978.
11. Weinberger, A., and Schumacher, H.R.: Experimental joint trauma: Synovial response to blunt trauma and inflammatory reaction to intra-articular injection of fat. J. Rheumatol., *8*:380–389, 1981.
12. Zarins, B., and Nemeth, V.A.: Acute knee injuries in athletes. Orthop. Clin. North Am., *16*:285–302, 1985.
13. Smith, R.W., and Reischl, S.F.: Treatment of ankle sprains in young athletes. Am. J. Sports Med., *14*:465–471, 1986.
14. Cass, J.R., and Morrey, B.F.: Ankle instability: current concepts, diagnosis and treatment. Mayo Clin. Proc., *59*:165–170, 1984.
15. Harrington, K.D.: Degenerative arthritis of the ankle secondary to longstanding lateral ligament instability. J. Bone Joint Surg., *61A*:354–361, 1979.
16. Ahrengart, L.: Periarticular heterotopic ossification after total hip arthroplasty: Risk factors and consequences. Clin. Orthop., *263*:49–58, 1991.
17. Garland, D.E.: A clinical perspective on common forms of acquired heterotopic ossification. Clin. Orthop., *263*:13–29, 1991.
18. Rush, P.J.: The rheumatic manifestations of traumatic spinal cord injury. Semin. Arthritis Rheum., *19*:77–89, 1989.
19. Yue, C.C., Regier, A., and Kushner, I.: Heterotopic ossification presenting as arthritis. J. Rheumatol., *12*:769–772, 1985.
20. Wright, V.: Post-traumatic osteoarthritis—A medicolegal minefield. Br. J. Rheumatol., *29*:474–478, 1990.
21. Julkunen, H., Rasanen, J.A., and Kataja, J.: Severe trauma as an etiologic factor in rheumatoid arthritis. Scand. J. Rheumatol., *3*:97–102, 1974.
22. Wisnieski, J.J.: Trauma and Reiter's syndrome: Development of "reactive arthropathy" in two patients following musculoskeletal injury. Ann. Rheum. Dis., *43*:829–832, 1984.
23. Olivieri, I., et al.: Trauma and seronegative spondyloarthropathy: Rapid joint destruction in peripheral arthritis triggered by physical injury. Ann. Rheum. Dis., *47*:73–76, 1988.
24. Larsson, L., Baum, J., and Mudholker, G.S.: Hypermobility: Features and differential incidence between the sexes. Arthritis Rheum., *30*:1426–1430, 1987.
25. Biro, F., Gewanter, H.L., and Baum, J.: The hypermobility syndrome. Pediatrics, *72*:701–706, 1983.
26. Arroyo, I.L., Brewer, E.J., and Giannini, E.H.: Arthritis/arthralgia and hypermobility of the joints in schoolchildren. J. Rheumatol., *15*:978–980, 1988.
27. Harinstein, D., et al.: Systemic joint laxity (the hypermobile joint syndrome) is associated with temporomandibular joint dysfunction. Arthritis Rheum., *31*:1259–1264, 1988.
28. Beighton, P.H., Grahame, R., and Bird, H.: Hypermobility of Joints. New York, Springer-Verlag, 1983.
29. Pitcher, D., and Grahame, R.: Mitral valve prolapse and joint hypermobility: Evidence for a systemic connective tissue abnormality? Ann. Rheum. Dis., *41*:352–354, 1982.
30. Grahame, R., et al.: A clinical and echocardiographic study of patients with the hypermobility syndrome. Ann. Rheum. Dis., *40*:541–546, 1981.
31. Al-Rawi, Z.S., and Al-Rawi, Z.T.: Joint hypermobility in women with genital prolapse. Lancet, *1*:1439–1441, 1982.
32. Handler, C.E., et al.: Mitral valve prolapse, aortic compliance, and skin collagen in joint hypermobility syndrome. Br. Heart J., *54*:501–508, 1985.
33. Schott, G.D.: Mechanisms of causalgia and related clinical conditions. Brain, *109*:717–738, 1986.
34. Schutzer, S.F., and Gossling, H.R.: The treatment of reflex sympathetic dystrophy syndrome. J. Bone Joint Surg., *66A*:625–629, 1984.
35. Rush, P.J., et al.: Severe reflex neurovascular dystrophy in childhood. Arthritis Rheum., *28*:952–956, 1985.
36. Goldsmith, D.P., et al: Nuclear imaging and clinical features of childhood reflex neurovascular dystrophy: Comparison with adults. Arthritis Rheum., *32*:480–485, 1989.

36a. Poplawski, Z.J., Wiley, A.M., and Murray, J.F.: Post-traumatic dystrophy of the extremities: a clinical review and trial of treatment. J. Bone Joint Surg., *65A*:642–655, 1983.

37. Silber, T.J., and Majd, M.: Reflex sympathetic dystrophy syndrome in children and adolescents: Report of 18 cases and review of the literature. Am. J. Dis. Child., *142*:1325–1330, 1988.
38. Katz, M.M., and Hungerford, D.S.: Reflex sympathetic dystrophy affecting the knee. J. Bone Joint Surg., *69B*:797–803, 1987.
39. Naides, S.J., Resnick, D., and Zvaifler, N.J.: Idiopathic regional osteoporosis: A clinical spectrum. J. Rheumatol., *12*:763–768, 1985.
40. Guenee, B., et al.: Type IV hyperlipoproteinemia in patients with algodystrophy. Clin. Exp. Rheumatol., *3*:49–52, 1985.
41. Phillips, H.O., and Grubb, S.A.: Familial multiple osteochondritis dissecans. J. Bone Joint Surg., *67A*:155–156, 1985.
42. Bradley, J., and Dandy, D.J.: Osteochondritis dissecans and other lesions of the femoral condyles. J. Bone Joint Surg., *71B*:518–522, 1989.
43. Lindholm, T.S., Osterman, K., and Vankka, E.: Osteochondritis

dissecans of the elbow, ankle and hip. Clin. Orthop., *148*:245–253, 1980.
44. Pappas, A.M.: Osteochondrosis dissecans. Clin. Orthop., *158*:59–69, 1981.
45. Bauer, M., Jonsson, K., and Linden, B.: Osteochondritis dissecans of the ankle: A 20-year follow-up study. J. Bone Joint Surg., *69B*:93–96, 1987.
46. Douglas, G., and Rang, M.: The role of trauma in the pathogenesis of the osteochondroses. Clin. Orthop., *158*:28–32, 1981.
47. Duthie, R.B., and Houghton, G.R.: Constitutional aspects of the osteochondroses. Clin. Orthop., *15B*:19–27, 1981.
48. Aeschlimann, A., and Kahn, M.F.: Tietze's syndrome: A critical review. Clin. Exp. Rheumatol., *8*:407–412, 1990.
49. Peyton, F.W.: Unexpected frequency of idiopathic costochondral pain. Obstet. Gynecol., *62*:605–608, 1983.
50. Kadzombe, E.A., and Robson, W.J.: Perichondritis. Lancet, *2*:1010–1011, 1988.
51. Wright, J.T.: Slipping-rib syndrome. Lancet, *2*:632–634, 1980.
52. Kawaik, K., et al.: Bone and joint lesions associated with pustulosis palmaris et plantaris. J. Bone Joint Surg., *70B*:117–122, 1988.
53. Benhamou, C.L., Chamot, A.M., and Kahn, M.F.: Synovitis—acne—pustulosis—hyperostosis—osteomyelitis syndrome (Sapho). A new syndrome among spondyloarthropathies? Clin. Exp. Rheum., *6*:109–112, 1988.
54. Ibbertson, H.K., et al.: The acromegalic rosary. Lancet, *1*:154–156, 1991.
55. Rosenthal, R.E., et al.: Osteomyelitis of the symphysis pubis: A separate disease from osteitis pubis. J. Bone Joint Surg., *64A*:123–128, 1982.
56. Wiley, J.J.: Traumatic osteitis pubis: the gracilis syndrome. Amer. J. Sports Med., *11*:360–363, 1983.
57. Rauschning, W.: Anatomy and function of the communication between knee joint and popliteal bursae. Ann. Rheum. Dis., *39*:354–358, 1980.
58. Stannard, M.W., and Fink, C.W.: Diagnosis of synovial cysts in children by magnetic resonance imaging. J. Rheumatol., *16*:540–541, 1989.
59. Lee, K.R., Cox, G.G., Neff, J.R., et al.: Cystic masses of the knee: Arthrographic and CT evaluation. AJR, *148*:329–334, 1987.
60. Sundaram, M., et al.: Magnetic resonance imaging of lesions of synovial origin. Skeletal Radiol., *15*:110–116, 1986.
61. Young, L., Bartell, T., and Logan, S.E.: Ganglions of the hand and wrist. South. Med. J., *81*:751–760, 1988.
62. Burk, D.L. Jr., et al.: Meniscal and ganglion cysts of the knee: MR evaluation. AJR, *150*:331–336, 1988.
63. Rosson, J.W., and Walker, G.: The natural history of ganglion in children. J. Bone Joint Surg., *71B*:707–708, 1989.
64. Schumacher, H.R., Jr., Dorwart, B.B., and Korzeniowski, O.M.: Occurrence of DeQuervain's tendinitis during pregnancy. Arch. Int. Med., *145*:2083–2084, 1985.
65. Rhoades, C.E., Gelberman, R.H., and Manjarris, J.F.: Stenosing tenosynovitis of the fingers and thumb. Clin. Orthop., *190*:236–238, 1984.
66. Anderson, B., and Kaye, S.: Treatment of flexor tenosynovitis of the hand ("trigger finger") with corticosteroids. Arch. Intern. Med., *151*:153–156, 1991.
67. Martens, M., et al.: Patellar tendinitis: Pathology and results of treatment. Acta Orthop. Scand., *53*:445–450, 1982.
68. Bodne, D., et al.: Magnetic resonance images of chronic patellar tendinitis. Skeletal Radiol., *17*:24–28, 1988.
69. Ray, J.M., Clancy, W.G., and Lemon, R.A.: Semimembranosus tendinitis: An overlooked cause of medial knee pain. Am. J. Sports Med., *16*:347–351, 1988.
70. Chard, M.D., and Hazleman, B.L.: Tennis elbow—A reappraisal. Br. J. Rheumatol., *28*:186–190, 1989.
71. Binder, A., et al.: Is therapeutic ultrasound effective in treating soft tissue lesions? Br. Med. J., *290*:512–514, 1985.
72. Bywaters, E.G.L.: Lesions of bursae, tendons and tendon sheaths. Clin. Rheum. Dis., *5*:883–925, 1979.
73. Strickland, R.W., Vukelja, S.J., Wohlgethan, J.R., and Canoso, J.J.: Hemorrhagic subcutaneous bursitis. J. Rheumatol., *18*:112–114, 1991.
74. Mysnyk, M.C., et al.: Prepatellar bursitis in wrestlers. Am. J. Sports Med., *14*:46–54, 1986.
75. Rasmussen, K.-J.E., and Fanø, N.: Trochanteric bursitis: treatment by corticosteroid injection. Scand. J. Rheumatol., *14*:417–420, 1985.
76. Larsson, L.-G., and Baum, J.: The syndromes of bursitis. Bull. Rheum. Dis., *36*:1–8, 1986.
77. Weinstein, P.S., Canoso, J.J., and Wohlgethan, J.R.: Longterm follow-up of corticosteroid injection for traumatic olecranon bursitis. Ann. Rheum. Dis., *43*:44–46, 1984.
78. Kerlan, R.K., and Glousman, R.E.: Tibial collateral ligament bursitis. Am. J. Sports Med., *16*:344–346, 1988.
79. Toohey, A.K., LaSalle, T.L., Martinez, S., and Polisson, R.P.: Iliopsoas bursitis: Clinical features, radiographic findings, and disease associations. Semin. Arthritis Rheum., *20*:41–47, 1990.
80. Underwood, P.L., McLeod, R.A., and Ginsburg, W.W.: The varied clinical manifestations of iliopsoas bursitis. J. Rheumatol., *15*:1683–1685, 1988.
81. Deutsch, A.L., and Mink, J.H.: Magnetic resonance imaging of musculoskeletal injuries. Radiol. Clin. North Am., *27*:983–1002, 1989.
82. Fleckenstein, J.L., et al.: Sports-related muscle injuries: Evaluation with MR imaging. Radiology, *172*:793–798, 1989.
83. Kretzler, H.H., Jr., and Richardson, A.B.: Rupture of the pectoralis major muscle. Am. J. Sports Med., *17*:453–458, 1989.
84. McClure, J.G.: Gastrocnemius musculotendinous rupture: a condition confused with thrombophlebitis. South. Med. J., *77*:1143–1145, 1984.
85. Johnson, K.A.: Tibialis posterior tendon rupture. Clin. Orthop., *177*:145–147, 1983.
86. Rosenberg, Z.S., et al.: Rupture of posterior tibial tendon: CT and MR imaging with surgical correlation. Radiology, *169*:229–235, 1988.
87. Wills, L.A., et al.: Achilles tendon rupture: a review of the literature comparing surgical versus nonsurgical treatment. Clin. Orthop., *207*:156–163, 1986.
88. Mathieson, J.R., Connell, D.G., Cooperberg, P.L., and Lloyd-Smith, D.R.: Sonography of the Achilles tendon and adjacent bursae. AJR, *151*:127–131, 1988.
89. Keene, J.S., Lash, E.G., Fisher, D.R., and Desmet, A.A.: Magnetic resonance imaging of Achilles tendon ruptures. Am. J. Sports Med., *17*:333–337, 1989.
90. Matsen, F.A., Winquist, R.A., and Klugmire, R.B.: Diagnosis and management of compartmental syndromes. J. Bone Joint Surg., *62A*:286–291, 1980.
91. Schwartz, J.T., et al.: Acute compartment syndrome of the thigh. J. Bone Joint Surg., *71A*:392–400, 1989.
92. Oh, S.J., Rollins, J.I., and Lewis, I.: Pentazocine-induced fibrous myopathy. JAMA, *231*:271–273, 1975.
93. D'Ambrosia, R., and Drez, D., Jr.: Prevention and Treatment of Running Injuries. Thorofare, New Jersey, Charles B. Slack, Inc., 1982.
94. Micheli, L.J.: Lower extremity overuse injuries. Acta Med. Scand. (Suppl., *711*:171–177, 1986.
95. Macera, C.A., et al.: Predicting lower-extremity injuries among habitual runners. Arch. Intern. Med., *149*:2565–2568, 1989.
96. Lane, N.E., Bloch, D.A., Wood, P.D., and Fries, J.F.: Aging, long-distance running, and the development of musculoskeletal disability. Am. J. Med., *82*:772–780, 1987.

97. Norfray, J.F., et al.: Early confirmation of stress fractures of joggers. JAMA, *243*:1647–1649, 1980.
98. Hoppmann, R.A., and Patrone, N.A.: A review of musculoskeletal problems in instrumental musicians. Semin. Arthritis Rheum., *19*:117–126, 1989.
99. Lockwood, A.H.: Medical problems of musicians. N. Engl. J. Med., *320*:221–227, 1989.
100. McDermott, F.T.: Repetition strain injury: a review of current understanding. Med. J. Aust., *144*:196–200, 1986.
101. Smythe, H.: The "repetitive strain injury syndrome" is referred pain from the neck. J. Rheumatol., *15*:1604–1608, 1988.
102. Dennett, X., and Fry, H.J.H.: Overuse syndrome: A muscle biopsy study. Lancet, *1*:905–908, 198.
103. Csuka, M.E., Brewer, B.J., Lynch, K.L., and McCarty, D.J.: Osteonecrosis, fractures, and protrusio acetabuli secondary to X-irradiation therapy for prostatic carcinoma. J. Rheumatol., *14*:165–170, 1987.
104. Libshitz, H.I., and Edeiker, B.S.: Radiotherapy changes of the pediatric hip. Am. J. Roentgenol., *137*:585–588, 1981.
105. Mayfield, J.K.: Postradiation spinal deformity. Orthop. Clin. North Am., *10*:829–844, 1979.
106. Tiliakos, N.A., and Wilson, C.H., Jr.: Ultrasound-induced arthritis (abstract). Arthritis Rheum., *26*:549, 1983.
107. Glick, R., and Parhami, N.: Frostbite arthritis. J. Rheumatol., *6*:456–460, 1979.
108. Carrera, G.F., Kozin, G., and McCarty, D.J.: Arthritis after frostbite injury in children. Arthritis Rheum., *22*:1082–1087, 1979.

90

Mechanical Disorders of the Knee

JAMES B. STIEHL

A mechanical disorder of the knee is defined as any condition interfering with normal joint motion or mobility. Such disorders include any intra-articular process or *internal derangement* blocking or limiting motion such as a torn meniscus, articular osteochondral fragment, or loose body. Conditions external to the joint leading to articular surface damage through altered joint kinematics are included also. Ligamentous disruption, patellar malalignment, and quadriceps or hamstring insufficiency are the most important of this group. Finally, knee osteoarthritis (OA), which ultimately results secondary to these problems, becomes an irreversible factor limiting normal joint function.

The pathomechanical basis of these disorders is due to abnormally increased stress at the cartilage articular surface accumulated over a long period. Whether this is a mechanical block, acting like a grain of sand in a fine bearing, or abnormal wear analgous to that occurring in an improperly balanced tire, the results are the same. The pathologic changes of OA with joint space narrowing, spurs, subchondral sclerosis, and joint deformity represent the final common pathway. This discussion will be limited to the common acquired conditions that are seen after maturity and are usually traumatic or degenerative in nature.

MENISCAL INJURY

Approximately two thirds of all derangements of the knee joint are due to lesions of the menisci.[1–6] These structures are triangular-shaped rings of fibrocartilage filling the space between the convex condyles of the femur and the flat posterior sloping tibial plateaus (Fig. 90–1). The collagen fibers are oriented circumferentially, allowing the meniscus to withstand tensile loading. This arrangement allows the translation of vertical compressive loads into circumferential or hoop stresses. The menisci enhance knee stability, improve joint congruency, and transmit between 50 and 70% of the load applied across the knee during axial loading.[7] Their nutrition comes from the joint fluid and from the blood vessels supplying their periphery. In the newborn, 50% of the periphery of the menisci is vascularized, but in adulthood only 10 to 30%, or 2 to 3 mm, has a blood supply.[8,9]

Meniscal injuries are commonly associated with traumatic ligamentous disruptions resulting from athletic injuries and falls during which abnormal excursion of the articular surfaces under load entraps the margin of the meniscus. The ligament damage typically occurs with exaggerated valgus and rotation causing anterior cruciate stretching or tearing as the tibia moves forward under the femoral condyle. A vertical longitudinal tear of the middle portion of the meniscus results as the femur and tibia contact in this abnormal position (Fig. 90–2). With a displaced bucket handle tear, the torn inner portion displaces toward the intercondylar notch as the knee reduces.[10–17]

Acute hemarthrosis accompanies over 80% of these traumatic injuries and is associated with pain and limited range of motion. Displaceable tears cause the sensation of "catching" and "popping," and the knee may be locked in a flexed position. The symptom of "buckling" or "giving way" is due to instability from the commonly associated anterior cruciate ligament (ACL) injury. Joint line tenderness is the hallmark of meniscal injury and results from chronic pinching of the meniscus in the joint, which tugs on the peripheral joint capsule, which has a rich nerve supply.[18–20]

Signs of meniscal entrapment include pain on forced flexion, the presence of a block to extension, and positive McMurray and Apley grind tests. The McMurray test is done with the patient in the supine position with

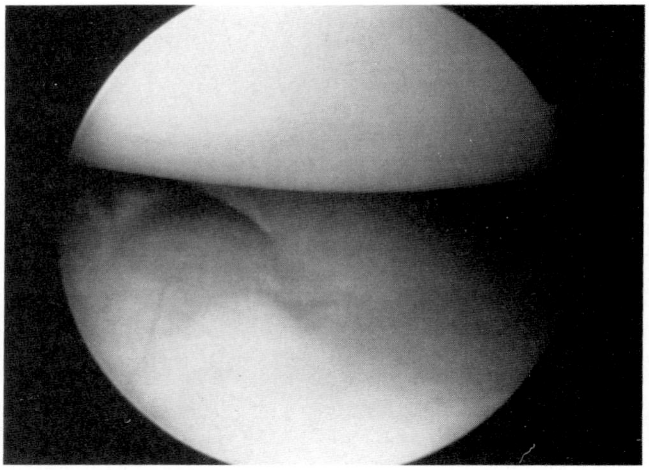

FIGURE 90–1. Arthroscopic view of normal lateral meniscus.

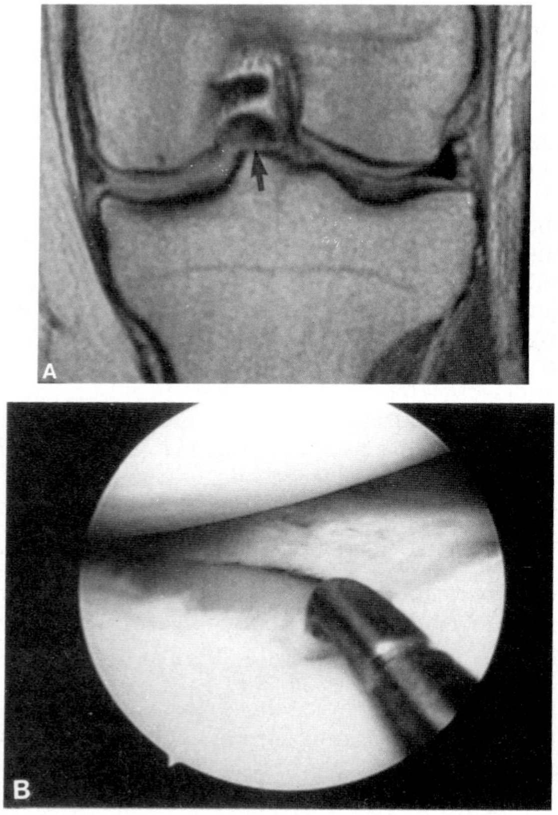

FIGURE 90–2. *A*, Magnetic resonance image of a displaced bucket handle tear (*arrow*) and absent meniscus sign. *B*, Arthroscopic view of verticle longitudinal medial meniscus tear with displaced bucket handle tear under probe.

the affected knee maximally flexed until the heel almost touches the buttock. The knee is then forcibly internally or externally rotated to impinge the lateral or medial meniscus. A palpable or audible snap in the joint constitutes a positive test. Pain may not be present in older tears. The Apley grind test is done with the patient prone. The tibia is flexed 90° and manually compressed on the knee joint. Rotation of the knee internally and externally will produce a "snap" consistent with a torn meniscus. A combination of joint line tenderness with one or both of signs correlates very well with subsequent diagnostic tests.[21]

Degenerative meniscal tears cause a horizontal cleavage. They usually occur in the posterior third of the meniscus and are frequently associated with OA (Fig. 90–3). Flap tears are common, most frequently occurring on the superior surface of the meniscus. Symptoms differ from verticle tears in that pain and injury are more subtle. An episode of squatting and twisting or a sudden misstep may be the only history. Effusion may be slight, but clinical findings of joint line tenderness and meniscal entrapment are usually present.

Dandy studied 1000 cases of symptomatic meniscal lesions with arthroscopy; 81% of the patients were men, most commonly with medial meniscus lesions of the right knee (56.5%). Of the medial meniscus tears, 75% were vertical, which were frequently locked; 23% were horizontal. Of the flap tears, superior flaps were six times more common than inferior flaps. Vertical tears occurred most frequently in the fourth decade, while horizontal tears were seen in the fifth. The common pattern seen in the lateral compartment was a vertical tear involving half the length and width of the meniscus. Myxoid degeneration consisting of a softening of the meniscal substance was seen in a small portion of the lateral tears. The patient experiences a deep-seated aching pain in the knee at night with localized swelling. In distinction from meniscal "cysts" or ganglions, there is significant destruction of the meniscus, which usually requires meniscectomy.[22]

Clinical findings are accurate in making a proper diagnosis in over 75% of cases. The diagnosis of meniscal pathology can be confirmed by arthrogram, magnetic resonance imaging (MRI), or diagnostic arthroscopy. In experienced hands, arthroscopy is nearly 100% accurate in identifying the morphology of derangement and is considered the gold standard. Double-contrast arthrography has been used for many years and has an accuracy of 60 to 90%, depending on the experience of the person interpreting the study. Most recently, MRI has been used with a diagnostic accuracy of 70 to 95%. It is noninvasive, offers excellent soft tissue contrast, and has multiplanar capabilities. It has certain advantages over arthroscopy in that lesions involving the posterior horn or inferior surface of the meniscus may be identified. Other lesions may be differentiated such as osteochondral fractures, osteochondritis dissecans, ligamentous injuries, and pigmented villonodular synovitis. The greatest value of MRI lies in its high negative predictive value; in few cases, use of MRI failed to result in

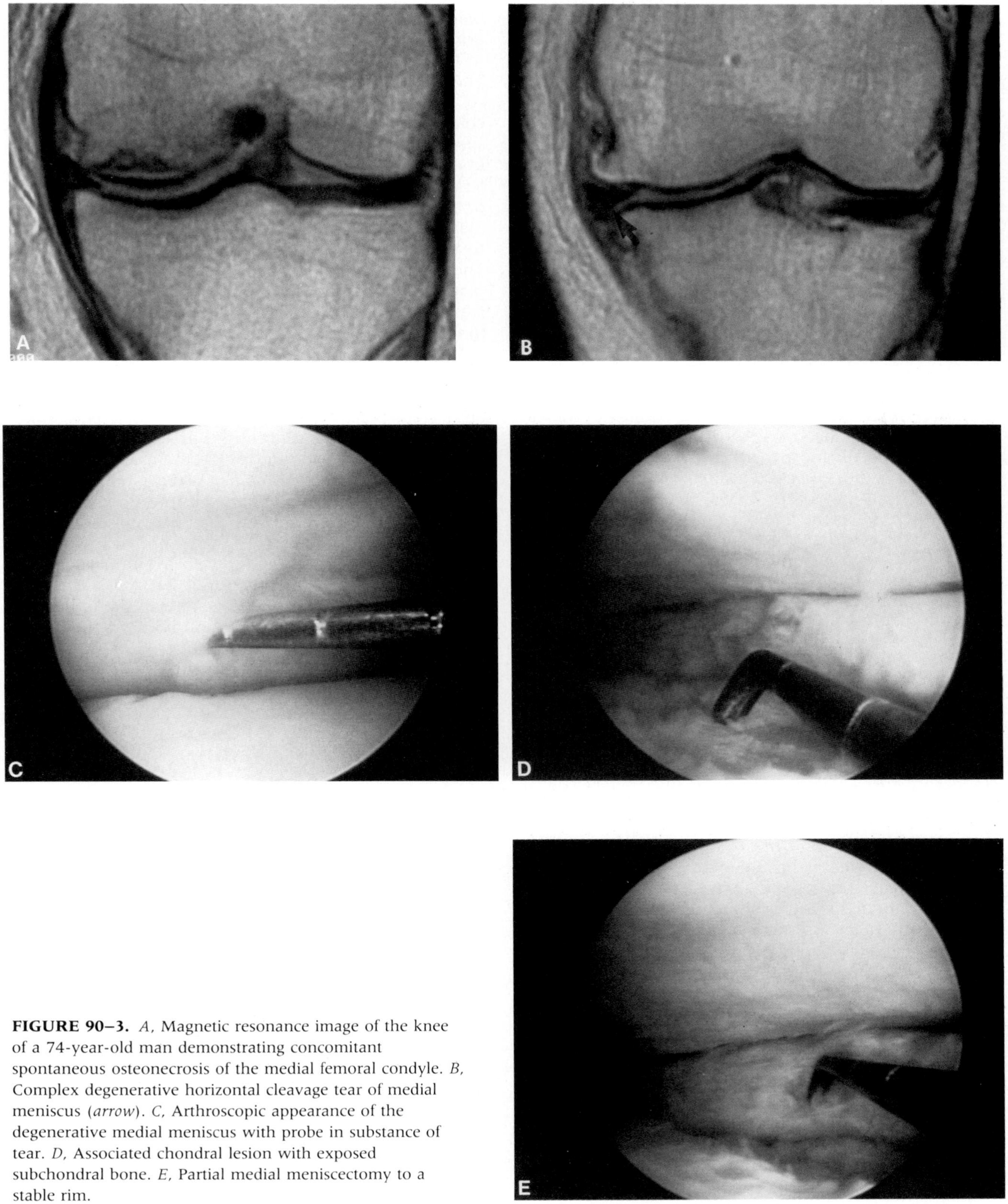

FIGURE 90–3. *A,* Magnetic resonance image of the knee of a 74-year-old man demonstrating concomitant spontaneous osteonecrosis of the medial femoral condyle. *B,* Complex degenerative horizontal cleavage tear of medial meniscus (*arrow*). *C,* Arthroscopic appearance of the degenerative medial meniscus with probe in substance of tear. *D,* Associated chondral lesion with exposed subchondral bone. *E,* Partial medial meniscectomy to a stable rim.

diagnosis of a tear. MRI is less accurate in diagnosing degenerative tears and will often result in identification of increased signal intensity where no lesion is found. This may represent a lesion predisposing to degenerative tears and structures such as the meniscofemoral ligaments and the bursa of the popliteal ligament, can be mistaken for meniscal tears on MRI.[23–30]

Operative arthroscopy is the standard diagnostic and treatment modality for meniscal lesions. Long-term outcome studies have not shown a distinct advantage over open meniscectomy, but patient recovery may be enhanced by the more limited approach. Access to the menisci is much easier with the arthroscope, and partial meniscectomy is possible. Arthroscopy is a major surgical procedure, and significant complications have been noted including infection, phlebitis, neurovascular injury, and anesthesia death. Conservative treatment therefore is warranted in most cases except when a "locked" meniscus causes great pain and limited motion. Because of the high diagnostic capability of clinical examination correlated with MRI, there is little place for "look see" diagnostic arthroscopy. This approach fails to find pathologic changes in a high proportion of cases.

Meniscectomy is the treatment of choice for detached and unstable fragments of meniscus. The long-term effects of this treatment include narrowing of the joint space, ridge formation, flattening of the femoral condyle, and predisposition to OA. Articular cartilage degeneration results from the loss of the 30 to 60% load transmission normally passing through the menisci. Partial meniscectomy, leaving the peripheral portion intact, had a less dramatic biomechanical effect. Leaving the meniscal rim intact after removing a torn bucket handle has resulted in significantly fewer long-term degenerative changes. Also fewer arthritic changes also were found in dogs after a partial meniscectomy. The standard arthroscopic technique at this time is partial meniscectomy debriding the meniscus to a stable rim.[31–33]

Because of the late arthritic changes after meniscectomy, meniscal repair has been advocated for vertical peripheral tears occurring in the vascular zone within 2 mm of the meniscosynovial junction. These tears must be short, and there should be no tear extending into the substance. Finally, associated ligamentous instability involving the ACL should be repaired at the same time.

The late results after meniscectomy are definitely related to the amount of pre-existing degenerative changes identified at the time of surgery by radiography and by arthroscopy. Excellent late functional results occur after meniscectomy if the articular cartilage is well preserved, but results are less satisfactory if significant arthritis was present. Nonetheless, locking and joint line pain are eliminated in most patients despite the arthritis.

LIGAMENTOUS INSTABILITY

Disruption of knee ligament alters the limits of joint motion. The normal kinematics of joint function are changed, with exaggerated stresses on the articular cartilage, leading to degenerative arthritis. Instability or abnormal motion resulting from a torn ligament can occur in the anterior, posterior, medial, or lateral direction. The four primary ligaments limiting this motion are the ACL, posterior cruciate, medial collateral, and fibular collateral. Each ligament provides restraint regarding its specific motion depending on the angle of flexion of the knee. As the knee extends, isolated ligament restraint lessens and the concerted function of several ligaments or secondary restraints increases. For example, the medial collateral ligament (MCL) is the primary restraint to valgus angulation with the knee in 30° of flexion. The MCL is also a secondary restraint to anterior displacement, which is controlled by the ACL. If the ACL is disrupted, the MCL then is one of several structures limiting anterior displacement.[34–38]

With major ligament disruption, rotational instability occurs. The femur rotates abnormally on the fixed tibia. This is an important clinical finding because the typical episode of buckling or "giving way" seen with functional instability reproduces this phenomenon. ACL disruption results in anterior displacement of the tibia, but anterolateral rotatory instability also occurs. The lateral tibial plateau rotates and subluxes anteriorly with knee extension and then reduces as the knee moves into flexion (the pivot shift sign).[39–41]

The diagnosis of ligamentous disruption is usually made by physical examination. Anesthesia may be needed if the injury is acute because of the associated pain and swelling. Combined with instrumented measurements such as the KT 1000 or stress radiographs, 90% diagnostic accuracy can be achieved. In most clinical grading systems, grade I laxity represents up to 5 mm of motion; grade II, 6 to 10 mm; grade III, 11 to 15 mm; and grade IV, greater than 15 mm. The opposite normal knee is used as the reference point.[42]

The most sensitive test of a torn ACL is the anterior drawer sign. This maneuver is performed with the knee flexed to 25° (Lachman's test) (Fig. 90–4). Posterior cruciate ligament integrity is best measured by the posterior drawer test, which is done with the knee flexed to 90°. Medial collateral ligament laxity is best tested using a valgus stress with the knee flexed 30°. Fibular collateral ligament integrity and lateral capsule laxity are tested using a varus stress with the knee flexed to 30°. It is important that the knee is first in neutral position before testing. In the 90° flexed position, one looks for posterior sag of the tibia compared to the opposite normal knee, which indicates posterior cruciate ligament disruption. The neutral position for varus, valgus tests in the coronal plane is the position in which the medial and lateral joint surfaces are in contact. Rotational tests include the pivot shift test, indicating anterior subluxation of the lateral tibial plateau secondary to ACL disruption; reverse pivot shift test, which is posterior subluxation of the lateral tibial plateau (secondary to posterolateral capsule disruption); and anteromedial subluxation (secondary to injuries of the anteromedial structures) (Fig. 90–5).[43–46]

The most common disabling knee injury in athletes

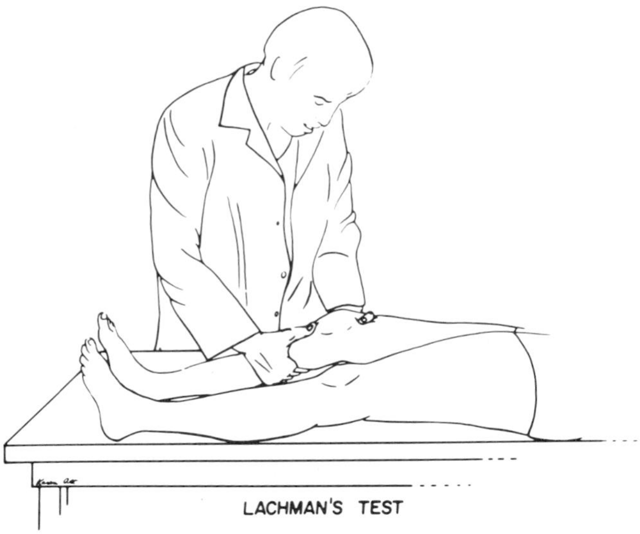

FIGURE 90–4. Lachman's test for anterior cruciate stability done with the knee at 25° flexion.

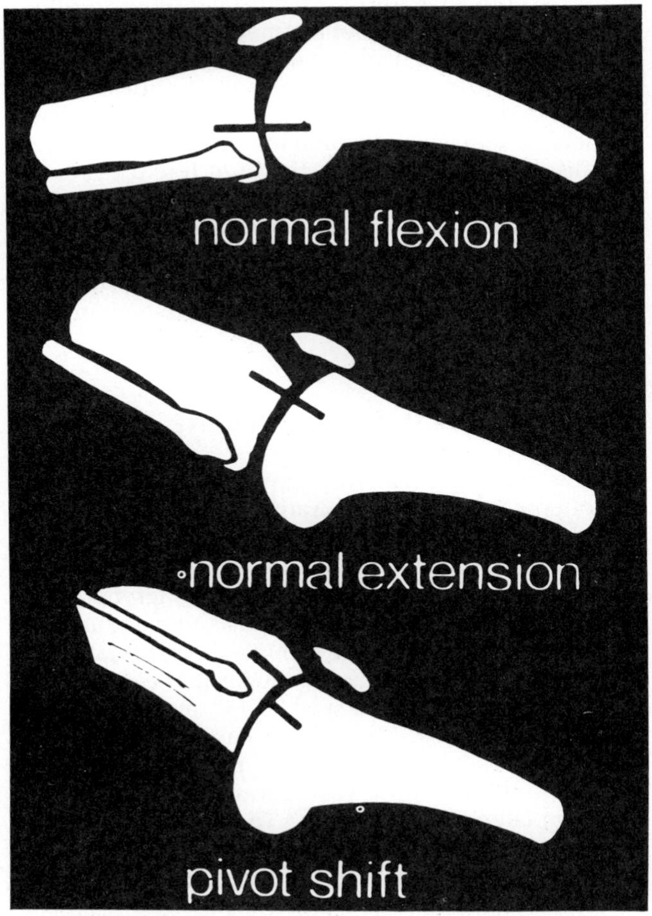

FIGURE 90–5. Principle of "pivot shift" phenomenon, anterior lateral tibial subluxation at full extension with reduction as the knee flexes past 20°.

is the ACL disruption. Over 70% of ACL injuries occur during sports activities and involve jumping and cutting motions during which abnormal valgus rotation forces cause disruption of the ligament. Severe swelling occurs within 2 to 6 hours. Over 80% of knees with traumatic hemarthrosis have acute ACL injuries. Most cases can be diagnosed by physical examination. Arthroscopy is reserved for cases with suspected associated damage such as torn menisci, osteochondral fractures, or loose bodies.[47–51]

Treatment of ACL injuries is based on the activity level and functional expectations of each individual. Patients with grade I or II laxity remain functionally stable after rehabilitation and modification of their activities. Those with grade IV knee laxity can be severely disabled whether the individual is athletic or not. Surgical reconstruction is usually recommended in such cases. Patients with grade III laxity fall into the "gray zone." Such knees may need surgical intervention if the patient wishes to be athletic, or if other associated ligaments are injured, or if there is a reparable meniscus. If doubt exists in the patient's mind regarding surgical reconstruction, then conservative measures are generally indicated. There is no conclusive evidence that surgical repair avoids late complications such as meniscal tear or degenerative arthritis.[52–57]

A medial collateral ligament injury usually heals satisfactorily without surgery, but there may be some late morbidity after unrepaired grade III disruptions. Treatment usually consists of a hinged cast or brace for 3 to 6 weeks. When MCL disruption is combined with ACL disruption, surgical repair is usually indicated. Not uncommonly, disruption of the medial retinaculum and vastus medialis is associated with patellar dislocation. Lateral ligamentous disruptions, like those of the medial ligaments, are usually associated with ACL disruption. Surgical repair of the fibular collateral and posterolateral structures (arcuate ligament complex and popliteus tendon) are generally recommended.[58,59]

Posterior cruciate ligament disruption is rare, occurring only 10% as frequently as ACL injury. Associated meniscal injuries are infrequent, but articular surface damage is not. This may result from the exaggerated pull of the quadriceps tendon on the patella to stabilize the knee in flexion. Many patients are only modestly impaired from this injury, but the incidence of late degenerative arthritis is high. Surgical repair is indicated when bone fragment is avulsed, enabling a stable fixation of the ligament. Repair of midsubstance tears are unsuccessful. Reconstructions are variably successful.[60–62]

Rehabilitation is important in the treatment of any knee injury. Normally, the hamstrings are two thirds as strong as the quadriceps, but after ACL injuries, the goal is to make the hamstring/quadriceps strength ratio 1 : 1. On the other hand, in posterior cruciate ligament injury, the goal is strengthening of the quadriceps maximally for knee stability. Similarly, after lateral ligament injuries with posterolateral instability, quadriceps strength is maximized and flexion exercises are eliminated to remove the detrimental effect of the biceps femoris.

OSTEOCHONDRITIS DISSECANS

Although the term denotes inflammation of bone and cartilage, osteochondritis dissecans presents with little inflammation. The condition occurs when an island of subchondral bone with its articular cartilage separates from the femoral condyle. This island, usually 1 to 2 cm in diameter, often "dissects" from the main condylar mass. It can be thought of as a small fracture that develops chronic nonunion. Eighty-five percent of these lesions are found in the knee joint, but they have been reported in many sites, including the femoral head, the dome of the talus, and the capitelum humeri.[63–65]

Osteochondritis dissecans is a condition of unknown origin in which 85% of the lesions appear on the medial or central portion of the medial femoral condyle and 15% occur laterally. These lesions are possibly shear fractures, but their occasional "mirror-image," bilateral occurrence suggests other anatomic or developmental causes. Prominent tibial spines have been associated with the condition and have been implicated as sites of impingement with rotation of the tibia against the condyles. The small bony island is probably alive at the time of separation or fracture. The edges of the bony fragment become necrotic, but the overlying articular cartilage, nourished by synovial fluid, remains alive. Studies on the blood supply of the condyles indicate a rich, anastomotic arterial network that makes localized infarction an unlikely cause. The lesion has been reported in families as an autosomal dominant condition.

This lesion is most common in adolescents and young adults, less common in patients in their 30s and 40s, and rare in the elderly, in whom degeneration overshadows the primary cause. Males are affected three times more than females. Shed or free fragments of bone loose in the knee joint are common in adults and rare in children. There are two types of lesions. One occurs in the skeletally immature individual, and healing almost always follows restriction of activity and splinting. The other occurs in the skeletally mature patient in whom there is a high incidence of fragment separation.

MRI can demonstrate the subchondral fracture but may not always permit detection of cartilage disruption. Arthroscopy is the best way to assess whether the lesion is a fragment in situ, a partially detached fragment, or a free body. Treatment of in situ lesions may be done by drilling the fragment in cases where healing is delayed. For the more usual partially detached fragment, bone grafts may be applied either directly under the articular cartilage or from a superior hole directed into the lesion using the arthroscope. Stabilization of free fragments includes inserting pins with the arthroscope. If a free fragment cannot be replaced, the free body is removed and the remaining bed is trephined to allow for fibrocartilaginous ingrowth and healing.[66–68]

Long-term followup studies have revealed that many patients with osteochondritis dissecans develop degenerative arthritis. Thirty-eight of 48 patients seen at an average of 33 years after diagnosis had arthritis. At least 20 years of observation are often required before arthritis is manifest. The arthritic process is accelerated in athletes.

TRAUMATIC CHONDRAL FRACTURES

Isolated cartilage fractures of the articular surface are not uncommon arthroscopic findings when meniscal pathology is suspected. Patients can usually describe an injury such as contact with an automobile dashboard or torsion during athletics. Symptoms usually include pain and chronic effusion, and there may be localized joint line tenderness. Terry has described three types of lesions: (1) stellate with central defect and radiating fissures, (2) flap with attached base, and (3) crater-type with exposed defect. In all cases, the underlying subchondral bone was exposed. Bony contact may be an important factor in these injuries. The tibial spine can be opposed to lesions on the medial femoral condyle, and in other cases, the lateral femoral condyle and tibial plateau lesions match in a weight-bearing position.

Treatment of these lesions remains controversial because of the limiting healing potential of damaged cartilage. Mankin has suggested that once a critical threshold of injury is reached with articular cartilage, permanent damage occurs and the occurrence of osteoarthritis is invariable. Thus, chondral fractures have a worse prognosis than typical meniscus tears. The long-term outcome of arthroscopically proven cases is unknown. These lesions are of interest relative to the pathophysiology of cartilage degeneration and illustrate the morbidity that may result from seemingly benign knee injuries.[69–72]

PATELLOFEMORAL MALALIGNMENT

Anterior knee pain is an important and common affliction often ascribed to chondramalcia patella, a morbid softening, fissuring degeneration process of the patellar cartilage. For the most part, however, this condition is primarily associated with patellar malalignment. The association between patellar crepitus and pain has been noted for many years. More recently, specific data have accumulated defining how malalignment can be studied and treated.[73] Using a specific 45° tangential radiograph of the patella, Merchant separated chondromalacia cases into two types: (1) those with normal alignment and (2) those with abnormal alignment resulting in lateral subluxation.[79] This problem has been further studied using tangential computed tomography with the knee in slight flexion. A classification scheme has evolved such that the direct arthroscopic appearance of the articular lesion can be correlated with findings of subluxation, subluxation and patellar tilt, patellar tilt alone, or normal alignment.[74]

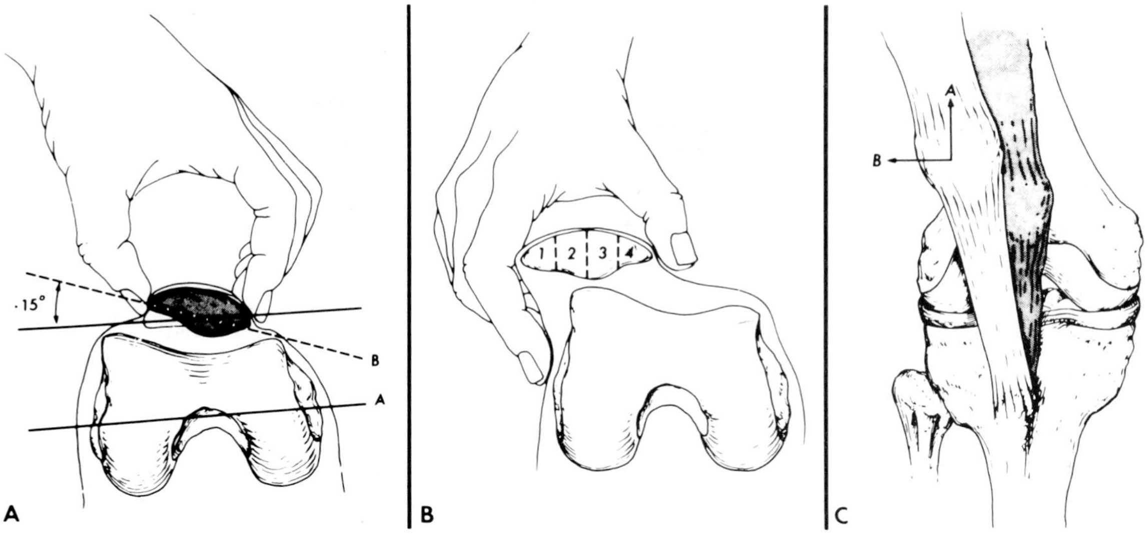

FIGURE 90–6. *A,* Passive patellar tilt indicates laxity of lateral ligamentous restraints. A patellar tilt of 0° or less indicates tight lateral retinacular ligaments. *B,* Passive lateral glide test demonstrates the ability to laterally displace the patella with the knee in full extension, subluxation beyond one half of its width indicates laxity of medial retinacular restraints. *C,* Increased "functional" Q angle is present if lateral excursion (B) exceeds proximal excursion (A).

The clinical evaluation of patellar alignment requires a detailed history of the onset and progression of patellar instability and pain. Bilateral pain and recurrent dislocation are usually associated with malalignment. A direct blow to the anterior knee does not cause malalignment. Symptoms consist of pain with activities involving knee flexion such as ascending or descending stairs, running, jumping, squatting, and progressive resistive exercise. Localized aching occurs after periods of immobility with the knee in the flexed position, such as watching television or working at a desk (the "movie sign"). Tenderness of the peripatellar muscle, tendon, and retinaculum may result from stretching of the lateral retinaculum when the extensor mechanism is abnormally aligned. This is to be distinguished from articular pain that is due to patellofemoral OA, which may be related to malalignment but can also be caused by trauma. Articular pain is usually increased by patellofemoral compression and is usually coupled with crepitus and effusion. Not all patients with crepitus have pain. Conversely, many have anterior knee pain without signs of chrondromalacia or crepitus.[75,76]

Physical examination of the knee may reveal noticeable tilting of the patella with active flexion and extension. Normally, the patella is firmly engaged in the trochlea at 30 to 40° of flexion. The passive patellar tilt test assesses patellar laxity when the lateral patellar edge is elevated from the femoral condyle. A 0° or a negative tilt angle usually reflects excessive lateral retinacular tightness. The passive patellar glide test estimates lateral patellar excursion. Lateral overhang exceeding half the width of the patellar usually indicates lax or torn medial patellofemoral restraints. The functional quadriceps (Q) angle measures the amount of lateral excursion compared with superior excursion as the patient contracts the quadriceps with the knee flexed 20°. If lateral excursion exceeds superior excursion, then an excessive lateral quadriceps vector exists. The overall alignment of the lower extremity should be assessed with the patient standing; look for anatomic variants that may increase the Q angle (i.e., the line of quadriceps pull from the patella and tibial tubercle) (Fig. 90–6). Vastus medialis

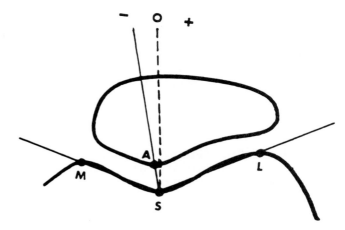

FIGURE 90–7. Merchant's angle of congruence measured from the sulcus angle MSL (mean = 137°) and SO, which bisects the sulcus angle. The congruence angle is ASO (mean = 6° and abnormal if greater than 4°).

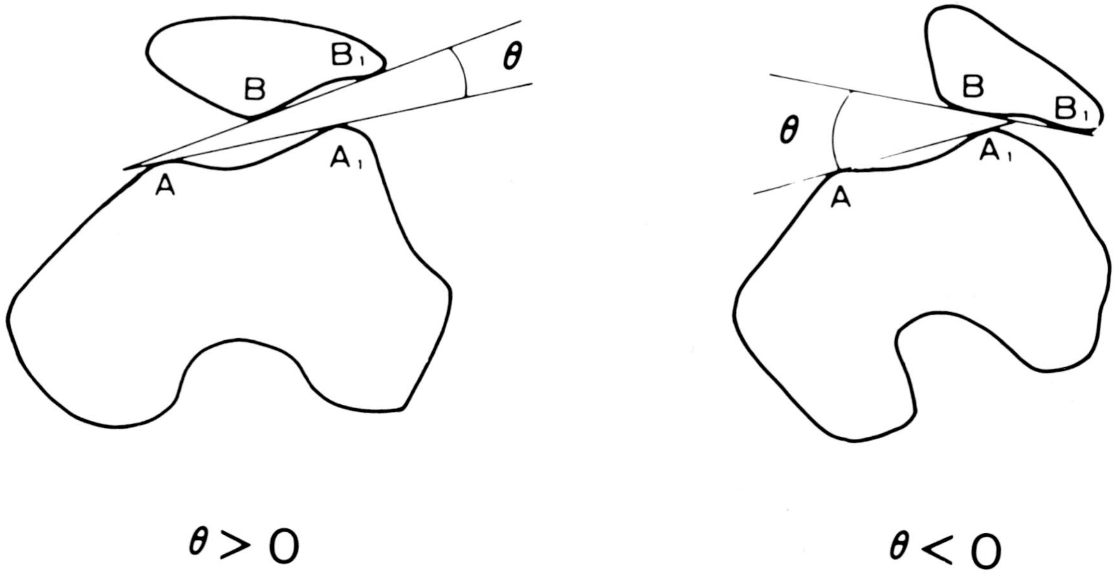

FIGURE 90–8. Angle of Laurin measures the lateral patellofemoral angle, where line A–A1 passes through the femoral condyles and B–B1 passes through the lateral patellar facet. The angle is positive if it opens laterally, and abnormal if it opens medially.

atrophy, laterally placed tibial tubercle, valgus deformity of the knee, and generalized laxity with forefoot pronation are findings associated with malalignment.[77]

Radiographic analysis of the patellofemoral joint includes the so-called "sunrise" (tangential) view of the patella. Merchant measured the angle of congruence on a standard tangential (axial) radiograph done with knee flexed 45°, and the x-ray beam directed at a 30° angle from the horizontal. This angle is made from a line of the bisected femoral trochlea and a line of the apex of the patella to the trochlear groove.[78] Aglietti believed that this angle of congruence should be less than 4°. It usually is negative (Fig. 90–7). Patellar tilt can be measured by the angle of Laurin, which measures the lateral patellofemoral angle with the knee in 20° of flexion. This angle measures the line of the lateral patellar facet compared with the line drawn across the lateral femoral trochlea. In the normal patellofemoral joint, if this angle opens laterally, it is positive. If there is abnormal patellar tilt, it opens medially and is negative (Fig. 90–8).[77–80]

Schutzer used computed tomography to define the normal patellar alignment. Using midpatellar transverse cuts at 0, 10, 20, and 30° of flexion, the patella enters the trochlea early in flexion of the knee with the angle of congruence equal to 0° at 10 and 20° of flexion. The patella is centered and upright without tilt beyond 10° of flexion.[80a] Computed tomography (if properly done) more accurately defines the normal patellofemoral relationship than do radiographs as they are obtained with the knee in near full extension where the subluxation occurs (Fig. 90–9). Standard radiographs must be taken with the knee in at least 20 to 30° of flexion and are less able to show the problem. Finally, technetium bone scintigraphy is helpful in identifying patellofemoral arthrosis and planning surgery.[81]

Arthroscopy is invaluable for assessing the extent of damage to the articular cartilage. Grading is done by the classification scheme of Outerbridge: stage 1, softening of the cartilage only; stage 2, fibrillation of less than 0.5 inch in width; stage 3, fibrillation or more than 0.5 inch in width; and stage 4, exposed bone.[82] Arthroscopic chondral debridement is indicated when recurrent effusion is caused by cartilage flaps and fibrillation. The underlying malalignment, however, must be corrected to prevent further progression of articular cartilage damage.

Patients may have varying degrees of patellar subluxation, tilt, or OA. Patients with subluxation alone may have transient episodes of instability more than pain. Osteoarthritis is not a prominent finding unless the patella has been damaged by dislocation. Patellar tilt without subluxation increases the risk of medial patellar OA from abnormal lessened contact and OA of the lateral

FIGURE 90–9. Radiographic evaluation of symptomatic patellar subluxation in a 38-year-old woman with patellofemoral arthrosis: *A*, Technetium bone scan demonstrates uptake in lateral patellofemoral joint. *B*, Hughston sunrise at 60° flexion shows no subluxation. *C*, Merchant's view at 30° flexion shows no subluxation. *D*, Computed tomography at 15° flexion shows significant subluxation.

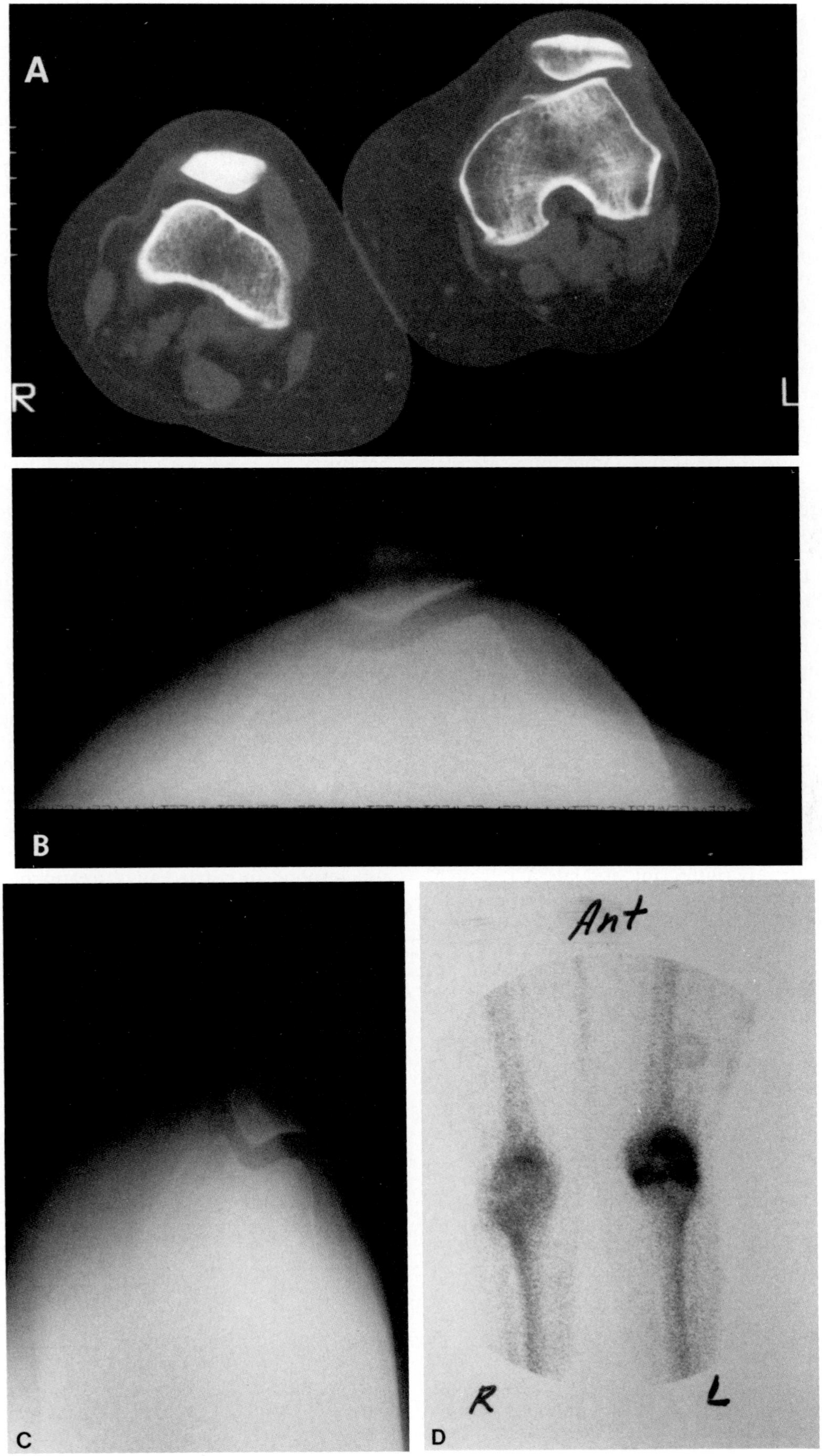
A
R
L
B
C
D
Ant
R
L

facet (lateral facet syndrome) because of increased pressure. There is lateral retinacular pain as the retinaculum is adaptively shortened and stretches as the knee flexes. The most symptomatic patients have both tilt and subluxation, which causes lateral facet syndrome, medial facet arthrosis, and instability. These patients have retinacular pain early in the course and have both articular breakdown and even patellar dislocation.[83,86]

Treatment of patellar malalignment is conservative initially. This includes exercises to stretch the retinaculum, hamstrings, and iliotibial band and to strengthen the quadriceps muscle, particularly the vastus medialis obliquus. Other modalities include elastic knee supports, anti-inflammatory medication, orthotics, and modification of activity. Short arc quadriceps exercises are important, and deep knee bends are to be avoided. Patients with crepitus and recurrent effusion are less likely to respond to this program. Other intra-articular pathology must be ruled out.[87]

Operative treatments aim at either correcting malalignment or reducing the symptoms of OA. For patellar subluxation, retinacular lateral release may be all that is needed, but the results of this intervention alone are inconsistent. Proximal medial advancement of the vastus medialis obliquus or even anteromedial transfer of the tibial tubercle may be needed to restore normal alignment. Patients with patellar tilt and no OA demonstrated by computed tomography will respond to lateral release alone. In patients with tilt and OA, lateral release and anteromedialization of the tibial tubercle are needed to reduce the forces on the patella.[88]

When degeneration of the articular cartilage reaches stage 3 or 4 on the lateral facet, lateral retinacular pain may resolve as the tension on the ligament shortens with cartilage loss. If bone scintigraphy is positive, articular damage is already significant, and lateral release is unlikely to be helpful. Patellectomy has been done in the past but often leaves the patient in chronic pain because of pre-existing damage to the femoral trochlea. Other problems include extensor lag and instability. Anterior tibial tubercle transfer by the Maquet procedure has been advocated, and significant relief of pain occurs if 10 to 15 mm of anterior transfer is done. This procedure has a significant complication rate including skin breakdown, infection, and nonunion of the graft. An alternative is the anteromedialization of the tibial tubercle described by Fulkerson: The tibial tubercle is advanced both anteriorly and medially for a distance of up to 17 mm. This procedure is for those cases with both OA and malalignment and has fewer reported complications. Accurate diagnosis is needed in treating these cases, and poorly planned procedures are likely to be ineffective or cause iatrogenic complications.[88–90]

SPONTANEOUS OSTEONECROSIS

The syndrome of osteonecrosis was defined by Ahlback and Bauer as sudden onset of pain in an older patient localized over the medial femoral condyle with a positive bone scan and the eventual development of a subchondral radiolucent lesion. Women over 60 years of age are most commonly affected. The onset of pain is so severe that many patients can describe the exact moment when it began. Night pain is common; activity only moderately increases pain. Exquisite tenderness exists over the medial femoral condyle and joint effusions are common. Early on, the hallmark is an intense uptake of bone-seeking radionuclide. These lesions also can be detected by MRI.[91,92]

The treatment and prediction of ultimate outcome depend on the radiographic features as well as the clinical picture. If bone scan and MRI findings are positive but standard radiographs are normal, the lesion is probably too small to be of consequence, and these patients can be treated with protracted protected weight bearing and analgesics. When the radiographic appearance is abnormal, these lesions can predictably be placed in one of two groups, depending on the size of the defect as a percentage of the affected condyle. If the lesion is less than 50% of the affected condyle, the prognosis is good and should be treated conservatively unless and until secondary degenerative changes occur. If medial compartment OA develops, high tibial osteotomy or unicondylar arthroplasty is indicated.[93–95]

In those cases involving more than 50% of the articular surface of the medial femoral condyle, there is a more progressive downhill course with bone loss and the development of contractures. Curretage of the lesion and proximal tibial osteotomy is not helpful. Unicondylar arthroplasty should be done early, once the clinical pattern is recognized. For severe cases, bicompartmental total arthroplasty may be needed.[96,97]

A similar condition has been recognized in the proximal tibial plateau, but these lesions are usually small and respond to conservative treatment. The cause of osteonecrosis of the knee remains unknown, but most authors regard it as a subchondral stress fracture as it more typically occurs in older osteoporotic women. Healing of these lesions is variable, and the ultimate outcome depends on the size of the lesion.[98]

OSTEOARTHRITIS

The cause of OA (see also Chapter 102) has been related to both injury and chronic occupational overuse. In one study, 4.5 times as many OA patients had a history of knee injury compared to controls. Obese people were at least 3.5 times more likely to have OA; individuals engaged in heavy manual labor were two to three times more likely to develop this condition. Long-distance running, on the other hand, was not likely to cause a higher incidence of OA, but such runners are not likely to be obese, and individuals with mechanical disorder or early OA probably exclude themselves and are not likely to become long-distance runners.[99]

Bony fracture is an important cause of late joint problems and OA. Elderly patients have generally poorer results after fracture treatment, either conservative or

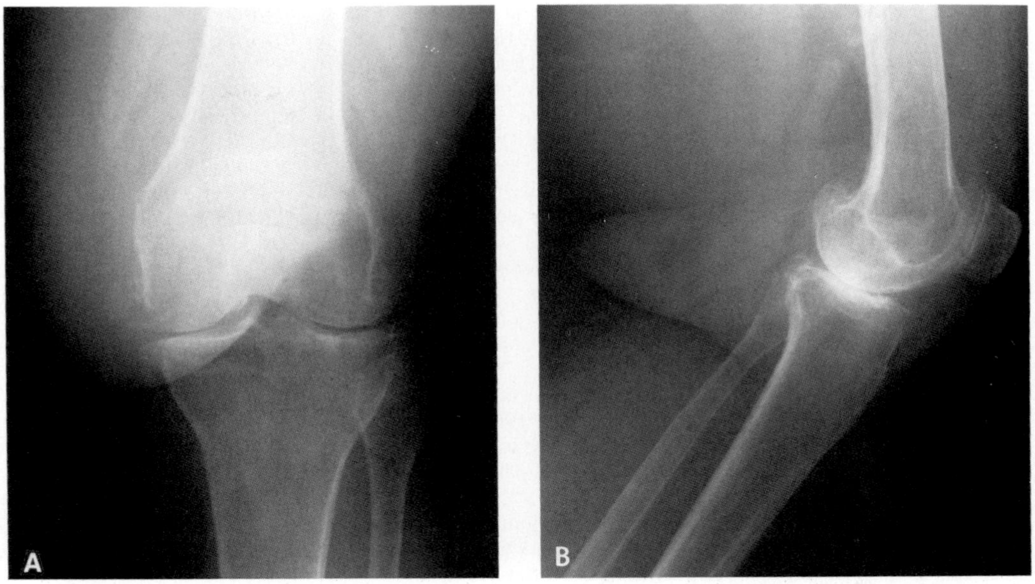

FIGURE 90–10. Anterior posterior (*A*) and lateral (*B*) radiograph demonstrating typical late findings of degenerative arthritis.

surgical. Violent injuries resulting in joint-comminuted and displaced fractures were found more likely to lead to OA. Also, most patients who were considered treatment failures developed arthritis early within the first 6 to 8 years. Anatomic restoration of articular congruity and joint alignment with early active and passive motion of the joint are the goals of early fracture treatment.[100]

From the foregoing discussion, the final common pathway of all mechanical disorders is secondary OA typified by cartilage loss, joint space narrowing, osteophyte formation, and angular deformity (Fig. 90–10). Clinical findings of importance include chronic pain unrelieved by nonsteroidal anti-inflammatory drugs, crepitus, joint line tenderness, significant loss in range of motion, and external varus or valgus deformity. Radiographically, it is important to define the degree of joint space narrowing. This can best be done with a 45° posteroranterior flexed weight-bearing radiograph, because the areas of increased contact of the articular surfaces and subsequently degeneration occur with the knee flexed 30 to 60°. If the joint space is narrowed more than 2 mm compared to the opposite normal side, then grade 3 or 4 degeneration of cartilage is likely to be present.[101]

The late treatment of knee OA is initially conservative and includes weight reduction, rest, restriction of activity, nonsteroidal anti-inflammatory medication, occasional injection of corticosteroids, and physical therapy. In cases for which this treatment is ineffective, alternatives include osteotomy to correct severe angular deformity and joint arthroplasty. With continued technical improvements, total joint replacement becomes an even more attractive salvage procedure in older patients.[102]

REFERENCES

1. Daniel, D., Daniels, E., and Aronson, D.: The diagnosis of meniscus pathology. Clin. Orthop., *163*:218–224, 1982.
2. Hamberg, P., Gillquist, J., and Lysholm, J.: Surture of new and old peripheral meniscus tears. J. Bone Joint Surg., *65A*:193–197, 1983.
3. Jones, R.E., Smith, E.C., and Resich, J.S.: Effects of medial meniscectomy in patients older than forty years. J. Bone Joint Surg., *60A*:783–786, 1978.
4. Noble, J., and Erat, K.: In defense of the meniscus. J. Bone Joint Surg., *62B*:7–11, 1980.
5. Sonne-Holm, S., Fledelius, I., and Ahn, N.: Results after meniscectomy in 147 athletes. Acta Orthop. Scand., *51*:303–309, 1980.
6. Hough, A.J., and Webber, R.J.: Pathology of the meniscus. Clin. Orthop., *252*:32–40, 1990.
7. Walker, P.S., and Erkman, M.J.: The role of the menisci in force transmission across the knee. Clin. Orthop., *109*:184–192, 1975.
8. Johnson, R.J.: Anatomy and biomechanics of the knee. *In* Operative Orthopaedics. Edited by M. Chapman. New York, Churchill Livingstone, 1983.
9. American Academy of Orthopaedic Surgeons Orthopaedic Knowledge Update, Vol. 1. Park Ridge, IL, A.A.O.S., 1982.
10. Arnold, J.A., et al.: Natural history of anterior cruciate tears. Am. J. Sports Med., 7:305–313, 1979.
11. Fetto, J.F., and Marshall, J.L.: The natural history and diagnosis of anterior cruciate ligament insufficiency. Clin. Orthop., *147*:29–38, 1980.
12. Grove, T.P. et al.: Non-operative treatment of the torn anterior cruciate ligament. J. Bone Joint Surg., *65A*:184–192, 1983.
13. Noyes, F.R. et al.: The symptomatic anterior cruciate-deficient knee: Part II. The results of rehabilitation activity modification and counseling on functional disability. J. Bone Joint Surg., *65A*:163–174, 1983.
14. Noyes, F.R. et al.: The symptomatic anterior cruciate-deficient

knee: Part I. The long term functional disability in athletically active individuals. J. Bone Joint Surg., *65A*:154–162, 1983.
15. Indelicato, P.A., and Bittar, E.S.: A perspective of lesions associated with ACL insufficiency of the knee. A review of 100 cases. Clin. Orthop., *198*:77–80, 1985.
16. Nicholas, J.A.: Injuries to the menisci of the knee. Orthop. Clin. North Am., *4*:647–664, 1973.
17. Bray, R.C., and Dandy, D.J.: Meniscal lesions and chronic anterior cruciate ligament deficiency. J. Bone Joint Surg., *71B*:128–130, 1989.
18. Warren, R.F., and Levi I.M.: Meniscal lesions associated with anterior cruciate ligament injury. Clin. Orthop., *172*:32–37, 1983.
19. DeHaven, K.E.: Diagnosis of acute knee injuries with hemarthrosis. Am. J. Sports Med., *8*:9–14, 1980.
20. Noyes, F.R. et al.: Arthroscopy in acute traumatic hemarthrosis of the knee. J. Bone Joint Surg., *62A*:687–695, 1980.
21. Fowler, P.J., and Lubliner, J.A.: The predictive value of five clinical signs in the evaluation of meniscal pathology. J. Arthros., *5*:184–186, 1989.
22. Dandy, D.J.: The arthroscopic anatomy of symptomatic meniscal lesions. J. Bone Joint Surg., *72B*:628–633, 1990.
23. Freiberger, R.H., and Kaye, J.J.: Arthrography. New York, Appleton-Century-Crofts, 1979.
24. Casscells, S.W.: The place of arthroscopy in the diagnosis and treatment of internal derangement of the knee: An analysis of 1000 cases. Clin. Orthop., *151*:135–142, 1980.
25. Curran W.P., and Woodward, E.P.: Arthroscopy: Its role in diagnosis and treatment of athletic knee injuries. Am. J. Sports Med., *8*:415–418, 1980.
26. Polly, D.W., Callaghan, J.J., Sikes, R.A., et al.: The accuracy of selective magnetic resonance imaging compared with the findings of arthroscopy of the knee. J. Bone Joint Surg., *70JA*:192–198, 1988.
27. Watanabe, A.T., Carter, B.C., Teitelbaum, G.P., and Bradley, W.G.: Common pitfalls in magnetic resonance imaging of the knee. J. Bone Joint Surg., *71A*:857–861, 1989.
28. Mink, J.H., and Deutsch, A.L.: Magnetic resonance imaging of the knee. Clin. Orthop., *244*:29–47, 1989.
29. Raunest, J., Oberle, K., Lochnert, J., and Hoetzinger, H.: The clinical value of magnetic resonance imaging in the evaluation of meniscal disorders. J. Bone Joint Surg., *73A*:11–29, 1991.
30. Glashow, J.L., Katz, R., Schneider, M., and Scott, W.N.: Double-blind assessment of the value of magnetic resonance imaging in the diagnosis of anterior cruciate and meniscal lesions. J. Bone Joint Surg., *71A*:113–119, 1989.
31. McGinty, J.B., and Freedman, P.A.: Arthroscopy of the knee. Clin. Orthop., *121*:173–180, 1976.
32. Watanabe, M.: Arthroscopy: The present state. Orthop. Clin. North Am., *10*:505–522, 1979.
33. O'Connor, R.L.: Arthroscopy. Philadelphia, J.B. Lippincott, 1977.
34. Torg, J.S., Conrad, W., and Kalen, V.: Clinical diagnosis of anterior cruciate ligament instability in the athlete. Am. J. Sports. Med., *4*:84–93, 1976.
35. Marshall, J.L., and Baugher, W.H.: Stability examination of the knee: A simple anatomic approach. Clin. Orthop., 146:78–83, 1980.
36. Marshall, J.L., Fetto, J.F., and Botero, P.M.: General orthopaedics: Knee ligament injuries: A standardized evaluation method. Clin. Orthop., *123*:115–129, 1977.
37. Hughston, J.C. et al.: Classification of knee ligament instabilities: Part I. The medial compartment and cruciate ligaments. J. Bone Joint Surg., *58A*:159–172, 1976.
38. Noyes, F.R., Grood, E.S., and Torzilli, P.A.: The definitions of terms for motion and position of the knee and injuries of the ligaments. J. Bone Joint Surg., *71A*:465–472, 1989.
39. Galway, H.R., and MacIntosh, D.L.: The lateral pivot shift: A symptom and sign of anterior cruciate ligament insufficiency. Clin. Orthop., *147*:45–50, 1980.
40. Slocum, D.B. et al.: Clinical test for anterolateral rotary instability of the knee. Clin. Orthop., *118*:63–69, 1976.
41. Jakob, R.P., Staubli, H.U., and Deland, J.T.: Grading the pivot shift. J. Bone Joint Surg., *69B*:294–299, 1987.
42. Harter, R.A., Osternig, L.R., and Singer, K.M.: Instrumented Lachman tests for evaluation of anterior laxity after reconstruction of the anterior cruciate ligament. J. Bone Joint Surg., *71A*:975–987, 1989.
43. Baker, C.L., Norwood, L.A., and Hughston, J.C.: Acute posterolateral rotatory instability of the knee. J. Bone Joint Surg., *65A*:614–618, 1983.
44. Hughston, J.C., and Norwood, L.A.: The posterolateral drawer test and external rotational recurvatum test for posterolateral rotatory instability of the knee. Clin. Orthop., *147*:82–87, 1980.
45. Hughston, J.C., and Barrett, G.R.: Acute anteromedial rotatory instability. J. Bone Joint Surg., *65A*:145–153, 1983.
46. Gurtler, R.A., Sjtine, R., and Toro, J.S.: Lachman test evaluated. Clin. Orthop., *216*:141–150, 1987.
47. Butler, J.C., and Andrews, J.R.: The role of arthroscopic surgery in the evaluation of acute traumatic hemarthrosis of the knee. Clin. Orthop., *228*:150–152, 1988.
48. Sandberg, R., and Balkfors, B.: Partial rupture of the anterior cruciate ligament. Clin. Orthop., *220*:176–178, 1987.
49. Bumberg, B.C., and McGinty, J.B.: Acute hemarthrosis of the knee: Indications for diagnostic arthroscopy. J. Arthros., *6*:221–225, 1990.
50. Kannus, P., and Jarvinen, M.: Long-term prognosis of nonoperatively treated acute knee distortions having primary hemarthrosis without clinical instability. Am. J. Sports Med., *15*:138–148, 1987.
51. Casteleyn, P.P., Handelberg, F., and Opdecan, P.: Traumatic hemarthrosis of the knee. J. Bone Joint Surg., *70B*:404–406, 1988.
52. Barrack, R.L., Buckley, S.L., Bruckner, J.D., et al.: Partial versus complete acute anterior cruciate ligament tears. J. Bone Joint Surg., *72JB*:622–627, 1990.
53. Noyes, F.R., Barber, S.D., and Mangine, R.E.: Bone–patellar ligament–bone and fascia latas allografts for reconstruction of the anterior cruciate ligament. J. Bone Joint Surg., *72A*:1125–1136, 1990.
54. Noyes, F.R., Bassett, R.W., Grood, E.S., and Butler, D.L.: Arthroscopy in acute traumatic hemarthrosis of the knee. J. Bone Joint Surg., *62A*:687–695, 1980.
55. Kannus, P., and Jarvinen, M.: Conservatively treated tears of the anterior cruciate ligament. J. Bone Joint Surg., *71A*:975–987, 1989.
56. Pattee, G.A., Fox, J.M., DelPizzo, W., and Friedman, M.J.: Four to ten year followup of unreconstructed anterior cruciate ligament tears. Am. J. Sports Med., *17*:430–435, 1989.
57. American Academy of Orthopaedic Surgeons Orthopaedic Knowledge Update. Vol. 3. Park Ridge, IL, A.A.O.S., 1990.
58. Kannus, P.: Long-term results of conservatively treated medial collateral ligament injuries of the knee joint. Clin. Orthop., *226*:103–112, 1988.
59. Sandberg, R., Balkfors, B., Nilsson, B., and Westlin, N.: Operative versus non-operative treatment of recent injuries to the ligaments of the knee. J. Bone Joint Surg., *69A*:1120–1126, 1987.
60. Clancy, W.G. et al.: Treatment of knee joint instability secondary to rupture of the posterior cruciate ligament. J. Bone Joint Surg., *65A*:310–322, 1983.
61. Torg, J.S., Barton, T.M., Pavlov, H., and Stine, R.: Natural his-

tory of the posterior cruciate ligament-deficient knee. Clin. Orthop., *246*:208–216, 1989.

62. Daniel, D., Stone, M.L., Barnett, P. and Sachs, R.: Use of the quadriceps active test to diagnose posterior cruciate-ligament disruption and measure posterior laxity of the knee. J. Bone Joint Surg., *70A*:386, 1988.
63. Aichroth, P.: Osteochondritis dissecans of the knee: A clinical survey. J. Bone Joint Surg., *53A*:440–447, 1971.
64. Fairbank, H.A.T.: Osteochondritis dissecans. Br. J. Surg., *21*:67–82, 1933.
65. Linden, B.: Osteochrondritis dissecans of the femoral condyles. J. Bone Joint Surg., *59A*:769–776, 1977.
66. Smillie, I.S.: Treatment of osteochondritis dissecans. J. Bone Joint Surg., *39B*:248–260, 1957.
67. Hughston, J.C., Hergenroeder, P.T., and Courtenay, B.G.: Osteochondritis dissecans of the femoral condyles. J. Bone Joint Surg., *66A*:1340–1348, 1984.
68. Stougaard, J.: Familial occurrence of osteochondritis dissecans. J. Bone Joint Surg., *46B*:542–543, 1964.
69. O'Donoghue, D.H.: Chondral and osteochondral fractures. J. Trauma, *6*:469–481, 1966.
70. Mankin, H.J.: Biochemical Changes in Articular Cartilage in Osteoarthritis. St. Louis, C.V. Mosby, 1976.
71. Zamber, D.W., Teitz, C.C., McGuire, D.A., et al.: Articular cartilage lesions of the knee. J. Arthros., *5*:258–268, 1989.
72. Terry, G.C., Flandry, R., Vanmanen, J.W., and Norwood, L.A.: Isolated chondral fractures of the knee. Clin. Orthop. *234*:170–177, 1988.
73. Haut, R.C.: Contact pressures in the patellofemoral joint during inpact loading on the human flexed knee. J. Orthop. Res., *7*:272–280, 1989.
74. Merchant, A.C.: Classification of patellofemoral disorders. J. Arthros., *4*:235–240, 1988.
75. Insall, J.: Current concepts review: Patellar pain. J. Bone Joint Surg., *64A*:147–152, 1982.
76. Kettelkamp, D.B.: Current concepts review: Management of patellar malalignment. J. Bone Joint Surg., *63A*:1344–1348, 1981.
77. American Academy of Orthopaedic Surgeons Orthopaedic Knowledge Update. Vol. 2. Park Ridge, IL, A.A.O.S., 1985.
78. Merchant, A.C. et al.: Roentgenographic analysis of patellofemoral congruence. J. Bone Joint Surg., *56A*:1391–1396, 1974.
79. Aglietti, P., Insall, J.N., Cerulli, G.: Patella pain and incongruence, I: Measurements of incongruence. Clin. Orthop., *176*:217–224, 1983.
80. Laurin, C.A. et al.: The abnormal lateral patellofemoral angle: A diagnostic roentgenographic sign of recurrent patellar subluxation. J. Bone Joint Surg., *60A*:55–60, 1978.

80a. Schutzer, S.F., Ramsby, G.R., Fulkerson, J.P.: Computed tomographic classification of patellofemoral pain patients. Ortho. Clin. N. Am.: *17*:235–248, 1986.

81. Inoue, M., Shino, K., Hirose, H., et al.: Subluxation of the patella, computed tomography analysis of patellofemoral congruence. J. Bone Joint Surg., *70A*:1331–1337, 1988.
82. Outerbridge, R.E.: The etiology of chordeo malecia pattelae. J. Bone Joint Surg., *43B*:752–757, 1961.
83. Johnson, R.P.: The lateral facet syndrome of the patella. Lateral restraint analysis and use of lateral resection. Clin. Orthop., *233*:61–71, 1988.
84. Ficat, R.P., and Hungerford, D.S. (eds.): Disorders of the Patellofemoral Joint: The Excessive Lateral Pressure Syndrome. Baltimore, Williams & Wilkins, 1977.
85. Larson, R.L.: Subluxation-dislocation of the patella. *In* The Injured Adolescent Knee. Edited by J.C. Kennedy. Baltimore, Williams & Wilkins, 1979.
86. Macnab, I.: Recurrent dislocation of the patella. J. Bone Joint Surg., *34A*:957–967, 1952.
87. Whitelaw, G.P., Rullo, D.J., Markowitz, H.D., et al.: A conservative approach to anterior knee pain. Clin. Orthop., *246*:234–237, 1989.
88. Fulkerson, J.P., and Shea, K.P.: Current concepts review: Disorders of patellofemoral alignment. J. Bone Joint Surg., *72A*:1424–1429, 1990.
89. Ferguson, A.B., Jr. et al.: Relief of patellofemoral contact stress by anterior displacement of the tibial tubercle. J. Bone Joint Surg., *61A*:159–172, 1979.
90. Maquet, P.G.J.: Biomechanics of the Knee: With Application to the Pathogenesis and the Surgical Treatment of Osteoarthritis. New York, Springer-Verlag, 1976.
91. Ahlback, S., Bauer, G.C.H., and Bohne, W.H.: Spontaneous osteonecrosis of the knee. Arthritis Rheum., *11*:705–733, 1968.
92. Rozing, P.M., Insall, J., and Bohne, W.H.: Spontaneous osteonecrosis of the knee. J. Bone Joint Surg., *62A*:2–7, 1980.
93. Pollack, M.S., Dalinka, M.K., Kressel, H.Y., et al.: Magnetic resonance imaging in the evaluation of suspected osteonecrosis of the knee. Skeletal Radiol., *16*:121–127, 1987.
94. Bauer, G.C.H.: Osteonecrosis of the knee. Clin. Orthop., *130*:210–217, 1978.
95. Lotke, P.A., Ecker, M.L., and Alavi, J.A.: Painful knees in older patients. J. Bone Joint Surg., *59A*:617–621, 1977.
96. Lotke, P.A., Abend, J.A., and Ecker, M.L.: The treatment of osteonecrosis of the medial femoral condyle. Clin. Orthop., *171*:109–115, 1982.
97. Muheim, G., and Bohne, J.G.: Prognosis in spontaneous osteonecrosis of the knee. J. Bone Joint Surg., *52B*:605–612, 1970.
98. Lotke, P.A., and Ecker, M.L.: Osteonecrosis-like syndrome of the medial tibial plateau. Clin. Orthop., *176*:148–153, 1983.
99. Kohatsu, N.D., and Schurman, D.J.: Risk factors for the development of osteoarthrosis of the knee. Clin. Orthop., *261*:242–250, 1990.
100. Volpin, G., Dowd, G.S.E., Stein, H., and Bentley, G.: Degenerative arthritis after intra-articular fractures of the knee. J. Bone Joint Surg., *72B*:634–638, 1990.
101. Messiah, S.S., Fowler, P.J., and Munro, T.: Anterior posterior radiographs of osteoarthritis of the knee. J. Bone Joint Surg., *72JB*:639–640, 1990.
102. Evarts, C.M., DeHaven, K., and Nelson, C.L.: Proximal tibial osteotomy for degenerative arthritis of the knee. Orthop. Clin. North Am., *2*:231–243, 1971.

91

Painful Feet

JOHN S. GOULD

Painful foot disorders have been classified according to relative anatomic areas, for example, metatarsalgia, arch strain, heel pain, with empiric efforts made to treat these nonspecific entities. The modern orthopedist evaluates the foot for biomechanical, vascular, neurogenic (local and referred), infectious, neoplastic, traumatic, developmental, and acquired disorders. Each area of the anatomy may be the source of the disorder, or a reflection of an underlying problem involving the skin, bursae, tendons, nerves, fasciae, blood vessels, joints, and bone.

Evaluation begins with the history and physical examination, includes the use of foot mirrors and footprint papers in the office, and may require noninvasive vascular analysis, nerve conduction studies and electromyography, plain radiographs, computed tomography (CT), magnetic resonance imaging (MRI), sophisticated gait analysis (force plate) examination, and routine or specialized laboratory tests. Management of the problems, of course, includes medical and surgical solutions, but also may involve simple or sophisticated pedorthic prescriptions, pedicare (nail, corn, and callus trimming), and physical therapy. The pedorthist (trained and certified in the fabrication of orthotic devices for the foot and the modification and custom design of shoes), the skilled foot-care nurse, and the physical therapist have collaborated with the orthopedist, rheumatologist, dermatologist, and peripheral vascular specialists to provide a multidisciplinary approach to optimal foot care.

PAINFUL TOES

Painful toes or areas of the toes may result from trauma or from an underlying acquired or congenital deformity, which becomes painful after contact with certain types of footwear.

ATHLETIC INJURIES

Various athletic injuries may also be associated with toe injuries. Acute or chronic trauma to toenails often occurs in skiers, who may bruise the nail to the great or long second toe in a new, hard boot. The subungual hematoma is obvious and requires treatment with a longer or better-fitting boot, and occasional drainage of the hematoma when exquisitely painful. More subtle, repetitive trauma occurs in tennis players, whose nails simply become white after a low-grade injury, and eventually slough (tennis toe). A similar injury occurs in ballet dancers.[1]

CORNS

Persons with fixed flexion contractures of the distal interphalangeal joint from an acquired hammer or mallet toe or from a congenital mallet toe can develop an apical corn on the tip of the toe. Shoes with a higher or increased depth of the toe box and lower heels will help, but loafers and fashionable shoes with the usual tapered toe cause pain. For flexion deformity of the distal joint, resection of the distal middle phalanx condyles, with or without formal fusion, resolves the problem.

Corns develop typically on the dorsum of the joints, which are acutely angled dorsally, as over a claw toe when contact is made with a hard shoe (Fig. 91–1). The underlying problem may be congenital clawing, or an acquired phenomenon associated with crowding of the second toe by the great toe in a bunion deformity, congenital overlapping of the fifth toe, and dislocation or subluxation of the metatarsophalangeal (MTP) joints from synovitis. The dorsum of the joint contacts the shoe, producing callus formation. As the callus grows, it causes pain on contact. Pedicare by trimming or "paring" or by abrading the corn with a pumice stone is

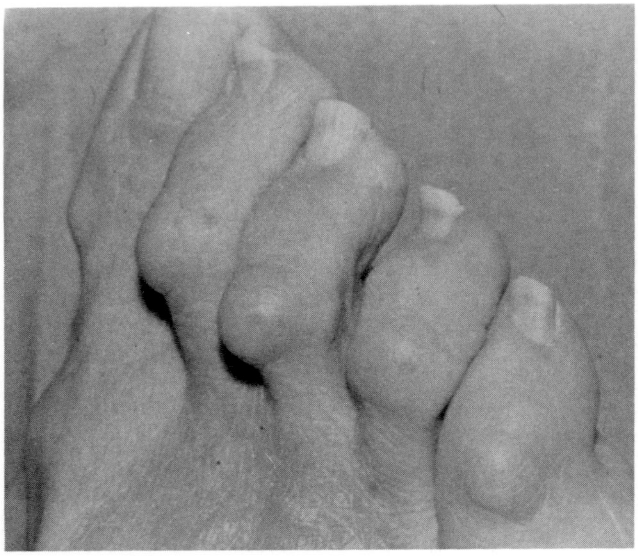

FIGURE 91–1. Claw toes with corns over proximal interphalangeal joints.

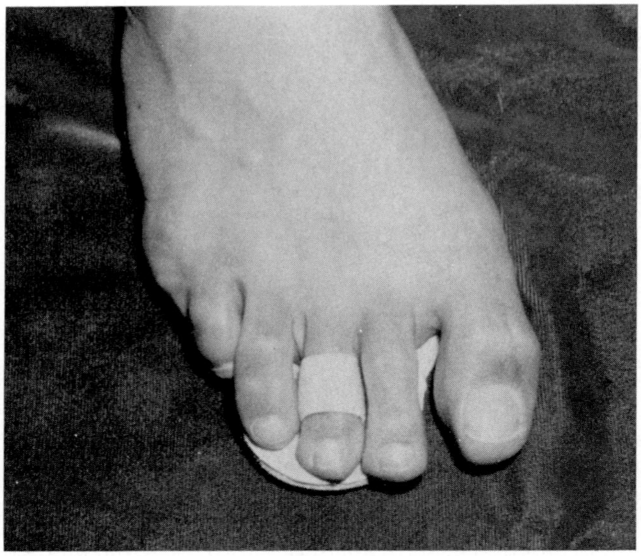

FIGURE 91–2. Use of a toe shield to correct a claw toe.

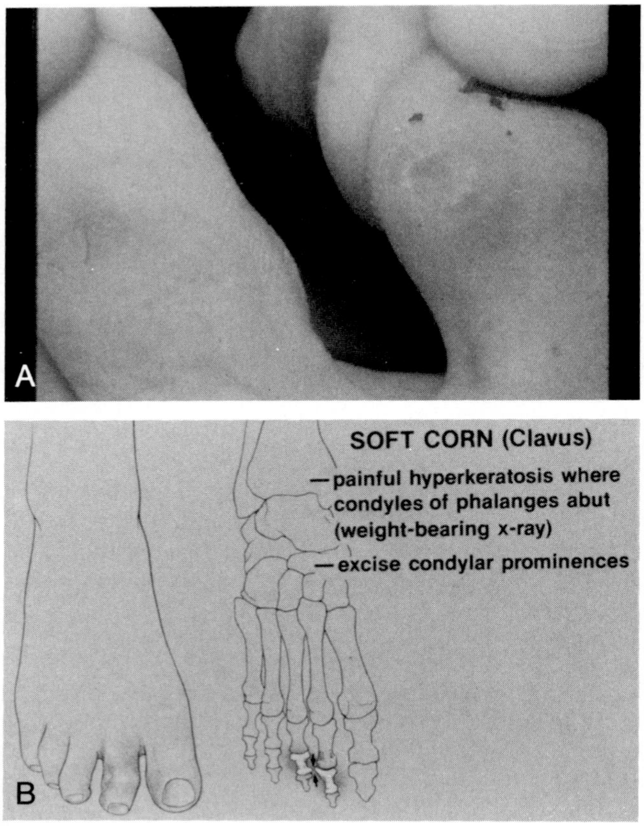

A
SOFT CORN (Clavus)
—painful hyperkeratosis where condyles of phalanges abut (weight-bearing x-ray)
—excise condylar prominences
B

FIGURE 91–3. *A*, Soft corn between toes secondary to contacting adjacent condyles. *B*, Artist's depiction of soft corn pathodynamics.

helpful; moleskin cutouts (corn pads), higher toe boxes in shoes, stretching the contacting area of shoe leather (use of the shoemakers' wand), and dynamic correction of a flexible deformity with a toe shield (Fig. 91–2) are all conservative approaches to the problem.[2] Surgical correction of bunions, overlapping toes, and claw toes may be needed. Joint resection, fusions, and dynamic corrections with tendon transfers may be indicated.

Soft corns (Fig. 91–3) develop between toes when contacting condyles of the adjacent toes cause extremely painful callus formation. Toe separators help, but simple condylectomies relieve the problem, which originated during toe crowding from certain footwear.[3] For soft corns deep in the 4/5 web, excision of the involved skin and extending the webbing more distally (partial syndactylization) is the treatment of choice.

INGROWN TOENAILS

Ingrown toenails may occur from inappropriate short trimming or may follow trauma with secondary infections. In mild cases, the nail grooves are gently packed with cotton to allow the nail to grow out normally. More refractory problems may require *partial matrixectomies* performed mechanically, chemically (phenol), or with lasers; or *wedge resections* of nail and matrix.[4] Recalcitrant cases are treated by *total matrixectomy*, with and without skin grafting, or by *excision of nail and distal phalanx tuft* (terminal Syme's procedure).

SYNOVITIS

"Jamming" and hyperextension injuries, particularly to the great toe joint, may occur on artificial athletic field surfaces (turf toe). Such traumatic synovitis is effectively treated with splinting, rest, and nonsteroidal anti-inflammatory drugs. Osteochondral fractures may be

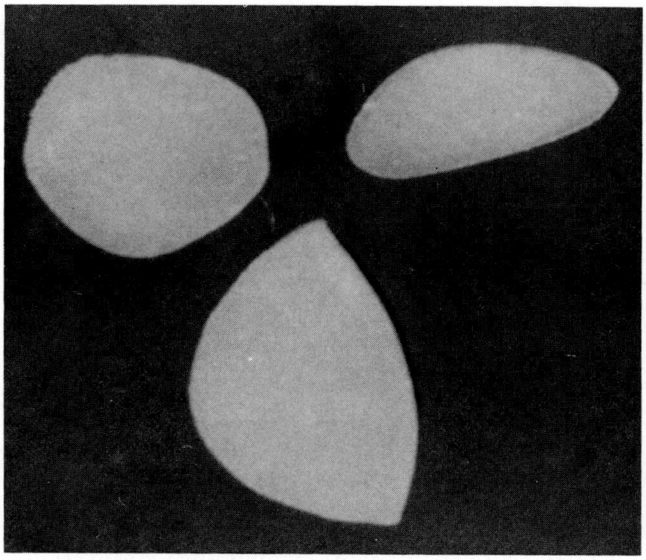

FIGURE 91–4. A variety of metatarsal felt pads may be shaped and cemented to the insole of the shoe behind painful lesions.

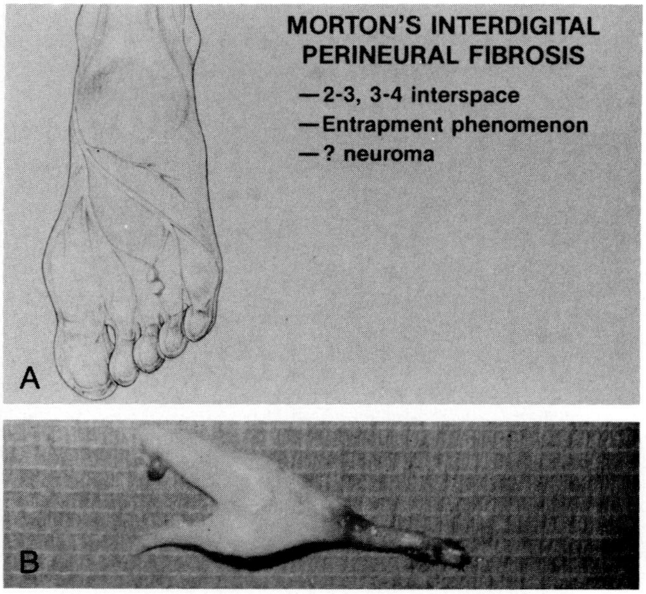

FIGURE 91–5. *A*, Artist's rendition of the thickened interdigital nerve (Morton's neuroma). *B*, The resected interdigital nerve. Note the marked enlargement of the nerve.

found in refractory cases and require surgical intervention.

MORTON'S NEUROMA

Toe pain emanating from the web space, particularly from compression of an interdigital nerve, occurs frequently in athletes or middle-aged patients. So-called Morton's neuroma,[5] pain from perineural fibrosis, results from compression of an interdigital nerve under the intermetatarsal ligament. The patient presents with shooting pain into the toes, or paresthesias or numbness in the involved toes and localized pain with compression of the metatarsal heads. Tenderness is specifically localized between the involved metatarsal heads, typically between the third and fourth, less frequently between the second and third. More specific findings include palpation of a mass, divergence of the toes, and a clicking sensation when the adjacent toes are flexed and extended. In acute cases, a metatarsal pad (Fig. 91–4) behind the involved heads may help. An association with a pronated foot may require longitudinal arch support as well. More resistant cases are treated with local corticosteroid injections; the most refractory cases require neurectomy (Fig. 91–5).[6] Simple division of the intermetatarsal ligament alone has had some recent interest.[7]

METATARSALGIA

Metatarsal pain, frequently plantar, may be isolated to a specific joint or generalized across the ball of the foot.[8] As already discussed, Morton's neuroma may present as pain in the metatarsal area. Other localized problems are delineated below.

BUNIONS

Hallux valgus, usually associated with *metatarsus primus varus*, or "splay" between the first and second metatarsals, is not in itself painful. However, patients seek medical help for the correction of appearance and for the relief of pain caused by footwear. Although some MTP joints become secondarily arthritic, the pain usually occurs over the medial prominence of the first metatarsal head, under the second metatarsal head, or over the proximal interphalangeal joint of the second toe. Unshod populations also develop bunion deformities but rarely request medical help, apparently because of lack of pain.[9] The medial first MTP pain may be secondary to an inflamed bursa (Fig. 91–6) or to pressure on the medial branch of the superficial peroneal nerve, which is stretched over the bunion and compressed. The painful corn over the second proximal interphalangeal joint has already been described. The callosity (intractable plantar keratosis) under the second metatarsal head is secondary to altered weight-bearing (Fig. 91–7). As the first metatarsal moves into varus at its joint with the first cuneiform, its head also moves dorsally, resulting in a transfer of weight to the second metatarsal head. This is known as a "transfer lesion," and it is further accentuated as the second MTP joint hyperextends. Biomechanically, with the toe now positioned dorsally, further downward force is exerted on the metatarsal head.

Bunion pain can be managed using a shoe with a wider toebox and increased depth (made on a bunion

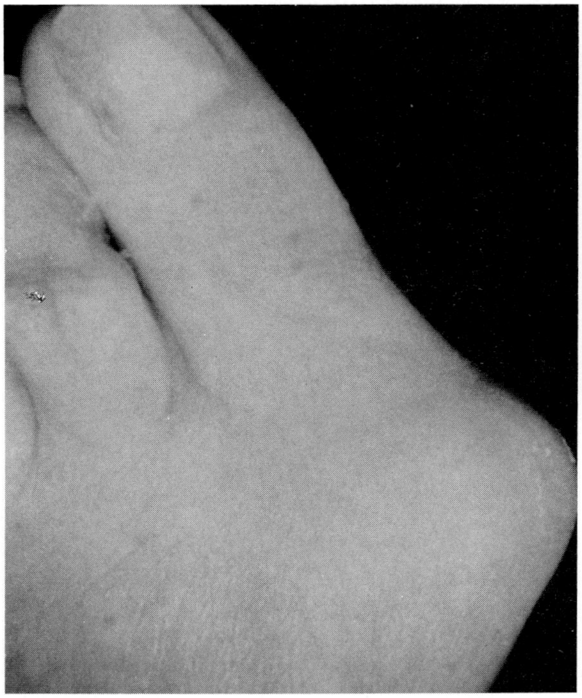

FIGURE 91–6. Bunion (hallux valgus) deformity with medial bursa.

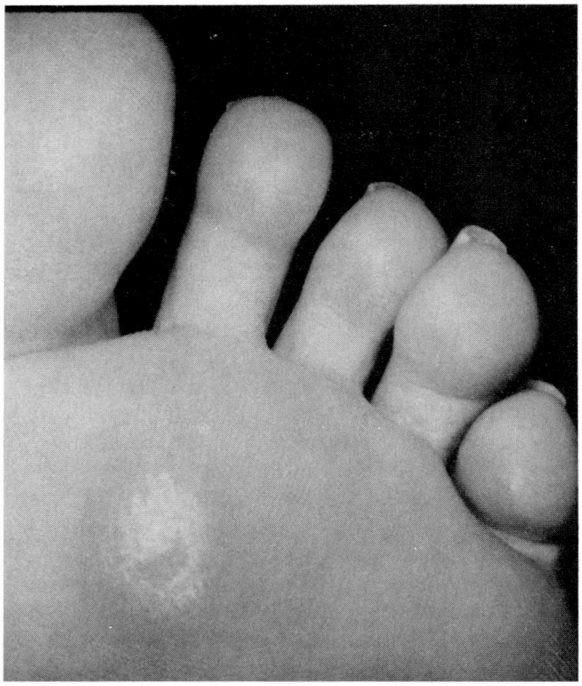

FIGURE 91–7. Intractable plantar keratosis (IPK) under second metatarsal head (transfer lesion).

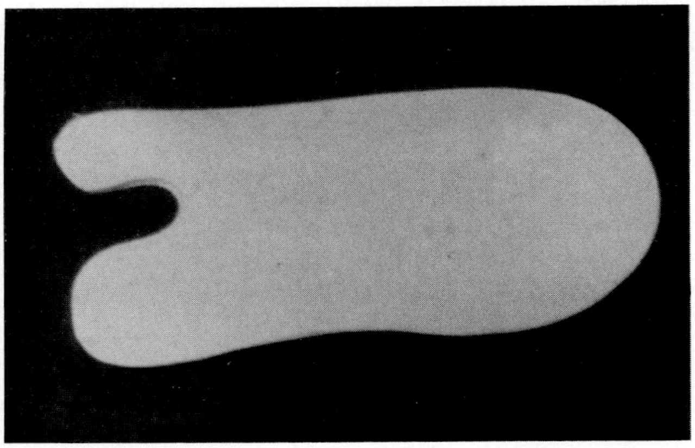

FIGURE 91–8. Total contact insert with relief around IPK.

last), and with a "total contact" insert increasing the thickness of the material proximal to the painful second metatarsal head, around it, and particularly under the first metatarsal head ("Morton's extension") (Fig. 91–8). Paring an associated callus is also helpful.

Treatment of more severe cases is by osteotomy, which moves the first metatarsal back to the neutral position, decreases the angle between the first and second metatarsals to less than 8° (normal), and depresses the first metatarsal head slightly plantarward. I perform a concentric-shaped osteotomy at the first metatarsal base.[9] Distally, the medial prominence of the first metatarsal is excised (ostectomy), the soft tissue is released laterally, and the capsule is imbricated medially with realignment of the sesamoids. The toe is thus realigned, and the bunion corrected. The deformity of the second toe is also corrected, often with a capsulectomy and tenotomy at the MTP joint. I resect the proximal phalanx distal condyles in a fixed deformity at the proximal interphalangeal joint, with a flexor to extensor tendon transfer. A transfer alone may be sufficient to correct a flexible deformity.

BUNIONETTE

A *bunionette* (tailor's bunion) is the reverse of the first MTP joint bunion, involving the fifth MTP joint. A bursa forms over the lateral prominence of the fifth metatarsal head. Again, a wider toebox and a moleskin cutout may help. Surgical correction can usually be accomplished by simple resection of the fifth metatarsal prominence. If splay between the fourth and fifth metatarsals is significant, an osteotomy (usually an oblique diaphyseal type) is done to narrow the foot, along with the ostectomy.

HALLUX RIGIDUS

Other painful afflictions around the hallux (great toe) include hallux rigidus, a degenerative arthritis of the first MTP joint, typically occurring in relatively young men, characterized by localized dorsal spurring on the

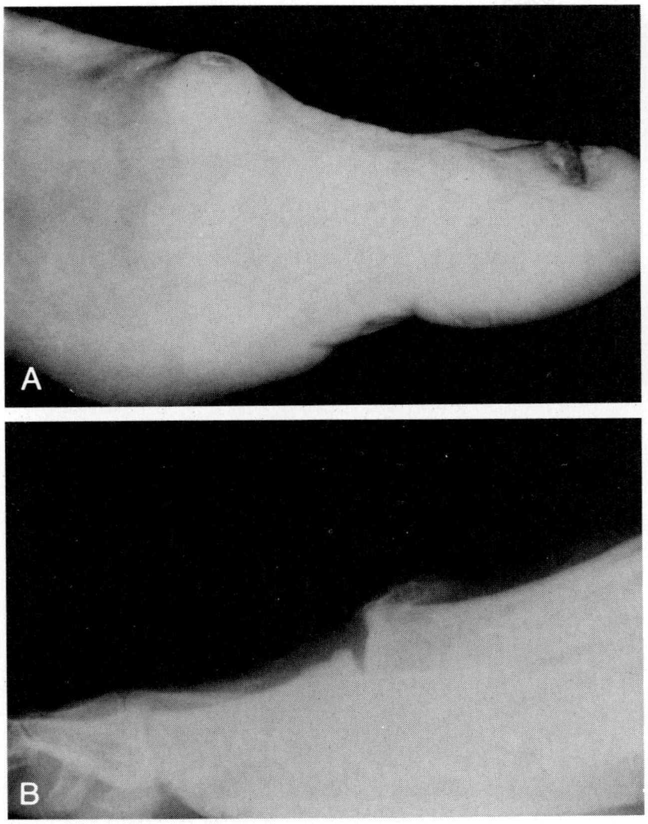

FIGURE 91–9. *A*, Clinical appearance of hallux rigidus. *B*, Radiograph of hallux rigidus. Note dorsal spurring at first MTP joint.

first metatarsal head (Fig. 91–9), but not generalized MTP joint arthritis. Dorsiflexion of the first MTP joint is limited, as is motion in the first cuneiform–first metatarsal joint, thought to be the primary source of the problem.

Traumatic arthritis or osteoarthritis of the first MTP joint also results in pain and loss of motion, but here the process is generalized. Primary osteoarthritis is common in this joint, but more frequently afflicts the first cuneiform–first metatarsal joint.

Conservative treatment includes NSAIDs and the use of stiff-soled shoes. An extended steel shank between the outsole and midsole or insole may be needed from the heel to the distal end of the sole. This eliminates the normal sole break and a rocker sole must be added to the shoe. This dramatically relieves the pain in most cases. If it does not, resection of the dorsal half of the first metatarsal head (cheilectomy) will allow increased motion and is the procedure of choice. More extensive arthritis is treated by hemiresection of the joint (Keller arthroplasty), prosthetic replacement, or arthrodesis.[10] The latter procedure is generally favored by most foot surgeons today, because pain, including transfer lesion pain, is relieved, and weight can again be borne on the first ray.

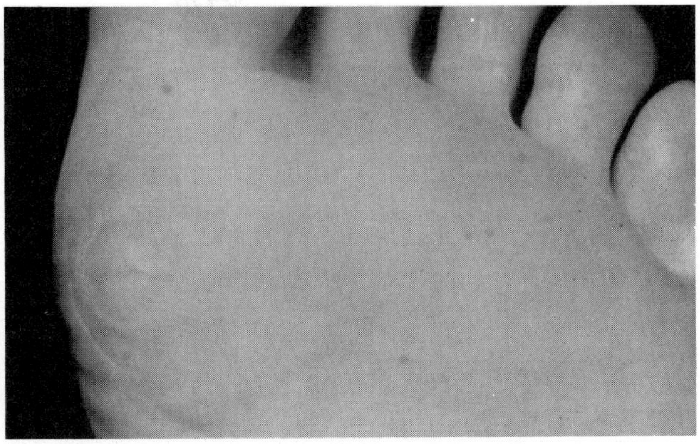

FIGURE 91–10. Callus (IPK) under tibial sesamoid.

SESAMOIDITIS

Pain under the great toe sesamoids may arise from prominence of the tibial sesamoid (Fig. 91–10), from chondromalacia, or from osteoarthritis between the sesamoid and its articulation with the plantar condyles of the metatarsal head. With a localized prominence under a single sesamoid, paring of the associated callus and a total contact insert under the painful area will help. Shaving the plantar surface of the prominent sesamoid is often sufficient, but a total sesamoidectomy is usually necessary when advanced chondromalacia or osteoarthritis has developed and nonoperative means have failed. This is not done frequently today because imbalance of alignment of the toe from disruption of one tendon of the flexor brevis may occur. One sesamoid can usually be safely removed, unless bunionectomy is required also. Here the balance is more delicate and sesamoidectomy should be avoided.

SYNOVITIS OF THE MTP JOINTS

Inflammation of the MTP joints can be significantly relieved by the use of an extended steel shank and rocker sole. In rheumatoid arthritis, the problem may be extensive with upward subluxation of the proximal phalanx, forward shift of the plantar fat pad under the toes, and significant loss of articular cartilage (Fig. 91–11). Clawing of the toes may occur, with development of calluses, corns, and adventitial bursae. In such cases the patient requires an extra-depth shoe, usually made with a pliable leather upper such as deerskin. Polyethylene foam (Plastazote) may be bonded to the leather and heat-molded to the patient's foot. A total contact insert is made with polyethylene foam of various grades (e.g., Plastazote, Pelite) (Fig. 91–12), built up behind the heads and relieved under them. In areas of breakdown or impending ulcer, the relieved area may be filled with a viscoelastic polymer, which is particularly effective in preventing tissue breakdown. An extended steel shank and rocker sole completes the prescription.[11] Surgical treatment (see Chapter 55) usually consists of resection

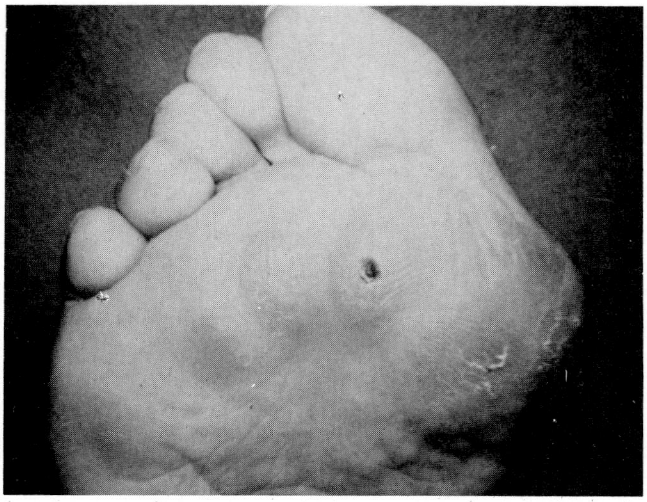

FIGURE 91–11. Plantar aspect of the rheumatoid foot.

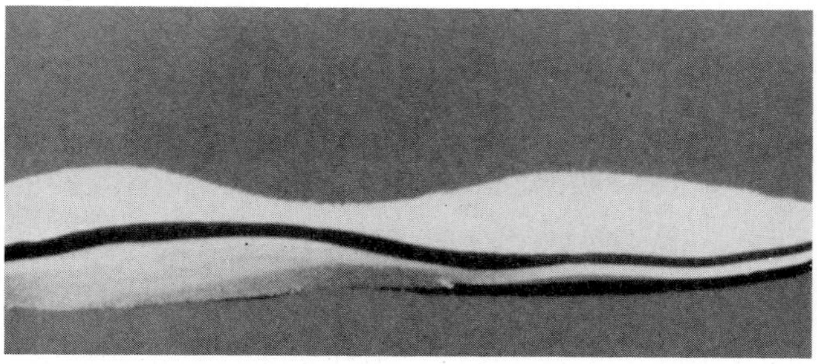

FIGURE 91–12. The total contact insert made with various grades of polyethylene foam (Plastazote). The device depicted here includes a middle layer of shear relieving micropore rubber.

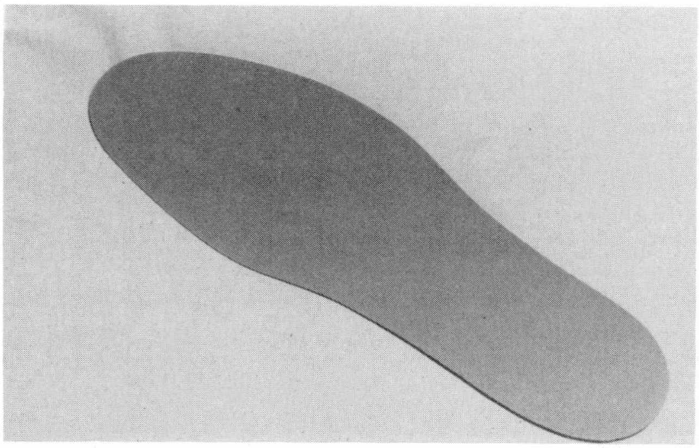

FIGURE 91–13. The micropore rubber insert.

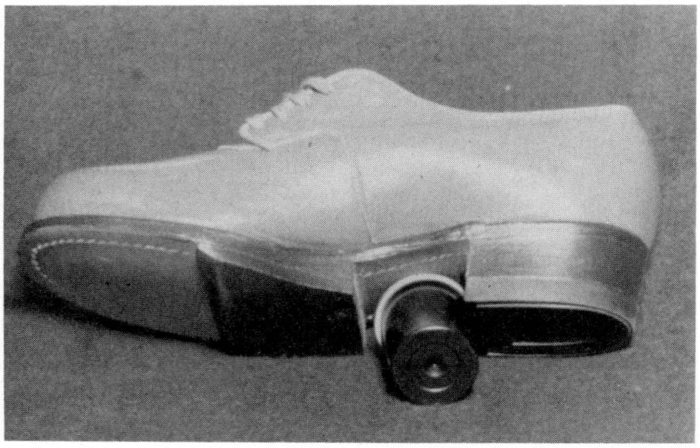

FIGURE 91–14. The metatarsal (Jones) bar.

of the metatarsal heads and, often, the proximal condyles of the proximal phalanges. The first MTP joint is resected, fused, or replaced with a prosthesis. I prefer the latter two approaches.[12]

METATARSAL PAIN ASSOCIATED WITH CAVUS DEFORMITY

Cavus deformity is discussed later in the section on the midfoot, but may be associated with pain in the metatarsal heads. In such cases, the flexible orthotic includes a total contact insert to diffuse the pressure both proximal to and over the metatarsal heads.

NONSPECIFIC PAIN IN THE METATARSALS

Patients with biomechanically normal feet may develop pain in the metatarsal area under certain circumstances, such as changes in walking surfaces (e.g., steel- or concrete-reinforced floors), hard running surfaces, use of shoes with poorly cushioned soles, and excessive wearing of high-heeled shoes. Recommendations include lower heels, an ankle strap, which will decrease forward shifting of the foot when in high heels; more cushioned soles (e.g., crepe rubber, or Vibram); mild rocker soles, which shift weight-bearing behind the metatarsal heads; and thin micropore rubber (Spenco) inserts (Fig. 91–13). Thicker inserts are not tolerated in ordinary depth shoes. Ready-made metatarsal pads sometimes help, and, traditionally, a metatarsal bar (Jones bar) (Fig. 91–14) is inserted on the sole to place weight-bearing behind the heads. The bar is less well tolerated than the mild rocker, and felt pads in normal shoes may become quite uncomfortable.

MIDFOOT AND LONGITUDINAL ARCH PAIN

FLAT FEET

Flexible flat feet (pes planus) are not necessarily painful, nor are congenitally relatively stiff flat feet, seen in various barefoot populations such as African blacks and South American Indians. However, hard surfaces, noncushioning shoes, weight gain, and other unknown factors may lead to complaints of pain in a pronated foot. The flat-footed marcher or runner does not necessarily develop pain more commonly than his companions with normal arches. The normal biomechanics of gait begins with heel strike, and then a supple phase where the foot pronates as a shock absorber with weight-bearing along its lateral border and then on all the metatarsal heads evenly. As the weight moves forward, the foot supinates, becomes more rigid, and toe-off is completed. If, in the foot-flat position, the longitudinal arch is flat or very low, but reforms as the patient goes up on his toes, the foot is functioning relatively normally.

If the arch does ache, an orthotic such as a Plastazote-lined device, reinforced (or "posted") in the arch with cork can be used. This device is comfortable, well tolerated, and can be worn in most shoes, including running shoes. If the medial leather of the shoe is too flexible, the orthotic will be less effective. Steel (Whitman plates) or hard plastic orthotics are more durable but often not well tolerated. I do not prescribe them. The hyperpronated foot[13] with excessive medial motion of the talar head at the talonavicular joint may also be a source of arch pain and is usually successfully treated with a semirigid, well-molded orthotic device.

THE COLLAPSED FOOT

Spontaneous unilateral collapse of the foot is a painful condition usually caused by rupture of the posterior tibial tendon.[14] From behind, the observer sees "too many toes" laterally. The patient cannot stand on tiptoes when standing on the involved foot. The condition usually begins with posterior tibial tendonitis. The sheath may be swollen and tender, but no fixed deformity has occurred. The patient cannot toe-up without pain. NSAIDs and a longitudinal arch orthotic device are often curative. If they are not, surgical decompression of the tendon sheath and subsequent use of the orthotic are sufficient. If rupture has occurred direct repair is rarely possible, and a tendon transfer using the flexor digitorum or the flexor hallucis longus is performed. An orthotic device is used postoperatively. In a chronic case subtalar arthritis has occurred, and a subtalar arthrodesis is the appropriate surgical maneuver. If midtarsal joint collapse has also occurred, a more extensive surgical reconstruction may be needed.

THE SPASTIC FLAT FOOT

A spastic flat foot is a rigid painful deformity. It is said to be due to inflammation of the subtalar joint, caused by a local or generalized condition. A tarsal coalition (usually calcaneonavicular or talocalcaneal) may become symptomatic and is often refractory to drugs and immobilization. Resection of the bar with soft tissue interposition is routinely performed for calcaneonavicular coalition, and is now attempted frequently for a talocalcaneal bar, because this can be well delineated by CT and three-dimensional imaging.[15] A subtalar arthrodesis is an effective salvage procedure.

THE CAVUS FOOT

The cavus or rigid high-arched foot is a significant problem for runners and distance walkers.[16] Normal talonavicular motion is impaired and the foot will not normally pronate after heel strike. This results in poor shock absorption and pain in the arch and over the dorsal midfoot. Better cushioned soles (crepe rubber) are useful, with a semirigid or flexible orthotic to cushion the foot. These help with normal rates of gait, but a symptomatic distance runner frequently has to find another source of exercise. Surgical procedures to lower the arch and relieve the accompanying varus heel have included release of the plantar fascia and osteotomies of the os calcis and metatarsals. Although the foot will be more comfortable and fit into a shoe better postoperatively, it is still rigid and unfit as a shock absorber.

STRESS FRACTURES

A metatarsal stress fracture must be suspected when a history of localized pain and tenderness follows an overuse situation such as running an increased distance and hiking. If plain films are normal, bone scintigraphy confirms the diagnosis. Periosteal reaction and eventual callus will be seen on later radiographs. A stiff-soled shoe, avoidance of the stress-provoking situation, and (possibly) casting are appropriate treatment.

HEEL PAIN

PLANTAR FASCIITIS

The plantar fascia is a static functional structure, described as a windlass mechanism. During toe-off it helps the arch to reform and the foot to become more rigid. Stress on this structure at its narrow proximal origin on the os calcis with repetitive microtrauma results in an inflammatory condition known as *plantar fasciitis*. Bone may form at this site (spur) secondary to the inflammatory response. On examination, there is point tenderness at the origin of the fascia, and hyperextension of the toes at the MTP joints increases the discomfort. Heel cutouts and heel cups along with local steroid injections constitute the most common treatment. I feel that these approaches are often either insufficient or, in the case of steroids, ill-advised. A heel cup encloses the plantar heel fat pad, providing a cushion around the inflamed area. A cutout may result in "window" edema, so it is usually filled with a viscoelastic polymer. The longitudinal arch is supported to relieve the tension on the plantar fascia. Hence, a combination of a posted longitudinal arch (cork and polyethylene foam liner), an attached heel cup, and filled cutout are effective treatment (Fig. 91–15). I avoid steroid injections, because they cause atrophy of fat, which in the heel can result in a new, far more pernicious, lesion.* NSAIDs are often helpful. If the problem is refractory to a conservative approach the

* *Editor's note.* I agree strongly with the author's view.

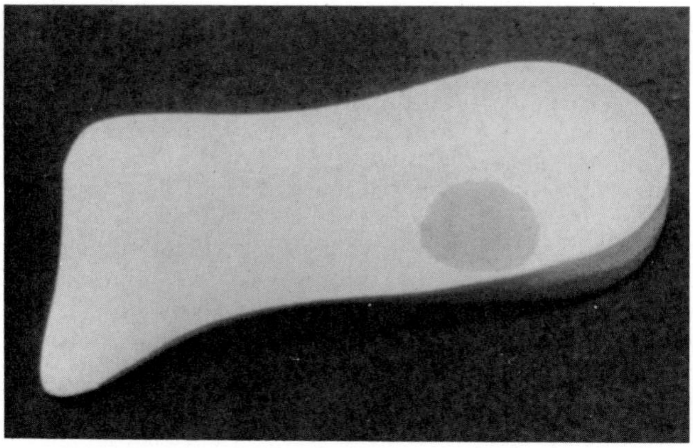

FIGURE 91–15. Combination of heel cup, longitudinal arch support, and cutout filled with viscoelastic polymer.

origin of the plantar fascia is released through a short longitudinal arch incision.

TARSAL TUNNEL SYNDROME (See Also Chapter 97)

Compression of the posterior tibial nerve, and its branches, the median and lateral plantar, results in heel and plantar foot pain. The laciniate ligament behind the medial malleolus, the superior and inferior fibrous edge of the abductor hallucis, deep fascia and varicosities[17] have each been implicated as the source of the compression. Compression of the calcaneal branch by local fascia and a motor branch of the abductor digiti minimi off the lateral plantar nerve,[18] under the origin of the plantar fascia, have also been implicated as causes of pain. Pain and paresthesias in the course of the nerves help with the diagnosis, as does localized tenderness and, specifically, a localized paresthesia with percussion (Tinel's sign). A nerve conduction study, particularly the sensory component, will confirm the diagnosis. A semirigid longitudinal arch orthotic with relief over the nerve medially will relieve acute conditions. Surgical decompression is done, but a determination of the site of the compression preoperatively, with a localizing Tinel's sign, carries a better prognosis for relief.

OTHER SOURCES OF HEEL PAIN

Other causes of heel pain include stress fractures of the os calcis, detected by plain radiographs, tomograms, or bone scintigraphy;[19] osteoid osteoma, characterized by night pain and relieved specifically with aspirin; and heel pad attrition and heel bruising (stone bruise). A fracture responds to immobilization, osteoid osteoma to excision, and heel pad attrition or bruising to polyethylene foam inserts and solid action cushion heels (SACH).

Painful bursae may occur behind the heel deep to the Achilles tendon. These lesions respond to cushioning, NSAIDs, occasional injections with steroids, and at times, surgical excision. Avascular necrosis of the tarsal navicular (Köhler's disease), the second metatarsal (Freiberg's infraction), and the apophysis of the os calcis are well-known sources of pain. Ordinary films demonstrating dense areas of bone are not conclusive for diagnosis. MRI scans can determine avascularity (see Chapter 6).

BURNING PAIN IN THE FOOT

The complaint of burning pain in the foot provides a diagnostic and therapeutic challenge. Dermatologic causes include a mixed fungal and bacterial infection (athlete's foot) or neurodermatitis.

A vasogenic cause may be a large- or, more typically, a small-vessel disease. If noninvasive vascular studies reveal satisfactory pulse pressures and pulse volume recordings in the toes, and if the skin of the foot has a purplish discoloration, empiric treatment may be initiated. This includes physical modalities such as contrast baths (alternating cold water and hot whirlpool), swimming pool walking, and medications to improve local perfusion. Controlled studies to determine the efficacy of these modalities are lacking despite promising anecdotal accounts.

Neurogenic causes may be local or referred. Local compressions and "neuromas" may be primary, traumatic, or iatrogenic.[20] Interdigital (Morton's) neuroma, pressure over the medial branch of the superficial peroneal or the saphenous nerve associated with a bunion, and tarsal tunnel syndrome have been described already. The superficial peroneal nerve is also vulnerable over the dorsum of the foot as it crosses potentially arthritic joints, such as the talonavicular, naviculocuneiform, or cuneiform-first metatarsal. Pressure from the joint below and the shoe above can account for the entrapment. The sural nerve may be compressed and entrapped with and after os calcis fractures, and all nerves are subject to damage from surgical procedures. Referred pain from lumbosacral spinal root compression can result in a burning pain in the appropriate dermatome. Although referred pain areas classically lack localized tenderness, the affected dermatomes may develop local hyperpathia.

Mechanical sources of pain are ruled out because nerve pain is typically not relieved by non-weight-bearing, and indeed, is often accentuated at night.

CONCLUSION

This review is brief but covers most causes of foot pain other than fractures and infection. All components of the anatomy, alone and in various combinations, may be involved. Medical, surgical, pedorthotic, and physical modalities may all be needed to provide relief. Definitive treatment may occasionally be surgical, as with an osteoid osteoma, but in general, nonoperative approaches are most appropriate initially. It is important, however, to carry out these approaches properly. If a patient fails to respond, the accuracy of the diagnosis must be reassessed and it must be determined that orthotic appliances or shoes have been properly prescribed and fabricated. Lastly, the physician must determine whether the patient has been compliant in following the prescribed program.

REFERENCES

1. Sammarco, G.J., and Miller, E.H.: Forefoot conditions in dancers. Foot Ankle, *3*:85–98, 1983.
2. Smith, R.W.: Calluses: Nonsurgical treatment. *In* The Foot Book. Edited by J.S. Gould. Baltimore, Williams & Wilkins, 1988.
3. Shereff, M.J.: Acquired disorders of the toes. *In* The Foot Book. Edited by J.S. Gould. Baltimore, Williams & Wilkins, 1988.
4. Dixon, G.L.: Treatment of ingrown toenail. Foot Ankle, *3*:254–260, 1983.
5. Morton, T.G.: A peculiar and painful affection of the fourth metatarsophalangeal articulation. Am. J. Med. Sci., *71*:37–45, 1876.
6. Mann, R.A., and Reynolds, J.C.: Interdigital neuroma—a critical clinical analysis. Foot Ankle, *3*:238–243, 1983.
7. Gauthier, G.: Thomas Morton's disease: A nerve entrapment syndrome. Clin. Orthop., *142*:90–92, 1979.
8. Scranton, P.E.: Metatarsalgia: A clinical review of diagnosis and management. Foot Ankle, *1*:229–234, 1981.
9. Mann, R.A., and Coughlin, M.J.: Hallux valgus and complications of hallux valgus. *In* Surgery of the Foot. Edited by R.A. Mann. St. Louis, The C.V. Mosby Co., 1986.
10. Gould, N.: Hallux rigidus: Cheilectomy or implant? Foot Ankle, *1*:315–320, 1981.
11. Gould, J.S.: Conservative management of the hypersensitive foot in rheumatoid arthritis. Foot Ankle, *2*:224–229, 1982.
12. Cracchiolo, A.: Rheumatoid arthritis of the foot and ankle. *In* The Foot Book. Edited by J.S. Gould. Baltimore, Williams & Wilkins, 1988.
13. Gould, N.: Graphing the adult foot and ankle. Foot Ankle, *2*:213–219, 1982.
14. Mann, R.A.: Tendon injuries. *In* Surgery of the Foot. Edited by R.A. Mann. St. Louis, The C.V. Mosby Co., 1986.
15. Herzenberg, J.E., Goldner, J.L., Martinez, S., and Silverman, P.M.: Computerized tomography of talocalcaneal tarsal coalition: A clinical and anatomic study. Foot Ankle, *6*:273–288, 1986.
16. Lutter, L.D.: Cavus foot in runners. Foot Ankle, *1*:225–228, 1981.
17. Gould, N., and Alvarez, R.: Bilateral tarsal tunnel syndrome caused by varicosities. Foot Ankle, *3*:290–292, 1983.
18. Baxter, D.E., and Thigpen, C.M.: Heel pain—operative results. Foot Ankle, *5*:16–25, 1985.
19. Graham, C.E.: Painful heel syndrome: Rationale of diagnosis and treatment. Foot Ankle, *3*:261–267, 1983.
20. Kenzora, J.E.: Symptomatic incisional neuromas on the dorsum of the foot. Foot Ankle, *5*:2–15, 1985.

92

Cervical Spine Syndromes

JOE G. HARDIN
JAMES T. HALLA

Neck pain is a common problem in individuals with and without well-defined rheumatic disorders. It occurs at some time in about 35% of the population.[1] Typically the pain is perceived not only in the neck itself, but also in other regions, such as the back of the head, the shoulder girdle, the arm, and the anterior chest. Pain originating from neck structures might be perceived exclusively in extracervical areas. In patients with unequivocal cervical trauma, cervical degenerative disc and joint disease, or inflammatory arthropathies, the origin of pain in the neck *might* be easy to establish, at least by inference. In individuals with pain but with none of these conditions, the cause is often impossible to establish with certainty. Fortunately, many of these pain syndromes are transient. The neck is an extraordinarily complex anatomic structure with many components that lend themselves poorly to diagnostic investigation.

It can be assumed that most pain derived from the cervical spine originates in one or more of a limited number of structures: joints (either synovial or cartilaginous), ligaments, neural tissue (especially nerve roots), muscle and tendons. Disease in one structure (i.e., a joint) often leads to symptoms in another (i.e., a nerve). Available diagnostic modalities can identify joints or neural tissue as a probable source of pain with relative ease. Recognition of pathology in muscle or ligament is much more difficult, a fact that accounts for the difficulty in precise identification of the nature of cervical pain in individuals with no underlying rheumatic disorders.

The functional anatomy of the cervical spine and structures related to it will first be addressed, followed by a review of cervical syndromes commonly encountered in otherwise normal individuals, syndromes associated with trauma, syndromes associates with degenerative disc and joint disease, and finally syndromes resulting from inflammatory arthropathies.

FUNCTIONAL ANATOMY

Emphasis here is on the spine, its articulations, and their relationship to neural structures. Individual cervical vertebrae and their components are illustrated in Figure 92–1. The atlas (C1) (Fig. 92–1A) is a ring of bone modified by articular facets anterolaterally. The superior facets articulate with the skull, forming relatively stable joints that permit only flexion-extension. The inferior facets articulate with their counterparts on the axis (C2) (Fig. 92–1B). A third C1-C2 articulation plays an important role in the motion occurring between these two vertebrae. This is the joint formed between the odontoid process of C2 and the anterior chamber of C1, the atlanto-odontoid articulation. This joint is stabilized by the transverse ligament of C1 behind the odontoid and by ligaments between the odontoid and the occiput. The head and C1 tend to move as a unit on C2 during cervical flexion. This motion stresses the stability of the atlanto-odontoid articulation and tends to force the odontoid posteriorly into the area occupied by the spinal canal. The three C1-C2 articulations contribute about 50% of the rotational motion of the cervical spine, and all three are synovial-lined joints.

Below the axis the remaining five cervical vertebrae (Fig. 92–1C) are relatively constant; their articulations account for the remaining motions permitted by the cervical spine. Anteriorly the vertebral body articulates with its counterpart via the cartilaginous intervertebral disc. During youth the disc is typical of others elsewhere in the spine with a dense outer anulus fibrosus and a central nucleus pulposus. Laterally near the interverte-

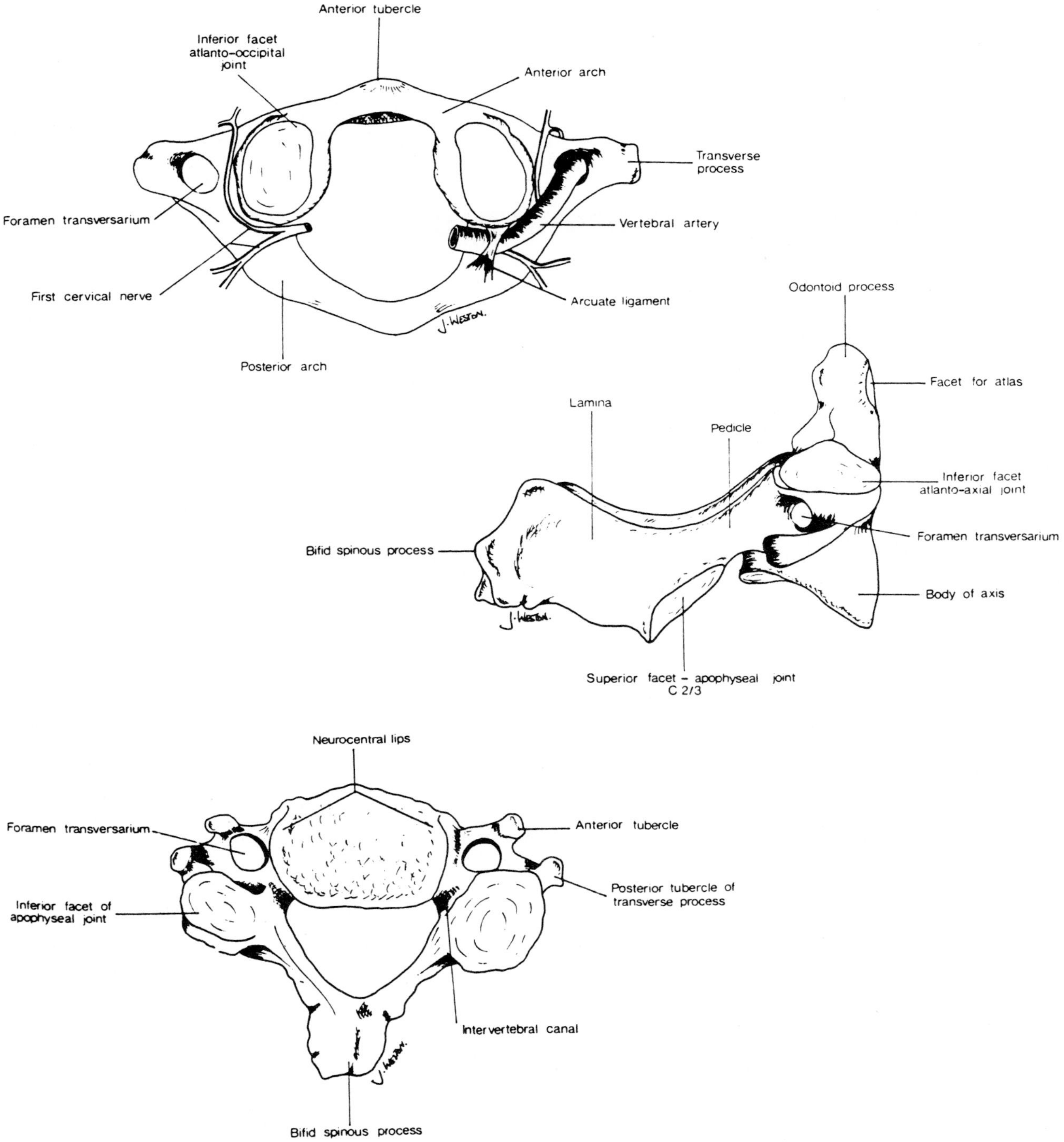

FIGURE 92–1. Atlas, axis and typical lower cervical vertebra: *A*, Atlas, superior aspect. *B*, Axis, lateral view. *C* Typical cervical vertebra, superior view. From Jeffreys, E.: Disorders of the Cervical Spine. Butterworths, 1980, p. 3.

bral neural foramina, the vertebral bodies are modified by superior uncinate processes (neurocentral lips) that articulate with a region of the vertebral bodies above them, forming the so-called "joints" of Luschka. The adult cervical disc loses its nucleus pulposus, and clefts develop at the site of the uncinate processes. With increasing age these clefts dissect medially, bisecting the disc but not forming a true synovial joint.[1] According to this observation Luschka's joints are mythical.[1]

The posterior elements of C2 and the lower five cervi-

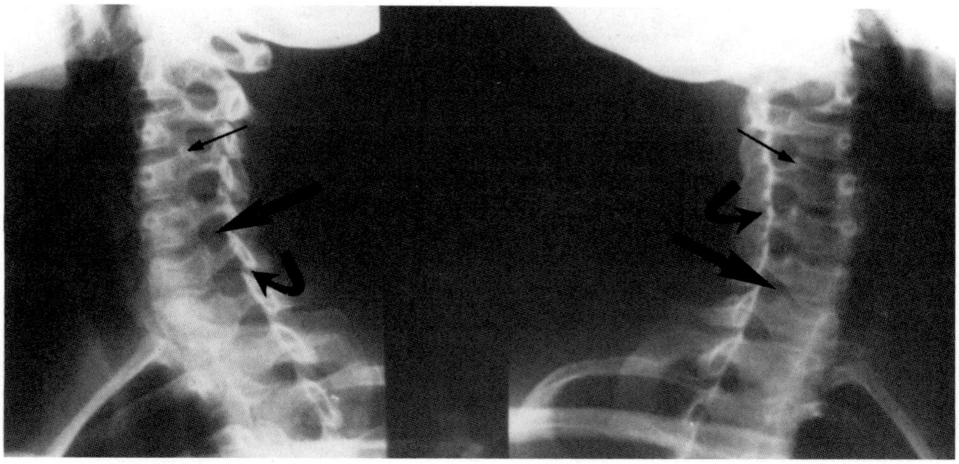

FIGURE 92–2. Right and left oblique views of the cervical spine demonstrating the intervertebral neural foramina (large arrows). Sites of the uncinate processes are indicated by small arrows; the facet joints are indicated by curved arrows.

cal vertebrae form the neural arch surrounding the spinal canal laterally and posteriorly. Laterally the narrow pedicles provide for the oval intervertebral neural foramina (Figure 92–2), and the transverse processes, extending anterolaterally from the pedicles, form shelves or gutters for the exiting nerves. Except for that of C7 each transverse process, including those of C1 and C2, are perforated by a foramen for the vertebral artery (foramen transversum). The intervertebral neural foramina are best viewed obliquely in the anterolateral plane. Posterior to the pedicle the neural arch flares inferiorly and superiorly to form the articular facets that lie considerably posterior to the articular facets of C1 and C2. The articulating surfaces of the facets face each other at an angle of about 45°. The facet (apophyseal) are true synovial joints. The posterior elements (lamina) of the neural arch complete the spinal canal.

Motions permitted by the cervical articulations vary with age, sex, and the observer measuring them. Average ranges are as follows: flexion-extension—106°; lateral flexion or bending—178°; and rotation—131°. Ranges in all directions decrease significantly with increasing age.[2]

The first cervical nerve exits superior to C1 posterior to the articular facet, and the second cervical nerve exits similarly superior and posterior to the superior articular facet of C2. All other cervical nerves pass anterolaterally through their respective gutters and posterior to the vertebral artery. After exiting the spinal canal the posterior and anterior nerve roots join within their dural sleeve in the gutter to form the cervical nerve, with the posterior root lying superior to the anterior root. Their position in the foramina and the uncinate processes serve to protect the roots from protrusion or herniation of disc material.

Important ligaments add support to the cervical spine below the C1-C2 articulations. The anterior longitudinal ligament is bound to the front of the vertebral bodies, its fibers blending loosely with the anulus fibrosus as it crosses the disc spaces. The reverse is true for the posterior longitudinal ligament, which is loosely bound to the posterior aspects of the vertebral bodies but more firmly attached to the discs. The posterior longitudinal ligament is much thicker in the cervical than in the thoracolumbar spine. The lamina or posterior aspects of the neural arch are bound to their inferior and superior counterparts by the tough elastic ligamenta flava, which extend anteriorly to blend with the capsules of the facet joints.

A large muscle mass occupies the posterolateral cervical area. Most of these muscles are attached to the spine and to the skull, especially the occiput. In concert with the sternomastoid and the anterior neck muscles they move the head and neck, support and stabilize the head and neck, and balance the head on the spine.

GENERAL APPROACHES TO CERVICAL SYMPTOMS

Most symptoms perceived in the neck region are transient and of uncertain cause. Many probably qualify as myofascial.[3] Symptoms are typically rapid in onset, are associated with limited or painful mobility of the neck and shoulder girdle, and seldom last longer than a week. The neurologic examination is normal; other physical findings are nonspecific and diagnostic imaging is not helpful. This syndrome is often referred to by patients as a "crick." In one study transcutaneous electrical nerve stimulation was superior to a collar or to manual therapy[4]; treatment is best regarded as symptomatic and nonspecific, however.

Symptoms persisting beyond 1 or 2 weeks or associated with certain other features must be taken more seriously. Other features suggesting a potentially serious or diagnosable cause include pain in other parts of the

TABLE 92–1. DISORDERS THAT SOMETIMES PRESENT WITH SYMPTOMS IN THE NECK REGION

Rheumatic Disease
Fibromyalgia
Polymyalgia rheumatica
Rheumatoid arthritis
Juvenile rheumatoid arthritis
Ankylosing spondylitis
Peripheral spondyloarthropathies
Crystal deposition diseases
Degenerative disc and joint diseases
Diffuse idiopathic skeletal hyperostosis
Trauma
Fractures-dislocations
Soft tissue injuries
Regional Cervical Disorders
Myofascial pain
Osteomyelitis
Septic discitis
Septic arthritis
Congenital and acquired torticollis syndromes
Other congenital disorders of the cervical spine
Cervical lymphadenitis
Hyoid bone syndrome
Neck-tongue syndrome
Longus colli muscle tendinitis
Facet joint synovial cyst
Thyroiditis
Thoracic outlet syndrome
Bone Diseases
Paget's disease
Osteomalacia
Osteoporosis
Metastatic tumor
Neuromuscular Disorders
Meningitis
Cerebral palsy and other spastic conditions
Paralysis of cervical muscles from any cause

body, neurologic symptoms, abnormal neurologic findings, fever, and palpable or audible cervical crepitus. Polymyalgia rheumatica, fibromyalgia, and some of the inflammatory arthropathies might begin or predominate in the cervical region, as outlined in Table 92–1.[5,6] Symptoms or signs in other areas of the body might suggest one of these conditions.

When the diagnosis is not apparent and the symptoms persist or seem potentially serious, further diagnostic efforts are indicated; these are listed in Table 92–2. The history and physical examination maneuvers are routine, but very important. Cervical spine radiographs—anteroposterior, lateral, right and left oblique, and flexion and extension views in the lateral projection—are usually indicated. The facets between C1 and C2 are generally visualized by a view taken through the open mouth. Conventional tomography can be helpful if a bony defect or spinal derangement is suspected but not well defined by routine radiography or radioisotopic scintigraphy. Electrodiagnostic studies might confirm or better define a suspected neurologic deficit. Computed tomography (CT), magnetic resonance imaging (MRI), and myelography are used to define the source of a neurologic sign or symptom. Which one or combination of the three to use is a matter of current controversy.

TABLE 92–2. USEFUL DIAGNOSTIC MANEUVERS IN PATIENTS WITH SYMPTOMS IN THE NECK REGION

History
Duration
Trauma
Pain or similar symptoms elsewhere
Pain related to head-neck motion or position
Referral pattern and nature of referred pain
Neurologic symptoms
Physical Examination
Abnormal head position
Neck motion and pain on motion
Spine tenderness
Tender or trigger points in neck area
Motor or sensory deficits or reflex abnormalities, especially in the arms
Diagnostic Imaging
Routine radiographs (with oblique views)
Radioisotope scanning
Conventional tomography
Computed tomography
Magnetic resonance imaging
Myelography
Electrodiagnostic Studies
Nerve conduction studies
Electromyography

NECK PAIN ASSOCIATED WITH TRAUMA

Fractures and dislocations of the cervical spine must be excluded in symptomatic patients with a recent history of cervical trauma. A number of terms are used interchangeably to refer to the typical soft tissue injury syndrome, including "whiplash," cervical "sprain" or "strain," and post-traumatic cervical syndrome. Although industrial or sports injuries might cause the problem in the United States, most such injuries result from automobile collisions from the rear, most often with the victim using a seat belt.[7] Medicolegal considerations can complicate and confound the clinical picture. The typical injury occurs as the head is first flexed and then forcibly hyperextended beyond its normal range of motion. Presumably the affected tissues include muscles, tendons, joints, ligaments, and perhaps nerve roots. The pathogenesis of the injury is not well understood. Usually the onset of pain begins within hours of the accident, and it predominates in the neck and medial aspects of the shoulder girdle. Headaches are common, and post-traumatic audiologic and vestibular dysfunction have been reported. Cervical radiographs can show loss of lordosis secondary to cervical muscle spasm.[7,8]

The natural history of the syndrome can be influenced by psychologic and medicolegal factors, and is highly variable. In one series it had resolved in 52% of patients at 8 weeks and in 87% at 5 months.[9] The relationship of these injuries to subsequent degenerative changes is uncertain. Therapy seems generally unsatisfactory, though immobilization is often recommended.[9] Collars, traction, other physical therapies and analgesic

TABLE 92–3. FEATURES ASSOCIATED WITH DEGENERATIVE CERVICAL SPINE DISEASE THAT LEND DIFFICULTY TO PRECISE DIAGNOSES

Symptoms can arise from the facet joints or anulus fibrosus.
Radiographic abnormalities are almost universal in the elderly population, most of whom are asymptomatic.
Diagnostic imaging abnormalities might correlate poorly with symptoms.
Distribution of diagnostic imaging abnormalities might correlate poorly with location of symptoms.
Neurologic physical findings are most often absent.
With age the ligamenta flava become inelastic and can buckle into the spinal canal, causing symptoms.
With age the posterior longitudinal ligament can further thicken, encroaching on the spinal canal and causing symptoms.
Lesions that appear to encroach on neural structures by diagnostic imaging might not cause symptoms.
By age 40 the nucleus puplosus is no longer present in the cervical discs (suggesting that it cannot herniate).[1]
The posterior longitudinal ligament and the uncinate processes provide formidable barriers to disc herniation.[1]
The lower cervical nerve roots exit below the disc level, apparently protecting them from herniation in any event.[1]
The anterior nerve roots are positioned too low in the intervertebral foramina to be vulnerable to osteophytic encroachment.[1]

agents can help symptomatically, though they do not seem to affect the course of the syndrome.*

DEGENERATIVE DISC AND JOINT DISEASES (INCLUDING DIFFUSE IDIOPATHIC SKELETAL HYPEROSTOSIS)

Although diffuse idiopathic skeletal hyperostosis (DISH) is usually readily identifiable from plain radiographs and typically produces few neck symptoms, degenerative disease of the spinal articulations can result in a confusing array of symptoms that are often difficult to explain. Confounding observations that can account for this difficulty are summarized in Table 92–3. Despite these difficulties diagnoses continue to be made, and the conditions often are treated successfully. In few cases, however, is the precise pathogenesis clearly understood. Four syndromes will be addressed: presumed herniation of the nucleus pulposus (HNP), presumed osteophytic neural and vascular encroachment, facet joint osteoarthritis, and DISH.

HERNIATION OF THE NUCLEUS PULPOSUS (HNP)

Disc ruptures, protrusions, and extrusions are used synonomously with this term. Much of the literature concerning cervical disc disease fails to distinguish between HNP and osteophytic encroachment on neural structures, apparently because the two often appear to occur together. A distinctive clinical syndrome might be apparent, however. The HNP syndrome occurs at a younger age than does the osteophytic one and more often affects men. Protrusion tends to occur acutely on one side and at one level (most often C6-C7), dorsolaterally (apparently compressing intrameningeal nerve roots) or intraforaminally (apparently compressing the exiting nerve roots). Most often there is no history of trauma sufficient to account for the event. Symptoms often begin with neck pain that progresses to involve the scapular area, anterior chest, or arm, depending on which root is affected. Hyperextension of the neck or deviation of the head toward the side of the HNP can aggravate the pain. Neurologic findings and other signs are often present, depending on the site of the lesion[10,11] (Table 92–4).

The diagnosis may be supported by electromyography and confirmed by myelography, MRI, or CT. The procedure of choice is a matter of opinion. Therapy is also a matter of opinion. Progressive neurologic deficits, signs of myelopathy, and intractable pain usually indicate surgery, however (see Chapter 52). Conservative therapy consists of intermittent or continuous cervical traction, bed rest, analgesics, and cervical collars for comfort.[12]

OSTEOPHYTIC DISEASE (SPONDYLOSIS)

Anterior osteophytes arising at the disc margins might imply more posterior disease, but themselves are typically asymptomatic. The uncinate processes enlarge with age, so that what appear to be osteophytes in that area radiographically might not be, but foraminal bony encroachment from that region is seen commonly, as is similar encroachment from facet joint osteophytes posteriorly. Only the facet osteophytes are in a position to impinge on a nerve root, and only the posterior root is vulnerable.[1] Posterior osteophytes from the vertebral bodies at the disc margins are common and can be sufficiently large to compress the spinal cord, though they too are most often asymptomatic. In general the lower cervical spine, especially C5-C6, is most prominently involved. Three overlapping syndromes can result from spondylitic osteophytic neural or vascular encroachment: nerve root compression (radiculopathy), spinal cord compression (myelopathy), and vertebral artery compression.

It might not be possible, even at surgery, to clearly distinguish between a radiculopathy due in an HNP and one due to osteophytic encroachment, and the reported clinical syndromes resulting from these events are similar, except as already mentioned. HNP tends to occur in younger patients, affecting a single root. Approaches to diagnosis and therapy are also similar.[11–14] A less dramatic, more ill-defined syndrome is more common than

* *Editor's note:* A 10-day course of prednisone (30 mg/day) together with the use of a collar has helped to shorten this syndrome's period of morbidity in my experience.

TABLE 92–4. CLINICAL TESTS FOR CERVICAL NERVE ROOT COMPRESSION

TEST	TECHNIQUE
Neck compression test	With the patient sitting, examiner laterally flexes, slightly rotates, and then compresses the patient's head with a force of about 7 kg. Positive result is pain or paresthesias in distribution of affected root.
Axial manual traction test	With the patient supine, examiner applies manual traction to neck with a force of 10–15 kg. Positive result is relief of radicular symptoms.
Shoulder abduction test	With patient sitting, the arm is actively abducted above the head. Positive result is relief of radicular symptoms.

Based on the results of myelography or magnetic resonance imaging, these tests are highly specific, but together have a sensitivity only in the range of 50%.[11]

the classic one usually reported in textbooks. Older patients commonly experience neck, shoulder area, and arm pain, often aggravated by neck motion, and sometimes associated with intermittent paresthesias. Sometimes tests listed in Table 92–4 are positive but neurologic deficits are absent. Plain cervical radiographs document neural foraminal osteophytic encroachment, often at several levels. More-expensive diagnostic studies are seldom indicated. Symptoms tend to respond to conservative therapy, perhaps improving with time alone. Intermittent cervical traction is frequently helpful. It is seldom possible to clearly document an association between a given osteophytic encroachment and the symptoms.

Bland and Boushey suggest that spondylitic myelopathy is more common than radiculopathy.[1] The syndrome is seen more often in older men and is typically gradual in onset. Leg symptoms predominate and spasticity is common. Radicular symptoms frequently accompany the myelopathy. A congenitally narrow spinal canal and posterior longitudinal ligament thickening or ossification might contribute to the compression. Myelography or MRI confirms the diagnosis, and surgical therapy is often indicated.[14,15]

Many symptoms can result from osteophytic compression of the vertebral artery, especially in the upper cervical region. These include autonomic symptoms, transient ischemic attacks, dizziness, vertigo, and headaches; symptoms are often related to cervical motion.[5] The association of cervical spondylosis with headache has been questioned, however.[16]

FACET JOINT OSTEOARTHRITIS

It is widely assumed but difficult to prove that neck discomfort in the older population is related to the radiographic findings of facet joint osteoarthritis (facet joint OA). In one follow-up study of 205 patients, such an association could not be documented.[17] A few patients with cervical OA have symptoms arising primarily from the C1-C2 facet joints, however. Patients with this syndrome tend to be older women complaining primarily of occipital pain. Crepitus in the upper cervical spine, occipital tender points, and a rotational head tilt deformity are common. These patients usually respond to conservative therapy, but surgical fusion is occasionally indicated for intractable pain.[18]

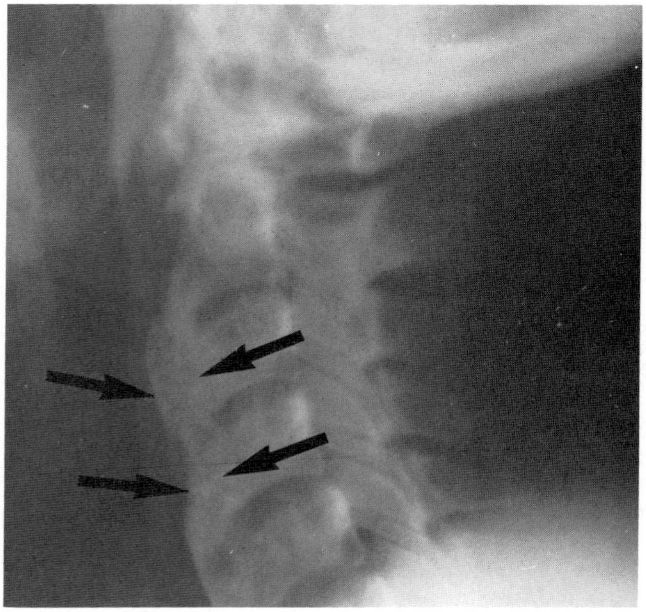

FIGURE 92–3. Cervical DISH. Arrows indicate the extent of the anterior longitudinal ligament ossification.

DIFFUSE IDIOPATHIC SKELETAL HYPEROSTOSIS (DISH)

The anterior longitudinal ligament of the cervical spine is commonly ossified in patients with DISH, and sometimes the ossification is luxuriant (Fig. 92–3). Although most often asymptomatic, extensive ossification can be associated with limited neck mobility, anterior cervical masses, and dysphagia from esophageal compression.[19] DISH has also been associated with ossification of the posterior longitudinal ligament, sometimes resulting in myelopathy with quadriplegia.[20]

INFLAMMATORY ARTHROPATHIES

Neck syndromes are common in the inflammatory arthropathies (Table 92–1), especially rheumatoid arthritis (RA).

RHEUMATOID ARTHRITIS (RA)

Neck pain occurs in half of the patients with RA, but half of these patients have normal cervical spine radiographs. Abnormalities of the rheumatoid cervical spine and its supporting structures occur in three patterns: (1) atlantoaxial (C1-C2) complex involvement with subluxation anteriorly or posteriorly with or without odontoid erosion; (2) C1-C2 lateral facet joint and/or atlanto-occipital joint involvement with lateral or rotatory subluxations; and (3) subaxial involvement with subluxation and/or spondylodiscitis.[21]

More than one pattern might be seen in any individual patient, and each pattern might be associated with a distinctive clinical profile. For example, involvement of the C1-C2 lateral facet joints, either unilaterally or bilaterally, is characterized by pain that parallels the degree of radiographic involvement, by restricted neck motion and by a nonreducible rotational head tilt (NRRHT) paralleling the degree of lateral mass collapse (Fig. 92–4). Neurologic symptoms are uncommon.[22,23]

Neck symptoms resulting from anteroposterior subluxations at the C1-C2 complex are less distinctive (Fig. 92–5). Anterior C1-C2 subluxation is the most frequent radiographic abnormality. The correlation between the degree of subluxation demonstrated radiographically and symptoms, especially neurologic symptoms, is poor, however.[24]

Subaxial involvement includes vertebral endplate erosions, disc space narrowing without osteophytes, spondylodiscitis, and subluxation. Subluxation, either at single or multiple levels, is not uncommon, but rarely causes symptoms unless accompanied by discitis.[21]

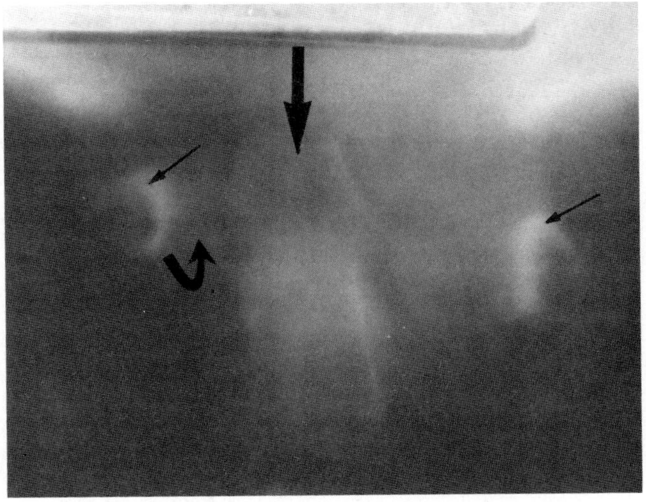

FIGURE 92–5. Conventional lateral tomography of C1-C2 area in a patient with severe rheumatoid arthritis. Small arrows indicate C1, and large arrow indicates the odontoid process. The spinal canal is to the left (curved arrow). This patient had severe C1-C2 anterior subluxation with no symptoms!

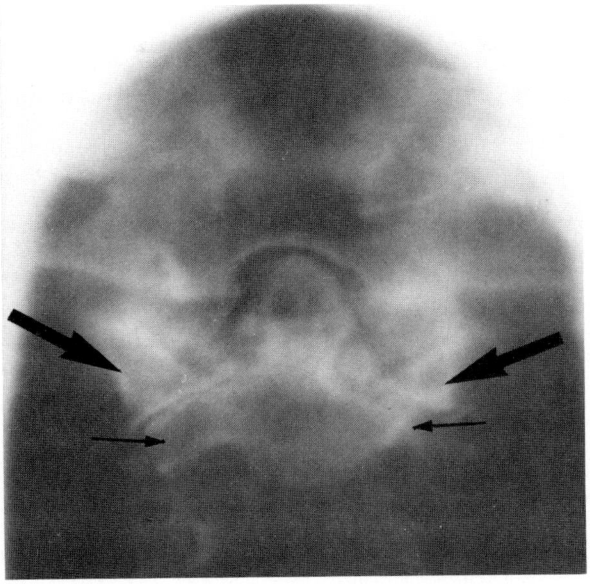

FIGURE 92–4. Conventional anteroposterior tomography of C1-C2 in a patient with severe rheumatoid arthritis. Large arrows indicate C1 lateral mass collapse; small arrows indicate C2 lateral mass collapse.

Treatment of neck pain in patients with RA should be guided by the radiographic pattern and by the nature of the symptoms. Sometimes no therapy is necessary, and conservative measures including physical therapy and drugs usually suffice. If pain is intractable, surgical fusion (occiput to C3) might give dramatic pain relief; this is especially true if the pain is due to C1-C2 lateral facet joint disease.[22,23]

JUVENILE RHEUMATOID ARTHRITIS (JRA)

Cervical spine involvement occurs in up to 50% of patients with JRA, and is most prominently associated with polyarticular disease, a positive rheumatoid factor, or both. Manifestations include loss of cervical lordosis; apophyseal joint erosions and ankylosis, especially in the upper cervical spine; failure of vertebral body growth; C1-C2 anterior subluxation; and lateral facet joint disease with NRRHT.[25,26]

Neck pain can be either the presenting feature or a later manifestation of adult-onset Still's disease. Because the childhood and adult forms of Still's disease are similar in presentation and course, radiographic similarities are not unexpected. Unlike the childhood form, the adult disease tends to involve both the upper and lower cervical segments.[27]

ANKYLOSING SPONDYLITIS (AS)

Neck pain in AS is common. As many as 5 to 10% of patients present with neck pain in the absence of back pain.[28] Neck pain usually correlates with radiographic changes, but can be present in their absence. Conversely, radiographic abnormalities without neck pain are sometimes seen. Cervical spine involvement usually accompanies disease in the thoracolumbar spine, though women might have a higher frequency of isolated cervical spine disease.[29]

Involvement of the C1-C2 complex occurs uncommonly; subluxation, usually anterior, and odontoid erosions are its usual manifestations.[30] Subluxations tend to occur in patients with longstanding disease and peripheral arthritis; they might be associated with neck pain and might have neurologic sequelae. The C1-C2 lateral facet joints might be the commonest source of severe neck pain in AS.[26]

Cervical spine fracture, usually with minor trauma, is another cause of neck pain in patients with AS and is easily overlooked. These patients tend to be older men (mean age: 55 years) with advanced disease (average duration: 25 years). Neurologic deficits are common and mortality is as high as 35%.[31]

Spondylodiscitis is another source of neck pain in patients with AS. This radiographic finding occurs in 1 to 28% of patients, usually during the first 10 years of disease. The more destructive the lesion, the more likely there is to be widespread spinal ankylosis.[32] Infectious spondylitis must be excluded.

REITER'S SYNDROME

Cervical spine involvement in Reiter's syndrome is uncommon; fewer than 6% of patients demonstrate radiographic abnormalities. Manifestations include C1-C2 subluxations, C1-C2 lateral facet joint disease including NRRHT, atlanto-occipital joint involvement, anterior longitudinal ligamentous ossificaion, and spondylitis.[33,34] All of these can be a source of neck pain.

PSORIATIC ARTHRITIS

Involvement of the cervical spine in psoriatic arthritis occurs in two patterns: a pattern similar to RA and a pattern similar to AS.[35] Neck pain is common and neurologic complications occur, especially in those patients with an RA-like pattern.[36]

CRYSTALLOPATHIES

As a group the crystallopathies rarely affect the cervical spine. Gout can produce neck symptoms in a variety of ways, however, including intradural deposition of urate, discitis, and subluxations.[37] Of a group of 85 patients with calcium pyrophosphate deposition disease, 10 had neck symptoms.[38] Radiographic abnormalities included disc space loss with vertebral sclerosis and osteophyte formation, facet joint abnormalities, and crystal deposition in synovial and ligamentous structures, including the ligamenta flava.

Crystal deposition, usually in the form of hydroxyapatite, can also occur in periarticular locations in the spine. Calcification within the longus colli muscle and tendon can be responsible for acute neck and occipital pain with or without dysphagia.[39] Hydroxyapatite crystal deposition has also been reported in the infraoccipital region, interspinous bursae, and ligamenta flava, and has been associated with neck pain and neurologic manifestations.[40]

REFERENCES

1. Bland, J.H., and Boushey, D.R.: Anatomy and physiology of the cervical spine. Semin. Arthritis Rheum., *20*:1–20, 1990.
2. O'Driscoll, S.L., and Tomenson, J.: The cervical spine. *In* Clinics in Rheumatic Diseases. Edited by V. Wright. Philadelphia, W.B. Saunders, 1982, pp. 617–630.
3. Travell, J.G., and Simons, D.G.: Myofascial Pain and Dysfunction. Baltimore, Williams & Wilkins, 1983, pp. 321–367.
4. Nordemar, R., and Thorner, C.: Treatment of acute cervical pain—A comparative group study. Pain, *10*:93–101, 1981.
5. Bland, J.H.: Disorders of the Cervical Spine. Philadelphia, W.B. Saunders, 1987, pp. 186–235.
6. Bland, J.H.: Cervical and thoracic pain including thoracic outlet syndrome and brachial neuritis. Curr. Opin. Rheumatol., *2*:242–252, 1990.
7. Bauer, W.: Neck pain. *In* Neck Pain. Edited by S.W. Weisel, H.L. Feffer, and R.H. Rothman. Charlottesville, VA, Michie Company, 1986, pp. 1–17.
8. Maimaris, C., Barnes, M.R., and Allen, M.J.: Whiplash injuries of the neck: A retrospective study. Br. J. Accident Surg., *19*:393–396, 1988.
9. Pennie, B.H., and Agambar, L.J.: Whiplash injuries. J. Bone Joint Surg., *72B*:277–279, 1990.
10. Ehni, G.: Cervical Arthrosis. Diseases of Cervical Motion Segments. Chicago, Year Book, 1984, pp. 44–77.
11. Viikari-Juntura, E., Porras, M., and Laasonen, E.M.: Validity of clinical tests in the diagnosis of root compression in cervical disc disease. Spine, *14*:253–257, 1989.
12. Johnson, E.W.: Conservative Management of cervical disc disease. *In* Seminars in Neurological Surgery. Cervical spondylosis. Edited by S.B. Dunsker. New York, Raven Press, 1981, pp. 145–153.
13. McLaurin, R.L.: Diagnosis and course of cervical radiculopathy. *In* Seminars in Neurological Surgery. Cervical spondylosis. Edited by S.B. Dunsker. New York, Raven Press, 1981, pp. 103–117.
14. Yu, Y.L., Woo, E., and Huang, C.Y.: Cervical spondylotic myelopathy and radiculopathy. Acta Neurol. Scand., *75*:367–373, 1987.
15. Magnaes, B., and Hauge, T.: Surgery for myelopathy in cervical spondylosis. Spine, *5*:211–214, 1980.
16. Edmeads, J.: The cervical spine and headache. Neurology, *38*:1874–1878, 1988.
17. Gore, D.R., Sepic, S.B., Gardner, G.M., et al.: Neck pain: A long-term follow-up of 205 patients. Spine, *12*:1–5, 1987.
18. Halla, J.T., and Hardin, J.G.: Atlantoaxial (C1-C2) facet joint osteoarthritis: A distinctive clinical syndrome. Arthritis Rheum., *30*:577–582, 1987.
19. Kritzer, R.O., and Rose, J.E.: Diffuse idiopathic skeletal hyperoxtosis presenting with thoracic outlet syndrome and dysphagia. Neurosurgery, *22*:1072–1074, 1988.
20. Pouchot, J., Watts, C.S., Esdaile, J.M., et al.: Sudden quadriplegia complicating ossification of the posterior longitudinal ligament and diffuse idiopathic skeletal hyperostosis. Arthritis Rheum., *30*:1069–1072, 1987.
21. Halla, J.T., Hardin, J.G., Vitek, J., et al.: Involvement of the cervical spine in rheumatoid arthritis. Arthritis Rheum., *32*:652–659, 1989.

22. Halla, J.T., Fallahi, S., and Hardin, J.G.: Nonreducible rotational head tilt and lateral mass collapse: a prospective study of frequency, radiographic findings, and clinical features in patients with rheumatoid arthritis. Arthritis Rheum., *25*:1316–1324, 1982.
23. Halla, J.T., and Hardin, J.G.: The spectrum of atlantoaxial (C1-C2) facet joint involvement in rheumatoid arthritis. Arthritis Rheum., *33*:325–329, 1990.
24. Weissman, B., Aliabadi, P., Weinfeld, M., et al.: Prognostic features of atlantoaxial subluxation in rheumatoid arthritis patients. Radiology, *144*:745–751, 1982.
25. Ansell, B., and Kent, P.: Radiological changes in juvenile chronic polyarthritis. Skeletal Radiol., *1*:129–144, 1977.
26. Halla, J.T., Fallahi, S., and Hardin, J.G.: Nonreducible rotational head tilt: A study of its clinical and radiographic features in patients with juvenile rheumatoid arthritis. Arch. Intern. Med., *143*:471–474, 1983.
27. Elkon, K., Hughes, G., Bywaters, E., et al.: Adult onset Still's disease: Twenty-five year follow-up and further studies of patients with active disease. Arthritis Rheum., *25*:647–654, 1982.
28. Hochberg, M., Borenstein, D., and Arnett, F.: The absence of back pain in classic ankylosing spondylitis. Johns Hopkins Med. J., *143*:181–183, 1978.
29. Wiesner, K., and Bryan, B.: Clinical and radiographic abnormalities in ankylosing spondylitis: A comparison of men and women. Radiology, *119*:293–297, 1976.
30. Sorin, S., Askari, A., and Moskowitz, R.: Atlantaaxial subluxation as a complication of early ankylosing spondylitis. Arthritis Rheum., *22*:273–276, 1979.
31. Murray, G., and Persellin, R.: Cervical fracture complicating ankylosing spondylitis. Am. J. Med., *70*:1033–1041, 1981.
32. Dihlmann, W.: Current radiodiagnositc concept of ankylosing spondylitis. Skeletal Radiol., *4*:179–188, 1979.
33. Melsom, R., Benjamin, J., and Barnes, C.: Spontaneous atlantoaxial subluxation: An unusual presenting manifestation of Reiter's syndrome. Ann. Rheum. Dis., *48*:170–172, 1989.
34. Halla, J., Bliznak, J., and Hardin, J.G.: Involvement of the craniocervical junction in Reiter's syndrome. J. Rheumatol., *15*:1722–1725, 1988.
35. Blau, R., and Kaufman, R.: Erosive and subluxing cervical spine disease in patients with psoriatic arthritis. J. Rheumatol., *14*:111–117, 1987.
36. Fam, A., and Cruickshank, B.: Subaxial cervical subluxation and cord compression in psoriatic spondylitis. Arthritis Rheum., *25*:101–106, 1982.
37. Resnick, D., and Niwayama, G.: Gouty arthritis. *In* Diagnosis of Bone and Joint Disorders. 2nd Ed. Philadelphia, W.B. Saunders, 1988, pp. 1618–1671.
38. Haselwood, D., and Wiesner, K.: Clinical, radiographic and pathologic abnormalities in calcium pyrophophate dihydrate deposition disease: Pseudogout. Radiology, *122*:1–15, 1977.
39. Resnick, D., and Niwayama, G.: Calcium hydroxyapatite crystal deposition disease. *In* Diagnosis of Bone and Joint Disorders. 2nd Ed. Philadelphia, W.B. Saunders, 1988, pp. 1733–1764.
40. Nakajima, K., Miyaoka, M., Sumie, H., et al.: Cervical radioculomyelopathy due to calcification of the ligamenta flava. Surg. Neurol., *21*:479–488, 1984.

93

Painful Temporomandibular Joint

DORAN E. RYAN

The temporomandibular joint (TMJ), like other central joints, is paired and cannot function alone. This rotating, sliding joint must function in total harmony with its counterpart on the opposite side of the horseshoe-shaped mandible. The articulating surfaces of the bone are not covered by hyaline cartilage as are most other joints of the body, but rather by an avascular fibrous connective tissue that may contain chondrocytes and hence is designated fibrocartilage.[1] The fifth cranial nerve, which supplies the muscles that move the joint, also provides sensory protection and innervates the overlying skin.

ANATOMIC FEATURES

This joint is complex, with an articulating fibrous connective tissue disc interposed between the temporal and the mandibular bones, separating the articular space into superior and inferior compartments. The articulating surface of the mandible is the anterosuperior surface of the condylar head. This surface measures approximately 16 to 20 mm mediolaterally and 8 to 10 mm anteroposteriorly. The disc is ovoid with distinct anterior, central, and posterior zones and is firmly attached to the medial and lateral poles of the condylar head. Its average measurements are 27.5 mm mediolaterally and 9 mm anteroposteriorly. The posterior band is its thickest part (3 mm). The central zone is only 1 mm thick, and the anterior band is about 2 mm thick. Chondrocytes can be found in the disc with aging, and cartilage will form when the disc is displaced and abnormal forces exerted.[1]

The fibrous capsule is frail, although its lateral surface is strengthened into a distinct temporomandibular ligament. The joint capsule is attached to the border of the temporal articulating surface and to the neck of the mandible. It is directly fused to the medial anterior and lateral circumference of the articulating disc. Posteriorly, however, the disc and the capsule become integrated into the posterior attachment, or "bilaminar zone." This area is generously innervated and vascularized, with large sinusoids that fill and empty during joint function. The zone is termed "bilaminar" because it splits, with one attachment on the posterior condyle neck and the other on the anterior wall of the auditory canal.

The only muscle directly attached to the TMJ is the lateral (external) pterygoid. It has two points of origin, the superior portion from the infratemporal crest and the undersurface of the greater wing of the sphenoid bone. Its bundles converge to attach to the capsular ligament and directly into the articular disc. The inferior portion of the muscle is larger and arises from the lateral surface of the pterygoid process, from the pyramidal process of the palatine bone, and from the maxillary tuberosity. Its bundles converge to insert on the condylar head and neck. As the head rotates and then translates, the interior belly of the muscle contracts, helping to pull the condyle forward and inferiorly along the posterior slope of the eminentia articularis. The superior belly of the muscle remains flaccid on opening, and the disc moves in concert with the head of the condyle by mechanical action. On closing, the superior belly of this muscle contracts to maintain the disc in proper relation to the head of the condyle.

SIGNS AND SYMPTOMS

Examination of the patient with TMJ symptoms begins when the patient enters the room. Note should be made of the posture, stride, and general carriage.

When did symptoms first appear and under what circumstances? Was the onset acute or insidious? Was there a specific incident, or did the patient simply wake up one morning with symptoms? How do the symptoms relate to time of day and physical activity? What can be accomplished to increase or decrease the severity of symptoms? Where are the symptoms located? Has treatment of any kind been instituted? If so, has the treatment helped?

The examiner should put the patient at ease and should watch mandibular function as the conversation proceeds, noting particularly thrusting, limited function, or deviation of the mandible. Once normal or abnormal function of the mandible has been established, specific voluntary movements are requested. The interincisal distance is measured at the midline with the patient's mouth open. A range of approximately 38 to 42 mm is normal, although this distance varies with sex and general physical build. Lateral excursions are requested, and measurements are made as the jaw moves into right lateral, left lateral, and protrusive positions. Normal lateral excursions are 5 to 10 mm, and normal protrusion is 4 to 6 mm. Function of the mandible is then ascertained while the joints are palpated. A smooth rotation followed by translation of the condylar head without pops, clicks, or crepitus is normal. At the same time, the examiner questions the patient about pain and determines local tenderness by digital pressure over the joint or through the external auditory canal.

A stethoscope is used to auscultate the joints during function; one should listen for the character of the noise, if noise is present. A pop or click signifies malposition of the disc, whereas grating or crepitus usually indicates bone-on-bone contact. The muscles of mastication are then palpated, beginning with the temporalis muscle and proceeding to the masseter, digastric, and medial and lateral pterygoid muscles. Accessory muscles of mastication such as the suprahyoid and infrahyoid, digastric, and sternocleidomastoid muscles are also palpated. Muscle spasm in the sternocleidomastoid or the hyoid muscles or in the muscles of mastication may occur in patients with limited mandibular function. Spasm in some or all of the vertebral muscles may cause the patient to have difficulty in moving the head.

Examination of the dentition follows, with special attention to the skeletal relationship of the arches, as well as the tooth–bone relationship. This determination is important because persons with a class II (retrognathia) skeletal and dental malocclusion have a slightly higher frequency of TMJ symptoms than patients with class I (normal) and class III (prognathic) skeletal relationships.[2] Finally, the patient is asked to point to the area of pain. The pointing finger frequently distinguishes between muscular disorders and internal joint derangements.

DIAGNOSTIC MODALITIES

RADIOGRAPHIC EXAMINATION

Roentgenograms of the painful TMJ give a wealth of information and are particularly useful in patients with possible internal joint derangements. Screening films are important, but definitive diagnosis should not be attempted using these alone. The most common views are the panoramic and the transcranial or transpharyngeal views in both opened and closed positions. These views reveal the general shape and condition of the bony condylar head, but they do not show its position relative to the glenoid fossa. It is possible to obtain these data with corrected tomograms. If the clinical examination and screening radiographic examination suggest internal joint derangement, further specific radiographic studies may be indicated.

ARTHROGRAPHY

Arthrography is an excellent secondary imaging procedure for investigating interarticular disease including disc displacement and disc perforations. Therapeutic potential of this invasive dynamic procedure has been demonstrated.[3–6] An iodized dye is injected into the inferior joint spaces or into both the inferior and superior spaces. If both joint spaces are injected, the disc will be outlined between the two pools of dye (Fig. 93–1). With a single inferior joint space injection, the disc is outlined by dye between the inferior compartment and the eminentia articularis (Fig. 93–2). As multiple sequential films are exposed with the patient opening and closing the mouth, the dye shifts from anterior to posterior as the condyle first rotates and then translates. In a person with an anterior displacement of the disc, the dye concentrates anterior to the condylar head. As the disc is captured by forward movement of the condyle, the dye flows rapidly posterior to the condylar head. At maximal joint opening, little dye is evident in the anterior portion of the inferior joint space. In the anterior closed lock, the disc is not recaptured, and a pool of dye remains in the anterior compartment of the inferior joint space, with the disc bunched superior to the dye concentrations and inferior to the eminentia articularis (Fig. 93–3).

Arthrographic views of the TMJ are recorded dynamically on videotape and are far easier to interpret because the action of the condylar head in relation to the disc and dye is viewed in its entirety. One can watch the immediate and rapid shift of dye from anterior to posterior as the disc is captured or the concentrated anterior pools of dye with forced displacement of the disc anterior to the articular eminence. In a static arthrogram, in which the disc is recaptured at midfunction, the series of pictures may well show abnormal position of the disc on two or three views, followed by normal position of the disc on the remaining views.

SCINTIGRAPHY

Single photon emission computed tomography (SPECT) is an excellent noninvasive technique for determining the presence or absence of TMJ disorders.[7] When internal joint derangement is present, condylar

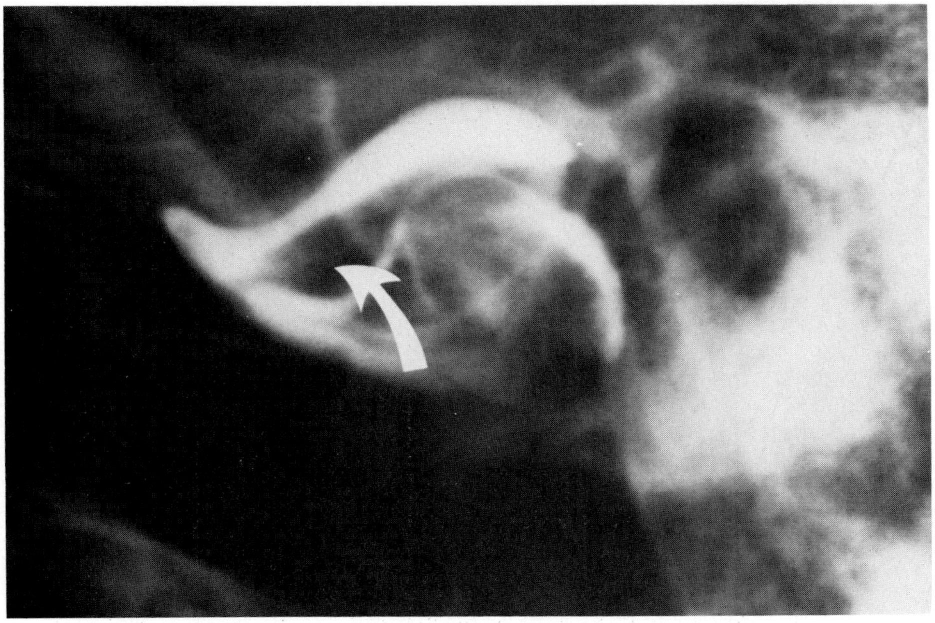

FIGURE 93–1. Disc *(arrow)* outlined by dye in both the superior and inferior joint compartments.

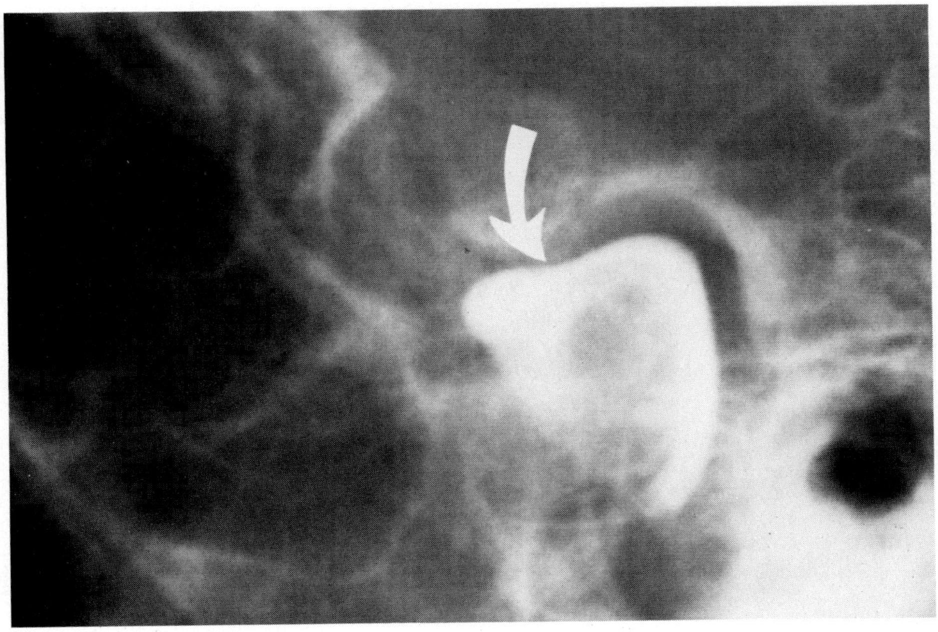

FIGURE 93–2. Disc *(arrow)* outlined by dye between the inferior joint compartment and the articular eminence.

remodeling takes place and bone scintiscans using ^{99m}Tc MDP are positive before either conventional radiographs or x-ray tomograms demonstrate joint space narrowing, bony sclerosis, or disc degeneration.[8] Radionuclide angiography is performed with 10 sequential 3-second anterior-view images of the head, followed by a 50,000-count image 3 hours later. Anterior, right-lateral, and left-lateral planar bone scintigrams (500,000 count) of the head are obtained using a large-field-of-view γ-camera equipped with a high-resolution collimator. A right lateral view demonstrates increased bone uptake over the right TMJ (Fig. 93–4). Tomographic studies in the coronal and transaxial planes can confirm the marked increase in radionuclide activity over the right TMJ (Figs. 93–5, 93–6). Quantitative analysis of the bone uptake over both joints and intervening bony structures also shows the sharp peak of increased activity over the right TMJ (Fig. 93–6, caused by subchondral bone changes from anterior displacement of the disc noted on clinical examination.

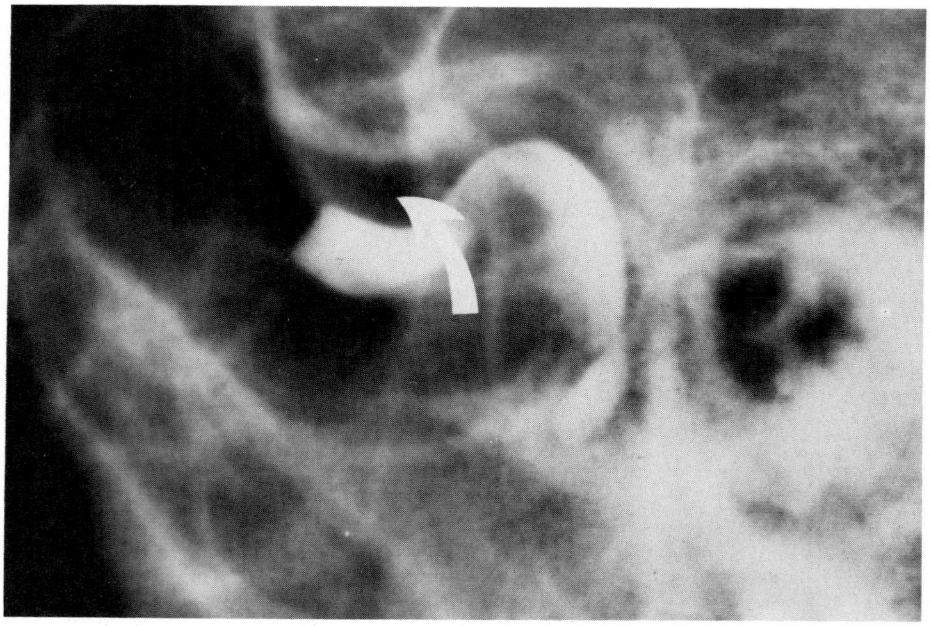

FIGURE 93–3. Disc bunching ahead of the condyle as the condyle head attempts to move anteriorly *(arrow)*.

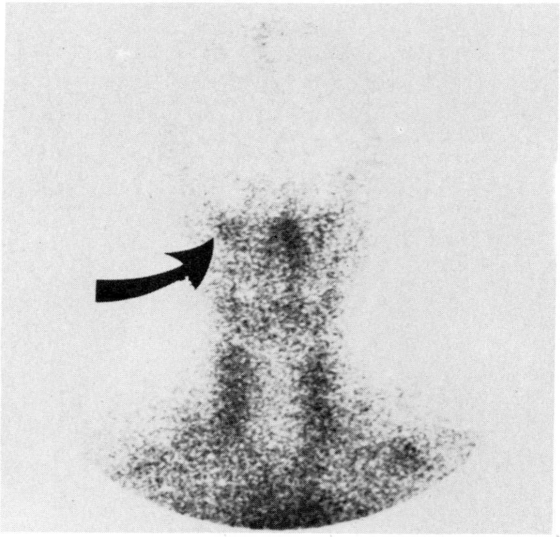

FIGURE 93–4. Increased radionuclide activity *(arrow)* over the right temporomandibular joint.

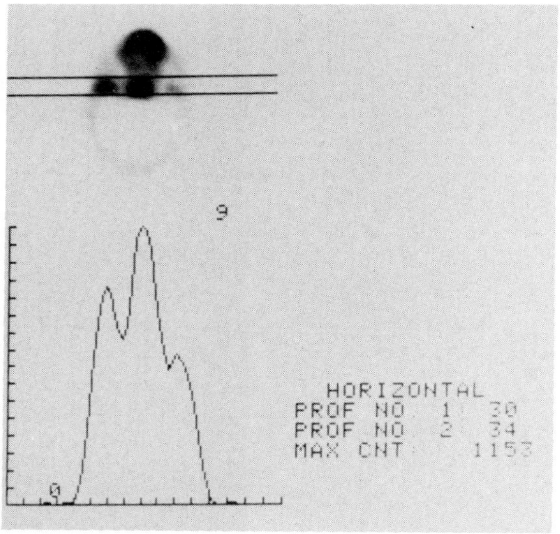

FIGURE 93–5. Coronal slice through the head of the TMJ joint showing a marked increase in activity on the right side *(arrow)*.

MAGNETIC RESONANCE IMAGING

The usefulness of high-resolution magnetic resonance imaging (MRI) obtained with surface coil for imaging of the disc and of replacement implants of the TMJ has been well documented.[9,10] Recent clinical and laboratory investigations with MRI have demonstrated joint inflammation,[11] adhesions, cartilaginous and osseous degeneration,[12] and musculotendinous abnormalities.[13]

In a normal TMJ, the condyle and eminence are easily visualized because of the high-intensity signal from the marrow spaces and the low-intensity signals from the cortical bone (Fig. 93–7). The posterior attachment, or bilaminar zone, is a mixed vascular and connective tissue structure with medium intensity and can therefore be distinguished from the low-intensity avascular disc (Fig. 93–7). In the anterior displaced disc of internal joint derangement, the disc will be located anterior to the condyle and below the articular eminence with the posterior attachment stretched over the condyle (Fig. 93–8).

MRI is a noninvasive, painless imaging technique

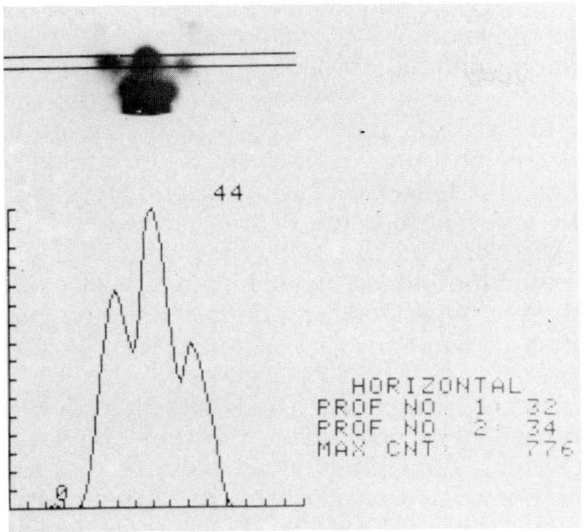

FIGURE 93–6. Transaxial slice in a single photon emission computed tomogram confirms increased radioactivity in the right temporomandibular joint (TMJ) (upper part of the figure). Quantitative analysis shows a sharp peak of activity in the right TMJ (lower part of the figure).

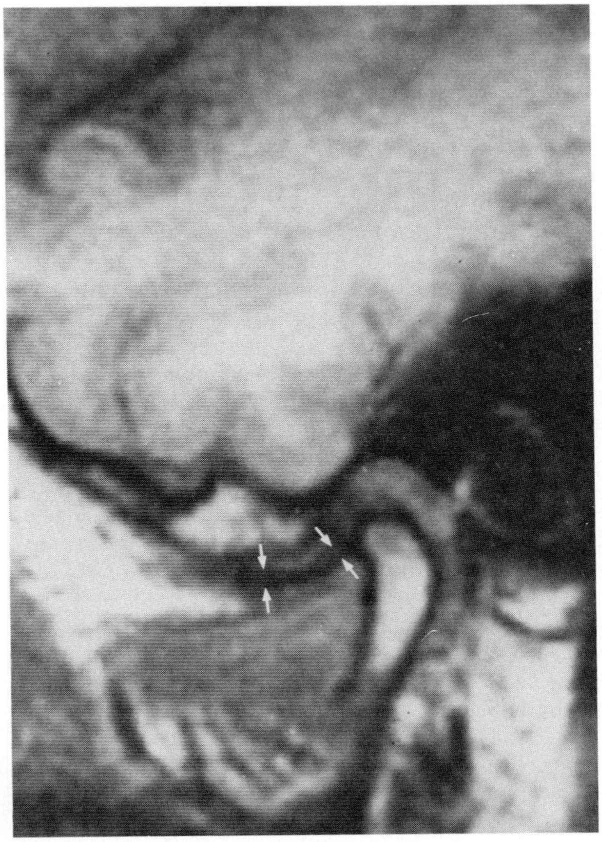

FIGURE 93–8. Magnetic resonance image of the left TMJ in closed position showing an anteriorly displaced disc *(arrows)*. (Courtesy Bruce Kneeland, MD, Medical College of Wisconsin, Milwaukee)

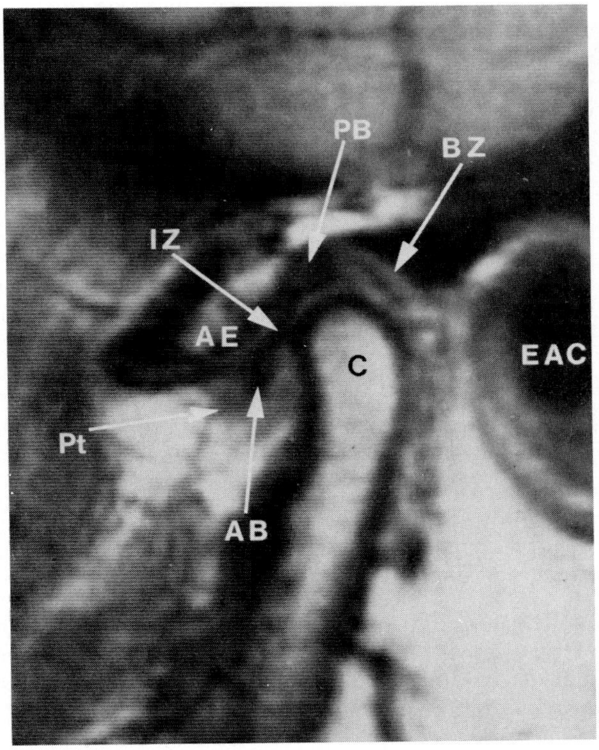

FIGURE 93–7. Magnetic resonance image of the left temporal temporomandibular joint in closed position. Condyle (C), articular eminence (AE), external auditory canal (EAC), bilaminar zone (BZ), posterior band of disc (PB), intermediate zone (IZ), anterior band of disc (AB), lateral pterygoid muscle (PT). (Courtesy Bruce Kneeland, MD, Medical College of Wisconsin, Milwaukee)

that does not use ionized radiation. Unfortunately MRI provides static images, which in its present state of development cannot reproducibly demonstrate perforations of the soft tissues of the TMJ. The long scanning time (8 to 12 minutes per image) make MRI a more expensive procedure than other imaging techniques, but as technology advances, MRI may well replace arthrograms for the diagnosis of internal joint derangement of the TMJ.

DIFFERENTIAL DIAGNOSIS AND TREATMENT

Determining the source of pain from the TMJ and its surrounding structures is complex because the maxillofacial region has the highest sensory innervation density in the body, and the cranial nerves do not follow the orderly segmentation typically found in other joints of the body. Because of this complicated innervation, the diagnosis of diseases of the TMJ joint can be difficult.

REFERRED OTALGIA AND ODONTALGIA

The symptom of earache is common with lesions of the TMJ. The auricle, external auditory canal, and tympanum are supplied by sensory fibers from the fifth, seventh, ninth, and tenth cranial nerves, in addition to the second and third cervical nerves. Earache caused by pain referred from other sites is more common than that resulting from disorders of the ear itself. Because the sensory innervation varies widely and overlaps, it is often difficult for the patient to localize the pain to a particular area of the ear. For these reasons, diagnosis of lesions of both the external and the inner ear is made mainly by clinical evaluation. If the patient's pain is localized within the meatus of the auditory canal and if pain is produced by palpation or passive movement of the auricle, a lesion of the external ear or auditory canal should be suspected. Diseases of the middle ear usually produce symptoms of hearing impairment, low-pitched tinnitus, and pain that varies from mild discomfort or pressure sensation, as seen with an early, acute serious or purulent otitis media, to a deep, boring pain, as seen late in these diseases. If the earache is modified in any way by movement of the lower jaw, and if the auricle, external auditory canal, and tympanic membrane appear normal on examination, the diagnosis of TMJ disease should be considered.

Pain of dental origin is commonly referred to the TMJ through the fifth cranial nerve, primarily the auriculotemporal branch. It is often difficult for the patient to determine whether the offending tooth is in the mandible or the maxilla, and the pain may be felt diffusely throughout the teeth, jaw, face, and head. Because of the variability and the diffuse nature of the pain, it is wise to consider all diffuse pain in the head and neck, including the oral cavity, to be of dental origin until proved otherwise. In most cases, clinical evaluation reveals a large carious lesion or a fractured tooth to be the source of pain. Palpation of the affected tooth with a tongue blade elicits pain and is thereby a dependable means of diagnosis. The surrounding soft tissues may also show signs of inflammation.

Radiographic Findings. In dental disease, radiographs are helpful and often diagnostic. The panoramic radiograph and the periapical radiograph taken in a dental office are most frequently used.

Laboratory Findings. Except in the case of acute infection, when the white blood cell count is elevated, the laboratory examination does not contribute to the diagnosis.

MYOFASCIAL PAIN DYSFUNCTION SYNDROME

As many as 85% of all patients seen with "TMJ syndrome" really have myofascial pain dysfunction (MPD) of the muscles of mastication. The TMJ is implicated because pain occurs when it is mobilized. The female/male sex ratio is 8:1, with an age range from puberty to 40 years, although it can occur at any age. The cardinal signs and symptoms of this syndrome include pain on movement of the jaw, limited ability to open the jaw, deviation of the open jaw toward the affected side, and clicking or popping heard in the TMJ during motion. Two negative findings are important: (1) No tenderness on palpation of the TMJ, and (2) normal bony radiographic findings.[14] Classically, the patient describes the pain by placing the whole hand over the affected side of the face. The description of pain varies from a sensation of pressure to severe and lancinating, occurring both spontaneously and in response to movement of the involved muscles. Pain occurs when chewing and when clenching the teeth. The pain is often more severe in the morning, on awakening, secondary to nocturnal bruxism. A period of emotional stress often precedes the onset of symptoms.

Clinical Findings. No pain is present in the TMJ during movement or on palpation of the condylar head. The "clicking" sometimes felt during early movement of the joint is related to spasm of the superior belly of the lateral pterygoid muscle. If clicking is detected during extreme excursion, a diagnosis of internal joint derangement should be considered. MPD is present in 50% of patients with internal joint derangements. It may be secondary to the joint dysfunction or may be primary and aggravating a previously asymptomatic disc displacement. At least one of the muscles of mastication is tender to palpation on the painful side, and when the patient bites, pain is experienced in the same muscles. If a tongue blade is placed between the incisors and the patient is asked to bite, the pain should decrease. If the tongue blade is placed on the posterior teeth, and the patient is asked to bite, the pain will probably increase.

Treatment. Initial treatment consists of muscle relaxants, anti-inflammatory drugs, moist heat, and a soft diet. If the symptoms persist for more than 2 weeks, the patient should be referred to a dentist for construction of an acrylic splint to help to disocclude the teeth. Because bruxism or clenching of the teeth is a primary cause of this syndrome, the splint may interrupt the cycle of jaw clenching and muscle spasm. Psychologic counseling may be indicated because emotional stress often initiates the problem. If these measures are not successful, physical therapy, biofeedback, hypnosis, and formal psychotherapy may be tried.

INTERNAL TEMPOROMANDIBULAR JOINT DERANGEMENT

By definition, this disorder is an abnormal relationship of the disc with the condyle when the teeth are in maximal occlusion.[15] The abnormal position of the disc is usually anteromedial because of the direction of contraction of the superior belly of the lateral pterygoid muscles toward the pterygoid plates. Internal derangements are subdivided into the following categories: (1) anteromedial displacement of the disc with reduction; (2) anteromedial displacement of the disc without reduction (close lock); and (3) perforation of the disc or the posterior attachment of the disc. These derangements are also classified by the amount of movement of

TABLE 93–1. INTERNAL TEMPOROMANDIBULAR JOINT DERANGEMENT

CLINICAL PROGRESSION OF DISEASE	PATHOPHYSIOLOGY
Clicking	Stretching of lateral attachment Stretching and loss of elasticity of posterior attachment
Clicking with intermittent locking	Thickening of posterior ridge of disc
Close lock	Metaplasia of disc tissue to cartilage or permanent deformation of disc
Crepitus	Perforation of posterior attachment

the mandible necessary to reposition or "capture" the disc, as evidenced by the clicking sound. Thus, *early, midphase*, or *late reductions* are classified by measurement of the interincisal opening. If the reduction occurs during the first 15 mm of interincisal opening, it is considered an early reduction; if it occurs during 15 to 30 mm of interincisal opening, it is a midphase reduction; and if it occurs after 30 mm, it is classified as a late reduction. If the patient can open the mouth only to 27 to 30 mm with deviation toward the affected side and no clicking is heard or palpated, a "close lock" must be considered. With close lock, the disc is wedged in front of the condyle and prevents forward motion of the mandible. The pathophysiologic features of the abnormality are compared with its unpredictable clinical progression (Table 93–1).[15–17] The disorder may progress in a period of several months to years, or it may not follow the full sequence of clinical events.

Clinical Findings. The ratio of women/men affected with the disorder is 8 : 1, and the condition is most commonly seen in the second, third, or fourth decade, but it can occur at any age. The cardinal signs and symptoms of internal joint derangement include pain on palpation of the condylar head, and popping, clicking, or crepitus in the TMJ. One also sees limited range of motion, as in close lock, deviation toward the affected side before the pop takes place, and finally, return to midline at maximal opening. Other, more variable symptoms include temporal or frontal headaches, retro-orbital pain, otalgia, tinnitus, dizziness, and varying degrees of myofascial pain dysfunction syndrome. A history of asymptomatic clicking is important, especially when the patient has limited and noiseless joint opening.

Radiographic Findings. Routine radiographic examination is not diagnostic. Arthrography is invaluable in the diagnosis of internal joint derangement and is the definitive test of choice. More recently, MRI has also become a valuable diagnostic tool.[9,10]

Treatment. Treatment depends on the severity of the condition. The patient with painless joint clicking is informed of the possible progression of the disease, but no treatment is indicated. If a patient has early clicking and pain, nonsurgical techniques are used, including splint therapy to recapture the disc followed by alteration of the occlusion to hold the position.[4,18,19] With late reduction or with nonreduction (close lock) of the disc or in patients unsuccessfully treated by nonsurgical means, a surgical procedure is indicated. If the disc is of normal shape and texture and is easily pulled posteriorly and laterally into a normal relationship with the condyle head, a diskoplasty is performed. The posterior and lateral attachments are shortened, and the disc is reattached to the condyle.[4,18] If the disc has undergone metaplasia or is scarred in an anteromedial position, a diskectomy is indicated with or without autogenous, homologous, or alloplastic replacement. Autogenous materials include ear cartilage,[20] temporalis myofascial or fascia flaps,[21] and dermal grafts.[22] Homologous materials include freeze-dried dura or fresh-frozen cartilage. A soft silicone implant can be used as an alloplastic replacement. Because a fibrous capsule is formed around the silicone implant in approximately 3 months, the implant can be removed either prophylactically or if it has become torn or perforated. The fibrous capsule then functions as a "disc-like" structure to separate the condyle from the temporal bone.[23] At present, fractured implants can be imaged *only* with MRI (Fig. 93–9).[10] Patients tolerate these surgical procedures well; diskoplasty is successful in 80 to 90%; the success rate of the diskectomy with implantation is between 70 and 90%. Good long-term results have been reported with diskectomy without replacement, but 97% showed flattening of the articular surface.[20] Zero to three percent of the patients treated may have an increase in symptoms.

Arthroscopic examination and surgery is now being used in the treatment of internal joint derangement.[24,25] Indications for arthroscopy of the TMJ include acute hemarthrosis, acute locking unresponsive to manipulation, and chronic scarring of the disc to the temporal bone. An arthroscope between 1.5 and 2.3 mm is introduced into the superior joint space, and changes such as synovial hypertrophy, hyperemia of the posterior attachment, disc dislocation, perforation of the disc, and adhesions of the disc to the temporal bone can be identified.[26] Surgically, adhesions can be lysed, the disc mobilized by sweeping the superior compartment, and mobile foreign bodies removed with copious irrigation. Corticosteroid esters, either triamcinolone or betamethasone, can be injected to decrease the inflammatory process and its accompanying pain.

DEGENERATIVE JOINT DISEASE

Unlike other diarthrodial joints, the articular surface of the TMJ is covered with fibrocartilage rather than with hyaline cartilage. The progression of degenerative disease in the TMJ also differs from that in other joints. Initially, erosion is seen in the subchondral bone, followed by thinning and destruction of the fibrocartilage, with some attempts at repair. Degenerative joint disease

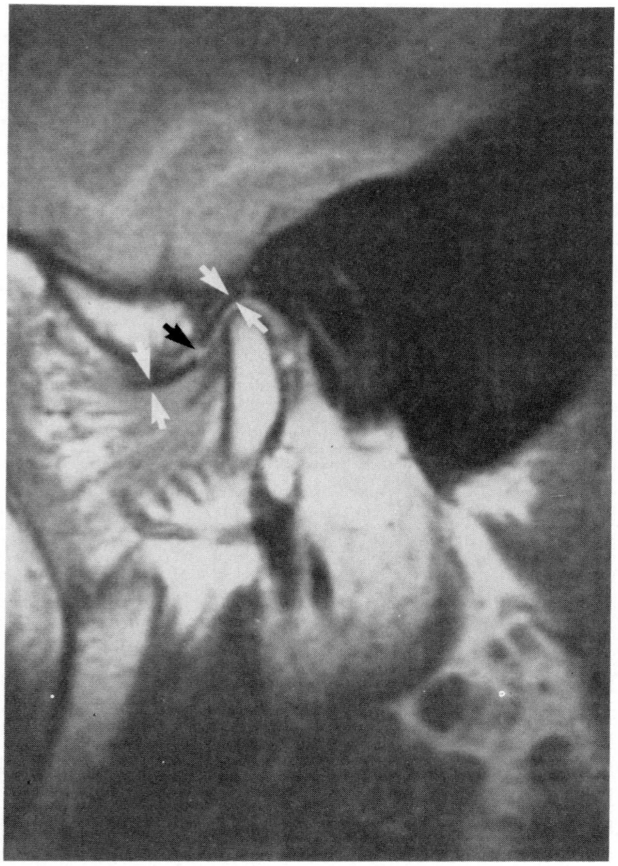

FIGURE 93–9. Magnetic resonance image showing a silicone implant *(white arrows)* with discontinuity *(black arrow)*, representing a fracture. (From Kneeland, J.B. et al.[8] Reprinted with permission of the Journal of Computer Assisted Tomography.)

is traditionally divided into primary and secondary types.[27] Primary disease is idiopathic, whereas secondary disease is related to trauma or, most important, to chronic internal joint derangement. In patients with primary disease, with an intact articular disc, the clinical course of pain and dysfunction is short and is usually followed by repair, with diminution or resolution of symptoms. In secondary disease, the disc is either destroyed or damaged beyond repair, symptoms become chronic, and natural repair is only partial.

Clinical Findings. The onset of this disorder is usually insidious. The initial symptom is stiffness of the involved joint. Pain on joint motion becomes worse by progressive activity during the day. Patients are least symptomatic on arising in the morning. Coarse crepitus is often felt in the affected joint late in the disease process, especially in secondary degenerative joint disease.[28]

Radiographic Findings. A screening radiograph is first obtained. Tomograms or CT can be used to delineate the extent of the bony changes if a surgical procedure is contemplated. Arthrograms are of great value in determining whether the disc is displaced or torn, a finding that determines therapy. Bone scanning with tomography is also of diagnostic value and can be used to evaluate the effectiveness of treatment. Early radiographic changes include thinning or loss of the cortical bone in the area of articulation. As the disease progresses, one sees a roughened and irregular bony surface, which can lead to loss of normal condylar anatomic features. Flattening of the superior and anterior aspects with anterior clipping of the condyle are evidence of natural repair, and cortical margins develop when repair is complete.

Treatment. Primary degenerative joint disease is usually a self-limiting process, often treated symptomatically and nonsurgically. If the disc remains intact, normal healing by fibrocartilaginous proliferation will take place on the condylar surface, and the disease generally runs its course in approximately 2 years. In secondary disease, in which the disc is destroyed or torn and displaced, the condition progresses, and surgical treatment is indicated. This treatment consists of diskoplasty with repair or diskectomy, smoothing of the articular surfaces, and placement of an implant between the condylar head and glenoid fossa. Corticosteroid injections have been used to create a "chemical smoothing" of the articular surfaces of the condyle with moderate success.[29]

RHEUMATOID ARTHRITIS

Involvement of the TMJ in rheumatoid arthritis (RA) varies from 1 to 60%. Affected women outnumber affected men 3 to 1. The disease usually affects both TM joints. Only the condylar head is affected, and the glenoid fossa is seldom involved. Initial bony destruction occurs in the neck of the condyle inferior to the fibrocartilaginous cover of the head. It then involves the cartilaginous surface and the subchondral spaces of the bone.[30] The disc is usually destroyed in the process.

Clinical Findings. Signs and symptoms of RA in the TMJ are similar to those in other affected joints. Pain and stiffness on arising in the morning are prominent features. These symptoms decrease with moderate activity, and stiffness recurs with inactivity. Pain becomes more severe during strenuous activity. On palpation there is tenderness over the joint, and limitation of motion becomes progressive as the disease develops. Later in the disease process, crepitus may be found.

Radiographic Findings. A screening radiograph is used for initial evaluation. Erosions of the neck and head, marginal proliferations of bone, flattening of the superior and anterior surfaces of the condylar head, and eventually, gross deformities are evident. Although not as diagnostic, limitation of joint excursions and narrowing of the joint space are also seen. More detailed evaluation can be accomplished by the use of tomography or corrected tomography. Tomographic bone scanning is diagnostic for RA, and arthrograms can be valuable in determining the status of the disc.

Laboratory Findings. Rheumatoid factor test is positive in 70 to 80% of patients, and other findings are identical to those described in Chapter 43.

Treatment. The usual treatment is conservative, as described in Chapter 47. With successful management of the systemic disease, symptoms of the TMJ usually subside. Rest is prescribed for the joints during the acute phase of the illness, along with mild exercises to maintain function. Occasionally, an acrylic splint is useful to remove the mandible from tooth function or to replace missing teeth, thereby decreasing trauma to the joint. Ankylosis is rare. If it does occur, the procedure of choice consists of creating a joint space, lining the joint space with silicone implant, and instituting motion soon after the operation. Occasionally, an alloplastic total joint replacement or a costochondral rib graft is necessary to maintain a functioning mandible.

GOUTY ARTHRITIS

Gout of the TMJ is rare but painful. As in other joints of the body, urate crystals precipitate in the synovial tissues and fluid. Left untreated, degenerative joint disease develops.[31,32]

Clinical and Laboratory Findings. Sudden onset of symptoms, frequently at night and for no apparent reason, is characteristic. A warm sensation over the joint is common, and the patient notes limitation of mandibular movement because of the acute pain and swelling. The patient may also experience headache, fever, and general malaise.

Radiographic Findings. In the acute phase of the disorder, no radiographic changes are seen. If the disease becomes chronic, radiographic changes resemble those of degenerative joint disease.

Treatment. Aspiration of the joint gives temporary symptomatic relief; medical management of the acute attack is uniformly successful (see Chapter 95).

OTHER DISEASES

The TMJ can be affected by any disease that involves the joints. Short- or long-term symptoms in this joint may be due to the deposition of calcium pyrophosphate dihydrate crystals, as discussed in Chapter 108. Crystal masses may occur in areas of chondroid metaplasia in the synovium as an isolated finding, resembling osteochondromatosis. Acute temporomandibular gout or pseudogout was thought to be precipitated by bruxism in one patient.[33]

Two other categories that cause extreme joint symptoms, only mentioned here, are trauma and either benign or malignant tumors. Trauma can cause pain and can limit movement in the TMJ, but diagnosis is straightforward, by history, examination, and standard facial radiographs. Tumors are rare. Pain usually occurs late in the course of the disease. Limited function and grossly abnormal radiographic changes often precede pain. Biopsy is needed for diagnosis, and treatment is determined by the nature of the lesion.

In summary, pain in the TMJ is often misdiagnosed and frequently attributed to a psychologic cause. With the introduction of arthrography, scintigraphy, and MRI, as well as a better understanding of the anatomy and physiology of this joint, most patients can now be helped.

REFERENCES

1. Dolwick, M.F., Aufdemorte, T.B., and Cornelius, J.D.: Histopathologic findings in TMJ internal derangements. J. Dent. Res., *63*:267 (Abstract 865), 1985.
2. Dworkin, S.F. et al.: Epidemiology of signs and symptoms in temporomandibular disorders: Clinical signs in cases and controls. J. Am. Dent. Assoc., *120*:273–281, 1990.
3. Bronstein, S.L., Tomasetti, B.J., and Ryan, D.E.: Internal derangement of the temporomandibular joint: Correlation of arthrographic and surgical findings. J. Oral Surg., *39*:572–584, 1982.
4. Dolwick, M.D.: Surgical management in internal derangements of the temporomandibular joint. *In* Internal Derangement of the Temporomandibular Joint. Edited by C.A. Helms, R.W. Katzberg, and M.F. Dolwick. San Francisco, Radiology Research and Education Foundation, 1983.
5. Katzberg, R.W.: Temporomandibular joint imaging. Radiology, *170*:297–307, 1989.
6. Schellhas, K.P.: Imaging of the temporomandibular joint. Oral Maxillofacial Surg. Clin. North Am., *1*:13–25, 1989.
7. Krasnow, A.Z. et al.: Comparison of high resolution MRI and SPECT bone scintigraphy for noninvasive imaging of the temporomandibular joint. J. Nucl. Med., *28*:1268–1274, 1987.
8. Collier, D. et al.: Detection of internal derangement of the temporomandibular joint by single photon emission computed tomography. Radiology, *149*:557–561, 1983.
9. Katzberg, R.W. et al.: Normal and abnormal temporomandibular joint: MR imaging with a surface coil. Radiology, *158*:183–189, 1986.
10. Kneeland, J.B. et al.: Magnetic resonance imaging of temporomandibular disc prosthesis: A case report. J. Comput. Assist. Tomogr., *11*:199–200, 1987.
11. Schellhas, K.P., and Wilkes, C.H.: Temporomandibular joint inflammation: Comparison of MR fast scanning to T1 and T2 weighted imaging techniques. A. J. R., *153*(1):93–98, 1989.
12. Schellhas, K.P., Wilkes, C.H., et al.: MR of osteochondritis dissecans and avascular necrosis in the mandibular condyle. A.J.R., *152*:551–560, 1989.
13. Schellhas, K.P.: MR imaging of muscles of mastication. A.J.R., *153*:847–855, 1989.
14. Laskin, D.M.: Etiology of pain dysfunction syndrome. J. Am. Dent. Assoc., *79*:147–153, 1969.
15. Dolwick, M.F., and Sanders, B.: TMJ internal derangement and arthrosis surgical atlas. 1st Ed. St. Louis, The C. V. Mosby Co., 1985, pp. 27–50.
16. Farrar, W.B.: Diagnosis and treatment of anterior dislocation of the articular disc. N. Y. J. Dent., *41*:348–351, 1971.

17. Scapino, R.P.: Histopathology associated with malposition of the human temporomandibular joint disc. Oral Surg., *55*:382–397, 1983.
18. McCarty, W.L., Jr., and Farrar, W.B.: Surgery for internal derangement of the temporomandibular joint. J. Prosthet. Dent., *42*:191–196, 1979.
19. McNeill, C. et al.: Craniomandibular (TMJ) disorders—the state of the art. J. Prosthet. Dent., *44*:434, 1980.
20. Hall, H.D., and Link, J.J.: Diskectomy alone and with ear cartilage interposition grafts in joint reconstruction. Oral Maxillofacial Surg. Clin. North Am., *2*:329–340, 1989.
21. Albert, T.W., and Merrill, R.G.: Temporalis myofascial flap for reconstruction of the temporomandibular joint. Oral Maxillofacial Surg. Clin. North Am., *1*:341–349, 1989.
22. Meyer, R.A.: Autogenous dermal grafts in reconstruction of the temporomandibular joint. Oral Maxillofacial Surg. Clin. North Am., *1*:351–361, 1989.
23. Eriksson, L., and Westesson, P.L.: Deterioration of temporary silastic implants in the temporomandibular joint: A clinical and arthroscopic follow-up study. Oral Surg., *62*:2–6, 1986.
24. Sanders, B.: Arthroscopic surgery of the temporomandibular joint: Treatment of internal derangement with persistent closed-lock. Oral Surg., *62*:361–372, 1986.
25. Sanders, B., and Buoncristiani, R.: Diagnostic and surgical arthroscopy of the TMJ: Clinical experience with 137 patients over 2 years. Craniomand. Disorders Facial Oral Pain, *1*:202–213, 1987.
26. Kaminishi, R.M., and Davis, C.L.: Temporomandibular joint arthroscopic observations of superior space adhesions. Oral Maxillofacial Surg. Clin. North Am., *1*:103–109, 1989.
27. Toller, P.A.: Osteoarthrosis of the mandibular condyle. Br. Dent. J., *134*:223–231, 1973.
28. Kreutziger, K.L., and Mahan, P.E.: Temporomandibular degenerative joint disease. I. Anatomy, pathophysiology and clinical description. Oral Surg., *40*:165–182, 1975.
29. Poswillo, D.: Experimental investigation of the effects of interarticular hydrocortisone and high condylectomy on the mandibular condyle. Oral Surg., *30*:161, 1970.
30. Ogus, H.: Rheumatoid arthritis of the temporomandibular joint. Br. J. Oral Surg., *12*:275–284, 1975.
31. Kleinman, H.Z., and Ewbank, R.L.: Gout of the temporomandibular joint: Report of three cases. Oral Surg., *27*:281–282, 1969.
32. Rodnan, G.P.: Gout and other crystalline forms of arthritis. Postgrad. Med., *58*:6, 1978.
33. Good, A.E., and Upton, L.G.: Acute temporomandibular arthritis in a patient with bruxism and calcium pyrophosphate deposition disease. Arthritis Rheum., *25*:353–355, 1982.

94

The Painful Back

DAVID B. LEVINE
JAMES M. LEIPZIG

Back pain is one of the most prevalent medical disorders in industrialized societies. Despite the aggressive research approach of the past decade, there remains no clear understanding of the exact etiology of the vast majority of cases of low-back pain.

The etiology of a painful back encompasses a wide range of possibilities, including degenerative, rheumatic, infectious, neoplastic, and traumatic considerations.

Physicians should plan an orderly approach to the patient with back pain. They should first attempt to determine whether the cause is primarily musculoskeletal, neurologic, or visceral. A differential diagnosis (Table 94–1) should then be established by medical history, physical examination, radiographs (as indicated), and laboratory analysis. Only then can a logical management plan be formulated.

EPIDEMIOLOGY

Low back pain is the major cause of industrial disability, with an estimated reported financial impact of 11 to 16 billion dollars annually in the United States.[1,8]

It is estimated that 80% of all people will experience at least one episode of back pain in their life-time,[2] with point prevalence ranging from 15 to 39%.[3] Seventy percent of patients with an episode of low back pain recover within 1 month, and 90% within 3 months. Only 4% of patients will have symptoms larger than 6 months.[2] This relatively small number of patients account for 85 to 90% of funds spent on the treatment and compensation for low back pain.[4] Only 50% of these chronically symptomatic patients return to work, according to one study.[2]

RISK FACTORS FOR LOW-BACK PAIN

Numerous studies have detailed risk factors associated with low-back pain. Age, sex, weight, ethnicity, cigarette smoking, occupation, vibrational exposure, repetitive heavy lifting, bending, prolonged sitting, the geometry of the lumbar spinal canal, and psychologic factors have all been implicated.[5,6,8,9] The risk of low-back pain increases until the age of 50; in men it then begins to decrease, but it continues to increase in women.[7] The increasing incidence in women over the age of 50 most likely reflects the added impact of osteoporosis-related conditions.

EMBRYOLOGY

The anlage of the spine forms in a right and left column on each side of the primitive notochord just anterior to the neural tube. At a later stage of development, the two halves fuse anteriorly and posteriorly around the developing spinal cord. A failure of this process accounts for the frequent incidence of fusion defects, various degrees of spina bifida when development fails posteriorly, and various degrees of platyspondylisis and butterfly vertebrae when it fails anteriorly, which occurs much less commonly than posterior failure.

The vertebral bodies are formed in a different plane, with the inferior portion of one sclerotome fusing with the subjacent superior part of another. Disturbances of this process result in such clinical entities as hemivertebrae and asymmetric segmentation.

The lateral halves of the vertebral body then fuse in the midline. Here, between the centra (the primordial vertebral body), the notochord undergoes mucoid degeneration, developing into a gelatinous mass of cells

TABLE 94–1. DIFFERENTIAL DIAGNOSIS OUTLINE FOR THE SYNDROME OF LOW-BACK PAIN

Anatomic Factors	Vertebra (alignment)
Vertebra (hard)	Paravertebra (muscular)
Body	Anterior
Neural arch	Posterior
Spinous process	Lateral
Lamina	*Etiologic Factors*
Facet	Traumatic
Pedicle	Acute
Transverse process	Chronic
Vertebra (soft	Congenital
Supraspinous ligament	Degenerative
Infraspinous ligament	Inflammatory
Ligamentum flavum	Infectious
Posterior longitudinal	Noninfectious
ligament	Neoplastic
Anterior longitudinal	Developmental
ligament	Metabolic
Intervertebral disc	Toxic
Minor ligaments	Psychoneurotic
Vertebra (articulation)	Nerves
Anterior (disc)	Primary (local)
Posterior (facets)	Primary (general)
Lateral (sacroiliac joints)	Coverings
Vertebra (orifices)	Vessels
Neural canal	Arterial
Intervertebral foramina	Venous
	Visceral organs

that becomes the nucleus pulposus. Defects in this process lead to defects in the cartilaginous endplates. The anulus fibrosus, which encloses the nucleus pulposus, originates in the mesenchyme, remaining as the cephalad and caudad portions of the sclerotome separate to form the vertebral bodies.

ANATOMY

The human spinal column comprises 33 vertebrae each composed of a cancellous body anteriorly and a neural arch posteriorly. The neural arch is connected to the body via the pedicles (Fig. 94–1). Arising from the neural arch are the transverse processes, the single midline posterior spinous process, and bilaterally, the superior and inferior articular processes (facets). The clinically important region of bone between the superior and inferior articular processes is termed the pars interarticularis.

The vertebrae are segmentally articulated anteriorly via the intervertebral disc, and posteriorly via the important apophyseal* (facet) joints, which are true diarthroidal (synovial) joints.

The intervertebral disc is a complex that includes the tough anulus fibrosus, a strong fibrocartilaginous outer ring of the disc. This structure is composed of concentrically arranged fibers of type 1 collagen, arranged in multiple and criss-crossed layers. The inner core of the disc is the nucleus pulposus, a viscous gel containing type 2 collagen and proteoglycan aggregates. Superiorly and inferiorly, the disc is bound by the cartilaginous endplate, which blends with the anulus fibrosus and the bony cortical endplate of the vertebral body.

The important ligamentous structures of the spine are the anterior longitudinal ligament, the narrow posterior longitudinal ligament, and the ligamentum flavum. There are also intertransverse ligaments and the interspinous ligaments. The anterior longitudinal ligament is a strong, broad structure that is firmly attached to the periosteum of the vertebral bodies but loosely draped over the intervertebral disc. In comparison, the posterior longitudinal ligament is a narrow structure that is intimately attached to the disc. It is, however, firmly attached only laterally, and is strong in the midline, thus providing an area of relative weakness just slightly lateral to midline.[10] It is this posterolateral site where most disc herniations occur. The ligamentum flavum (yellow ligament) is an elastic interlaminar ligament that spans from the deep, mid-aspect of the superior lamina to the anterior edge of the inferior lamina. This

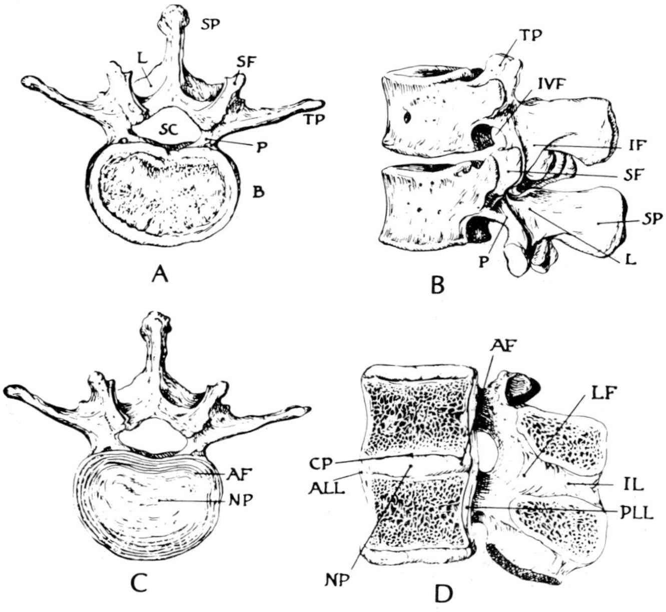

FIGURE 94–1. Anatomy of the lumbar vertebrae and their articulations. *A*, Superior view of a stripped lumbar vertebra. *B*, Lateral view of two articulated lumbar vertebrae. *C*, Superior view of a horizontal section of a lumbar disc. *D*, Lateral view of a sagittal section of two articulated lumbar vertebrae. B, body of the vertebra; SC, spinal column; IVF, intervertebral foramen; IF, inferior articular facet; SF, superior articular facet; P, pedicle; TP, transverse process; SP, spinous process; L, lamina; AF, anulus fibrosus; NP, nucleus pulposus; CP, cartilage plate; ALL, anterior longitudinal ligament; PLL, posterior longitudinal ligament; LF, ligamentum flavum; IL, interspinous ligament.

* *Editor's note: Zygapophyseal* was the original name used by the Greeks to describe these joints. The word means "scale" or "balance"; this word was used because the paired joints were reminiscent of the ancient instrument for weighing.

structure is clinically important when gaining surgical access to the spinal canal.

NEUROANATOMY

At birth the spinal cord extends to the caudal end of the dural (thecal) sac at about the level of the third sacral segment. It retracts superiorly as the spine grows in length to reach the final adult position at the level of the first lumbar vertebra.

The nerve roots of the lumbosacral plexus are drawn up with the spinal cord within the dura, forming the cauda equina. The filum terminale is a slender filament that anchors the distal end of the spinal cord to the coccyx. Each nerve root leaves the spinal canal inferior to its corresponding vertebral segment, except in the cervical spine, where there are eight cervical nerves (and seven cervical vertebrae), and the nerves exit superior to the vertebral level. Each nerve root is in intimate relationship with several parts of the vertebra and discs as it passes from the dural sac to the periphery. In the lower lumbar spine, each nerve root, together with a sheath of dura, becomes separated from the remainder of the cauda equina at the level of the superior aspect of the disc, courses laterally as it passes distally across its corresponding vertebral body, and reaches the intervertebral foramen at a point opposite its disc of the same numerical designation. In the foramen, it is held against the medial and inferior surface of the pedicle, lying in a groove called the sulcus nervi spinalis. Anteriorly lies the vertebral body; inferiorly lies the disc; and posteriorly, shielded by the ligamentum flavum, lies the inferior facet. Therefore, pathologic or traumatic disturbances of any of these structures can obstruct and compress the nerve root. An area of specific interest is the sinuvertebral nerve, a recurrent branch of the spinal nerve that branches just distal to the dorsal root ganglion. It has an inferior and superior division, which eventually supplies the posterior longitudinal ligament, the dura, the periosteum, the annulus fibrosus, and the epidural vessels.[10] Dysfunction of this nerve might be a key factor in the etiology of back pain.

VASCULAR SUPPLY

The vertebral column receives a segmental arterial supply. From these segmental vessels arise neural branches that enter via the intervertebral foramen, with twigs supplying the ganglia, roots, and dura. The blood supply to the cord is complex and is beyond the scope of this chapter. The artery of Adamkiewicz, however, deserves mention because it arises from segmental vessels of the upper lumbar or lower thoracic levels. It ascends along the anterior median sulcus, usually on the left side, to anastamose with the anterior spinal artery. This artery, at times, can supply up to two-thirds of the lower spinal cord.[12] Its disruption, whether due to trauma, surgery, or vasculitis, can be disastrous.

The venous drainage of the vertebral column is clinically important. There is an external and an internal venous plexus, the latter being more important. The internal venous plexus is valveless, lying in two columns just medial to the pedicles, and is referred to as Batson's plexus. It drains through interforaminal veins into segmental intercostal or lumbar veins, and thence to the azygous and caval systems. Because the veins are valveless, drainage from the pelvis, under the "pumping" influence of changing interabdominal and interthoracic pressure, provides a route for the metastatic spread of tumor from lower pelvic neoplasms.[13]

BIOMECHANICS

The spine is formed as one long curve, with its convexity directed posteriorly. With the assumption of vertical posture, the sagittal curves develop. Lordosis in the cervical spine develops with head control at the age of 3 months. Lumbar lordosis develops with bipedal stance. Because of the immobility of the thoracic segment, in part due to the attached ribs, the thoracic kyphosis persists. The sagittal curves improve spinal stability by allowing the weight of the trunk to be carried directly over its base, and also provide a shock-absorbing mechanism. The lordotic curves are entirely functional and can be reversed by bending forward, in contrast to the structural thoracic kyphosis.

Both Nachemson and Anderson have measured lumbar disc pressures in different body positions[14,15] (Fig. 94–2). These studies show that lumbar disc pressure is highest in the forward leaning position, with disc pressure being more than 100% greater than in the standing position. Disc pressure is lowest in the reclining supine position. These data have implications for the rehabilitation and back school setting.

The spinal kinematics enable flexibility in three planes of motion. The cervical spine allows both rotation and flexion-extension, with approximately 50% of rotation occurring at the C1-C2 level. The greatest amount of flexion-extension occurs at C5-C6, also the level with the highest incidence of disc disease. Because of the coronal orientation of the thoracic facet joints and the bony rigidity imposed by the ribs and sternum, thoracic motion is restricted, with the greatest motion occuring in the sagittal plane (flexion-extension). In the lumbar spine, the facet joints assume a sagittal orientation. Here, lateral bending exceeds rotation by 3 to 4 times, and flexion-extension increases from L1 to L5.

Because of the relative fixed attitude of the pelvis, the lumbosacral junction is subject to a high level of stress. Axial compression or lateral bend can result in flexion, rotation, or shear forces. With increased lordosis of the lumbosacral junction, the shear force at the L5-S1 level is increased; this is one factor in the etiology of spondylithesis, which is discussed in detail later in the chapter.

MEDICAL HISTORY

A general appraisal should include sex, age, race, economic and social background, family and past medical history, and the presence of workman's compensation

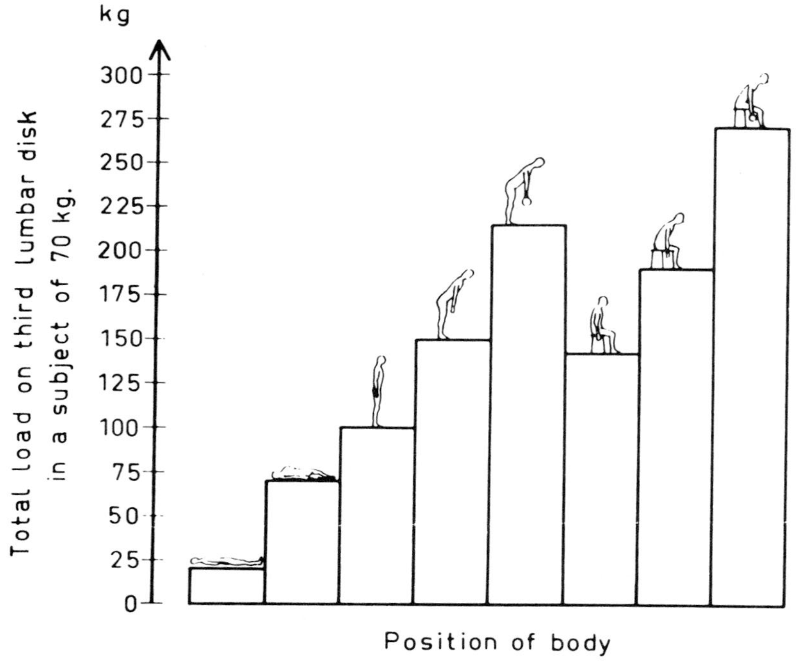

FIGURE 94–2. Total load on the L3 disk in different positions in a subject weighing 70 kg. Positions shown are (1) reclining (relaxed, supine), (2) reclining (lateral decubitus), (3) standing upright, (4) standing and 20° forward leaning without and (5) with a 20-kg load in arms, (6) sitting upright, arms and back unsupported, (7) sitting and 20° forward leaning without and (8) with a 20-kg load in arms. (From Nachemson, A.: Acta Orthop. Scand., *36*:426, 1965).

or ongoing litigation. The patient's type of work, recreation, and daily habits should also be determined.

The chronology, the inciting event, the character, and the pattern of the pain should be ascertained. The presence of ongoing litigation or workman's compensation is correlated with a poor prognosis and should be determined.[16] One should determine if the pain has remained the same, worsened, or lessened. Is the pain intermittent, or are there periods of amelioration or exacerbation? Is there pain at night? Night pain might indicate a neoplastic process. In addition, the patient should be questioned with regard to any treatment he or she has received.

The medical history determines if the pain pattern is of a radicular or nonradicular nature. Radicular pain is defined as pain secondary to a lesion of the spinal nerve root, which radiates from the back into the dermatome that that nerve root supplies.[17] Ask the patient to trace the pain pattern on his own extremity, and to complete a pain drawing. Nonradicular pain radiates into a nondermatomal pattern, and therefore indicates that the pain is not due to nerve root irritation. The pain might be due to a lesion of the spinal motion segment, such as facet arthrosis, or other causes, such as paraspinal muscle sprain or involvement of the spinal ligaments or lumbodorsal fascia.[18]

PHYSICAL EXAMINATION

A general physical examination, including examination of the heart, lungs, lymph nodes, and vasculature, as well as a general orthopaedic assessment, should be performed in each case with assessment of the hips, knees, and upper extremities.

The patient's stance and posture are then evaluated. It should be noted whether the iliac crests are level, whether the spine is straight or curved, and whether the patient lists to one side. A lateral deviation in the spinal column (scoliosis) is generally compensated by an opposite deviation elsewhere in the spine. Full compensation signifies that the first thoracic vertebra is centered over the sacrum. If the spine is uncompensated, then the first thoracic vertebra is not centered, and the patient has a list. This is measured by dropping a plumbline (using a tape measure) from the first thoracic spinous process, and observing whether or not it falls in the midgluteal cleft or to the right or left of the cleft (Fig. 94–3). This distance should be measured and recorded.

Scoliosis can be structural or functional. A structural scoliosis is associated with structural changes of the vertebral column and thoracic rib cage, and can be detected by viewing the back as the patient bends forward. Other signs of scoliosis are pelvic obliquity or unequal shoulder heights. A functional, nonstructural scoliosis can (1) be secondary to leg-length discrepency, which should be corrected with an appropriate leg block or lift, (2) due to an acute back sprain, or (3) due to the muscle spasm associated with an acutely herniated lumbar disc.

The contour of the spine should be observed in the forward lean posture. Viewed from the side, there should be a gentle, smooth contour to the spine. An abrupt or angular bend to the thoracic spine might indicate a structural kyphotic deformity (Fig. 94–4). When the patient is bending forward and then again standing upright, the motion of the spine should be observed.

The lordotic curve of the lumbar spine should first flatten and then reverse slightly as the degree of forward bending increases. If it does not do so, motion will be limited, even though the patient is able to touch the floor. The other motions of the spine—flexion, extension, and lateral bend—should then be measured. At this point, the back should be palpated. This is facilitated by having the patient lie prone with a pillow under the abdomen, which will reverse the lumbar lordosis. The paraspinal musculature is palpated for the presence of spasm, tenderness, or trigger points. The spinous processes are palpated, as are the interspinal spaces. In a patient with an acute lumbar disc herniation, palpation of the corresponding interspinous ligament might produce a sharp pain that might radiate down the extremity.[19]

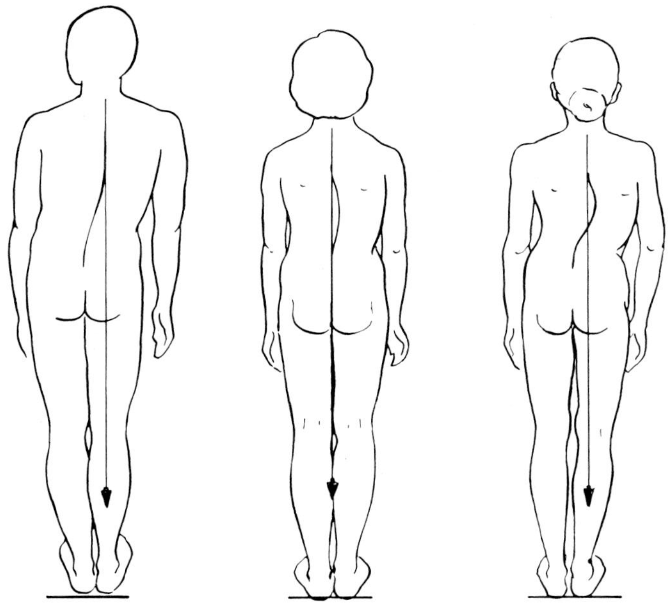

A B C

FIGURE 94–3. Compensated and uncompensated deviations of posture. *A,* A plumb line dropped from the first thoracic spinal process indicates a right list. *B,* A compensated right thoracolumbar scoliosis. *C,* An uncompensated right thoracic, left lumbar scoliosis with right list. List or decompensation causes prominence of the hip opposite the direction of the list.

NEUROLOGIC EXAMINATION

The neurologic examination includes standard motor, sensory, and reflex tests, which should be performed while keeping in mind the specific nerve root that is being tested. The examiner should be able to determine, in the case of a herniated lumbar or cervical disc, which nerve root is involved. In the lumbar spine, the nerve roots exit *below* the numbered vertebra. The nerve root then exits the foramen by passing just below the pedicle, at an angle of approximately 45°. Because the lumbar discs lie just below this level, a lateral disc herniation will involve the next lower segmental nerve root (Fig. 94–5). For example, a disc herniation at the L4–L5 level will involve the L5 nerve root. There is some overlap in nerve distribution, and the examination might not always show classic changes.

Because the cervical spine has eight nerve roots and seven vertebrae, the nerve roots exit *above* the numbered vertebra—for example, the C6 nerve root exits above C6. At this level, however, the intervertebral disc lies at the level of the lower-numbered nerve root. Therefore, a disc herniation will compress the next

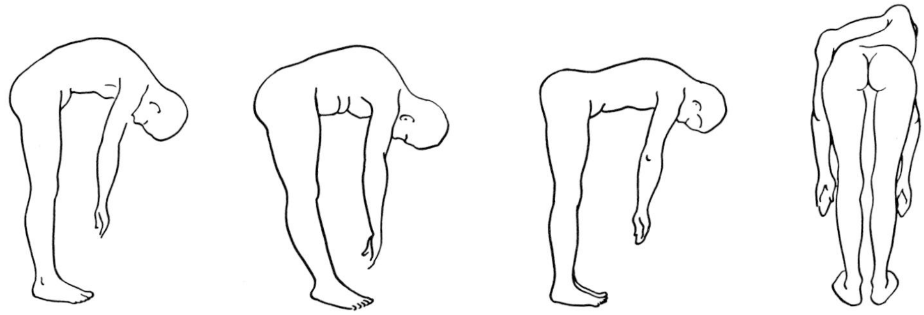

A B C D

FIGURE 94–4. Forward bending. *A,* Normally on forward bending, one sees an even contour of the spine when the spine is viewed laterally. *B,* An accentuation of the thoracic kyphosis indicates a thoracic round back, especially when the apex of the curve is sharp and angular. *C,* A persistence of the angular lordotic curve in the position of forward bending indicates that the lumbar spine has lost its flexibility. The flexion is all taking place at the hip joints. *D,* When viewed posteriorly, minor degrees of structural scoliosis can readily be detected in the position of forward bending. The convex rotation of the thoracic vertebrae is easily recognized because it is accentuated by the rib deformity or hump. Similar rotation of the lumbar segment is more difficult to detect.

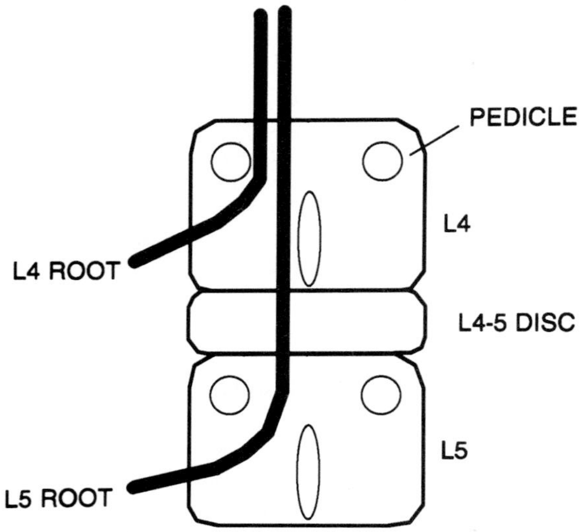

FIGURE 94–5. Schematic drawing of a lumbar vertebra motion segment with an exiting and traversing nerve root. A disc herniation will compress the lower numbered nerve root (in this example L5) because the upper nerve root (L4) has exited the neural foramen.

lower numbered nerve root—that is, a C5–C6 disc herniation (laterally) will involve the C6 nerve root. By keeping these anatomic details in mind while performing the neurologic examination, one can generally pinpoint the exact level of neurologic involvement in most cases with radicular involvement.

Another part of the neurologic examination is the evaluation of gait. The patient should be observed during ambulation for the presence of a list (as previously described), antalgic or coxalgic gait, foot drop, shuffling gait, or balance disorders. The toe and heel walk should be observed, which are gross measures of L4 and S1 function, respectively. Running in place on the toes can demonstrate subtle weakness that is only apparent with fatigue.

Rectal examination is especially important in patients with coccygeal pain in order to rule-out masses. After trauma, rectal sphincter tone is noted, along with perirectal sensation (S5 nerve root).

SPECIAL TESTS—SCIATIC TENSION TESTS

The *straight leg raising test of Laseque* is one of the most useful maneuvers in the analysis of low-back disorders (Fig. 94–6). The test places tension on the sciatic nerve, therefore stretching the roots of the lumbosacral plexus. In addition, it flattens the lumbar spine by placing tension on the hip extensor musculature and the hamstrings. By definition, a "positive" straight leg raise (SLR), an indicator of nerve root irritation, produces radicular symptoms (pain, numbness, tingling, or a combination of these) down the leg below the knee, and should reproduce the patient's radicular symptoms. Hamstring tightness with leg raising does not constitute a positive SLR. The SLR can also be performed while the patient is seated. This can be helpful in the differentiation of nonorganic low-back pain from organic low-back pain. In some patients with a positive SLR in the supine position, a seated SLR, in which the patient usually doesn't realize what is being tested, can be negative. A *crossover test* is the presence of elicited radicular symptoms down the involved leg when an SLR is performed on the contralateral leg. This test is the most sensitive clinical indicator of a herniated intervertebral disc. The *bowstring test* is the presence of tenderness in the popliteal fossa while the fossa is palpated during an SLR maneuver. This is another indicator of sciatic nerve tenderness.

The *iliac compression test* is pathognomonic of sacroiliac disease. It is most easily performed with the patient lying on his or her side. The examiner applies firm pressure against the uppermost iliac crest. A positive result is elicited when pain is produced in the region of the involved sacroiliac joint. Another sign of sacroiliac joint pain is a positive *flexion abduction external rotation* (*FABER*) test. Pain in the sacroiliac joint with forced, maximal hip flexion abduction external rotation constitutes a positive result.

ORGANIC VERSES NONORGANIC PAIN

Because of the complex nature of low-back pain, especially that associated with psychosocial factors, it is important that the physical examination be used to screen for nonorganic causes of low-back pain. Much work has been performed to try to determine an accurate means to test for nonorganic low-back pain. Waddell et al. published an approach to this problem in 1980, describing a series of maneuvers to help differentiate organic from nonorganic low-back pain.[20] Organic pain is defined as pain that follows neuroanatomy, whereas nonorganic pain is pain that cannot be explained by

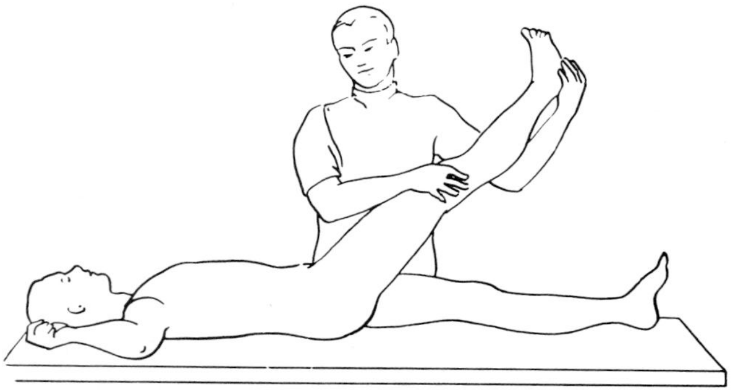

FIGURE 94–6. Straight leg raising test. The leg being tested should be relaxed and should rest in the examiner's hand. The knee is fully extended and is kept from flexing by gentle pressure against the patella.

pathologic involvement of anatomic structures. The reader is referred to this paper for complete details.

The distraction test, pinch test, axial loading test, and over-reaction test are the keys. The *distraction test* refers to performing a known positive test—for example, the straight leg raise test—while the patient is being distracted—for example, performing the test in the seated position and observing for a negative response. The *pinch test* is positive when pinching the lumbar skin produces deep tenderness over a wide, nonanatomic area. *Axial loading* is performed by vertically loading the spine by pressing down on the skull, and is positive when back pain is produced. *Over-reaction* during examination should also be noted, and should lead the examiner toward determining a nonorganic basis for the pain. The unifying concept of the tests of Waddell et al. is that they detect divergence from neuroanatomic explanation. These tests should be performed when the clinical situation warrants them.

DIAGNOSTIC AND IMAGING MODALITIES

A multitude of diagnostic and imaging modalities are now available. The advent of magnetic resonance imaging (MRI) was the single most important advance. Each of the available modalities has its strong points and its limitations, and should be used judiciously. An unfortunate contemporary trend is to use MRI alone, without a good physical examination or without plain radiographs. This approach is wasteful in terms of dollars and can often lead to misdiagnosis and mistreatment.

RADIOGRAPHS

Standard radiographic evaluation of the back includes an anteroposterior (AP) and a lateral view (Fig. 94–7). Oblique views will outline the facet joints and the pars interarticularis and should be ordered as the clinical situation warrants (Fig. 94–8). Although routine radiographic examination is often performed as part of an initial evaluation of the back, this practice has been criticized. Nachemson stated that in only 1 of 1000 patients do routine lumbar radiographs affect the diagnosis, prognosis, or treatment in initial evaluations.[21] Fry-

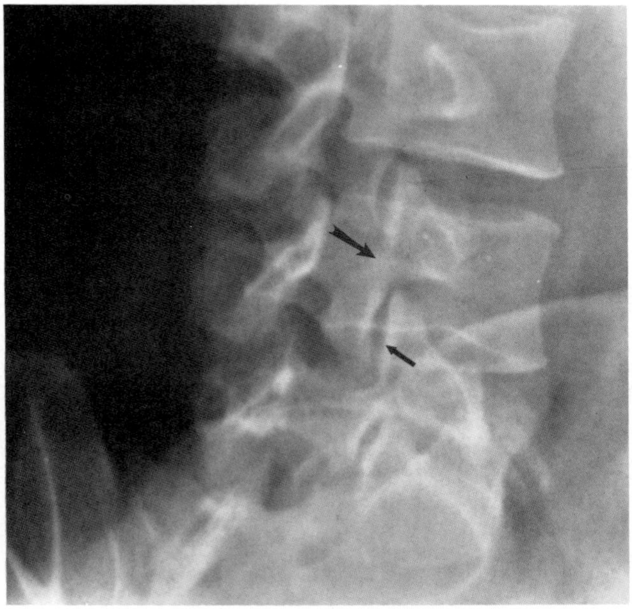

FIGURE 94–8. Forty-five degree oblique view of the lumbosacral spine. This view demonstrates the pars intra-articularis (large arrow) as well as the facet joint (small arrow), and is important in the diagnosis and evaluation of spondylosysis and spondylolisthesis.

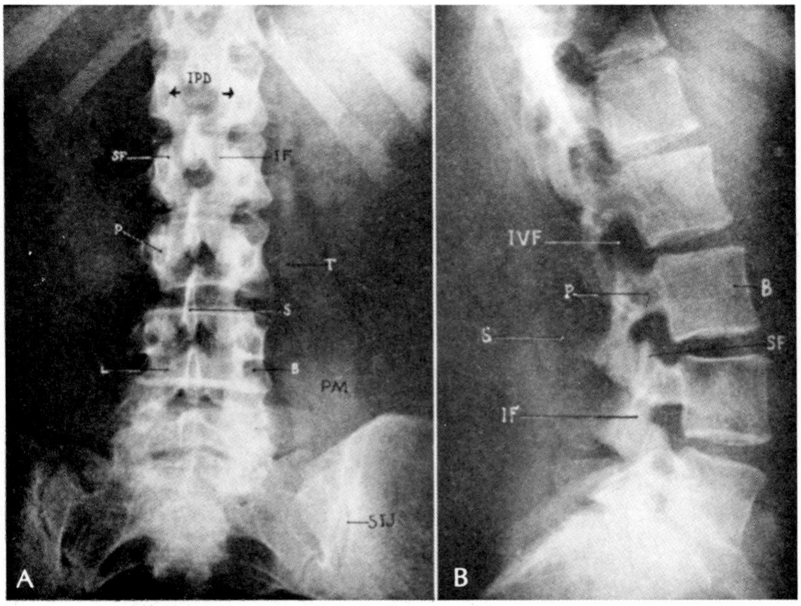

FIGURE 94–7. Roentgenographs of the normal spine. *A*, Anteroposterior and *B*, lateral films of the lumbar spine. Note the detail of most of the lumbar spine, but the obscurity of the lumbosacral region. B, body; D, disc space; I, isthmus, or pars interarticularis; IF, inferior facet; IVF, intervertebral foramen; L, lamina; P, pedicle; PM, psoas margin; S, spinous process; SF, superior facet; SIJ, sacroiliac joint; T, transverse process; IPD, interpedicular diameter.

moyer et al. found a similar frequency of Schmorl's nodes, vacuum sign, disc space narrowing between L3 and L4 and between L5–S1, and the presence of transitional vertebrae in groups of patients with and without low-back pain.[21] Only the presence of disc degeneration at the L4–L5 level and the presence of traction spurs at that level were associated with the presence of low-back pain. Another study found no correlation between the presence of disc degeneration and spondylosis in patients with and without low-back pain and sciatica.[22] Particular indications for low-back radiographs are a suspicion of trauma, infection, neoplasm, metabolic disorder,[4] or persistant back-pain that is not resolving on follow-up evaluation. Such radiographic evaluation should be performed if symptoms persist longer than 4 to 6 weeks, especially if no previous radiographs have been obtained.

MAGNETIC RESONANCE IMAGING (MRI)

At this time MRI is the most accurate means of evaluating the intervertebral disc. MRI produces high-resolution axial, coronal, and sagittal images of the spine, utilizing magnetic properties of tissues (Fig. 94–9), without the use of invasive techniques or ionizing radiation. The quality of MRI has improved significantly in the past several years because of both software and hardware advances.

Varying the pulse sequence parameters (T_1 and T_2), taking advantage of different proton relaxation times, allows for physiologic assessment of the tissues being studied. In T_1 images, the neural structures will appear white, with fluid (e.g., cerebrospinal fluid) appearing gray. In T_2 images, the neural structures will be gray and the cerebrospinal fluid will appear white, thus giving a mylogram-like image.[25] As degenerated intervertebral

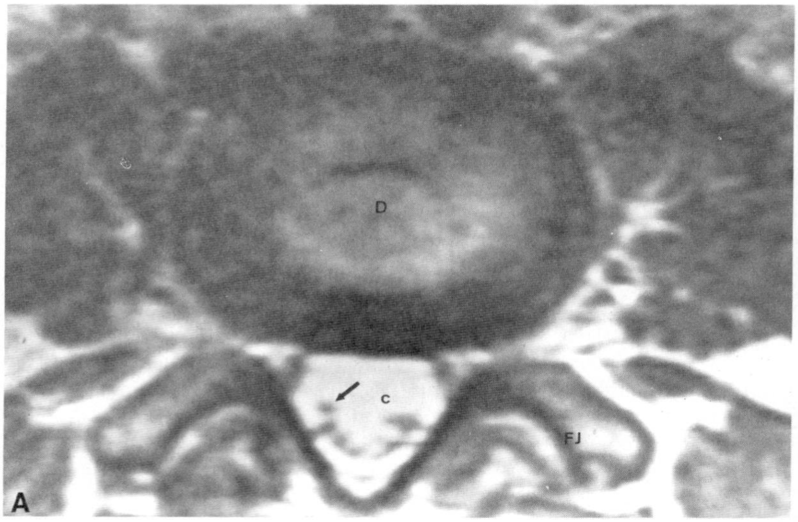

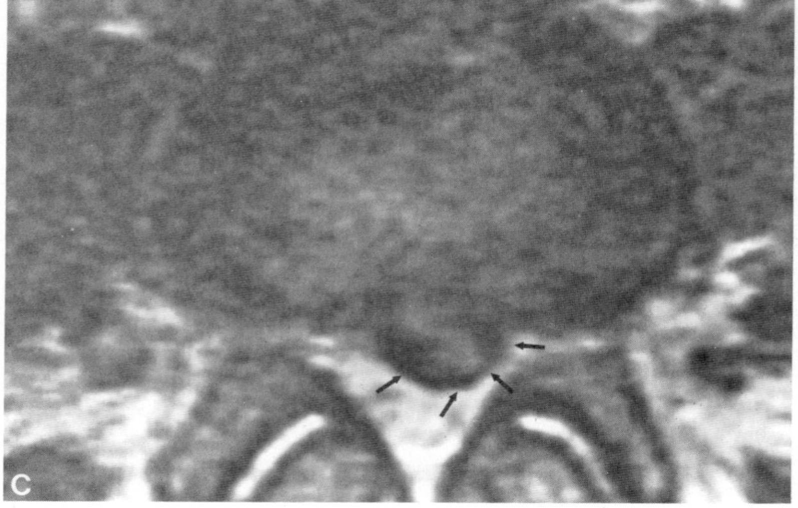

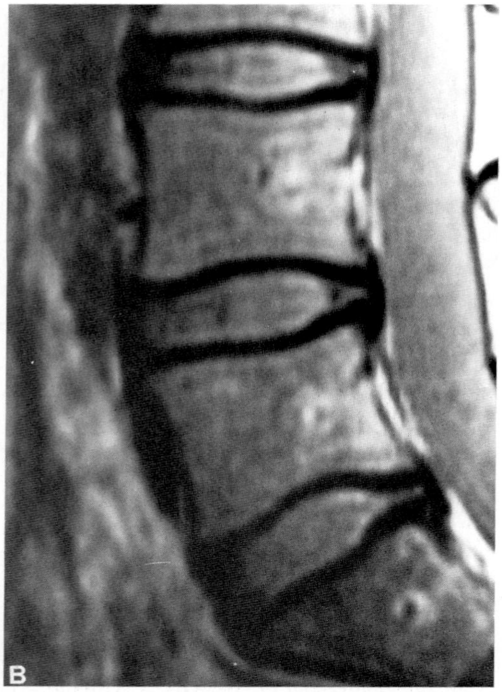

FIGURE 94–9. *A*, Axial MRI image through the L4–L5 disc demonstrates normal facet joints, intact posterior longitudinal ligament, and cauda equina. Note individual nerve rootlet (arrow) demonstrated as low-intensity signal within the cauda equina. D, disc; C, cauda equina; FJ, facet joint. *B*, Sagittal MRI image of the lumbosacral spine demonstrating mild disc degeneration at the L4–L5 and L5–S1 level with no compression of the cauda equina. *C*, Axial MRI image at the L4–L5 level demonstrating a large central and left-sided herniated nucleus pulposus with cauda equina compression and impingement of the left L5 nerve root. This lesion presented clinically with left-sided sciatica.

discs undergo dessication, the water content of a degenerated disc is decreased, and will give a decreased signal on the T_2-weighted image. Also, the T_2 scan is an excellent means for evaluation of interspinal disorders such as spinal cord tumors, syringomyelia, and other abnormalities.

The recent development of paramagnetic contrast agents has aided the evaluation for disc reherniation versus peridiscal scar in the postsurgical patient. Gadolinium-DPTA is administered as an intravenous injection.[26] This agent relies on the principle that disc material is avascular, whereas peridiscal fibrous tissue contains capillaries with abnormal junctional membranes. Following injection of gadolinium-DPTA, there is consistent enhancement of the peridiscal fibrous tissue within 15 minutes, whereas disc tissue, representing a recurrent disc herniation, will not be enhanced.[25] The effect is diminished after approximately 30 minutes, and therefore the test depends highly on technique. In one study, patients with a nonenhancing lesion on their gadolinium-DPTA MR scan, which was thought to be a recurrent disc herniation, underwent surgical exploration; 100% of them had a recurrent disc herniation.[27]

Because of the high sensitivity of the images, overreading of the scans is possible. A current study found a high incidence of abnormal MRI scans in asymptomatic subjects.[23] This study found abnormalities on 57% of scans in asymptomatic subjects over the age of 60 (36% with herniated nucleus pulposus and 21% with spinal stenosis), and 20% of subjects less than 60 years old were found to have a herniated nucleus pulposus. Therefore, it is essential that the history and physical findings be correlated with the MRI scan. Diagnoses based solely on the MRI will lead to misdiagnosis and overdiagnosis.

COMPUTED TOMOGRAPHY (CT)

CT allows excellent imaging of bony anatomy of the spine, especially in the axial plane, and is felt to be the single best diagnostic tool for evaluation of the facet joints and lateral recesses.[25] Because the neural elements are not well visualized with CT scans, the modality is often combined with myelography (CT-myelography) (Fig. 94–10). One study found that adding myelography to the CT scan increased accuracy in the diagnosis of herniated lumbar discs from 71.4 to 76%.[31] New technology utilizes three-dimension imaging capability along with the CT-myelogram (Fig. 94–11). We think that the CT scan, combined with myelography, is best obtained when evaluating bony elements, such as in fracture, deformity, or stenosis. The MRI scan, which is a better examination of soft tissues, is the single best test for the diagnosis of herniated lumbar discs. An important point is that in the cervical spine, because the bony elements (osteophytes) are often an important factor in symptoms, the CT-myelogram is often superior to the MRI scan.

As with MRI scans, abnormal CT scans are seen in the asymptomatic subject. Wiesel et al. demonstrated a prevalence of 35.4% for abnormal CT scans of the lower back, irrespective of age, in asymptomatic individuals.[28]

MYELOGRAPHY

Myelography involves the injection of a radiopaque contrast agent into the subarachnoid space, followed by radiographs, to study the neural elements (Fig. 94–12).

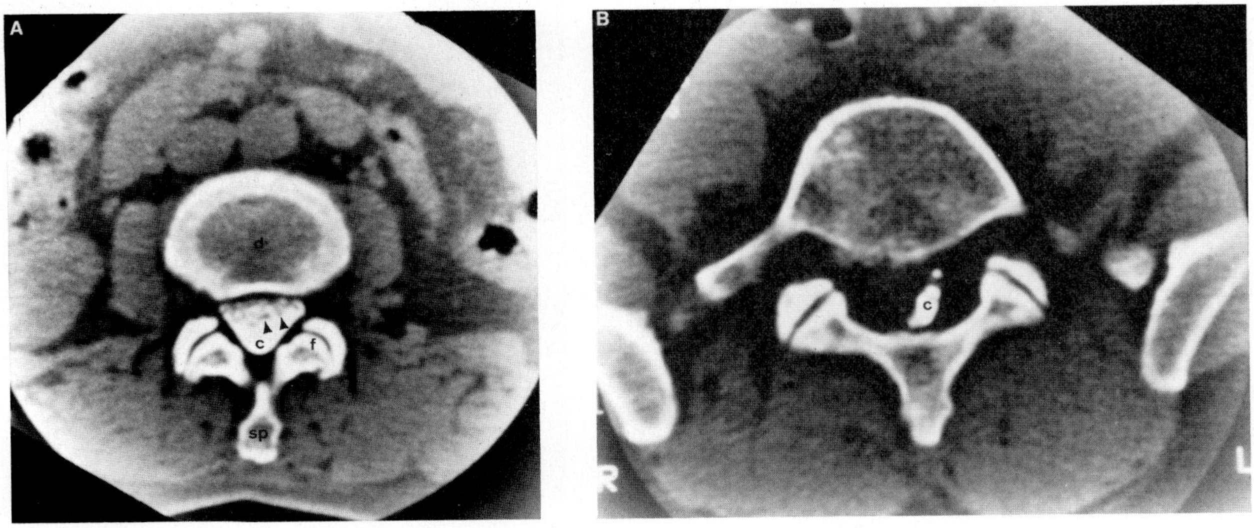

FIGURE 94–10. *A*, Axial CT-myelographic image of an L4–L5 disc space. The architecture of the facet joints is well visualized, along with the normal cauda equina with enclosed nerve rootlets (arrow). d, disc; c, cauda equina; f, facet joint; sp, spinous process. *B*, Axial CT-myelographic view of an L5–S1 disc space with a large herniated nucleus pulposus on the right side with severe compression of the cauda equina. c, compressed cauda equina.

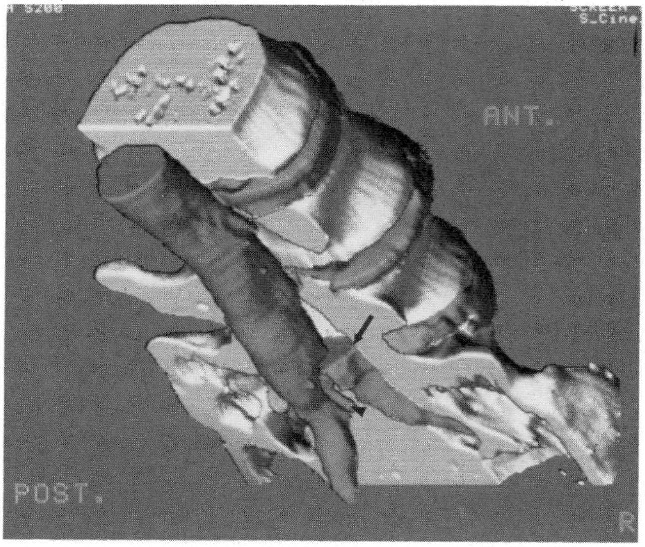

FIGURE 94–11. Three-dimensional CT-myelographic construct. Graphic demonstration of a herniated lumbar disc (large arrow) with nerve root compression (arrowhead).

Currently, Omnipaque is the agent of choice. This is a water-based, nonionic agent, which is associated with a lower complication rate than the older oil-based agents such as Pantopaque. Major complications with Pantopaque are spinal headaches, seizures, and arachnoditis, all of which are less frequent with metrizimide.[25] As noted previously, myelography is often obtained in conjunction with CT. Myelography alone has been found to be superior to CT alone in the diagnosis of herniated lumbar intervertebral discs and spinal stenosis. Bell et al. found myelography to be superior to CT scans in both of these situations (83% vs. 72% and 93% vs. 89%, respectively).[29] It is generally accepted, however, that CT in conjunction with myelography is superior to either of these modalities separately.[30,31]

DISCOGRAPHY

Discography was introduced in 1948 by Lindblom as a technique for imaging the intervertebral disc[32] (Fig. 94–13). Its popularity diminished with the advent of myelography and computed tomography. Currently, the indications for discography are controversial. A discogram is performed by directly injecting contrast agent into the disc space being studied. The discogram is both a functional and a radiologic study. During disc injection, the patient is questioned regarding reproduction (provocation) of his or her symptoms, with provocation being evidence of disc pathology.

A British study found a high degree of success (89%) for operations on patients whose discograms showed both disc abnormality and provocation of symptoms, whereas only 52% of patients had significant relief of symptoms when the discogram showed abnormalities without provocation of symptoms.[33] Another study found discography only to be 64% accurate for a diagnosis of herniated nucleus pulposus even with a positive provocation test.[30] Frazel et al. reported an infection (discitis) rate of 0.7 to 2.7% following discography, emphasizing the invasive nature of their study.[34] Despite criticism, there is still strong support for discography because it is a reliable method for imaging the disc and the anulus fibrosis, and because any extravasation of contrast medium within the anular fissures indicates disc degeneration or herniation. Sensitivity is increased with the addition of computed tomography (the CT-discogram), with accuracy rates for the diagnosis of herniated intervertebral discs reported to be 91%.[30] Compared to CT, myelography, CT-myelography, and discography alone, the CT-discogram was reported to be the most accurate test for the diagnosis of foraminal disc herniations.[30]

In another study, CT-discography was found to be accurate in 93% of cases, revealing disc herniation in 18 of 177 discs for which the MRI was negative.[35] Currently, we are investigating the use of combined CT-discography with CT-myelography (disco-CT-myelography) for the diagnosis of recurrent herniated lumbar intervertebral disc versus postoperative scarring.

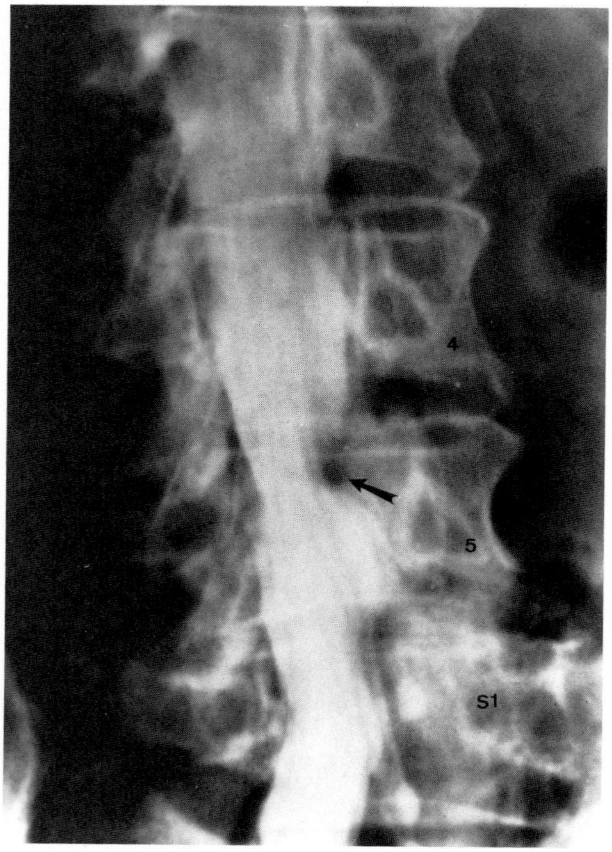

FIGURE 94–12. Myelogram with herniation of the L4–L5 disc. This AP myelographic view demonstrates a herniated nucleus pulposus at the L4–L5 level with indentation of the myelographic contrast agent (arrow).

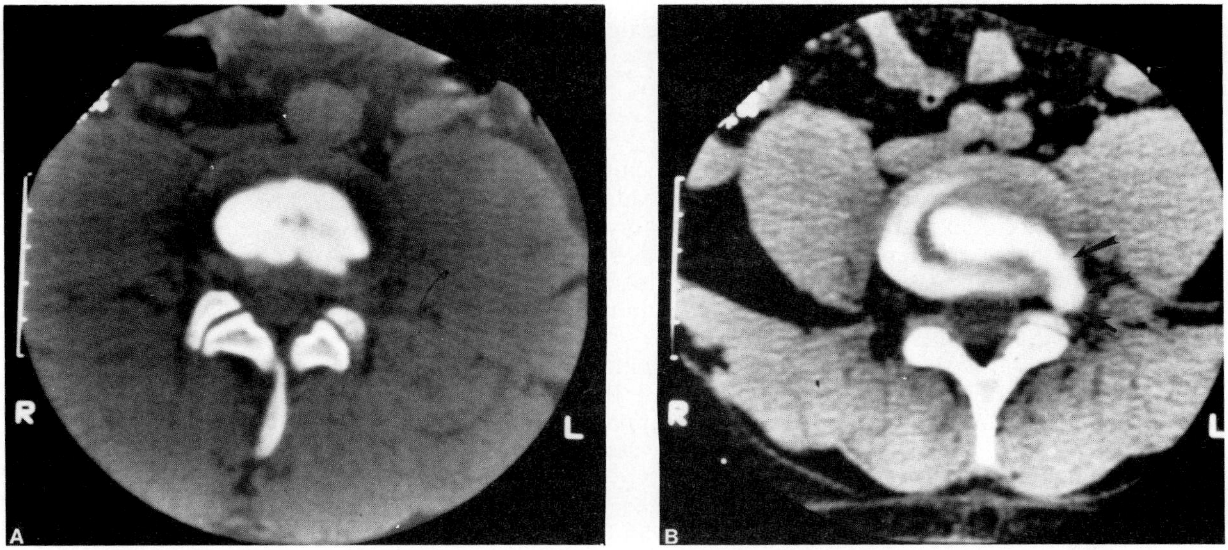

FIGURE 94–13. *A*, Normal CT-discogram. Dye within the disc is well-contained with regular borders and no leakage of dye. *B*, CT-discogram with large foraminal herniated disc. Note leakage of dye directly into the left neural foramen (arrow). This patient presented with weakness and severe radiating leg pain.

THERMOGRAPHY

Thermography is a noninvasive technique that relies on infrared radiation to image the structural cause of low-back pain or sciatica. This modality assumes that stimulation of nociceptive nerves will bring coexistent vasodilation and hence increased blood flow and increased heat. The usefulness of this modality in the diagnosis of radiculopathy has been seriously questioned,[36] and we do not advocate its use in this setting. Thermography might be useful in the evaluation of reflex sympathetic dystrophy,[37] and can be used to monitor the effect of sympathetic blocks.

ELECTROMYOGRAPHY

Electromyography (EMG) involves the measurement of action potentials in muscle fibers, and is performed by placing recording electrodes (needles) into the muscle being tested. EMG therefore tests whether a muscle is innervated or denervated. The procedure is painful. EMG examination helps to identify patients with nerve root compression and to localize the level of the involved nerve root, but does have its limitations. As the test measures reinnervation and denervation, there is a delay of 3 to 4 weeks before muscle cell membranes are sufficiently hypersensitive to generate positive sharp waves and fibrillation potentials. Therefore, it is recommended that one wait at least 4 weeks from the onset of suspected nerve compression until the test is obtained. In addition, the muscles of the lower extremity generally have motor nerves coming from more than one level, making interpretation of the EMG difficult. EMG was 78 to 92% accurate in identifying a root lesion at the correct level in one study.[38] A negative result with EMG does not rule out radiculopathy.

SOMATOSENSORY EVOKED CORTICAL POTENTIALS (SSEP)

This modality involves the stimulation of peripheral nerves with measurement of the generated electrical potentials in the scalp. It was first described by Dawson in 1947.[19] This examination is obtained when evaluation of spinal cord function is desired, but its main indication is in intraoperative monitoring of spinal cord function during cord manipulation, as in scoliosis or kyphosis surgery.

CLINICAL ENTITIES

The spectrum of disorders presenting with back pain is broad. In this section we shall review several major commonly encountered clinical entities.

ACUTE BACK PAIN

Acute low-back pain is frequently encountered. In most cases the etiology is unclear, yet is felt to primarily concern soft tissue. Symptoms are often self-resolving. Of patients with acute low-back pain, 70% will have complete resolution of symptoms within 2 to 4 weeks, and 90% will be asymptomatic by 3 months.[2]

The determination of the presence or absence of radicular pain is important. Of patients with low-back pain, only 10% have a radicular component.[4] Radiculopathy implies nerve root involvement and directs investigation toward the intervertebral discs.

ACUTE BACK SPRAIN

Acute back sprain is a soft-tissue injury. The inciting event is usually specific, such as lifting a heavy load or an automobile accident. Pain is primarily in the lower back. Muscle spasm and tenderness is significant, but sciatica is not present. Pain might be referred to the buttocks and posterior thigh, but sciatica (i.e., pain radiating below the knee) is absent.

Treatment consists of rest, restriction of activities, nonsteroidal anti-inflammatory medication, and the use of muscle relaxants. Oral narcotics are appropriate in selected cases. If symptoms persist past a few days, often a lumbosacral corset can be helpful.

Prolonged bed rest is not advised because of the well-known deleterious effects of prolonged immobilization. A 1986 study showed that 2 days of bed rest was as effective as 1 week,[39] whereas Waddell stated that prolonged bed rest is harmful.[40] In the absence of neurologic findings, diagnostic testing can be safely delayed for 4 to 6 weeks.[4] Several theories for the cause of this condition have been advanced. Some have suggested that partial rupture of the anulus fibrosus, specifically the deep fibers, is the pathologic event responsible in acute low-back sprain. This event will indirectly result in nerve root irritation through chemical or inflammatory stimulation, rather than through mechanical means, as will be discussed later. Any anular disruption, whether it be posterior or posterolateral, will cause pain mediated via the sinuvertebral nerve, a recurrent sensory branch of the spinal nerve. Other etiologic possibilities include tears of the superficial anular fibers, supraspinous ligament tears, or partial tears or rupture of other musculoligamentous or musculotendinous structures. Minute endplate fractures have also been postulated as a possible cause of symptoms.

McNab and McCulloch feel strongly that acute back sprain is simply a facet joint sprain, a condition secondary to a degenerated disc, and should be treated like any other sprain.

Whatever the cause of an acute back sprain, the sprain's natural history favors resolution. A "grass roots" basic approach to management should be followed, because the patient will likely improve despite treatment!

INTERVERTEBRAL DISC HERNIATION

Disc herniations are classified anatomically as prolapsed, extruded, or sequestered (Fig. 94–14). a *prolapsed* disc bulges but remains contained by the anulus fibrosus. An *extruded* disc ruptures through the anulus but is contained by the posterior longitudinal ligament. A *sequestered* disc ruptures through both the anulus and the posterior longitudinal ligament, becoming a free fragment within the spinal canal.[43]

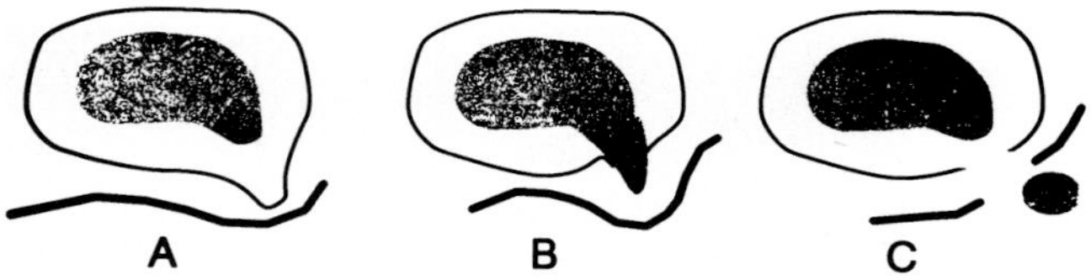

FIGURE 94–14. *A*, Protruded nucleus pulposus with bulging of the posterior longitudinal ligament (PLL) and intact anulus fibrosus. *B*, Extruded nucleus pulposus with rupture of the anulus fibrosus but containment by the PLL. *C*, Sequestered nucleus pulposus with rupture of the anulus fibrosus and the PLL, with the disc fragment lying free within the spinal canal.

Although any disc can herniate, those at L4–L5 and L5–S1 do so most often (90% of the time).[4] Onset of symptoms can follow a sneeze, heavy lifting, or sudden movement; often there is no identifiable inciting event.

The classic picture is that of an otherwise healthy person in the third to fifth decade of life who develops intense radicular pain into the involved extremity. Most patients will give a history of antecedent bouts of low-back pain, which are considered to represent ongoing instability or disc degeneration.[41] Back pain might be present at the time of acute presentation. Radicular pain is accompanied by numbness and paresthesiae. The patient cannot stand straight (lists), which is often associated with a limp. Examination reveals positive results with the straight leg raising test and sciatic notch tenderness; neurologic examination yields inconsistent findings. Decreased sensation, objective weakness, and reflex loss are variable. It is important in the initial evaluation to inquire about bladder and bowel function; incontinence, retention, or feelings of pressure could indicate *cauda equina syndrome*, an urgent indication for surgical decompression.

Treatment

A classic study by Weber of 281 patients with herniated lumbar discs randomized to surgical discectomy or conservative treatment found the surgically treated group to have better results at 1 and 4 years.[42] After 4 years, however, the surgically treated patients no longer had significantly better results. This study should be kept in mind when planning the care of any patient with a herniated lumbar disc.

Conservative Management

Opinions vary regarding conservative management of a patient with a herniated lumbar disc. Prolonged bedrest was once advised for periods of 2 to 3 weeks.[42,44] The detrimental physical and psychologic effects of prolonged immobilization are now well known.[45] A conservative approach now includes 3 to 7 days of bed rest along with anti-inflammatory medication. This notion is supported by a recent study showing that 2 days of bed rest was as effective as 7 days.[48] The use of narcotic medication is sometimes necessary but best avoided. Some authors recommend epidural corticosteroid injections for relief of radicular pain; others do not feel that these injections are beneficial. The use of epidural steroid injections in this setting is therefore empirical and based on individual anecdotal experience.[46,47] Following resolution of acute pain and radiculopathy, mobilization and rehabilitation is heeded. Bending and the lifting of heavy weights are proscribed. A physical therapy program including back "education," flexibility exercises, postural control, and trunk strengthening is initiated. Pain relief coinciding with conservative management is probably due to subsidence of nerve root edema and inflammation, as well as to limited repair of superficial layers of the anulus fibrosus and the richly innervated posterior longitudinal ligament. Herniated disc material is never completely resorbed, but partial resorption allows for some relief of nerve compression and extremity pain. The formation of secondary osteophytes might allow stabilization of the abnormal segment to occur.[49,50]

Surgical Management

A progressive neurologic deficit or cauda equina syndrome is an absolute indication for surgical excision of the herniated disc.[43] Relative indications include persistent pain lasting 3 to 5 months that markedly interferes with the patient's lifestyle, intolerable pain, and a severe postural list.[43,50] Surgical management gives faster results than conservative management, but the results of either approach do not differ after 4 years.[42] Surgical disc excision does not improve a static neurologic deficit, whether sensory or motor. Therefore, such a deficit should not be considered an indication for surgery.[42] The major indication for disc excision in most cases is intolerable and intractable pain that interferes with the activities of daily living.

Classic Discectomy. Standard discectomy involves an incision 3 to 5 cm in length. The lamina cranial and caudal to the level are exposed; a limited laminotomy is performed, followed by incision of the anulus fibrosus and posterior longitudinal ligament, with removal and excision of the disc fragment. With proper patient selection, good to excellent results can be expected in 88 to 95% of cases.[51,52]

Microdiscectomy. Here a discectomy is performed with the use of an operating microscope or other means of magnification. A smaller skin incision is used with less muscular dissection and a smaller laminotomy or laminectomy than with conventional discectomy. Proponents of the procedure claim a faster rehabilitation due to lessened surgical trauma; critics of the procedure refer to the greater infection rate, the increased chance of missing a disc fragment because of the limited exposure, and the risk of missing lateral nerve root stenosis, which might coexist with the disc herniation. Most surgeons routinely use magnification loupes for discectomy. The use of an operating microscope affords better magnification and illumination, but sacrifices surgical exposure. Its use depends on the individual surgeon's experience and training.

Chemonucleolysis. Chemonucleolysis refers to the intradiscal injection of a lysing agent.[43] The technique was approved for general use by the United States Food and Drug Administration in 1983.[19] Its popularity has diminished markedly in the wake of reports of neurologic complications. Selection criteria are essential if good results are to be expected. Candidates should have a prolapsed intervertebral disc with sciatic complaints but no evidence of disc sequestration or concommitant spinal stenosis. Contraindications are the presence of a sequestered fragment, previous chymopapain injection, allergy to papaya or its derivatives, herniation at more than one level, pregnancy, or the presence of bladder or bowel dysfunction.[19,43,50]

In carefully selected patients, chemonucleolysis produces success rates of 79 to 88%.[53] Complications include anaphylaxis, paresis, paraplegia, transverse myelitis, and Guillain-Barré syndrome. The neurologic complication rate is approximately 0.06%.[43] The incidence of transverse myelitis might be increased if discography has been performed along with the chymopapain injection.[52,53] The role of chymopapain injections remains controversial.

Percutaneous Discectomy. Percutaneous discectomy is a relatively new procedure in which an automated cutting-suction cannula is inserted into the disc in the same manner that discography or chymopapain injection is performed. The instrument is then made to resect and remove disc material, thereby decompressing the nucleus pulposus. Indications for this procedure are the same as with chemonucleolysis, and therefore are rather limited. Anatomic constraints can make operation at the L5–S1 level difficult. One recent study reported good results in only 50% of carefully selected patients.

OTHER CONDITIONS PRODUCING LOW-BACK PAIN

INFECTIONS

Pott's Disease (Tuberculosis)

Tuberculosis of the spine is a secondary infection, with the primary lesion in the lung, gastrointestinal tract, or other area. Symptoms can vary considerably. The classic presentation is back pain and a gibbus. Back pain might be present for several months before other changes occur. Systemic signs, especially unexplained weight loss, should make one suspicious. Night pain, fever, or history of pulmonary tuberculosis can be helpful in making the diagnosis. Paraplegia and deformity (kyphosis) are possible complications. Tests for elevation

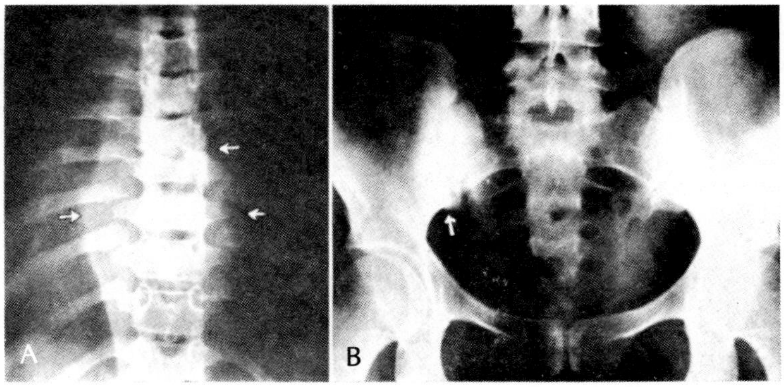

FIGURE 94–15. Tuberculosis of the spine. *A*, Tuberculous spondylitis; note the abscess (arrow). Destruction of the sixth dorsal intervertebral disc space has occurred. This case is too high to cause pain in the lower back. When involvement is in the lumbar spine, the abscesses frequently follow the plane of the psoas muscle, and roentgenographs show distention of the muscle border. *B*, Sacroiliac tuberculosis; note the sclerosis and irregularity (arrow) of the right sacroiliac joint.

of the erythrocyte sedimentation rate and skin testing for tuberculosis are helpful diagnostically.

Radiographs usually demonstrate destruction of the vertebral body (Fig. 94–15). MRI is an extremely valuable tool for visualizing a soft-tissue abscess. Bone scans are also helpful. Definitive diagnosis is made via direct aspiration for smear and culture. Anterior surgery might be required for debridement and fusion, which has the advantage of slightly decreasing the amount of residual kyphosis.

The disease can also involve the sacroiliac joints. Radiographic evidence of bone destruction is the most important diagnostic finding.

An important consideration regarding tuberculosis of the spine is human immunodeficiency virus (HIV) infection. Three of five patients with spinal tuberculosis seen at an inner-city New York hospital between 1987 and 1989 tested positive for HIV. The purified protein derivative (PPD) test for each of these patients was negative. In such high-risk patients, a high index of suspicion must be maintained. The authors of this study found MRI exceedingly useful in the early diagnosis of these problems.

Pyogenic Spinal Infections

The most common pyogenic infections are vertebral osteomyelytis and septic discitis. Epidural abscess is occasionally seen.

Vertebral Osteomyelitis. Approximately 50% of cases of vertebral osteomyelitis are secondary to Staphylococcus; Streptococcus, Proteus, and E. coli account for most of the remainder of cases.[54] The major presenting symptom is back pain. Neurologic involvement with paresis or complete paraplegia might be present. Genitourinary manipulation, diabetes, or immunosuppression due to chemotherapy can contribute to this problem.[55] Treatment goals are resolution of the infection, drainage of any soft-tissue abscesses, restoration of stability, and decompression of neural elements. Surgical management addresses each of these goals. Relief of pain, stabilization, and decompression are usually accomplished through the anterior approach. Autogenous bone grafts are incorporated in the presence of sepsis.[55]

Discitis. This pyogenic infection of the intervertebral disc can be a consequence of hematogenous spread or secondary to an invasive procedure such as discography, chymopapain injection, or excision of a herniated nucleus pulposus. In children, discitis is a relatively benign disease with rapid resolution. There is controversy about whether childhood discitis represents a true bacterial infection.[56] The disease is much more serious in adults.

Presenting symptoms include relentless back pain, usually localized and persisting at night. Muscle spasm, point tenderness, and sciatic nerve irritation might be present.[57] Paresis or paraplegia occurs in up to 40% of cases.[54]

Diagnosis is confirmed by laboratory and imaging data. An elevated erythrocyte sedimentation rate is a good indicator that can also be used to follow the clinical course. Blood cultures are rarely positive, but direct needle aspiration yields positive cultures in up to 70% of cases.[54] Radiographic changes occur after 2 to 6 weeks and consist of loss of disc space height followed by irregular endplate destruction and eventual sclerotic reaction (Fig. 94–16). The technetium-99m MDP bone scintigram is positive at the time of clinical presentation, but MRI might be even more sensitive, showing an increased disc signal on the T_2-weighted image. Unlike bone scintigraphy, MRI pinpoints the abnormality to the involved disc.[54]

The treatment in children is cast immobilization and rest. Antibiotics are only used if there is other evidence of a bacterial infection such as a high fever or extreme pain. In children, needle aspiration is often not necessary. Rapid resolution is seen in most cases.[56]

Treatment in adults requires prolonged intravenous antibiotics (2 to 3 months), along with strict immobilization in a cast or well-fitting brace. Patients who do not respond to this regimen will require anterior disc space debridement and fusion.

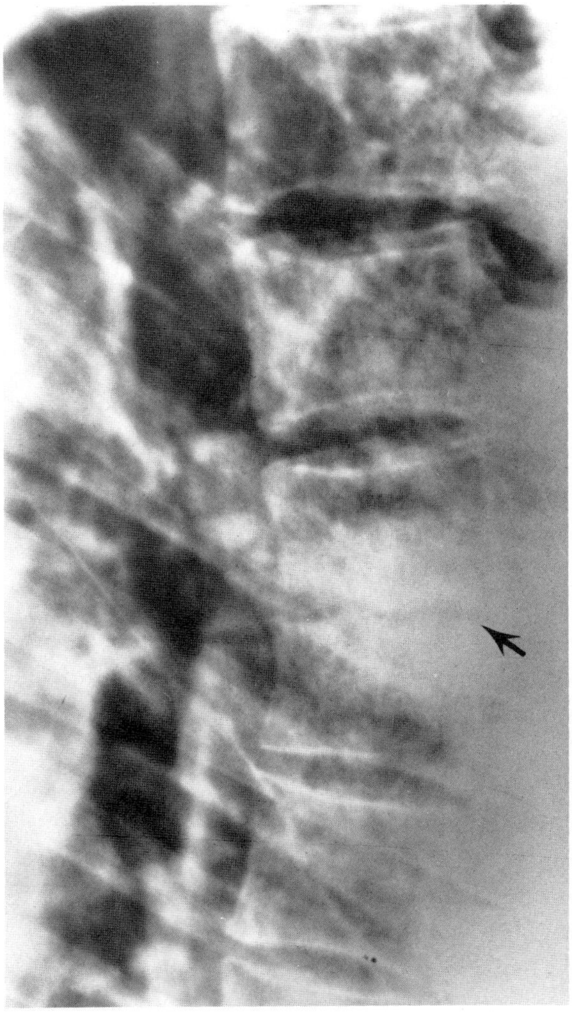

FIGURE 94–16. Discitis. Lateral radiograph of the thoracic spine demonstrating irregular vertebral body endplate destruction with sclerotic reaction and loss of disc space height.

Epidural Abscess. This unusual condition presents with the same picture as other spine infections. Neurologic impairment might be present because of associated epidural compression. Surgical drainage is required, which is often performed by a neurosurgeon.

SPINAL FRACTURES

Fractures of the spine secondary to trauma are an obvious cause of back pain. These injuries vary considerably and are usually due to high-energy trauma. In the ambulatory setting, thoracic or lumbar compression fractures related to osteoporosis are common (Fig. 94–17). Diagnosis is made on the basis of back pain of recent onset with vertebral body wedging seen on radiographs. Care must be taken so that a wedge compression fracture due to a primary or secondary malignancy is not missed.

NEOPLASTIC DISEASE

The spine is a common site of metastases from pelvic and abdominal neoplasms. Hematogenous extension to the spine is via Batson's plexus. Breast, kidney, thyroid, and lung carcinoma often metastasize to the spine. Primary malignancies of the spine include multiple myeloma, chordoma, and osteogenic sarcoma.

Benign neoplastic tumors producing spinal pain include osteoid osteoma, osteoblastoma, and aneurysmal bone cyst. Treatment for each of these conditions should be individualized by an orthopedic spine surgeon.

SPINAL STENOSIS

This important subject is discussed in Chapter 96.

PREGNANCY

Low-back pain occurs in 48 to 56% of pregnant women and is severe in one-third of cases.[61,62] Symptoms usually begin between the fifth and seventh months. Disc herniations can occur, although they are rare.[63]

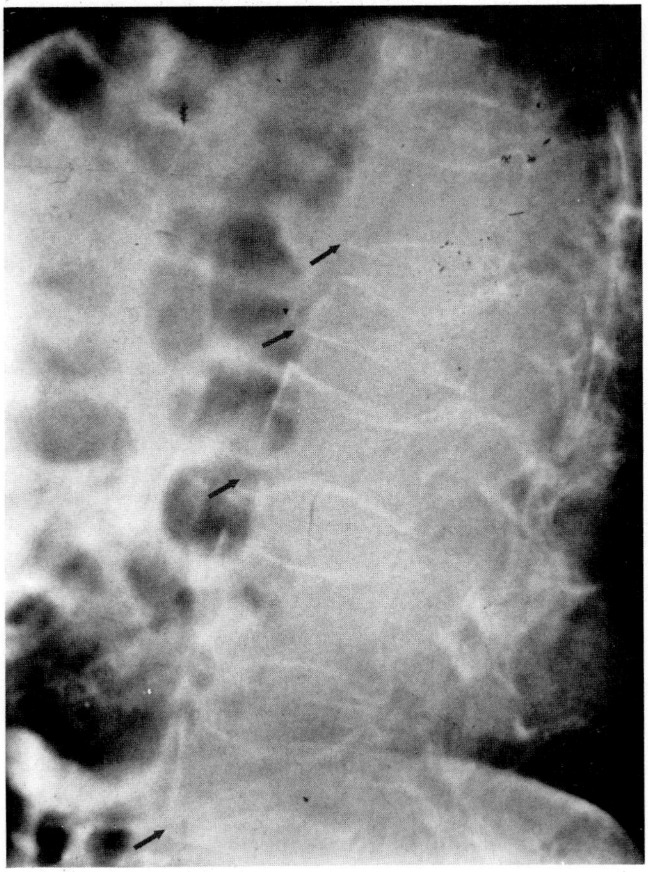

FIGURE 94–17. Osteoporotic lumbar spine with compression fractures. Severe osteoporosis with multiple compression fractures. In the thoracic spine these lead to the characteristic kyphosis.

The cause of pregnancy-induced back pain is unclear. Increased lumbar lordosis, pelvic ligamentous laxity secondary to the hormone relaxin, the heavy weight of the fetus anterior to the weight-bearing sagittal axis of the body, and direct pressure on the spine and neural elements by the gravid uterus have all been cited as contributing factors.

Conservative treatment should be used, because the clinical course is usually benign. Although symptoms can persist into the first year post partum, resolution is usual. Radiographs and surgery should be avoided during pregnancy. Likewise, most medications should be avoided, although acetaminophen is nonteratogenic and is felt to be safe during both pregnancy and lactation.[61]

Conservative treatment includes rest, abdominal and pelvic floor muscle exercises, a cushion behind the lower back when supine, and possibly a special lumbosacral corset designed for the pregnant patient. The patient should be reassured that the condition is benign and that resolution is expected.

SCOLIOSIS

There is no evidence that scoliotic curves of 45° or less at the end of growth are responsible for any increased risk for pain, decreased self-image, or respiratory deficit compared with the population at large.[64,65] A review of adult patients showed that back pain occurred in 59% of patients with scoliosis, which was similar to the incidence of pain in the general population.[66] Pain does become a factor in the adult when the curve exceeds 45%, and it is associated with facet joint sclerosis. Interestingly, nerve root compression is unusual in adult scoliosis, occuring in only 2.2% of patients in one series.[66]

Treatment for the adult with painful scoliosis is the same as for other adults with back pain, and includes physical therapy, muscle strengthening, nonsteroidal anti-inflammatory agents, weight loss, cessation of smoking and corsets. Surgical indications are refractory, debilitating back pain or radiculopathy, and documented progression of the curve.[67]

RHEUMATIC DISEASE

Back pain can be a feature of several rheumatic diseases, including rheumatoid arthritis, psoriatic arthritis, and especially ankylosing spondylitis. These topics are covered in detail in Chapters 44, 62, and 60.

SPONDYLOLITHESIS AND SPONDYLOLYSIS

Spondylolysis refers to a defect of the pars interarticularis; spondylolithesis refers to a forward slippage of one vertebra on another. A spondylolytic defect is best seen on an oblique radiographic view, whereas as lateral view is needed to appreciate a spondylolithesis (Fig. 94–18).

Spondylolithesis and spondylolysis are classified ac-

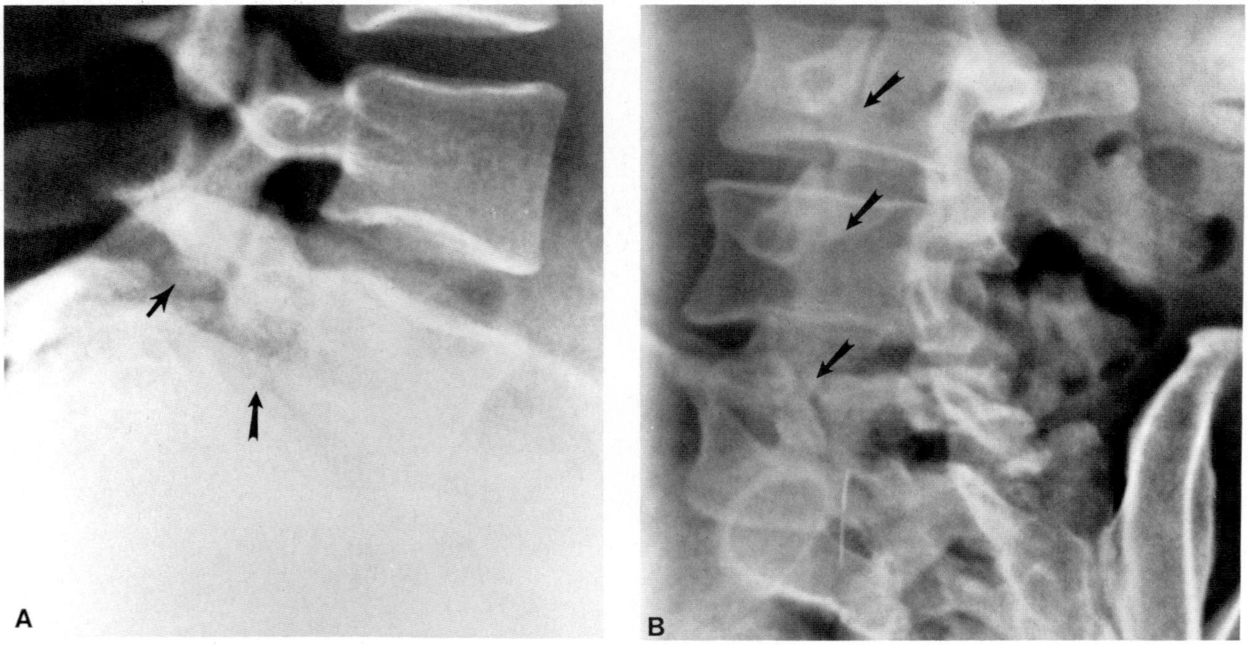

FIGURE 94–18. *A*, Lateral radiograph of the lumbosacral articulation demonstrating a spondylolithesis at L5–S1 of less than 25% (grade 1). Upper arrow demonstrates the pars intra-articularis defect. *B*, Oblique radiographic view demonstrating a large defect of the pars interarticularis (arrows) in this patient with spondylolysis.

cording to a scheme devised by Wiltse, Newman, and McNab.[68] The *dysplastic* type (type 1) refers to a congenital deficiency of either the superior sacral facet or the arch of L5. The *isthmic* type (type 2), which is the most common, involves a lesion of the pars interarticularis, usually of L5, which permits a forward slippage of L5 on S1. This can be a lytic or stress fracture of the pars, an elongated but intact pars interarticularis, or an acute pars fracture. An important type of spondylolithesis is type 3, *degenerative* spondylolithesis. This is usually seen at the L4–L5 level, and is secondary to degenerative disc disease and degenerative disease of the facet joints, leading to segmental instability. The remaining types are type 4, *traumatic*, which involves an acute fracture elsewhere than the pars, and type 5, *pathologic*, which involves a pathologic change such as tumor of the pedicles.

Treatment of symptomatic spondylolysis and spondylolithesis often involves arthrodesis of the involved segment, using the technique of an intertransverse (or lateral) fusion.

COCCYDYNIA

Pain in the coccygeal region is of multifaceted etiology. Common causes include direct trauma, postpartum status, having undergone spinal surgery, and pelvic or lower gastrointestinal tumors.

Most patients are satisfactorily treated with conservative measures. Nonsteroidal anti-inflammatory agents, a sitting cushion, and local corticosteroid infiltration are often used. Rarely is coccygectomy required. The results of coccygectomy vary according to cause. Good results can be expected in up to 75% of patients if the coccydynia is secondary to trauma or postpartum changes, but results are poor if the pain is spontaneous or follows spinal surgery.

In summary, conservative treatment of coccydynia usually yields good results. Careful examination, including rectal examination, must be performed. One should strongly suspect intrapelvic neoplasm. Proctologic, gynecologic, or urologic evaluation might be indicated.

VASCULAR DISEASE

Buttock, groin, and thigh pain, especially when brought on by walking and relieved by rest, might be due to stenosis of the aortic bifurcation or the iliac or femoral arteries. Palpation of the peripheral and femoral arteries should be a part of the routine evaluation of a painful back.

HIP JOINT DISEASE

The pain from arthritic hips or trochanteric bursa might be confused with back pain or sciatica. Palpation of the greater trochanters and determination of the range of motion of the hips is part of the back evaluation.

REFERRED PAIN FROM VISCERAL STRUCTURES

A lesion in one of the pelvic organs or the retroperitoneum can cause pain referred to the back. One mechanism is direct nerve compression by the lesion. The most common condition in women is a retroverted uterus, but disease of the ovaries or fallopian tubes might also be the cause. In men, referred low-back pain is usually the result of a prostatic lesion. Renal or ureteral calculi cause back and flank pain and are usually easily diagnosed. A dissecting aortic aneurysm classically causes severe back pain.

REFERENCES

1. Frymoyer, J.W., and Cats-Baril, W.: Predictors of low back pain disability. Clin. Orthop., *221*:85, 1987.
2. Berquist-Ullman: Acute low back pain in industry. Acta Orthop. Scand. Suppl., *170*:170, 1977.
3. Deyo, R.A., and Tsui-Wu, Y.J.: Descriptive epidemiology of low back pain and its related medical care in the United States. Spine, *12*:264, 1987.
4. Kahanowitz, N.: The lumbar spine. *In* Orthopaedic Knowledge Update III. Edited by Stephen J. Lipson. Chicago, American Academy of Orthopaedic Surgeons, 1990.
5. Frymoyer, J.W., et al.: Epidemiologic studies of low back pain. Spine, *5*:419, 1980.
6. Kelsey, J.L., and Hardy, R.J.: Driving of motor vehicles as a risk factor for acute herniated lumbar intervertebral discs. Am. J. Epidemiol., *102*:63, 1975.
7. Biering-Sorensen, F.: Low back trouble in a general population of 30-, 40-, 50-, and 60-year old men and young women: Study design, representativeness and basic results; Dan. Med. Bull., *29*:289, 1982.
8. Frymoyer, J.W., et al.: Risk factors in low back pain. J. Bone Joint Surg., *65A*:213, 1983.
9. Porter, R.W., Hibbert, C., and Wellman, P.: Backache and the lumbar spinal canal. Spine, *5*:99, 1980.
10. Bell, G.R., Yang-Hing, K., Kirkaldy-Willis, W.H.: Anatomy of Low Back Pain. *In* The Lumbar Spine. Edited by J.N. Weinstein and S.W. Wiesel. Philadelphia, W.B. Saunders, 1990.
11. Arnold, C.C.: Interosseous hypertension: A possible cause of low back pain? Clin. Orthop., *115*:30, 1976.
12. Williams, P.L., and Warwich, R.: Gray's Anatomy. Philadelphia, W.B. Saunders, 1980.
13. Parke, W.W.: Applied anatomy of the spine. *In* The Spine. Edited by R. Rothman and F.A. Simeone. Philadelphia, W.B. Saunders, 1982.
14. Nachemson, A.: The load on lumbar discs in different positions of the body. Clin. Orthop., *45*:107, 1966.
15. Anderson, B.J., et al.: The sitting posture: An electromyographic and discometric study. Orthop. Clin. North Am., *6*:105, 1975
16. Deyo, R.A.: Occupational back pain. Spine, State of the Art Reviews *2*:1, 1987.
17. Watkins, R.G., and Collis, J.J. Jr.: Lumbar Discectomy and Laminectomy. Rockville, MD, Aspen Publications, 1987.
18. van Akkerveelken, P.F.: Pain Patterns and Diagnostic Blocks. *In* The Lumbar Spine. Edited by J.N. Weinstein and S.W. Wiesel. Philadelphia, W.B. Saunders, 1990.
19. Levine, D.B.: The Painful Back in Athletic and Allied Disorders. 11th Ed. Philadelphia, Lea & Febiger, 1989.
20. Waddell, G., et al.: Nonorganic physical signs in low back pain. Spine, *5*:2, 1980.

21. Frymoyer, J.W., et al.: Spine radiographs in patients with low back pain. J. Bone Joint Surg., *60A*:1048, 1984.
22. Witt, I., Vestergaard, A., and Rosenblint, A.: A comparative analysis of x-ray findings of the lumbar spine in patients with and without lumbar pain. Spine, *19*:298, 1984.
23. Boden, S.D., et al.: Abnormal magnetic resonance scans of the lumbar spine in asymptomatic subjects. J. Bone Joint Surg., *72A*:1178, 1990.
24. Modic, M.T., et al.: Imaging of degenerative disc disease. Radiology, *168*:177, 1988.
25. Borenstein, D.G., and Wiesel, S.W.: Low Back Pain. Philadelphia, W.B. Saunders, 1989.
26. Hoefle, M., et al.: Lumbar spine: Postoperative MR imaging with Gd-DTPA. Radiology, *167*:817, 1988.
27. Delamarter, R.: Personal communication, 1990.
28. Wiesel, S.W., et al.: A study of computer-assisted tomography: The incidence of positive CT scans in an asymptomatic group of patients. Spine, *9*:549, 1984.
29. Bell, G.R., et al.: A study of computer-assisted tomography: Comparison of metrizamide myelography and computed tomography in the diagnosis of herniated lumbar discs and spinal stenosis. Spine, *9*:552, 1984.
30. Jackson, R.P., et al.: The neuroradiographic diagnosis of lumbar herniated nucleus pulposus. I. A comparison of computed tomography (CT), myelography, CT-myelography, discography, and CT-discography. Spine, *14*:1356, 1989.
31. Jackson, R.P., et al.: The neuroradiographic diagnosis of lumbar herniated nucleus pulposus. II. A comparison of computed tomography (CT), myelography, CT-myelography, discography, and CT-discography. Spine, *14*:1362, 1989.
32. Lindblom, K.: Diagnostic puncture of intervertebral discs in sciatica. Acta Orthop. Scand., *17*:231, 1948.
33. Calhoun, E., et al.: Provocation discography as a guide to planning operations on the spine. J. Bone Joint Surg., *70B*:267, 1988.
34. Frazel, R.D., Osti, O.C., and Vernon-Roberts, B.: Discitis after discography. J. Bone Joint Surg. 69-B, *1*:26, 1987.
35. Bernard, T.: Lumbar discography followed by computed tomography: Refining the diagnosis of low back pain. Spine, *115*:690, 1990.
36. Frymoyer, J.W., and Haugh, L.D.: Thermography: A call for scientific studies to establish its diagnositic efficacy. Orthopedics, *9*:699, 1986.
37. Vematsu, S., et al.: Thermography and electromyography in the differentiated diagnosis of chronic pain syndromes and reflex sympathetic dystrophy. Electromyogr. Clin. Neurophysiol., *21*:165, 1982.
38. Borenstein, D.G., and Wiesel, S.W.: Low Back Pain, Medical Diagnosis and Comprehensive Management. Philadelphia, W.B. Saunders, 1989.
39. Deyo, R.A., Diehl, A.K., and Rosenthal, M.: How many days of bed rest for acute low back pain?; N. Engl. J. Med., *315*:1064, 1986.
40. Waddell, G.: A new clinical model for the treatment of low-back pain. Spine, *12*:632, 1987.
41. McNab, I., and McCulloch, J.: Backache. Baltimore, Williams & Wilkins, 1990.
42. Weber, H.: Lumbar disc herniation: A controlled, prospective study with 10 years of observation. Spine, *8*:131, 1983.
43. Eismont, F.J., and Currier, B.: Surgical management of lumbar intervertebral disc disease. J. Bone Joint Surg., *71A*:1266, 1989.
44. Bell, G.R., and Rothman, R.H.: The conservative management of sciatica. Spine, *9*:54, 1984.
45. Nachemson, A.L.: Advances in low back pain. Clin. Orthop., *200*:266, 1985.
46. Saal, J.A., and Saal, J.S.: Nonoperative treatment of herniated lumbar intervertebral disc with radiculopathy: An outcome study. Spine, *14*:431, 1989.
47. Cuckler, J.M., et al.: The use of epidural steroids in the treatment of lumbar pain. J. Bone Joint Surg., *67A*:63, 1985.
48. Deyo, R.A., Diehl, A.K., and Rosenthal, M.: How many days of bed rest for acute back pain? A randomized clinical trial. N. Engl. J. Med., *315*:1064, 1986.
49. Nachemson, A.: Lumbar spine instability: A critical update and symposium summary. Spine, *10*:290, 1985.
50. Mooney, V., Brown, M., and Modic, M.: New Perspectives In Low Back Pain. Chicago, American Academy of Orthopaedic Surgeons, 1989.
51. Silvers, H.R.: Microsurgery versus standard lumbar discectomy. Neurosurgery, *22*:837, 1988.
52. Andrews, D.W., and Layne, M.H.: Retrospective analysis of microsurgical and standard lumbar discectomy. Spine, *15*:329, 1990.
53. McDermott, J.J., et al.: Chymodiactin for patients with herniated lumbar intervertebral disc(s): An open-label multicenter study. Spine, *10*:242, 1985.
54. Leong, J.C.Y., and Fraser, R.D.: Spinal Infections in the Lumbar Spine. Philadelphia, W.B. Saunders, 1990.
55. Lifeso, R.M.: Pyogenic spinal sepsis in adults. Spine, *15*:1265, 1990.
56. Scoles, P.V., and Quinn, T.P.: Intervertebral discitis in children and adolescents. Clin. Orthop., *162*:31, 1982.
57. McCain, G.A., et al.: Septic discitis. J. Rheumatol., *8*:100, 1981.
58. Nachemson, A.: A long term follow-up study of non-treated scoliosis. J. Bone Joint Surg., *50A*:203, 1969.
59. Nachemson, A.: A long term follow-up study of nontreated scoliosis. Acta Orthop. Scand., *39*:466, 1977.
60. Ellinas, P.A., and Rosner, F.: Pott's disease in urban populations: A report of five cases and a review of the literature. N.Y. State J. Med., *90*:585, 1990.
61. Anderson, G.B.J.: Low back pain in pregnancy. *In* The Lumbar Spine. Philadelphia, W.B. Saunders, 1990.
62. Fast, A., et al.: Low-back pain in pregnancy. Spine, *12*:368, 1987.
63. O'Connell, J.E.A.: Lumbar disc protrusion in pregnancy. J. Neurol. Neurosurg. Psychiatry, *23*:138, 1960.
64. Winter, R.B.: Natural history of spinal deformity. *In* Scoliosis and Other Spinal Deformities. Edited by David B. Bradford. Philadelphia, W.B. Saunders, 1987.
65. Nachemson, A.: A long term follow-up study of nontreated scoliosis. J. Bone Joint Surg., *50A*:203, 1969.
66. Kostuik, J.P., and Bentivoglio, J.: The incidence of pain in adult scoliosis. Spine, *6*:268, 1981.
67. Kostuik, J.P.: Adult scoliosis. *In* The Lumbar Spine. Edited by James N. Weinstein and Sam W. Wiesel. Philadelphia, W.B. Saunders, 1990.
68. Wiltse, L.L., Newman, P.H., and McNab, I.: Classification of spondylolisthesis. Clin. Orthop., *117*:23, 1976.
69. Bayne, O., Bateman, J.E., and Cameron, H.: The influence of etiology on the results of coccygetcomy. Clin. Orthop., *190*:266, 1984.

95

Spinal Stenosis

J. DESMOND O'DUFFY
MICHAEL J. EBERSOLD

Spinal stenosis is an anatomic term that implies pressure on the spinal cord or cauda equina by a narrowed spinal canal.[1–6] Typically such compression occurs in the cervical and lumbar spine in persons over age 50. In each case the end result is a disorder of gait. The two clinical syndromes of spinal stenosis are cervical myelopathy caused by cervical spondylosis,[5,6] and caudal compression with neurogenic claudication caused by lumbar stenosis.[1,2–4,7] Each of these syndromes is a manifestation of regional osteoarthritis. Whether these patients have more extensive nonspinal osteoarthritis than age-matched controls is not known.

HISTORY

An early description of lumbar spinal stenosis appeared in 1893 by the London surgeon Sir William Arbuthnot Lane.[8] His patient, a 35-year-old servant, complained of "weakness of her back and insecurity of her legs" and had reduced sensation in her feet. Lane noted an unusual convexity of the lumbar spine. At laminectomy he observed that the spine of L5 was "buried" as a consequence of spondylolisthesis. Since he noted that the neural arch was intact he assumed that the listhesis was degenerative. The idea that spondylolisthesis, with or without a defect in the neural arch, might cause sciatica was later developed by Junghanns,[9] MacNab,[10] and Stewart.[11]

"Congenital stricture of the spinal canal" was the term used by M.A. Sarpyener, a Turkish orthopedic surgeon, who in 1945 described 12 children with severe and varied neurologic sequelae to a congenital narrowing of the spinal canal.[12] In 1954 Verbiest, a Dutch surgeon, described patients having "signs of disturbance of the cauda equina, i.e., bilateral radicular pains, and disturbances of sensation and impairment of motor power in the legs" upon standing and walking, with relief of symptoms upon recumbence.[1] Verbiest used myelography to demonstrate extradural compression. Van Gelderen had antedated (1948) Verbiest's description and had proposed that a hypertrophied ligamentum flavum was responsible.[13] In contrast, Verbiest championed the contribution of congenital narrowing of the lumbar vertebral canal even though the mean age in his seven patients was 51 years.[1] The debate over the relative contributions of congenital narrowing versus hypertrophic changes persists. The history of lumbar stenosis has been reviewed by Kirkaldy-Willis.[3]

Verbiest's descriptions of lumbar stenosis coincided with reports from English neurologists of spondylotic cervical myelopathy.[6,14–16] Just as lumbar disc protrusion entered the medical consciousness ahead of lumbar stenosis, so had Stookey described cervical disc protrusion[17] many years before cervical myelopathy caused by advanced cervical spondylosis was proposed by Brain and colleagues.[6]

CERVICAL SPONDYLOSIS WITH MYELOPATHY

ETIOLOGY AND PATHOLOGY

After decades of attrition caused by trauma and central dehydration, one or more cervical discs degenerates. At the adjacent posterior margins of the vertebral bodies, posterior protrusions of exostotic bone and degenerated anulus fibrosus and disc cause "spondylotic bars" compressing the cord anteriorly.[5,15,18] Thickening of the ligamentum flavum encroaches on the cord from behind.[5] The lateral corticospinal tracts are demyelinated at and below the level of compression, whereas the ascending dorsal sensory columns are demyelinated above this level.[5] Frequently there are deep indentations of the cord by several spondylotic bars (Fig. 95–1). Because the bars can extend into the intervertebral foramina, the cervical nerve roots often become compressed. This compression results in fibrosis of the dural sleeves of the nerve roots. The theory that the myelopathy is due to ischemia is disputed.[18]

Nurick discussed the various contributions to such a squashed cervical cord.[15,16] As with lumbar stenosis, controversy exists regarding the relative importance of a congenitally narrow canal versus the end results of degenerative disc disease, that is, osteophytes, subluxations, thickened yellow ligament, and impaired blood supply through the anterior spinal artery.[15,19] Hindering a resolution of this conflict are the imprecision of radiographic measurements and the considerable overlap between the anteroposterior (AP) spinal diameters of patients with cord compression and those of controls. Thus the mean minimum AP diameter of myelopathic cervical spines, as determined radiologically by Nurick, was 14.6 mm, whereas that of controls was 16.2 mm.[15] The average AP diameter of the cervical cord itself in the normal adult is about 10 mm.

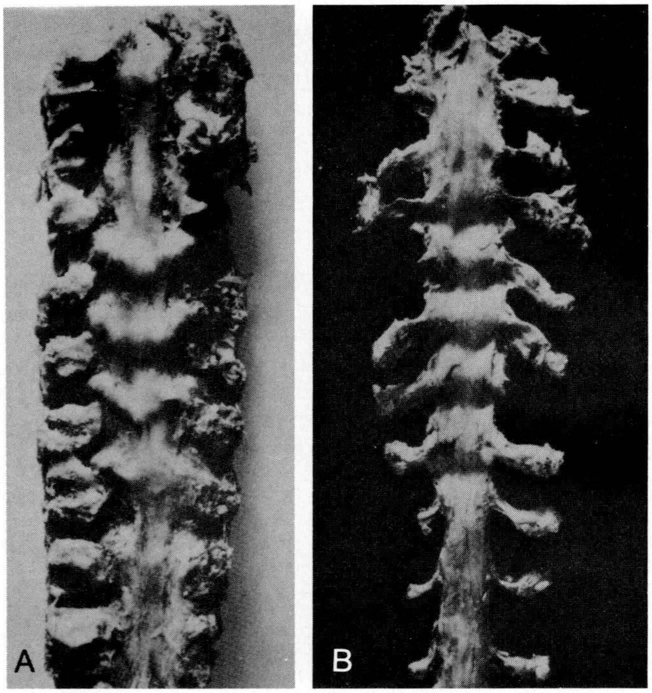

FIGURE 95–1. *A,* Posterior aspect of bodies of cervical vertebrae showing transverse bosses and bars. *B,* Same patient showing indentations of anterior cervical cord and nerve roots corresponding to the bosses and bars. From Wilkinson, M.: Pathology: Cervical myelopathy. *In* Cervical Spondylosis. Edited by M. Wilkinson. Philadelphia, W.B. Saunders, 1971, pp. 49–51.

INCIDENCE

The peak age at onset of symptoms is in the range of 40 to 60 years.[14,16] Males predominate in a ratio of 60:40, and to an even greater extent beyond age 60. Although cervical disc degeneration is present in 50% of persons at age 45 and in over 90% after age 60, only a few patients with spondylosis develop cervical myelopathy.[14,19] Among a group of 51 patients with cervical spondylosis followed for over 6 years, none developed symptoms or signs of cord compression.[14] Those who did develop cord symptoms and signs seldom recalled previous discrete episodes of cervical radiculopathy.

SYMPTOMS AND SIGNS

The clinical manifestations of spondylotic cervical myelopathy are presented in Table 95–1. Typically the patient has a spastic gait, hyper-reflexia in the lower limbs, and Babinski signs. There may be upper and/or lower motor neuron signs in the upper extremities depending on the site of compression.[5,14,19] Neck pain may be absent, but restricted neck motion is usual. Cervical radicular pains are often present. Disturbances of sensation can include dysesthesias and clumsiness in the hands, while impaired vibration and joint-position sense can occur in the lower extremities. Weakness and wasting of the small muscles of the hands are common. The site of the lesion can sometimes be deduced from the pattern of upper motor neuron change. Thus, absence of biceps deep tendon reflexes combined with hyperactive triceps tendon reflexes can signify cord compression at C6. Fasciculations can be seen in upper extremity muscles, especially in the small muscles of the hands. Urinary in-

TABLE 95–1. SYMPTOMS AND SIGNS OF MYELOPATHY CAUSED BY SPONDYLOTIC CERVICAL MYELOPATHY IN 32 PATIENTS*

TYPE	PERCENT
Motor	
Hyper-reflexia	87
Babinski sign	54
Spastic gait	54
Sphincter disturbance	49
Arm weakness	31
Paraparesis	21
Quadriparesis	10
Brown-Sequard	10
Hand atrophy	13
Fasciculation	13
Sensory	
Vague sensory level	41
Proprioceptive loss	39
Cervical dermatome sensory loss	33
Pain	
Radicular, arm	41
Cervical pain	26

* From Lundsford, L.D., Bissonette, D.J., and Zarub, D.S.: Anterior surgery for cervical disc disease. Part 2: Treatment of cervical spondylotic myelopathy in 32 cases. J. Neurosurg., *53*:12–19, 1980.

continence is uncommon. While there is usually no history of discrete neck trauma, sometimes sudden worsening of neurologic signs may follow a mild neck injury.[14]

DIAGNOSIS

Roentgenograms of the cervical spine show narrowed disc spaces and osteophytes, especially at C5-6 and C6-7 (Fig. 95–2A). Oblique views show encroachment of intervertebral foramina by spurs of Luschka joints. The myelogram suggests distortion of the cord with interruptions in the column of radiocontrast material, often with complete subarachnoid block. Computed tomography (CT) with myelography reveals cross-sectional anatomy (Fig. 95–2C). This is the diagnostic procedure of choice. Its limitations are discussed by Penning et al.[46] Although the diagnosis might be suspected by CT or magnetic resonance imaging (MRI), myelographic features remain most helpful. MRI is a useful noninvasive test that can *rule out* nonspondylotic causes of cord compression. The corkscrew shape of the cervical cord that is compressed at several levels is seen well in T_2-weighted images (Fig. 95–2B) and gives an approximate sense of the amount of impingement into the subarachnoid space and consequently on the cord itself. Scoliosis can lead to a false MRI impression of a narrowed cervical cord; otherwise, MRI is almost as useful in determining the presence of spinal stenosis as myelography and is more helpful in determining if there is a tumor causing cord compression. Nevertheless, myelography and water-soluble contrast and postmyelographic CT scanning is still the gold standard for defining the extent of extradural compression. MRI is especially useful in detecting tumors that might mimic stenosis. Cerebrospinal fluid (CSF) from below the block might show protein content above 50 mg/dl.[19]

Myelography can usually distinguish cervical cord tumors, cervical disc herniation, and arteriovenous malformations from spondylotic myelopathy. However, multiple sclerosis, amyotrophic lateral sclerosis, and neurosyphilis, as well as subacute combined degeneration of the cord with vitamin B_{12} deficiency, must also be considered in the differential diagnosis.

NATURAL HISTORY

Most authors describe an indolent course with little progression of disability from the time of diagnosis.[14,15] Lees and Turner followed 44 of 51 well-documented, and mostly unoperated on, patients for 5 or more years.[14] An injury often preceded the onset of symptoms, and the indolent course was punctuated at long intervals by one or more episodes of neurogenic exacerbation. Disability in these 44 patients, although rated "severe" in over half, did not change appreciably during observation.[14] Nevertheless, Nurick, while extolling the virtues of nonoperative measures, found that about 20% of their patients worsened.[16]

TREATMENT

Because the neurologic status might not change much after surgical laminectomy or anterior decompression, and because the conservative measures of physiotherapy and the use of a cervical collar are of unproven benefit, controversy exists over the value of an operation in spondylotic myelopathy.[5,14,20] A laminectomy, which is usually multilevel, decompresses the cord and results in improvement in 56 to 61% of patients.[5,16] Multilevel foraminotomies to decompress nerve roots are usually done also. Anterior fusion did not relieve symptoms in the series of Lunsford et al.,[20a] but the decision to decompress anteriorly or posteriorly de-

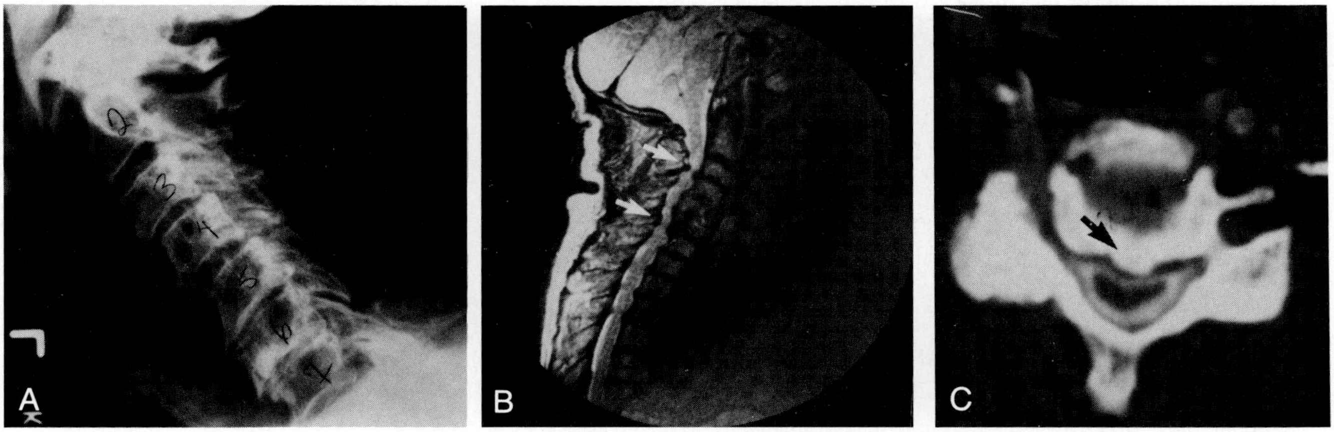

FIGURE 95–2. *A,* Cervical spondylosis, showing disc degeneration at C5-C6 and C6-C7, and mild subluxation C3 and C4. *B,* MRI T_2-weighted image with CSF (appearing white) showing beaded stenosis worst at C3-C4 and C6-C7 (arrows). *C,* CT-metrizamide myelogram showing a spondylotic bar (arrow) protruding posteriorly that resulted in squashed canal contents at C4-C5.

pends on the radiographic site of the lesion. The reasons that there is less enthusiasm for cervical than for lumbar procedures include (1) the risk of paralysis in cervical decompression, (2) the possibility of a vascular component unresponsive to decompression, and (3) the fact that cervical cord decompression in some patients might need both anterior and posterior decompression for optimal results.

Surgical results do not appear to be influenced by the age of the patient, but patients left with "stable" cervical spines appeared to fare better than those left with an increased range of movement.[20] The upper extremity sensory symptoms may improve less than the gait disturbance. Appropriate guidelines for extensive laminectomy are not yet defined. When patients are told of the uncertain results of surgical treatment, some decline. At present the best surgical candidates are those with demonstrated recent progression in gait disturbance.

LUMBAR STENOSIS

DEFINITION

The definition of lumbar stenosis invokes a description of symptoms and myelographic findings, because there are no widely acceptable criteria based on the AP diameter of the spinal canal.[3,4,21] This diameter may range from 10 to 15 mm in symptomatic patients.[21] It is generally agreed that there is "an incongruity between the capacity and the contents of the lumbar spinal canal [that] may give rise to compression of the roots of the cauda equina".[7] The clinical syndrome consists of symptoms of compression of the roots of the cauda equina.[1,3,22,23] These symptoms are intermittent claudication brought on by walking and pain or paresthesias in the legs evoked by standing and accentuated by exercise, but relieved by sitting or lying down.[1,10,22,24–26] The diagnosis is confirmed by demonstrating a blockage to the flow of myelographic contrast material and by the surgical finding of compression of the caudal sac.

PATHOPHYSIOLOGY (Table 95–2)

The laminae and facets are dense and thickened, creating difficulty in performing spinal puncture.[27] The pathology is diagrammatically shown in Figure 95–3, in which a normal-sized spinal canal is compared with a congenitally narrow one and with the more-commonly encountered canal that is compromised by hypertrophic

TABLE 95–2. CAUSES OF LUMBAR STENOSIS

Degenerative
Lumbar spondylosis with or without spondylolisthesis
Iatrogenic (previous fusion)
Paget's disease of the bone
Congenital
Narrow lumbar canal
Achondroplasia

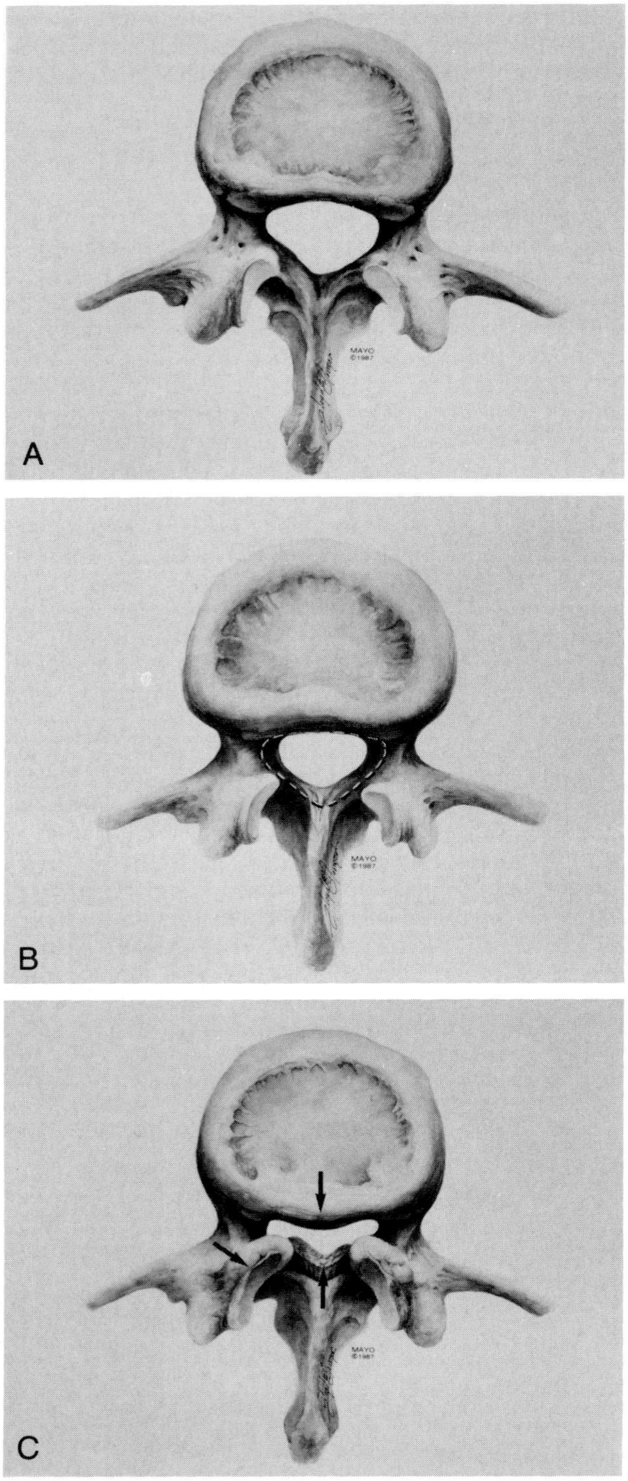

FIGURE 95–3. Types of lumbar spinal canal. *A,* Normal. *B,* Congenital narrowing. Stippled line shows normal dimensions. *C,* Hypertrophy of ligamentum flavum, apophyseal joints, and vertebral body (arrows). This is the most common pathology in lumbar stenosis.

changes. Facet joint hypertrophy is the leading cause of lumbar stenosis.[47] Synovial cysts from the hypertrophic apophyseal joints may be encountered. Degeneration of discs, although not the immediate cause of radiculopathies, along with apophyseal joint disease contributes to the syndrome.[22,27] The ligamentum flavum, which should not exceed 4 mm in thickness, may be up to 7 or 8 mm thick.[3,22] The apophyseal joint hypertrophy is the key to narrowing of the lateral recesses and contributes to the spondylolisthesis that occurs in at least one third of patients.[26] Lumbar stenosis has been described in achondroplasia,[28] in Paget's disease of the bone, in diffuse intervertebral skeletal hyperostosis,[29] and after surgical lumbar fusion.[25] In one study calcium pyrophosphate crystals were encountered in four patients, but all had previously undergone surgery.[30] Because the dura is not normally opened at laminectomy, the nerve roots are seldom seen. In one patient who died after laminectomy there was segmental demyelination from compressions of the roots of the cauda equina at regular intervals in accordance with the myelographic findings.[26] This finding and the abnormal electromyographic findings at rest suggest that mechanical pressure rather than ischemia causes the symptoms.[26] Proof of ischemia as a cause of symptoms is lacking.[23,31]

SYMPTOMS AND SIGNS

The cardinal symptom is neurogenic claudication.[1,3,23,26] This "pseudoclaudication" is usually bilateral and consists of discomfort or weakness in the buttocks, thighs, legs, and calves brought on by standing or walking and relieved by sitting or lying down.[3,22,23,25,26] The symptoms and signs are listed in Table 95–3. Patients describe "numbness" or "tingling" and "weakness" in the legs,[23,26] which symptoms are relieved by adopting a flexed position.[26] To alleviate symptoms patients will lean against a wall or, more typically, lean forward on a shopping cart or a church pew (Fig. 95–4). In advanced cases not only is the pain provoked by standing and walking a brief distance, but it may come on even when patients are lying supine. Lying on one side, curled in a fetal position, relieves the pain.

Neurogenic claudication differs from vascular claudication. In vascular claudication leg pain is provoked by walking and is relieved by standing, whereas in neurogenic claudication the symptoms are provoked by standing as well as by walking, and paresthesias often accompany the pain.[23] Typically, symptoms come on after walking 100 to 200 yd (90 to 180 m) and usually are felt in the entire lower extremities.[26] Sometimes the symptoms are confined to either above or below the knee; in the case of one-sided lateral recess stenosis, they may be unilateral. Patients often describe their symptoms with a sweeping downward motion of the hands, indicating buttock to heel sciatica. Seldom do patients experience acute radicular symptoms with aggravation by a Valsalva maneuver. If they do, they are probably experiencing discogenic sciatica. Hip stiffness is absent, but spinal stenosis has been confused with hip disease.[24]

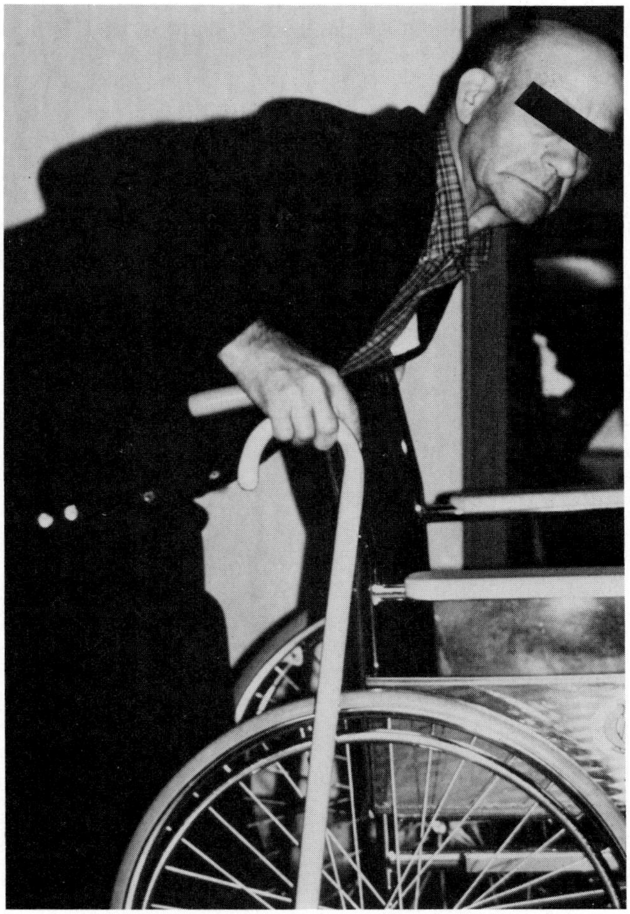

FIGURE 95–4. Typical posture of patient with severe lumbar stenosis (simian stance).

TABLE 95–3. SYMPTOMS AND SIGNS OF LUMBAR STENOSIS

	NEUROGENIC CLAUDICATION	VASCULAR CLAUDICATION
Distribution	Buttock, thigh or calf (often, the entire leg)	Buttock (aortoiliac) or calf (femoropopliteal)
Symptoms	Cramping pain, numbness, loss of power	Cramping, pain
Inciting factors	Exercise in the erect position, prolonged standing	Exercise in any posture
Relieving factors	Bending forward, sitting or lying down	Standing or sitting
Pulses	Usually normal	Diminished or absent
Electromyogram	Abnormal	Normal

Most patients experience lumbar pain that is mechanical and mild.[22,25,26] In our series, only 19% previously had well-defined discogenic sciatica.[26] Patients often complain of leg weakness[3] and may actually fall down. In contrast to other causes of cauda equina compression, sphincter disturbances are rare.

CLINICAL SIGNS

On examination few physical signs are present.[26,31] Pedal pulses are normal unless atherosclerosis coexists with lumbar stenosis as it does in about 9% of patients.[26] Deep tendon reflexes were reduced at the ankle in 29 of 68 (43%) and at the knee in 12 of 68 (18%) patients.[26] Mild, often unilateral, weakness in the lower limbs is found in about one third of patients and usually in the distribution of L5 and S1 roots. This weakness is best evoked by attempts to walk on the heels and toes, respectively. Straight leg raising should not evoke back pain in the Lasègue test.[23,26] Range of motion of the lumbar spine, which is difficult to estimate in any age group, may be reduced or normal.[3,26] The best test is to provoke the symptoms by having the patient stand up or walk for a few minutes and noticing if he adopts a flexed position. Typically, standing up for several minutes will cause the patient to bend forward and lean on the nearest support. Continuous walking for several minutes should induce leg distress (see Fig. 95–4). Occasionally, rechecking the deep tendon reflexes after the symptoms develop will show a reduction as compared with sitting.[23] The frequency of coexisting severe osteoarthritis in the limb joints has not been studied in patients with lumbar stenosis.

The differential diagnosis of lumbar stenosis is (1) vascular claudication caused by atherosclerosis, (2) osteoarthritis of the hips,[24] knees, or both, (3) lumbar disc disease with radiculopathy, and (4) chronic neurologic disease, that is, intraspinal tumor or arteriovenous malformation, multiple sclerosis, and peripheral neuropathy.

LABORATORY FINDINGS

Electromyography (EMG) can be diagnostically helpful by showing evidence of chronic neurogenic changes in the distribution of several lumbosacral nerve roots, often bilaterally.[26] The muscles supplied by the L5 and S1 nerve roots are most commonly affected. In our series, 34 of 37 patients (92%) undergoing EMG showed neurogenic abnormalities compatible with nerve root compression. However, all of our patients had complete blocks on Pantopaque myelography and thus had advanced disease.[26] Although testing of somatosensory evoked potentials (SEP) has been proposed as a more sensitive test than EMG, in a study proposing this test only 1 of 11 patients tested by EMG had a positive EMG, while all 11 had abnormal SEPs.[32] At the Mayo Clinic, EMG is done in only half of spinal stenosis patients presenting for surgery,[26] and SEP is omitted.

If the CSF is examined below the level of myelographic block, the CSF protein will be elevated, whereas it is usually normal if measured above a block.[23]

RADIOLOGY

Plain radiographs of the lumbar spine show dense bony structures and one or more degenerative discs.[26] The oblique views show narrowing and sclerosis of apophyseal joints. Chondrocalcinosis is occasionally seen.[30] Over one third of patients have spondylolisthesis, typically L4 on L5.[1,26] This results from partial subluxation of the apophyseal joints. The myelogram is usually done at L2 and typically is technically difficult.[25] *Myelography is the most important diagnostic test and, in our opinion, is indicated when laminectomy is being considered.* The distal flow of contrast material is blocked either completely or subtotally in the usual position of myelography, that of spinal extension (Fig. 95–5A).[1,27] Flexion of the spine, however, will usually allow the iodinated contrast material to flow (Fig. 95–5B).[22,23,26] About 30% of spinal stenosis patients have multilevel block.[26,27] An hourglass deformity signifies the dual contribution from the apophyseal joints and ligamentum flavum behind and from the degenerated disc in front of the cauda equina (Fig. 95–5A).[3]

Water-soluble agents such as the nonionic Iopamidol are now preferred over iophendylate (Pantopaque), which was not readily absorbed and had to be removed after the procedure lest it cause arachnoiditis.[33,34] Because important stenotic or neoplastic lesions at higher levels, typically in the cervical canal, can coexist with lumbar stenosis, *complete myelography is advised.*[25,26]

CT[4,36–39] and MRI[40,41] are used by some in place of myelography, but in our opinion CT is better used as a complement to the myelogram. Myelography does not allow good visualization of the neural foramina of the spinal canal and lateral recesses, especially at the levels below a block.[35] For this reason, CT, with its ability to show a cross section of bone and soft tissues, has gained favor.[4,36–39] Although CT is widely used, is noninvasive, can show inadequate previous operations, and distinguishes scar from block, its contribution to the diagnosis is controversial.[36,37] Many CT study reports have had serious flaws in design.[36] The problems with relying on CT alone for a diagnosis of lumbar stenosis include lack of clear guidelines for defining stenosis,[38] false positive interpretations,[37] and the fact that CT may not visualize the spinal canal above L3.[26] *Of our 68 patients, 6 (9%) had stenosis only at L1, L2, or both,*[26] *that is, sites that are not routinely examined on CT of the lumbosacral spine.* In one prospective study of surgically treated patients in whom an attempt was made to compare diagnostic techniques, water-soluble contrast myelography proved superior to CT.[36] At present, CT is combined with myelography to enhance diagnosis.[35] CT allows inspection of the lateral recesses and neural foramina, areas that are poorly seen with myelography.[35] Although MRI has also been proposed as a diagnostic test,[40] its expense and unproven diagnostic validity in the lumbar canal[41] place it second to CT myelography.

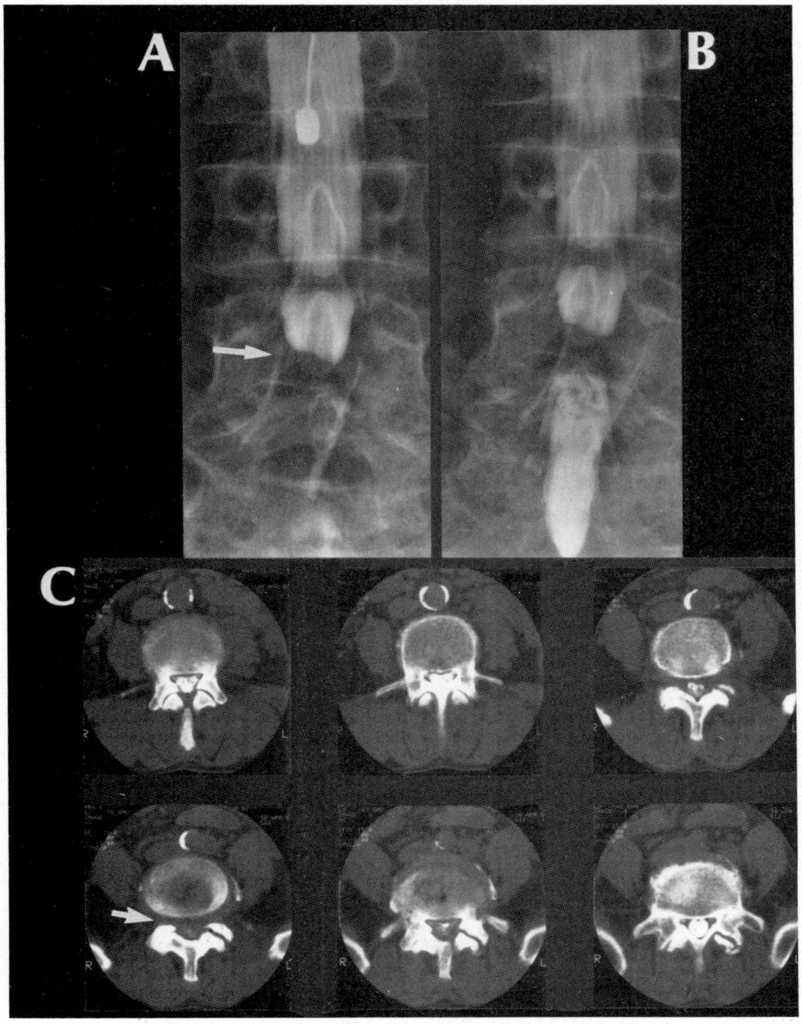

FIGURE 95–5. *A*, Iopamidol myelogram done via needle introduced at L2. Spine is in extension. There is complete block at L4-L5 (upper arrow). *B*, Needle is removed and patient is allowed to flex his spine. Iopamidol now flows beyond the block. *C*, Postmyelographic CT sequence from L3-L4 (top left) through L5 (bottom right). Note the hypertrophic apophyseal joints and the disappearance of contrast at L4-L5 (arrow, bottom left).

TREATMENT

There is little evidence that conservative treatment with bracing, exercises, and analgesics is effective. Patients find that using a short cane or walker and wearing padded shoes help. Only those patients with severely restricted activities and who are otherwise in good health are offered surgery. Myelography is done only as a prelude to planned surgery. *Patients are told to expect little or no improvement in back pain.*

Surgery is extensive.[7] Most patients require bilateral laminectomy at two or three levels.[26] The average operation is a three-level procedure, while the range in levels operated is from one to five.[26] Foraminotomies for lateral recess stenosis may be needed, in which case, owing to the width of the laminectomy, the medial part of the hypertrophied facet joint is trimmed, that is, a hemifacetectomy is performed. A few patients also need to have large discs or disc fragments removed.[26]

Adding to the difficulty of surgery is the thickness and density of the bones and ligaments.[3,7,22,25] The surgeon notices absence of dural fat and dural pulsations as well as a ligamentum flavum that is up to 8 mm thick.[3,22,25] Indications for fusion are not clearly defined. When spondylolisthesis of L4 on L5 is so advanced that it has slipped forward by a half or more of its AP diameters, that is, grade-2 slip or more, then laminectomy is combined with lateral interbody fusion.[42] A recent trend is the combination of laminectomy and fusion in patients with lesser degrees of subluxation.

RESULTS

In a mean followup of 4 years, two thirds of the 68 patients at the Mayo Clinic in a 30-month period reported excellent to good relief of their lower limb symptoms while about one third reported little or no improvement.[26] Causes of the disappointing results in the minority appear to be restenosis,[43] inadequate unroofing of the spinal canal, or an increase in mechanical back pain from instability[44,45] especially if a spondylolisthetic slip was worsened.[3,45] Nevertheless, at present there is more enthusiasm for surgical treatment of lumbar stenosis than there is for operation for cervical myelopathy.

REFERENCES

1. Verbiest, H.: A radicular syndrome from developmental narrowing of the lumbar vertebral canal. J. Bone Joint Surg., *36B*:230–237, 1954.
2. Jones, R.A.C., Thomson, J.L.G.: The narrow lumbar canal. J. Bone Joint Surg., *50B*:595–605, 1960.
3. Kirkaldy-Willis, W.J., et al.: Lumbar spinal stenosis. Clin. Orthop. *99*:30–50, 1974.
4. Uden, A., et al.: Myelography in the elderly and the diagnosis of spinal stenosis. Spine, *10*:171–174, 1985.
5. Wilkinson, M.: Pathology: cervical myelopathy. *In* Cervical Spondylosis. Its Early Diagnosis and Treatment. Edited by M. Wilkinson. Philadelphia, W.B. Saunders, 1971, pp. 49–55.
6. Brain, W.R., Knight, G.C., and Bull, J.W.D.: Discussion on rupture of the intervertebral disc in the cervical region. Proc. R. Soc. Med., *41*:509–516, 1948.
7. Epstein, J.A., Epstein, B.S., and Lavine, L.: Nerve root compression associated with narrowing of the lumbar spinal canal. J. Neurol. Neurosurg. Psychiatry, *25*:165–176, 1962.
8. Lane, W.A.: Case of spondylolisthesis associated with progressive paraplegia; laminectomy. Lancet, *1*:991, 1893.
9. Junghanns, H.: Spondylolisthesen ohne spalt im 3 weischengelenkstuck (Pseudospondylolisthesen). Arch. Orthop. Trauma Surg., *29*:118–127, 1930.
10. MacNab, I.: Spondylolisthesis with an intact neural arch: The so-called pseudo-spondylolisthesis. J. Bone Joint Surg., *32B*:325–333, 1950.
11. Stewart, T.D.: Spondylolisthesis without separate neural arch (pseudospondylolisthesis of Junghanns). J. Bone Joint Surg., *17*:640–648, 1935.
12. Sarpyener, M.A.: Congenital stricture of the spinal canal. J. Bone Joint Surg., *27*:70–79, 1945.
13. Van Gelderen, C.: Ein Orthotisches (Lurdotisches) Kaudasyndrom. Acta Psychiatr. Neurol., *23*:57–68, 1948.
14. Lees, F., and Turner, J.W.A.: Natural history and prognosis of cervical spondylosis. Br. Med. J. *2*:1607–1610, 1963.
15. Nurick, S.: The pathogenesis of the spinal cord disorder associated with cervical spondylosis. Brain, *95*:87–100, 1972.
16. Nurick, S.: The natural history and the results of surgical treatment of the spinal cord disorder associated with cervical spondylosis. Brain, *95*:101–108, 1972.
17. Stookey, B.: Compression of the spinal cord due to ventral extradural cervical chondromas. Arch. Neurol. Psychiatry, *20*:275–291, 1928.
18. Dunsker, S.B.: Cervical spondylotic myelopathy: Pathogenesis and pathophysiology. *In* Seminars in Neurological Surgery. Cervical Spondylosis. Edited by Stewart Dunsker. New York, Raven Press, 1980, pp. 119–134.
19. Rowland, L.P.: Cervical spondylosis. *In* Merritt's Textbook of Neurology. 7th Ed. Edited by L.P. Rowland. Philadelphia, Lea & Febiger, 1984, pp. 310–312.
20. Adams, C.B.T., and Logue, V.: Studies in cervical spondylotic myelopathy, Parts I, II and III. Brain, *94*:557–594, 1971.

20a. Lunsford, L.D., Bissonette, D.J., and Zarub, D.S.: Anterior surgery for cervical disc disease. Part 2: Treatment of cervical spondylotic myelopathy in 32 cases. J. Neurosurg., *53*:12–19, 1980.

21. Naylor, A.: Factors in the development of the spinal stenosis syndrome. J. Bone Joint Surg., *61B*:306–309, 1979.
22. Yamada, H., et al.: Intermittent cauda equina compression due to narrow spinal canal. J. Neurosurg., *37*:83–88, 1972.
23. Blau, J.N., and Logue, V.: Intermittent claudication of the cauda equina. Lancet, *1*:1081–1086, 1961.
24. Bohl, W.R., and Steffee, A.D.: Lumbar spinal stenosis: A cause of continued pain and disability in patients after total hip arthroplasty. Spine, *4*:168–173, 1979.
25. Pennal, G.F., and Schatzker, J.: Stenosis of the lumbar spinal canal. Clin. Neurosurg., *18*:86–105, 1971.
26. Hall, S., et al.: Lumbar spinal stenosis: Clinical features, diagnostic procedures and results of surgical treatment in 68 patients. Ann. Intern. Med., *103*:271–275, 1985.
27. Ehni, G.: Significance of the small lumbar canal: Cauda equina compression syndromes due to spondylosis. Part 1. J. Neurosurg., *31*:490–494, 1969.
28. Pyeritz, R.E., Sack, G.H., and Udvarhelyi, G.B.: Cervical and lumbar laminectomy for spinal stenosis in achondroplasia. Johns Hopkins Med. J., *146*:203–209, 1980.
29. Karpman, R.R., et al.: Lumbar spinal stenosis in a patient with diffuse idiopathic skeletal hypertrophy syndrome. Spine, *7*:598–603, 1982.
30. Ellman, M.H., et al.: Calcium pyrophosphate dihydrate deposition in lumbar disc fibrocartilage. J. Rheumatol. *8*:955–958, 1981.
31. Ciric, I., and Mikhael, M.A.: Lumbar spinal lateral recess stenosis. Neurol. Clin., *3*:417–423, 1985.
32. Keim, H.A., et al.: Somatosensory evoked potentials as an aid in the diagnosis and intraoperative management of spinal stenosis. Spine, *10*:338–355, 1985.
33. Herkowitz, H.N., et al.: Metrizamide myelography and epidural venography. Spine, *7*:55–64, 1982.
34. McIvor, G.W.D., and Kirkaldy-Willis, W.H.: Pathologic and myelographic changes in the major types of lumbar spinal stenosis. Clin. Orthop., *115*:72–76, 1976.
35. McAfee, P.C., et al.: Computed tomography in degenerative spinal stenosis. Clin. Orthop., *161*:221–234, 1981.
36. Bell, G.R., et al.: A study of computer-assisted tomography: Comparison of metrizamide myelography and computed tomography in the diagnosis of herniated lumbar disc and spinal stenosis. Spine, *9*:552–556, 1984.
37. Wiesel, S.W., et al.: A study of positive CAT scans in an asymptomatic group of patients. Spine, *9*:549–551, 1984.
38. Hammerschlag, S.B., Wolpert, S.M., and Carter, B.L.: Computed tomography of the spinal canal. Radiology, *121*:361–367, 1976.
39. Sheldon, J.J., Russin, L.A., and Gargano, F.P.: Lumbar spinal stenosis. Radiographic diagnosis with special reference to transverse axial tomography. Clin. Orthop., *115*:53–67, 1976.
40. Modic, M.T., et al.: Lumbar herniated disc disease and canal stenosis. Prospective evaluation by surface coil MR, CT and myelography. Am. J. Neuroradiol., *7*:709–717, 1986.
41. Han, J.S., et al.: NMR imaging of the spine. A.J.R., *141*:1137–1145, 1983.
42. Onofrio, B.: Personal communication, May, 1987.
43. Levy, W.J., Dohn, D.F., and Duchesneau, P.M.: Recurrence of lumbar canal stenosis. A decade after decompressive laminectomy. Surg. Neurol., *17*:96–98, 1982.
44. Shenkin, H.A., and Hack, C.J.: Spondylolisthesis after multiple bilateral laminectomies and facetectomies for lumbar spondylosis. J. Neurosurg., *50*:45–47, 1979.
45. Johnsson, K.E., Willner, S., and Johnsson, K.: Postoperative instability after decompression for lumbar stenosis. Spine, *11*:107–110, 1987.
46. Penning, L., Wilmink, J.T., van Woerden, H.H., and Knol, E.: CT myelographic findings in degenerative disorders of the cervical spine: Clinical significance. Am. J. Radiol., *146*:793–801, 1986.
47. Penning, L., and Wilmink, J.T.: Posture dependent bilateral compression of L4 or L5 nerve roots in facet hypertrophy. A dynamic CT-myelographic study. Spine, *12*:488–500, 1987.

96

Fibrosing Syndromes—Diabetic Stiff Hand Syndrome, Dupuytren's Contracture, and Plantar Fasciitis

WILMER L. SIBBITT, JR.

Fibrosis is the invasion and replacement of normal tissue by increased quantities of collagen. In some instances normal connective tissue is replaced or infiltrated by tissue with different biologic properties. Fibrosis can interfere with normal function by distorting the anatomy and increasing tissue stiffness.[1–3] A *fibrosing (sclerosing) disease* is characterized by an over-accumulation that interferes with function. A partial list of diseases characterized clinically by fibrosis is shown in Table 96–1.

PATHOGENESIS OF FIBROSIS

Fibrosis can be induced by a number of mechanisms, including tissue injury, vascular ablation, chronic inflammation, alterations in collagen type, and chemical modifications of existing collagen. The cellular and molecular events leading to fibrosis are identical to those of normal healing, which creates new collagenous tissue in response to injury.

HEALING

Normal healing is characterized by four distinct phases: (1) initial tissue injury; (2) secondary inflammation; (3) tissue proliferation; and (4) tissue remodeling (Table 96–2). During the initial injury, types I and III collagens are exposed, resulting in platelet adhesion, aggregation, and release of soluble factors that enhance fibroblast proliferation, promote leukocyte chemotaxis, and increase capillary permeability.

Neutrophils, eosinophils, mast cells, lymphocytes, and monocytes migrate to the site of injury during the local inflammatory reaction. Macrophages (from blood monocytes), fibroblasts, and the infiltrating cells secrete a variety of factors that induce fibroblast and endothelial cell proliferation.[5] These factors include EGF, PDGF, FGF, TGF, IL-1, GM-CSF, M-CSF, TNF, and various prostaglandins.[6,7] Monocytes and macrophages might be most central to the formation of new connective tissue in normal healing, whereas mast cells and activated lymphocytes might be more important in the fibrotic diseases vis a vis normal healing.[8]

Fibroblasts and capillary endothelial cells derived from local tissue invade the injured area 24 to 48 hours after the migration of blood leukocytes. Migrating fibroblasts exude extracellular strand-like arrays, which firmly anchor the fibroblast to the surrounding tissues and which sense the direction of external stresses. The activated fibroblasts secrete collagen, fibronectin, reticulin, and proteoglycans, creating a stabilizing matrix in the area of injury. Remodeling of the extracellular matrix begins immediately by fibroblast-mediated resorption of existing collagen and secretion of new collagen, particularly along the aforementioned lines of mechanical stress.

CONTRACTION OF CONNECTIVE TISSUE

Contraction of the developing connective tissue is mediated by epithelial cells in the early wound, and by fibroblasts and fibroblast-derived myofibroblasts in mature granulation tissue. *Myofibroblasts* are contractile cells containing large amounts of the protein myosin.[9] The contractures and distorted microscopic and macroscopic anatomy of the fibrosing diseases are mediated by the contraction of myofibroblasts in the maturing granulation tissue.[10]

ABNORMALITIES OF COLLAGEN

In certain diseases, fibrosis can be manifested by an increase in the total amount of tissue collagen. Increased local production of collagen is usually implicated, but increased collagen content can also occur from a relative resistance of resident collagen to collagenase. Increased local production of collagen occurs in the presence of chronic inflammatory diseases, in areas of massive tissue necrosis, and in the presence of chronic vascular insufficiency. Macroscopic and microscopic vascular ablation has been increasingly recognized as a major mechanism for the induction of fibrosis. Hypoxia in areas of injury can stimulate the production of collagen by fibroblasts. Vascular ablation can also be a critical mechanism of fibrosis in progressive systemic sclerosis and Dupuytren's contracture.

Changes in the ratio of type I to type III collagen are common in the fibrosis induced by inflammatory diseases. For example, pulmonary fibrosis is not characterized by an increase in total tissue collagen, but rather by an increase in type I collagen relative to that of type III.[11] In Dupuytren's contracture, both total collagen and type III collagen were increased in early lesions, whereas type I predominated in late lesions. Post-translational chemical changes of collagen such as glycosylation and cross-linking can change the hydrophilic characteristics, tensile strength, and resistance to collagenase, resulting in passive collagen accumulation.

The number of diseases associated with fibrosis is large and beyond the scope of this chapter (Table 96–1). Progressive systemic sclerosis and scleroderma variants are discussed in great detail in Chapters 73 and 74 and will be mentioned only in relationship to regional fibrosing diseases of the musculoskeletal system.

TABLE 96–1. FIBROSING DISEASES

Skin and musculoskeletal system
Progressive systemic sclerosis
Morphea
Graft-host reaction
Diabetic stiff-hand syndrome
Dupuytren's contracture
Aponeurotic plantar fibrosis
Knuckle pads (Garrod's nodules)
Plantar fasciitis
Keloids
Lungs
Pulmonary fibrosis
Chronic pleural reaction
Cardiovascular system
Constrictive pericarditis
Vascular plaques
Intimal proliferation
Gastrointestinal system
Chronic active hepatitis
Primary biliary cirrhosis
Sclerosing cholangitis
Esophageal stricture
Collagenous colitis
Genitourinary system
Nephritis
Nephrosclerosis
Interstitial cystitis
Peyronie's disease
Other
Pseudotumor
Retroperitoneal fibrosis
Reidel's struma
Cancer
Sjögren's syndrome

DUPUYTREN'S CONTRACTURE

PATHOLOGY AND BIOCHEMISTRY

Dupuytren's contracture is characterized by nodular thickening of the palmar fascia and flexor contracture of the digits (Fig. 96–1). This disorder was first described by Felix Plater in 1614, and later was given a full and accurate description by the French surgeon Baron Guillaume Dupuytren, among others.[12–14] Although usually an incidental finding, Dupuytren's contracture can be both deforming and disabling.

Dupuytren's contracture is an active fibrotic process characterized by the proliferation of fibroblasts and the accelerated production of collagen in and around the palmar fascia.[15–17] The fibrotic tissue coalesces into palmar nodules, cords, and bands composed of contractile

TABLE 96–2. THE NORMAL HEALING PROCESS

PHASE	EVENT(S)	TIME AFTER INJURY (DAYS)
1 Tissue injury	Exposure of hidden proteins	0
Platelet activation	Release of mediators	0
Coagulation	Release of chemoattractants	0–2
2 Secondary inflammation	Neutrophils and eosinophils	1–4
	Monocytes	2–6
3 Tissue proliferation	Fibroblast migration	3–7
	Vascular ingrowth	6–10
	Collagen secretion	2–21
4 Tissue remodeling	Modification by proteases	3–21
	Collagen cross-linking	7–72

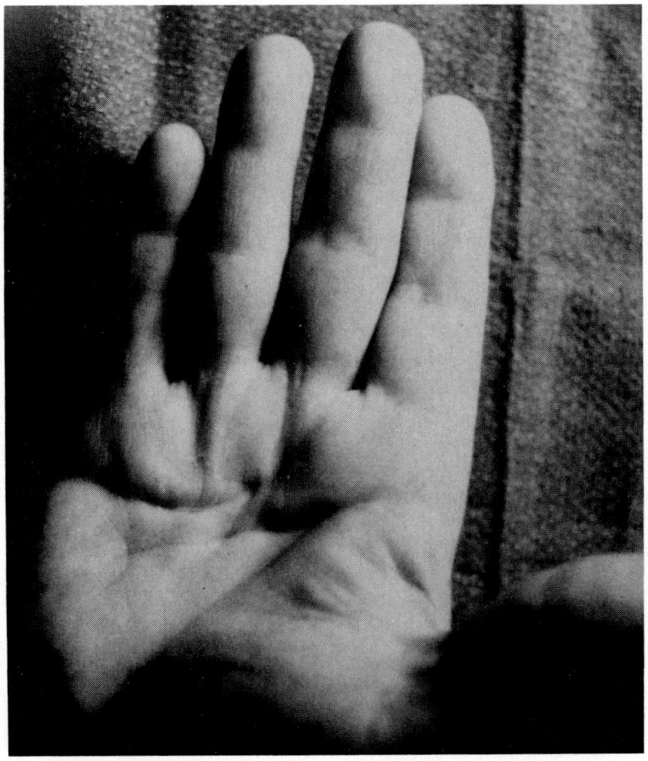

FIGURE 96–1. *Dupuytren's contracture.* This is an early stage of Dupuytren's contracture characterized by a puckering of the skin and the presence of nodular thickening of the palmar fascia. The contracture of the 4th metacarpophalangeal joint is in an incipient stage, but should progress with time. Similar lesions might be present in the plantar fascia (plantar fibromatosis).

TABLE 96–3. ASSOCIATIONS WITH DUPUYTREN'S CONTRACTURE

Intrinsic associations
Male gender
Northern European descent
Increasing age
Family history
Chromosomal abnormalities
Disease associations
Diabetes mellitus
Epilepsy
Anticonvulsant therapy
Plantar fasciitis
Peyronie's disease
Plantar fibrosis (Ledderhose's disease)
Knuckle pads (Garrod's nodules)
Carpal tunnel syndrome
Trigger finger
Rheumatoid arthritis
Eosinophilic fasciitis
Extrinsic associations
Injury to palmar aspect of hand
Pulmonary tuberculosis
Alcoholism
Cigarette smoking
Human immunodeficiency virus

connective tissue. Nodules are usually confined to the palmar aponeurosis, whereas the bands and cords are long fibrotic structures extending into the digital fascia.[18] Typically, the palmar aponeurosis, the flexor tendons, the neurovascular bundles, the skin, and the periarticular structures are all entrapped by the fibrotic process, resulting in pain, deformity, and loss of function.

Dupuytren's diathesis consists of Dupuytren's contracture, nodules in the plantar fascia (Ledderhose disease), Peyronie's disease, and pads in the popliteal fossa, shoulder, knuckles, and other areas (Garrod's nodules). Affected individuals usually have more severe disease and tend to have postsurgical recurrences.

Dupuytren's contracture is characterized by three stages. *The early (proliferative) stage* begins with the clinical appearance of a palmar nodule without contracture. Endothelial cell swelling, proliferation of the layers of basal laminae, microvascular occlusion, and fibroblast hypertrophy are prominent. *The active phase* is characterized by dimpling of the overlying skin, continued growth of existing nodules, and the development of thickened cords and bands in the fascia.[19] Contractile myofibroblasts are present throughout the lesion, and dense connective tissue accumulates in the nodules and cords. Vascular elements are increasingly confined to the periphery of the lesions. *The advanced (residual) stage* is characterized by rigid, disabling contractures and atrophy of the muscles of the hand and forearm. The thickened cords and nodules of the advanced stage consist mainly of type I collagen and are largely avascular.[19]

ETIOLOGY

Heredity and pre-existing systemic diseases are strongly associated with the development of Dupuytren's contracture[20] (Table 96–3). Northern Europeans, especially Celts, have a prevalence of 25% in populations greater than 60 years old, and 40% in those aged 80 and older. An autosomal dominant hereditary pattern may be present in this group, with 68% of first-degree relatives affected. Dupuytren's disease has been increasingly recognized in African and Asian populations, although with a lesser prevalence.[21] Men develop the condition 2 to 10 times more often than women, but the prevalence in women older than 75 approaches that of men the same age. Chromosomal abnormalities and mosaicism has been described, further implicating a genetic basis for this disorder.[1]

Dupuytren's contracture is often associated with chronic metabolic and inflammatory disease, occurring in up to 42% of diabetic patients.[22] Whether the metabolic derangements or genetic patterns create this association is unclear. Injury to the palmar structures, epilepsy, anticonvulsant therapy, hepatic disease, carpal tunnel syndrome, trigger finger, alcoholism, cigarette smoking, chronic pulmonary tuberculosis, human immunodeficiency virus, eosinophilic fasciitis, and rheumatoid arthritis have all been associated with Dupuytren's disease.[19,23–25] Age, total alcohol consumption, gender, and previous hand injuries, but not chronic liver disease, are most closely associated with Dupuytren's disease.[26] Occupation, including manual labor, was not related to the development of this disorder.

CLINICAL FINDINGS

Patients note decreased mobility in the affected fingers and might complain of pain in the palm or digits.[23] Both hands are often affected, and identical lesions can occur on the palmar surface of the feet.[24] The ring finger is most commonly involved, but the fifth, third, and second digits, in decreasing frequency, can also be affected. A nodular thickening is present in the palmar fascia on examination. Unlike nodules associated with flexor tenosynovitis, the nodules of Dupuytren's contracture are less discrete, do not move in the exact track of the tendon, and typically dimple the overlying skin (Fig. 96–1).

Congenital flexion deformity, post-traumatic scar, immobilization contracture, Volkmann's ischemic contracture (wrist and PIP flexed), primary joint contracture, tenosynovitis, fibrosarcoma (no contracture), and plantar fasciitis should be excluded by appropriate history and physical findings. In Dupuytren's contracture, the restriction of the flexor tendons is not altered by flexing the wrist (as in congenital or spastic contractures) or by flexing the metacarpophalangeal joints (as in contracture of the intrinsic muscles). If any question remains concerning the identity of the process, a magnetic resonance (MR) study might delineate the presence of the Dupuytren's fibrotic mass with angular traction on the tendon apparatus (Fig. 96–2).

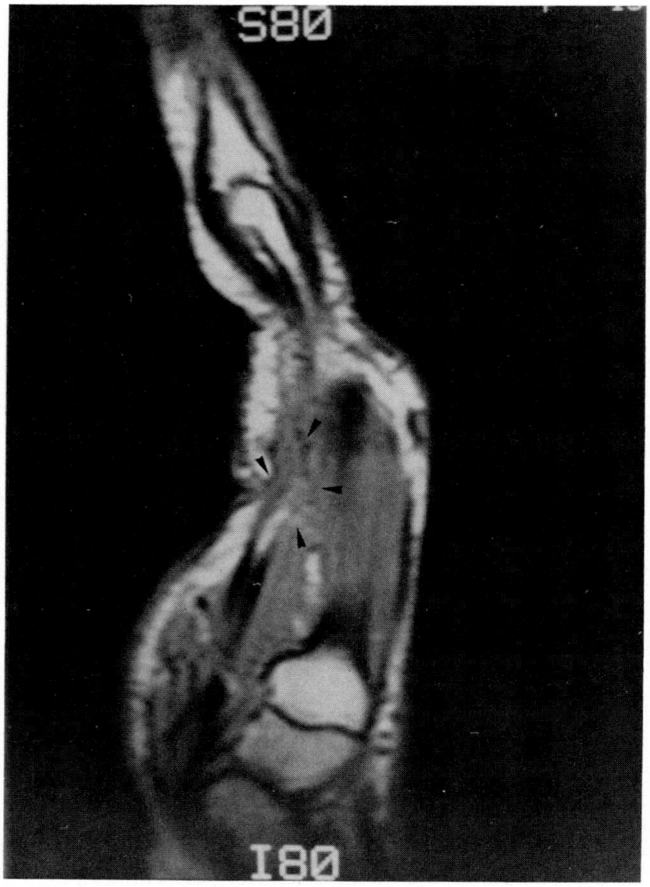

FIGURE 96–2. *Dupuytren's contracture.* A magnetic resonance (MR) image of the patient's hand shown in Figure 96–1 demonstrates the invading mass of connective tissue extending along the palmar fascia into the adjoining structures. The contractile mass of tissue has enmeshed the flexor digitorum profundus and superficialis tendons and exerts traction, resulting in an angular deformity of the tendon and a clinical contracture. Courtesy of Randy R. Sibbitt, M.D.

THERAPY

Reassurance, local heat, range-of-motion exercises, splinting, and an intralesional long-acting corticosteroid injection might alleviate the symptoms and improve function for patients with an early, painful lesion without significant contracture.[23,26] In patients with disabling contractures, surgery might be necessary to remove the mass of hypertrophied connective tissue from the flexor tendon and affected digits.[27] If a contracture greater than 10° is present in the proximal interphalangeal joint, some authors recommend early release to prevent permanent deformity.[19] Surgical approaches to the treatment of Dupuytren's contracture are necessarily cautious, because the fibrotic tissue often affects the neurovascular bundles as well as the fascia and tendons. Surgical procedures include nodule excision, fasciotomy, regional fasciotomy, and radical fasciotomy.[19,23,26,28] Complication rates associated with such treatment approach 20% and include flexion contractures, hematoma, skin necrosis, infection, reflex sympathetic dystrophy, and nodule recurrence.[19]

SYNDROME OF LIMITED JOINT MOBILITY

The syndrome of limited joint mobility (SLJM) should be considered in the context of other diabetes-associated lesions of the hand and upper extremity (Table 96–4). These musculoskeletal disorders constitute a spectrum of pathologic changes resulting from active fibrosis (Dupuytren's contracture, tenosynovitis), passive fibrosis (nonenzymatic glycosylation), motor neuropathy (neuropathic contractures), and autonomic disturbance (reflex sympathetic dystrophy).[29] SLJM and diabetic sclerodactyly remain the most insidious and underdiagnosed of the diabetic complications affecting the upper extremity, despite the high frequency of these disorders in both adult and juvenile diabetic populations.

Diabetic contractures, including those of SLJM, have been recognized in one form or another for over a cen-

TABLE 96–4. DIABETIC COMPLICATIONS INVOLVING THE UPPER EXTREMITY

CONDITION	TYPICAL JOINTS INVOLVED	COMMENTS
Syndrome of limited joint mobility	MCP, PIP, wrists, other joints	Decreased range of motion of the small joints. Often associated with sclerodactyly
Diabetic sclerodactyly	Distal digits, but can extend to entire hand	Thickened, waxy skin
Reflex sympathetic dystrophy (RSD)	Contracture and edema of the entire hand, occasionally entire arm	More often bilateral (42%) than in other conditions (5%); bone scan is positive
Adhesive capsulitis	Contracture of shoulder	Often associated with RSD or bicipital or supraspinatus tenosynovitis
Dupuytren's contracture	3rd, 4th, and 5th MCP and PIP contractures	Palpably thickened palmar fascia, dimpling of skin, associated with plantar fibromatosis
Flexor tenosynovitis	Any digit, but especially 2nd, 3rd, and 4th digits	Presence of painful trigger finger, thickened tendon sheath, nodule on tendon in area of pulley
Carpal tunnel syndrome	MCP and PIP contractures	Prominent pain, wasting of thenar musculature, positive Tinel's and Phelan's signs; slowed nerve conduction
Diabetic neuropathy	Variable contractures	Dysesthesias, pain, loss of proprioception and fine touch; abnormal nerve conduction
Aseptic necrosis of humoral head	Shoulder contractures	Pain, loss of motion, radiographic changes delayed

MCP = metacarpophalangeal joint; PIP = proximal interphalangeal joint; RSD = reflex sympathetic dystrophy

tury.[26–31] SLJM is characterized by decreased range of motion of the joints of the hands and wrists in a patient with diabetes mellitus without apparent underlying joint disease.[32] Synonyms include cheiroarthropathy, diabetic stiff hand syndrome, and waxy contractures of diabetes.[1] *Diabetic sclerodactyly* often accompanies SLJM. Together these disorders constitute a passive fibrotic syndrome closely resembling limited forms of scleroderma.

The early stages of SLJM are usually asymptomatic, although accompanying aching, neuropathy, or vascular phenomena can occur. Later, when the contractures become more severe, the patient might complain of difficulty using the hands. When the contractures are severe, SLJM can be disabling because of decreased grip and impaired digital agility.

By definition, SLJM is a complication of diabetes mellitus, and must be distinguished from other diabetic and nondiabetic contractures. In normal populations, the range of motion of the small joints of the hands varies considerably, but decreases with aging.[33,34] Because of these normal age-related changes, decreased range of motion of the joints in a younger individual with diabetes has far greater significance than similar changes in an older individual. SLJM is most common in patients with type I diabetes, but it is also frequent in type II patients[35,36]; 32 to 40% of all insulin-dependent diabetics might eventually be affected.[35] SLJM appears to affect all racial groups with diabetes, although concomitant nephropathy, neuropathy, and retinopathy might occur more often in caucasians.[37] SLJM is associated with increasing age, duration of diabetes, the presence of Dupuytren's contracture, retinopathy, neuropathy, and cigarette smoking.[38–40]

CLINICAL FINDINGS

SLJM is characterized by the presence of contractures involving the small joints of the hands, including the proximal and distal interphalangeal joints and the metacarpophalangeal joints (Fig. 96–3). Patients usually have a prominent "prayer sign" indicating the presence of contractures of the interphalangeal and metacarpophalangeal joints. Decreased extension at the wrists and metacarpophalangeal joints is the most reliable prognostic measure of disability. Some patients also have decreased range of motion in the shoulders and other large joints.[41]

SLJM is often accompanied by *diabetic sclerodactyly*, a thickening and rigidity of the skin of the distal digits resembling scleroderma. This process usually begins distally, but can affect the wrist, elbows, and neck. Conditions often confused with SLJM and diabetic sclerodactyly include scleroderma, reflex sympathetic dystrophy, diabetic neuropathy, Dupuytren's contracture, and flexor tenosynovitis with or without trigger finger.

Because SLJM is closely associated with the presence of retinopathy, nephropathy, and neuropathy, patients with classic diabetic complications should be carefully examined for limited joint movement. Other than the presence of elevated blood glucose and glycosylated hemoglobin, laboratory evaluation is not useful. Antinuclear antibodies and rheumatoid factor are not found in true SLJM, but might be found in diabetes associated

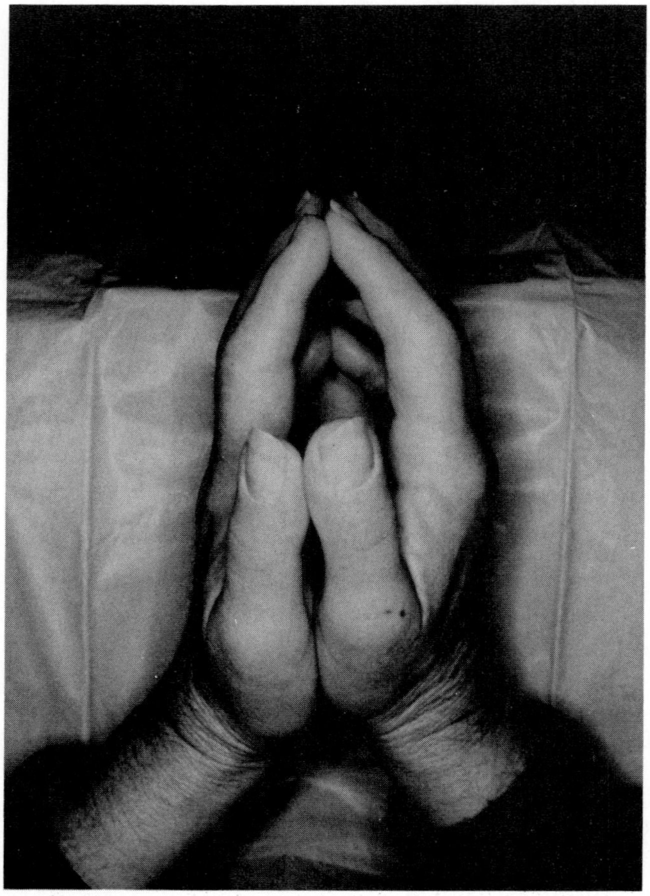

FIGURE 96–3. *Syndrome of limited joint mobility (SLJM).* This diabetic patient is suffering from contractures of the metacarpophalangeal, proximal interphalangeal, and distal interphalangeal joints, resulting in a prominent "prayer sign." The skin is also thickened and has lost much of its fine wrinkles, simulating true sclerodactyly.

with scleroderma or lupus-like autoimmune syndromes. SLJM might be associated with restrictive pulmonary disease consistent with a generalized alteration of collagen.[29,32]

PATHOLOGY

The etiology of SLJM and diabetic sclerodactyly is unknown, but probably relates to the same underlying mechanisms that induce other diabetic complications.[42] Biopsies from patients with SLJM show extensive fibrosis with markedly increased amounts of collagen in the dermis. This collagen has increased cross-linking and glycosylation, both of which can result in resistance to normal collagenase-mediated collagen turnover with subsequent passive accumulation. The basement membrane of microvessels are thickened, endothelial cells demonstrate degenerative changes, binuclear fibroblasts are present, and muscle fibers reveal vacuolization and mitochondrial degeneration.[43] These changes might be related to the increased hydration of connective tissue associated with polyol accumulation and its metabolic consequences (Fig. 96–4).[44] SLJM might also be related to neuropathy, especially carpal tunnel syndrome.[45] Diabetic microsvasculopathy of the digits is closely associated with SLJM and diabetic sclerodactyly, and could promote fibrosis through chronic ischemia, analogous to that occurring in progressive systemic sclerosis.[46]

TREATMENT

Treatment remains controversial and unsatisfactory. As with other diabetic complications, strict control of blood glucose is indicated.[32] Range of motion exercises are essential to maintain strength and flexibility, but do not reverse established contractures. Aldose reductase inhibitor agents can be effective, but are still undergoing randomized trials.[31,32] Penicillamine and aminoguanidine, which inhibit cross-linking of collagen, are possible therapies. Both are toxic and cannot be generally recommended.[29]

PLANTAR FASCIITIS

THE PAINFUL HEEL

Painful heel is a common musculoskeletal complaint. *Plantar fasciitis* refers specifically to a syndrome characterized by pain and stiffness involving the heel and plantar surface of the foot with maximum tenderness localized at the insertion of the plantar fascia on the calcaneal tuberosity. This disorder is characterized by local inflammation and fibrosis.[47] Radiologic studies often reveal small calcifications anterior to the calcaneal tuberosity and the presence of an exuberant anterior calcaneal osteosis (spur) (Fig. 96–5). The calcaneal ostosis of plantar fasciitis is really an extension of the calcaneal tuberosity.

Disorders that must be differentiated from plantar fasciitis include Achilles tendinitis/tenosynovitis, Achilles tendon rupture, calcaneal apophysitis, posterior tibial and flexor hallucis longus tendonitis/tenosynovitis, calcaneal periostitis, calcaneal osteomyelitis, stress fracture, and nonanterior calcaneal spur or ostosis (Table 96–5).

ETIOLOGY

Plantar fasciitis is responsible for over 15% of all complaints in clinics specializing in care of the foot. Plantar fasciitis is most commonly related to noninflammatory conditions including obesity,[48] excessive pronation,[49] increasing age,[50] metabolic bone disease,[51] and overuse, particularly long-distance running.[52,53] Plantar fasciitis can also be associated with inflammatory diseases (Table 96–6), including Reiter's syndrome, ankylosing spondylitis, rheumatoid arthritis, Dupuytren's contracture, lupus, gout, and others.[1] Plantar fasciitis and

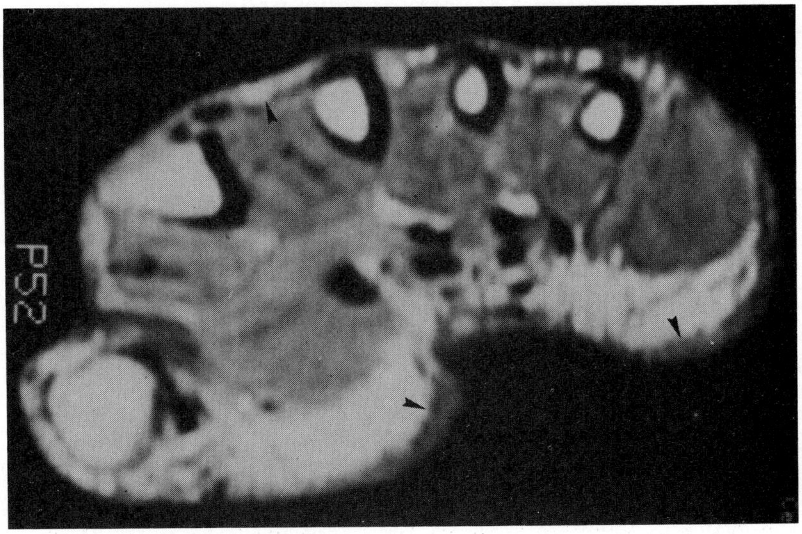

FIGURE 96–4. *Syndrome of limited joint mobility (SLJM).* This MR image of the hand of the patient shown in Figure 96–3 demonstrates thickened dermal connective tissue resembling that of progressive systemic sclerosis. The dermis also is characterized by increased proton density, suggesting accentuated hydration of the resident connective tissue. Courtesy of Randy R. Sibbitt, M.D.

other inflammatory heel disorders are often a hallmark of the seronegative spondylarthropathies.

Plantar fasciitis is most often induced by excessive repetitive stress applied to the foot, resulting in torsion and tension on the plantar fascia. These stresses particularly damage the flexible flat foot, which has a tendency to pronate (evert) at the talonavicular or naviculocuneiform joints. Excessive pronation of the foot increases tension across the plantar fascia after heel strike and before toe-off, which can result in a microscopic avulsion or tear in a portion of the fascial fibers. Continued stress to the fascial apparatus eventually results in chronic inflammation and replacement with connective tissue elements.

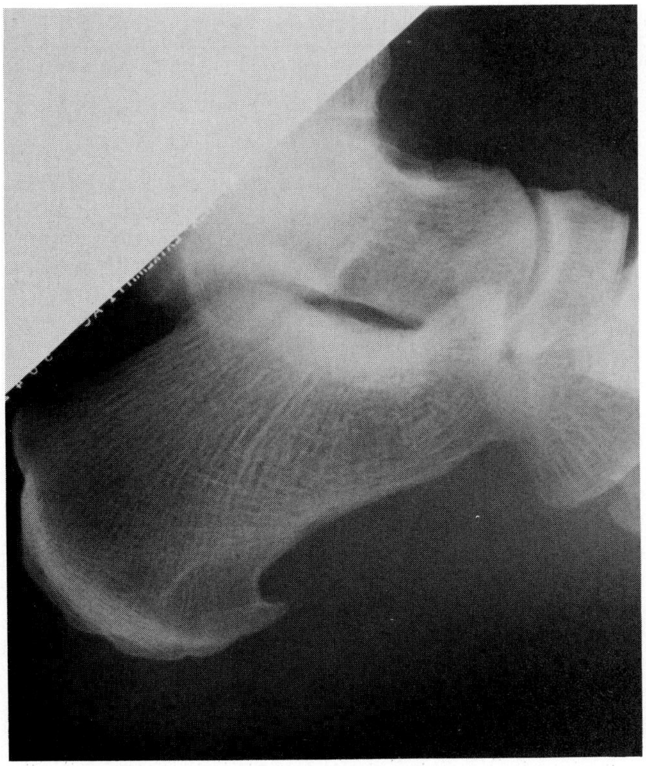

FIGURE 96–5. *Plantar fasciitis.* This patient, a long-distance runner, continued to run despite severe calcaneal pain secondary to plantar fasciitis. A large calcaneal hyperostosis extends anteriorly, following the plantar fascia. The patient responded to 8 months of abstinence from long-distance running and eventually was able to resume running at reduced distances with the use of antipronator running shoes. Courtesy of Randy R. Sibbitt, M.D.

PATHOLOGY

Histopathologically plantar fasciitis is characterized by collagen degeneration, angiofibroblastic hyperplasia, chondroid metaplasia, and calcification of degenerated matrix. Periosteal inflammation is almost ubiquitous, frequently resulting in the growth of an anterior calcaneal spur along the course of the fascia. The presence of an anterior heel spur on a radiograph is not necessary for the diagnosis of plantar fasciitis, but often it is confirmatory. The presence of such a spur implies that the process has already become chronic (Fig. 96–5). The anterior calcaneal ostosis remains after symptoms of pain have resolved, indicating that the inflammation and injury, not the ostosis, is the cause of pain in these patients.

DIAGNOSIS

Inflammatory conditions, particularly seronegative spondylarthropathy, should be excluded by clinical, radiologic, and laboratory examination. Other causes of heel pain should be excluded (Table 96–6). The patient should be questioned about overuse, particularly long-

TABLE 96–5. INTRINSIC CAUSES OF HEEL PAIN

DISORDER	COMPLAINTS	DIAGNOSTIC SIGNS
Plantar fasciitis	Plantar foot, anterior heel	Tenderness over calcaneal tuberosity; anterior spur
Achilles tendon		
Tendosynovitis*	Tendon, posterior heel	Diffuse tenderness and swelling along tendon
Tendonitis	Tendon, posterior heel	Diffuse tenderness along tendon and calcaneal insertion
Subtendinous bursitis	Tendon, posterior heel	Tenderness and swelling superior to posterior calcaneus
Subcutaneous bursitis	Tendon, posterior heel	Tenderness and swelling inferior to posterior calcaneus
Rupture	Weakness, pain often not present	Tenderness and defect in tendon in area of rupture
Calcaneal apophysitis (enthesopathy)	Posterior heel	Tenderness at insertion of Achilles tendon; x-ray "whiskering"
Calcaneal stress fracture	Heel	Stress fracture, x ray
Flexor hallucis longus tendonitis or tenosynovitis	Anterior superior heel and posterior medial malleolus into plantar foot	Tenderness and swelling posterior to medial malleolus into plantar foot
Tibialis posterior tendonitis or tenosynovitis	Anterior superior heel and posterior medial malleolus into plantar foot	Tenderness and swelling posterior to medial malleolus into plantar foot
Calcaneal periostitis or erosion	Tenderness in heel	Radiologic diagnosis; inflammatory arthritis; bone scan positive
Osteomyelitis	Heel pain	Radiologic diagnosis; bone scan positive; gallium or indium scan positive
Calcaneal spur	Heel pain	Nonanterior calcaneal ostosis; pain directly over ostosis
Tarsal tunnel syndrome	Heel and midfoot	Neurologic abnormalities in heel and plantar foot

* The Achilles tendon lacks a true tenosynovium, but a false synovial sheath, associated with tendon inflammation, can develop.

TABLE 96–6. CONDITIONS ASSOCIATED WITH PLANTAR FASCIITIS

Inflammatory conditions
- *Frequent*
  - Reiter's syndrome
  - Ankylosing spondylitis
  - Psoriatic arthritis
  - Intestinal arthropathies
  - Behçet's disease
- *Less common*
  - Rheumatoid arthritis
  - Systemic lupus erythematosus

Structural abnormalities
- Pes valgus
- Increased pronation
- Flexible "flat foot"
- *Overuse*
  - Long-distance running
  - Prolonged walking or standing
  - Aerobic dance
  - Other endurance exercise

Other
- Diabetes mellitus
- Gout
- Obesity
- Calcaneal spurs
- Dupuytren's contracture
- Achilles tendonitis
- Metabolic bone disease

distance running. The structure and motion of the foot, ankle, knee, and hip should be carefully examined for a tendency to pronate. Neurologic dysfunction should be considered, and tarsal tunnel syndrome should be excluded (see also Chapter 97).

THERAPY

Treatment should first be directed at reducing torsion and injury to the plantar fascia and its bony insertion. Long-distance running and other activities contributing to overuse should be suspended until the symptoms have completely resolved, a process that typically requires months. Obesity should be corrected. The patient should be reassured that rest is best. If the patient is a compulsive exerciser, another endurance exercise with less associated foot trauma such as bicycling or swimming should be substituted. Continued abuse of the foot will result in chronic, intractable pain and the development of a hyperostosis on the calcaneus.

Nonsteroidal anti-inflammatory drugs are often effective in diminishing the pain and stiffness of plantar fasciitis, but are not curative. If a month-long trial of rest and nonsteroidal drugs has not markedly improved the patient's symptoms, injection of the plantar fascia with corticosteroids might temporarily improve symptoms. Injection of the plantar fascia is best accomplished through a lateral or medial approach, not through the plantar surface of the foot. If corticosteroid flows back along the needle track, atrophy of the plantar skin and calcaneal fat pad might occur, resulting in bone-on-skin in the critical weight-bearing pressure point of the heel. As usual with soft tissue injections, preparations of corticosteroids containing fluorine should be avoided and the suspension should be diluted with local anesthesia (at least 5:1).

If these measures are ineffective, orthotic devices can be constructed to reduce the tension in the plantar fascia. These devices, the simplest of which is the varus wedge, may consist of a plastic heel cup and medial arch support or may be customized from plaster foot moldings and adjusted to the appropriate degree of correction. Prolonged use of these devices is required before permanent improvement is noted.

Finally, for cases resistant to conservative therapy, surgical intervention may be considered. Both fasciectomy and fasciotomy (fascial release) have been successful,[1] although these procedures can increase the instability of the foot. The symptomatic effectiveness of surgical therapy might be related to hypesthesia of the heel secondary to oblation of the lateral plantar nerve. This type of surgical therapy does not alter the forces that induced the fasciitis originally, except at the point of fascial insertion. Because of this, surgery for plantar fasciitis should be considered only when prolonged rest, anti-inflammatory drugs, and orthotic devices have failed after a minimum trial of 6 months.

REFERENCES

1. Sibbitt, W.L. Jr.: Fibrosing syndromes: Diabetic stiff hand syndrome, Dupuytren's contracture, and plantar fasciitis. *In* Arthritis and Allied Conditions. Edited by D.J. McCarty. Philadelphia, Lea & Febiger, 1989, pp. 1473–1485.
2. Jimenez, S.A.: Other fibrosing syndromes. Curr. Opin. Rheumatol., *1*:516–522, 1989.
3. Wooldridge, W.E.: Four related fibrosing diseases. Postgrad. Med., *84*:269–274, 1988.
4. Eckersley, J.R.T., and Dudley, H.A.F.: Wounds and wound healing. Br. Med. Bull., *44*:423–436, 1988.
5. Kahaleh, M.B., DeLustro, F., Bock, W., and LeRoy, E.C.: Human monocyte modulation of endothelial cells and fibroblast growth: Possible mechanism for fibrosis. Clin. Immunol. Immunopathol., *39*:242–255, 1986.
6. Turk, C.W., Dohlman, J.G., and Goetzl, E.J.: Immunological mediators of wound healing and fibrosis. J. Cell. Physiol. Suppl., *5*:89–93, 1987.
7. Libby, P., Friedman, G.B., and Salomon, R.N.: Cytokines as modulators of cell proliferation in fibrotic diseases. Am. Rev. Resp. Dis., *140*:1114–1117, 1989.
8. Atkins, F.M., and Clark, R.A.F.: Mast cells and fibrosis. Arch. Dermatol., *123*:192–193, 1987.
9. Vande Berg, J.S., and Rudolph, R.: Cultured myofibroblasts: A useful model to study wound contraction and pathological contracture. Ann. Plast. Surg., *14*:111–120, 1985.
10. Tomasek, J.J., Schultz, R.J., Episalla, C.W., and Newman, S.A.: The cytoskeleton and extracellular matrix of the Dupuytren's disease "myofibroblast": An immunofluorescence study of a nonmuscle cell type. J. Hand Surg., *11A*:365–371, 1986.
11. Kirk, J.M.E., Da Costa, P.E., Turner-Warwick, M., et al.: Biochemical evidence for an increased and progressive deposition of collagen in lungs of patients with pulmonary fibrosis. Clin. Sci., *70*:39–45, 1986.
12. Elliot, D.: The early history of contracture of the palmar fascia. Part 1: The origin of the disease; the curse of the MacCrimmons; the hand of benediction; Cline's contracture. J. Hand Surg., *13B*:246–253, 1988.
13. Elliot, D.: The early history of contracture of the palmar fascia. Part 2: The revolution in Paris; Guillaume Dupuytren; Dupuytren's disease. J. Hand Surg., *13B*:371–378, 1988.
14. Elliot, D.: The early history of contracture of the palmar fascia. Part 3: The controversy in Paris and the spread of surgical treatment of the disease throughout Europe. J. Hand Surg., *14*:25–31, 1989.
15. Gonzalez, S.M., and Gonzalez, R.I.: Dupuytren's disease. West. J. Med., *152*:430–433, 1990.
16. Hill, N.A., and Hurst, L.C.: Dupuytren's contracture. Hand Clinics, *5*:349–357, 1989.
17. Murrel, G.A.C., and Hueston, J.T.: Aetiology of Dupuytren's contracture. Aust. N. Z. J. Surg., *60*:247–252, 1990.
18. Strickland, J.W., and Bassett, R.L.: the isolated digital cord in Dupuytren's contracture: Anatomy and clinical significance. J. Hand Surg., *10A*:118–124, 1985.
19. Legge, J.W.H.: Dupuytren disease. Surg. Annu., *45*:355–368, 1985.
20. Mikusev, I.E.: New facts about the pathogenesis of Dupuytren's contracture. Acta Chir. Plast., *31*:1–14, 1989.
21. Srivastava, S., and Nancarrow, J.D.: Dupuytren's disease in patients from the Indian sub-continent. Report of ten cases. J. Hand Surg., *14*:32–34, 1989.
22. Pal, B., Griffiths, I.D., Anderson, J., and Dick, W.C.: Association of limited joint mobility with Dupuytren's contracture in diabetes mellitus. J. Rheumatol., *14*:582–585, 1987.
23. Bradlow, A., and Mowat, A.G.: Dupuytren's contracture and alcohol. Ann. Rheum. Dis., *45*:304–307, 1986.
24. Bower, M., Nelson, M., and Gazzard, B.G.: Dupuytren's contractures in patients infected with HIV. Br. Med. J., *300*:164–165, 1990.
25. Kaklamanis, P., Vayopoulos, G., Aroni, K., and Meletis, J.: Eosinophilic fasciitis with thrombocytopenia and Dupuytren's contracture. Scand. J. Rheumatol., *19*:245–247, 1990.
26. Attali, P., Ink, O., Pelletier, G., et al.: Dupuytren's contracture, alcohol consumption, and chronic liver disease. Arch. Intern. Med., *147*:1065–1067, 1987.
27. McGrouther, D.A.: La Maladie de Dupuytren. To incise or excise? J. Hand Surg., *13B*:368–369, 1988.
28. Hill, N.A.: Dupuytren's contracture. J. Bone Joint Surg., *67A*:1439–1443, 1985.
29. Kapoor, A., and Sibbitt, W.L. Jr.: Diabetic contractures: The syndrome of limited joint mobility. Semin. Arthritis Rheum., *18*:168, 1989.
30. Cambell, R.R., Hawkins, S.J., Maddison, P.J., and Reckless, J.P.D.: Limited joint mobility in diabetes mellitus. Ann. Rheum. Dis., *44*:93–97, 1985.
31. Eaton, R.P.: Aldose reductase inhibition and the diabetic syndrome of limited joint mobility: Implications for altered collagen hydration. Metabolism, *35*:119–121, 1986.
32. Eaton, R.P., Sibbitt, W.L. Jr., and Harsh, A.: The effect of an aldose reductase inhibiting agent on limited joint mobility in diabetes mellitus. JAMA, *253*:1437–1471, 1985.
33. Larkin, J.G., and Frier, B.M.: Limited joint mobility and Dupuytren's contracture in diabetic, hypertensive, and normal populations. Br. Med. J., *292*:1494, 1986.
34. Wright, V.: The rheology of joints. Br. J. Rheumatol., *25*:243–252, 1986.
35. Slama, G., Letanoux, M., Thibult, N., et al.: Quantification of

early subclinical limited joint mobility in diabetes mellitus. Diabetes Care, *8*:329–332, 1985.
36. Pal, B., Anderson, J., Dick, W.C., and Griffiths, I.D.: Limitation of joint mobility and shoulder capsulitis in insulin- and non–insulin-dependent diabetes mellitus. Br. J. Rheumatol., *25*: 147–151, 1986.
37. Akanji, A.O., Bella, A.F., and Osotimehin, B.O.: Cheiroarthropathy and long term diabetic complications in Nigerians. Ann. Rheum. Dis., *49*:28–30, 1990.
38. Jennings, A.M., Milner, P.C., and Ward, J.D.: Hand abnormalities are associated with the complications of diabetes in type 2 diabetes. Diabetic Med., *6*:43–47, 1989.
39. Eadington, D.W., Patrick, A.W., Collier, A., and Frier, B.M.: Limited joint mobility, Dupuytren's contracture and retinopathy in type 1 diabetes: Association with cigarette smoking. Diabetic Med., *6*:152–157, 1989.
40. Pal, B., Griffiths, I.D., Anderson, J., and Dick, W.C.: Association of limited joint mobility with Dupuytren's contracture in diabetes mellitus. J. Rheumatol., *14*:582–585, 1987.
41. Sukenik, S., Weitzman, S., Buskila, D., et al.: Limited joint mobility and other rheumatological manifestation in diabetic patients. Diabetes Metab. Rev., *13*:187–192, 1987.
42. Beacom, R., Gillespie, E.L., Middleton, D., et al.: Limited joint mobility in insulin dependent diabetes mellitus: Relationship to retinopathy, peripheral nerve function and HLA status. Q. J. Med., *56*:337–344, 1985.
43. Ceruso, M., Lauri, G., Bufalini, C., et al.: Diabetic hand syndrome. J. Hand Surg., *13A*:765–770, 1988.
44. Eaton, R.P.: The collagen hydration hypothesis: A new paradigm for the secondary complications of diabetes mellitus. J. Chronic Dis., *39*:763–766, 1986.
45. Chaudhuri, K.R., Davidson, A.R., and Morris, I.M.: Limited joint mobility and carpal tunnel syndrome in insulin-dependent diabetes. Br. J. Rheumatol., *28*:191–194, 1989.
46. Mitchell, W.S., Winocour, P.H., Gush, R.J., et al.: Skin blood flow and limited joint mobility in insulin-dependent diabetes mellitus. Br. J. Rheumatol., *28*:195–200, 1989.
47. LeMelle, D.P., Kisilewicz, P., and Janis, L.R.: Chronic plantar fascial inflammation and fibrosis. Clin. Podiatr. Med. Surg., *7*:385–389, 1990.
48. Hills, J.J. Jr., and Cutting, P.J.: Heel pain and body weight. Foot Ankle, *9*:254–256, 1989.
49. Kwong, P.K., Kay, D., Voner, R.T., and White, M.W.: Plantar fasciitis. Mechanics and pathomechanics of treatment. Clin. Sports Med., *7*:119–126, 1988.
50. Williams, P.L.: The painful heel. Br. J. Hosp. Med., *38*:562–563, 1987.
51. Paice, E.W.: Nutritional osteomalacia presenting with plantar fasciitis. J. Bone Joint Surg., *69B*:38–40, 1987.
52. Messier, S.P.: Etiologic factors associated with selected running injuries. Med. Sci. Sports Exercise, *20*:501–505, 1988.
53. Warren, B.L.: Predicting plantar fasciitis in runners. Med. Sci. Sports Exercise, *19*:71–73, 1987.

97

Nerve Entrapment Syndromes

NORTIN M. HADLER

The major peripheral nerves of healthy individuals, with the few exceptions discussed later here, withstand compromise in spite of their length and soft tissue shielding. Blunt trauma, fractures, and lacerations are the usual culprits and are the purview of trauma surgeons. Rheumatologists, however, often care for the systemically ill in whom the soft-tissue shielding of the peripheral nerves and the nerves themselves are often involved in synovitis and vasculitis, respectively. The challenge is to discern the symptoms and signs of peripheral neuropathy in a more general inflammatory setting.

THE CLINICAL PRESENTATION

This chapter considers entrapment neuropathies of the major peripheral nerves as they course through the upper and lower extremities. The chapter focuses on those lesions likely to present to the rheumatologist; rare and exceptional sites of compression neuropathy require a more encyclopedic treatment.[1] The differential diagnosis of peripheral compression neuropathies includes more proximal neurologic disease. Cervical and lumbar radiculopathies are discussed in Chapters 92, 94, and 95, thoracic outlet syndrome and diseases of the brachial plexus in Chapter 99, and complementary essays are readily available.[2,3] Rather than re-emphasize the hallmarks of these confounding diagnoses, the distinctive features of peripheral entrapment neuropathies are emphasized here. Several of these features are common to all peripheral entrapment neuropathies and are discussed in the following paragraphs.

1. Dysesthesias are characteristic; they are often localized to the sensory distribution of the involved nerve.

2. The discomfort is variously described as burning, tingling, "pins and needles," or even "itchy" skin. Sometimes an aching pain is noted in the muscles, even the proximal muscles, innervated by the involved nerve.

3. The discomfort is not prominently use related. Tenderness in the distribution of the dysesthesias is not a feature; on the contrary, dysesthesias occurring at night and at rest plague these patients. The response is to attempt to rub or move the distal extremity, leading to further dismay if the patient has coincident inflammatory arthritis.

4. *Tinel's sign* is elicited by tapping the nerve at the site of entrapment. Focal tenderness is usually present but nonspecific, particularly in the setting of synovitis. The more specific response is to elicit pain and dysesthesias radiating into the sensory distribution of the nerve distal to the point of damage. The sign is useful both in the clinical diagnosis of entrapment neuropathy and in the localization of the compression.

5. The dysesthesias and associated symptoms reflect the greater vulnerability of the sensory fibers in the peripheral nerve to compressive damage. The process, however, rarely progresses to severe hypesthesia such that traditional testing with a pin is clearly abnormal. More-subtle tests of tactile compromise such as sensory thresholds are unreliable in the hands of many experienced investigators. Regardless, a normal sensory examination does not militate against the diagnosis of an entrapment neuropathy.

6. With severe and prolonged compression, the motor function of the nerve is compromised as well. In instances of insidiously progressive compression, such as some patients with rheumatoid arthritis (RA), motor compromise may be present with insignificant dysesthesias. In the upper extremity, motor compromise is manifest as clumsiness and decreased hand function. In the lower extremity, a gait disorder may eventuate. Atrophy and weakness becomes evident in muscles innervated by the compressed nerve.

7. Discerning entrapment neuropathies in the setting of rheumatoid or other inflammatory arthritis is obviously particularly difficult. With many idiopathic entrapments, particularly those occurring after subtle trauma, the involvement is often unilateral. Idiopathic carpal tunnel syndrome is an important exception. Symmetry of proliferative synovitis, however, can lead to symmetric entrapment neuropathies. Discerning the historical features of entrapment neuropathy among the more familiar inflammatory complaints is crucial. Inspecting the distal musculature is important, seeking asymmetry in the typical pattern of periarticular muscle atrophy, both between and within hands and feet, that might provide a clue to a peripheral neuropathy.

8. Although the patient may perceive that the involved distal extremity is "swollen," objective swelling or vasomotor phenomena are unusual in entrapment neuropathies, and their presence should lead to a restructuring of the differential diagnosis.

9. Entrapment neuropathies should be treated conservatively, unless symptoms become recalcitrant or weakness or atrophy supervenes. Atrophy is often obscured in the setting of inflammatory synovitis. Before considering surgical decompression, the physician should attempt to confirm the clinical diagnosis of entrapment and localize the compression by electroneurography.[4] The sensitivity of these techniques varies depending on the lesion; for some, such as carpal tunnel syndrome, it can approach 90%.

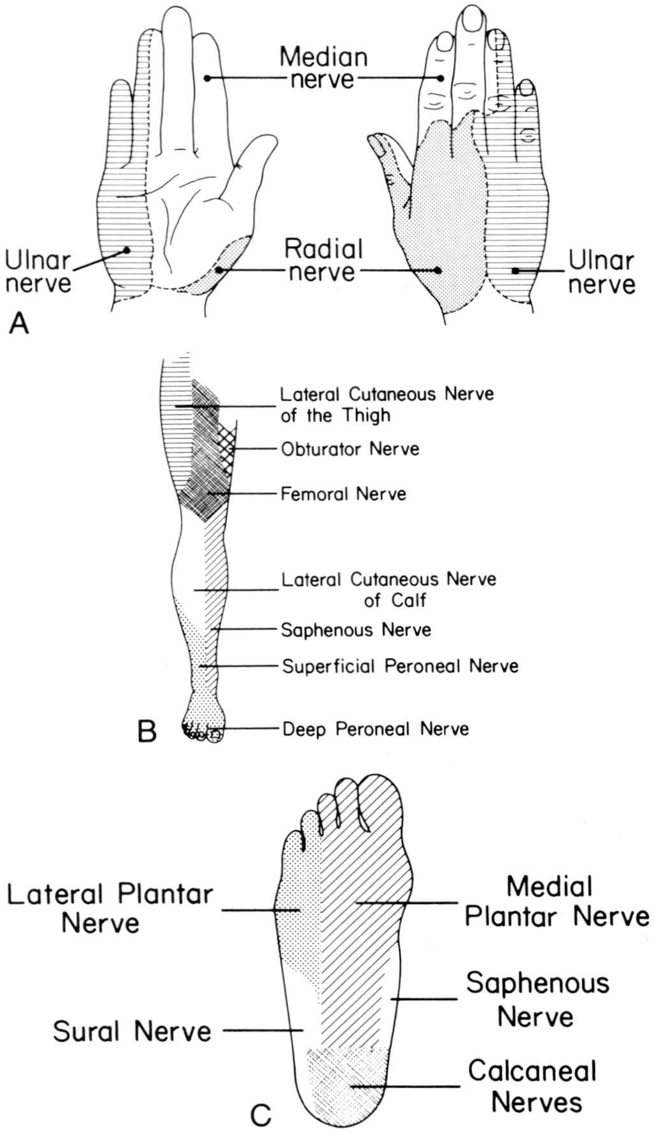

FIGURE 97–1. Distribution of the cutaneous nerves to the extremities. *A*, Sensory innervation of the palm and dorsum of the hand. *B*, Sensory innervation of the anterior aspect of the leg. *C*, Cutaneous innervation of the sole.

ENTRAPMENT NEUROPATHIES OF THE UPPER EXTREMITY

The three major nerves of the upper extremity course through the arm, protected from external compression short of that consequent to a humeral fracture or similar trauma. At the elbow, all three are at risk. Their course is more superficial at the elbow, even subcutaneous; they traverse synovial reflections that can proliferate in RA, and they are sandwiched at points between long bones and muscles. At the wrist, they again are at risk for all of the preceding reasons except that the sandwich is between bony prominences and tendons. Each nerve is considered separately in the following sections.

MEDIAN NERVE

The median nerve approaches the antecubital fossa lying medial to the brachial artery and separates from the artery at the artery's bifurcation. The nerve passes between the two heads of the pronator teres (the ulnar artery is deep to this muscle) and courses through the forearm lying between the flexores digitorum superficialis and profundus. It then passes through the carpal tunnel just beneath the transverse carpal ligament deep to the tendon of the palmaris longus. The median nerve supplies all the superficial and deep muscles of the volar forearm except the flexor carpi ulnaris. It also supplies nearly all the muscles of the thenar eminence: the abductor pollicis brevis, the oppenens pollicis, and the superficial head of the flexor pollicis brevis. The sensory distribution is illustrated in Figure 97–1A.

Entrapment neuropathy of the median nerve is the most common of entrapment neuropathies. In fact, it is the most common peripheral neuropathy. Regardless of the clinical setting, the most common site of compression is within the carpal tunnel. Thus, the carpal tunnel syndrome is the prototype entrapment neuropathy most likely to exhibit all of the preceding clinical features. Motor compromise involves the thenar eminence, with weakness and atrophy best detected by inspecting the contour of the abductor pollicis brevis (Fig.

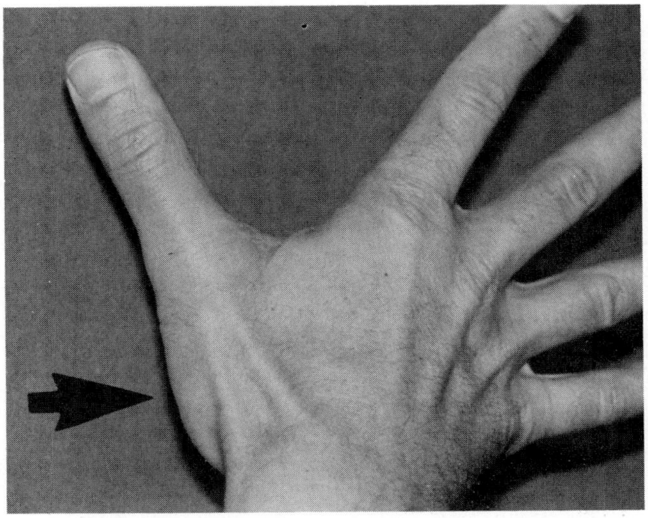

FIGURE 97–2. The lateral contour of the thenar eminence is the abductor pollicis brevis. Abduction against resistance allows one to assess the power of this muscle and inspect its bulk as a bulge (arrow). Since the innervation of this muscle is exclusively the median nerve, weakness and atrophy are specific signs of median neuropathy.

97–2). There is less uniformity of opinion regarding the sensitivity of provocative tests and the sensory examination. Some clinicians,[5] including me, find the Tinel's and Phalen's signs (symptoms reproduced on flexion at the wrist) useful, whereas most clinicians find sensory examinations very insensitive and provocative tests with a blood pressure cuff useless.[6] When systematically compared with standard electrodiagnostic tests, Tinel's is the only sign with sufficient positive predictive value to be clinically useful.[7]

Management of idiopathic carpal tunnel syndrome begins with splinting the wrist in the neutral position, particularly at night. In those with persistent symptoms in spite of splinting, steroid injection into the carpal tunnel provides complete relief in the majority, although up to 78% will relapse within 18 months.[8] In cases severe enough to undergo carpal tunnel release, the pressure to which the nerve is subjected is increased.[9] Thenar atrophy is a consensus indication for surgical intervention; recalcitrant symptoms, particularly atypical symptoms, call for perspicacity, judgment, and unequivocal electroneurographic confirmation of the diagnosis. It is important to emphasize that valid idiopathic carpal tunnel syndrome is not prevalent; its incidence approximates 1/1000/year.[10] Furthermore, it is not a consequence of performing repetitive motions if the elements of usage are comfortable and it does not occur in endemic form.[11]

Carpal tunnel syndrome can complicate RA, even early in the course and with bilateral involvement. Here, too, steroid injection can prove palliative with two provisos: first, thenar muscle atrophy secondary to median nerve compression can be obscured by that caused by articular inflammation, mandating close observation and ready recourse to surgical consultation. Second, injection therapy by the usual volar route carries greater risk of nerve infiltration and damage because of anatomic distortion secondary to articular destruction. Injecting the proximal radiocarpal joint by the dorsal approach carries no such risk and may produce the same end result.

The differential diagnosis of carpal tunnel syndrome is broad and lengthy, but aside from pregnancy, most associated entities are exceedingly rare. Nonetheless, consideration and, on occasion, appropriate laboratory tests are germane because interventions vary considerably. Myxedema, tuberculous wrist, and gout are examples of medically treatable entities. Amyloid, multiple myeloma, and perhaps, diabetic or uremic involvement may not respond even to carpal tunnel release.

The median nerve is only rarely subjected to compression at sites other than the carpal tunnel. Compression between the heads of the pronator teres is suspected by a localizing Tinel's sign, confirmed by electrodiagnosis, and can be treated by constraining forceful pronation.[12] Such a proximal median neuropathy may compromise the long flexors to the digits; the patient may be unable to flex distal interphalangeal joints as confirmed in the clinical test of opposing the tips of the first and second digits to the thumb to form a circle.

ULNAR NERVE

The ulnar nerve parts from the brachial artery in the middle of the arm. It courses dorsally, piercing the medial intermuscular septum, and it lies in the condylar groove behind the medial epicondyle at the elbow. The nerve then courses in a volar direction, and 2 cm into the forearm, it enters the "cubital tunnel," the floor of which is the medial ligament of the elbow joint; the roof is the aponeurosis of the flexor carpi ulnaris muscle. It courses beneath this muscle and lies subcutaneous and lateral to the ulnar artery in the distal half of the forearm. The ulnar nerve enters the wrist superficial to the flexor retinaculum (here called the *pisohamate ligament*) between the pisiform and the hook of the hamate and deep to the superficial volar carpal ligament in a conduit called *Guyon's canal*. The ulnar nerve supplies the flexor carpi ulnaris and, with the median, the profundus in the forearm. In the palm it supplies the muscles of the hypothenar eminence, all the interossei, the third and fourth lumbricals, the adductor pollicis, and part of the flexor pollicis brevis. Its cutaneous distribution is shown in Figure 97–1.

The ulnar nerve is at risk of compression at the condylar groove, in the cubital tunnel, and in Guyon's canal. Furthermore, all three sites are potential targets of proliferative synovitis in RA. The presentation can have all the features of compression neuropathy, but it is notoriously variable. Insidiously progressive atrophy can occur with little discomfort and even little sensory loss, the so-called "tardy ulnar palsy." Discerning early motor compromise is difficult and particularly challeng-

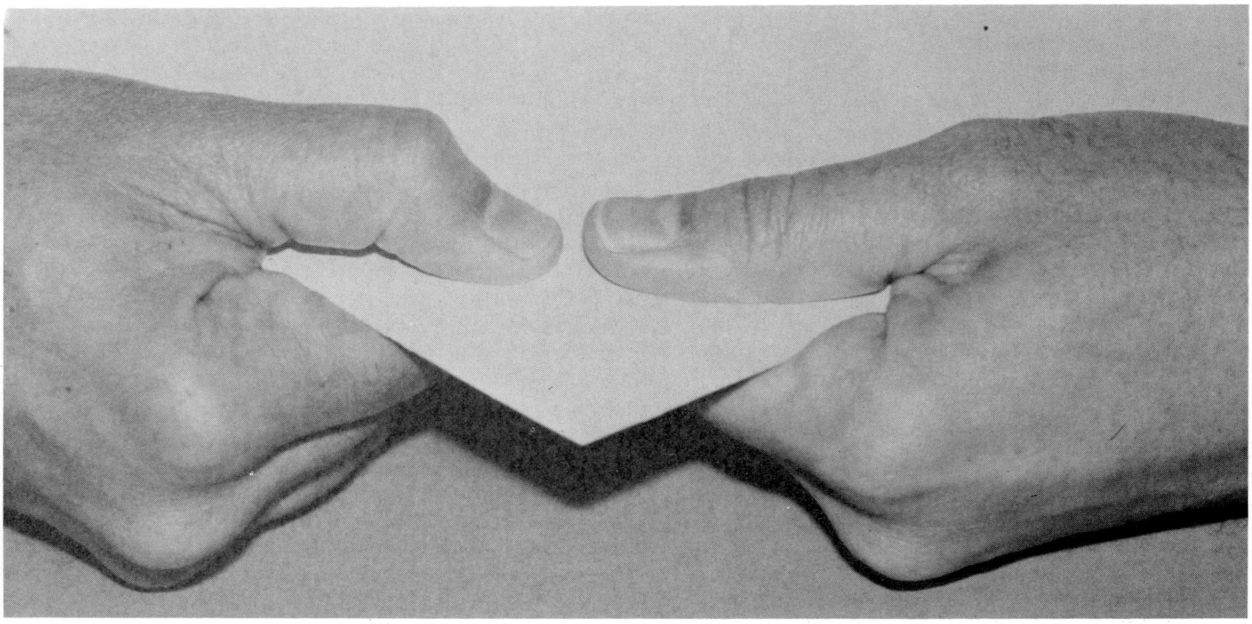

FIGURE 97–3. Froment's sign is the inability to maintain extension of the interphalangeal joint of the thumb during forceful pinching. It is a subtle sign of intrinsic muscle compromise in ulnar palsy.

ing in the setting of RA. Weakness in apposition of the fourth and fifth digits and *Froment's sign* (Fig. 97–3) can be helpful along with inspection of the hypothenar eminence for atrophy. Localization of the site of the compressive lesion can be challenging, particularly because the sensitivity of electrodiagnostic testing for ulnar neuropathy does not equal that for median neuropathies.

Ulnar neuropathies must be distinguished from lesions that involve the lower trunk of the brachial plexus. In these cases, the symptoms often extend proximal to the elbow. Pancoast tumors must be sought; a Horner syndrome may offer a clue. "Thoracic outlet syndrome" is an often abused and often tenuous concept.[3] In an undisputed *axonopathic* form of neurogenic thoracic outlet syndrome, there is weakness and atrophy of median and ulnar innervated muscles of the hand and forearm with sensory disturbance in the ulnar, but *not* the median, distribution.

In the setting of RA, treatment of ulnar neuropathies includes injections of corticosteroids into the elbow or wrist joints to decrease the synovitis. Such maneuvers are of unproven benefit, however, in idiopathic ulnar neuropathies. In the absence of joint deformities, conservative management focuses on preventing trauma to the nerve at the elbow with padding and by restricting flexion. The decision to attempt "decompression" or nerve transposition will tax the judgment of any surgeon.

RADIAL NERVE

The radial nerve leaves the axilla, passes posterior to the humerus, through the lateral intermuscular septum just distal to the deltoid insertion to lie superficially in the lateral arm. The nerve then passes between the brachialis and brachioradialis to the front of the lateral epicondyle near where it divides into two branches. The deep branch, the posterior interosseous nerve, passes into the supinator muscle through the arcade of Frohse and courses within the muscle in the supinator canal, from which it emerges to supply the extensor muscles of the digits and some of the wrist. The superficial radial nerve passes over the supinator and pronator teres muscles and descends along the lateral border of the forearm to provide the sensory distribution of the radial nerve (see Fig. 97–1).

The radial nerve is at risk of compression on the humerus as it courses through the radial groove. Generally, compression is the result of prolonged improper positioning during anesthesia or sleeping on the arm, often when inebriated or sedated ("Saturday night palsy") and results in wristdrop; sensory involvement is variable.

The posterior interosseous nerve is at risk of entrapment at the elbow by the proliferative synovitis of RA. Entrapment is manifest by weakness in the finger extensors more than in the wrist extensors and needs to be distinguished from compromise in the integrity of extensor tendons by dorsal synovitis at the wrist. Neither lesion produces a sensory deficit. It has been argued,[13] though not convincingly, that entrapment of the posterior interosseus nerve in the arcade of Frohse or in the supinator canal is common and mimics lateral epicondylitis ("tennis elbow"). Such a clinical hypothesis would suggest surgical remediation, but electrodiagnosis should be a prerequisite.

The superficial radial nerve is subject to external

trauma, often resulting in distressing dysesthesias. Rarely, rupture of a rheumatoid elbow effusion can similarly compromise the nerve.[14]

ENTRAPMENT NEUROPATHIES OF THE LOWER EXTREMITY

Compression or entrapment of the peripheral nerves in the absence of external force occurs less frequently in the lower extremity than in the upper. Lower extremity entrapment neuropathy is seldom recognized in RA. Nonetheless, there are a few examples that are themselves important and enter into a differential diagnosis relevant to rheumatologic practice.

FEMORAL NERVE

The femoral nerve exits the pelvis beneath the medial aspect of the inguinal ligament to supply the quadriceps and the skin of the anterior thigh (see Fig. 97–1B). It terminates at the saphenous nerve, which courses through the subsartorial canal before emerging through the fascia above the knee to supply the cutaneous innervation of the medial leg (see Fig. 97–1). Aside from trauma and hematomas, femoral or saphenous entrapment is exceedingly rare. Saphenous entrapment is seen occasionally as a consequence of scarring from surgery on the venous system.

LATERAL CUTANEOUS NERVE OF THE THIGH

The lateral cutaneous nerve of the thigh exits the pelvis either through or beneath the lateral inguinal ligament. The nerve is purely sensory (see Fig. 97–1). Compression causes burning paresthesias and hyperpathia along the lateral aspect of the thigh, the syndrome of *meralgia paresthetica*, or *Bernhardt's disease* (*meralgia* derives from the Greek for pain in the thigh). The symptoms are worsened by standing and walking or by prolonged adduction or extension of the leg. The pathogenesis is thought to be entrapment of the nerve either at the inguinal ligament or when it pierces the fascia to reach the skin.[15] The differential diagnosis includes an L3 radiculopathy or a femoral neuropathy, though both ofthese cause more anterior symptoms and rarely hyperesthesia. Rarely, retroperitoneal compression of the lumbar plexus by lymphoma or other neoplasms can provoke meralgia paresthetica. The diagnosis is based on the clinical features because there is no reliable electrodiagnostic test. Treatment is conservative because spontaneous regression of symptoms is the rule. Attempts should be made to eliminate compression by tight garments; weight loss is often advised. Surgical decompression has been disappointing.[16]

SCIATIC NERVE

The sciatic nerve exits the pelvis through the sciatic notch and lies between the greater trochanter and the ischial tuberosity deep to the gluteus maximus muscle. It courses deep to the hamstrings and supplies the posterior thigh muscles. In the pelvis it is at risk for compression by neoplasms and inflammatory lesions such as a tubo-ovarian abscess. It is at some risk at the pyriform fossa, particularly with prolonged sitting on a hard surface or in a wheelchair. The "pyriformis syndrome" is a tenuous and controversial explanation for sciatica that invokes entrapment by the pyriformis muscle.[17] Aside from overt trauma, the nerve is well cushioned throughout its course once it exits the pelvis, and compression from a gluteal abscess,[18] for example, is exceedingly rare. Sciatic neuropathy as a manifestation of trochanteric bursitis has seldom been convincingly demonstrated.[19] In the upper popliteal fossa, the sciatic nerve divides into the common peroneal nerve and the tibial nerve.

Common Peroneal Nerve

The common peroneal nerve courses obliquely around the lateral aspect of the proximal fibula to pass through the superficial head of the peroneus longus muscle in the "fibular tunnel." On emerging, it divides into the superficial (musculocutaneous) and deep (anterior tibial) peroneal nerves. The former courses beside and supplies the peroneal muscles and supplies cutaneous innervation to the lateral and distal portion of the leg and dorsum of the foot (see Fig. 97–1B). The deep peroneal nerve runs in the anterior compartment of the leg between the tibialis anterior and extensor hallucis longus muscles and tendons. It passes beneath the extensor retinaculum at the ankle and supplies most of the ankle and toes and the skin between the first and second toes.

The common peroneal nerve is peculiarly susceptible to compression in its superficial course around the fibula. Plaster casts and leg braces are frequent culprits, although prolonged pressure, prolonged squatting, and even habitual leg crossing have been implicated when no other explanation is patent. The syndrome includes footdrop and sensory compromise. The deep peroneal nerve can be compressed in the very rare anterior tibial syndrome. After trauma, or even excessive exercise, this compartment can become inflamed to the point of which timely surgical decompression is mandatory.

Tibial Nerve

The tibial nerve branches in the popliteal fossa to give off the sural nerve, which descends in the midline of the calf and passes behind the lateral malleolus to supply the skin over the lateral ankle and foot (see Fig. 97–1C). The tibial nerve continues through the popliteal fossa and deep to the gastrocnemius to emerge at the medial aspect of the Achilles tendon. It then passes deep to the flexor retinaculum at the medial malleolus to enter the sole. This retinaculum forms the roof of the tarsal tunnel, which also contains the tendons of the tibialis posterior, flexor digitorum longus, and flexor hallucis longus muscles, as well as the posterior tibial artery and veins. The tibial nerve branches from the tarsal tunnel into two plantar nerves and calcaneal sensory branches. The tibial nerve supplies the flexors of the ankle and toes and provides cutaneous innervation (see Fig. 97–1C).

The tibial nerve is at risk of entrapment beneath the flexor retinaculum, the tarsal tunnel syndrome. Although this syndrome is most often described after trauma, rheumatoid synovitis and focal lesions[20] are also frequent settings. Paresthesias and, to a lesser extent, pain are the presenting complaints with the features previously listed. Occasionally, specific muscular atrophy can be discerned, though this is usually obscured by rheumatoid foot deformities. The distribution of paresthesias and a Tinel's sign suggest the diagnosis, which can be confirmed electrodiagnostically. The plantar and digital nerves are also subject to compression neuropathy, but specific diagnosis and differentiation from the tarsal tunnel syndrome is difficult if not elusive. Initial treatment is conservative with systemic and local anti-inflammatory agents and orthotic devices. Surgical decompression is technically demanding and reserved for the rare patient with recalcitrant symptoms or compromised muscle strength.[21]

REFERENCES

1. Gelberman, R.H. (ed.): Operative Nerve Repair and Reconstruction. Philadelphia, J.B. Lippincott, 1991.
2. Frymoyer, J.W., Ducker, T.B., Hadler, N.M., et al. (eds.): The Adult Spine. Principles and Practice. New York, Raven Press, 1991.
3. Hadler, N.M., and Bunn, W.B. (eds.): Occupational Problems in Medical Practice. New York, Delacorte, 1990.
4. Kimura, J.: Electrodiagnosis in Diseases of Nerve and Muscle: Principles and Practice, 2nd Ed. Philadelphia, F.A. Davis, 1989.
5. Pfeffer, G.B., and Gelberman, R.H.: The carpal tunnel syndrome. *In* Clinical Concepts in Regional Musculoskeletal Illness. Orlando, FL, Grune & Stratton, 1987.
6. Golding, D.N., Rose, D.M., and Selvarajah, K.: Clinical tests for carpal tunnel syndrome: An evaluation. Br. J. Rheum., *25*:388–390, 1986.
7. Katz, J.N., Larson, M.G., Sabra, A., et al.: The carpal tunnel syndrome: Diagnostic utility of the history and physical examination findings. Ann. Intern. Med., *112*:321–327, 1990.
8. Gelberman, R.H., Aronson, D., and Weisman, M.H.: Carpal tunnel syndrome: Results of a prospective trial of steroid injection and splinting. J. Bone Joint Surg., *62A*:1181–1184, 1980.
9. Gelberman, R.H. et al.: The carpal tunnel syndrome: A study of carpal canal pressures. J. Bone Joint Surg., *63A*:380–383, 1981.
10. Stevens, J.C., Sun, S., Beard, C.M., et al.: Carpal tunnel syndrome in Rochester, Minnesota, 1961–1980. Neurology, *38*:134–138, 1988.
11. Hadler, N.M.: The roles of work and of working in disorders of the upper extremity. Baillire's Clin. Rheumatol., *3*:121–141, 1989.
12. Morris, H.H., and Peters, B.H.: Pronator syndrome: Clinical and electrophysiological features in seven cases. J. Neurol. Neurosurg. Psychiatr., *39*:461–464, 1976.
13. Roles, N.C., and Mauldsley, R.H.: Radial tunnel syndrome. J. Bone Joint Surg., *54B*:499, 1972.
14. Fernandes, L., Goodwill, C.J., and Srivatsa, S.R.: Synovial rupture of rheumatoid elbow causing radial nerve compression. Br. Med. J., *2*:17, 1979.
15. Jefferson, D., and Eames, R.A.: Subclinical entrapment of the lateral femoral cutaneous nerve: An autopsy study. Muscle Nerve, *2*:145–151, 1979.
16. Macnicol, M.F., and Thompson, W.J.: Idiopathic meralgia paresthetica. Clin. Orthop. Rel. Res., *254*:270–274, 1990.
17. Jankiewicz, J.J., Hennrikus, W.L., and Houkom, J.A.: The appearance of the pyriformis muscle syndrome in computed tomography and magnetic resonance imaging: A case report and review of the literature. Clin. Orthop. Rel. Res., *262*;205–209, 1991.
18. Shames, J.L., and Fast, A.: Gluteal abscess causing sciatica in a patient with systemic lupus erythematosus. Arch. Phys. Med. Rehab., *70*:410–411, 1989.
19. Crisci, C., Baker, M.K., Wood, W.J., et al.: Trochanteric sciatic neuropathy. Neurology, *39*:1539–1541, 1989.
20. Erickson, S.J., Quinn, S.F., Kneeland, J.B., et al.: MR imaging of the tarsal tunnel and related spaces: Normal and abnormal findings with anatomic correlation. Am. J. Roentgenol., *155*:323–328, 1990.
21. Mackinnan, S.E., and Dellon, A.L.: Homologies between the tarsal and carpal tunnels: Implications for treatment of the tarsal tunnel syndrome. Contemp. Orthop., *14*:75, 1987.

98

Tumors of Joints and Related Structures

JUAN J. CANOSO

Every practicing rheumatologist is bound to encounter, sooner or later, benign or malignant tumors that lie in, or adjacent to, articular tissues. The challenge is to identify these lesions from the overwhelmingly more common inflammatory or degenerative diseases. Prototypical situations exist in which knowledge of pathology, proficiency in physical examination, and expertise in the use of imaging techniques may lead to early diagnosis. A few examples in point follow:

1. A chronically swollen joint in a patient with normal laboratory tests including the erythrocyte sedimentation rate (ESR). Although this clinical presentation suggests the late effects of mechanical damage, psoriatic arthritis, thorn synovitis, and rarely chronic infection, it is also characteristic of pigmented villonodular synovitis, synovial hemangiomas, lipoma arborescens, and synovial chondromatosis.
2. Popliteal "cysts" that do not soften with knee flexion: The differential diagnosis here includes tense-packed cysts (knee disease should be apparent in these patients), ganglia, popliteal artery aneurysms, popliteal artery wall cysts, and unfortunately, sarcomas.
3. Eccentric swellings that do not conform to the anatomic locations of bursal, tenosynovial, or meniscal structures. This should constitute a major red flag because a sarcomatous growth may be present. Two examples are worth mentioning: A young man was referred with a refractory tennis elbow. Surprisingly, full passive elbow extension could not be achieved, and a questionable bulge was palpable between the olecranon process and the lateral epicondyle. The eventual diagnosis was clear cell sarcoma. A middle-aged man presented with a slow-growing swelling in his hand; a fleshy mass was palpable deep in the first interosseal space, and a sarcomatous growth was suspected. Pulmonary metastases were present. The diagnosis was synovial sarcoma.
4. Knee hemarthrosis in an older patient in absence of trauma, anticoagulation, or crystals in synovial fluid: The possibility of metastatic tumor synovitis should be considered in this patient, or synovial hemangioma, especially if the hemarthrosis is recurrent.
5. A finger lump: In addition to ganglia, one must consider nodular pigmented synovitis and fibroma of the tendon sheath.
6. An expanding nodule attached to fascia or tendon: Clear cell sarcoma and epithelioid sarcoma should be considered in the differential diagnosis.

Fortunately, the diagnosis of these lesions has been facilitated by techniques such as arthroscopy, computed tomography (CT), and especially magnetic resonance imaging (MRI).

BENIGN TUMORAL CONDITIONS

Benign tumoral conditions comprise a heterogeneous group of disorders of joints, bursae, and tendon sheaths. They include pigmented villonodular synovitis (PVS), which is a chronic inflammatory lesion of unknown origin, synovial chondromatosis, and other cartilaginous metaplasias of the subsynovial tissue, vascular malformations, fat growths, and fibromas.

PIGMENTED VILLONODULAR SYNOVITIS

The term *pigmented villonodular synovitis (PVS)* denotes a group of interrelated tumorous disorders that involve the lining of joints, bursae, and tendon sheaths.[1–11]

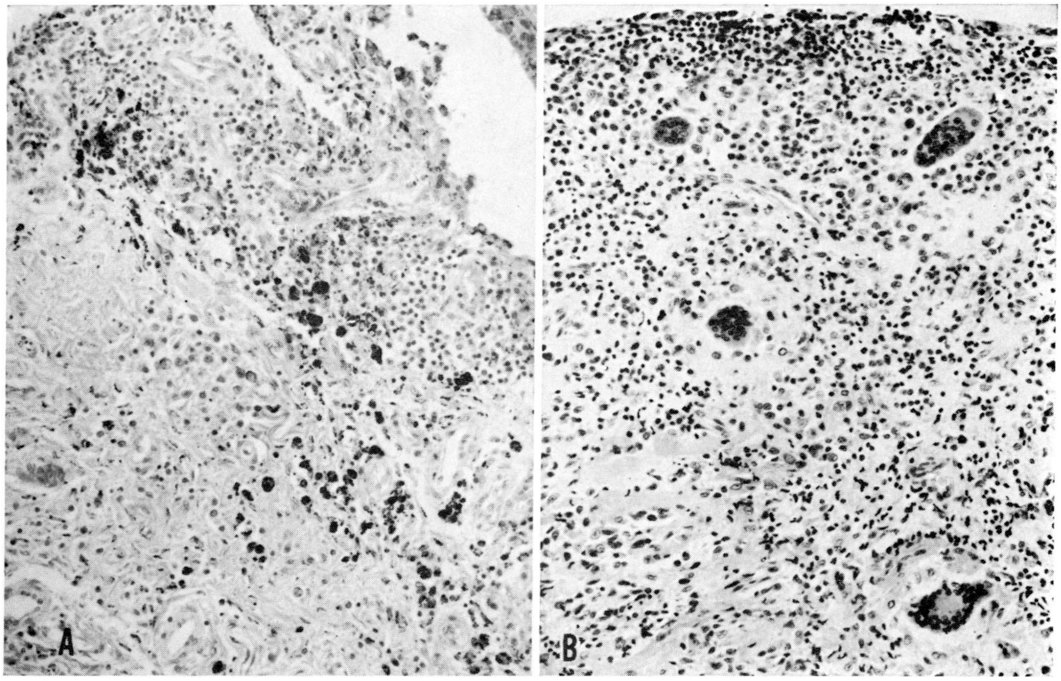

FIGURE 98–1. Circumscribed nodular synovitis; photomicrographs of a nodular lesion. *A*, Large deposits of hemosiderin pigment in richly cellular connective tissue stroma. *B*, Multinucleated giant cells amid dense infiltrate of small round cells and large cells with pale, spindle-shaped nuclei (× 175).

These lesions, often locally aggressive but not metastasizing, consist of villous or nodular growths covered by a thin layer of synovial lining cells. The connective tissue stroma contains a heterogeneous, variably dense collection of cells, collagen bundles, and blood vessels. The cellular infiltrate consists of polyhedral, histiocytic-like cells, lipid-laden cells appearing as foam cells on routine histologic preparations, hemosiderin-laden cells, and multinucleated giant cells (Fig. 98–1). Early lesions are highly vascular; old lesions are less vascular, exhibit more fibrosis and hyalinization, and may contain cholesterol crystals.[1,12] The color of the lesion, ranging from yellow to tan to dark brown, depends on the proportion of lipids and hemosiderin. In several cases involving the soft tissues of the hand[13] or the temporomandibular joint, PVS has co-existed with synovial chondromatosis.[14,15] Bony invasion may result from direct penetration through vascular foramina. The invading tissue carries its own blood supply, so there appears to be no attachment of the diseased tissue to the cavitary walls.[16] Bone involvement may also occur through the chondro-osseous junction at the articular margin and pressure erosion.[17,18]

Electronmicroscopic studies in both villous and nodular forms usually revealed a predominance of cells resembling fibroblasts (synovial type-B cells) and a lesser number of cells resembling both macrophages (synovial type-A cells) and intermediate cells, consistent with a derivation from normal synovial.[19–22] The iron tends to be deposited within lysosomal bodies (siderosomes) in deep type-B cells. PVS is largely confined to humans, although a typical case was reported in a dog in association with a retroperitoneal B-cell lymphoma.[23]

Clinical Findings

Involvement of the affected joint, tendon sheath, or bursa may be either diffuse or localized. The condition is typically monotropic and lacks systemic symptoms or findings. Rarely, two or more joints are affected.[24–26] Several cases have been observed in association with rheumatoid arthritis (RA)[5,6,19,25,27] or psoriatic arthritis.[28] It is unclear whether this is a true association or a detection bias. The patient's ESR is usually normal,[4,5] except in cases associated with RA or other systemic diseases.

PVS is classified according to location (articular, tenosynovial, or bursal) and to lesional type, (diffuse or nodular). Distinguishing between these two types may be difficult in some cases.

Articular, Diffuse. This condition occurs chiefly in young adults, equally in both sexes.[4,5,29] The joint usually affected is the knee; much less commonly involved are the hip, ankle, shoulder, elbow, carpus, hand, and tarsal joints. Rare locations include the temporomandibular joint[14,15,30,31] and the vertebral facet joint.[32] The principal symptom is pain, which may be mild and intermittent for a long period, and the principal sign is gradual swelling of the joint that is due to synovial proliferation and effusion. In the knee, focal masses are usually palpable, and a popliteal cyst often develops.[21,33] The joint fluid is usually sanguineous or dark brown, not viscous, and does not usually clot. One report noted an average of 26% neutrophils. Red blood cell counts have varied from 43,000 to 1,780,000/mm^3. Mucin clot tests varied from fair to good.[34] The glucose content was normal. Intra- and extracellular lipid droplets producing Maltese crosses on polarizing microscopy have been reported.[35] The frequency of this finding is unknown.

Roentgenographic examination shows increased amounts of joint fluid and sometimes lobulation and thickening of the synovial tissues. Lack of osteopenia, absence of heterotopic calcification, and mild spur formation and characteristic. Bony erosions in PVS occur as subchondral or para-articular cysts, each surrounded by a well-defined sclerotic line. These may be multilocular and may involve both sides of the joint (Fig. 98–2). The differential diagnosis[36] of cystic lesions affecting both sides of a joint includes osteoarthritis, RA, hemophilia, gout, and calcium pyrophosphate dihydrate (CPPD) crystal deposition. Intraosseous ganglia, chondroblastoma, and metastatic carcinoma generally affect only one side of the joint. In capacious joints such as the knee, erosions are rare, and when they occur, usually involve the patella.[25,37] In tighter joints such as the hip, elbow, and shoulder, as well as on occasion the wrist, finger, and temporomandibular joint, cyst formation is pronounced and one may see considerable concentric joint space narrowing.[38] Many PVS lesions have been erroneously considered malignant, based on the extent of bone destruction.[39–42] Arthrograms demonstrate recesses and filling defects but, the same appearance can be observed in RA and synovial hemangioma. Although the findings are not pathognomonic, MRI is very useful in the diagnosis of PVS. Many previously misdiagnosed cases are being uncovered as MRI is used in the evaluation of patients with protracted monoarticular disease. MRI findings in PVS include synovial proliferation with focal decrease of signal intensity in both T1- and T2-weighted pulse sequences as a result of hemosiderin accumulation, joint effusion, and a full display of the articular, bursal, and osseous involvement.[33,43] A similar focal decrease in signal intensity may occur as a result of flowing blood and calcification. In isolation MRI findings are insufficient to distinguish PVS from other forms of hemosideric synovitis such as chronic trauma, hemophilia, and cases of RA. These and other conditions must be excluded on clinical, laboratory, and roentgenographic grounds. *A diagnosis of PVS requires demonstration of the characteristic pathologic changes on tissue obtained arthroscopically or by open biopsy, plus the exclusion of mycobacterial and fungal infection* by the use of appropriate tissue stains and cultures.

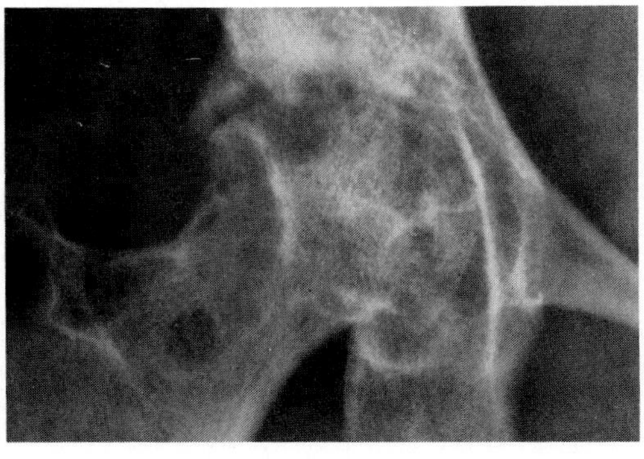

FIGURE 98–2. Cartilage narrowing and cystic erosive changes in the acetabulum and femoral head and neck from pigmented villonodular synovitis.

Articular, Circumscribed (Nodular). Localized involvement of the synovium occurs less frequently than in the diffuse form of the disease, with a ratio of 1:4.[5,44,45] Here again, the knee is most commonly affected, and the patient is usually an adult with symptoms for many months or years. Symptoms are often episodic and consist of pain, swelling, locking, and "giving way" of the joint, mimicking a meniscal lesion.[10,11] Acute symptoms may follow torsion and infarction of tissue.[46] Small-to-moderate effusions and occasional limited range of joint motion are found. The synovial fluid is less likely to be sanguineous. Roentgenograms usually show no abnormalities. The true nature of the process is not suspected until one or more nodular growths are found on an MRI study, arthroscopy, or at operation.

Tenosynovial, Circumscribed (Nodular). This type is by far the most common form of this disorder. It is 10 times more common than circumscribed nodular synovitis.[5,22] It is the second most common soft-tissue tumor of the hand, outnumbered only by ganglia.[47] The majority of patients are young or middle-aged adults. Women are affected more often than men and the incidence is higher in the dominant hand. The fingers are most frequently involved more often the index or middle, on the volar (60%) or dorsal or lateral aspect where a firm, slow-growing, painless nodular mass develops. Less often, the lesion is found near a metacarpophalangeal joint, wrist, ankle, or toe. Larger lesions may cause extensive pressure erosion of adjacent bone. The origin of lesions arising in sites devoid of tendon sheaths, such as the lateral or dorsal aspect of fingers, is controversial. The differential diagnosis includes foreign body granulomas, tendinous xanthomas, necrobiotic granulomas, and fibromas of the tendon sheath.[9]

Tenosynovial, Diffuse. Diffuse involvement of the tendon sheaths of the wrist and foot may occur. Such lesions may become quite large and may erode neighboring bone.[1,48–50]

Bursal. This uncommon lesion, usually diffuse, may be found in a deep bursa such as the iliopsoas,[51] the gastrocnemius-semimembranosus with[21,33] or without[1] concomitant disease in the knee joint, the suprapatellar (an unusual case in which this bursa was separate from the joint),[52] the anserine,[1,53] and an unspecified ankle region bursa.[1] No instances have been described involving subcutaneous bursae.

Pathogenesis

Whether PVS represents a true neoplasm of synovial tissue, a proliferative reaction to recurrent hemarthrosis, or an inflammatory reaction to an unidentified microbial agent is still not clear. The nodular growth pattern, the relative lack of inflammatory cells, the frequent erosion of adjacent bone by these lesions, and their recurrence after synovectomy, have been thought to favor the theory of a benign neoplasm. A neoplastic origin is supported by cytogenetic studies in a case of diffuse PVS and one of nodular tenosynovitis.[54] Although the local destruction may be extensive, there are only sporadic observations of well-documented metastasizing lesions.[9,42]

Similarities between PVS and the findings in hemophilia and intra-articular hemangioma have led many to consider that the lesion might result from recurrent hemarthrosis.[55] In support of this view, changes resembling those of the human disease have been experimentally produced in dogs and in rhesus monkeys by repeated intra-articular injection of blood and colloidal iron.[56,57] Moreover, multiple lesions in children have been associated with cutaneous or synovial hemangiomas,[58,59] suggesting a pathogenetic role of recurrent hemarthrosis. No evidence of vascular malformation, however, exists in most instances of PVS, and foam cells do not occur in hemosideric synovitis induced experimentally[57] or in hemophilic joints.[60] A related hypothesis is that recurrent lipohemarthrosis could explain the deposition of both hemosiderin and lipids. This view is supported by the finding that, in over 50% of patients, acute or repetitive local trauma seemingly precedes the appearance of the lesion.[5] In contrast to hemophilic synovitis in which the siderosomes occur in type-A cells and are surrounded by damaged organelles, iron deposits are found in type-B cells in PVS, without evidence of local damage.[61]

A microbial cause of the lesion has been sought but not found. Cultures are routinely negative. Tubular structures resembling myxovirus nucleoprotein were found in only one of many cases studied by electron microscopy.[62] There is an obvious need to reinvestigate a possible microbial cause with newer sensitive techniques such as the polymerase chain reaction on synovial fluid or tissue samples. The possibility remains that the lesion as defined histopathologically may result from more than one causative mechanism.[21]

Treatment

Although PVS is considered to be a benign lesion usually confined to a single joint or soft tissue structure, the results of surgical treatment are often disappointing. Resection of nodular synovitis of tendon sheath has a recurrence rate of approximately 20%, presumably owing to incomplete removal of the lesion. A followup study of patients with PVS affecting large joints treated with various methods—including arthroscopic synovectomy, synovectomy and arthroplasty, adjuvant external beam radiotherapy, and arthrodesis—the probability of being disease free at 25 years after the initial procedure was only 65%.[29] Recurrences occurred only in the knee (25%). Surprisingly, the failure rate was approximately the same in patients with a solitary pedunculated nodule as in those with diffuse villonodular disease. No recurrences were noted after hip, shoulder and elbow surgery, although the number of cases affecting the latter two joints was too small to allow definitive conclusions. Interestingly, bone involvement had no bearing on disease recurrence. Best results were obtained with complete synovectomy and with prosthetic joint replacement. In the hip,[63] complete synovectomy (achieved by dislocating the joint) may be effective in early lesions in which the joint space is preserved and no erosions are present. Because bone erosion is present in most cases, however, the usual treatment consists of total hip replacement in conjunction with synovectomy. Arthrodesis may be performed in patients who are young and very active. The treatment of recurrent PVS is unsatisfactory. Arthroscopic surgical procedures[10] have the advantage of low morbidity, and they can be repeated easily if necessary. Another possibility is the use of total joint replacement or arthrodesis if the initial, failed procedure was a synovectomy. Radiotherapy with an external beam, advocated in the past, lacks convincing benefit.[29] Finally, the intra-articular administration of the radioisotope yttrium-90 silicate, which may be effective in early cases as an alternative to synovectomy, had disappointing results in patients with failed synovectomy.[64–66] Chronic pain and limitation of joint motion are frequent sequelae of the disease.[67]

SYNOVIAL CHONDROMATOSIS

Synovial chondromatosis is a condition characterized by multiple cartilaginous nodules within the joint space. A similar disorder may occur in joint capsule, tendon sheath, bursa, or para-articular connective tissue.[2,68–72] The nodules may be buried in the synovial membrane (Fig. 98–3), may be pedunculated, or may lie free within the synovial cavity.[73,74] These cartilage nodules may calcify or even ossify, leading to the term *osteochondromatosis*. The origin of the disorder is unknown. The lesion is benign and rarely undergoes malignant change.[75]

Synovial chondromatosis occurs most often as a monoarticular disturbance in young or middle-aged adults and is more common in men than in women. Pediatric cases are rare.[76–78] There is a report of familial chondromatosis[79] in which familial calcium pyrophosphate deposition disease as a predisposing factor could not be excluded.

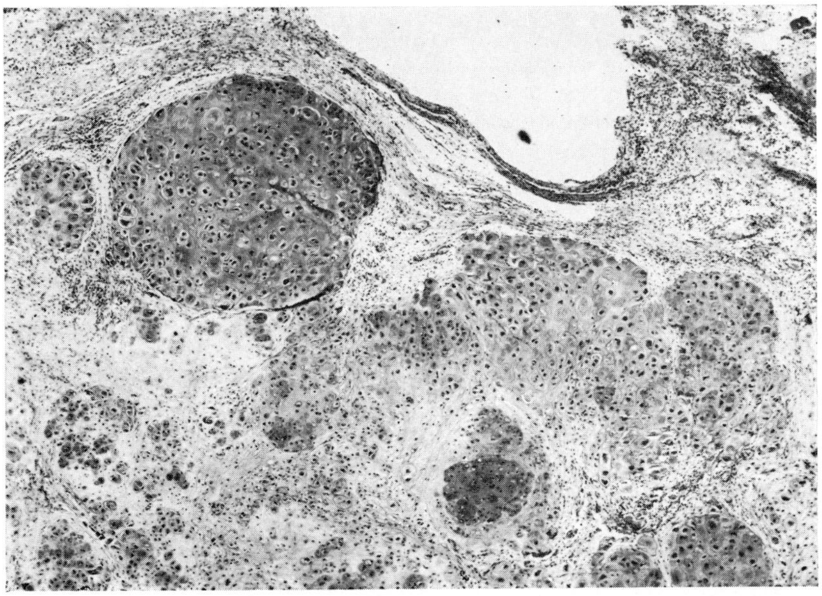

FIGURE 98–3. Synovial chondromatosis; photomicrograph of synovium showing several small islands of cellular cartilage lying just beneath the surface of the membrane (×25).

Articular. The joint most frequently involved is the knee, followed by the hip, elbow, ankle, shoulder, and wrist.[68,72,78] Osteochondromatosis of the temporomandibular joint, sometimes in association with pigmented villonodular synovitis,[14,15] has also been reported.[14,15,80,81] In uncommon cases of multiple joint involvement, both knees or both hips are usually affected.[78]

Clinical Findings

Patients may have pain, swelling, and limited joint motion, or they may be asymptomatic, with the lesion discovered by accident. Even in patients with free intracavitary nodules, locking of the joint is uncommon.[68,69] Examination often reveals the presence of loose bodies and increased amounts of synovial fluid, which is viscous and normal in all other characteristics. Compression neuropathies may occur.[82]

The diagnosis, usually established by roentgenographic examination, discloses multiple stippled calcifications within the confines of the joint capsule in approximately 90% of patients (Fig. 98–4). Pressure erosions are frequent, particularly in the femoral neck and proximal humerus, and may lead to a pathologic fracture.[78,83] The joint otherwise appears normal.

The differential diagnosis of synovial chondromatosis includes several other conditions associated with loose joint bodies, such as severe osteoarthritis with intra-articular osteophytic fragments, osteochondritis dissecans, neuropathic arthropathy, and the "Milwaukee" shoulder.[84] Synovial calcification mimicking osteochondromatosis can also occur in CPPD crystal deposition disease.[85]

Extra-articular. Synovial chondromatosis may occur in tendon sheaths[86–88] bursae such as the ischial,[89] the iliopsoas,[70] the anserine,[70] the gastrocnemius-semimembranosus[69,70,90] (in patients with or without concurrent articular disease), an adventitious deep bursa,[91] and the prepatellar.[92] Moreover, chondromatosis may involve the soft tissue of the extremities without an apparent connection with synovial structures.[88]

Pathogenesis

Gross examination of the affected joint reveals variably large and compact clusters of flat or pedunculated cartilaginous nodules protruding from the thickened synovial membrane, as well as loose bodies within the joint cavity. Microscopic study reveals cartilaginous masses with chondrocytes arranged in small clusters within the masses, separated into lobules by acellular septa (Fig. 98–4). An imperceptible transition between subsynovial fibrocytes and fully developed chondrocytes has been shown by electron microscopy.[93] Early calcification occurs in the perilacunar matrix. In extensively calcified masses, a fatty marrow is frequently found in the center. Pedunculated or free bodies exhibit similar findings. The differentiation from chondrosarcoma may be difficult. In malignancy, the cloning pattern of chondrocytes, which are now arranged in sheaths, is lost; there are myxoid changes in the matrix and crowding of cells with spindling of the nuclei at the periphery. Necrosis may be present, and bone erosion is not by pressure but by permeation with filling of marrow spaces.[75]

Detailed analysis of histologic findings in loose bodies and synovial membrane has permitted a reconstruction of the natural history of the disease.[74] At first, cartilage metaplasia occurs in the subsynovial tissue in a multifocal fashion (phase I). In a later stage, some of the growing nodules become pedunculated and are finally released as loose joint bodies, whereas others remain buried in the membrane (phase II). Finally, the synovial

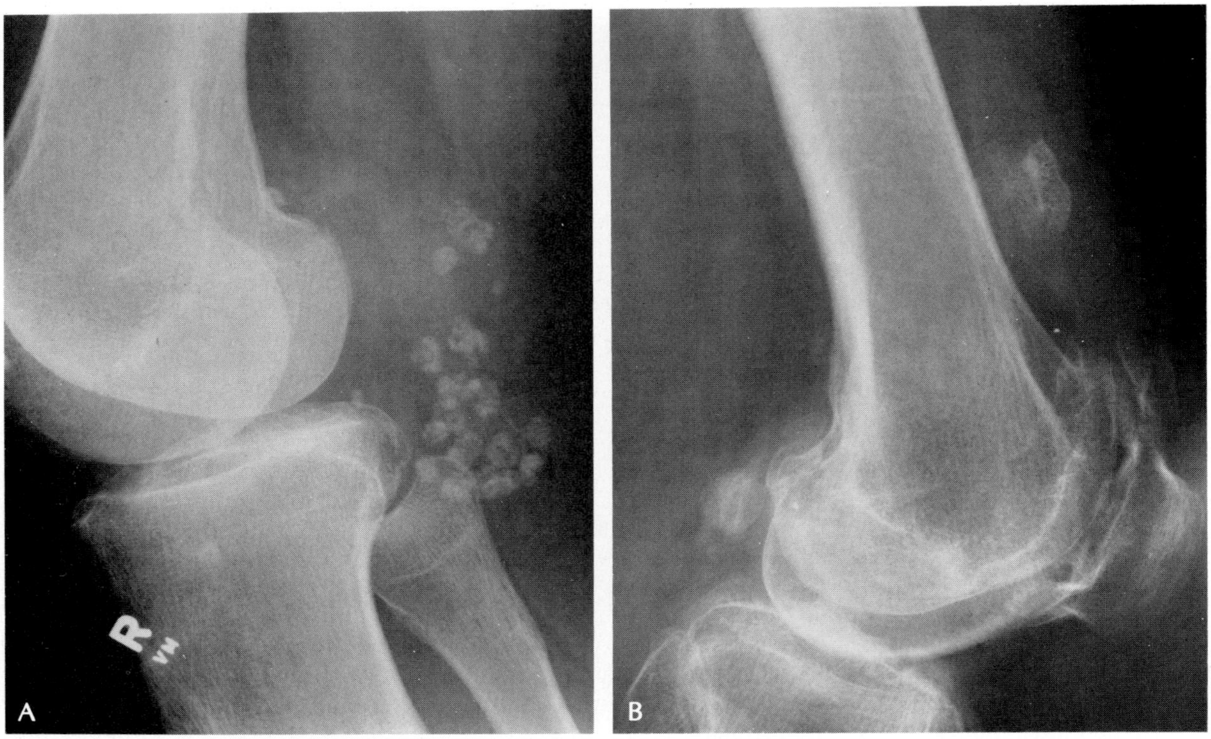

FIGURE 98–4. *A,* Primary synovial osteochondromatosis with multiple loose bodies extruded into a Baker's cyst. *B,* Advanced degenerative joint disease with effusion and secondary osteochondromatosis.

membrane resumes its normal morphologic features, probably by resorption of residual foci of cartilaginous metaplasia, while the loose bodies undergo further remodeling (phase III). Calcification and ossification of the nodules can occur either before or after their release into the joint cavity. Although this notion of pathogenesis has found general acceptance, an opposite interpretation has been suggested based on arthroscopic and histologic findings:[94] In four patients with a short history of knee pain and crepitation in whom myriad cartilaginous bodies were found at arthroscopy, the synovial membrane was normal. Minor trauma, according to this hypothesis, dislodged chondrocytes from the cartilage surface; free chondrocytes proliferate in synovial fluid, and each clone becomes surrounded by a chondroid matrix; these nodules may then be taken up by the synovium.

Treatment

When the condition is suspected, arthroscopy or arthrotomy should be undertaken to remove the loose bodies, to determine the condition of the synovial membrane and remove the involved tissue, and to assess the integrity of the articular cartilage.[72,95] Open synovectomy, however, involves major operative trauma and is often followed by considerable stiffness that may require prolonged physiotherapy or even manipulation under anesthesia. As arthroscopic experience has accrued,[90,96] it is becoming clearer that the results of arthroscopic surgery are at least equal to surgical synovectomy, but with far less morbidity. Although some authors have advocated the removal of loose bodies only, the additional removal of any abnormal synovial tissue appears prudent. Arthroscopic surgery is emerging as the treatment of choice at any stage of the disease.[90] More than one arthroscopic procedure may be needed. Provided that no significant osteoarthritis is present, an asymptomatic joint can be expected in almost all patients.

INTRACAPSULAR, EXTRASYNOVIAL CHONDROMA

Intracapsular, extrasynovial chondroma is an unusual lesion that occurs most frequently in the knee.[71,97] The patient has discomfort and a firm mass distal to the patella and deep to the patellar tendon. Lateral radiographs reveal a calcified lesion within the infrapatellar fat pad. Treatment is surgical excision.

HEMANGIOMA

Joint and tendon sheath hemangiomas represent an unusual location of the most common type of benign soft tissue tumors in infancy and childhood.[9,98] Articular hemangiomas occur most often in adolescents or in young adults, many of whom have had symptoms since childhood; this feature suggests that the lesion may represent a congenital vascular malformation. The knee joint usually is affected.[2] The lesion, which may grow as a pedunculated nodule or as a diffuse process, histologically corresponds to a cavernous (massively engorged capillary vessels) hemangioma in most cases. Nodular lesions often originate in the infrapatellar fat pad.[99] Wider seated or diffuse hemangiomas often merge with extra-articular hemangiomas usually involving neighboring muscle.[100–102] The usual history is one of recurrent hemarthrosis. Chronic limb pain[99,103] and bland, nonhemorrhagic effusions may also occur. In some cases, a doughy mass decreases in size with compression or elevation of the limb. Hemangiomas may be seen in the overlying skin. In extensive lesions with large arteriovenous shunting, the leg may be hypertrophic, including increased length, and a high cardiac output state may be created. The *Klippel-Trenaunay syndrome* is characterized by port-wine cutaneous angiomatous nevi, varicose veins, and a hypertrophic leg.[104,105] In the *Parkes-Weber syndrome* the same findings are associated with arteriovenous fistulas. Large vascular tumors may be complicated by a consumption coagulopathy known as the *Kasabach-Merritt syndrome*;[106] this complication is extremely rare in articular hemangiomas.[107]

Roentgenographic examination is usually normal in nodular angiomas. Phleboliths, often present in larger angiomas, are helpful in the differential diagnosis of articular and para-articular masses. Recurrent hemangiomatous bleeding may lead to enlarged epiphyses, joint space narrowing, and enlargement of the intercondylar notch resembling hemophilic arthropathy.[108] When hemangioma is suspected in a patient with recurrent hemarthrosis, arthroscopy without the use of a tourniquet usually reveals the nature of the lesion. It may be difficult to distinguish localized hemangiomas with a marked synovial reaction from pigmented villonodular synovitis. Indeed, there are several reports of concurrence of the two lesions.[58,59] In patients with a large limb and varicosities or when a doughy compressible mass is present, arteriography and MRI are extremely helpful to reveal both the nature and anatomic distribution of the lesion.

Surgical excision, usually simple and effective in patients with a circumscribed hemangioma, is often unsatisfactory in patients with diffuse involvement of the synovial membrane and regional soft tissues. In these cases, parts of the lesion may be missed, or the process may be so extensive as to render full resection unrealistic. Amputation is sometimes required.

Hemangiomas may also occur in tendon sheaths, involving both the tendon itself and the surrounding structures. A soft compressive swelling, which decreases as the limb is elevated and increases when a tourniquet is placed proximal to the mass is usually noted. Roentgenographic examination frequently reveals many phleboliths. The hand, forearm, and ankle are the sites favored by this lesion, which is treated by surgical excision.

FAT TUMORS

Lipomas, tumors composed of mature fat, occur rarely in joints and tendon sheaths. Articular lipomas have been found predominantly in the knee joint in relation to the subsynovial fat on either side of the patellar ligament or the anterior surface of the femur.[2] Tendon sheath lipomas may occur in the hand, wrist, feet, and ankles.[109] Extensor tendons are affected more often than flexor tendons, and involvement may be bilateral.

Additional lipomatous growths include the synovial hyperplasia (including subsynovial fat) seen near the affected articular surfaces in osteoarthritis,[110,111] a condition known as *lipoma arborescens*, and *Hoffa's disease*. Lipoma arborescens[2,111–113] is a rare condition of unknown origin in which villous proliferation involves the entire synovial lining of a joint, most prominently in cases affecting the knee in the suprapatellar pouch. Each villus consists of mature stromal fat lined by flattened synovium. Lipoma arborescens occurs in males predominantly. It is usually found in the knee and is bilateral in approximately 20% of cases. Rarely, it involves the wrist, the hip, or occurs in multiple joints. If osteoarthritis coexists, it is usually mild, suggesting a fortuitous association. In a typical case a knee has been swollen for years, with episodic inflammation after trauma. Laboratory studies are normal including the ESR. The diagnosis may be suggested by a lobulated, low-density mass seen in the suprapatellar pouch on lateral roentgenograms of the knee. CT, MRI, or arthrographic examination reveals sharply marginated filling defects. Synovectomy is curative. The term *Hoffa's disease*[114] designates the traumatic inflammation of the infrapatellar fat pad. Patients are in pain, and the usual finding is swelling in the infrapatellar region, deep to the patellar tendon. The differential diagnosis includes pretendinous bursitis, deep infrapatellar bursitis, and intracapsular, extrasynovial chondroma.

FIBROMA

Intra-articular fibroma is rare,[115] but fibroma of a tendon sheath is frequent.[9,116] The great majority of fibromas occur in the fingers, hand, and wrist, and consist of a firm, lobulated, painless nodule usually measuring 1 to 2 cm in diameter, firmly attached to tendon or tendon sheath. Flexion may be limited. The nodules, which are composed of myofibroblasts, fibroblasts, and dense collagen, are frequently divided by narrow clefts. The lesion is benign, but recurrences have been noted in 24% of cases after local excision.

MALIGNANT NEOPLASMS OF JOINTS

Malignant neoplasms of joints may be either primary or secondary. Primary intra-articular tumors are very rare and are represented by synovial sarcomas and chondrosarcomas that originate in synovial chondromatosis.[75] Far more frequently, synovial sarcomas arise in the vicinity of large joints, particularly the knee.[9] Other malignant tumors with an origin in the fascial tissues of the extremities include clear cell sarcoma of tendons and aponeuroses[117] and epithelioid sarcoma.[118] Secondary involvement of joints occurs as a complication of the contiguous spread of malignant bone tumors, metastases of carcinoma, leukemia, or lymphoma. Rheumatic manifestations of hematologic malignant diseases are discussed in Chapter 87.

SYNOVIAL SARCOMA

Clinical Findings

Synovial sarcoma is a malignant and histologically complex neoplasm generally found *near* a large joint.[9,119–121] The tumor seldom originates within the joint itself[122] (Table 98–1). Synovial sarcoma occurs most often in adolescents or in young adults, although it has been observed at all ages from birth to 80 years. A slight preponderance is seen in men. The lower limb (thigh/knee > foot > lower leg/ankle > hip/groin) is more commonly the site of primary involvement than the upper limb (shoulder > elbow/upper arm > hand). Other primary sites have included the buttocks, abdominal wall, retroperitoneum, chest, neck, face, orbit, mouth, larynx, pharynx, esophagus, and mediastinum.[9,123] The characteristic history is that of a slowly growing, often painless mass that, in the case of a deeply situated lesion, may reach a considerable size before detection. Infrequently, pain or tenderness is the first manifestation of the disease.

The typical roentgenographic appearance of synovial sarcoma is that of a nonspecific para-articular soft tissue mass of homogenous water density, possibly lobulated, with a sharp, discrete border. Less often, the mass is irregular in outline and is not clearly separable from the surrounding tissues. In 30% of patients, the tumor contains small (rarely large) foci or amorphous calcification.[9,120,124] In 10 to 20% of patients, secondary involvement of contiguous bone produces a periosteal reaction, surface erosion, or bone invasion.

Although the rate of growth and the rapidity of metastatic spread vary, the disease characteristically follows a malignant course. The mass grows centrifugally, and compression of the surrounding tissues forms a pseudocapsule that is often perforated by fingers of tumor cells, leading to satellite lesions. As is true for other soft tissue sarcomas, synovial sarcoma spreads by direct extension along tissue planes, muscle bundles, nerves, and by way of the vascular system. Invasion of regional lymph nodes occurs in approximately 20% of cases. The most common site of visceral metastasis is the lung, in which the lesions appear as multiple large densities or as a diffuse infiltrate; cavitary metastases are rare.[125] The pleura, diaphragm, pericardium, and skin may also be involved. Bone marrow deposits are seen in approximately 20% of cases. Osteolytic lesions are more common than sclerotic changes radiographically.

TABLE 98–1. CHARACTERISTICS OF MALIGNANT SYNOVIAL TUMORS[9,139,143,146,150]

	SYNOVIAL SARCOMA	CLEAR CELL SARCOMA OF TENDONS AND APONEUROSES	EPITHELIOID SARCOMA
Age			
Median	26.5	27	26
Greatest prevalence	15–35	20–40	15–35
Sex, male/female	1.2:1	1:1	2:1
Clinical features	Deep mass related to joints; most frequent in lower extremities	Deep-seated nodule adherent to tendon or aponeurosis Most frequent in foot and ankle	Slow-growing nodule in finger, hand, forearm, knee, lower leg Rare in other locations Central necrosis common; ulceration
Radiologic calcification	30%	Occasional	Not seen
Histology	Biphasic (epithelial cells, spindle cell stroma); monophasic; undifferentiated*	Nests or fascicles of fusiform or rounded cells with clear cytoplasm	Large ovoid to plump spindle cells arranged in a nodular pattern
Immunohistochemistry	Cytokeratin	S-100 protein	Cytokeratin
Electron microscopy	Basal lamina, zonulae adherentes, desmosomes	Melanosomes or premelanosomes	Zonulae adherentes, desmosomes, watertight junctions
Histologic grade†	2 or 3; 1	2 or 3	2 or 3
Metastases	Lung, lymph nodes, bone marrow	Lung, lymph nodes, bones	Lymph nodes, lung, skin
Recurrence rate	28–49%	50%	76%
5-Year survival	25–63%	30%	NA

* In all types, a biphasic cellular pattern is required in at least one portion of the neoplasm.

† Grade is determined by a combined assessment of cellularity, cellular anaplasia or pleomorphism, mitotic activity, expansive or infiltrative growth, and necrosis[9]

NA = not available; S-100 protein = a neuroectodermal marker.

Histopathologic Findings

The gross appearance of synovial sarcoma depends on its place of origin, the duration and rapidity of its growth, and its cellular composition. The color of the tumor varies from a pale gray-yellow to a deep red, usually the result of hemorrhage. The tumor may feel uniformly firm when spindle cell elements predominate, or it may be soft and contain cystic spaces filled with mucoid secretions when epithelial cells predominate.

Synovial sarcomas are pleomorphic tumors. The classic type is characterized by a biphasic cellular pattern that includes epithelial cells arranged in nests, tubules and acini, and a stroma of spindle cells and abundant reticulin fibers with the appearance of a fibrosarcoma (Fig. 98–5). Other tumors are monophasic, most commonly of the spindle-cell type (fibrous synovial sarcoma) and less commonly of the epithelial cell type, in which the cells are arranged in sheaths and cords in a tenuous reticular stroma. Finally, an undifferentiated type is also recognized. Calcification may occur in any of the four types of synovial sarcoma; it may consist of small elements, usually in the periphery of the tumor, or it may occupy large areas. Mast cell infiltrates are frequently found in the spindle cell areas of the tumor. Synovial sarcomas exhibit prominent vascularity, and vascular invasion is often apparent. A purely intra-arterial synovial sarcoma is on record.[126]

Regardless of the type, the diagnosis of synovial sarcoma requires the presence of a biphasic cellular pattern in at least one portion of the primary or recurrent tumor. The most distinctive histologic feature of synovial sarcoma is the presence of clefts and cystic spaces, lined by cuboidal or columnar cells and containing a mucin-rich secretion that stains intensely with periodic acid-Schiff, mucicarmine, colloidal iron, and alcian blue and is resistant to hyaluronidase. A second type of mucinous material, present in the spindle cell areas, is sensitive to hyaluronidase.

Immunocytochemical studies have proven helpful in differentiating synovial sarcoma from other soft tissue tumors of similar histopathology.[127] They have also provided intriguing information regarding histogenesis.[9,127] Cytokeratin, an epithelial marker, can be detected in the epithelial cells and spindle cells in biphasic and most monophasic synovial sarcomas, allowing the exclusion of fibrosarcoma, malignant schwannoma, and hemangiopericitoma. On further study of intermediate filaments in various types of spindle cell sarcomas, cytokeratins 8 and 18 were widespread, while cytokeratins 8 and 18 and desmoplakins (specific proteins of the

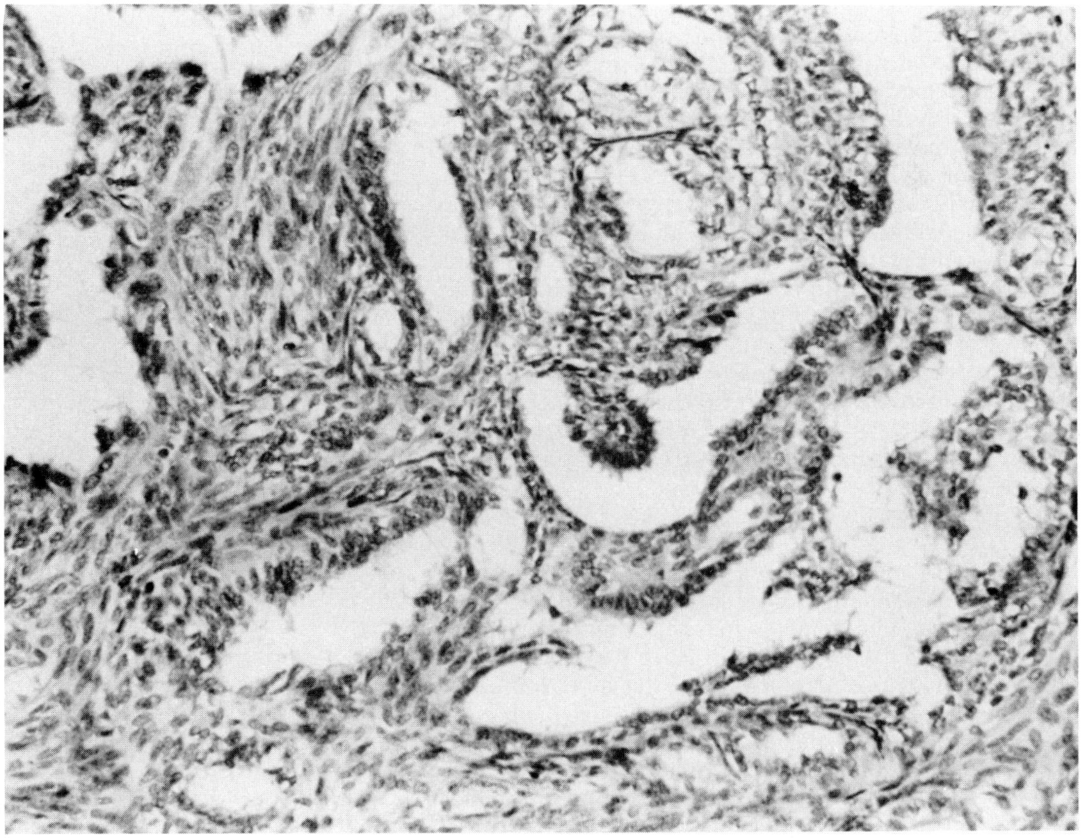

FIGURE 98–5. Biphasic synovial sarcoma. Note the irregular spaces lined with columnar cells, in addition to the spindle-cell stroma ($\times$ 100).

desmosomal junctions) were restricted to the glandular component of synovial sarcoma.[128] Vimentin, an intermediate filament associated with mesenchymal cells and mesenchymal cell tumors, is present in the spindle cells of both biphasic and monophasic tumors.

The ultrastructural characteristics of these tumors help in the differential diagnosis when epithelial markers are not expressed and are intriguing in terms of histogenesis.[129] The epithelial cells have a well-defined ovoid nucleus and abundant mitochondria, a prominent Golgi complex, and smooth and rough endoplasmic reticulum. Cellular arrangements in clusters and grandlike structures are frequent, and microvilli are present on the apical cell surfaces facing pseudoglandular spaces. Epithelial cells enclosing glandlike lumina are connected by junctional complexes, desmosomes and zonulae adherentes, which are not present in normal synovial tissue. Furthermore, most observations have revealed the presence of a continuous basal lamina at the epithelial–stromal junction, a structure also absent from normal synovial tissue. The spindle cells generally resemble fibroblasts but have less cytoplasm and a less-developed endoplasmic reticulum than do fibroblasts. The contact between neighboring cells in monophasic sarcomas is tighter than in the stroma of the biphasic type.[127]

The random location of synovial sarcoma in relation to joints, the lack of effect of hyaluronidase on the tinctorial characteristics of the mucinous material, and the presence of cytokeratin and ultrastructural findings that do not occur in normal synovial tissue raise important questions regarding tumor histogenesis. The presence of cytokeratins in synovial and other sarcomas does not necessarily prove an epithelial derivation of these tumors. Some vascular smooth muscle cells, fetal striated muscle cells, and cultured mesenchymal cells such as transformed fibroblasts and smooth muscle cells also contain cytokeratins.[128] Synovial sarcomas probably arise from primitive mesenchymal cells (the arthrogenic mesenchyma) with an inherent or acquired ability to undergo epithelial cellular differentiation.[9,127,129] A primary event in tumor development may be a reciprocal translocation involving the chromosomes X and 18, t(X; 18) (p11.2;q11.2), shown by chromosome analysis in monophasic (spindle cell type) as well as biphasic synovial sarcomas.[130,131]

Diagnosis

Synovial sarcoma should be suspected when a deep-seated swelling or a palpable mass develop in the vicinity of a joint in a young patient. Plain roentgenograms of the region are useful to determine the general characteristics of the mass and the possible presence of phleboliths, amorphous calcification, or bone abnormalities. Sonography is important to exclude cystic lesions such as a Baker's cyst, a meniscal cyst, or a ganglion. If the mass is solid, the next question is to determine if the lesion is benign or malignant.[126,132] Because no clinical or imaging procedures can reliably distinguish the two, a biopsy is always necessary.[133] MRI is the most efficient means of defining the exact location of the tumor and the possible involvement of neighboring structures in transverse and sagittal views.[43,134–138] CT may be required if the integrity of cortical bone is in question. Then the biopsy is performed.[133] Fine-needle aspiration biopsy, and needle biopsy are helpful to document local or distant metastases or in suspected recurrence. A primary diagnosis, however, requires excisional or incisional biopsy. Excisional biopsies imply the "shelling out" of the entire tumor and are used exclusively in small lesions. Incisional biopsies, in which only part of the tumor is removed, are used in masses greater than 3 cm in diameter. Tissue manipulation should be minimal to avoid tumor spread. Because frozen sections (which are useful to determine adequacy of the sample) are suboptimal to distinguish the various types of soft tissue sarcoma, a definitive diagnosis rests on the interpretation of permanent sections. A chest CT and a bone scan are obtained routinely to detect metastatic disease, which if present, may alter the treatment of the primary tumor.

Prognosis and Treatment

Adverse prognostic factors in synovial sarcoma include older age, male sex, proximal tumors, deep tumors, large tumors (greater than 5 cm in diameter), absence of extensive calcification, evidence of nodal involvement, invasion of neurovascular structures or bone, and a high mitotic rate of the tumor.[139–144]

Because of the pattern of tumor spread, en-block excision of the tumor and the entire muscle compartment, or radical amputation in which the joint proximal to the involved compartment is desarticulated are often required. With these procedures, the rate of local recurrence is less than 20%.[133] Alternatively, one of several limb-sparing procedures may be considered. A frequently used approach is wide local excision in which the tumor is removed along with several centimeters of normal tissue in all directions, along with lymphadenectomy, given the frequent nodal involvement in synovial sarcoma. The procedure may be preceded by or (usually) followed by radiotherapy, often in association with adjuvant chemotherapy. In a randomized trial of amputation compared with limb-sparing surgery in which all patients received postoperative radiotherapy and chemotherapy, the rate of local recurrence was extremely low (0 of 16 amputated patients and 4 of 27 treated with limb-sparing surgery), and the survival at 5 years was 83% and 88%, respectively.[145] Although various drugs have been used in adjuvant chemotherapy, a proven combination includes doxorubicin, cyclophosphamide, and high-dose methotrexate. Local recurrences and isolated pulmonary metastases may be treated surgically. The response rate of disseminated disease to chemotherapy (partial plus complete responses) is about 30%.

CLEAR CELL SARCOMA OF TENDONS AND APONEUROSES

Clear cell sarcoma[9,117,146] is a peculiar neoplasm that affects young individuals, more frequently women (Table 98–1). Clinically, it presents as a deep, painless, slow-growing mass intimately associated to tendons or aponeuroses. In approximately 75% of cases, the site of lesion is in the lower extremity, predominantly the foot or ankle, and less frequently the knee or thigh. Most of the remaining lesions occur in the upper extremity.

The tumor is peculiarly composed of compact nests and fascicles of round or fusiform pale- (glycogen) staining cells with vesicular nuclei and prominent nucleoli. Because intracellular melanin is found in nearly half the cases, and because melanosomes and the neuroectodermal protein S-100 are virtually always present, a neuroectodermal derivation of clear cell sarcoma appears certain.[9,147,148] Prognosis is generally poor, particularly when the tumor mass is 5 cm or more in diameter. Local recurrences are common, and lymph node, lung and bone metastases occur in most cases.[9,149,150] Treatment of this lesion includes radical excision or amputation, combined with radiotherapy and adjuvant chemotherapy. Lymph node excision should be included, because regional node involvement occurs in about 30% of cases.

EPITHELIOID SARCOMA

This distinctive sarcoma occurs predominantly in young adults (Table 98–1)[118], usually in the hand, wrist, forearm, and lower leg. The lesion may arise in the subcutis or deeper tissues such as tendon, tendon sheaths, and deep fascia. Superficial lesions have a predilection for the fingers, forearms, and tibial regions and develop as raised, slow-growing, woody nodules that weeks or months later become ulcerated. Understandably, these lesions tend to be confused with necrotizing infectious granulomas, ulcerating squamous cell carcinomas, necrobiosis lipoidica, granuloma annulare, and rheumatoid nodules. Deep lesions tend to be larger and are firmly attached to the fibrous structure on which they grow; although initially they may be interpreted as nodular tendinitides, subsequent growth suggests a sarcomatous origin. Microscopically, the tumor includes large, acidophilc polygonal cells and spindle cells arranged in irregular nodules where central necrosis is frequent.[9,118] Immunohistochemical stains are positive for cytokeratin and vimentin and negative for the S-100 protein.[151,152] Electronmicroscopy reveals polygonal and spindle-shaped cells with interdigitating cellular processes. Maculae adherentes and desmosomes are present, but a basal lamina is absent.[9] Epithelioid sarcoma is a tumor with a tendency to recur, sometimes repeatedly, over many years. Metastases develop in 45% of cases, predominantly to regional lymph nodes and lung. Treatment of this legion is similar to that of synovial sarcoma.

SYNOVIAL ANGIOSARCOMA

Angiosarcomas usually involve skin, soft tissues, the heart, or the liver. Primary synovial angiosarcoma is truly exceptional.[153]

INVOLVEMENT OF JOINTS BY PRIMARY BONE TUMORS

Metaphyseal bone tumors, chiefly osteosarcoma, fibrosarcoma, and chondrosarcoma, often invade joints.[154] Ewing's sarcoma usually involves the diaphysis, but cases that originate in the epiphysis may involve a joint.[155] Articular (hyaline) cartilage is thought to act as a barrier to local tumor angiogenesis.[156] Tumor penetration eventually occurs, however, whether peripherally beneath the joint capsule, at the bone attachment of intracapsular ligaments such as the cruciate ligaments of the knee, or across cartilage itself. Bland synovial effusions may indicate early invation of the joint.[157]

CARCINOMATOUS SYNOVITIS

That metastases to synovium are clinically rare is surprising given the high frequency of disseminated carcinomas and the rich vascular supply of synovial tissue. Knees are most commonly affected.[158,159] Other evidence of disseminated tumor is usually present, but, rarely, joint metastases are the first indications of malignant disease or of tumor dissemination.[158,160,161] Radiographic studies of such joints demonstrate lytic lesions of the patella, femur, or tibia, but patients with early cases may lack abnormal findings.[160,161]

Bone scanning may reveal increased local radionuclide uptake.[162,163] Multiple focal lesions of increased activity throughout the skeleton provide further evidence of metastatic disease. Synovial fluid is hemorrhagic, with 100 to 8000 WBCs/mm^3, predominantly mononuclear cells. The fluid of one patient exhibited eosinophilia.[161] Tumor cells are found in synovial fluid in 80% of patients;[158,160,162,163] arthrotomy or closed synovial biopsy reveals carcinomatous involvement of the synovium. Arthroscopy is valuable in the diagnosis of synovial metastases when the results of other tests are inconclusive.

METASTASES TO BONES OF THE HANDS AND FEET

Bone metastasis of the hands and feet is an unusual form of "arthritis" occurring in patients with disseminated carcinoma. Metastases occur in small bones, particularly the distal phalanges and the tarsal bones. Clinically, these resemble paronychia or gout. Lytic lesions, sometimes with pathologic fractures, are usually present.[164–168]

METASTASES TO SHOULDERS

Bone metastasis in renal cell carcinoma exhibit a curious predilection for the clavicle, acromion, and proximal humeral head.[169] Painful lytic lesions in these areas should direct attention to the kidney. An instance of nasopharyngeal carcinoma metastatic to both acromioclavicular joints is on record.[170]

LYMPHOMA

Musculoskeletal manifestations of lymphoma, both Hodgkin's[171] and non-Hodgkin's,[172,173] include pain caused by bone metastasis[174] or primary involvement of bone hypertrophic osteoarthropathy in patients with intrathoracic lesions and very rarely arthritis caused by lymphomatous synovial infiltration. The latter is usually monoarticular,[175,176] but polyarticular cases may resemble RA.[173,177]

NONMETASTATIC SYNDROMES

The nonmetastatic syndromes comprise a variety of conditions.[178–180]

HYPERTROPHIC OSTEOARTHROPATHY

The well-known association of intrathoracic tumors and hypertrophic osteoarthropathy is discussed separately (see Chapter 88). It can be considered the prototype of tumor-associated arthritis; its onset often leads to the discovery of an unsuspected intrathoracic malignant process.[181,182]

PANCREATIC CANCER WITH ARTHROPATHY AND FAT NECROSIS

Panniculitis resembling erythema nodosum sometimes accompanied by synovitis and serositis is a well-known accompaniment of pancreatic carcinoma, particularly of the acinar cell type, as well as of pancreatitis. The pancreatitis is often clinically silent. Its pathogenesis includes fat necrosis in subcutaneous tissue, bone marrow, and subsynovial fat, as a result of high levels of circulating pancreatic lipase.[183–188] The synovitis can occur without panniculitis, sometimes migratory over a period of months or years. Involvement of marrow fat may produce pathologic features.

CANCER ARTHRITIS

Several observers have described a syndrome resembling RA with typical or atypical features,[189–191] having its onset a few months before the discovery of a tumor. The atypical form is characterized by explosive onset, asymmetry of joint involvement, sparing of wrists and small joints of the hand, absence of subcutaneous nodules, and seronegativity. All patients in one series were in their fifth decade or older. Removal or successful treatment of the tumor was associated with remission of the arthritis in approximately half these patients. Remission was more frequent in the atypical than in the typical RA-like arthritis. The validity of these associations has not been definitely established by epidemiologic methods.

Supporting evidence of a casual association between carcinoma and rheumatic disease has been provided by individual observations, in which removal of carcinoma has been followed by complete clinical and serologic remission of the syndrome.

The tumors involved included lung carcinoma,[192,193] esophageal carcinoma,[194,195] gastric carcinoma,[196] colonic carcinoma,[197] breast carcinoma,[198] and ovarian dysgerminoma.[199,200]

HYPERURICEMIA AND GOUT

The degree of hyperuricemia in patients with carcinoma correlates with extensiveness of the disease, involvement of the liver, and presence of hypercalcemia. Gout occurred in only 5 of 70 patients studies. In 2 of these patients, the gout preceded the tumor.[201] The frequency of hyperuricemia and gout in a cancer patient population remains to be elucidated. Hyperuricemia has been noted in association with cisplatin therapy.[202] Interestingly, hypouricemia has also been described in association with disseminated carcinoma.[203]

CARCINOID ARTHROPATHY

This peculiar form of arthropathy characterized by arthralgias, juxta-articular demineralization, erosions, and subchondral cysts was observed in four of five consecutive patients with the carcinoid syndrome.[204,205]

LYMPHOMATOID GRANULOMATOSIS

Arthralgia may be associated with this peculiar lymphoproliferative disorder, which is characterized by angiodestructive lymphoreticular proliferative granulomata. A case presenting with the polyarthritis has been recorded.[206]

MULTICENTRIC RETICULOHISTIOCYTOSIS

An association may well be present between multicentric reticulohistiocytosis and cancer; 28% of the 82 cases in one review had an associated neoplasm.[207]

PALMAR FASCIITIS AND POLYARTHRITIS ASSOCIATED WITH CARCINOMA

Medsger et al.[208] have described a unique syndrome of palmar fasciitis and polyarthritis in six patients with ovarian carcinoma predominantly of the endometrioid type. Other tumors may also produce this syndrome.[209] The palmar changes ranged from diffuse globular swelling with warmth and erythema to typical Dupuytren's contractures, including plantar nodular fasciitis. The shoulders and the metacarpophalangeal and proximal interphalangeal joints were most frequently involved, exhibiting painful and limited motion and flexor contractures. Morning stiffness was prominent. Although

TABLE 98–2. RHEUMATOLOGIC SYNDROMES ASSOCIATED WITH NONHEMATOLOGIC MALIGNANT DISEASES

BY DIRECT EXTENSION OR METASTATIC
Primary bone tumors
Carcinomatous (metastatic) synovitis
Metastases to small bones
NONMETASTATIC (PARANEOPLASTIC)
Articular
Hypertrophic osteoarthropathy
Subcutaneous nodules, arthritis, and serositis (fat necrosis) in pancreatic cancer (as in pancreatitis)
Cancer arthritis
Hyperuricemia and gout; hypouricemia
Carcinoid arthropathy
Multicentric reticulohistiocytosis
Palmar fasciitis and polyarthritis associated with carcinoma
Coincidental arthritis of any type
Muscular
Polymyositis (dermatomyositis)
Eaton-Lambert syndrome
Carcinoid myopathy
Type II muscle fiber atrophy
Coincidental myopathy of any type
Cutaneous
Carcinoid "scleroderma"
AS COMPLICATIONS OF THERAPY
Aseptic necrosis of bone
Septic arthritis
Corticosteroid myopathy
Chemotherapy-induced fibrotic syndromes
Interleukin-1–induced polyarthritis

two of these patients had carpal tunnel syndrome, none had Raynaud's phenomenon, dermal or pulmonary fibrosis, or evidences of myositis. In five patients, the articular symptoms preceded the diagnosis of malignant disease by several months to 2 years. In the remaining patient, the articular symptoms preceded tumor recurrence. In all patients, the ovarian tumor was extensive and gave evidence of intra- and extraperitoneal spread. The median survival time after diagnosis of the tumor was 6 months. The pathogenesis of this syndrome, which resembles reflex sympathetic dystrophy, remains unexplained.

OTHER RHEUMATOLOGIC SYNDROMES

Polymyositis (dermatomyositis) and other muscle syndromes associated with tumors are discussed in Chapter 72. Other nonmetastatic rheumatologic or neuromuscular syndromes associated with malignant disease are listed in Table 98–2.

COMPLICATIONS OF CANCER TREATMENT

Tumor involvement of joints is occasionally suggested when a patient is receiving corticosteroid or immunosuppressive therapy, which alone can be associated with secondary joint manifestations. These manifestations include aseptic necrosis of bone (see Chapters 37 and 100), septic arthritis (see Chapters 115 and 116), and steroid myopathy (see Chapters 37 and 111). In addition, chemotherapy with bleomycin can give rise to a fibrotic syndrome resembling systemic sclerosis (see Chapter 73), and cases of chronic polyarthritis have followed interleukin-2 infusions.[210]

REFERENCES

1. Jaffe, H.L., Lichtenstein, L., and Sutro, C.J.: Pigmented villonodular synovitis, bursitis and tenosynovitis. Arch. Pathol., *31*:731–765, 1941.
2. Jaffe, H.L.: Tumors and Tumorous Conditions of the Bones and Joints. Philadelphia, Lea & Febiger, 1958.
3. Granowitz, S.P., D'Antonio, J., and Mankin, H.L.: The pathogenesis and long-term end results of pigmented villonodular synovitis. Clin. Orthop., *114*:335–351, 1976.
4. Docken, W.P.: Pigmented villonodular synovitis: A review with illustrative case reports. Semin. Arthritis Rheum., *9*:1–22, 1979.
5. Myers, B.W., Masi, A.T., and Feigenbaum, S.L.: Pigmented villonodular synovitis and tenosynovitis: A clinical epidemiology study of 166 cases and literature review. Medicine, *59*:223–238, 1980.
6. Rao, A.S., and Vigorita, V.J.: Pigmented villonodular synovitis (Giant-cell tumor of the tendon sheath and synovial membrane). J. Bone Joint Surg., *66A*:76–94, 1984.
7. Flandry, F., and Hughston, J.C.: Current concepts review. Pigmented villonodular synovitis. J. Bone Joint Surg., *69A*:942–949, 1987.
8. Goldman, A.B., and DiCarlo, E.F.: Pigmented villonodular synovitis. Diagnosis and differential diagnosis. Radiol. Clin. North Am., *26*:1327–1347, 1988.
9. Enzinger, F.M., and Weiss, S.W.: Soft Tissue Tumors. Second Ed. St. Louis, Mosby, 1988.
10. Bentley, G., and McAuliffe, T.: Pigmented villonodular synovitis. Ann. Rheum. Dis., *49*:210–211, 1990.
11. Klompmaker, J. et al.: Pigmented villonodular synovitis. Arch. Orthop. Trauma Surg., *109*:205–210, 1990.
12. Rosenthal, D.I., Coleman, P.K., and Schiller, A.L.: Pigmented villonodular synovitis: Correlation of angiographic and histologic findings. AJR, *135*:581–583, 1980.
13. Dahlin, D.C., and Salvador, A.D.: Cartilaginous tumors of the soft tissues of the hands and feet. Mayo Clin. Proc., *49*:721–726, 1974.
14. Raibley, S.O.: Villonodular synovitis with synovial chondromatosis. Oral Surg., *44*:279–284, 1977.
15. Takagi, M., and Ishikawa, G.: Simultaneous villonodular synovitis and synovial chondromatosis of the temporomandibular joint. Report of a case. J. Oral Surg., *39*:699–701, 1981.
16. Scott, P.M.: Bone lesions in pigmented villonodular synovitis. J. Bone Joint Surg., *50B*:306–311, 1968.
17. Goldberg, R.P., Weissman, B.N., Naimark, A., and Braunstein, E.: Femoral neck erosions: Sign of hip synovial disease. AJR, *141*:107–111, 1983.
18. Dorwart, R.H., Genant, H.K., Johnston, W.H., and Morris, J.M.: Pigmented villonodular synovitis of synovial joints: Clinical, pathologic and radiologic features. AJR, *143*:877–885, 1984.
19. Reginato, A., Martinez, V., Schumacher, H.R., and Torres, J.: Giant cell tumor associated with rheumatoid arthritis. Ann. Rheum. Dis., *33*:333–341, 1974.

20. Ghadially, F.N., Lalonde, J.M., and Dick, C.E.: Ultrastructure of pigmented villonodular synovitis. J. Pathol., *127*:19–26, 1979.
21. Schumacher, H.R., Lotke, P., Athreya, B., and Rothfuss, S.: Pigmented villondular synovitis: Light electron microscopic studies. Semin. Arthritis Rheum., *12*:32–43, 1982.
22. Ushijima, M., Hashimoto, H., Tsuneyoshi, M., and Enjoji, M.: Pigmented villonodular synovitis. A clinicopathologic study of 52 cases. Acta Pathol. Jpn., *36*:317–326, 1986.
23. Somer, T., Sittnikow, K., Henriksson, K., and Saksela, E.: Pigmented villonodular synovitis and plasmacytoid lymphoma in a dog. J. Am. Vet. Med. Assoc., *197*:877–879, 1990.
24. Wendt, R.G., et al.: Polyarticular pigmented villonodular synovitis in children: Evidence for a genetic contribution. J. Rheumatol., *13*:921–926, 1986.
25. Flandry, F., McCann, S.B., Hughston, J.C., and Kurtz, D.M.: Roentgenographic findings in pigmented villonodular synovitis of the knee. Clin. Orthop., *247*:208–219, 1989.
26. Jamieson, T.W., et al.: Bilateral pigmented villonodular synovitis of the wrists. Orthop. Rev., *19*:432–436, 1990.
27. Torisu, T., and Watanabe, H.: Pigmented villonodular synovitis occurred in a rheumatoid patient. Clin. Orthop., *91*:134–140, 1973.
28. Archer-Harvey, J.M., Henderson, D.W., Papadimitriou, J.M., and Rozenbilds, M.A.M.: Pigmented villonodular synovitis associated with psoriatic polyarthropathy: An electron microscopic and immunocytochemical study. J. Pathol., *144*:57–68, 1984.
29. Schwartz, H.S., Unni, K.K., and Pritchard, D.J.: Pigmented villonodular synovitis. A retrospective review of affected large joints. Clin. Orthop. *247*:243–255, 1989.
30. Curtin, H.D., Williams, R., Gailla, L., and Meyers, E.N.: Pigmented villonodular synovitis of the temporomandibular joint. Comput. Radiol., *7*:257–260, 1983.
31. Dawiskiba, S., et al.: Diffuse pigmented villonodular synovitis of the temporomandibular joint demonstrated by fine-needle aspiration cytology. Diagn. Cytopathol., *5*:301–304, 1989.
32. Karnezis, T.A., McMillan, R.D., and Ciric, I.: Pigmented villonodular synovitis in a vertebra. A case report. J. Bone Joint Surg., *72A*:927–930, 1990.
33. Steinbach, L.S., et al.: MRI of the knee in diffuse pigmented villonodular synovitis. Clin. Imaging, *13*:305–316, 1989.
34. Ropes, M.W., and Bauer, W., Synovial Fluid Changes in Joint Disease. Cambridge, MA, Harvard University Press, 1953.
35. Ugai, K., Kurosaka, M., and Hirohata, K.: Lipid microspherules in synovial fluid of patients with pigmented villonodular synovitis. Arthritis Rheum., *31*:1442–1446, 1988.
36. Bullough, P.G., and Bansal, M.: The differential diagnosis of geodes. Radiol. Clin. North Am., *26*:1165–1184, 1988.
37. Zwass, A., Abdelwahab, I.F., and Klein, M.J.: Case report 463. Skeletal Radiol., *17*:81–84, 1988.
38. Abrahams, T.G., Pavlov, H., Bansal, M., and Bullough, P.: Concentric joint space narrowing of the hip associated with hemosiderotic synovitis (HS) including pigmented villonodular synovitis. Skeletal Radiol., *17*:37–45, 1988.
39. Nilsonne, U., and Moberger, G.: Pigmented villonodular synovitis of joints. Histological and clinical problems in diagnosis. Acta Orthop. Scand., *40*:448–460, 1969.
40. Jergesen, H., E., and Mankin, H.J.: Diffuse pigmented villonodular synovitis of the knee mimicking primary bone neoplasm. A report of two cases. J. Bone Joint Surg., *60A*:825–829, 1978.
41. Andersen, J.A., and Ladefoged, C.: A case of aggressive pigmented villonodular synovitis. Acta Orthop. Scand., *59*:467–470, 1988.
42. Nielsen, A.L., and Kiaer, T.: Malignant giant cell tumor of synovium and locally destructive pigmented villonodular synovitis. Ultrastructural and immunohistochemical study and review of the literature. Hum. Pathol., *20*:765–771, 1989.
43. Kransdorf, M.J., et al.: Soft-tissue masses: Diagnosis using MR imaging. AJR, *153*:541–547, 1989.
44. Granowitz, S.P., and Mankin, H.: Pigmented villonodular synovitis of the knee. Report of five cases. J. Bone Joint Surg., *49A*:122–128, 1967.
45. Lowenstein, M.B., Smith, J.R.V., and Cole, S.: Infrapatellar fat pad villonodular synovitis. Arthrographic detection. AJR, *135*:279–282, 1980.
46. Howie, C.R., Smith, G.D., Christie, J., and Gregg, P.J.: Torsion of localized pigmented villonodular synovitis of the knee. J. Bone Joint Surg., *67B*:564–566, 1985.
47. Shenag, S.M.: Benign skin and soft-tissue tumors of the hand. Clin. Plast. Surg., *14*:403–412, 1987.
48. Schajowicz, F., and Blumenfeld, I.: Pigmented villonodular synovitis of the wrist with penetration into bone. J. Bone Joint Surg., *50B*:312–317, 1968.
49. Hansen, P., Nielsen, P.T., and Wahlin, A.B.: Pigmented villonodular synovitis of the extensor tendon sheaths in a child. J. Hand Surg., *13B*:313–314, 1988.
50. Sherry, C.S., and Harms, S.E.: MR evaluation of giant cell tumors of the tendon sheath. Mag. Reson. Imaging, *7*:195–201, 1989.
51. Weisser, J.R., and Robinson, D.W.: Pigmented villonodular synovitis of the iliopectineal bursa. J. Bone Joint Surg., *33A*:988–992, 1951.
52. El-Khoury, G.Y., Corbett, A.J., and Summers, T.B.: Case report 303. Skeletal Radio., *13*:164–168, 1985.
53. Present, D.A., Bertoni, F., and Enneking, W.F.: Case report 384. Skeletal Radiol., *15*:236–240, 1986.
54. Ray, R.A., et al.: Cytogenetic evidence of clonality in a case of pigmented villonodular synovitis. Cancer, *67*:121–125, 1991.
55. Hawley, W.L., and Ansell, B.M.: Synovial hemangioma presenting as monoarticular arthritis of the knee. Arch. Dis. Child, *56*:588–560, 1981.
56. Roy, S., and Ghadially, F.N.: Synovial membrane in experimentally produced chronic hemarthrosis. Ann. Rheum. Dis., *28*:402–414, 1969.
57. Singh, R., Grewal, D.S., and Chakravarti, R.N.: Experimental production of pigmented villonodular synovitis in the knee and ankle joints of Rhesus monkeys. J. Pathol., *98*:137–142, 1969.
58. Bobechko, W.P., and Kostuik, J.P.: Childhood villonodular synovitis. Can. J. Surg., *11*:480–486, 1968.
59. Juhl, M., and Krebs, B.: Arthroscopy and synovial hemangioma or giant cell tumour of the knee. Arch. Orthop. Trauma Surg., *108*:250–252, 1989.
60. Duthie, R.B., and Rizza, C.R.: Rheumatological manifestations of the hemophilias. Clin. Rheum. Dis., *1*:53–93, 1975.
61. Morris, C.J., Blake, D.R., Wainwright, A.C., and Steven, M.M.: Relationship between iron deposits and tissue damage in the synovium: An ultrastructural study. Ann. Rheum. Dis., *45*:21–26, 1986.
62. Molnar, Z., Stern, W.H., and Stoltzner, G.H.: Cytoplasmic tubular structures in pigmented villonodular synovitis. Arthritis Rheum., *14*:784–787, 1971.
63. Gitelis, S., Heligman, D., and Morton, T.: The treatment of pigmented villonodular synovitis of the hip. A case report and review of the literature. Clin. Orthop., *239*:154–160, 1989.
64. Robert D'Eshoughes, J., Delcambre, B., and Delbart, P.: Pigmented villonodular synovitis and radioisotopic synoviorthesis. (French.) Lille Med., *20*:438–446, 1975.
65. O'Sullivan, M.M., Yates, D.B., and Pritchard, M.H.: Yttrium 90 synovectomy. A new treatment for pigmented villonodular synovitis. Br. J. Rheumatol., *26*:71–72, 1987.
66. Franssen, M.J.A.M. et al.: Treatment of pigmented villonodular

synovitis of the knee with yttrium-90 silicate: Prospective evaluations by arthroscopy, histology, and 99mTc pertechnetate uptake measurements. Ann. Rheum. Dis., *48*:1007–1013, 1989.

67. Donde, R, and Funding, J.: Pigmented villonodular synovitis. A follow-up study. Scand. J. Rheumatol, *9*:172–174, 1980
68. Murphy, F.P., Dahlin, D.C., and Sullivan, C.R.: Articular synovial chondromatosis. J. Bone Joint Surg., *44A*:77–86, 1962.
69. Milgram, J.W.: Synovial osteochondromatosis. A histopathological study of thirty cases. J. Bone Joint Surg., *59A*:792–801, 1977.
70. Sim, F.H., Dahlin, D.C., and Ivins, J.C.: Extra-articular synovial chondromatosis. J. Bone Joint Surg., *59A*:492–495, 1977.
71. Karlin, C.A., et al.: The variable manifestations of extraarticular synovial chondromatosis. AJR, *137*:731–735, 1981.
72. Maurice, H., Crone, M., Watt, I.: Synovial chondromatosis. J. Bone Joint Surg., *70B*:807–811, 1988.
73. Milgram, J.W.: The classification of loose bodies in human joints. Clin. Orthop., *124*:282–291, 1977.
74. Milgram, J.W.: The development of loose bodies in human joints. Clin. Orthop., *124*:292–303, 1977.
75. Bertoni, F., Unni, K.K., Beabout, J.W., and Sim, F.H.: Chondrosarcomas of the synovium. Cancer, *67*:155–162, 1991.
76. Carey, R.P.L.: Synovial chondromatosis of the knee in childhood. A report of two cases. J. Bone Joint Surg., *59A*:444–447, 1983.
77. Pelker, R.R., Drennan, J.C., and Ozonoff, M.B.: Juvenile synovial chondromatosis of the hip. J. Bone Joint Surg., *65A*:552–554, 1983.
78. Norman, A., Steiner, G.C.: Bone erosion in synovial chondromatosis. Radiology, *161*:749–752, 1986.
79. Steinberg, G.G., Desai, S.S., Malhorta, R., and Hickler, R.: Familial synovial chondromatosis. J. Bone Joint Surg., *71B*:144–145, 1989.
80. Dolan, E.A., Vogler, J.B., and Angelillo, J.C.: Synovial chondromatosis of the temporomandibular joint diagnosed by magnetic resonance imaging: Report of a case. J. Oral. Maxillofac. Surg., *47*:411–413, 1989.
81. Rosati, L.A., and Stevens, C.: Synovial chondromatosis of the temporomandibular joint presenting as an intracranial mass. Arch. Otolaryngol. Head Neck Surg., *116*:1334–1337, 1990.
82. Jones, J.R., Evans, D.M., and Kaushik, A.: Synovial chondromatosis presenting with peripheral nerve compression. Report of two cases. J. Bone Joint Surg., *12B*:25–27, 1987.
83. Szypryt, P., Twining, P., Preston, B.J., and Howell, C.J.: Synovial chondromatosis of the hip joint presenting as a pathologic fracture. Br. J. Radiol., *59*:339–401, 1986.
84. McCarty, D.J. et al.: "Milwaukee shoulder"—Association of microspheroids containing hydroxyapatite crystals, active collagenase, and neutral protease with rotator cuff defects: I. Clinical aspects. Arthritis Rheum., *24*:464–473, 1981.
85. Ellman, M.H., Krieger, M.I., and Brown, N.: Pseudogout mimicking synovial chondromatosis. J. Bone Joint Surg., *57A*:863–865, 1975.
86. DeBenedetti, M.J., and Schwinn, C.P.: Tenosynovial chondromatosis of the hand. J. Bone Joint Surg., *61A*:889–903, 1979.
87. Cremone, J.C., Wolff, T.W., and Wolfort, F.G.: Synovial chondromatosis of the hand. Plast. Reconst. Surg., *69*:871–874, 1982.
88. Catalano, F., Fanfani, F., and Taccardo, G.: Tumoral and pseudotumoral cartilaginous lesions of the soft tissues of the hand. (French.) Ann. Chir. Main, *7*:314–321, 1988.
89. Pope, T.L., Jr. et al.: Idiopathic synovial chondromatosis in two unusual sites: Inferior radioulnar joint and ischial bursa. Skeletal Radiol., *16*:205–208, 1987.
90. Coolican, M.R., and Dandy, D.J.: Arthroscopic management of synovial chondromatosis of the knee. Findings and results in 18 cases. J. Bone Joint Surg., *71B*:498–500, 1989.
91. Milgram, J.W., and Keagy, R.D.: Bursal osteochondromatosis: A case report. Clin. Orthop., *144*:269–271, 1979.
92. Wilner, D.: Radiology of Bone Tumors and Allied Disorders. Vol. 4. Philadelphia, W.B. Saunders, 1982, p. 3941.
93. McCarthy, E.F., and Dorfman, H.D.: Primary synovial chondromatosis. An ultrastructural study. Clin. Orthop., *168*:178–186, 1982.
94. Kay, P.R., Freemont, A.J., and Davies, D.R.A.: The aetiology of multiple loose bodies. Snow storm knee. J. Bone Joint Surg., *71B*:501–504, 1989.
95. Shpitzer, T., Ganel, A., and Engelberg, S.: Surgery for synovial chondromatosis. 26 cases followed up for 6 years. Acta Orthop. Scand., *61*:567–569, 1990.
96. Okada, Y. et al.: Arthroscopic surgery for synovial chondromatosis of the hip. J. Bone Joint Surg., *71B*:198–199, 1989.
97. Nuovo, M.A., Desai, P., Shankman, S., and Present, D.: Intracapsular paraarticular chondroma of the knee. Bull. Hosp. Jt. Dis., *50*:189–194, 1990.
98. Watson, W.L., and McCarthy, W.D.: Blood and lymph vessel tumors. A report of 1056 cases. Surg. Gynecol. Obstet., *71*:569–585, 1940.
99. Ryd, L., and Stenstrom, A.: Hemangioma mimicking meniscal injury. A report of 10 years of knee pain. Acta Orthop. Scand., *60*:230–231, 1989.
100. Seimon, L.P., and Hekmat, F.: Synovial hemangioma of the knee. J. Pediatr. Orthop., *6*:356–359, 1986.
101. Aalberg, J.R.: Synovial hemangioma of the knee. Acta Orthop. Scand., *61*:88–89, 1990.
102. Visuri, T.: Recurrent spontaneous hemarthrosis of the knee associated with a synovial and juxta-articular hemangiohamartoma. Ann. Rheum. Dis., *49*:554–556, 1990.
103. Ehrlich, M.G., and Zaleske, D.J.: Pediatric orthopedic pain of unknown origin. J. Pediatr. Orthop., *6*:460–468, 1986.
104. Stringel, G., and Dastous, J.: Klippel-Trenaunay syndrome and other causes of lower limb hypertrophy: Pediatric surgical implications. J. Pediatr. Surg., *22*:645–650, 1987.
105. Sooriakumaran, S., and Lal Landham, S.: The Klippel-Trenaunay syndrome. J. Bone Joint Surg., *73B*:169–170, 1991.
106. El-Dessouky, M., Azmy, A.F., Raine, P.A.M., and Young, D.G.: Kasabach-Merritt syndrome. J. Pediatr. Surg., *23*:109–111, 1988.
107. Larsen, E.C., Zinkham, W.H., Eggleston, J.C., and Zitelli, B.J.: Kasabach-Merritt syndrome: Therapeutic considerations. Pediatrics, *79*:971–980, 1987.
108. Resnick, D., and Oliphant, M.: Hemophilia-like arthropathy of the knee associated with cutaneous and synovial hemangiomas. Radiology, *114*:323–326, 1975.
109. Sullivan, C.R., Dahlin, D.C., and Bryan, R.S.: Lipoma of the tendon sheath. J. Bone Joint Surg., *38A*:1275–1280, 1956.
110. Placeo, F., and Tassi, D.: Clinical considerations regarding 62 cases of posttraumatic lipoma arborescens of the knee, with or without a meniscal lesion. (Italian) Minerva Chir., *8*:316–322, 1953.
111. Hallel, T., Lew, S., and Bansal, M.: Villous lipomatous proliferation of the synovial membrane (lipoma arborescens). J. Bone Joint Surg., *70A*:264–270, 1988.
112. Armstrong, S.J., and Watt, I.: Lipoma arborescens of the knee. Br. J. Radiol., *62*:178–180, 1989.
113. Hubscher, O., Costanza, E., and Elsner, B.: Chronic monoarthritis due to lipoma arborescens. J. Rheumatol., *17*:861–862, 1990.
114. Hoffa, A.: The influence of the adipose tissue with regard to the pathology of the knee joint. JAMA, *43*:795–796, 1904.
115. Ogata, K., and Ushijima, M.: Tendosynovial fibroma arising

from the posterior cruciate ligament. Clin. Orthop., *215*:153–155, 1987.
116. Chung, E.B, and Enzinger, F.M.: Fibroma of tendon sheath. Cancer, *44*:1945–1954, 1979.
117. Enzinger, F.M.: Clear-cell sarcoma of tendons and aponeuroses. An analysis of 21 cases. Cancer, *18*:1163–1174, 1965.
118. Enzinger, F.M.: Epithelioid sarcoma. A sarcoma simulating a granuloma or a carcinoma. Cancer, *26*:1029–1041, 1970.
119. Haagensen, C.D., and Stout, A.P.: Synovial sarcoma. Ann. Surg., *120*:826–842, 1944.
120. Cadman, N.L., Soule, E.H., and Kelly, P.: Synovial sarcoma. An analysis of 134 tumors. Cancer, *18*:613–627, 1965.
121. Soule, E.H.: Synovial sarcoma. Am. J. Surg. Pathol., *10*(Suppl. 1):78–82, 1986.
122. McClain, R., Buckwalter, J., and Platz, C.E.: Synovial sarcoma of the knee: Missed diagnosis despite biopsy and arthroscopic synovectomy. J. Bone Joint Surg., *72A*:1092–1094, 1990.
123. Witkin, G.B., Miettinen, M., and Rosai, J.: A biphasic tumor of the mediastinum with features of synovial sarcoma. A report of four cases. Am. J. Surg. Pathol., *13*:490–499, 1989.
124. Horowitz, A.L., Resnick, D., and Caird Watson, R.: The roentgen features of synovial sarcomas. Clin. Radiol., *24*:481–484, 1973.
125. Traweek, S.T., Rotter, A.J., Swartz, W., and Azumi, N.: Cystic pulmonary metastatic sarcoma. Cancer, *65*:1805–1811, 1990.
126. Leeson, M.C., Malaei, M., and Makley, J.T.: Leiomyosarcoma of the popliteal artery. A report of two cases. Clin. Orthop., *253*:225–230, 1990.
127. Ordoñez, N.G., Mahfouz, S.M., and Mackay, B.: Synovial sarcoma: An immunohistochemical and ultrastructural study. Hum. Pathol., *21*:733–749, 1990.
128. Miettinen, M.: Keratin subsets in spindle cell sarcomas. Am. J. Pathol., *138*:505–513, 1991.
129. Ghadially, F.N.: Is synovial sarcoma a carcinosarcoma of connective tissues? Ultrastruct. Pathol., *11*:147–151, 1987.
130. Reeves, B.R., et al.: Characterization of the translocation between chromosomes X and 18 in human synovial sarcomas. Oncogene, *4*:373–378, 1989.
131. Nojima, T. et al.: Morphological and cytogenic studies of a human synovial sarcoma xenotransplanted into nude mice. Acta Pathol. Jpn., *40*:486–493, 1990.
132. Toolanen, G. et al.: Sonography of popliteal masses. Acta Orthop. Scand., *59*:294–296, 1988.
133. Chang, A.E., Rosenberg, S.A., Glatstein, E.J., and Antman, K.H.: Sarcomas of soft tissues. In Cancer: Principles & Practice of Oncology. 3rd Ed. Vol. 2, Edited by V.T. DeVita, Jr., S. Hellman, and S.A. Rosenberg. Philadelphia, Lippincott, 1989, pp. 1345–1398.
134. Chang, A.E., et al.: Magnetic resonance imaging versus computed tomography in the evaluation of soft tissue tumors of the extremities. Ann. Surg., *205*:340–348, 1987.
135. Mahajan, H., Lorigan, J.G., and Shirkhoda, A.: Synovial sarcoma: MR imaging. Mag. Reson. Imaging, *7*:211–216, 1989.
136. Burk, D.L. Jr., Mitchell, D.G., Rifkin, M.D., and Vinitski, S.: Recent advances in magnetic resonance imaging of the knee. Radiol. Clin. North Am., *28*:379–393, 1990.
137. Wetzel, L.H., and Levine, E.: Soft-tissue tumors of the foot: Value of MR imaging for specific diagnosis. AJR, *155*:1025–1030, 1990.
138. Morton, M.J. et al.: MR imaging of synovial sarcoma. AJR, *156*:337–340, 1991.
139. Varela-Durán, J., and Enzinger, F.M.: Calcifying synovial sarcoma. Cancer, *50*:345–352, 1982.
140. Tsujimoto, M., et al.: Multivariate analysis for histologic prognostic factors in soft tissue sarcomas. Cancer, *62*:994–998, 1988.
141. Tsujimoto, M., et al.: Histological changes in recurrent soft tissue sarcomas: Analysis of 65 patients. Jpn. J. Clin. Oncol., *18*:135–142, 1988.
142. Alvegard, T.A., and Berg, N.O.: Histopathology peer review of high-grade soft tissue sarcoma: The Scandinavian Sarcoma Group experience. J. Clin. Oncol., *7*:1845–1851, 1989.
143. Rooser, B., Willén, H., Hugoson, A., and Rydholm, A.: Prognostic factors in synovial sarcoma. Cancer, *63*:2182–2185, 1989.
144. Jensen, O.M. et al.: Histopathological grading of soft tissue tumours. Prognostic significance in a prospective study of 278 consecutive cases. J. Pathol., *163*:19–24, 1991.
145. Rosenberg, S.A., et al.: The treatment of soft tissue sarcomas of the extremities. Ann. Surg., *196*:305–315, 1982.
146. Chung, E.B., and Enzinger, F.M.: Malignant melanoma of soft parts. A reassessment of clear cell sarcoma. Am. J. Surg. Pathol., *7*:405–413, 1983.
147. Mii, Y., et al.: Neural crest origin of clear cell sarcoma of tendons and aponeuroses. Virchows Arch. [A], *415*:51–60, 1989.
148. Swanson, P.E., and Wick, M.R.: Clear cell sarcoma. An immunohistochemical analysis of six cases and comparison with other epithelioid neoplasms of soft tissue. Arch. Pathol. Lab. Med., *113*:55–60, 1989.
149. Chinoi, R.F., and Jadav, J.: Clear cell sarcomas of the tendon sheath. An experience of 22 cases seen over 16 years. Indian J. Cancer, *26*:164–174, 1989.
150. Sara, A.S., Evans, H.L., and Benjamin, R.S.: Malignant melanoma of soft parts (clear cell sarcoma). A study of 17 cases, with emphasis on prognostic factors. Cancer, *65*:367–374, 1990.
151. Chase, D.R., Weiss, S.W., Enzinger, F.M., and Langloss, J.M.: Keratin in epithelioid sarcoma. An immunohistochemical study. Am. J. Surg. Pathol., *8*:435–441, 1984.
152. Daimaru, Y., Hashimoto, H., Tsuneyoshi, M., and Enjoji, M.: Epithelial profile of epithelioid sarcoma. Immunohistochemical analysis of eight cases. Cancer, *59*:134–141, 1987.
153. Case 43-1983. N. Engl. J. Med., *309*:1042–1049, 1983.
154. Simon, M.A., and Hecht, J.D.: Invasion of joints by primary bone sarcomas in adults. Cancer, *50*:1649–1655, 1982.
155. McGirr, E.E., and Edmonds, J.P.: Ewing's sarcoma presenting as monoarthritis. J. Rheumatol., *11*:534–536, 1984.
156. Folkman, J., and Klagsburn, M.: Angiogenic factors. Science, *235*:442–447, 1987.
157. Lagier, R.: Synovial reaction caused by adjacent malignant tumors. Anatomopathological study of three cases. J. Rheumatol., *4*:65–72, 1977.
158. Fam, A.G., Kolin, A., and Lewis, A.J.: Metastatic carcinomatous arthritis and carcinoma in the lung: A report of two cases diagnosed by synovial fluid cytology. J. Rheumatol., *7*:98–104, 1980.
159. Murray, G.C., and Persellin, R.H.: Metastatic carcinoma presenting as monoarticular arthritis: A case report and review of the literature. Arthritis Rheum., *23*:95–100, 1980.
160. Weinblatt, M.E., and Karp, G.I.: Monoarticular arthritis: Early manifestations of a rhabdomyosarcoma. J. Rheumatol., *8*:685–688, 1981.
161. Goldenberg, D.L., Kelley, W., and Gibbons, R.B.: Metastatic adenocarcinoma of synovium presenting as acute arthritis: Diagnosis by closed synovial biopsy. Arthritis Rheum., *18*:107–110, 1975.
162. Khan, F.A., Garterhouse, W., and Khan, A.: Metastatic bronchogenic carcinoma: An unusual cause of localized arthritis. Chest, *67*:738–739, 1975.
163. Speerstra, F. et al.: Arthritis caused by metastatic melanoma. Arthritis Rheum., *25*:223–226, 1982.
164. Colson, G.M., and Willcox, A.: Phalangeal metastases in bronchogenic carcinoma. Lancet, *1*:100–102, 1948.
165. Vaezy, A., and Budson, D.C.: Phalangeal metastases from bronchogenic carcinoma. JAMA, *239*:226–227, 1978.

166. Amadio, P.C., and Lombardi, R.M.: Metastatic tumors of the hand. J. Hand Surg., *12A*:311–316, 1987.
167. Zindrick, M.R.: Metastatic tumors of the foot. Clin. Orthop., *170*:219–225, 1982.
168. Besser, E., et al.: Bone tumors of the hand. A review of 300 cases documented in the Westphalian Bone Tumor Register. Arch. Orthop. Trauma Surg., *106*:241–247, 1987.
169. Ritch, P.S., Hansen, R.M., and Collier, D.: Metastatic renal cell carcinoma presenting as shoulder arthritis. Cancer, *51*:968–972, 1983.
170. Rozboril, M.B., Good, A.E., Zarbo, R.J., and Schultz, D.A.: Sternoclavicular joint arthritis: An unusual presentation of metastatic carcinoma. J. Rheumatol., *10*:499–502, 1983.
171. Barton, A., and Hickling, P.: Synovial involvement in Hodgkin's disease. Br. J. Rheumatol., *25*:391–392, 1986.
172. Rice, D.M. et al.: Primary lymphoma of bone presenting as monoarthritis. J. Rheumatol., *11*:851–854, 1984.
173. Dorfman, H.D., Siegel, H.L., Perry, M.C., and Oxenhandler, R.: Non-Hodgkin's lymphoma of the synovium simulating rheumatoid arthritis. Arthritis Rheum., *30*:155–161, 1987.
174. Newcomer, L.N. et al.: Bone involvement in Hodgkin's disease. Cancer, *49*:338–342, 1982.
175. Mariette, X. et al.: Monoarthritis revealing non-Hodgkin's T cell lymphoma of the synovium. Arthritis Rheum., *31*:571–572, 1988.
176. Savin, H. et al.: Seronegative symmetric polyarthritis in Sezary syndrome. J. Rheumatol., *18*:464–467, 1991.
177. Seleznick, M.J., Aguilar, J.L., Rayhack, J., et al.: Polyarthritis associated with cutaneous T cell lymphoma. J. Rheumatol., *16*:1379–1382, 1989.
178. Caldwell, D.S., and McCallum, R.M.: Rheumatologic manifestations of cancer. Med. Clin. North Am., *70*:385–417, 1986.
179. Benedek, T.G.: Neoplastic associations of rheumatic diseases and rheumatic manifestations of cancer. Clin. Geriatr. Med., *4*:333–355, 1988.
180. Schwarzer, A.C., and Schrieber, L.: Rheumatic manifestations of neoplasia. Curr. Opin. Rheumatol., *1*:545–550, 1989.
181. Schumacher, H.R., Jr.: Articular manifestations of hypertrophic pulmonary osteoarthropathy in bronchogenic carcinoma. Arthritis Rheum., *19*:629–636, 1976.
182. Martinez-Lavin, M.: Digital clubbing and hypertrophic osteoarthropathy: A unifying hypothesis. J. Rheumatol., *14*:6–8, 1987.
183. Good, A.E. et al.: Acinar pancreatic tumor with metastatic fat necrosis. Dig. Dis. Sci., *21*:978–987, 1976.
184. Mullin, G.T. et al.: Arthritis and skin lesions resembling erythema nodosum in pancreatic disease. Ann. Intern. Med., *68*:75–87, 1968.
185. Simkin, P.A. et al.: Free fatty acids in the pancreatic arthritis syndrome. Arthritis Rheum., *26*:127–132, 1983.
186. Wilson, H.A. et al.: Pancreatitis with arthropathy and subcutaneous fat necrosis. Arthritis Rheum., *26*:121–126, 1983.
187. Halla, J.T., Schumacher, H.R., Jr., and Trotter, M.E.: Bursal fat necrosis as the presenting manifestation of pancreatic disease: Light and electron microscopic studies. J. Rheumatol., *12*:359–364, 1985.
188. Marhaug, G., Hvidsten, D.: Arthritis complicating acute pancreatitis—A rare but important condition to be distinguished from juvenile rheumatoid arthritis. Scand. J. Rheumatol., *17*:397–399, 1988.
189. Mackenzie, A.H., and Sherbel, A.L.: Connective tissue syndromes associated with carcinoma. Geriatrics, *18*:745–753, 1963.
190. Sheon, R.P., Kirsner, A.B., Tangsintanapas, P., et al.: Malignancy in rheumatic disease: Interrelationships. J. Am. Geriatr. Soc., *25*:20–27, 1977.
191. Strandberg, B.: Rheumatoid arthritis and cancer arthritis. Scand J. Rheumatol. [suppl.], *5*:1–14, 1974.
192. Litwin, S.D., Allen, J.C., and Kunkel, H.G.: Disappearance of the clinical and serological manifestations of rheumatoid arthritis following a thoracotomy for a lung tumor. Arthritis Rheum., *9*:865, 1966.
193. Bradley, J.D., and Pinals, R.S.: Carcinoma polyarthritis: Role of immune complexes in pathogenesis. J. Rheumatol., *10*:826–828, 1983.
194. Cayla, J., Rondier, J., Leger, J.M., and Giraudon, C.: Esophageal carcinoma revealed by acute polyarthritis. (French.) Rev. Rhum. Mal. Osteoartic., *48*:595–600, 1981.
195. Burki, F., and Treves, R.: Polyarthritis and esophageal carcinoma. (French.) Rev. Rhum. Mal. Osteoartic., *53*:547–549, 1986.
196. Chaun, H., Robinson, C.E., Sutherland, W.H., and Dunn, W.L.: Polyarthritis associated with gastric carcinoma. Can. Med. Assoc. J., *131*:909–911, 1984.
197. Simon, R.D., and Ford, L.E.: Rheumatoid-like arthritis associated with colonic carcinoma. Arch. Intern. Med., *140*:698–700, 1980.
198. Chan, M.K., Hendrickson, C.S., and Taylor, K.E.: Polyarthritis associated with breast carcinoma. West J. Med., *137*:132–133, 1982.
199. Kahn, M.F. et al.: Systemic lupus erythematosus and ovarian dysgerminoma: Remission of the systemic lupus erythematosus after extirpation of the tumor. Clin. Exp. Immunol., *1*:355–359, 1966.
200. Bennett, R.M., Ginsberg, M.H., and Thomsen, S.: Carcinomatous polyarthritis: The presenting symptoms of an ovarian tumor and association with a platelet activating factor. Arthritis Rheum., *19*:953–958, 1976.
201. Ultman, J.E.: Hyperuricemia in disseminated neoplastic disease other than lymphomas and leukemias. Cancer, *15*:122–129, 1962.
202. Nanji, A.A., Mikhael, N.Z., and Stewart, D.J.: Increase in serum uric acid level associated with cisplatin therapy. Arch. Intern. Med., *145*:2013–2014, 1985.
203. Ramsdell, C.M., and Kelley, W.N.: The clinical significance of hypouricemia. Ann. Intern. Med., *78*:239–242, 1973.
204. Plonk, J.W., and Feldman, J.M.: Carcinoid arthropathy. Arch. Intern. Med., *134*:651–654, 1974.
205. Crisp, A.J.: Carcinoid arthropathy. (Letter.) Br. J. Radiol., *56*:782, 1983.
206. Bergin, C., Stein, H.B., Boyko, W., et al.: Lymphomatoid granulomatosis presenting as polyarthritis. J. Rheumatol. *11*:537–539, 1984.
207. Nunnink, J.C., Krusinski, P.A., and Yates, J.W.: Multicentric reticulohistiocytosis and cancer: A case report and review of the literature. Med. Pediatr. Oncol., *13*:273–279, 1985.
208. Medsger, T.A., Jr., Dixon, J.A., and Garwood, V.F.: Palmar fasciitis and polyarthritis associated with ovarian carcinoma. Ann. Intern. Med., *96*:424–431, 1982.
209. Pfinsgraff, J., et al.: Palmar fasciitis and arthritis with malignant neoplasms: A paraneoplastic syndrome. Semin. Arthritis Rheum., *16*:118–125, 1986.
210. Massarotti, E.M., Liu, N.Y., Mier, J., and Atkins, M.B.: Chronic inflammatory arthritis following treatment with interleukin-2 (IL-2) for malignancy. Am. J. Med. (in press).

99

Painful Shoulder and the Reflex Sympathetic Dystrophy Syndrome

FRANKLIN KOZIN

Evolutionary development of the prehensile upper extremity and upright posture in man was accompanied by structural changes in the shoulder girdle and its musculature. Unlike the weight-bearing lower extremity, which remained firmly fixed to the axial skeleton, the upper extremity became loosely joined to the trunk at the small sternoclavicular joint. The result was a tremendous increase in mobility, providing a wide range of efficient hand function. This freedom of motion was achieved only by sacrificing stability.

EVOLUTIONARY CHANGES

The origins of the upper limb and shoulder girdle can be traced to the lateral fin folds of early fish[1-3] The first true pectoral girdle is found in later fish where it is attached to the skull and butresses the bilateral pectoral fins and their cartilaginous radials (limb forerunners). As these structures were adapted for weight bearing and terrestrial locomotion in amphibians and reptiles, the shoulder girdle separated from the skull and migrated to a more caudal position to provide increased support. Failure of scapular separation and descent in human ontogeny is reflected in congenital anomalies such as Sprengel's deformity.

Acquisition of prehensile function in mammals and upright posture in primates evoked new changes in the shoulder. The greatest change occurred in the structure and position of the scapula. The scapular spine appeared, creating the infraspinous and supraspinous segments, and gradually the infraspinous segment elongated. The distal end of the scapular spine, the acromion, enlarged in size and mass to accommodate a growing deltoid muscle. With these changes, the scapula migrated from its lateral position on the chest wall to a posterior position and, at the same time, rotated, maintaining the anterior and lateral planes of arm movement. A new bone, the clavicle, developed and assumed its present position in the shoulder girdle, where it functions primarily as a buttress to prevent medial and forward displacement of the scapula and arm. The humerus elongated and twisted along its shaft, bringing the hand into a more functional position relative to the arm and trunk.

Parallel modifications evolved in the shoulder musculature. The scapulohumeral muscles, including the supraspinatus, infraspinatus, teres major and minor, subscapularis, and deltoid, which subserve arm rotation and elevation, underwent the most pronounced changes. The deltoid muscle doubled in relative mass and its insertion on the humerus migrated distally. These factors increased its leverage and established the deltoid muscle as a prime abductor and extendor of the arm. The lower fibers of the deltoid gave rise to a new muscle not found in lower animals, the teres minor. It and the other short rotator muscles formed the musculotendinous (rotator) cuff of the shoulder, so important in stabilizing the joint. Less-pronounced changes occurred in the axioscapular (trapezius, rhomboids, levator scapulae) and axiohumeral (pectoralis major and minor, latissimus dorsi) muscles, which help to suspend the arm and to fix the scapula during movement.

FUNCTIONAL ANATOMY

Normal shoulder motion is the result of complex, integrated movement in four separate joints: the glenohumeral, acromioclavicular, sternoclavicular, and scapu-

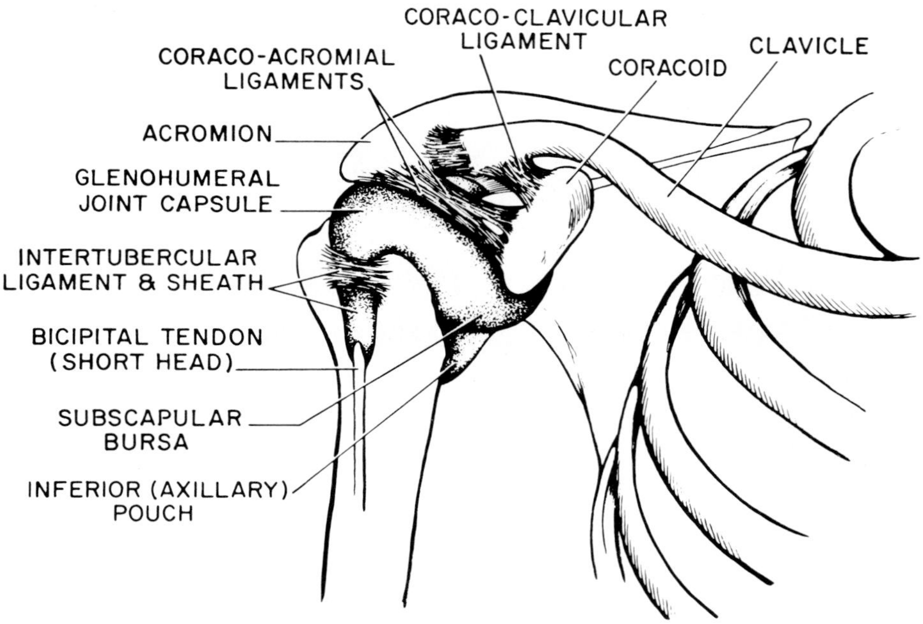

FIGURE 99–1. The glenohumeral joint capsule and surrounding structures.

lothoracic joints. This last structure, although not a true joint anatomically, is concerned with scapular motion around the thoracic wall. The three diarthrodial joints allow movement of the shoulder girdle as a whole and a wide range of glenohumeral motion. Although these joints are considered individually, all four joints normally move simultaneously and synchronously to produce smooth, uninterrupted shoulder motion or "scapulothoracic rhythm."

The sternoclavicular joint unites the shoulder girdle to the trunk and is formed by the first rib, the clavicle, and the manubrium sterni. A fibrocartilaginous disc is interposed between the bones to provide stability and to ensure a smooth articulation. A thick, fibrous capsule and several surrounding ligaments strengthen this important joint. The acromioclavicular joint also has an intra-articular fibrocartilaginous disc, but unlike that of the sternoclavicular joint, it is inconstant and often rudimentary and may predispose the joint to degenerative arthritis.[1] Adjacent to this joint is the coracoacromial arch (Fig. 99–1), which consists of the acromion and coracoacromial ligaments and protects the humeral head and rotator cuff superiorly. The sternoclavicular and acromioclavicular joints allow the clavicle to rotate along its long axis and permit elevation or depression (as in shrugging the shoulders) and extension for flexion (as in forward or backward thrusting of the shoulders) of the entire shoulder girdle (Fig. 99–2).[1–4] These movements are essential to full elevation of the arm in abduction or extension.

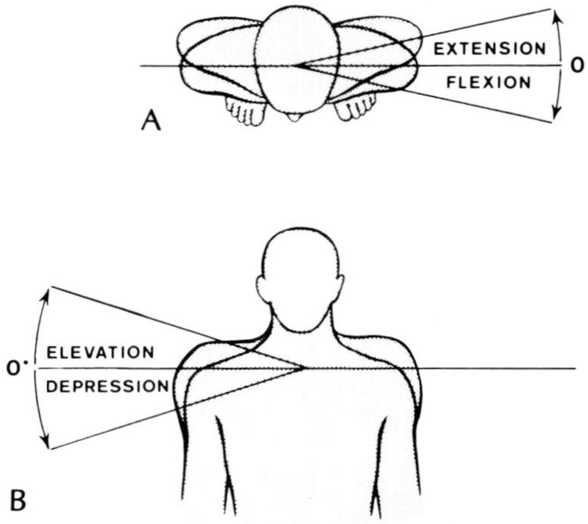

FIGURE 99–2. *A* and *B*, Movements of the sternoclavicular and acromioclavicular joints.

The glenohumeral joint is formed by the articulation of the humerus and scapula at the shallow glenoid fossa, which is deepened by an encircling rim of fibrocartilage, the labrum glenoidale or glenoid lip. The articular capsule is loose and redundant inferiorly (Fig. 99–3); its surface area is twice that of the humeral head.[1,5] Anteriorly, it is usually thickened into two or three glenohumeral ligaments that support the humerus at its least stable point.[6] The coracohumeral ligament and the long bicipital tendon, which passes through the capsule and functions as an accessory ligament,[2] further support the joint. Despite this organization, most of the dynamic stability of the joint is derived from the surrounding short rotator muscles of the humerus, the supraspinatus superiorly, the infraspinatus and teres minor posteriorly, and the subscapularis anteriorly. The relative position of these muscles may change with glenohumeral motion,[7] although no stabilizing structures are present inferiorly. The short rotator muscle tendons insert radially on the proximal humerus (Fig. 99–4); they are joined by loose connective tissue to form a layer, the

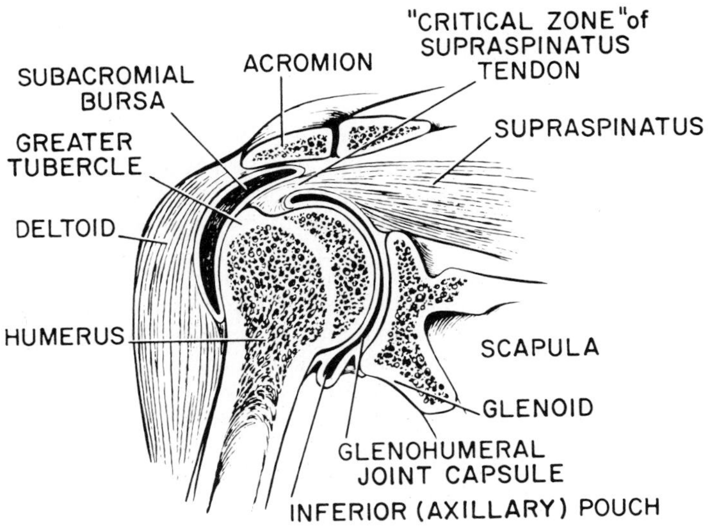

FIGURE 99–3. Coronal section of the shoulder, illustrating the relationships of the glenohumeral joint, the joint capsule, the subacromial bursa, and the rotator cuff (supraspinatus tendon).

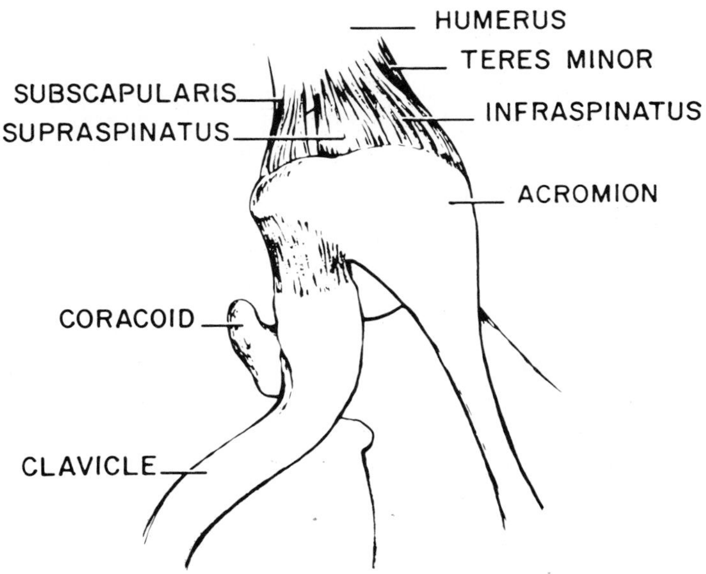

FIGURE 99–4. The musculotendinous (rotator) cuff viewed from above.

rotator cuff, that is closely applied to the underlying capsule. Overlying the rotator cuff, and separated from it by the subacromial bursa, is a second layer of muscle composed of the deltoid and teres major (Fig. 99–3). Thus, the joint capsule is supported and protected by two musculotendinous layers: the inner rotator cuff and the outer deltoid and teres minor.

Normal movement in the glenohumeral joint is accompanied by scapulothoracic motion. During the initial 30 to 60° of humeral elevation, that is, abduction or extension, scapular motion is variable and apparently unique to each individual.[3] Thereafter, depending on the precise plane in which it is studied, the ratio of glenohumeral to scapulothoracic movement is constant and ranges from 1.25 to 2.00; in other words, for every degree of glenohumeral motion there is 0.5 to 0.8° of scapulothoracic motion.[3,8] It is possible to fix or to immobilize the scapula and still elevate the arm 90° actively or 120° passively, when further movement is blocked by the acromion. This movement results in a significant loss of power, however, and is not physiologically important.[3,9]

The chief muscles producing glenohumeral joint motion are the deltoid, pectoralis major and minor, teres major, latissimus dorsi, and those in the rotator cuff.[10] Abduction is accomplished by the rotator cuff muscles acting with the deltoid and, occasionally, the long head of the biceps. The down-and-in action of the rotator muscles and the up-and-down action of the deltoid muscle produce a "force couple," in which the off-setting vertical forces stabilize the humeral head within the glenoid while the lateral forces cause abduction.[3,6,9] During abduction, maximum forces on the glenohumeral joint are attained at 90° of elevation.[11] The chief adductors are the pectoralis major and latissimus dorsi, with assistance from deltoid. Internal and external rotation are produced by the short rotator (cuff) muscles and the latissimus dorsi and deltoid muscles, respectively. Flexion is due primarily to the action of the pectoralis major and deltoid muscles, although both heads of the biceps muscle also are active, and extension is produced by the deltoid, pectoralis major, and latissimus dorsi muscles.

Many of our daily activities require the arm to be used in forward flexion and elevation, especially in the scapular plane.[12] These movements are produced by the concerted function of the supraspinatus, infraspinatus, and deltoid muscles. When these muscles are paralyzed by loss of suprascapular and axillary nerve function, the shoulder is essentially immobile.[13] The supraspinatus and deltoid contribute equally to the force of these movements.[12]

ASSESSMENT OF THE PATIENT

A detailed medical history and physical examination are essential in all patients with shoulder complaints to determine whether these symptoms arise from local injury, from systemic disease, or from pain referred from another location.[1,14,15] Particular attention should be given to a patient's occupation or avocation; the presence of chronic illness, particularly diabetes mellitus (see following); and general mental attitude. Impairment of shoulder motion can lead to significant disability,[16] especially in the elderly.

The shoulder is examined with the patient standing or sitting and undressed to the waist, to permit a thorough inspection and comparison of both sides. Joint swelling, abnormality of bony structure, such as inequality or malposition, or muscle fasciculation or atrophy may be apparent. Atrophy of the infraspinatus or supraspinatus muscles, detected as diminished fullness of the respective scapular fossae, usually indicates chronically painful shoulders or tear of the rotator cuff. Arthritis involving the synovial joints of the shoulder may produce soft tissue or bony swelling or effusions; in the glenohumeral joint, an effusion may be detected by swelling along the bicipital tendon as it traverses the bicipital groove. Fullness or fluctuance beneath the deltoid muscle suggests subacromial (subdeltoid) bursitis. The patient's posture should be noted.

Shoulder motion is evaluated next. The normal shoulder is capable of a wide range of movement including abduction and adduction (raising or lowering the arm in the coronal plane), flexion and extension (backward or forward movement of the arm in the sagittal plane), internal and external rotation, circumduction, and other remarkable combinations of these motions (Fig. 99–5). Movements of the shoulder girdle as a unit include elevation and depression, as in shrugging, or extension and flexion, as in protrusion (Fig. 99–2). Active range of motion may be determined quickly and accurately by asking the patient to perform the following movements, keeping in mind that minor variations of the "normal range" exist, depending on the age and sex of the patient: (1) raise both arms to the side until the hands touch overhead, return them to the side, and cross them in front (abduction and adduction); (2) extend both arms forward until the hands touch overhead and extend them behind the back (flexion and extension); (3) place both hands behind the neck (external rotation) and behind the back, as high as possible (internal rotation) (Fig. 99–6); and (4) shrug and protrude the shoulders (sternoclavicular and acromioclavicular joints). Careful observation during these movements is essential because patients with shoulder pain often learn to achieve full abduction or extension by hunching the shoulder to reverse the normal scapulohumeral rhythm.

Assessment of passive shoulder motion may provide additional diagnostic clues when active movements are limited. As with active motion, particular attention is given to abduction and rotation because these movements are frequently the best indicators of early glenohumeral disease. Passive abduction is measured by fixing the scapula with one hand while the other supports the arm at the partially flexed elbow and abducts it; normally, 90 to 120° of abduction is possible. Shoulder abduction is significantly reduced in normal, healthy older subjects.[16a] To measure passive rotation, the arm is abducted with the elbow flexed to 90° and is slowly rotated (Fig. 99–5B); a 180° arc can usually be achieved.

Patients who complain of pain during arm elevation, usually from 60 to 120° of abduction or extension (a "painful arc"), should be assessed with several specific maneuvers. The *impingement sign* is elicited by immobilizing the scapula while forcibly elevating the arm. Subjects with the impingement syndrome experience pain when the greater tuberosity impinges against the coracoacromial arch;[17] on occasion, concomitant popping or "clunking" can be palpated or heard. Injection of 3 to 10 mL 1% xylocaine beneath the acromium may produce relief during this maneuver, thereby conferring some specificity to this test.[17] The *supraspinatus test* is performed by placing the arm in 90° of abduction and internal rotation and by angling the arm 30° forward to isolate the supraspinatus muscle. Muscle strength is tested against resistance to indicate weakness or pain in the supraspinatus. A *subluxability test* also may be useful, especially in elderly individuals with poorly localized pain. Patients are asked to lie supine with the shoulder over the edge of the examination table; the shoulder is then tested for ease of subluxation.[18] During this test, the glenoid lip should be palpated to disclose tenderness, which may be the only physical finding in tears of this structure.

Assessment of resisted movements in the arm may help isolate the painful structure(s). Thus, pain on resisted abduction suggests supraspinatus tendinitis; pain on resisted external rotation, subscapularis tendinitis. This approach may be helpful in diagnosis of difficult

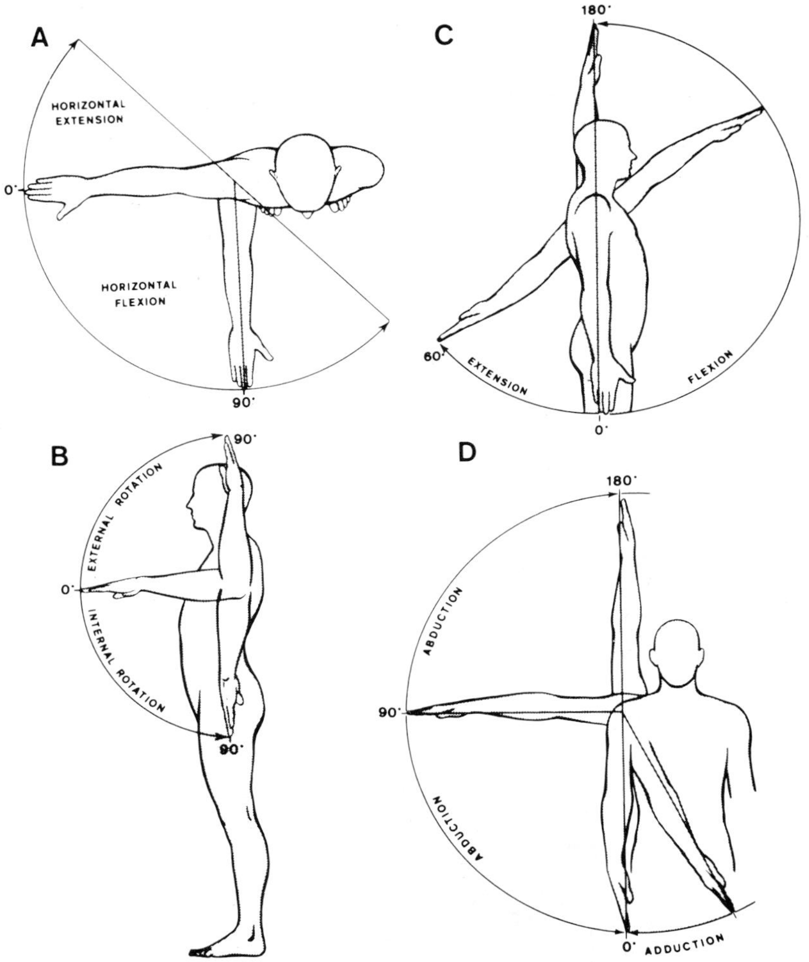

FIGURE 99–5. Movements of the shoulder. *A*, "Horizontal" flexion and extension. *B*, Internal and external rotation. *C*, "Vertical" flexion and extension. *D*, Abduction and adduction.

shoulder problems, especially when pain is not reproduced by simple active range of motion.

Finally, the shoulder must be palpated to determine the exact site of tenderness and to identify areas of increased heat, swelling, fluctuation, muscle spasm or atrophy, or, on occasion, frank tears within the rotator cuff. Although shoulder pain may be deep and widely radiating, the patient often suggests the diagnosis by identifying a specifically painful point.

RADIOLOGIC EXAMINATION

Certain studies that should be considered in many patients with shoulder pain are discussed in this section.

PLAIN RADIOGRAPHY

Proper positioning is essential in visualizing specific structures such as the glenohumeral, sternoclavicular, and acromioclavicular joints, the scapula and clavicle, the humeral head or greater tuberosity, and the bicipital groove. Arthritis changes, fractures and dislocation, and soft-tissue calcification may be identified and localized more readily when the appropriate projection is used. Although of little direct benefit in the diagnosis of soft-tissue lesions such as tendinitis, bursitis, or rotator cuff tears, plain radiography may show degenerative changes in the tuberosities or the humeral head and avulsion fractures at tendon insertions, which frequently accompany these conditions (Fig. 99–7). Soft-tissue xeroradiography may be of considerable value in the recognition of soft-tissue lesions and localized areas of tendon calcification.[19,20]

ARTHROGRAPHY

Contrast studies of the glenohumeral joint are helpful in diagnosing adhesive capsulitis, bicipital tenosynovitis or tendon rupture, rotator cuff tears, and shoulder dislocations.[21–24] The normal arthrogram demonstrates the bicipital sheath, the redundant inferior joint capsule, and the subscapular bursa (Fig. 99–8A). The cartilage of the glenoid lip appears as a negative shadow. Because no communication normally exists between the joint cavity and the subacromial bursa, the bursa is not visible.

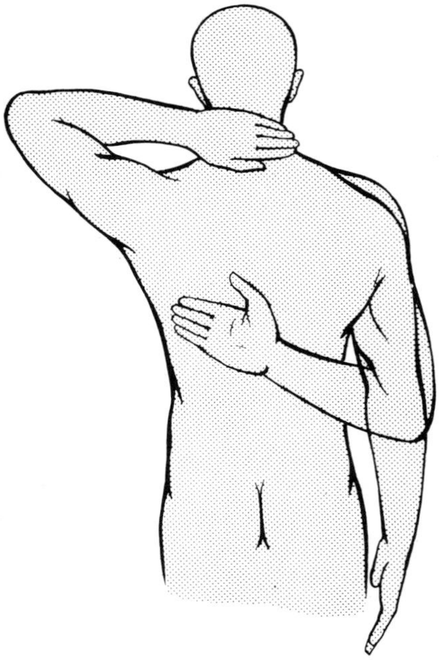

FIGURE 99–6. Internal and external rotation of the shoulder (active).

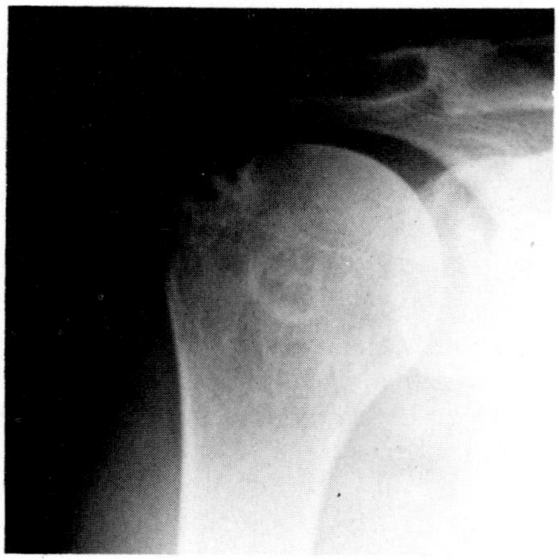

FIGURE 99–7. Plain radiograph of the shoulder, illustrating humeral cysts and sclerosis, particularly about the greater tuberosity.

Complete rotator cuff tears (full-thickness tears) are seen readily as extravasation of contrast material into the subacromial bursa or, occasionally, soft tissues (Fig. 99–8B). Incomplete tears (partial-thickness tears) are more difficult to recognize, although they may be suggested by irregularities or mall clefts in the rotator cuff. Bicipital tendon tenosynovitis or rupture may produce irregularity in the bicipital sheath or leakage of the contrast material into the soft tissues of the upper arm. Shoulder dislocations and subluxations that tear the capsule away from the glenoid lip may be demonstrated by excessive capsule laxity (ballooning) or by leakage of dye.

The arthrogram in adhesive capsulitis is characteristic. Joint volume is reduced, and the normal anterior and inferior pouches are obliterated. As a result, *the volume of contrast material that can be injected is reduced from the usual 15 to 35 mL to only 5 to 10 mL.*

Double-contrast arthrography, in which a small amount of radiopaque contrast material and a larger amount of air are instilled into the glenohumeral joint, improves the resolution of the rotator cuff structures and the articular cartilage,[22] and it may cause less joint irritation than other methods.[25] Although it appears to be extremely sensitive,[26] this technique is more difficult to perform and to interpret than the conventional method.[27] When this technique is combined with tomography (arthrotomography), it is possible to visualize abnormalities of the glenoid lip effectively and to diagnose avulsion or tears of the cartilaginous rim.[28,29]

Subacromial bursography is used with increasing frequency, particularly for diagnosis of adhesive subacromial bursitis, in which the bursal volume is reduced from 4 to 6 mL to 1 to 2 mL,[30] and in the shoulder impingement syndrome discussed later in this chapter.[24,30]

SCINTIGRAPHY

Inflamed joints can be readily detected by scintigraphy,[31,32] and it may be useful in mildly or even noninflammatory articular disease.[31,33] Studies in adhesive capsulitis[34] and polymyalgia rheumatica[33] show abnormal shoulder uptake, but such findings must be interpreted cautiously because increased local radioactivity is common in patients without symptoms or radiographic abnormalities relating to the shoulder,[35,36] or in patients with injury of the rotator cuff.[37]

ULTRASONOGRAPHY

High-resolution ultrasonography has evolved over the past decade as a rapid, inexpensive means of detecting partial or complete rotator cuff tears.[38] Initial reports were very encouraging, with sensitivity and specificity approximating 90%, but later studies suggest a sensitivity in the range of 58 to 68% and a specificity in the range of 43%.[39,40,40a] These discrepancies may be attributed to positioning artifacts, experience with the technique, or other factors.[40b]

COMPUTED TOMOGRAPHY

Computed tomography (CT) is useful for evaluating the unstable shoulder. This technique may be preferable to arthrography or arthrotomography.[41,42] CT may be useful for assessing rotator cuff integrity,[43] especially when combined with arthrography.[44]

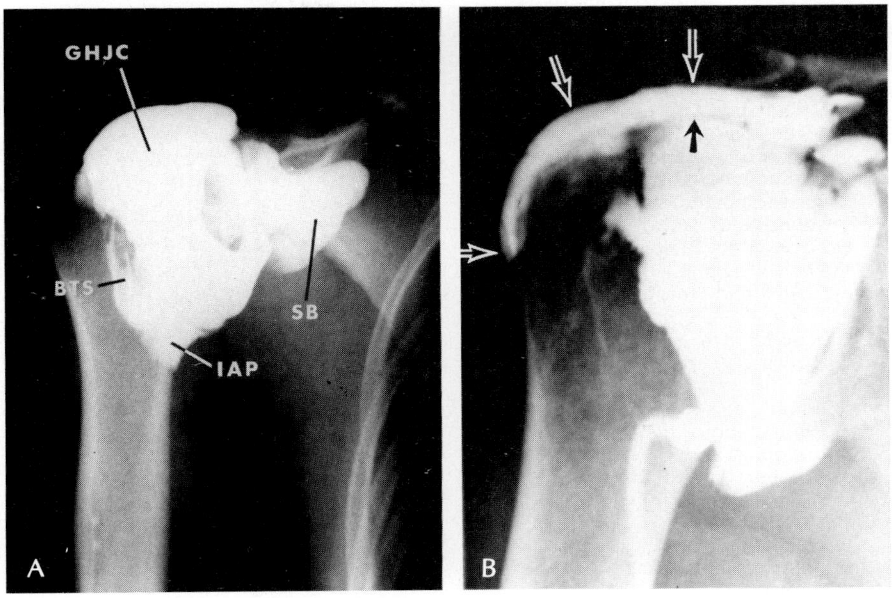

FIGURE 99–8. *A*, Arthrogram of the normal shoulder, showing the glenohumeral joint capsule (GHJC), the subscapular bursa (SB), the inferior axillary pouch (IAP), and the bicipital tendon sheath (BTS). *B*, Arthrogram of the shoulder in a patient with a complete rotator cuff rupture, demonstrating contrast in the subacromial bursa (arrows).

MAGNETIC RESONANCE IMAGING

Insufficient data exist for critical analysis of the role of magnetic resonance imaging (MRI) in the diagnosis of shoulder pain. Published studies and recent experience leave little doubt that it is rapidly becoming an important adjunct for the assessment of shoulder problems.[45] MRI provides superb anatomic detail of the structures about the shoulder,[46,47] but it is still not clearly the method of choice in the diagnosis of adhesive capsulitis or in distinguishing rotator cuff tendinitis from tear.

PAINFUL SHOULDER

Shoulder pain is among the most common complaints in medical practice and may occur in up to 25% of elderly subjects.[47a,47b] In the older age groups, shoulder pain often leads to significant disability.[47b] Such pain may be caused by local problems within the shoulder region or by remote disorders, especially heart, lung, and cervical spinal disease, or systemic conditions. A variety of classifications has been devised to aid in differential diagnosis; it seems most useful to divide shoulder pain into two broad etiologic categories: intrinsic (local) and extrinsic (remote and systemic) disorders (Table 99–1). Intrinsic conditions, which account for most shoulder complaints, are emphasized here. Extrinsic disorders may account for up to 20% of shoulder pain.[48]

IMPINGEMENT SYNDROME

The coracoacromial arch (Fig. 99–1) protects the humeral head and the rotator cuff from direct trauma. The arch is rigid and may limit full arm elevation. The impingement syndrome occurs when the supraspinatus tendon and the subacromial bursa are caught between the humerus and the overlying coracoacromial arch.[17,49] Repeated impingement may result in attrition of rotator cuff tendons or frank rotator cuff tears. A number of sports appear to increase the incidence of impingement.[50]

Jobe has emphasized the importance of age in distinguishing the cause of impingement.[50a] In younger individuals, shoulder problems are typically seen in "overhead" athletics (baseball, football, tennis, swimming). The mechanical stress of these activities results in microtrauma and ultimately in anterior instability, subluxation, impingement, and rotator cuff tear. In the older individual (over age 35), shoulder disorders are more likely to be associated with degenerative changes.

Subjects with the impingement syndrome often complain of a painful arc in the range of 60 to 120° of arm elevation. The impingement sign, described previously in this chapter, is a specific test for diagnosis.[17] Radiographs often show bony spurs on the undersurface of the acromion,[46] although the frequency of this finding varies considerably.[51,52] Subacromial bursography demonstrates reduced volume and abnormal configuration of the bursa.[53]

Neer proposes three stages of impingement.[49] *Stage 1* typically is seen in subjects younger than 25 years who are active athletically or frequently use their arm overhead. The subacromial bursa demonstrates edema and hemorrhage. *Stage 2* affects individuals ages 25 to 40 and presumably results from repeated or subacute impingement. Thickening and fibrosis are present in the bursa and rotator cuff. In *Stage 3*, subjects are older, usually over 40 years, and have chronic impingement. Degenerative changes or frank tears in the rotator cuff may be present. Calcific deposits are often observed in the rotator cuff tendons or bursa.[52]

TABLE 99–1. DIFFERENTIAL DIAGNOSIS OF THE PAINFUL SHOULDER

Intrinsic Disorders
Impingement Syndrome
Specific Lesions of the Rotator Cuff
Degenerative tendinitis
Calcific tendinitis
Subacromial bursitis
Rotator cuff rupture
Lesions of the Bicipital Tendon
Adhesive Capsulitis ("Frozen Shoulder")
Fibrositis and Fibromyalgia
Arthritis
Degenerative
"Milwaukee shoulder"
Neurotrophic
Traumatic and Athletic Injuries
Subluxation or dislocation
Neurologic
Peripheral neuropathy
Brachial plexus injury
Postural Effects
Infection
Neoplasia, Benign and Malignant
Extrinsic Disorders
Inflammatory Conditions
Rheumatoid arthritis
Spondyloarthritides
Myopathies
Polymyalgia rheumatica
Avascular Necrosis
Metabolic and Endocrine
Gout and pseudogout
Diabetes mellitus
Hyperparathyroidism
Other
Neurologic
Cervical nerve root compression (C4, C5, C6)
Lesions of the spinal cord
"Viscerosomatic" and referred pain
Peripheral neuropathy
Neurovascular
Thoracic outlet syndrome
Axillary arterial and venous thrombosis
Reflex Sympathetic Dystrophy Syndrome(s)

Conservative therapy is sufficient to control symptoms and limit progression in earlier or milder cases.[17,52] Surgical intervention with acromioplasty or bursectomy may be necessary in later or more severe cases.[49,54,55] Significant reduction in pain was found in athletic individuals who required surgery; however, only 40% of subject were able to return to their preinjury level of function.[56]

DEGENERATIVE TENDINITIS ("SUPRASPINATUS SYNDROME")

Origin and Pathogenesis

Degenerative changes in the rotator cuff tendons appear to represent the normal aging process.[15] Twenty-five percent of unselected subjects have attritional changes in the rotator cuff by their fifth decade, and the incidence increases progressively thereafter.[15] The supraspinatus tendon is affected most frequently, especially in the so-called critical zone of Codman, a site approximately 1 to 2 cm medial to the tendon's insertion at the greater tuberosity. Several factors may combine to explain the increased susceptibility of this region:[57,58] (1) it is a relatively avascular zone where the osseous and tendinous blood supplies anastomose;[58a] (2) the few blood vessels in this area are compressed when the arm is hanging down normally;[57] and (3) repeated impingement of this area may occur between the acromion and the humeral head during abduction. In contrast, the vascular supply of the other flat tendons of the rotator cuff is greater, nonanastomotic, and unimpeded by arm motion.[57] These observations also may explain the high frequency of degenerative tendinitis in subjects with repeated occupational stresses to the shoulder, such as carpenters, painters,[15] and welders,[59] or with a compromised neurologic or vascular supply, such as alcoholics and diabetics.[15,60,61] Experimentally, it is difficult to tear a normal tendon, but it is easy to tear an ischemic tendon.

Clinical Features

The patient with degenerative tendinitis is most likely to be a man in his fifth decade or older, to work as a laborer, and to localize his complaints to the dominant side. The condition is generally asymptomatic until provoked by minor trauma or exertion; however, careful questioning often elicits a history of recurrent shoulder problems.

The patient complains of a dull ache in the shoulder that is not easily localized. It may be more severe at night and may interfere with sleep. On examination, active shoulder movements are restricted, especially abduction. A painful arc from 70 to 100° of abduction is characteristic, probably reflecting supraspinatus involvement because at this range supraspinatus activity is maximal and the greatest force is applied across the glenohumeral joint.[3,8,10,11] Many patients learn to avoid this painful arc by reversing the scapulohumeral rhythm, that is, by hunching their shoulder to position the scapula before initiating glenohumeral motion. Often, passive movements are normal because force across the joint is minimal when the arm is supported. Weakness is uncommon unless the pain is chronic, the pain is of more than 3 weeks' duration, or an associated rotator cuff tear is present. In patients with severe pain, it may be necessary to inject an anesthetic agent into the rotator cuff before attempting to assess strength.[62] Palpation is helpful in identifying the source of pain. Tenderness over the bicipital groove suggests bicipital tendinitis. Subscapularis tendinitis may be detected by tenderness at its insertion on the lesser tuberosity. Similarly, tenderness localized to the superior or inferolateral aspects of the greater tuberosity suggests supraspinatus tendinitis or injuries of the infraspinatus or teres minor tendons, respectively. Location of the area of maximal tenderness is important in guiding therapy.[63]

Radiologic Examination

A radiograph of a shoulder with an early tendon lesion generally is normal. In patients with chronic disease, degenerative changes such as bony fragments, pseudocysts, sclerosis, and osteophytes may develop in the greater tuberosity and the humeral head (Fig. 99–7).[1,15] Unless the disorder has progressed to a frank rotator cuff tear, the arthrogram is usually normal, although small irregularities on the undersurface of the tendon may be noted.

The treatment of this disorder is discussed later in this chapter, under "Bursitis."

CALCIFIC TENDINITIS (See also Chapter 110)

Origin and Pathogenesis

Many have assumed that tendon calcification occurs as a consequence of degenerative tendinitis.[1,15,64] Yet considerable evidence from studies in experimental animals,[65,66] as well as from observations of patients with uremia,[67] hypervitaminosis D,[68] and multiple sites of "calcific periarthritis,"[69,70] suggests that calcium deposits in tendon may occur in the apparent absence of local degeneration. A controlled study found a two- to threefold greater prevalence of calcific tendinitis in shoulders of subjects with adult-onset diabetes mellitus and insulin-dependent diabetes mellitus. Bilateral involvement was common.[70a]

Most studies of the pathogenesis of this condition have focused on local factors that predispose tendons to calcification. Although the precise mechanism still remains uncertain, a number of hypotheses have evolved.[71–76] Altered tendon physiologic features, possibly produced by changes in blood flow, minor trauma, or mild inflammation, may promote a direct interaction between tendon matrix and calcium ion.[71,72] Phospholipids and various proteins have been implicated in the process of calcification in bone,[77–80] and they may subserve this function in tendon as well. The resultant calcium complex then may react with phosphorus, to produce a series of intermediate salts until hydroxyapatite is formed.[74] This crystalline substance has been identified in shoulder tendons,[1,81] just as in other forms of calcific periarthritis.[69] Four histologic phases have been described in "primary" calcific tendinitis that occurs typically in the aforementioned critical zone.[82,83] These phases are: (1) "precalcific," in which metaplastic fibrocartilage is observed within the tendon; (2) "calcific," in which deposits of calcium are found within a fibrocartilaginous nodule in a close relationship with matrix vesicles, without reactive changes; (3) "resorptive," in which reactive changes consist of phagocytic cells and increased vascularity; and (4) "repair," which is characterized by the appearance of abundant mesenchymal cells within the tendon. The natural history of primary calcific deposits is spontaneous resorption. The majority of patients in a recent study had no reactive or reparative changes associated with tendon calcification.[83] "Secondary" calcification occurs at the torn edges of the rotator cuff or in a degenerated tendon insertion into the greater trochanter, that is, an enthesopathy distal to the critical zone. Such calcific deposits do not resorb spontaneously and elicit little repair reaction.

Once deposited, the calcified material exists in two states, or possibly phases, that seem to correlate with the clinical stage of the condition. In the chronic stage, the deposits are usually hard and dry (inspissated), with a gritty consistency; in the acute stage, the material is creamy white and paste-like (hydrated).[15,83] No differences in the scanning electron microscopic or x-ray diffraction appearance of the crystal deposition these different states were found.[83a]

Clinical Features

The prevalence of calcific tendinitis is high, occurring in 2.7 to 8.0% of the general population.[84] The highest incidence appears to be in the fifth decade, and the association with various chronic diseases, particularly diabetes mellitus, is strong.[15,60] Unlike degenerative tendinitis, this condition is seen in both sexes equally and often affects subjects in sedentary occupations.[1,15,84] Like degenerative tendinitis, the supraspinatus tendon is most commonly involved (approximately 50% of cases), followed by the infraspinatus, teres minor, and subscapularis tendons and the subacromial bursa. Multiple sites of calcification and bilateral involvement are also common.[1,70,84]

Three clinical states are recognized and resemble those of the other crystal-induced arthritides (see Chapters 106–111).[1,15,85] The first, asymptomatic stage is found incidentally on radiographs usually obtained for other reasons.[84] Little or no inflammatory reaction is present, possibly because the calcium deposit is small and located in the avascular critical zone.[1] Radiologically, the borders of the deposit are smooth. The calcium may be resorbed spontaneously, often correlating with symptoms of pain and inflammation. The borders of the calcific deposit appear scalloped. Other symptoms develop later. These stages might be likened to acute or "tophaceous" gout, both clinically and pathologically, because granulomatous reaction with chronic inflammation and giant cells is present as part of the resorptive process.[15,82] Chronic symptoms and physical signs are indistinguishable from those of degenerative tendinitis, previously described, and the course of the disorder is characterized by exacerbations and remissions. The acute stage resembles the acute gouty or pseudogouty attack: pain is sudden and severe, often following minimal trauma or effort. This diffuse pain may radiate into the subdeltoid (bursa) area; a few patients develop features of a reflex sympathetic dystrophy in the ipsilateral hand.[1,15] Because the rotator cuff muscles are in spasm, the arm is held rigidly in a neutral or an adducted position. Even the slightest movement evokes a painful outcry. Complete examination of the patient is virtually impossible, although gentle palpation may reveal a point of maximal tenderness. As in acute gout and pseu-

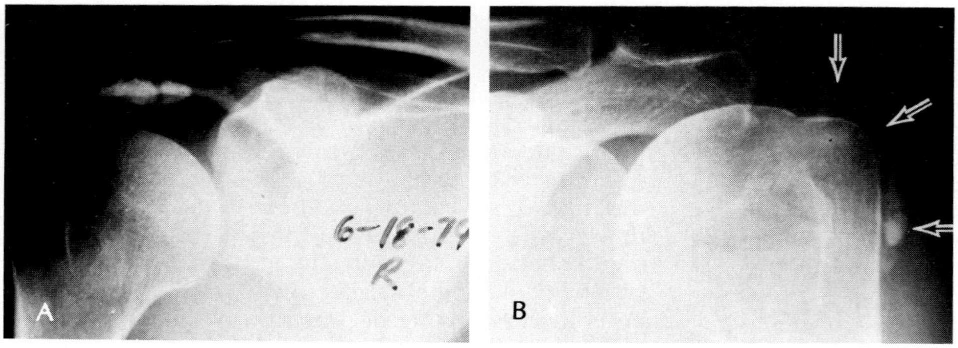

FIGURE 99–9. Plain radiographs of the shoulder in a patient with calcification in the supraspinatus tendon, *A*, and in the subacromial bursa, *B*. Note the calcium extending into the subdeltoid area in *B* (arrows).

dogout, colchicine therapy often has dramatic results. The relation of calcific tendinitis to a more advanced form of crystal-induced shoulder disease. Milwaukee shoulder, is uncertain.

Standard radiographs show the typical ovoid calcific deposit (Fig. 99–9A), although special views may be needed to identify the exact site of calcification.[86] Rupture into the subacromial bursa is noted in about 5% of cases (Fig. 99–9B).[84] When rupture occurs, the calcium salt is usually rapidly resorbed. Such rupture may leave a hole in the rotator cuff, designated as a tear.

The treatment of this disorder is discussed in the following section, "Bursitis."

BURSITIS

Origin and Pathogenesis

A number of bursae or thin-walled, usually closed sacs lined with synovial tissue strategically placed to minimize friction between moving parts are found in the shoulder region. The largest and most constant is the subacromial bursa, located between the rotator cuff inferiorly and the deltoid and teres major muscles superiorly (Fig. 99–3). Its lateral extension beneath the deltoid muscle is termed the subdeltoid bursa. Other bursae include the subscapular and supracoracoid and those found in relation to the insertion of various muscles, such as the trapezius, pectoralis major, teres major, and latissimus dorsi muscles. Except for the systemic arthritides, which may affect the bursae primarily, bursitis of the shoulder area is usually secondary to traumatic, degenerative, or calcific disease in the rotator cuff. The subacromial bursa is most commonly involved because of its large size and its anatomic position.

Clinical Features

Symptoms of subacromial bursitis or "deal-runner's shoulder" are similar to those of the primary disease. Pain and tenderness may extend distally to the superior third of the arm because of the subdeltoid extension of the bursa. Active and passive abduction are usually reduced, but active motion is disproportionately limited, probably because of the added force of the contracting abductor muscles on the bursa.

Depending on the primary disease, plain radiographs may demonstrate bony changes,[87,88] calcific deposits,[84] or actual enlargement of the bursa. An arthrogram may show a communication with the glenohumeral joint capsule when bursitis is caused by complete rupture of the rotator cuff.[23,62,89] Bursography may be useful in demonstrating the impingement syndrome, adhesive bursitis, or rotator cuff tears.[30]

Treatment

Treatment of degenerative or calcific tendinitis and subacromial bursitis is directed at pain relief, maintenance of maximal shoulder function, prevention of complications such as adhesive capsulitis or the reflex sympathetic dystrophy syndrome, early rehabilitation, and education of the patient in methods of avoiding recurrent attacks.[1,15] The vast number of therapeutic programs that have been advocated attest to their lack of specificity and to the unavailability of a uniformly successful program.

Basic conservative treatment is outlined in Table 99–2. There are few data regarding efficacy or cost-effectiveness of different treatments for patients with a painful shoulder. Conservative measures including analgesics, physiotherapy, and nonsteroidal anti-inflammatory drugs (NSAIDs) are not uniformly successful.[89a] Patients with more prolonged symptoms at the time of presentation or with involvement of their dominant shoulder are more likely to have persistent or recurrent pain. In this group especially, early subacromial corticosteroid injection is more cost-effective than physiotherapy alone or combined with NSAIDs.[89b] Rest of the acutely painful shoulder is essential. Immobilization of the arm in partial adduction with a sling may help. Salicylate or other NSAIDs in adequate doses are useful for their analgesic and anti-inflammatory properties,[90] although convincing evidence of their beneficial effect is lacking.[91,92] Concomitant administration of simple analgesics, such as acetaminophen or propoxyphene, or narcotic analgesics may be required. Muscle relaxants are of doubtful value. Any of a variety of local physical

TABLE 99–2. CONSERVATIVE TREATMENT PROGRAM FOR PAINFUL SHOULDER*

1. Limited use of extremity during acute painful period
   - Complete rest for hyperacute symptoms
   - Arm in adduction sling; hand and forearm elevated
2. Anti-inflammatory and analgesic agents
   - Salicylates and other nonsteroidal anti-inflammatory drugs
   - Acetaminophen and propoxyphene derivatives
   - Narcotic analgesics for severe pain
3. Physical Therapy
   - Heat or cold (cold for acute conditions; heat for subacute or chronic symptoms)
     - Home: heating pad, hot packs, ice packs
     - Physician's office or hospital: ultrasound, hydrocollator packs
   - Exercises
     - Initially, as acute pain subsides: passive range of motion
     - Later, when pain is mild to moderate: pendulum swinging (Codman); active exercises with resistance or assistance
4. Treatment of associated or underlying condition
5. Psychologic support in the form of reassurance and encouragement
6. Education for self-help and avoidance of provocative activities

* Objectives: Relief of pain and muscle spasm, maintenance and restoration of motion, and prevention of secondary changes.

modalities that provide heat or cold to the affected area may assist in reducing pain. These modalities include moist hot-packs, such as hydrocollator packs, ultrasonography,[93,94] other such methods,[95] or simple ice packs.[93] These techniques may raise the local pain threshold,[93] promote local blood flow, enhance tissue repair,[96,97] reduce muscle spasm, or simply exert a placebo effect.[98,99] Controlled studies suggest that some of these approaches have no effect.[100] Treatment with local radiotherapy, dimethyl sulfoxide (DMSO),[101] or acupuncture,[98] although recommended by some, does not appear to be any more effective than treatment with the other measures discussed and is not recommended.

Early mobilization of the painful extremity is important in minimizing disability and the risk of adhesive capsulitis or reflex dystrophy. Passive movements immediately after local heat or cold applications or 1 to 2 hours after analgesic drug administration may be instituted. These movements may be extended gradually, and active exercises may be started as symptoms subside. Often, the simple pendulum exercise of Codman, which uses the effect of gravity, is a good starting point. The trunk is flexed at the hips and lumbar spine, and the arm allowed to hang in approximately 90° of flexion; as the patient swings the body, the arm moves back and forth like a pendulum. This exercise is done first in the sagittal plane (flexion-extension) and later in the coronal plane (abduction-adduction). Eventually, full, active range-of-motion exercises can be encouraged, with or without assistance or resistance.[102]

Failure of these basic measures to control symptoms and to restore movement requires a more aggressive approach. The usual first step is the local instillation of corticosteroids. One should mix 25 to 100 mg hydrocortisone acetate or equivalent amounts of the newer preparations with 5 to 10 mL 1% procaine and inject into the point(s) of maximal tenderness. Local corticosteroids are not without potentially serious side effects, however.[97,103–105] In addition to the possible complication of systemic adsorption and the risk of infection,[106] intratendinous or peritendinous corticosteroids may interfere with healing,[107] may reduce the tensile strength of unaffected tendon, and ultimately may cause tendon rupture.[108] A transient, 24- to 48-hour increase in symptoms may follow local injection.[109] Little critical evidence suggests that corticosteroid injections are more or even equally effective as the basic conservative measures.[110] Empirically, however, when conservative treatment fails to produce satisfactory results, corticosteroid injections may be useful. Systemic administration of corticosteroids or adenocorticotrophic hormone (ACTH) has also been advocated, but it should be reserved for the most difficult therapeutic problems, in view of serious potential side effects. Operative intervention for degenerative tendinitis is rarely necessary.

In most cases, considerable improvement occurs within 2 to 6 weeks of therapy. Persistence of pain beyond this time should suggest a serious rotator cuff tear, and a thorough re-evaluation, including arthrographic study or MRI is indicated. After improvement, the physician should make every effort to identify the source(s) of shoulder trauma, such as employment or avocational abuse, and to suggest appropriate modifications in these activities to prevent recurrence.

Calcific tendinitis or bursitis presents a special problem. Acute symptoms probably represent a form of crystal-induced synovitis, so local corticosteroids early in the disease appear justified,[81] especially if conservative therapy, including NSAIDs, proves ineffective within the initial 24 to 72 hours of symptoms. Spontaneous resolution occurs in at least 30 to 40% of such patients, however. In those with chronic symptoms or recurrent attacks, removal of the calcific deposit may be indicated, achieved by needling the affected area, with or without concomitant instillation of corticosteroids and local anesthetics.[1,111] On occasion, surgical removal of the deposit is useful in providing relief,[83] but this procedure should be delayed as long as possible because recovery with resorption of the deposits is the rule in most patients.[1,84]

RUPTURE OF THE ROTATOR CUFF

Origin and Pathogenesis

Because of its critical role in stabilizing the glenohumeral joint, the musculotendinous (rotator) cuff may be torn by a variety of forces applied to the joint.[1,15,112] In younger individuals, as considerable force is necessary, tears usually follow direct trauma, unexpected falls on an outstretched arm, or the extreme stress of modern athletics. Much less force is required in older individuals, possibly as a result of pre-existent degenerative tendinitis and decreased vascularity that weakens the tendon structure. In such patients, tears are usually idiopathic or follow minor falls or the lifting of a weight with the arm fully extended or abducted.

Lesions of the rotator cuff are divided into complete or partial tears. Complete tears involve the full thickness of the cuff and the overlying subacromial bursa. As in degenerative tendinitis, the supraspinatus tendon is affected most commonly. Partial tears produce incomplete rents in the cuff, usually on the undersurface of the tendon near its insertion, and communication with the subacromial bursa does not occur.

Both conditions are more common than generally believed; partial tears are found in as many as 30% of cadavers.[1,15] The condition frequently goes unrecognized because the clinical and radiographic features of other forms of rotator cuff disease are so similar.

Clinical Features

The classic history of a fall or direct shoulder trauma in a patient complaining of shoulder pain and limitation of motion generally suggests the diagnosis of rotator cuff tear. Often, however, a specific event is not apparent, even after careful questioning. Persistence of symptoms in the shoulder of a patient who was previously diagnosed as having tendinitis, bursitis, or "strain" for more than 6 to 8 weeks should suggest a rotator cuff tear, especially in an older patient.

Acute full-thickness rupture produces immediate pain and muscle spasm. Weakness of the arm may be marked within hours to days of the injury, and both pain and weakness may persist for many months. On examination, motion is limited by pain and muscle spasm; in mild cases, pain may be present during active abduction in an arc between 70 and 100°. Local infiltration of an anesthetic agent abolishes pain, but not weakness. Although this finding is not entirely specific, it is suggestive of a rotator cuff tear. Frequently, the *drop arm sign* is positive: the arm is passively abducted to 90°, but it falls to the side when no longer supported by the examiner.[15,113] The patient cannot usually hold the arm in abduction at 90°, or the arm collapses to the side with just a little push downward by the physician. Occasionally, the actual tear can be palpated directly by an experienced examiner.

Diagnosis of the small complete tear or partial tear is more difficult. Persons engaged in overhead work, such as paperhangers and painters, or in lifting with extended arms, such as nurses and waitresses, appear to be predisposed to those lesions, just as they are to degenerative tendinitis. Although shoulder pain or discomfort is often present, it may be minimal. Frequently, the only complaint or physical finding is weakness in elevation of the arm, an important clue to diagnosis.

The symptoms and signs of rotator cuff rupture are similar to those of older "degenerative diseases" of the rotator cuff, but persistent pain and, especially, weakness in arm elevation, often with early (2 to 4 weeks) muscle atrophy, suggest this diagnosis. Full-thickness tears can be present for years without any symptoms, especially in the elderly person who demands little from his body.

Radiologic Examination

The plain radiograph in rotator cuff ruptures in younger individuals is usually normal. That it is abnormal in as many as 60% of older individuals may reflect pre-existent degenerative tendinitis.[87,88] Changes consist of erosion, sclerosis, pseudocysts, and osteophytes about the greater tuberosity at the site of insertion of the supraspinatus tendon. These changes are indistinguishable from those of degenerative tendinitis (Fig. 99–7). The severity of radiographic change may help predict which patient has a torn rotator cuff.[113a] Narrowing of the space between the humeral head and the acromion is a useful radiologic sign of superior subluxation of the humerus. This condition may be so extreme as to produce a "pseudoarticulation."

Complete ruptures of the rotator cuff may be confirmed by arthrography.[21,62,89] Leakage of contrast material into surrounding soft tissues or into the subacromial bursa is diagnostic of this condition (Fig. 99–8B). In partial ruptures, however, the arthrogram is normal, although, rarely, small irregularities or clefts are seen.[112] Partial rotator cuff tears or degenerative changes in the cuff are best visualized by double-contrast arthrography[22] or bursography.[30] MRI imaging may prove to be very useful in demonstrating a partial or complete rotator cuff tear, but available data are not conclusive.

Treatment

Early surgical repair of the acute, complete rupture, before granulation tissue forms and the edges of the torn capsule retract or calcify, appears to provide the best long-term result.[1,15,88,113–115] Treatment of patients with chronically torn rotator cuffs remains an unresolved problem.[54,115] Conservative therapy, as outlined in Table 99–2, may be effective, especially when supplemented with local corticosteroid injection.[116] Sixty percent of patients so treated show significant improvement,[115] although this figure may depend on which factors are assessed.[110] Newer surgical approaches have produced satisfactory results with reduction in pain and improvement in function in the majority of patients.[54,117–120] Although the greater size of the tear,[103,121,122] longer duration of symptoms,[117] or greater severity of symptoms[120] has been reported to adversely affect outcome, agreement on these issues is lacking.[118] Only one third of professional athletes who require surgical repair of a torn rotator cuff return to professional competition.[119] It should be emphasized that complete pain relief or return to full function are uncommon after surgery.[120–122]

BICIPITAL SYNDROMES

Origin and Pathogenesis

The long head (tendon) of the biceps brachii extends from its origin on the supraglenoid tubercle and posterior rim of the glenoid lip, through the articular capsule and intertubercular (bicipital) groove, and inserts on the posterior portion of the radial tuberosity. Within the joint capsule, the tendon functions as an accessory ligament and prevents upward and outward displacement of the humeral head. The tendon remains ensheathed in synovial tissue as it leaves the articular capsule until it traverses the bicipital groove (Fig. 99–1). The biceps supinates the forearm and assists in abduction and flexion of the arm.

The following four conditions are included in the category of bicipital syndromes: (1) tendinitis and tenosynovitis, (2) elongation of the tendon, (3) rupture, and (4) dislocation and subluxation.[15] Bicipital tendinitis or tenosynovitis is usually produced by constant friction within the intertubercular groove that causes attrition and inflammation of the tendon and its sheath. When these attritional changes are severe, the tensile strength of the tendon is lost, and elongation occurs. This condition may progress to frank rupture following even minimal effort. Dislocation or subluxation of the bicipital tendon is usually related to a congenitally shallow intertubercular groove or to traumatic disruption of the intertubercular ligaments that hold the tendon in the groove (Fig. 99–1).

Clinical Features

Bicipital tendinitis produces pain in the anterior shoulder that may radiate along the biceps into the forearm. Limitation of abduction or internal rotation may be present. Occasionally, a history of repetitive arm movements can be elicited, but it is not generally possible to identify a specific cause. On examination, several signs are useful in differential diagnosis. Manual side-to-side displacement of the bicipital tendon ("twanging") or simple palpation of the tendon in the bicipital groove during arm rotation may be associated with marked tenderness, indicating bicipital tendinitis. Pain along the course of the tendon produced by resisted supination of the forearm (Yergason's supination sign) or by resisted flexion at the elbow also suggests bicipital tendinitis. When elongation has occurred, pain may be minimal, but bicipital weakness is prominent. Absence of a palpable tendon and loss of normal bicipital contraction during resisted supination confirm this diagnosis. This syndrome can be differentiated from frank rupture, which causes persistent swelling of the biceps in the upper arm; in acute rupture, extravasation of blood is noted in the upper arm. Dislocation and subluxation are recognized by palpation of the tendon as it snaps or slides in and out of the bicipital groove.

Radiologic Examination

Radiographic studies of the shoulder in this condition are usually normal. Special views of the bicipital groove may show irregularity or osteophytes of the tuberosities in tendinitis or a shallow groove in a case of subluxation of the tendon. Arthrograms are rarely abnormal, but they may demonstrate irregularity or blockage of contrast medium within the tendon sheath. Ultrasonography may be useful in assessing this condition,[40,123] although data are incomplete.

Treatment

The initial program consists of the measures outlined in Table 99–2. In resistant cases, local instillation of corticosteroids into the tendon sheath is indicated and often produces a good result. Operative intervention is rarely necessary, but in persistent cases it may prove beneficial.[124] When a lax, elongated tendon does not respond to conservative therapy, resection of the intraarticular portion of the tendon with fixation of the distal end may restore useful function.

Pain from a dislocating or subluxing tendon may also respond to a conservative program and exercises. Surgical treatment may be necessary, however, to fix the tendon within the groove or to the proximal humerus. In acute bicipital rupture in younger patients, early surgical repair is indicated. If several weeks have passed or if the patient is elderly, a conservative approach may be better.

ADHESIVE CAPSULITIS

This disorder is also known as frozen shoulder, scapulohumeral periarthritis, periarthritis of Duplay, periarthritis of the shoulder, and check-rein shoulder.

Origin and Pathogenesis

Adhesive capsulitis is an entity once thought to be unique to the shoulder, although a similar process in the wrist suggests that other joints may be affected.[124a] It is characterized by pain and stiffness in the absence of any recognized intrinsic abnormality, although it may complicate any of the conditions previously discussed. In addition to following local soft tissue injuries, adhesive capsulitis may result from such problems as other trauma, coronary artery disease, chronic lung disease, pulmonary tuberculosis, diabetes mellitus, and cervical spinal syndromes.[34,125,126a,126b] The common denominator appears to be prolonged immobility of the arm.[1,127] A third factor, the "periarthritic personality," has been suggested as a necessary component for the development of the full syndrome, but psychologic testing of a large group of patients has failed to confirm this hypothesis.[34] A possible immunologic basis for adhesive capsulitis and an association of this syndrome with HLA-B27 have not been confirmed.[128–131]

The pathologic findings have been described by several investigators.[1,23] The joint capsule is thickened and is loosely adherent to the underlying humeral head; the normal capsular folds are obliterated. Microscopic changes include proliferation of synovial lining cells, fibrosis, and a mild, chronic inflammatory cell infiltrate. Such findings are inconstant, and at least 20% of cases have a normal histologic appearance.[23] As in other immobilized joints,[132] biochemical studies of the joint capsule have shown diminished glycosaminoglycan and water content.[132,133]

Clinical Features

Adhesive capsulitis is more common in women than in men, occurs in the fifth decade or later, and bears no relation to occupation.[1,15,34] The associated clinical conditions have already been enumerated. Both shoulders may be affected simultaneously or successively in some patients.[1,134]

The patient characteristically complains of the insidious onset of a diffusely painful and stiff shoulder. A specific precipitating event is rarely identified. The patient is unable to sleep because of pain and, perhaps as a result, is often anxious and irritable; hence the "periarthritic personality." Objective findings include diffuse tenderness about the glenohumeral joint and restricted active and passive motion in all planes. Injection of anesthetic agent locally may reduce pain but fails to improve mobility.

Three phases of the disease have been described.[1,134] The first, characterized primarily by pain and by gradually increasing stiffness, usually last 2 to 9 months. In the second phase, pain is less severe, and the patient often describes a vague discomfort in the shoulder, but stiffness is marked ("frozen shoulder"). This phase persists from 4 to 12 months. The final phase, lasting an additional 5 to 26 months, is one of gradual recovery of function ("thawing") and resolution of pain. *The natural progression of a frozen shoulder is a thaw.* The majority of patients are often fully improved within 12 to 18 months of the onset of this disorder,[15,127,134] although symptoms may persist for many more months.[15,134]

Radiologic Examination

Except for localized osteopenia in the shoulder after 1 to 2 months of disuse, the plain radiograph in adhesive capsulitis is generally normal.[23,135] An arthrogram may be useful in differentiating this disorder from other painful conditions, however.[21,24] The joint capsule typically appears contracted, with absence of the normal inferior reflection (axillary pouch), bicipital tendon sheath, and subscapular bursa.[15,21,24,89] The injectable volume of contrast material may be reduced by 60 to 90%. One report demonstrated some volume loss in 67% of cases, but marked volume loss (≥50%) was found in only 43%.[136] Intra-articular adhesions were not observed. It has been suggested that scintigraphy of the shoulder may be helpful in the diagnosis of adhesive capsulitis and related conditions and in predicting response to local corticosteroid injection.[31,126] Confirmatory studies and further characterization of scintigrams in normal shoulders,[36,112] as well as in injured shoulders,[37] are needed before this approach can be recommended, however. Over 90% of patients with adhesive capsulitis were reported to have abnormal scintigrams, but a number of them were found to have rotator cuff tears, indicating a mixed population.[137]

Treatment

The best treatment of adhesive capsulitis is prevention. Early mobilization of the shoulder(s) in any painful condition or chronic illness is essential, although this approach may not be effective in patients with hemiparesis.[30,138] Once the disorder is established, little critical evidence suggests that any therapeutic approach shortens the natural course of the disease. A conservative program should be instituted as early as possible (Table 99–2); however, if symptoms persist or worsen, a variety of therapeutic techniques have been advocated. These include local corticosteroid injections,[104,127,139,140] stellate ganglion blockade,[140] systemic corticosteroids or ACTH, antidepressant medications,[141] and exercises combined with transcutaneous nerve stimulation.[142]

In the patient with a resistant case or in those who have had symptoms for several months, I have achieved good to excellent responses with injection into the joint of a mixture containing 2.5 to 3.0 mL 1% procaine, 20 to 40 mg of prednisolone tertiary butyl acetate microcrystalline suspension, and 20 mL sterile saline solution, using maximum pressure on the injecting syringe, followed immediately by exercises.[143] A similar procedure, termed *infiltration brisement*, has been used successfully by others,[85] and simple pressure distension during arthrography appears to yield similar gratifying results.[144,145] Unfortunately, none of these regimens have been studied under controlled conditions. Manipulation of the shoulder under general anesthesia has been used in refractory cases with varied success,[146] but this form of therapy remains controversial because of the risk of considerable soft tissue damage, shoulder dislocation, or even humeral fracture.[85]

FIBROSITIS (FIBROMYALGIA)

Fibrositis, a poorly defined entity of unknown cause, appears to be most common in women between the ages of 35 and 50 years who are anxious and often fatigued. An aching pain, usually aggravated by stress or cold, damp weather, is reported in soft tissues between the shoulder and neck. Frequently, painful trigger points or actual small nodules can be found on careful palpation. Treatment by injection of local anesthetic agents with or without corticosteroids may be helpful, especially when accompanied by considerable reassurance and support. This condition is more fully discussed in Chapter 82.

ARTHRITIS

Although arthritis is an uncommon cause of isolated shoulder pain,[97] each of the shoulder girdle joints and bursae can be affected by the various arthritides described in this book. By far the most frequent is degenerative arthritis, which is found in the shoulders of approximately 30% of elderly subjects.[15] This disorder is almost always asymptomatic and is an incidental radiographic abnormality,[147,148] but unless it is considered in the differential diagnosis of shoulder pain, especially in patients of advanced age, error in diagnosis and treatment may occur.

Acromioclavicular Joint

The acromioclavicular joint is particularly prone to degenerative arthritis because of its rudimentary intra-articular disc,[1] which apparently has a protective function, and because of the repeated stresses to which this joint is exposed during overhead arm movements. The patient usually complains of shoulder pain, but often cannot localize it specifically; sleeping on the affected side may increase the pain. That elevation of the arm above shoulder level produces pain is an important clue to diagnosis because rotator cuff lesions cause pain at or below this level.

Inspection of the shoulder may reveal a distorted contour with prominence of the affected joint. Direct palpation over this area elicits tenderness. Active shrugging of the shoulder, passive adduction and flexion of the arm across the chest, and forcing of the humerus by passively raising the arm against a fixed clavicle isolate the movement of this join and aid in diagnosis when pain or crepitus is found. Confirmation of the diagnosis by plain radiography is helpful, but degenerative changes, although frequently present, are often asymptomatic.

Treatment consists of the standard conservative approach (Table 99–2) and restriction of the patient's movements to a painless, and usually functional, arc. Occasionally, intra-articular corticosteroid injections are of benefit. In difficult cases, arthroplasty may be necessary; this procedure generally provides a satisfactory result. Osteolysis of the distal clavicle may resemble acute arthritis of the acromioclavicular joint. This condition may follow traumatic shoulder injuries[149] or repeated minor traumas such as occur in weight lifters or those who work with arms extended.[150]

Sternoclavicular Joint

Arthritis in this small but important joint is rare. Post-traumatic arthritis, degenerative arthritis, and rheumatoid arthritis (RA) are the most common forms, although this joint is also affected in ankylosing spondylitis and related diseases. Two unusual forms of arthritis, *pustulotic arthro-osteitis*, reported in Japanese patients, and *sternoclavicular hyperostosis*, appear to involve the sternoclavicular joint particularly frequently. These entities are probably identical, differing only in the frequency of associated pustular lesions of the palms and soles.[151–153]

Patients often complain of pain, tenderness, and swelling of the sternoclavicular joint, although a careful history and examination may disclose an inflammatory polyarthritis. Maximal pain in the sternoclavicular joint is present during the midrange of arm elevation or on protrusion of the shoulders. Pustular lesions are found on the palms and soles in many patients.

Laboratory studies are normal or nonspecific, and synovial tissue is moderately inflamed in this condition.[154] The plain radiograph is often difficult to interpret because of overlying shadows. Scintigraphy may help localize the site of inflammation, and polytomography or CT may be necessary to identify erosive changes. Changes resembling diffuse idiopathic skeletal hyperostosis (DISH) or ankylosing spondylitis may be present elsewhere.[153]

Conservative treatment with NSAIDs or intra-articular corticosteroids is usually sufficient for symptomatic relief. Concomitant use of antibacterial agents may be of benefit.[154]

Several other disorders may affect the sternoclavicular joint, as noted.[155] Erosive changes occur in polymyalgia rheumatica (see Chapter 81) with variable frequency.[156,157] These also respond to conservative measures or treatment of the underlying condition. Surgical intervention is required occasionally, especially in post-traumatic arthritis.[158]

Glenohumeral Joint

Degenerative arthritis of the glenohumeral joint, which is uncommon, generally involves the glenoid rather than the humeral side of the joint.[1,159] This feature may be due to its nonweight-bearing nature, although considerable force is exerted across the joint.[1] On occasion, ischemic (avascular) necrosis or neurotropic arthropathy, usually secondary to syringomyelia, causes identical symptoms. Pain is rarely severe, and the patient is more likely to be concerned by the cosmetic appearance of the joint, such as after fracture and malunion, or by the restricted motion. Functional limitation can usually be overcome by increased movement in accessory joints and by avoidance of painful motion. Examination discloses a crepitant joint with diminished mobility, but minimal pain. Radiography may reveal an old fracture site or characteristic changes of osteoarthritis. Severe degenerative arthropathy is often associated with calcium pyrophosphate or basic calcium phosphate crystal deposits in synovial tissues or in shoulder joint cartilage; the shoulder is not involved in primary generalized osteoarthritis.

Again, treatment is conservative and symptomatic for the most part. Arthrodesis or arthroplasty may be indicated in certain instances, but the results, except pain relief, are less than ideal.

Milwaukee shoulder is a form of advanced degenerative arthritis involving the glenohumeral joint[160] as well as other large joints.[161] Patients are usually elderly women who complain of weakness and loss of motion in the dominant shoulder, but who are in little pain. Massive rotator cuff tears are present. Microcrystalline basic calcium phosphates are found in synovial fluids and have been implicated in the pathogenesis of this syndrome (see Chapter 110). This arthropathy resembles *dislocation, or cuff-tear, arthropathy* in some respects,[162,163] and both conditions seem related to shoulder joint instability. This condition may be associated with stress fractures of the acromion.[164]

OTHER "INTRINSIC" CAUSES OF SHOULDER PAIN

Athletic and Other Traumatic Injuries

A detailed discussion of traumatic injuries to the shoulder, whether produced by blunt or by penetrating forces, is beyond the scope of this chapter. Although such injuries are diagnosed with relative ease from the patient's medical history, cautious examination is essential to avoid overlooking associated soft tissue, bony, or neurovascular complications.[164a]

In addition to many of the conditions discussed previously, trauma may result in capsular ruptures with or without associated hemarthrosis, subluxation or dislocation, fractures, tendon avulsion (especially in adolescents), nerve injuries, and a variety of sprains and contusions. Obviously, knowledge of the type and mechanism of injury provides important clues to diagnosis; several of the more common injuries are considered briefly. Chronic repetitive trauma may lead to advanced degenerative changes in the glenohumeral joint.[165]

Falls. During unexpected falls, the arm is usually extended to cushion the impact, thereby transmitting the force upward to the shoulder and either anteriorly, as in backward falls, or posteriorly, as in forward falls. As a result, the rotator cuff or the joint capsule itself can be torn, or if sufficient force is applied, subluxation (dislocation), neurovascular injury or actual fracture may be present.

Dislocation of the glenohumeral joint is common, especially in athletic young men. Anterior dislocation occurs in 95% of these cases because the humeral head is usually thrust forward against the weak anteroinferior portion of the joint capsule. Posterior dislocations, although rare, are more likely to be overlooked.

Acute dislocation is readily diagnosed. The patient provides a history of recent injury followed by sudden, severe pain in the shoulder. He supports the injured arm at the forearm with the elbow angled outward. The deltoid muscle is often tense on palpation. A depression is observed on palpation just inferior to the acromion. Neurovascular injuries may accompany shoulder dislocation in up to 25% of cases;[166] careful examination of the neurologic and vascular systems is essential whether dislocation is suspected. Characteristic radiographic changes are present, although special views may be required.

Treatment consists of closed reduction within the first hours after dislocation. Thereafter, increasing restriction in shoulder motion may necessitate surgical repair.

Recurrent or habitual dislocations may follow the acute dislocation, especially in subjects under 20 years of age. Each subsequent dislocation may require less and less force, so even routine tasks, such as combing the hair, may cause it. A number of reasons for recurrent dislocation have been proposed, including an incompetent glenoid labrum, poor capsular ligament development, an enlarged humeral head, or a shallow glenoid fossa. A number of surgical approaches have been advocated for this problem.[1]

Direct Impact. The shoulder girdle is a prime target for falling objects, in part because of the protective flexion reflex of the neck and head. Depending on the point of impact, fractures, severe contusions, or nerve root or neurovascular injuries may occur.

Throwing. The overhead throw in baseball or football is a complex, coordinated series of movements. The shoulder girdle acts first as a base and then as a fulcrum to support and propel the object. The throw has four phases: (1) the preparation, in which the arm is extended, abducted, and externally rotated; (2) the phase of forward flexion and release; (3) the follow-through; and (4) the braking phase. Shoulder pain may result from repeated impingement, as well as from injury during the braking phase, because the joint capsule and rotator cuff are maximally stretched to prevent humeral dislocation. Tears may result, and when they occur repeatedly or are not allowed to heal, a periosteal reaction and, later, osteophytes develop.

The underhand throw, as in softball, bowling, or curling, is not as forceful, and injuries to the shoulder are far less common. Because this motion brings the anterior capsular mechanism and the bicipital apparatus into play, injuries to these structures may result. They are rarely serious, and rest is sufficient for complete healing in most cases.

Golfing. Usually considered a "safe" sport, golfing may result in injuries to the shoulder girdle. The most common injuries, resulting from recurrent stress at or superior to the horizontal plane, are those of the acromioclavicular joint. Symptoms and findings relating to this joint have previously been discussed; rest and other conservative measures are usually adequate.

Contact Sports. The causes of injury in the various contact sports such as football, hockey, basketball, and soccer are apparent. In addition to those injuries already discussed, fracture and dislocation, subluxation, and soft-tissue tears are common.

Congenital and Developmental Anomalies

Many bony, muscular, and articular anomalies of the shoulder region have been recognized.[1,167,168] Although they rarely cause serious pain, they may produce functional or cosmetic problems requiring medical intervention.

The most common congenital anomaly of the shoulder, *Sprengel's deformity*, or congenital elevation of the scapula, is often associated with other skeletal and soft tissue abnormalities. It is caused by a failure of the scapula to descend normally during ontogeny. Surgical treatment is arduous and is often less than satisfactory, and it is warranted only if the deformity produces serious functional disability or psychologic problems.[167]

Another congenital anomaly that occasionally produces shoulder pain is the Klippel-Feil syndrome, or congenital brevicollis, in which failure of segmentation or fusion of two or more cervical vertebrae may be associated with a cervical rib, other bony abnormalities, or an anomalous nerve and blood supply to the head, neck, and upper extremities.

Posture

Poor posture, a frequent cause of shoulder and neck pain, often goes unrecognized. It may result from working in a slumped position, from spinal malformation such as kyphosis or spondyloarthritis, from psychologic difficulties, from chronic illness with reduced muscle tone, or from a combination of these and other factors. Whatever the cause, abnormal posture places undue stress on the suspensory or mooring muscles of the upper extremity, especially the trapezius, rhomboid, and latissimus dorsi muscles. It may be difficult to identify this cause of shoulder pain because symptoms often develop hours after the patient has left work, and only a careful medical history reveals the source. Chronic aberrant posture is readily apparent. The patient complains of pain in the shoulder girdle, although this pain may radiate widely.

Correction of work or living habits, postural instruction, and physiotherapy usually produce improvement, but braces or supports are occasionally required.

NEUROLOGIC CAUSES OF SHOULDER PAIN

Brachial Plexus Injuries

Trauma is the most common cause of isolated brachial plexus lesions.[1,169,170] These injuries may result from penetrating wounds such as stab or gunshot wounds; blunt trauma, as from falling objects; external pressure, such as from backpacks; or stretch injuries, either obstetric or from machines. Surgery and radiotherapy also may produce brachial plexus injuries.[171] The clinical picture varies, depending on the specific site and branch affected; however, loss of motor function, rather than pain, is usually the predominant complaint. Involvement of cervical roots 5 and 6 is common and produces weakness in the deltoid, biceps, and rotator cuff muscles, so abduction and rotation of the arm are altered. When pain does occur in brachial plexus injuries, it often has a burning or causalgic quality, which represents an adverse prognostic sign.

Peripheral Neuropathy

Localized peripheral nerve lesions are usually traumatic in origin, but other factors may contribute to or produce them directly, such as vasculitis, metabolic derangements, heavy-metal toxicity, and vitamin deficiencies.[1] As with brachial plexus injury, peripheral neuropathies generally result in loss or decrease in motor function, but rarely in pain. The *suprascapular nerve* may be *entrapped* during scapular fractures or by compression of the nerve as it traverses the notch of the scapula.[1,172,173] Lesions of the axillary nerve are most often produced by blunt or penetrating trauma,[174] as well as by traumatic shoulder dislocation. Injuries of the suprascapular nerve, which supplies the infraspinatus and supraspinatus muscles, or of the axillary nerve, which supplies the deltoid muscle, weaken abduction but do not eliminate it.

Neuralgic Amyotrophy (Brachial Plexitis, Parsonage-Turner Syndrome)

This rare disorder has received scant attention in the literature in the United States.[14,175] It appears to be an actual peripheral neuropathy with "causalgic" features in patients recovering from a variety of serious illnesses. Characteristically, the patient has sudden pain in and about the shoulder, followed in several days to weeks by muscle weakness or paralysis, again usually in the shoulder region. Spontaneous recovery generally occurs, and no specific treatment exists.

EXTRINSIC CAUSES OF SHOULDER PAIN

Few causes of shoulder pain are truly extrinsic, except referred pain. A variety of systemic inflammatory or metabolic diseases is considered under this category because shoulder pain or disability is a single manifestation of the broader disease process. Such diseases in fact produce intrinsic shoulder lesions.

Arthritis

Virtually all forms of generalized arthritis can, and often do, affect the shoulder girdle joints and the bursae. RA and osteoarthritis are most common. These and the other arthritides are discussed elsewhere and need not be considered here. Over 90% of unselected patients with RA have had shoulder pain, and 30 to 40% have erosive disease in the glenohumeral, acromioclavicular, and sternoclavicular joints.[147,176,177] Similarly, radiographic evidence of osteoarthritis in these joints is common, especially in patients with osteoarthritis in other joints.[147]

Avascular Necrosis

Avascular (ischemic, aseptic) necrosis of the humeral head is rarely an isolated finding in the shoulder. It usually occurs in patients with other diseases, as discussed in Chapter 100.

Polymyalgia Rheumatica

Polymyalgia rheumatica, a chronic systemic disease of unknown origin, primarily affects individuals in their sixth decade or older and is discussed in Chapter 81. Pain and stiffness occur in both the shoulder and the pelvic girdles, but symptoms may be present in only one girdle. Erosive changes may be present in the sternoclavicular joints.[156,157]

Muscular Diseases

Polymyositis, the muscular dystrophies, and various other myopathies frequently affect the upper limb girdle muscles. Pain is rarely a major symptom, but weakness and disability may cause the patient to seek medical attention.

Metabolic Diseases

Diabetes Mellitus. The prevalence of certain disorders of the shoulder, such as degenerative and calcific tendinobursitis,[60,61,146,178] degenerative arthritis,[60] and adhesive capsulitis,[125,126] is increased in patients with diabetes mellitus. Limitation of shoulder mobility has been found in 50% of unselected diabetic patients.[179] Adhesive capsulitis was diagnosed in 19% of these patients (versus 5% of normal and control subjects). Adhesive capsulitis often is associated with *cheirarthropathy* in diabetic subjects. The latter condition is characterized by waxy skin, skin and connective tissue induration, and finger flexion contractures.[180] The recent observation of improved joint mobility following aldose reductase administration[181] supports the hypothesis that reversible metabolic changes in periarticular connective tissues account for the joint changes observed in diabetes mellitus (see Chapter 115).

Gout and Pseudogout. Crystal-induced synovitis may occur in any of the shoulder girdle joints. Gouty arthritis is rare,[182] whereas pseudogout is seen in 25 to 50% of affected subjects, at least by the radiographic findings of calcium pyrophosphate deposition (see Chapter 109).[183]

Hyperparathyroidism. Patients with hyperparathyroidism may develop a number of musculoskeletal complaints. In addition to a distinct hyperparathyroid arthropathy, these patients may have pseudogout, resorption of the distal clavicle, or formation of cystic brown tumors in the clavicle, humerus, or other long bones. With the greater use of biochemical screening studies and the earlier recognition of this disease, articular complications are far less common than formerly.

Other Disorders. Shoulder arthropathy may be found in patients with other metabolic diseases including hemachromatosis, alkaptonuria, ochronosis, Wilson's disease, and amyloidosis.

Neurologic Diseases

Perception of pain at a site remote from the area of irritation is considered referred pain. Attention was focused on this cause of pain by the classic experiments of Kellgren and Lewis, who injected hypertonic saline solution into interspinous ligament or specific muscle groups and mapped out the location and extent of resulting pain. These researchers found that pain frequently radiated distally, but always within the same sensory root segment. The various causes of neurologic pain discussed under the category of "extrinsic" are all examples of referred pain.

Cervical Nerve Root Compression. Compression of a cervical nerve root is commonly a result of degenerative arthritis or spondylopathy. Other causes include spinal infection, especially tuberculosis, primary or secondary neoplasms, spondyloarthritis, fractures, subluxations, or congenital anomalies.

Because the fifth and sixth cervical vertebrae are usually affected, complaints of shoulder and neck stiffness and aching are common. Pain may be increased by moving the neck and by coughing and sneezing, which stretch the affected nerve root. Objective evidence of motor or sensory nerve involvement, or changes in tendon reflexes, and of muscle wasting provides clues to diagnosis.

Radiographic evidence of degenerative arthritis is common in subjects beyond the age of 50 years and must be interpreted cautiously unless definite neuroforaminal encroachment is present. In patients with a herniated disc, the plain radiograph may be entirely normal, and diagnosis depends on myelographic or CT study.

These and other features of the cervical syndrome, which represents the most common extrinsic cause of shoulder pain, are discussed fully in Chapter 92.

Spinal Cord Lesions. Other lesions of the cervical spine and of the spinal cord itself may cause pain to be referred to the shoulder. These lesions include traumatic injuries; infections such as tuberculosis, herpes zoster, and poliomyelitis; syringomyelia; tumors; and various vascular anomalies. Patients with herpes zoster also may lack shoulder abduction when the C5-C6 nerve roots are affected.

Viscerogenic (Viscerosomatic) Pain. Pain is referred to the shoulder from deeper somatic or visceral structures by intrasegmental transmission. Most common are lesions along the course of the phrenic nerve, originating from C4 primarily, with fibers from C3 and C5, or from the diaphragm, which it supplies. The diaphragm can be irritated by many conditions involving the mediastinum, and pericardium, the inferior pulmonary segments, the liver, and especially the biliary tract. Other visceral diseases that refer pain to the shoulder are myocardial ischemia, pulmonary infarction or neoplasm, perforated intra-abdominal or pelvic viscera, peptic

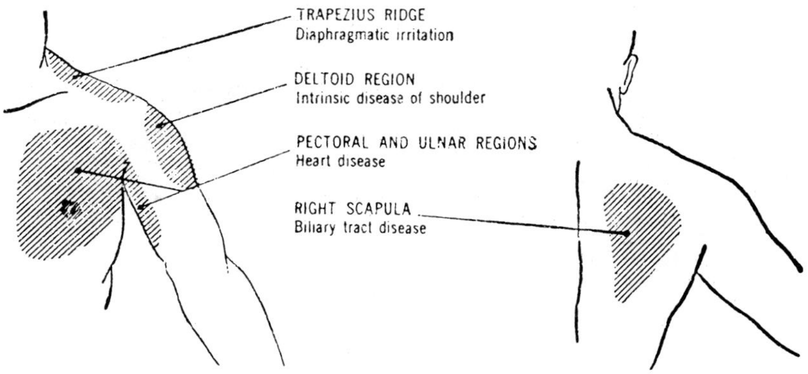

FIGURE 99–10. Sites of reference about the shoulder in viscerogenic pain. (From Morgan. Courtesy of Modern Medicine.)

esophagitis or esophageal spasm, and dissecting aortic aneurysm (Fig. 99–10). Referred pain to the shoulder may be the sole symptom of serious distant disease.

THORACIC OUTLET SYNDROME(S)

The region through which the neurovascular supply of the upper extremity exits the neck and thorax to enter the axilla constitutes the thoracic outlet.[184,185] It actually represents a series of narrow, fixed passages, each of which affords opportunity for compression of the neurovascular bundle. Symptoms and signs vary, depending on the nature and position of the obstruction. The manifestations include a cervical rib, anomalies of the first rib, interscalene muscle compression, and other rarer entities collectively termed the thoracic outlet syndrome.

ANATOMY AND PATHOPHYSIOLOGY

The anatomic relationships of the thoracic outlet are complex but are considered briefly.[1,184] The clavicle conveniently divides the region into three segments, supraclavicular, retroclavicular, and infraclavicular. Each is associated with certain structural or functional abnormalities that may compress the neurovascular bundles.

In the supraclavicular segment, in the posterior triangle of the neck, the subclavian artery and the brachial plexus lie between the anterior and posterior scalenic muscle masses. The subclavian vein is situated in front of the anterior scalene muscle here and therefore is separated from the artery and the plexus; it joins them at the level of the clavicle. Two major sources of neurovascular compression are seen in this segment. Interscalenic compression, also known as *scalenus anterior syndrome*, or Naffziger's syndrome, is caused by minor variations in the size, contour, or sites of insertion of the scalene muscles, with resultant narrowing of the already small interscalenic triangle. The presence of a cervical rib, found in approximately .6% of the population,[184] may also compromise the neurovascular supply

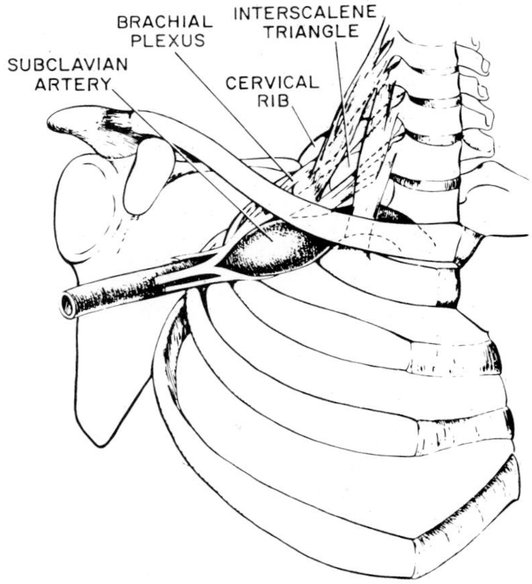

FIGURE 99–11. Thoracic outlet syndrome produced by a cervical rib; poststenotic dilatation of the subclavian artery is present.

in this segment by angulating the bundle or by narrowing the interscalene triangle (Fig. 99–11).

In the retroclavicular space, the neurovascular bundle, now joined by the subclavian vein, passes between the clavicle anteriorly and the first or thoracic rib posteriorly (Fig. 99–11). Compression in this segment is produced by a variety of conditions that narrow this space, such as clavicular fracture or its complications of malunion or exuberant callus formation, congenital anomalies of the clavicle or first rib, external pressure from heavy weights or packs, and poor posture. These conditions are termed the *costoclavicular disorders*.

The infraclavicular segment of the neurovascular bundle is situated behind (beneath) the pectoralis minor tendon and the clavipectoral fascia and in front of the subscapularis, from which it is separated by abundant areolar tissue. The considerable variation in the structural relationships of this region that occurs with nor-

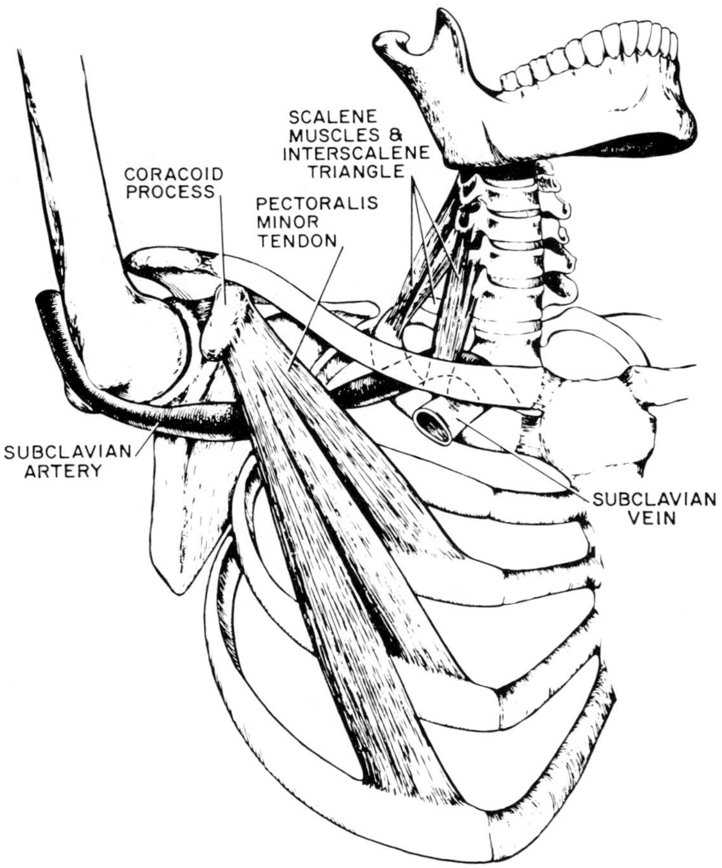

FIGURE 99–12. Thoracic outlet syndrome produced by hyperabduction maneuver; note compression beneath the pectoralis minor tendon.

mal arm motion may result in neurovascular compression, the so-called clavipectoral disorders. The most common is the hyperabduction syndrome, in which the neurovascular bundle is pulled around the pectoralis minor tendon during abduction, to create a pulley-like effect (Fig. 99–12). This hyperabducted position was well known to soldiers in the past as a method of controlling upper extremity bleeding. It is usually seen in patients who sleep with arms hyperabducted, that is, folded under the head, or who are engaged in occupations requiring this position for prolonged periods, such as automobile mechanics and painters.

Clinical Features

Symptoms of the thoracic outlet syndrome may be variable and intermittent, depending on the role of fixed anatomic abnormalities, shoulder movement, or combinations of these factors.[184–186] Pain in the shoulder or arm is characteristic of the syndrome, although it is present in only 70% of patients.[186] When neural in origin, the pain is segmental in distribution, usually in the ulnar segment because it roots, C8 and T1, are lowermost and more readily compressed, and is often described as a dull aching or burning sensation. This pain is almost always associated with paresthesias and numbness. Objective findings include diminished sensation, muscle weakness, or atrophy. When the pain is vascular in origin, it is vague and poorly localized and is described as a fullness or numbness. One may see associated objective findings of edema, color and temperature change, Raynaud's phenomenon, and dilatation of the superficial veins of the arm, shoulder, and neck.

A careful medical history may reveal typical patterns of aggravation and relief of symptoms. For example, symptoms present on awakening may be produced by placing the hands beneath the head or pillow during sleep. Occupation may be a factor when symptoms develop during the day or early evening in those who work overhead, such as automobile mechanics and painters. Symptoms that occur on weekends or vacations may be traced to sporting habits, as with backpackers who compress their costoclavicular space with heavy shoulder weights. Certain large-breasted women also may experience compressive symptoms as a consequence of brassiere-strap pressure.[187] Although poor upper back and neck posture have long been recognized to contribute to compression of the neurovascular bundle, a particular group of subjects with long necks and low-set shoulders that appears to be at increased risk has been described.[188]

The presenting complaint may represent a complication of neurovascular compression. A cool, cyanotic, or pallid extremity, with or without Raynaud's phenomenon, ulceration, or frank gangrene, may occur consequent to arterial obstruction or thrombosis. Postobstructive arterial dilatation may be recognized as a supraclavicular mass. Venous obstruction produces edema, an increased girth in the affected arm, dilation and tortuosity of superficial veins, or venous thrombosis (Paget-Schroetter syndrome).

Diagnosis and Differential Diagnosis

Diagnosis depends on a thorough medical history and physical examination to reveal the typical clinical features of neurovascular compression.[184,185] Several special tests may be helpful in confirming the diagnosis and in localizing the site of obstruction. The *Adson maneuver*, which narrows the interscalene triangle, is performed with the patient holding his breath in full inspiration and then fully extending his neck and rotating it toward the side examined. The *costoclavicular maneuver* diminishes the costoclavicular space and is effected by bracing the shoulders posteriorly and inferiorly, the exaggerated military posture. The *hyperabduction maneuver* for hyperabduction syndrome is performed by abducting the arms 180° in external rotation. A positive test result reproduces the patient's symptoms and obliterates or dampens the radial artery pulse. Because the radial pulse is often reduced in normal subjects during these maneuvers;[185,186,189] this sign alone is insufficient for diagnosis.

Other studies may be useful in diagnosis and differential diagnosis. The plain radiograph of the chest, cervical spine, and entire shoulder area may disclose specific bony abnormalities, such as cervical rib or clavicular fracture, that explain the patient's symptoms. Doppler studies, venography, arteriography, and plethysmography may be useful as well, especially when performed during the foregoing postural maneuvers.[186,189,190] Determination of nerve conduction velocities across the thoracic outlet, elbow, and wrist may also help in diagnosis and differential diagnosis, but must be interpreted cautiously.[191] Somatosensory-evoked potentials across the thoracic outlet (Erb's point) may reveal poorly formed waves, supporting the diagnosis.[192]

Depending on whether neurologic or vascular signs predominate, several conditions may enter into the differential diagnosis. Some of these are listed in Table 99–3. When the thoracic outlet syndrome is suspected, it is essential that the diagnosis be established promptly, so appropriate therapy can be initiated.

TABLE 99–3. DIFFERENTIAL DIAGNOSIS OF THORACIC OUTLET SYNDROME

Primarily Neurologic Symptoms
Cervical spine syndromes
Spinal cord tumors
Syringomyelia
Entrapment neuropathy
Ulnar nerve (elbow)
Medial nerve (carpal tunnel)
Peripheral neuropathy
Brachial plexus neuropathy
Herpes zoster and postherpetic neuralgia
Primarily Vascular Symptoms
Arterial
Granulomatous arteritis, Takayasu's disease
Atherosclerosis
Embolic disease
Arterial aneurysms
Raynaud's phenomenon or disease
Venous
Thrombophlebitis
Obstruction, benign or malignant
Neurovascular Symptoms
Reflex sympathetic dystrophy syndrome

Treatment

Unless the disorder is complicated by serious obstructive vascular disease or neurologic findings, initial therapy of the thoracic outlet should be conservative. Reassurance, education, and postural retraining to reduce thoracic outlet compression are of prime importance and are sufficient in most patients.[185,186,193] Usually, these measures are combined with physiotherapy to reduce muscle spasm and to strengthen the suspensory muscles, such as the rhomboid, levator scapulae, and trapezius muscles. In patients with severe or refractory disease, operative intervention is indicated. Careful preoperative assessment is imperative, however, because more than one site of obstruction may be present.

REFLEX SYMPATHETIC DYSTROPHY SYNDROME

The unusual complex of symptoms constituting reflex sympathetic dystrophy syndrome (RSDS) was first isolated by S. Weir Mitchell and his colleagues Moorehouse and Keen during the American Civil War,[194] although several cases with similar features had been reported earlier. Later, Mitchell introduced the term *causalgia*, derived from the Greek words for "heat" and "pain," to describe the peculiar burning pain so characteristic of this disorder.[195–197] Unfortunately, the confusing array of terms and designations for the syndrome that appeared in the years following Mitchell's classic studies created considerable uncertainty as to its very nature and existence (Table 99–4).

The exact prevalence of RSDS is unknown. Data from several studies suggest that it is frequent in patients with coronary artery disease (5 to 20%),[198,199] in patients with hemiplegia (12 to 21%),[200,201] in patients with Colles' fracture (.2 to 11%),[202–204] and in patients with peripheral nerve injury (3%) or other forms of traumatic injury (.5%).[205] Although emphasis on early mobilization following fractures, myocardial infarction, and stroke has reduced the frequency of this complication, it has not been eliminated.[200,203,206]

TABLE 99–4. SYNONYMS FOR THE REFLEX SYMPATHETIC DYSTROPHY SYNDROME

Causalgia, major or minor
Acute atrophy of bone
Sudeck's atrophy
Sudeck's osteodystrophy
Peripheral acute thromphoneurosis
Traumatic angiospasm
Traumatic vasospasm
Post-traumatic osteoporosis
Postinfarctional sclerodactyly
Shoulder-hand syndrome
Shoulder-hand-finger syndrome
Reflex dystrophy
Reflex neurovascular dystrophy
Reflex sympathetic dystrophy
Algodystrophy
Algoneurodystrophy

TABLE 99–5. CONDITIONS ASSOCIATED WITH THE REFLEX SYMPATHETIC DYSTROPHY SYNDROME

Trauma, major or minor
Fractures, especially Colles' fracture
Primary central nervous system disorders
Cerebrovascular disease with hemiplegia
Hemiplegia of other causes
Convulsive disorders (?)
Spinal cord lesions
Cervical spine disease, such as arthritis or discogenic disorders
Peripheral neuropathy
Herpes zoster with postherpetic neuralgia
Ischemic heart disease
Painful lesions of the rotator cuff
Pulmonary tuberculosis
Antituberculous drug administration
Barbiturate and other anticonvulsive drug administration
Hysterical personality (?)

ORIGIN

Many diseases, precipitating events, or drugs have been associated with RSDS (Table 99–5). They are thought to provoke the syndrome though reflex neurologic mechanisms, although their exact role in its pathogenesis remains obscure. It is difficult, if not impossible, to determine the relative frequency of these factors in initiating the syndrome because of selection factors in reported series. In surgical practice, trauma is clearly the most common precipitant, especially fractures or peripheral nerve injuries. In medical practice, although trauma, often minor, still ranks as the leading provocative event, myocardial ischemia, cervical spinal or spinal cord disorders, and a variety of cerebral lesions are also common. These findings are shown in Table 99–6, in which several studies are compared. Two points are worthy of note. First, in over 25% of patients, a definitive precipitating event could not be identified. Second, cervical discogenic disease is so common in this age group that its significance remains uncertain; before considering this as an "associated disease," definite evidence of nerve root impingement should be present.

CLINICAL FEATURES

Both sexes are affected equally in RSDS except when the provocative cause is sex-related, such as myocardial ischemia in men. No predilection exists for the dominant side. In medical practice, the syndrome is far more common in patients over the age of 50 years (Table 99–6), probably because of the foregoing disease associations. Children and younger individuals are not spared.[215–220]

The fully developed syndrome is usually characterized by pain and swelling in the distal extremity, trophic skin changes, and signs and symptoms of vasomotor instability (Table 99–7). The pain is often severe and burning, or causalgic, and it generally involves the entire hand or foot. Other sites are less commonly affected; the syndrome may be segmental in distribution, involving one or two rays of the hand or foot (radial form),[221,222,222a] knee,[223–225] or hip,[226,227] or a portion of bone (zonal form), such as part of the femoral head.[221] Patients may wrap an extremity in wet dressings to protect it and to reduce the pain. Objective examination may disclose an exquisitely tender hand or foot, which the patient withdraws at the slightest touch. Tenderness is generalized, but is most severe in the periarticular tissues.[228] Tenderness may be further characterized by *allodynia*, pain due to "non-noxious stimuli" (light touch), or *hyperpathia*, pain persisting or increasing after mild or light pressure.[229,230] Several investigators have suggested that the presence of severe, burning pain, allodynia, and hyperpathia may be sufficient for diagnosis.[231,232] Pitting or nonpitting edema is usually present and is localized to the painful and tender region; again, this feature appears to be more pronounced in the periarticular areas.[228,230] When RSDS occurs in the upper extremity, the patient may have associated pain and limitation of motion in the ipsilateral shoulder (*shoulder-hand syndrome*) (Fig. 99–13).

Vasomotor or sudomotor disturbances vary from patient to patient or within the same patient at different times. Occasionally, frank Raynaud's phenomenon occurs, but vasodilation or vasoconstriction is more common. Locally, increased sweating, hyperhidrosis, may be noted or reported by the patient and is an important diagnostic sign. Dystrophic changes in the skin gradually develop (Table 99–7). Ultimately, atrophy of the skin and of the subcutaneous tissue produces a shiny, thinned appearance. Contractures of the fingers and palmar fascia, Dupuytren's contracture, may eventually occur, leaving a claw-like, deformed hand.

RSDS may be complicated by a severe movement disorder characterized by focal dystonia and increased muscle tone and reflexes.[232a,232b] These may be quite painful. RSDS often is complicated by myofascial pain proximal to the involved site (hip or shoulder girdle), causing patients to be concerned about ascending RSDS.

TABLE 99–6. ESTIMATED FREQUENCY OF ASSOCIATED CONDITIONS IN THE REFLEX SYMPATHETIC DYSTROPHY SYNDROME

STUDY	NO. OF PATIENTS	AGE	BILATERAL INVOLVEMENT (%)	FRACTURE	PERIPHERAL NERVE INJURY	OTHER TRAUMA	MYOCARDIAL ISCHEMIA	CENTRAL NERVOUS SYSTEM DISEASE	SPINAL INJURY OR DISCOGENIC DISEASE	IDIOPATHIC OR MISCELLANEOUS CONDITIONS
Acquaviva et al.[207]*	585	51	10	216	23	179	3	16	0	148
Evans[206]	57	—	—	12	1	26	0	1	2	15
Johnson and Pannozzo[209]	76	59†	18	6	0	15	10	18	13	14
Kozin et al.[210]	11	56	18	0	0	1	1	2	3	4
Kozin et al.[197]	32‡	—	—	4	3§	10§	0	6	2	7
Pak et al.[206]	140	54	—	28	0	40	12	3	3	43
Patman et al.[211]	113	44†	—	41	0	57	0	0	0	15
Rosen and Graham[212]	73	63	30	1	0	5	27	9	14	17
Steinbrocker and Argyros[139]	146	>50	25	0	0	15	30	11	29	61
Subbarao and Stillwell[213]	125	54¶	10	31	24	25	4	6	0	35
Thompson[214]	17	>50	47	0	0	1	2	7	1	6
Totals										
Number	1375	—	—	339	51	374	89	79	67	376
Percentage	—	—	23	25	4	27	6	6	5	27

* Patients diagnosed as "algodystrophy"; number with "definite" diagnosis uncertain.
† Estimated average age.
‡ Definite and probable diagnosis.
§ Two patients had peripheral nerve injury associated with fractures.
¶ Median age.

TABLE 99–7. REVISED CLASSIFICATION AND CLINICAL CRITERIA FOR THE REFLEX SYMPATHETIC DYSTROPHY SYNDROME

DEFINITE
1. Pain associated with allodynia or hyperpathia
2. Tenderness
3. Vasomotor and sudomotor changes
   - Cool, pallid extremity (vasospasm)
   - Warm, erythematous extremity (hyperemia)
   - Hyperhidrosis or hypertrichosis
4. Dystrophic skin changes
   - Shiny skin with loss of normal wrinkling
   - Atrophy
   - Scaling
   - Nail changes (color, friable)
   - Thickened palmar/plantar fascia
5. Swelling (pitting or nonpitting edema)

PROBABLE
1. Pain and allodynia
2. Vasomotor or sudomotor changes
3. Swelling

POSSIBLE
1. Vasomotor or sudomotor changes
2. Swelling

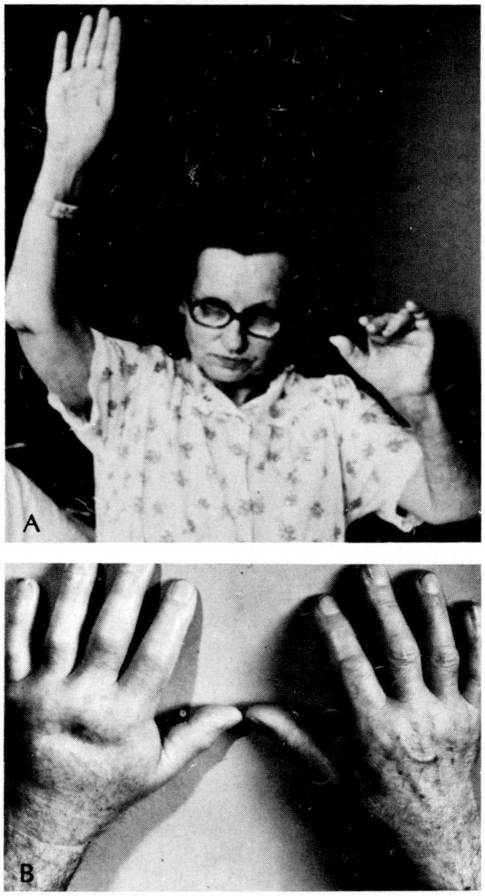

FIGURE 99–13. *A*, A patient with shoulder-hand syndrome who has limited shoulder motion and diffuse swelling of the hand. *B*, Note the flexion contractures of the hands and the presence of pitting edema.

The clinical course of RSDS has been divided into three overlapping stages.[233,234] The first, "acute" stage lasts 3 to 6 months and is characterized primarily by pain, tenderness, swelling, and vasomotor disturbances. In the second, "dystrophic" stage, these features resolve completely or partially, and trophic changes develop in the skin. This phase persists an additional 3 to 6 months. A third, "atrophic" stage then gradually evolves, in which skin and subcutaneous tissue atrophy and contractures predominate. Once this stage occurs, substantial reversal is uncommon, and the patient is left with a shiny, cool, contracted, and usually painless extremity.

Although staging of this syndrome is useful, it is often difficult to distinguish specific stages in an individual patient. More often, fluctuation between the first two stages occurs for weeks or months, until the atrophic and contractural changes gradually supervene. Therapy during the "active" period (stages 1 and 2) is essential; therapy during the last stage is rarely of benefit.

Incomplete (partial, limited, abortive, circumscribed) forms of this syndrome exist.[235] These types may include such diverse conditions as transient painful osteoporosis or osteolysis,[223,226,236] juvenile osteoporosis,[237,238] major or minor causalgia, segmental causalgia as in postherpetic syndromes, adhesive capsulitis or frozen shoulder, and idiopathic carpal tunnel syndrome or Dupuytren's contracture, especially when associated with a painful shoulder. Until the pathogenic mechanisms are understood and until more specific diagnostic tests are developed, the relation of these conditions to the reflex sympathetic dystrophy syndrome must remain uncertain. The incomplete category also includes patients who do not manifest all four clinical features evident in the classic syndrome (Table 99–6).[210] My colleagues and I have proposed criteria that allow such patients to be distinguished clinically and to be compared with others having overlapping symptoms or signs (Table 99–7).[210]

Bilateral involvement is generally thought to be present in 18 to 50% of patients (Table 99–6). Careful analysis of a small group of patients with the fully developed syndrome, however, has disclosed bilateral changes in all instances by clinical and radiologic methods.[210,239] This finding supports the concept that the syndrome is, in fact, "reflex" and is mediated by central neurologic mechanisms.

Laboratory studies, such as blood count and erythrocyte sedimentation rate, and other special studies are usually normal or show changes consistent with other associated conditions. The prevalence of hyperlipoproteinemia may be increased.[240,241] Unless the patient has had a specific nerve injury, electromyography and nerve condition velocity studies are normal.[211,242] Thermography,[242–245] as well as skin potential measurements,[246] have been advocated as diagnostic tests for this disorder. Diagnosis depends on the clinical and radiologic features (see following). Differential diagnosis includes local injury or inflammation, infection, or early RA and scleroderma. Either reflex sympathetic dystrophy syndrome or a condition that resembles it, termed *palmar fasciitis and arthritis*, may develop as a paraneoplastic syndrome.[247–249]

RADIOLOGIC FEATURES

Radiologic features include those evident on plain roentgenograms as well as those requiring newer radiographic techniques.[197,218,221,228,239,250–253]

Plain Radiography

The characteristic radiographic appearance of the reflex sympathetic dystrophy syndrome is a patchy or mottled osteopenia (Fig. 99–14), a finding recognized since the early descriptions of Sudeck[254,255] and Kienbock.[256] This appearance is not found in all cases,[210,212,228] however, nor is it pathognomonic of the syndrome because it may be present in simple disuse osteopenia, such as from hemiparesis or immobilization, or in other conditions.[250] Its patchy character is caused by irregular resorption of cancellous or trabecular bone.[250,253] In addition, fine-detail radiographic techniques have disclosed resorption of subperiosteal, intracortical, endosteal, and subchondral and marginal bone.[243] Subchondral bone resorption produces a form of "erosive" articular disease manifested either as cortical breaks, surface erosions, as may be seen in early RA, or a peculiar fragmentation of marginal bone, "crumbling" erosion (Fig. 99–14).[228,253] Late in the course of the illness, diffuse osteopenia occurs and gives the radiograph a ground-glass appearance.

In adults, once these changes are established, they appear to be irreversible, although this feature may depend on the duration of the disease.[252] In children, the potential for healing appears to be greater.[218]

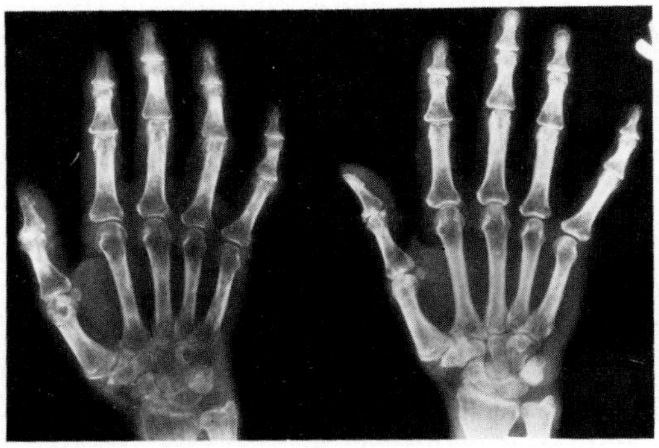

FIGURE 99–14. Fine-detail radiographs of a patient with the reflex sympathetic dystrophy syndrome illustrating progressive osteopenia at three months (right) and eight months (left) after the onset of symptoms.

Quantitative Bone Mineral Analysis

In RSDS, one sees an average loss of one third of the entire bone mineral content or cortical thickness in the affected extremity.[253] Treatment halts progression of the osteopenia, but it does not reverse it.

Scintigraphic Studies

The use of technetium-99m (^{99m}Tc) as the pertechnetate, which depends on the local blood pool, demonstrates increased periarticular uptake in the affected extremity (Fig. 99–15).[210,228,229,257–260] Frequently, uptake in the contralateral extremity is also increased, suggesting subclinical bilateral involvement.[202,229] Technetium-99m–labeled diphosphonate or polyphosphate uptake, which depends on local blood flow immediately after injection and on adsorption to bone later on, is also increased in the metaphysial regions of the bones on the affected, and to a lesser extent, on the contralateral side. In several reported cases, diminished radionuclide uptake was found in the affected extremity.[210,261] Scintigraphy may also be valuable in detecting incipient or subclinical reflex dystrophy.[262]

Rapid-sequence imaging immediately after radionuclide injection often demonstrates enhanced uptake in the affected extremity in patients with this syndrome,[210,239] and these findings indicate increased local blood flow.[253,263]

A number of studies have confirmed the value of scintigraphy in the diagnosis,[210,239,257,258,264] and possibly in the therapy,[210] of this syndrome. Studies are abnormal in 68 to 87% of subjects,[210,264] as well as in virtually all patients with transient osteoporosis syndromes, which often are clinically indistinguishable from RSDS. Radionuclide scans returned to normal in certain patients after successful treatment with systemic corticosteroids[210] or calcitonin[264a,264b] but not after treatment with NSAIDs.[264a] Demongeat et al. suggested three different stages of RSDS based on analysis of scintigraphic changes.[264b]

PATHOLOGY AND PATHOPHYSIOLOGY

The skin and subcutaneous tissues are usually normal or exhibit minor, nonspecific changes. Dupuytren's contracture is frequently present. Affected bone is hyperemic, and prominent osteoclastic activity is seen in the areas of patchy osteoporosis.[233,254,255,265] Fibrosis of the surface of affected cartilage may be observed.[265] Synovial tissue is abnormal in adhesive capsulitis.[197] The histologic changes consist of proliferation of synovial lining cells and small blood vessels, synovial edema, and subsynovial fibrosis (Fig. 99–16). Little or no inflammatory cell infiltrate is present.

Any explanation of the pathophysiologic features of the reflex sympathetic dystrophy syndrome must account for its peculiar clinical features, such as nonsegmental pain, trophic skin changes, and vasomotor insta-

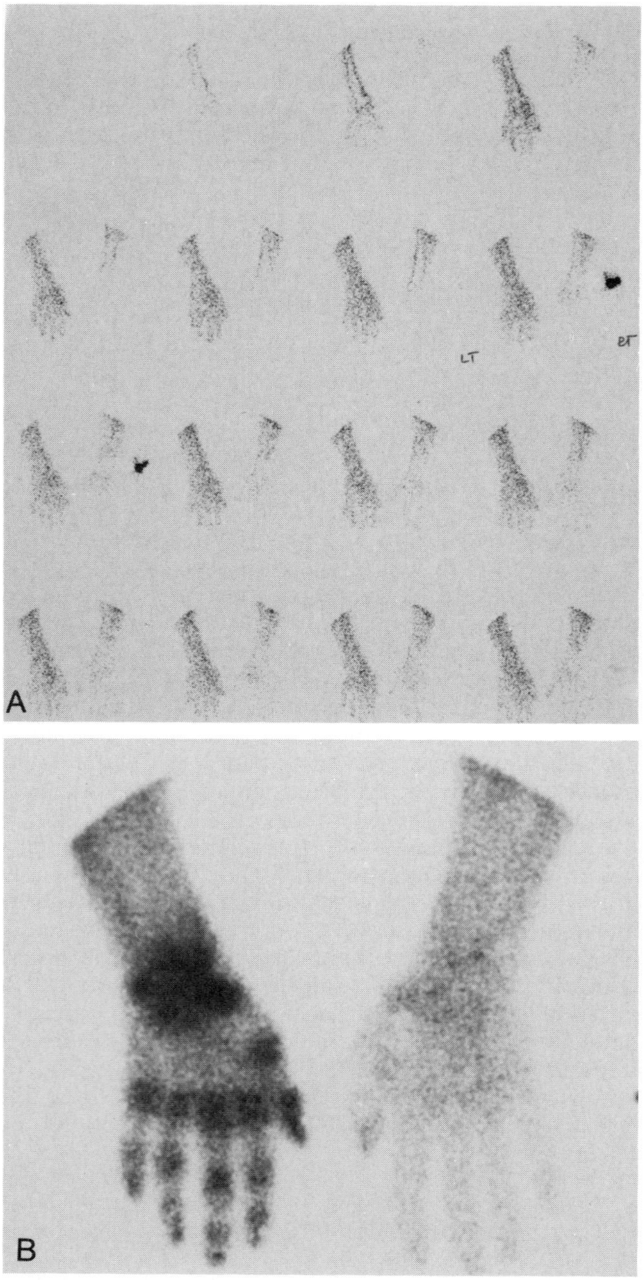

FIGURE 99–15. A three-phase bone scintigram in a patient with reflex sympathetic dystrophy syndrome affecting the left hand is illustrated. *A*, The characteristic changes are shown in the flow study in which there is more rapid accumulation of radionuclide in the left hand, and *B*, in the 2.5-hour delayed bone scan in which increased radionuclide is present in the periarticular tissues.

bility, its radiographic findings of patchy osteopenia, and its evidence of increased local blood flow.[233,243,266,267] Although a number of theories have been proposed, most suggest a disturbance of autonomic nervous system regulation to explain these diverse findings. Little true evidence of autonomic nerve dysfunction exists, however.

Moberg attributes RSDS primarily to a mechanical disturbance of venous and lymphatic flow.[268] He suggests that shoulder and hand movements are essential for fluid removal from the extremity, and any interference in this mechanism produces edema, further limitation of motion, disuse osteopenia, and, eventually, contracture formation. A second factor, sympathetic nervous system stimulation, occasionally contributes to the pain and limitation of motion when the syndrome is initiated by a traumatic, usually painful, injury. Although intriguing, especially with regard to the shoulder-hand syndrome, this hypothesis fails to account for the syndrome after painless, nonimmobilizing events, such as drug ingestion,[269,270] after myocardial ischemia with pain in the opposite arm,[212] or in isolated regions, for example, the hand or the patella.[223]

Theories supporting the primary involvement of the sympathetic nervous system are more popular and have been reviewed recently.[223,224] These may be divided into either the peripheral or the central hypothesis, depending on the site of injury. The central hypothesis was favored by De Takats and Steinbrocker and their co-workers,[234,235,265,271] who championed the theory of Livingston,[272] who originally proposed that a painful peripheral stimulus produced excessive, repetitive excitation of the internuncial neuron pool in the spinal cord. Spread of these impulses to adjacent areas in the spinal cord then activates efferent autonomic and motor nerves and results in increased blood flow, vasomotor changes, and other "dystrophic" changes in bone and soft tissues. These factors, in turn, produce further sensory input and establish a vicious cycle between central and peripheral mechanisms of pain and response. Livingston's theory may explain the RSDS in any location and may be extended to precipitants other than pain because changes in the central regulatory mechanism may be caused by drugs, stroke, or other provocative stimuli.

Noordenhos and others have offered an intriguing variant of this mechanism.[273] Two types of nerve fibers are suggested to exist: small fibers that carry the painful impulse and large fibers that inhibit this transmission. Normally, a delicate balance exists under central control, but a shift in this balance may result in excessive pain, either real or imagined, and may establish the vicious cycle already described. The beneficial effects of selective large-fiber stimulation in certain patients with causalgia support this proposal.[274,275]

More recently, the gate-control theory of pain, which combines many features of the aforementioned mechanisms, has achieved prominence.[276,277] In this model, a dynamic balance that exists between large, inhibitory and small, effector neurons is influenced by cognitive and perceptual processes in the central nervous system. Because the sympathetic nervous system impulses also feed into the same receptor center(s), stimulation of efferent sympathetic fiber may produce RSDS, by ascending "painful" sources such as trauma; by descending

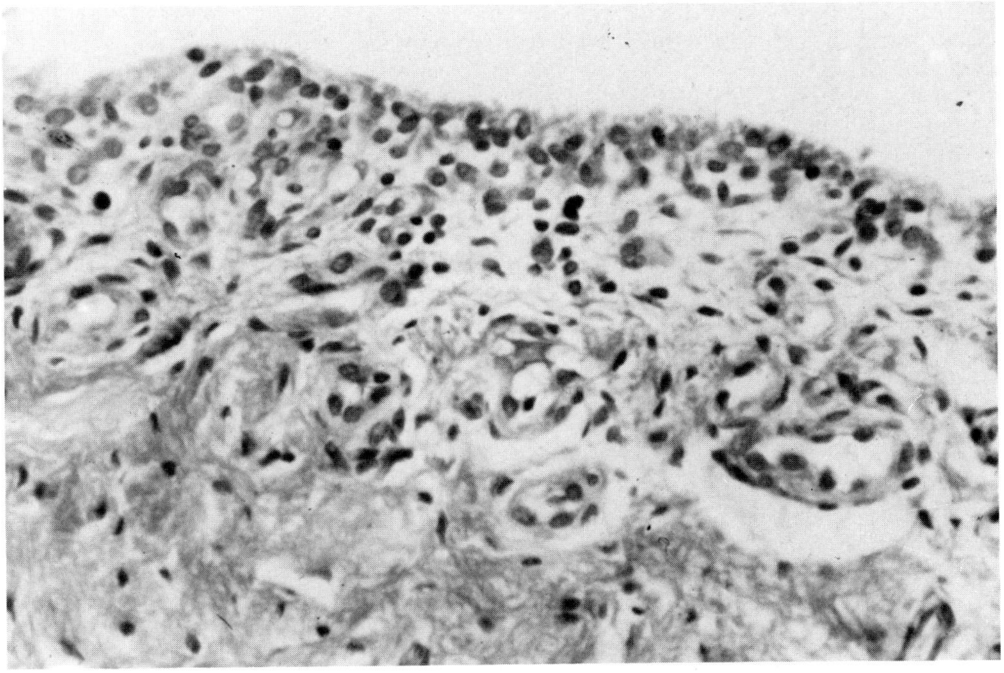

FIGURE 99–16. Photomicrograph of synovium of a metacarpophalangeal joint from a patient with the reflex sympathetic dystrophy syndrome, illustrating synoviocyte and vascular proliferation.

cognitive or perceptual mechanisms such as stroke, drugs, or trauma; or by direct irritation of the receptor center(s) such as by stroke, drugs, or cervical spine or spinal cord lesions.

Roberts extended this view by proposing that nociceptive inputs may excite wide-dynamic-range neurons in the spinal cord, causing these neurons to become sensitized to subsequent afferent input.[231] Afferent stimuli may be initiated by sympathetic nerves to produce a painful state or to maintain a painful state following injury. Alternatively, increased sympathetic activity may lower the threshold of nociceptor or mechanoreceptor function.

TREATMENT

Because the natural history of RSDS is to variable and unpredictable, results of the usual therapeutic approaches are difficult to interpret. Therapy appears to have little relation to the initiating or provocative event, the severity of trauma, or the stage of disease. It is generally thought that the earlier the institution of therapy, the better the result.[206,212] Rosen and Graham examined this problem carefully and found that only 20% of patients symptomatic for 6 months or longer had a good or excellent response to treatment, as compared with 43% of those with symptoms of shorter duration.[212] The overall response rate was poor, however; over 50% of their patients had significant pain or disability 2 to 6 years later. Other authors suggest that most patients recover in 6 to 24 months.[278,279]

Clearly, avoidance of the syndrome is the best treatment. Early mobilization following trauma[280] or myocardial infarction[199] may be helpful in this regard, although even this concept is controversial.[138,281] Once the disease process is established, a number of therapeutic approaches have been advocated, including exercises, various physical therapeutic techniques, sympathetic blockade, local or systemic corticosteroids, vasodilator drugs, α- or β-adrenergic drugs, and continuous elevation of the involved extremity. None are specific; all are most effective when used early. Unfortunately, even today, prolonged delays in recognition of the syndrome and in institution of therapy are common.[211]

The basic treatment program should consist of analgesic medications, local heat or cold packs, and exercises of the affected and contralateral extremities to improve motion. A favorable result may be expected in a majority of patients with these conservative measures if treatment is started early in the course of the disease,[206,209] especially in children.[215,220] More aggressive therapy is indicated if a satisfactory result is not obtained within 1 to 4 weeks. The most effective therapeutic measures are sympathetic blockade and administration of systemic corticosteroids.

Sympathetic blockade represents a rational attempt to block the vicious cycle of pain at an accessible site in the efferent pain pathway. Results of this approach are variable, although the patient may have partial or transient relief of pain.[208,211,282] Satisfactory control of symptoms, defined as a 50% relief of pain or a significant reduction in disability, can be expected in only 14 to 25% of patients,[142,172,199,208,211,283] although several authors report response rates as high as 50 to 100%.[204,282,284] My own experience with stellate ganglion blockade has been discouraging,[210] and Patman et al. found that all 41 causalgic patients treated with sympathetic blockade later required surgical sympathectomy.[211] Frequently, a series of daily or alternateday sympathetic blocks are required;[282] this approach should be abandoned if 3 to 5 successive blocks fail to provide lasting symptomatic relief. Patients who benefit from sympathetic blockade appear to be excellent candidates for surgical sympathectomy. Results of this procedure appear to be rewarding, both in reduction of pain and in restoration of motion.[208,211,285]

Other methods for interrupting sympathetic tone appear to be effective as well, including regional intravenous reserpine,[286–288] or guantehidine, which is not approved by the United States Food and Drug Administration,[83,289–291] or oral phenoxybenzamine.[292] β-Adrenergic blocking agents have been beneficial in some,[293,294] but not all,[286] patients.

Systemic corticosteroids are effective in controlling RSDS,[197,200,210,212,295–297] although the use of these agents is not without controversy.[298] Studies of high-dose corticosteroid treatment, using sensitive, quantifiable methods of assessment, showed improvement in a majority of patients with a reflex dystrophy.[197,210,296] These findings have been confirmed.[266] Although not all patients had a complete recovery, most experienced marked, lasting pain relief and restoration of function. Furthermore, progression of osteopenia appeared to be reduced in adults,[197] as well as reversed in a child.[218] Patients with positive scintigraphic evidence of the disease appeared to respond best to corticosteroids.[210]

Initial therapy should consist of 60 to 80 mg prednisone or an equivalent preparation daily *in 4 divided doses*. In 1 to 2 weeks, one can rapidly reduce the dose, with the aim of discontinuing corticosteroids entirely after 3 to 4 weeks of treatment. One often sees a mild, "poststeroid" exacerbation, which usually resolves within 10 days.[197,210] Occasionally, patients require retreatment, in which case a longer period of high-dose therapy, lasting 2 to 4 weeks, and a more gradual tapering program, lasting 4 to 8 weeks, are indicated. Rarely, a maintenance dose of prednisone, 5 to 10 mg on alternate days or 5 mg daily, is required to control symptoms permanently. Lower doses have been used successfully.[266] Intravenous injection of corticosteroids into the affected extremity may be an effective approach.[299]

Unlike the interruption of sympathetic pathways, no currently known theoretic mechanisms explain the efficacy of corticosteroids in RSDS. It is possible that these agents interfere with the action of peripheral mediators, which perhaps are prostaglandin-like substances, or they may modulate the transmission of neural impulses in the gate-control system or the internuncial pool.

Other agents, including griseofulvin and calcitonin, have been used effectively in patients with algodystrophy;[261] it is not clear whether all patients with this diagnosis fulfill the rigorous criteria of RSDS.

Recent studies employing transcutaneous nerve stimulation in patients with causalgia following nerve injuries have been encouraging,[300,301] although this technique has failed on occasion.[286] Again, the best responses were obtained in patients symptomatic for brief periods before treatment.

REFERENCES

1. DePalma, A.F.: Surgery of the Shoulder. 3rd ed. Philadelphia, J.B. Lippincott, 1983.
2. Boileau Grant, J.C., and Basmajian, J.V.: Grant's Method of Anatomy. 7th ed. Baltimore, Williams & Wilkins, 1965.
3. Inman, V.T., Saunders, J.B., and Abbott, L.C.: Observations on the function of the shoulder joint. J. Bont Joint Surg., *26*:1–30, 1944.
4. Conway, A.M.: Movements in the sternoclavicular and acromioclavicular joints. Phys. Ther. Rev., *41*:421–432, 1975.
5. Rothman, R.H., Marvel, J.P., and Heppenstall, R.B.: Anatomic considerations in the glenohumeral joint. Orthop. Clin. North Am., *6*:341–352, 1975.
6. Saha, A.K.: Dynamic stability of the glenohumeral joint. Acta Orthop. Scand., *42*:491–505, 1971.
7. Turkel, S.J. et al.: Stabilizing mechanisms preventing anterior dislocation of the gleno-humeral joint. J. Bone Joint Surg., *63A*:1208, 1981.
8. Poppen, N.K., and Walker, P.S.: Forces at the glenohumeral joint in abduction. Clin. Orthop., *135*:165–170, 1978.
9. Lucas, D.B.: Biomechanics of the shoulder joint. Arch. Surg., *107*:425–432, 1973.
10. Basmajian, J.V.: Muscles Alive: Their Functions Revealed by Electromyography. Baltimore, Williams & Wilkins, 1962, pp. 161–178.
11. Poppen, N.K., and Walker, P.S.: Normal and abnormal motion of the shoulder. J. Bone Joint Surg., *58A*:195–201, 1976.
12. Howell, S.M., Imobersteg, A.M., Seger, D.H., and Marone, P.J.: Clarification of the role of the supraspinatus muscle in shoulder function. J. Bone Joint Surg., *68A*:398–404, 1986.
13. Colachis, S.C., Jr., and Strohm, B.R.: Effect of suprascapular and axillary nerve blocks on muscle force in upper extremity. Arch. Phys. Med. Rehabil., *52*:22–29, 1971.
14. Booth, R.E., and Marvel, J.P.: Differential diagnosis of shoulder pain. Orthop. Clin. North Am., *6*:353–379, 1975.
15. Moseley, H.F.: Shoulder Lesions. 3rd ed. Edinburgh, Churchill Livingstone, 1969.
16. Badley, E.M., Wagstaff, S., and Wood, P.H.N.: Measures of functional ability (disability) in arthritis in relation to impairment of range of joint movement. Ann. Rheum. Dis., *43*:563–569, 1984.

16a. Bassey, E.J., Morgan, K., Dallosso, H.M., and Ebrahim, S.B.J.: Flexibility of the shoulder joint measured as a range of abduction in a large representative sample of men and women over 65 years of age. Eur. J Appl. Physiol., *58*:353–360, 1989.

17. Neer, C.S.: Anterior acromoplasty for the chronic impingement syndrome in the shoulder. J. Bone Joint Surg., *54A*:41–50, 1972.
18. Jobe, F.W., and Jobe, C.M.: Painful athletic injuries of the shoulder. Clin. Orthop., *173*:117–124, 1983.
19. Gerster, J.C. et al.: Tendon calcification in chondrocalcinosis. Arthritis Rheum., *20*:717–722, 1977.
20. Reichmann, S. et al.: Soft tissue xeroradiography of the shoulder joint. Acta Radiol. (Diagn.), *21*:572–576, 1975.
21. Freiberger, R.H., and Kaye, J.J.: Arthrography. New York, Appleton-Century-Crofts, 1979.
22. Goldman, A.B., and Ghelman, B.: The double-contrast shoulder arthrogram. Radiology, *127*:655–663, 1978.
23. Neviaser, J.S.: Adhesive capsulitis of the shoulder: A study of

the pathological findings in periarthritis of the shoulder. J. Bone Joint Surg., *27*:211–222, 1945.
24. Reeves, B.: Arthrographic changes in frozen and post-traumatic stiff shoulders. Proc. R. Soc. Med., *59*:827–830, 1966.
25. Hall, F.M. et al.: Morbidity from shoulder arthrography: Etiology, incidence, and prevention. Am J. Roentgenol., *136*:59–62, 1981.
26. Mink, J.H., Harris, E., and Rappaport, M.: Rotator cuff tears: Evaluation using double-contrast shoulder arthrography. Radiology, *157*:621–623, 1985.
27. Resnick, D.: Shoulder arthrography. Radiol. Clin. North Am., *19*:243–253, 1981.
28. Braunstein, E.M., and O'Connor, G.: Double-contrast arthrotomography of the shoulder. J. Bone Joint Surg., *64A*:192–195, 1982.
29. McGlynn, F.J., El-Khoury, G., and Albright, J.P.: Arthrotomography of the glenoid labrum in shoulder instability. J. Bone Joint Surg., *64A*:506–518, 1982.
30. Lie, S., and Mast, W.A.: Subacromial bursography. Radiology, *144*:626–630, 1982.
31. Bekerman, C. et al.: Radionuclide imaging of the bones and joints of the hand: A definition of normal and a comparison of sensitivity using ^{99m}Tc-pertechnetate and ^{99m}Tc-diphosphonate. Radiology, *118*:653–659, 1976.
32. Maxfirld, W.S., Weiss, T.E., and Shirler, S.E.: Synovial membrane scanning in arthritic disease. Semin. Nucl. Med., *2*:50–70, 1972.
33. O'Duffy, J.D., Wahner, H.W., and Hunder, G.G.: Joint imaging in polymyalgia rheumatica. Mayo Clin. Proc., *51*:519–531, 1976.
34. Wright, V., and Haq, A.M.M.M.: Periarthritis of the shoulder. I. Aetiological considerations with particular reference to personality factors. Ann. Rheum. Dis., *35*:213–219, 1976.
35. Genoe, G.A., and Moeller, J.A.: Normal shoulder variations in the technetium 99m polyphosphate bone scan. South. Med. J., *67*:659–662, 1974.
36. Sebbs, J.I., Vasinrapee, P., and Friedman, B.I.: The relationship between radiographic findings and asymmetrical radioactivity in the shoulder. Radiology, *120*:139–142, 1976.
37. Stodell, M.A. et al.: Radio-isotope scanning in the painful shoulder. Rheumatol. Rehabil., *19*:163–166, 1980.
38. Hodler, J., Fretz, C.J., Terrier, F., and Gerber, C.: Rotator cuff tears: Correlation of sonographic and surgical findings. Radiology, *169*:791–794, 1988.
39. Brandt, T.D., Cardone, B.W., Grant, T.H., et al.: Rotator cuff sonography: A reassessment. Radiology, *173*:323–327, 1989.
40. Miller, C.L., Karasick, Kurtz, A.B., and Fenlin, J.M.: Limited sensitivity of ultrasound for the detection of rotator cuff tears. Skeletal Radiol., *18*:179–183, 1989.
40a. Vick, C.W., and Bell, S.A.: Rotator cuff tears: Diagnosis with sonography. Am. J. Roentgenol., *154*:121–123, 1990.
40b. Middleton, W.D.: Status of rotator cuff sonography. Radiology, *173*:307–309, 1989.
41. Deutsch, A.L. et al.: Computed and conventional arthrotomography of the glenohumeral joint: Normal anatomy and clinical experience. Radiology, *153*:603–609, 1984.
42. Rafii, M. et al.: Athlete shoulder injuries. CT arthrographic findings. Radiology, *162*:559–564, 1987.
43. Beltran, J. et al.: Rotator cuff lesions of the shoulder: Evaluation by direct sagittal CT orthography. Radiology, *160*:161–165, 1986.
44. Wilson, A.J., Totty, W.G., Murphy, W.A., and Hardy, D.C.: Shoulder joint: Arthrotomographic CT and long-term follow-up with surgical correlation. Radiology, *173*:329–333, 1989.
45. Zlatkin, M.B., Iannotti, J.P., Roberts, M.C., et al.: Rotator cuff tears: Diagnostic performance of MR imaging. Radiology, *172*:223–229, 1989.
46. Meyer, S.J.F., and Dalinka, M.K.: Magnetic resonance imaging of the shoulder. Semin. Ultrasound, CT, MR, *11*:253–266, 1990.
47. Holt, R.G., Helms, C.A., Steinbach, L., et al.: Magnetic resonance imaging of the shoulder: Rationale and current applications. Skeletal Radiol., *19*:5–14, 1990.
47a. Chard, M.D., and Hazelman, B.L. Shoulder disorders in the elderly (a hospital study). Ann. Rheum. Dis., *46*:684–687, 1987.
47b. Chakravarty, K.K., and Webley, M.: Disorders of the shoulder: An often unrecognized cause of disability in elderly people. Br. Med. J., *300*:848–849, 1990.
48. Anderson, B.C., and Kaye, S.: Shoulder pain: Differential diagnosis. West. J. Med., *138*:268–269, 1983.
49. Neer, C.S.: Impingement lesions. Clin. Orthop., *173*:70–77, 1983.
50. Penny, J.N., and Welch, R.P.: Shoulder impingement syndromes in athletes and their surgical management. Am. J. Sports Med., *9*:11–15, 1981.
50a. Jobe, F.M., and Bradley, J.P.: The diagnosis and nonoperative treatment of shoulder injuries in athletes. Clin. Sports Med., *8*:419–437, 1989.
51. Cone, R.O., Resnick, D., and Danzig, I.: Shoulder impingement syndrome: Radiographic evaluation. Radiology, *150*:29–33, 1984.
52. Hardy, D.C., Vogler, J.B., III, and White, R.H.: The shoulder impingement syndrome: Prevalence of radiographic findings and correlation with response to therapy. Am. J. Roentgenol., *147*:557–561, 1986.
53. Strizak, A.M. et al.: Subacromial bursography. J. Bone Joint Surg., *64A*:196–201, 1982.
54. Ha'eri, G.B., and Wiley, A.M.: Advancement of the supraspinatus muscle in the repair of ruptures of the rotator cuff. J. Bone Joint Surg., *63A*:232–238, 1981.
55. Post, M., and Cohen, J.: Impingement syndrome. A review of late stage II and early stage III lesions. Clin. Orthop., *207*:126–132, 1986.
56. Tibone, J.E. et al.: Shoulder impingement syndrome in athletes treated by an anterior acromioplasty. Clin. Orthop., *198*: 134–140, 1985.
57. Rathburn, J.B., and Macnab, I.: The microvascular pattern of the rotator cuff. J. Bone Joint Surg., *52B*:540–553, 1970.
58. Rothman, R.H., and Parke, W.W.: The vascular anatomy of the rotator cuff. Clin. Orthop., *41*:176–186, 1965.
58a. Lohr, J.F., and Uhthoff, H.K.: The microvascular pattern of the supraspinatus tendon. Clin. Orthop., *254*:35–38, 1990.
59. Herberts, P. et al.: Shoulder pain in industry: An epidemiological study on welders. Acta Orthop. Scand., *52*:299–306, 1981.
60. Campbell, H.L., and Feldman, F.: Bone and soft tissue abnormalities in the upper extremity in diabetes mellitus. Am. J. Roentgenol., *124*:7–16, 1975.
61. Trapp, R.G., Soler, N.G., and Spencer-Green, G.: Musculoskeletal abnormalities of the upper extremities and neck in insulin dependent diabetics: sympatomatology and physical findings. (Abstract.) Arthritis Rheum., *26*:547, 1983.
62. Kerwein, G.A., Roseberg, B., and Sneed, W.R.: Aids in differential diagnosis of the painful shoulder syndrome. Clin. Orthop., *20*:11–20, 1961.
63. Kessel, L., and Wastson, M.: The painful arc syndrome: clinical classification as a guide to management. J. Bone Joint Surg., *59B*:166–172, 1977.
64. Pedersen, H.E., and Key, J.A.: Pathology of calcareous tendinitis and subdeltoid bursitis. Arch. Surg., *62*:50–63, 1951.
65. McClure, J., and Gardner, D.L.: The production of calcification

in connective tissue and skeletal muscle using various chemical compounds. Calcif. Tissue Res., *22*:129–135, 1976.

66. Selye, H., Goldie, I., and Strebel, R.: Calciphylaxis in relation to calcification in periarticular tissues. Clin. Orthop., *28*:151–158, 1963.
67. Parfitt, A.M. et al.: Disordered calcium and phosphorus metabolism during maintenance hemodialysis. Am. J. Med., *51*:319–330, 1971.
68. Christensen, W.K., Liebman, C., and Sosman, M.C.: Skeletal and periarticular manifestations of hypervitaminosis. D. Am. J. Roentgenol., *65*:27–41, 1951.
69. McCarty, D.J., and Gatter, R.A.: Recurrent acute inflammation associated with focal apatite crystal deposition. Arthritis Rheum., *9*:804–819, 1964.
70. Pinals, R.S., and Short, C.L.: Calcific periarthritis involving multiple sites. Arthritis Rheum., *9*:566–574, 1966.

70a. Mavrikakis, M.E., Drimis, S., Kontoyannis, D.A. et al.: Calcific shoulder perarthritis (tendinitis) in adult onset diabetes mellitus: A controlled study. Ann. Rheum. Dis., *48*:211–214, 1989.

71. Luben, R.A., and Wadkins, C.L.: Studies of the relationship of proton production and calcification of tendon matrix in vitro. Biochemistry, *10*:2183, 1971.
72. Luben, R.A., Sherman, J.K., and Wadkins, C.L.: Studies of the mechanism of biological calcification. IV. Ultrastructural analysis of calcifying tendon matrix. Calcif. Tissue Res., *11*:39–55, 1973.
73. Urist, M.R., Moss, M.J., and Adams, J.M.: Calcification of tendon: A triphasic local mechanism. Arch. Pathol., *77*:594–608, 1964.
74. Fisher, L.W., and Termine, J.D.: Noncollagenous proteins influencing the local mechanisms of calcification. Clin. Orthop., *200*:362–385, 1985.
75. Addadi, L., and Weiner, S.: Interactions between acidic proteins and crystals: Stereochemical requirements in biomineralization. Proc. Natl. Acad. Sci. USA, *82*:4110–4114, 1985.
76. Poole, A.R., and Rosenberg, L.C.: Chondrocalcin and the calcification of cartilage. Clin. Orthop., *208*:114–118, 1986.
77. de Bernard, B.: Glycoproteins in the local mechanism of calcification. Clin. Orthop., *162*:233–244, 1982.
78. Neuman, W.F. et al.: Blood:bone disequilibrium. VI. Studies of the solubility characteristics of brushite:apatite mixtures and their stabilization by noncollagenous proteins of bone. Calcif. Tissue Int., *34*:149–157, 1982.
79. Termine, J.D., Eanes, E.D., and Conn, K.M.: Phosphoprotein modulation of apatite crystallization. Calcif. Tissue Int., *31*:247–251, 1980.
80. Yaari, A.M., Shapiro, I.M., and Brown, C.E.: Evidence that phosphatidylserine and inorgnaic phosphate may mediate calcium transport during calcification. Biochem. Biophys. Res. Comm., *105*:778–784, 1982.
81. Quigley, T.B.: The nonoperative treatment of symptomatic calcareous deposits in the shoulder. Surg. Clin. North Am., *6*:1495–1503, 1963.
82. Lippmann, R.K.: Observations concerning the calcific cuff deposit. Clin. Orthop., *20*:49–60, 1961.
83. McKendry, R.J.R. et al.: Calcifying tendinitis of the shoulder: Prognostic value of clinical, histologic, and radiologic features in 57 surgically treated cases. J. Rheumatol., *9*:75–80, 1982.

83a. Gartner, J., and Simons, B.: Analysis of calcific deposits in calcifying tendinitis. Clin. Orthop., *254*:111–120, 1990.

84. Bosworth, B.M.: Calcium deposits in the shoulder and subacromial bursitis: a survey of 12,122 shoulders. JAMA, *116*: 2477–2482, 1941.
85. Simon, W.H.: Soft tissue disorders of the shoulder. Orthop. Clin. North Am., *6*:521–539, 1975.
86. ViGario, G.D., and Keats, T.E.: Localization of calcific deposits in the shoulder. Am. J. Roentgenol., *108*:806–811, 1970.
87. Kotzen, L.M.: Roentgen diagnosis of rotator cuff tear: Report of 48 surgically proven cases. Am. J. Roentgenol., *112*:507–511, 1971.
88. Wolfgang, G.L.: Surgical repair of tears of the rotator cuff or the shoulder. J. Bone Joint Surg., *56A*:14–26, 1974.
89. Killoran, J.R., Marcone, R.C., and Freiberger, R.H.: Shoulder arthrography. Am. J. Roentgenol., *103*:658–668, 1968.

89a. Chard, M.D., Sattelle, L.M., and Hazelman, B.L.: The long-term outcome of rotator cuff tendinitis—A review study. Br. J. Rheumatol., *27*:385–389, 1988.

89b. Dacre, J.E., Beeney, N., and Scott, D.L.: Injections and physiotherapy. Ann. Rheum. Dis., *48*:322–325, 1989.

90. Soave, G. et al.: Indoproten versus indomethacin in acute painful shoulder and other soft-tissue rheumatic complaints. J. Int. Med. Res., *10*:99–103, 1982.
91. Bulgen, D.Y. et al.: Frozen shoulder: Prospective clinical study with an evaluation of three treatment regimens. Ann. Rheum. Dis., *43*:353–360, 1984.
92. Ward, M.C., Kirwan, J.R., Norris, P., and Murray, N.: Paracetamol and diclofenac in the painful shoulder syndrome. (Letter.) Br. J. Rheumatol., *25*:412, 1986.
93. Benson, T.B., and Copp, E.P.: The effects of therapeutic forms of heat and ice on the pain threshold of the normal shoulder. Rheumatol. Rehabil., *13*:101–104, 1974.
94. Berry, H. et al.: Clinical study comparing acupuncture, physiotherapy, injection and oral-anti-inflammatory therapy in shoulder-cuff lesions. Curr. Med. Res. Opin., *7*:121–126, 1980.
95. Binder, A., Parr, B., and Fitton-Jackson, S.: Pulsed electromagnetic field therapy of persistent rotator cuff tendinitis. A double-blind controlled assessment. Lancet *1*:695–698, 1984.
96. Harvey, W. et al.: The stimulation of protein synthesis in human fibroblasts by therapeutic ultrasound. Rheumatol. Rehabil., *14*:237, 1975.
97. Richardson, A.T.: The painful shoulder. Proc. R. Soc. Med., *68*:731–736, 1975.
98. Moore, M.E., and Berk, S.N.: Acupuncture for chronic shoulder pain: An experimental study with attention to the role of placebo and hypnotic susceptibility. Ann. Intern. Med., *84*:381–384, 1976.
99. Hashish, I., Harvey, W., and Harris, W.: Anti-inflammatory effects of ultrasound therapy: Evidence for a major placebo effect. Br. J. Rheumatol., *25*:77–81, 1986.
100. Downing, D., and Weinstein, A.: Ultrasound therapy of subacromial bursitis: A double blind trial. (Abstract.) Arthritis Rheum., *26*:S87, 1983.
101. Symposium: DMSO in musculoskeletal conditions. Ann. N.Y. Acad. Sci., *141*:493, 1967.
102. McMillan, J.A.: Therapeutic exercise for shoulder disabilities. J. Am. Phys. Ther. Assoc., *46*:1052–1060, 1966.
103. Fitzgerald, R.H.: Intrasynovial injection of steroids: Uses and abuses. Mayo Clin. Proc., *51*:655–659, 1976.
104. Roy, S., and Oldham, R.: Management of painful shoulder. Lancet, *1*:1322–1324, 1976.
105. Steinbrocker, O., and Neustadt, D.H.: Aspiration and Injection Therapy in Arthritis and Musculo-Skeletal Disorders. Hagerstown, MD, Harper & Row, 1972.
106. Koehler, B.E., Urowitz, M.B., and Killinger, D.W.: The systemic effect of intra-articular corticosteroid. J. Rheumatol., *1*:117–125, 1974.
107. Asboe-Hansen, G.: Influence of corticosteroids on connective tissue. Dermatologica, *152*:127–132, 1976.
108. Sweetham, R.: Corticosteroid arthropathy and tendon rupture. J. Bone Joint Surg., *51B*:397–398, 1969.
109. McCarty, D.J., and Hogan, J.: Inflammatory reaction after intrasynovial injection of microcrystalline adrenocorticosteroid esters. Arthritis Rheum., *7*:359–367, 1964.
110. Darlington, L.G., and Coombs, E.N.: The effects of local steroid

injection for supraspinatus tears. Rheumatol. Rehabil., *16*:172–179, 1977.
111. Comfort, T.H., and Arafiles, R.P.: Barbotage of the shoulder with image-intensified fluoroscopic control of needle placement for calcific tendinitis. Clin. Orthop., *135*:171–178, 1978.
112. Nixon, J.E., and DiStefano, V.: Ruptures of the rotator cuff. Orthop. Clin. North Am., *6*:423–447, 1975.
113. Neviaser, J.S.: Ruptures of the rotator cuff of the shoulder. Arch. Surg., *102*:483–485, 1971.
113a. Norwood, L.A., Barrack, R., and Jacobson, K.E.: Clinical presentation of complete tears of the rotator cuf. J. Bone Joint Surg., *71A*:499–505, 1989.
114. Bakalim, G., and Pasila, M.: Rotator cuff tears. Acta Orthop. Scand., *46*:751–757, 1975.
115. Samilson, R.L., and Brider, W.F.: Symptomatic full thickness tears of the rotator cuff: An analysis of 292 shoulders in 276 patients. Orthop. Clin. North Am., *6*:449–466, 1975.
116. Weiss, J.J.: Intra-articular steroids in the treatment of rotator cuff tear: reappraisal by arthrography. Arch. Phys. Med. Rehabil., *62*:555–557, 1981.
117. Post, M., Silver, R., and Singh, M.: Rotator cuff tear: Diagnosis and treatment. Clin. Orthop., *173*:78–91, 1983.
118. Hawkins, R.J., Misamore, G.W., and Hobeika, P.E.: Surgery for full-thickness rotator-cuff tears. J. Bone Joint Surg., *67A*:1349–1355, 1985.
119. Tibone, J.E. et al.: Surgical treatment of tears of the rotator cuff in athletes. J. Bone Joint Surg., *68A*:887–891, 1986.
120. Ellman, H., Hanker, G., and Bayer, M.: Repair of the rotator cuff. End-result of factors influencing reconstruction. J. Bone Joint Surg., *68A*:1136–1144, 1986.
121. Gore, D.R., Murray, M.P., Sepic, S.B., and Gardner, G.M.: Function after surgical repair of full-thickness rotator cuff tears. Long-term follow-up of fifty-one patients. Orthop. Trans., *9*:466–467, 1985.
122. Cofield, R.H., and Lanzer, W.L.: Rotator cuff repair, results related to surgical pathology. Orthop. Trans., *9*:466, 1985.
123. Middleton, W.D. et al.: US of the biceps tendon apparatus. Radiology, *157*:211–215, 1985.
124. Neviaser, T.J. et al.: The four-in-one arthroplasty for the painful arc syndrome. Clin. Orthop., *163*:107–112, 1983.
124a. Maloney, M.D., Sauser, D.D., Hanson, E.C., et al.: Adhesive capsulitis of the wrist: Arthrograhpic diagnosis. Radiology, *167*:187–190, 1988.
125. Bridgeman, J.F.: Periarthritis of the shoulder and diabetes mellitus. Ann. Rheum. Dis., *31*:69, 1972.
126a. Withrington, R.H., Girgis, F.L., and Seifert, M.H.: A comparative study of the aetiological factors in shoulder pain. Br. J. Rheumatol., *24*:24–26, 1985.
126b. Wright, M.G., Richards, A.J., and Clarke, M.B.: ^{99m}Tc-pertechnetate scanning in capsulitis. Lancet, *2*:1265–1266, 1975.
127. Lee, P.N., et al.: Periarthritis of the shoulder, trial of treatments investigated by multivariate analysis. Ann. Rheum. Dis., *33*:116–119, 1974.
128. Bulgen, D.Y. et al.: Immunological studies in frozen shoulder. Ann. Rheum. Dis., *37*:135–138, 1978.
129. Bulgen, D.Y., Hazelman, B.L., and Voak, D.: HLA-B27 and frozen shoulder. Lancet, *1*:1042–1044, 1976.
130. Noy, S. et al.: HLA-B27 and frozen shoulder. Tissue Antigens, *17*:251, 1981.
131. Seignalet, J. et al.: Lack of association between HLA-B27 and frozen shoulder. Tissue Antigens, *18*:364, 1981.
132. Akeson, W.H. et al.: The connective tissue response to immobility: Biochemical changes in periarticular connective tissue of the immobilized rabbit knee. Clin. Orthop., *93*:356–362, 1973.
133. Lundberg, B.J.: Glycosaminoglycans of the normal and frozen shoulder-joint capsule. Clin. Orthop., *69*:279–284, 1970.
134. Reeves, B.: The natural history of the frozen shoulder syndrome. Scand. J. Rheumatol., *4*:193–196, 1975.
135. Wright, V., and Haq, A.M.M.M.: Periarthritis of the shoulder. II. Radiological features. Ann. Rheum. Dis., *35*:220–226, 1976.
136. Ha'eri, G.B., and Maitland, A.: Arthroscopic findings in the frozen shoulder. J. Rheumatol., *8*:149–152, 1981.
137. Binder, A.I. et al.: Frozen shoulder: An arthrographic and radionuclear scan assessment. Ann. Rheum. Dis., *43*:365–369, 1984.
138. Brockelhurst, J.C. et al.: How much physical therapy for patients with stroke? Br. Med. J., *1*:1307–1310, 1978.
139. Steinbrocker, O., and Argyros, T.G.: Frozen shoulder: Treatment by local injections of depot corticosteroids. Arch. Phys. Med. Rehabil., *55*:209–213, 1974.
140. Williams, N.E. et al.: Treatment of capsulitis of the shoulder. Rheumatol. Rehabil., *14*:236, 1975.
141. Tyler, M.A.: Treatment of the painful shoulder syndrome with amitriptyline and lithium carbonate. Can. Med. Assoc. J., *111*:137–140, 1974.
142. Rizk, T.E. et al.: Adhesive capsulitis (frozen shoulder): A new approach to its management. Arch. Phys. Med. Rehabil., *64*:29–33, 1983.
143. Kozen, F.: Painful shoulder and the reflex sympathetic dystrophy syndrome. *In* Arthritis and Allied Conditions, 9th ed. Edited by D.J. McCarty. Philadelphia, Lea & Febiger, 1979, pp. 1322–1355.
144. Older, M.W.H., McIntyre, JL., and Lloyd, G.J.: Distension arthrography of the shoulder joint. Can. J. Surg., *19*:203–207, 1976.
145. Gilula, L.A., Schoenecker, P.C., and Murphy, W.A.: Shoulder arthrography as a treatment modality. Am. J. Roentgenol., *131*:1047–1048, 1978.
146. Thomas, D., Williams, R.A., and Smith, D.S.: The frozen shoulder: A review of manipulative treatment. Rheumatol. Rehabil., *19*:173–179, 1980.
147. McNair, M.M. et al.: A clinical and radiological study of rheumatoid arthritis with a note on the findings in osteoarthrosis. I. The shoulder joint. Clin. Radiol., *20*:269–277, 1969.
148. Zanca, P.: Shoulder pain: Involvement of the acromioclavicular joint. Am. J. Roentgenol., *112*:493–506, 1971.
149. Quinn, S.F., and Glass, T.A.: Post-traumatic osteolysis of the clavicle. South. Med. J., *76*:307–308, 1983.
150. Kaplan, P.A., and Resnick, D.: Stress-induced osteolysis of the clavicle. Radiology, *158*:139–140, 1986.
151. Sonozaki, H. et al.: Clinical features of 53 cases with pustulotic arthro-osteitis. Ann. Rheum. Dis., *40*:541–553, 1981.
152. Nilsson, B.E., and Uden, A.: Skeletal lesions in palmar-plantar pustulosis. Acta Orthop. Scand., *55*:366–370, 1984.
153. Sartoris, D.J. et al.: Sternocostoclavicular hyperostosis: A review and report of 11 cases. Radiology, *158*:125–128, 1986.
154. Chigira, M. et al.: Sternoclavicular hyperostosis. A report of nineteen cases, with special reference to etiology and treatment. J. Bone Joint Surg., *68A*:103–112, 1986.
155. Kofold, H., Thomsen, P., and Lindenberg, S.: Serous synovitis of the sternoclavicular joint. Differential diagnostic aspects. Scand. J. Rheumatol., *14*:61–64, 1985.
156. Paice, E.W., Wright, F.W., and Hill, A.G.S.: Sternoclavicular erosions in polymyalgia rheumatica. Ann. Rheum. Dis., *42*:379–383, 1983.
157. Healey, L.A.: Long-term follow-up of polymyalgia rheumatica: Evidence for synovitis. Semin. Arthritis Rheum., *13*:322–336, 1984.
158. Pierce, R.: Internal derangement of the sternoclavicular joint. Clin. Orthop., *141*:247–250, 1979.
159. Meachim, G.: Effect of age on the thickness of adult articular cartilage at the shoulder joint. Ann. Rheum. Dis., *30*:43–46, 1971.

160. McCarty, D.J. et al.: "Milwaukee shoulder"—Association of microspheroids containing hydroxyapatite crystals, active collagenase, and neutral protease with rotator cuff defects. I. Clinical aspects. Arthritis Rheum., *24*:464–473, 1981.
161. Halverson, P.B., McCarty, D.J., Cheung, H.S., and Ryan, L.M.: Milwaukee shoulder syndrome: Eleven additional cases with involvement of the knee in seven (basic calcium phosphate crystal deposition disease). Semin. Arthritis Rheum., *14*:36–44, 1984.
162. Samilson, R.L., and Preito, V.: Dislocation arthropathy of the shoulder. J. Bone Joint Surg., *65A*:456–460, 1983.
163. Neer, C.S., II, Craig, E.V., and Fukuda, H.: Cuff-tear arthropathy. J. Bone Joint Surg., *65A*:1232–1244, 1983.
164. Dennis, D.A., Ferlic, D.C., and Clayton, M.L.: Acromial stress fractures associated with cuff-tear arthropathy. J. Bone Joint Surg., *68A*:937–940, 1986.
164a. Perry, J., and Glousman, R.E.: Biomechanics of the athletic arm. *In* The Upper Extremity in Sports Medicine. Edited by Nicholson and Hershman. St. Louis, C.V. Mosby, 1990.
165. Hellmann, D.B., Helms, C.A., and Genant, H.K.: Chronic repetitive trauma: A cause of atypical degenerative joint disease. Skeletal Radiol., *10*:236–242, 1983.
166. Pasila, M. et al.: Recovery from primary shoulder dislocation and its complications. Acta Orthop. Scand., *51*:257–262, 1980.
167. Chung, S.M.K., and Nissenbaum, M.M.: Congenital and developmental defects of the shoulder. Orthop. Clin. North Am., *6*:381–392, 1975.
168. Tachdjian, M.O.: Pediatric Orthopedics. Philadelphia, W.B. Saunders, 1972.
169. Leffert, R.D.: Brachial plexus injuries. N. Engl. J. Med., *291*:1059–1067, 1974.
170. Meyer, R.D.: Treatment of adult and obstetrical brachial plexus injuries. Orthopedics, *9*:899–903, 1986.
171. Clodius, L., Uhlschmid, G., and Hess, K.: Irradiation plexitis of the brachial plexus. Clin. Plast. Surg., *11*:161–165, 1984.
172. Garcia, G., and McQueen, D.: Bilateral suprascapular-nerve entrapment syndrome. J. Bone Joint Surg., *63A*:491–492, 1981.
173. Ganzhorn, R.W. et al.: Suprascapular nerve entrapment. J. Bone Joint Surg., *63A*:492–494, 1981.
174. Berry, H., and Bril, V.: Axillary nerve palsy following blunt trauma to the shoulder region: A cervical and electrophysiological review. J. Neurol. Neurosurg. Psychiatry, *45*:1027–1032, 1982.
175. Gathier, J.C., and Bruyn, G.W.: Neuralgic amyotrophy. *In* Handbook of Clinical Neurology. Vol. 8. Diseases of Nerves. Part II. Edited by P.J. Vinkin and G.W. Bruyn. New York, American Elsevier, 1970, pp. 77–85.
176. Petersson, C.J.: Painful shoulders in patients with rheumatoid arthritis: Prevalent clinical and radiological features. Scand. J. Rheumatol., *15*:275–279, 1986.
177. Kalliomaki, J.L., Viitanen, S.-M., and Virtama, P.: Radiological findings of sternoclavicular joints in rheumatoid arthritis. Acta Rheumatol. Scand., *14*:223–240, 1968.
178. Kaklamanis, P. et al.: Calcificaiton of the shoulders and diabetes mellitus. N. Engl. J. Med., *293*:1266–1267, 1975.
179. Pal, B., Anderson, J., Dick, W.C., and Griffiths, I.D.: Limitation of joint mobility and shoulder capsulitis in insulin- and non-insulin-dependent diabetes mellitus. Br. J. Rheumatol., *25*:147–151, 1986.
180. Fisher, L., Kurtz, A., and Shipley, M.: Association between cheiroarthropathy and frozen shoulder in patients with insulin-dependent diabetes mellitus. Br. J. Rheumatol., *25*:141–146, 1986.
181. Eaton, R.P.: Aldose reductase inhibition and the diabetic syndrome of limited joint mobility: Implications for altered collagen hydration. Metabolism, *35*(Suppl. 1):119–121, 1986.
182. Hadler, N.M. et al.: Acute polyarticular gout. Am. J. Med., *56*:715–719, 1974.
183. Okazaki, I. et al.: Pseudogout: clinical observations and chemical analysis of deposits. Arthritis Rheum., *19*:293–306, 1976.
184. Rosati, L.M., and Lord, J.W.: Neurovascular Compression Syndromes of the Shoulder Girdle. New York, Grune & Stratton, 1961.
185. Tyson, R.R., and Kaplan, G.F.: Modern concepts of diagnosis and treatment of the thoracic outlet syndrome. Orthop. Clin. North Am., *6*:507–519, 1975.
186. Dunant, J.H.: The diagnosis of thoracic outlet syndrome. *In* Pain in the Shoulder and Arm. Edited by J.M. Greep et al. The Hague, Martinus Nijhoff, 1979.
187. De Sliva, M.: The costoclavicular syndrome: A "new cause." Ann. Rheum. Dis., *45*:916–920, 1986.
188. Swift, T.R., and Nichols, F.T.: The droopy shoulder syndrome. Neurology, *34*:212–215, 1984.
189. Gergoudis, R., and Barnes, R.W.: Thoracic outlet arterial compression: Prevalence in normal persons. Angiology, *31*:538–541, 1980.
190. Stallworth, J.M., Quinn, G.J., and Aiken, A.F.: Is rib resection necessary for relief of thoracic outlet syndrome? Ann. Surg., *185*:581–589, 1979.
191. Wilborn, A.J., and Lederman, R.J.: Evidence for a conduction delay in thoracic outlet syndrome is challenged. N. Engl. J. Med., *310*:1052, 1984.
192. Yiannikas, C., and Walsh, J.C.: Somatosensory evoked response in the diagnosis of thoracic outlet syndrome. J. Neurol. Neurosurg. Psychiatry, *46*:234, 1983.
193. Stallworth, J.M., and Horne, J.B.: Diagnosis and management of thoracic outlet syndrome. Arch. Surg., *119*:1149–1151, 1984.
194. Mitchell, S.W.: Injuries of Nerves and Their Consequences. Philadelphia, J.B. Lippincott, 1872.
195. Richards, R.L.: The term 'causalgia.' Med. Hist., *11*:97–99, 1967.
196. Mitchell, S.W., Moorehouse, G.R., and Keen, W.W.: Gunshot Wounds and Other Injuries of Nerves. Philadelphia, J.B. Lippincott, 1864.
197. Kozin, F. et al.: The reflex sympathetic dystrophy syndrome. I. Clinical and histologic studies: Evidence for bilaterality, response to corticosteroids, and articular involvement. Am. J. Med., *60*:321–331, 1976.
198. Johnson, A.C.: Disabling changes in the hands resembling sclerodactylia following myocardial infarction. Ann. Intern. Med., *19*:443–456, 1943.
199. Russek, H.I.: Shoulder-hand syndrome following myocardial infarction. Med. Clin. North Am., *42*:1555–1556, 1958.
200. Davis, S.W. et al.: Shoulder-hand syndrome in a hemiplegic population: 5-year retrospective study. Arch. Phys. Med. Rehabil., *58*:353–356, 1977.
201. Eto, F. et al.: Shoulder-hand syndrome as a complication of hemiplegia. Jpn. J. Geriatr., *12*:245–251, 1977.
202. Bacorn, R.W., and Kurtzke, J.F.: Colles' fracture: A study of two thousand cases from the New York State Workman's Compensation fund. J. Bone Joint Surg., *35A*:643–658, 1953.
203. Cooney, W.P., Dobyns, J.H., and Linscheid, R.L.: Complications of Colles' fracture. J. Bone Joint Surg., *62A*:613–619, 1980.
204. Dunningham, T.H.: The treatment of Sudeck's atrophy in the upper limb by sympathetic blockade. Injury, *12*:139–144, 1981.
205. Plewes, L.W.: Sudeck's atrophy in the hands. J. Bone Joint Surg., *38B*:195–203, 1956.
206. Pak, T.J. et al.: Reflex sympathetic dystrophy—A review of 140 cases. Minn. Med., *53*.:507–511, 1970.
207. Acquaviva, P. et al.: Reflex dystrophies: Background and etiological factors. Rev. Rhum. Mal. Osteoartic., *49*:761–766, 1982.

208. Evans, J.A.: Reflex sympathetic dystrophy: Report on 57 cases. Ann. Intern. Med., *26*:417–426, 1947.
209. Johnson, E.W., and Pannozzo, A.N.: Management of shoulder-hand syndrome. JAMA, *195*:152–154, 1966.
210. Kozin, F. et al.: The reflex sympathetic dystrophy syndrome (RSDS) III. Scintigraphic studies, further evidence for the therapeutic efficacy of systemic corticosteroids, and proposed diagnostic criteria. Am. J. Med., *70*:23–30, 1981.
211. Patman, R.D., Thompson, J.E., and Perrson, A.V.: Management of post-traumatic pain syndromes: Report of 113 cases. Ann. Surg., *177*:780–786, 1973.
212. Rosen, P.S., and Graham, W.: The shoulder-hand syndrome: Historical review with observations on seventy-three patients. Can. Med. Assoc. J., *77*:86–91, 1957.
213. Subbarao, J., and Stillwell, G.K.: Reflex sympathetic dystrophy syndrome of the upper extremity: Analysis of total outcome of management of 125 cases. Arch. Phys. Med. Rehabil., *62*:549–554, 1981.
214. Thompson, M.: Shoulder-hand syndrome. Proc. R. Soc. Med., *54*:679–682, 1961.
215. Bernstein, B.H. et al.: Reflex neurovascular dystrophy in childhood. J. Pediatr., *93*:211–215, 1978.
216. Carron, H., and McCue, F.: Reflex sympathetic dystrophy in a ten year old. South. Med. J., *65*:631–632, 1972.
217. Fermaglich, D.R.: Reflex sympathetic dystrophy in children. Pediatrics, *60*:881–883, 1977.
218. Kozin, F., Houghton, V., and Ryan, L.N.: The reflex sympathetic dystrophy in a child. Pediatrics, *90*:417–419, 1977.
219. Matles, A.I.: Reflex sympathetic dystrophy in a child: A case report. Bull. Hosp. Joint. Dis., *32*:193–197, 1971.
220. Ruggeri, S.B. et al.: Reflex sympathetic dystrophy in children. Clin. Orthop., *103*:225–230, 1982.
221. Lequesne, M. et al.: Partial transient osteoporosis. Skeletal Radiol., *2*:1–30, 1977.
222. Helms, C.A., O'Brien, E.T., and Katzberg, R.W.: Segmental reflex sympathetic dystrophy syndrome. Radiology, *35*:67–68, 1980.
222a. Laukaitis, J.P., Varma, V.M., and Borenstein, D.G.: Reflex sympathetic dystrophy localized to a single digit. J. Rheumatol., *16*:402–405, 1989.
223. Corbett, M., Colston, J.R., and Tucker, A.K.: Pain in the knees associated with osteoporosis of the patella. Am. Rheum. Dis., *36*:188–191, 1977.
224. Kim, H.J. et al.: Reflex-sympathetic dystrophy of the knee following meniscectomy: Report of three cases. Arthritis Rheum., *22*:177–181, 1979.
225. Tietjen, R.: Reflex sympathetic dystrophy of the knee. Clin. Orthop., *209*:234–243, 1986.
226. Gaucher, A. et al.: The diagnostic value of ^{99m}Tc-diphosphonate bone imaging in transient osteoporosis of the hip. J. Rheumatol., *6*:774, 1979.
227. Langloh, N.D. et al.: Transient painful osteoporosis of the lower extremities. J. Bone Joint Surg., *55A*:1188–1227, 1973.
228. Kozin, F. et al.: The reflex sympathetic dystrophy syndrome. II. Roentgenographic and scintigraphic evidence of the bilaterality and periarticular accentuation. Am. J. Med., *60*:332–338, 1976.
229. International Association on the Study of Pain. Subcommittee on Taxonomy Pain Terms: A list with definitions and notes on usage. Pain, *6*:249–252, 1979.
230. Tahmoush, A.J.: Causalgia: Redefinition as a clinical pain syndrome. Pain, *10*:187–197, 1981.
231. Roberts, W.J.: A hypothesis on the physiological basis for causalgia and related pains. Pain, *2400*:297–311, 1986.
232. Kozin, F.: The reflex sympathetic dystrophy syndrome. Bull. Rheum. Dis., *36*:1–8, 1986.
232a. Schwartzman, R.J., and Kerrigan, J.: The movement disorder of reflex sympathetic dystrophy. Neurology, *40*:57–61, 1990.
232b. Bobberecht, W., Van Hess, J., Adriaensen, H., and Carton, H.: Painful muscle spasm complicating algodystrophy: central or peripheral disease? J. Neurol. Neurosurg. Psych., *51*:563–567, 1988.
233. Miller, D.S., and de Takats, G.: Post-traumatic dystrophy of the extremities. Surg. Gynecol. Obstet., *125*:558–582, 1941.
234. Steinbrocker, O., and Argyros, T.G.: The shoulder-hand syndrome: Present status as a diagnostic and therapeutic entity. Med. Clin. North Am., *42*:1533–1553, 1958.
235. Steinbrocker, O., Spitzer, N., and Friedman, H.H.: The shoulder-hand syndrome in reflex dystrophy of the upper extremity. Ann. Intern. Med., *29*:22–52, 1947.
236. Naides, S.J., Resnick, D., and Zvaifler, N.J.: Idiopathic regional osteoporosis: A clinical spectrum. J. Rheumatol., *12*:763–768, 1985.
237. Dent, C.E., and Friedman, M.: Idiopathic juvenile osteoporosis. Q. J. Med., *34*:177–210, 1965.
238. Jowsey, J., and Johnson, K.A.: Juvenile osteoporosis: Bone findings in seven patients. J. Pediatr., *81*:511–517, 1972.
239. Kozin, F. et al.: Bone scintigraphy in the reflex sympathetic dystrophy syndrome. Radiology, *138*:437–443, 1981.
240. Amor, B. et al.: Algodystrophies et hyperlipemies. Rev. Rhum. Mal. Osteoartic., *47*:353–358, 1980.
241. Pinals, R.S., and Jabbs, J.M.: Type IV hyperlipoproteinemia and transient osteoporosis. Lancet, *2*:929, 1972.
242. Uematsu, S. et al.: Thermography and electromyography in the differential diagnosis of chronic pain syndromes and reflex sympathetic dystrophy. Electromyogr. Clin. Neurophysiol., *21*:165–182, 1981.
243. Sylvest, J. et al.: Reflex dystrophy: Resting blood flow and muscle temperature as diagnostic criteria. Scand. J. Rehabil. Med., *9*:25–29, 1977.
244. Ecker, M.A.: Contact thermography in diagnosis of reflex sympathetic dystrophy. *In* Thermography. Edited by A. Fischer. Philadelphia, W.B. Saunders, 1984.
245. Hendler, N., Uematsu, S., and Long, D.: Thermographic validation of physical complaints in "psychogenic pain" patients. Psychosomatics, *23*:283–287, 1982.
246. Cronin, K.D., and Kirsner, R.L.G.: Diagnosis of reflex sympathetic dysfunction: Use of skin potential response. Anaesthesia, *37*:847–852, 1982.
247. Pfinsgraff, J. et al.: Palmar fasciitis and arthritis with malignant neoplasms: A paraneoplastic syndrome. Semin. Arthritis Rheum., *16*:118–125, 1986.
248. Medsger, T.A., Dixon, J.A., and Garwood, V.F.: Palmar fasciitis and polyarthritis associated with ovarian carcinoma. Ann. Intern. Med., *96*:424–431, 1982.
249. Michaels, R.M., and Sorber, J.A.: Reflex sympathetic dystrophy as a probable paraneoplastic syndrome: Case report and literature review. Arthritis Rheum., *27*:1183–1185, 1984.
250. Allman, R.M., and Brower, A.C.: Circulatory patterns of deossification. Radiol. Clin. North Am., *19*:553–569, 1981.
251. Herrmann, L.G., Reincke, H.G., and Caldwell, J.A.: Posttraumatic painful osteoporosis: A clinical and roentgenological entity. Am. J. Roentgenol., *47*:353–361, 1942.
252. Jones, G.: Radiological appearances of disuse osteoporosis. Clin. Radiol., *20*:345–353, 1969.
253. Genant, H.K. et al.: The reflex sympathetic dystrophy syndrome: A comprehensive analysis using fine-detail radiography, photon absorptiometry and bone and joint scintigraphy. Radiology, *117*:21, 1975.
254. Sudeck, P.: Über die akute (reflektorishe) Knockenatrophie nach Entzundungen und Verletzungen an den Extrematation

and ihre Klinischen Ersheinungen. Fortschr. Gebd. Roentgen., *5*:277–293, 1901–1902.

255. Sudeck, P.: Über die akute entzundlicke Knockenatrophie. Arch. Klin. Chir., *62*:147–156, 1900.
256. Keinbach, R.: Über akute knochenatrophie bie Enuyndungprocessen an den Extrematatun (Falschlich sagenannage inactivatats atrophie die Knochen) und ihre Diagnose nach dem Roentgen-Bild. Wien Med. Wochenschr., *5*:1345–1360, 1901.
257. Holder, L.E., and MacKinnon, S.E.: Reflex sympathetic dystrophy in the hands: Clinical and scintigraphic criteria. Radiology, *152*:517–522, 1984.
258. MacKinnon, S.E., and Holder, L.E.: The use of three-phase radionuclide bone scanning in the diagnosis of reflex sympathetic dystrophy. J. Hand Surg., *9A*:556–563, 1984.
259. Charkes, N.D.: Skeletal blood flow: Implications for bone-scan interpretation. J Nucl. Med., *21*:91–98, 1980.
260. McKinstry, P. et al.: Relationship of 99m Tc-MDP uptake to regional osseous circulation in skeletally immature and mature dogs. Skeletal Radiol., *8*:115–121, 1982.
261. Doury, P., Dirheimer, Y., and Pattin, S.: Algodystrophy. New York, Springer-Verlag, 1981.
262. Carlson, D.H., Simon, H., and Wegner, W.: Bone scanning and diagnosis of reflex sympathetic dystrophy secondary to herniated lumbar discs. Neurology, *27*:791–793, 1977.
263. Deutsch, S.D., Gandsman, E.J., and Spraragen, S.C.: Quantative regional blood-flow analysis and its clinical application during routine bone-scanning. J. Bone Joint Surg., *63A*:295–305, 1981.
264. Simon, H., and Carlson, D.H.: The use of bone scanning in the diagnosis of reflex sympathetic dystrophy. Clin. Nucl. Med., *5*:116–121, 1980.

264a. Rico, H., Merono, E., Gomez-Castresana, F., et al.: Scintigraphic evaluation of reflex sympathetic dystrophy: Comparative study of the course of the disease under two therapeutic regimes. Clin. Rheumatol., *6*:233–237, 1987.

264b. Demangeat, J.-L., Constantinesco, A., Brunot, B., et al.: Three-phase bone scanning in reflex sympathetic dystrophy of the hand. J. Nucl. Med., *29*:26–32, 1988.

265. Arlet, J. et al.: Histopathology of bone and cartilage lesions in reflex sympathetic dystrophy of the knee: Report of 16 cases. (French.) Rev. Rhum. Mal. Osteoartic., *48*:315–321, 1981.
266. Christensen, K., Jensen, E.M., and Noer, I.: The reflex dystrophy syndrome: Response to treatment with systemic corticosteroids. Acta Chir. Scand., *148*:653–655, 1982.
267. Stolte, B.H., Stolte, J.B., and Leyten, J.F.: De pathofysiologie van het shoulder-handsyndroom. Med. Tijdschr. Geneeskd., *114*:1208–1209, 1980.
268. Moberg, E.: The shoulder-hand-finger syndrome. Surg. Clin. North Am., *40*:367–373, 1960.
269. Good, A.E., Green, R.A., and Zorafonetis, C.J.D.: Rheumatic symptoms during tuberculosis therapy: A manifestation of isoniazid toxicity. Ann. Intern. Med., *63*:800–807, 1965.
270. van der Korst, J.K., Colenbrauder, H., and Cats, A.: Phenobarbital and the shoulder-hand syndrome. Ann. Rheum. Dis., *25*:553–555, 1966.
271. DeTakats, G.: Reflex sympathetic dystrophy of the extremities. Arch. Surg., *34*:939–956, 1937.
272. Livingston, W.K.: Pain Mechanisms. New York, Macmillan, 1943.
273. Noordenhos, W.: Pain. Amsterdam, Elsevier, 1959.
274. Meyer, G.A., and Fields, H.L.: Causalgia treated by selective large fibre stimulation of peripheral nerve. Brain, *95*:163–168, 1972.
275. Richlin, D.M. et al.: Reflex sympathetic dystrophy: Successful treatment by transcutaneous nerve stimulation. J. Pediatr., *93*:84–86, 1978.
276. Melzack, R.: The Puzzle of Pain. New York, Basic Books, 1973.
277. Melzack, R., and Wall, P.D.: Pain mechanisms: A new theory. Science, *150*:971–979, 1965.
278. Doury, P. et al.: Algodystrophy with hypofixation of technetium 99m pyrophosphate on bone scintigraphy. (French.) Sem. Hop. Paris, *57*:1325–1327, 1981.
279. van der Korst, J.B.: Shoulder-pain as a rheumatologic problem. *In* Pain in the Shoulder and Arm. Edited by I.M. Green et al. The Hague, Martinus Nijhoff, 1979.
280. Frykman, G.: Fracture of the distal radius including sequelae—Shoulder-hand-finger syndrome, disturbance in the distal radioulnar joint, and impairment of nerve function. Acta Orthop. Scand., *108*(Suppl.1):1–153, 1967.
281. Lind, K.: A synthesis of studies on stroke rehabilitation. J. Chronic Dis., *35*:133–149, 1982.
282. Steinbrocker, O., Neustadt, D., and Lapin, L.: Sympathetic block compared with corticotropin and cortisone therapy. JAMA, *153*:788–791, 1953.
283. Drucker, W.R. et al.: Pathogenesis of post-traumatic sympathetic dystrophy. Am. J. Surg., *97*:454–465, 1979.
284. Wang, J.K., Johnson, K.A., and Ilstrup, D.M.: Sympathetic blocks for reflex sympathetic dystrophy. Pain. *23*:13–17, 1985.
285. Buker, R.H. et al.: Causalgia and transthoracic sympathectomy. Am. J. Surg., *124*:724–727, 1972.
286. Benzon, H.T., Chomka, C.M., and Brunner, E.A.: Treatment of reflex sympathetic dystrophy with regional intravenous reserpine. Anesth. Analg., *59*:500–502, 1980.
287. Chuinard, R.G. et al.: Intravenous reserpine for treatment of reflex sympathetic dystrophy. South. Med. J., *74*:1481–1484, 1981.
288. Chuinard, R.G. et al.: Intravenous reserpine for treatment of reflex sympathetic dystrophy. South. Med. J., *74*:1481–1484, 1981.
289. Hannington-Kiff, J.G.: Relief of Sudeck's atrophy by regional intravenous guanethidine. Lancet, *1*:1132–1134, 1977.
290. Hannington-Kiff, J.G.: Relief of causalgia in limbs by regional intravenous guanethidine. Br. Med. J., *2*:367–368, 1979.
291. Bonelli, S., Conocente, F., et al.: Regional intravenous guanethidine vs. stellate ganglion block in reflex sympathetic dystrophies: A randomized trial. Pain, *16*:297–307, 1983.
292. Ghostine, S.Y. et al.: Phenoxybenzamine in the treatment of causalgia. A report of 40 cases. J. Neurosurg., *60*:1263–1268, 1984.
293. Simson, G.: Propranolol for causalgia and Sudeck's atrophy. JAMA, *227*:327, 1974.
294. Visitsunthorn, U., and Prete, P.: Reflex sympathetic dystrophy of the lower extremity. West. J. Med., *135*:62–66, 1981.
295. Glick, E.N., and Helal, B.: Post-traumatic neurodystrophy: treatment by corticosteroids. Hand, *8*:45–48, 1976.
296. Mowat, A.G.: Treatment of the shoulder-hand syndrome with corticosteroids. Ann. Rheum. Dis., *33*:120–123, 1974.
297. Russek, H.I. et al.: Cortisone treatment of shoulder-hand syndrome following acute myocardial infarction. Arch. Intern. Med., *91*:487–492, 1953.
298. Glick, E.N.: Reflex dystrophy (algoneurodystrophy): reults of treatment by corticosteroids. Rheumatol. Rehabil., *1*:84–88, 1973.
299. Poplawski, E.J., Wiley, A.M., and Murray, J.F.: Post-traumatic dystrophy of the extremities. J. Bone Joint Surg., *65A*:642–649, 1983.
300. Prough, D.S. et al.: Efficacy of oral nifedipine in the treatment of reflex sympathetic dystrophy. Anesthesiology, *62*:796–799, 1985.
301. Wall, P.D., and Sweet, W.H.: Temporary abolition of pain in man. Science, *155*:108–109, 1967.

100

Osteonecrosis

JOHN PAUL JONES, JR.

The terms *osteonecrosis, avascular (aseptic) necrosis,* and *osseous ischemia* indicate death of the cellular constituents of both bone and bone marrow. A minimum of 2 hours of complete ischemia and total anoxia is needed to cause irreversible osteocytic necrosis.[1] Although the cause is multifactorial, intravascular coagulation[2] is the most likely final common pathway in the early pathogenesis.

PATHOPHYSIOLOGIC FEATURES

TRAUMATIC (MACROVASCULAR) DAMAGE

Post-traumatic osteonecrosis is caused by disruption of the *arterial* blood supply to bone. It usually involves those vulnerable bones covered extensively by cartilage, with few vascular foramina and limited collateral circulation. For example, because blood to the superolateral two thirds of the femoral head comes almost entirely from the lateral epiphyseal branches of the medial femoral circumflex artery, this area is particularly susceptible to osteonecrosis. The only other blood available to the femoral head flows through the ligamentum teres (medial epiphyseal artery), which has limited anastomoses with these lateral epiphyseal vessels. Intracapsular femoral neck fractures interrupt most blood flow through the subsynovial retinacular vessels, including these important lateral epiphyseal arteries; 78% of post-fracture femoral head specimens were partially or totally avascular on histologic examination.[3] Late segmental collapse of the articular surface occurred in about 30% of displaced fractures and 10% of hip dislocations without fractures, because dislocations usually rupture the ligamentum teres. Hemarthrosis with intracapsular tamponade may aggravate ischemia in undisplaced fractures.[4,5] Necrosis can also be produced in immature animals as a result of arterial, rather than venous, intracapsular tamponade.

Several other bones have precarious vascularity. For example, the body of the talus is particularly vulnerable to osteonecrosis, which occurred after 54% of talar neck fractures.[6] Four-part fractures of the proximal humerus[7] may impair humeral head vascularity, primarily arising from the ascending branch of the anterior circumflex artery,[8] often resulting in osteonecrosis. A fracture propagating (in microseconds) through intraosseous arteries during a partial systolic ejection could also potentially result in instantaneous arterial intravasation of marrow fat and tissue thromboplastin directly into the subchondral capillary trap, triggering focal intravascular coagulation, thrombosis, and necrosis.[9,10]

NONTRAUMATIC (MICROVASCULAR) DAMAGE

Intravascular Coagulation (Thrombosis)

There is histologic evidence of intraosseous thromboses in very early osteonecrosis.[10–12] Thrombosis of the *microcirculation* of susceptible intraosseous end organs appears to be the genesis of nontraumatic osteonecrosis, and it results from a combination of at least three factors (Virchow's triad): (1) stasis, (2) hypercoagulability, and (3) endothelial damage. The initial lesion is localized to the *subchondral* bone, which has a vulnerable microanatomy facilitating stasis. Terminal arteries with few collaterals supply subchondral areas, which favor embolic occlusion and thrombosis, especially with localized vasoconstriction, or possibly, vasospasm (Raynaud's phenomenon). Intramedullary pressure and blood flow are reduced in the fatty subchondral bone of epiphyseal regions with long, narrow arcades of subchondral end capillaries.[9] Relative stasis also occurs in sinusoids and the central venous sinus.

Hypercoagulability[13] occurs under local conditions of increased procoagulant activities, decreased anticoagulant activities, vasoconstriction (neural, metabolic, and humeral) of the subchondral arteriolar bed, and decreased fibrinolysis.[14] For example, protein C and S deficiencies, antithrombin III deficiency, hyperviscosity, hyperlipemia, hyperfibrinogemia, polycythemia, lupus coagulant, thrombocytosis, elevated plasminogen activator inhibitor, and other platelet activating factors most likely produce a decreased threshold resistance to thrombogenesis and osteonecrosis.

The surface/volume ratio of the subchondral capillary bed results in a marked increase of endothelial cells in direct contact with blood. In the perturbed state, subchondral endothelial cells can be thrombogenic through the synthesis of von Willebrand factor antigen (vWF:Ag), plasminogen activator inhibitor-1 (PAI-1), and especially tissue factor (thromboplastin), a high-affinity, cell-surface receptor for factor VII.[15] This functional bimolecular complex mediates the initial proteolytic activation of the extrinsic coagulation cascade.

Endothelial damage of subchondral capillaries and sinusoids, with release of tissue factor (thromboplastin), is the most likely event triggering platelet aggregation and fibrin thrombosis, with progressive involvement of venules, veins, arterioles, and occasionally, extraosseous arteries.[16] In children, thrombosis of the *subchondral* vessels on the epiphyseal side of the growth plate (physis) also may occur.

Confirmatory Evidence

Several human and animal models can trigger intravascular coagulation and produce osteonecrosis (Fig. 100–1). The earliest case of osteonecrosis, affecting both humeral (Fig. 100–2) and femoral heads, with subchondral fat embolism (Fig. 100–3A) and disseminated intravascular coagulation (DIC), occurred 18 hours after anaphylactic shock.[10] Subchondral fibrin thrombi (Fig. 100–3B) and peripheral interadipocytic hemorrhage resulting from secondary fibrinolysis and reperfusion of necrotic vessels were found.

Additional evidence relating fat embolism and DIC to osteonecrosis is derived from studies of the generalized Shwartzman phenomenon.[17] Rabbits given endotoxin developed hyperlipemia, fatty liver, systemic fat embolism, and DIC with fibrin thrombosis.[18–20] Fifty-one osteonecrotic lesions, including the humeral (Fig. 100–4) and femoral heads, complicated DIC in eight children.[21–25] Collateral histologic studies revealed ischemia and fibrin thrombi within the microvasculature adjacent to necrotic bone.[26] Osteonecrosis in those same patients with systemic lupus erythematosus (SLE) who are not receiving corticoids may also involve the Shwartzman-like phenomenon.[27]

Two animal models (type III hypersensitivity, immune-complex mediated) also suggest intravascular coagulation as the final common pathway. Two to three hours after antigen injection into rabbit knees,[28] focal areas of subchondral bone were found to be devoid of secondary and tertiary branches of the epiphyseal arteries. At 1 to 2 weeks, occlusions of subchondral vessels were observed adjacent to avascular subchondral bone. In another study,[29] a combination of serum sickness

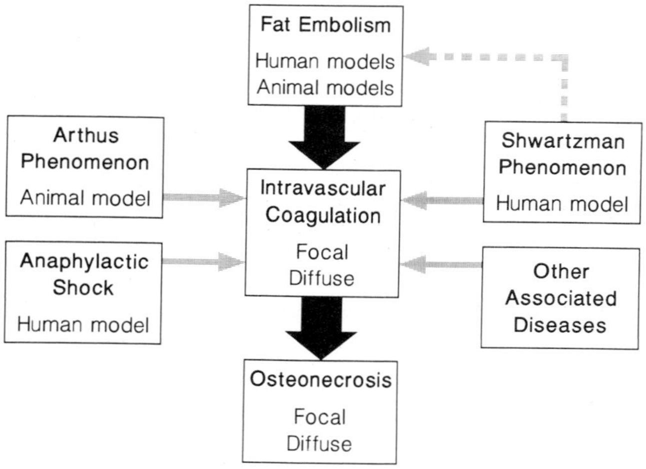

FIGURE 100–1. Flowchart depicting intravascular coagulation as the final common pathway producing osteonecrosis, not only in diseases associated with fat embolism, especially alcoholism and hypercortisonism, but also in an animal model using an immune complex, delayed hypersensitivity reaction (Arthus phenomenon), and human models employing either an endotoxic reaction (Shwartzman phenomenon) or an immediate antigen–antibody reaction producing anaphylactic shock, as well as other associated diseases that can directly trigger intravascular coagulation.

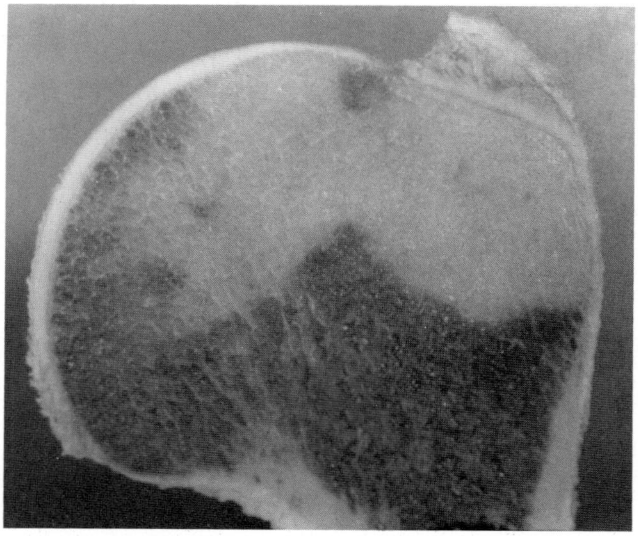

FIGURE 100–2. Coronal section of left humeral head in a patient who expired 18 hours after developing anaphylactic shock. Disseminated intravascular coagulation had resulted in fibrin thromboses of vessels, with necrosis of hematopoietic and adipocytic marrow tissue (nonviable light areas) and secondary fibrinolysis and interadipocytic hemorrhage of adjacent marrow (viable dark areas). This classic distribution of osteonecrosis was also seen in this patient's right humeral head and both femoral heads.

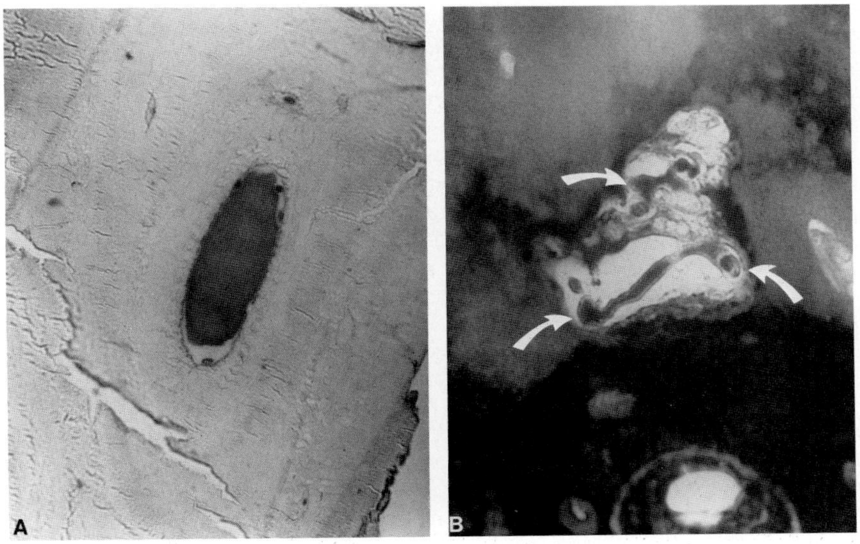

FIGURE 100–3. *A*, Photomicrograph of subchondral bone from humeral head showing pyknotic-appearing endothelial cell nuclei within a Haversian canal that is completely occluded by a deformed fat embolus (S.B. Doty modification of osmium-potassium dichromate technique stain ×400). *B*, Photomicrograph of humeral head at the tidemark revealing subchondral capillaries occluded with multiple fibrin thrombi (arrows) (phosphotungstic acid-hematoxylin stain ×200).

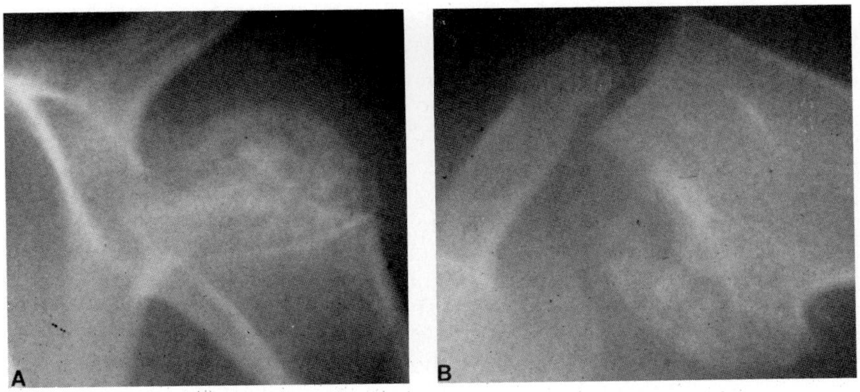

FIGURE 100–4. Radiographic views (*A,B*) of left shoulder demonstrating osteonecrosis with hypoplasia, irregularity, and fragmentation of the capital humeral epiphysis. This 22-month-old girl had recovered from disseminated intravascular coagulation following infection with Hemophilus influenzae at age 2 months. (Courtesy of Louise S. Acheson.)

and high-dose corticoids produced arterial interruptions and necrotic lesions in 70% of rabbit femurs.

Extensive bone infarctions probably result from a consumptive coagulopathy in SLE,[30] dysbaric syndromes,[31] pancreatitis,[32] pregnancy,[33,34] Leriche syndrome,[35,36] meningococcemia,[37] malignancy, chemotherapy, and other conditions.[38–40]

Intravascular Coagulation (Hemorrhage)

Subchondral fibrin-platelet thrombosis is usually followed by some degree of endogenous fibrinolysis (Fig. 100–2). Reperfusion of these necrotic vessels is postulated to result in marrow hemorrhage (Fig. 100–5) adjacent to the area of infarction. Ischemia-reperfusion injuries could cause lipid damage to endothelial cell membranes by oxygen free radicals, also potentiating microfocal bleeding. There is extravasation of erythrocytes between marrow adipocytes, hemosiderin deposition, and deposition of eosinophilic amorphous mate-

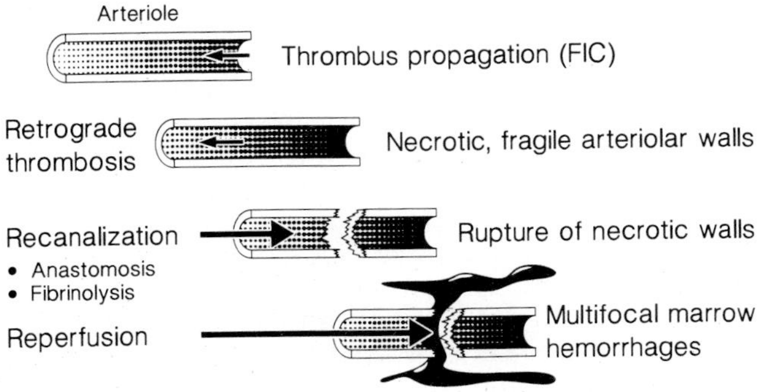

FIGURE 100–5. Probable mechanism for the development of focal intramedullary hemorrhages resulting from focal intravascular coagulation (FIC) of sinusoids and capillaries and retrograde fibrin-platelet thrombosis with fibrinolysis and rupture of necrotic arteriolar walls with reperfusion.

rial between adipocytes.[10,11,41] In one study,[42] core biopsies of 16 intact femoral heads in steroid-treated patients showed multifocal marrow hemorrhages with damaged or ruptured blood vessels in the hemorrhagic areas.

Experimentally,[43,44] between 1 and 2 hours of arterial or venous marrow ischemia resulted in sinusoidal distension and rupture, with interadipocytic hemorrhage followed by a plasma-like fluid (plasmostasis) appearing between the fat cells. After a few days the affected capillaries and sinusoids sometimes disappeared altogether.

Intravascular coagulation is not the cause of osteonecrosis, but it is always an intermediary event triggered by a variety of factors.

Fat Embolism

Osteonecrosis associated with fat embolism of bone[9] was first demonstrated clinically in 1965 and experimentally in 1966. In one epidemiologic study 89% of 269 patients with nontraumatic osteonecrosis had disorders known to be complicated by disturbed fat metabolism or fat embolism.[45]

Fat emboli may arise from a fatty liver (*mechanism A*), destabilization and coalescence of plasma lipoproteins (*mechanism B*), and/or disruption of fatty bone marrow or other adipose tissue depots (*mechanism C*) (Fig. 100–6). Fat embolism occurs in several disorders associated with osteonecrosis (Table 100–1).

Absolute Fat Overload. An absolute overload[46,47] of intraosseous fat emboli, with inadequate clearance of procoagulants and intravascular coagulation, appears to be the most common underlying cause of nontraumatic osteonecrosis,[48] especially in alcoholism and hypercortisonism, which now account for about two thirds of all cases. A critical *ischemic threshold* of subchondral fat overload with intravascular free fatty acid generation and endothelial injury from chemical (toxic) vasculitis can be related to the dose or duration of intraosseous fat embolism. There is a cumulative alcohol or corticoid dose-related osteonecrosis response.[49,50]

Experimental Confirmation. Studies have been conducted in corticosteroid-treated rabbits from nine laboratories.[16] In summary, all instances involved hyperlipemia, fatty liver, pulmonary fat embolism, systemic fat embolism, and subchondral fat embolism of the femoral (and humeral) heads (Fig. 100–7). Focal osteocyte death in the femoral heads occurred in six of the eight series studied. Corticosteroids caused hyperlipemia, especially increased very-low-density, pre-B lipoproteins, after 4 to 7 days, and fatty liver. Systemic fat embolism to the subchondral arterioles and capillaries of the femoral heads occurred after 2 to 3 weeks. Significant bone marrow necrosis occurred as early as 3 weeks. Increased intrafemoral head pressure with decreased blood flow occurred after 6 to 8 weeks.

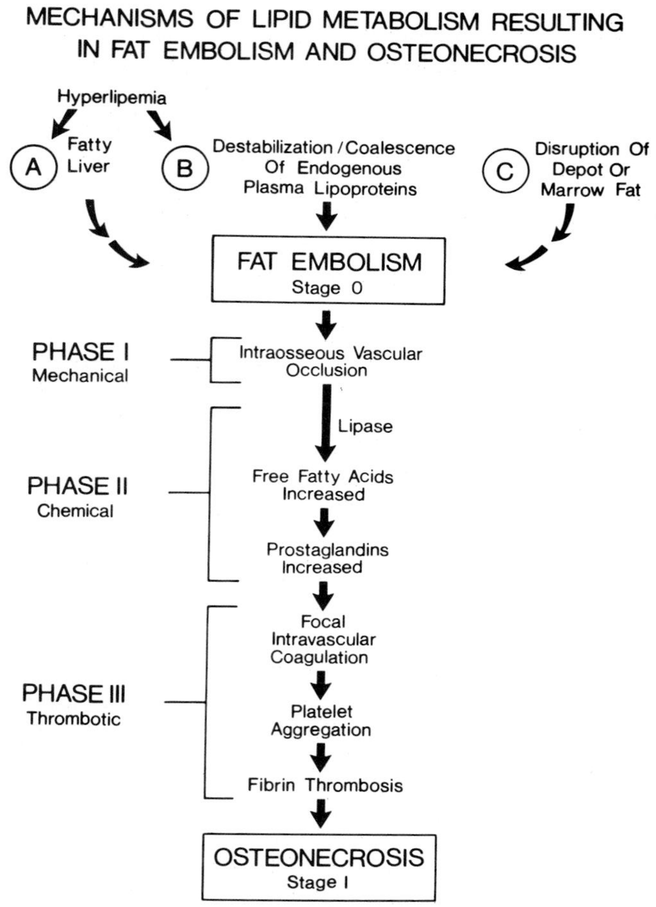

FIGURE 100–6. Schematic representation of three mechanisms potentially capable of producing intraosseous fat embolism and triggering a process leading to focal intravascular coagulation and osteonecrosis. (From Jones, J.P., Jr.: Fat embolism and osteonecrosis. Orthop. Clin. North Am., *16*:595, 1985.)

TABLE 100–1. CONDITIONS ASSOCIATED WITH OSTEONECROSIS RELATED TO FAT EMBOLISM

CONDITION	SUSPECTED MECHANISM*		
Alcoholism	A		
Carbon tetrachloride poisoning	A		
Diabetes mellitus	A	B	
Dysbaric phenomena		B	C
Hemoglobinopathies			C
Hypercortisonism (or Cushing's syndrome)	A		
Hyperlipemia (type II or IV)	A	B	
Obesity	A	B	
Oral contraceptives (estrogen)	A	B	
Pancreatitis		B	C
Pregnancy	A	B	
Unrelated fractures			C

* A = fatty liver; B = coalescence of plasma lipoproteins; C = disruption of fatty bone marrow.

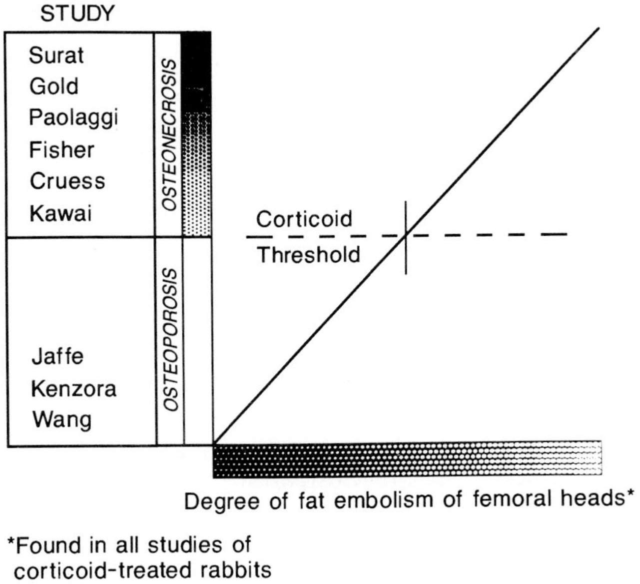

FIGURE 100–7. Hypothetical dose–response curve relating the degree of fat embolism of the femoral heads of corticoid-treated rabbits in various experimental studies to osteoporosis and a threshold beyond which progressively more severe osteocytic necrosis occurs.[193–201]

Extravascular Lipid Migration. There is rapid centrifugal movement of intravascular macromolecules into the peripheral osteocytic lacunae of the osteon.[51] Discontinuous capillaries with relatively large gap junctions (transcapillary clefts) are found in the marrow and relatively large molecules can pass between osteoblasts surrounding the capillaries in Haversian systems.[52]

Intravascular labeled fat extended circumferentially through canaliculi to become deposited within individual osteocytic lacunae.[9] This lipid most likely reached the osteocytes by traversing the space of Neumann between the cell-process membrane and the lacunar-canalicular collagen matrix wall. Entrapment of fat emboli is most likely to occur in the relatively low-pressure and low-flow subchondral (and subperiosteal) capillary beds, which normally terminate at the tidemark, the boundry between calcified and noncalcified cartilage. An accumulation of lipid in subchondral osteocytes subsequently becomes necrotic, both experimentally[53] and clinically[54] in alcoholism and hypercortisonism. Steroid-induced lipid-accumulating osteocytes differ ultrastructurally from ischemic osteocytes.[55]

Relative Fat Overload. *Osteoporosis.* A dose and duration of intraosseous (subperiosteal and subchondral) fat embolism below the ischemic threshold and insufficient to trigger intravascular coagulation may cause decreased bone formation. In corticoid-treated rabbits both, fat embolism and osteoporosis were observed in the femoral heads in all nine studies.[16] Moreover, lipid-clearing agents prevented corticoid-induced osteoporosis.[56] Unfortunately, long-term heparin therapy given to prevent intravascular coagulation itself causes osteoporosis. Hypertriglyceridemia, increased lipolytic activity, and cell toxicity may occur in hemodialysis patients receiving heparin.[57,58] Histomorphometric studies from 68 of 77 (89%) osteonecrosis patients showed coexistent osteoporosis.[59]

For example, massive bone marrow necrosis occurred with DIC complicating pregnancy.[60] Perhaps transient osteoporosis of the hip in pregnancy[61] is related to early osteonecrosis.[62] Scintigraphy and magnetic resonance imaging (MRI) studies performed early in both conditions are similar. Rapid and complete fibrinolysis could result in transient hypervascularity, edema, and osteoporosis, rather than persistent fibrin-platelet thrombosis and osteonecrosis.

The sequence of intraosseous fat embolism, endothelial cell necrosis, extravascular lipid migration, reduced osteoblastic activity, and fatty osteocytic necrosis has recently been confirmed in space-flight rats.[63,64] The stress of weightlessness may cause endogenous hypercortisonism with increased adrenal weight[65] and increased catecholamine and corticosterone secretion.[66]

POPULATION AT RISK

DYSBARISM-RELATED OSTEONECROSIS

Fossilized evidence (64 to 100 million years) of osteonecrosis has been discovered in the humeral heads and vertebral bodies of deep-diving mosasaur lizards and turtles.[67] Virtually identical humeral head lesions have been found in those humans exposed to changes in atmospheric pressure in the course of their occupations, principally compressed-air workers and divers.

No direct evidence indicates that the cause of bone and marrow necrosis is the embolism or compression of vessels by gas bubbles, as is generally believed.[68] A single rapid decompression has been shown to cause gas embolism, fat embolism,[69] DIC,[31] and osteonecrosis.[70] Recompression therapy for decompression sickness eliminates gas emboli, but fat emboli remain. Intravascular fat may augment DIC. Decreased antithrombin III activity, prolonged prothrombin time, increased fibrin degradation products, and accelerated platelet and fibrinogen turnover are associated with dysbarism.[71] Dysbaric osteonecrosis has been produced experimentally, particularly in obese mice subjected to multiple hyperbaric exposures.[72]

Compressed-Air Workers (Tunnel or Caisson)

Thirteen percent (164 of 1269) of hyperbaric workers had bone lesions.[73] The risk of decompression sickness is minimal at working pressures below 11 psig; pressures greater than 17 psig increased its incidence and the risk of osteonecrosis.[74] Thirty-eight percent of 977 lesions in 383 compressed-air workers appeared in the lower femoral shaft, as compared to 54% of 114 lesions in 60 commercial divers; however, 12% of the lesions developed in the femoral head in the compressed-air workers, as compared to only 0.9% in the divers.[75]

Divers

Advances in diving research now permit safe underwater operations in depths to 1600 feet. Four groups of divers are considered: (1) skin divers, in whom osteonecrosis is nonexistent, and sport scuba divers, in whom it is virtually nonexistent; (2) U.S., British, French, Japanese, and Canadian navy divers, who have a 1 to 3% incidence of osteonecrosis, using standard tables; (3) commercial divers, who have a 4.2% overall and a 1.2% juxta-articular incidence; and (4) Hawaiian and Japanese diving fishermen, who have a 50 to 65% incidence of lesions.

OSTEONECROSIS ASSOCIATED WITH OTHER CONDITIONS

Hypercortisonism

Both endogenous (Cushing's disease) and exogenous hypercortisonism can cause osteonecrosis.[76] The at-risk threshold for the adult is generally considered to be about 2000 mg prednisone or its equivalent. About 4% of patients with inflammatory bowel disease[77] and about 5% of adults with SLE[78] treated with steroids develop osteonecrosis. Osteonecrosis in patients with SLE who are not taking corticosteroids is rare and may be associated with Raynaud's phenomenon, thrombotic thrombocytopenic purpura, and/or anti-cardiolipin antibodies. The capitellum, carpal scaphoid, and capitate, metacarpal and metatarsal heads, distal femoral condyles, patella, talus, and tibial plateau, as well as the femoral and humeral heads, have been involved in osteonecrosis in lupus patients.

Hemodialysis patients not receiving corticosteroids may develop lytic subchondral cysts resulting from amyloidosis, which may be confused with osteonecrosis.[79] Osteonecrosis occurred in 299 of 2285 (13%) patients from 18 renal-transplant centers.[80] Cyclosporin A use has reduced the dose of prednisone needed and also reduced the incidence of osteonecrosis.

Alcoholism

An elevated plasma cortisol concentration may occur in alcohol-induced pseudo-Cushing's syndrome.[81] Alcoholics under age 50 also have an increased thrombotic tendency and reduced fibrinolytic activity.[82] Alcohol-induced fatty liver is conceivably the most common source of continuous, low-grade, and relatively asymptomatic showers of systemic fat emboli.[9,83] In 26 alcoholic patients with osteonecrosis of the femoral head, 38 hips showed elevated intraosseous pressures in the early stages.[84] Of 38 alcoholics with osteonecrosis, 24 (63%) had type II or type IV hyperlipemia and biopsy-proven fatty livers.

Hyperlipemia

Although the most dramatic elevations of serum triglycerides occur in types I and V, osteonecrosis is most common in type II and IV hyperlipemia, where elevated soluble fibrin complexes are found.[85,86] Eight family members had type IV hyperlipidemia and osteonecrosis of the femoral heads.[87] Hyperlipemia is often accompanied by osteonecrosis in obesity, diabetes, and rarely, in hypothyroidism.[88] Hyperlipemia also occurs in the nephrotic syndrome with DIC. Fat embolism and coagulation activation may occur in obese type II diabetic patients.[89]

Pregnancy

Osteonecrosis can develop in pregnancy, usually in the third trimester or early postpartum period,[90] often in association with hypercoagulability.[91] Plasma lipid levels increase after the third month of gestation, when adrenocortical activity is elevated. Fatty liver may occur in the third trimester[92] and is associated with osteonecrosis.[9] These patients commonly have DIC[93] with low fibrinogen levels, elevated prothrombin and partial thromboplastin times, fibrin split products, and decreased antithrombin III. Osteonecrosis has also been linked to the use of oral contraceptives.[45]

Hemoglobinopathies

Osteonecrosis in sickle cell anemia and its variants, including sickle trait, have been considered to be due solely to plugging of intraosseous vessels by sickled erythrocytes, but fibrin deposition and impaired fibrinolysis occur at the same time as erythrocyte sequestration.[94,95] Although dense (dehydrated, irreversibly sickled) erythrocytes are decreased 70% during painful crises in those sickle cell patients with marrow abnormalities detected by MRI,[96] it is doubtful that these dense red cells, which are selectively sequestered in the microcirculation during vaso-occlusive events, can by themselves cause osteonecrosis, because they apparently produce stasis without thrombosis.[97] Several other factors, however, activate the coagulation system and produce thrombosis in the hemoglobinopathies, including fat embolism, thrombocytosis, elevated factor VIII, lowered factor V and plasminogen, hyperviscosity, hyperfibrinogenemia, and elevated serum fibrin split products.

Early osteoarthritis (OA) of the hip developed in 30 of 95 (35%) hips in adults with childhood osteonecrosis resulting from hemoglobinopathies. Five hips had no definite deformity in the femur or acetabulum but developed OA which perhaps was due to abnormal subchondral bony remodeling.[98]

Obesity

Obesity is a risk factor for both osteonecrosis[9] and primary osteoarthritis.[99,100] Osteocytic necrosis can be found in arthrosis.[101] With advancing age there is an increase in the intracellular and extracellular lipids of human articular cartilage[102] and an association between lesion severity, total lipid content, and fatty acid levels.[103] Lipid readily enters cartilage and rapidly appears in chondrocytes, which may become necrotic.[104] Obese mice can develop enlarged fatty livers and either osteonecrosis[72] or increased osteoarthritis (OA).[105] Histologic sections of human femoral heads with OA have revealed fat in the vascular spaces of subchondral bone.[106]

Subchondral hypoxia[107,108] probably stimulates osteoblastic new bone formation in subchondral regions with fractional osteocytic necrosis because hyperoxia downregulated osteoblastic activity in subchondral areas with dead (revascularizing) bone.[109] If the revascularization process targets fractional necrosis of the subchondral plate, there may be overzealous capillary penetration through the tidemark. Such exaggerated remodeling could potentially result in hypervascularity and increased enchondral ossification of the subchondral plate in obese patients who develop primary (idiopathic) osteoarthrosis.

PATHOGENESIS OF NONTRAUMATIC OSTEONECROSIS

I have divided the pathophysiology of osteonecrosis into five stages: 0, I, II, III, and IV. Thermal injuries, chemotherapy, and radiation cause osteonecrosis by direct cytotoxicity and obliterative endarteritis. Necrosis is also caused by occlusive vascular disease with thrombosis. I speculate that, particularly in hypercortisonism, intraosseous fat embolism (stage 0) may trigger a three-phase process leading to focal intravascular coagulation and focal osteonecrosis (stage I) (Fig. 100–6).

Stage I lesions show dead bone marrow and dead bony trabeculae *without repair.* Repair starts in stage II with recanalization of thrombosed vessels and revascularization (resorption, followed by reossification) but without subchondral collapse or articular incongruity. Late segmental collapse initiates stage III, which is usually followed by stage IV and *secondary* (OA).

STAGE 0

Phase 1: Mechanical (Intraosseous Vascular Occlusion) Obstruction

The dynamics of intraosseous fat embolism were originally studied experimentally using Lipiodol (iodized oil, U.S.P.).[110] In other studies, the injection of depot fat produced hypoxemia and pulmonary edema. A biphasic response consisting of an early mechanical insult and a later chemical one was suggested. Subchondral hypoxia and perivascular edema were thought likely to occur after intraosseous vascular occlusion also.

Phase 2: Chemical (Inflammatory) Vasculitis

Neutral marrow fat itself produces little or no thrombotic reaction in the isolated venous segment, but neutral embolic fat is indirectly thrombogenic through its ability to generate free fatty acids.[111,112] The complete breakdown of intraosseous fat emboli required up to 5 weeks experimentally,[110] producing a latent period between the mechanical and chemical phases.

Oleic acid is the main fatty acid in neutral trioleum, the most abundant marrow fat. Free oleic acid caused a marked stripping of capillary endothelium, passive congestion, and edema formation shown by time-lapse cinemicrography in dogs.[113] Oleic acid also produced local thrombosis when injected into an isolated vein segment. Marked platelet aggregation and fibrin deposition occurred in the vicinity of the fat.[114] Oleic acid injected into the pulmonary circulation of dogs produced intravascular coagulation, deposition of labeled fibrinogen and platelets, and secondary thrombocytopenia.[115]

Free fatty acids produced a rapid endothelial sloughing, exposure of the subendothelial collagen, and release of tissue factor (thromboplastin) considered the decisive trigger of intravascular coagulation. Free fatty acids lead directly to increased production of prostaglandins, which can cause intramedullary edema and increased intraosseous pressure. Twofold to threefold elevations in unbound free fatty acids and plasma prostaglandins began 1 to 2 weeks after giving corticoids to rabbits.[116] Elevated total serum lipids and free fatty acids, intraosseous fat emboli, and increased prostaglandin content were found in the necrotic femoral heads of steroid-treated rabbits in another study. The PGE_2-like activity was increased 8-fold and 16-fold, after 30 and 90 days of prednisolone administration, respectively.[117]

Phase 3: Thrombotic (Focal Intravascular Coagulation) Occlusion

A relatively common subclinical form of fat embolism is associated with intravascular coagulation, platelet aggregation, and fibrin thrombi.[118] Intravascular coagulation may be precipitated by endothelial damage and fat embolism. Elevated plasma lipids may accelerate blood clotting, increasing platelet adhesiveness and aggregation. Intraosseous fat embolism, intravascular coagulation (thrombosis *and* hemorrhage), and osteonecrosis (traumatic and nontraumatic) have been shown to coexist in humans.[10]

Laboratory Tests. Early detection of focal intravascular coagulation (stage 0, phase 3) is enhanced in patients at high risk of ischemic end organ damage by using a triple test screen of plasma fibrino-peptide A, D-dimer fibrin fragments and antithrombin III.[9,10]

Prevention and Treatment. Prevention requires avoidance of known causative factors. Further studies are necessary to determine if prompt anticoagulation will prevent impending osteonecrosis. Experimentally, aprotinin (Trasylol) prevented steroid-induced osteonecrosis by inhibiting tissue kallikrein activity and platelet aggregation, preventing contact activation of intravascular coagulation.[117]

DIAGNOSIS AND MANAGEMENT OF OSTEONECROSIS

I will focus on management of lesions affecting the juxta-articular or epiphyseal regions because metadiaphyseal lesions, such as calcified intramedullary fat necrosis or bone infarction, are neither symptomatic nor disabling.

STAGE 1 LESION

The patient is asymptomatic, with no physical or radiographic findings. Histologically, localized stage I lesions show dead bone marrow and dead trabeculae, without any evidence of repair. The generalized stage I lesion occurs with physiologic death of the skeleton, as seen in certain archeologic specimens (Fig. 100–8).

Pathologic Features

Under light microscopy hematopoietic marrow cells and capillary endothelial cells are the first to appear necrotic, followed by adipocytic necrosis. More than 200 biopsy specimens of early lesions showed interstitial edema, necrosis of fatty and hematopoietic marrow, and rupture of lipocytes, producing large, fatty cysts and liquefaction necrosis, amorphous debris, sinusoidal distension, and arteriolar thrombosis.[11] Marrow changes occurred before alterations in the trabeculae were noted. The presence or absence (empty lacunae) of osteocyte nuclei was variable as a result of wide variations in autolytic rates after functional death. At the margin of the necrotic sequestrum in early osteonecrosis, sinusoids may be enlarged and contain lipid droplets, and there may be hemorrhagic marrow lesions with hemosiderin-filled macrophages.[10,119] With thrombosis of the subchondral capillary and sinusoidal bed, it is likely that arteriolar-venular shunts open, resulting in venous congestion and increased venous-outlet resistance. Inflammatory marrow edema progresses within the rigid bony compartment, further aggravating the pre-existing ischemic perfusion damage.

Interstitial edema probably occurs very rapidly after fat embolism and fibrin thrombosis.[120] Cytokine mediators such as interleukin-1 (IL-1) and tumor necrosis factor (TNF) may cause a nonspecific secondary inflammatory response to a severe ischemic insult. Neutrophil activation and protease release induces vascular damage, cellular destruction, increased vascular permeability, and probable intraosseous edema. Cytokines also increase tissue factor (thromboplastin) exposure, decrease thrombomodulin expression, and increase secretion of PAI-1, further aggravating microvascular thrombosis. With venous thrombosis venous drainage is deficient, intraosseous pressure is increased, and marrow perfusion is decreased.

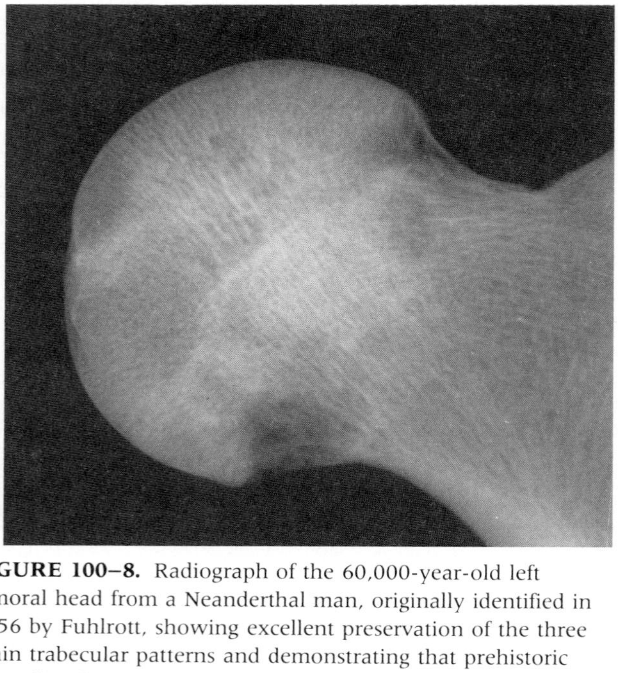

FIGURE 100–8. Radiograph of the 60,000-year-old left femoral head from a Neanderthal man, originally identified in 1856 by Fuhlrott, showing excellent preservation of the three main trabecular patterns and demonstrating that prehistoric bone that dies and undergoes natural mummification (dehydration without fossilization), *without repair,* does not spontaneously collapse. (Courtesy of Paul Dann.)

Laboratory Tests

Stage-I lesions are rarely discovered. Elevated plasma fibrinopeptide A was found in two stage I patients with evidence of systemic fat embolism and arterial interruptions detected by superselective angiography.[16] Another stage I patient had elevated D-dimer fibrin fragments and decreased antithrombin III.[10]

The duration of the stage I lesion is only about a week. During this time the diagnosis of osteonecrosis can be established and subsequently confirmed by biopsy with a combination of *decreased* radionuclide uptake on ^{99m}Tc-methylene diphosphonate scintigrams, and either normal (false-negative), *decreased* signal intensity (without bands or rings), or a diffuse edema pattern (decreased T1-weighting; increased T2-weighting) on MRI.

Because osteonecrotic damage is selective, radiographs should concentrate on the shoulder, hip, and knee joints with two rotational views of each shoulder, and an anteroposterior and lateral projection of each hip and knee. Conventional radiography is not satisfactory for early diagnosis of osteonecrosis, because death of bone and marrow, *without repair,* produces no radiologic abnormality. Therefore, computed tomography (CT), even with multiplanar reconstructions, will not show any abnormalities in stage I.

Scintigraphy. A photon-deficient "cold" lesion provides the best evidence for a stage I lesion.[121] Such cold lesions commonly occur immediately after sickle cell crises or decompression sickness[122] and represent acute bone infarctions. Decreased uptake is best found within 48 hours of symptoms of a vaso-occlusive crisis.[123] Acute bone infarcts less than 1 week old are also usually photopenic on both ^{99m}Tc-sulfur colloid and ^{67}Ga-citrate images.[124,125]

Scintigraphy performed within 4 weeks of femoral neck fractures may show diminished femoral head uptake.[126] This was the finding in 25 of 45 (55%) hips; whereas repeat scintigraphy at 4 months showed decreased activity in 5 of 40 (12%) hips, and these underwent late segmental collapse.[127] Recently, bone marrow scintigraphy with ^{99m}Tc-nanocolloid has been found to be a sensitive method for diagnosing post-traumatic osteonecrosis, using the normal side for comparison.[128]

Interpretation of technetium ^{99m} methylene diphosphonate scintigrams is based on asymmetric radioisotope uptake, so diagnosis becomes more difficult in patients with bilateral involvement. Osteonecrosis on the less affected side is often overlooked. Single photon emission computed tomography (SPECT) may better find photon-deficient areas in the femoral heads during the early avascular phase.[129,130]

Magnetic Resonance Imaging. Because of false-negative studies, MRI is not as useful as scintigraphy for stage I lesions.[131–133] These lesions can appear normal on MRI for at least 3 days after a known ischemic event.[134,135] Probably the earliest MRI finding of osteonecrosis is the edema pattern with diffusely decreased signal intensity (hypointensity) on T1 weighting and hyperintensity on T2 weighting, often extending into the intertrochanteric region. This pattern suggests increased free water content, which may be located either in capillaries and sinusoids in the form of vascular congestion or hyperemia, in the interstitial space in the form of edema, or within ischemic and swollen cells (hydropic degeneration).

An identical marrow edema pattern occurs early in transient osteoporosis[136,137] and in sickle cell crisis.[138] The conversion to an edema pattern with sickle cell crises correlated with acute infarction. Some children may have transient bone marrow edema, rather than irreversible osteonecrosis.[139]

In MRIs acquired with a T1-weighted, spin-echo pulse sequence, the normal bone marrow is characterized by a signal of high intensity reflecting its high content of hydrogen-rich marrow fat.[140] Normally, high signal intensity (white) appears on coronal images of the humeral and femoral heads. Fat cells may remain viable appearing for 2 to 5 days. In stage I the necrotic zone will retain high signal intensity (isointense with viable marrow fat) if the nonviable fat cells and fatty cysts have not yet saponified. However, the necrotic zone will have homogeneous low signal intensity on T1-weighting if liquefaction and coagulation necrosis and saponification have resulted in degradation of the pre-existing fat into amorphous granular debris. Heterogeneous hypointensity most likely occurs when only a portion of the nonviable fat undergoes saponification.

Intraosseous Pressure and Venography. Elevations of intraosseous pressure in perinecrotic regions and intramedullary stasis with venous obstruction are well documented in early osteonecrosis.[11,141] Even if the major arterial and venous circulation appears normal, the capillary and sinusoidal microcirculation may be thrombosed and destroyed, and the contrast media is not absorbed but diffuses slowly through the medullary space.[142]

Digital Subtraction and Superselective Angiography. If the scintigram and/or MRI is abnormal, superselective angiographic studies may reveal an abrupt interruption of the medial femoral circumflex artery or absence of its lateral epiphyseal (superior retinacular) branches.[16,143,144] Angiography showed obstruction of the superior retinacular artery in Perthes disease.[145]

Microvascular Cartography. Evidence of early global devascularization of the femoral head was observed when technetium-labeled microspheres of serum albumin with a mean diameter of 40 μm (embolic scintigraphy) were combined with subtraction superselective arteriography of the medial femoral circumflex artery.[146] Nontraumatic osteonecrosis began in six of eight stage I lesions with global arterial ischemia (total devascularization of the femoral head).

Biopsy

A biopsy should be obtained to confirm the diagnosis if the scintigram or MRI is abnormal. A trephine is introduced into the subchondral bone of the femoral or humeral head under radiographic control, and the tissue is examined both microscopically and microroentgenographically. A histochemical method for identification of lactate dehydrogenase activity in viable osteocytes in fresh calcified and decalcified sections is recommended.[147]

STAGE II LESION

The patient with a stage II lesion is usually asymptomatic and still has no physical findings. The bony lesion shows repair *without* collapse.

Pathologic Features

A lag period occurs before repair begins, during which, collateral circulation is presumably stimulated and fibrinolysis occurs. Angiogenesis may be stimulated by growth factors such as those from platelets[148]. Osteoclast migration may be stimulated by necrotic collagen degradation products. Spontaneous revascularization of segmental necrotic lesions of the femoral head from the cancellous region is possible, within certain limits (15

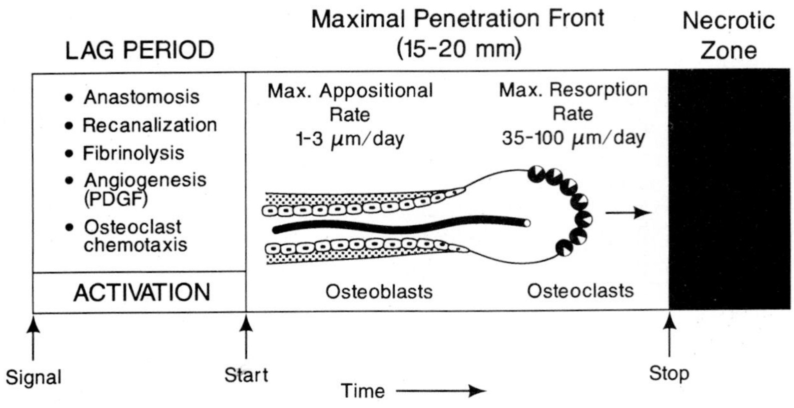

FIGURE 100–9. Chronologic concept of various components causing an activation lag period, which is followed by generation and penetration of a revascularization front (cutting cone) into the necrotic bone. Maximal penetration of the overall front is finite in cancellous, and especially in cortical (subchondral), bone. A subchondral zone of residual necrosis usually remains if the trabecular lesion is greater than 15 to 20 mm in diameter. (PDGF = platelet-derived growth factor.)

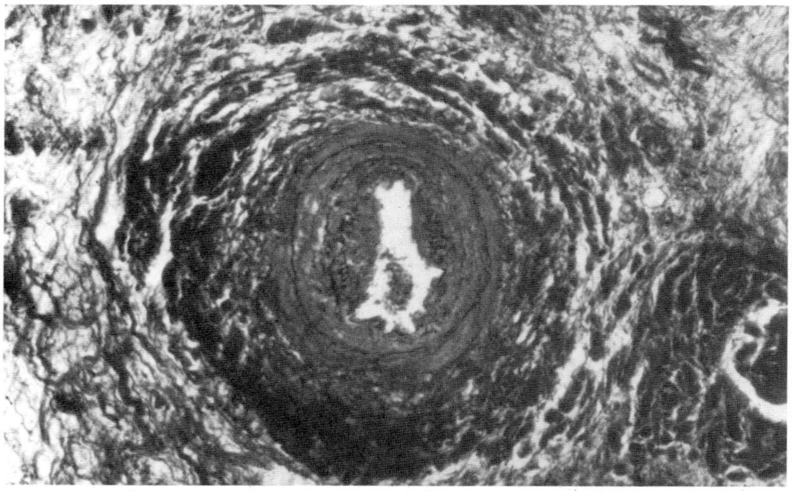

FIGURE 100–10. Photomicrograph of a lateral epiphyseal artery within a necrotic femoral head specimen demonstrating intraluminal, transthrombotic *recanalization* and intimal hyperplasia with residual partial occlusion. (Courtesy of Yoichi Sugioka.)

to 20mm) (Fig. 100–9). Repair can begin only along the perimeter of the avascular bone, at the junction of the ischemic zone surrounding the dead area and the viable area with intact circulation (the *hyperemic* zone). Primitive, undifferentiated mesenchymal cells and capillary buds containing endothelial cells proliferate and differentiate to fibroblasts, which begin synthesizing collagen. Subsequently, these mesenchymal cells differentiate to osteoblasts. The dead trabeculae are partially or completely resorbed by osteoclasts and are replaced or covered with new appositional bone, resulting in thickened, reinforced trabeculae. Reossification usually occurs distal to the revascularization and resorption front. The revascularization front includes osteoclasts, fibroblasts, and capillaries. Intimal thickening and myointimal cell proliferation with subendothelial fibrosis following endothelial cell injury or recanalization can result in narrowing of the arterial lumen (Fig. 100–10).

Radiographic Features. Radiographic changes produced by infarcted bone and marrow vary according to location. Areas of focal demineralization beneath an intact articular surface first appear on conventional radiographic examination as less dense areas, the result of subchondral bone resorption (radiolucency) and surrounding appositional new bone formation (radiosclerosis) (Fig. 100–11). Metaphyseal lesions often appear as irregular lucencies or linear or mottled densities.[149] Shaft or diaphyseal lesions often show serpentine calcification. No evidence of secondary subchondral fracture exists; the radiolucent "crescent" sign is not yet seen. It is important to precisely determine the size (and approximate volume) of juxta-articular lesions by using a radiographic staging system.[150]

Magnetic Resonance Imaging. MRI is the most sensitive, specific, low-risk, noninvasive test for the localization of osteonecrosis in stage II. Eventual bilaterality occurs in 80 to 95% of nontraumatic lesions.[151] In one study, biopsies were available in 55 of 90 patients with suspected osteonecrosis; MRI was 96% accurate when compared with biopsy findings. Isotopic studies and CT scans correlated with biopsy findings in 71% and 54%, respectively.[152] In another study, MRI suggested osteonecrosis in 26 hips; Only 4 of 13 MRI-positive hips with normal radiographs had abnormal technetium di-

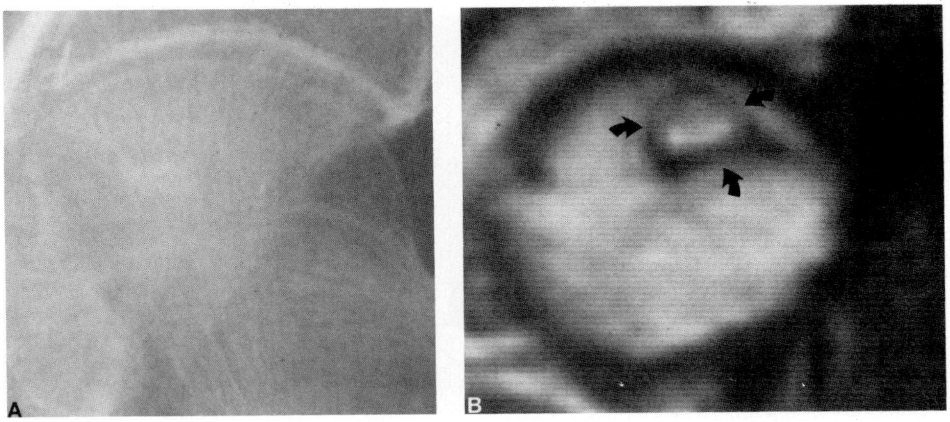

FIGURE 100–11. A focal stage II lesion is silently undergoing repair without collapse. *A*, It is not visualized in a normal-appearing plain radiograph of the femoral head. *B*, Magnetic resonance imaging with T1 weighting demonstrated a single reparative ring of low-intensity signal (arrows) in the superolateral femoral head. The central, residual necrotic nidus is isointense with the normal high-intensity, perinecrotic region.

phosphonate scintigrams.[153] The results of MRI in 20 patients were compared with bone scintigraphy in 12 patients and with conventional radiographs in 14 patients; MRI gave abnormal results in 5 cases with normal scintiphotos.[154]

In general stage II lesions show either rings (focal smaller lesions) (Fig. 100–11) or bands (larger lesions) (Fig. 100–12) or subchondral crescents of low signal intensity, representing the combined revascularization and reossification front surrounding the necrotic zone. Once an enlarging revascularization (repair) front begins penetrating into the necrotic zone, there is a further delay before a discrete band is obvious on MRI. In stage II, a repair front appears as a *single band* or ring of decreased signal intensity on T1 weighting (Fig. 100–13). This band is composed of viable tissue without fat cells and includes two parts, a resorption front, which is usually proximal, and a formation front, which is usually more distal.

These two parts may be visualized with T2 weighting, the pathognomonic *double-line sign* (Fig. 100–14). The high-intensity proximal part of this sign most likely represents granulation tissue with inflammatory edema and hyperemia (the resorption front), and the low-intensity distal band represents thickened trabeculae (Fig. 100–15). Lesions either stay the same size or get smaller; they do not enlarge.

Adjacent vertebral bodies can be similarly affected with precollapse (stage II) lesions[155] (Fig. 100–16) and can be associated with both degenerative disc disease and osteonecrosis of the femoral heads.[2] Four additional patients showed bands of decreased intensity on T1 weighting and increased intensity on T2 weighting in vertebrae, similar to the MRI findings in osteonecrosis of the hip.[156] Abnormalities in the cartilaginous end plates may precede histologic changes in the nucleus pulposis and anulus fibrosus. Impaired diffu-

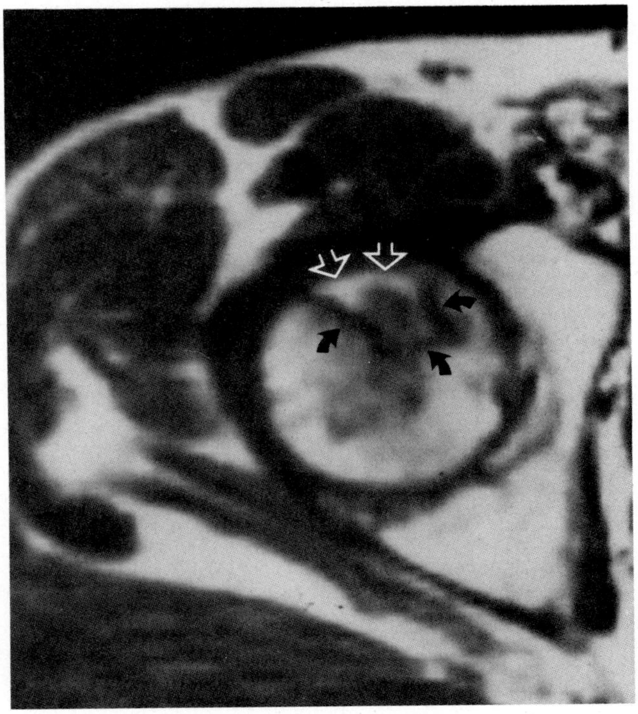

FIGURE 100–12. Magnetic resonance image (T1 weighted) of femoral head in axial plane showing a classic, reparative lesion without collapse (stage II) that is surrounded by a dark band (black arrows), the revascularization front. Heterogeneous signal intensity in the necrotic segment results from residual, dead, unsaponified adipocytes in the anterior third of the lesion (white arrows). This patient had alcoholism with pancreatitis and diabetes.

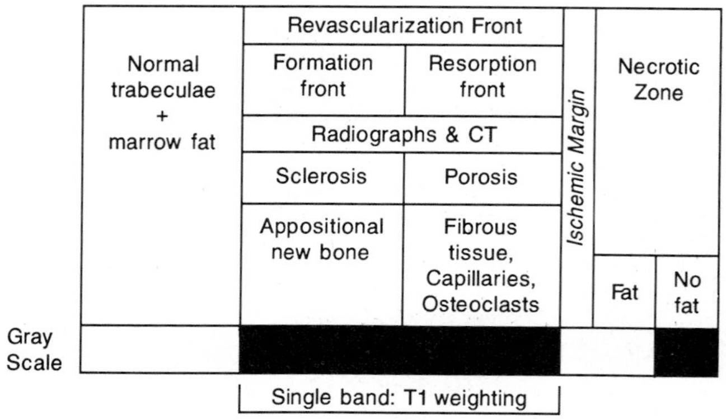

FIGURE 100–13. Gray-scale analysis of various components of stage II lesion using magnetic resonance imaging with *T1 weighting* (short TR/TE). The single band (or ring) usually represents the combined revascularization (resorption and formation) front, appearing as porosis and sclerosis on radiographs and computed tomography (CT). The necrotic zone will have high signal intensity, and erroneously will appear normal, if the dead fat has not yet saponified, and low intensity if it has already undergone liquefaction and coagulation necrosis and become amorphous debris. The stage I lesion has no discernible revascularization front (no single band).

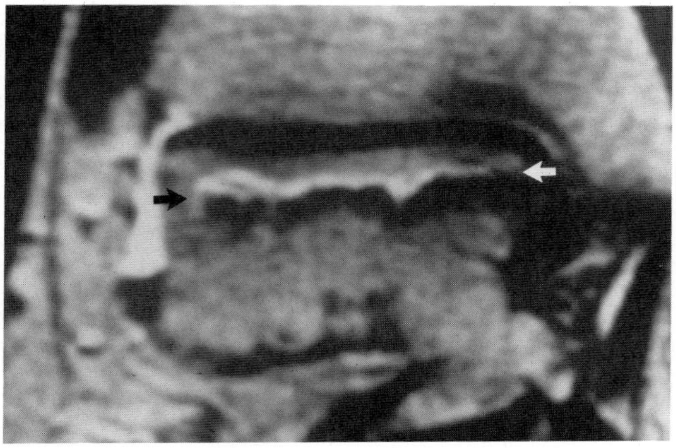

FIGURE 100–14. The pathognomonic *double-line sign* (arrows) is obvious on this T2 weighted (TR/TE, 2400/20) magnetic resonance image, appearing as a transverse double band (compare with Fig. 100–16) across the dome of the body of the right talus, immediately beneath the ankle mortise. This patient has morbid obesity, diabetes, and hyperlipemia.

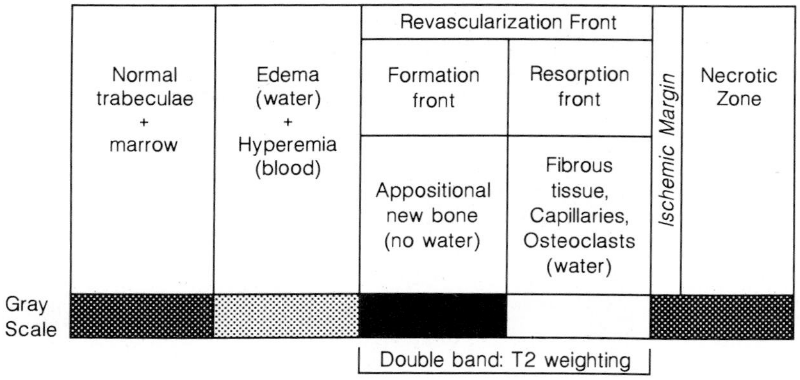

FIGURE 100–15. Gray-scale analysis of various components of stage II lesions using magnetic resonance imaging with *T2 weighting* (long TR/TE). The pathognomonic double band usually represents the revascularization front with a proximal (white: high signal intensity) resorption front with hyperemia (blood and edema), and a distal (black: low-intensity signal) formation front. Marrow edema (water) often appears distal to the revascularization front in the form of intermediate-to-high signal intensity. The stage I lesion often shows an edema pattern (high intensity, T2 weighting) but has no discernible revascularization front (no double line sign).

sion of oxygen[157] and nutrients[158] into the intervertebral disc across necrotic vertebral end plates could be important in the pathogenesis of discogenic vertebral sclerosis[159,160] and osteoarthrosis.[161]

Scintigraphy. With revascularization, ^{99m}Tc-MDP (methylene diphosphonate) is localized along mineralization fronts of newly formed bone on the 2-hour delayed images.[162] Stage II lesions show increased radionuclide uptake.[163] In the transition from a stage I "cold" lesion to a stage II "hot" lesion is an intermediate, virtually pathognomonic stage II *"cold–hot" lesion* in which the revascularization front surrounds the necrotic zone (Fig. 100–17). This cold–hot lesion must be defined because it is prone to collapse into stage III; it is best visualized by SPECT scintigrams.

Single Photon Emission Computed Tomography. The advantage of SPECT over planar imaging is that "cold" spots are not obscured by overlying or contiguous "hot" areas.[129] In stage II lesions, osteonecrosis is diagnosed by SPECT when an area of no uptake or an area of diminished uptake is surrounded by an area of increased uptake[164] (Fig. 100–17).

Computed Tomography with Multiplanar Reconstructions. Although the possibility of articular collapse (stage III lesion) can be directly evaluated by arthroscopy of the shoulder, knee or hip,[165] CT with mul

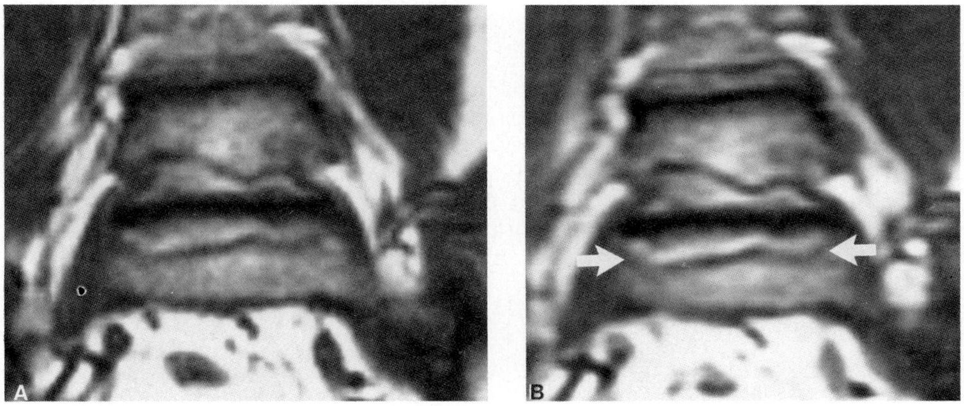

FIGURE 100–16. *A,* T1-weighted (TR/TE, 600/20) magnetic resonance image of the lumbosacral spine demonstrating transverse single-banded revascularization fronts involving the inferior L5 and superior S1 vertebral bodies. *B,* T2 weighting (TR/TE, 2000/20) reveals an obvious double-banded (resorption/formation) front (arrows) within the superior aspect of S1, (compare with Fig. 100–14). This vertebral end plate necrosis was associated with (and perhaps caused) degenerative disc disease at L5-S1. This former U.S. Navy diver also had a focal stage II lesion in his left femoral head and stage IV postcollapse osteonecrosis involving his right hip. (Courtesy of Paul Swenson.)

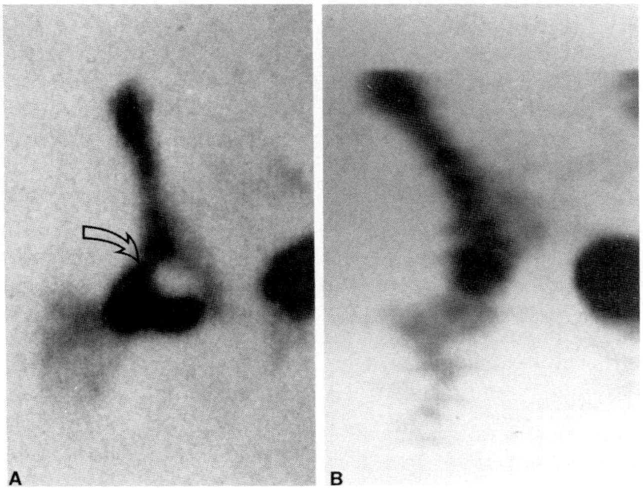

FIGURE 100–17. Single photon emission computed tomography (SPECT) image of a partially revascularized precollapse femoral head lesion (stage II) with a *photopenic* superomedial necrotic zone surrounded by a hyperemic (resorptive) margin with increased radionuclide uptake. *A,* A transitional cold–hot (C/H) lesion of this magnitude has a poor prognosis, because it is especially vulnerable to collapse near the superolateral chondro-osseous junction (arrow). *B,* SPECT image of a diffusely hot (H), but much smaller, femoral head lesion (stage II), which as a much better prognosis, because it has repaired without collapsing.

tiplanar reconstructions (CT/MPR) is noninvasive and also sensitive to small changes of contour (subchondral collapse) and differences in radiographic density. With conventional transaxial CT, it is difficult to evaluate the superior pole of the femoral head because of a partial volume effect. Unsuspected osteonecrosis of the contralateral hip was found by CT/MPR in 16% of patients (9/55), most of whom had stage II lesions.[166]

Superselective Angiography. When performed in hips with stage II to III lesions, superselective angiography (SSA) indicates hypervascularity[167] of the femoral head by probable reconstituted (recanalized) lateral epiphyseal vessels about a subchondral zone of devascularization. Ultimately, there may also be some collateral circulation of the lateral epiphyseal vessels derived from the uninvolved lateral femoral circumflex arterial tributaries, the inferior gluteal vessels, and the obturator artery and its medial epiphyseal branches traversing the ligamentum teres. These are known to anastomose with lateral epiphyseal (superior retinacular) vessels to a limited extent.

Noninvasive Treatment

Unfortunately, improved diagnosis of stage I to II lesions has not been translated into treatment strategies that consistently prevent the ultimate collapse of a juxta-articular lesion. Conservative non-weight bearing is generally ineffective. Only 6% of lesions remained clinically stable in one series of hips, while progressive femoral collapse occurred in 67%.[168] Small focal lesions (IIA) measuring 5 to 15 mm in diameter may spontaneously heal,[9,169] especially if they are localized in the central portion of the bone; 20 to 22 (91%) such lesions did not collapse.[170]

Electrical Stimulation. None of 12 hips in stage II collapsed when treated noninvasively with pulsing electromagnetic fields (PEMF).[171] In another study[172] only 26% of stage II lesions progressed with PEMF treatment. There is no indication, however, that either intraosseous electrical coils[173] or capacitive coupling gave better results than decompression and grafting alone.[174]

Invasive Treatment

Core decompression is a controversial procedure.[175] It may be more useful than non-weight bearing alone in precollapse lesions.[176,177] Others, however, believe that once nontraumatic osteonecrosis has occurred, core decompression will not significantly influence the subsequent course of the disease.[178]

In one series,[141] radiographic evidence of progression occurred in 51 of 139 (36%) bones 32 months after core decompression. My analysis of nine studies showed that 218 of 369 (59%) of the core decompressions performed in precollapse stages failed to prevent progressive collapse. Because of the deleterious effects on the distribution of stress to the femoral head, core biopsy decompression without cortical grafting is discouraged.[179]

To augment intrinsic revascularization, the necrotic zone in the femoral head is excavated. Although vascularized bone grafts have been successfully performed in animals,[180] the incidence of postoperative collapse in humans has varied from 25%[181] to 100%.[182]

STAGE III LESIONS

Often, the patient remains asymptomatic until the articular surface undergoes late segmental *collapse,* when a stage II lesion converts to stage III. The patient reports symptoms of acute joint pain, and occasionally spasm, usually aggravated by weight bearing and relieved by rest. Joint tenderness and slight limitation of motion are often present, especially internal rotation of the hip in flexion.

Pathologic Features

Late segmental collapse is a result of the repair process. If repair were prevented entirely, the necrotic femoral head would not collapse, because dead bone (stage I) is essentially as strong as living bone (Fig. 100–8). In stage III lesions, however, the radiolucent revascularization front has resorbed subchondral bone, as well as calcified and uncalcified articular cartilage. Intracapital fractures begin in a focal area of osteoclastic resorption at the chondro-osseous junction (Fig. 100–18). Stress risers are created by focal resorption of the subchondral plate. The low elastic modulus of this region may reduce its ability to resist deformation.[183]

Impulse loading leads to shear-induced microfractures of the pre-existing necrotic trabeculae, beginning at the stress risers, which propagate into the femoral head. In post-traumatic osteonecrosis, these intracapital fractures usually propagate deeper into the femoral head. Finally, the anterosuperior portion of the femoral head or the central portion of the humeral head buckles and collapses. Fibrocartilaginous metaplasia often occurs beneath the subchondral fracture, blocking further revascularization. This metaplasia probably develops as a result of micromotion or terminal hypoxia at the revascularization front. Perinecrotic intraosseous arteries may show concentric intimal proliferation and thickening with narrowed lumens, probably resulting from endothelial denudation and/or recanalization. Microangiography of postcollapse specimens may reveal extraosseous interruption of superior retinacular arteries with newly formed branches arising from their stumps.[184]

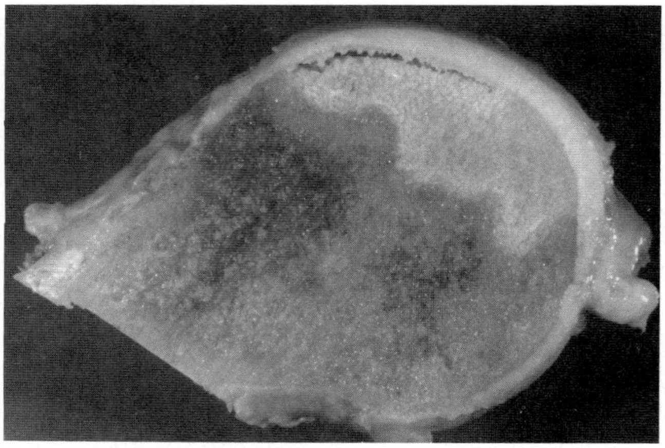

FIGURE 100–18. Gross sagittal section of right femoral head showing a stage III postcollapse lesion with an extensive subchondral fracture (radiolucent crescent) with incomplete detachment of the overlying cartilage, and a dark zone of revascularization, especially in the region of the lateral epiphyseal vessels. This patient had morbid obesity, diabetes, fatty liver, arterial fat embolism, increased free fatty acids, and intravascular coagulation.

Radiographic Features

Radiographic examination, particularly external rotation views of the shoulder and lateral views of the hip, indicate architectural failure and structural collapse. A unipolar or bipolar subchondral fracture is often apparent. A positive, radiolucent, crescent (meniscus) sign indicates a stage III lesion. Once a break has occurred in the smooth, spherical articular cartilage and in subchondral bone, the necrotic lesion is *irreversible,* inevitably progressing to further collapse, with articular incongruity and secondary degenerative changes. On axial MRIs of the femoral head, the collapse usually begins in the lateral revascularization front (low-intensity band) of the lateral epiphyseal vessels (Fig. 100–19).

The presence on plain radiographs of an intravertebral vacuum cleft in a partially collapsed vertebra is con-

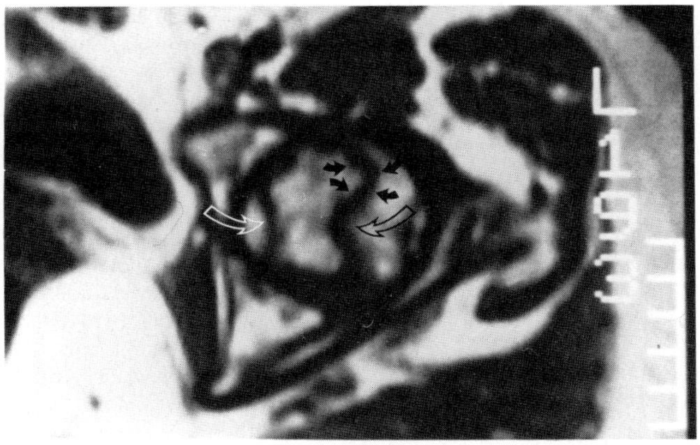

FIGURE 100–19. Magnetic resonance image of necrotic femoral head in axial plane showing two dark, vertically oriented bands on T1 weighting. The shorter medial band (white arrow) represents the revascularization front originating from the medial epiphyseal artery of the ligamentum teres; the longer and wider lateral band (black open arrow) is the repair front generated by lateral epiphyseal arteries. Between these two bands is an area of heterogeneous hyperintensity—the residual, yet unrepaired necrotic tissue. This femoral head collapsed (stage III) in the resorptive, anterior portion of the lateral front (between black closed arrows).

sidered virtually pathognomonic of osteonecrosis.[185] These have been recently studied by MRI.[186]

Treatment

The humeral or femoral head cannot be saved at this point. The humeral head can be replaced by a metal prosthesis held in the humeral shaft by a stem (hemiarthroplasty) if the glenoid is normal.[187] Using a varus or valgus trochanteric osteotomy,[188] smaller necrotic areas can be moved so that maximal stress may fall on the uninvolved surface of a femoral head. If the lesion involves less than 25% of the femoral head and is confined entirely to the anterosuperior quadrant, a transtrochanteric rotational osteotomy may be successful. Although excellent results were obtained in 98 of 128 (77%) hips in one study, progressive collapse in the newly created weight-bearing area occurred in 25 hips in which the lesions had been more extensive.[189,190] To avoid acetabular protrusio, total hip replacement is indicated for patients with extensive involvement of the femoral head even when the acetabulum grossly appears normal. Co-existent osteoporosis or osteomalacia, however, accelerates mechanical failure in young patients.[191]

STAGE IV LESIONS

Patients with stage IV lesions have continuous joint pain, limpness, stiffness, and weakness. Physical findings include tenderness, deformity, crepitation, contracture, and limited motion.

Pathologic Features

As subchondral collapse continues, joint destruction occurs with advanced changes typical of *secondary* osteoarthritis, including a narrowed, incongruous joint space, diffuse hypertrophy with extensive marginal osteophytic proliferation, and degenerative cyst formation of either side of the joint. Malignant fibrous histiocytomas and osteogenic sarcomas have been associated (rarely) with intramedullary bone infarcts.[192]

Treatment

Total joint replacement is the recommended treatment for stage IV lesions.

REFERENCES

1. James, J., and Steijn-Myagkaya, G.L.: Death of osteocytes. Electron microscopy after in vitro ischaemia. J. Bone Joint Surg., *68B*:620–624, 1986.
2. Jones, J.P., Jr.: Intravascular coagulation and osteonecrosis. Clin. Orthop., (in press), 1991.
3. Calandruccio, R.A., and Anderson, W.E., III: Post-fracture avascular necrosis of the femoral head. Correlation of experimental and clinical studies. Clin. Orthop., *152*:49–84, 1980.
4. Harper, W.M., Barnes, M.R., and Gregg, P.J.: Femoral head blood flow in femoral neck fractures. An analysis using intraosseous pressure measurement. J. Bone Joint Surg., *73B*:73–75, 1991.
5. Wingstrand, H., Stromqvist, B., Egund, N., et al.: Hemarthrosis in undisplaced cervical fractures. Tamponade may cause reversible femoral head ischemia. Acta Orthop. Scand., *57*:305–308, 1986.
6. Canale, S.T.: Fractures of the neck of the talus. Orthopedics, *13*:1105–1115, 1990.
7. Fourrier, P., and Martini, M.: Post-traumatic avascular necrosis of the humeral head. Int. Orthop., *1*:187–190, 1977.
8. Gerber, C., Schneeberger, A.G., and Vinh, T.-S.: The arterial vascularization of the humeral head. J. Bone Joint Surg., *72A*:1486–1494, 1990.
9. Jones, J.P., Jr.: Fat embolism and osteonecrosis. Orthop. Clin. North Am., *16*:595–633, 1985.
10. Jones, J.P., Jr.: Fat embolism, intravascular coagulation and osteonecrosis. Clin. Orthop., (in press), 1991.
11. Ficat, R.P., and Arlet, J.: Ischemia and Bone Necrosis. Baltimore, Williams & Wilkins, 1980.
12. Spencer, J.D., and Brookes, M.: Avascular necrosis and the blood supply of the femoral head. Clin. Orthop., *235*:127–140, 1988.
13. Joist, J.H.: Hypercoagulability: Introduction and perspective. Semin. Thromb. Hemost., *16*:151–157, 1990.
14. Muller-Berghaus, G.: Pathophysiologic and biochemical events in disseminated intravascular coagulation: Dysregulation of procoagulant and anticoagulant pathways. Semin. Thromb. Hemost., *15*:58–87, 1989.
15. Morrissey, J.H., Fakhrai, H., and Edgington, T.S.: Molecular cloning of the cDNA for tissue factor, the cellular receptor for the initiation of the coagulation protease cascade. Cell, *50*:129–135, 1987.
16. Jones, J.P., Jr.: Osteonecrosis. *In* Arthritis and Allied Conditions: A Textbook of Rheumatology. 11th Ed. Edited by D.J. McCarty. Lea & Febiger, Philadelphia, 1989, pp. 1545–1562.

17. Brozna, J.P.: Shwartzman reaction. Semin. Thromb. Hemost., *16*:326–332, 1990
18. Allardyce, D.B., and Groves, A.C.: Intravascular coagulation, hyperlipemia, and fat embolism: Their association during the generalized Shwartzman phenomenon in rabbits. Surgery, *66*:71–79, 1969.
19. Halleraker, B.: Fat embolism and intravascular coagulation. Acta Pathol. Microbiol. Immunol. Scand., *78*:432–436, 1970.
20. Hirsch, R.L., McKay, D.G., Travers, R.I., and Skraly, R.K.: Hyperlipidemia, fatty liver, and bromsulfophthalein retention in rabbits injected intravenously with bacterial endotoxins. J. Lipid Res., *5*:563–568, 1964.
21. Acheson, L.S.: Disturbances of bone growth in a child who survived septic shock. J. Fam. Pract., *23*:321–329, 1986.
22. Barre, P.S., Thompson, G.H., and Morrison, S.C.: Late skeletal deformities following meningococcal sepsis and disseminated intravascular coagulation. J. Pediatr. Orthop., *5*:584–588, 1985.
23. Fernandez, F., Pueyo, I., Jimenez, J.R., et al.: Epiphysiometaphyseal changes in children after severe meningococcic sepsis. Am. J. Radiol., *136*:1236–1238, 1981.
24. Patriquin, H.B., Trias, A., Jecquier, S., and Marton, D.: Late sequelae of infantile meningococcemia in growing bones of children. Radiology, *141*:77–82, 1981.
25. Robinow, M., Johnson, F., Nanagas, M.T., and Mesghali, H.: Skeletal lesions following meningococcemia and disseminated intravascular coagulation. Am. J. Dis. Child., *137*:279–281, 1983.
26. Grogan, D.P., Love, S.M., Ogden, J.A., et al.: Chondroosseous growth abnormalities after meningococcemia. A clinical and histopathological study. J. Bone Joint Surg., *71A*:920–928, 1989.
27. Philips, M.R., Abramson, S.B., and Weissmann, G.: Neutrophil adhesion and autoimmune vascular injury. Clin. Aspects Autoimmunity, *3*:6–15, 1989.
28. Mahowald, M.L., Majeski, P.J., and Ytterberg, S.R.: Microvascular pathology of antigen induced arthritis. Arthritis Rheum., *31*(Suppl.):S91, 1988.
29. Matsui, M.: Experimental osteonecrosis in the rabbit with serum sickness treated by high dose glucocorticosteroid. Clin. Orthop., (in press), 1991.
30. Nagasawa, K., Ishii, Y., Mayumi, T., et al.: Avascular necrosis of bone in systemic lupus erythematosus: Possible role of haemostatic abnormalities. Ann. Rheum. Dis., *48*:672–676, 1989.
31. Kitano, M., and Hayashi, K.: Acute decompression sickness—Report of an autopsy case with widespread fat embolism. Acta Pathol. Jpn., *31*:269–276, 1981.
32. Lasson, A., and Ohlsson, K.: Consumptive coagulopathy, fibrinolysis and protease-antiprotease interactions during acute human pancreatitis. Thromb. Res., *41*:167–183, 1986.
33. Aarnoudse, J.G., Houthoff, H.J., Weits, J., et al.: A syndrome of liver damage and intravascular coagulation in the last trimester of normotensive pregnancy. A clinical and histopathological study. Br. J. Obstet. Gynecol., *93*:145–155, 1986.
34. Liebman, H.A., McGehee, W.G., Patch, M.J., and Feinstein, D.I.: Severe depression of antithrombin III associated with disseminated intravascular coagulation in women with fatty liver of pregnancy. Ann. Intern. Med., *98*:330–345, 1983.
35. Bick, R.L.: Disseminated intravascular coagulation and related syndromes: A clinical review. Semin. Thromb. Hemost., *14*:299–338, 1988.
36. Hughes, E.C., Jr., Schumacher, H.R., and Sbarbaro, J.L., Jr.: Bilateral avascular necrosis of the hip following Leriche syndrome. J. Bone Joint Surg., *53A*:380–382, 1974.
37. Duncan, J.S., and Ramsay, L.E.: Widespread bone infarction complicating meningococcal septicaemia and disseminated intravascular coagulation. Br. Med. J., *288*:111–112, 1984.
38. Marymont, J.V., and Kaufman, E.E.: Osteonecrosis of bone associated with combination chemotherapy without corticosteroids. Clin. Orthop., *204*:150–153, 1986.
39. Laso, F.J., Gonzalez-Diaz, M., Paz, J.I., and DeCastro, S.: Bone marrow necrosis associated with tumor emboli and disseminated coagulation. Arch. Int. Med., *143*:2220–2225, 1983.
40. Harigaya, K., Watanabe, S., Watanabe, Y., et al.: Multiple bone marrow necrosis and disseminated intravascular coagulation. Arch. Pathol. Lab. Med., *101*:652–654, 1977.
41. Shiobara, H., Ashizawa, M., Usui, H., et al: Changes detected in the femoral heads of autopsy patients with systemic lupus erythematosus. Clin. Orthop. Surg. (Jpn.), *11*:1074–1081, 1976.
42. Saito, S., Inoue, A., and Ono, K.: Intramedullary haemorrhage as a possible cause of avascular necrosis of the femoral head. The histology of 16 femoral heads at the silent stage. J. Bone Joint Surg., *69B*:346–351, 1987.
43. Rutishauser, E., Rohner, A., and Held, D.: Experimentelle Untersuchungen uber die Wirkung der Ischamie auf den Knochen und das Mark. Virchows Arch. [A], *333*:101–118, 1960.
44. Oberling, F., Cazenzve, J.P.: Experimental bone marrow fat necrosis. Virchows Arch. [A], *376*:133–143, 1977.
45. Jacobs, B.: Epidemiology of traumatic and nontraumatic osteonecrosis. Clin. Orthop., *130*:51–67, 1978.
46. Shaprio, S.C., Rothstein, F.C., Newman, A.J., et al.: Multifocal osteonecrosis in adolescents with Crohn's disease: A complication of therapy? J. Pediatr. Gastroenterol. Nutr., *4*:502–506, 1985.
47. Haber, L.M., Hawkins, E.P., Seilheimer, D.K., and Slaeem, A.: Fat overload syndrome. An autopsy study with evaluation of the coagulopathy. Am. J. Clin. Pathol., *90*:223–227, 1988.
48. Jones, J.P., Jr.: Etiology and pathogenesis of osteonecrosis. Semin. Arthroplasty, (in press), 1991.
49. Felson, D.T., and Anderson, J.J.: Across-study evaluation of association between steroid dose and bolus steroids and avascular necrosis of bone. Lancet, *8358*:902–905, 1987.
50. Matsuo, K., Hirohata, T., Sugioka, Y., et al.: Influence of alcohol intake, cigarette smoking and occupational status on idiopathic osteonecrosis of the femoral head. Clin. Orthop., *234*:115–123, 1988.
51. Montgomery, R.J., Sutker, B.D., Bronk, J.T., et al.: Interstitial fluid flow in cortical bone. Microvasc. Res., *35*:295–307, 1988.
52. Doty, S.B.: Morphological evidence of gap junctions between bone cells. Calcif. Tissue Int., *33*:509–512, 1981.
53. Kawai, K., Tamaki, A., and Hirohata, K.: Steroid-induced accumulation of lipid in the osteocytes of the rabbit femoral head. A histochemical and electron microscopic study. J. Bone Joint Surg., *67A*:755–763, 1985.
54. Muratsu, H., Shimizu, T., Kawai, K., and Hirohata, K.: Alcohol-induced accumulations of lipids in the osteocytes of the rabbit femoral head. Trans. Ortho. Res. Soc., *15*:402, 1990.
55. Usui, Y., Kawai, K., and Hirohata, K.: An electron microscopic study of the changes observed in osteocytes under ischemic conditions. J. Orthop. Res., *7*:12–21, 1989.
56. Wang, G.J., Chung, K.C., Shen, W.J., and Stamp, W.G.: Preventing steroid induced osteoporosis in the femoral head using lipid clearing agents. Trans. Orthop. Res. Soc., *14*:457, 1989.
57. Schrader, J., Andersson, L.O., Armstrong, V.W., et al.: Lipolytic effects of heparin and low molecular weight heparin and their importance in hemodialysis. Semin. Thromb. Hemost., *16*:41–45, 1990.
58. Wessel-Aas, T., Blomhoff, J.P., Wirum, E., and Nilson, T.: Hemodialysis and cell toxicity in vitro related to plasma triglycerides, post-heparin lipolytic activity and free fatty acids. Acta Med. Scand., *216*:75–83, 1984.
59. Arlot, M.E., Bonjean, M., Chavassieux, P.M., and Meunier, P.J.:

Bone histology in adults with aseptic necrosis. Histomorphometric evaluation of iliac biopsies in seventy-seven patients. J. Bone Joint Surg., *65A*:1319–1327, 1983.
60. Szasz, I., Morrison, R.T., Lyster, D.M., and Naiman, S.C.: Bone scintigraphy in massive disseminated bone necrosis. Clin. Nucl. Med., *6*:97–100, 1981.
61. Brodell, J.D., Burns, J.E., Jr., and Heiple, K.G.: Transient osteoporosis of the hip of pregnancy. Two cases complicated by pathological fracture. J. Bone Joint Surg., *71A*:1252–1257, 1989.
62. McGuigan, L., and Fleming, A.: Osteonecrosis of the humerus related to pregnancy. Ann. Rheum. Dis., *42*:597–599, 1983.
63. Doty, S.B., Morey-Holton, E.R., Durnova, G.N., and Kaplansky, A.S.: Cosmos 1887: Morphology, histochemistry, and vasculature of the growing rat tibia. FASEB, *4*:16–23, 1990.
64. Doty, S.B.: Combined cytochemistry and morphometry to determine bone cell response to hypogravity. Bull. Am. Soc. Gravit. Space Biol., *4*:37, 1990.
65. Grindeland, R.E., Popova, I.A., Vasques, M., and Arnaud, S.B.: Cosmos 1887 mission overview: Effects of microgravity on rat body and adrenal weights and plasma constituents. FASEB, *4*:105–109, 1990.
66. Coomes, R.K., Sebastian, L.A., Stump, C.S., et al.: Influence of two methods of head down suspension (HDS) on the stress response of rats: Preliminary results. Bull. Am. Soc. Gravit. Space Biol., *4*:86, 1990.
67. Martin, L.D., and Rothschild, B.M.: Paleopathology and diving mosasaurs. Am. Scientist, *77*:460–467, 1989.
68. Gregg, P.J., and Walder, D.N.: Caisson disease of bone. Clin. Orthop., *210*:43–54, 1986.
69. Giertsen, J.C., Sandstad, E., Morild, I., et al.: An explosive decompression accident. Am. J. Forensic Med. Pathol., *9*:94–101, 1988.
70. James, C.C.M.: Late bone lesions in caisson disease. Three cases in submarine personnel. Lancet, *2*:6–8, 1945.
71. Philp, R.B.: A review of blood changes associated with compression-decompression: Relationship to decompression sickness. Undersea Biomed. Res., *1*:117–148, 1974.
72. Chryssanthou, C.P.: Dysbaric osteonecrosis in mice. Undersea Biomed. Res., *3*:67–83, 1976.
73. Zhang, L.D., Kang, J.F., and Xue, H.L.: Distribution of lesions in the head and neck of the humerus and the femur in dysbaric osteonecrosis. Undersea Biomed. Res., *17*:353–358, 1990.
74. Jones, J.P., Jr., and Behnke, A.R., Jr.: Prevention of dysbaric osteonecrosis in compressed-air workers. Clin. Orthop., *130*:118–128, 1978.
75. Decompression Sickness Panel, and Medical Research Council: Aseptic bone necrosis in commercial divers. Lancet, *8243*:384–388, 1981.
76. Alexakis, P.G., and Wallack, M.: Idiopathic osteonecrosis of the femoral head associated with a pituitary tumor. J. Bone Joint Surg., *71A*:1412–1414, 1989.
77. Vakil, N., and Sparberg, M.: Steroid-related osteonecrosis in inflammatory bowel disease. Gastroenterology, *96*:62–67, 1989.
78. Diaz-Jouanen, E., Abud-Mendoza, C., Inglesias-Gamarra, A., and Gonsalez-Amaro, R.: Ischemic necrosis of bone in systemic lupus erythematosus. Early and late onset subgroups. Orthop. Rev., *14*:303–309, 1985.
79. Ross, L.V., Ross, G.J., Mesgarzadeh, M., et al.: Hemodialysis-related amyloidomas of bone. Radiology, *178*:263–265, 1991.
80. Ibels, L.S., Alfrey, A.C., and Huffer, W.E.: Aseptic necrosis of bone following renal transplantation: Experience in 194 transplant recipients and review of the literature. Medicine (Baltimore) *57*:25–45, 1978.
81. Lamberts, S.W.J., Klijn, J.G.M., de Jong, F.H., and Birkenhager, J.C.: Hormone secretion in alcohol-induced pseudo-Cushing's syndrome. JAMA, *242*:1640–1643, 1979.
82. Lee, K., Nielsen, J.D., Zeeberg, I., and Gormsen, J.: Platelet aggregation and fibrinolytic activity in young alcoholics. Acta Neurol. Scand., *62*:287–292, 1980.
83. Horowitz, I., Klingenstein, R.J., Levy, R., and Zimmerman, M.J.: Fat embolism syndrome in delirium tremens. Am. J. Gastroenterol., *68*:476–480, 1977.
84. Hungerford, D.S., and Zizic, T.M.: Alcoholism associated ischemic necrosis of the femoral head: Early diagnosis and treatment. Clin. Orthop., *130*:144–153, 1978.
85. Mielants, H., Veys, E.M., DeBuggare, A., and van der Jeught, J.: Avascular necrosis and its relation to lipid and purine metabolism. J. Rheumatol., *2*:430–436, 1975.
86. Carvalho, A.C., Lees, R.S., Vaillancourt, R.A., et al.: Intravascular coagulation in hyperlipidemia. Thromb. Res., *8*:843–857, 1976.
87. Palmer, A.K., Hensinger, R.N., Costenbader, J.M., and Bassett, D.R.: Osteonecrosis of the femoral head in a family with hyperlipoproteinemia. Clin. Orthop., *155*:166–171, 1981.
88. Seedat, Y.K., and Randeree, M.: Avascular necrosis of the hip joints in hypothyroidism. S. Afr. Med. J., *49*:2071–2072, 1975.
89. Van Wersch, J.W.J., Westerhuis, L.W.J.J.M., and Venekamp, W.J.R.R.: Coagulation activation in diabetes mellitus. Haemostasis, *20*:263–269, 1990.
90. Cheng, N., Burssens, A., and Mulier, J.C.: Pregnancy and post-pregnancy avascular necrosis of the femoral head. Arch. Orthop. Traum. Surg., *100*:199–210, 1982.
91. Gore, M., Eldon, S., Trofatter, K.F., et al.: Pregnancy induced tissue plasminogen activator and increased levels of the fast-acting tissue plasminogen activator inhibitor. Am. J. Obstet. Gynecol., *156*:674–680, 1987.
92. Watson, W.J., and Seeds, J.W.: Acute fatty liver of pregnancy. Obstet. Gynecol. Surv., *45*:585–593, 1990.
93. Minakami, H., Oka, N., Sato, T., et al.: Preeclampsia: A microvesicular fat disease of the liver? Am. J. Obstet. Gynecol., *159*:1043–1047, 1988.
94. Rickles, F.R., and O'Leary, D.S.: Role of coagulation system in pathophysiology of sickle cell disease. Arch. Intern. Med., *133*:635–641, 1986.
95. Beurling-Harbury, C., and Schade, S.G.: Platelet activation during pain crisis in sickle cell anemia patients. Am. J. Hematol., *31*:237–241, 1989.
96. Mankad, V.N., Williams, J.P., Harpen, M.D., et al.: Magnetic resonance imaging of bone marrow in sickle cell disease: Clinical, hematologic, and pathologic correlations. Blood, *75*:274–283, 1990.
97. Billett, H.H., Nagel, R.L., and Fabry, M.E.: Evolution of laboratory parameters during sickle cell painful crisis: Evidence compatible with dense red cell sequestration without thrombosis. Am. J. Med. Sci., *296*:293–298, 1988.
98. Hernigou, P., Galacteros, F., Bachir, D., and Goutallier, D.: Deformities of the hip in adults who have sickle-cell disease and had avascular necrosis in childhood. A natural history of fifty-two patients. J. Bone Joint Surg., *73A*:81–92, 1991.
99. Davis, M.A., Ettinger, W.H., and Neuhaus, J.M.: Obesity and osteoarthritis of the knee: evidence from the national health and nutrition examination survey (NHANES I). Semin. Arthritis Rheum., *20*:34–41, 1990.
100. van Saase, J.L.C.M., Vandenbroucke, J.P., van Romunde, L.K.J., and Valkenburg, H.A.: Osteoarthritis and obesity in the general population. A relationship calling for an explanation. J. Rheumatol., *15*:1152–1158, 1988.
101. Wong, S.Y.P., Evans, R.A., Needs, C., et al.: The pathogenesis of osteoarthritis of the hip. Evidence of primary osteocyte death. Clin. Orthop., *214*:305312, 1987.

102. Bonner, W.M., Jonsson, H., Malanos, C., and Bryant, M.: Changes in the lipids of human articular cartilage with age. Arthritis Rheum., *18*:461–473, 1975.
103. Lippiello, L., Walsh, T., and Feinhold, M.: Lipids in the pathogenesis of osteoarthrosis. Trans. Orthop. Res. Soc., *15*:211, 1990.
104. Ghadially, F.N., Mehta, P.N., and Kirkaldy-Willis, W.H.: Ultrastructure of articular cartilage in experimentally produced lipoarthrosis. J. Bone Joint Surg., *52A*:1147–1158, 1970.
105. Sokoloff, L., Mickelsen, O., Silverstein, E., et al.: Experimental obesity and osteoarthritis. Am. J. Physiol., *198*:765770, 1960.
106. Kenzora, J.E., and Glimcher, M.J.: Osteonecrosis. *In* Textbook of Rheumatology. Edited by W.N. Kelley, E.D. Harris, Jr., S. Ruddy, and C.B. Sledge, Philadelphia, W.B. Saunders, 1981, p. 1755–1779.
107. Heppenstall, R.B.: Fracture healing. *In* Fracture Treatment and Healing. Edited by R.B. Heppenstall. Philadelphia, W.B. Saunders, 1980, pp. 35–64.
108. Kiaer, T., Pedersen, N.W., Kristensen, K.D., and Starklint, H.: Intraosseous pressure and oxygen tension in avascular necrosis and osteoarthritis of the hip. J. Bone Joint Surg., *72B*:1023–1030, 1990.
109. Jones, J.P., Jr., Lewis, R.H., Lewis, T., et al.: The effect of hyperbaric oxygen on osteonecrosis. Undersea Biomed. Res., *18*(suppl.):82, 1991.
110. Jones, J.P., Jr., and Sakovich, L.: Fat embolism of bone. A roentgenographic and histological investigation, with use of intra-arterial Lipiodol, in rabbits. J. Bone Joint Surg., *48A*:149–164, 1966.
111. Soloway, H.B., and Robinson, E.F.: The coagulation mechanism in experimental pulmonary fat embolism. J. Trauma, *12*:630–631, 1972.
112. Saldeen, T.: The importance of intravascular coagulation and inhibition of the fibrinolytic system in experimental fat embolism. J. Trauma, *10*:287–298, 1970.
113. King, E.G., Wagner, W.W., Jr., Ashbaugh, D.G., et al.: Alterations in pulmonary microanatomy after fat embolism. In vivo observations via thoracic window of the oleic acid-embolized canine lung. Chest, *59*:524–533, 1971.
114. Sikorski, J.M.: Venous thrombosis produced by the local injection of fat. J. Bone Joint Surg., *65B*:340–345, 1983.
115. King, E.G. et al.: Consumption coagulopathy in the canine oleic acid model of fat embolism. Surgery, *69*:533–541, 1971.
116. Gold, E.W., Fox, O.D., Weissfeld, S., and Curtis, P.H.: Corticocosteroid-induced avascular necrosis: An experimental study in rabbits. Clin. Orthop., *135*:272–280, 1978.
117. Surat, A.: Isolation of prostaglandin E2-like material from osteonecrosis induced by steroids and its prevention by kallikrein-inhibitor, aprotinin. Prostaglandins Leukotrienes Med., *13*:159–167, 1984.
118. Bradford, D.S., Foster, R.R., and Nossel, H.L.: Coagulation alterations, hypoxemia, and fat embolism in fracture patients. J. Trauma, *10*:307–321, 1970.
119. Hauzeur, J.P., and Pasteels, J.L.: Pathology of bone marrow distant from the sequestrum in nontraumatic aseptic necrosis of the femoral head. *In* Bone Circulation and Bone Necrosis. Edited by J. Arlet and B. Mazieres. Heidelberg, Germany, Springer-Verlag, 1990, pp. 73–76.
120. Bierre, A.R., and Koelmeyer, T.D.: Pulmonary fat and bone marrow embolism in aircraft accident victims. Pathology, *15*:131–135, 1983.
121. Sy, W.M., Westring, D.W., and Weinberger, G.: "Cold" lesions on bone imaging. J. Nucl. Med., *16*:1013–1016, 1975.
122. Macleod, M.A., McEwan, A.J.B., and Pearson, R.R.: Functional imaging in the early diagnosis of dysbaric osteonecrosis. Br. J. Radiol., *55*:497–500, 1982.
123. Koren, A., Garty, I., and Katzuni, E.: Bone infarction in children with sickle cell disease: Early diagnosis and differentiation from osteomyelitis. Eur. J. Pediatr., *142*:93–97, 1984.
124. Armas, R.R., and Goldsmith, S.J.: Gallium scintigraphy in bone infarction: correlation with bone imaging. Clin. Nucl. Med., *9*:1–3, 1984.
125. Sebes, A.J.: Diagnostic imaging of bone and joint abnormalities associated with sickle cell hemoglobinopathies. AJR, *152*:1153–1159, 1989.
126. Grieff, J., Lanng, S., Hoilund-Carlsen, P.F., et al.: Early detection by 99mTc-Sn-pyrophosphate scintrigraphy of femoral head necrosis following medial femoral neck fractures. Acta Orthop. Scand., *51*:119–125, 1980.
127. Bauer, G.C.H., Ceder, L., Hansson, L.I., et al.: Dynamics of post-traumatic necrosis of the femoral head studied with 99m-TcDMP imaging techniques. Trans. Orthop. Res. Soc., *7*:189, 1982.
128. Tawn, D.J., and Watt, I.: Bone marrow scintigraphy in the diagnosis of post-traumatic avascular necrosis of bone. Br. J. Radiol., *62*:790–795, 1989.
129. Collier, B.D., Carrera, G.F., Johnson, R.P., et al.: Detection of femoral head avascular necrosis in adults by SPECT. J. Nucl. Med., *25*:979–987, 1985.
130. Greyson, N.D., Lotem, M.M., Gross, A.E., and Houpt, J.B.: Radionuclide evaluation of spontaneous femoral osteonecrosis. Radiology, *142*:729–735, 1982.
131. Beltran, J., Herman, L.J., Burk, J.M., et al.: Femoral head avascular necrosis: MR imaging with clinical-pathologic and radionuclide correlation. Radiology, *166*:215–220, 1988.
132. Robinson, H.J., Jr., Hartleben, P.D., Lung, G., and Schreiman, J.: Evaluation of magnetic resonance imaging in the diagnosis of osteonecrosis of the femoral head: Accuracy compared with radiographs, core biopsy, and intraosseous pressure measurements. J. Bone Joint Surg., *71A*:650–662, 1989.
133. Henderson, R.C., Renner, J.B., Sturdivant, M.C., and Greene, W.B.: Evaluation of magnetic resonance imaging in Legg-Perthes disease: A prospective, blinded study. J. Pediatr. Orthop., *10*:289–297, 1990.
134. Lang, P., Jergesen, H.E., Genant, H.K., et al.: Magnetic resonance imaging of the ischemic femoral head in pigs. Dependency of signal intensities and relaxation times on elapsed time. Clin. Orthop., *244*:272–280, 1989.
135. Speer, K.P., Spritzer, C.E., Harrelson, J.M., and Nunley, J.A.: Magnetic resonance imaging of the femoral head and acute intracapsular fracture of the femoral neck. J. Bone Joint Surg., *72A*:98–103, 1990.
136. Wilson, A.J., Murphy, W.A., Hardy, D.C., and Totty, W.G.: Transient osteoporosis: Transient bone marrow edema? Radiology, *167*:757760, 1988.
137. Bloem, J.L.: Transient osteoporosis of the hip: MR imaging. Radiology, *167*:757–760, 1988.
138. Rao, V.M., Fishman, M., Mitchell, D.G., et al.: Painful sickle cell crisis: Bone marrow patterns observed with MR imaging. Radiology, *161*:211–215, 1986.
139. Pay, N.T., Singer, W.S., and Bartal, E.: Hip pain in three children accompanied by transient abnormal findings on MR images. Radiology, *171*:147–149, 1989.
140. Jergesen, H.E., Heller, M., and Genant, H.K.: Magnetic resonance imaging in osteonecrosis of the femoral head. Orthop. Clin. North Am., *16*:705–716, 1985.
141. Zizic, T.M., and Hungerford, D.S.: Avascular necrosis of bone. *In* Textbook of Rheumatology. 2nd Ed. Edited by Kelley, W.N., et al. Philadelphia, W.B. Saunders, 1985, pp. 1689–1710.
142. Schulte, L.A.M., and Ludwig, W.: The venous pattern in femoral head necrosis. Digital subtraction angiography and phlebography in 5 patients. Acta Orthop. Scand., *59*:396–399, 1988.

143. Atsumi, T.: Hemodynamic study of the idiopathic necrosis of femoral head using superselective angiography. J. Jpn. Orthop. Assoc., *57*:353–372, 1983.
144. Camargo, F.P., Godoy, R.M., Jr., and Tovo, R.: Angiography in Perthes' disease. Clin. Orthop., *191*:216–220, 1984.
145. Theron, J.: Angiography in Legg-Calve-Perthes disease. Radiology, *135*:81–92, 1980.
146. Steib, J.P., Moyses, B., Wenger, J.J., et al.: A study of the microcirculation in bone in aseptic necrosis of the femoral head using radioactive microspheres. French J. Orthop. Surg., *2*:12–18, 1988.
147. Wong, S.Y.P., Dunstan, C.R., Evans, R.A., and Hills, E.: The determination of bone viability: A histochemical method for identification of lactate dehydrogenase activity in osteocytes in fresh calcified and decalcified sections of human bone. Pathology, *14*:439–442, 1982.
148. Antoniades, H.N., and Williams, L.T.: Human platelet-derived growth factor: structure and function. Fed. Proc., *42*:2630–2634, 1983.
149. Munk, P.L., Helms, C.A., and Holt, R.G.: Immature bone infarcts: Findings on plain radiographs and MR scans. AJR, *52*:547–549, 1989.
150. Steinberg, M.E., and Steinberg, D.R.: Osteonecrosis. *In* Textbook of Rheumatology. 3rd Ed. Edited by Kelley, W.N. et al. Philadelphia, W.B. Saunders, 1989, pp. 1749–1773.
151. Stulberg, B.N., Bauer, T.W., Belhobek, G.H., et al.: A diagnostic algorithm for osteonecrosis of the femoral head. Clin. Orthop., *249*:176–182, 1989.
152. Mitchell, M.D. et al.: Avascular necrosis of the hip: Comparison of MR, CT, and scintigraphy. AJR, *147*:67–71, 1986.
153. Bassett, L.W. et al.: Magnetic resonance imaging in the early diagnosis of ischemic necrosis of the femoral head: Preliminary results. Clin. Orthop., *214*:237–248, 1987.
154. Totty, W.G. et al.: Magnetic resonance imaging of the normal and ischemic femoral head. AJR, *143*:1273–1280, 1984.
155. Bullough, P.G., and Vigorita, V.J.: Atlas of Orthopaedic Pathology With Clinical and Radiologic Correlations. Baltimore, University Park Press, 1981, pp. 7–8.
156. deRoos, A., Kressel, H., Spritzer, C., and Dalinka, M.: MR imaging of marrow changes adjacent to end plates in degenerative lumbar disk disease. AJR, *149*:531–534, 1987.
157. Kofoed, H., and Levander, B.: Respiratory gas pressures in the spine. Measurements in goats. Acta Orthop. Scand., *58*:415–418, 1987.
158. Urban, J.G.P., Holm, S., Maroudas, A., and Nachemson, A.: Nutrition of the intervertebral disc. Clin. Orthop., *129*:101–114, 1977.
159. Pope, T.L., Jr., Want, G., and Whitehill, R.: Discogenic vertebral sclerosis: A potential mimic of disc space infection or metastatic disease. Orthopedics, *13*:1389–1397, 1990.
160. Katz, M.E., Teitelbaum, S.L., Gilula, L.A., et al.: Radiologic and pathologic patterns of end-plate-based vertebral sclerosis. Invest. Radiol., *23*:447–454, 1988.
161. Modic, M.T., Steinberg, P.M., Ross, J.S., et al.: Degenerative disc disease: Assessment of changes in vertebral body marrow with MR imaging. Radiology, *166*:193–199, 1988.
162. Einhorn, T.A., Vigorita, V.J., and Aaron, A.: Localization of technetium-99m methylene diphosphonate in bone using microautoradiography. J. Orthop. Res., *4*:180–187, 1986.
163. Greyson, N.D., Lotem, M.M., Gross, A.E., and Houpt, J.E.: Radionuclide evaluation of spontaneous femoral osteonecrosis. Radiology, *142*:729–735, 1982.
164. Stulberg, B.N., Levine, M., Bauer, T.W., et al.: Multimodality approach to osteonecrosis of the femoral head. Clin. Orthop., *240*:181–193, 1989.
165. Eriksson, E., Arvidsson, I., and Arvidsson, H.: Diagnostic and operative arthroscopy of the hip. Orthopedics, *9*:169–176, 1986.
166. Magid, D. et al.: Computed tomography with multiplanar reconstructions in the assessment in staging of avascular necrosis of the femoral head. Radiology, *157*:751–758, 1985.
167. Heuck, A., Reiser, M., Schmucker, F., et al.: Selective digital subtraction arteriography in necrosis of the femoral head. Skeletal Radiol., *16*:270–274, 1987.
168. Musso, E.S., Mitchell, S.N., Schink-Ascani, M., and Bassett, C.A.L.: Results of conservative management of osteonecrosis of the femoral head. A retrospective review. Clin. Orthop., *207*:209–215, 1986.
169. Daley, B.J., Bonfiglio, M., Brand, R.A., and Boyer, D.W., Jr.: Aseptic necrosis of the femoral head with a forty-year followup. J. Bone Joint Surg., *73A*:134–136, 1991.
170. Ohzono, K., Saito, M., Takaoka, K., et al.: Natural history of nontraumatic avascular necrosis of the femoral head. J. Bone Joint Surg., *73B*:68–72, 1991.
171. Bassett, C.A.L., Schink-Ascani, M., and Lewis, S.M.: Effects of pulsed electromagnetic fields on Steinberg ratings of femoral head osteonecrosis. Clin. Orthop., *246*:172–185, 1989.
172. Aaron, R.K., Lennox, D., Bunce, G.E., and Ebert, T.: The conservative treatment of osteonecrosis of the femoral head. A comparison of core decompression and pulsing electromagnetic fields. Clin. Orthop., *249*:209–218, 1989.
173. Trancik, T., Lunceford, E., and Strum, D.: The effect of electrical stimulation on osteonecrosis of the femoral head. Clin. Orthop., *256*:120–124, 1990.
174. Steinberg, M.E., Brighton, C.T., Bands, R.E., and Hartman, K.M.: Capacitive coupling as an adjunctive treatment for avascular necrosis. Clin. Orthop., *261*:11–18, 1990.
175. Colwell, C.W., Jr.: The controversy of core decompression of the femoral head for osteonecrosis. Arthritis Rheum., *32*:797–800, 1989.
176. Hungerford, D.S.: The role of core decompression in the treatment of ischemic necrosis of the femoral head. Arthritis Rheum., *32*:801–806, 1989.
177. Stulberg, B.N., Bauer, T.W., and Belhobek, G.H.: Making core decompression work. Clin. Orthop., *261*:186–195, 1990.
178. Learmonth, I.D., Maloon, S., and Dall, G.: Core decompression for early atraumatic osteonecrosis of the femoral head. J. Bone Joint Surg., *72B*:387–390, 1990.
179. Penix, A.R., Cook, S.D., Skinner, H.B., et al.: Femoral head stress following cortical bone grafting for aseptic necrosis: A finite element study. Clin. Orthop., *173*:159–165, 1983.
180. del Pino, J.G., Knapp, K., Castresana, F.G., and Benito, M.: Revascularization of femoral head ischemic necrosis with vascularized bone graft: A CT scan experimental study. Skeletal Radiol., *19*:197–202, 1990.
181. Gilbert, A., Judet, H., Judet, J., and Ayatti, A.: Microvascular transfer of the fibula for necrosis of the femoral head. Orthopedics, *9*:885–890, 1986.
182. Rindell, K., Tallroth, K., and Lindholm, T.S.: Radiographic changes of the revascularized femoral head. Eur. J. Radiol., *10*:9–14, 1990.
183. Brown, T.D., and Vrahas, M.S.: The apparent elastic modulus of the juxtarticular subchondral bone of the femoral head. J. Orthop. Res., *2*:32–38, 1984.
184. Atsumi, T., Kuroki, Y., and Yamano, K.: A microangiographic study of idiopathic osteonecrosis of the femoral head. Clin. Orthop., *246*:186–194, 1989.
185. Resnick, D., Niwayama, G., Guerra, J., et al.: Spinal vacuum phenomena: Anatomical study and review. Radiology, *139*:341–348, 1981.
186. Naul, L.G., Peet, G.J., and Maupin, W.B.: Avascular necrosis

of the vertebral body: MR imaging. Radiology, *172*:219–222, 1989.

187. Cruess, R.L.: Experience with steroid-induced avascular necrosis of the shoulder and etiologic considerations regarding osteonecrosis of the hip. Clin. Orthop., *130*:86–93, 1978.
188. Canadell, J., Aguilella, L., Azcarate, J.R., and Valenti, J.R.: The place of intertrochanteric osteotomy in the treatment of idiopathic necrosis of the head of the femur. Int. Orthop., *10*:41–46, 1986.
189. Kotz, R.: Avascular necrosis of the femoral head: A review of the indications and results of Sugioka transtrochanteric rotational osteotomy. Int. Orthop., *5*:53–58, 1981.
190. Sugioka, Y., Katsuki, I., and Hotokebuchi, T.: Transtrochanteric rotational osteotomy of the femoral head for the treatment of osteonecrosis: Follow-up statistics. Clin. Orthop., *169*:115–126, 1982.
191. Cabanela, M.E.: Bipolar versus total hip arthroplasty for avascular necrosis of the femoral head. A comparison. Clin. Orthop., *261*:59–62, 1990.
192. Breen, T.F., and Healy, W.L.: Malignant fibrous histiocytoma arising in medullary long bone infarcts. A case report. Orthopedics, *10*:1169–1173, 1987.
193. Surat, A.: Isolation of prostaglandin E2-like material from osteonecrosis induced by steroids and its prevention by kallikrein inhibitor, aprotinin. Prostaglandins Leukotrienes Med., *13*: 159–167, 1984.
194. Gold, E.W., Fox, O.D., Weissfeld, S. et al.: Corticosteroid-induced avascular necrosis: An experimental study in rabbits. Clin. Orthop., *135*:272–280, 1978.
195. Paolaggi, J.B., LeParc, J.M., Durigon, M. et al.: Early alterations of bone and marrow after high doses of steroids: Results in two animal species. In Arlet, J., Ficat, R.O., and Hungerford, D.S. (eds.): Bone Circulation. Baltimore, Williams and Wilkins, 1984, pp. 42–47.
196. Fisher, D.E., Bickel, W.H., Holley, K.E. et al.: Corticosteroid-induced aseptic necrosis. II. Experimental study. Clin. Orthop., *84*:200–206, 1972.
197. Cruess, R.L., Ross, D., and Crawshaw, E.: The etiology of steroid-induced avascular necrosis of bone. A laboratory and clinical study. Clin. Orthop., *113*:178–183, 1975.
198. Kawai, K., Tamki, A., and Hirohata, K.: Steroid-induced accumulation of lipid in the osteocytes of the rabbit femoral head. A histochemical and electron microscopic study. J Bone Joint Surg., *67A*:755–763, 1985.
199. Jaffe, W.L., Epstein, M., Heyman, N. et al.: The effect of cortisone on femoral and humeral heads in rabbits. An experimental study. Clin. Orthop., *82*:221–228, 1972.
200. Kenzora, J.E.: The effect of high dose corticosteroids on kidney, liver and bone tissues of rabbits. Unpublished data, 1978.
201. Wang, G.-J., Sweet, D.E., Reger, S.I. et al.: Fat-cell changes as a mechanism of avascular necrosis of the femoral head in cortisone-treated rabbits. J. Bone Joint Surg., *59A*:729–735, 1977.

SECTION IX

Osteoarthritis

101

Pathology of Osteoarthritis

AUBREY J. HOUGH, JR.

One purpose for studying a disease is to gain insight into its causation. Osteoarthritis (OA), despite widespread occurrence in the adult population, offers formidable obstacles to the acquisition of such understanding. The very name *osteoarthritis* is a misnomer, because it implies an inflammatory process. The term, however, has been used in the English-speaking world for several generations, and neither the pathologically more accurate term *degenerative joint disease* nor the European term *osteoarthrosis* have displaced it. Osteoarthritis also suffers from a lack of consensus regarding its definition. It is not a single disease entity but a common reaction pattern of joint tissues to several types of injury. Its cause involves the interaction of mechanical and biologic factors. Different classification schemes of OA are based on these putative mechanical and biologic factors.[1–5] Osteoarthritis is defined here as an *inherently noninflammatory disorder of movable joints characterized by deterioration of articular cartilage and by the formation of new bone at the joint surfaces and margins.* The relationship between cartilaginous and bony changes has long been a source of contention. The nature of this relationship bears on the explanation of the pathologic changes seen in OA.

OSTEOARTHRITIS AND REMODELING

Remodeling is defined as the gradual alteration of the internal and external architecture of the skeleton in response to mechanical loading.[6] The removal of bone from certain sites coincides with the simultaneous formation of new bone elsewhere.[7] Remodeling of bone explains changes in the shape of the joints with age and in OA.[8] In experimental models, these forces can produce resorption of calcified cartilage in areas of decreased pressure and necrobiosis of chondrocytes in areas of increased pressure.[9]

Accounts of early OA usually maintain that fibrillation of articular cartilage precedes the development of other lesions. Biopsies of cartilage in early OA show that fibrillation is the earliest gross change seen (Fig. 101–1).[10] Similar changes are seen in early OA induced by partial meniscectomy in rabbits.[11] Cartilaginous changes, however, may not be first as the adjacent bony structure changes may precede them.[7] The relationships between the cartilaginous and bony changes are complex, and the hypotheses relating them have been summarized by Sokoloff.[6,7] Osteoarthritis can be viewed as a degeneration of articular cartilage progressively leading to denudation of the joint surface. If this chondrogenic theory were valid, little or no concomitant remodeling of bone would occur. Osteoarthritis of the hip in which eburnation ensues without deforming osteophytes is termed *concentric.* Such a pattern does occur, but rarely,[12] and results from inflammatory lysis of cartilage rather than from mechanical overloading.[13,14] In keeping with this hypothesis, the extent of remodeling in surgically resected femoral heads is generally greater in OA (coxa magna) than in rheumatoid arthritis (RA).[15] Similar lack of remodeling in ochronotic arthropathy is due to the intrinsic metabolic deterioration of cartilage.[16]

A second hypothesis is that cartilage fibrillation (Fig. 101–2A) sets in motion a cascade of events leading to secondary bony remodeling of the joint. This concept is very difficult to substantiate from the cartilage pathology alone because other morphologic events often occur in cartilage or simultaneously in other tissues. For instance, age-related remodeling[17,18] in the osteochondral junction may coexist with surface fibrillation. Remodeling of the basal calcified cartilage is more apparent in non–weight-bearing areas of the joint[19,20] in contrast to fibrillation, which is more prominent in the weight-bearing areas. Thus, direct causal relationships

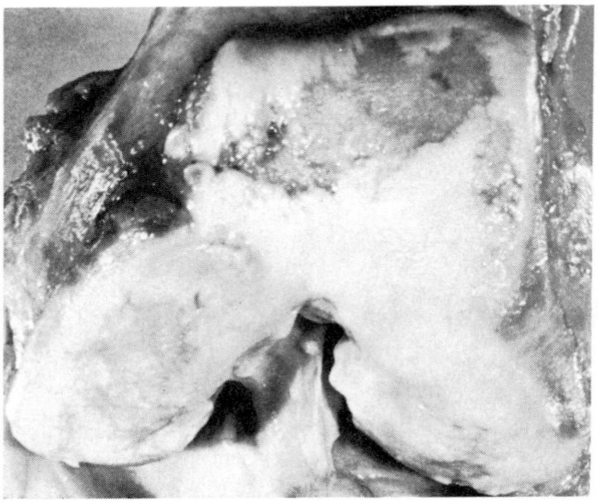

FIGURE 101–1. Osteoarthritis of the knee. Large areas of erosion of articular cartilage are present on the patellar facet and on the condyles of the femur. These erosions occupy principally the central portions of the joint surfaces and spare the marginal regions. The cartilage at the eroded edges is fibrillated. The irregular elevations at the periphery of the surfaces are osteophytic.

between these two early changes are difficult to establish. Microfractures of the calcified cartilage, however, may presage the development of later cartilage degeneration.

A third hypothesis proposes that OA is a consequence of increased stiffness of subchondral bone.[6] Radin et al., have postulated that microfractures of subchondral bone precede cartilage damage[21] because bone, rather than cartilage, absorbs most of the energy of impact loading transmitted through the extremities. Repair of these microfractures results in a net increase in bone stiffness, causing the overlying cartilage to absorb a greater proportion of the transmitted energy. This repartition of forces eventually is postulated to result in degeneration of the articular cartilage. Although this hypothesis has a distinct biomechanical logic, there are, as with the previous two hypotheses, certain limitations: the microfractures of the subchondral bony trabeculae may actually be a protective mechanism to maintain normal joint function because their numbers are decreased in OA joints as compared to normal.[22] This view holds that the remodeling of the subchondral trabeculae into thicker structures is the primary event rather than the microfractures.[23] One source of the confusion is the failure to distinguish between microfractures of the subchondral bony plate itself and those occurring at some distance in the trabecular bone. The former are clearly involved in the formation of subchondral pseudocysts (Fig. 101–3). The latter are variously influenced by the systemic state of the skeleton and the extent of remodeling activities.[22,23]

These degenerative and remodeling events are intertwined to the extent that identification of a unique initial event in the process of OA, if one exists, has not been possible. The same processes that culminate in destruction of the osteoarticular junction and the abrasion of the cartilage surface also result in proliferation of new cartilage and bone at or near the joint surface (Fig. 101–4). Although the exact cause of this proliferation has not been established, the generation of new cartilage in defects in the joint surface that penetrate into the subjacent bone marrow has been documented in experimental models.[24,25] In advanced OA, islands of cartilaginous proliferation are interspersed with new bone formation in the subchondral bone marrow,[26] representing abortive attempts at repair of infractions of the joint surface.

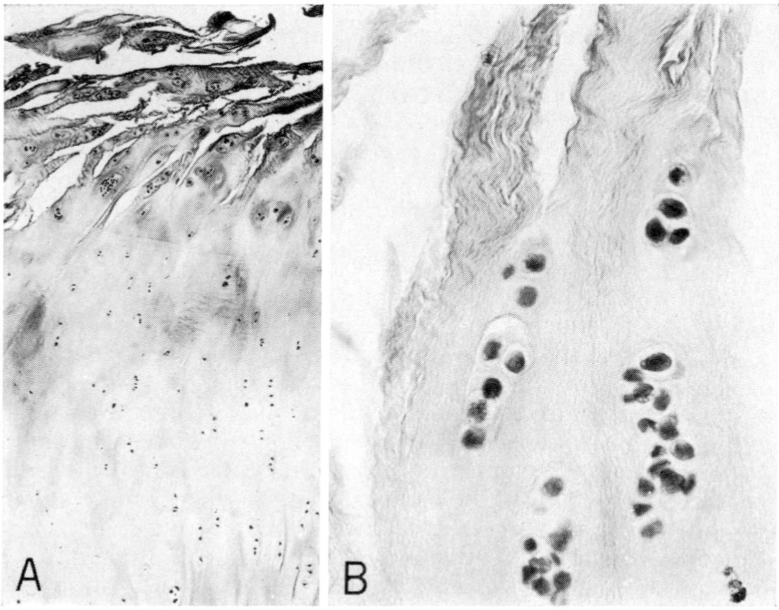

FIGURE 101–2. Fibrillation of articular cartilage. *A*, The most superficial dehiscences are oriented parallel to the surface and then arch downward in a more vertical direction. This pattern corresponds to the fibrous planes of the cartilage. (Hematoxylin and eosin stain, × 40.) *B*, Higher magnification (×240) of the fibrillated edge. The collagen fibrils at the surface have been "unmasked" from the hyaline matrix and appear frayed. Clusters of chondrocytes have proliferated to form so-called brood capsules.

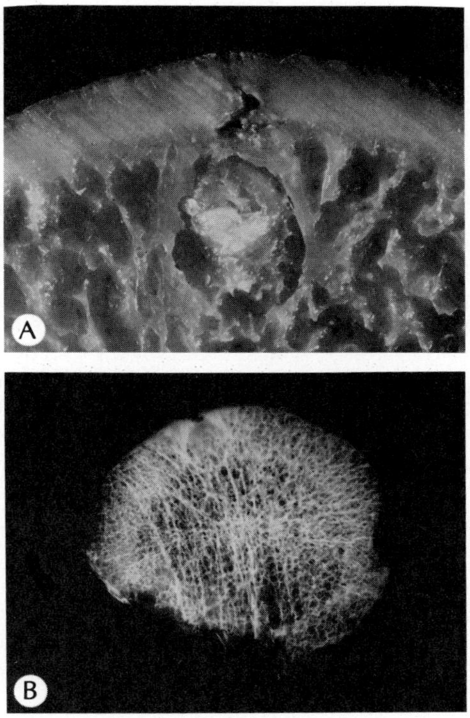

FIGURE 101–3. Relationship between a pseudocyst and a microfracture of the subchondral plate. This fortuitous slab section is from a recently fractured femoral head of a 77-year-old woman. Although moderate fibrillation is present elsewhere in the cartilage surface, the sole pseudocyst is located immediately beneath the minute discontinuity in the otherwise intact cartilage and osteochondral junction. *A*, Gross appearance (approximately × 4). *B*, Roentgenogram, showing the gap in the subchondral plate and the sclerotic wall of the "cyst."

The marginal osteophyte represents a proliferative response to joint injury (Fig. 101–4). Although osteophytes are conspicuous features of advanced OA, it would be erroneous to conclude that they represent merely a late change in the evolution of the joint lesions. Periarticular bone remodeling appears early in the course of experimental canine OA, parallel to changes in the composition of articular cartilage. Osteoarthritis represents not so much the inability of the joint surface to initiate repair but rather the failure of repair to restore function.[6]

ARTICULAR CARTILAGE

MICROSCOPIC CHANGES

Many changes have been observed microscopically in articular cartilage from early OA, but opinions differ about which is the earliest. Correlation of these early changes with biochemical and cell biologic information has been difficult, which is due to regional variations of osteoarthritic changes within cartilage.

Focal Chondromucoid Degeneration

Bennett, Waine, and Bauer concluded that focal swelling of the cartilage matrix associated with increased affinity for hematoxylin constituted the initial event in the process of OA.[27] This superficial mucoid transformation is associated with an increased number of chondrocytes adjacent to the alteration.

Focal Loss of Metachromasia

Loss of metachromatic staining material, presumably chondroitin sulfate, from all but the deepest portion of the radial zone of articular cartilage, has been proposed[7] as the histologic counterpart of chondromalacia followed by OA. Decreased metachromasia is accompanied by a loss of affinity for hematoxylin, in contrast to the view of Bennett et al.[27] This theory is supported by evidence that the hyaluronic acid[28] and proteoglycan[29] content of cartilage is reduced in early OA. Furthermore, severity of histologic change in cartilage correlated with proteoglycanase activity in human OA.[30] Serum keratan sulfate levels were increased in patients with hypertrophic OA.[31]

Proliferation of Chondrocytes

Small clusters of chondrocytes are common at the margin of minute fissures in the surface of the cartilage. These chondrocytes have proliferated in response to the dehiscence of the tissue (Fig. 101–2).

Diminution of Chondrocytes

Once adulthood is reached, the unit number of chondrocytes changes little in articular cartilage with aging.[32] In OA, however, chondrocyte loss is found in all layers of articular cartilage. Relics of disintegrated cells are often seen associated with microscars. Similar changes occurred in experimental OA in foxhounds.[33]

Fatty Degeneration

Fine fat deposits in the interterritorial matrix represent an early degenerative change in cartilage; these may become larger, forming coarse droplets at the "capsule" of the chondrocytes. The content of triglyceride and complex lipids increases with age in the cells and in cartilage matrix even before fibrillation. Increased arachidonic acid, the precursor of prostaglandins, is confined to the tangential layer.[7]

Alteration of Collagen Fibrils

In aging articular cartilage, the general architecture and appearance of the collagen fibrils are preserved, although looser packing and occasional fragmentation are sometimes seen in the superficial layers. The aforementioned microscars increase in numbers as OA evolves. Some of the fragmented fibrils in these areas

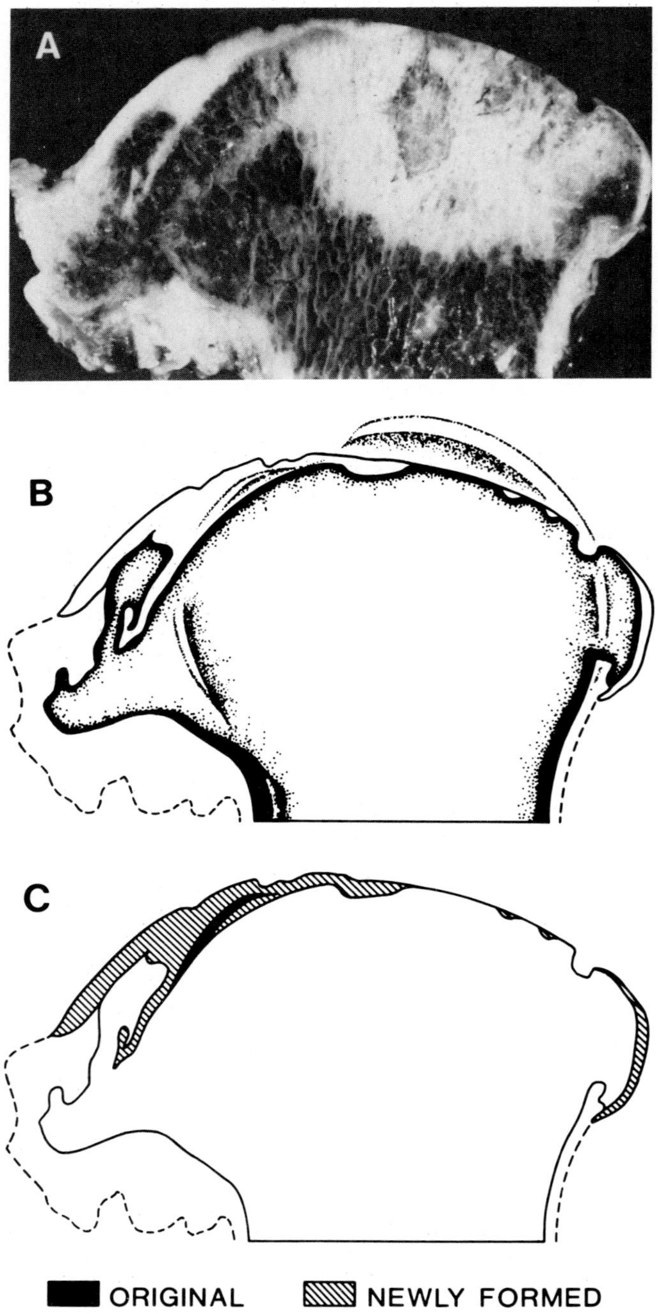

FIGURE 101–4. Advanced osteoarthritis of the head of the femur. *A*, The contour has been deformed both by abrasion of the bearing surface and by formation of marginal osteophytes. The large inferomedial spur at the left has grown not only to the side but also into the original joint cartilage. Subchondral pseudocysts approach the eroded surface through slender crevices. The pallor of the eburnated zone reflects the condensation of bony trabeculae and compact fibrous tissue, in contrast to the darker, vascular hematopoietic marrow. *B*, Schematic representation of the remodeling. The outline of the gross specimen is superimposed on a best-fit contour of a normal femoral head of corresponding size. Bone appears black; cartilage, white outlined by a solid line. The broken line demarcates retinacular synovium. The loss of substance affects both articular cartilage and the immediately subjacent bone. *C*, Newly formed cartilage as deduced from the difference in the corresponding outlines in *B*. Only a minute residue of the original cartilage (black) persists at the base of the inferomedial osteophyte. The bulk of the cartilage must have therefore formed in the retinaculum or the subchondral bone marrow.

have a larger diameter. A progressive radial reorientation of the collagen fibrils has been noted by electron microscopy and by x-ray diffraction. Although amianthoid (asbestos-like) degeneration of the matrix has been described as a late feature of OA,[34] this process typically occurs in costal and other extra-articular cartilage rather than in joint cartilage.

Surface Irregularities

Age-dependent irregularities in the surface of articular cartilage have been proposed to evolve into fibrillation.[35] Although several types of evidence support this concept, the data are inconclusive because the various analytic procedures used themselves may involve technical artifacts.

Weichselbaum's Lacunar Resorption

Focal dissolution of matrix by chondroclastic cells in the cartilage lacunae was once regarded as a feature of OA (Fig. 101–5) but is more characteristic of RA. (See Chapter 41.) Evidence that cytokines, particularly in-

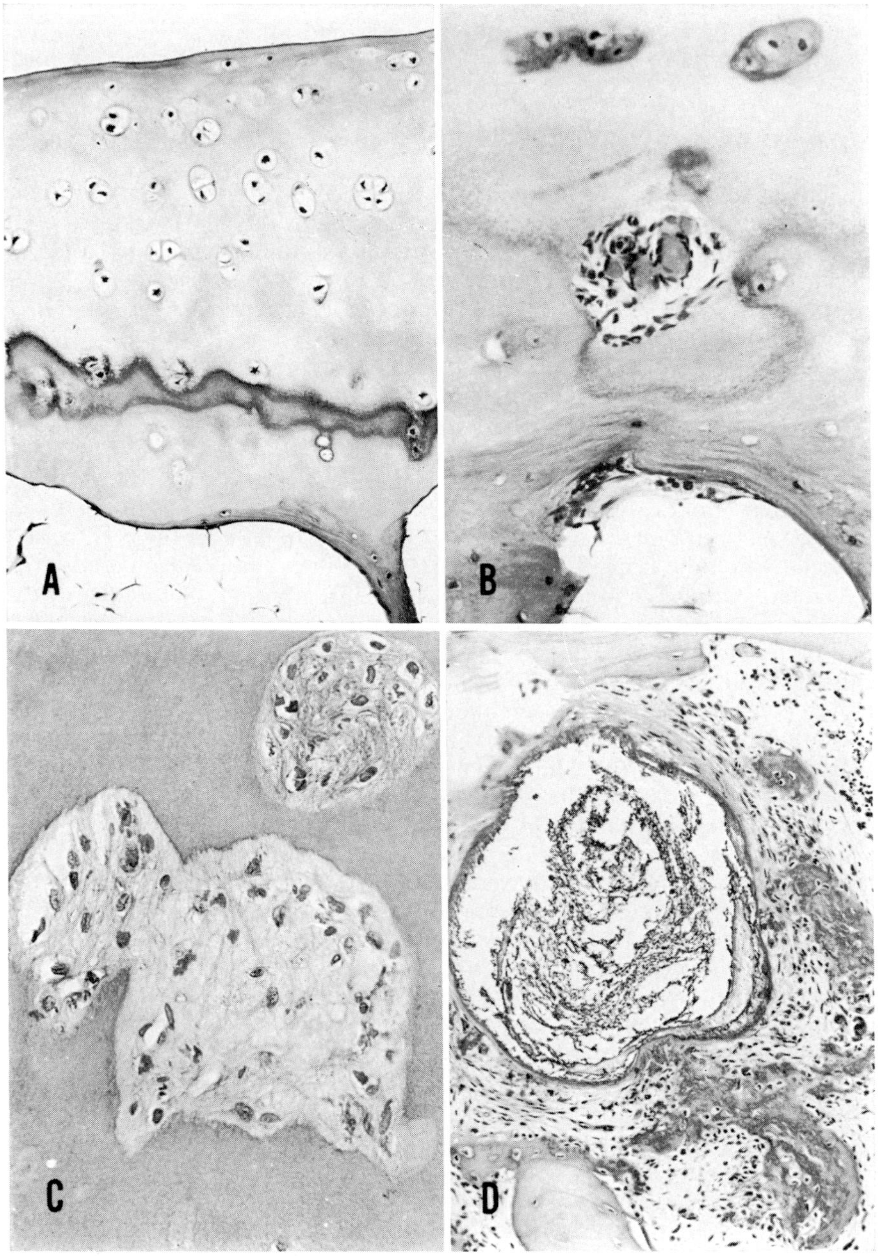

FIGURE 101–5. Miscellaneous remodeling and degenerative changes; all sections are stained with hematoxylin and eosin. *A*, Reduplication of calcification "tidemark" (×95). *B*, Vascularization of base of articular cartilage; the dark-stained material in the capsules of the chondrocytes is calcific (×183). *C*, Weichselbaum's lacunar resorption; small, geographic areas of hyaline cartilage are replaced by loose-textured, cellular fibrous tissue (×210). *D*, Early subchondral "cystic" degeneration; a small true cyst, filled with mucoid material, has a fibrous border. New bone formation is seen in the adjacent marrow (×90).

terleukin-1 (IL-1),[36] can stimulate chondrocytes to release matrix-destroying proteases[30] supports the observation that lacunar resorption is a significant pathologic process in cartilage destruction regardless of disease specificity.

GROSS CHANGES

Localized areas of softening of the cartilage are associated with a fine, velvety disruption of the surface. In these areas, one sees a dehiscence of the cartilage along the axis of the matrix collagen. In disruption confined to the surface tangential layer, the process is referred to as *flaking*; when the process extends to the deeper radial layer, it is described as *fibrillation* (Fig. 101–2). Because these minute discontinuities in the surface are readily stained grossly by India ink,[37] they lend themselves to quantitative study. Abrasion of the fibrillated cartilage takes place with progressive denudation of the underlying bony cortex (Fig. 101–1). The sites of predilection for destruction of the joint surface are those subject to greatest load bearing or shearing stress. Earliest fibrillation, however, is often present in regions with presumably low compressive stress, such as the infrafoveal portion of the femoral head. In the patella, the central facets are the sites most prone to erosion.[38] Although not a weight-bearing joint, the patella is subjected to enormous loads by leverage when the knee is flexed, such as stair climbing or squatting.

LATE HISTOLOGIC CHANGES

In fibrillated regions, continuity of the surface of the articular cartilage is disrupted. The height of the fronds is in the range of 20 to 150 μm.[39] Ground-substance metachromasia is reduced, and the matrix has a fibrillary, disheveled appearance. Birefringence of collagen fibrils is increased. Clusters of chondrocytes, long known as *brood capsules*, are located close to the margins of the clefts (Fig. 101–2B). The proliferative and proteoglycan-producing activities of these cells have been amply documented by autoradiography. Little or no collagen is seen within the clones, and it must be presumed that chondrolytic enzymes, including collagenases, have been generated to remove matrix to make room for the new cells (see Chapter 102).

The fate of these cellular clusters has been the subject of debate. Although small areas of necrobiosis are seen, these are not necessarily limited to the cell clusters. The clustered cells are active metabolically. Focal proliferation of chondrocytes is also seen in deeper areas, where severe lesions have disrupted the surrounding matrix. The matrix in these areas has a pale, myxoid appearance. Evidence indicates that type II collagen degradation products are present in OA cartilage[40] and that unusual types of collagens develop in the pericellular matrix.[41] This could be a manifestation of proteoglycan depletion exposing collagen to enzymatic degradation.

Mitrovic et al. described increases in biosynthetic activity of articular chondrocytes in the same joint even at some distance from the sites of overt damage to the cartilage.[42] This judgment is based on advanced lesions in which the bulk of the cartilage is of a new and immature type. Reparative cartilage is typically composed of a mixed hyaline and fibrocartilaginous tissue with more conspicuous fibrillary collagen and less intense staining for proteoglycan. Osteophytes are covered by a combination of a fibrocartilaginous surface with areas of overt fibrous tissue. In many cases secondary degenerative change and fibrillation are superimposed on the reparative cartilage, further complicating the histologic appearance. As a result the histochemical features of the matrix are heterogeneous.[43,44]

Reduplication of the tidemark is exaggerated in the vicinity of the fibrillated cartilage and, more remotely, at the margin of the joint.[7] Several types of degenerative change in the calcified zone have been described.[45] Calcium-containing crystals are deposited in the territorial matrix of the adjacent chondrocytes as forward remodeling occurs. These crystals appear as basophilic granules in demineralized sections (Fig. 101–5B) and within or around matrix vesicles in electron micrographs.[17] The activities of matrix vesicle enzymes increase progressively along with histologic features of OA.[46]

BONE

New bone formation occurs in two separate locations in relation to the joint surface: in exophytic growths at the margins of the articular cartilage and in the immediately subjacent bone marrow (Fig. 101–4). Marginal osteophytes have two patterns of growth. One consists of a protuberance into the joint space, while the other develops within capsular and ligamentous attachments to the joint margins. In each circumstance the direction of the osteophyte is governed by the lines of mechanical force exerted on the area of growth, generally corresponding to the contour of the joint surface from which the osteophyte protrudes. The osteophyte consists in large part of bone that merges imperceptibly with the other cortical and cancellous tissue of the subchondral bone. The osteophyte is capped by a layer of hyaline and fibrocartilage continuous with the adjacent synovial lining. In advanced lesions, the landmarks are obliterated because the osteophytic surface itself undergoes degeneration. Proliferative tissue frequently occupies the fovea of the ligamentum teres and extends down along the femoral neck to form buttress osteophytes. These buttress osteophytes may obscure the normal boundary between the femoral head and the femoral neck. In most surgical specimens of the femoral head removed for OA, the combination of degenerative and proliferative activity has destroyed virtually all of the native articular cartilage.

The proliferation of bone in the subchondral tissue is most marked in areas denuded of their cartilaginous covering.[47] In these regions, the articulating surface consists of bone that has been rubbed smooth. The glistening appearance of this polished sclerotic surface suggests ivory, hence the name *eburnation*. Nubbins of newly proliferated cartilage usually protrude through minute gaps in the eburnated bone.[26] Proliferation of new bone at these sites is an integral part of the eburnation. Many of the osteocytes in the eburnated zones die, as indicated by empty lacunae. Frictional heat is the most likely cause for their death.

"Cystic" areas of rarefaction of bone are commonly seen immediately beneath eburnated surfaces in the hip joint (see Fig. 101–2). Such structures are much less frequent in other joints. The cystic areas occur on both femoral and acetabular sides of the joint. The lesions are most frequently present on the superolateral weight-bearing surface. In severe instances they may involve other regions of the hip as well.[48] In a few cases, these lesions appear roentgenographically before narrowing of the joint space has given evidence of cartilage destruction. The lesions only infrequently contain pockets of mucoid fluid and thus are not truly cystic (see Fig. 101–5D). The trabeculae in the affected areas disappear, and the bone marrow undergoes fibromyxoid degeneration. Fragments of dead bone, cartilage, and amorphous debris are often interspersed within them. In time, the entire area is encircled by a rim of reactive new bone and compact fibrous tissue (see Fig. 101–5D). Minute gaps in the overlying articular cortex, resulting from microfractures, are commonly seen at the apex of the pseudocysts (Fig. 101–3). These findings are consistent with an intrusion of pressure, if not of synovial fluid, from the joint cavity through a defect in the articular cortex into the subchondral bone marrow. Intra-articular pressures exceeding 1000 mm Hg occur in hip joints with effusions.[49] The increased pressure is dissipated radially into the adjacent bone marrow, compresses the medullary blood vessels, and thereby leads to the retrogressive changes. This mechanism is not contradicted by observations that the intraosseous pressure is normal in osteoarthritic femoral heads at the time of arthroplasty. In these specimens, bulk pressures, rather than localized gradients, are measured. Furthermore, internal remodeling compensates for the presumptive pressure gradients. The "punched out" lesions observed roentgenographically in gout and the bone "cysts" in hemophilic arthropathy correspond pathologically to the pseudocysts in OA, except the specific exudates of the former also lie within the degenerated marrow space.

New bone formation also occurs in the form of focal enchondral ossification of the base of the articular cartilage.[45] Such metaplasia is a component of the remodeling process through which bone is added to a portion of the articular cortex while other areas of the joint undergo resorption of bone. The osteochondral junction is juxtaposed to a zone of calcified cartilage. During the period of active skeletal growth, this osteochondral junction has an epiphysis-like function that permits actual enlargement of the bone through sequential ossification of the calcified cartilage. In adults the interface between calcified and noncalcified hyaline articular cartilage is demarcated by a thin, undulating, hematoxyphilic line known as the *tidemark* (see Fig. 101–5A). In older persons this line is usually transformed into several parallel discontinuous ones whose presence is clear evidence of the progression of calcification front into the articular cartilage.[17] The possibility that the progression of the basilar calcification might lead to thinning of the articular cartilage (senile atrophy) has not been substantiated by careful studies.[18]

The role of osteonecrosis in the generation of OA has also been the subject of considerable discussion. Much of the deformity in symptomatic OA results from collapse of the joint surface. Localized areas of necrosis are seen frequently in this location, and occlusion of minute intramedullary arteries has been demonstrated by angiography. Small secondary infarcts of eburnated bone are seen in approximately 6 to 14% of surgically resected femoral heads.[26,50,51]

Wong, Evans, Needs, and co-workers used histochemical staining for lactate dehydrogenase to show that the osteocytes of many bone trabeculae in OA are nonviable.[52] Nevertheless, Streda's suggestion that all OA of the hip is secondary to osteonecrosis exceeds the evidence.[53] The new bone formation of the remodeling process is accompanied by increased vascularity and is the basis for scintigraphic studies using bone-seeking radionuclides in this disorder.[54]

CHONDROCALCINOSIS

The frequency of chondrocalcinosis, especially in the older age group (see also Chapters 108 and 109), has generated divergent opinions on the relationship of the condition to OA.[55] Calcium pyrophosphate dihydrate (CPPD) crystal deposition has been variously considered to have no relationship to OA;[56] to favor its development[57] or its inflammatory manifestations;[58] to result from OA or other derangement of articular cartilage metabolism in the aged;[59] or to be yet another but separate manifestation of articular aging distinct from OA. The significance of basic calcium phosphate (BCP)[60] versus CPPD crystals in synovial fluid has also been debated. Correlation of joint fluid and radiographic findings led to the suggestion[61] that BCP crystals are a feature of OA whereas CPPD crystals are a consequence of aging per se.

The experience of Sokoloff and Varma[62] indicates that meniscal chondrocalcinosis is present in roughly half of knees treated surgically for OA after age 68. The risk for meniscal calcinosis in surgically removed knees was sixfold that of an age- and sex-adjusted postmortem population. Felson, Anderson, Naimark, et al. found a lower but significant association between OA of the knee and chondrocalcinosis using radiographic assessment in an epidemiologic study.[63] By contrast, CPPD crystals were rarely found in femoral heads removed for OA.[5] Chondrocalcinosis also is relatively infrequent in fractured hips below the age of 85. The view of Pritzker et al.[55] that BCP crystals in OA synovial fluid arise predominantly from abrasion of the eburnated surface or the remodeling basal cartilage, whereas CPPD crystals are part of the meniscocalcinosis, is attractive from the pathologist's perspective. Why the meniscus is the predominant site of involvement in OA of the knee, while the hyaline articular cartilages are largely spared, remains a matter of conjecture.[64] Ordinarily, the deposition of CPPD in the OA knee engenders no inflammatory reaction. Deposits of lipid are associated with CPPD deposits and are also present in the adjacent chondrocytes.[65] The role of this lipid material in the deposition of crystals is unclear.

In contrast to the articular chondrocytes that are degenerate at sites of CPPD crystal deposition,[56] meniscal fibrochondrocytes apparently remain metabolically active in the presence of these crystals.[66] Several observers have noted that joint mice are more frequent in OA specimens with chondrocalcinosis than in those without crystal deposition. Basic calcium phosphate crystal deposition is characteristically associated with more severe arthropathy with occasional Charcot-like breakdown of joints[67,68] (see Chapter 109).

SOFT TISSUE

During recent years the inflammatory manifestations of OA have aroused discussion.[69–72] Although by definition OA is inherently not an inflammatory condition,

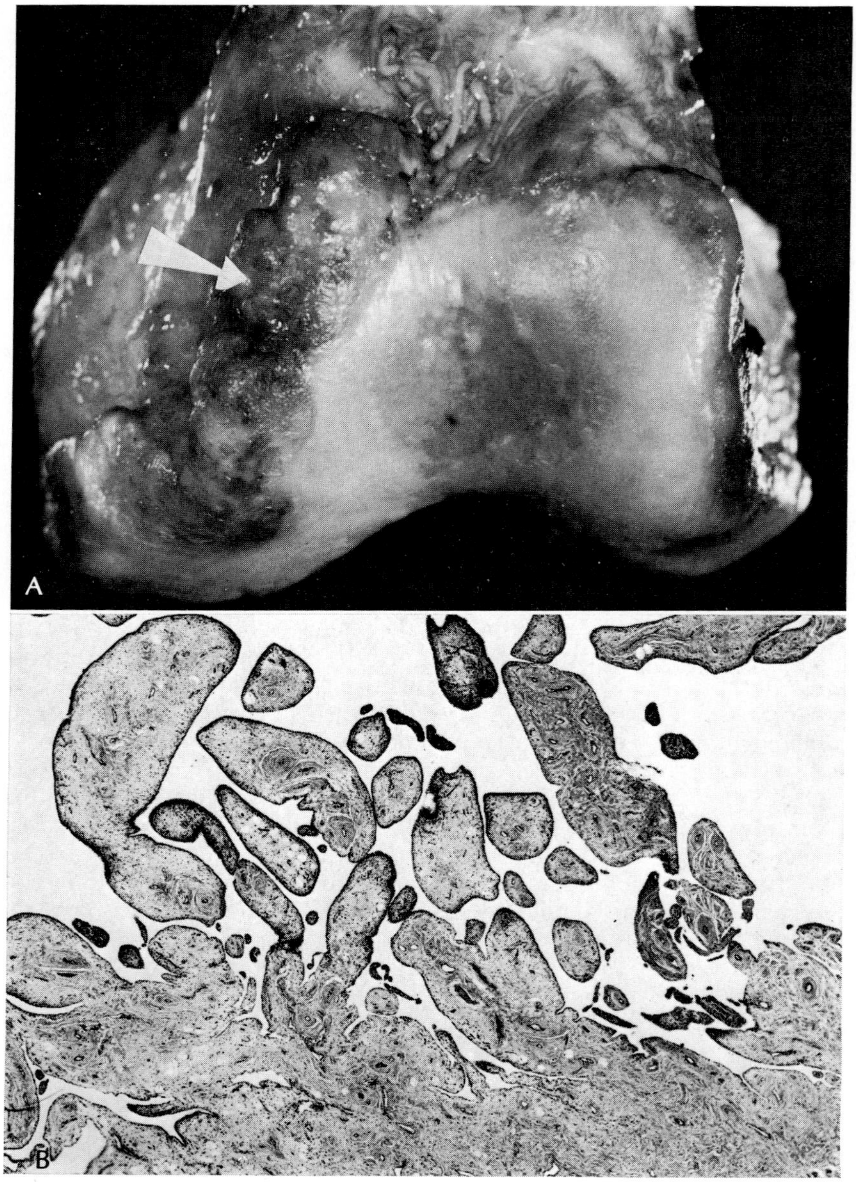

FIGURE 101–6. Synovial hypertrophy in severe osteoarthritis. The patient is a 63-year-old man whose left knee had been enlarged for 23 years following an automobile accident. *A*, A massive osteophyte (arrow) is seen at the medial border of the articular surface. The adjacent synovial tissue has undergone prominent papillary thickening. *B*, Histologically, the villous processes are made up of compact fibrous tissue not infiltrated by inflammatory cells. (Hematoxylin and eosin stain, ×16.)

some degree of synovial villous hypertrophy and fibrosis are seen in the majority of symptomatic cases (Fig. 101–6). A moderate focal chronic synovitis has been described in about one fifth of surgically resected specimens.[51] This synovitis is characterized by hyperplasia and enlargement of synovial lining cells and by mild lining infiltration of lymphocytes and mononuclear cells.[72] The infiltrate is generally mild and heterogeneous with respect to immunopathology.[73] Polyclonal B cells compose part of the infiltrate, and extracellular deposits of C3 have also been described.[7] Fibronectin is deposited in exudative foci.[74] Other tissue changes such as hemosiderin deposition,[75] foreign body reaction to joint detritus, and xanthoma-like changes around fat necrosis may be seen. Very occasionally, the inflammation is severe enough to raise a question of RA. Immunopathologic studies, however, show significant qualitative differences in the infiltrates characterizing the two diseases. Synovial macrophages are more frequent in RA,[76,77] as are cells bearing activation antigens.[76] The mean nuclear density of cellularity is higher in RA, and immunoglobulin-producing plasma cells, common in RA, are rare in OA synovia.[72] Immunoblasts are not seen in the synovial fluid in OA.[78] Helper/suppressor (CD4/CD8) ratios vary between upper and lower synovial regions in RA but are uniform throughout the synovium in OA.[72] These findings clearly differentiate the inflammatory infiltrates in OA and RA. Synovial inflammation in OA is probably a secondary phenomenon. Similar, relatively low-grade synovial inflammatory responses occur in other joint diseases of nonphlogistic origin, such as acromegaly.[79]

Autosensitization to joint detritus is an attractive consideration in the genesis of the inflammatory reaction. This theory is supported by experimental induction of immunity to homologous collagens and proteoglycans in rabbits.[80] Additional supportive evidence for autosensitization is the finding of autoantibodies against both native and denatured type II collagen in 50% of OA cartilage extracts.[81] Analysis of DNA restriction enzyme patterns of T-lymphocytes from OA synovia show an oligoclonal pattern of T-cell receptor β-chain gene rearrangements, suggesting a response by a limited number of T-cell clones.[82] Such a response may indicate a response to released indigenous articular cartilage proteins. Additional evidence for an immune response in certain types of OA is the finding of immunoglobulin-complement complexes deposited in the superficial zones of OA articular cartilage.[83] Deposits in articular cartilage in RA were quantitatively greater and granular in nature as opposed to the nongranular nature of the OA deposits. Whether the deposits in OA are a primary phenomenon or merely a response to matrix damage is not known.

Another possible mechanism for the inflammatory changes in the synovium involves response to CPPD or BCP crystals.[70] Both species occur in the synovium, in cartilage and in the synovial fluid (see Chapters 5, 109, and 110). Crystals have been proposed as one method of activation of cytokines, particularly IL-1.[83] Interleukin-1 stimulates synovial cells and articular chondrocytes to release neutral proteases capable of destroying cartilage matrix.[36,84,85] Human OA cartilage is enriched with partially degraded type II collagen,[40] indicating that this mechanism may be of significance in perpetuating articular destruction.

Other soft tissues also participate in the OA complex of degenerative changes. Minute tears in capsular tissue appear as slender, fibrovascular seams disrupting the principal axes of the collagen bundles. Secondary osteochondromatosis occurs at times but is much more characteristic of neuropathic arthropathy than of OA. The ligamentum teres commonly disintegrates. In the knee joint, the cruciate ligaments and menisci also become frayed. Substantial clinical and experimental[86] evidence suggests that meniscectomy leads to OA, but no correlation has been found in autopsy material between tears or other lesions of the semilunar cartilages and OA.[87] Fibrillation and fibrosis of the synovial surface and even mild cartilaginous metaplasia of patellar tendon may occur. Analysis of hand and knee radiographs of 150 subjects who had undergone unilateral meniscectomy 19 or more years earlier showed a striking correlation between degeneration in the finger joints and in both the operated and opposite knee.[88] Degeneration was more severe, however, on the operated side and was independent of age and sex. This study suggests that a predisposition to primary OA influences the development of secondary degeneration and makes a clear distinction between these two subsets of the disease more difficult. Cooke[89] similarly found evidence of generalized or polyarthritis in 62% of those patients requiring surgery for severe hip or knee OA. Thus, although meniscectomy resulted in OA, underlying or systemic factors may have contributed to its severity.

Amyloid deposits have been reported in the joint capsule in OA, but they also occur in joint capsules and articular cartilage of normal joints and in the intra-articular discs of older individuals.[90–93] Amyloid or amyloid-like materials, however, have been described in several different tissues of aged individuals.[94] Any claim for specificity for amyloid in cartilage requires a considerably more discriminatory technique than screening by green birefringence after congo red staining, the usual histochemical method.

A progressive increase in the amount of fibrous tissue separating the synovial capillaries from the joint space has been described as an age-related finding, but it is unlikely that this condition interferes with the nourishment of the cartilage. Hyaline sclerosis of minute vessels is a common, although focal, in joints even of young individuals is a finding not directly related to OA. Periarticular muscle undergoes atrophy; type 2 myofibers are affected primarily.[95]

COMPARATIVE PATHOLOGY OF OSTEOARTHRITIS

Osteoarthritis occurs widely in the vertebrate kingdom, regardless of the position of the species in the taxonomic scale. Osteophytic lesions, sometimes leading to ankylosis, were common in certain giant dinosaurs 100 million years ago (see Chapter 1). The disorder has been observed in large and small mammals, in animals that swim (cetaceans) rather than bear their weight on their extremities, and also, to a mild degree, in birds. It is of considerable economic importance in livestock commerce, the horse-racing industry, and veterinary practice.

In small laboratory animals, it has been possible to study a number of pathogenetic concepts of OA. The importance of genetic factors has been established in mice.[96] The inheritance appears to be polygenic and the overall behavior, recessive. No evidence suggests major sex linkage. Male mice consistently develop more severe OA than do females. Obesity is not an important factor.[97] In laboratory rodents, the knee and elbow joints are commonly affected severely but the hips rarely. That heritable biochemical defects are major factors in the development of OA is suggested by the frequency of OA lesions in blotchy (BLO) mice, in which a mutant gene leads to inadequate cross linking of collagen.[98] In the STR/ORT mouse, widely studied for its predisposition to OA, Walton attributed knee joint changes to spontaneous patellar subluxation.[99] Surgical containment of the subluxation prevented the development of OA. Susceptibility to OA in these animals seems attributable to abnormal mechanical loading rather than to a cartilage metabolic abnormality. Although impressive, these data are difficult to reconcile with Sokoloff's observations[7] that lesions in STR/1N mice were not confined to the knee but were more generalized. More generalized cartilage degeneration has been observed in guinea pigs as well.[100] Genetic factors influencing the development of OA may be influenced at many levels: local and generalized, mechanical and metabolic.

The genetic aspect of the disorder is also manifested by variable susceptibility of different species to its development. Rats, for example, are generally resistant, whereas another rodent, *Mastomys natalensis*, develops a severe generalized OA by the age of 2 years. Another desert rodent, the Mediterranean sand rat (*Psammomys obesus*) develops a severe degenerative spondylosis with disc thinning and anterior vertebral hyperostosis reminiscent of human hyperostotic spondylosis.[101] Genetic contributions are also found in certain breeds of cattle and swine. The fundamental pathogenetic problem is whether these genetic factors are local and articular, related to the configuration and mechanical forces exerted on the joint, as in the dysplastic hips of German shepherd dogs, or whether they are more generalized metabolic properties of the articular tissues.

DEGENERATIVE DISEASE OF THE SPINAL COLUMN

Degenerative changes in the spine affect two discrete but interrelated articular systems: the amphiarthroses (discs) and the diarthrodial (zygoapophyseal or facet) joints. The former develop changes with increasing age characterized by loss of ground substance metachromasia[7] and matrix water content,[102] increased vascularization of the hyaline cartilage end plates[103] and disorderly and attenuated collagen fibrils.[7] In many individuals such degeneration leads to disc herniation and to breakdown of the cartilaginous end plates with the development of spinal osteochondrosis.[103] The prominent osteochondral osteophytes that develop in this condition have led to the wide use of the term *spondylosis deformans* (see Chapters 94 and 95). The cervical[104] and lumbar spines[103] are most susceptible to the clinical manifestations of this condition. The diarthrodial joints develop OA changes similar to those in peripheral joints.

This distinction in terms should not lead to the conclusion that the two processes are unrelated, because the pathologic findings in the joints are similar. The nucleus pulposus becomes fissured and deformed, and similar cracks appear in the anulus fibrosus. Fibrillary disintegration of the hyaline cartilage plates, through which the disc is attached to the vertebral bodies, cannot be distinguished histologically from the changes in diarthrodial OA. Eburnation of the subchondral bony plate develops in like manner. Marginal osteophytes arise under the mechanical stimulus of horizontal pulsion of the anulus fibrosus and its periosteal attachments as a result of collapse and spreading out of the nucleus pulposus. Traction forces by spinal muscles on the tendinous insertions in this region also have been implicated in this disorder. Furthermore, intervertebral disc disease shifts a greater proportion of the compressive and torsional loads on the apophyseal facet joints,[103] contributing to further degenerative changes.

Another feature of spinal osteochondrosis[103] is the development of nodules of cartilaginous and fibrous tissue beneath the subchondral plate of the vertebral bodies called Schmorl's nodes, which are usually attributed to the displacement of a nucleus pulposus into a vertebral body.[105] These islands are often surrounded by a shell of bone and, except for their greater content of cartilage, are reminiscent of the subchondral "cysts" in OA peripheral joints. Schmorl's nodes are not a pathognomonic feature of vertebral osteoporosis, because they occur commonly in degenerative disc disease not associated with osteopenia.

Although the marginal osteophytes develop most often on the anterolateral aspects of the vertebral bodies, posterior osteophytic protrusions occur and may affect the spinal cord and its roots. In the cervical region, spondylosis constitutes a hazard among older patients because of the resultant spinal stenosis. In the lumbar region, spinal stenosis develops with encroachment of osteophytes on the spinal canal and is due to degenerative spondylolisthesis associated with apophyseal OA.[103] Osteophytes in the Luschka (uncovertebral, neurocentral) joints have been shown by anatomic and angiographic means to compromise the neighboring vertebral arteries (see Chapter 92). The narrowing of the vascular lumen is most marked during rotation of the head and provides the basis for the posterior cervical sympathetic or *Barré-Liéou* syndrome.

Osteoarthritis does not characteristically lead to ankylosis; however, in at least three forms of segmental disease of the senescent spine, bony bridges unite the vertebral bodies. The proclivity for ankylosis may be related to the inherent limited mobility of the intervertebral disc.

HYPEROSTOTIC SPONDYLOSIS

The best known entity goes by several names: *hyperostotic spondylosis, senile ankylosing hyperostosis of Forestier and Rotes-Querol* or *spondylorrheostosis*. Hyperostotic spondylosis nominally is distinguished from ordinary spondylosis by the absence of disc degeneration.[7] The distal thoracic spine is the site of predilection.[103] The ankylotic bridges are located on the anterolateral portions of the vertebral bodies and extend into the anterior longitudinal ligaments (Fig. 101–7). The appearance has often led to confusion with ankylosing spondylitis. In some instances the vertebral lesion is accompanied by excessive osteophyte formation in peripheral joints. From this feature comes still another term for this condition, *diffuse idiopathic skeletal hyperostosis (DISH)*.[106] Currently, no consensus exists as to the definition of the DISH syndrome.

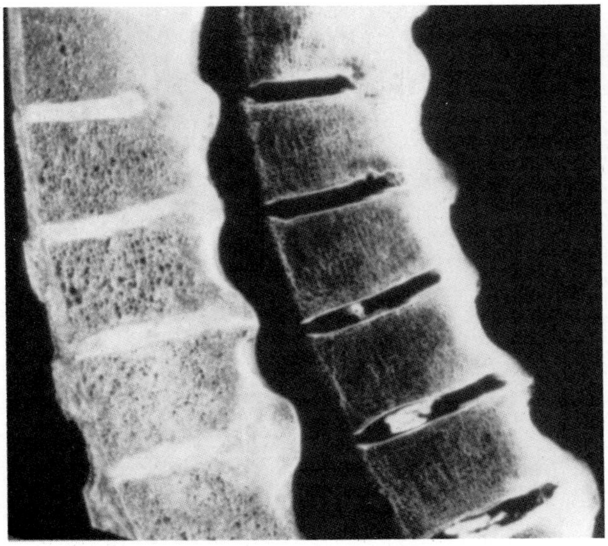

FIGURE 101–7. Hyperostotic spondylosis in the thoracic spine of an elderly male. Unlike the lesions of ankylosing spondylitis (Marie-Strümpell arthritis), the vertebral bodies do not manifest a "squared" appearance. Ossification has developed in the intervertebral discs, and the disc space is also narrowed anteriorly. Ossification in the anterior longitudinal ligament has blended with a hyperostotic response of the anterior vertebral bodies forming a continuous bony bridge (×0.5). (Courtesy of W.A. Gardner.)

ANKYLOSIS

Ankylosis may accompany severe spondylosis in man and other species. The disc space is narrowed. Destructive changes are present in the cortex of the anterior portion of the vertebral bodies.[103,104] Dense new bone formation is seen in the anterior longitudinal ligament. The appearance suggests that the ligament is first avulsed from the osteophyte and then repaired.

OTHER SEGMENTAL DISEASE

Several patterns of dorsal protrusion and bridging of cervical vertebrae (posterior spondylotic osteophytes) may cause life-threatening cervical myelopathy.[104] The relation of physiologic vertebral ligamentous ossification to the preceding disorder and to hyperostotic spondylosis is uncertain. It occurs in 7% of Japanese[107] and 0.3% of U.S. adults.[108] These lesions are asymptomatic in individuals with large spinal canals, but they require surgical decompression when spinal canals are small and myelopathy has developed.[109]

Baastrup's syndrome, an OA-like change that is due to bursitis between the distal portions of "kissing" lumbar dorsal, spinous processes,[103] is usually associated with severe spondylosis.

SPECIAL FORMS OF OSTEOARTHRITIS

HEBERDEN'S NODES

Despite the relative antiquity of the description of Heberden's nodes and their frequency, comparatively little information is available on their histopathology. They are marginal osteophytes of the distal interphalangeal joints. In more advanced cases these lesions are indistinguishable from those arising in OA remodeling in other sites (Fig. 101–8). Ossific transformation of the tendinous insertion into the joint capsule creates the exophytosis. In other instances mucoid transformation of the periarticular fibroadipose tissue is associated with proliferation of myxoid fibroblasts and cyst formation. Hyaluronic acid has been found in the cyst fluid. This finding is not a unique anatomic feature of Heberden's nodes. Indistinguishable changes may be present in other OA joints in other species. The process has certain morphologic similarities to ganglion formation or to cystic degeneration of the semilunar cartilages and to the subchondral pseudocysts of OA. Unilateral sparing from Heberden nodes after hemiplegia has been reported.[110] This observation suggests the possibility of neurovascular contributions to the development of the lesion but does not exclude a biomechanical explanation. The association of the para-articular mucous cysts of the distal interphalangeal joints with osteophytes has been emphasized because they are likely to recur following excision unless the osteophytes are also removed (see Chapter 49).

The term *erosive OA* (see Chapter 103) has been applied to a disorder resembling in its predilection for the distal and proximal interphalangeal joints, but in which a distinct inflammatory component exists.[111] A nonspecific, chronic synovial lymphocytic and mononuclear cell infiltrate is present. The nosologic status of the disorder is uncertain. One possibility is that this entity simply represents OA with a prominent, detritic synovitis. In a few cases, the lesion is disseminated to other joints and has been reported to evolve into RA.[112] Such "RA" patients, however, are generally seronegative and show a much greater tendency toward osteophyte formation than patients with seropositive RA. Bony ankylosis may occasionally occur in the finger joints in association with Heberden's nodes, especially of the inflammatory type (see Chapter 103).

GENERALIZED FORMS OF OSTEOARTHRITIS

The generalized forms of OA are variants that have in common a marked tendency to polyarticular involvement. With the exception of endemic arthritis, all have degrees of heritability.

PRIMARY GENERALIZED OSTEOARTHRITIS

Primary generalized osteoarthritis (GOA) was first defined as an entity by Kellgren, Lawrence, and Bier.[113] Conspicuous features of the disorder included a preponderance in middle-aged women, Heberden node forma-

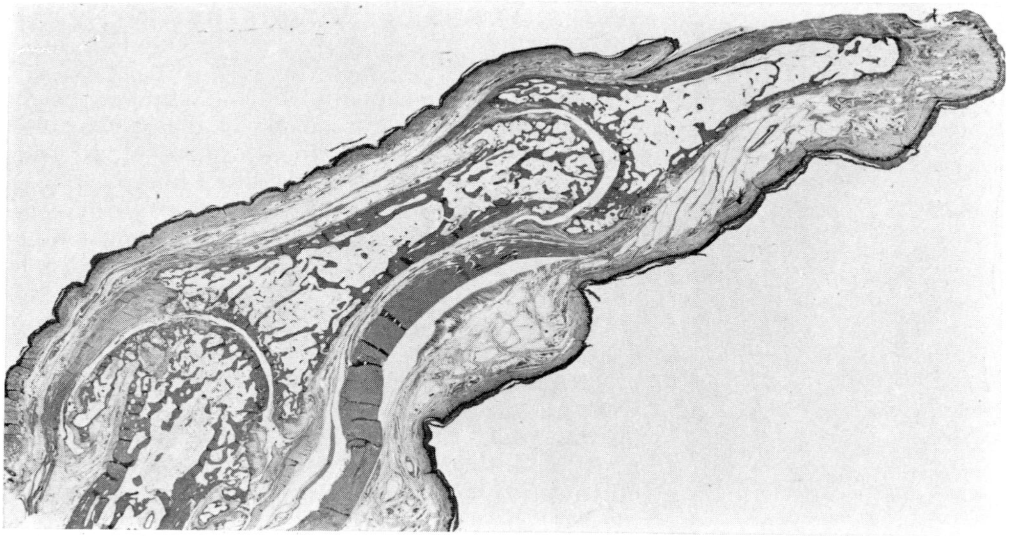

FIGURE 101–8. Heberden's node. The articular cartilage has completely disappeared from the surfaces of the distal interphalangeal joint. Bony osteophytes, directed toward the base of the finger, are present on the dorsal and palmar aspects of both articulating surfaces. Advanced osteoarthritic changes also are present in the proximal interphalangeal joint and form a so-called Bouchard node (Hematoxylin and eosin stain, ×20.)

tion, and involvement of the first carpometacarpal and knee joints. Hip joints were affected less commonly. Key features of the syndrome included signs of articular inflammation and radiologic evidence that proliferation of adjacent bone rather than erosion of articular cartilage was the primary event in the genesis of the lesions. The description of the syndrome was based on limited anatomic material, a situation not entirely corrected by succeeding studies. The status of GOA remains controversial.[114] Most patients with this pattern of disease do not present for surgical intervention. Thus, the condition is far more common in rheumatologic than in orthopedic practice. Some studies have confirmed an association of GOA with OA of the hips,[51,88,115] whereas others have denied this relationship.[116] From the obverse viewpoint, patients requiring hip and knee surgery for localized OA are significantly more likely to have generalized disease as well.[89] When hip disease is associated with Heberden's nodes, particularly in patients with inflammatory features, it is of the concentric type[13,14] rather than the more common deforming type. Some authors maintain that this pattern is only a part of the GOA syndrome.[89] A genetic predisposition to the development of GOA is suggested by the increased frequency of HLA-A1,B8.[117]

OSTEOARTHRITIS CAUSED BY HERITABLE COLLAGEN DEFECTS

Recently, other forms of polyarticular OA associated with mutant type II collagens have been described in several unrelated families[118–120] (see Chapters 11, 102 and 103). These disorders produce precocious generalized OA with accentuated involvement of weight-bearing joints. In one family a mild spondylodysplasia with truncal shortening was present,[118] and in two others more severe manifestations of spondyloepiphyseal dysplasia were noted.[119,120] In the mildly spondylodysplastic family, a single point mutation at residue 519 in the triple helical domain substituted cysteine for arginine, producing abnormal post-translational overmodification.[121] The abnormal collagen has been isolated from cartilage remaining on a surgically excised femoral head from an affected family member[122] in which about one quarter of the α-1(II) chains contained the substitution. In a more severely dysplastic family, an entire exon coding for 36 amino acids was deleted from the type II triple helical domain[120] with a calculated effect that 90% of the type II collagen homotrimers would be abnormal in the heterozygous state. All three affected families showed definite or probable autosomal dominant inheritance[118–120] with an age-dependent penetrance approaching 100%. Population studies for generalized OA with Heberden's nodes have suggested an OA in a single gene that is dominant in males and recessive in females.[113] Whether point mutations or partial deletions in the type II procollagen gene are responsible for large numbers of cases of idiopathic OA is unknown. The usual pattern in generalized OA, however, does not include a clinically detectable spondyloarthropathy (see Chapter 103).

OCHRONOTIC ARTHROPATHY

Alkaptonuria eventually results in a generalized degeneration of joints similar to OA (see Chapter 112). Several differences are notable, however. External remodeling is less prominent than in idiopathic OA.[16] Destructive spinal changes are marked. This includes a calcification or ossification of the nucleus pulposus of the intervertebral discs and breakdown of the vertebral endplates. Osteophyte production is not a conspicuous feature of the spondylopathy. In many cases the spinal disease is so severe as to imitate that of a mucopolysaccharidosis (see Chapter 87). The pigmented cartilage is extremely brittle, so that comminution with a resultant detritic synovitis is prominent. Pigmented cartilage fragments are found in the synovial fluid. Reactive "polyps" of the synovium containing these fragments are common and may be mistaken for "loose bodies" on radiographs. A complicating feature is that both calcium pyrophosphate and BCP crystals have been identified in ochronotic cartilage.

GOUT

The arthropathy of gout develops as a consequence of the deposition of monosodium urate monohydrate crystals in and around joint tissues (see Chapters 105 and 106). Mono-, oligo-, and polyarticular forms occur. The character of the lesions depends on the amount, location, and duration of the deposits. Tophaceous deposits can cause massive disorganization of articular structures, and acute inflammatory episodes are a hallmark of the disease, but the most common lesion is OA. The urate crystals are deposited not only on and in the surface of the articular cartilage but also in the subchondral marrow. Chondrocytes are characteristically necrotic and often surrounded by an oxyphilic matrix in areas of urate crystal deposition. Urate crystals are quite soluble in neutral buffered 4% formaldehyde, the routine histologic fixative. If tissue confirmation of gout is required, fixation in 95% alcohol should be employed.[123]

ENDEMIC OSTEOARTHRITIS

The term *endemic OA* encompasses special types of noninflammatory deforming joint disease occurring frequently in certain geographically confined areas.[124] Although these disorders have certain features in common with generalized OA, they differ from the latter in producing stunted growth. Despite extensive research in several different countries, workers continue to speculate on the cause of these disorders. Two types currently receiving attention are discussed here.

KASHIN-BECK DISEASE

Kashin-Beck disease, formerly known as *endemic osteoarthrosis deformans*, affects approximately 2 million persons in northern China, North Korea, and adjacent regions of Siberia.[125] The changes first appear during childhood and develop with variable severity in different affected individuals. The early changes consist of a zonal necrosis of the articular and epiphyseal chondrocytes.[124] Profound deformity is the result in many affected individuals. Two basic schools of thought on the cause of the disorder have emerged. One is that the soil and water of the region are deficient in selenium. The other is that mycotoxins, particularly those of *Fusarium sp.* are involved through contamination of grain. Some clinical and experimental evidence justifies both viewpoints, but neither is conclusive at present.

MSELENI DISEASE

Mseleni disease, common in northern Zululand, has been described more recently than Kashin-Beck disease. The disorder is polyarticular and noninflammatory, and the hip is particularly susceptible. In surgically resected femoral heads, eburnation was absent. The joint surface was instead covered by a combination of regenerated and degenerated cartilage.[126] Some investigators have proposed that the disorder is heterogeneous, in part being hereditary spondyloepiphyseal dysplasia.[127] Patients with Mseleni joint disease are more likely to show histologic evidence of osteopenia, osteomalacia, and osteoclast failure, but abnormalities in calcium metabolism are not thought to be causal.[128] Generalized OA of the usual sort seen in predominantly European populations occurs less frequently in black Africans.[129,130]

HEMOPHILIC ARTHROPATHY

Joint disease following recurrent hemarthroses of the hemophilias may be considered as a type of OA. Like ordinary OA, erosion of articular cartilage occurs early, accompanied by eburnation of bone and marginal osteophyte formation. Unlike the subchondral pseudocysts of OA, those in hemophilic arthropathy are filled with hemorrhagic material. The synovium usually contains such immense quantities of hemosiderin that it appears reddish-brown grossly, but only minute quantities can be detected in articular chondrocytes.[131,132] How the iron reaches the chondrocytes is unknown because excessive iron is not detectable in the matrix.[131] In advanced lesions the destruction of the joint is more profound than that seen in OA, with disintegration and fibrous ankylosis as the end results. Although hemophilic arthropathy may affect any combination of joints, the larger peripheral joints are particularly prone to severe involvement.[133]

The pathogenesis of the cartilage destruction is not understood, although it is somehow related to recurrent articular hemorrhage (see Chapter 86). Two general hypotheses are entertained. One is that chondrolytic enzymes are released from hemosiderin-laden synovial macrophages.[134] A second hypothesis is that cartilage damage is due to toxic products of hemoglobin degradation such as free radicals created by ionic iron from degraded hemoglobin. Iron may also chelate with proteoglycans and alter the elastic properties of the matrix.[131,132]

OSTEOARTHRITIS ASSOCIATED WITH OTHER HERITABLE OSTEOARTICULAR DISEASES

A number of types of multiple epiphyseal dysplasia have been described.[135] In these rare conditions, epiphyseal growth and maturation of variable portions of the axial and appendicular skeleton are defective. Many affected persons die in infancy,[135] but precocious OA develops with great frequency in those who survive childhood. In many instances the OA has supervened in joints where the contiguous bone is markedly deformed. In some instances the anatomic changes are indistinguishable from those of banal OA; in others, eburnation is absent, and the articular surface is covered by a shaggy reparative cartilage.[136] Similar changes are seen on the surface of femoral heads removed from children with spastic cerebral palsy. Osteoarthritis has been reported in patients with a rare form of heritable osteochondrosis of the digits. The nail-patella syndrome (hereditary osteo-onychodysplasia, Turner-Kieser syndrome, iliac horn syndrome) is also frequently complicated by OA.

Osteoarthritis commonly follows congenital hip dysplasia in humans (see Chapter 53), possibly caused by elevated pressure resulting from the distribution of forces over the reduced contact area of the dysplastic femoral head.[137] The hereditary contribution to the incidence of this condition is the subject of debate. Its frequency is increased in conditions with oligohydramnios,[138] pointing toward an acquired defect in utero, but other studies suggest a more generalized connective tissue defect in some cases.[139] In dogs, however, the evidence supports a strong genetic contribution. Certain breeds, such as German shepherds, commonly develop it, whereas others, such as American greyhounds, do not. Shepherd dogs are also prone to dysplasia and secondary OA of the elbows. The condition is of considerable economic importance in work dogs.

LOCALIZED FORMS OF OSTEOARTHRITIS

MALUM COXAE SENILIS

Several childhood hip abnormalities lead to premature OA degeneration in adult life. Such disorders include congenital hip dysplasia, Legg-Perthes disease, slipped capital femoral epiphysis, and congenital coxa vara. At times there is such a clear history that a pathogenetic sequence seems certain. In other patients, however, no precursor state is evident. These patients are sometimes felt to have had a forme fruste of congenital hip dysplasia.[140] This retrospective view may be questioned because subluxation has been documented only as a late manifestation of the joint deformity.

CHONDROMALACIA PATELLAE

The term *chondromalacia patellae* is used loosely to describe a clinically distinctive, post-traumatic softening of the articular cartilage of the patella in young persons (see Chapter 90). The anatomic lesions resemble those of early OA, although subtle differences have been described by some authors.[7] Changes involve the cartilage and the subchondral bone.[141] Softening, swelling, and increased water content of cartilage have all been reported in the early stages of chondromalacia. In a minority of patients, a significant inflammatory component may be present secondary to irritation of synovium from detachment of cartilage fragments (detritic synovitis).

NEUROPATHIC ARTHROPATHIES

Neuropathic arthropathies comprise articular degenerations with varying morphologies according to the duration and type of the underlying sensory defects.[142] Collectively, these are called "Charcot joints" owing to their description by J.M. Charcot in 1868 (see Chapter 83). The changes resemble those of severe OA but are profoundly destructive. Extensive detritic synovitis is characteristic and is frequently accompanied by secondary osteochondromatosis. The pathogenesis of these lesions is complex, with damaged neurovascular reflexes, sensory denervation, and metabolic factors all having advocates (see Chapter 83). In the diabetic foot, the most frequent site of Charcot joints in the United States, the landmarks of the tarsal bones are often obliterated by fusion,[143] indicating extensive remodeling. Some authors have proposed that subtle sensory deprivation contributes to the acceleration of some cases of idiopathic OA.[144] The similarity of Charcot joints and severe examples of CPPD crystal arthropathy is described in Chapter 109.

ASSOCIATED OSTEONECROSIS

Osteoarthritis as a late sequela of previous bone infarction (osteonecrosis) has been the subject of a large body of literature (see also Chapter 100). The epiphyseal ends of the bones are involved primarily in osteonecrosis, because they receive a discrete arterial supply distinct from that to the remainder of the bone.[145] The femoral and humeral heads are the most frequent sites of osteonecrosis. Articular cartilage derives nutrition from synovial fluid so infarction is limited to the subchondral bone, which fractures and collapses, leading to loss of the normal congruency of the joint surface. Proliferative remodeling leads to osteophyte formation. As the disorder progresses, the articular cartilage may slough, leading to exposure of bone and further remodeling. Osteonecrosis principally begins in only one articular member of a joint, but in later stages, secondary degeneration involves the mating articular surface. Although overt OA may ensue, eburnation is usually not a conspicuous feature. Ordinary OA of the hip may be associated with areas in which the osteocytes of underlying subchondral bone are necrotic.[52] The preponderance of evidence, however, suggests that such necrosis is a secondary event[26,50,51] and that ischemic necrosis of bone is an infrequent cause of ordinary OA.

A special form of osteonecrosis of the medial femoral condyle develops in elderly persons,[146] leading to "gonarthrosis." The sudden onset of symptoms (pain) may have been precipitated by a segmental fracture with depression of the articular cortex. Others have associated the disorder with medial meniscus tears.[147] Osteoarthritis has been described as a late consequence of this disorder. Thus, when segmental infarction occurs in OA of the knee,[148] it probably is a secondary phenomenon, as in the hip.

Osteonecrosis is a common occupational disease in sandhogs, pearl divers, and submariners. Dysbaric release of dissolved gases from the adipose tissue in the bone marrow is responsible for the death of bone tissue. Despite this association, a history of acute painful attacks (bends) often cannot be elicited. Several cases of authentic associated OA have been reported, but in most published accounts, eburnation has not been documented.

BIOCHEMICAL PATHOLOGY OF OSTEOARTHRITIS

Understanding of the biochemical changes in OA has made rapid advances in recent years,[149] as discussed in Chapter 102. The principal pitfalls in interpreting biochemical data are the problems of sampling variability and of discriminating changes associated with OA[13,25,28–30,149] from those associated with aging.[7,12,150–152] When living tissue is required for metabolic studies, the source is frequently surgically resected femoral heads. Sampling of reparative rather than degenerated native cartilage from such specimens probably accounts for the major discrepancies noted between biochemical data from articular cartilage obtained from necropsy[153] with that from surgically resected specimens (see Chapter 102). Similar variability can be introduced by using fractured femoral heads as a source of control cartilage because such tissue undergoes secondary changes following injury.[154] The knee joint is recommended for study by some authors for this reason. Although the destructive process commonly is "unicompartmental," the other condyle is not immune from the complex processes that are in part proliferative. Finally, biochemical properties in nonarticular cartilages show significant differences in some parameters.[7] Thus, such findings are difficult to extrapolate to the pathobiology of articular cartilage.

Advances in the cell and molecular biology of cartilage collagens provide insight into the changes in structural proteins occurring in OA.[155] Type VI collagen is normally found in very small amounts in the pericellular domains[149] of normal cartilage but increases markedly in early experimental OA.[40] Immunohistochemical techniques are necessary to localize collagens and other proteins to specific areas[149] because biochemical findings from fibrillated articular cartilage may differ considerably from those in nondegenerated areas. Classification of changes as due to chronological aging rather than degeneration requires that the tissue be histologically normal.

IMMUNOPATHOLOGY OF OSTEOARTHRITIS

Inflammatory mediators have been explored as possible factors in the generation or prolongation of some types of OA.[36,84,85] The identification of low levels of immunoglobulins in cartilage in primary (generalized) OA[82] and the demonstration of specificity for type II collagen antibodies in some cases of OA[80] provide evidence of immune activation. Interleukin-1 activation of cartilage[31,36] and synovial proteases have assumed an important role in the potentiation of cartilage destruction.[149] The ability of chondrocytes to resorb their pericellular matrix has long been recognized (Fig. 101–4C). To accept without reservation the concept that chondrocytes contain the "seeds of their own destruction" secreted in response to IL-1 would discount the contribution of biomechanical forces to OA and exceed the evidence. Nevertheless, IL-1 probably plays a role in the promotion of joint destruction in OA[149] and in crystal-induced arthritis[156] and may promote the deposition of certain types of amyloid.[157]

ROLE OF ARTICULAR CARTILAGE REPAIR

The persistent erosion of articular cartilage in OA has long aroused interest in the limited ability of this tissue to grow.[3] By all measures the metabolic activity of hyaline cartilage is low. Experimentally induced gaps in articular cartilage show little tendency to repair if they do not penetrate into the vascularized bone marrow, leading to a common view that failure of cartilage repair is responsible for the irreversible development of OA.[7]

Such dogma deserves serious reconsideration. Chondrocytes are capable of brisk mitotic and metabolic activities in vitro.[158] Their release from surrounding matrix by enzymes provides a stimulus to cell division in vivo as illustrated by proliferating cell clones near areas of matrix fibrillation (Fig. 101–2). Thymidine incorporation[159] and biosynthetic activities of chondrocytes[149] are increased in OA. Although their rate of repair is low, it may be significant over the extended periods required for the development of OA.

The more obvious mechanism of cartilage repair lies in the proliferation and differentiation from pluripotential cells in the subchondral bone marrow. The fibrocartilaginous covering of osteophytes illustrates repair by this mechanism and foci of hyaline and fibrocartilage[12] develop in the fibro-osseous granulation tissue[160] forming beneath metallic joint prostheses. Wedge osteotomies designed to redistribute forces in OA hips have resulted in radiologic widening of the joint space and in a few instances in fibrocartilaginous recovering of joint spaces.

EXPERIMENTAL INDUCTION

Numerous animal models of OA have been developed.[161,162] Some directly damage articular cartilage. Small surgically induced defects do not usually produce OA. Larger defects deforming this joint contour, however, may result in OA and direct damage to cartilage by heat, freezing,[163] or other physical agents may also cause OA. Synovitis induced by intrasynovial instillation of irritants may eventuate in osteoarthritic changes, but these may have acted on the cartilage as well.[7] Subluxation of the patella and hip dislocation have produced early remodeling and later OA. Surgical interruption of the cruciate ligaments, usually the anterior, are frequently used to induce OA in a relatively short time.[28,33] Partial meniscectomy is used in a similar way in rabbits.[11,164] Prolonged compression of the articular cartilages for even a few days causes death of chondrocytes, which may be followed by OA. This sequence is presumably due to prevention of percolation of interstitial fluids into the cartilage.[7] Restriction of joint motion was found in older studies to lead to degeneration resembling OA, but one problem with such studies is that it is difficult to restrict joint mobility without altering joint loading.[7] Others have found that motion in the absence of weight bearing does not maintain normal articular cartilage.[165] In humans immobilized for long periods, contracture and fibrous ankylosis develop rather than OA.[166]

Repetitive impact loading has been used to induce degenerative changes resembling early OA, in animal models.[21] Supporting the hypothesis that damage to the subchondral bone results in eventual destruction of cartilage in OA.[22,23] Intra-articular instillation of abrasive particles such as carborundum induce superficial degeneration of articular cartilage and a foreign body reaction in the synovium. The similarity to the pattern of synovitis induced by cartilage detritus is apparent.[7] Enzymes such as papain induce degenerative changes and low-grade synovitis when injected into rabbit joints. Eburnation follows.[7] A variety of experimental manipulations that directly affect the viability of articular chondrocytes or the integrity of the surrounding matrix can result in OA-like disease. Other procedures placing abnormal mechanical stresses on joints can induce remodeling of articular contours. The application of any of these models to human disease requires discretion.

CONCEPTS OF PATHOGENESIS

The clinical and experimental pathology of OA suggests certain concepts about pathogenesis.

CONCEPT: PRIMARY VERSUS SECONDARY OSTEOARTHRITIS

Osteoarthritis frequently develops in joints with clearcut pre-existing structural abnormalities, classified as secondary OA. In primary OA no trauma or other predisposition can be identified, and aging or intrinsic alterations of the articular tissues are presumed to be responsible. Differences in the conformation of OA joints in ochronotic[16] or postinflammatory arthropathies suggest that intrinsic cartilage damage is also responsible for concentric OA, while mechanical overloading is responsible for the much more common varieties in which joint remodeling is conspicuous. In the hip joint the patterns of cartilage loss and osteophyte development have been proposed as representative of the original causal abnormalities.[167] Use of surgically resected femoral heads to support such causal explanations is quite difficult, owing to the advanced nature of the changes in such specimens.[51] Stulberg et al. have proposed that a pre-existing structural basis for OA of the hip can be identified in 85% of cases.[140] The entire issue is controversial,[114] because others report a much lower percentage of pre-existing conditions[14,51,115] and recognize primary OA of the hip as the dominant entity.[89] The hypothesis that primary OA itself can potentiate secondary OA further complicates the discussions.[88]

CONCEPT: ORIGIN IN BONE OR IN CARTILAGE

If the earliest events in the progression to OA occur in articular cartilage, then the bone remodeling results from the loss of energy-absorbing function of the cartilage. The osteophytes in common OA can thus be viewed as an attempt to redistribute the increased transmitted forces over a greater surface area. If the primary alteration is in the subchondral bone,[21–23] then the cartilage changes represent a failure of cartilage repair to compensate for the remodeling, including that of calcified cartilage[17] occurring as a consequence of aging.[8,18] Evidence that bony changes underlie the deterioration of cartilage includes (1) articular cartilage has little measurable impact-absorbing function; (2) microfractures and subchondral trabecular sclerosis precede measurable changes in the cartilage; and (3) cartilage is mechanically more susceptible to impact loading, producing deformation of subchondral bone, than to shearing stresses.[21] Osteophytes, the most conspicuous features of established OA of the hip, develop very early concomitant with radiologic evidence of joint space narrowing.[168] Similar early remodeling changes are present in experimental OA.[11] The pathogenesis of OA likely involves an interaction between intrinsic cartilage metabolism and extrinsic mechanical factors. Their relative contribution may vary in different joints and in different forms of OA. This subject is considered in further detail in Chapter 102.

CONCEPT: SYSTEMIC CONTRIBUTIONS TO OSTEOARTHRITIS

Several systemic factors have been considered already in relation to OA including age, metabolic and genetic influences, obesity, and exercise. A salient feature of OA is a strong association with advancing age.[12,169] This may suggest either that a series of cumulative insults is required to produce disease or that time-dependent molecular alterations occur independently of environmental insults. Some degree of deterioration of the articular surface occurs linearly with increasing age,[12] but the rate is greater in some joints than others. The changes in surgically resected OA hip specimens are far outside the normal distribution of changes seen in natural aging, suggesting that other local or systemic factors are of etiologic importance.[170]

Metabolic Factors

The increased prevalence of OA in patients with several different types of metabolic disease (e.g., ochronosis and acromegaly) has suggested that systemic factors are important (see Chapter 103). Fasting levels of growth hormone were higher in patients with primary OA than in control subjects in one study.[171] Diabetes is associated with neuropathic joint disease,[172] ankylosing hyperostosis, and other manifestations of the DISH syndrome,[173] which can be confused with OA. Important sex differences in humans OA exist; multiple joint involvement is far more frequent in women.[113,174] In men, OA of hips, wrist, and spine[175] is more frequent. The influence of endocrinopathies on the development of rheumatic disease is discussed in Chapter 114.

OSTEOPOROSIS

Although both osteoporosis and OA are diseases of the aging skeleton, they do not frequently coexist. The age-corrected incidence of OA is decreased in individuals with osteoporosis.[176]

GENETIC FACTORS

Genetic factors contributing to OA in other species may have systemic, metabolic, or, as in the dysplasias local effects (see Chapter 103). Data regarding inheritance of Heberden's nodes have been interpreted as reflecting involvement of a single gene, dominant in females and recessive in males.[7] In other studies polygenic, but recessive, inheritance for OA in other peripheral and spinal joints has been postulated.[7] Increased frequency of certain HLA antigens in GOA patients suggests a genetic component.[117] The contribution of inherited abnormalities in collagens[118–122] to the overall incidence of primary OA remains uncertain.

OBESITY

Obesity is accepted as a definite contributory factor. It seems self-evident that excessive weight imposes a mechanical burden on the joints undergoing abrasion, but several studies indicate that the situation is not so simple. In mice, obesity itself does not have an important effect on OA.[98,177] Some human data support an association of OA of the knee with obesity,[178] while other studies deny it.[179] Heberden's nodes are apparently not associated with obesity.[179] The caveat that patients with OA are likely to exercise less and thus become obese is well worthy of consideration.[175] Spondylosis was more common in obese persons than in those of normal weight.[180] Because joints involved in such studies are often not weight bearing, constitutional effects of obesity may be as important as biomechanical considerations.

LIGAMENTOUS LAXITY

A variety of postural abnormalities of joints associated with laxness of the ligamentous structures also predispose patients to OA. Severe joint hypermobility occurring in states such as the Marfan and Ehlers-Danlos syndromes is associated with OA.[172] Some other states, such as the Larsen syndrome, combine multiple congenital joint dislocations and epiphyseal dysplasias.[135] Other studies have implicated an increased frequency of OA, especially of the knee and shoulder, occurring with idiopathic joint hypermobility.[180]

CONCEPT: MECHANICAL FACTORS IN OSTEOARTHRITIS

Mechanical factors have been proposed as evocative of OA in specific joints. Elbow OA of foundry workers using long tongs to lift hot metals and "coal miner's back" are two such examples. Vibratory trauma has been implicated in the cause of OA of the hands and feet in some studies[181] but not others.[182] Osteoarthritis of the knee was more common in a study in individuals whose occupations involve heavy labor.[183]

The occurrence of OA in runners was not increased over control populations.[184,185] Other types of athletic activity may not be as uninfluential. Retired soccer players, for example, had more OA of the hips than an age- and weight-matched control group.[186] Single injuries probably do not cause OA unless they are severe enough to disorganize the joint surface or its major stabilizing structures (see Fig. 101–6).

Direct evidence for the mechanical abrasion of cartilage from the joint surface is provided by the shards of cartilage found in the synovial fluid and synovium in OA. In ochronosis, such joint detritus is a dominant feature of the disease and incites significant immune and inflammatory response in the synovium.[187] The actual mechanical basis of the abrasion injuries in common OA is still unclear.

One cause of increased cartilage abrasion could be decreased or disordered joint lubrication.[7] The articular cartilage of animal joints oscillated in vitro in the absence of synovial fluid undergoes rapid frictional destruction. Instillation of testicular hyaluronidase also leads to in vitro scoring of joint surfaces. Although the depolymerization of synovial mucin could account for the friction, it is possible that the hyaluronidase may also have acted directly on the cartilage matrix. The subject of joint lubrication has attracted much interest in recent years. Hyaluronidase abolishes the viscosity of synovial fluid but not its lubricating ability.[188,189] Under conditions reproducing the joint loading occurring during walking, however, Roberts, Unsworth, and Mign[190] found that friction on human femoral heads increased after hyaluronidase digestion of synovial fluid.

The volume, hyaluronate content, and relative viscosity of synovial fluid are usually normal OA, although other studies have shown diminished polymerization of synovial mucin and a reduction of the hyaluronate content.[7] The contradictory data arise in part because truly normal synovial fluids are not readily obtained for comparison. In the absence of joint disease, the amount of synovial fluid within joints is small, and many joints aspirated have low-grade synovitis.[7] The synovial fluid contains a lubricating glycoprotein called *lubricin*,[189,191] but its role in OA is still unclear.[192] In a synthetic bearing test system, no deficiency in the boundary-lubricating ability of synovial fluid was found in OA.[193]

Measurement of the stresses acting on diarthrodial joints has not been achieved directly. Estimates, however, have been made using artificial models,[194] with analyses conducted of the rate and magnitude of the excursion of the center of gravity.[195] The computation of moments from roentgenograms provides a clinical approximation of the distribution and magnitude of compressive loading of the hip and knee and underlies the design for osteotomy in the treatment of OA.

The elastic properties and strength of the articular cartilage are components in its resistance to "wear and tear." Although simple walking may appear nonstressful, loads on the hip, knee, and ankle are several times body weight during portions of each step.[195] The elasticity of articular cartilage, measured either as stiffness or as recovery from deformation, is not altered in aging unless fibrillation is also present.[177]

The stiffness of the underlying bone has been considered as a factor in the development of OA,[21,23] and the decreased stiffness of osteoporotic bone may explain why OA is less common in osteoporotic patients.[196] Some evidence, however, from studies of comparative pathology of OA suggests that deficiency of mineralized bone may adversely affect cartilage.[96] Such deficiency of mechanical support may contribute to the arthropathy seen in hyperparathyroidism.[177] Conversely, osteopetrosis, a rare condition characterized by a markedly increased stiffness of bone, favors the development of premature OA.[197] The cause and effect relationship, however, is still unclear because fractures with deformity also characterize the disorder.

Paget's disease produces significant bone deformation that may extend into the subchondral osteoarticular junction and produce irregularities at the joint surface. The hip is frequently the site of mixed patterns of Paget's disease and OA.[198] Protrusio acetabuli develops in approximately 25% of such patients, a far higher frequency than in OA without Paget's disease.

CONCLUSIONS

Understanding the pathogenesis of OA requires reconciliation of apparently divergent biomechanical and biochemical concepts about the initial events in the evolution. The nature of the lesions and numerous lines of experimental work seem to reaffirm an interdependence between mechanical "wear and tear" processes and an altered metabolic state of articular tissues.[4,6–8] The synthesis of these concepts is discussed in Chapter 102. The pathologic findings in OA do not establish that the disease is an inevitable concomitant of aging[12] or that the lesions, once developed, have no biologic potential for repair. Advances in our understanding continue, and their significance is illustrated by discussions of "chondroprotection" related to use of certain nonsteroidal anti-inflammatory drugs.[199]

REFERENCES

1. Gardner, D.L.: The nature and causes of osteoarthrosis. Br. Med. J., *286*:418–424, 1983.
2. Moskowitz, R.W.: Primary osteoarthritis: Epidemiology, clinical aspects, and general management. Am. J. Med., *83*(Suppl. 5A):5–10, 1987.
3. Bland, J.H., and Cooper, S.M.: Osteoarthritis: A review of the cell biology involved and evidence for reversibility, management rationally related to known genesis and pathophysiology. Semin. Arthritis Rheum., *14*:106–133, 1984.
4. Howell, D.S.: Pathogenesis of osteoarthritis. Am. J. Med., *80*(Suppl. 4B):24–28, 1986.
5. Hamerman, D.: Osteoarthritis. Orthop. Rev., *17*:353–360, 1988.
6. Sokoloff, L.: Osteoarthritis as a remodeling process. J. Rheumatol., *14*(Suppl. 14):7–10, 1987.
7. Hough, A.J., and Sokoloff, L.: Pathology of osteoarthritis. *In* Arthritis and Allied Conditions. 11th Ed. Edited by D.J. McCarty. Philadelphia, Lea & Febiger, 1989, pp. 1571–1594.
8. Bullough, P.G.: The geometry of diarthrodial joints, its physiologic maintenance and the possible significance of age-related changes in geometry-to-load distribution and the development of osteoarthritis. Clin. Orthop. Rel. Res., *156*:61–66, 1981.
9. Thompson, R.C. Jr., and Bassett, C.A.L.: Histological observations on experimentally induced degeneration of articular cartilage. J. Bone Joint Surg., *52A*:435–443, 1970.
10. Soren, A., Cooper, N.S., and Waugh, T.R.: The nature and designation of osteoarthritis determined by its histopathology. Clin. Exp. Rheumatol., *6*:41–46, 1988.
11. Malemud, C.J., Goldberg, V.M., and Moskowitz, R.W.: Pathological, biochemical, and experimental therapeutic studies in meniscectomy models of osteoarthritis in the rabbit—Its relationship to human joint pathology. Br. J. Clin. Pract., *43*(Suppl):21–31, 1986.
12. Sokoloff, L.: Aging and degenerative diseases affecting cartilage. *In* Cartilage. Vol. 3. Edited by B.K. Hall. New York, Academic Press, 1987.
13. Fabry, G., and Mulier, J.C.: Biochemical analyses in osteoarthritis of the hip: A correlative study between glycosaminoglycan loss, enzyme activity and radiologic signs. Clin. Orthop., *153*:253–264, 1980.
14. Solomon, L.: Patterns of osteoarthritis of the hip. J. Bone Joint Surg., *58B*:176–183, 1976.
15. Ilardi, C.F., and Sokoloff, L.: The pathology of osteoarthritis:

Ten strategic questions for pharmacologic management. Semin. Arthritis Rheum., *11*(Suppl. 1):3–7, 1981.

16. Lagier, R.: The concept of osteoarthrotic remodeling as illustrated by ochronotic arthropathy of the hip: An anatomicoradiological approach. Virchows Arch. [A], *385*:293–298, 1980.
17. Bullough, P.G., and Jagannath, A.: The morphology of the calcification front in articular cartilage. J. Bone Joint Surg., *65B*:72–78, 1983.
18. Lane, L.B., and Bullough, P.G.: Age-related changes in the thickness of the calcified zone and the number of tidemarks in adult human articular cartilage. J. Bone Joint Surg., *62B*:372–375, 1980.
19. Meachim, G., and Allibone, R.: Topographical variation in the calcified zone of upper femoral articular cartilage. J. Anat., *139*:341–352, 1984.
20. Clark, J.M., and Huber, J.D.: The structure of the human subchondral plate. J. Bone Joint Surg., *72B*:866–873, 1990.
21. Radin, E.L. et al.: Response of joints to impact loading: III. Relationship between trabecular microfractures and cartilage degeneration. J. Biomech., *6*:51–57, 1973.
22. Fazzalari, N.L., Vernon-Roberts, B., and Darracott, J.: Osteoarthritis of the hip. Possible protective and causative roles of trabecular microfractures in the head of the femur. Clin. Orthop., *216*:224–233, 1987.
23. Koszyca, B., Fazzalari, N.L., and Vernon-Roberts, B.: Microfractures in coxarthrosis. Acta Orthop. Scand., *61*:307–310, 1990.
24. Cheung, H.S. et al.: *In vitro* synthesis of tissue specific type II collagen by healing cartilage: 1. Short term repair of cartilage in mature rabbits. Arthritis Rheum., *23*:211–219, 1980.
25. Furukawa, T. et al.: Biochemical studies on repair cartilage resurfacing experimental defects in the rabbit knee. J. Bone Joint Surg., *62A*:79–89, 1980.
26. Milgram, J.W.: Morphologic alterations in the subchondral bone in advanced degenerative arthritis. Clin. Orthop., *173*:293–312, 1983.
27. Bennett, G.A., Waine, H., and Bauer, W.: Changes in the Knee Joint at Various Ages. New York, Commonwealth Fund, 1942.
28. Manicourt, D.H., and Pita, J.C.: Progressive depletion of hyaluronic acid in early experimental osteoarthritis in dogs. Arthritis Rheum., *31*:538–544, 1988.
29. Heinegard, D., Inerot, S., Olsson, S.E., and Saxne, T.: Cartilage proteoglycans in degenerative joint disease. J. Rheumatol., *14*(Suppl. 14):110–112, 1987.
30. Ehrlich, M.G.: Degradative enzyme systems in osteoarthritic cartilage. J. Orthop. Res., *3*:170–184, 1985.
31. Sweet, M.B.E., Coelho, A., Schnitzler, C.M., et al.: Serum keratan sulfate levels in osteoarthritis patients. Arthritis Rheum., *31*:648–652, 1988.
32. Vignon, E., Arlot, M., and Vignon, G.: Etude de la densite cellulaire due cartilage de la tete femoral en function de l'age. Rev. Rhum. Mal. Osteoartic., *43*:403–405, 1976.
33. Pidd, J.G., Gardner, D.L., and Adams, M.E.: Ultrastructural changes in the femoral condylar cartilage of mature American foxhounds following transection of the anterior cruciate ligament. J. Rheumatol., *15*:663–669, 1988.
34. Ghadially, F.N., Lalonde, J.M., and Yong, N.K.: Ultrastructure of amianthoid fibers in osteoarthritic cartilage. Virchows Arch. [B], *31*:81–86, 1979.
35. Longmore, R.B., and Gardner, D.L.: The surface structure of ageing human articular cartilage: A study by reflected light interference microscopy (RLIM). J. Anat., *126*:353–365, 1978.
36. Arner, E.C., and Pratta, M.A.: Independent effects of interleukin-1 on proteoglycan breakdown, proteoglycan synthesis and prostaglandin E_2 release from cartilage in organ culture. Arthritis Rheum., *32*:288–297, 1989.
37. Meachim, G.: Light microscopy of Indian ink preparations of fibrillated cartilage. Ann. Rheum. Dis., *31*:457–464, 1972.
38. Meachim, G.: Age-related degeneration of patellar articular cartilage. J. Anat., *134*:365–371, 1982.
39. Minns, R.J., Steven, F.S., and Hardinge, K.: Osteoarthritic articular cartilage lesions of the femoral head observed in the scanning electron microscopy. J. Pathol., *122*:63–70, 1977.
40. Dodge, G.R., and Poole, A.R.: Immunohistochemical detection and immunohistochemical analysis of type II collagen degradation in human normal, rheumatoid, and osteoarthritic articular cartilages and in explants of bovine articular cartilage cultured with Interleukin 1. J. Clin. Invest., *83*:647–661, 1989.
41. McDevitt, C.A. et al.: Experimental osteoarthritic articular cartilage is enriched in guanidine-soluble type VI collagen. Biochem. Biophys. Res. Commun., *157*:250–255, 1988.
42. Mitrovic, D. et al.: Metabolism of human femoral head cartilage in osteoarthrosis and subcapital fracture. Ann. Rheum. Dis., *40*:18–26, 1981.
43. Christensen, S.B., and Reimann, I.: Differential histochemical staining of glycosaminoglycans in the matrix of osteoarthritic cartilage. Acta Pathol. Microbiol. Scand., *88*:61–68, 1980.
44. Getzy, L. et al.: Factors influencing metachromatic staining in paraffin-embedded sections of rabbit and human articular cartilage: A comparison of the safranin O and toluidine blue techniques. J. Histotechnol., *5*:111–116, 1982.
45. Revell, P.A. et al.: Metabolic activity in the calcified zone of cartilage: Observations on tetracycline labelled articular cartilage in human osteoarthritic hips. Rheumatol. Int., *10*:143–147, 1990.
46. Einhorn, T.A., et al.: Matrix vesicle enzymes in human osteoarthritis. J. Orthop. Res., *3*:160–169, 1985.
47. Christensen, P. et al.: The subchondral bone of the proximal tibial epiphysis in osteoarthritis of the knee. Acta Orthop. Scand., *53*:889–896, 1982.
48. Resnick, D., Niwayama, G., and Coutts, R.D.: Subchondral cysts (geodes) in arthritic disorders: Pathologic and radiographic appearance of the hip joint. AJR, *128*:799–806, 1977.
49. Termansen, N.B. et al.: Primary osteoarthritis of the hip: Interrelationship between interosseous pressure, x-ray changes, clinical severity and bone density. Acta Orthop. Scand., *52*:215–222, 1981.
50. Ilardi, C.F., and Sokoloff, L.: Secondary osteonecrosis in osteoarthritis of the femoral head: A pathological study. Hum. Pathol., *15*:79–83, 1984.
51. Meachim, G. et al.: An investigation of radiological, clinical, and pathological correlations in osteoarthrosis of the hip. Clin. Radiol., *31*:565–574, 1980.
52. Wong, S.Y.P., Evans, R.A., Needs, C., et al.: The pathogenesis of osteoarthritis of the hip. Evidence for primary osteocyte death. Clin. Orthop., *214*:305–312, 1987.
53. Streda, A.: Participation of osteonecrosis in the development of severe coxarthrosis. Acta Univ. Carol. [Med. Monogr.] (Praha), *46*:103–153, 1971.
54. Christensen, S.B., and Arnoldi, C.C.: Distribution of 99m Tc-phosphate compounds in osteoarthritic femoral heads. J. Bone Joint Surg., *62A*:90–96, 1980.
55. Pritzker, K.P.H., and Cheng, P.T.: Which comes first—crystals or osteoarthritis? J. Rheumatol., *10*:38–39, 1983.
56. Pritzker, K.P., Cheng, P.T., and Renlund, R.C.: Calcium pyrophosphate crystal deposition in hyaline cartilage: Ultrastructural analysis and implications for pathogenesis. J. Rheumatol., *15*:828–835, 1988.
57. Menkes, C.J., Decraemer, W., Poste, M., and Forest, M.: Chondrocalcinosis and rapid destruction of the hip. J. Rheumatol., *12*:130–133, 1985.
58. Gordon, G.V., Villanueva, C., Schumacher, H.R., and Gohel, V.:

Autopsy study correlating degree of osteoarthritis, synovitis and evidence of articular calcification. J. Rheumatol., *11*:681–686, 1984.

59. Dieppe, P.A., and Watt, I.: Crystal deposition in osteoarthritis: An opportunistic event? Clin. Rheum. Dis., *11*:367–392, 1985.
60. Gibilisco, P.A., Schumacher, H.R., Hollander, J.L., and Coper, K.A.: Synovial fluid crystals in osteoarthritis. Arthritis Rheum., *28*:511–515, 1985.
61. Halvorsen, P.B., and McCarty, D.J.: Patterns of radiographic abnormalities associated with basic calcium phosphate and calcium pyrophosphate dihydrate deposition in the knee. Ann. Rheum. Dis., *45*:603–605, 1986.
62. Sokoloff, L., and Varma, A.A.: Chondrocalcinosis in surgically resected joints. Arthritis Rheum., *31*:750–756, 1988.
63. Felson, D.T., Anderson, J.J., Naimark, A., et al.: The prevalence of chondrocalcinosis in the elderly and its association with knee osteoarthritis: The Framingham Study. J. Rheumatol. *16*:1241–1245, 1989.
64. Hough, A.J., and Webber, R.J.: The pathology of the meniscus. Clin. Orthop., *252*:32–40, 1990.
65. Ohira, T., Ishikawa, K., Masuda, T., et al.: Histologic localization of lipid in the articular tissues in calcium pyrophosphate dihydrate crystal deposition disease. Arthritis Rheum., *31*:1057–1062, 1988.
66. Boivin, G., and Lagier, R.: An ultrastructural study of articular chondrocalcinosis in cases of knee osteoarthritis. Virchows Arch. [A], *400*:13–29, 1983.
67. Halverson, P.B., McCarty, D.J., Cheung, H.S., and Ryan, L.M.: Milwaukee shoulder syndrome: Report of eleven additional cases with concomitant involvement of the knee is seven instances. Semin. Arthritis Rheum., *14*:36–40, 1984.
68. Halverson, P.B., Garancis, J.C., and McCarty, D.J.: Histopathologic and ultrastructural studies of Milwaukee shoulder syndrome—A basic calcium phosphate crystal arthropathy. Ann. Rheum. Dis., *43*:734–741, 1984.
69. Arnoldi, C.C., Reimann, I., and Bretlau, P.: The synovial membrane in human coxarthrosis. Light and electron microscope studies. Clin. Orthop., *148*:213–220, 1979.
70. Doyle, D.V.: Tissue calcification and inflammation in osteoarthritis. J. Pathol., *136*:199–216, 1982.
71. Goldenberg, D.L., Egan, M.S., and Cohen, A.S.: Inflammatory synovitis in degenerative joint disease. J. Rheumatol., *9*:204–209, 1982.
72. Kennedy, T.H., Plater-Zyberk, C., Partridge, T.A., et al.: Morphometric comparison of synovium from patients with osteoarthritis and rheumatoid arthritis. J. Clin. Pathol., *41*:847–852, 1988.
73. Fritz, P. et al.: Beitrage zum enzymhistochemischen Nachweis von Immunoglobulinen in Gelenkkapsel bei chronischer Polyarthritis und entzundlich aktivierter Arthrose. Z. Rheumatol., *39*:331–342, 1980.
74. Scott, D.L. et al.: Significance of fibronectin in rheumatoid arthritis and osteoarthrosis. Ann. Rheum. Dis., *40*:142–153, 1981.
75. Ogilvie-Harris, D.J., and Fornasier, V.L.: Synovial iron deposition in osteoarthritis and rheumatoid arthritis. J. Rheumatol., *7*:30–49, 1980.
76. Helbig, B., Gross, W.L., Borisch, B., et al.: Characterization of synovial macrophages by monoclonal antibodies in rheumatoid arthritis and osteoarthritis. Scand. J. Rheumatol. [Suppl.], *76*:61–66, 1988.
77. Geiler, G., and Riedel, V.: Detection by the PAP technique of lysozyme containing synoviocytes and their quantity in rheumatoid arthritis and osteoarthrosis. Histochem. J., *17*:562–563, 1985.
78. Eghtedari, A.A., Bacon, P.A., and Collins, A.: Immunoblasts in synovial fluid and blood in the rheumatic diseases. Ann. Rheum. Dis., *39*:318–322, 1980.
79. Johanson, N.A. et al.: Acromegalic arthropathy of the hip. Clin. Orthop., *173*:130–139, 1982.
80. Champion, B.R., Sell, S., and Poole, A.R.: Immunity to homologous collagens and cartilage proteoglycans in rabbits. Immunology, *48*:605–616, 1983.
81. Jasin, H.E.: Autoantibody specificities of immune complexes sequestered in articular cartilage of patients with rheumatoid arthritis and osteoarthritis. Arthritis Rheum., *28*:241–248, 1985.
82. Stamenkovic, I., Stegagno, M., Wright, K.A., et al.: Clonal dominance among T-lymphocyte infiltrates in arthritis. Proc. Natl. Acad. Sci. (USA), *85*:1179–1183, 1988.
83. Vetto, A.A., Mannik, M., Zatarain-Rios, E., et al.: Immune deposits in articular cartilage of patients with rheumatoid arthritis have a granular pattern not seen in osteoarthritis. Rheumatol. Int., *10*:13–20, 1990.
84. Hamerman, D., and Klagsbrun, M.: Osteoarthritis. Emerging evidence for cell interactions in the breakdown and remodeling of cartilage. Am. J. Med., *78*:495–499, 1985.
85. Collier, S., and Ghosh, P.: The role of plasminogen in interleukin-1 mediated cartilage degradation. J. Rheumatol., *15*:1129–1137, 1988.
86. Lanzer, W.L., and Komenda, G.: Changes in articular cartilage after meniscectomy. Clin. Orthop., *252*:41–48, 1990.
87. Fahmy, N.R., Williams, E.A., and Noble, J.: Meniscal pathology and osteoarthritis of the knee. J. Bone Joint Surg., *65B*:24–28, 1983.
88. Doherty, M., Watt, I., and Dieppe, P.A.: Influence of primary generalized osteoarthritis on development of secondary osteoarthritis. Lancet, *2*:8–11, 1983.
89. Cooke, T.D.V.: The polyarticular features of osteoarthritis requiring hip and knee surgery. J. Rheumatol., *10*:288–290, 1983.
90. Egan, M.S. et al.: The association of amyloid deposits and osteoarthritis. Arthritis Rheum., *25*:204–208, 1983.
91. Goffin, Y.A., Thoua, Y., and Potvliege, P.R.: Microdeposition of amyloid in the joints. Ann. Rheum. Dis., *40*:27–33, 1981.
92. Ladefoged, C.: Amyloid in osteoarthritis hip joints: A pathoanatomical and histological investigation of femoral head cartilage. Acta Orthop. Scand., *53*:581–586, 1982.
93. Ladefoged, C., Christensen, H.E., and Sorensen, K.H.: Amyloid in osteoarthritis hip joints: Deposition in cartilage and capsule. Acta Orthop. Scand., *53*:587–590, 1982.
94. Castano, E.M., and Frangione, B.: Human amyloidosis, Alzheimer disease and related disorders. Lab. Invest., *58*:122–132, 1988.
95. Sirca, A., and Sucec-Michieli, M.: Selective type II fibre muscular atrophy in patients with osteoarthritis of the hip. J. Neurol. Sci., *44*:149–159, 1980.
96. Wigley, R.D. et al.: Degenerative arthritis in mice: Study of age and sex frequency in various strains with a genetic study of NZB/B1, NZY/B1, and hybrid mice. Ann. Rheum. Dis., *36*:249–253, 1977.
97. Walton, M.: Obesity as an aetiological factor in the development of osteoarthrosis. Gerontology, *25*:165–172, 1979.
98. Silberberg, R.: Epiphyseal growth and osteoarthrosis in blotchy mice. Exp. Cell. Biol., *45*:1–8, 1977.
99. Walton, M.: Patella displacement and osteoarthrosis of the knee joint in mice. J. Pathol., *127*:165–172, 1979.
100. Bendele, A.M., and Hulman, J.F.: Spontaneous cartilage degeneration in guinea pigs. Arthritis Rheum., *31*:561–565, 1988.
101. Moskowitz, R.W., Ziv, I., Denko, C.W., et al.: Spondylosis in sand rats: A model of intervertebral disc degeneration and hyperostosis. J. Orthop. Res., *8*:401–411, 1990.
102. Andersson, G.B.J.: Measurements of loads on the lumbar spine.

In American Academy of Orthopaedic Surgeons Symposium on Low Back Pain. Edited by A.A. White, III, and S.L. Gordon. St. Louis, C.V. Mosby, 1982, pp. 220–251.
103. Bullough, P.G., and Boachie-Adjei, O.: Atlas of Spinal Diseases. Philadelphia, Lippincott, 1988, pp. 77–97.
104. Boushey, D.R., and Bland, J.H.: Pathology. *In* Disorders of the Cervical Spine. Philadelphia, W.B. Saunders, 1987, pp. 64–73.
105. Hilton, R.C., Ball, J., and Benn, R.T.: Vertebral endplate lesions (Schmorl's nodes) in the dorsolumbar spine. Ann. Rheum. Dis., *35*:127–132, 1976.
106. Resnick, D. et al.: Diffuse idiopathic hyperostosis (DISH) (ankylosing hyperostosis of Forestier and Rotes-Querol). Semin. Arthritis Rheum., *7*:153–187, 1978.
107. Ono, K. et al.: Ossified posterior longitudinal ligament: A clinicopathological study. Spine, *2*:128–138, 1978.
108. Firooznia, H. et al.: Calcification and ossification of posterior longitudinal ligament of spine. NY State J. Med., *82*:1193–1198, 1982.
109. Miyasaka, K. et al.: Myelopathy due to ossification or calcification of the ligamentum flavum: Radiologic and histologic evaluations. Am. J. Neurol. Radiol., *4*:629–632, 1983.
110. Goldberg, R.P., Zulman, J.I., and Genant, H.K.: Unilateral primary osteoarthritis of the hand in monoplegia. Radiology, *135*:65–66, 1980.
111. Utsinger, P.D. et al.: Roentgenologic, immunologic, and therapeutic study of erosive (inflammatory) osteoarthritis. Arch. Intern. Med., *138*:693–697, 1978.
112. Ehrlich, G.E.: Pathogenesis and treatment of osteoarthritis. Compr. Ther., *5*:36–40, 1978.
113. Kellgren, J.H., Lawrence, J.S., and Bier, F.: Genetic factors in generalized osteoarthritis. Ann. Rheum. Dis., *22*:237–255, 1963.
114. Buchanan, W.W., and Park, W.M.: Primary generalized osteoarthritis: Definition and uniformity. J. Rheumatol., *10*(Suppl. 9):4–6, 1983.
115. Stewart, I.M., Marks, J.S., and Hardinge, K.: Generalized osteoarthrosis and hip disease. *In* Epidemiology of Osteoarthritis. Edited by J. Peyron. Paris, Geigy, 1981.
116. Yazici, H. et al.: Primary osteoarthrosis of the knee or hip. JAMA, *231*:1256–1260, 1975.
117. Pattrick, M., Manhire, A., Ward, A.M., et al.: HLA-A, B antigens and α1-antitrypsin phenotypes in nodal generalized osteoarthritis and erosive osteoarthritis. Ann. Rheum. Dis., *48*:470–475, 1989.
118. Knowlton, R.G., Katzenstein, P.L., Moskowitz, R.W., et al.: Genetic linkage of a polymorphism in the Type II procollagen gene (COL2A1) to primary osteoarthritis associated with mild chondrodysplasia. N. Engl. J. Med., *322*:526–530, 1990.
119. Palotie, A., Vaisanen, P., Ott, J., et al.: Predisposition to familial osteoarthrosis linked to type II collagen gene. Lancet, *1*:924–927, 1989.
120. Lee, B., Vissing, H., Ramirez, F., et al.: Identification of the molecular defect in a family with spondyloepiphyseal dysplasia. Science, *244*:978–980. 1989.
121. Ala-Kokko, L., Baldwin, C.T., Moskowitz, R.W., and Prockop, D.J.: Single base mutation in the type II procollagen gene (COL2A1) as a cause of primary osteoarthritis associated with a mild chondrodysplasia. Proc. Natl. Acad. Sci. (USA), *87*:6565–6568, 1990.
122. Eyre, D.R., Weis, M.A., and Moskowitz, R.W.: Cartilage expression of a type II collagen mutation in an inherited form of osteoarthritis associated with a mild chondrodysplasia. J. Clin. Invest., *87*:357–361, 1991.
123. Bancroft, J.D., and Stevens, A.: Theory and Practice of Histological Techniques. 3rd Ed. Edinburgh, Churchill-Livingstone, 1990, p. 262–263.
124. Sokoloff, L.: Endemic forms of osteoarthritis. Clin. Rheum. Dis., *11*:187–202, 1985.
125. Sokoloff, L.: The history of Kashin-Beck disease. NY State J. Med., *89*:343–351, 1989.
126. Sokoloff, L., Fincham, J.E., and du Toit, G.T.: Pathological features of the femoral head in Mseleni disease. Hum. Pathol., *16*:117–120, 1985.
127. Solomon, L.: Distinct types of hip disorder in Mseleni joint disease. S. Afr. Med. J., *69*:15–17, 1986.
128. Schnitzler, C.M., Pieczkowski, W.M., Fredlund, V., et al.: Histomorphometric analysis of osteopenia associated with endemic osteoarthritis (Mseleni joint disease). Bone, *9*:21–27, 1988.
129. Valkenburg, H.A.: Osteoarthritis in some developing countries. J. Rheumatol., *10*:(Suppl. 10):20–22, 1983.
130. Adebajo, A.O.: Pattern of osteoarthritis in a west African teaching hospital. Ann. Rheum. Dis., *50*:20–22, 1991.
131. Hough, A.J., Banfield, W.G., and Sokoloff, L.: Cartilage in hemophilic arthropathy: Ultrastructural and microanalytical studies. Arch. Pathol. Lab. Med., *100*:91–96, 1976.
132. Rippey, J.J. et al.: Articular cartilage degradation and the pathology of hemophilic arthropathy. S. Afr. Med. J., *53*:345–351, 1978.
133. Steven, M.M. et al.: Hemophilic arthritis. Q. J. Med., *58*:181–197, 1986.
134. Mainardi, C.L. et al.: Proliferative synovitis in hemophilia: Biochemical and morphological observations. Arthritis Rheum., *21*:137–144, 1978.
135. Yang, S.S.: The skeletal system. *In* Textbook of Fetal and Perinatal Pathology. Edited by J.S. Wigglesworth and D.B. Singer. London, Blackwell, 1991, pp. 1197–1200.
136. Stanescu, V., Stanescu, R., and Maroteaux, P.: Articular degeneration as a sequela of osteochondrodysplasia. Clin. Rheum. Dis., *11*:239–270, 1985.
137. Hadley, N.A., Brown, T.D., and Weinstein, S.L.: The effects of contact pressure elevations and aseptic necrosis on the long-term outcome of congenital hip dislocation. J. Orthop. Res., *8*:504–513, 1990.
138. Smith, D.W.: Recognizable patterns of human deformation. Identification and management of mechanical effects on morphogenesis. Major Probl. Clin. Pediatr., *21*:1–21, 1981.
139. Uden, A. et al.: Inguinal hernia in patients with congenital hip dislocation. Acta Orthop. Scand. *59*:667–668, 1988.
140. Stulberg, S.D. et al.: Unrecognized childhood hip disease: A major cause of osteoarthritis of the hip. *In* The Hip. St. Louis, C.V. Mosby, 1975, pp. 221–228.
141. Goodfellow, J., Hungerford, D.S., and Wood, C.: Patello-femoral joint mechanics and pathology: 2. Chondromalacia patellae. J. Bone Joint Surg., *58B*:291–299, 1976.
142. Brower, A.C., and Allman, R.M.: The neuropathic joint: A neurovascular bone disorder. Radiol. Clin. North Am., *19*:571–580, 1981.
143. Raju, U.B., Fine, G., and Partemian, J.O.: Diabetic neuroarthropathy (Charcot's joint). Arch. Pathol. Lab. Med., *106*:349–351, 1982.
144. Connor, B.L., Palmoski, M.J., and Brandt, K.D.: Neurogenic acceleration of degenerative joint lesions. J. Bone Joint Surg., *67A*:562–572, 1985.
145. Brighton, C.T.: Morphology and biochemistry of the growth plate. Rheum. Dis. Clin. North Am., *13*:75–100, 1987.
146. Bauer, G.C.H.: Osteonecrosis of the knee. Clin. Orthop., *130*:210–217, 1978.
147. Norman, A., and Baker, N.D.: Spontaneous osteonecrosis of the knee and medial meniscus tears. Radiology, *129*:653–656, 1978.
148. Ahuja, S.A., and Bullough, P.G.: Osteonecrosis of the knee: A

clinicopathological study in twenty-eight patients. J. Bone Joint Surg., *60A*:191–197, 1978.

149. McDevitt, C.A., and Miller, R.R.: Biochemistry, cell biology, and immunology of osteoarthritis. Curr. Opin. Rheum., *1*:303–314, 1989.
150. Theocharis, D.A., Kalpaxis, D.L., and Tsiganos, C.P.: Cartilage keratan sulphate: Changes in chain length with aging. Biochim. Biophys. Acta, *841*:131–134, 1985.
151. Laver-Rudich, Z., and Silbermann, M.: Cartilage surface charge. A possible determinant in aging and osteoarthritic processes. Arthritis Rheum., *28*:660–670, 1985.
152. Eyre, D.R., Dickson, I.R., and Van Ness, K.: Collagen cross-linking in human bone and articular cartilage. Age-related changes in the content of mature hydroxypyridinium residues. Biochem. J., *252*:495–500, 1988.
153. Santer, V., White, R.J., and Roughley, P.J.: Proteoglycans from normal and degenerate cartilage of adult human tibial plateau. Arthritis Rheum., *24*:691–700, 1981.
154. Hirotani, H., and Ito, T.: The fate of the articular cartilage in intracapsular fractures of the femoral neck. Arch. Orthop. Unfallchir., *86*:195–199, 1976.
155. Mayne, R.: Cartilage collagens. What is their function, and are they involved in articular disease? Arthritis Rheum., *32*:241–246, 1989.
156. DiGiovine, F.S., Malawista, S.E., Nuki, G., and Duff, G.W.: Interleukin 1 (IL-1) as a mediator of crystal arthritis. Stimulation of T cell and synovial fibroblast mitogenesis by urate crystal-induced IL-1. J. Immunol., *138*:3213–3218, 1987.
157. Sipe, J.D. et al.: The role of interleukin 1 in acute phase serum amyloid A (AA) and serum amyloid P (SAP) biosynthesis. Ann. NY Acad. Sci., *389*:137–150, 1982.
158. Sokoloff, L.: *In vitro* culture of joints and articular tissues. *In* The Joints and Synovial Fluid. Vol. 2. Edited by L. Sokoloff. New York, Academic Press. 1980, pp. 1–26.
159. Hirotani, H., and Ito, T.: Chondrocyte mitosis in the articular cartilage of femoral heads with various diseases. Acta Orthop. Scand., *46*:979–986, 1975.
160. Milgram, J.W., and Rana, N.A.: The pathology of the failed cup arthroplasty. Clin. Orthop., *158*:159–179, 1981.
161. Adams, M.E., and Billingham, M.E.: Animal models of degenerative joint disease. Curr. Top. Pathol., *71*:265–297, 1982.
162. Moskowitz, R.W.: Experimental models of osteoarthritis. *In* Osteoarthritis. Edited by R.W. Moskowitz et al. Philadelphia, W.B. Saunders, 1984, pp. 109–128.
163. Simon, W.H., Lane, J.M., and Beller, P.: Pathogenesis of degenerative joint disease produced by *in vivo* freezing of rabbit articular cartilage. Clin. Orthop., *155*:259–268, 1981.
164. Lanzer, W.L., and Komenda, G.: Changes in articular cartilage after meniscectomy. Clin. Orthop., *252*:41–48, 1990.
165. Palmoski, M.J., Colyer, R.A., and Brandt, K.D.: Joint motion in the absence of normal loading does not maintain normal articular cartilage. Arthritis. Rheum., *23*:325–334, 1980.
166. Enneking, W.F., and Horowitz, M.: The intra-articular effects of immobilization on the human knee. J. Bone Joint Surg., *54A*:973–985, 1972.
167. Resnick, D.: Patterns of migration of the femoral head in osteoarthritis of the hip: Roentgenographic-pathologic correlation and comparison with rheumatoid arthritis. AJR, *124*:62–74, 1975.
168. Wroblewski, B.M., and Charnley, J.: Radiographic morphology of the osteoarthritic hip. J. Bone Joint Surg., *64B*:568–569, 1982.
169. Anderson, J. and Felson, D.: Factors associated with knee osteoarthritis (OA) in a national survey. The Framingham study. Arthritis Rheum., *29*:526, 1986.
170. Byers, P.D., Contempomi, C.A., and Farkas, T.A.: Postmortem study of the hip joint: III. Correlations between observations. Ann. Rheum. Dis., *35*:122–126, 1976.
171. Waine, H. et al.: Association of osteoarthritis and diabetes mellitus. Tufts Fol. Med., *7*:13–19, 1961.
172. Schumacher, H.R., Jr.: Secondary osteoarthritis. *In* Osteoarthritis, Diagnosis and Management. Edited by R.W. Moskowitz et al. Philadelphia, Saunders, 1984, pp. 235–264.
173. Boachie-Adjei, O., and Bullough, P.G.: Incidence of ankylosing hyperostosis of the spine (Forestier's disease) at autopsy. Spine, *12*:739–743, 1987.
174. Davis, M., Ettinger, W.H., Neuhaus, J.M., et al.: Sex differences in osteoarthritis of the knee. The role of obesity. Am. J. Epidemiol., *127*:1019–1030, 1988.
175. Peyron, J.G.: The epidemiology of osteoarthritis. *In* Osteoarthritis. Diagnosis and Management. Edited by R.W. Moskowitz et al. Philadelphia, W.B. Saunders, 1984, pp. 9–27.
176. Pogrund, H., Rutenberg, M., Makin, M., et al.: Osteoarthritis of the hip joint and osteoporosis: A radiological study in a random population sample in Jerusalem. Clin. Orthop., *164*:130–135, 1982.
177. Sokoloff, L.: The Biology of Degenerative Joint Disease. Chicago, University of Chicago Press, 1969.
178. Davis, M.A., Neuhaus, J.M., and Ettinger, W.H.: Body fat distribution and osteoarthritis. Am. J. Epidemiol., *132*:701–707, 1990.
179. Goldin, R.H. et al.: Clinical and radiological survey of the incidence of osteoarthrosis among obese patients. Ann. Rheum. Dis., *35*:349–353, 1976.
180. Bird, H.A., Tribe, C.R., and Wright, V.: Joint hypermobility leading to osteoarthritis and chondrocalcinosis. Ann. Rheum. Dis., *37*:203–211, 1978.
181. Bovenzi, M., Petronio, L., and DiMarino, F.: Epidemiological survey of shipyard workers exposed to hand-arm vibration. Int. Arch. Occup. Environ. Health, *46*:251–266, 1980.
182. Burke, M.D., Fear, E.C., and Wright, V.: Bone and joint changes in pneumatic drillers. Ann. Rheum. Dis., *36*:276–279, 1977.
183. Lindberg, H., and Montgomery, F.: Heavy labor and the occurrence of gonarthrosis. Clin. Orthop., *214*:235–236, 1987.
184. Lane, N.E., Bloch, D.A., Hubert, H.B., et al.: Running, osteoarthritis and bone density: Initial 2-year longitudinal study. Am. J. Med., *88*:452–459, 1990.
185. Konradsen, L., Berg-Hansen, E.-M., and Sondergaard, L.: Long distance running and osteoarthrosis. Am. J. Sports Med., *18*:379–381, 1990.
186. Klunder, K.B., Rud, B., and Hansen, J.: Osteoarthritis of the hip and knee in retired football players. Acta Orthop. Scand., *51*:925–927, 1980.
187. Konttinen, Y.T., Hoikka, V., Landtman, M., et al.: Ochronosis: A report of a case and a review of literature. Clin. Exp. Rheumatol., 7:435–444, 1989.
188. Davis, W.H., Jr., Lee, S.L., and Sokoloff, L.: A proposed model boundary lubrication by synovial fluid: Structuring of boundary water. J. Biomech. Eng., *101*:185–192, 1979.
189. McCutchen, C.W.: Lubrication of joints. *In* The Joints and Synovial Fluid. Vol. 1. Edited by L. Sokoloff. New York, Academic Press, 1978, pp. 438–483.
190. Roberts, B.J., Unsworth, A., and Mign, N.: Modes of lubrication in human hip joints. Ann. Rheum. Dis., *41*:217–224, 1982.
191. Swann, D.A., Silver, F.H., Slayter, H.S., and Stafford, W.: The molecular structure and lubricating activity of lubricin isolated from bovine and human synovial fluids. Biochem. J., *225*:195–201, 1985.
192. Swann, D.A., Bloch, K.J., Swindell, D., and Shore, E.: The lubricating activity of human synovial fluids. Arthritis Rheum., *27*:552–556, 1984.
193. Davis, W.H., Jr., Lee, S.L., and Sokoloff, L.: Boundary lubricat-

ing ability of synovial fluid in degenerative joint disease. Arthritis Rheum., *21*:754–760, 1978.

194. Rushfeldt, R.D., Mann, R.W., and Harris, W.H.: Improved techniques for measuring *in vitro* the geometry and pressure distribution in the human acetabulum: II. Instrumental endoprosthesis measurement of articular surface pressure distribution. J. Biomech., *14*:315–323, 1981.
195. Paul, J.P.: Joint kinetics. In The Joints and Synovial Fluid. Vol. 2. Edited by L. Sokoloff. New York, Academic Press, 1980, pp. 139–176.
196. Dequeker, J.: The relationship between osteoporosis and osteoarthritis. Clin. Rheum. Dis., *11*:271–296, 1985.
197. Milgram, J.W., and Jasty, M.: Osteopetrosis: A morphological study of twenty-one cases. J. Bone Joint Surg., *64A*:912–929, 1982.
198. Altman, R.D., and Collins, B.: Musculoskeletal manifestations of Paget's disease of bone. Arthritis Rheum., *23*:1121–1127, 1980.
199. Lane, N.E. et al.: Osteoarthritis in the hand: A comparison of handedness and hand use. J. Rheumatol., *16*:637–642, 1989.

102

Etiopathogenesis of Osteoarthritis

DAVID S. HOWELL
JEAN-PIERRE PELLETIER

Osteoarthritis (OA) is defined here as a complex of interactive degradative and repair processes in cartilage, bone, and synovium, with secondary components of inflammation. The etiopathologic processes involved are complex, and their relative importance continues to be debated. Our goal in this chapter is to survey some of the most relevant and newer reports in the scientific literature related to the etiopathogenesis of OA.[1–12]

By currently held concepts, two general pathways lead to OA.[1] The first involves fundamentally defective cartilage with biomaterial properties directly or indirectly leading to OA. Thereby, a matrix of cartilage fails under normal loading of the joint. The first type II collagen gene defect recently described (see following) exemplifies this pathway. Ochronotic cartilages that fail under normal loading as a result of deleterious pigment deposition, represent another example. Osteoarthritis ensues following biomechanical failure. The second and by far most prevalent cause of OA is based on the concept of a major role of physical forces causing damage to normal articular cartilage matrix.[1] Two subpathways are involved here. First, direct injury of the matrix. Second, chondrocytes imbedded in the matrix are injured by the same forces.[1–5] In the course of time these chondrocytes react to injury by elaborating degradative enzymes and developing inappropriate repair responses.[2–5] Much recent research implicates enzymatic breakdown of the cartilage as a key feature of disease progression. Repeated microtrauma or single events of macrotrauma may be causative. In addition, badly transmitted physical forces of normal intensity that are due to a variety of causes constitute an important subgroup. For normal force transmission, there is a slight normal incongruity in the articular surfaces, and there is an optimal distribution of force transmission during normal locomotor cycles.[6]

Various types of joint injury produce altered joint contours resulting in localized sites of concentrated force transmission and resultant cartilage damage. Some of these changes consist of wounding of the cartilage per se or of stimulation of subchondral bone remodeling and gradual development of altered contours[6,7] (see following).

Various developmental etiologies can lead to abnormal distribution of force transmission, even without antecedent injury.[8–10] Examples include abnormal bone development from growth plate failures, including "pistol grip" deformities of the hip,[8] shallowness or bony ridge formation of the acetabulum,[1] tilted position of the femoral head on the femoral neck,[10] and genu varus or genus valgus, as well as unequal limb length. In addition to abnormal joint contours, joint instability can cause abnormal force transmission. Examples include ligamentous laxity from heritable disorders of collagen structure, as well as degenerated or torn menisci or ruptured ligaments (see following).[2–5]

EFFECTS OF AGING, EXERCISE, AND DISUSE

Hyaline articular cartilage can be encroached on from below by subchondral bone remodeling and tidemark reduplication. These accelerate sharply in the decade beyond the age of 50 years. Furthermore, progression of OA lesions in articular cartilage over several years was best predicted by a parameter of bone remodeling and vascular penetration.[13,14] Resultant changes in cartilage surface contours and changes of congruence affect force disturbance.[15] Increased severity of OA of the hand correlated positively with iliac crest biopsy histomorphometric measurements, indicating increased bone density.[16] Atrophy that is due to disuse or immobilization causes cartilage to become a weaker biomaterial, making it vulnerable to injury during subsequent exercise. For example, one hind limb of a dog was immobilized for several weeks, and severe OA lesions in the immobilized knee were then produced by treadmill exercise.[17] Untoward effects of disuse also were demonstrated by biomechanical studies.[18] The tensile modulus of canine knee articular cartilage was reduced after 1 month of immobilization.[18] These findings provide insight on the factor of joint motion in the etiology of OA. Pain per se can lead to reflex muscle tightening, reduced activity of a limb, and partial atrophy.

NEUROGENIC CONTROL

Altered locomotor or stereognostic control as it changes with aging or disease is another factor, especially control of the opposing muscle groups surrounding afflicted joints.

Destabilization of the stifle (knee) joint by anterior cruciate ligament section in the Pond-Nuki dog model causes a mild OA lesion in the early stages, which progresses to severe disease by 3 years. In the first few weeks, this lesion can be magnified by sectioning posterior nerve roots at the spinal cord level governing stereognostic control of the involved limb.[19] Gait analyses have shown that smooth attenuation of loading forces on heel strike were impaired in OA patients compared to normal persons.[20]

Stereognostic control of loading force attenuation is an important regulatory mechanism, because it can be potentially modified by conservative physical therapy and gait control.[21]

PROPERTIES OF INDIVIDUAL JOINTS

Each joint contains specific characteristic growth and development changes that can increase its vulnerability to OA. For example, in the knee, a developmental varus deformity predisposes the medial tibiofemoral compartment to injury, while valgus deformity unduly loads the lateral compartment. Qualitative structural differences can also be important. For example, in chondromalacia and patellofemoral compartment OA, there is frequently a lateral pull on the patella stemming from faulty tendon alignment. Large differences in biomechanical properties were found in the patellar versus the femoral cartilage components in one study.[22] Thus each joint has a unique distribution of mechanical forces in relation to its anatomic characteristics. These, as well as the unique biomechanical properties of its tissues, determine its ability to function normally over time.

Joint instability caused by loose joint capsules and ligaments following injury in accidents and the like is a major factor leading to OA. Similarly, hyperelasticity such as the Ehlers-Danlos or joint hypermobility syndromes increase the risk of OA in several joints. Osteoarthritis and associated chondrocalcinosis in the knee have been associated with the latter syndrome.[23]

Finally, diseases causing shortening of one leg may shift weight-bearing forces and lead to OA of the opposite limb.

METABOLISM IN ARTHRITIC CARTILAGE

Evidence has accumulated favoring an important role of metabolic changes in chondrocytes, with pathologic elaboration of factors causing matrix degradation.[24–27] Moreover, the regulation of chondrocytic function involves message systems between adjacent chondrocytes, as well as synovial cells and chondrocytes, in amplification of cartilage breakdown. Thus, development of secondary inflammation and, to some extent, immunologic changes have been documented.

In the normal joint there is a balance between continuous processes of cartilage matrix degradation and repair. These functions are performed almost solely by resident chondrocytes dispersed in their lacunae throughout the matrix and lasting a lifetime under normal conditions. Chondrocytes function in response to cytokine and growth factor signals and to direct physical stimuli in a complex manner. The end result is a change in the rate of synthesis versus that of enzymatic breakdown of the cartilage matrix, both around the cells and at same distance. Both autocrine and paracrine actions have been demonstrated in chondrocytes and in synovial lining cells as well. In OA, there is a disruption of this homeostatic state. In most sites of OA change the anabolic processes of these cells become deficient relative to their catabolic effects. Focal repair responses are inadequate to maintain normal matrix integrity. At the time of appearance of OA lesions histologically, the matrix has reached the critical point where its viscoelastic properties become insufficient to withstand joint loads normally and progressive cartilage loss may follow. Biomechanical factors assume a more prominent role.

To understand the pathologic cellular mechanisms involved, normal chondrocyte-mediated homeostasis has been studied intensively over the last few years. Cytokine enhancement of enzymatic degradation of cartilage matrix and growth factor stimulation of cartilage matrix synthesis have been studied.[28,29]

MECHANISMS OF CARTILAGE DEGRADATION

Biochemical changes in OA affect several cartilage components, including its major matrix constituents, proteoglycan and collagen (Fig. 102–1). The proteoglycans are probably the first to be affected, because they are progressively depleted in parallel with the severity of the disease. At a certain stage of evolution of the OA lesion, the chondrocytes appear unable to compensate fully for proteoglycan loss by increased synthesis, resulting in a net loss of matrix. The structure of the proteoglycan remaining in the cartilage changes in different ways according to different investigators. In our view, hyaluronic acid content of OA cartilage is decreased

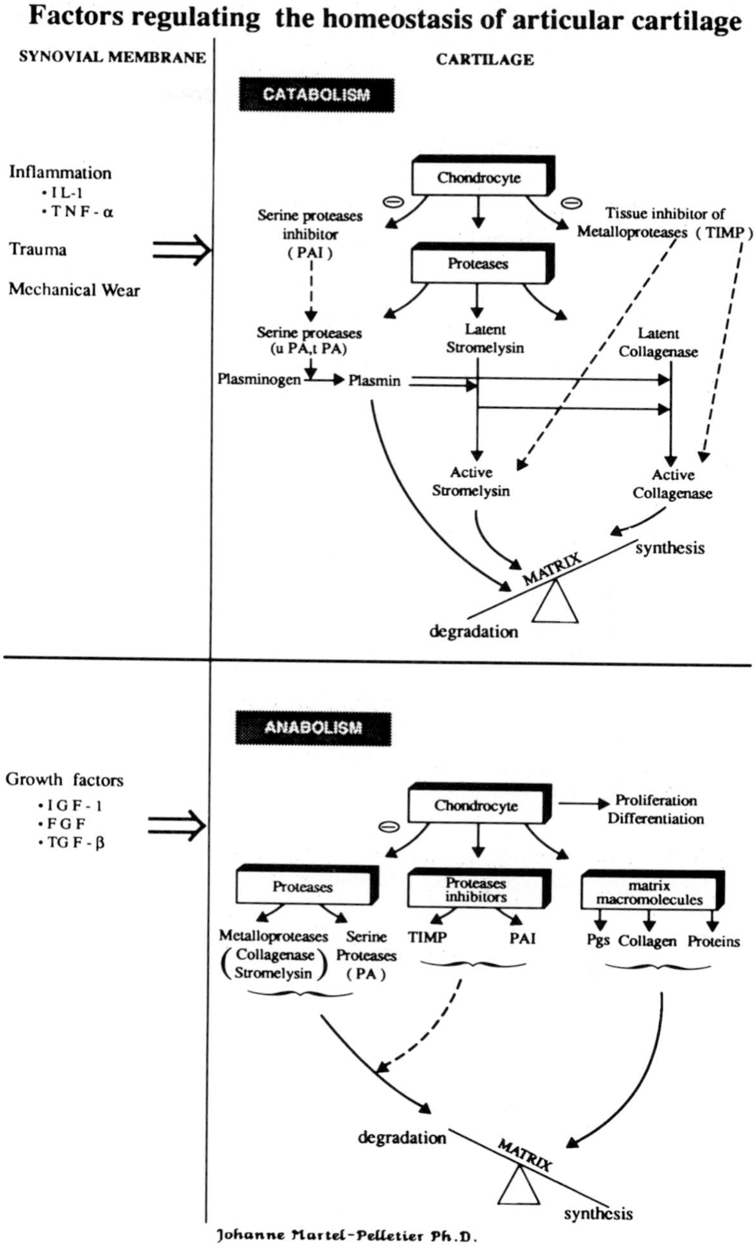

FIGURE 102–1. Factors regulating the homeostasis of articular cartilage matrix.

with diminution in the size of the proteoglycan aggregates. As a result of facilitated diffusion of linear polymers favoring loss of proteoglycan breakdown products from cartilage, a selective retention of normal components of the aggregates occurs; that is, most of the retained monomers are capable of aggregation. Degradation products of the proteoglycan monomers with cleavage at several sites along the molecules have been demonstrated.[30–32] The decreased proteoglycan content of the matrix in association with damaged collagen structure leads to functional loss of normal matrix physiologic properties.[33] Antibodies to epitopes near the collagenase cleavage site on type II collagen fibers have shown specific collagenase cleavage.[34]

ROLE OF PROTEASES AND PROTEASE INHIBITORS

In addition to the mechanical factors already discussed, enzymatic pathways are involved in OA cartilage matrix degradation.[27] Enzymatic processes resemble a cascade similar to that of the coagulation or complement systems. In rheumatoid arthritis (RA), the synovium is the most abundant source of degradative enzymes, but in OA chondrocytes seem to be the prime source of enzymes responsible for cartilage matrix catabolism. Enzyme families identified as playing a big role in OA pathophysiology include metalloproteases, serine proteases, and thiol proteases. A role for still other enzymes, however, cannot be ruled out.

Among the metalloproteases, collagenase and proteoglycanases play a predominant role. Collagenase appears to be responsible for breakdown of the collagen type II network in OA, as first suggested by Ehrlich.[58] It has been identified in situ in OA cartilage and its activity correlated with the histologic severity of OA cartilage lesions.[35] Two forms of proteoglycanase have been identified in human articular cartilage. Stromelysin has been reported in neutral and in acid form.[36] Stromelysin seems to be confined to the acid pH form. The so-called neutral form of this enzyme could be a gelatinase (Woessner and Gunja-Smith, unpublished observations). Nevertheless, both forms are active at the pH found in cartilage, and both were increased in OA cartilage. As with collagenase, their level also correlated with the histologic severity of OA lesions.[37] Furthermore, active stromelysin can mimic ex vivo and in vitro the breakdown of the proteoglycan monomer core protein, including hyaluronate-binding region (HABR) cleavage seen in OA.[30–32] Histochemical studies[37] suggested a relationship between the level of the acid form and the severity of degradation of pericellular proteoglycan. Degradation of type IX collagen—a glycoprotein with both collagenous and noncollagenous domains that plays an important role in cartilage matrix stability by linking type II collagen and proteoglycan—also occurred through the action of stromelysin.[38] Interestingly, stromelysin is also implicated in the enzymatic cascade responsible for the activation of procollagenase.[39] This enzyme thus may have a dual role in OA pathophysiology.

Metalloprotease biologic activity is controlled by physiologic inhibitors and activators. Two inhibitors of metalloproteases have been identified: tissue inhibitor of metalloprotease-1 (TIMP-1) and TIMP-2. TIMP-1 is present in cartilage and is synthesized by chondrocytes.[40] In OA cartilage there is an imbalance between the amount of TIMP-1 and metalloprotease activity, which is due to a relative deficiency of inhibitor.[41] This finding could explain the increased level of active metalloproteases found in OA cartilage. Enzymes from the serine protease and thiol-dependent protease families, such as plasminogen activator (PA)–plasmin system and cathepsin B, have been suggested as possible activators of metalloproteases (reviewed in 27). Activation of latent (inactive) collagenase involves a cascade of events starting with cleavage of the amino terminal end by a protease such as plasmin and an additional proteolytic cleavage by stromelysin at the c-terminal end for full activation.[42,43] The detailed molecular changes during activation of collagenase have been recently reviewed.[42]

Serine Proteases

A role for the PA–plasmin system in latent metalloprotease activation was first suggested by in vitro studies showing that this system could activate RA synovial collagenase.[44] Later studies showed that complete collagenase activation requires, in conjunction with plasmin, the presence of active stromelysin.[39,42] Plasminogen activator has been found in human cartilage, and the synthesis of both tissue- and urokinase-type by chondrocytes was stimulated markedly by interleukin-1 (IL-1).[45]

The role of PA in cartilage metabolism is still not fully understood, but it may directly digest connective tissue glycoprotein.[46] As stromelysin and collagenase are synthesized as latent enzymes in cartilage and can be converted to their active forms by plasmin, PA and plasminogen could be important members of the enzyme cascade involved in cartilage degradation.

Few studies have addressed in the in vivo involvement of PA–plasmin in OA. Osteoarthritis cartilage was shown to contain increased plasmin activity and plasminogen activator (urokinase type) levels. A direct, positive correlation was found between the level of plasmin activity and active collagenase activity.[47]

Several physiologic serine protease inhibitors have been found in cartilage also,[48–50] and their level of plasminogen activator inhibitor (PAI-1) is decreased in OA cartilage.[47,51] This, combined with the increased level of PA, may explain, at least in part, the increased level of biologically active metalloproteases found in OA tissue.

Thiol Proteases

The degradation of cartilage extracellular matrix macromolecules, as shown by ultrastructural and microscopic examination, often occurs in the perilacunar area where the matrix pH is in the acid range. At first, cathepsin D was thought to be a prime candidate causing this matrix degradation,[52] but as reported by Hembry, Knight, Dingle, et al.,[53] although cathepsin D is elevated in OA cartilage, it does not seem to be involved in cartilage matrix resorption. Cathepsin B, however, another lysosomal enzyme, likely does play an important role in cartilage degradation, particularly in the pericellular area. This enzyme, in addition to having a direct degradative effect on both collagen and proteoglycans, may also be a metalloprotease activator.[54] Only in vitro studies support this notion so far. The maximal activity of cathepsin B is at pH 6.0, but it can exert proteolytic activity for a limited time at neutral pH.[55]

As in several human enzyme systems, the proteolytic effect of cathepsin B is regulated by specific inhibitors. Two such inhibitors, with molecular weights of 67 and 16 kilodaltons (kd) have been found in articular cartilage.[50] In diseased cartilage such as in OA, cathepsin B levels are increased, with a concomitant decrease in cysteine protease inhibitory activity.[56] This imbalance, may be an important contributing factor in OA cartilage degradation.

Other Proteases

Although lysosomes of cultured chondrocytes contain exo-B-n-D-hexosaminidase and exo-B-d-glucuronidases capable of degrading oligosaccharides, no enzyme capable of cleaving the chains of chondroitin sulfate and releasing sulfated oligosaccharides has been found in adult cartilage. A hyaluronidase has been isolated from adult articular cartilage, but it was not active at physiologic pH of cartilage matrix.[57]

The cationic protein lysozyme is abundant in cartilage, where it can regulate the size of proteoglycan aggregates.[58] The presence of aggregates appears to reduce the vulnerability of proteoglycan to enzymatic attack. After a minute amount of neutral protease attacks a proteoglycan monomer, it may clip selectively the HA-binding region. Such degraded fragments can rapidly diffuse from cartilage in organ culture, leaving behind the normal proteoglycan still capable of aggregation.[59] This important finding may explain why so few breakdown products of proteoglycans have been found in OA cartilage; as soon as degradation occurs, the products are either further degraded by chondrocyte enzymes, or they rapidly diffuse into the synovial fluid. Furthermore, proteoglycan degradation products have been identified in synovial fluid of OA patients.[60] A hallmark sugar of cartilage proteoglycan degradation, keratan sulfate, has been found significantly elevated in the sera of patients with OA.[61]

CYTOKINES AND OSTEOARTHRITIS

Since the discovery of humoral factors such as cytokines, which can regulate connective tissue metabolism (anabolism and catabolism), questions have arisen concerning their involvement in the pathophysiology of various rheumatic diseases. Their role in the tissue destruction of joint diseases such as RA and OA has been the subject of numerous studies, as summarized elsewhere.[27–29,62] There is strong evidence that some cytokines are involved in RA pathophysiology; their role in OA, however, has not been studied as extensively. An association between cytokines and the in vivo changes in the OA joints is very likely however (reviewed in 27). The concept that cytokines may play a role in cartilage degradation began with the work of Fell and Jubb.[63] Using an organ culture system, those authors showed that a mediator from synovial membrane induced the catabolism of co-incubated cartilage. Most studies on cytokines in OA have focused on IL-1 and tumor necrosis factor (TNF), because these are believed to be the main cytokines linked to the disease process.

SYNOVIUM

A cartilage catabolic factor in human arthritic synovial fluid identified as IL-1 was first reported by Wood, Ihrie, Dinarello, and Cohen.[64] Herman, Appel, and Hess[65] also isolated a cartilage catabolic factor from OA synovium that was probably IL.

Similarly, Sabiston and Adams[66] found such a factor in canine synovium from an experimental OA model. Synovial explants from human OA knees in culture synthesized increased amounts of both isoforms of IL-1 (α and β); IL-1β predominated, and its production was greatly enhanced by lipopolysaccharide (LPS) stimulation.[67] TNF-α was detected only at low level and only occasionally in the culture medium of LPS-stimulated synovial membrane explants. Immunostaining of OA synovium[67] revealed the presence of significant amounts of both isoforms of IL-1 located mainly in macrophages and synovial lining cells (Fig. 102–2A). TNF-α was detected only occasionally and only in trace amounts. This finding is in accordance with the study of Hopkins and Meager[68] showing a significant level of TNF-α in most of the synovial fluid samples from RA patients but in only a few of the samples from OA patients. Inflammatory changes observed in OA synovium[69] could very well be induced by cytokines, among other factors because injection of IL-1 into the ankle joints of normal rats induced a chronic synovitis, characterized by the presence of mononuclear cells and fibrosis.[70] Cytokines in the synovial fluid are believed to originate from an increased synthesis by the membrane, but this is certainly not the primary cause of the synovitis. Synovial inflammation in OA is almost certainly secondary and related to multiple factors, including the release of cartilage matrix breakdown products and microcrystals.[27]

Interleukin-1 and TNF-α can increase the synthesis of proteases such as the metalloproteases and plasminogen activators. Such cytokines are probably responsible for increasing protease synthesis in OA synovium. Metalloproteases such as stromelysin have been identified in these synovia (Fig. 102–2B); their production correlated with the severity of inflammation, which in turn correlated positively with the level of synovial fluid IL-1.[64] Because synoviocytes can secrete IL-1, it is tempting to speculate that autocrine stimulation may also play a role in the regulation of synoviocyte enzyme synthesis. On the other hand, the ability of IL-1 to stimulate type I collagen synthesis by fibroblasts[71] may increase the amount of fibrosis frequently seen in OA synovium.[69] Of particular importance and clinical relevance is the increased synthesis of prostaglandins by synovial cells exposed to IL-1 or TNF-α.[72,73] This effect could be responsible for several symptoms observed in OA.

The possible role of IL-6 in OA has not yet been defined. Several studies have reported the presence of IL-6 in arthritic tissues. IL-6 levels, measured by the proliferation of B 9.9 hybridoma cell assay (HGF), was detected in the synovial fluid of patients with various arthropathies, including both OA and RA,[74] with higher levels noted in the latter. IL-6 did not stimulate prostaglandin or collagenase production, either by synovial fibroblasts or chondrocytes.[52] Because IL-6 can activate, B and T cells in vivo, however,[75] it might contribute to the immunologic phenomena observed in OA synovium.

CARTILAGE

Direct evidence supporting the involvement of IL-1 or TNF-α in OA cartilage degradation is still very scarce. RNA coding for IL-1α and IL-1β, as well as IL-1 activity,

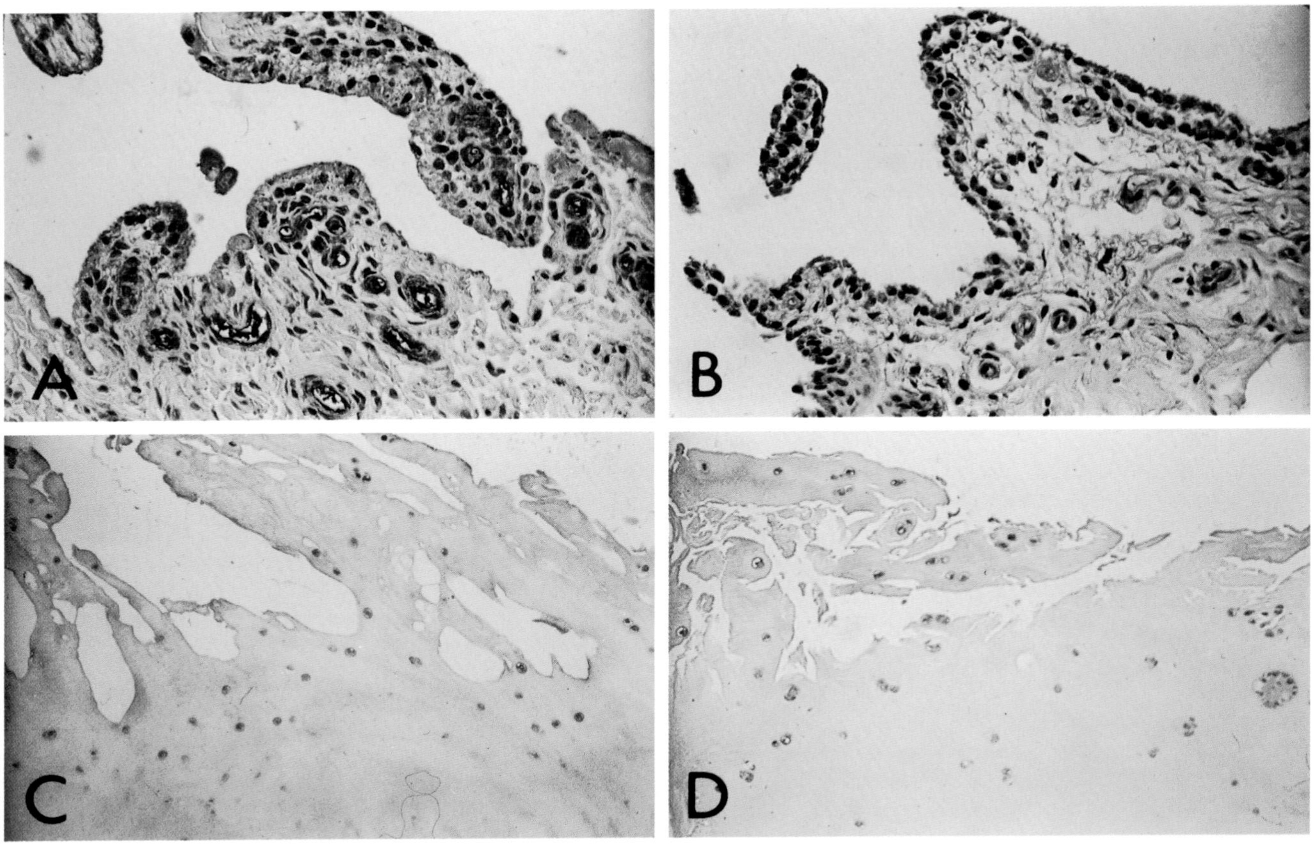

FIGURE 102–2. Immunohistochemical localization of interleukin-1 (IL-1) and stromelysin in human osteoarthritis knee synovium and cartilage. The tissues were reacted with a monoclonal antibody against human stromelysin (generously provided by Scott Wilhelm, Miles Inc.) or human recombinant IL-1, followed by the avidin-biotin-peroxidase complex method. *A*, In osteoarthritic synovium, IL-1 was identified in the lining cells as well as in the infiltrating macrophages and in the blood vessel cells. *B*, Stromelysin was located mainly in synovial lining cells. In osteoarthritic cartilage, IL-1, *C*, and stromelysin, *D*, were identified primarily in the cytoplasma of chondrocytes located in fibrillated areas (J.-P. Pelletier and J. Martel-Pelletier, personal observations).

was seen in human and bovine cartilage chondrocytes.[76] Under resting conditions, normal human cartilage chondrocytes in culture produced both isoforms of IL-1 (α and β), and LPS stimulation increased predominantly the production of IL-1β.[67] Immunohistochemical studies (personal observations) of normal human cartilage showed the presence of IL-1 in a very small number of chondrocytes and only from the superficial layer. In OA cartilage, a strong positive staining of chondrocytes, IL-1 (Fig. 102–2C) and TNF-α[67] in the upper half of the cartilage in both chondrocytes and the extracellular matrix, as well as stromelysin (Fig. 102–2D) and collagenase strongly suggest that they are secreted by chondrocytes. However, a major question arises as to how and in what manner chondrocytes are induced to produce cytokines. Whether this represents an autocrine and/or a paracrine stimulation is not yet known and requires further investigation.

The changes observed in OA cartilage are numerous and involve morphologic and synthetic changes of chondrocytes as well as biochemical and structural alterations of the extracellular matrix. Because IL-1 and TNF-α induce resorption of cartilage both in vitro[45,77] and in vivo,[78] their involvement in the etiology of OA seems very likely. Much evidence supports their involvement in modulating chondrocytic synthetic pathways, including matrix macromolecules.[79,80] The increased minor type collagen in OA cartilage strongly suggests an influence of IL-1, because this cytokine stimulated chondrocyte collagen type I and III synthesis and decreased the synthesis of types II and IX.[79] Such changes could result in inappropriate matrix repair and lead to further cartilage erosion. Similarly, some of the decreased proteoglycan synthesis found in the OA cartilage lesions may be induced by IL-1.[80]

The inhibition–activation of metalloproteases in OA

tissue could very well be modulated by cytokines also. For instance, the imbalance in TIMP-1 and metalloprotease levels found in OA cartilage[41] could be mediated by IL-1, because this cytokine decreased in vitro TIMP-1 synthesis in parallel with increased metalloprotease synthesis in articular chondrocytes.[81] The PA system is similarly modulated by IL-1. The in vitro effect of IL-1 on articular cartilage showed a dose-dependent increase in PA synthesis,[45] and a decreased PAI-1 level.[81] These in vitro effects of IL-1 on cartilage complement the ex vivo findings in OA cartilage and stress the role of this cytokine in OA pathophysiology. Furthermore, the profound effect of IL-1 on PAI-1, in combination with the PA enhancement, is a powerful mechanism boosting the generation of both plasmin and metalloprotease activation. Along with its role as an enzyme activator, plasmin could be involved in cartilage matrix degradation by direct proteolysis of the proteoglycan monomer.[82] Interleukin-1 may be involved in proliferative events in OA, such as osteophyte formation, by stimulating the proliferation of human osteoblast-like cells, leading to increased periarticular bone formation.[83]

Chondrocytes isolated from human normal and OA cartilage spontaneously released IL-6, and histochemical study revealed the in situ presence of this cytokine in human OA cartilage.[84] The involvement of IL-6 in the proliferation of chondrocytes as well as clones is plausible because it increased human OA chondrocyte proliferation.[84] This may be another example of autocrine chondrocyte stimulation occurring in OA.

GROWTH FACTORS

Cartilage extracellular matrix structure plays an integral role in the function of this tissue (Fig. 102–1). Matrix homeostasis is controlled by chondrocytes through a balanced regulation of synthesis and degradative events, with the rate of new matrix synthesis being equal to the rate of matrix degradation. Both processes are controlled by a variety of extracellular messenger proteins, termed *growth factors* or *cytokines*. Growth factors, such as insulin-like growth factor (IGF-1) and transforming growth factor-β (TGF-β), are generally associated with the stimulation of connective tissue synthesis, whereas cytokines such as IL-1 and TNF-α are usually associated with the stimulation of molecules leading to matrix degradation.

Some growth factors can counteract the effect of cytokines TGF-α, produced by various cell types including bone cells, macrophages, and synovial fibroblasts can at least partially reverse IL-1–induced suppression of aggregating proteoglycan synthesis and stimulation of metalloprotease secretion.[85] TGF-β stimulated collagen transcription and inhibited collagenase mRNA levels in synoviocytes.[86] Furthermore, TGF-β induced the synthesis of TIMP-1 and PAI by connective tissue cells,[87] further controlling the degradative effects of IL-1. Other cytokines, such as γ-interferon, also opposed the action of IL-1 on metalloprotease secretion and proteoglycan depletion from cartilage.[88] Thus, the net effects of multiple growth factors and cytokines regulate the synthesis enzymes, inhibitors, and matrix macromolecules in favor of synthesis or degradation, providing homeostatic control over tissue remodeling.

One of the first cartilage-stimulating growth factors identified were the somatomedins or insulin-like growth factors.[89] Two major classes of somatomedins have been described: somatomedin-C (Sm-C), now generally called *insulin-like growth factor 1 (IGF-1)*[90] and *insulin-like growth factor-II (IGF-II)*.[91] IGF-1 stimulated articular chondrocyte mitotic activity[92] as well as proteoglycan and collagen synthesis.[93] Like other peptide growth factors, IGF-1 exerts its cellular effects by interacting with specific cell surface receptors. IGF-1 receptors have been identified on chondrocytes.[94] The role of IGF-1 in serum from OA patients[95] remains unknown. Normal and rheumatoid synovial fluid stimulation of chondrocyte proteoglycan synthesis appeared to be attributable to the presence of IGF-1.[96] The decreased responsiveness of articular chondrocytes to somatomedin in pathologic conditions could contribute to the development of OA.[97]

Fibroblast growth factor (FGF) has been identified in synovial fluid of patients with different forms of arthritis.[98] It has been isolated from multiple tissues in two forms: acidic and basic. Basic FGF (bFGF) has greater potency.[99] FGF stimulated mitotic activity in articular cartilage chondrocytes[100] but did not stimulate the synthesis of glycosaminoglycans.[101] Although no role for bFGF in the etiopathogenesis of OA has been found, it is of potential therapeutic interest, because, administered intra-articularly, it promoted the healing of articular cartilage in a rabbit knee model.[102]

Connective tissue–activating peptide III (CTAP III) from platelets stimulated glycosaminoglycan synthesis in cultured chondrocytes, which might affect repair processes in cartilage next to extravasating synovial sites.[103]

INFLAMMATORY RESPONSES—A DIFFERENT PERSPECTIVE

In most patients with OA, focal or scattered sites of synovial inflammation have been detected, considered an epiphenomenon by most investigators.[104–107] Such inflammation is initiated by mechanical and enzymatic breakdown of OA cartilage, producing wear particles and soluble cartilage-specific degraded macromolecules. When such molecules are released into the synovial space, they are taken up by lining synovial macrophages or, like keratan sulfate, escape into the blood (see preceding discussion). Stimulation of proinflammatory peptide secretion by the synovial lining cells follows. Proteoglycan[108] and collagen,[109] as well as other components are released into synovial fluid from cartilage. Secondary stimulation of macrophages to release proinflammatory products has also been reported. For example, cyanogen bromide peptide CB11 of type II collagen stimulated output of IL-1 from human monocytes.[110] As mentioned, IL-1 and TNF-α have been detected in OA synovial fluids.[2] Nonmyelinated sensory neurons in the synovium are believed to respond to these inflammatory changes, releasing substance P and K (reviewed in 111). In in vitro studies, these neuropeptides stimulated monocytes to secrete IL-1 and TNF-α; interleukin VI;[112] products of arachidonic acid;[113] the oxidative burst;[114] and chemotaxis.[115] Substance P has been detected in inflamed human tissues.[116]

IMMUNOLOGIC RESPONSES IN OSTEOARTHRITIS

The immune system during embryonic and postnatal development receives little exposure to cartilage cell surface antigens and matrix components, because of their avascular shielded location.[117,118] Nevertheless, humoral and cell-mediated immune responses may develop to multiple cartilage antigens in patients with OA.[117,118] In patients with OA of the hip, Cooke and co-workers found IgG, IgA, IgM, and C′ (see preceding discussion) in the surface layer of articular cartilage. That such patients had a higher frequency of polyarthritis than those without such deposits suggested an etiopathologic immune response in at least one or more subsets of OA.[119]

Variable evidence for activation of cell-mediated immune response to proteoglycans by mononuclear cells from OA patients was found by Herman and Appel.[117]

MINERAL DEPOSITION AND ITS RELATIONSHIP TO OSTEOARTHRITIS

Several mechanisms have been hypothesized to relate deposition in cartilage and joint capsules of calcium pyrophosphate dihydrate (CPPD) and other types of crystals to the development of OA.[120,121] In many patients such crystal deposition appears to precede development of clinical or radiographic evidence of OA. Crystal deposition could predispose cartilage to degenerative changes as in gout. In other patients, OA appeared first, which might predispose to crystal deposition.[120] As both chondrocalcinosis and OA are common in the elderly,[122] such correlations must be interpreted cautiously.

A destructive arthropathy in patients with articular chondrocalcinosis[123] appeared more frequently when generalized OA and chondrocalcinosis coexisted.[124] Synovial and knee radiographs from 59 patients with symptomatic OA were analyzed by Halverson and McCarty.[125] The presence of basic calcium phosphate (BCP) alone or BCP and CPPD crystals together correlated with radiographic evidence of joint degeneration. CPPD crystals alone correlated with patient age but not with joint degeneration. Under certain conditions hydroxyapatite crystal aggregates and CPPD crystals have been found to be phlogistic in both in vivo animal models and in vitro cell culture systems.[126–128]

HERITABLE PRIMARY OSTEOARTHRITIS

Premature onset of primary OA was studied clinically and genetically in three generations of an nonconsanguineous family.[129] Clinical and radiologic changes of OA began in the second and third decades of life and involved multiple joints. Pedigree studies indicated an autosomal dominant trait that was pinpointed to alleles of the type II procollagen (COL2A1) gene of chromosome 12 based on study of restriction fragment length polymorphism (RFLP) on samples of leucocytic DNA.[130] The arthritis was apparently caused by a mutation introducing a cysteine into the triple-helical domain of type II procollagen$_2$ chains at position 519 in place of arginine.[131] Although there was mild chondrodysplasia as a result of this mutation, because all cartilages were affected in most of the OA joints, radiographic analysis suggested that matrix failure in the hips and other joints was the cause of the OA rather than secondary changes of bony shape resulting from growth plate disturbance. *Stickler's syndrome* is an opthalmologic disorder associated with OA for which there is also evidence of a type II collagen gene mutation.[132] Many chondrodysplastic syndromes lack such collagen gene mutations.[133] These studies represent a breakthrough in identifying a specific cause of cartilage matrix failure in terms of structural genetic mutation in the most prevalent structural molecule, type II collagen.

SYSTEMIC HORMONES FROM A CLINICAL PERSPECTIVE

Augmented levels of circulating growth hormones were reported in postmenopausal patients with OA in comparison to age-matched controls.[134,135] Growth hormone excess appears to be the cause of thickened cartilage, marginal bone thickening, and reduced joint motion as well as splitting and erosion of cartilage in acromegaly. Secondary inflammation and joint effusions also seem to be caused by synovial uptake of wear particles, as described previously. Acromegalic arthropathy may represent a response to cartilage injury caused by abnormal physical forces resultant from cartilage overexpansion as well as possibly poor biomaterial properties.

It remains questionable whether estrogen deprivation in the menopause correlates with onset of Heberden's and Bouchard's nodes in the genetically defined groups studied by Stecher.[136]

Interestingly, a group of patients with OA who were euglycemic, as compared with control subjects without OA, showed low IGF-1 elevated growth hormone, and reduced insulin levels in their serum.[137]

DIET

Dietary influences on OA remain uncertain. This is a subject extremely difficult to assess because of uncontrollable variables, especially in humans. Factors such as ingestion of a fungus in food have been suggested as causing the OA in Kashin-Beck disease.[11,138] Diets supplemented with ascorbic acid appeared protective against cartilage injury in a guinea pig OA model.[139] The low-calorie Oriental diets have been proposed as an explanation for the low incidence of OA of the hip in Chinese subjects, but little data are available to support this notion.[140]

CONCLUSION

Expanded research in biomechanics and cell biology has led to increased understanding of the etiopathology of OA. Although some of the factors bearing on this disorder are becoming clearer, many additional etiological variables certainly remain to be discovered. Methods are lacking to assess the relative importance of the multiple factors discussed here with respect to disease severity and rate of progression.

REFERENCES

1. Byer, P.D., Bayliss, M.T., Maroudas, A., et al.: Hypothesizing about joints. *In* Studies in Joint Disease 2. Edited by A. Maroudas and E.J. Holborow. London, Pitman, 1983, pp. 241–276.
2. Dieppe, P.: Osteoarthritis and related disorders. *In* Oxford Textbook of Medicine. Edited by D.J. Weatherall and J.G.G. Ledingham. New York, Oxford University Press, 1987, pp. 1676–1684.
3. Mankin, H.J., Brandt, K.D., and Shulman, L.E.: Workshop on etiopathogenesis of osteoarthritis: Proceedings and recommendations. J. Rheumatol., *13*:1130–1160, 1986.
4. Hamerman, D.: The biology of osteoarthritis. N. Engl. J. Med., *320*:1322–1329, 1989.
5. Howell, D.S.: Pathogenesis of osteoarthritis. *In* Inflammatory Disease and the Role of Voltaren. Edited by J.J. Calabro and G.E. Ehrlich. Am. J. Med., *80*:24–28, 1986.
6. Burr, D.B., and Radin, E.L.: Trauma as a factor in the initiation of osteoarthritis. *In* Cartilage Changes in Osteoarthritis. Edited by K.D. Brandt. Ciba-Geigy, 1990, pp. 73–80.
7. Radin, E.L., and Rose, R.M.: Role of subchondral bone in the initiation and progression of cartilage damage. Clin. Orthop. Rel. Res., *213*:34–40, 1986.
8. Harris, W.H.: Idiopathic osteoarthritis of the hip: A twentieth century myth? J. Bone Joint Surg., *59B*:121, 1977.
9. Day, W.H., Sawson, S.A., and Freeman, M.A.: Contact pressures in the loaded human cadaver hip. J. Bone Joint Surg., *57B*:302–313, 1975.
10. Murray, R.O.: The aetiology of primary osteoarthritis of the hip. Br. J. Radiol., *50*:81–83, 1965.
11. Sokoloff, L.: Endemic forms of osteoarthritis. Clin. Rheum. Dis., *11*:187–202, 1985.
12. Bullough, P.G., and Jagannath, A.: The morphology of the calcification front in articular cartilage. J. Bone Joint Surg., *65B*:72–78, 1983.
13. Hutton, C.W., Watt, I., and Dieppe, P.A.: Technetium-99m HMDP bone scanning in osteoarthritis: A predictor of joint progression. Br. J. Radiol., *59*:807–808, 1986.
14. Hutton, C.W., Higgs, E.R., Jackson, P.C., et al.: 99m Tc HMDP bone scanning in generalized nodal osteoarthritis: The four-hour bone scan image predicts radiographic change. Ann. Rheum. Dis., *45*:617–621, 1986.
15. Bullough, P.G., Goodfellow, J., and O'Connor, J.: The relationship between degenerative changes and load-bearing in the human hip. J. Bone Joint Surg., *55B*:746–758, 1973.
16. Gevers, G., Dequeker, J., Geusens, P., et al.: Physical and histomorphological characteristics of iliac crest bone differ according to the grade of osteoarthritis at the hand. Bone, *10*:173–177, 1989.
17. Palmoski, M.J., and Brandt, K.D.: Running inhibits the reversal of atrophic changes in canine knee cartilage after removal of a leg cast. Arthritis Rheum., *24*:1329–1337, 1981.
18. Setton, L.A., Zimmerman, J.R., Mow, V.C., et al.: Effects of disuse on the tensile properties and composition of canine knee joint cartilage. Trans. Orthop. Res. Soc., *15*:155, 1990.
19. O'Connor, B.L., Palmoski, M., and Brandt, K.D.: Neurologic acceleration of degenerative joint lesions. J. Bone Joint Surg., *67A*:562–572, 1985.
20. Yang, K.H., Riegger, C.L. Rodgers, M.M., et al.: Diminished lower limb deceleration as a factor in early stage osteoarthritis. Trans. Orthop. Res. Soc., *14*:52, 1989.
21. Radin, E.L.: Role of muscles in protecting athletes from injury. *In* Physical Activity in Health and Disease. Edited by P.O. Astrand, and G. Grimby. Acta Med. Scand. Symposium, Series No. 2(Suppl. 711), 143–147, 1986.
22. Froimson, M.I., Athanasiou K.A., Kelley, M.A., et al.: Mismatch of cartilage properties at the patellofemoral joint. Trans. Orthop. Res. Soc., *15*:152, 1990.
23. Bird, H.A., Tribe, C.R., and Bacon, P.A.: Joint hypermobility leading to osteoarthrosis and chondrocalcinosis. Ann. Rheum. Dis., *37*:203–211, 1978.
24. Mankin, H.J., and Treadwell, B.V.: Osteoarthritis: An 1987 update. Bull. Rheum. Dis., *36*:1–10, 1986.
25. Sokoloff, L.: Osteoarthritis as a remodeling process. J. Rheumatol., *14*:7–10, 1987.
26. Pelletier, J.P., and Martel-Pelletier, J. (Chairpersons): Proceedings of the Symposium on Osteoarthritis: Update on diagnosis and therapy. J. Rheumatol., *18* (Suppl. 27), 1991.
27. Pelletier, J.P., Roughley, P.J., DiBattista, J.A., et al.: Are cytokines involved in osteoarthritic pathophysiology? Semin. Arthritis Rheum., *20*:12–25, 1991.
28. Arend, W.P., and Dayer, J.M.: Cytokines and cytokine inhibitors or antagonists in rheumatoid arthritis. Arthritis Rheum., *33*:305–315, 1990.
29. Verschure, P.J., and Van Noorden, C.J.F.: The effects of interleukin-1 on articular cartilage destruction as observed in arthritic diseases, and its therapeutic control. Clin. Exp. Rheumatol., *8*:303–313, 1990.
30. Martel-Pelletier, J., Pelletier, J.P., and Malemud, C.J.: Activation of neutral metalloprotease in human osteoarthritic knee cartilage: Evidence for degradation in the core protein of sulphated proteoglycan. Ann. Rheum. Dis., *47*:801–808, 1988.
31. Campbell, I.K., Roughley, P.J., and Mort, J.S.: The action of human articular cartilage metalloproteinase on proteoglycan and link protein. Similarities between products of degradation *in situ* and *in vitro*. Biochem. J., *237*:117–122, 1986.
32. Tyler, J.A.: Chondrocyte-mediated depletion of articular cartilage proteoglycans *in vitro*. Biochem. J., *225*:493–507, 1985.
33. Dodge, G.R., and Poole, A.R.: Immunohistochemical detection and immunochemical analysis of type II collagen degradation in human normal, rheumatoid, and osteoarthritic articular cartilages and in explants of bovine articular cartilage cultured with interleukin 1. J. Clin. Invest., *83*:647–661, 1989.
34. Pelletier, J.P. et al.: Collagenolytic activity and collagen matrix breakdown of the articular cartilage in the Pond-Nuki dog model of osteoarthritis. Arthritis Rheum., *26*:866–874, 1983.

35. Pelletier, J.P. et al.: Collagenase and collagenolytic activity in human osteoarthritic cartilage. Arthritis Rheum., *26*:63–68, 1983.
36. Woessner, J.F., Jr., and Selzer, M.G.: Two latent metalloproteases of human articular cartilage that digest proteoglycans. J. Biol. Chem., *259*:3633–3638, 1984.
37. Pelletier, J.P., Martel-Pelletier, J., Cloutier, J.M., and Woessner, J.F., Jr.: Proteoglycan-degrading acid metalloprotease activity in human osteoarthritic cartilage and the effect of intraarticular steroid injections. Arthritis Rheum., *30*:541–548, 1987.
38. Okada, Y. et al.: Degradation of type IX collagen by matrix metalloproteinase 3 (stromelysin) from human rheumatoid synovial cells. FEBS Lett., *244*:473–476, 1989.
39. Murphy, G. et al.: Stromelysin is an activator of procollagenase: A study with natural and recombinant enzymes. Biochem. J., *248*:265–268, 1987.
40. Dean, D.D., and Woessner, J.F., Jr.: Extracts of human articular cartilage contain an inhibitor of tissue metalloproteinases. Biochem. J., *218*:277–280, 1984.
41. Dean, D.D. et al.: Evidence for metalloproteinase and metalloproteinase inhibitor (TIMP) imbalance in human osteoarthritic cartilage. J. Clin. Invest., *84*:678–685, 1989.
42. Woessner, J.F., Jr.: Matrix metalloproteinases and their inhibitors in connective tissue remodelling. FASEB Journal, *5*:2145–2154, 1991.
43. Nagase, H., Enghild, J.J., and Suzuki, K.: Stepwise activation mechanisms of the precursor of matrix metalloproteinase 3 (stromelysin) by proteinases and (4-aminophenyl) mercuric acetate. Biochemistry, *29*:5783–5789, 1990.
44. Werb, Z., Mainardi, C.L, Vater, C.A., and Harris, E.D., Jr.: Endogenous activation of latent collagenase by rheumatoid synovial cells. Evidence for a role of plasminogen activator. N. Engl. J. Med., *296*:1017–1023, 1977.
45. Campbell, I.K. et al.: Recombinant human interleukin-1 stimulates human articular cartilage to undergo resorption and human chondrocytes to produce both tissue- and urokinase-type plasminogen activator. Biochem. Biophys. Acta., *967*:183–194, 1988.
46. Quigley, J.P.: Phorbol ester-induced morphological changes in transformed chick fibroblasts: Evidence for direct catalytic involvement of plasminogen activator. Cell, *7*:131–141, 1979.
47. Martel-Pelletier, J., Cloutier, J.M., and Pelletier, J.P.: Role of plasminogen activators and their inhibitors in the enzymatic degradation of human osteoarthritic cartilage. (Abstract.) Arthritis Rheum., *33*:S31, 1990.
48. Andrews, J.L., and Ghosh, P.: Low molecular weight serine proteinase inhibitors of human articular cartilage. Isolation, characterization, and biosynthesis. Arthritis Rheum., *33*:1384–1393, 1990.
49. Pavia, M., Towle, C.A., and Treadwell, B.V.: IL-1 activated chondrocytes synthesize an inhibitor of plasminogen activator. (Abstract.) Trans. Orthop. Res. Soc., *15*:238, 1990.
50. Killackey, J.J., Roughley, P.J., and Mort, J.S.: Proteinase inhibitors of human articular cartilage. Coll. Rel. Res., *3*:419–430, 1983.
51. Poole, A.R.: Enzymatic degradation: cartilage destruction. In Cartilage changes in osteoarthritis. Edited by K.D. Brandt. Indianapolis, Indiana University School of Medicine. Ciba Geigy, 63–72, 1990.
52. Sapolsky, A.I., Altman, R.D., Woessner, J.F., Jr., and Howell, D.S.: The action of cathepsin D in human articular cartilage on proteoglycans. J. Clin. Invest., *52*:624–633, 1973.
53. Hembry, R.M., Knight, C.G., Dingle, J.T., and Barrett, A.J.: Evidence that extracellular cathepsin D is not responsible for the resorption of cartilage matrix in culture. Biochem. Biophys. Acta., *714*:307–312, 1982.
54. Eeckhout, Y., and Vaes, G.: Further studies on the activation of procollagenase, the latent precursor of bone collagenase. Effects of lysosomal cathepsin B, plasmin and kallikrein, and spontaneous activation. Biochem. J., *166*:21–31, 1977.
55. Mort, J.S., Recklies, A.D., and Poole, A.R.: Extracellular presence of the lysosomal proteinase cathepsin B in rheumatoid synovium and its activity at neutral pH. Arthritis Rheum., *27*:509–515, 1984.
56. Martel-Pelletier, J., Cloutier, J.M., and Pelletier, J.P.: Cathepsin B and cysteine protease inhibitors in human osteoarthritis. J. Orthop. Res., *8*:336–344, 1990.
57. Stack, M.T., and Brandt, K.D.: Identification and characterization of articular cartilage hyaluronidase (HAase). Arthritis Rheum., *25* (Suppl.):S100, 1982.
58. Woessner, J.F., Jr., and Howell, D.S.: Hydrolytic enzymes in cartilage. *In* Studies in Joint Disease. Vol. 2. Edited by A. Maroudas and E.J. Holborow. Turnbridge Wells, England, Pitman Medical Books, 1983.
59. Carney, S.L., Billingham, M.E.J., Muir, H., and Sandy, J.D.: Demonstration of increased proteoglycan turnover in cartilage explants from dogs with experimental osteoarthritis. J. Orthop. Res., *2*:201–206, 1984.
60. Witter, J.P., Roughley, P.J., Caterson, B., and Poole, A.R.: The isolation and characterization of proteoglycan fragments derived from articular cartilage in human arthritic synovial fluid. (Abstract.) Trans. Orthop. Res. Soc., *9*:313, 1984.
61. Thonar, E.J.M. et al.: Quantification of keratan sulfate in blood as a marker of cartilage metabolism. Arthritis Rheum., 1367–1376, 1985.
62. Larrick, J.W., and Kunkel, S.L.: The role of tumor necrosis factor and interleukin-1 in the immunoinflammatory response. Pharm. Res., *5*:129–139, 1988.
63. Fell, H.B., and Jubb, R.W.: The effect of synovial tissue on the breakdown of articular cartilage in organ culture. Arthritis Rheum., *20*:1359–1371, 1977.
64. Wood, D.D., Ihrie, E.J., Dinarello, C.A., and Cohen, P.L.: Isolation of interleukin-1-like factor from human joint effusions. Arthritis Rheum., *26*:975–983, 1983.
65. Herman, J.H., Appel, A.M., and Hess, E.V.: Modulation of cartilage destruction by select nonsteroidal anti-inflammatory drugs. *In vitro* effect on the synthesis and activity of catabolism-inducing cytokines produced by osteoarthritic and rheumatoid synovial tissue. Arthritis Rheum., *30*:257–265, 1987.
66. Sabiston, C.P., and Adams, M.E.: Production of catabolin by synovium from an experimental model of osteoarthritis. J. Orthop. Res., *7*:519–529, 1989.
67. Martel-Pelletier, J., Cloutier, J.M., and Pelletier, J.P.: Cytokines, interleukin-1 and the tumor necrosis factor in human osteoarthritic tissues. (Abstract.) Trans. Orthop. Res. Soc., *15*:111, 1990.
68. Hopkins, S.J., and Meager, A.: Cytokines in synovial fluid: II. The presence of tumor necrosis factor and interferon. Clin. Exp. Immunol., *73*:88–92, 1988.
69. Haraoui, B. et al.: Synovial membrane histology and immunopathology in rheumatoid arthritis and osteoarthritis: *In-vivo* effects of antirheumatic drugs. Arthritis Rheum., *34*:153–163, 1991.
70. Stimpson, S.A., Dalldorf, F.G., Otterness, I.G., and Schwab, J.H.: Exacerbation of arthritis by IL-1 in rat joints previously injured by peptidoglycan-polysaccharide. J. Immunol., *140*:2964–2969, 1988.
71. Krane, S.M., Dayer, J.M., Simon, L.S., and Byrne, M.S.: Mononuclear cell-conditioned medium containing mononuclear cell factor (MCF), homologous with interleukin 1, stimulates collagen and fibronectin synthesis by adherent rheumatoid synovial

cells: Effects of prostaglandin E_2 and indomethacin. Coll. Rel. Res., *5*:99–117, 1985.

72. Dayer, J.M. et al.: Human recombinant interleukin-1 stimulates collagenase and protaglandin E_2 production by human synovial cells. J. Clin. Invest., *77*:645–648, 1986.
73. Dayer, J.M., Beutler, B., and Cerami, A.: Cachectin/tumor necrosis factor stimulates collagenase and prostaglandin E_2 production by human synovial cells and dermal fibroblasts. J. Exp. Med., *162*:2163–2168, 1985.
74. Guerne, P.A. et al.: Synovium as a source of interleukin 6 *in vitro*. Contribution to local and systemic manifestations of arthritis. J. Clin. Invest., *83*:585–592, 1989.
75. Kishimoto T.: The biology of interleukin-6. Blood, *74*:1–10, 1989.
76. Ollivierre, F. et al.: Expression of IL-1 genes in human and bovine chondrocytes: A mechanism for autocrine control of cartilage matrix degradation. Biochem. Biophys. Res. Commun., *141*:904–911, 1986.
77. Saklatvala, J.: Tumor necrosis factor alpha stimulates resorption and inhibits synthesis of proteoglycan in cartilage. Nature, *322*:547–549, 1986.
78. Henderson, B., and Pettipher, E.R.: Arthritogenic actions of recombinant IL-1 and tumor necrosis factor alpha in the rabbit: Evidence for synergistic interactions between cytokines *in vivo*. Clin. Exp. Immunol., *75*:306–310, 1989.
79. Goldring, M.B. et al.: Interleukin-1 suppresses expression of cartilage-specific types II and IX collagens and increases types I and III collagens in human chondrocytes. J. Clin. Invest., *82*:2026–2037, 1988.
80. Tyler, J.A.: Articular cartilage cultured with catabolin (pig interleukin-1) synthesizes a decreased number of normal proteoglycan molecules. Biochem. J., *227*:869–878, 1985.
81. Martel-Pelletier, J., Zafarullah, M., Kodama, S., and Pelletier, J.P.: *In vitro* effects of interleukin-1 on the synthesis of metalloproteases, TIMP, plasminogen activators and inhibitors in human articular cartilage. J. Rheumatol., *18*:80–84, 1991.
82. Mochan, E., and Keler, T.: Plasmin degradation of cartilage proteoglycan. Biochem. Biophys. Acta., *800*:312–315, 1984.
83. Bunning, R.A. et al.: The effect of interleukin-1 on connective tissue metabolism and its relevance to arthritis. Agent Actions, *18*(Suppl.):131–152, 1986.
84. Guerne, P.A. et al.: Interleukin-6 and joint tissues. Ann. NY Acad. Sci., *557*:558–561, 1989.
85. Chandrasekhar, S., and Harvey, A.K.: Transforming growth factor-beta is a potent inhibitor of IL-1 induced protease activity and cartilage proteoglycan degradation. Biochem. Biophys. Res. Commun., *157*:1352–1359, 1988.
86. Lafyatis, R. et al.: Transforming growth factor-β production by synovial tissues from rheumatoid patients and streptococcal cell wall arthritic rats: Studies on secretion by synovial fibroblast-like cells and immunohistologic localization. J. Immunol., *143*:1142–1148, 1989.
87. Overall, C.M., Wrana, J.L., and Sodek, J.: Independent regulation of collagenase, 72 kDa progelatinase and metalloendoproteinase inhibitor expression in human fibroblasts by transforming growth factor-beta. J. Biol. Chem., *264*:1860–1869, 1989.
88. Andrews, H.J., Bunning, R.A., Dinarello, C.A., and Russell, R.G.: Modulation of human chondrocyte metabolism by recombinant human interferon gamma: *In vitro* effects on basal and IL-1 stimulated proteinase production, cartilage degradation and DNA synthesis. Biochem. Biophys. Acta., *1012*:128–134, 1989.
89. Van Wyk, J.J. et al.: The somatomedins: A family of insulin-like hormones under growth hormone control. Recent Prog. Horm. Res., *30*:259–318, 1974.
90. Klapper, D.G., Svoboda, M.E., and Van Wyk, J.J.: Sequence analysis of somatomedin-C: Confirmation of identity with insulin-like growth factor I. Endocrinology, *112*:2215–2217, 1983.
91. Rinderknecht, E., and Humbel, R.E.: Primary structure of human insulin-like growth factor II. FEBS Lett., *89*:283–286, 1978.
92. Osborn, K.D., Trippel, S.B., and Mankin, H.J.: Growth factor stimulation of adult articular cartilage. J. Orthop. Res. 7:35–42, 1989.
93. Guenther, H.L., Froesch, E.R., Guenther, H.E., and Fleisch, H.: Effect of insulin-like growth factor on collagen and glycosaminoglycan synthesis by rabbit articular chondrocytes in culture. Experientia, *38*:979–981, 1982.
94. Trippel, S.B., Van Wyk, J.J., Foster, M.B., and Svoboda, M.E.: Characterization of a specific somatomedin-C receptor on isolated bovine growth plate chondrocytes. Endocrinology, *112*:2128–2136, 1983.
95. Denko, C.W., Boja, B., and Moskowitz, R.W.: Growth-promoting peptides-insulin-like growth factor-1, insulin growth hormone in diffuse idiopathic skeletal hyperostosis. (Abstract.) Arthritis Rheum., *32*:S84, 1989.
96. Schalkwijk, J. et al.: Insulin-like growth factor stimulation of chondrocyte proteoglycan synthesis by human synovial fluid. Arthritis Rheum., *32*:66–71, 1989.
97. Joosten, L.A. et al.: Chondrocyte unresponsiveness to insulin-like growth factor I. A novel pathogenetic mechanism for cartilage destruction in experimental arthritis. Agents and Actions, *26*:193–195, 1989.
98. Hamerman, D., Taylor, S., Kirschenbaum, I., et al.: Growth factors with heparin binding affinity in human synovial fluid. Proc. Soc. Exp. Biol. Med., *186*:384–389, 1987.
99. Kato, Y. et al.: Differential and synergistic actions of somatomedin-like growth factors, fibroblast growth factor and epidermal growth factor in rabbit costal chondrocytes. Eur. J. Biochem., *125*:685–690, 1983.
100. Sachs, B.L., Goldberg, V.M., Moskowitz, R.W., and Malemud, C.J.: Response of articular chondrocytes to pituitary fibroblast growth factor (FGF). J. Cell Physiol. *112*:51–59, 1982.
101. Kato, Y., and Gospodarowicz, D.: Sulfated proteoglycan synthesis by confluent cultures of rabbit costal chondrocytes grown in the presence of fibroblast growth factor. J. Cell Biol. *100*:477–485, 1985.
102. Cuevas, P., Burgos, J., and Baird, A.: Basic fibroblast growth factor (FGF) promotes cartilage repair *in vivo*. Biochem. Biophys. Res. Commun., *156*:611–618, 1988.
103. Castor, C.W., and Jurisson, M.L.: Influence of mediators of human chondrocyte function. *In* Degenerative Joint Disease. International Congress Series 668. Edited by G. Verbruggen and E.M. Vey, Amsterdam, Excerpta Medica, pp. 125–136, 1985.
104. Lindblad, S., and Hedfors, E.: Arthroscopic and immunohistologic characterization of knee joint synovitis in osteoarthritis. Arthritis Rheum., *30*:1081–1088, 1987.
105. Evans, C.H., Mazzocchi, R.A., Nelson, D.D., and Rubach, H.E.: Experimental arthritis induced by intra-articular injection of allogenic cartilaginous particles into rabbit knees. Arthritis Rheum., *27*:200–207, 1984.
106. Schumacher, R.: The role of inflammation and crystals in the pain of osteoarthritis. *In* Pain in Osteoarthritis. Edited by R.D. Altman. Semin. Arthritis Rheum., *18*(52):81–85, 1989.
107. Jasin, H.E.: Immune mechanisms in osteoarthritis. Edited by R.D. Altman. Semin. Arthritis Rheum., *18*(52):86–90, 1989.
108. Witter, J.P., Roughley, P.J., Webber, C., et al.: The immunologic detection and characterization of cartilage proteoglycan degradation in synovial fluids of patients with arthritis. Arthritis Rheum., *30*:519–529, 1987.
109. Cheung, H.S. Ryan, L.M., Kozin, B., and McCarty, D.J.: Identifi-

cation of collagen subtypes in synovial fluid sediments from arthritic patients. Am. J. Med., *68*:73–79, 1980.

110. Goto, M., Yoshinoya, S., Miyamoto, T., et al.: Stimulation of interleukin-1α and interleukin-1β release from human monocytes by cyanogen bromide peptides of type II collagen. Arthritis Rheum., *31*:1508–1514, 1988.

111. Konttinen, Y.T., Gronblad, M., Hukkanen, M., et al.: Pain fibers in osteoarthritis: A review. *In* Pain in Osteoarthritis. Edited by R.D. Altman. Semin. Arthritis Rheum., *18*(2):35–40, 1989.

112. Lotz, M., Vaughan, J.H., and Carson, D.A.: Effect of neuropeptides on production of inflammatory cytokines by human monocytes. Science, *241*:1218–1221, 1988.

113. Hartung, H.P., Wolters, K., and Toyka, K.V.: Substance P: Binding properties and studies on cellular responses in guinea pig macrophages. J. Immunol., *136*:3856–3863, 1986.

114. Hartung, H.P., and Toyka, K.V.: Activation of macrophages by substance P.: Induction of oxidative burst and thromboxane release. Eur. J. Pharmacol., *89*:301–305, 1983.

115. Ruff, M., Schiffmann, E., Terranova, V., and Pert, C.B.: Neuropeptides are chemoattractants for human tumor cells and monocytes: A possible mechanism for metastasis. Clin. Immunol. Immunopathol., *37*:387–396, 1985.

116. Payan, D.G., McGillis, J.P., and Goetzl, E.J.: Neuroimmunology. Adv. Immunol., *39*:299–323, 1986.

117. Herman, J.H., and Appel, A.M.: Immunologic modulation of cartilage metabolism. *In* Proteases: Their involvement in OA. Edited by J.P. Pelletier. J. Rheumatol., *14S*14:83–85, 1987.

118. Jasin, H.E.: Autoantibody specificities of immune complexes sequestered in articular cartilage of patients with rheumatoid arthritis and osteoarthritis. Arthritis Rheum., *28*:241–248, 1985.

119. Cooke, T.D.: Which comes first: Inflammation or osteoarthritis? Relationship of immune deposits in articular cartilagenous tissues to synovitis in osteoarthritis. *In* Clinical Pathological Osteoarthritis Workshop. Edited by T.D.V. Cooke, I. Dwosh, and J. Cossairt. J. Rheumatol., *10*(Suppl. 9):55–56, 1983.

120. Ryan, L.M., and McCarty, D.J.: Calcium pyrophosphate crystal deposition disease; pseudogout, articular chondrocalcinosis. *In* Arthritis and Allied Conditions. 11th Ed. Edited by D.J. McCarty. Philadelphia, Lea & Febiger, 1989, pp. 1711–1736.

121. Terkeltaub, R.A., Ginsberg, M.H., and McCarty, D.J.: Pathogenesis and treatment of crystal induced inflammation. *In* Arthritis and Allied Conditions. 11th Ed. Edited by D.J. McCarty. Philadelphia, Lea & Febiger, 1989, pp. 1691–1710.

122. Doherty, M., and Dieppe, P.: Crystal deposition disease in the elderly. Clin. Rheum. Dis., *12*:97–116, 1986.

123. Richards, A.J., and Hamilton, E.B.: Destructive arthropathy in chondrocalcinosis articularis. Ann. Rheum. Dis., *33*:196–203, 1974.

124. Gerster, J.C., Vischer, T.L., and Fallet, G.H.: Destructive arthropathy in generalized osteoarthritis with articular chondrocalcinosis. J. Rheumatol., *2*:265–269, 1975.

125. Halverson, P.B., and McCarty, D.J.: Patterns of radiographic abnormalities associated with basic calcium phosphate and calcium pyrophosphate dihydrate crystal deposition in the knee. Ann. Rheum. Dis., *45*:603–605, 1986.

126. Ali, S.Y.: Apatite-type crystal deposition in arthritic cartilage. Scan. Electron Microscopy, *4*:1555–1566, 1985.

127. McCarty, D.J., and Cheung, H.S.: Prostaglandin (PG) E_2 generation by cultured canine synovial fibroblast exposed to microcrystals containing calcium. Ann. Rheum. Dis., *44*:316–320, 1985.

128. Howell, D.S., and Dean, D.D.: Biology and biochemistry of the growth plate. *In* Disease of Bone. Edited by F. Coe and M. Favus. Philadelphia, W.B. Saunders, (in press), pp. 1–120.

129. Katzenstein, P.L., Malemud, C.J., Pathria, M.N., et al.: Early-onset primary osteoarthritis and mild chondrodysplasia. Radiographic and pathologic studies with an analysis of cartilage proteoglycans. Arthritis Rheum., *33*:674–684, 1990.

130. Knowlton, R.G., Katzenstein, P.L., Moskowitz, R.W., et al.: Genetic linkage of a polymorphism in the type II procollagen gene (COL2A1) to primary osteoarthritis associated with mild chondrodysplasia. N. Engl. J. Med., *322*:526–530, 1990.

131. Ala-Kokko, L., Baldwin, C.T., Moskowitz, R.W., et al.: Single base mutation in the type II procollagen gene (COL2A1) as a cause of primary osteoarthritis associated with mild chondrodysplasia. Clin. Res., *328*:317A, 1990.

132. Francomano, C.A., Liberfarb, R.M., Hirose, T., et al.: The Stickler syndrome: Evidence for close linkage to the structural gene for type II collagen. Genomics, *1*:293–296, 1987.

133. Wordsworth, P., Ogilvie, D., Priestley, L., et al.: Structural and segregation analysis of the type II collagen gene (COL2A1) in some heritable chondrodysplasias. J. Med. Genet., *25*:521–527, 1988.

134. Dequeker, J., Burssens, A., Creytens, G., and Bouillon, R.: Ageing of bone: its relation to osteoporosis and osteoarthrosis in post-menopausal women. Frontiers Horm. Res., *3*:116–130, 1975.

135. Cronin, M.E.: Rheumatic aspects on endocrinopathies. *In* Arthritis and Allied Disorders. 11th Ed. Edited by D.J. McCarty. Philadelphia, Lea & Febiger, 1989, pp. 1842–1859.

136. Stecher, R.M.: Heberden oration: Heberden's nodes; clinical description of osteoarthritis of finger joints. Ann. Rheum. Dis., *14*:1–10, 1955.

137. Denko, C.W., Boja, B., and Moskowitz, R.W.: Growth-promoting peptides—insulin, insulin-like growth factor-1, growth hormone—in osteoarthritis. J. Rheumatol., (in press).

138. Sokoloff, L.: The history of Kashin-Beck disease. NY State J. of Med., *89*:343–351, 1989.

139. Schwartz, E.R., Leveille, C.R., Stevens, J.W., and Oh, W.H.: Proteoglycan structure and metabolism in normal and osteoarthritic cartilage of guinea pigs. Arthritis Rheum., *24*:1528–1539, 1981.

140. Axelsson, I., Pita, J.C., Howell, D.S., et al.: Kinetics of proteoglycans and cells in growth plate of normal, diabetes and malnourished rats. Acta Paediatr. Scand. Suppl. *332*:39, 1985.

103

Clinical and Laboratory Findings in Osteoarthritis

ROLAND W. MOSKOWITZ

Osteoarthritis (OA) is a slowly evolving articular disease characterized by the gradual development of joint pain, stiffness, and limitation of motion. The terms *degenerative joint disease* or *osteoarthrosis* may be more precise because degeneration of cartilage is the most prominent pathologic change. Both experimental[1] and clinical[2] studies have shown mild-to-moderate synovitis, however. Some favor a particular form of nomenclature, but at present, the terms *osteoarthritis, osteoarthrosis,* and *degenerative joint disease* are used interchangeably. Although this disease is often benign, severe degenerative changes may cause serious disability. Newer concepts of pathogenesis suggest that OA is not an inevitable sequence of aging itself and raise the possibility of rational preventive and therapeutic methods in the future.

CLASSIFICATION

Classification of OA is difficult because of its varying forms of presentation. Increasing support exists for the concept that OA may represent several disease subsets leading to similar clinical and pathologic alterations, rather than being one specific disorder. The disease is classified as *primary* or idiopathic when it occurs in the absence of any known underlying predisposing factor. In contrast, *secondary* OA is that form of the disease following an identifiable underlying local or systemic pathogenetic factor. The distinctions on which this simple classification is based may be artificial, however. Studies on OA of the hip, for example, show that many cases of "primary" OA are actually secondary to anatomic abnormalities that result in articular incongruity and premature cartilage degeneration, such as congenital hip dysplasia and slipped capital femoral epiphysis of childhood.[3]

Classification criteria for OA of the knee,[4] hand,[5] and hip[6] have been developed by the American College of Rheumatology (ACR).[7] Although classification criteria should not be used as diagnostic criteria, because sensitivity and specificity are not 100%, they are valuable in standardization of reporting series of cases, in performing investigational studies, and in improving consistency in communication.[7] Alternative sets of criteria may be used under different circumstances. For example, criteria not involving radiographs can be used in screening in an office practice. Clinical trials in which radiographs are obtained routinely and in which other parameters are frequently quantified allow use of criteria based on clinical examination, laboratory tests, and radiographs. Criteria based on clinical examination alone are useful for population surveys and other epidemiologic studies. Difficulties inherent in development of classification criteria of clinical OA are related to imprecisely defined clinical symptomatology, disparity between pathologic and clinical findings, absence of specific diagnostic tests, and differences in criteria related to different joints involved. Altman suggests use of checklists (see Tables 103–1 to 103–3) to simplify the task of using various parameters for classification purposes.[7]

To increase sensitivity and specificity in parallel, classifications have been developed that use surrogate variables when the primary variables are not available.[4,6] Although the algorithms give high sensitivity and specificity, their complexity requires an understanding of and familiarization with the sophisticated methods used, making them less practical for everyday use.

Various forms of the disease, such as primary generalized OA, erosive inflammatory OA, diffuse idiopathic skeletal hyperostosis (DISH), and chondromalacia pa-

TABLE 103–1. CHECKLIST FOR CLASSIFICATION OF OSTEOARTHRITIS OF THE KNEE

CLINICAL
_____ **1.** Knee pain for most days of prior month
_____ **2.** Crepitus on active joint motion
_____ **3.** Morning stiffness of the knee ≤30 minutes
_____ **4.** Age ≥38 years
_____ **5.** Crepitus; bony enlargement of knee
_____ **6.** No crepitus; bony enlargement

Osteoarthritis present* _____ 1, 2, 3, 4 or
_____ 1, 2, 3, 5 or
_____ 1, 6

CLINICAL AND RADIOGRAPHIC
_____ **1.** Knee pain for most days of prior month
_____ **2.** Radiographc osteophytes at the joint margins
_____ **3.** Synovial fluid of osteoarthritis (at least 2: clear, viscous, WBC <2,000 cells/mL)
_____ **4.** Synovial fluid not available; age ≥40 years
_____ **5.** Morning stiffness of the knee ≤30 minutes
_____ **6.** Crepitus on active joint motion

Osteoarthritis present* _____ 1, 2 or
_____ 1, 3, 5, 6 or
_____ 1, 4, 5, 6

* Minimum criteria for classification.
WBC = white blood cell.
(From Altman, R.D.[7])

TABLE 103–2. CHECKLIST FOR CLASSIFICATION OF OSTEOARTHRITIS OF THE HAND

_____ **1.** Hand pain, aching, or stiffness for most days of prior month
_____ **2.** Hard tissue enlargement of ≥2 of 10 selected hand joints
_____ **3.** MCP swelling in ≤2 joints
_____ **4.** Hard tissue enlargement of >1 DIP
_____ Deformity of ≥1 of 10 selected hand joints

Osteoarthritis present* _____ 1, 2, 3, 4 or
_____ 1, 2, 3, 5

Note: Second and third DIP may be counted in both item no. 2 and item no. 4. Ten selected hand joints include second and third DIP, second and third PIP, and first CMC of both hands.
* Minimum criteria for classification.
CMC = carpometacarpal joint; DIP = distal interphalangeal joint; MCP = metacarpophalangeal joint; PIP = proximal interphalangeal joint.
(From Altman, R.D.[7])

tellae, have different clinical, pathologic, and radiologic findings and are generally considered distinct syndromes. Alternatively, because of fundamental ignorance in pathogenesis, these syndromes may merely reflect various clinical extremes of the disease. A working classification of OA based on known anatomic and etiologic mechanisms is presented in Table 103–4.

PRIMARY OSTEOARTHRITIS

Interpretation of data regarding the natural history of primary OA is complicated by the different case-finding techniques, whether clinical, radiologic, or pathologic,

TABLE 103–3. CHECKLIST FOR CLASSIFICATION OF OSTEOARTHRITIS OF THE HIP

CLINICAL
_____ **1.** Hip pain for most days of the prior month
_____ **2.** Hip internal rotation ≤15°
_____ **3.** Hip internal rotation >15°
_____ **4.** ESR ≤45 mm/h
_____ **5.** ESR not available; Hip flexion ≤115°
_____ **6.** Morning stiffness of the hip of ≤60 minutes
_____ **7.** Age >50 years

Osteoarthritis present* _____ 1, 2, 4 or
_____ 1, 2, 5 or
_____ 1, 3, 6, 7

CLINICAL AND RADIOGRAPHIC
_____ **1.** Hip pain for most days of the prior month
_____ **2.** ESR ≤20 mm/h
_____ **3.** Radiographic femoral and/or acetubular osteophytes
_____ **4.** Radiographic hip joint space narrowing

Osteoarthritis present* _____ 1, 2, 3 or
_____ 1, 2, 4 or
_____ 1, 3, 4

* Minimum criteria for classification.
ESR = erythrocyte sedimentation rate.
(From Altman, R.D.[7])

TABLE 103–4. CLASSIFICATION OF OSTEOARTHRITIS

- Primary (Idiopathic)
  - Peripheral joints
  - Spine
    - Apophyseal joints
    - Intervertebral joints
  - Subsets
    - Generalized osteoarthritis
    - Erosive inflammatory osteoarthritis
    - Diffuse idiopathic skeletal hyperostosis
    - Chondromalacia patellae
- Secondary
  - Trauma
    - Acute
    - Chronic (occupational, sports)
  - Underlying joint disorders
    - Local (fracture, infection)
    - Diffuse (rheumatoid arthritis)
  - Systemic metabolic or endocrine disorders
    - Ochronosis (alkaptonuria)
    - Wilson's disease
    - Hemochromatosis
    - Kashin-Beck disease
    - Acromegaly
    - Hyperparathyroidism
  - Crystal deposition disease
    - Calcium pyrophosphate dihydrate (pseudogout)
    - Basic calcium phosphate (hydroxyapatite-octacalcium phosphate-tricalcium phosphate)
    - Monosodium urate monohydrate (gout)
  - Neuropathic disorders (Charcot joints)
    - Tabes dorsalis
    - Diabetes mellitus
  - Intra-articular corticosteroid overuse
  - Miscellaneous
    - Bone dysplasia (multiple epiphyseal dysplasia; achondroplasia)
    - Frostbite

used in many of the reported studies. Moreover, studies focused on different joints cannot be compared, even when similar case-finding methods are used. Variations that are due to interobserver error may be significant, despite the use of essentially identical protocols. Nevertheless, sufficient data permit a reasonable approximation of the natural course of the disease.

EPIDEMIOLOGIC FEATURES

A comparison of epidemiologic surveys undertaken to characterize the prevalence and clinical characteristics of OA requires close attention to variations in analytic techniques and populations studied[8] (see Chapter 3). Such variations may have a major impact on the data obtained. Studies derived from autopsy analyses, for example, define earlier disease manifestation than clinical studies based on symptoms that develop later. In clinical surveys, disease definitions must be clear, and the use of prospective or retrospective techniques must be taken into account. Data obtained from roentgenographic studies depend on the number and location of joints studied.[9] Surveys of hospitalized patients, in contrast to those in the general population, are narrow in scope, but they may be useful in identifying certain disease subsets.

Prevalence

Autopsy studies show that degenerative joint changes begin in the second decade.[10] By age 40, 90% of all persons have such changes in their weight-bearing joints, even though clinical symptoms are generally absent. Roentgenographic manifestations of the disease are common in the third decade, and involvement increases progressively with age. A roentgenographic survey showed OA in approximately 52% of an adult English population.[11] When minimal disease was excluded, the prevalence of OA was about 20%. In persons age 55 to 64 years, 85% of these studied had some degree of OA in one or more joints. Studies in a Dutch population demonstrated that, by 40 years of age, 10% of the population had distal interphalangeal OA and 20% had metatarsophalangeal disease.[12]

Signs and symptoms suggestive of OA of the knee were evaluated in 682 elderly people.[13] The frequency of signs and symptoms and their degree of severity remained constant in the seventh, eighth, and ninth decades, suggesting that OA of the knee was indeed common in the elderly but not inevitably progressive. In contrast to these observations, however, OA of the knee in 1424 subjects over age 63 (Framingham heart study cohort) increased progressively with age.[14] This difference might be related to the diagnostic use of roentgenographic, in addition to clinical, findings. Of interest in studies of the Framingham population was an unexplained negative association of OA with smoking![15]

Studies of OA prevalence have also been carried out as part of the National Health and Nutrition Examination Survey II (NHANES II).[16] Including mild disease, OA was described in individuals aged 75 to 79 in 84% of hands, 51% of feet, 13.8% of knees, and 3.1% of hips; fortunately, only a fraction of these cases were symptomatic. In addition to the high prevalence figures noted, the survey confirmed an increasing incidence of OA with age. This striking increase of OA with aging is consistent with other studies and, when individuals with severe grades of OA only are considered, the increase with age is exponential.[11]

Sex, Race, and Heredity

Men and women were equally affected by OA in one study when all ages were considered.[17] Under age 45, prevalence was greater among men, whereas prevalence was greater in women than in men after age 55. Moderate and severe grades of OA were seen to a greater extent in women than in men. In radiographic studies in Great Britain on population samples from the age of 15 years,[18] the number of joints involved and severity were similar in men and women to age 54; thereafter, the disease was more severe and more generalized in women. The pattern of joint involvement was also similar in men and women under age 55, but in older persons, distal interphalangeal, proximal interphalangeal, and first carpometacarpal joints were more frequently affected in women, and hips were more commonly affected in men. The sex difference in patterns of joint involvement suggests that, although the same basic etiologic mechanisms may be involved in osteoarthritis in both sexes, the pattern in men may be affected by trauma, occupational stress, and mechanical factors. Clinical symptoms appear to be more common in women.

Differences in the prevalence of OA in black and white races have been noted, particularly when patterns of joint involvement are analyzed.[19,20] The differences can often be attributed to variations in occupation and life-style. Differences in certain predisposing genetic factors, such as congenital subluxation of the hip, may also play a role.

Southern Chinese,[21] South African blacks,[22] and East Indians[23] have a lower incidence of OA of the hip than European or American whites. In the Chinese, the hip joint may be protected by the extreme range of motion required for frequent squatting. A decreased frequency of predisposing factors such as rheumatoid arthritis (RA), congenital dysplasia of the hip, and slipped capital femoral epiphysis, all believed to be uncommon in the Chinese, may also explain some of the differences.[21] In contrast, Japanese have a high incidence of secondary OA of the hip, related to antecedent congenital hip disease, especially dislocation or acetabular dysplasia.[24] Painful arthropathy of the hips described in the black population around Mseleni in southern Africa appears to be the result of two distinct abnormalities: protrusio acetabuli, affecting mainly women and increasing in frequency with age; and hip dysplasia, which does not increase in frequency with age.[25] Degenerative joint disease was *more* prevalent in Native Americans than in the general population.[17]

Genetic factors in generalized OA have been evaluated.[18,26,27] Patients with generalized OA comprised two clinical groups, differentiated by involvement of the distal interphalangeal joints of the hands (i.e., Heberden's nodes). Nodal generalized OA was more common in women and had an inheritance pattern consistent with a single autosomal gene, dominant in females and recessive in males.[28] Generalized OA in the absence of Heberden's nodes, "non-nodal OA," showed polygenic inheritance.

Four studies have analyzed the frequencies of human leukocyte antigen (HLA) in patients with OA;[29–33] an increased frequency of HLA-A1BB and HLA-B8 were described. Compared with reference populations, an independently increased frequency of the HLA-A1B8 and MZ α_1-antitrypsin phenotypes were observed.[34] A restriction fragment length polymorphorism (RFLP) study demonstrated that one allele of the gene for type II procollagen (COL2A1), the precursor of the major protein of cartilage, is inherited in individuals with a precocious form of primary OA associated with mild chondrodysplasia.[35] Hull and Pope reported an increased frequency of a closely situated restriction fragment polymorphorism (BamHI) for collagen 2A1 in a population of women with OA.[36] A single base mutation of the type II procollagen gene, representing the first direct evidence for a genetic etiology has been found in familial patients with a primary generalized form of OA.[37]

Climate

Geographic studies in Northern Europe and America suggest that OA is less frequent farther north.[19] The prevalence of OA may be lower in Alaskan Eskimos[38] and less prevalent in Finland than in the Netherlands.[39] Studies comparing populations in Jamaica and Great Britain, however, revealed an equal frequency in the two climates.[19] Factors such as race, culture, and environment complicate comparisons of climatic effects on disease prevalence. Symptoms may be less severe in a warmer climate, related perhaps to higher temperatures, greater amounts of sunshine, and lighter-weight clothes.

Obesity, Body Somatotype, and Bone Density

The role of *obesity* in the etiology of OA remains controversial. Some experimental[40] and clinical[41,42] studies suggest that obesity itself is not a factor in the induction or aggravation of degenerative joint disease; other studies have demonstrated an increased frequency of OA in the obese, particularly in weight-bearing joints.[43–45]

The role of systemic and metabolic factors in the association of obesity with knee OA was examined in 3885 American adults as part of the national HANES I study.[46] Obesity was observed to be associated with both bilateral and unilateral OA but more strongly with the former. Controlling for metabolic factors such as serum cholesterol, serum uric acid, diabetes, and blood pressure, no significant reduction in the association between obesity and knee OA was observed, thereby failing to support a metabolic link between obesity and knee OA.[46] Another study noted that obesity at a younger age predicted the development of OA in later years.[47] This might be explained by increased forces across the joint as a result of obesity or, alternatively, by metabolic factors linked with obesity that themselves cause OA.

Obese persons have an increased incidence of OA in non–weight-bearing joints, such as the sternoclavicular and distal interphalangeal joints.[44] It has been suggested that obesity in OA patients may be secondary to the relative inactivity brought on by joint pain and limitation of motion.[41]

In addition to the possible biomechanical effects of obesity in the origin of OA, a *metabolic* role for fat in disease pathogenesis has been suggested.[48] Studies in strains of mice that develop OA showed that diets enriched with lard, a saturated fat, increased the frequency and severity of the degenerative lesions. When unsaturated fat was fed to achieve the same body weight, however, no adverse effect was noted. Perhaps obesity in humans is related to OA not only through its biomechanical effects, but also as a result of still obscure metabolic changes in cartilage.

OA has been associated with specific somatotypes; its prevalence is greater in stout individuals than in thin ones.[49] Patients with OA of the hip or femoral neck fractures were compared; 94% of the former were endomorphic mesomorphs, whereas the majority of patients with fractures were ectomorphic.[50]

Bone density is associated with OA. In studies of the femoral head, a diminished bone mass was associated with femoral neck fracture; increased bone mass, on the other hand, showed a positive correlation with osteoarthritis.[51–53] Reduction in bone mass increases the shock-absorbing capacity of subchondral bone and protects articular cartilage against stress. Conversely, stiffer, denser subchondral bone increases the mechanical forces acting though cartilage, with a resultant predisposition to degenerative change, according to the hypothesis formulated by Radin.[54]

Increased ligamentous laxity correlated positively with joint degeneration. Patients with joint hypermobility had an increased prevalence of generalized OA compared to age- and sex-matched control subjects.[55] Conversely, when patients with OA were evaluated, the prevalence of generalized joint hypermobility was higher than in matched control subjects. Synovial effusions and chondrocalcinosis were common in patients with hypermobility syndrome.

Occupation and Sports

Stress related to occupation or sports activities has been implicated in the induction of OA. In one study, OA of the hips, knees, and shoulders was more common in miners than in porters or clerks.[56] Dock workers showed a higher prevalence of OA of the fingers, elbows, and knees than age-matched civil servants.[57] The joints in the right hand are more commonly involved than those in the left hand. Repetitive manual work performed by women in a weaving factory confirmed that the right hand was more severely involved; this study also noted that the pattern of hand and finger lesions could be directly related to the type of work done by each group, and the joints used most repetitively were also the most involved by disease.[58] Prolonged or repeated, heavy overuse of joints has been related to an increased frequency of OA in bus drivers[27] and foundry workers.[59]

Some studies, however, have failed to show a consistent relationship between OA and the trauma related to overuse. Pneumatic-hammer drillers had no increased risk of elbow disease. The prevalence of OA in shipyard laborers, all of whom had been working for decades in heavy industry, was compared to that in white-collar workers and in a random population sample.[60] All groups were males of the same age. OA of the hip occurred in about 3% of both the laborers and their white-collar controls.

Williams, Cope, Gaunt, et al.[61] described seven patients with painful, palpably enlarged metacarpophalangeal joints characterized radiographically by severe OA abnormalities that included joint space loss, osteophytes, and cysts. All patients with this so-called *Missouri metacarpal syndrome* had similar backgrounds of heavy manual labor involving sustained gripping motions of both hands for 30 years or more.

The role of physical activity, both work and leisure time, was evaluated as part of a study of risk factors in the development of knee OA.[62] OA patients were two to three times more likely than controls to have performed heavy work, and almost five times more likely to have had a significant knee injury. The development of OA of dominant versus nondominant hands in a series of patients aged 53 to 75 was evaluated.[63] OA was found in 133 of 134 subjects; no radiologic or clinical differences were found between dominant and nondominant hands. Twenty-six individuals with heavier life-time hand use had somewhat greater clinical and radiographic evidence of OA.

Involvement of millions of individuals in aerobic exercise of various sorts, especially running, has intensified interest in the possible relationships of joint overuse to OA. An older study showed no increase in OA of the hip in Finnish running champions as compared to age- and sex-matched controls.[64] A later study comparing knee roentgenograms of long-distance runners aged 50 to 72 years to those of community controls revealed a statistically significant increase in knee sclerosis in women but not in men and no differences in joint-space narrowing, crepitus, joint stability, or symptomatic OA.[65] A study of men who ran many miles per week over many years showed no evidence of premature OA in the lower extremities.[66] The effects of habitual running on development of premature OA were studied in Danes who had been running for an average of 40 years at mileage levels comparable to recreational runners of today.[67] No differences in joint alignment, range of motion, or complaints of pain were found between runners and nonrunners; roentgenographic cartilage thickness and osteophyte formation also did not differ. Unfortunately, these studies represent *retrospective* investigations of the prevalence of OA in self-selected individuals with a demonstrated ability to maintain active running. Selection bias cannot be excluded in any of these studies; that is, individuals with a predisposition to OA (because of obesity, habitus, or metabolic or structural connective tissue abnormalities) may not have chosen this particular form of exercise. In addition, individuals who developed OA early may have discontinued running. Further longitudinal studies of a prospective nature should provide more definitive information regarding the relationship, if any, of increased susceptibility to OA and running or other exercise programs.

Many studies have suggested that OA is common in soccer players.[68,69] Many of these studies, however, used osteophytes alone as an indication of OA. In summary, there is no evidence suggesting that exercise is deleterious to normal joints when the criterion used in the loss of roentgenographic joint space.[64]

SYMPTOMS AND SIGNS

The symptoms of OA are localized to the affected joints (Table 103–5). Involvement of many joints may suggest a systemic form of arthritis. Frequently, little or no correlation exists between the joint symptoms and the extent or degree of pathologic or radiologic change. Only about 30% of persons with roentgenographic evidence of OA complained of pain at the relevant sites.[70] Except for lumbar apophyseal joints, persons with radiographic OA were predisposed to develop related symptoms.[11] Similarly, a positive correlation between clinical symptoms and roentgenographic evidence of OA of the knee was noted.[71] Some of the apparent disparity between symptoms and radiologic abnormalities may relate to the roentgenologic definition of OA. For example, the use of osteophytes alone as a diagnostic feature has been questioned. Long-term radiographic studies of the hip and knee suggest that the presence of osteophytes does not imply later development of other structural changes of OA, such as joint space narrowing, subchondral bone cysts, and eburnation.[72] Correlation of symptoms with these more definitive structural abnormalities might well provide evidence of a positive interrelationship.

The cardinal symptom of OA is pain, which at first occurs after joint use and is relieved by rest. The pain is usually aching in character and is poorly localized. As the disease progresses, pain may occur with minimal motion or even at rest. In advanced cases, pain may awaken the patient from sleep because of the loss of protective muscular joint splinting, which during the waking hours limits painful motion. Because cartilage has no nerve supply and is insensitive to pain, the pain in OA must arise from noncartilaginous intra-articular and periarticular structures. The pain is usually multi-

TABLE 103–5. CLINICAL PROFILES OF OSTEOARTHRITIS

FACTOR	CHARACTERISTICS AND OCCURRENCE
Age	Usually advanced; symptoms uncommon before age 40, unless due to secondary cause
Joint involvement	Commonly, distal interphalangeal, proximal interphalangeal, first carpometacarpal, hip, knee, first metatarsophalangeal joints and lower lumbar and cervical vertebrae Rarely, metacarpophalangeal, wrist, elbow, or shoulder joints, except after trauma
Joint effusion	Little or none
Onset	Usually insidious
Systemic manifestations	Rare
True bony ankylosis	Uncommon
Symptoms	Pain on motion (early); pain at rest (later); pain aggravated by prolonged activity, relieved by rest; localized stiffness of short duration ("gelling") relieved by exercise; possibly painful muscle spasm; limitation of motion; "flares" associated with crystal-induced synovitis
Signs	Localized tenderness; crepitus and crackling on motion; mild joint enlargement with firm consistency from proliferation of bone and cartilage; synovitis (less common), gross deformity (later)

factorial and may result from elevation of the periosteum accompanying marginal body proliferation, pressure on exposed subchondral bone, venous engorgement with intramedullary hypertension, trabecular microfractures, involvement of intraarticular ligaments, capsular distension, and pinching or abrasion of synovial villi. Additional contributory factors may be synovitis and capsulitis. Although prostaglandins released from synovial tissues and chondrocytes may theoretically contribute to pain response, a parallel between the inflammatory response and joint fluid prostaglandin concentrations has not been described.[73] Periarticular tissues, such as tendons and fascia, are supplied with sensory nerves and are an important source of pain. Muscle spasms around the joint or pressure on contiguous nerves may be more painful than the pain of articular origin. Frequently, as with other types of joint disease, the pain is intensified just before weather changes.

Factors associated with pain and OA were evaluated as part of a community health study.[74] Findings confirmed previously described discrepancies between radiologic evidence of OA and joint pain, although pain prevalence increased significantly with increasing levels of maximum grade OA. Pain prevalence was higher for women than men for all OA grades in hand radiographs. Education and income were both significant predictors of the presence of hand or knee pain. A disproportionate number of subjects with painful hand joint OA had no high school diploma. Income was also lower among those with hand pain than those without.

OA is sometimes associated with acute or subacute inflammation. This response is most common in erosive (inflammatory) OA of the hands, but it may occur in other peripheral joints. When seen in peripheral joints other than the hands, such inflammatory "acute flares" have been attributed to various degrees of trauma or to crystal-induced synovitis in response to calcium pyrophosphate or other crystals.[75]

Stiffness on awakening in the morning and after periods of inactivity during the day is a common complaint. Such stiffness is of short duration, rarely lasting for more than 15 minutes. *Articular gelling,* a transient stiffness lasting only for several flexion-extension cycles, is extremely common, especially in the lower extremity joints of elderly patients. This occurs often in the absence of other symptoms of OA and follows prolonged inactivity. The initial few steps of a grandparent going to the television set to change the channel is a familiar example. The physiologic basis for gelling is poorly understood. Gelling needs to be distinguished from the more prolonged stiffness associated with inflammation (see Chapter 4). Limitation of motion develops as the disease progresses, owing to joint surface incongruity, muscle spasm and contracture, capsular contracture, and mechanical block from osteophytes or loose bodies. In weight-bearing joints, abrupt *giving way* may occur. Objectively, joints may show *localized tenderness,* especially if synovitis is present. *Pain on passive motion* may be a prominent finding even without local tenderness. *Crepitus,* a crackling or grating sound as the joint is moved, may result from cartilage loss and joint surface irregularity. Enlargement of the joint may be caused by secondary synovitis, an increase in synovial fluid, or marginal proliferative changes in cartilage or bone (osteophytes). Osteophytes can be readily palpated along the margins of the affected joint. Late stages of the disease are associated with gross deformity and subluxation resulting from cartilage loss, collapse of subchondral bone, formation of bone cysts, and gross bony overgrowth. Although these symptoms and signs are common to OA in general, the clinical picture and course depend on the particular joint involvement.

SPECIFIC JOINT INVOLVEMENT

Heberden's Nodes

One of the most common manifestations of primary OA, *Heberden's nodes,*[76] (Figs. 103–1, 103–2), represents cartilaginous and bony enlargement of the dorsolateral and dorsomedial aspects of the distal interphalangeal joints of the fingers, often associated with flexion and lateral deviation of the distal phalanx. Simi-

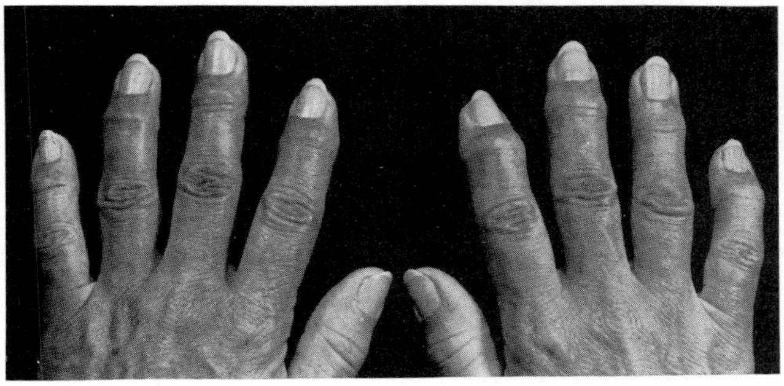

FIGURE 103–1. Typical Heberden's nodes, the cardinal sign of primary osteoarthritis. Note their characteristic position at the distal interphalangeal joints. The proximal interphalangeal joints may be involved later.

lar nodes may be seen in the proximal interphalangeal joints, where they are called *Bouchard's nodes* (Fig. 103–3). Heberden's nodes may be single, but they usually are multiple. They begin most often after age 45 years, but can begin in the third decade of life. Women are affected much more frequently than men, at a ratio of approximately 10:1.[77] Heredity plays a large part in the origin of these lesions, particularly in the female side of the family, in mothers, daughters, and sisters.[78] Heberden's nodes were twice as common in mothers and three times as common in sisters of affected women than in the general population.[28] Stecher postulated a single autosomal gene, sex-influenced, dominant in females and recessive in males, with complete penetrance by age 70, because all who have this gene develop the lesions. Although idiopathic Heberden's nodes undoubtedly have a genetic origin, the exact mode of transmission remains open to question because several

FIGURE 103–2. Close-up view of Heberden's nodes (arrows) affecting the index and middle fingers.

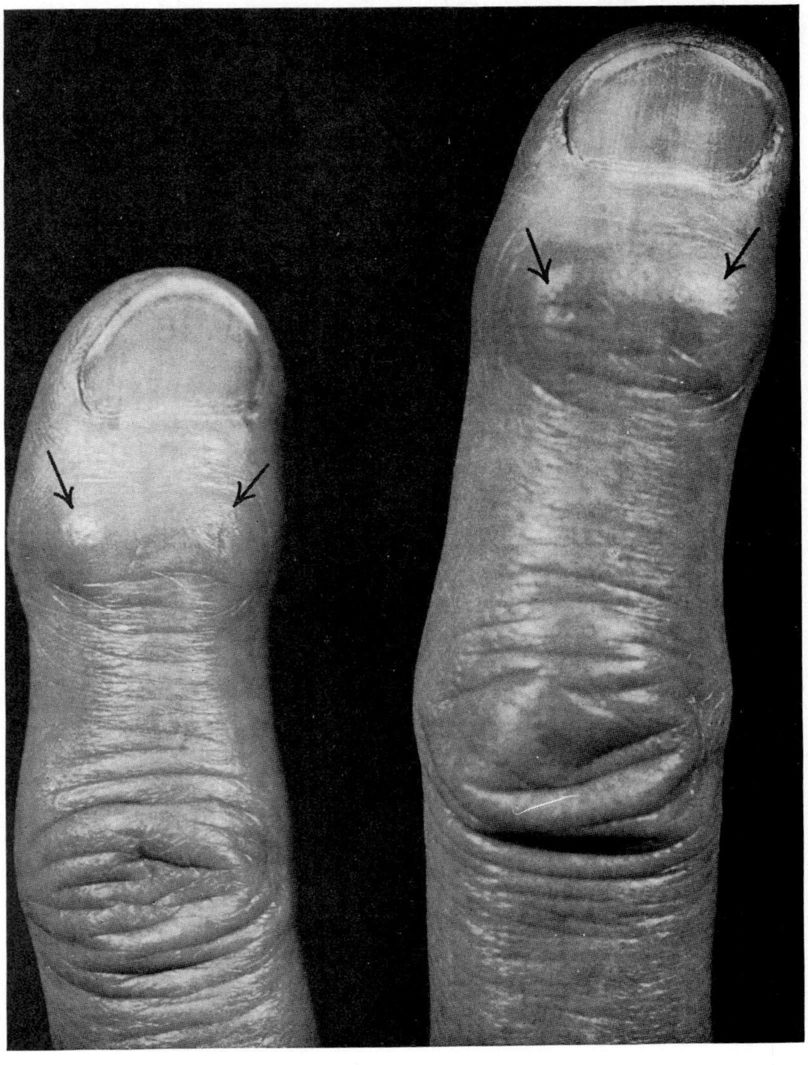

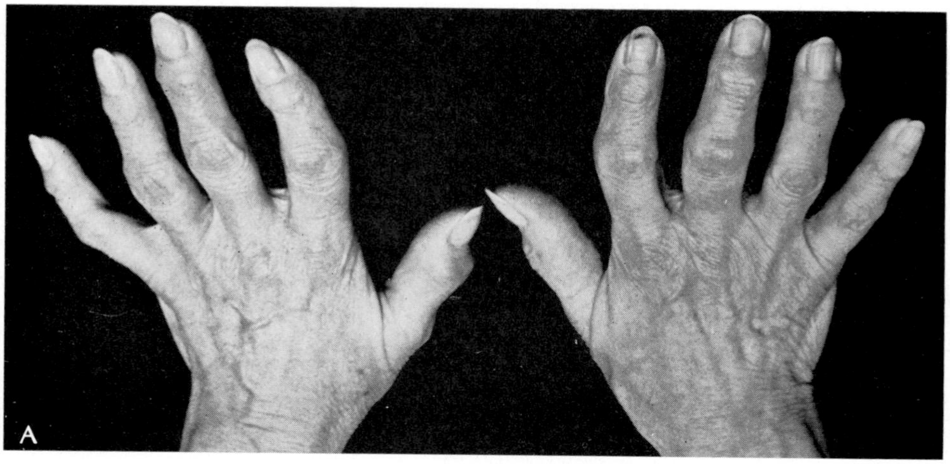

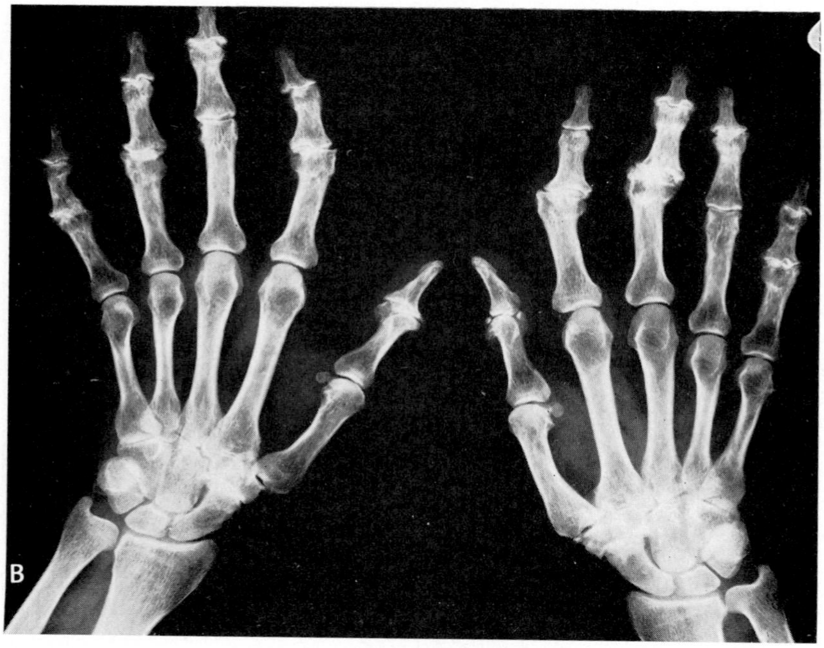

FIGURE 103–3. *A*, Primary osteoarthritis of the hands with marked proximal interphalangeal joint involvement (Bouchard's nodes), as well as distal interphalangeal joint involvement (Heberden's nodes). *B*, Roentgenographic appearance of the same hands.

genetic patterns fit the available data. The demonstration of gene-related abnormalities for type II collagen in OA[35–37] promises further clarification of inheritance patterns.

Clinically, Heberden's nodes may develop gradually with little or no pain and may progress essentially unnoticed for months or years. In other cases, they appear rapidly with redness, swelling, tenderness, and aching, particularly after use. Afflicted individuals may complain of paresthesias and loss of dexterity. Many joints may be involved almost simultaneously, or one or two joints may be involved for a long time before others develop similar changes. The swollen joints may feel either soft and fluctuant or hard. Small, gelatinous cysts may appear, generally on the dorsal aspects of the joint or just proximal to it. These cysts, which are often attached to tendon sheaths and resemble ganglia, may recede spontaneously or may persist indefinitely. At times, they precede the appearance of Heberden's nodes themselves. The cysts' cause is uncertain. Studies have demonstrated communication of the cysts with the distal interphalangeal joint space.[79] This communication may later be pinched off, but at some stage in development the cysts are in direct communication with the joint space. As stated, the *proximal interphalangeal joints* of the fingers may also be involved, usually after several distal joints are affected. Horizontal deviation of the distal and proximal interphalangeal joints may lead to a

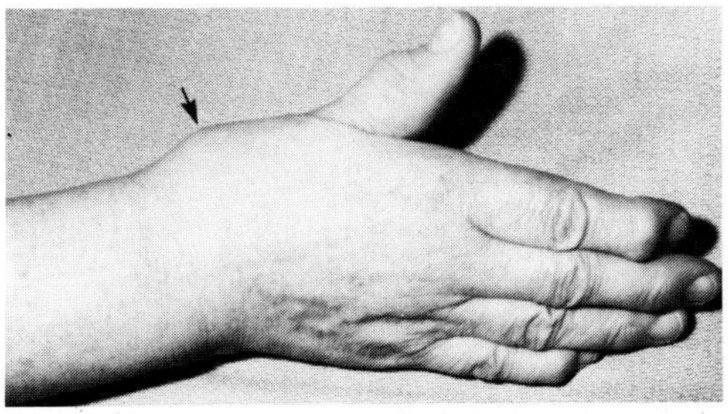

FIGURE 103–4. Severe osteoarthritis of the first carpometacarpal joint leads to a prominent squaring (shelf sign) at the base of the thumb (arrow). Heberden's nodes are also seen.

snake-like configuration of the fingers. Metacarpophalangeal joint involvement is rare; when it does occur, it involves the joints of the second and third fingers.

Carpometacarpal and Trapezioscaphoid Joints. Degenerative changes involving the first carpometacarpal joint are often present. Pain and localized tenderness may suggest a stenosing tenosynovitis. The patient often has a tender prominence at the base of the first metacarpal bone, and the joint in this area may have a squared appearance (shelf sign) (Fig. 103–4). Motion is often limited and painful. Radiographic examination may reveal subluxation of the base of the first metacarpal bone in addition to joint space narrowing and osteophyte formation.

Osteoarthritic changes in the *trapezioscaphoid joint* of the wrist are common.[80] Such changes may occur in association with OA of the first carpometacarpal and distal interphalangeal joints, or they may be an isolated finding. Symptoms and signs include pain in the wrist and thumb base, radial and volar swelling, and tenderness over the scaphoid bone.

Metatarsophalangeal Joints. One of the most common sites of primary OA is the first metatarsophalangeal joint of the foot; OA at the other metatarsophalangeal joints occurs to a lesser degree. The onset is usually insidious, with gradual progression of swelling and pain. Symptoms may be aggravated by wearing tight shoes. A sudden increase in swelling and pain may accompany inflammation of the bursa at the medial aspect of the joint (bunion). The irregular contour of the involved joint can be felt. Foot symptoms may also result from OA of the subtalar and other tarsal joints. Pain of subtalar origin is aggravated by inversion and eversion of the foot, and symptoms may make walking difficult.

Acromioclavicular Joint

OA of the acromicoclavicular joint is common and frequently overlooked as a cause of shoulder pain and disability. Symptoms are usually poorly localized to the joint, and shoulder motion is nearly normal, although painful. Tenderness localized to the joint is the key finding. Roentgenographic changes of degeneration are often minimal. OA of the *manubriosternal joint* is rare, but it may result in chest pain and tenderness.

Temporomandibular Joints

OA produces symptoms of crepitus, stiffness, and pain in chewing (see Chapter 93). Similar symptoms may be caused by disturbances in temporomandibular joint dynamics (temporomandibular dysfunction syndrome), rather than by structural degenerative change. The patient may complain of joint noise and pain, masticatory muscle tenderness, limited motion, and deviation of the jaw to the affected side. The distinction between OA and other causes of jaw pain are discussed in detail in Chapter 93.

Knee

The knee joint is frequently affected by primary OA, with involvement of one or more of its three compartments (medial femorotibial, lateral femorotibial, and patellofemoral) (Fig. 103–5). Symptoms consist of pain on motion, relieved by rest; stiffness, particularly after sitting or rising in the morning; and crepitus on motion. Little objective change might be found on examination. At times, the patient has localized tenderness over various aspects of the joint and pain on passive motion. Marginal osteophytes may be seen and felt. These are often more prominent on physical examination than they are on roentgenography. Mild synovitis and joint effusion may be present. Crepitus can often be detected when the examiner's hand is held over the patella as the knee is flexed. Pain may be elicited by the examiner, by holding the patella tight against the femur with the quadriceps relaxed and then requesting that the patient contract this muscle. Limitation of joint motion, usually extension, on both active or passive motion may be noted. Muscle atrophy about the knee may occur rapidly, especially with disuse. Disproportionate degenerative changes localized to the medial or lateral compartment of the knee may lead to secondary genu varus or, much less commonly, to genu valgus with joint instability and subluxation. Instability is further aggravated by laxity of the collateral ligaments. Isolated patellofemoral compartment or tricompartmental involvement should alert the clinician to underlying calcium pyrophosphate dihydrate (CPPD) crystal deposition. Joint fluid basic calcium phosphate (BCP) crystals were associated with lateral tibiofemoral disease in patients with concomitant (Milwaukee) shoulder joint disease.[81] Ike et al. found erosions of the articular cartilage of the lateral compartment arthroscopically in all patients with lateral tibiofemoral joint space narrowing by roentgenographic examination, and all had CPPD deposits.[82] They also found medial meniscal degeneration and cartilage erosions in all patients with medial tibiofemoral compartment narrowing. Although chondrocalcinosis was significantly associated with OA after controlling for age,

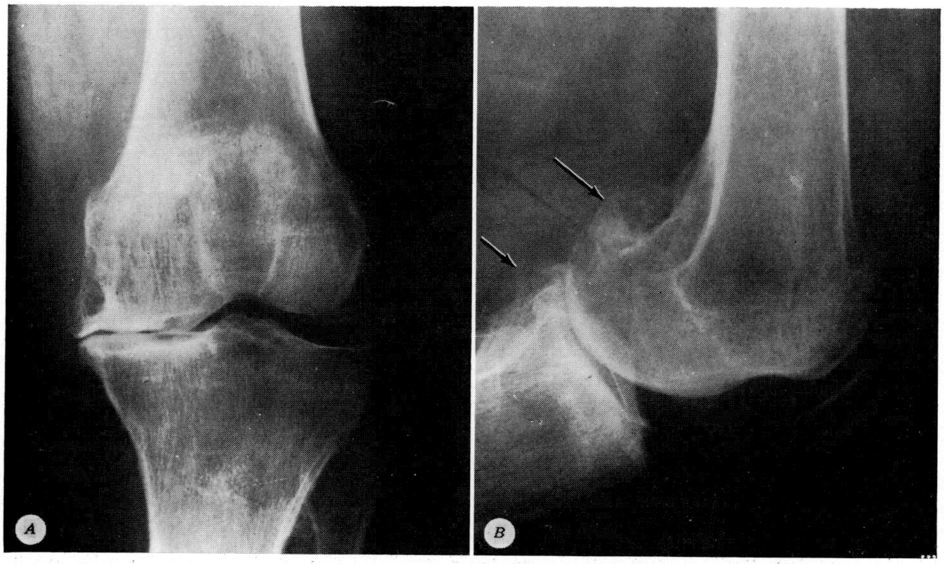

FIGURE 103–5. *A*, Osteoarthritis of the knee; medial joint space narrowing is prominent and is associated with subchondral bony sclerosis (eburnation) and osteophyte formation. *B*, Lateral view of the same knee; large osteophytes can be seen at the posterior aspects of the femur and tibia (arrows).

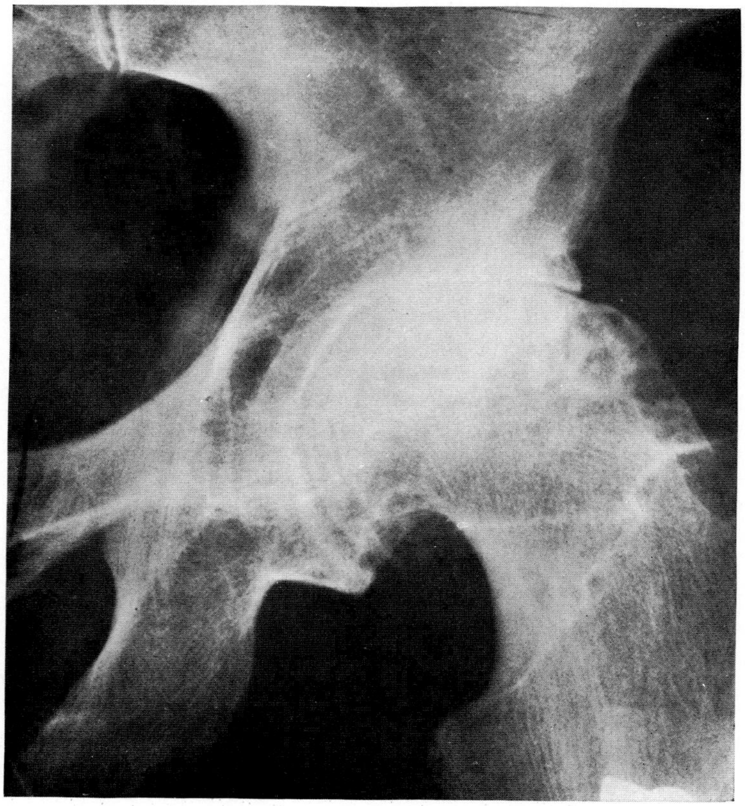

FIGURE 103–6. Osteoarthritis of the hip. Note the almost complete loss of articular cartilage, flattening of the femoral head, and small cystic areas in the head and neck of the femur. Subchondral bone is sclerotic.

both OA and chondrocalcinosis increased independently with age as well.[83]

Hip. OA of the hip, also known as malum coxae senilis or morbus coxae senilis, may be disabling (Fig. 103–6). Symptoms usually first appear in older individuals. This condition occurs more frequently in men than in women and may be unilateral or bilateral. In a study of the natural history of hip OA, Evarts noted that over 8 years, 10% of patients with unilateral hip degeneration developed bilateral disease.[84]

Data on the frequency of right and left hip involvement in unilateral disease are conflicting. One study of 54 patients with idiopathic OA of the hip noted that the two sides were affected with equal frequency when disease was unilateral.[85] Another study of 175 patients found that 13% of men and 29% of women had unilateral disease.[86] The latter patients had a significant predilection for a particular side; 20 right and 10 left hips were involved, a 2:1 ratio. In those with the onset of symptoms after age 60, the ratio of right to left hip involvement was even more marked, 7:1.

The main symptom of OA of the hip is insidious pain followed by a characteristic limp (*antalgic gait*). Pain in the "hip" may often not originate there, and pain actually arising in the hip joint may be referred to other areas. True hip pain is usually felt on its outer aspect, the groin, or along the inner aspect of the thigh. It may be referred to the buttocks or sciatic region and is often referred down the obturator nerve to the knee. Occasionally, most of the pain is in the knee, and its true origin is overlooked. The degree of pain varies widely and does not always correlate with the extent of cartilaginous and osseous changes. *Trochanteric bursitis*, caused by inflammation of the bursa over the greater trochanter, produces pain and tenderness at the lateral aspect of the hip; symptoms and physical findings may simulate those seen in patients with OA of the hip. Pain is exaggerated by weight bearing, and a mild limp is common, however, *hip motion is normal, in contrast to the invariable limitation of motion seen in OA of the hip joint.* Localized tenderness over the bursa is characteristic. Rapid relief of symptoms following bursal injection with local corticosteroids and procaine is diagnostically helpful.

Stiffness is common and increases after inactivity. Examination reveals varying degrees of limited motion. The leg is often held in external rotation with the hip flexed and adducted. *Severe backache* may result from the compensatory lordosis accompanying flexion contracture. Functional shortening of the extremity may occur. The gait is frequently awkward with shuffling or waddling. Sitting is difficult, as is rising from this position, owing to limitation of motion.

In addition to characteristic involvement of joints, noted previously, primary OA was opined to occur in sites generally considered "protected." Sixteen patients with elbow OA unassociated with nodal- or crystal-related degenerative changes were reported.[87] Elbow OA appeared to affect primarily middle-aged men and was commonly associated with metacarpophalangeal OA. In another report, the unrecognized association of nodal OA of the fingers with OA of interphalangeal joints of the toes was emphasized.[88]

Spine. (See Chapters 93, 95 and 96.) OA of the spinal joints is common (Fig. 103–7). It often results from degenerative changes in the intervertebral fibrocartilaginous discs, from damage to vertebral bodies, or from degeneration in the posterior apophyseal articulations themselves. Disc narrowing may cause subluxation of the posterior apophyseal joints (see Chapter 93). Lipping or spur formation (osteophytosis) on the vertebral bodies is a prominent finding (Fig. 103–8). Anterior spurs are most prevalent. Although usually asymptomatic, large anterior osteophytes in the cervical spine may give rise to symptoms of dysphagia.[89] Respiratory symptoms such as hoarseness, coughing, and aspiration may be noted. Joint space narrowing, bony sclerosis, and spur formation are often seen in apophyseal joints. Some authors make a distinction between degenerative changes involving the discs and vertebral bodies, for which they use the term *spondylosis*, and degenerative changes of the apophyseal joints, which are classified as

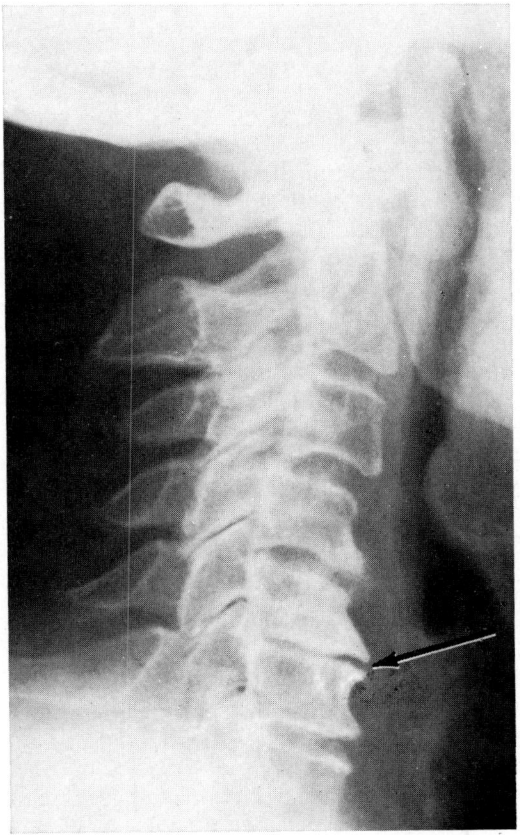

FIGURE 103–7. Osteoarthritis changes in the lower cervical spine. Spur formation is prominent. Note the marked narrowing of the intervertebral disc between C5 and C6 vertebrae (arrow) and subluxation of C3-C4.

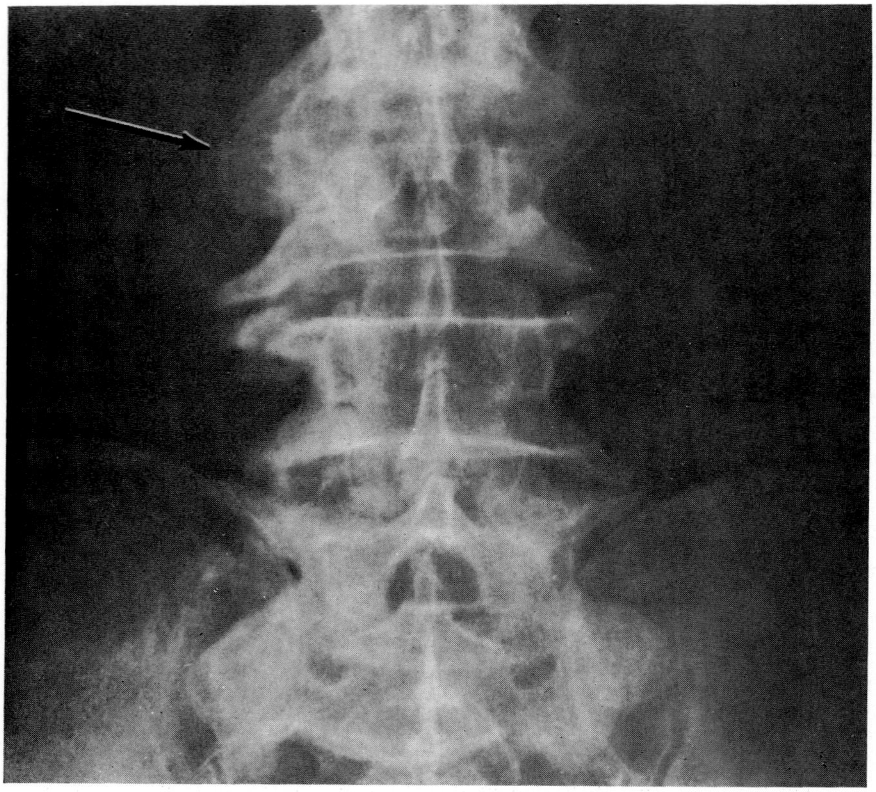

FIGURE 103–8. Osteoarthritis of the lumbar spine. Note the marked osteophyte formation with bridging of spurs between L2 and L3 on the right (arrow).

true OA, because radiologic abnormalities more closely resemble those seen in other diarthrodial joints.

Degenerative changes of all types are most frequent in the areas of the lordotic and kyphotic apices, C5, T8, and L3 to L4, and correlate in general with the areas of maximal spine motion. In some older individuals, however, osteophytes may extend along the entire length of the spine, with prominent involvement of the thoracic region (Fig. 103–9). These osteophytes may be striking, and coalescence with fusion may occur (Fig. 103–10). Forestier et al. have suggested the name *ankylosing hyperostosis* for these severe cases, which may be associated with moderate-to-several spinal limitation.[90] The frequent extraspinal manifestations of "Forestier's disease" have led to the term *diffuse idiopathic skeletal hyperostosis* (DISH),[91,92] discussed later in this chapter.

Symptoms of spinal OA include localized pain and stiffness and radicular pain. Localized pain has been assumed to originate in paraspinal ligaments, joint capsules, and periosteum. Such changes may explain spontaneous fluctuations of symptoms in the presence of persistent or progressive cartilage degeneration and spur formation. Spasm of paraspinal muscles is common and may be a major cause of pain. Radicular pain may be due to compression of nerve roots, or it may represent pain referred along dermatomes related to the primary local lesion.

Nerve root compression causing neuropathy is common. This disorder may result from impingement on the

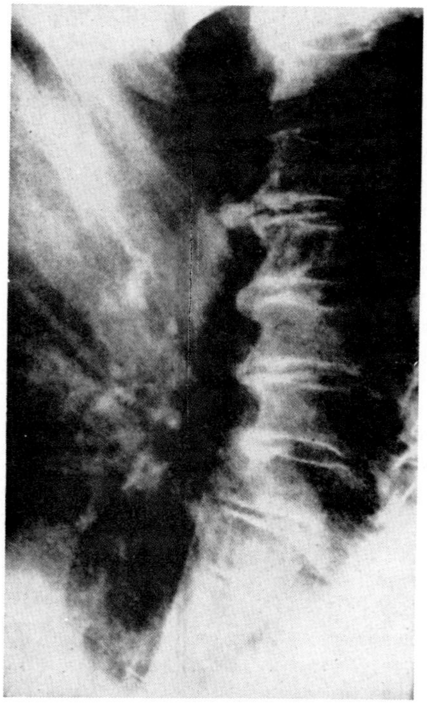

FIGURE 103–9. Osteoarthritis of the thoracic spine. Note the pronounced exostoses at the anterior vertebral margins and the narrowed intervertebral disc spaces.

nerve root by spurs that compromise the foraminal space (Fig. 103–11), by lateral prolapse of a degenerated disc, or by foraminal narrowing from apophyseal joint subluxation. Pressure on nerve roots may cause radicular pain, paresthesias, and reflex and motor changes in the distribution of the involved root. Neurologic complications of this type occur most frequently in the neck because of its small spinal canal and intervertebral foramina, but they can occur in other areas of the spine. Nerve root compression in the dorsal spine may result in radicular pain radiating around the chest wall in a girdle distribution. This must be differentiated from symptoms caused by other disorders. Involvement of nerve roots in the lumbosacral area is associated with low back pain and neurologic signs and symptoms, which frequently allow localization of specific nerve root compression. Involvement of the L3 or L4 nerve roots is associated with a diminished or absent patellar reflex; an absent ankle jerk indicates involvement of the S1 nerve root. Sensory loss over the anteromedial aspect of the leg is consistent with L4 nerve root compression. A lesion at L5 causes sensory changes at the anterolateral aspect of the leg and the medial aspect of the foot and weakness of dorsiflexion of the foot and great toe. S1 nerve root compression results in sensory changes at the posterolateral aspect of the calf and the lateral foot. Gastrocnemius muscle weakness may be evident.

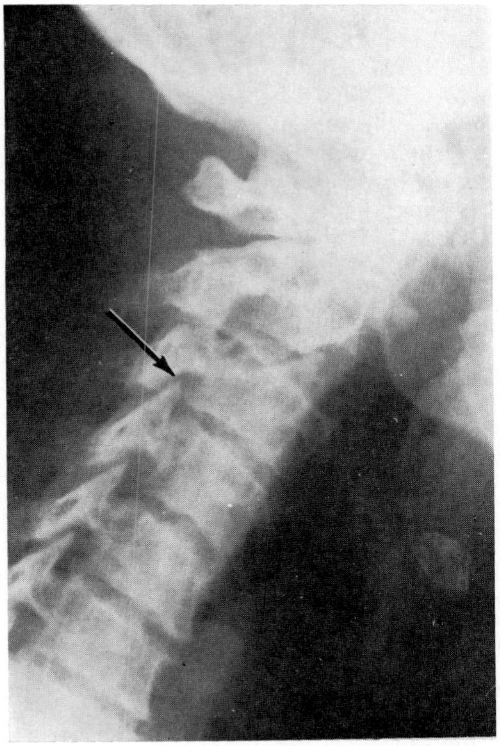

FIGURE 103–11. Osteoarthritis of cervical spine, oblique radiologic view. The foraminal space between C3 and C4 (arrow) is compromised by marked posterior spur formation.

Further neurologic symptoms may be associated with cervical OA if large posterior spurs or protruded discs compress the spinal cord. In these cases, upper-motor-neuron and other long-tract signs may be observed. Compression of the anterior spinal artery may produce a central cord syndrome. The blood supply to the brain may be compromised if large spurs compress the vertebral arteries. The spectrum of clinical signs and symptoms is similar to that in basilar artery insufficiency. Exacerbations are often associated with postural neck changes from compression of vertebral arteries by osteophytes. Angiographic studies of carotid and vertebral arteries are diagnostically helpful.

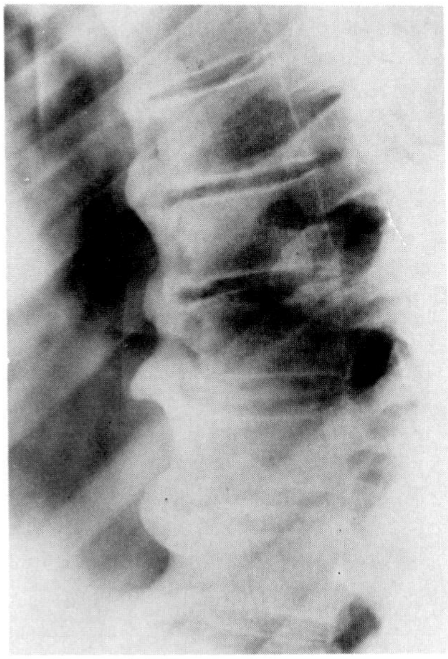

FIGURE 103–10. Florid hyperostosis of the spine in a patient with Forestier's disease (diffuse idiopathic skeletal hyperostosis). A flowing mantle of ossification from ligamentous calcification and coalescence of osteophytes is seen at the anterior aspect of the spine. (Courtesy of Dr. Donald Resnick.)

OA of the atlantoaxial joint has been described in 31 patients.[93] Radiologic signs consisted of joint space narrowing, marginal cortical thickening, and osteophyte formation. Involvement of the lateral atlantoaxial joint, the articulation of the atlas with the odontoid, or mixed involvement was found. Patients complained of occipital pain, stiffness of the shoulder, and paresthesias of the fingers. Conservative treatment provided satisfactory relief of symptoms, except in one patient who required a transoral atlantoaxial fusion.

Spinal cord lesions as a result of OA of the dorsal spine are rare. Spinal cord compression is not seen in patients with lumbosacral lesions because the spinal cord ends at the level of L1, but *cauda equina syndrome* with sphincter dysfunction may develop.

Spinal stenosis (Chapter 95) may produce symptoms in the lower back and the lower extremities. Pain may be constant or intermittent. It is often worsened by exercise, simulating intermittent claudication. Hyperextension of the spine often exacerbates symptoms; relief is noted with flexion. The patient may stand with knees, hips, and lumbar spine flexed (simian stance). Sensory change may be present, and motor power in the legs may be diminished. Stenosis is usually caused by combined anatomic abnormalities because congenital narrowing alone is generally asymptomatic.[94] Commonly associated causes include degenerative spurs, disc herniation, ligamentous hypertrophy, and spondylolisthesis. Trauma, postoperative fibrosis, Paget's disease, and fluorosis are less commonly associated.

Radiologic evidence of degenerative disease in the spine may be extensive but may still bear little relation to the patient's symptoms. On the other hand, severe symptoms may develop with minor spur formation if the spur is located in a critical area. Roentgenographic changes of marginal lipping, sclerosis of the articular margins, and narrowing have been found in sacroiliac joints with increasing age, but it is unlikely that such changes lead to symptoms.

LABORATORY FINDINGS

No specific diagnostic laboratory abnormalities exist in primary OA (Table 103–6). The erythrocyte sedimentation rate, routine blood counts, urinalyses, and blood chemical determinations are normal in patients with primary disease but are important in excluding other forms of arthritis considered in the differential diagnosis, and they may identify systemic metabolic disorders associated with secondary OA. For example, patients with associated CPPD crystal deposition disease may have evidence of underlying primary hyperparathyroidism with elevation of serum calcium and an increase in serum parathyroid hormone level. Patients with Paget's disease exhibit elevated serum alkaline phosphatase levels and increased urinary hydroxyproline excretion. In patients with joint disease associated with ochronosis, the presence of homogentisic acid metabolites in the urine darkens the urine on standing or causes a false-positive Benedict's test result for glycosuria.

Much interest has been directed toward study of proteoglycan components in synovial fluid or serum as a measure of cartilage degradation.[95–98] The search for such "markers" has been advanced by the availability of monoclonal or polyclonal antibodies raised against various cartilage and bone macromolecules. Among these potential markers, keratan sulphate (KS) has had the greatest study, both in experimental models and in humans.[95–98] Serum KS concentrations were shown to be increased in patients with OA or RA as compared to normals or patients with fibromyalgia syndrome;[95] but no correlation between the level of KS and the joint score or the duration of disease was found, in either OA or RA. Studies in patients with anterior cruciate ligament rupture or meniscal tears reported elevations of proteoglycan epitopes in synovial fluid.[97]

Attention has also been directed toward serum hyaluronate concentrations in the presence of degenerative and inflammatory joint disease.[99,100] Hyaluronate levels were elevated in patients with OA and were even higher in patients with RA.[99] Inflamed synovium is probably the main source of these elevated concentrations, which may result from decreased hepatic clearance, increased release from synovial tissue, or increased synthesis.[99,100]

Measurements of urinary pyridinium cross links were also suggested as an indicator of cartilage and bone collagen degradation in both OA and RA.[101]

Study of serum or synovial fluid "markers" is complicated by some factors including slow release of macromolecular substances from cartilage, presence of similar macromolecular compounds in tissues other than joints, and difficulties in separating out the effects of synthesis versus degradation in contributing to serum level. Accordingly, use of serum markers for diagnostic and prognostic purposes remains investigational.[102]

TABLE 103–6. LABORATORY AND RADIOLOGIC FINDINGS IN PRIMARY OSTEOARTHRITIS

LABORATORY TESTS	RESULTS
Erythrocyte sedimentation rate	Usually normal
Routine blood counts	Normal
Rheumatoid factor	Negative
Antinuclear antibody	Negative
Serum calcium, phosphorus, alkaline phosphatase, serum protein electrophoresis	Normal
Synovial fluid analysis	Good viscosity with normal mucin clot; modest increase in leukocyte number Presence of fibrils and debris (wear particles)
RADIOLOGIC FINDINGS	**CAUSES**
Narrowing of joint space	Articular cartilage ulceration
Subchondral bony sclerosis (eburnation)	New bone formation
Marginal osteophyte formation	Proliferation of cartilage and bone
Bone cysts and bony collapse	Subchondral microfractures
Gross deformity with subluxation and loose bodies	Ligamentous laxity as a result of mechanical forces

Synovial fluid in primary OA is "noninflammatory" with no abnormalities other than a slight increase in white cells. Viscosity is good, and the mucin clot formed after addition of glacial acetic acid is normal. Synovial fluid fibrils, morphologically indistinguishable from sloughed collagen fibers, are often seen. The collagen fibers seen in synovial fluid in OA appear to be type II, derived from articular hyaline cartilage.[103] CPPD or BCP crystals may be present. Cholesterol crystals have been identified by light microscopy in synovial fluids of patients with recurrent OA knee effusions.[104] Although evidence of altered cellular and humoral immune mechanisms has been described,[105–107] its significance remains to be determined. Immune complexes have been detected in hyaline articular cartilage of OA joints but not in synovial fluid.[108]

Histologic examination of the synovium in primary OA reveals nonspecific changes of chronic mild inflammation, particularly in more advanced disease.

SCINTIGRAPHY

Bone and joint scintigraphy using technetium 99m (^{99m}Tc) as the pertechnetate has been of limited diagnostic value,[109] but studies using 4-hour ^{99m}Tc coupled with bone-seeking diphosphonates correlated with radiographic abnormalities in OA of hand joints.[110,111] Abnormalities predicted the development of radiographic signs, and joints abnormal on scintigraphy showed the greatest progression in followup studies. Some joints were abnormal on either roentgenogram or scan alone, and others showed a marked disparity in the degree of abnormality on radiographic evaluation compared with isotopic evaluation. These discrepancies suggested that scintigraphy offered a different way of assessing OA changes, perhaps useful in evaluating response to therapeutic strategies. Expanded studies may further define its role in the evaluation of OA.

Intraosseous phlebography reveals impaired drainage from the juxta-articular bone marrow.[112,113] Venous stasis and engorgement are generally associated with intramedullary hypertension. Thermography, a method of constructing photographic images of surface temperatures, may be normal or, in the presence of mild synovitis, may show a pattern of heat emission. Arthrography may be useful in differential diagnosis. The role of these techniques in the routine diagnosis of OA remains limited and poorly defined. They usually add little to observations evident on routine physical examination.

ROENTGENOGRAPHIC APPEARANCE

The roentgenographic appearance may be normal if the pathologic changes leading to clinical symptoms are sufficiently mild. Many gradations of abnormality may be noted as the disease progresses (Table 103–6). *Joint space narrowing* occurs as a result of degeneration and disappearance of articular cartilage. *Subchondral bony sclerosis* (eburnation) is noted as increased bone density. *Marginal osteophyte formation* takes place as a result of proliferation of cartilage and bone. *Cysts*, varying in size from several millimeters to several centimeters, are seen as translucent areas in periarticular bone. Gross *deformity* and *subluxation* and *loose bodies* may occur in advanced cases.

Although osteophytes are usually regarded as a manifestation of OA, the use of this feature alone in diagnosis has been questioned, as noted earlier in this chapter. Osteophytes correlate with aging and are not necessarily an early sign of OA.[72,114] The diagnosis of OA of the peripheral joints may be more validly based on radiologic findings of structural abnormalities in cartilage (decreased joint space) or in subchondral bone (cysts and eburnation) or in both.

The origin of the subchondral "detritus" cysts has been explained as follows: (1) a failure in the bone remodeling process, in which local osteoclastic activity outstrips that of osteoblasts; or (2) the result of pressure transmitted from the joint surface to subarticular bone through cracks in the subchondral plate (trabecular microfractures). The cysts may contain fluid, nonspecific detritus, or a primitive mesenchymal tissue that undergoes fibrosis. *These cysts may be prominent even in joints with adequately preserved joint space when seen radiographically.*

Ankylosis in OA is uncommon. It is seen occasionally in OA of the hands, especially in its erosive inflammatory form.

Osteophytes are usually located on the anterior and anterolateral borders of the vertebral bodies and are best visualized on lateral roentgenograms. The amount of bony overgrowth varies. Spurs arising from the posterior margins of the vertebral bodies or from the margins of the articular facets are less common but are of greater clinical importance, owing to their proximity to neural structures. Narrowing of intervertebral joint spaces results from disc degeneration; this is most frequent and usually most marked in the lower cervical and lower lumbar regions. Sclerosis of adjacent bone is common, and one sometimes sees wedging of the anterior borders of the vertebral bodies. Apophyseal joints may show joint space narrowing, sclerosis, and associated spur formation. Osteoporosis is not a component of OA.

Many of the previously mentioned radiologic abnormalities may be visualized on routine posteroanterior and lateral views. Oblique views of the cervical and lumbar spine should be performed routinely, if degenerative changes involving intervertebral foramina and apophyseal joints are to be accurately delineated. Myelography may be of help when symptoms are severe and a surgical procedure is contemplated. Computed tomography (CT) scanning is particularly useful diagnostically in patients with OA of the spine, especially when spinal stenosis or lumbar facet disease is suspected (see Chapter 95). Diagnostic evaluation of disc herniation is enhanced, especially when the procedure is combined with myelography. Magnetic resonance imaging (MRI) promises to provide significant advances in noninvasive diagnostic imaging of both the spinal and peripheral articulations (Chapter 6).

Roentgenographic study of Heberden's and Bouchard's nodes reveals joint space narrowing, bony sclerosis, and cyst formation. Spur formation, best seen radiologically on routine posteroanterior views, is prominent and appears to develop at the attachments of the flexor and extensor tendons to the distal phalanx. In some patients, however, spurs may be directed anteroposteriorly rather than mediolaterally, and lateral views with the fingers spread may be necessary to demonstrate changes. Although the nodes may feel hard, only minimal spur formation may be visible radiographically, and the enlargement may consist of soft tissue and cartilage. OA of metacarpophalangeal joints is uncommon, but *hook-like osteophytes* were noted on the radial side of the head of the metacarpal bones in 7 of 100 patients with nodal OA.[115] These changes, seen primarily in patients over 65 years of age, may result from tension on capsular ligaments caused by contraction of interosseous muscles at the radial side of the metacarpal head.

Anteroposterior views of the pelvis should be obtained routinely when OA of the hip is suspected. This view is especially informative in that the hips, sacroiliac joints, symphysis pubis, and pelvic bones are visualized. Special views of the hips, including lateral views and tomograms, may be of value when pathologic changes are suspected but not seen by routine techniques. Advanced disease may demonstrate striking abnormalities such as *protrusio acetabuli* (arthrokatadysis), a condition in which the floor of the acetabulum is displaced medially by the head of the femur, so that the femoral head may bulge into the pelvis ("Otto's pelvis").

Although OA changes of the knee are usually readily seen on routine anterposterior and lateral views, special views are often helpful. *Tunnel views* taken with the knee in flexion expose the intercondylar notch and enable one to identify loose bodies, intra-articular spurs, and changes in the tibial spines. Tunnel views may best reveal loss of the joint space.[116] Their effectiveness in delineating cartilage loss may relate to the visualization of a more posterior portion of the femoral condyles, where cartilage loss may be significant. *"Skyline"* (Hughston) views taken from above allow more detailed study of the patellofemoral compartment. Films obtained when the patient is *bearing weight* allow optimal demonstration of genu varus or genu valgus and medial or lateral compartment narrowing. Roentgenograms of the contralateral joint are helpful in evaluating observed changes.

Newer imaging modalities including CT, MRI, and ultrasonographic techniques may provide additional information regarding degenerative joint changes.[117–119] Macroradiographic examination of joints using quantitative microfocal assessments provides fine detail of early lesions.[120,121] On a practical level, these elaborate, costly techniques provide little additional information for routine diagnosis of OA, but they are helpful in differentiating other lesions such as internal joint derangements, avascular necrosis, and pigmented villonodular synovitis.

VARIANT FORMS

The clinical, radiologic, and pathologic findings in certain patients with primary OA are sufficiently different from those usually seen to warrant consideration of these cases as distinct symptom complexes.[91,92,122–126] One such group, characterized by diffuse polyarticular involvement, has been termed *primary generalized osteoarthritis*.[122] A second group demonstrating similar features has been given the name *ankylosing hyperostosis* or *diffuse idiopathic skeletal hyperostosis*.[91,92,126] A third group, characterized by inflammatory synovitis of interphalangeal joints of the hands in association with juxta-articular bone erosions, has been termed *erosive inflammatory osteoarthritis*.[123–125] Finally, a fourth group of patients may exhibit evidence of *chondromalacia patellae* with variable degrees of progression of full forms of osteoarthritic change.[127,128]

Primary Generalized Osteoarthritis

This pattern of "nodal" OA occurs predominantly in middle-aged women.[122] Distal and proximal interphalangeal joints and first carpometacarpal joints are sites of predilection and are often affected in succession. Other peripheral joints including knees, hips, and metatarsophalangeal joints are frequently involved, as are joints of the spine. An acute inflammatory phase commonly precedes chronic articular symptoms. The erythrocyte sedimentation rate is normal or slightly elevated; serum rheumatoid factor is absent. Although the overall pattern of radiologic changes is similar to that usually seen in localized OA, certain differences are notable. Articular facets, neural arches, and spinous processes of the vertebral column are often enlarged, leading to the radiologic designation of "kissing spines." Knee films show marked joint space narrowing with "molten wax" osteophytes as opposed to ordinary, sharply pointed osteophytes. Patients with advanced cases show radiologic changes in excess of the clinical findings. Joint function is often only mildly affected despite severe anatomic changes.

The concept of primary generalized OA as a distinct subset is still controversial. This form may simply reflect more severe disease differentiated only by polyarticular involvement.

In some patients with generalized OA, chondrocalcinosis has been noted.[75,129,130] Studies have demonstrated the presence of diffuse deposits of CPPD crystals.[131,132] A familial form of chondrocalcinosis associated with "apatite" crystal deposition has been described in patients exhibiting symptoms indistinguishable from those seen in generalized OA alone.[133] Synovial fluid BCP crystals (apatite-type) correlated well with the severity of radiographic joint degeneration, and synovial fluid CPPD crystals correlated with patient age but not with degeneration.[134]

Erosive Inflammatory Osteoarthritis

Erosive inflammatory[123,125] OA is another variant of "nodal" disease and involves primarily the distal and proximal interphalangeal joints. The metacarpophalangeal joints may also be involved. The disease is usually hereditary. Painful inflammatory episodes eventually lead to joint deformity and sometimes to ankylosis. Postmenopausal women are most frequently affected. Acute flares may occur for years, but eventually, the affected joints often become asymptomatic. Gelatinous cysts, variably painful and tender, may develop over the involved joints. Inflammation and swelling may be sufficiently severe to suggest a diagnosis of RA. Roentgenographic examination reveals loss of joint cartilage, spur formation, and subchondral bony sclerosis. Bony erosions are prominent. Bony ankylosis, commonly seen, may be the result of synovial inflammation and pannus formation, healing of denuded cartilage surfaces, or coalescence of adjacent osteophytes. Studies of synovium may reveal an intense proliferative synovitis, often indistinguishable from that of RA. The erythrocyte sedimentation rate is usually normal or only slightly elevated. In one study of this disorder,[124] later changes more characteristic of RA were noted in 15% of cases.

Rheumatoid factor and antinuclear antibodies are absent. The presence of abnormal immune mechanisms has been suggested, however, by the demonstration of immune complexes in involved synovium.[135] Synovial fluid and synovial specimens from patients with erosive osteoarthritis have increased numbers of Ia^+ T-lymphocytes, similar to those seen in specimens from patients with RA.[136] These findings are not present in patients with OA of other types. Evidence of sicca syndrome in patients with erosive OA suggests the presence of some immunologic abnormality.[137,138] Such individuals may well represent a subset of erosive inflammatory OA with an autoimmune background.

Premature development of erosive OA of the hands was described in patients with chronic renal failure. The prevalence of grade 3 or 4 OA changes was three times greater in renal failure patients under age 65 than in the control population; erosions of subchondral bone were characteristic findings.[139]

Diffuse Idiopathic Skeletal Hyperostosis; Ankylosing Hyperostosis

DISH is characterized by an unusual type of florid hyperostosis of the spine, with large spurs or marginal bony proliferations in the form of anterior osseous ridges.[91,92,126] Fusion of these ridges often has a flowing appearance (Fig. 103–10). Ossification occurs in the connective tissue surrounding the spine, such as the anterior longitudinal ligament and peripheral disc margins. A predilection exists for involvement of the dorsal spine, although all levels of the spine may be affected. Lesions are most marked at the anterior and right lateral aspects of the vertebral column. The observation of left-sided vertebral bridging in patients with situs inversus suggests that the descending thoracic aorta plays a role in the location of vertebral calcification.[140] Although most common in older patients, the disease has been noted in younger persons. Despite extensive anatomic abnormalities, pain is often minimal or absent, and spinal motion is only moderately limited. Physiologic vertebral ligamentous calcification is probably a variant of this same process.[141]

Subsequent studies have further defined the clinical and pathologic features of this syndrome[91,92] and have demonstrated extraspinal manifestations.[91] Resnick and co-workers defined specific criteria for vertebral involvement, to allow differentiation of this disorder from degenerative disc disease or ankylosing spondylitis.[142] The criteria include flowing ossification along the anterolateral aspect of at least four contiguous vertebral bodies; preservation of disc height; absence of vacuum phenomena or vertebral body marginal sclerosis; and absence of apophyseal joint ankylosis or sacroiliac joint erosions, sclerosis, or fusion. Frequently, radiolucency is apparent between the abnormal calcification and the underlying vertebral body. Extraspinal manifestations include irregular new bone formation or "whiskering," large bony spurs, seen particularly on the olecranon process and the calcaneus (Fig. 103–12), and severe ligamentous calcification, seen mainly in the sacrotuberous, iliolumbar (Fig. 103–13), and patellar ligaments. Periarticular osteophytes were conspicuous.

Spinal stiffness is a prominent clinical complaint despite surprising maintenance of spinal motion with minimal pain. Dysphagia related to severe cervical osteophytosis has been reported. Peripheral joint symptoms include pain in involved elbows, ilium, shoulders, hips, knees, and ankles. Heel pain related to a calcaneal spur is common. The diffus radiographic findings involving both spinal and extraspinal structures have led to the suggestion that this disorder represents an "ossifying diathesis," rather than merely a localized disorder of the spine.

Hyperglycemia is the commonest laboratory abnor-

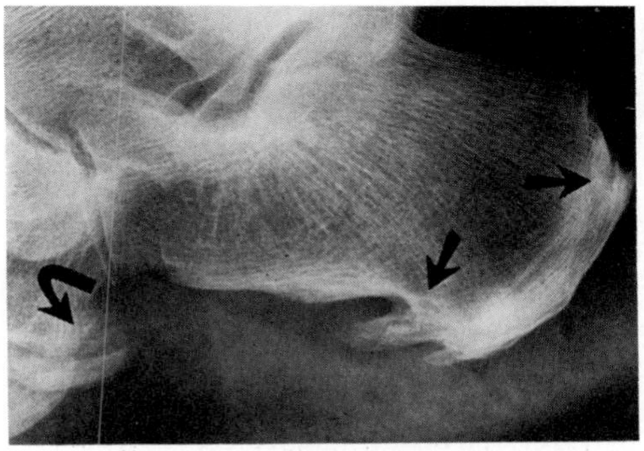

FIGURE 103–12. Diffuse idiopathic skeletal hyperostosis. The calcaneus demonstrates large, irregular spurs at its posterior and plantar aspects (straight arrows). Associated irregularity at the area of the cuboid and fifth metatarsal bones is seen (curved arrow). (Courtesy of Dr. Donald Resnick.)

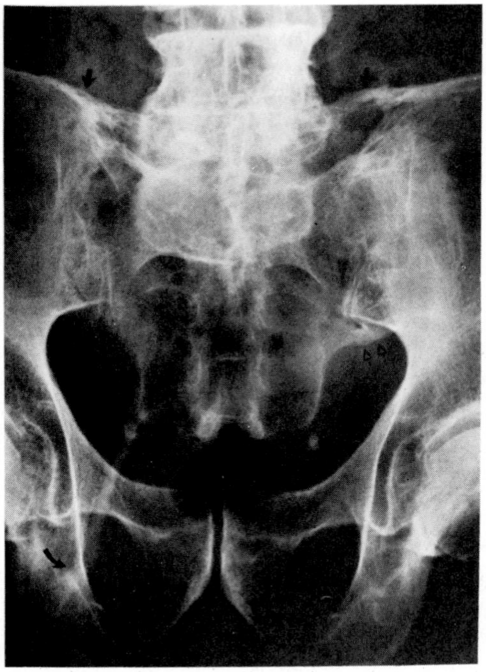

FIGURE 103–13. Radiogram of the pelvis in a patient with diffuse idiopathic skeletal hyperostosis reveals iliolumbar (straight arrow) and sacrotuberous (curved arrow) ligament ossification and para-articular sacroiliac osteophyte formation (open arrows). (From Resnick D., et al.[91]).

mality noted in patients with this syndrome, with an incidence of abnormal glucose tolerance tests about twice that seen in an age-, sex-, and weight-matched populations. In a recent study, diabetes mellitus was present in 40% of these patients.[143] Growth hormone and somatomedin (insulin-like growth factor) levels are normal in DISH, but insulin levels have been shown to be elevated.[144–146]

The etiopathogenesis of DISH is unknown. In one report, 16 of 47 patients with this syndrome were HLA-B27 positive.[147] In other studies, however, a statistically significant increase in HLA-B27 has not been confirmed. Studies of Pima Indians have shown this syndrome to be present in 50% of all individuals, with a 20% frequency of HLA-B27.[148] No significant association was seen, however, with B-locus antigens when Pima Indians with the syndrome were compared to age-matched control subjects. Patients with DISH have increased levels of serum vitamin A.[149] Of special interest in this regard is the observation that patients receiving high doses of synthetic vitamin A derivatives, retinoids, develop an ossification disorder resembling DISH.[150,151] Radiographic features may simulate vertebral and extravertebral manifestations of DISH syndrome, or may be limited to extraspinal tendon and ligament calcification with minimal or absent vertebral involvement. In a limited report, five patients with DISH syndrome were noted to have elevated plasma and urine fluoride levels.[152] Abnormal levels of fluoride were, however, not noted in other studies.[92,153]

A syndrome characterized by *ossification of the posterior longitudinal ligament* has been described, occurring mainly in Japanese.[154] It has been estimated that over 4000 patients in Japan are afflicted with this disorder. Roentgenographic study of the spine reveals lumpy or linear bony masses across one or more disc spaces, sometimes extending from the superior cervical spine to the thoracic region. Ankylosing hyperostosis of the type seen in DISH may be associated. Clinical manifestations may be severe because of spinal cord compression.

Chondromalacia Patellae

This disorder is characterized by degenerative changes of the cartilage of the patella and is included in those conditions associated with OA changes in the knee (see Chapter 90). Although in the past it was identified as a specific entity, chondromalacia patellae is now thought to result from many conditions affecting the knee that lead to cartilage degeneration.[127,128] The malacic changes are considered to be simply the final common pathway through which articular cartilage of the patella degenerates. The specific conditions effecting these changes—such as primary meniscal disease, knee laxity, or abnormal patellar positions such as patella alta—may lead to a similar end stage complex of symptoms. The syndrome is often associated with repeated trauma, as occurs in recurrent lateral subluxation of the patella. Radiologic changes may be limited or absent. Pain is present about the patella and is aggravated by activity such as ascending or, particularly, descending stairs. Paradoxically, vague knee pain may occur after periods of inactivity in the flexed position, such as watching a movie. The disease is typically seen in young adults, especially women, and may be a precursor to the development of patellofemoral compartment OA.

Although the findings described in the foregoing discussion support the existence of various forms of OA, the validity of classifying these as distinct symptom complexes or entities remains open to question. OA may affect many joints in any given patient, so generalized involvement may merely reflect one end of the spectrum of clinical severity. Inflammation may occur in early OA, whether localized or generalized, and its use as a differentiating characteristic is not definitive. In some patients, it is difficult to rule out the coexistence of seronegative RA and OA.[124] Ankylosing hyperostosis has many characteristics that distinguish it from the more common forms of OA. The pathologic changes may be indistinguishable, however, especially in early disease.

PROGNOSIS

The outlook for patients with primary OA is variable, depending on the extent and site of the disease. Involvement of the distal interphalangeal joints, for example, may be associated with a moderate amount of pain, but usually causes little limitation of function unless fine finger motion is required occupationally, such as in typing or in playing musical instruments. Involvement of weight-bearing joints, on the other hand, may lead to marked disability. Similarly, OA of the cervical spine may not only give rise to distressing symptoms but may also lead to severe objective neurologic deficits and disability.

Studies of disease progression in specific joints suggest that not all cases of OA inevitably deteriorate.[42,155] In a study of 6321 patients who had undergone roentgenographic examination of the colon, 4.7% had OA of the hip.[156] Only half of these patients with roentgenographic evidence of hip OA actually needed treatment, and 20% were entirely free of symptoms.

Occasional patients may develop a rapidly progressive, destructive OA of the hip.[157–159] Severe changes are seen both in the acetabulum and in the femoral head. Degenerative pseudocysts and lack of osteophyte formation are characteristic findings. Synovitis noted at operation is of a low grade. Such rapid deterioration of hip joints may be associated with use of nonsteroidal anti-inflammatory drugs (NSAIDs).[160–163] Such an association, if real, might be related to increased joint use permitted by the analgesic action of these drugs, to a direct effect of these drugs on cartilage with inhibition of proteoglycan synthesis, or both.[164] As noted, similar rapid destructive changes have been described unrelated to the use of analgesic agents,[157–159] and the overall clinical experience with these agents over many years in the treatment of various forms of arthritis is reassuring.

Some studies of the natural course of OA of the knee suggest a worse prognosis than in disease of the hip.[114] Most patients worsened during the 10- to 18-year period of followup, with increased pain, deformity, and instability and decreased function. Most patients were unable to use public transportation because of pain on walking. Marked radiologic deterioration was noted, usually limited to the compartment first affected. Varus deformity and early development of pain were unfavorable prognostic factors. Other data suggest that OA of the knee affects only a limited portion of the population and is not inevitably progressive.[18]

The incidence and progression of various radiographic features were examined in a study of the natural history of hand OA.[165] These features increased with age, although their rate of progression slowed as disease severity increased. The earliest radiographic signs of OA were joint space narrowing and possible osteophytes regardless of age. Approximately 10 to 20 years elapsed before any of the radiographic features progressed one grade and even longer before OA progressed from intermediate to late stages. Slowing of OA progression at higher levels of severity has important implications when assessing outcome variables in clinical trials.

Treatment may retard the progression of the disease and is of further value in protecting the contralateral joints exposed to increased stress. Patients should be reassured that the general outlook is favorable and disability is uncommon, in contrast to the threat of crippling seen in patients with RA. Patients should be told that involvement of certain joints may be associated with localized pain, stiffness, and limitation of motion. OA is certainly not always benign.

DIFFERENTIAL DIAGNOSIS

The differentiation of primary OA from other disorders of the musculoskeletal system depends on a correlation of clinical, laboratory, and roentgenographic findings. OA may be confused with other forms of arthritic disease because pain, stiffness, and limitation of motion are common features in all these disorders. Differential diagnosis is further complicated by the high radiologic prevalence of OA in the general population that often bears no relation to the musculoskeletal complaints of a given patient.

In most patients, the diagnosis is simple. In others, however, atypical disease presentation and behavior may require extensive differential diagnostic considerations. Examples of such presentations include OA occurring in an atypical site such as the shoulder, association with a significant inflammatory element, coexistence with other entities such as CPPD crystal deposition, precocious occurrence in young individuals, and OA of the spine with neurologic findings that simulate other underlying neurologic disorders.

RA can usually be differentiated on the basis of its more inflammatory nature and the characteristic pattern of joint involvement. If RA begins as monarticular disease of the knee or hip, however, differentiation from OA may be difficult without prolonged followup study. An increase in the erythrocyte sedimentation rate, a positive test for rheumatoid factor, and synovial fluid analysis are helpful (see Chapter 5). RA may be particularly difficult to differentiate from erosive OA. The pattern of joint involvement is of diagnostic value because the latter is limited mainly to the distal and proximal interphalangeal joints of the hands; RA usually affects the metacarpophalangeal and the wrist and carpal joints and peripheral joints elsewhere. *Joints afflicted with active seropositive RA rarely develop osteophytes.* Some patients with Heberden's nodes or erosive OA may later develop RA, in which case osteophytes *precede* rheumatoid involvement, and a careful clinical history is necessary to identify the presence of a "mixed" arthritis. Mixed disease may also be present but RA leads to secondary degenerative change, but bony overgrowth occurs only in "burned out" disease, and even then, osteophyte formation is abortive. Proximal or distal interphalangeal joint involvement in juvenile RA or psoriatic arthritis is frequently accompanied by nodal formation in these joints.

Rheumatic syndromes characterized by involvement of the distal interphalangeal joints of the hands, such as psoriatic arthritis, Rieter's syndrome, and the arthritis of chronic ulcerative colitis, may be confused with OA of the nodal type. The associated clinical findings of the underlying disease in these patients usually suffice to clarify the diagnosis. Pseudogout syndrome, or chondrocalcinosis articularis, may simulate OA when low-grade arthralgias result from the presence of CPPD crystals in synovial fluid. The pattern of arthritis is clearly different in these patients; the metacarpophalangeal joints, wrists, elbows, shoulders, knees, hips, and ankles are often affected (see Chapter 108). Symptoms related to early manifestations of localized joint disorders such as osteonecrosis, pigmented villonodular synovitis, and chronic infectious arthritis may be mistakenly attributed to degenerative changes seen as coincidental radiographic findings. Neurologic symptoms secondary to spinal OA must be differentiated from those that result from other neurologic disorders. The symptoms of OA of the cervical spine may simulate those of multiple sclerosis, syringomyelia, amyotrophic lateral sclerosis, progressive spinal atrophy, and spinal cord tumors.

SECONDARY OSTEOARTHRITIS

The term *secondary OA* describes those cases that follow a recognizable underlying local or systemic factor, some of which are noted in Table 103–4. A diagnosis of secondary OA should be considered, particularly when the disease develops at an early age.

ACUTE TRAUMA

Joint degeneration may follow acute injury. The history includes the injurious event followed by redness, soft tissue swelling, and pain over the involved joint. In several months, the inflammatory changes subside and are replaced by a hard, painless enlargement. The deformity is localized to the injured joint. The anatomic changes are similar to those seen in primary OA. Injury of this nature involving the distal interphalangeal joints of the hands may lead to traumatic Heberden's nodes.[77] Acute trauma to any of the interphalangeal joints of the hands may lead to the common "baseball finger" (Fig. 103–14).

CHRONIC TRAUMA

An increased prevalence of OA is associated with chronic trauma related to certain occupations. Although exposure of a joint to subtle chronic trauma, or microtrauma, has been suggested as an etiologic factor in the development of primary OA, the relationship between trauma and joint changes, as described previously, seems more clear-cut and supports the classification of such lesions as secondary.

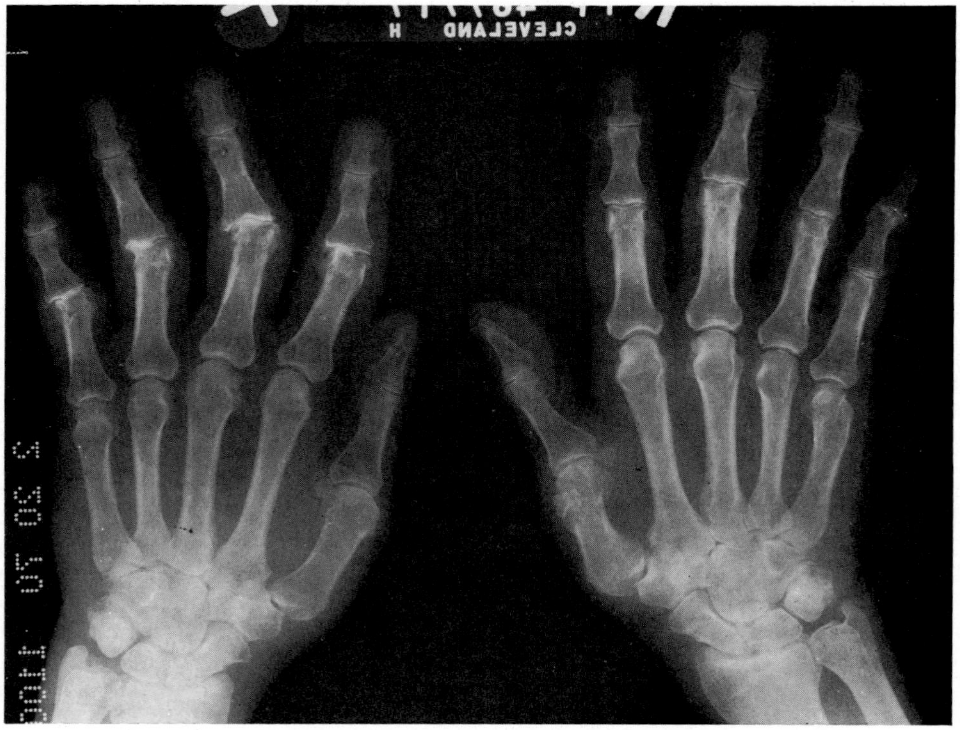

FIGURE 103–14. Secondary osteoarthritis of the second, third, fourth, and fifth proximal interphalangeal joints of the left hand ("baseball fingers") in a patient with recurrent episodes of acute trauma while a semiprofessional baseball player.

OTHER JOINT DISORDERS

Such disorders may be either local or diffuse. Secondary localized OA may follow local joint disorders of other causes, such as fractures, aseptic necrosis, or acute or chronic infection. Early-age OA in the knee may be the result of torn menisci, patellar dislocation, strain resulting from obesity, or poor mechanics as a result of genu varus, or tibial torsion. Localized OA of the hip may follow childhood disorders such as congenital dysplasia of the hip, slipped capital epiphysis, and Legg-Calvé-Perthes disease. OA of the midfoot or hindfoot may result in patients with congenital calcaneonavicular and talocalcaneal coalition.

Diffuse secondary degenerative changes may supervene in patients with RA, in patients with bleeding dyscrasias in whom repeated hemarthroses may occur, or in dwarfs with achondroplasia.

SYSTEMIC METABOLIC OR ENDOCRINE DISORDERS

OA changes may follow several metabolic or endocrine disorders (see also Chapters 112 and 114).

Alkaptonuria (Ochronosis)

This inherited metabolic disease, associated with an absence of homogentisic acid oxidase and characterized by excretion of homogentisic acid in the urine and by a binding of its metabolic products to connective tissue components, is associated with generalized OA.[166] Tissue deposition of brown-black pigment, or ochronosis, is seen primarily in cartilage, skin, and sclera. Degenerative disease of the spine occurs frequently; calcification of numerous intervertebral discs is a characteristic finding. Arthritis of peripheral joints such as hips, knees, and shoulders is less common and develops later. Tissue damage may involve an inhibitory effect of homogentisic acid on chondrocyte growth.[167]

Wilson's Disease

Hepatolenticular degeneration, or Wilson's disease, is an inherited disorder characterized by excessive retention of copper, with degenerative changes in the brain and hepatic cirrhosis. Premature OA has been described as one component of associated articular manifestations of this disorder.[168,169] In a small series of patients, copper was demonstrated in cartilage.[169]

Hemochromatosis

This chronic disease is associated with excessive deposition of iron and fibrosis in a variety of tissues. Although it can result from long-term overingestion of iron and from multiple transfusions, the disease is most often idiopathic. OA changes occur in 20 to 50% of patients.[170,171] Hands, knees, and hips are most commonly involved, although virtually any joint, including those in the feet, can be affected. Involvement of the second and third metacarpophalangeal joints of the hands is particularly characteristic. Synovial tissue shows a striking deposition of iron, most prominently in the synovial lining cells. Roentgenograms reveal joint space narrowing and irregularity, subchondral sclerosis, cystic erosions, bony proliferation, and at times, subluxation. Chondrocalcinosis with deposits of CPPD is seen in up to 60% of patients.

Kashin-Beck Disease

This disorder, characterized by disturbances in growth and maturation in children, is endemic in eastern Siberia, northern China, and northern Korea.[172] Abnormalities in enchondral bone growth lead to dystrophic changes in epiphyseal and metaphyseal areas. Severe secondary OA involves the peripheral joints and the spine. Various causes have been suggested, including a relation to a fungus ingested with cereal grains, iron excess, or selenium deficiency.[173]

Acromegaly

Hypersecretion of growth hormone by the anterior pituitary gland in adults leads to a slowly progressive overgrowth of soft tissue, bone, and cartilage. Peripheral and spinal OA is common. Peripheral joint symptoms occur in about 60% of patients.[174] Most commonly involved are the knees, hips, shoulders, and elbows. Carpal tunnel syndrome is frequently seen. Backache is common, but back motion is often normal or increased because of the thickened intervertebral discs and the laxity of acromegalic ligaments. Early, increased cartilage thickness gives wide joint spaces on roentgenograms. Later, joint space narrowing, osteophyte formation, and subchondral sclerosis occur. Prominent new bone formation is similar to that seen in DISH syndrome and may bear a relationship to increased levels of serum growth hormone.[175,176]

Hyperparathyroidism

Increased levels of parathyroid hormone, whether primary or secondary, can produce many rheumatic problems. It has been postulated that degenerative changes result from damage to cartilage related either to CPPD crystal deposition or to subchondral bony erosion from the resorptive effects of parathyroid hormone. Roentgenograms classically show subperosteal bone resorption, cystic or sclerotic changes in bones, and chondrocalcinosis.

CRYSTAL DEPOSITION DISEASE

Generalized OA has been reported in patients with idiopathic articular chondrocalcinosis.[177] Large joints of the lower limbs and intervertebral joints of the lumbar spine are especially involved. Although a destructive arthropathy has been described in patients with articular chondrocalcinosis,[178] these changes appear to be much more common when generalized OA and chondrocalcinosis coexist.[179] Weight-bearing joints are frequently affected, but involvement of non-weight-bearing joints such as the elbow, shoulder, wrist, and metacarpophalangeal joints also occurs.

Several mechanisms have been postulated to relate the increased association of CPPD crystal deposition to OA.[180,181] In certain patients, obvious crystal deposition antedates significant OA; alterations in calcium matrix in these patients may predispose them to degenerative changes. In other patients, OA is present for a prolonged period and crystal deposition disease occurs later in the disorder. Whether changes in cartilage matrix as a result of OA may favor the deposition of these crystals is still unclear.

An association between BCP (apatite-type) crystal deposition and OA has been described.[134,182,183] The disease in patients with identifiable BCP crystals in synovial fluid is similar to other forms of OA, except the presence of crystals correlates with more severe roentgenographic change. Whether apatite crystals are a result of or a cause of OA is unknown. Severe degenerative changes of the shoulder in association with BCP crystal deposition have been described by Halverson and McCarty and colleagues and termed *Milwaukee shoulder*.[182,183,184] Similar changes have been seen on other joints, such as the knee.[134,184]

NEUROPATHIC DISORDERS

Severe OA occurs in association with neuropathic disorders, as first described by Charcot.[185] The loss of proprioceptive or pain sensation, or both, relaxes the normal protective mechanisms of the joint and leads to articular instability and an exaggerated response to normal daily stresses. Although first described in patients with tabes dorsalis, similar lesions may be seen in other diseases associated with neuropathy including diabetes mellitus, syringomyelia, meningomyelocele, and peripheral nerve section (see Chapter 83).

OVERUSE OF INTRA-ARTICULAR CORTICOSTEROID THERAPY

The development of localized OA has been ascribed to the repeated use of intra-articular injections of adrenal corticosteroids.[186] In these patients, pain relief may allow overuse of already damaged joints and may thereby promote degenerative change. Studies have demonstrated a direct, deleterious effect of corticosteroids on cartilage, suggesting a second mechanism for the development of those degenerative changes.[187]

MISCELLANEOUS ASSOCIATIONS

OA, often polyarticular, is associated with several *bone dysplasias*. These disorders are uncommon and include multiple epiphyseal dysplasia, spondyloepiphyseal dysplasia, and osteo-onychodystrophy, or nail-patella syndrome. Mechanisms for OA are related to the severe distortion of articulating bone. The primary defects leading to bone dysplasia and the possible contributions of the primary metabolic defect are as yet unknown.

Severe cold injury with *frostbite* may lead to premature OA when cold exposure occurs before epiphyseal closure.[188] Joint pain may begin months to years later.

Symptoms and signs, laboratory findings, and roentgenographic abnormalities of secondary OA are generally similar to those seen in the primary form of the disease. Additional findings related to associated underlying disease state are also present. The management of secondary OA is similar to that of the primary form of the disease.

REFERENCES

1. Moskowitz, R.W., Goldberg, V.M., and Berman, L.: Synovitis as a manifestation of degenerative joint disease: An experimental study. Arthritis Rheum., *19*:813, 1976.
2. Goldenberg, D.L., Egan, M.S., and Cohen, A.S.: Inflammatory synovitis in degenerative joint disease. J. Rheumatol., *9*:204–209, 1982.
3. Murray, R.O., The aetiology of primary osteoarthritis of the hip. Br. J. Radiol., *38*:810–824, 1965.
4. Altman, R. et al.: Development of criteria for the classification and reporting of osteoarthritis. Classification of osteoarthritis of the knee. Arthritis Rheum., *29*:1039–1049, 1986.
5. Altman, R., Alarcon, G., Appelrouth, D., et al.: The American College of Rheumatology criteria for classification and reporting of osteoarthritis of the hand. Arthritis Rheum., *33*:1601–1610, 1990.
6. Altman, R., Alarcon, G., Appelrouth, D., et al.: Criteria for classification and reporting of osteoarthritis of the hip. Arthritis Rheum., *34*:505–515, 1991.
7. Altman, R.: Classification of disease: Osteoarthrits. Semin. Arthritis Rheum., *20*(Suppl. 2):40–47, 1991.
8. Peyron, J.G.: Epidemiologic and etiologic approach of osteoarthritis. Semin. Arthritis Rheum., *8*:288–306, 1979.
9. Bland, J.H et al.: A study of inter- and intra-observer error in reading plain roentgenograms of the hands: "To err is human." Am. J. Roentgenol., *105*:853–859, 1969.
10. Lowman, E.W.: Osteoarthritis. JAMA, *157*:487–488, 1955.
11. Lawrence, J.S., Brenner, J.M., and Bier, F.: Osteoarthrosis. Prevalence in the population and relationship between symptoms and x-ray changes. Ann. Rheum. Dis., *25*:1–24, 1966.
12. Van Saase, J.L.C.M., Van Romunde, L.K.J., Cats, A., et al.: Epidemiology of osteoarthritis: Zoetermeer survey. Comparison of radiological osteoarthritis in a Dutch population with that in 10 other countries. Ann. Rheum. Dis., *48*:271–280, 1989.
13. Forman, M., Malamet, R., and Kaplan, D.: A survey of osteoarthritis of the knee in the elderly. J. Rheumatol., *10*:283–287, 1983.
14. Felson, D. et al.: The prevalence of knee osteoarthritis (OA) in the elderly: The Framingham study. Arthritis Rheum., *30*:914–915, 1987.
15. Felson, D., Anderson, J.J., Naimark, A., et al.: Does smoking protect against osteoarthritis? Arthritis Rheum., *32*:166–172, 1989.
16. Lawrence, R.C., Hochberg, M.C., Kelsey, J.L., et al.: Estimates of the prevalence of selected arthritic and musculoskeletal diseases in the United States. J. Rheumatol., *16*:427–441, 1989.
17. Roberts, J., and Burch, T.A.: Prevalence of osteoarthritis in

adults by age, sex, race, and geographic area, United States—1960–1962. [National Center for Health Statistics: vital and health statistics: Data from the national health survey.] United States Public Health Service Publication No. 1000, Series 11, No. 15, 1966. Washington, D.C.: United States Government Printing Office.
18. Kellgren, J.H., Lawrence, J.S., and Bier, F.: Genetic factors in generalized osteo-arthrosis. Ann. Rheum. Dis., *22*:237–255, 1963.
19. Bremner, J.M., Lawrence, J.S., and Miall, W.E.: Degenerative joint disease in a Jamaican rural population. Ann. Rheum. Dis., *27*:326–332, 1968.
20. Solomon, L., Beighton, P., and Lawrence, J.S.: Rheumatic disorders in the South African Negro. Part II. Osteoarthrosis. S. Afr. Med. J., *49*:1737–1740, 1975.
21. Hoaglund, F.T., Yau, A.C.M.C., and Wong, W.L.: Osteoarthritis of the hip and other joints in Southern Chinese in Hong Kong. J. Bone Joint Surg., *55A*:645–657, 1973.
22. Solomon, L., Beighton, P., and Lawrence, J.S.: Rheumatic disorders in the South African Negro, Part II. Osteo-arthrosis. S. Afr. Med. J., *49*:1737–1740, 1975.
23. Mukhopadhaya, B., and Barooah, B.: Osteoarthritis of hip in Indians: An anatomical and clinical study. Indian J. Orthop., *1*:55–62, 1967.
24. Hoaglund, F.T., Shiba, R., Newberg, A.H., and Leung, K.Y.K.: Diseases of the hip. A comparative study of Japanese oriental and American white patients. J. Bone Joint Surg., *67*:1376–1383, 1985.
25. Solomon, L. et al.: Distinct types of hip disorder in Mseleni joint disease. S. Afr. Med. J., *69*:15–17, 1986.
26. Lawrence, J.S.: Hypertension in relation to musculoskeletal disorders. Ann. Rheum. Dis., *34*:451–456, 1975.
27. Lawrence, J.S.: Generalized osteoarthrosis in a population sample. Am. J. Epidemiol., *90*:381–389, 1969.
28. Stecher, R.M., Hersh, A.H., and Hauser, H.: Heberden's nodes: Family history and radiographic appearance of large family. Am. J. Hum. Genet., *5*:46–60, 1953.
29. Doherty, M., Pattrick, M., and Powell, R.: Nodal generalised osteoarthritis is an autoimmune disease. Ann. Rheum. Dis., *49*:1017–1020, 1990.
30. Lawrence, J.S., Gelsthorpe, K., and Morell, G.: Heberden's nodes and HLA markers in generalised osteoarthritis. J. Rheumtaol., *10*:(Suppl. 9):32–33, 1983.
31. Brodsky, A., Appelboan, T., Govaerts, A., and Famey, J.P.: Antigens HLA et nodosites d'Heberden. Acta Rheumatologica, *3*:95–103, 1979.
32. Ercilla, M.G., Brancos, M.A., Breysse, Y., et al.: HLA antigens in Forestier's disease, ankylosing spondylitis, and polyarthrosis of the hands. J. Rheumatol., *4*(Suppl. 3):89–93, 1977.
33. Benavides, G., Cervantes, A., Silva, B., et al.: HLA and Heberden's nodes in Mexican mestizos. Clin. Rheumatol., *4*:97–98, 1985.
34. Pattrick, M., Manhire, A., Ward, A.M., and Doherty, M.: HLA-A, B antigens and α_1-antitrypsin phenotypes in nodal generalised osteoarthritis and erosive osteoarthritis. Ann. Rheum. Dis., *48*:470–475, 1989.
35. Knowlton, R.G., Katzenstein, P.L., Moskowitz, R.W., et al.: Genetic linkage of a polymorphism in the type II procollagen gene (COL2A1) to primary osteoarthritis with mild chondrodysplasia. N. Engl. J. Med., *322*:526–530, 1990.
36. Hull, R., and Pope, F.M.: Osteoarthritis and cartilage collagen genes. Lancet, *1*:1337–1338, 1989.
37. Ala-Kokko, L., Baldwin, C.T., Moskowitz, R.W., and Prockop, D.J.: Single base mutation in the type II procollagen gene (COL2A1) as a cause of primary osteoarthritis associated with a mild chondrodysplasia. Proc. Natl. Acad. Sci. USA, *87*:6565–6568, 1990.
38. Blumberg, B.S. et al.: A study of the prevalence of arthritis in Alaskan Eskimos. Arthritis Rheum., *4*:325–341, 1961.
39. Lawrence, J.S., DeGraff, R., and Laine, V.A.I.: Degenerative joint disease in random samples and occupational groups. *In* The Epidemiology of Chronic Rheumatism, Vol. 1. Edited by J.H. Kellgren, M.R. Jeffrey and J. Ball. Oxford, Blackwell, 1963.
40. Sokoloff, L. et al.: Experimental obesity and osteoarthritis. Am. J. Physiol., *198*:765–770, 1960.
41. Goldin, R.H. et al.: Clinical and radiological survey of the incidence of osteoarthrosis among obese patients. Ann. Rheum. Dis., *35*:349–353, 1976.
42. Seifert, M.H., Whiteside, C.G., and Savage, O.: A 5-year follow-up of fifty cases of idiopathic osteoarthritis of the hip. Ann. Rheum. Dis., *28*:325–326, 1969.
43. Kellgren, J.H.: Osteoarthrosis in patients and population. Br. Med. J., *2*:1–6, 1961.
44. Kellgren, J.H., and Lawrence, J.S.: Osteo-arthrosis and disk degeneration in an urban population. Ann. Rheum. Dis., *17*:388–397, 1958.
45. Leach, R.E., Baumgard, S., and Broom, J.: Obesity: Its relationship to osteoarthritis of the knee. Clin. Orthop., *93*:271–273, 1973.
46. Davis, M.A., Ettinger, W.M., and Neuhaus, J.M.: The role of metabolic factors and blood pressure in the association of obesity with osteoarthritis of the knee. J. Rheumatol., *15*:1827–1832, 1988.
47. Felson, D.T., Anderson, J.J., Naimark, A., et al.: Obesity and knee osteoarthritis: The Framingham osteoarthritis study. Ann. Intern. Med., *109*:18–24, 1988.
48. Silberberg, M., and Silberberg, R.: Osteoarthritis in mice fed diets enriched with animal or vegetable fat. Arch. Pathol., *70*:385–390, 1960.
49. Acheson, R.M., Collart, A.N.: New Haven survey of joint diseases XIII. Relationship between some systemic characteristics and osteoarthrosis in a general population. Ann. Rheum. Dis., *34*:379–387, 1975.
50. Solomon, L., Schnitzler, C.M., and Browett, J.P.: Osteoarthritis of the hip: The patient behind the disease. Ann. Rheum. Dis., *41*:118–125, 1982.
51. Foss, M.V.L., and Byers, P.D.: Bone density, osteoarthrosis of the hip and fracture of the upper end of the femur. Ann. Rheum. Dis., *31*:259–264, 1972.
52. Roh, Y.S., Dequeker, J., and Mulier, J.C.: Bone mass in osteoarthrosis, measured in vivo by photon absorption. J. Bone Joint Surg., *56*:587–591, 1974.
53. Weintroub, S. et al.: Osteoarthritis of the hip and fractures of the proximal end of the femur. Acta Orthop. Scand., *53*:261–264, 1982.
54. Radin, E.L. et al.: Effects of mechanical loading on the tissues of the rabbit knee. J. Orthop. Res., *2*:221–234, 1984.
55. Bird, H.A., Tribe, C.R., and Bacon, P.A.: Joint hypermobility leading to osteoarthrosis and chondrocalcinosis. Ann. Rheum. Dis., *37*:203–211, 1978.
56. Schlomka, G., Schroter, G., and Ocherwal, A.: Uber der bedeutung der beruflischer Belastung fur die entsehung der degenerativen Gelenkleiden. Z. Gesamte. Inn. Med., *10*:993–999, 1955.
57. Partridge, R.E.H., and Duthie, J.J.R.: Rheumatism in dockers and civil servants: A comparison of heavy manual and sedentary workers. Ann. Rheum. Dis., *27*:559–568, 1968.
58. Hadler, N.M. et al.: Hand structure and function in an industrial setting. Influence of three patterns of sterotyped repetitive usage. Arthritis Rheum., *21*:210–220, 1978.
59. Mintz, G., and Fraga, A.: Severe osteoarthritis of the elbow in foundry workers. Arch. Environ. Health, *27*:78–80, 1973.

60. Lindberg, H., and Danielson, L.G.: The relationship between labor and coxarthrosis. Clin. Orthop., *191*:159–161, 1984.
61. Williams, W.V., Cope, R., Gaunt, W.D., et al.: Metacarpophalangeal arthropathy associated with manual labor (Missouri metacarpal syndrome). Arthritis Rheum., *30*:1362–1381, 1987.
62. Kohatsu, N.D., and Schurman, D.J.: Risk factors for the development of osteoarthrosis of the knee. Clin. Orthop., *261*:242–246, 1990.
63. Lane, N.E., Bloch, D.A., Jones, H.H., et al.: Osteoarthritis in the hand: A comparison of handedness and hand use. J. Rheumatol., *16*:637–642, 1989.
64. Puranen, J. et al.: Running and primary osteoarthrosis of the hip. Br. Med., J., *2*:424–425, 1975.
65. Lane, N.E. et al.: Long-distance running, bone density, and osteoarthritis. JAMA, *255*:1147–1151, 1986.
66. Panush, R.S. et al.: Is running associated with degenerative joint disease? JAMA, *255*:1155–1154, 1986.
67. Konradsen, L., Hansen, E.-M.B., and Sondergaard, L.: Long distance running and osteoarthrosis. Am. J. Sports Med., *18*:379–381, 1990.
68. Brodelius, A.: Osteoarthrosis of the talar joints in footballers and ballet dancers. Acta Orthop. Scand., *30*:309–341, 1961.
69. Solonen, K.A.: The joints of the lower extremities of football players. Ann. Chir. Gynaecol. Fenn., *55*:176, 1966.
70. Cobb, S., Merchant, W.R., and Rubin, T.: The relation of symptoms to osteoarthritis. J. Chronic Dis., *5*:197–204, 1957.
71. Gresham, G.E., and Rathey, U.K.: Osteoarthritis in knees of aged persons: Relationship between roentgenographic and clinical manifestations. JAMA, *233*:168–170, 1975.
72. Hernborg, J., and Nilsson, B.E.: The relationship between osteophytes in the knee joint, osteoarthritis and aging. Acta Orthop. Scand., *44*:69–74, 1973.
73. Tokunaga, M. et al.: Change of prostaglandin E level in joint fluids after treatment with flurbioprofen in patients with rheumatoid arthritis and osteoarthritis. Ann. Rheum. Dis., *40*:462–465, 1981.
74. Carman, J.W.: Factors associated with pain and osteoarthritis in the Tecumseh community health study. Semin. Arthritis Rheum., *18*(Suppl. 2):10–13, 1989.
75. Schumacher, H.R. et al.: Osteoarthritis, crystal deposition, and inflammation. Semin. Arthritis Rheum., *11*(Suppl.):116–119, 1981.
76. Heberden, W.: Commentaries on the History and Cure of Diseases, 2nd ed. London, T. Payne, 1803.
77. Stecher, R.M., and Hauser, H.: Heberden's nodes: Roentgenological and clinical appearance of degenerative joint disease of fingers. Am. J. Roentgenol., *59*:326–327, 1948.
78. Stecher, R.M.: Heberden's nodes: Heredity in hypertrophic arthritis of finger joints. Am. J. Med. Sci., *201*:801–809, 1941.
79. Eaton, R.G., Dobranski, A.I., and Littler, J.W.: Marginal osteophyte excision in treatment of mucous cysts. J. Bone Joint Surg., *55A*:570–574, 1973.
80. Patterson, A.C.: Osteoarthritis of the trapezioscaphoid joint. Arthritis Rheum., *18*:375–379, 1975.
81. Halverson, P.B., Cheung, H.S., and McCarty, D.J.: Milwaukee shoulder syndrome (MSS): Description of predisposing factors. Arthritis Rheum., *30*:S131, 1987.
82. Ike, R.W., Arnold, W.J., and Simon, C.: Correlations between radiographic (XR) changes, meniscal chondrocalcinosis and other intra-articular (IA) abnormalities (ABN) in patients (PT) with osteoarthritis of the knee (OAK) undergoing arthroscopy (AR). Arthritis Rheum., *30*:S131, 1987.
83. Felson, D.T., Anderson, J.J., Naimark, A., et al.: The prevalence of chondrocalcinosis in the elderly and its association with knee osteoarthritis: The Framingham study. J. Rheumatol., *16*:1241–1245, 1989.
84. Evarts, C.M.: Challenge of the aging hip. Geriatrics, *24*:112–119, 1969.
85. Meachim, G., et al.: An investigation of radiological, clinical and pathological correlations in osteoarthrosis of the hip. Clin. Radiol., *31*:565–574, 1980.
86. Macys, J.R., Bullough, P.G., and Wilson, P.D., Jr.: Coxarthrosis: A study of the natural history based on a correlation of clinical, radiographic, and pathologic findings. Semin. Arthritis Rheum., *10*:66–80, 1980.
87. Doherty, M., and Preston, B.: Primary osteoarthritis of the elbow. Ann. Rheum. Dis., *48*:743–747, 1989.
88. McKendry, R.J.R. Nodal osteoarthritis of the toes. Arthritis Rheum., *16*:126–134, 1986.
89. Prince, D.S., et al.: Osteophyte-induced dysphagia: Occurrence in ankylosing hyperostosis. JAMA, *234*:77–78, 1975.
90. Forestier, J., Jacqueline, F., and Rotes-Querol, J.: Ankylosing Spondylitis: Clinical Considerations, Roentgenology, Pathologic Anatomy, Treatment. Springfield, IL, Charles C. Thomas, 1956.
91. Resnick, D., Shaul, S.R., and Robins, J.M.: Diffuse idiopathic skeletal hyperostosis (DISH): Forestier's disease with extraspinal manifestations. Radiology, *115*:513–524, 1975.
92. Utsinger, P.D., Resnick, D., and Shapiro, R.: Diffuse skeletal abnormalities in Forestier disease. Arch. Intern. Med., *136*:763–768, 1976.
93. Harata, S., Tohno, S., and Kawagishi, T.: Osteoarthritis of the atlanto-axial joint. Int. Orthop., *5*:277–282, 1981.
94. Arnoldi, C.C., Brodsky, A.E., and Cauchoix, J.: Lumbar spinal stenosis and nerve root entrapment syndromes—Definition and classification. Clin. Orthop., *115*:4–5, 1976.
95. Mehraban, F., Finegan, C.K., and Moskowitz, R.W.: Serum keratan sulfate. Quantitative and qualitative comparisons in inflammatory versus noninflammatory arthritides. Arthritis Rheum., *34*:383–392, 1991.
96. Witter, J., Roughley, P.J., Webber, C., et al.: The immunologic detection and characterization of cartilage proteoglycan degradation products in synovial fluids of patients with arthritis. Arthritis Rheum., *30*:519–529, 1987.
97. Lohmander, L.S., Dahlberg, L., Ryd, L., and Heinegard, D.: Increased levels of proteoglycan fragments in the knee joint after injury. Arthritis Rheum., *32*:1434–1442, 1989.
98. Thonar, E.J.-M.A., Lenz, M.E., Klintworth, G.K., et al.: Quantification of keratan sulfate in blood as a marker of cartilage catabolism. Arthritis Rheum., *28*:1367–1376, 1985.
99. Goldberg, R.L., Huff, J.P., Lenz, M.E., et al.: Elevated plasma levels of hyaluronate in patients with osteoarthritis and rheumatoid arthritis. Arthritis Rheum., *34*:799–807, 1991.
100. Paimela, L., Heiskanen, A., Kurki, P., et al.: Serum hyaluronate level as a predictor of radiologic progression in early rheumatoid arthritis. Arthritis Rheum., *34*:815–821, 1991.
101. Siebel, M.J., Duncan, A., and Robins, S.P.: Urinary hydroxypyridinium crosslinks provide indices of cartilage and bone involvement in arthritic diseases. J. Rheumatol., *16*:964–970, 1989.
102. Brandt, K.D.: A pessimistic view of seriologic markers for diagnosis and management of osteoarthritis. Biochemical, immunologic and clinicopathologic barriers. J. Rheumatol., *16*(Suppl. 18):39–42, 1989.
103. Cheung, H.S. et al.: Identification of collagen subtypes in synovial fluid sediments from arthritic patients. Am. J. Med., *68*:73–79, 1980.
104. Fam, A.G. et al.: Cholesterol crystals in osteoarthritic joint effusions. J. Rheumatol., *8*:273–280, 1981.
105. Stastny, P. et al.: Lymphokines in the rheumatoid joint. Arthritis Rheum., *18*:237–243, 1975.
106. Moskowitz, R.W., and Kresina, T.F.: Immunofluorescent analy-

sis of experimental osteoarthritic cartilage and synovium: Evidence for selective deposition of immunoglobulin and complement in cartilaginous tissues. J. Rheumatol., *13*:391–396, 1986.
107. Kresina, T.F., Malemud, C.J., and Moskowitz, R.W.: Analysis of osteoarthritic cartilage using monoclonal antibodies reactive with rabbit proteoglycan. Arthritis Rheum., *29*:863–871, 1986.
108. Cooke, T.D.V. et al.: Identification of immunoglobulins and complement in rheumatoid articular collagenous tissues. Arthritis Rheum., *18*:541–551, 1975.
109. Tanaka, S. Ito, T., Hamamoto, K., and Torizuka, K.: Clearance of technetium pertechnetate from the hip joint with arthrosis deformans. Am. J. Roentgenol. Radium Ther. Nucl. Med., *118*:870–875, 1973.
110. Hutton, C.W. et al.: ^{99m}Tc HMDP bone scanning in generalised nodal osteoarthritis. I. Comparison of the standard radiograph and four hour bone scan image of the hand. Ann. Rheum. Dis., *45*:617–621, 1986.
111. Hutton, C.W. et al.: ^{99m}Tc HMDP bone scanning in generalised nodal osteoarthritis. II. The four hour bone scan image predicts radiographic change. Ann. Rheum. Dis., *45*:622–626, 1986.
112. Arnoldi, C.C. et al.: Intraosseous phlebography, intraosseous pressure measurements and ^{99m}Tc-polyphosphate scintigraphy in patients with various painful conditions in the hip and knee. Acta Orthop. Scand., *51*:19–28, 1980.
113. Arnoldi, C.C., Linderholm, H., and Müssbichler, H.: Venous engorgement and intraosseous hypertension in osteoarthritis of the hip. J. Bone Joint Surg., *54B*:409–421, 1972.
114. Hernborg, J.S., and Nilsson, B.E.: The natural course of untreated osteoarthritis of the knee. Clin. Orthop., *123*:130–137, 1977.
115. Swezey, R.L., Peter, J.B., and Evans, P.L.: Osteoarthritis of the metacarpophalangeal joint: Hook-like osteophytes. Arthritis Rheum., *12*:405–410, 1969.
116. Resnick, D., and Vint, V.: The "tunnel" view in assessment of cartilage loss in osteoarthritis of the knee. Radiology, *137*:547–548, 1980.
117. Martel, W., Adler, R.S., Chan, K., et al.: Overview: New methods of imaging osteoarthritis. J. Rheumatol., *18*:(Suppl. 27):32–37, 1991.
118. Li, K.C., Higgs, J., Alsen, A.M., et al.: MRI in osteoarthritis of the hip: Gradations of severity. Magnet. Reson. Imag., *6*:229–236, 1988.
119. Bongartz, G., Bock, E., Horbach, T., and Requardt, H.: Degenerative cartilage lesions of the hip-magnetic resonance evaluation. Magnet. Reson. Imag., *7*:179–186, 1989.
120. Buckland-Wright, J.C., MacFarlane, D.G., Lynch, J.A., and Clark, B.: Quantitative microfocal radiographic assessment of progression in osteoarthritis of the hand. Arthritis Rheum., *33*:57–65, 1990.
121. Buckland-Wright, J.C., and Bradshaw, C.R.: Clinical applications of high-definition microfocal radiography. Br. J. Radiol., *62*:209–217, 1989.
122. Kellgren, J.H., and Moore, R.: Generalized osteoarthritis and Heberden's nodes. Br. Med. J., *1*:181–187, 1952.
123. Crain, D.C.: Interphalangeal osteoarthritis. JAMA, *175*:1049–1053, 1961.
124. Ehrlich, G.E.: Inflammatory osteoarthritis: II. The superimposition of RA. J. Chronic Dis., *25*:635–643, 1972.
125. Ehrlich, G.E.: Inflammatory osteoarthritis: I. The clinical syndrome. J. Chronic Dis., *25*:317–328, 1972.
126. Forestier, J., and Lagier, R.: Ankylosing hyperostosis of the spine. Clin. Orthop., *74*:65–83, 1971.
127. DeHaven, K.E., Dolan, W.A., and Mayer, P.J.: Chondromalacia patellae in athletes. Am. J. Sports Med., *7*:1–5, 1979.
128. Goodfellow, J.W., Hungerford, D.S., and Woods, C.: Patellofemoral mechanics and pathology: II. Chondromalacia patellae. J. Bone Joint Surg., *58B*:291–299, 1976.
129. Dieppe, P.A., et al.: Mixed crystal deposition disease in osteoarthritis. Br. Med. J., *1*:150–152, 1978.
130. Doyle, E.V., Huskisson, E.C., and Willoughby, D.A.: A histological study of inflammation in osteoarthritis: The role of calcium phosphate crystal deposition. Ann. Rheum. Dis., *38*:192, 1979,
131. Alexander, G.M. et al.: Pyrophosphate arthropathy: A study of metabolic associations and laboratory data. Ann. Rheum. Dis., *41*:377–381, 1982.
132. Dieppe, P.A. et al.: Pyrophosphate arthropathy: A clinical and radiological study of 105 cases. Ann. Rheum. Dis., *41*:371–376, 1982.
133. Marcos, J.C. et al.: Idiopathic familial chondrocalcinosis due to apatite crystal deposition. Am. J. Med., *71*:557–564, 1981.
134. Halverson, P.B., and McCarty, D.J.: Patterns of radiographic abnormalities associated with basic calcium phosphate and calcium pyrophosphate dihydrate crystal deposition in the knee. Ann. Rheum. Dis., *45*:603–605, 1986.
135. Ohno, O., and Cooke, T.D.: Electron microscopic morphology of immunoglobulin aggregates and their interaction in rheumatoid articular collagenous tissues. Arthritis Rheum., *21*: 516–517, 1978.
136. Utzinger, P.D., and Fite, F.L.: Immunologic evidence for inflammation (I) in osteoarthritis (OA): High percentage of Ia^+ T lymphocytes (L) in the synovial fluid (SL) and synovium (S) of patients with erosive osteoarthritis (EOA). Arthritis Rheum., *25*:S44, 1982.
137. Singleton, P.T., Cervantes, A.G., and McKoy, J.: Sicca complex and erosive osteoarthritis: Immunologic implications of a new osteoarthritis subset. Arthritis Rheum., *25*:S33, 1982.
138. Shuckett, R., Russell, M.L., and Gladman, D.D.: Atypical erosive osteoarthritis and Sjögren's syndrome. Ann. Rheum. Dis., *45*:281–288, 1986.
139. Duncan, I.J.S., Hurst, N.P., Sebben, R., et al.: Premature development of erosive osteoarthritis of hands in patients with chronic renal failure. Ann. Rheum. Dis., *49*:378–382, 1990.
140. Bahrt, K.M., Nashal, D.J., and Haber, G.: Diffuse idiopathic skeletal hyperostosis in a patient with situs inversus. Arthritis Rheum., *26*:811–812, 1983.
141. Smith, C.F., Pugh, D.G., and Polley, H.F.: Physiologic vertebral ligamentous calcification: Aging process. Am. J. Roentgenol., *74*:1049–1058, 1955.
142. Resnick, D. et al.: Diffuse idiopathic skeletal hyperostosis (DISH) [ankylosing hyperostosis of Forestier and RotesQuerol]. Semin. Arthritis Rheum., *7*:153–187, 1978.
143. Robbes-Ruy, E., Rojo-Mejia, A., Harrison-Garcin Calderon, J., and Discoya-Arbanil, J.: Diffuse idiopathic skeletal hyperostosis: Clinical and radiologic manifestations in 50 patients. Arthritis Rheum., *25*:S101, 1982.
144. Littlejohn, G.O., and Smythe, H.A.: Marked hyperinsulinemia after glucose challenge in patients with diffuse idiopathic skeletal hyperostosis. J. Rheumatol., *8*:965–968, 1981.
145. Littlejohn, G.O.: Insulin and new bone formation in diffuse idiopathic skeletal hyperostosis. Clin. Rheum., *4*:294–300, 1985.
146. Denko, C.W., Boja, B., and Moskowitz, R.W.: Growth-promoting peptides—Insulin-like growth factor-1, insulin, growth hormone in diffuse idiopathic skeletal hyperostosis. Arthritis Rheum., *32*(Suppl.):S84, 1989.
147. Shapiro, R., Utsinger, P.D., and Wiesner, K.B.: The association of HLA-B27 with Forestier's disease (vertebral ankylosing hyperostosis). J. Rheumatol., *3*:4–8, 1976.
148. Spagnole, A., Bennett, P., and Terasaki, P.: Vertebral ankylosing hyperostosis (Forestier's disease) and HLA antigens in Pima Indians. Arthritis Rheum., *21*:467–472, 1978.

149. Abiteboul, M. et al.: Hyperostose vertébral ankylosante et métabolisme de la vitamine A. Rev. Rhum., *9*:8–9, 1981.
150. Pittsley, R.A., and Yoder, F.W.: Retinoid hyperostosis. N. Engl. J. Med., *308*:1012–1025, 1983.
151. Di Giovanna, J.J., Helfgott, R.K., Gerber, H.L., and Peck, G.L.: Extraspinal tendon and ligament calcification associated with long-term therapy with etretinate. N. Engl. J. Med., *315*: 1177–1182, 1986.
152. Mills, D.M. et al.: Association of diffuse idiopathic skeletal hyperostosis and fluorosis (Abstract.) Arthritis Rheum., *26*(Suppl.):S11, 1983.
153. Utsinger, P.D.: A clinical and laboratory analysis of 200 patients with DISH. Clin. Exp. Rheumatol. (in press).
154. Ono, K. et al.: Ossified posterior longitudinal ligament, a clinicopathologic study. Spine, *2*:126–138, 1977.
155. Nilsson, B.E., Danielsson, L.G., and Hernborg, S.A.J.: Clinical feature and natural course of coxarthrosis and gonarthrosis. Scand. J. Rheumatol., *43*(Suppl.):13–21, 1982.
156. Jorring, K.: Osteoarthritis of the hip. Epidemiology and clinical role. Acta Orthop. Scand., *51*:523–530, 1980.
157. Edelman, J., and Owen, E.T.: Acute progressive osteoarthropathy of large joints: Report of three cases. J. Rheumatol., *8*:482–485, 1981.
158. Keats, T.E., Johnstone, W.H., O'Brien, W.M.: Large joint destruction in erosive osteoarthritis. Skeletal Radiol., *6*:267–269, 1981.
159. Bouvier, M., Bonvoisin, B., Colson, F., and David, P.H.: Les coxarthroses destructices rapides. Etude radioclinique de neuf cas. Ann. Radiol., *28*:549–553, 1985.
160. Moskowitz, R.W.: Use of nonsteroidal antiinflammatory drugs in rheumatology: A review. Semin. Arthritis Rheum., *15*:1–10, 1986.
161. Ronningen, H., and Langeland, N.: Indomethacin treatment in osteoarthritis of the hip joint. Acta Orthop. Scand., *50*:169–174, 1979.
162. Newman, N.M., and Ling, R.S.M.: Acetabular bone destruction related to non-steroidal anti-inflammatory drugs. Lancet, *2*:11–13, 1985.
163. Rashad, S., Revell, P., Hemingway, A., et al.: Effect of nonsteroidal anti-inflammatory drugs on the course of osteoarthritis. Lancet, *2*:519–522, 1989.
164. Palmoski, M.J., and Brandt, K.D.: Effect of some nonsteroidal anti-inflammatory drugs on proteoglycan metabolism and organization in canine articular cartilage. Arthritis Rheum., *23*:1010–1020, 1980.
165. Kallman, D.A., Wigley, F.M., Scott, W.W., Jr., et al.: The longitudinal course of hand osteoarthritis in a male population. Arthritis Rheum., *33*:1323–1332, 1990.
166. O'Brien, W.M., La Du, B.N., and Bunim, J.J.: Biochemical, pathologic and clinical aspects of alcaptonuria, ochronosis and ochronotic arthropathy: Review of world literature (1584–1962). Am. J. Med., *34*:813–838, 1963.
167. Angeles, A.P., Badger, R., Bruber, H.E., and Seegmiller, J.E.: Chondrocyte growth inhibition induced by homogentisic acid and its partial prevention with ascorbic acid. J. Rheumatol., *16*:512–517, 1989.
168. Golding, D.N., Walshe, J.M.: Arthropathy of Wilson's disease: Study of clinical and radiological features in 32 patients. Ann. Rheum. Dis., *36*:99–111, 1977.
169. Menerey, K.A., Eider, W., Brewer, G.J., et al.: The arthropathy of Wilson's disease: Clinical and pathologic features. J. Rheumatol., *15*:331–337, 1988.
170. Hamilton, E., et al.: Idiopathic hemochromatosis. Q. J. Med., *145*:171–182, 1968.
171. Schumacher, H.R.: Articular cartilage in the degenerative arthropathy of hemochromatosis. Arthritis Rheum., *25*: 1460–1468, 1982.
172. Nesterov, A.I.: The clinical course of Kashin-Beck disease. Arthritis Rheum., *7*:29–40, 1964.
173. Wei, X.W., Wright, G.C., and Sokoloff, L.: The effect of sodium selenite on chondrocytes in monolayer culture. Arthritis Rheum., *29*:660–664, 1986.
174. Bluestone, R. et al.: Acromegalic arthropathy. Ann. Rheum. Dis., *30*:243–258, 1971.
175. Littlejohn, G.O., Hall, S., Brand, C.A., et al.: New bone formation in acromegaly. Clin. Exp. Rheum., *4*:99–104, 1986.
176. Bijlsma, J.W.J., and Duursma, S.A.: Serum concentrations of somatomedins and growth hormone in relation to bone metabolism in acromegaly and thyroid dysfunction. Clin. Exp. Rheum., *4*:105–110, 1986.
177. Atkins, C.J. et al.: Chondrocalcinosis and arthropathy: Studies in haemochromatosis and in idiopathic chondrocalcinosis. Q. J. Med., *39*:71–82, 1970.
178. Richards, A.J., and Hamilton, E.B.D.: Destructive arthropathy in chondrocalcinosis articularis. Ann. Rheum. Dis., *33*: 196–203, 1974.
179. Gerster, J.C., Vischer, T.L., and Fallet, G.H.: Destructive arthropathy in generalized osteoarthritis with articular chondrocalcinosis. J. Rheumatol., *2*:265–269, 1975.
180. Hernborg, J., Linden, B., and Nilsson, B.O.E.: Chondrocalcinosis: A secondary finding in osteoarthritis of the knee. Geriatrics, *32*:123–126, 1977.
181. Wilkins, E., Dieppe, P., Maddison, P., and Evison, G.: Osteoarthritis and articular chondrocalcinosis in the elderly. Ann. Rheum. Dis., *42*:280–284, 1983.
182. McCarty, D.J. et al.: "Milwaukee shoulder"—Association of microspheroids containing hydroxyapatite crystals, active collagenase, and neutral proteases with rotator cuff defects. I. Clinical aspects. Arthritis Rheum., *24*:464–473, 1981.
183. Halverson, P.G. et al.: "Milwaukee shoulder"—Association of microspheroids containing hydroxyapatite crystals, active collagenase, and neutral protease with rotator cuff defects. II. Synovial fluid studies. Arthritis Rheum., *24*:474–483, 1981.
184. Halverson, P.B. et al.: Milwaukee shoulder syndrome: Eleven additional cases with involvement of the knee in seven (basic calcium phosphate crystal deposition disease). Semin. Arthritis Rheum., *14*:36–44, 1984.
185. Charcot, J.M.: Sur quelques arthropathies qui paraissent dépendre d'une lésion du cerveau ou de la moelle épinière: arthrites dans l'hémiplégie de cause cérébrale. Arch. Physiol. Norm. Pathol., *2*:379–400, 1868.
186. Gottlieb, N.L., and Risken, W.G.: Complications of local corticosteroid injections. JAMA, *243*:1547–1548, 1980.
187. Moskowitz, R.W. et al.: Experimentally induced corticosteroid arthropathy. Arthritis Rheum., *13*:236–243, 1970.
188. Glick, R., and Parhami, N.: Frostbite arthritis. J. Rheumatol., *6*:456–460, 1979.

104

Management of Osteoarthritis

THOMAS J. SCHNITZER

The past decade has seen significant advances in our understanding of the biochemical basis of cartilage metabolism and in new, more sensitive noninvasive imaging methods, which have permitted the earlier definition of changes in joints affected by osteoarthritis (OA). Despite these advances, clinicians are faced with the same treatment dilemmas: How to provide improved function and symptomatic relief with the fewest untoward effects? Although no striking therapeutic advances have been made, a better understanding of disease pathophysiology interventions aimed at specific steps in the process has become possible. Perhaps more important, it is now possible to monitor the effects of such interventions in more specific ways, allowing refinement of therapy. The approach to treatment of OA is discussed in relation to the paradigm presented in Fig. 104–1. This model is supported by evidence presented here and in earlier chapters and serves to permit an understanding of how various therapeutic modalities and interventions may affect the disease.

It is important to differentiate the disease *process* from the *outcome* of the process.[1,2] To the clinician, the outcome of the process is considered the disease. It is the clinical condition that is apparent and of which the patient complains. However, what must be kept in mind is that the clinical condition is the end result of several different processes that have taken place over time. Treatment of the patient must address the symptomatic complaints and attempt to interfere with the ongoing processes driving the pathologic condition. Prevention of OA will eventually be accomplished by interventions affecting the processes leading to the development of disease before the onset of symptoms. This is not yet possible, because there are no diagnostic "markers" permitting definition of the preclinical stage of OA. Identification of such markers may permit prevention of those processes ultimately leading to joint damage rather than attempting to promote repair, reduce inflammation, and alleviate symptoms when the disease process is relatively advanced.

THE DIAGNOSTIC CHALLENGE

The first step in approaching a patient suspected of having OA is accurate diagnosis. Because of the extremely high prevalence of OA,[3,4] particularly in individuals over the age of 65 years, radiographic and even clinical evidence of OA may often be found in patients complaining of pain in and around their joints that is due to a variety of other unrelated conditions. The clinician must make certain that the symptoms are indeed a result of OA and not a consequence of concomitant disease.[5]

The disorders that may present in a manner similar to OA are numerous and in many instances location specific. The knees, fingers, and hips are the most frequently symptomatic diarthrodial joints in OA.[3,4] Osteoarthritis can be mimicked by inflammatory arthropathies, particularly seronegative spondyloarthropathies, typically asymmetric and affecting large joints; crystal-induced arthropathies, especially pseudogout in the elderly with a predilection for knees and other large joints; osteonecrosis of the hip or knee, particularly in populations with relevant risk factors; fibromyalgia; anserine bursitis; tensor fascia lata syndrome; and a wide range of soft tissue injuries. Radiculopathies can manifest pain in either the hip or the knee. In sum, the diagnosis of symptomatic OA can be made only after exclusion of other conditions and when supported by appropriate clinical signs and symptoms, laboratory data, and radiographic findings. These other conditions

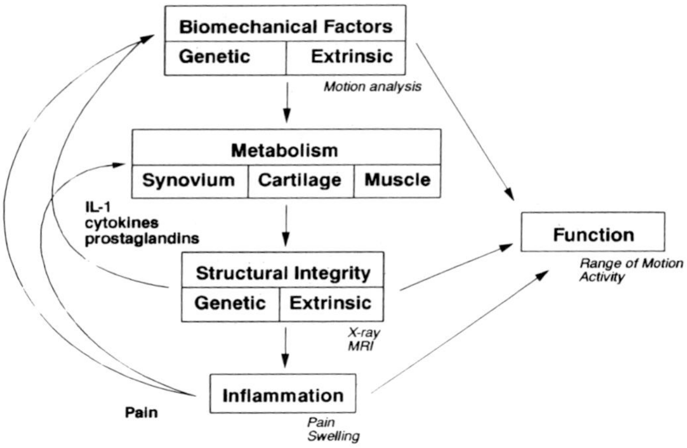

FIGURE 104–1. Conceptual overview of pathophysiology of osteoarthritis. Those items in italics represent clinical parameters of the processes that are used by physicians to define the condition. IL-1 = interleukin-1; MRI = magnetic resonance imaging.

can often exist together with symptomatic OA, of course.

ANALGESIC INTERVENTION

Pain relief is the primary goal of most OA patients. To treat effectively any painful condition, a comprehensive understanding of pain mechanisms is desirable. Unfortunately, little is known about the cause of pain in OA.

As cartilage is aneural, pain must originate from stimulation of sensory receptors in the adjacent synovial tissue, bone, or surrounding connective tissues. It is likely that a number, if not all, of these sites are involved in producing the pain, explaining the varying nature of the quality of pain perceived by different patients or in the same patient at different times. Microfractures of the underlying bone in involved joints have been well described.[5a] tendons and ligaments are subject to abnormal loads; muscles are fatigued by overuse. A significant degree of synovial inflammation often occurs, leading to pain as well.

The role of simple analgesic agents as the sole therapeutic intervention is still poorly defined. Brandt and colleagues found that acetaminophen was as effective as an over-the-counter dose or anti-inflammatory dose of ibuprofen for relief of pain in patients with relatively mild OA of the knee in a 1-month blinded trial.[5b] Other studies also suggest that pure analgesic agents are of similar benefit to nonsteroidal anti-inflammatory drugs (NSAIDs) when used over the short term.[6–8] Unfortunately, the lack of placebo group prevents definitive conclusions to be drawn from any of these studies.

The major value of simple analgesic agents such as acetaminophen or propoxyphene is their relative freedom from serious side effects commonly encountered with the NSAIDs. Interruption of the pain pathway would be expected to have a direct effect on biomechanical factors important in the evolution of the disease process. Whether such alterations are beneficial or detrimental probably is highly dependent on the individual situation: Lack of any painful feedback may lead to overuse and rapid joint destruction, whereas in other circumstances pain reduction could lead to reduced muscle spasm with improved biomechanics and more normal joint loading.

Further controlled studies using simple analgesic agents in defined populations of patients with OA are clearly needed. These agents will continue to play an important role in the treatment of patients with OA, particularly patients who need short-term pain relief and who may have exhibited an intolerance to use of NSAIDs.

NONSTEROIDAL ANTI-INFLAMMATORY AGENTS

NSAIDs have been widely used in OA for over three decades, but the rationale for their use is poorly understood. Their ultimate value in patients with OA is a matter of debate.[9–11] Some clinicians feel that they may be detrimental to cartilage, leading to more rapid joint destruction. These compounds were, after all, developed for their ability to suppress synovitis in classic animal models. Subsequently, all except nonacetylated salicylates and phenylbutazone were found to be potent in vitro inhibitors of prostaglandin synthesis. All are mild-to-moderate analgesic agents.

As a consequence of their demonstrated efficacy in animal and human inflammatory arthritides, these agents were tested in patients with OA. A very large number of clinical trials has clearly demonstrated the efficacy of NSAIDs in the short-term symptomatic relief of pain in OA. No significant differences in efficacy are apparent among different NSAIDs or classes of NSAIDs. The clinical improvement observed may be entirely secondary to the analgesic effects of these agents or to a reduction in the accompanying synovitis. Because of the chronic course and fundamentally degenerative nature of OA, long-term studies may be more relevant. In the limited number of such studies, the major finding has been how few people continue on therapy for long periods; patients stop therapy for lack of efficacy or, more importantly, because of side effects resulting from toxicity.[12]

It is clear that biochemical alterations in cartilage occur well before clinical disease is evident.[13,14] Once symptoms are present, considerable structural damage usually has already occurred, with evidence of degradative processes involving all aspects of the cartilage matrix. At the same time, there is evidence of attempts at cartilage repair. Therefore, treatment initiated at this point should inhibit the destructive processes while promoting cartilage anabolic activity. With this notion in mind, several new drugs have been developed (see following), and the concept of "chondroprotective agents" has emerged.[9] And many of the available NSAIDs have been examined in vitro and in vivo for their effects on cartilage metabolism.[11,15–19] Significant differences were found among NSAIDs, but the clinical relevance of these differences is still unclear. Additional work in humans needs to be undertaken using new, more sophisticated means of following cartilage metabolism and integrity. Such pharmacologic intervention may have no effect on the underlying factors responsible for initiating and perpetuating the metabolic disturbances, particularly if these are secondary to biomechanical alterations or genetic molecular abnormalities.

In Vitro Metabolic Studies

An extensive literature details the direct effects of various NSAIDs on anabolic and catabolic processes in cartilage, both in vitro and ex vivo. These studies, using different animal systems, were stimulated by observations that the most commonly used NSAID, aspirin, inhibited proteoglycan synthesis and under certain conditions led to enhanced cartilage destruction.[18–20] Numerous studies have confirmed this observation. Although some other NSAIDs shared this property, others did not. Some actually stimulated sulfate incorporation into glycosaminoglycans, a reflection of increased proteoglycan synthesis.[16,17] Relatively few studies have looked at effects of NSAIDs on the metabolism of hyaluronic acid, the other major component of cartilage extracellular matrix. Available studies demonstrated heterogeneity of their effects; some NSAIDs inhibited whereas others stimulated hyaluronate synthesis.[21]

Besides stimulating cartilage matrix synthesis, inhibition of the degradative processes is important. NSAIDs also vary in their ability to interfere with catabolic processes.[10] Cartilage matrix proteoglycans can be degraded in vitro by various enzymes, including metalloproteinases and serine proteases. Some NSAIDs are more effective inhibitors of these enzymes than others.[15–17] Cartilage matrix integrity may be compromised by mediators such as interleukin-1 (IL-1), proteolytic enzymes, or free oxygen radicals produced by synoviocytes or by mononuclear cells. These molecules can be targeted for intervention. Certain NSAIDs interfere with both the synthesis and activity of several of these mediators.[10,22,23]

Interpretation of many of these studies is difficult because of differences in species, experimental conditions, and drug concentrations. Few studies have examined *net* matrix production, which is the bottom line. Because of technical considerations, either the anabolic or the catabolic effects are examined in isolation. Compounds that reduce synthesis but in parallel reduce degradation may be more beneficial than compounds enhancing both processes. The ratio between the two, the net change, unfortunately has not often been addressed.

Human and In Vivo Animal Studies

Several reports have suggested that the use of indomethacin or other NSAIDs in OA produced an accelerated destruction of affected joints.[24–26] The controversy regarding the potential harmful effects of NSAIDs in OA remains, despite several excellent studies demonstrating no difference in progression of radiographic changes between patients treated with NSAIDs, analgesic agents, or placebo.[27,28] That some patients with OA demonstrate rapid joint destruction is irrefutable, but this probably relates more to the nature of the disease rather than to its treatment.[28]

To demonstrate effects of NSAIDs on cartilage integrity, animal studies have been conducted using various experimental models of OA.[10,11,18,19,29] These have largely confirmed the in vivo findings. Many NSAIDs caused an increased rate of loss of cartilage matrix integrity. Others were associated with stabilization of the degradative process and even a stimulation of matrix regeneration. Interpretation of these data is again confounded by the extreme variability in results in different species and because the animal models used represent disease that differs significantly in cause and possibly in mechanism from that seen in humans. *Uncritical extrapolation of these findings to human OA is not warranted.* Studies of NSAID effects on human OA cartilage are extremely limited.[30] Available results have generally confirmed those seen in animal studies, but again, interpretation is limited by the tremendous variability in the condition of clinical samples and the lack of any true controls. Because of these studies, however, concern remains regarding the long-term use of most if not all NSAIDs in patients with OA. Despite this concern, long-term NSAID use has not been associated with accelerated disease in most patients and has remained the mainstay of symptomatic medical therapy.

CHONDROPROTECTIVE AGENTS

The concept of enhancing net cartilage matrix production by stimulating chondrocyte synthesis while decreasing its degradation led to the term *chondroprotective*. Compounds have been developed with this goal in mind, rather than as anti-inflammatory agents.[17] These compounds are all highly sulfated proteins with a strong negative charge. Two, SP-54 and glycosaminoglycan polysulfate (Arteparon), relatively low molecular weight heparinoids, are inhibitors of a wide range of proteolytic enzymes as might be expected. A third, glycosaminoglycan-peptide complex (Rumalon) represents a partially purified extract of bovine cartilage and bone marrow. It is also highly negatively charged but of higher molecular weight (range 10,000 to 2,000,000 daltons).

These compounds stimulate proteoglycan synthesis significantly in vitro and are also potent inhibitors of the metalloproteinases important in proteoglycan degradation.[17,31,32] They have consistently produced amelioration of cartilage lesions in animal models of OA.[31–35] Ex vivo studies confirmed their ability to prevent progressive changes and to maintain cartilage integrity. Arteparon and Rumalon have been used extensively outside the United States in the treatment of human OA. A number of studies have described efficacy of these compounds,[36–39] but they have lacked sufficient methodologic rigor to convince most clinical investigators of their validity.

INTRA-ARTICULAR THERAPY

MICROCRYSTALLINE ADRENAL CORTICOSTEROID ESTERS

The intrasynovial injection of microcrystalline adrenocorticosteroid esters was introduced by Hollander in 1951 shortly after the first synthesis of compounds E and F.[40–42] Despite their widespread use in the treatment of OA, only clinical judgment guides the clinician in issues such as the choice of the optimal steroid preparation or the maximum frequency for injection of involved joints. There are few well-controlled studies providing evidence of efficacy of this treatment. Furthermore, controversy still surrounds the potential deleterious effects of such therapy. As in use of potents NSAIDs, pain relief might be accompanied by overuse of an already damaged joint, leading to accelerated degeneration.

The use of hydrocortisone acetate, the initial crystal preparation, provided only a few days of symptomatic relief. To prolong the duration of action, several less soluble microcrystalline steroid compounds were synthesized. Triamcinolone hexacetonide is the least soluble and produced the most long-lived effects. No controlled studies, however, have demonstrated the superiority of any particular corticosteroid preparation in OA or have defined either a minimally effective or optimum dosage. Existing guidelines are based on clinical judgment, supported by long-standing patterns of use in both rheumatoid arthritis (RA) and OA (see Chapter 39).[41,42] Pharmacokinetic data support the relatively short synovial half-life of soluble hydrocortisone (1 to 2 hours), a longer half-life for triamcinolone acetonide (2 days), and the still longer half-life (4 to 5 days) for triamcinolone hexacetonide.[43] Systemic absorption from the synovial fluid does occur, at a rate slower than after oral administration and directly related to the aqueous solubility of the crystals injected. Suppression of the hypothalamic–pituitary axis can occur, particularly when multiple joints are injected simultaneously or if injections are given at close intervals over long periods.[44] Even single injections of large doses cause transient reversible depression of endogenous corticosteroid production.[41]

The clinical efficacy of intra-articular corticosteroid therapy was described by Hollander[45] but rigorously documented in only three controlled trials,[46–48] all focusing on OA of the knee. Although the study design of each was different, the results were surprisingly similar and consistent with the uncontrolled findings of Hollander recorded 30 years earlier. Compared to placebo, corticosteroid injections were associated with definite but limited improvement, primarily decreased pain but with little if any alteration in function parameters.* Pain relief was short-lived, most marked 1 to 2 weeks after treatment with loss of efficacy by 4 weeks. The response to placebo was consistently great, with 35 to 45% of patients improving after injection with saline or vehicle alone. In the study by Dieppe, Sathapatayavongs, Jones, et al.,[46] no correlation was found between the therapeutic response and synovial fluid cell count or radiographic grade. Response was associated with a fall in the thermographic index, suggesting either an anti-inflammatory effect of the steroids and/or an effect on synovial permeability, this result supported by other data.[49] Although used in many different joints, injection of the knee was associated with the highest success rate. Corticosteroid crystal injection of OA of the hip is more difficult technically. It had limited usefulness and was sometimes associated with significant worsening of symptoms.[50]

Recognized complications of intra-articular steroid therapy are primarily limited to infection and flares of inflammation in the injected joint shortly after treatment.[41,42] Iatrogenic infection is an exceedingly rare event, even without strict surgical aseptic technique. From the data of Hollander and others, the infection rate is less than 0.01%, in the range of 1/10,000 to 1/50,000. Acute pain and swelling, the "postinjection flare," occurs in 2 to 5% of patients 6 to 12 hours after injection. This is a dose-related, neutrophil-dependent, crystal-induced arthritis. The condition is self-limited, resolves in 24 hours without specific therapy. If the inflammation does not subside within this time, aspiration and culture must be done to rule out infection.

Early reports linking intra-articular steroids to accelerated joint destruction have spurred concern over this possibility. Reports of deleterious effects, however, have been anecdotal and uncontrolled.[50] No firm evidence exists that intra-articular steroid treatment hastens joint deterioration. In largely historical data from Philadelphia[45] and Aberdeen[51] involving over 250,000 injections in 8,000 patients and 80,000 injections, respectively, the incidence of rapid joint destruction was less than 1%, even with repeated injection over many years into the same joints. Most rheumatologists are reluctant, however, to inject a given joint more than three to four times a year.

Numerous studies have attempted a better understanding of the effects of intra-articular steroids on cartilage and synovial metabolism.[52–57] Animal studies have shown a strong species-specific response, with rabbits demonstrating progression of degenerative lesions, whereas cartilages of dogs and primates were relatively protected by these compounds. Corticosteroids were potent inhibitors of collagen and proteoglycan synthesis by chondrocytes in vitro with a reduction

* *Editor's note*: As expressed in previous editions of this book, I rarely use corticosteroid crystals to treat OA. They may provide a stopgap therapy in an elderly frail patient with hip or knee disease. The use of a drug that inhibits reparative cellular processes to treat a disease that is fundamentally degnerative fails to make much sense to me.

in matrix production. But they produce an equally impressive reduction of catabolic processes with inhibition of degradative metalloproteinases. As with NSAID therapy, the net effect of corticosteroid treatment may depend on the net effects between these two processes. Short-term treatment may indeed lead to decreased matrix degradation by reducing synovial inflammation and by the release of degradative enzymes and mediators from synoviocytes and inflammatory cells as well as reduction of endogenous chondrocyte catabolic activity. Longer term treatment may be detrimental because of depressed chondrocyte synthetic activity.

HYALURONATE AND OTHER THERAPIES

Peyron and Balazs[58] in 1975 first reported the clinical use of high molecular weight hyaluronic (HA) in the treatment of OA with beneficial results in a double-blind, placebo-controlled study of 28 patients. Further studies,[59,60] many in Japan and Italy, also report efficacy after use of various HA preparations. A 63-patient multicenter, double-blind, placebo-controlled randomized clinical trial with sodium HA demonstrated decreased pain, both at rest and on movement in the treated group.[61] Pain reduction at rest was significant over the 6-month period of the trial. Other parameters such as activities of daily living showed no significant differences between the two groups. Comparison of studies is confounded by different study designs, the varying frequency of joint injections, the concomitant use of NSAIDs and analgesics, and the different outcome parameters used. Further well-controlled clinical trials are needed in light of the reported beneficial responses without significant adverse effects.

Animal studies confirm those in humans.[62,63] HA has been widely used in equine OA with improved function. Experiments in dog models of OA have demonstrated the value of HA therapy, with reduced progression of disease and in improved histopathologic appearance of the joint. The mechanism of the beneficial effect of HA is unknown. Although highly viscous in concentrated solutions, it has a very short half-life after injection into joints and hence does not function as a lubricant but rather may have direct, more long-lasting effects on chondrocyte or synovial metabolism.

Other compounds with anti-inflammatory properties have been injected into OA joints. Orgotein, a metalloprotein enzyme isolated from bovine liver, is the best characterized and has been investigated in Europe as well as the United States. Orgotein acts as a superoxide dismutase, catalyzing the conversion of the superoxide free radical anion to oxygen and hydrogen peroxide, thereby reducing the highly reactive free radicals generated by inflammatory cells in the synovium or synovial fluid. Such free radicals are potent mediators of inflammation and of tissue injury. They can degrade collagen and hyaluronate.[64] Several studies have reported short-term efficacy in clinical use.[65,66] Evidence exists for longer term symptomatic benefit, although the magnitude of the placebo response was considerable and the use of analgesic agents during the trial weakens its conclusions.[67]

JOINT LAVAGE

Joint lavage with physiologic saline in patients with OA of knee or shoulder joints has been used, primarily by orthopedic surgeons. This procedure is undoubtedly effective at removing cartilage fragments and other wear particles with at least short-term symptomatic improvement. Controlled trials comparing tidal lavage with medical management have shown clinical benefit,[68,69] but another study demonstrated no better improvement than with injections of isotonic saline.[70] These results suggested a placebo effect of arthrocentesis per se. Larger, controlled studies are needed, with particular attention to defining the study population as to stage and extent of cartilage damage. This procedure may be of benefit to patients with more advanced disease, defined arthroscopically rather than radiographically.

PHYSICAL MEDICINE

BIOMECHANICAL INTERVENTIONS

Biomechanical factors often play a primary role in the etiology and progression of OA (see Fig. 104–1). Few conservative therapeutic approaches have been directed toward altering these factors, to a large extent because of the technical difficulty of quantifying primary biomechanical abnormalities. The development of computerized motion analysis now permits such studies, providing quantitative data relative to altered weight bearing in affected OA joints. Prodromos, Andriachhi, and Galante[71] demonstrated increased loads across medial compartments of the knee in patients with OA and varus deformity. Those patients with the highest abnormal loads before high tibial osteotomy had the poorest clinical and biomechanical outcomes. These data support the primary importance of reducing abnormal mechanical loading of affected joints. The mechanism by which this can be accomplished early in the disease process is an important area of current research.

The ability to reproducibly quantify biomechanical parameters has already permitted the evaluation of several simple nonsurgical interventions directed toward reducing load in affected joints. Under static conditions,[72] the use of a wedged insole changes the angle of the lower extremity and reduces the medial force at the knee. This resulted in an improved clinical outcome in an uncontrolled study.[73] NSAID therapy resulted in increased stride length, knee flexion, and walking speed.[73] Interestingly, these changes did not correlate with decreased pain, suggesting that the measured biomechanical effects of these agents were not due simply to analgesia. Other studies, using computerized gait analysis, have confirmed the efficacy of NSAIDs, particularly by altering joint-loading patterns, in a manner different from that seen with simple analgesic agents.[74,75] Such quantifiable and reproducible assessment provides a rational theoretic basis for analysis of the results of the numerous procedures advocated for OA.

THERAPEUTIC EXERCISE

Patients with OA have reduced muscle strength, particularly in those muscle groups around involved joints, decreased flexibility, weight gain, limitation in their ability to carry out activities of daily living, and often compromised mobility.[76,77] Knee OA occurs typically in obese persons, especially obese women. This problem is compounded by the decreased physical activity associated with advancing disease. These findings are largely explained by a decreased mobility that is due to limitations imposed by the disease. Such decrease in physical activity leads to deconditioning and loss of aerobic capacity. Furthermore, OA patients are biomechanically inefficient, requiring higher energy expenditures than normal persons for everyday tasks such as walking.[78] Together with muscle weakness, this may explain the poor endurance of these patients. As discussed, alterations in gait to improve biomechanical efficiency may be important in the therapeutic approach to OA patients.

The goals of an integrated exercise program are increased physical and psychosocial function and an increased feeling of well-being. The immediate objectives include increasing joint motion, enhancing muscle strength, increasing aerobic capacity, and reaching optimal body weight. Exercises are usually undertaken in a specified order: initial warm-up and range of motion, followed by muscle strengthening, an aerobic program, and then cooling down with stretching.[79,80] Properly conducted, this program is beneficial and does not to lead to further joint damage in patients with OA.[81] Obviously, patients with acute painful joint swelling and those having significant cardiovascular disease should not enter such a program.

Few studies have evaluated the efficacy of this treatment. The beneficial effects of aerobic exercise are now amply documented.[81] Patients with RA undergoing a 12-week aerobic exercise program significantly increased their aerobic capacity compared to a control group and tolerated the exercise well. The exercised patients also showed significant improvement in their physical activity and in psychosocial factors, with decreased depression and anxiety. Thus, an exercise program provides significant multifaceted benefit to arthritic patients.

Increasing muscle strength is thought to protect a damaged joint by reducing load and providing a more efficient "shock absorber." Muscle strength may be increased by isometric (static), isokinetic (constant rate of movement with variable force [Kinetron, Cybex]), or isotonic (variable rate of movement) exercise. Exercises done under static conditions (isometric) increase intra-articular pressure less than the other types and may be preferred in patients with evidence of joint effusion.[82] Although exercise programs have been widely prescribed for decades, only two studies examined their benefit in OA. The benefit of a relatively simple exercise program documented that the improvements seen at the end of 12 weeks were maintained by exercises done at home.[83] Improvement was seen in pain, endurance, range of motion, and maximum weight lift. A more sophisticated isometric exercise program resulted in increased maximum force, endurance, and speed of knee extension, and a decrease in pain and walking time, with enhanced stair-climbing ability and decreased dependency.[84] In similar studies, patients with long-standing OA had significant pain relief to the point of being able to stop entirely their use of NSAIDs and analgesic agents.[84] Additional studies are needed to examine the applicability of this approach to all patients with OA.

HEAT AND COLD THERAPY

The use of heat or cold to treat joint pain has long been advocated and an extensive literature exists on the subject. Early studies[85–87] done by Hollander documented that intra-articular temperature in OA was often increased. Local application of heat to the joint surface results in a paradoxic, probably reflex, decrease in the intra-articular temperature; conversely, local cold elevates joint temperatures. Application of ultrasound (diathermy) produces deep heating of tissues. Heat may facilitate muscle relaxation and has been postulated to have an analgesic effect.[88] Although no definitive study has proven the efficacy of either heat or cold, the subjective improvements felt by the patients will guarantee the continued use of modalities.

ENVIRONMENTAL MEASURES

As part of any comprehensive rehabilitation program, evaluation of the environmental milieu of the patient and alterations in simple physical and social factors may be of equal importance to pharmacologic intervention.[80] Increasing chair height, elevating toilet seats, reducing the need to use stairs by changing bedroom locations, and the use of aids in the kitchen can improve the function as well as the mental well-being of OA patients. Occupational therapy assessments should include a consideration of the home environment as well as the more traditional review of activities of daily living. Psychosocial issues such as the effect of OA on sexuality, mood, and employment should be openly discussed, with appropriate referral if needed.

SURGICAL THERAPY

Successful total hip joint replacement surgery by Charnley over 30 years ago heralded a new era in the treatment of OA.[89] By providing a dramatic improvement in function and pain relief, this approach has permitted many patients to enjoy a more productive, meaningful life. The development and introduction of many new prostheses for the hip and knee and for the shoulder, elbow, hand, foot, and ankle (Chapters 49–55). The indications for joint replacement have remain unchanged: severe pain unsuccessfully controlled by medical management or functional limitations severe enough to prevent normal daily activities. Age is another consideration. Replacement of major weight-bearing joints is reserved primarily for patients over the age of 60 years because the failure rate of prostheses increases with time as well as with the biomechanical demands made on them. With people living longer and remaining physically active longer, it remains important to give a conservative program every chance before resorting to surgery.

The major limitation of joint replacement surgery is failure of the prosthesis. Short-term complications primarily relate to the risk of infection. In the longer term, the risk of infection remains but is exceeded by the rate of loosening of the prosthesis with attendant pain. Such loosening is believed to be due to "stress shielding" and secondary remodeling of bone. Newer designs permit fixation by bone ingrowth into the prosthesis rather than by cement. The use of growth factors to stimulate bony ingrowth, the use of biomaterials for prosthesis, and the possibility of cartilage transplantation are discussed in Chapter 106.

FUTURE DIRECTIONS

Prevention of OA is of course preferred to treatment of established disease. By the time pain occurs, significant irreversible damage has already occurred to the joint cartilage. Treatment with analgesics and anti-inflammatory agents may provide symptomatic relief, delaying more definitive surgical intervention. However, the basic mechanism behind the cause of the joint deterioration has not been addressed.

Detection of early changes in cartilage structure and function would provide an opportunity for intervention before irreversible changes take place. Serum markers of cartilage metabolism have been defined, and their significance is being investigated.[90–92] More sensitive imaging modalities, such as magnetic resonance imaging, may approach the level of sensitivity necessary to detect the changes seen in the earliest phases of OA. Sophisticated computerized opticokinetic motion analysis systems[71] permit definition of the biomechanical alterations in gait associated with all stages of disease.[71] A combination of these approaches will be necessary to better understand OA.

REFERENCES

1. McAlindon, T., and Dieppe, P.: The medical management of osteoarthritis of the knee: An inflammatory issue? Br. J. Rheum., *29*:471–473, 1990.
2. Doherty, M.: Letters to the editor. Ann. Rheum. Dis., *49*:339, 1990.
3. Wood, P.H.N.: Osteoarthrosis in the community. Clin. Rheum. Dis., *2*:495–507, 1976.
4. VanSaase, J.L.C.M., VanRomunde, L.K.J., Cats, A., et al.: Epidemiology of osteoarthritis: Zoetermeer survey. Comparison of radiological osteoarthritis in a Dutch population with that in 10 other populations. Ann. Rheum. Dis., *48*:271–280, 1989.
5. Wright, V.: Osteoarthritis. Diagnosis is not as simple as it seems. Br. Med. J., *299*:1476–1477, 1989.

5a. Burr, D.B. and Radin, E.L.: Trauma as a factor in the initiation of osteoarthritis. Cartilage Changes in Osteoarthritis. Edited by Kenneth D. Brandt. Indianapolis, Indiana University School of Medicine, 1990, pp. 73–80.

5b. Bradley, J.D., Brandt, K.D., Katz, B.P. et al.: Comparison of an anti-inflammatory dose of ibuprofen, an analgesic dose of ibuprofen, and acetominophen in the treatment of patients with osteoarthritis of the knee. N. Engl. J. Med., *325*:87–91, 1991.

6. Doyle, D.V., Dieppe, P.A., Scott, J., and Huskisson, E.C.: An articular index for the assessment of osteoarthritis. Ann. Rheum. Dis., *40*:75–78, 1981.
7. Bradley, J., Brandt, K.D., Katz, B.P., and Ryan, S.I.: Analgesic vs. nonsteroidal antiinflammatory drug (NSAID) treatment of osteoarthritis (OA). Arthritis Rheum., *32*(Suppl.):138, 1989.
8. Huskisson, E.C., Doyle, D.V., and Lanham, J.G.: Drug treatment of osteoarthritis. Clin. Rheum. Dis., *11*:421–430, 1985.
9. Doherty, M.: Leader. Chondroprotection by non-steroidal anti-inflammatory drugs. Ann. Rheum. Dis., *48*:619–621, 1989.
10. Pelletier, J.P., and Martel-Pelletier, J.: The therapeutic effects of NSAID and corticosteroids in osteoarthritis: To be or not to be. J. Rheum., *16*:266, 1989.
11. Brandt, K.D.: The mechanism of action of nonsteroidal anti-inflammatory drugs. J. Rheum., *18*(Suppl.):120–121, 1991.
12. CSM Update: Non-steroidal anti-inflammatory drugs and serious gastrointestinal adverse reactions—1. Br. Med. J., *292*:614, 1986.
13. Muir, H.: Current and future trends in articular cartilage research and osteoarthritis. *In* Articular Cartilage Biochemistry. Workshop Conference Hoechst-Werk Albert. Edited by K.E. Kuettner, T. Schleyerbach, and V.C. Hascall. New York, Raven Press, 1985, pp. 423–440.
14. Bayliss, M.T.: Proteoglycan structure in normal and osteoarthrotic human cartilage. *In* Articular Cartilage Biochemistry. Workshop Conference Hoechst-Werk Albert. Edited by K.E. Kuettner, T. Schleyerbach, and V.C. Hascall. New York, Raven Press, New York, 1985, pp. 295–310.
15. Lentini, A., Ternai, B., and Ghosh, P.: Inhibition of human leukocyte elastase and cathepsin G by non-steroidal antiinflammatory compounds. Biochem. Int., *15*:1069–1078, 1987.
16. Ghosh, P.: Anti-rheumatic drugs and cartilage. Bailliere's Clin. Rheum., *2*:309–338, 1988.
17. Burkhardt, D., and Ghosh, P.: Laboratory evaluation of antiarthritic drugs as potential chondroprotective agents. Semin. Arthritis Rheum., *17*(Suppl. 1):3–34, 1987.
18. Brandt, K.D.: Effects of nonsteroidal anti-inflammatory drugs on chondrocyte metabolism in vitro and in vivo. Am. J. Med., *83*(Suppl. 5A):29–33, 1987.
19. Brandt, K.D., and Slowman-Kovacs, S.: Nonsteroidal antiinflammatory drugs in treatment of osteoarthritis. Clin. Orthop. Related Res., *213*:84–91, 1986.
20. Palmoski, M.J., and Brandt, K.D.: Effects of some nonsteroidal antiinflammatory drugs on proteoglycan metabolism and organization in canine articular cartilage. Arthritis Rheum., *23*:1010–1020, 1980.
21. Carlin, G., Djursater, R., Smedegard, G., and Gerdin, B.: Effect of anti-inflammatory drugs on xanthine oxidase and xanthine oxidase induced depolymerisation of hyaluronic acid. Agents Actions, *16*:377–384, 1985.

22. Herman, J.H., Appel, A.M., and Hess, E.V.: Modulation of cartilage destruction by select nonsteroidal antiinflammatory drugs. In vitro effect on the synthesis and activity of catabolism-inducing cytokines produced by osteoarthritic and rheumatoid synovial tissue. Arthritis Rheum., *30*:257–263, 1987.
23. Pelletier, J.P., and Martel-Pelletier, J.: Evidence for the involvement of interleukin 1 in human osteoarthritic cartilage degradation: Protective effect of NSAID. J. Rheum., *16*:19–27, 1989.
24. Ronningen, H., and Langeland, N.: Indomethacin treatment in osteoarthritis of the hip joint. Acta Orthop. Scand., *50*:169–174, 1979.
25. Newman, N.M., and Ling, R.S.M.: Acetabular bone destruction related to nonsteroidal anti-inflammatory drugs. Lancet, *2*(8445):11–13, 1985.
26. Rashad, S., Hemingway, A., Rainsford, K., et al.: Effect of nonsteroidal anti-inflammatory drugs on the course of osteoarthritis. Lancet, *2*(8662):519–521, 1989.
27. Hodgkinson, R., and Woolf, D.: A five-year clinical trial of indomethacin in osteoarthritis of the hip. Practitioner, *210*:392–396, 1973.
28. Doherty, M., Holt, M., MacMillan, P., et al.: A reappraisal of 'analgesic hip.' Ann. Rheum. Dis., *45*:272–276, 1986.
29. Colombo, C., Butler, M., Hickman, L., et al.: A new model of osteoarthritis in rabbits: II. Evaluation of anti-osteoarthritic effects of selected antirheumatic drugs administered systemically. Arthritis Rheum., *26*:1132–1139, 1983.
30. McKenzie, L.S., Horsburgh, B.A., Ghosh, P., and Taylor, T.K.F.: Effect of anti-inflammatory drugs on sulphated glycosaminoglycan synthesis in aged human articular cartilage. Ann. Rheum. Dis., *35*:487–495, 1976.
31. Golding, J., and Ghosh, P.: Drugs for osteoarthrosis: II. The effects of a glycosaminoglycan polysulphate ester (arteparon) on proteoglycan aggregation and loss from articular cartilage of immobilized rabbit knee joints. Curr. Ther. Res., *34*:67–80, 1983.
32. Altman, R.D., Dean, D.D., Muniz, O.E., and Howell, D.S.: Therapeutic treatment of canine osteoarthritis with glycosaminoglycan polysulfuric acid ester. Arthritis Rheum., *32*:1300–1307, 1989.
33. Altman, R.D., Dean, D.D., Muniz, O.E., and Howell, D.S.: Prophylactic treatment of canine osteoarthritis with glycosaminoglycan polysulfuric acid ester. Arthritis Rheum., *32*:759–766, 1989.
34. Carreno, M.R., Muniz, O.E., and Howell, D.S.: The effect of glycosaminoglycan polysulfuric acid ester on articular cartilage in experimental osteoarthritis: Effects on morphological variables of disease severity. J. Rheum., *13*:490–497, 1986.
35. Olijhoek, G., Drukker, J., van der Linden, T.J., and Terwindt-Rouwenhorst, E.A.W.: Drug effects on arthrosis. Comparison in rabbits of 3 modes of action. Acta Orthop. Scand., *52*:186–190, 1988.
36. Rejholec, V.: Clinical trials of anti-osteoarthritic agents. Scand. J. Rheum., *81*(Suppl.):28–31, 1990.
37. Rejholec, V.: Long-term studies of antiosteoarthritic drugs: An assessment. Semin. Arthritis Rheum., *17*(Suppl. 1):35–53, 1987.
38. Katona, G.: A clinical trial of glycosaminoglycan-peptide complex ('Rumalon') in patients with osteoarthritis of the knee. Cur. Med. Res. Opin., *10*:625–633, 1987.
39. Gramajo, R.J., Cutroneo, E.J., Fernandez, D.E., et al.: A single-blind, placebo-controlled study of glycosaminoglycan-peptide complex ('Rumalon') in patients with osteoarthritis of the hip or knee. Cur. Med. Res. Opin., *11*:366–373, 1989.
40. Hollander, J.L., Brown, E.M., Jr., Jessar, R.A., and Brown, C.Y.: Hydrocortisone and cortisone injected into arthritic joints. JAMA, *14*:1631–1635, 1951.
41. Gray, R.G., Tenebaum, J., and Gottlieb, N.L.: Local corticosteroid injection treatment in rheumatic disorders. Semin. Arthritis Rheum., *10*:231–254, 1981.
42. Gray, R.G., and Gottlieb, N.L.: Intra-articular corticosteroids. An updated assessment. Clin. Orthop. Related Res., *177*:235–263, 1983.
43. Derendorf, H., Mollmann, H., Gruner, A., et al.: Pharmacokinetics and pharmacodynamics of glucocorticoid suspensions after intra-articular administration. Clin. Pharmacol. Ther., *39*:313–317, 1986.
44. O'Sullivan, M.M., Rumfeld, W.R., Jones, M.K., et al.: Cushing's syndrome with suppression of the hypothalamic-pituitary-adrenal axis after intra-articular steroid injections. Ann. Rheum. Dis., *44*:561–563, 1985.
45. Hollander, J.L.: Intra-articular hydrocortisone in arthritis and allied conditions. A Summary of two years' clinical experience. J. Bone Joint Surg., *5A*:983–990, 1953.
46. Dieppe, P.A., Sathapatayavongs, B., Jones, H.E., et al.: Intra-articular steroids in osteoarthritis. Rheumatol. Rehabil., *19*:212–217, 1980.
47. Wright, V., Chandler, G.N., Morison, R.A.H., and Hartfall, S.J.: Intra-articular therapy in osteo-arthritis. Comparison of hydrocortisone acetate and hydrocortisone tertiary-butylacetate. Ann. Rheum. Dis., *19*:257–259, 1960.
48. Friedman, D.M., and Moore, M.E.: The efficacy of intraarticular steroids in osteoarthritis: A double-blind study. J. Rheumatol., *7*:850–856, 1980.
49. Eymontt, M.J., Gordon, G.V., Schumacher, H.R., and Hansell, J.R.: The effects on synovial permeability and synovial fluid leukocyte counts in symptomatic osteoarthritis after intraarticular corticosteroid administration. J. Rheumatol., *9*:198–203, 1982.
50. Bentley, G., and Goodfellow, J.W.: Disorganisation of the knees following intra-articular hydrocrortisone injections. J. Bone Joint Surg., *51B*:498–502, 1969.
51. Balch, H.W., Gibson, J.M.C., El-Ghobarey, A.F., et al.: Repeated corticosteroid injections into knee joints. Rheumatol. Rehabil., *16*:137–140, 1977.
52. Moskowitz, R.W., Davis, W., Sammarco, J., et al.: Experimentally induced corticosteroid arthropathy. Arthritis Rheum., *13*:236–243, 1970.
53. Behrens, F., Shepard, N., and Mitchell, N.: Alteration of rabbit articular cartilage by intra-articular injections of glucocorticoids. J. Bone Joint Surg., *57*:70–76, 1975.
54. Gibson, T., Burry, H.C., Poswillo, D., and Glass, J.: Effect of intra-articular corticosteroid injections on primate cartilage. Ann. Rheum. Dis., *36*:74–79, 1976.
55. Pelletier, J.P., and Martel-Pelletier, J.: Protective effects of corticosteroids on cartilage lesions and osteophyte formation in the Pond-Nuki dog model of osteoarthritis. Arthritis Rheum., *32*:181–193, 1989.
56. Pelletier, J.P., Martel-Pelletier, J., Cloutier, J.M., and Woessner, J.F., Jr.: Proteoglycan-degrading acid metalloprotease activity in human osteoarthtritic cartilage, and the effect of intraarticular steroid injections. Arthritis Rheum., *30*:541–548, 1987.
57. Williams, J.M., and Brandt, K.D.: Triamcinolone hexacetonide protects against fibrillation and osteophyte formation following chemically induced articular cartilage damage. Arthritis Rheum., *28*:1267–1274, 1985.
58. Peyron, J.G., and Balazs, E.A.: Preliminary clinical assessment of Na hyaluronate injection into human arthritic joints. Pathologie-Biologie, *22*:731–735, 1974.
59. Punzi, L., Schiavon, F., Ramonda, R., et al.: Intra-articular hyaluronic acid in the treatment of inflammatory and noninflammatory knee effusions. Cur. Therap. Res., *43*:643–647, 1988.
60. Namiki, O., Toyoshima, H., and Morisaki, N.: Therapeutic effect of intra-articular injection of high molecular weight hyaluronic acid on osteoarthritis of the knee. Internatl. J. Clin. Pharmacol. Therap. Toxicol., *20*:501–507, 1982.
61. Dixon, A. St.J., Jacoby, R.K., Berry, H., and Hamilton, E.B.D.: Clinical trial of intra-articular injection of sodium hyaluronate in

patients with osteoarthritis of the knee. Curr. Med. Res. Opin., *11*:205–213, 1988.
62. Auer, J.A., Fackelman, G.E., Gingerich, D.A., and Fetter, A.W.: Effect of hyaluronic acid in naturally occurring and experimentally induced osteoarthritis. Am. J. Vet. Res., *41*:568–574, 1980.
63. Schiavinato, A., Lini, E., Guidolin, D., et al.: Intraarticular sodium hyaluronate injections in the Pond-Nuki experimental model of osteoarthritis in dogs: II. Morphological findings. Clin. Orthop. Rel. Res., *241*:286–299, 1989.
64. McCord, J.M.: Free radicals and inflammation: Protection of synovial fluid by superoxide dismutase. Science, *185*:529–531, 1974.
65. Lund-Olsen, K., and Menander, K.B.: Orgotein: A new anti-inflammatory metalloprotein drug: Preliminary evaluation of clinical efficacy and safety in degenerative joint disease. Curr. Ther. Res., *16*:706–717, 1974.
66. Gammer, W., and Broback, L.-G.: Clinical comparison of orgotein and methylprednisolone acetate in the treatment of osteoarthrosis of the knee joint. Scand. J. Rheumatol., *13*:108–112, 1984.
67. McIlwain, H., Silverfield, J.C., Cheatum, D.E., et al.: Intra-articular orgotein in osteoarthritis of the knee: A placebo-controlled efficacy, safety, and dosage comparison. Am. J. Med., *87*:295–300, 1989.
68. Reardon, E.V., Tuggle, C.J., Clough, J.D., and Segal, A.M: A prospective study of the use of tidal lavage (irrigation) in patients with arthritis of the knee. Arthritis Rheum., *32*(Supl. 4):S139, 1989.
69. Arnold, W.J. et al.: Tidal irrigation versus medical management in patients with osteoarthritis of the knee: Results of a single blind randomized multicenter study. Arthritis Rheum., *32*(Suppl. 4):S138, 1989.
70. Dawes, P.T., Kirlew, C., and Haslock, I.: Saline washout for knee osteoarthritis: Results of a controlled study. Clin. Rheumatol., *6*:61–63, 1987.
71. Prodromos, C.C., Andriachhi, T.P., and Galante, J.O.: A relationship between gait and clinical changes following high tibial osteotomy. J. Bone Joint Surg., *67A*:1188–1194, 1985.
72. Yasuda, K., and Sasaki, T.: The mechanics of treatment of the osteoarthritic knee with a wedged insole. Clin. Orthopaed. Rel. Res., *215*:162–172, 1987.
73. Sasaki, T., and Yasuda, K.: Clinical evaluation of the treatment of osteoarthritic knees using a newly designed wedged insole. Clin. Orthopaed. Rel. Res., *221*:181–187, 1987.
74. Blin, O., Pailhous, J., Lafforgue, P., and Serratrice, G.: Quantitative analysis of walking in patients with knee osteoarthritis: A method of assessing the effectiveness of non-steroidal anti-inflammatory treatment. Ann. Rheum. Dis., *49*:990–993, 1990.
75. Schnitzer, T.J., Andriacchi, T.P., Fedder, D., and Lindeman, M.: Effect of NSAIDs on knee loading in patients with osteoarthritis (OA). Arthritis Rheum., *33*(Suppl.):S92, 1990.
76. Nordesjo, L.-O., Nordgren, B., Wigren, A., and Kolstad, K.: Isometric strength and endurance in patients with severe rheumatoid arthritis or osteoarthrosis in the knee joints. A comparative study in healthy men and women. Scand. J. Rheumatol., *12*:152–156, 1983.
77. Semble, E.L., Loeser, R.F., and Wise, C.M.: Therapeutic exercise for rheumatoid arthritis and osteoarthritis. Semin. Arthritis Rheum., *20*:32–40, 1990.
78. Minor, M.A., Hewett, J.E., Webel, R.R., et al.: Exercise tolerance and disease related measures in patients with rheumatoid arthritis and osteoarthritis. J. Rheumatol., *15*:905–911, 1988.
79. Pothier, B., and Allen, M.E.: Kinesiology and the degenerative joint. Rheum. Dis. Clin. North Am., *16*:989–1002, 1990.
80. Hicks, J.E., and Nicholas, J.J.: Treatments utilized in rehabilitative rheumatology. *In* Handbook of Rehabilitative Rheumatology. Atlanta, GA, American Rheumatism Association, 1988, pp. 32–79.
81. Minor, M.A., Hewett, J.E., Webel, R.R., et al.: Efficacy of physical conditioning exercise in patients with rheumatoid arthritis. Arthritis Rheum., *32*:1396–1405, 1989.
82. Jayson, M.I.V., and Dixon, A. St.J.: Intra-articular pressure in rheumatoid arthritis of the knee: III. Pressure changes during joint use. Ann. Rheum. Dis., *29*:401–408, 1970.
83. Chamberlain, M.A., Care, G., and Harfield, B.: Physiotherapy in osteoarthrosis of the knees. A controlled trial of hospital versus home exercises. Int. Rehab. Med., *4*:101–106, 1982.
84. Fisher, N., Pendergast, D., Gresha, G., and Calkins, E.: Muscle rehabilitation: Its effect on muscular and functional performance of patients with knee osteoarthritis. Arch. Phys. Med. Rehab., *72*(6):367–379, 1991.
85. Hollander, J.L., and Horvath, S.M.: Changes in joint temperature produced by disease and by physical therapy. Preliminary report. Arch. Intern. Med., *30*:437–440, 1949.
86. Horvath, S.M. and Hollander, J.L.: Intra-articular temperature as a measure of joint reaction. Arch. Phys. Med., *3*:437–440, 1949.
87. Clarke, G.R., Willis, L.A., Stenner, L., and Nichols, P.J.R.: Evaluation of physiotherapy in the treatment of osteoarthrosis of the knee. Rheumatol. Rehab., *13*:190–197, 1974.
88. Feibel, A., and Fast, A.: Deep heating of joints: A reconsideration. Arch. Phys. Med. Rehabil., *57*:513–514, 1976.
89. Charnley, J.: Low friction arthroplasty of the hip. Theory and practice. Berlin, Springer, Verlag, 1979.
90. Thonar, E.J.-M.A., Williams, J., Sweet, M.B.E., et al.: Serum kertan sulfate concentration as a measure of the catabolism of cartilage proteoglycans. *In* Monoclonal Antibodies, Cytokines, Arthritis: Mediators of Inflammation and Therapy. Edited by T. Kressina. New York, Marcel Dekker, 1991, pp. 373–398.
91. Lohmander, L.S., Dahlberg, L., Ryd, L., and Heinegard, D.: Increased levels of proteoglycan fragments in knee joint fluid after injury. Arthritis Rheum., *32*:1434–1442, 1989.
92. Campion, G.V., Delmas, P.D., and Dieppe, P.A.: Serum and synovial fluid osteocalcin (bone GLA protein) levels in joint disease. Br. J. Rheum., *28*:393–398, 1989.

SECTION X

Metabolic Bone and Joint Diseases

105

Clinical Gout and the Pathogenesis of Hyperuricemia

DENNIS J. LEVINSON
MICHAEL A. BECKER

> *Asa, King of Judah: 917–876 B.C.*
> "But in the time of his old age he was diseased in his feet."
> *Kings, 15:23*

Gout is a heterogeneous group of diseases resulting from tissue deposition of monosodium urate or uric acid crystals from extracellular fluids supersaturated with respect to this end product of human purine metabolism. The limited range of clinical manifestations of urate deposition includes recurrent attacks of a unique type of acute inflammatory arthritis (acute gout); accumulation of potentially destructive crystalline aggregates (tophi), especially in connective tissue structures; uric acid urolithiasis; and infrequently, renal impairment (gouty nephropathy). *Hyperuricemia* (supersaturation for urate in serum) is the pathogenetic common denominator through which diverse etiologic influences predispose to crystal deposition and the potential for clinical events. Although hyperuricemia is a necessary underlying feature of gout, it is in the majority of instances insufficient for expression of the disorder. Thus, the distinction between hyperuricemia, a biochemical aberration, and gout, a disease state, is essential. Recognition of this distinction, in conjunction with increasing evidence that hyperuricemia and gout are, at worst, only weak risk factors for the development of chronic renal insufficiency, has promoted conservatism in the use of drug therapy to treat asymptomatic hyperuricemia and even the early stages of gout.

HISTORY OF GOUT

Gout is among the most illustrious and well-described diseases of man, and it is probably not coincidental that contemporary understanding of the pathogenesis of hyperuricemia and gout is quite extensive. The distinctive clinical features of gouty arthritis were recognized by Hippocrates in the fifth century B.C. and were described in the oldest known medical text.[1] The Roman physicians Galen (who was the first to describe gouty tophi) and Celsus recognized that gout afflicted the rich and powerful, especially those who were most overindulgent. An inherited tendency to gout (gouty diathesis) was also suspected by the Romans two millennia before the inclusion of gout among the first group of "inborn errors of metabolism" by Sir Archibald Garrod in 1909.[2] The medieval concept that gout arises as a consequence of poisonous "noxa" appears to be the basis for the term *gout,* which is from the Latin *"guta"*, meaning "a drop." In view of the contemporary understanding of gout as monosodium urate crystal deposition disease, the term reflects a certain prescience.

A relationship between gout and uric acid has long been recognized. Van Leeuwenhoek, the Dutch microscopist, sketched needle-shaped crystals obtained from a gouty tophus in 1679,[3] and, a century later, Scheele, a Swedish chemist, identified urolithic (uric) acid in a urinary calculus.[4] In 1797, the British chemist Wollaston identified urate as the major constituent of a gouty tophus.[5] The demonstration of excess uric acid in the acidified serum from patients with gout using a "thread test" provided the basis for Alfred Baring Garrod's remarkably clear and accurate postulates concerning gouty pathogenesis (1859, 1863) and was also a pioneering achievement in the new science of clinical chemistry.[6] Garrod described asymptomatic hyperuricemia, the relationship of hyperuricemia to gout, the cause and effect relationship between urate crystal deposition and gouty inflammation, and roles for increased uric acid formation and impaired renal uric acid excretion among patients with gout. Surprisingly, this work was largely forgotten until monosodium urate crystals were specifically identified in the synovial fluid of patients with acute gouty arthritis by McCarty and Hollander in 1961.[7]

Since the 1960s, sophisticated biochemical, isotopic, and cell biologic studies of the pathophysiology of hyperuricemia and gout have resulted in a unified concept of gout centering on the role of urate crystal deposition. Concomitantly, this period has witnessed development of highly successful management modalities based on rational therapeutics and the availability of multiple classes of agents to achieve the major aims of therapy in gout: treatment of acute inflammation; prevention of recurrent attacks of arthritis and urinary tract stones; and reversal of hyperuricemia. These therapeutic achievements are the culmination of nearly 1,000 years of medical intervention in gout, dating to the introduction of colchicine in the Middle Ages.

DEFINITION OF HYPERURICEMIA

Physical, chemical and epidemiologic definitions of hyperuricemia have been proposed. Solubility product considerations dictate that at the sodium concentrations prevailing in extracellular fluids, serum at 37° C is supersaturated for monosodium urate at concentrations greater than about 6.5 mg/dL (Fig. 105–1).[8] Above this theoretic limit of solubility, increasing risks for gout and urinary tract stones have been documented. In most population groups tested, application of the specific uricase-spectrophotometric serum uric acid assay has established upper limits of normal (mean + 2 SD) of about 7.0 mg/dL in adult men and 6.0 mg/dL in premenopausal women.[9,10] Nevertheless, hyperuricemia defined by the solubility of urate is preferable to population-defined hyperuricemia, because the distribution of serum urate values is not symmetric about the mean but is skewed so that the majority of values falling outside 2 SD from the mean are high.

Automated enzymatic methods rely on the production of H_2O_2 generated in the oxidation of urate by uricase and constitute the most common and convenient procedures now used for measurement of serum and urinary uric acid values.[11] These methods are subject to minor nonspecific interference, but, with proper standardization, they are sufficiently accurate for routine clinical practice and represent a considerable improvement on prior colorimetric methods, which have largely been abandoned.

Serum urate values in children are lower than those in adults, and, during male puberty, values rise into the adult male range.[12,13] The lower serum urate values in women of reproductive age compared to their male counterparts have been ascribed to effects of estrogenic compounds on renal urate clearance.[14,15] With the onset of menopause, serum urate values in women approach or equal those of men of corresponding age, and this physiologic change is accompanied by an increase in the incidence of gout.

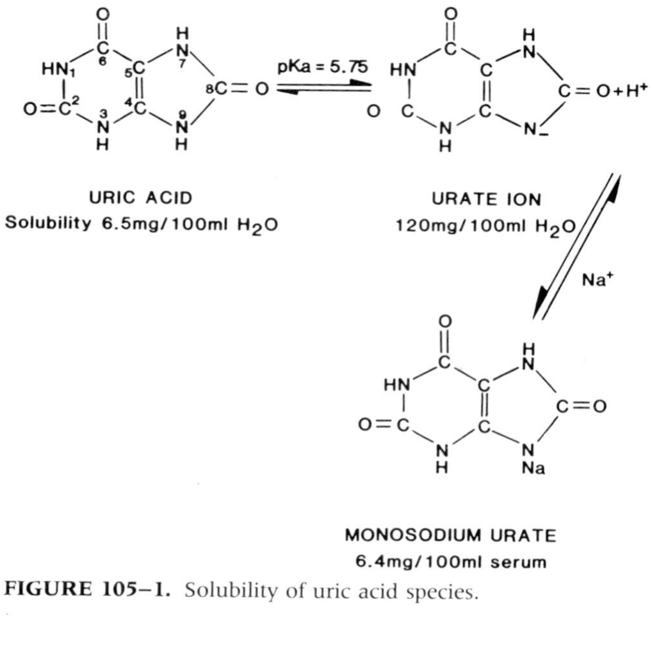

FIGURE 105–1. Solubility of uric acid species.

ASYMPTOMATIC HYPERURICEMIA

The term *asymptomatic hyperuricemia* is applied to the state in which the serum urate concentration is abnormally high but symptoms have not occurred. In men, primary hyperuricemia frequently begins at puberty, while in women, it is usually delayed until menopause. Once developed, asymptomatic hyperuricemia frequently lasts a lifetime, but gout may develop in hyperuricemic individuals at any point. The prevalence of asymptomatic hyperuricemia among adult American males has been estimated at 5 to 8%. Management of hypertension and congestive heart failure with diuretics has expanded an already large population of individuals with asymptomatic hyperuricemia, particularly among elderly women.

Few studies have assessed the risks of asymptomatic hyperuricemia. In a cohort of 2046 initially healthy men followed for 15 years with serial measurements of serum urate concentrations, the annual incidence rate of gout was 4.9% for a serum urate of 9 mg/dL or more.[16] In contrast, the incidence rate was only 0.5% for values between 7.0 and 8.9 mg/dL, and 0.1% for values below 7.0 mg/dL. Throughout this prospective study, there was no evidence of renal deterioration attributable to hyperuricemia. This finding was confirmed by a study of 3693 subjects enrolled in a hypertension detection and followup program.[17] Therapy with thiazide-type diuretics increased both serum urate and creatinine concentrations. However, lowering urate values with drug therapy did not influence creatinine values. In addition, the incidence of gouty attacks in subjects at risk was only 2.7% over a 5-year period. Fessel concluded that hyperuricemia is of no clinical importance with respect to renal outcomes until serum urate levels reach at least 13 mg/dL in men and 10 mg/dL in women, limits beyond which little information is available.[18] Urolithiasis was rare among previously asymptomatic hyperuricemic individuals, with an annualized incidence rate of 0.4% compared to 0.9% in gouty patients. In the Framingham study, gout developed in only 12% of patients with urate levels between 7 and 7.9 mg/dL over a period of 14 years.[19] Values greater than 9 mg/dL had a sixfold greater predictive value but represented only 20% of the gouty population.

The available data thus do not justify therapy for most patients with asymptomatic hyperuricemia. Nevertheless, hyperuricemia does predispose individuals to both articular gout and nephrolithiasis. Once a hyperuricemic individual experiences one of these complications, the asymptomatic phase is ended, and medical management of hyperuricemia may be indicated. (See Chapter 104 on the management of hyperuricemia and gout).

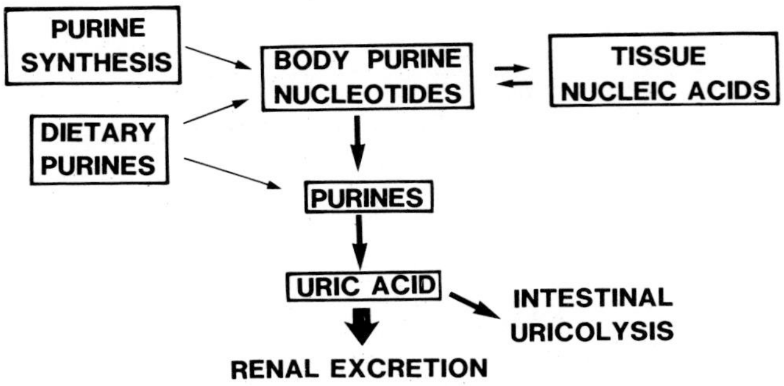

FIGURE 105–2. Schematic illustrating human purine metabolism.

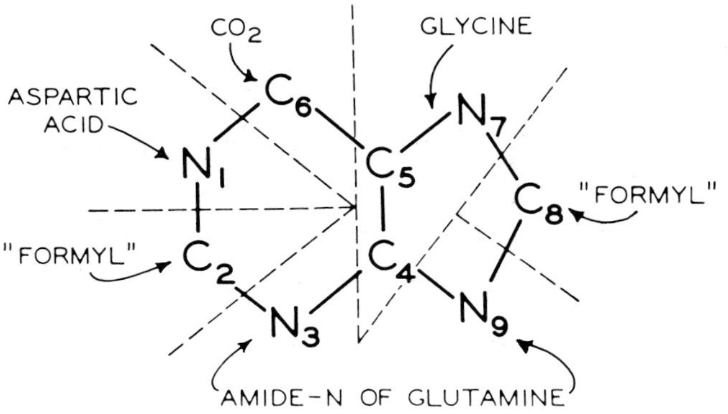

FIGURE 105–3. Precursors of purine ring.

PATHOGENESIS OF HYPERURICEMIA AND GOUT

Among mammalian species, only man and the great apes excrete uric acid as the end product of purine metabolism, reflecting the lack of the enzyme uricase, which catalyzes the degradation of uric acid to the readily excretable compound, allantoin.[20] Uric acid is a weak organic acid ($pK_{a1} = 5.75$) that is sparingly soluble (about 6.5 mg/dL) both in the unionized acid form prevalent in normal urine and in the ionized urate form at the pH and sodium concentration of other extracellular fluids (Fig. 105–1).[21] The combination of lack of uricase and the solubility properties of uric acid condition humans to the deposition of urate from supersaturated (hyperuricemic) body fluids, with the consequent risk of clinical sequelae (gout). The magnitude of this problem is dramatized as, at least among normal adult white men, mean serum urate concentrations are within 1 mg/dL of the theoretic limit of urate solubility in serum.[10] The factors determining who will develop hyperuricemia and, among this group, who will develop gout are diverse and are best understood in the context of how purine compounds are normally metabolized (Fig. 105–2) and the physiologic mechanisms maintaining uric acid homeostasis.

PURINE METABOLISM IN MAN

Net contributions to body pools of purine compounds are provided only by dietary purine ingestion and the endogenous pathway of purine nucleotide synthesis de novo. The latter is a sequence of 10 enzymatic reactions by which small molecule precursors of uric acid are incorporated into a purine ring (Fig. 105–3) synthesized on a ribosephosphate backbone donated by 5-phosphoribosyl 1-pyrophosphate (PRPP) (Figure 105–4).[22] This pathway requires 6 moles of adenosine triphosphate (ATP) for generation of each mole of inosinic acid, the first purine nucleotide in the pathway. A complex network of purine interconversion reactions ensures efficient reuse of preformed purines, so that much of the cellular energy that would otherwise be consumed in synthesis of new purines is conserved. Foremost among these are the single-step salvage reactions, involving the two enzymes adenine and hypoxanthine-guanine phosphoribosyltransferase (APRT and HGPRT), which catalyze conversion of the respective purine bases directly to the corresponding nucleotides by reaction with PRPP.[23]

Together, purine base salvage and de novo purine synthesis pathways provide alternative but concerted means for adjusting the production of purine nucleotides to needs. The molecular mechanisms effecting this regulation have been defined.[24,25] Control of purine synthesis de novo (Fig. 106–4) is exerted in large part in a regulatory domain encompassing the first reaction uniquely committed to the pathway, catalyzed by amidophosphoribosyltransferase (amidoPRT),[24] and the preceding PRPP synthetase reaction in which PRPP is

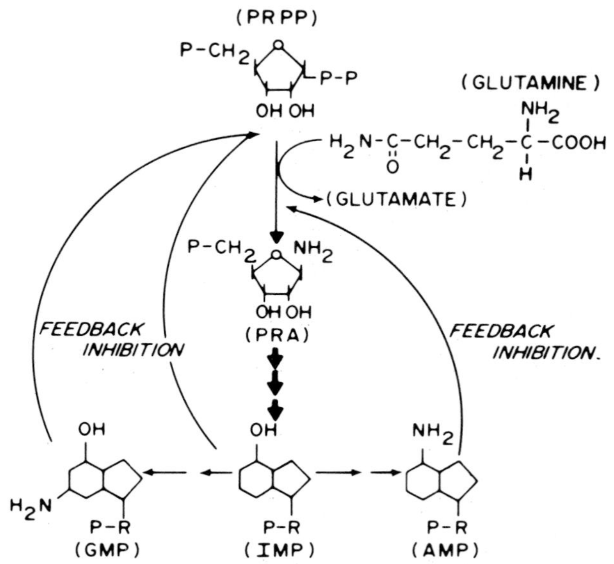

FIGURE 105–4. Regulation of purine nucleotide synthesis. AMP = adenosine monophosphate; GMP = guanosine monophosphate; IMP = inosine 5^1-monophosphate; PRA = phosphoribosylamine; PRPP = phosphoribosylpyrophosphate.

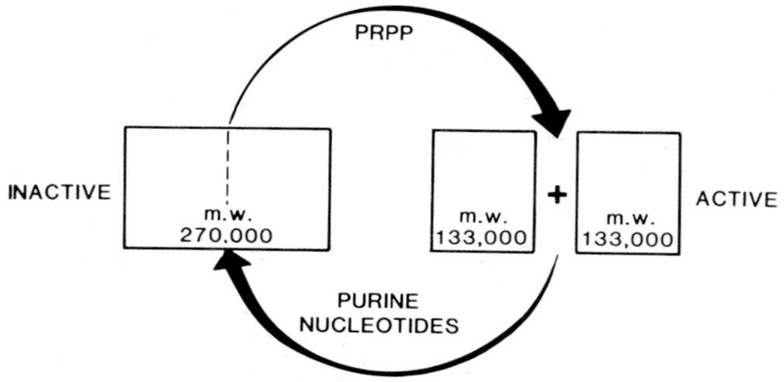

ENZYMATIC ABNORMALITIES LEADING TO PURINE OVERPRODUCTION IN MAN

FIGURE 105–5. Schematic illustrating the control of human amidophosphoribosyltransferase. PRPP = phosphoribosylpyrophosphate.

generated.[25] The allosteric regulatory properties of amidoPRT reflect an antagonistic interaction at the level of the enzyme between PRPP and pathway end products.[24,26–28] AmidoPRT activity is inhibited by purine nucleotides, and this feedback inhibition is reversed by PRPP.[26,27] Concentrations of PRPP in normal cells are below the apparent affinity constant of amidoPRT for PRPP,[26,29] suggesting that availability of this compound is the basis of rate limitation at the amidoPRT reaction. AmidoPRT can assume two subunit conformations (Fig. 105–5).[24,28] The active 133-kilodalton (kd) monomer can be reversibly converted into an inactive 270-kd dimer by addition to purine nucleotides, and this effect is blocked by increasing concentrations of PRPP. This molecular mechanism provides a structural basis for control of amidoPRT activity and has been demonstrated in vivo[28] as well as in purified preparations of the enzyme.[24]

An additional level of inhibitory control is exerted by the purine nucleotides on the activity of PRPP synthetase (Fig. 105–4), but this enzyme is less sensitive than amidoPRT to nucleotide inhibition.[25,30] Moreover, PRPP synthetase activity is also inhibited by pyrimidine and, perhaps, pyridine nucleotides, products of pathways that also require PRPP.[29,31] Overall, the dual regulation of purine nucleotide production is admirably suited to maintain both fine and broad control over changes in end product availability: the former by alterations in amidoPRT subunit structure and activity in response to small changes in purine concentrations,[24,25,28,30] and the latter by changes in the activity of PRPP synthetase in response to larger variations in concentrations of the nucleotide products of several metabolic pathways.[25,30–32]

Adenine and guanine nucleotides are intracellular building blocks for RNA and DNA, and purine compounds are also essential in energy metabolism and intercellular signaling, including neural transmission. On the catabolic side of purine metabolism (Fig. 105–2), purine nucleotides are degraded through purine nucleoside and purine base forms, with ultimate irreversible oxidation of unreclaimed hypoxanthine to xanthine and xanthine to uric acid, a reaction sequence catalyzed by xanthine oxidase (Fig. 105–6).[20]

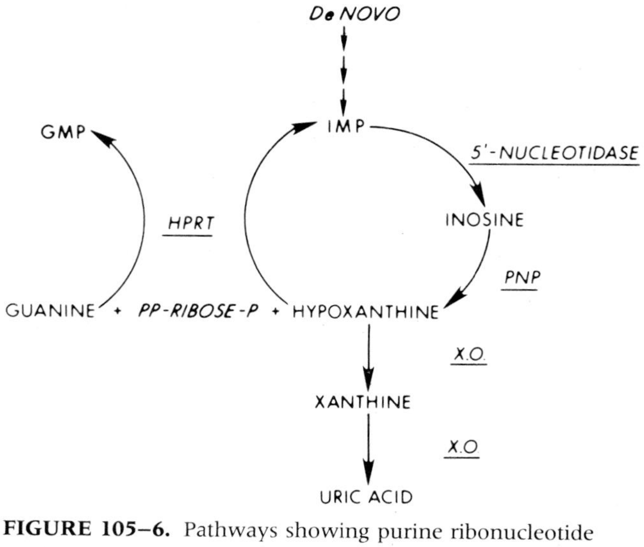

FIGURE 105–6. Pathways showing purine ribonucleotide catabolism, salvage of purine bases, and oxidation to uric acid. GMP = guanosine monophosphate; HPRT = hypoxanthine-guanine phosphoribosyltransferase; IMP = inosine 5^1-monophosphate; PNP = purine nucleoside phosphorylase; XO = xanthine oxidase.

URIC ACID HOMEOSTASIS IN NORMAL AND GOUTY INDIVIDUALS

Uric acid, synthesized mainly in the liver, is released into the circulation, where only a small percentage (less than 4% under physiologic conditions)[33–35] is bound nonspecifically to albumin or to a specific urate-binding globulin.[36] The vast majority of circulating urate is thus readily available for filtration at the glomerulus and for participation in a complex series of renal uric acid handling mechanisms, as discussed later. When tracer doses of isotopically labeled uric acid (e.g., [^{15}N] urate) are given intravenously to normal individuals at steady state, the size and dynamics of the miscible pool of uric acid can be quantitated and the overall contribution of renal excretion to uric acid disposal can be estimated from the isotopic enrichment of urinary uric acid.[37–40] The miscible urate pool in normal men averages about 1200 mg, and mean turnover of this pool is approximately 700 mg/day.[40–42] In women, the average urate pool size is about 600 mg, and the turnover rate of the pool is also about 0.6 pools/day. In both sexes, urinary uric acid excretion accounts for approximately two thirds of the uric acid turned over daily, with degradation by gut bacteria of uric acid secreted into the intestine (intestinal uricolysis) accounting for nearly all of the additional urate disposed of by extrarenal routes.[38,39,43]

Uric acid pool size is enlarged in all untreated patients with gout regardless of the magnitude of urinary uric acid excretion. (Uric acid pools in gout patients are usually in the range of 2000 to 4000 mg in the absence of evident tophi but may reach 30,000 mg or more in tophaceous gout.)[37,38,44] In hyperuricemic or gouty patients, extrarenal uric acid disposal is invariably normal or increased (to as much as 50% of total daily excretion), excluding impaired intestinal uricolysis as a mechanism of hyperuricemia.[39] Although many patients with gout have rates of turnover of the uric acid pool that overlap the normal range,[40] increased rates of turnover are uniformly found in patients who show excessive rates of incorporation of radioactively labeled precursor molecules (such as [^{14}C] glycine) into urinary uric acid (a measure of purine nucleotide and uric acid synthesis)[41,45,56] and daily urinary uric acid excretion clearly exceeding that of normal individuals.[39,41,44]

These findings provided the first evidence of heterogeneity in the mechanisms accounting for uric acid accumulation, hyperuricemia, and the consequent predisposition to urate crystal deposition in gout.[39,41,46] Additional study has confirmed that excessive production and diminished renal excretion of uric acid, operating singly or in combination, are the major abnormalities demonstrable among hyperuricemic individuals with or without gout.[47] Whether the hyperuricemia occurs exclusive of a coexisting disease or aberrant physiologic state (primary hyperuricemia) or is a consequence of one of the conditions listed in Table 105–1 (secondary hyperuricemia), one or both of these mechanisms underlie the development of hyperuricemia.

TABLE 105–1. CAUSES OF HYPERURICEMIA IN MAN

INCREASED PURINE BIOSYNTHESIS OR URATE PRODUCTION

- Inherited enzymatic defects
  - Hypoxanthine-guanine phophoribosyltransferase deficiency
  - Phosphoribosylpyrophosphate synthetase overactivity
  - Glucose-6-phosphatase deficiency
- Clinical disorders leading to purine overproduction
  - Myeloproliferative disorders
  - Lymphoproliferative disorders
  - Polycythemia vera
  - Malignant diseases
  - Hemolytic disorders
  - Psoriasis
  - Obesity
  - Tissue hypoxia
  - Glycogenesis III, V, VII
- Drugs or dietary habits
  - Ethanol
  - Diet rich in purines
  - Pancreatic extract
  - Fructose
  - Nicotinic acid
  - Ethylamino-1,3,4-thiadiazole
  - 4-Amino-5-imidazole carboxamide riboside
  - Vitamin B_{12} (patients with pernicious anemia)
  - Cytotoxic drugs
  - Warfarin

DECREASED RENAL CLEARANCE OF URATE

- Clinical disorders
  - Chronic renal failure
  - Lead nephropathy
  - Polycystic kidney disease
  - Hypertension
  - Dehydration
  - Salt restriction
  - Starvation
  - Diabetic ketoacidosis
  - Lactic acidosis
  - Obesity
  - Hyperparathyroidism
  - Hypothyroidism
  - Diabetes insipidus
  - Sarcoidosis
  - Toxemia of pregnancy
  - Bartter's syndrome
  - Chronic beryllium disease
  - Down's syndrome
- Drugs or dietary habits
  - Ethanol
  - Diuretics
  - Low doses of salicylates
  - Ethambutol
  - Pyrazinamide
  - Laxative abuse (alkalosis)
  - Levodopa
  - Methoxyflurane
  - Cyclosporine

Distinction in individual patients between uric acid overproduction and impaired renal uric acid excretion as the basis of hyperuricemia has therapeutic as well as investigative significance and is warranted in most patients with gout and perhaps all who have normal renal function. The most practical approach to achieving this distinction is measurement of daily urinary uric acid excretion. This determination is best made on 2 consecutive days 5 days after initiation of an isocaloric purine-free diet and at least 10 days after medications affecting uric acid production or excretion have been discontinued. (Indomethacin and colchicine do not alter uric acid production or excretion and may be given during the study period, but radiologic contrast agents should be avoided because of their uricosuric effects).[48] Under these conditions of steady state with regard to uric acid metabolism, urinary excretion of uric acid represents a minimal estimate of the rate of uric acid synthesis (uncorrected for extrarenal uric acid disposal), which, in groups of white men, averages about 425 mg/day with an SD of 75 to 80 mg/day.[41,49] Excretion of urinary uric acid in excess of 600 mg/day (mean + 2 SD) is interpreted as indicative of uric acid overproduction.

The strict dietary control necessary for the accuracy of this determination is difficult to achieve in ambulatory patients. Measurement of daily urinary uric acid excretion during normal dietary intake is an alternative approach frequently used. Excretion in excess of 1000 mg/day is regarded as clearly excessive. Values between 800 and 1000 mg/day are deemed equivocal, requiring retesting under closer dietary control.[47,50] Women, children, noncaucasian males, and obese or very large individuals are groups for which normal values are not readily available. For such persons, daily urinary uric acid excretion exceeding about 12 mg/kg body weight most likely represents uric acid overproduction.

OVERPRODUCTION OF URIC ACID

Excessive daily urinary uric acid excretion is demonstrable in 10 to 15% of patients with gout and primary hyperuricemia and in most patients whose hyperuricemia reflects increased cell turnover (e.g., a myelo- or lymphoproliferative disease) or a toxic state or pharmacologic intervention resulting in increased uric acid production (Table 105–1).[47] In vivo isotopic labeling studies applied to such individuals almost invariably confirm the presence of increased purine nucleotide and uric acid synthesis (Fig. 105–7)[41,47] The consistency of this relationship renders the highly accurate but cumbersome and expensive isotopic procedures unnecessary in this group.

In some circumstances, however, rates of uric acid synthesis are increased as determined isotopically in patients with normal or even reduced daily urinary uric acid excretion values.[41] These discrepancies usually reflect increased extrarenal contributions to uric acid disposal such as with deposition of urate in the tophi of patients with extensive tophaceous gout or with increased intestinal uricolysis in patients with renal insufficiency. Failure to confirm a strong suspicion of uric acid overproduction by urinary uric acid excretion measurements in patients with tophi or renal insufficiency should prompt consideration for direct measurement of rates of purine nucleotide synthesis either by in vivo labeling or by measurement of rates of purine synthesis

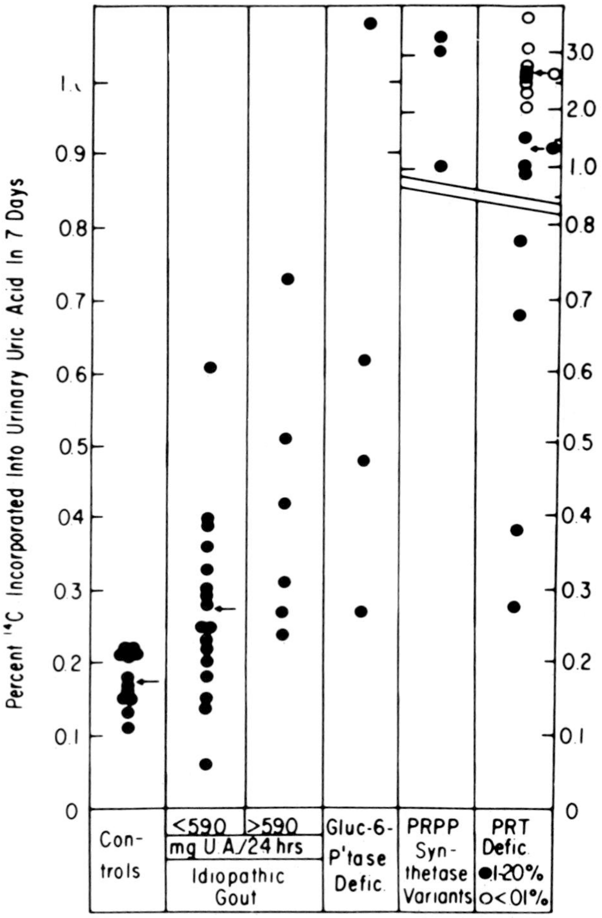

FIGURE 105–7. Summary of ^{14}C-glycine incorporation values in control and gouty subjects (From Wyngaarden, J.B., and Kelley, W.N.[47]) PRPP = phosphoribosylpyrophosphate; PRT = phosphoribosyltransferase.

de novo in fibroblasts cultured from skin biopsy material. The latter method provides a sensitive and reliable means for detecting purine overproduction in patients with primary hyperuricemia.[51,52] These alternatives to daily urinary uric acid excretion studies are also valuable in detecting the occasional patient whose cryptic uric acid overproduction is accompanied by impaired renal uric acid disposal but who has neither tophi nor overt reduction in glomerular filtration rate.

Persistent uric acid overproduction in patients with gout and primary hyperuricemia indicates excessive rates of purine synthesis de novo. In keeping with the proposed scheme for regulation of the rate of this pathway, involving antagonistic interaction of PRPP and purine nucleotides on amidoPRT activity (Fig. 105–4),[24,25] altered balance in the availability of these small molecule effectors has been identified under several circumstances in which inherited or acquired hyperuricemia is associated with uric acid overproduction. In these instances, either increased PRPP availability or diminished purine nucleotide concentrations (or both) constitute the immediate stimuli for excessive purine nucleotide and uric acid production. Although an amidoPRT with decreased response to nucleotide inhibition or increased response to PRPP could also result in purine overproduction,[51,52] defects in this enzyme have yet to be confirmed among gouty individuals.

INCREASED PRPP AVAILABILITY

A wealth of biochemical, pharmacologic, and clinical data support the role of PRPP as a critical component in the regulation of purine synthesis and thus of uric acid production.[29,47] Increased PRPP availability as the driving force for excessive rates of purine synthesis de novo is best exemplified in the two X chromosome-linked inborn errors of purine metabolism, HGPRT deficiency[53,54] and PRPP synthestase superactivity (Figs. 105–4, 105–8).[55,56] In both of these disorders, uric acid overproduction, hyperuricemia, and hyperuricosuria occur in conjunction with increased PRPP levels but not with a decrease in purine nucleotide concentrations.[25,32,56–58] A unique or contributing role for increased PRPP availability in uric acid overproduction has also been suggested in several other proposed or established enzymatic defects or metabolic states (Fig. 105–8), but the associations remain to be more fully delineated.

HGPRT Deficiency

HGPRT catalyzes the salvage reactions of the purine bases hypoxanthine and guanine with PRPP (Figs. 105–4, 105–6) to form the respective mononucleotides IMP and GMP.[23] The presence of HGPRT activity in all cells suggests a "housekeeping" function, and there appears to be relatively little regulation of the expression of the HGPRT gene evident in cell types examined to date.[59] Despite alternative routes of purine nucleotide synthesis, however, HGPRT function is clearly not redundant, as revealed by the consequences of inherited deficiency of the enzyme.

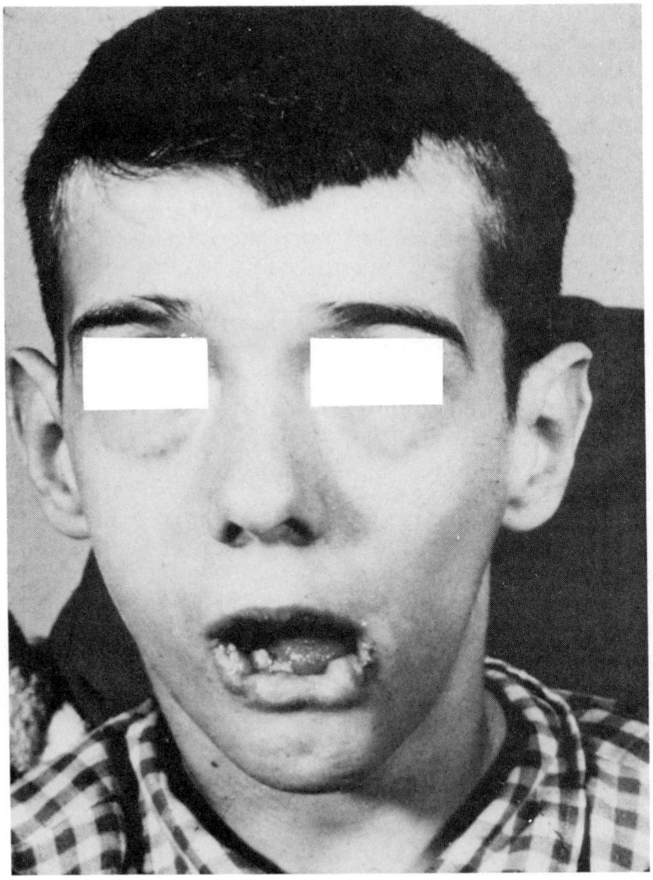

FIGURE 105–9. Lesch-Nyhan syndrome. Note the mutilation of the lower lip. (Courtesy of J. Edwin Seegmiller)

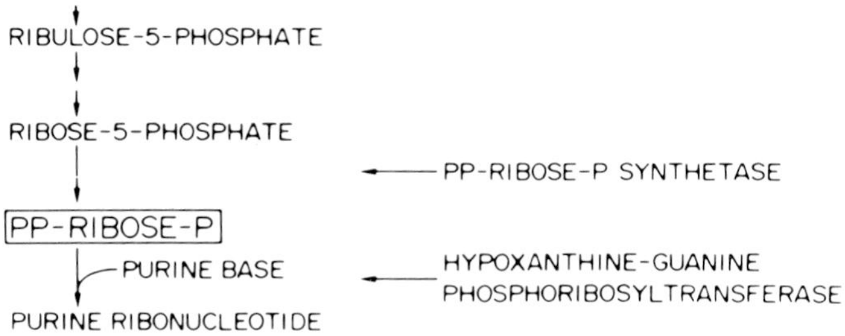

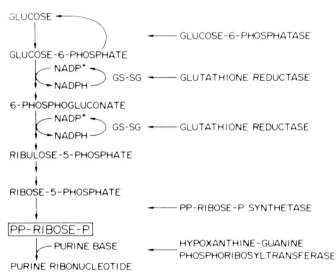

FIGURE 105–8. Enzymatic defects that may result in increased phosphoribosylpyrophosphate. NADP = nicotinamide-adenine dinucleotide phosphate; NADPH = reduced nicotinamide-adenine dinucleotide phosphate.

Deficiency of HGPRT is expressed in two clinical forms, only one of which appears among hemizygous affected males in a single family. In general, those phenotypes correlate with the presence or absence of residual HGPRT activity. The Lesch-Nyhan syndrome[60] appears in infancy or early childhood in conjunction with complete HGPRT deficiency (Fig. 105–9).[53] This is a dramatic and devastating disorder in which the clinical consequences of hyperuricemia and hyperuricosuria (most frequently uric acid urolithiasis) are usually secondary in importance to a neurobehavioral constellation that includes most or all of the following features: choreoathetosis, spasticity, varying degrees of mental retardation, and compulsive self-mutilation. How the neurologic features of the syndrome relate to the inherited defect in purine metabolism is uncertain. Nevertheless, comparatively high levels of HGPRT activity are found in the basal ganglia of the normal brain,[57] and abnormalities in the dopaminergic neurotransmitter pathway from the substantia nigra to the putamen and caudate nucleus have been identified in brains of Lesch-Nyhan syndrome patients,[61] implicating these regions of the brain despite the minimal histologic damage found at necropsy.

Partial deficiencies of HGPRT are associated with clinical manifestations directly correlated with severe uric acid overproduction, hyperuricemia, and hyperuricosuria: gouty arthritis and/or uric acid urolithiasis, appearing in males in late adolescence or early adulthood.[54,57] Neurobehavioral defects are not often a feature of partial HGPRT deficiency, even though residual enzyme activity may be less than 1% that of normal. At the other end of the spectrum, residual HGPRT activities of up to 60% have been reported among affected males in certain families, but closer examination has usually revealed kinetic defects in HGPRT resulting in more severely reduced HGPRT function under conditions occurring in intact cells.[62,63]

Expression of HGPRT deficiency is virtually restricted to males, reflecting the fact that the HGPRT gene maps to the long arm of the X chromosome (Xq26).[64] Extensive analyses of normal and mutant human HGPRT genes, cDNAs, and enzymes have revealed marked heterogeneity in the precise structural defects associated with enzyme deficiencies and with the distinctive clinical phenotypes.[62,65–68] HGPRT is undetectable both enzymatically and immunochemically in the cells of the majority of patients with Lesch-Nyhan syndrome.[69,70] HGPRT gene transcripts (mRNAs) can, however, be detected at normal or reduced abundance in most instances, and a wide range of genetic defects characteristic of these families have been precisely defined by molecular cloning of the respective HGPRT cDNAs.[67,68] Nucleotide deletions, additions, and, most frequently, base transitions have been revealed in these studies.[67,68] The identification of multiple sites of mutation leading to severe enzyme deficiency has shed some light on the relationship of HGPRT primary structure and enzymatic function.[59] Moreover, recent technologic advances have permitted development of oligonucleotide-specific hybridization analysis for detection of carriers and prenatal diagnosis of affected fetuses in individual families.

Partial deficiencies of HGPRT are most often accompanied by a residual HGPRT protein,[59,65,66] allowing the possibility of characterization of mutation by protein analysis as well as by the cloning techniques necessary for analysis of severe enzyme deficiencies. Protein chemical analyses of HGPRT isolated from the cells of patients with partial enzyme deficiency (and even a few with Lesch-Nyhan syndrome) have been achieved by means of enzyme purification and peptide sequencing.[59,65] These studies have revealed amino acid substitutions correlated with varying degrees of enzyme deficiency, providing further insight into enzyme structure–function relationships.[59]

The study of HGPRT deficiency has reached a high level of sophistication, particularly at the level of basic cell biology and molecular genetics.[59,71] It seems likely that current model systems designed to transfer human HGPRT DNA into nervous systems of experimental animals will ultimately yield the ability to attempt genetic correction of Lesch-Nyhan syndrome.[72,73] Given the available analytic expertise, measurement of HGPRT activity should be undertaken in patients with demonstrated primary uric acid overproduction and is especially important in those families with childhood onset of symptoms and a neurologic syndrome.

Despite the structural heterogeneity underlying HGPRT deficiency and the consequent variability in the magnitude of the derangement in purine synthesis, the biochemical mechanism of purine nucleotide and uric acid overproduction is unitary (Fig. 105–4). PRPP availability is increased as a result of decreased use of this compound in the salvage of hypoxanthine and guanine.[58] Overall synthesis of PRPP is not increased and purine nucleotide concentrations are not diminished.[32,58] Accumulation of PRPP activates amidoPRT, the rate-determining reaction of purine synthesis de novo and thus, accelerates the pathway.[26] Once the excessive purine nucleotide products of the pathway are converted into hypoxanthine or guanine, failure of purine base reuse means that these purine bases are directed to formation of uric acid (Fig. 105–6).[32,74,75] The inability to salvage hypoxanthine and guanine not only contributes to hyperuricemia but also precludes the salvage synthesis of purine nucleotide feedback inhibitors of purine synthesis de novo, that would normally modulate the rate of the pathway.[32,75]

Purine nucleoside phosphorylase deficiency, an enzyme defect resulting in inherited immunodeficiency disease, also results in purine overproduction as a consequence of impaired PRPP use in purine base salvage.[76] This disorder, however, is accompanied by hypouricemia because purine nucleoside phosphorylase activity is required for formation of hypoxanthine and guanine, without which only limited amounts of uric acid can be produced.

PRPP Synthetase Superactivity

This enzyme catalyzes synthesis of PRPP from ribose-5-phosphate and ATP in a reaction dependent on inorganic phosphate (Pi) and Mg^{2+} as activators. The reaction is subject to inhibition by a variety of phosphorylated compounds, including purine and pyrimidine nucleotides (Fig. 105–10).[31,77,78] In common with HGPRT deficiency, PRPP synthetase superactivity is inherited as an X chromosome-linked trait,[79,80] which is expressed in two clinical phenotypes. The more severe phenotype involves neurodevelopmental impairment in association with more severe kinetic derangement in enzyme function and more aberrant PRPP and purine metabolism in the affected individuals and their cells in culture.[81] Among the kinetic alterations resulting in PRPP synthetase superactivity are (1) catalytic defects in which maximal reaction velocity is increased but substrate, activator, and inhibitor responsiveness are nor-

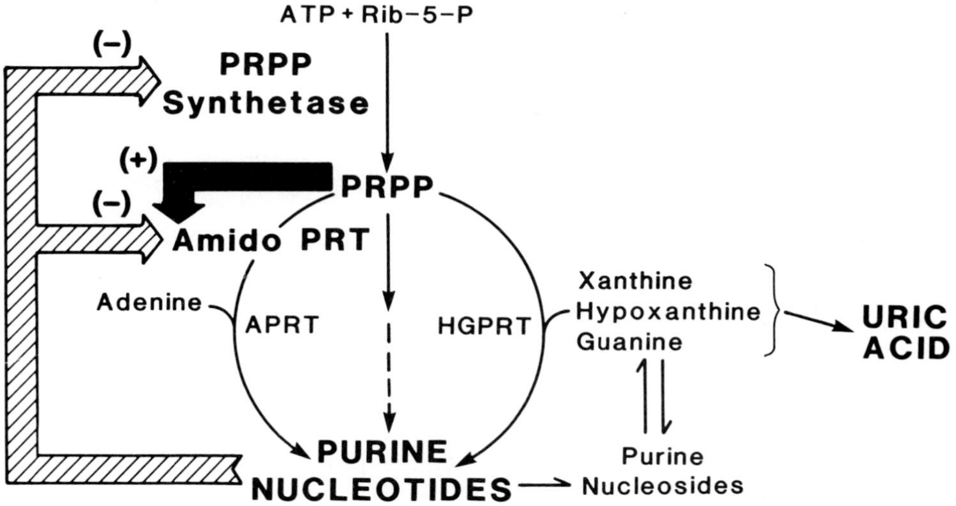

FIGURE 105–10. Control of phosphoribosylpyrophosphate (PRPP) synthetase activity by substrates and phosphorylated inhibitors. Purine nucleotide inhibition (−) of PRPP synthetase and amidophosphoribosyltransferase (amidoPRT) is indicated by hatched arrow, and allosteric activation (+) of amidoPRT by PRPP is indicated by the dark arrow. APRT = adenine phosphoribosyltransferase; ATP = adenosine triphosphate; HGPRT = hypoxanthine-guanine phosphoribosyltransferase.

mal;[78,82,83] (2) regulatory defects involving impaired responsiveness to purine nucleotide inhibitors, sometimes accompanied by increased activation by Pi; [81,84–86] (3) combined catalytic and regulatory defects; [87] and (4) increased affinity for the substrate ribose-5-phosphate.[51]

In all affected individuals, purine and uric acid overproduction results from increased PRPP availability, which is, in turn, a consequence of increased PRPP synthesis.[32,85] In this regard, PRPP synthetase superactivity differs from HGPRT deficiency in which increased PRPP concentrations result from impaired use in purine base salvage and rates of PRPP synthesis are normal. Families with regulatory or combined kinetic defects in PRPP synthetase generally have higher rates of PRPP production and, consequently, greater acceleration of purine nucleotide and uric acid synthesis.[32] Affected hemizygous male members of such families are likely to show infantile or early childhood symptoms and signs of uric acid overproduction in conjunction with neurodevelopmental impairment, most frequently sensorineural deafness.[81,82,87,88] Heterozygous female carriers in these families may develop gout during the reproductive period, sometimes in association with deafness.[82,87] In contrast, in families with catalytic defects alone, clinical presentation is almost always restricted to affected males in whom gout and uric acid urolithiasis, without neurologic defects, become evident in early childhood.[51,82,83,89]

The evidence that PRPP synthetase superactivity results from structural mutation in the PRPP synthetase gene is strong but, to date, indirect. Recently, a family of human PRPP synthetase genes has been identified and cloned.[90–92] These genes code for highly homologous proteins that appear to be independently active isoforms. Two of the PRPP synthetase genes map to the X chromosome but to different regions.[90,91] Preliminary evidence suggest that mutations in the coding region of the PRPP synthetase 1 gene (which is located on the long arm of the X chromosome at Xq22-q24)[91] underlie the diminished purine nucleotide feedback responsiveness leading to enzyme overactivity in at least certain families with the more severe clinical phenotype.[93]

PRPP Availability in Other States of Purine Overproduction and/or Gout

Together, HGPRT deficiency and PRPP synthetase superactivity account for only a small proportion (10 to 15%) of patients with primary uric acid overproduction.[47] Other enzyme defects that may shed light on additional members of this group of individuals as a consequence of increased PRPP production have been studied (Fig. 105–8).

In patients with glucose-6-phosphatase deficiency (glycogen storage disease, type I; Von Gierecke's disease), hyperuricemia appears as early as infancy and gout has been reported by the end of the first decade. Patients surviving into adulthood with this autosomal recessive disorder may then suffer tophaceous gout and gouty renal disease as major clinical problems unless effective management is instituted.[94]

The pathophysiology of hyperuricemia in glucose-6-phosphatase-deficient patients is multifactorial, involving both purine nucleotide and uric acid overproduction, confirmed by in vivo isotopic labeling,[94] and involving impaired renal uric acid excretion that is due to lacticacidemia and ketonemia.[95] Dual mechanisms through which increased PRPP production may contribute to the hyperuricemia of this disease have been proposed. First, glucose-6-phosphate accumulation, resulting from the inherited enzyme deficiency, may provide increased hepatic substrate for and stimulation of the oxidative branch of the pentose phosphate pathway, which leads to increased ribose-5-phosphate and ultimately, PRPP synthesis.[95] Second, diminished concentrations of inhibitory purine nucleotides occurring in the livers of patients with this disease during recurrent episodes of hypoglycemia may result in activation of amidoPRT and PRPP synthetase by release of one or both of these enzymes from nucleotide feedback inhibition.[28] The extent to which these possibly potentiating mechanisms play roles in purine nucleotide overproduction in glucose-6-phosphatase deficiency in man is uncertain, but results with human and animal experimental models indicate that both are tenable.[28,95]

Increased PRPP production as a consequence of enhanced oxidative pentose phosphate pathway production of ribose-5-phosphate has also been hypothesized to explain hyperuricemia in some gout patients without glucose-6-phosphatase deficiency. Increased concentrations and rates of production of ribose-5-phosphate and PRPP were shown in fibroblasts cultured from two patients with documented purine nucleotide and uric acid overproduction.[52] Also, a high frequency of overactive, electrophoretically variant forms of glutathione reductase has been reported in red blood cell lysates from patients with gout.[96] Activity of glutathione reductase promotes reduction of glutathione and oxidation of reduced nicotinamide adenine dinucleotide phosphate (NADPH) to nicotinamide adenine dinucleotide phosphate (NADP) a cofactor in the first two reactions of the oxidative pathway. Because the rate of operation of the pathway depends at least in part on the regulation of glucose-6-phosphate dehydrogenase activity by the ratio [NADPH]/[NADP], increased glutathione reductase activity could provide a tenable mechanism for excessive PRPP synthesis and purine nucleotide and uric acid overproduction.

Purine overproduction, however, was not demonstrated in the initial report of variant glutathione reductase activity,[96] and several subsequent studies have failed to confirm either abnormal enzyme activity or electrophoretically altered glutathione reductase in hemolyates from gouty patients.[97,98] In addition, experimental evidence linking rates of the oxidative and nonoxidative pathways of pentose phosphate generation to control of rates of PRPP and purine nucleotide synthesis under physiologic conditions, although suggestive, has not been definitive.

Decreases in Purine Nucleotide Concentrations

Although deficiency of HGPRT might be expected to result in reduced intracellular purine nucleotide concentrations (Fig. 105–4), such reductions have not been found in extracts of HGPRT-deficient cells.[32,58,75] Nevertheless, circumstances in which uric acid overproduction results from nucleotide depletion have been identified (Fig. 105–11). These circumstances have in common net degradation of ATP as a consequence of increased ATP consumption or impaired ATP regeneration.[99] In conditions in which the availability of Pi, oxygen, glucose, or fatty acids are restricted, optimal rates of ATP synthesis may be impaired, and severe ATP depletion and accompanying hyperuricemia may ensue, especially if the demands for ATP consumption are increased. Net ATP degradation results in accumulation of ADP and AMP, which are rapidly converted to uric acid through the intermediates adenosine, inosine, hypoxanthine, and xanthine. Thus, increases in any or all of these intermediates accompanying excessive uric acid levels in serum or urine provide evidence in support of this mechanism of hyperuricemia.[100–106]

The effects of rapid administration of fructose in man provides an experimental model for this mechanism.[107]

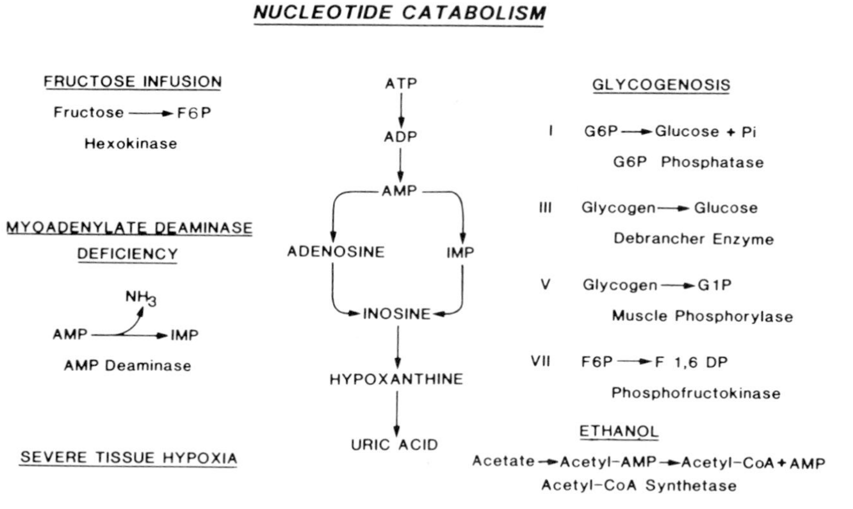

FIGURE 105–11. Disorders resulting in accelerated adenine nucleotide catabolism. ADP = adenosine diphosphate; AMP = adenosine monophosphate; ATP = adenosine triphosphate; F6P = fructose-6-phosphate, F 1, 6DP = fructose-1,6-diphosphate; G6P = glucose-6-phosphate, G1P = glucose-1-phosphate; IMP = inosine 5[1]-monophosphate.

Fructose phosphorylation in the liver uses ATP, and the accompanying Pi depletion limits regeneration of ATP from ADP, which, in turn, serves as substrate for the catabolic pathway to uric acid formation.[99] Thus, within minutes after fructose infusion, plasma (and later urinary) inosine, hypoxanthine, xanthine, and uric acid concentrations are increased.[107] In conjunction with purine nucleotide depletion, rates of purine synthesis de novo are accelerated, thus potentiating uric acid production.[102] Evidence from these studies and from fructose administration to rats confirms that the increased purine synthetic rate is accompanied by increased PRPP levels, presumably as a result of release of nucleotide inhibition of PRPP synthetase.[28,102] In addition, the distribution of amidoPRT in hepatic tissue is shifted toward the active monomeric form (Fig. 105–5) as might be predicted from the acceleration of purine synthesis de novo.[28]

Among the clinical states associated with net ATP degradation and consequent hyperuricemia are glycogen storage diseases, type III (debrancher deficiency), type V (myophosphorylase deficiency), and type VII (muscle phosphofructokinase deficiency) in which mild exercise provokes "myogenic hyperuricemia" and hyperuricosuria as a consequence of impaired glucose availability for regeneration of ATP from ADP in muscle.[104] Strenuous exercise or prolonged training in otherwise normal individuals may result in muscle hypoxia leading to muscle adenylate depletion and generation of hypoxanthine.[99] This purine base is then transported to the liver for conversion to uric acid, ultimately contributing more to the ensuing hyperuricemia than the accompanying hyperlacticacidemia and dehydration. In glucose-6-phosphatase deficiency, hypoglycemia or glucagon administration result in reduced hepatic ATP concentrations and purine catabolism contributing to multifactorial hyperuricemia.[95]

Hyperuricemia resulting at least in part from net ATP degradation is encountered quite commonly in two additional situations. First, in acutely ill patients with diseases such as adult respiratory distress syndrome (ARDS) myocardial infarction, or status epilepticus, tissue hypoxia may impair ATP synthesis from ADP in mitochondria, resulting in ADP catabolism and high plasma and urinary concentrations of inosine, hypoxanthine, xanthine, and uric acid.[100,101] The fact that these findings are associated with a poor prognosis in such patients suggests that significant hypoxia is required for activation of the purine catabolic pathway. Second, alcohol consumption results in accelerated conversion of ATP to AMP and enhanced production of uric acid and its immediate precursors when the rate of ATP use in ethanol metabolism via acetate to form acetyl coenzyme A (CoA) exceeds the capacity for ATP regeneration.[103,105] This mechanism can play a major role in the hyperuricemia associated with ethanol ingestion, along with renal uric acid retention in the course of dehydration and metabolic acidosis.

EXCRETION OF URIC ACID

In normal persons, approximately two thirds of the uric acid produced daily is excreted by the kidney, one third is eliminated by the gastrointestinal tract, and less than 1% is excreted in sweat.[43,108,109] In gouty patients, decreased renal clearance commonly leads to hyperuricemia despite increased gastrointestinal urate excretion.

CONTROL OF URIC ACID EXCRETION BY THE KIDNEY

Renal excretion of uric acid is a complicated physiologic function (Fig. 105–12); the component mechanisms have been defined since the mid-1970s as a result of pharmacologic and physiologic studies in experimental animals and in humans. Despite essentially free filtration of urate at the glomerulus, renal clearance of uric acid in normal subjects is only 7 to 10% that of creatinine or inulin clearances.[110] (The function [Curate/Ccreatinine × 100] is referred to as fractional urate excretion or FEurate, expressed as a percentage). This discrepancy implies that at least 90 to 93% of filtered urate is subjected to tubular reabsorption. Available animal studies indicate that the major site of uric acid reabsorption is in the proximal renal tubule and is facilitated by an active transport process independent of nonionic diffusion or passive forces.[111–113]

Evidence that a two-component system, involving

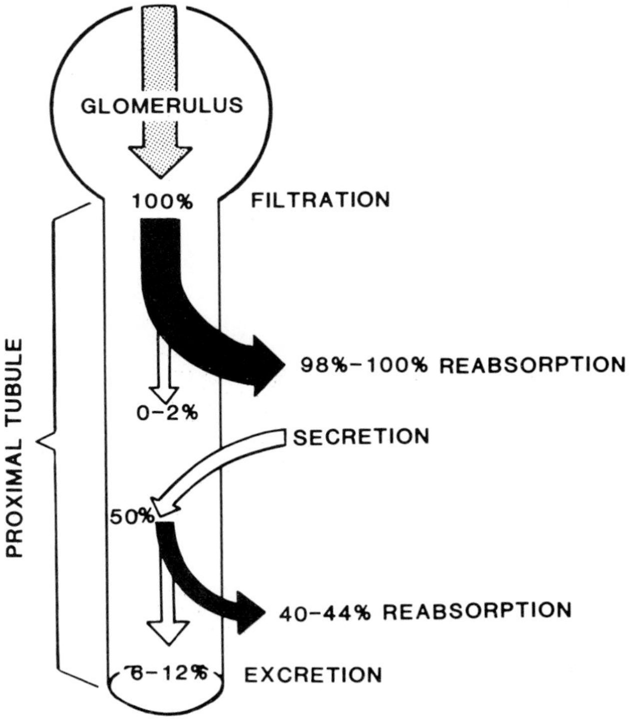

FIGURE 105–12. Four-component model illustrating bidirectional urate transport by the kidney. Tubular secretion and reabsorption are shown as a percentage of filtered urate.

glomerular filtration and proximal tubular reabsorption, was insufficient to define renal urate handling completely came from two sources. First, an otherwise healthy man was identified in whom marked hypouricemia was accompanied by a urate clearance that was 146% that of inulin clearance.[114] In this individual with an apparent selective defect in uric acid reabsorption, tubular urate secretion was postulated. The existence of this mechanism also appeared to explain the second experimental observation: the paradoxic effects of salicylates and probenecid on uric acid excretion.[115] In low doses, these drugs decrease uric acid excretion, but high doses result in uricosuria.[116] These phenomena were best explained by hypothesizing inhibition of tubular secretion at low doses and inhibition of both secretion and reabsorption at higher doses. Subsequently, tubular secretion as a third mechanism of renal uric acid handling was confirmed after urate loading, mannitol diuresis, and large doses of probenecid both in normal subjects and in animal studies employing micropuncture techniques.[117–119] The latter method has identified the proximal nephron as the major site of tubular secretion, and a study in man has shown that the proximal but not the distal nephron can transport urate from plasma to tubular fluid.[120] Finally, urate secretion in man appears to be mediated by a transport system shared with other organic acids such as salicylates, acetoacetate, lactate, β-hydroxybutyrate, branched-chair ketoacids, and pyrazinoic acid, the major metabolite of pyrazinamide.[121]

Pyrazinamide virtually abolishes uric acid excretion in man as a result of potent inhibition of tubular secretion of urate.[122] However, the fact that administration of this drug also abolishes the uricosuria of Wilson's disease[123] and Hodgkin's disease[124] as well as the uricosuric response to probenecid,[125] benzbromarone,[126] intravenous furosemide,[127] or volume expansion[128] has caused even the three-component model of renal urate handling to be reassessed. As a consequence of studies in humans and in Cebus monkeys, a four-component model incorporating extensive postsecretory reabsorption of secreted urate at a site either co-extensive with or distal to the secretory site has been proposed.[126,129,130] In fact, hyporuricemic individuals have been studied who have enhanced fractional excretion of urate, a normal response to pyrazinamide, and reduced uricosuric responses to benzbromarone or probenecid, findings most easily interpreted as reflecting an isolated defect in postsecretory reabsorption of uric acid.[131–133] Further documentation of the four-component model of urate handling, and quantitation of the flux of uric acid by the individual transport mechanisms, will require studies beyond the scope of in vivo pharmacologic manipulation. The discovery of postsecretory reabsorption has rendered invalid the pyrazinamide suppression test, formerly used to distinguish the relative contributions to urinary uric acid excretion of secreted and filtered but nonreabsorbed uric acid.[126,129]

DECREASED URIC ACID EXCRETION IN GOUT

A reduction of uric acid clearance may contribute to hyperuricemia in as many as 90% of patients with primary gout. Over a wide range of filtered urate loads, most gouty subjects have a lower FEurate than nongouty subjects (Fig. 105–13).[134] Simkin has shown that gouty individuals excrete on average 41% less uric acid than normal subjects for any given plasma concentration of urate.[134] Patients with primary hyperuricemia also have a greater increment in plasma urate concentrations in response to exogenous purines, a finding attributed to decreased urate clearances.[135] Gouty subjects require urate levels 2 to 3 mg/dL higher than nongouty subjects in order to achieve equivalent uric acid excretion rates.[134,136]

Decreased urate clearance in primary gout could be due to reduced urate filtration, enhanced uric acid reabsorption, or decreased urate secretion. The filtered load of urate could be decreased as a result of increased urate binding to plasma proteins. This defect has been proposed in the hyperuricemia of the Maoris of New Zealand and in a few gouty subjects, but this requires confirmation. Both increased reabsorption and decreased secretion of uric acid have been proposed as the basis for the lower urate clearances observed in patients with primary gout. To date, there is no compelling experimental evidence to affirm enhanced tubular reabsorption of uric acid as one mechanism. In contrast, diminished renal urate secretion per nephron has been implicated in the hyperuricemia of primary gout not associated with overproduction of uric acid.[137] Studies employing the uricosuric response to benzbromarone, a drug that selectively inhibits reabsorption of secreted

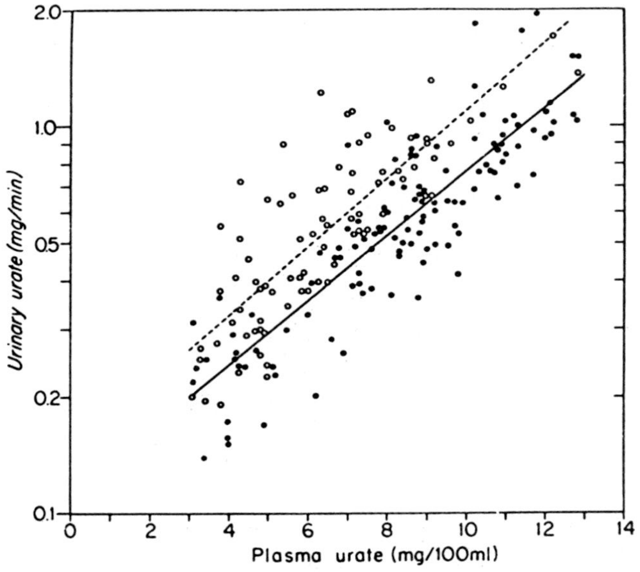

FIGURE 105–13. Urate excretion at various plasma urate concentrations in gouty (solid symbols) and nongouty (open symbols) subjects. (From Simkin, P.A.[134])

urate, to measure minimum tubular secretory rate are reported to show decreased secretion of uric acid in such patients compared to controls or to gouty subjects with overproduction hyperuricemia.[126] To date, no alteration in postsecretory reabsorption has been documented.

CLINICAL DESCRIPTION OF GOUT

Acute gouty arthritis, intercritical gout, and chronic tophaceous gout represent the three classic stages in the natural history of progressive urate crystal deposition disease. Contemporary management modalities are highly efficient in interrupting the progression of the disorder and in reducing the frequency of acute gouty arthritis and urolithiasis. Thus, gout only infrequently unfolds in the classic manner at present, and this is largely among noncompliant individuals and patients in whom the management scheme has not been appropriately communicated or the diagnosis of gout has not been made. Of special concern with regard to the latter circumstance is the recently noted rising incidence of gout among elderly women, often with mild renal insufficiency, osteoarthritic nodes, atypical and mild joint inflammation, and tophaceous deposits resembling rheumatoid nodules.

ACUTE GOUTY ARTHRITIS

> The patient goes to bed and sleeps quietly till about two in the morning when he is awakened by a pain which usually seizes the great toe, but sometimes the heel, ankle, or instep. The pain resembles that of a dislocated bone . . . and is immediately preceded by a chillness and slight fever in proportion to the pain which is mild at first but grows gradually more violent every hour; sometimes resembling a laceration of ligaments, sometimes the gnawing of a dog, and sometimes a weight and constriction of the parts affected, which becomes so exquisitely painful as not to endure the weight of the clothes nor the shaking of the room from a person walking briskly there-in. (From Sydenham quoted in Copeman, W.S.C.[138])

The acute gouty attack, so vividly described by Sydenham, lasts from a few days to several weeks in untreated patients. With multiple recurrences, shorter intervals, separate attacks, and polyarticular involvement are more frequent. Chronic inflammation with superimposed acute exacerbations may progress to a crippling arthritis. Various studies, heavily weighted to male patients, cite the peak age of onset of gouty arthritis to be between the fourth and sixth decades,[139–141] but, in women, initial episodes often arise in the sixth to eighth decades. Onset before age 30 should raise suspicion of a specific enzyme defect or, occasionally, intrinsic renal disease.

In older series describing the natural history of gout in men, fully 90% of patients experienced acute attacks at the base of the great toe (podagra) at some time during the course of their disease, and the first metatarsophalangeal joint was involved in about 50% of first attacks.[139,140] Reductions in these figures are the case now, given the truncated history of the joint disease under appropriate therapy and the recognition of atypical joint involvement in women. Although it is generally accepted that about 80% of initial attacks are monarticular, polyarticular first attacks are more common in elderly women and in patients with gout accompanying myeloproliferative disorders or the use of cyclosporine. In a recent series of 92 women with gout, 70% had had polyarticular attacks, and 35% gave no history of preceding monarthritis.[142] Other common initial sites of involvement include the instep, ankle, heel, knee, wrist, fingers, and elbows (olecranon bursa). Rarely involved sites include the shoulders, sternoclavicular joints, hips, spine, and sacroiliac joints. Conceptually, acute gout remains predominantly a disease of the lower extremity, and the more distal the site of involvement, the more typical the attack. Although urate-induced inflammation in unusual joints and soft tissue sites is often preceded by typical attacks in the usual distal joints, initial appearance in the former locations can cause diagnostic confusion.

Trivial episodes of pain ("petite attacks") lasting only hours and sometimes recurrent over several years may precede the first dramatic gouty attack. The initial attack of gout often occurs with explosive suddenness, typically awakening the patient, or becoming apparent as a foot is placed on the floor on arising. The skin over the affected joint soon becomes reddened and warm; extreme tenderness of the affected joint and periarticular tissues are noted (Fig. 105–14). The slightest pressure produces exquisite pain. Fever, leukocytosis, and elevation of the erythrocyte sedimentation rate often occur. The skin over the joint may desquamate as the episode subsides.

The course of untreated acute gout is variable. Mild attacks may subside in several hours or may persist for only a few days and not reach the intensity described by Sydenham. Severe attacks may last many days to several weeks.

On recovery, the patient re-enters an asymptomatic phase termed *the intercritical period.* Even though the attack may have been incapacitating, with excruciating pain and swelling, resolution is usually complete, and the patient is once again well. This freedom from symptoms during the intercritical period is an important feature in the diagnosis of acute arthritis as gout.

Provocative or Possible Etiologic Factors

Factors capable of provoking episodes of acute gouty arthritis include trauma, surgery, alcohol ingestion, starvation, overindulgence in foods with high purine

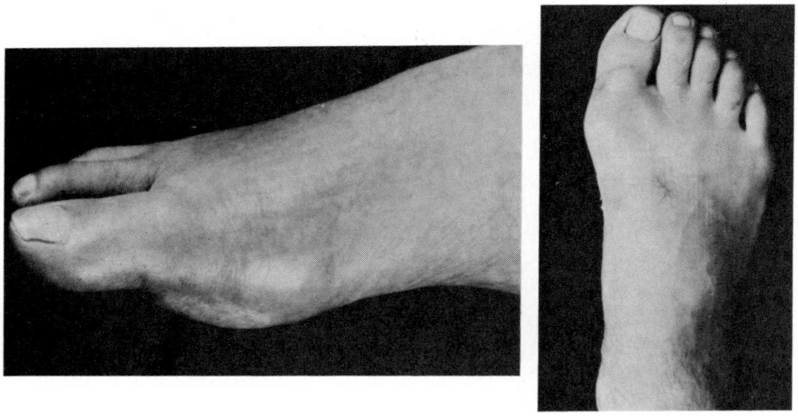

FIGURE 105–14. Acute gouty arthritis of the first metatarsophalangeal joint. (From Dieppe, P.A. et al. (Eds.): Gout. *In* Slide Atlas of Rheumatology. London, Gower Medical Publishing Ltd., 1985.)

content, and ingestion of drugs that cause changes in urate concentrations. The precise relationship of these factors to the attacks remains speculative. For example, the first metatarsophalangeal joint as a primary weight-bearing area is subject to considerable microtrauma. It is tenable that degenerative changes of the bunion joint, perhaps in conjunction with locally elevated urate concentrations as proposed by Simkin, render this site unusually susceptible to urate crystal deposition.[143] Each of the other factors is capable of provoking disturbances in extracellular urate concentrations. Alcohol binges, acute overeating, or starvation can induce marked rises in serum urate and acute attacks. The administration of drugs—such as thiazide diuretics for the treatment of hypertension, cyclosporin for immunosuppression,[144] or uricosuric agents or allopurinol for treatment of hyperuricemia—can result in gout with either elevated or lowered urate concentrations, and intravenous hyperalimenation is capable of provoking attacks of gout in predisposed individuals despite the associated hypouricemia.[145] Finally, surgery and acute trauma may predispose to gout as a consequence of the stress response with the attendant hyperuricosuria and hyperuricemia.[146]

INTERCRITICAL GOUT AND RECURRENT EPISODES

The intervals between gouty attacks are also called *the intercritical periods*. A clear and detailed history of an acute arthritic attack followed by a completely asymptomatic interval before a recurrence is valuable in pointing toward the diagnosis of gout. During this period, aspiration of a previously inflamed joint can frequently corroborate the diagnosis of gout. For example, in an untreated gouty population, 36 of 37 synovial fluid aspirates obtained during intercritical periods yielded urate crystals if the joint aspirated had been subject to past gouty attacks.[147] By comparison, the yield was only 22% without a prior history of involvement in the specific joint and 50% in patients on urate-lowering medication. The presence of crystals deposited in joints during the intercritical period corroborates the view that the stages of clinical gout represent arbitrary designations reflecting only the state of inflammation and the size of urate accumulations at a specific point in time. That is, by the time of the first attack of gouty arthritis, clinically inapparent crystal aggregates are likely to be present in the great majority of gout patients. Nevertheless, the duration of the intercritical period is variable. Without therapy, most gouty patients will experience a second episode within 2 years. In Gutman's series, 62% of patients had recurrences within the first year, and 78% within 2 years, with only 7% free of recurrences for 10 years or more.[148]

As the disease progresses in the untreated patient, acute attacks occur with increasing frequency and are often polyarticular, more severe, longer lasting, and occasionally associated with a febrile course. Although affected joints may continue to recover completely, bony erosions may develop. In one series, one third of patients with late polyarticular attacks reported that their initial attack was also polyarticular.[149] Joints may flare in sequence, in a migratory pattern, or as in pseudogout, several neighboring joints may be involved simultaneously in a cluster attack.[150] Frequently, periarticular sites such as bursae and tendons are also involved.

Eventually, the patient may suffer chronic polyarticular gout without pain-free intercritical periods. Gout at this stage may be confused with rheumatoid arthritis (RA), especially if tophi are mistaken for rheumatoid nodules. On occasion, the disease may progress from initial podagra to a RA-like chronic deforming arthritis without remissions but with synovial thickening and the early development of nodules (tophi). Unlike RA, in which polyarticular inflammation is most often synchronous, inflamed gouty joints are frequently out of phase: a flare in one joint may coincide with subsidence of inflammation in another joint. Conversely, subcutaneous nodules in patients with "rheumatoid nodulosis" are easily confused with tophi.[151] Up to 30% of patients with tophaceous gout have low serum titers of rheumatoid factor.[152] In a study of 160 patients with RA, hyperuricemia was found in 7.5%, a finding that was correlated inversely with disease activity.[153] Coexistence of gout and RA is rare, and the appropriate diagnosis is best established by demonstrating the presence or absence of urate crystals by aspiration of affected joints or tophaceous deposits.

CHRONIC TOPHACEOUS GOUT

Chronic tophaceous gout (Fig. 105–15) is characterized by the identifiable deposition of solid urate (tophi) in connective tissues, including articular structures, with ultimate development of a destructive arthropathy, often with secondary degenerative changes. The identification of tophi with or before the initial gouty attack is rare in primary gout. This situation has, however, been observed in 0.5% of subjects with gout secondary to myeloproliferative disease,[154] and in patients with type 1 glycogen storage disease,[155] and the Lesch-Nyhan syndrome.[156] In Gutman's series, the rate of urate deposition in joint tissue correlated with both the duration and degree of hyperuricemia.[157] In patients without tophi, the mean serum urate concentration was 9.2 mg/dL. Values of 10 to 11 mg/dL were found in subjects with minimal-to-moderate deposits, and patients with extensive tophaceous deposits had urate concentrations in excess of 11 mg/dL. In untreated patients, the interval from the gouty attack to the beginning of chronic arthritis or visible tophi is highly variable, ranging from 3 to 42 years with an average of 11.6 years.[158] A retrospective analysis of 1165 patients in the pretreatment era found that 70% were free of demonstrable tophi 5 years after the first gouty attack; at 10 years only 50% remained without tophi, and, by 20 years, this proportion had declined to 28%.[157] The percentage of patients with severe tophaceous gout reached appreciable proportions (24%) 20 years after the first attack. In a population of 4110 gouty Japanese subjects followed for 19 years, only 9.2% had tophaceous deposits.[159]

Tophaceous gout is often associated with an early age of onset, a long duration of active but untreated disease, frequent attacks, high serum urate values, and a predilection for upper extremity and polyarticular episodes.[160] A prospective study of 106 consecutive gouty men in a Veterans Administration (VA) hospital substantiated these observations, including episodes of polyarticular gout in 40% of patients.[161] Characteristics of the arthritis included asymmetric, ascending joint involvement in which chronic inflammation was typical. Although ethanol consumption and diuretic use were frequently associated with gout in this population, suboptimal management was considered to be a major factor in the progression from monarticular gout to polyarticular status.

A second group of more compliant patients is also prone to develop polyarticular and tophaceous gout. Of 60 consecutive gouty patients seen in a rheumatology unit, 15% were elderly women (mean age 82 years), all of whom were on diuretic therapy and most of whom had tophi in osteoarthritic interphalangeal joint nodes (Fig. 105–16).[162] In another series of 149 gout patients, 17% were found to have gout in joints affected with nodal osteoarthritis.[163] Mean age was 71 years, gender was evenly distributed, and the mean urate concentration was 11 mg/dL. Diuretics were being used by 72% of these patients, and impaired renal function was present in 60%. The combination of diuretic-induced hyperuricemia and nodal osteoarthritis appears to predispose the elderly to tophaceous gout arising in nodal tissue.[164] The clinical features of this group of patients, in which women are clearly overrepresented (impostumous gout),[165] set it apart from the classically described group of middle-aged male patients with tophaceous gout who have a high associated incidence of hypertension, obesity, and ethanol abuse.

The helix of ear is a classic location for tophaceous deposits, which take the form of small white excrescences (Fig. 105–17). Other sites of predilection include the olecranon and prepatellar bursae, ulnar surfaces of the forearm, and Achilles tendons. Deposits may produce irregular and often grotesque tumescences on the hands or feet with accompanying joint destruc-

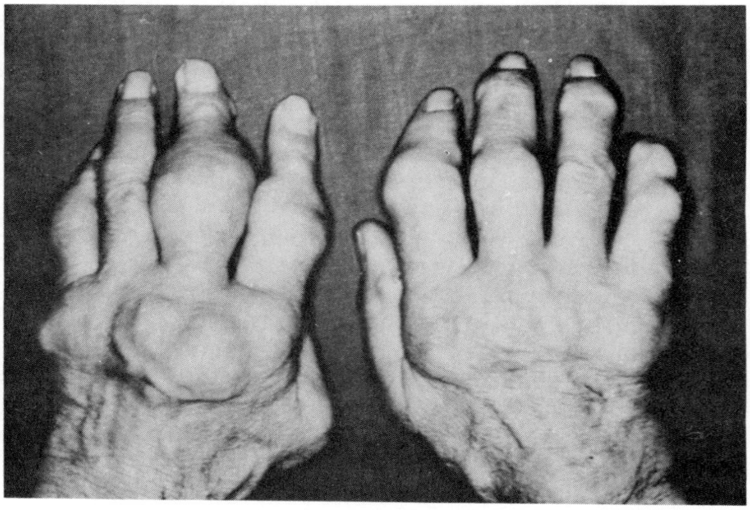

FIGURE 105–15. Chronic tophaceous gout with grotesque tumescences of hands. (From Dieppe, P.A. et al. (Eds.): Gout. *In* Slide Atlas of Rheumatology. London, Gower Medical Publishing Ltd., 1985.)

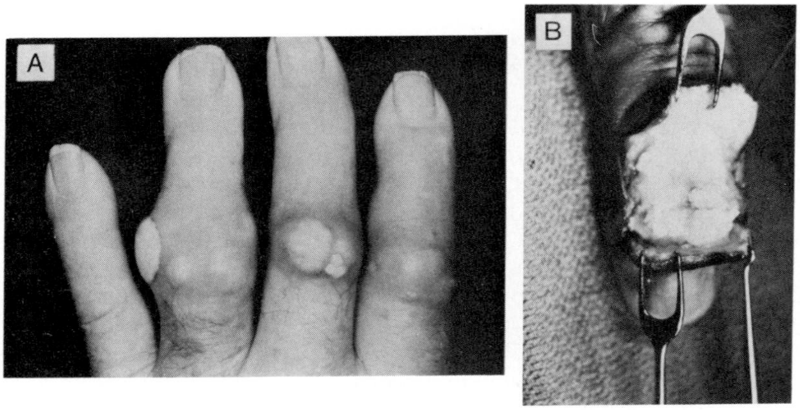

FIGURE 105–16. *A*, Impostumous gout involving osteoarthritic joints of an elderly woman on diuretic therapy for hypertension. *B*, Note the extensive urate deposits in periarticular tissue from a similar patient. (Courtesy of Dr. Michael Jablon.)

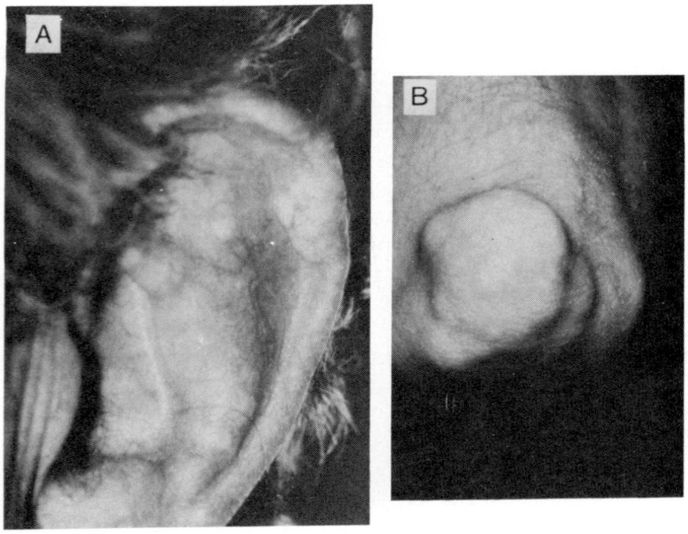

FIGURE 105–17. *A*, Tophus in helix of ear. *B*, Olecranon bursa.

tion and crippling (Figs. 105–15, 105–16). The tense, shiny skin overlying the tophus may ulcerate and extrude white, chalky material composed of needle-shaped (acicular) urate crystals (Fig. 105–18). Ulcerated tophi rarely become secondarily infected. Bony ankylosis is also unusual.[166]

The process of tophus formation advances insidiously, the patient often noting progressive stiffness and aching of affected joints. Tophi or a secondary degenerative process may limit joint mobility by mechanical destruction of the joints and adjacent structures. Likewise, the axial skeleton does not escape urate crystal deposition, which may mimic a tumor or protruded disc.[167] Tophaceous involvement of the sacroiliac joint and aseptic necrosis of the hip have been reported as manifestations of gout.[168,169] Monosodium urate crystals have been identified in avascular bone, although no cases of avascular necrosis of the femoral head were found in a systematic study of 138 gouty patients.[170]

As tophi and perchance, renal disease advance, acute attacks recur less frequently and are milder; late in the

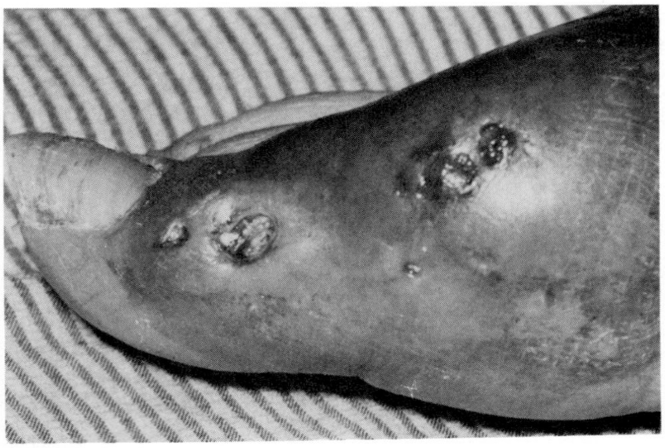

FIGURE 105–18. Ulcerated tophi. (Courtesy of Dr. Ira Melnicoff.)

illness, they may disappear entirely or may be superimposed on indolently inflamed joints. Virtually all parenchymal organs except the brain have been sites of tophus formation in one or another report.[171,172]

The availability of uricosuric agents and allopurinol has resulted in a significant decline in visible tophi and chronic gouty arthritis.[173] Before the introduction of these drugs, tophaceous deposits were found in as many as 70% of gouty patients;[174,175] more recent surveys report frequencies of less than 5%.[176] In some population groups, however, residual frequencies of tophaceous gout approaching 50% have been reported.[161] Factors such as noncompliance, poor physician–patient communication, misdiagnosis, aggressive management of hypertension with diuretics, especially in the elderly, and use of cyclosporine in transplant recipients make it unlikely that the frequency of tophaceous gout will continue to decline substantially in the future.

UROLITHIASIS AND GOUT

Uric acid stones account for 5 to 10% of all renal stones in the United States and Europe[177,178] and 75% of renal stones in Israel.[179] The overall prevalence of uric acid stones in the adult United States population is estimated to be 0.01%,[180] but in a series of 1258 patients with primary gout and 59 patients with secondary gout prevalence of renal lithiasis was 22 and 42%, respectively.[181] Fourteen years later, when the primary gout population had increased to 2038, the prevalence of uric acid stone disease was 23%.[182] Over 80% of calculi in these gouty patients were composed entirely of uric acid, with the remainder containing calcium oxalate or calcium phosphate, often with a central nidus of uric acid. The several hundred-fold higher incidence of uric acid stones in gout patients is accompanied by a 10- to 30-fold increased incidence of calcium oxalate stones.[183] Renal stones antedated arthritis in 40% of subjects with primary gout, and, in fact, occurred more frequently than arthritis as a first manifestation before the fourth decade.[182] When the prevalence of urolithiasis was related to serum urate values in the Framingham study, 12.7% of male subjects with urate values between 7 and 7.9 mg/dL and 40% of subjects with urate values greater than 9 mg/dL gave a history of renal stones.[19] The incidence of urolithiasis increased from 0.2%/year in normouricemic controls and 0.3%/year in asymptomatic hyperuricemic subjects to 0.9%/year in patients with gout.[18] About one third of nongouty hyperuricemic patients who developed uric acid stones give a family history of gout.[181]

In studies of gouty individuals, higher prevalence rates of uric acid urolithiasis are associated with increased uric acid excretion. In gouty patients excreting more uric acid than 1100 mg/day, the prevalence of stones was 50%, or 4.5-fold greater than in patients excreting less than 300 mg/day.[181] Many clinical circumstances result in hyperuricosuria, including inherited enzymatic defects and hematologic disorders that lead to accelerated purine biosynthesis, diets high in purine content,[135] and the administration of uricosuric drugs (which cause only a transient increase in uric acid excretion). The increase in uric acid excretion seen in patients ingesting large amounts of dietary purines may contribute to the development of calcium oxalate stones.[183] Low urine volume may be a predisposing factor to the development of uric acid calculi in patients with ileostomies or colostomies[184] as well as in people living in hot, arid climates.[179]

Because the hydrogen ion concentration in urine is a critical determinant of uric acid solubility, the excretion of a persistently acid urine is another predisposing factor to the development of uric acid stones. For example, at pH 5.0, the limit of solubility of uric acid in urine is 15 mg/dL, but if the pH is increased to 7.0, solubility increased to 200 mg/dL because 95% of uric acid is present as the more soluble urate ion.[185] Low urinary pH is a well-documented characteristic of patients with primary gout, in general, and in gout patients with uric acid stones, in particular.[181,182,186]

The low urinary pH of patients with uric acid calculi has been ascribed by some investigators to a defect in ammonium excretion and by others to an increase in titratable acidity.[187–189] These conflicting suggestions have not been thoroughly evaluated because other variables have not been adequately controlled. These include age, reduced nephron mass,[190] and diets high in protein and purines.[186,191] One hypothesis offered to explain the defect in ammonium excretion observed in gouty patients suggests that a deficiency of renal glutaminase activity results in reduced glutamine use for ammonium production by the kidney.[192] In direct assays, however, renal-glutaminase activity is normal in gouty subjects.[193]

Substances that may affect both uric acid solubility and crystal growth are important as additional factors to consider in the pathogenesis of uric acid and calcium oxalate stones in patients with idiopathic hyperuricosuria. Regarding uric acid solubility, the presence of a nondialyzable mucoprotein in urine, which retards uric acid precipitation, has been suggested.[194] No difference was found, however, in the amount of this substance in urine from patients with urolithiasis and healthy controls. Heterogeneous nucleation of calcium oxalate crystals can occur either on monosodium urate or uric acid seed crystals in patients with hyperuricosuria.[195] In addition, a glycoprotein-containing carboxyglutamic acid (nephrocalcin) has been isolated from kidney and urine.[196] This protein appears to inhibit calcium oxalate crystal growth and clearly warrants further study in stone formers and normal individuals.

KIDNEY DISEASE IN GOUT

Apart from arthritis and tophus formation, renal disease is the most frequently reported clinical association of hyperuricemia.[197–199] Hyperuricemia may affect the kidney through (1) deposition of urate crystals in the renal interstitium, referred to as *urate nephropathy*; (2) deposition of uric acid crystals in the collecting tubules, an entity referred to as *uric acid nephropathy*; and (3) uric acid urolithiasis. The distinction between the first two entities is often unclear and the term *gouty kidney* has been used for both. Urate nephropathy is not uncommon, by pathologic criteria at least, in patients with gout, regardless of the accompanying excretion of uric acid. In contrast, both uric acid nephropathy and urolithiasis are more common in patients with excessive uric acid production and excretion. In fact, acute uric acid nephropathy with accompanying acute renal tubular damage and an obstructive uropathic clinical picture is very uncommon except in patients with malignancy and hyperuricemia treated by radiation or chemotherapy, or with inherited enzyme defects resulting in increased purine nucleotide production. In addition to these direct effects of hyperuricemia, other causes of renal dysfunction such as hypertension, diabetes mellitis, alcohol abuse, nephrotoxic drug therapy, and lead nephropathy are also prevalent in the gouty population. The isolation of hyperuricemia or gout as primary risk factors for progressive renal disease is thus exceedingly difficult.

Urate nephropathy, if progressive at all, is only slowly progressive and does not materially reduce life expectancy.[18,200] The incidence of proteinuria in gout patients varies from 15 to 20%.[110,201] Hypertension is at least as common as proteinuria.[198] It is not entirely clear whether hypertension is the result of hyperuricemia and urate nephropathy or whether it is a cause of renal dysfunction observed in gouty patients.[202] The experience of the Mt. Sinai group suggests that uncontrolled hypertension is responsible for a significant amount of the renal dysfunction observed in gout patients,[201] and other studies support this concept.[18,203]

In past decades various authors have reported significant impairment of renal function in patients with gout ranging from 10 to 40%.[197,198] In the experience of Talbott and Terplan, renal failure was the eventual cause of death in 18 to 25% of their patients.[198] Recent evaluations have de-emphasized a causal relation between hyperuricemia, gout, and renal disease.[18,203] The incidence of renal disease is probably no higher than that of subjects of comparable age and similar degrees of hypertension, obesity, and primary renal disease.

PREVALENCE AND INCIDENCE OF GOUT

Although the prevalence of gout varies worldwide, it is similar in Europe (0.3%) and North America (0.27%).[204,205] A prevalence of 0.2% was found in Framingham, among 5127 subjects (2283 men and 2844 women), mean age 44 years.[19] Fourteen years later the prevalence had increased to 1.5% (mean age, 58 years): 2.8% in men and 0.4% in women. Among 4663 Parisian men age 40 to 44 years, the prevalence was 1.1% in the age group 35 to 39 and 2% in men 40 to 44 years.[206] The prevalence of gout is much higher among the islanders of the Mariana Islands and the Maori of New Zealand.[207,208] In this latter group the prevalence of gout is 10.3% in men and 4.3% in women. The prevalence of gout is related to the serum urate levels. (Table 105–2).[19]

Over 90% of patients with primary gout are men, and the age of peak incidence in men is earlier than that of affected women, who rarely develop the disorder before menopause.[141,209] Higher percentages of women have been reported in series that included patients with secondary gout complicated by renal disease or diuretic therapy.[142,162] Gout is uncommon before the third decade. In the Framingham study, the cumulative incidence rate in men appeared to be approaching a plateau at about age 58 years, although only one third of patients with urate levels 8 mg/dL or more had developed gout.[19] A few patients with persistently normal serum urate levels were reported to have gout, but this was not confirmed by crystal identification.

DIAGNOSIS OF GOUTY ARTHRITIS

The diagnosis of gout should be established on firm criteria to ensure that expensive and toxic medications are not prescribed unnecessarily. Available data do not

TABLE 105–2. PREVALENCE OF GOUTY ARTHRITIS IN RELATION TO SERUM URIC ACID LEVEL (ADMITTED AT A MEAN AGE OF 44 AND FOLLOWED FOR 14 YEARS)

	MEN: GOUTY ARTHRITIS DEVELOPED IN			WOMEN: GOUTY ARTHRITIS DEVELOPED IN		
SERUM URIC ACID LEVEL (MG/DL)	Total Examined (N)	n	Percentage	Total Examined (N)	n	Percentage
6	1281	8	0.6	2665	2	0.08
6–6.9	790	15	1.9	151	5	3.3
7–7.9	162	27	16.7	23	4	17.4
8–8.9	40	10	25.0	4	0	0
±9	10	9	90.0	1	0	0
Total	2283	69	2.8	2844	11	0.4

(From Hall, A.P., Barry, P.E., Dawber, T.R., and McNamara, P.M.[19])

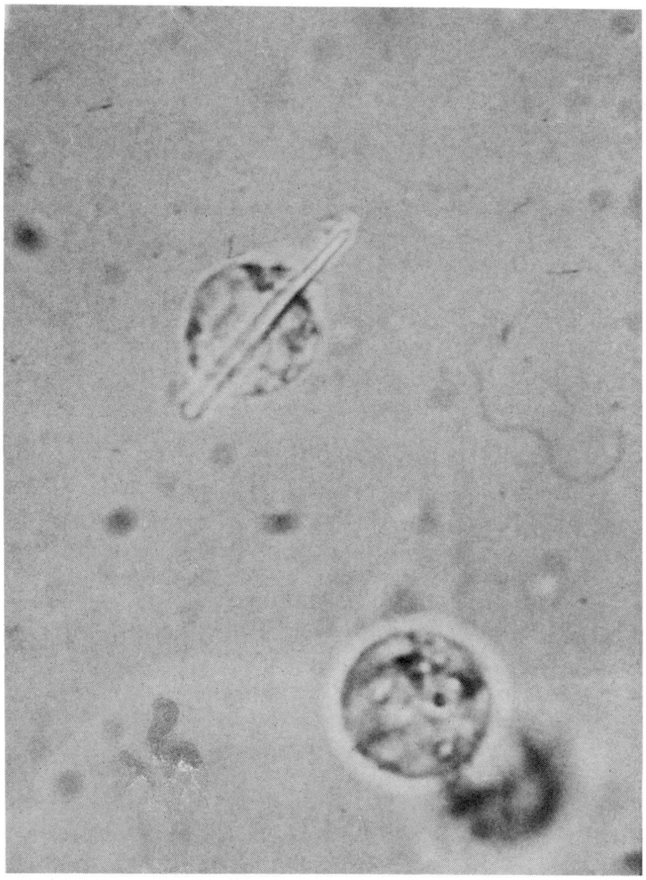

FIGURE 105–19. Polymorphonuclear leukocyte containing a phagocytized monosodium urate crystal.

support therapeutic intervention for the great majority of patients with asymptomatic hyperuricemia. A definitive diagnosis of gout is established by demonstration of intracellular monosodium urate crystals in synovial fluid neutrophils by polarized compensated light microscopy (Fig. 105–19) (see Chapter 5 on synovial fluid examination). In a study conducted by the American College of Rheumatology Subcommittee on Diagnostic and Therapeutic Criteria, the sensitivity of this technique in patients with gouty arthritis and an acutely inflamed joint was 84.4% and specificity for gout was absolute (100%).[210] It is, however, important to recall the occasional patient in whom acute gouty arthritis coexists with another type of joint disease such as acute septic arthritis or acute calcium pyrophosphate dihydrate (CPPD) crystal deposition disease (pseudogout).

Extracellular urate crystals are identifiable in synovial fluid from previously affected joints in 70 to 97% of gouty patients during asymptomatic intervals.[147,211] In one study documenting this point, only 1 of 19 asymptomatic hyperuricemic controls and 2 of 9 patients with renal failure but no history of acute arthritis had extracellular urate crystals demonstrable.[211] In another study, crystals were identified in only 1 of 31 subjects with asymptomatic hyperuricemia, and in none of six patients with renal failure.[212] Thus, extracellular urate crystals in synovial fluid are common during intercritical gout, but this test may be of lesser sensitivity and specificity for gout than is the case for intracellular urate crystal identification during episodes of acute arthritis.

Demonstration of urate crystals in tophi is nearly as specific for gout as synovial fluid crystal identification. Because, however, tophi are found in less than 10% of patients with gout, this diagnostic test is of limited sensitivity. In the absence of the means to identify urate crystals or a negative polarized light microscopic study, the following combination of findings can be useful in diagnosing gout: (1) a classic history of monarticular arthritis followed by an intercritical period completely free of symptoms; (2) rapid resolution of synovitis after colchicine therapy; and (3) hyperuricemia.[210] Criteria for improvement resulting from colchicine therapy are major subsidence of objective joint inflammation within 48 hours and no recurrence of inflammation in any joint for at least 7 days.[213] Arthritis alone in a hyperuricemic patient is insufficient to establish the diagnosis. Pseudogout (CPPD) and basic calcium phosphate (BCP) crystal-induced inflammation are diseases difficult to differentiate from acute gout. Self-limited attacks of acute inflammation in the first metatarsophalangeal joint (pseudopodagra), resulting from transient amorphous calcific deposits have been described in premenopausal women.[214] Septic arthritis and cellulitis are additional processes that often need careful exclusion in the clinical setting suggesting acute gouty arthritis. The resemblance of gouty inflammation to cellulitis points up the diffuse, periarticular nature of gouty inflammation, which differentiates this process from primary synovitic disorders such as RA.

ROENTGENOGRAPHIC FINDINGS IN GOUT

The major value of radiographic examination during the initial attack of gout is to exclude other types of arthritis. At this stage, the findings related to gout are nonspecific, usually in the form of soft tissue swelling. The radiographic hallmarks of longstanding gout are those of an asymmetric, inflammatory, erosive arthritis often accompanied by soft tissue nodules but with retention of normal bone and periarticular density and joint spaces.

Sharply "punched-out," round, or oval defects situated in the marginal areas of the joint and surrounded by a sclerotic border suggest gout (Fig. 105–20). Bony (intracellular) tophaceous lesions almost always antedate subcutaneous tophi and may be seen in joints that have never been clinically inflamed.[160] In about 40% of patients with gouty erosions in bone, an elevated margin extends outward into the soft tissue covering the tophaceous nodule.[215] This "overhanging margin" of bone, which may result from bony resorption beneath the enlarging tophus and periosteal apposition of the involved cortex, helps to distinguish gouty erosions

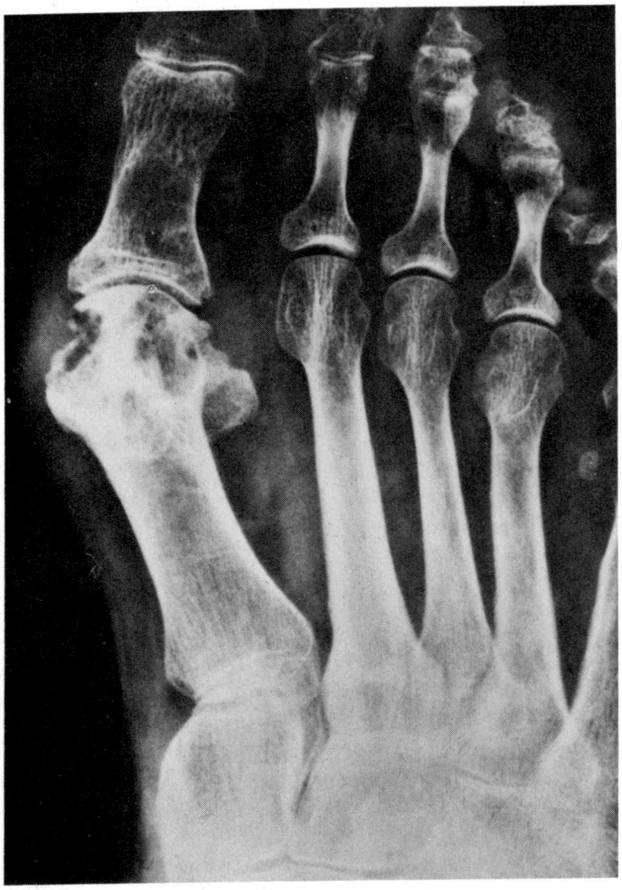

FIGURE 105–20. Radiographic features of gout. Marginal erosions with sclerotic borders, osseous cysts, and overhanding margins are seen. (From Dieppe, P.A., et al. (Eds.): Gout. *In* Slide Atlas of Rheumatology. London, Gower Medical Publishing Ltd., 1985.)

from the "pocketed" erosions seen in RA. Bony erosions occur relatively late in gout, and many patients with repeated acute attacks show neither bone nor soft tissue lesions. Another feature useful in distinguishing gout from RA is the infrequency of periarticular osteopenia in the former.

Bony erosions caused by deposits of urate crystals are related to both the duration and severity of the disease. In patients with advanced chronic tophaceous gout, joint destruction may be extensive. Bony ankylosing with obliteration of joint space has been observed but is rare except in the interphalangeal joints of the hands and feet and in the intercarpal region.[166] In fact, the presence of a relatively normal joint space in an articulation with extensive erosions is an important radiologic characteristic of gout.

Tophi in soft tissues are typically deposited in an asymmetric distribution reflected radiographically as nodular swellings particularly frequent in the feet, hands, ankles, elbows, and knees.[216] Soft tissue prominence about the dorsum of the foot and calcaneus are also characteristic. Calcification of tophi is unusual (Fig. 105–21).[217] Soft tissue tophi are often accompanied by erosions in adjacent bone with typical "overhanging margins," helping to distinguish urate crystal aggregates from nodular lesions associated with other types of arthritic and metabolic disorders.

Dodds and Steinbach found that 10 of 31 patients with gout had meniscal calcification of the type usually associated with CPPD crystal deposits.[218] In another study, calcification of one or more menisci was found in only 2 of 43 patients (5%) with gout, roughly the incidence of chondrocalcinosis observed in elderly populations.[219] Because of the high incidence of gout in patients with pseudogout (5%) and vice versa, the presence of cartilage calcification in a patient with gout should suggest that CPPD and pseudogout may also be present.

Subchondral lesions are occasionally observed near the sacroiliac joints in patients with chronic tophaceous gout (Fig. 105–22). Sclerotic punched-out lesions were found in the sacroiliac joints of seven of 95 gouty patients.[220] In six patients, tophaceous deposits were pres-

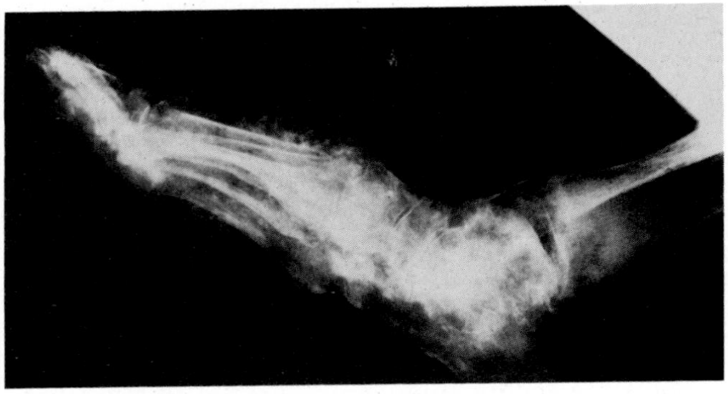

FIGURE 105–21. Calcified soft tissue prominence over the dorsum of the foot, and destruction of the talocalcaneus joint in a 63-year-old man with polyarticular tophaceous gout. (Courtesy of Dr. David Tartof.)

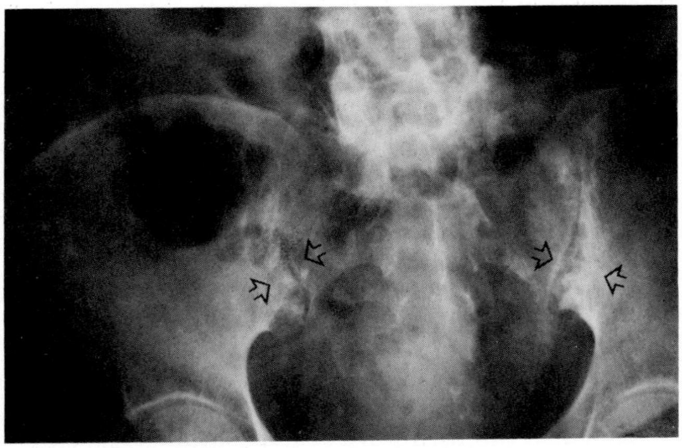

FIGURE 105–22. Sacroiliac joint showing scalloped erosions and adjacent bony sclerosis. (Courtesy of Dr. Nancy Brown.)

ent in the extremities, and in two, urate crystals were documented in these cystic spaces at autopsy. In a prospective radiologic survey of 143 gout patients, 24 individuals with tophi developed sacroiliac changes, which included sclerosis and irregulatory of joint margins, focal osteoporosis, and cysts with sclerotic rims.[221]

Uric acid stones are radiolucent and appear radiologically as "filling defects." Cysteine, xanthine, and 2,8-dihydroxyadenine stones are also radiolucent, but most radiolucent stones are composed of uric acid. Uric acid stones or gravel may be white or pink ("brick dust") as a result of absorption of a pigment that has not been identified. Patients with brick dust urine may present with what they believe to be hematuria. Radiopaque stones also occur with greatly increased frequency in gouty subjects and are composed largely of calcium oxalate. These stones often contain a small amount of uric acid, which probably serves as a nidus for the deposition of calcium oxalate by epitaxial overgrowth.

HEREDITY IN GOUT

Inherited influences have long been suspected in gout. English observers reported gout in family members of 38 to 81% of patients.[222] In series reported from the United States, familial incidence figures have ranged from 6 to 18%.[223] Among hyperuricemic relatives of gout patients, the incidence of gout averaged 20% in five series reviewed by Smyth.[224] In family members of gouty probands, asymptomatic hyperuricemia ranged from 25 to 27%.[225,226] A convincing example of hereditary influence is provided by consideration of patients with gout or hyperuricemia discovered early in life. In a study of 21 subjects with a mean age of 28 years, but without identifiable inherited enzyme defects, a family history of gout was noted in 71%.[227]

Although some studies of restricted populations (i.e., racially selected, geographically isolated, or families of gouty probands) show a bimodal distribution of serum urate values, supporting a single dominant gene hypothesis,[204,228–230] abundant data indicate that serum urate concentration is controlled by multiple genes. A study of Blackfeet and Pima Indians showed strong polygenic hereditary influences on serum urate and suggested both autosomal dominant and X-linked transmission patterns.[231] Additional studies have also favored multifactorial inheritance, demonstrating a prevalence of high urate values without evidence of bimodality.[10,19] In general, polygenic control is more prominent the greater the population heterogeneity. Thus, within limited groups of individuals, a single gene may influence urate values to the relative exclusion of other influences that may express themselves in broader populations in the form of apparent gene interaction.

PATHOLOGIC FEATURES OF GOUT

The most frequent sites of monosodium urate crystal deposition are cartilage, epiphyseal bone, periarticular structures, and the kidney. Although organs such as the liver, spleen, voluntary muscle, and nerve tissue are characteristically spared, crystal deposits have been described at one time or another in most organs other than brain.[232] Crystal aggregates produce local necrosis, and unless the tissue is avascular, a foreign body reaction ensues with proliferation of fibrous tissues. Tophi thus consist of a multicentric deposit of urate crystals and intercrystalline matrix, together with a foreign body reaction.[233] In the early stage of crystallization, needle-shaped urate crystals may be clustered radially in a sporulated form (resembling beach-balls) embedded beneath the synovial lining cells.[234] Affected joints may develop cartilaginous degeneration, synovial proliferation, erosion of marginal bone, or rarely, ankylosis (Fig. 105–23).[166] No joint is exempt, although those of the lower extremities are more commonly involved. The significance of the rich proteoglycan matrix of tophi is uncertain.[235] It is important to recall that urate crystals

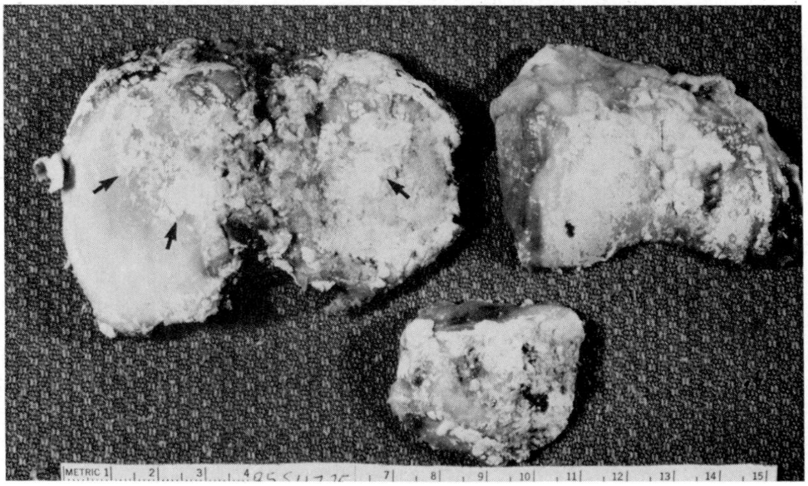

FIGURE 105–23. Encrusted urate deposits on eroded articular cartilage of the tibial plateau (*arrows*), and fragments of the femoral condyle. (Courtesy of Dr. Mitchell Krieger.)

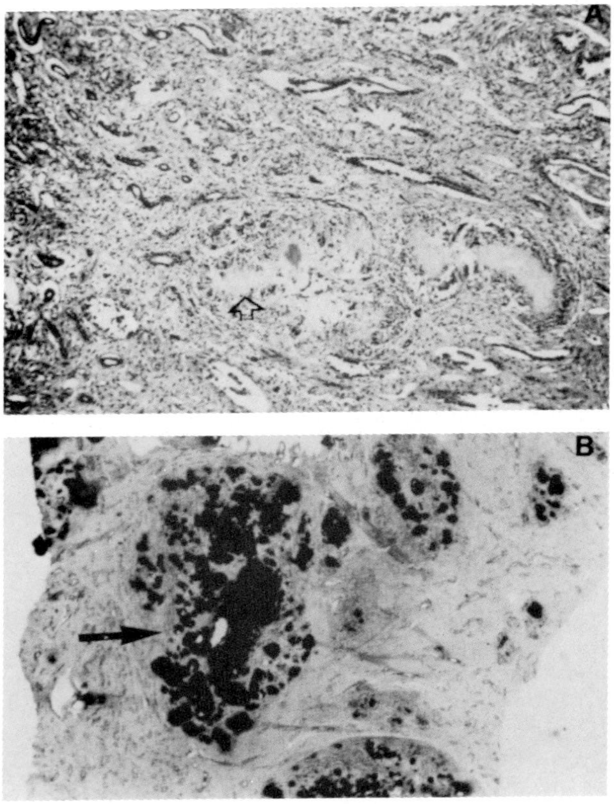

FIGURE 105–24. *A*, Urate deposits in the medulla of the kidney fixed in alcohol (hematoxylin and eosin stain, x100). *B*, Same deposit stained with methenamine silver (x375). (Courtesy of Dr. Wellington Jao.)

are water soluble, and nonaqueous fixation is necessary to preserve urate deposits in histologic sections.

The only distinctive histologic feature of urate nephropathy is the presence of urate crystals and a surrounding giant cell reaction (Fig. 105–24). Crystal deposition in the kidney may be associated with interstitial or vascular changes or both. That some of the vascular changes may be related to concomitant hypertension emphasizes the difficulty of attributing pathologic changes to a single factor. In a review of 191 gout patients in whom clinical information and postmortem renal tissue permitted adequate evaluation, all but three showed either urate crystals or pyelonephritic or vascular changes.[198] These features were present in variable proportion and severity. Vascular lesions included arterial and arteriolar sclerosis and, in 11 instances, findings of malignant hypertension. Kidneys from 30 patients revealed both well-developed vascular changes and pyelonephritis with extensive structural alterations and urate deposits.

Some exceptions were found to the correlation of clinical severity and renal pathology. A few patients with severe tophaceous gout showed only minimal clinical evidence of renal insufficiency, and other patients with severe renal disease had only minimal articular disease. In the latter type of patient, renal disease may have caused premature death, such as portrayed in a few reports of "gouty nephrosis" occurring without clinical evidence of gout.[232,236] In the rare patients with this syndrome, however, serum urate concentrations have not been reported.

A number of mechanisms have been proposed to explain the various pathologic findings reported in urate nephropathy. The renal lesions may stem from deposition of uric acid in collecting tubules with resultant obstruction, atrophy of the more proximal tubules, and secondary necrosis and fibrosis.[47] The associated interstitial inflammatory process has been attributed to complicating pyelonephritis.[237] Other studies have shown that tubular damage is an early structural abnormality associated with an interstitial reaction; this finding suggests a relationship between the interstitial and tubular changes.[238] The epithelial cells of Henle's loop show early atrophy and dilation, occasionally associated with brown pigment degeneration of the epithelium.[238] In kidneys without tophi, this reaction usually spares the medulla and the juxtamedullary cortex. Thus, the changes ascribed to chronic pyelonephritis may reflect an infectious origin or may be a manifestation of urate nephropathy. According to Gonick, Rubini, Gleason, and Sommers, a distinctive glomerulosclerosis in urate nephropathy also exists with uniform fibrillar thickening of glomerular capillary basement membranes, which differs from that of nephrosclerosis or diabetic glomerulosclerosis.[238] Heptinstall does not believe that this lesion is distinctive.

HYPERURICEMIA AND GOUT AS CONSEQUENCE OF DRUGS, TOXINS, ABNORMAL PHYSIOLOGIC STATES, OR OTHER DISEASES

The mechanisms underlying secondary hyperuricemia are precisely those responsible for primary hyperuricemia, although in the former case, activation of the abnormal metabolism is associated with a drug therapy, environmental factor, or associated disease process. Gout arises in these contexts as a consequence of urate crystal deposition and the identical attendant consequences as in primary gout, although, in some instances, the pace of clinical manifestations may be accelerated.

DRUGS

Diuretic therapy is one of the most frequent causes of secondary hyperuricemia. Diuretics were implicated in 20% of the hyperuricemic men admitted to a VA hospital.[240] Fifty percent of the new cases of gout in the Framingham study developed in subjects taking thiazides or ethacrynic acid.[19] Surveillance of the Framingham study population years later showed that 20% of men and 25% of women reported taking antihypertensive medications, and the mean serum urate concentration was 0.8 mg/dL higher for this group than for the untreated subjects.[241] Similar increments were observed in a short-term study of 358 mildly hypertensive subjects treated with very low doses of hydrochlorothiazide.[242] Other series reported increments in urate concentrations of 1.3 to 1.8 mg/dL during chronic thiazide administration.[17,243]

The primary mechanism of urate retention among diuretic-treated patients appears to be enhanced tubular reabsorption of both sodium and uric acid because urate excretion is unchanged when volume depletion is prevented with intravenous saline.[127,244] In addition, furosemide and diazoxide can induce hyperlacticacidemia sufficient to suppress tubular secretion of urate. Neither of these mechanisms represents a direct drug effect on bidirectional urate transport. Spironolactone may decrease the renal clearance of uric acid but has no consistent effect on urate values.[245] The recently recognized substantial prevalence of tophaceous gout among elderly women receiving chronic diuretic therapy attests to the importance of recognizing this consequence of drug therapy in an increasingly elderly population.

A wide variety of other drugs can induce hyperuricemia. Renal uric acid retention as a result of ingestion of low doses of salicylates (less than 2g/day) has been discussed earlier.[116] Suppression of tubular secretion of urate occurs at the resulting concentrations of free salicylate in tubular urine. Doses of aspirin exceeding about 3g/day result in suppression of both reabsorption and secretion, and the consequent net effect is uricosuria. The antituberculous drugs pyrazinamide[246] and ethambutol[247] decrease the renal clearance of uric acid, as does nicotinic acid,[248] but the last of these drugs and warfarin may also stimulate purine synthesis de novo.[249] Hyperuricemia and gout occur frequently in transplant patients using the immunosuppressive agent cyclosporine.[250,251] The degree of hyperuricemia and the severity of gout associated with this drug is often unusual, with early progression to polyarticular attacks and tophaceous deposits. Impaired renal urate excretion is the basis of cyclosporine-induced hyperuricemia, but the mechanisms of this effect are complex. Acute cyclosporine nephrotoxicity is a prerenal process, altering filtration and promoting urate retention as a result of increased tubular reabsorption.[251,252] Chronic cyclosporin-induced renal insufficiency is primarily characterized by interstitial fibrosis and arteriolar damage leading to a decreased filtered load of urate and adoptive declines in urate tubular handling mechanisms. In addition, a direct effect of cyclosporine on tubular urate transport remains a possibility, and the hyperuricemic effect appears to be potentiated by simultaneous administration of diuretics.[251]

TOXINS

As previously discussed, ethanol can result in hyperuricemia either as a consequence of enhanced nucleotide catabolism with excessive uric acid production or of dehydration and lacticacidemia leading to reduced renal uric acid excretion.[103,105,253] Epidemiologic studies show a strong correlation between serum urate levels and habitual alcohol intake, and gouty individuals consume more alcohol then nongouty counterparts.[253–255] In most large series of gout patients, heavily weighted toward a predominance of men, the proportion of patients who abuse alcohol ranges from 30 to 50%.

An increased incidence of gout is found in patients with chronic lead nephropathy (saturnine gout), and reduced renal clearance of uric acid is the primary mechanism of hyperuricemia.[256] In Australia,[257] leaded paint has provided the major source of lead exposure in contrast to the case in the southeastern United States, where the toxic exposure results from lead contamination during distillation or storage of unbonded alcohol, or "moonshine."[256,258] Although a reciprocal relationship between lead excretion after intravenous chelation with ethylenediamine tetra-acetic acid (EDTA) and creatinine clearance was described in a group of gouty patients, a later controlled study failed to confirm this relationship and questioned the importance of lead intoxication as a primary factor for decreased urate clearance in gouty patients.[259] In the latter study, nongouty "moonshiners" had lead stores comparable to gouty ingestors of moonshine, who, in turn, had no greater renal impairment than a group of patients with gout but no history of lead exposure. Factors other than lead nephropathy, such as obesity, alcohol consumption, and hypertension appear to be the major factors contributing to the decreased urate clearances in patients with gout, even those exposed to lead.

ABNORMAL PHYSIOLOGIC STATES

Total caloric restriction results in hyperuricemia, largely attributed to reduced renal urate clearance.[260,261] Urate retention correlates best with ketosis, especially concentrations of β-hydroxybutyrate and acetoacetate.[262] Carbohydrate, protein, or purine refeeding causes a prompt increase in urinary uric acid excretion and return of serum urate to control values,[255] but ketosis persists if a fat diet succeeds a fast. If starvation is attended by nucleotide depletion, excessive uric acid production may contribute to the associated hyperuricemia. Attacks of gout may occur during periods of starvation, usually in patients with a prior history of hyperuricemia or gout.

Hyperuricemia is common in uremic patients, but gouty arthritis is unusual and occurs in less than 1% of uremic individuals. Among 882 patients with chronic renal insufficiency, Sarre and Mertz found only two instances complicated by gouty arthritis.[263] In another study, 17 cases were reported among 1600 patients with chronic renal disease of long duration.[264] Extremely high serum urate values are unusual in chronic renal failure, owing in part to increased fractional excretion of uric acid. This results from persistence of tubular secretory capacity even as glomerular filtration rate falls, and reduced tubular uric acid reabsorptive capacity at glomerular filtration rates less than 10 mL/min.[265] In addition, extrarenal disposal of uric acid assumes a major role in urate homeostasis as renal function deteriorates, reaching up to 50% of total uric acid disposal.[266] The rarity of gout associated with uremia has been attributed to a shortened life span and a decreased ability to respond to an inflammatory stimulus.

Recurrent attacks of acute inflammatory arthritis or periarthritis occur in patients with chronic renal failure treated with long-term hemodialysis. Although the clinical features of these episodes in the setting of hyperuricemia often suggest gouty arthritis,[267] tissue and synovial fluid examination may show crystals of BCP (apatite), or of calcium oxalate[268] rather than urate crystals.

OTHER DISEASES

In a series of patients with leukemia, myeloid metaplasia, polycythemia vera, and multiple myeloma, increased cell turnover and nucleic acid turnover resulted in hyperuricemia in 66% of 113 men and 69% of 73 women.[269] Gouty arthritis was noted in 10 patients, an incidence similar to the 3.7 and 4.5% incidence of gouty arthritis reported in other series of patients with myeloproliferative and lymphoproliferative diseases.[140,270] In myeloid metaplasia, the incidence of gout, often complicated by early development of tophaceous deposits, may be as great as 27%, the longer survival of patients with this disorder perhaps accounting for the high incidence.

Mean urate excretion of 634 mg/24 hours was found in a group of 27 patients with gout and hematoproliferative diseases in comparison to a value of 497 mg/24 hours in a control group.[270] In these conditions, the miscible pool of uric acid is enlarged and uric acid turnover accelerated.[44] Peak incorporation of labeled precursors into uric acid and urinary purines occurs earlier than normal, indicating rapid turnover of newly synthesized nucleotides.[271] A secondary peak of urinary uric acid labeling after 1 to 2 weeks reflects the rapid turnover of cells of the abnormal hematopoietic line.

Hyperuricemia is also a relatively common finding in secondary polycythemias,[272,273] hemoglobinopathies,[274] pernicious anemia (especially after vitamin B_{12} therapy),[275] and chronic hemolytic states.[276] Occasionally, disseminated carcinomas with rapid cell turnover are accompanied by hyperuricemia.[277] Among patients with homozygous sickle cell disease, the frequency of hyperuricemia ranges from 26 to 39%, principally among patients in the third decade of life who have reduced renal urate secretory capacity.[274] Excessive urinary uric acid excretion, increased precursor labeling of urinary uric acid, and increased fractional excretion of uric acid in younger patients with sickle cell anemia also suggest excessive production of uric acid in this population.[278,279] Gouty arthritis is, however, unusual in patients with sickle cell anemia, probably because of shortened life span.[280]

Hyperuricemia is frequent in patients with hyperparathyroidism.[281,282] In most studies, however, hypertension, obesity, and renal disease have obscured the significance of elevated serum urate levels.[282,283] Shelp, Steele, and Rieselbach infused 14 volunteers with parathyroid hormone and did not alter the renal excretion of uric acid.[284] In large series of patients with primary hyperparathyroidism, the incidence of gouty arthritis is reported to be 3 to 9%,[281,285] but polarization of synovial fluid to detect and differentiate urate and calcium pyrophosphate crystals (pseudogout) was not performed in these earlier studies. An association between psoriasis and hyperuricemia is postulated to result from increased epidermal cell turnover, but not all studies confirm the association. The disparate prevalence rates (0 to 50%)[286,287] may reflect differences in disease severity or individual differences in bidirectional urate transport.[288] The pattern of labeled glycine incorporation into urinary uric acid in psoriatic individuals is consistent with accelerated nucleic acid turnover, presumably in the cells of psoriatic plaques.[286] An association of sarcoidosis, psoriasis, and gout is regarded by some authors as a syndrome[289] but may represent a chance occurrence.

Hyperuricemia has also been reported in patients with Down's syndrome,[290] cystinuria,[291] primary oxaluria,[292] Paget's disease of bone,[293] and Bartter's syndrome,[294] and episodes of gouty arthritis have been noted in the latter two of these conditions. Uric acid nephrolithiasis is described in cystinuria. Reduced renal uric acid clearance has been proposed in Bartter's syndrome,[294] Down's syndrome,[280] and in hyperoxaluria.[282]

DISORDERS ASSOCIATED WITH HYPERURICEMIA AND GOUT

Gout and hyperuricemia occur with increased frequency in several important disorders in which no cause–effect relationship has been established. Primary management of potentially serious disorders such as hypertension should not be withheld or delayed because of concern over the degree of hyperuricemia or the frequency of gouty attacks, issues that can most often be readily managed.

OBESITY

A strong positive correlation between body weight and serum urate concentration has been documented, but the relationship is both complex and multifactorial.[295–301] In a study of 73,000 obese women, the crude relative risk for gout was 2.56, and women who were 85% above desirable body weight[302] had gout 1.56 times more frequently than women weighing within 10% of ideal body weight. In the Framingham study, the correlation between uric acid levels and weight was particularly marked in the age group 35 to 44 years, with lower correlations seen in older age groups.[303] In another study, 52% of gouty patients were more than 20% over ideal body weight.[259] The fact that 85% were hypertensive and 48% had abnormal glucose tolerance tests and hyperlipidemia points out the multiplicity of variables relating to obesity and its metabolic complications. An elevated ponderal index and decreased fractional excretion of uric acid have also been reported among hyperuricemic Maori men.[304] Obesity has several effects on urate metabolism including decreased renal urate clearance and increased uric acid production.[305] Weight reduction is associated with a modest lowering of serum urate concentration and a decrease in the rate of purine synthesis de novo.[299]

HYPERLIPIDEMIA

An association between hypertriglyceridemia and hyperuricemia is well established.[299,306] Up to 80% of individuals with hypertriglyceridemia have hyperuricemia, and 50 to 75% of gouty patients have hypertriglyceridemia. Confounding the interpretation of these relationships are other variables observed in this population, including obesity and excessive alcohol intake. In one study of 40 gouty subjects, a correlation was found between the ponderal index and serum triglycerides.[307] Fasting triglyceride values were, however, not significantly higher than those of obese controls. The 17 gouty subjects in this study who drank excessive alcohol had higher triglyceride values than those who abstained. Another study reported a 1.6-fold increase in the frequency of hypertriglyceridemia independent of alcohol intake in a group of obese gouty patients whose hyperuricemia was normalized with either allopurinol or probenecid.[308] In 108 gouty Japanese men, hyperlipoproteinemia was seen in 56% and appeared to be independent of both alcohol intake and obesity.[309] Additional observations demonstrate a correlation between 24-hour urinary uric acid excretion and serum triglyceride levels.[310] Finally, no change was found in levels of serum urate or uric acid excretion when triglycerides were acutely elevated in three gouty subjects receiving intravenous intralipid.[311] Although hypertriglyceridemia and hyperuricemia may coexist independent of other risk factors, a common metabolic defect remains elusive.

HYPERTENSION

Hyperuricemia is reported in 22 to 38% of untreated hypertensive patients, and increases to 47 to 67% when therapy and renal disease are included.[312–314] The prevalence of gout in the hypertensive population is between 2 and 12%. Although the prevalence of hyperuricemia in the general population increases with increasing blood pressure, no consistent relationships emerge. In the Tecumseh study, no correlation was found between urate concentration and age, sex, anthropometric data, or level of blood pressure.[315] Likewise, only 1% of blood pressure variation could be accounted for by serum urate values in the Israeli ischemic heart study of 10,000 men aged 40 years or older.[316] Conversely, among patients with classic gout, 25 to 50% have hypertension that is unrelated to the duration of gout and is more common in obese patients.[140,197,317]

Causal factors relating hyperuricemia and hypertension are unclear. Renal urate clearances, which depend on tubular secretory and postsecretory reabsorption rates, are reported to be inappropriately low relative to glomerular filtration rates in both adult and childhood essential hypertension.[312,313,318] This process may be regulated in part, by renal blood flow. A recent study has documented reduced renal blood flow and increased renal vascular resistance and total peripheral resistance in subjects with essential hypertension and hyperuricemia.[202] In contrast, glomerular filtration rates, cardiac output, and intravascular volume were not specifically affected in this group. The authors suggest that hyperuricemia in patients with essential hypertension reflects early nephrosclerosis. The importance of this relationship should not be overlooked in the management of gout because untreated hypertension may contribute to renal morbidity in these patients.

ATHEROSCLEROSIS

Since the early description of an increased frequency of hyperuricemia in a group of young patients with coronary heart disease, the issue of hyperuricemia as an independent risk factor for atherosclerosis has been a subject of controversy.[319] Additional reports have noted a relationship of hyperuricemia and atherosclerosis,[320,321] but no clear association was found in the Tecumseh study when adjustments were made for age, sex, and relative weight.[315] Serum urate values did not differ significantly in the coronary heart disease group from the mean value of the entire population. Using multivariate analysis of risk factors at the thirteenth biennial evaluation of the original Framingham cohort, serum urate values did not add independently to the prediction of coronary heart disease.[241] Analysis of this population, segregated by diuretic use, showed that among gouty men who had never received diuretics, a 60% excess of coronary artery disease was present.[322] Alcohol intake, systolic blood pressure, and body mass index were higher in the gouty subjects. Among the Polynesians, hypertension, diabetes mellitus, and atherosclerosis are correlates of obesity rather than of hyperuricemia.[208] Thus, in hyperuricemic patients, a tangled web of coronary risk factors such as obesity, hypertension, insulin resistance, and hypertriglyceridemia contribute to the observed association between elevated urate values and atherosclerosis.

HYPOURICEMIA

It is difficult to arrive at a precise value below which the serum concentration of urate is abnormally low. The problem arises because of the different methods used to determine urate values and the non-Gaussian distribution of these values in the population. Using a conservative estimate, a serum urate concentration of 2 mg/dL or less was found in 0.8% of hospitalized patients[323,324] and 1.0% of the residents of Tecumseh.[10] Hypouricemia may result from diminished uric acid production, excess uric acid excretion, or a combination of these mechanisms. A pathologic consequence of hyporuricemia itself is not recognized, and no therapy is required. Rather, the clinical significance of hypouricemia is determined by the underlying causal condition.

Inherited deficiencies of xanthine oxidase and purine nucleoside phosphorylase result in hypouricemia. Hereditary xanthinuria is an autosomal recessive disorder characterized by the virtual absence of xanthine oxidase activity in conjunction with hypouricemia, hypouricaciduria, elevated urinary hypoxanthine and, especially, xanthine excretion, and recurrent urinary xanthine stones.[325] A crystal deposition myopathy has also been reported in xanthinuric patients. Treatment with the xanthine oxidase inhibitor allopurinol also results in elevation of urinary hypoxanthine and xanthine excretion and may result in hypouricemia (See Chapter 105 on treatment of gout). Purine nucleoside phosphorylase deficiency is associated with T-cell dysfunction and an immunodeficiency state.[76]

Hypouricemia that is due to enhanced renal clearance of uric acid may occur in Wilson's disease, Fanconi's syndrome, lymphomas, and carcinomas, especially small cell carcinoma of the lung associated with inappropriate secretion of antidiuretic hormone.[326] Severe liver disease may cause hypouricemia, perhaps as a result of decreased purine biosynthesis.

A long list of medications in addition to uricosuric drugs may reduce serum urate levels. In a series of over 6000 consecutive urate determinations, the agents most frequently associated with hyporuricemia were aspirin, x-ray contrast media, and glycerylguaiacolate.[323] Enhanced fractional excretion of uric acid and lowering of serum urate values is a common metabolic consequence of total parenteral nutrition, most likely as a result of the high glycine content of the infusion solution.[145]

Finally, hypouricemia has been noted in several healthy adults with an isolated defect in the bidirectional tubular transport of uric acid.[114,131–133] Isolated tubular defects that result in hypouricemia include diminished reabsorption of filtered urate, a defect in postsecretory reabsorption, and a defect characterized by urate clearances in excess of glomerular filtration rates resulting from deficient reabsorption of uric acid throughout the nephron. Hypouricemia detected during routine laboratory testing may be the initial clue leading to the proper diagnosis of one of these conditions.

REFERENCES

1. Hippocrates: The genuine works of Hippocrates. Vols. 1, 2. Translated and annotated by Francis Adams. New York, Wood, 1886.
2. Garrod, A.E.: The Inborn Factors in Disease: An Essay. New York, Oxford University Press, 1931.
3. McCarty, D.J.: A historical note: Leeuwenhoek's description of crystals from a gouty tophus. Arthritis Rheum., *13*:414–418, 1970.
4. Scheele, K.W.: Examen chemicum calculi urinarii. Opuscula, *2*:73, 1776.
5. Wollaston, W.H.: On gouty and urinary concretions. Philos. Trans. R. Soc., *87*:386–415, 1797.
6. Garrod, A.B.: Treatise on Gout and Rheumatic Gout (Rheumatoid Arthritis). 3rd Ed. London, Longmans, Green & Co., 1876.
7. McCarty, D.J., and Hollander, J.L.: Identification of urate crystals in gouty synovial fluid. Ann. Intern. Med., *54*:452–460, 1961.
8. Allen, D.J., Milosovich, G., and Mattock, A.M.: Inhibition of monosodium urate crystal growth. Arthritis Rheum., *8*:1123–1133, 1965.
9. Emmerson, B.J., and Sandilands, P.: The normal range of plasma urate levels. Aust. Ann. Med., *12*:46–52, 1963
10. Mikkelsen, W.M., Dodge, H.J., and Valkenburg, H.: The distribution of serum uric acid values in a population unselected as to gout or hyperuricemia. Tecumseh, Michigan, 1959–1960. Am. J. Med., *39*:242–251, 1965.
11. Price, C.P., and James, D.R.: Analytical reviews in clinical biochemistry: The measurement of urate. Ann. Clin. Biochem., *25*:484–498, 1988.
12. Harkness, R.A., and Nicol, A.D.: Plasma uric acid levels in children. Arch. Dis. Child., *44*:773–778, 1969.
13. Munan, L., Kelley, A., and Petitclerc, C.: Serum urate levels between ages 10 and 14: Changes in sex trends. J. Lab. Clin. Med., *90*:990–996, 1977.
14. Wolfson, W.Q. et al.: The transport and excretion of uric acid in man: 5. A sex difference in urate metabolism. J. Clin. Endocrinol., Metab., *9*:749–767, 1949.
15. Anton, F.M. et al.: Sex differences in uric acid metabolism in adults. Evidence for a lack of influence of estradiol 17 (E_2) on the renal handling of urate. Metabolism., *35*:343–348, 1986.
16. Campion, E.W., Glynn, R.J., and DeLabry, L.O.: Asymptomatic hyperuricemia. Risks and consequences in the normative aging study. Am. J. Med., *82*:421–426, 1987.
17. Langford H.G. et al.: Is thiazide-produced uric acid elevation harmful? Analysis of data from the hypertension detection and follow-up program. Arch. Intern. Med., *147*:645–649, 1987.
18. Fessel, J.W.: Renal outcomes of gout and hyperuricemia. Am. J. Med., *67*:74–82, 1979.
19. Hall, A.P., Barry, P.E., Dawber, T.R., and McNamara, P.M.: Epidemiology of gout and hyperuricemia: A long term population study. Am. J. Med., *42*:27–37, 1967.
20. Hitchings, G.H.: Uric acid: Chemistry and synthesis. *In* Uric Acid: Handbook of Experimental Pharmacology. Vol. 51. Edited by W.N. Kelley and I.M. Weiner. New York, Springer-Verlag, 1978.
21. Loeb, J.N.: The influence of temperature on the solubility of monosodium urate. Arthritis Rheum., *13*:189–192, 1972.
22. Holmes, E.W.: Regulation of purine biosynthesis de novo. *In* Uric Acid: Handbook of Experimental Pharmacology. Vol. 51. Edited by W.N. Kelley and I.M. Weiner. New York, Springer-Verlag, 1978.
23. Arnold, W.J.: Purine salvage enzymes.
24. Holmes, E.W., Wyngaarden, J.B., and Kelley, W.N.: Human glutamine phosphoribosylpyrophosphate amidotransferase: Two molecular forms interconvertible by purine nucleotide and phosphoribosylpyrophosphate. J. Biol. Chem., *248*:144–150, 1973.
25. Becker, M.A., and Kim, M.: Regulation of purine synthesis *de novo* in human fibroblasts by purine nucleotides and phosphoribosylpyrophosphate. J. Biol. Chem., *262*:14531–14537, 1987.
26. Holmes, E.W. et al.: Human glutamine phosphoribosylpyro-

phosphate amidotransferase: Kinetic and regulatory properties. J. Biol. Chem., *248*:144–150, 1973.
27. Wood, A.W., and Seegmiller, J.E.: Properties of 5-phosphoribosyl-1-pyrophosphate amidotransferase from human lymphoblasts. J. Biol. Chem., *248*:138–143, 1973.
28. Itakura, M., Sabina, R.L., Heald, P.W., and Holmes, E.W.: Basis for the control of purine biosynthesis by purine ribonucleotides. J. Clin. Invest., *67*:994–1002, 1981.
29. Becker, M.A., Raivio, K.O. and Seegmiller, J.E.: Synthesis of phosphoribosylpyrophosphate in mammalian cells. Adv. Enzymol., *49*:281–306, 1979.
30. Yen, R.C.K., Raivio, K.O., and Becker, M.A.: Inhibition of phosphoribosylpyrophosphate synthesis by 6-methylthionisoinate. J. Biol. Chem., *256*:1839–1845, 1981.
31. Fox, I.H., and Kelley, W.N.: Human phosphoribosylpyrophosphate synthetase: Distribution, purification, and properties. J. Biol. Chem., *246*:5739–5748, 1971.
32. Becker, M.A., Losman, M.J., and Kim, M.: Mechanisms of accelerated purine nucleotide synthesis in human fibroblasts with superactive phosphoribosylpyrophosphate synthetases. J. Biol. Chem., *262*:5596–5602, 1987.
33. Kovarsky, J., Holmes, E.W., and Kelley, W.N.: Absence of significant urate binding to human serum proteins. J. Lab. Clin. Med., *93*:85–91, 1979.
34. Kelton, J.G. et al.: A method for monitoring dialysis patients and a tool for assessing binding to serum proteins in vivo. Ann. Intern. Med., *89*:67–70, 1978.
35. Holmes, E.W., and Blondet, P.: Urate binding to serum albumin: Lack of influence of renal clearance of uric acid. Arthritis Rheum., *22*:737–739, 1979.
36. Alvsaker, J.O.: Genetic studies in primary gout: Investigations on the plasma levels of the urate binding α_1-α_2-globulin in individuals from two gouty kindreds. J. Clin. Invest., *47*:1254–1261, 1968.
37. Benedict, J.D., Forsham, P.H., and Stetten, D.W., Jr.: The metabolism of uric acid in the normal and gouty human studied with the aid of isotopic uric acid. J. Biol. Chem., *181*:183–193, 1949.
38. Sorensen, L.B.: Degradation of uric acid in man. Metabolism, *8*:687–703, 1959.
39. Sorensen, L.B.: The pathogenesis of gout. Arch. Intern. Med., *109*:379–390, 1962.
40. Scott, J.T. et al.: Studies of uric acid pool size and turnover rate. Ann. Rheum. Dis., *28*:366–373, 1969.
41. Seegmiller, J.E., Grayzel, A.I., Laster, L., and Little, L.: Uric acid production in gout. J. Clin. Invest., *40*:1304–1314, 1961.
42. Wyngaarden, J.B.: Gout. Adv. Metab. Disord., *2*:1–78, 1965.
43. Wyngaarden, J.B., and Stetten, D.W., Jr.: Uricolysis in normal man. J. Biol. Chem., *203*:9–21, 1953.
44. Bishop, C., Garner, W., and Talbot, J.H.: Pool size, turnover rate, and rapidity of equilibration of injected isotopic uric acid in normal and pathological subjects. J. Clin. Invest., *30*:879–888, 1951.
45. Benedict, J.D., Roche, M., Yu, T-F., and Bien, E.J.: Incorporation of glycine nitrogen into uric acid in normal and gouty man. Metabolism, *1*:3–12, 1952.
46. Wyngaarden, J.B.: Overproduction of uric acid as the cause of hyperuricemia in primary gout. J. Clin. Invest., *36*:1508–1515, 1957.
47. Wyngaarden, J.B., and Kelley, W.N.: Gout and Hyperuricemia. New York, Grune & Stratton, 1976.
48. Postlethwaite, A.E., and Kelley, W.N.: Uricosuric effect of radiocontrast agents. Ann. Intern. Med., *74*:845–852, 1971.
49. Becker, M.A., Meyer, L.J., and Seegmiller, J.E.: Gout with purine overproduction due to increased phosphoribosylpyrophosphate synthetase activity. Am. J. Med., *55*:232–242, 1973.
50. Berger, L., and Yu, T-F.: Renal function in gout. An analysis of 524 gouty subjects including long-term follow-up studies. Am. J. Med., *59*:605–613, 1975.
51. Becker, M.A.: Patterns of phosphoribosylpyrophosphate and ribose-5-phosphate concentration and generation in fibroblasts from patients with gout and purine overproduction. J. Clin. Invest., *57*:308–318, 1976.
52. Henderson, J.F., Rosenbloom, F.M., Kelley, W.N., and Seegmiller, J.E.: Variations in purine metabolism in cultured skin fibroblasts from patients with gout. J. Clin. Invest., *47*:1511–1516, 1968.
53. Seegmiller, J.E., Rosenbloom, F.M., and Kelley, W.N.: Enzyme defect associated with sex linked human neurological disorder and excessive purine synthesis. Science, *155*:1682–1684, 1967.
54. Kelley, W.N., Rosenbloom, F.M., Henderson, J.F., and Seegmiller, J.E.: A specific enzyme defect in gout associated with overproduction of uric acid. Proc. Natl. Acad. Sci. U.S.A., *57*:1735–1739, 1967.
55. Sperling, O. et al.: Altered kinetic property of erythrocyte phosphoribosylpyrophosphate synthetase in excessive purine production. Rev. Eur. Etud. Clin. Biol., *17*:703–706, 1972.
56. Becker, M.A., Meyer, L.J., Wood, A.W., and Seegmiller, J.E.: Purine overproduction in man associated with increased phosphoribosylpyrophosphate synthetase activity. Science, *179*:1123–1126, 1973.
57. Kelley, W.N. et al.: Hypoxanthine-guanine phosphoribosyltransferase deficiency in gout. Ann. Intern. Med., *70*:155–206, 1969.
58. Rosenbloom, F.M. et al.: Biochemical basis of accelerated purine biosynthesis *de novo* in human fibroblasts lacking hypoxanthine-guanine phosphoribosyltransferase. J. Biol. Chem., *243*:1166–1173, 1968.
59. Wilson, J.M., Young, A.S., and Kelley, W.N.: Hypoxanthine-guanine phosphoribosyltransferase deficiency: The molecular basis of the clinical syndromes. N. Engl. J. Med., *309*:900–910, 1983.
60. Lesch, M., and Nyhan, W.L.: A familial disorder of uric acid metabolism and central nervous system function. Am. J. Med., *36*:561–570, 1964.
61. Lloyd, K.G. et al.: Biochemical evidence of dysfunction of brain neurotransmitters in the Lesch-Nyhan syndrome. N. Engl. J. Med., *305*:1106–1111, 1981.
62. Benke, P.J., Herrick, N., and Hebert, A.: Hypoxanthine-guanine phosphoribosyltransferase variant associated with accelerated purine synthesis. J. Clin. Invest., *52*:2234–2240, 1973.
63. Sweetman, L. et al.: Diminished affinity for purine substrates as a basis for gout with mild deficiency of hypoxanthine-guanine phosphoribosyltransferase. Adv. Exp. Med. Biol., *76A*:319–325, 1977.
64. Seravelli, E. et al.: Further data on the cytologic mapping of the human X chromosome with man-mouse cell hybrids. Cytogenet. Cell Genet., *16*:219–222, 1976.
65. Wilson, J.M. et al.: Human hypoxanthine-guanine phosphoribosyltransferase. Purification and characterization of mutant forms of the enzyme. J. Biol. Chem., *256*:10306–10312, 1981.
66. Wilson, J.M. et al.: A molecular survey of hypoxanthine-guanine phosphoribosyltransferase deficiency in man. J. Clin. Invest., *77*:188–195, 1986.
67. Davidson, B.L., Tarle, S.A., Palella, T.D., and Kelley, W.N.: Molecular basis of hypoxanthine-guanine phosphoribosyltransferase deficiency in ten subjects determinant by direct sequencing of amplified transcripts. J. Clin. Invest., *84*:342–346, 1989.
68. Davidson, B.L. et al.: Identification of 17 independent mutations responsible for human hypoxanthine-guanine phosphoribosyltransferase (HPRT) deficiency. Am. J. Hum. Genet., (in press).

69. Upchurch, K.S. et al.: Hypoxanthine phosphoribosyltransferase deficiency. Association of reduced catalytic activity with reduced levels of immunologically detectable enzyme protein. Proc. Natl. Acad. Sci. U.S.A., *72*:4142–4146, 1975.
70. Ghangas, G.S., and Milman, G.: Radioimmune determination of hypoxanthine phosphoribosyltransferase crossreacting material in erythrocytes of Lesch-Nyhan patients. Proc. Natl. Acad. Sci. U.S.A., *72*:4147–4150, 1975.
71. Patel, P.I., Framson, P.E., Caskey, C.I., and Chinault, A.C.: Fine structure of the human hypoxanthine phosphoribosyltransferase gene. Mol. Cell. Biol., *6*:393–403, 1986.
72. Palella, T.D. et al.: Herpes simplex virus-mediated human hypoxanthine-guanine phosphoribosyltransferase gene transfer into neuronal cells. Mol. Cell. Biol., *8*:457–460, 1988.
73. Wolf, J.A., and Friedmann, T.: Approaches to gene therapy in disorders of purine metabolism. Rheum. Dis. Clin. North Am., *14*: 1988.
74. Edwards, N.L., Recker, D., and Fox, I.H.: Overproduction of uric acid in hypoxanthine-guanine phosphoribosyltransferase deficiency. Contribution by impaired purine salvage. J. Clin. Invest., *63*:922–930, 1979.
75. Hershfield, M.S., and Seegmiller, J.E.: Regulation of *de novo* purine synthesis in human lymphoblasts: Similar rates during growth by normal cells and mutants deficient in hypoxanthine-guanine phosphoribosyltransferase. J. Biol. Chem., *252*:6002–6010, 1977.
76. Thompson, L.F., Willis, R.C., Stoop, J.W., and Seegmiller, J.E.: Purine metabolism in cultured fibroblasts from patients deficient in hypoxanthine phosphoribosyltransferase, purine nucleoside phosphorylase, or adenosine deaminase. Proc. Natl. Acad. Sci. U.S.A., *75*:3722–3736, 1978.
77. Fox, I.H., and Kelley, W.N.: Human phosphoribosylpyrophosphate synthetase: Kinetic mechanism and end-product inhibition. J. Biol. Chem., *247*:2126–2131, 1972.
78. Becker, M.A., Kostel, P.J., and Meyer, L.J.: Human phosphoribosylpyrophosphate synthetase: Comparison of purified normal and mutant enzymes. J. Biol. Chem., *250*:6822–6830, 1975.
79. Zoref, E., deVries, A., and Sperling, O.: Metabolic cooperation between human fibroblasts with normal and with superactive phosphoribosylpyrophosphate synthetase. Nature, *260*:786–788, 1976.
80. Yen, R.C.K., Adams, W.B., Lazar, C., and Becker, M.A.: Evidence for X-linkage of human phosphoribosylpyrophosphate synthetase. Proc. Natl. Acad. Sci. U.S.A., *75*:482–485, 1978.
81. Becker, M.A. et al.: Inherited superactivity of phosphoribosylpyrophosphate synthetase: Association of uric acid overproduction and sensorineural deafness. Am. J. Med., *85*:383–390, 1988.
82. Becker, M.A. et al.: Phosphoribosylpyrophosphate synthetase superactivity: A study of five patients with catalytic defects in the enzyme. Arthritis Rheum., *29*:880–888, 1986.
83. Becker, M.A., Losman, M.J., Itkin, P., and Simkin, P.A.: Gout with superactive phosphoribosylpyrophosphate synthetase due to increased enzyme catalytic rate. J. Lab Clin. Med., *99*:485–511, 1982.
84. Sperling, O., Persky-Brosh, S., Boer, P., and deVries, A.: Human erythrocyte phosphoribosylpyrophosphate synthetase mutationally altered in regulatory properties. Biochem. Med., *7*:389–395, 1973.
85. Zoref, E., deVries, A., and Sperling, O.: Mutant feedback resistant phosphoribosylpyrophosphate synthetase associated with purine overproduction and gout. J. Clin. Invest., *56*:1093–1099, 1975.
86. Becker, M.A., Losman, M.J., Wilson, J., and Simmonds, H.A.: Superactivity of phosphoribosylpyrophosphate synthetase due to altered regulation by nucleotide inhibition and inorganic phosphate. Biochem. Biophys. Acta., *882*:168–176, 1986.
87. Becker, M.A. et al.: Variant human phosphoribosylpyrophosphate synthetase altered in regulatory and catalytic functions. J. Clin. Invest., *65*:109–120, 1980.
88. Simmonds, H.A., Webster, D.R., Lingam, S., and Wilson, J.: An inborn error of purine metabolism, deafness and neurodevelopmental abnormality. Neuropediatrics, *16*:106–108, 1985.
89. Akaoka, I. et al.: A gouty family with increased phosphoribosylpyrophosphate synthetase activity: Case reports, family studies, and kinetic studies of the abnormal enzyme. J. Rheumatol., *8*:563–574, 1984.
90. Taira, M. et al.: Localization of human phosphoribosylpyrophosphate synthetase subunit I and II genes (PRPS 1 and PRPS 2) to different regions of the X chromosome and assignment of two PRPS-related genes to autosomes. Somatic Cell Mol. Genet., *15*:29–37, 1989.
91. Becker, M.A. et al.: Cloning of cDNAs for human phosphoribosylpyrophosphate synthetases 1 and 2 and X chromosome localization of PRPS 1 and PRPS 2 genes. Genomics, *8*:555–561, 1990.
92. Taira, M. et al.: A human testis-specific mRNA for phosphoribosylpyrophosphate synthetase that initiates from a non-AUG codon. J. Biol. Chem., *265*:16491–16495, 1990.
93. Roessler, B.J. et al.: Identification of distinct PRS1 mutations in two patients with X-linked phosphoribosylpyrophosphate synthetase superactivity. Adv. Exp. Med. Biol., (in press).
94. Alepa, F.P., Howell, R.R., Klinenberg, J.R., and Seegmiller, J.E.: Relationships between glycogen storage disease and tophaceous gout. Am. J. Med., *42*:58–66, 1967.
95. Green, H.L. et al.: ATP depletion, a possible role in the pathogenesis of hyperuricemia in glycogen storage disease, type I. J. Clin Invest., *62*:321–328, 1978.
96. Long, W.K.: Glutathione reductase in red blood cells: Variant associated with gout. Science, *155*:712–713, 1967.
97. Wasserzing, O., Szeinberg, A., and Sperling, O.: Altered physical properties of glutathione reductase in G-6PD deficiency. (Abstract.) Hum. Hered., *27*:220, 1977.
98. Breven, J., Hardwell, T.R., Hickling, P., and Whittaker, M.: Effect of treatment on erythrocyte phosphoribosylpyrophosphate synthetase and glutathione reductase activity in patients with primary gout. Ann. Rheum. Dis., *45*:941–944, 1986.
99. Fox, I.H., Palella, T.D., and Kelley, W.N.: Hyperuricemia: A marker for cell energy crisis. N. Engl. J. Med., *317*:111–112, 1987.
100. Woolliscroft, J.O., Colfter, H., and Fox, I.H.: Hyperuricemia in acute illness: A poor prognostic sign. Am. J. Med., *72*:58–62, 1982.
101. Woolliscroft, J.O., and Fox, I.H.: Increased body fluid purine levels during hypotensive events. Evidence for ATP degradation. Am. J. Med. *81*:472–478, 1986.
102. Raivio, K.O. et al.: Stimulation of human purine synthesis *de novo* by fructose infusion. Metabolism, *24*:861–869, 1975.
103. Faller, J., and Fox, I.H.: Ethanol-induced hyperuricemia. Evidence for increased urate production by activation of adenine nucleotide turnover. N. Engl. J. Med., *307*:1598–1602, 1982.
104. Mineo, I. et al.: Myogenic hyperuricemia: A common pathophysiological feature of glycogenesis types III, V, and VII. N. Engl. J. Med., *317*:75–80, 1987.
105. Puig, J.G., and Fox, I.H.: Ethanol-induced activation of adenine nucleotide turnover: Evidence for a role of acetate. J. Clin. Invest., *74*:36–41, 1984.
106. Fox, I.H.: Adenosine triphosphate degradation in specific disease. J. Lab. Clin. Med., *106*:101–110, 1985.
107. Fox, I.H., and Kelley, W.N.: Studies on the mechanism of fruc-

tose-induced hyperuricemia in man. Metabolism, *21*:713–721, 1972.

108. Buzard, J., Bishop, C., and Talbott, J.H.: The fate of uric acid in the normal and gouty human being. J. Chronic Dis., *2*:42–49, 1955.
109. Sorenson, L.B.: The elimination of uric acid in man studied by means of ^{14}C-labelled uric acid. Scand. J. Clin. Lab. Invest. [Suppl.], *12*:1–214, 1960.
110. Gutman, A.B., and Yu, T-F.: Renal function in gout: With a commentary on the renal regulation of urate excretion, and the role of the kidney in the pathogenesis of gout. Am. J. Med., *23*:600–622, 1957.
111. Greger, R., Lang, F., and Deetjen, P.: Handling of uric acid by the rat kidney: 2. Microperfusion studies on bidirectional transport of uric acid in the proximal tubule. Pfluegers Arch., *335*:257–265, 1972.
112. Greger, R., Lang, F., and Deetjen, P.: Handling of uric acid by the rat kidney: 1. Microanalysis of uric acid in proximal tubular fluid. Pfluegers Arch., *324*:279–287, 1971.
113. Roch-Ramel, F., and Weiner, I.M.: Excretion of urate by the kidneys of Cebus monkeys: A micropuncture study. Am. J. Physiol., *224*:1369–1374, 1973.
114. Praetorius, E., and Kirk, J.E.: Hypouricemia: With evidence for tubular elimination of uric acid. J. Lab. Clin. Med., *35*:865–868, 1950.
115. Gutman, A.B., and Yu, T-F: A three component system for regulation of renal excretion of uric acid in man. Trans. Assoc. Am. Physicians, *74*:353–365, 1961.
116. Yu, T-F., and Gutman, A.B.: Study of the paradoxical effects of salicylate in low, intermediate and high dosage on the renal mechanism for excretion of urate in man. J. Clin. Invest., *38*:1298–1315, 1959.
117. Weiner, I.M., and Fanelli, G.M., Jr.: Renal urate excretion in animal models. Nephron, *14*:33–47, 1975.
118. Kessler, R.H., Hierholzer, K., and Gurd, R.S.: Localization of urate transport in the nephron of mongrel and dalmation dog kidney. Am. J. Physiol., *197*:601–603, 1959.
119. Mudge, G.H., McAlary, B., and Berndt, W.O.: Renal transport of uric acid in the guinea pig. Am. J. Physiol., *214*:875–879, 1968.
120. Podevin, R. et al.: Etude chezl'homme de la cinatigue d'apparition dans l'urine de l'acide urique $2^{14}C$. Nephron, *5*:134–140, 1968.
121. Weiner, I.M., and Mudge, G.H.: Renal tubular mechanisms for excretion of organic acids and bases. Am. J. Med., *36*:743–762, 1964.
122. Yu, T-F., et al.: Effect of pyrazinamide and pyrazinoic acid on urate clearance and other discrete renal functions. Proc. Soc. Exp. Biol. Med., *96*:264–267, 1957.
123. Wilson, D.M., and Goldstein, N.P.: Renal urate excretion in patients with Wilson's disease. Kidney Int., *4*:331–336, 1973.
124. Bennett, J.S., Bond, J., Singer, I., and Gottlieb, A.J.: Hypouricemia in Hodgkin's disease. Ann. Intern. Med., *76*:751–756, 1972.
125. Meisel, A.D., and Diamond, H.S.: Inhibition of probenecid uricosuria by pyrazinamide and para-aminohippurate. Am. J. Physiol., *232*:F222–F226, 1977.
126. Levinson, D.J., and Sorensen, L.B.: Renal handling of uric acid in normal and gouty subjects: Evidence for a 4-component system. Ann. Rheum. Dis., *39*:173–179, 1980.
127. Steele, T.H., and Oppenheimer, S.: Factors affecting urate excretion following diuretic administration in man. Am. J. Med., *47*:564–574, 1969.
128. Manuel, M.A., and Steele, T.H.: Pyrazinamide suppression of the uricosuric response to sodium chloride infusion. J. Lab Clin. Med., *83*:417–427, 1974.
129. Diamond, H.S., and Paolino, J.S.: Evidence for a post-secretory reabsorptive site for uric acid in man. J. Clin. Invest., *52*:1491–1499, 1973.
130. Puig, G.J.: Renal handling of uric acid in normal subjects by means of the pyrazinamide and probenecid tests. Nephron, *35*:183–186, 1983.
131. Sorensen, L.B., and Levinson, D.J.: Isolated defect in postsecretory reabsorption of uric acid. Ann. Rheum., Dis., *39*:180–183, 1980.
132. Smetana, S.S., and Bar-Khayim, Y.: Hypouricemia due to renal tubular defect. A study with the probenecid-pyrazinamide test. Arch. Intern. Med., *145*:1200–1203, 1985.
133. Tofukm, Y., Kuroda, M., and Takeda, R.: Hypouricemia due to renal urate wasting. Nephron, *30*:39–44, 1982.
134. Simkin, P.A.: Urate excretion in normal and gouty men. Adv. Exp. Med. Biol., *76B*:41–45, 1977.
135. Zollner, N., and Griebsch, A.: Diet and gout. Adv. Exp. Med. Biol., *41B*:435–442, 1974.
136. Levinson, D.J., Decker, D.E., and Sorensen, L.B.: Renal handling of uric acid in man. Ann. Clin. Lab. Sci., *12*:73–77, 1982.
137. Rieselbach, R.E., Sorensen, L.B., Shelp, W.D., and Steele, T.H.: Diminished renal urate secretion per nephron as a basis for primary gout. Ann. Intern. Med., *73*:359–366, 1970.
138. Copeman, W.S.C.: A Short History of the Gout. Los Angeles, University of California Press, 1964, p. 35.
139. Delbarre, F., Braun, S., and St. George-Chaumet, F.: La goutte: Problemes cliniques, biologiques et therapeutiques. Sem. Hop. Paris, *43*:623–633, 1967.
140. Grahame, R., and Scott, J.T.: Clinical survey of 354 patients with gout. Ann. Rheum. Dis., *29*:461–468, 1970.
141. Harth, M., and Robinson, C.E.G.: Gouty arthritis in a D.V.A. Hospital: A retrospective study. Med. Serv. J. Canada, *18*:671–674, 1962.
142. Meyers, O.L., and Monteagudo, F.S.E.: Gout in females. An analysis of 92 patients. Clin. Exp. Rheumatol., *3*:105–109, 1985.
143. Simkin, P.A.: The pathogenesis of Podagra. Ann. Intern. Med., *86*:230–233, 1977.
144. Kohl, L.E., Thompson, M.E., and Griffith, B.P.: Gout in the heart transplant recipient. Physiologic puzzle and therapeutic challenge. Am. J. Med., *87*:289–294, 1989.
145. Derus, C.L., Levinson, D.J., Bowman, B., and Bengoa, J.M.: Altered fractional excretion of uric acid during total parenteral nutrition. J. Rheumatol., *114*:978–981, 1987.
146. Bartles, E.C.: Gout as a complication of Surgery. Surg. Clin. North Am., *38*:845–848, 1957.
147. Pascual, E.: Persistence of monosodium urate crystals and low-grade inflammation in the synovial fluid of patients with untreated gout. Arthritis Rheum., *34*:141–145, 1991.
148. Gutman, A.B.: Gout and gouty arthritis. *In* Textbook of Medicine. Edited by P.B. Beeson and W. McDermott. Philadelphia, W.B. Saunders, 1958, p. 595.
149. Raddatz, D.A., Mahowald, M.L., and Bilka, P.J.: Acute polyarticular gout. Ann. Rheum. Dis., *42*:117–122, 1983.
150. McCarty, D.J.: Crystal-induced inflammation: Syndromes of gout and pseudogout. Geriatrics, *18*:467–478, 1963.
151. Ginsberg, M.H., and Genant, H.K., Yu, T-F., and McCarty, D.J.: Rheumatoid nodulosis: An unusual variant of rheumatoid disease. Arthritis Rheum., *18*:49–58, 1975.
152. Kozin, F., and McCarty, D.J.: Rheumatoid factors in the serum of gouty patients. Arthritis Rheum., *20*:1559–1560, 1977.
153. Agudelo, C.A., Turner, R.A., Panetti, M., and Pisko, E.: Does hyperuricemia protect from rheumatoid inflammation. Arthritis Rheum., *27*:443–448, 1984.
154. Yu, T-F.: Secondary gout associated with myeloproliferative diseases. Arthritis Rheum., *8*:765–771, 1965.

155. Smythe, C.M., and Cutchin, J.H.: Primary juvenile gout. Am. J. Med., *32*:799–804, 1962.
156. Wood, M.H. et al.: The Lesch-Nyhan syndrome: Report of three cases. Aust. N.Z. Med. J., *1*:57–64, 1972.
157. Gutman, A.B.: The past four decades of progress in the knowledge of gout with an assessment of the present status. Arthritis Rheum., *16*:431–445, 1973.
158. Hench, P.S.: Diagnosis of gout and gouty arthritis. J. Lab. Clin. Med., *22*:48–55, 1936.
159. Nishioka, N., and Mikanagi, K.: Clinical features of 4,000 gouty subjects in Japan. Adv. Exp. Med. Biol., *122A*:47–54, 1980.
160. Nakayama, D.A. et al.: Tophaceous gout: A clinical and radiographic assessment. Arthritis Rheum., *27*:468–471, 1984.
161. Lawry, G.V., II, Fan, P.T., and Bluestone, R.: Polyarticular versus monoarticular gout: A prospective comparative analysis of clinical features. Medicine, *67*:335–343, 1988.
162. Macfarlane, D.G., and Dieppe, P.A.: Diuretic-induced gout in elderly women. Br. J. Rheumatol., *24*:155–157, 1985.
163. Lally, E.V., Zimmerman, B., Ho, G., Jr., and Kaplan, S.R.: Urate-mediated inflammation in nodal osteoarthritis. Clinical and roentgenographic correlations. Arthritis Rheum., *32*:86–90, 1989.
164. Simkin, P.A., Campbell, P.M., and Larson, E.B.: Gout in Heberden's nodes. Arthritis Rheum., *26*:94–97, 1983.
165. Doherty, M., and Dieppe, P.A.: Crystal deposition disease in the elderly. Clin. Rheum. Dis., *12*:97–116, 1986.
166. Good, A.E., and Rapp, R.: Bony ankylosis. A rare manifestation of gout. J. Rheumatol., *5*:335–337, 1978.
167. Varga, J., Giampaola, C., and Goldenberg, D.L.: Tophaceous gout of the spine in a patient with no peripheral tophi: Case report and review of the literature. Arthritis Rheum., *28*:1312–1315, 1985.
168. McCallum, D.E., Mathews, R.S., and O'Neil, M.T.: Aseptic necrosis of the femoral head. Associated diseases and evaluation of treatment. Southern Med. J., *63*:241–253, 1970.
169. Hunder, G.G., Worthington, J.W., and Bickel, W.H.: Avascular necrosis of the femoral head in a patient with gout. JAMA, *203*:101–103, 1968.
170. Stockman, A., Darlington, L.G., and Scott, J.T. Frequency of chondrocalcinosis in the knees and avascular necrosis of the femoral head in gout: A controlled study. Ann. Rheum. Dis., *39*:7–11, 1980.
171. Lichtenstein, L., Scott, H.W., and Levin, M.H.: Pathologic changes in gout: Survey of 11 necropsied cases. Am. J. Pathol., *32*:871–895, 1956.
172. Stark, T.W., and Hirokawa, R.H.: Gout and its manifestations in the head and neck. Otolaryngol. Clin. North Am., *15*:659–664, 1982.
173. Yu, T-F., Milestones in the treatment of gout. Am. J. Med., *56*:676–685, 1974.
174. Bauer, W., and Klemperer, F.: Gout. *In* Diseases of Metabolism. 2nd Ed. Edited by G. Duncan. Philadelphia, W.B. Saunders, 1947, p. 611.
175. Bartels, E.C., and Matossian, G.S.: Gout: Six-year follow up on probenecid (Benemid) therapy. Arthritis Rheum., *2*:193–202, 1959.
176. O'Duffy, J.D., Hunder, G.G., and Kelly, P.J.: Decreasing prevalence of tophaceous gout. Mayo Clin. Proc., *50*:227–228, 1975.
177. Herring, L.J.: Observations on the analysis of ten thousand calculi. J. Urol., *88*:545–562, 1962.
178. Prien, E.L.: Crystallographic analysis of urinary calculi: A 23-year survey study. J. Urol., *89*:917–924, 1963.
179. Atsmon, A., DeVries, A., and Frank, M.: Uric acid lithiasis. Amsterdam, Elsevier, 1963.
180. Boyce, W.H., and Garvey, F.K., and Strawcutter, H.E.: Incidence of urinary calculi among patients in general hospitals, 1948 to 1952. JAMA, *161*:1437–1444, 1956.
181. Yu, T.-F., and Gutman, A.B.: Uric acid nephrolithiasis in gout: Predisposing factors. Ann. Intern. Med., *67*:1133–1148, 1967.
182. Yu, T.-F.: Urolithiasis in hyperuricemia and gout. J. Urol., *126*:424–430, 1981.
183. Coe, F.L., and Kavalach, A.G.: Hypercalciuria and hyperuricosuria in patients with calcium nephrolithiasis. N. Engl. J. Med., *291*:1344–1350, 1974.
184. Clarke, A.M., and McKenzie, R.G.: Ileostomy and the risk of urinary uric acid stones. Lancet, *2*:395–397, 1969.
185. Klinenberg, J.R., Goldfinger, S.F., and Seegmiller, J.E.: The effectiveness of the xanthine oxidase inhibitor allopurinol in the treatment of gout. Ann. Intern. Med., *62*:639–647, 1965.
186. Plante, G.E., Durivage, J., and Lemieux, G.: Renal excretion of hydrogen in primary gout. Metabolism, *17*:377–385, 1968.
187. Henneman, P.H., Wallach, S., and Dempsey, E.F.: The metabolic defect responsible for uric acid stone formation. J. Clin. Invest., *41*:537–542, 1962.
188. Gutman, A.B., and Yu, T.-F.: Urinary ammonium excretion in primary gout. J. Clin. Invest., *44*:1474–1481, 1965.
189. Brazel, U.S., Sperling, O., Frank, M., and DeVries, A.: Renal ammonium excretion and urinary pH in idiopathic uric acid lithiasis. J. Urol., *92*:1–5, 1964.
190. Wrong, O., and Davis, H.E.F.: The excretion of uric acid in renal disease. Q. J. Med., *28*:259–313, 1959.
191. Falls, W.F., Jr.: Comparison of urinary acidification and ammonium excretion in normal and gouty subjects. Metabolism., *21*:433–445, 1972.
192. Gutman, A.B., and Yu, T.-F.: An abnormality of glutamine metabolism in primary gout. Am. J. Med., *35*:820–831, 1963.
193. Pollak, V.E., and Mattenheimer, H.: Glutaminase activity in the kidney in gout. J. Lab. Clin. Med., *66*:564–570, 1965.
194. Sperling, O., De Vries, A., and Kedem, O.: Studies on the etiology of uric acid lithiasis: 4. Urinary non-dialyzable substances in idiopathic uric acid lithiasis. J. Urol., *94*:286–292, 1965.
195. Coe, F.L., Lawton, R.L., Goldstein, R.B., and Tembe, V.: Sodium urate accelerates precipitation of calcium oxalate in vitro. Proc. Soc. Exp. Biol. Med., *149*:926–929, 1975.
196. Nakagawa, Y., Abram, V., and Coe, F.L.: Isolation of calcium oxalate crystal growth inhibitor from rat kidney and urine. Am. J. Physiol., *247*:F765–F772, 1984.
197. Barlow, K.A., and Beilin, L.J.: Renal disease in primary gout. Q. J. Med., *37*:79–96, 1968.
198. Talbott, J.H., and Terplan, K.L.: The kidney in gout. Medicine, *39*:405–468, 1960.
199. Wyngaarden, J.B.: The role of the kidney in the pathogenesis and treatment of gout. Arthritis Rheum., *1*:191–203, 1958.
200. Reif, M.C., Constantiner, A., and Levitt, M.F.: Chronic gouty nephropathy: A vanishing syndrome? N. Engl. J. Med., *304*:535–536, 1981.
201. Yu, T.-F., and Berger, L.: Renal disease in primary gout: A study of 253 gout patients with proteinuria. Semin. Arthritis Rheum., *4*:293–305, 1975.
202. Messerli, F.H. et al.: Serum uric acid in essential hypertension: An indictor of renal vascular involvement. Ann. Intern. Med., *93*:817–821, 1980.
203. Berger, L., and Yu, T.-F.: Renal function in gout: 4. An analysis of 524 gouty subjects including long-term follow-up studies. Am. J. Med., *59*:605–613, 1975.
204. Lawrence, J.S.: Heritable disorders of connective tissue. Proc. R. Soc. Med., *53*:522–526, 1960.
205. Wyngaarden, J.B.: Gout. *In* The Metabolic Basis of Inherited Diseases. Edited by J.B. Stanbury, D.S. Fredrickson, and J.B. Wyngaarden. New York, McGraw-Hill, 1960, pp. 679–760.
206. Zalokar, J., Lellouch, J., and Claude, J.R.: Goutte et uricemia

dans une population de 4663 hommes jeumes actifs. Semin. Hop. Paris, *13–14*:664–670, 1981.

207. Lennane, G.A.Q., Rose, B.S., and Isdale, I.C.: Gout in the Maori. Ann. Rheum. Dis., *19*:120–125, 1960.
208. Prior, I.A.M., Rose, B.S., Harvey, H.P., and Davidson, F.: Hyperuricemia, gout and diabetic abnormality in Polynesian people. Lancet, *1*:333–338, 1966.
209. Turner, R.E., Frank, M.J., VanAusdal, D., and Bollet, A.J.: Some aspects of the epidemiology of gout: Sex and race incidence. Arch. Intern. Med., *106*:400–406, 1960.
210. Wallace, S.L. et al.: Preliminary criteria for the classification of the acute arthritis of primary gout. Arthritis Rheum., *20*:895–900, 1977.
211. Rouault, T., Caldwell, D.S., and Holmes, E.W.: Aspiration of the asymptomatic metatarsophalangeal joint in gout patients and hyperuricemic controls. Arthritis Rheum., *25*:209–212, 1982.
212. Weinberger, A. et al.: Frequency of intra-articular monosodium urate (MSU) crystals in asymptomatic hyperuricemic subjects. Adv. Exp. Med. Biol., *195A*:431–434, 1986.
213. Wallace, S.L., Bernstein, D., and Diamond, H.: Diagnostic value of colchicine therapeutic trial. JAMA, *199*:525–528, 1967.
214. Fam, A.G., and Rubenstein, J.: Hydroxyapatite Pseudopodagra: A syndrome of young women. Arthritis Rheum., *32*:741–747, 1989.
215. Martel, W.: The overhanging margin of bone: A roentgenologic manifestation of gout. Radiology, *91*:755–756, 1968.
216. Vyhnanek, L., Lavicka, J., and Blahos, J.: Roentgenological findings in gout. Radiol. Clin., *29*:256–264, 1960.
217. Talbott, J.H.: Gout. 3rd Ed. New York, Grune & Stratton, 1967.
218. Dodds, W.J., and Steinbach, H.L.: Gout associated with calcification of cartilage. N. Engl. J. Med., *275*:745–749, 1966.
219. Good, A.E., and Rapp, R.: Chondrocalcinosis of the knee with gout and rheumatoid arthritis. N. Engl. J. Med., *277*:286–290, 1967.
220. Malawista, S.E., Seegmiller, J.E., Hathaway, B.E., and Sokoloff, L.: Sacroiliac gout. JAMA, *194*:954–956, 1965.
221. Alarcon-Segovia, D.A., Cetina, J.A., and Diaz-Jouanen, E.: Sacroiliac joints in primary gout: Clinical and roentgenographic study of 143 patients. AJR, *118*:438–443, 1973.
222. Cohen, H.: Gout and other metabolic disorders producing joint disease. *In* Textbook of the Rheumatic Diseases. Edited by W.S.C. Copeman. Edinburgh, Livingstone, 1955, pp. 182–186.
223. Neel, J.V.: The clinical detection of the genetic carriers of inherited disease. Medicine, *26*:115–153, 1947.
224. Smyth, C.J.: Hereditary factors in gout: A review of recent literature. Metabolism, *6*:218–229, 1957.
225. Smyth, C.J., Cotterman, C.W., and Freyberg, R.H.: The genetics of gout and hyperuricemia—An analysis of nineteen families. J. Clin. Invest., *27*:749–759, 1948.
226. Hauge, M., and Harvald, B.: Hereditary in gout and hyperuricemia. Acta Med. Scand., *152*:247–257, 1955.
227. Calabrese, G., Simmonds, H.A., Cameron, J.S., and Davies, P.H.: Precocious familial gout with reduced fractional urate clearance and normal purine enzymes. Q. J. Med., *78*:441–445, 1990.
228. Laskarzewski, P.M. et al.: Familial hyper- and hypouricemia in random and hyperlipidemic recall cohorts. The Princeton School District Family Study. Metabolism, *32*:230–243, 1983.
229. Decker, J.L., Jane, J.J., Jr., and Reynolds, W.E.: Hyperuricemia in a male Filipino population. Arthritis Rheum., *5*:144–155, 1962.
230. Burch, T.A., O'Brien, W.M., Need, R., and Kurland, L.T.: Hyperuricemia and gout in the Mariana Islands. Ann. Rheum., Dis., *25*:114–119, 1966.
231. O'Brien, W.M., Burch, T.A., and Bunim, J.J.: Genetics of hyperuricemia in Blackfeet and Pima Indians. Ann. Rheum. Dis., *25*:117–119, 1966.
232. Talbott, J.H.: Gout. 2nd Ed. New York, Grune & Stratton, 1964.
233. Fiechtner, J.J., and Simkin, P.A.: Urate spherulities in gouty synovia. JAMA, *245*:1533–1536, 1981.
234. Weinberger, A. et al.: Spherulite crystals in synovial tissue of a patient with recurrent monarthritis. Clin. Exp. Rheum., *2*:63–65, 1984.
235. Perricone, E., and Brandt, K.D.: Enhancement of urate solubility by connective tissue: 1. Effect of proteoglycan aggregates and buffer cation. Arthritis Rheum., *21*:453–460, 1978.
236. Brown, J., and Mallory, G.K.: Renal changes in gout. N. Engl. J. Med., *243*:325–329, 1950.
237. Fineberg, S.K., and Altschul, A.: The nephropathy of gout. Ann. Intern. Med., *4*:1182–1194, 1956.
238. Gonick. H.C., Rubini, M.E., Gleason, I.O., and Sommers, S.C.: The renal lesion in gout. Ann. Intern. Med., *62*:667–674, 1965.
239. Heptinstall, R.H.: Diabetes mellitus and gout. *In* Pathology of the Kidney. 2nd Ed. Boston, Little, Brown, 1974, pp. 963–975.
240. Paulus, H.E. et al.: Clinical significance of hyperuricemia in routinely screened hospitalized men. JAMA, *211*:277–281, 1970.
241. Brand, F.N. et al.: Hyperuricemia as a risk factor of coronary heart disease: The Framingham Study. Am. J. Epidemiol., *121*:11–18, 1985.
242. Maroko, P.R., McDevitt, J.T., Fox, M.J. et al.: Antihypertensive effectiveness of very low doses of hydrochlorothiazide: Results of the PHICOG Trial. Clin. Ther., *11*:94–119, 1989.
243. Bryant, M.J. et al.: Hyperuricemia induced by administration of chlorthalidone and other sulfonamide diuretics. Am. J. Med., *33*:408–420, 1962.
244. Steele, T.H.: Evidence for altered renal urate reabsorption during changes in volume of the extracelluar fluid. J. Lab Clin. Med., *74*:288–299, 1969.
245. Roos, J.C., Boer, P., Peuker, K.H., and Dorhout Mees, E.J.: Changes in intrarenal uric acid handling during chronic Spironolactone treatment in patients with essential hypertension. Nephron, *32*:209–213, 1982.
246. Weiner, I.M., and Tinker, J.P.: Pharmacology of pyrazinamide metabolic and renal function studies related to the mechanism of drug-induced urate retention. J. Pharmacol. Exp. Ther., *180*:411–434, 1972.
247. Postlethwaite, A.E., Bartel, A.G., and Kelley, W.N.: Hyperuricemia due to ethambutol. N. Engl. J. Med., *286*:761–763, 1972.
248. Gershon, S.L., and Fox, I.H.: Pharmacologic effects of nicotinic acid on human purine metabolism. J. Lab. Clin. Med., *84*:179–186, 1974.
249. Menon, R.K. et al.: Warfarin administration increases uric acid concentration in plasma. Clin. Chem., *32*:1557–1559, 1986.
250. Gores, P.F., Fryd, D.S., Sutherland, D.E.R., et al.: Hyperuricemia after renal transplantation. Am. J. Surg., *156*:397–400, 1988.
251. Lin, H.Y., Rocher, L.L., McQuillan, M.A., et al.: Cyclosporine-indued hyperuricemia and gout. N. Engl. J. Med., *321*:287–292, 1989.
252. Gupta, A.K., Rocher, L.L., Schmaltz, S.P., et al.: Short-term changes in renal function, blood pressure and electrolyte levels in patients receiving cyclosporine for dermatologic disorders. Arch. Intern. Med., *151*:356–362, 1991.
253. Saker, B.M., Tofler, O.B., Burvill, M.J., and Reilly, K.A.: Alcohol consumption and gout. Med. J. Aust., *1*:1213–1216, 1967.
254. Evans, J.G., Prior, I.A.M., and Harvey, H.P.B.: Relation of serum uric acid to body bulk, haemoglobin, and alcohol intake in two South Pacific Polynesian populations. Ann. Rheum. Dis., *27*:319–324, 1968.
255. MacLachlan, M.J., and Rodnan, G.P.: Effects of food, fast and

alcohol on serum uric acid and acute attacks of gout. Am. J. Med., *42*:38–57, 1967.

256. Ball, G.V., and Sorensen, L.B.: Pathogenesis of hyperuricemia in saturnine gout. N. Engl. J. Med., *280*:1199–1202, 1969.
257. Emmerson, B.T.: Chronic lead neuropathy: The diagnostic use of calcium EDTA and the association with gout. Aust. Ann. Med., *12*:310–324, 1963.
258. Halla, J.T., and Ball, G.V.: Saturnine gout. A review of 42 patients. Semin. Arthritis Rheum., *11*:307–314, 1982.
259. Reynolds, P.P., Knapp, M.J., Baraf, H.S.B., and Holmes, E.W.: Moonshine and lead. Relationship to the pathogenesis and hyperuricemia in gout. Arthritis Rheum., *26*:1057–1064, 1983.
260. Cristofori, F.C., and Duncan, G.G.: Uric acid excretion in obese subjects during periods of total fasting. Metabolism, *13*:303–311, 1964.
261. Drenick, E.J., Swendseid, M.E., Blahd, W.H., and Tuttle, S.G.: Prolonged starvation as treatment for severe obesity. JAMA, *187*:100–105, 1964.
262. Goldfinger, S., Klinenberg, J.R., and Seegmiller, J.E.: Renal retention of uric acid induced by infusion of beta-hydroxybutyrate and acetoacetate. N. Engl. J. Med., *272*:351–355, 1965.
263. Sarre, H., and Mertz, D.P.: Sekundare Gicht bei Neireninsuffizenz. Klin. Wochenschr., *43*:1134–1140, 1965.
264. Richet, G., Mignon, F., and Ardaillou, R.: Goutte secondaire der nephropathies choniques. Presse Med., *73*:633–638, 1965.
265. Steele, T.H., and Rieselbach, R.E.: The contribution of residual nephrons within the chronically diseased kidney to urate homeostasis in man. Am. J. Med., *43*:876–886, 1967.
266. Sorensen, L.B., and Levinson, D.J.: Origin and extrarenal elimination of uric acid in man. Nephron, *14*:7–20, 1975.
267. Caner, J.E.Z., and Decker, J.L.: Recurrent acute (gouty) arthritis in chronic renal failure treated with periodic hemodialysis. Am. J. Med., *36*:571–582, 1964.
268. Reginato, A.J. et al.: Arthropathy and cutaneous calcinosis in hemodialysis oxalosis. Arthritis Rheum., *29*:1387–1396, 1986.
269. Lynch, E.C.: Uric acid metabolism in proliferative diseases of the marrow. Arch. Intern. Med., *109*:639–653, 1962.
270. Gutman, A.B., and Yu, T.-F.: Secondary gout. (Abstract.) Ann. Intern. Med., *56*:675, 1962.
271. Laster, L., and Muller, A.F.: Uric acid production in a case of myeloid metaplasia associated with gouty arthritis studied with N^{15}-labelled glycine. Am. J. Med., *15*:857–861, 1953.
272. Martinez-Lavin, M. et al.: Coexistent gout and hypertrophic osteoarthropathy in patients with cyanotic heart disease. J. Rheumatol., *11*:832–834, 1984.
273. Ross, E.A. et al.: Renal function and urate metabolism in late survivors with cyanotic congenital heart disease. Circulation, *73*:396–400, 1986.
274. Diamond, H.S. et al.: Hyperuricosuria and increased tubular secretion of urate in sickle cell disease. Am. J. Med., *59*:796–802, 1975.
275. Sears, W.G.: The occurrence of gout during the treatment of pernicious anemia. Lancet, *1*:24, 1933.
276. Paik, C.H., Alavi, I., Dunea, G., and Weiner, L.: Thalassemia and gouty arthritis. JAMA, *213*:296–297, 1970.
277. Ultmann, J.: Hyperuricemia in disseminated neoplastic disease other than lymphomas or leukemias. Cancer, *15*:122–129, 1962.
278. Diamond, H.S., Meisel, A.D., and Holden, D.: The natural history of urate overproduction in sickle cell anemia. Ann. Intern. Med., *90*:752–757, 1979.
279. Ball, G.V., and Sorensen, L.B.: The pathogenesis of hyperuricemia and gout in sickle cell anemia. Arthritis Rheum., *13*:846–848, 1970.
280. Espinoza, L.R., Spillberg, I., and Osterland, C.K.: Joint manifestations of sickle cell disease. Medicine, *53*:295–305, 1974.
281. Mallette, L.E., Bilezikian, J.P., Heath, D.A., and Aurback, G.D.: Primary hyperparathyroidism: Clinical and biochemical features. Medicine, *53*:127–145, 1974.
282. Scott, J.T., Dixon, A.St.J., and Bywaters, E.G.L.: Association of hyperuricemia and gout with hyperparathyroidism. Br. Med. J., *1*:1070–1073, 1964.
283. Castrillo, J.M., Diaz-Curiel, M., and Rapado, A.: Hyperuricemia in primary hyperparathyroidism: Incidence and evolution after surgery. Adv. Exp. Med. Biol., *165A*:151–157, 1984.
284. Shelp, W.D., Steele, T.H., and Rieselbach, R.E.: Comparison of urinary phosphate, urate and magnesium excretion following parathyroid hormone administration to normal man. Metabolism, *18*:63–70, 1969.
285. Dent, C.E.: Some problems of hyperparathyroidism. Br. Med. J., *2*:1419, 1495, 1962.
286. Eisen, A.Z., and Seegmiller, J.E.: Uric acid metabolism in psoriasis. J. Clin. Invest., *40*:1486–1494, 1961.
287. Lambert, J.R., and Wright, V.: Serum uric acid levels in psoriatic arthritis. Ann. Rheum. Dis., *36*:264–267, 1977.
288. Puig, T.G. et al.: Uric acid metabolism in psoriasis. Adv. Exp. Med. Biol., *195A*:411–416, 1986.
289. Zimmer, J.G., and Demis, D.J.: Associations between gout, psoriasis, and sarcoidosis: With consideration of their pathologic significance. Ann. Intern. Med., *64*:786–796, 1966.
290. Pant, S.S., Maser, H.W., and Krane, S.M.: Hyperuricemia in Down's syndrome. J. Clin. Endocrinol. Metab., *28*:472–478, 1968.
291. Meloni, C.R., and Canary, J.J.: Cystinuria with hyperuricemia. JAMA, *200*:257–259, 1967.
292. Aponte, G.E., and Fetter, T.R.: Familial idiopathic oxalate nephrocalcinosis. Am. J. Clin. Pathol., *24*:1363–1373, 1954.
293. Altman, R.D., and Collins, B.: Musculoskeletal manifestations of Paget's disease of bone. Arthritis Rheum., *23*:1121–1127, 1980.
294. Meyer, W.J., III, Gill, J.R., Jr., and Barter, F.C.: Gout as a complication of Barter's syndrome: A possible role for alkalosis in the decreased clearance of uric acid. Ann. Intern. Med., *83*:56–59, 1975.
295. Brauer, G.W., and Prior, I.A.M.: A prospective study of gout in New Zealand Maoris, Ann. Rheum Dis., *37*:466–472, 1978.
296. Fessel, W.J., and Bar, G.D.: Uric acid, lean body weight and creatine interactions. Results from regression analysis of 78 variables. Semin. Arthritis Rheum., *7*:115–121, 1977.
297. Fessel, W.J., Siegelaub, A.B., and Johnson, E.S.: Correlates and consequences of asymptomatic hyperuricemia. Arch. Intern. Med., *132*:44–54, 1973.
298. Glynn, R.J., Campion, E.W., and Silbert, J.E.: Trends in serum uric acid levels 1961–1980. Arthritis Rheum., *26*:87–93, 1983.
299. Scott, J.T.: Obesity and hyperuricaemia. Clin. Rheum. Dis., *3*:25–35, 1977.
300. Sturge, R.A. et al.: Serum uric acid in England and Scotland. Ann. Rheum. Dis., *36*:420–427, 1977.
301. Seidell, J.C. et al.: Overweight and chronic illness—A retrospective cohort study with a follow-up of 6–17 years, in men and women of initially 20–50 years of age. J. Chronic Dis., *39*:585–593, 1986.
302. Bray, G.A.: Complications of obesity. Ann. Intern. Med., *103*:1052–1062, 1985.
303. Kannel, W.B., and Gordon, T.: Physiological and medical concomitant of obesity: The Framingham Study. *In* Obesity in America. Edited by G.A. Bray. Bethesda, MD: National Institutes of Health, DHEW No. (NIH) 79–359, 1979.
304. Gibson, T. et al.: Hyperuricemia, gout and kidney function in New Zealand Maori Men. Br. J. Rheumatol., *23*:276–282, 1984.
305. Emmerson, B.T.: Alteration of urate metabolism by weight reduction. Aust. N.Z. J. Med., *3*:410–412, 1973.

306. Barlow, K.A.: Hyperlipidemia in primary gout. Metabolism, *17*:289–299, 1968.
307. Gibson, J.T., and Grahame, R.: Gout, hypertriglyceridemia, and alcohol consumption. Ann. Rheum. Dis., *3*:109–110, 1974.
308. Naito, H.K., and Mackenzie, A.H.: Secondary hypertriglyceridemia and hyperlipoproteinemia in patients with primary asymptomatic gout. Clin. Chem., *25*:371–375, 1979.
309. Jiao, S., Kameda, K., Matsuzawa, Y., and Tarui, S.: Hyperlipoproteinemia in primary gout: Hyperlipoproteinemic phenotype and influence of alcohol intake and obesity in Japan. Ann. Rheum. Dis., *45*:308–313, 1986.
310. Matsubara, K., Matsuzawa, Y., Jiao, S., et al.: Relationship between hypertriglyceridemia and uric acid production in primary gout. Metabolism, *38*:698–701, 1989.
311. Fox, I.H. et al.: Hyperuricemia and hypertriglyceridemia: Metabolic basis for the association. Metabolism, *34*:741–746, 1985.
312. Cannon, P.J. et al.: Hyperuricemia in primary and renal hypertension. N. Engl. J. Med., *275*:457–464, 1966.
313. Breckenridge, A.: Hypertension and hyperuricemia. Lancet, *1*:15–18, 1966.
314. Dollery, C.T., Duncan, H., and Schumer, B.: Hyperuricemia related to treatment of hypertension. Br. Med. J., *2*:832–835, 1960.
315. Myers, A.R., Epstein, F.H., Dodge, H.J., and Mikkelson, W.M.: The relationship of serum uric acid to risk factors in coronary heart disease. Am. J. Med., *45*:520–528, 1968.
316. Kahn, H.A. et al.: The incidence of hypertension and associated factors. The Israel ischemic heart disease study. Am. Heart J., *84*:171–182, 1972.
317. Rapado, A.: Relationship between gout and arterial hypertension. Adv. Exp. Med. Biol., *41B*:451–459, 1974.
318. Prebis, J.W., Gruskin, A.B., Polinsky, M.S., and Baluarte, H.J.: Uric acid in childhood essential hypertension. J. Pediatr., *98*:702–707, 1981.
319. Gertler, M., Garn, S.M., and Levine, S.A.: Serum uric acid in relation to age and physique in health and in coronary artery disease. Ann. Intern. Med., *34*:1421–1431, 1931.
320. Dreyfuss, F.: The role of hyperuricemia in coronary heart disease. Chest, *38*:332–334, 1960.
321. Hansen, O.E.: Hyperuricemia, gout and atherosclerosis. Am. Heart J., *72*:570–572, 1966.
322. Abbott, R.D., Brand, F.N., Kannel, W.B., and Castelli, W.P.: Gout and coronary heart disease, The Framingham Study. J. Clin. Epidemiol., *41*:237–242, 1988.
323. Ramsdell, M.C., and Kelley, W.N.: The clinical significance of hypouricemia. Ann. Intern. Med., *78*:239–242, 1973.
324. Van Peenen, H.J.: Causes of hypouricemia. Ann. Intern. Med., *78*:977–978, 1973.
325. Holmes, E.W., and Wyngaarden, J.B.: Hereditary xanthinuria. *In* The Metabolic Basis of Inherited Diseases. 5th Ed. Edited by J.B. Stanbury et al. New York, McGraw-Hill, 1983, pp. 1192–1201.
326. Dwosh, I.L., Roncari, D.A.K., Marliss, E., and Fox, I.H.: Hypouricemia in disease. A study of different mechanisms. J. Lab. Clin. Med., *90*:153–161, 1977.

106

Management of Hyperuricemia

ROBERT L. WORTMANN

Hyperuricemia is a common clinical state with many possible causes. Progress in the understanding of purine metabolism, knowledge of the potential consequences of this condition, and the availability of excellent therapeutic measures have rendered hyperuricemia one of the most rationally manageable conditions in medicine. Because of these factors, the treatment of hyperuricemia should be safe, effective, and satisfying for both patient and physician.

GENERAL PRINCIPLES

Hyperuricemia refers to an elevated serum urate concentration. This laboratory finding is present in 2% of adult males in the United States,[1] and 17% in France.[2] The incidence of hyperuricemia was 13.2% in a large series of hospitalized adult male patients.[3] Hyperuricemia does not represent a specific disease, nor is it an indication for therapy. Rather, the finding of hyperuricemia is an indication to determine its origin, and a decision to treat this condition is based on the cause and the consequences in each hyperuricemic patient. Rational management requires that the physician answer the following questions: (1) Is the individual truly hyperuricemic? (2) What is the cause of the hyperuricemia? (3) Should the serum urate concentration be lowered?

DEFINITION OF HYPERURICEMIA (see also Chapter 105)

Hyperuricemia is defined as a serum urate concentration greater than 7.0 mg/dL measured by the specific uricase method. The physicochemical saturation of urate in plasma occurs at this concentration, and in epidemiologic studies of healthy adults not selected for gout or hyperuricemia, 95% of the individuals had serum urate concentrations below this value.[4]

Because the decision to treat hyperuricemia is usually a commitment to therapy for life, it is essential to document that the hyperuricemia is real and sustained. Certainly, the decision should not be based solely on the result of one test. Serum urate concentrations vary with age and sex, fluctuate throughout the day in some individuals, and may be subject to seasonal variation. Other factors, such as recent weight loss, heavy physical exertion, or renal functional impairment, may alter the serum urate concentration. The ingestion of many substances, such as alcohol, diuretics, or salicylates in doses under 2 g/day, may cause hyperuricemia.

WORKUP OF HYPERURICEMIA

The finding of hyperuricemia by itself is not an indication for treatment. The finding of hyperuricemia is, however, an indication to determine its cause. Hyperuricemia may be easily explained and judged clinically insignificant, or it may reflect a serious medical problem. Knowledge of the cause helps one to decide whether and how the condition should be treated. Fortunately, the cause can be easily determined in 70% of patients by means of medical history and physical examination alone.[3]

Traditionally, hyperuricemia has been classified as either primary or secondary. Primary hyperuricemia refers to an elevated serum urate concentration, the cause of which is not understood; or if the cause is known, as for example, hypoxanthine-guanine phosphoribosyltransferase deficiency, hyperuricemia is its first manifestation. Secondary hyperuricemias are those ascribed to some other disorder or therapy in which the basic defect is understood. A more practical classification of hyperuricemia is based on the underlying pathophysiologic features. As reviewed in Chapter 105, hyperuricemia results from urate overproduction, from decreased uric acid excretion, or from a combination of these two mechanisms.

A 24-hour urinary uric acid measurement can be obtained to determine whether hyperuricemia in a given patient is the consequence of overproduction or of decreased excretion.[5] On a purine-free diet, normal men excrete 164 to 588 mg uric acid/day.[6] Hyperuricemic individuals who excrete more than 600 mg uric acid/day while on a purine-free diet are hyperuricemic because of purine overproduction, and those excreting less than 600 mg are most often hyperuricemic because of inadequate excretion. If the assessment is performed while the patient is on a regular diet, then a value of 800 mg/24 hours can be used.

Interpretation of 24-hour urine uric acid excretion requires attention to three factors. First, the foregoing values were determined in subjects with normal renal function. Because impaired renal function decreases the amount of urate filtered in the glomeruli, less uric acid appears in the urine. Consequently, a 24-hour urinary uric acid value of less than 600 mg, or less than 800 mg with regular diet, does not necessarily rule out urate overproduction in a patient with renal failure. On the other hand, elevated values in the presence of renal failure are strong evidence of purine overproduction. Second, it is essential to know the method employed by the laboratory to measure the uric acid in urine. The normal values given previously are for the specific uricase method. If a colorimetric method is employed, then drugs and chromogens normally found in urine can cause spuriously high values. These normal chromogens are increased in patients with renal failure. Fortunately, automated specific enzymatic methods are used in most laboratories today. Third, one must ascertain that the patient is not taking a uricosuric agent at the time of urine collection. Corticosteroids, ascorbic acid, salicylates in doses greater than 2 g/24 hours, and other agents (Table 106–1) promote urate excretion and interfere with the interpretation of results.

It is useful to know whether the hyperuricemia is due to overproduction or to decreased excretion because it narrows the list of conditions that may have caused the hyperuricemia (Table 106–2). If such a factor or disease is identified, the hyperuricemia should be considered secondary, and initial attempts at management should be directed to treating or eliminating the primary cause. In addition, knowing whether hyperuricemia is due to overproduction or to decreased excretion may help in the choice of an antihyperuricemic drug, if one is indicated.

TABLE 106–1. DRUGS WITH URICOSURIC ACTIVITY

Acetohexamide	Glycopyrrolate
Adrenocorticotropic hormone (ACTH) and glucocorticoids	Halofenate
Allopurinol	Irtemazole
Ascorbic acid	Meclofenamate
Azauridine	Merbarone
Benzbromarone	Phenylbutazone
Calcitonin	Phenolsulfonphathalein
Chlorprothixene	Probenecid
Citrate	Salicylates
Dicumarol	Sulfinpyrazone
Diflunisal	Roentgenographic contrast agents
Estrogens	Zoxazolamine
Glyceryl guaiacolate	

TREATMENT

Today, there is hardly any indication that specific urate-lowering drugs should be used to treat asymptomatic hyperuricemia. If the serum urate concentration can be lowered by treating an underlying disease or by removing a causal factor, however, such steps should be taken. Exactly when hyperuricemia should be treated in symptomatic patients remains the subject of much debate. Clearly, antihyperuricemic therapy is indicated in patients who suffer from frequent attacks of acute gouty arthritis or tophi. The use of specific urate-lowering drugs to treat hyperuricemia in patients who have had only a single episode of gouty arthritis is controversial.

Treatment with antihyperuricemic medicines is costly, inconvenient, and potentially toxic. Moreover, because these drugs are prescribed for life, they should not be used without definite indication. The decision to treat should be based on the needs of each patient, with the potential benefit-to-risk ratio weighed individually.*

COMPLICATIONS OF ASYMPTOMATIC HYPERURICEMIA

Hyperuricemia can lead to gouty arthritis and renal disorders and was considered to be a risk factor for coronary artery disease in the past. Because of the fear of these consequences, for many years specific urate-lowering drugs were prescribed for the treatment of asymptomatic hyperuricemic individuals. Obviously, if evidence existed that maintaining serum urate concentrations within normal limits prevented renal failure or heart disease, there would be no debate over the treatment of this condition. Little data exist concerning the benefits of treating asymptomatic hyperuricema, however, and such treatment is no longer recommended, except in rare circumstances. The rationale for this position is provided by considering the complications of hyperuricemia that could develop if therapy is withheld.

GOUT

The risk of gouty arthritis rises both with increasing severity of hyperuricemia and with age.[1,7] In most cases, gout develops only after 20 or more years of sus-

* *Editor's note.* A mistake made in the treatment of a chronic disease is a chronic mistake.

TABLE 106–2. CLASSIFICATION OF HYPERURICEMIA (SEE ALSO TABLE 106–1)

	PRIMARY CAUSES	SECONDARY CAUSES

Overproduction
(24-hour urinary uric acid concentration greater than 600 mg on purine-restricted diet; 800 mg on unrestricted diet)
	Idiopathic
	Hypoxanthine-guanine phosphoribosyltransferase deficiency
	Increased phosphoribosylpyrophosphate synthetase activity
		Hemolytic process
		Myeloproliferative disease
		Lymphoproliferative disorder
		Psoriasis
		Paget's disease
		Exercise
		Glucose-6-phosphatase deficiency
		Glycogen storage disease types III, V, VII
		Artifactual
		  Nonspecific method to measure uric acid
		  Patient taking uricosuric agent

Underexcretion
(24-hour urinary uric acid concentration less than 600 mg on purine-restricted diet; 800 mg on unrestricted diet)
	Idiopathic	Renal insufficiency
		Hypertension
		Acidosis
		Drug ingestion
		  Salicylates (<2 g/24 hr)
		  Diuretics
		  Alcohol
		  Cyclosporine
		  Levodopa
		  Phenylbutazone (<200 mg/24 hr)
		  Ethambutol
		  Pyrazinamide
		  Nicotinic acid
		  Nitroglycerin (intravenous)
		Sarcoidosis
		Lead intoxication
		Berylliosis

tained hyperuricemia. Although certain individuals may be at high risk for developing gouty arthritis, treatment of asymptomatic hyperuricemia simply to prevent the first episode of acute gouty arthritis is not indicated. No evidence indicates that structural kidney damage occurs before the first attach of gouty arthritis,[8] nor are tophi identifiable prior to that occurrence. Moreover, first attacks of gout are easily treated. It is best to withhold antihyperuricemic therapy until arthritis becomes manifest and the diagnosis is confirmed; this form of therapy is long term, and the drugs used are potentially toxic. The cost of the medication and the generally poor compliance in the treatment of asymptomatic problems both reinforce this position.[9]

RENAL DISEASE

Chronic renal disease is an important potential consequence of hyperuricemia. Hyperuricemia can affect the kidneys in three ways (see Chapter 105): (1) urate nephropathy, e.g., deposition of sodium urate crystals in the medullary interstitium and pyramids associated with a giant-cell inflammatory response; (2) nephrolithiasis; and (3) uric acid nephropathy, a reversible form of acute renal failure caused by the precipitation of uric acid crystals in the tubules, collecting ducts, pelvis, and ureters, and obstructing the flow of urine.

The risk of renal failure from hyperuricemia alone is low. One study of 113 patients with asymptomatic hyperuricemia and of 193 normouricemic control subjects followed for 8 years found that azotemia, defined as a serum creatinine greater than 1.6 mg/100 mL in males and 1.3 mg/100 mL in females, occurred in 1.8 and 2.1%, respectively.[10] Urate nephropathy leading to renal failure is difficult to document and is rarely encountered.[11] Thus, azotemia attributable to hyperuricemia alone is infrequent, mild, and probably of little clinical significance.

Even in patients with gout, strong evidence indicates that hyperuricemia alone is rarely damaging to renal function.[12] Long-term followup of renal clearance in 149 gouty patients suggested that various, independently coexisting diseases with associated nephropathy have the most significant impact on renal function, with aging itself a second important factor.[13] Studies of renal hemodynamics in 624 gouty patients confirmed that hyperuricemia alone did not adversely affect renal function. Associated cardiovascular disease, especially hypertension, independently occurring intrinsic renal disease, and aging did correlate with decreased renal function, however. Reduced inulin clearance was attributed to hyperuricemia only in patients with extensive tophaceous deposits, and even in this group, renal dysfunction was greater in patients with associated hypertensive vascular disease.[14]

The relationship between hyperuricemia and nephrolithiasis is complex.[15] Renal stones are 1000 times more prevalent in patients with primary gout than in the general population, but uric acid nephrolithiasis occurs in patients without manifestations of gout, only 20% of whom are hyperuricemic.[16,17] Moreover, some nongouty patients with calcium oxalate stones also have hyperuricosuria.[18,19]

In gouty patients, the risk of nephrolithiasis is related to the magnitude of the urinary uric acid excretion and, to a lesser degree, to the extent of serum urate elevation.[20] Such data are not available for individuals with asymptomatic hyperuricemia, but the risk of nephrolithiasis in such patients was assessed in one study. The rate of stone formation was 2.8 times higher in asymptomatic hyperuricemic individuals than in normouricemic control subjects; 1 stone per 295 asymptomatic hyperuricemic patients per year, as opposed to 1 stone per 825 control subjects per year.[10] This risk is sufficiently low to justify withholding therapy until the occurrence of the first stone.

Acute uric acid nephropathy is rare and occurs almost exclusively in patients receiving chemotherapy for hematologic malignancies. It is of little or no concern in the context of asymptomatic hyperuricemia, and its treatment is discussed later in this chapter.

CARDIOVASCULAR DISEASE

Hyperuricemia is associated with excess mortality from all causes as well as cardiovascular disease.[21] However, hyperuricemia itself cannot be labeled a direct risk factor for cardiovascular disease;[22,23] and it is best considered an indicator. In patients with essential hypertension, hyperuricemia most likely reflects early renal vascular involvement (nephrosclerosis),[24] and persistence of hyperuricemia following myocardial infarction is a sign of a poor prognosis.[25] No evidence indicates that lowering the serum urate concentration in either an asymptomatic hyperuricemic person or a patient with gout prevents cardiac disease.

In conclusion, little indication exists to screen asymptomatic individuals for hyperuricemia, and such screening is not recommended.[26] If hyperuricemia is encountered, however, its cause should be determined. The available data suggest that (1) renal function is not adversely affected by elevated serum urate concentrations; (2) renal disease accompanying hyperuricemia is often related to poorly controlled hypertension; (3) correction of hyperuricemia has no apparent effect on renal function; and (4) hyperuricemia is not an independent risk factor for coronary artery disease. For these reasons and because of the inconvenience, cost, and potential toxicity of antihyperuricemic drugs, it is reasonable not to treat, but merely to observe, patients with asymptomatic hyperuricemia, regardless of the serum urate level. Correction of causal factors, if the condition is secondary, and control of associated problems such as obesity, hypercholesterolemia, diabetes, and particularly hypertension are definitely indicated.

SYMPTOMATIC HYPERURICEMIA

GOUT

The most common indication for lowering the serum urate concentration is articular gout. Because treatment is costly, long-term, and potentially toxic, and because the differential diagnosis of acute monoarticular arthritis is extensive, accurate diagnosis must precede therapy. The finding of negatively birefringent crystals in polymorphonuclear leukocytes in synovial fluid or in subcutaneous tophi by compensated polarized light microscopy is definitive. The triad of acute monoarticular arthritis, hyperuricemia, and a dramatic response to colchicine is presumptive evidence of gouty arthritis in the absence of crystal identification. Criteria defining a colchicine "response" have been established as major subsidence of objective joint inflammatory changes within 48 hours of colchicine therapy and no recrudescence of inflammatory joint manifestations within 7 days.[27] Nevertheless, one should perform joint aspiration to search for crystals whenever possible until the diagnosis is proved.

Much debate exists concerning the appropriate moment to begin antihyperuricemic therapy in the course of gout. All authors agree that hyperuricemia should be treated in patients with recurrent attacks of gout, tophi, classic radiographic changes (bone tophi), or gout combined with nephrolithiasis:[28] Some maintain that the first attack of acute gouty arthritis is sufficient indication to initiate therapy. Others argue that first attacks are easily, inexpensively, and effectively treated, and these physicians postpone urate-lowering therapy. Some individuals experience only a single gouty episode and may not have another for up to 42 years (mean 11.4 years).[29] In the Framingham study, 25% of the patients with acute gouty arthritis had only a single attack in 12 years of observation.[1]

A gouty patient should be educated about the disease and the logic and risks of therapy. Weight control is recommended for obese patients, and meticulous attention should be given to blood pressure control. A 24-hour urinary uric acid measurement helps determine the cause of the hyperuricemia and aids in selecting the most appropriate urate-lowering agent.[5,30] This measurement also influences the decision of whether to start antihyperuricemic therapy after a first gouty attack because the prevalence of renal stones in gouty subjects correlates with the amount of urinary uric acid. One study reported that 35% of patients excreting 700 to 900 mg uric acid/24 hours had nephrolithiasis; 50% of patients excreting more than 1100 mg/24 hours had renal stones.[20]

If urate-lowering therapy is withheld from the patient with gout, a definite risk of destruction to bone and cartilage exists from the sustained hyperuricemia. All patients with gout have deposits of monosodium urate in their tissues. If hyperuricemia is not controlled, these deposits enlarge and are radiographically evident before subcutaneous tophi are found. In a study of patients with intercritical gout, 42% without subcutaneous tophi had radiographic changes characteristic of bony tophi.[31] One could not predict from the frequency of acute attacks, the history of therapy, or the serum urate levels at the time of evaluation which patient would show bony changes. Thus, if urate-lowering therapy is withheld from patients with gout, radiographic assessment is useful in defining the severity of the disease and in providing useful information concerning the advisability of treatment.[32] Furthermore, colchicine should not be given for prophylaxis if urate-lowering therapy is not employed. Such therapy would prevent acute attacks but would not alter the deposition of crystals, and, therefore, tissue damage would proceed without the usual clinical signs.

Before giving specific antihyperuricemic agents, the following criteria apply: (1) all signs of acute inflammation should be absent; (2) the patient should be counseled regarding factors capable of precipitating an acute attack and its prevention; (3) treatment with prophylactic colchicine should be started; (4) the patient should be advised that additional episodes of gouty arthritis are possible; and (5) he should be provided with anti-inflammatory medication with instructions concerning dosage, should such an episode occur.

The goal of antihyperuricemic therapy is the reduction of the total body urate pool. The serum urate concentration, which reflects this pool, is lowered with either a uricosuric agent or a xanthine oxidase inhibitor. Because any sudden increase or decrease in the serum urate concentration can prolong or trigger an acute attack, such therapy should be withheld until all signs of inflammation have resolved completely. Low doses of colchicine, 0.6 mg 1 to 3 times/day, are successful in preventing acute gouty attacks.[33] Prophylactic colchicine is most effective if started at least a week before the first dose of the urate-lowering agent is given and if continued until the serum urate concentration has been under control and the patient has been free of acute gouty attacks for 3 to 6 months. The use of prophylactic colchicine is generally well-tolerated and safe. Only an occasional patient will experience gastrointestinal side effects at these dosages. Neuromuscular toxicity may occur but is rare. This manifests as a subacute myopathy with associated axonal neuropathy and elevated serum creatine kinase levels, usually occurs in individuals with renal insufficiency, and is reversible within 3 to 4 weeks after the drug is discontinued.[34]

Antihyperuricemic therapy, regardless of the agent employed, should be entirely successful, but it can succeed only if the dosage is adequate. Dosage is adequate when it is sufficient to maintain the serum urate concentration below 5.0 mg/dL. Extracellular fluid is saturated with urate at a concentration of approximately 6.4 mg/dL, and if the serum urate concentration remains above this level, tissue deposition of urate crystals will continue. A reduction of the serum urate concentration from 9.5 to 8.0 mg/dL, for example, will not reduce the total body urate pool but will only retard the rate at which it increases.

Lack of compliance is almost certainly the reason for poor control of symptoms after 6 to 12 months of therapy. Supportive evidence for this assumption is provided by results of a randomized study that compared continuous versus intermittent therapy with allopurinol. Intermittent administration was clearly less effective in controlling symptoms of gout.[35] Poor compliance may result from the difficulty many patients have taking medications for asymptomatic conditions[9] or may relate to alcohol use.[36] In a study of 38 patients on long-term allopurinol therapy, recurrent gout attacks continued in 20 of 21 heavy drinkers but in less than one third of those who consumed moderate amounts or no alcohol. Although the effects of alcohol on purine metabolism and uric acid excretion can be implicated,[37] it is more likely that poor compliance with treatment was the major contributing factor.

In general, patients should continue to take the prescribed antihyperuricemic agent indefinitely once treatment is initiated. It may be possible, however, to discontinue these agents eventually, presumably after the total body urate pool has been sufficiently reduced. Unfortunately it is very difficult to determine when this has been achieved, and data on the subject are quite limited. Allopurinol therapy was discontinued in one group of 33 patients after a mean of 93 weeks of treatment. Although serum urate levels rose to pretreatment levels within 1 week of discontinuing the medication, recurrent gouty attacks developed in only 12 patients after up to 210 weeks of followup.[38]

Results appear more favorable if the duration of treatment is longer. In one report 10 patients with tophaceous gout treated for a mean of 7.2 years had no problems for at least 33 months after discontinuing allopurinol.[39] No recurrence of gouty attacks was noted in five patients followed for 5 years after discontinuing allopurinol after a mean treatment interval of 12 years.[40] Radiographic progression did occur in one of those patients, however. Until more data are available, it is still recommended that once initiated, antihyperuricemic therapy be continued indefinitely.

NEPHROLITHIASIS

Medical prophylaxis of either uric acid or calcium stones in hyperuricemic patients is effective. Both types of stones occur in association with hyperuricosuria. The chemical composition of the stone should be identified whenever possible. Regardless of the nature of the calculi, patients should dilute their urine by ingesting fluid sufficient to produce a daily urine volume greater than 2 L. Alkalinization of the urine with sodium bicarbonate or acetazolamide may be justified for patients with uric acid stones because this process increases the solubility of uric acid. At pH 5.0, urine is saturated at a uric acid concentration of 15 mg/dL; at pH 7.0, saturation occurs with 200 mg/dL.[8]

Specific treatment of uric acid calculi is achieved by reducing urinary uric acid concentration with allopurinol, an inhibitor of xanthine oxidase. Allopurinol is also useful in reducing the recurrence of calcium oxalate stones in gouty subjects and in nongouty individuals with hyperuricemia or hyperuricosuria because uric acid may nucleate calcium stones.[19,41] Potassium citrate (30 to 80 mEq/day orally in divided doses) has been used successfully and can provide an alternative to allopurinol therapy for patients with uric acid stones alone or coexistent with calcium stones.[42]

URIC ACID NEPHROPATHY

This reversible form of acute renal failure is a result of the precipitation of uric acid in renal tubules and collecting ducts resulting in obstruction.[43] Uric acid nephropathy may follow sudden urate overproduction with marked hyperuricosuria, dehydration, and acidosis. Autopsy studies have demonstrated intraluminal uric acid precipitates accompanied by dilated proximal tubules and normal glomeruli. Work in animals suggests that the primary early pathogenetic events include obstruction of the collecting ducts by un-ionized uric acid and obstruction of the distal renal vasculature. This form of acute renal failure develops most often in patients undergoing an aggressive or "blastic" phase of leukemia or lymphoma prior to or during cytotoxic therapy, but it has also been observed in patients with disseminated adenocarcinoma, after vigorous exercise with heat stress, following epileptic seizures, and after corticosteroid therapy for anaphylaxis.[44]

Uric acid nephropathy is important because it is often preventable and because immediate, appropriate therapy reduces the mortality rates associated with this condition from 47% to practically nil. In addition to hyperuricemia, ranging from 12 to 80 mg/dL,[45] and oliguria, the distinctive clinical finding is probably the urinary uric acid concentration. In most forms of acute renal failure with decreased urine output, uric acid excretion is normal or reduced, and the ratio of uric acid to creatinine is less than 1.0. A ratio of uric acid to creatinine greater than 1 in a random urine sample or in a 24-hour specimen may be diagnostic of uric acid nephropathy.[46]

Factors that favor uric acid precipitation should be reversed, and uric acid production should be blocked. Vigorous hydration by the intravenous route and furosemide administration are used to promote urine flow to 100 mL/hour or more. Acetazolamide, 240 to 500 mg every 6 to 8 hours, and sodium bicarbonate, 89 mEq/L, given intravenously, maximize the likelihood of achieving an alkaline urine.[47] It is important to monitor the patient's urine frequently to ensure that the pH remains above 7.0 and to watch for signs of circulatory overload.

In addition, antihyperuricemia therapy is administered to reduce the amount of urate that reaches the kidney. Allopurinol, which inhibits the production of urate and thereby decreases the concentration of urinary uric acid, is given in a single dose of 8 mg/kg. If renal insufficiency persists, subsequent daily doses should be reduced to 100 to 200 mg because oxipurinol, the active metabolite of allopurinol, is retained in this setting[48] (see the section on allopurinol in this chapter). Limited experience with urate oxidase, the enzyme that degrades uric acid to allantoin, has been reported.[49] Despite these measures, dialysis may be required. Hemodialysis should be employed because it is 10 to 20 times more effective than peritoneal dialysis in removing uric acid.[45]

THERAPEUTIC TECHNIQUES

DIET

Dietary considerations now play a minor role in the treatment of hyperuricemia, despite a fascinating history and abundant literature on the subject.[50] Strict restriction of purine intake reduces the mean serum urate concentration by only 1.0 mg/dL and urinary uric acid excretion by 200 to 400 mg/day.[51] Fortunately, modern therapeutic agents render attention to dietary purines rarely necessary.

Dietary counseling is important, however, and it should address the use of alcohol and associated medical problems such as obesity, hyperlipidemia, diabetes, or hypertension. Heavy alcohol consumption should be discouraged. An episode of excessive alcohol ingestion can cause temporary hyperlacticacidemia, elevate the serum urate concentration, and provoke an attack of gouty arthritis.[52] Long-term alcohol use increases uric acid production, hyperuricemia, and hyperuricosuria.[37,53]

URICOSURIC AGENTS

Candidates for uricosuric agents are gouty patients who meet all the following criteria: (1) hyperuricemia attributable to decreased uric acid excretion (less than 800 mg uric acid/24-hour urine specimen while the patient is on a regular diet; or less than 600 mg on a purine-restricted diet); (2) age under 60 years; (3) satisfactory renal function (a creatinine clearance greater than 80 mL/min is ideal, but it should be at least 50 mL/min); and (4) no history of nephrolithiasis.

Uricosuric agents reduce the serum urate concentration by enhancing the renal excretion of uric acid. This process occurs by the partial inhibition of proximal tubular reabsorption of filtered and secreted urate from the luminal side of the tubule at a site distal to the point of uric acid secretion.[54] If employed at a dosage sufficient to maintain the serum urate concentration at around 5.0 mg/100 mL, which is well below the level at which urate is saturated in extracellular fluid, these agents not only prevent urate deposition, but also allow dissolution of existing tophi.[55]

During the initial treatment period, the patient has a negative urate balance, and urinary uric acid excretion is elevated above pretreatment levels. Once the excess urate has been mobilized and excreted, urinary uric acid values return to original levels. At this point, the patient excretes uric acid at the pretreatment rate, but at a lower serum urate concentration.[56] Early in the course of treatment, before a steady state is re-established, how-

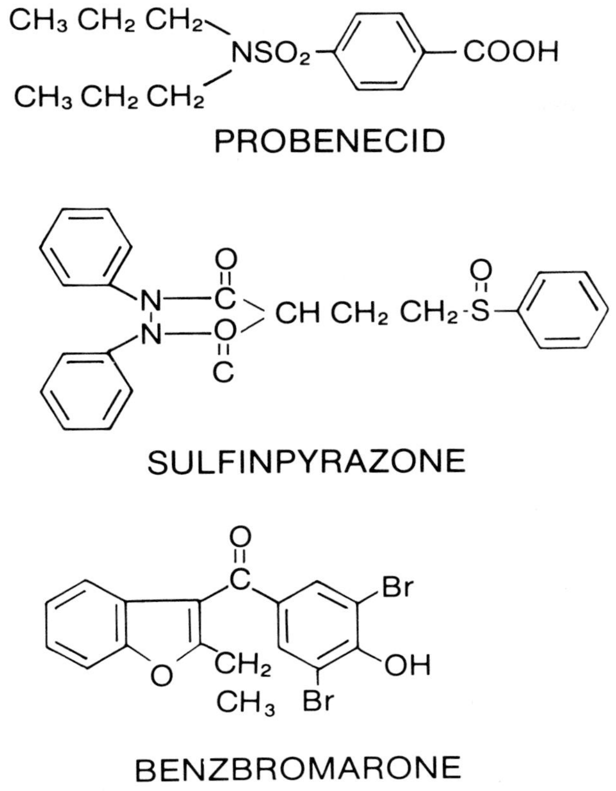

FIGURE 106–1. Structures of uricosuric agents effective in the treatment of hyperuricemia.

ever, the risk of developing renal calculi is as high as 9%.[55]

Uricosuric agents may be effective in 70 to 80% of patients. In addition to drug intolerance, failure to control a serum urate concentration can be attributed to poor compliance, concomitant salicylate ingestion, or impaired renal function. Salicylates block the uricosuric effects of these agents, possibly by inhibiting urate secretion.[57] These agents lose effectiveness as the creatinine clearance falls, and they are completely ineffective when glomerular filtration reaches 30 mL/min.[58]

Figure 106–1 illustrates the chemical structures of the three uricosuric agents discussed in the following paragraphs.

Probenecid

The "era of hypouricemic therapy" began in 1949 with the introduction of probenecid and the observations that sustained use of this agent controlled hyperuricemia, could mobilize tophi, and was well tolerated.[55,59] Probenecid is readily absorbed in the gastrointestinal tract. Its half-life ranges from 6 to 12 hours, is dose dependent[60] and is prolonged by allopurinol.[61] This drug is extensively bound to plasma proteins, is largely confined to extracellular fluid, and is rapidly metabolized, with less than 5% of the administered dose recoverable in the urine in 24 hours.[55,61] Probenecid increases the half-life of penicillin, ampicillin, dapsone, acetazolamide, indomethacin, and sulfinpyrazone by decreasing renal excretion, of rifampin by impairing hepatic uptake, and of heparin by retarding its metabolism.[62]

Therapy is begun at 250 mg twice a day and is increased as necessary up to 3.0 g/day. A dose of 1 g/day is appropriate for about 50% of patients.[55] Because the half-life is 6 to 12 hours, probenecid should be taken in two to three evenly spaced doses.

The potential complications of probenecid most likely to occur early in the course of therapy include precipitation of acute gouty arthritis and nephrolithiasis. Gouty arthritis is prevented by the use of prophylactic colchicine. Nephrolithiasis is prevented by starting therapy at low doses and by increasing the dose at a rate of 0.5 g every 1 to 2 weeks, by liberally ingesting fluids, and possibly by alkalinizing the urine. Hypersensitivity, skin rash, and gastrointestinal complaints are the major side effects. Serious toxicity is rare, but hepatic necrosis[63] and the nephrotic syndrome have been reported.[64,65]

Sulfinpyrazone

This analogue of a uricosuric metabolite of phenylbutazone possesses no anti-inflammatory activity and is a potent uricosuric agent. It is well absorbed through the gastrointestinal tract, with peak serum levels observed within an hour. The half-life of this agent is 1 to 3 hours.[66] Sulfinpyrazone is 98% bound to plasma proteins and is largely distributed in extracellular fluids. Although 20 to 45% of this drug is excreted unchanged in the urine, the majority is excreted as the parahydroxyl metabolite, which is also uricosuric.[67] In addition to the uricosuric properties, sulfinpyrazone has antiplatelet activity, mediated by thromboxane synthesis inhibition, rather than by its urate-lowering effect.[68]

Sulfinpyrazone therapy is initiated at a dose of 50 mg twice a day. The usual maintenance level is 300 to 400 mg/day in 3 or 4 divided doses, but 800 mg/day may be required for satisfactory results.

Sulfinpyrazone has side effects similar to those of probenecid, and the drug is generally well tolerated. Bone marrow suppression can occur but is rare.[69] Because of the rapid absorption and extreme potency of this drug, renal calculi are potentially more common early in the course of its use than with probenecid.

Benzbromarone

Benzbromarone is a halogenated uricosuric agent currently available outside the United States. This agent is debrominated in the liver and is excreted free or in the conjugated form primarily in the bile. Although a weak inhibitor of xanthine oxidase activity in vitro, the drug acts in vivo by inhibiting the tubular reabsorption of uric acid.[70]

Benzbromarone is effective and is well tolerated at daily doses of 25 to 120 mg.[71] This agent has been effective in patients with serum creatinine concentrations greater than 2.0 mg/dL and therefore my be useful for patients with renal insufficiency.[72]

INHIBITORS OF URIC ACID SYNTHESIS

Another approach for controlling the patient's serum urate concentration is the use of agents that decrease uric acid formation. Such agents are effective in the treatment of all types of hyperuricemia but are specifically indicated for the following: (1) patients with gout and (a) evidence of urate overproduction (24-hour urinary uric acid greater than 800 mg on a general diet; 600 mg on a purine-restricted diet); (b) nephrolithiasis; (c) renal insufficiency (creatinine clearance less than 80 mL/min); (d) tophaceous deposits; (e) age over 60 years; or (f) inability to take uricosuric agents because of ineffectiveness or intolerance; (2) patients with nephrolithiasis of any type and urinary uric acid excretion greater than 600 mg/24 hours; (3) patients with renal calculi composed of 2,8-dihydroxy-adenine; and (4) patients with, or at risk for, acute uric acid nephropathy.

The most widely used compound in this group is allopurinol, which inhibits xanthine oxidase. Oxipurinol, the major metabolite of allopurinol, is available outside the United States. Although useful in some patients who are sensitive to allopurinol,[73,74] the clinical utility of this drug is limited by its poor absorption from the gastrointestinal tract.[75] Thiopurinol, which probably inhibits de novo purine synthesis,[76] has had limited clinical use.

Allopurinol

This analogue of hypoxanthine originally synthesized to be an antitumor agent is a potent competitive inhibitor of xanthine oxidase.[77] It is also a substrate for the enzyme.[78] Oxypurinol, an analogue of xanthine, is the major metabolite of allopurinol and also effectively inhibits xanthine oxidase[79] (Fig. 106–2).

Allopurinol is completely absorbed from the gastrointestinal tract and has a half-life of 3 hours or less. Most oxypurinol formed is excreted unchanged in the urine and has a half-life of 14 to 28 hours.[80] Oxypurinol excretion is enhanced by uricosuric agents and is reduced by renal insufficiency.[81,82]

By inhibiting xanthine oxidase, these compounds block the conversion of hypoxanthine to xanthine and of xanthine to uric acid. The administration of allopurinol leads to decreases in serum urate concentration and in the urinary excretion of uric acid in the first 24 hours, and a maximum reduction occurs within 4 days to 2 weeks.[83] This change is accompanied by excretion of increased quantities of hypoxanthine and xanthine, which are the more readily excreted.[84] Total purine excretion declines by 10 to 60% of pretreatment levels when allopurinol is taken.[75,84] This decline results from increased salvage of hypoxanthine to inosine 5′-monophosphate and from the concomitant reduction in the rate of de novo purine biosynthesis, the metabolic consequences of allopurinol conversion to allopurinol ribonucleotides[85] (Fig. 106–3). Allopurinol is also a potent inhibitor of de novo pyrimidine biosynthesis,[86] but the significance of this observation is uncertain.

Between 100 and 800 mg/day allopurinol is required to control the serum urate concentration adequately, and the dose for a specific patient depends on the severity of the tophaceous disease and on renal function. The average effective dose for most individuals is 300 mg/day.[87] The failure of a 400-mg dose to produce an adequate antihyperuricemic effect is rare and should cause one to question the patient's compliance. Allopurinol is effective in patients with renal insufficiency,[48] but the dose should be reduced because of the prolonged half-life of oxypurinol.[82] Therapy may be initiated at a low dose and may gradually be increased to minimize precipitation of acute gouty attacks or to find the lowest effective dose, but this regimen is not necessary for most patients. Because of the long half-life of oxypurinol, allopurinol need be taken only once a day.

Allopurinol is clinically effective. Resolution of tophi is generally obvious, the frequency of gouty attacks is reduced, and the patient's functional status improves when the serum urate concentration has been controlled for 6 to 12 months.

Side effects, serious complications, and toxicity of allopurinol are unusual. Prophylactic colchicine is 85% effective in preventing episodes of acute arthritis that might be triggered by a sudden fall in serum urate concentration induced by allopurinol.[33] Because of the increased concentrations of oxypurines in the urine, xanthine renal calculi are possible. This complication is exceedingly uncommon, having been reported only in

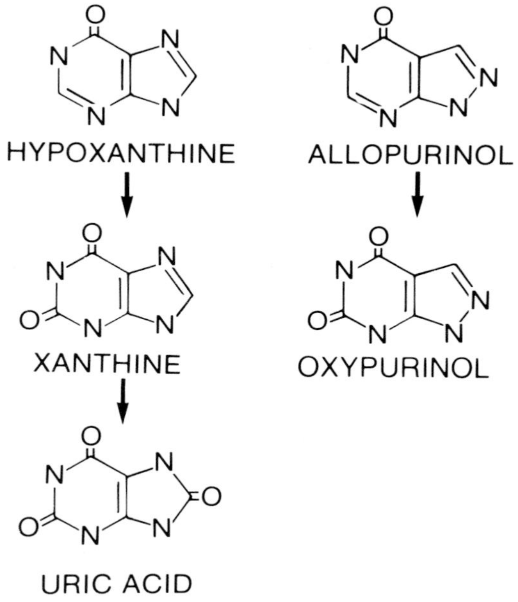

FIGURE 106–2. Xanthine oxidase catalyzes the conversion of hypoxanthine to xanthine, of xanthine to uric acid, and of allopurinol to oxypurinol. Note the structural similarity of hypoxanthine to allopurinol and of xanthine to oxypurinol.

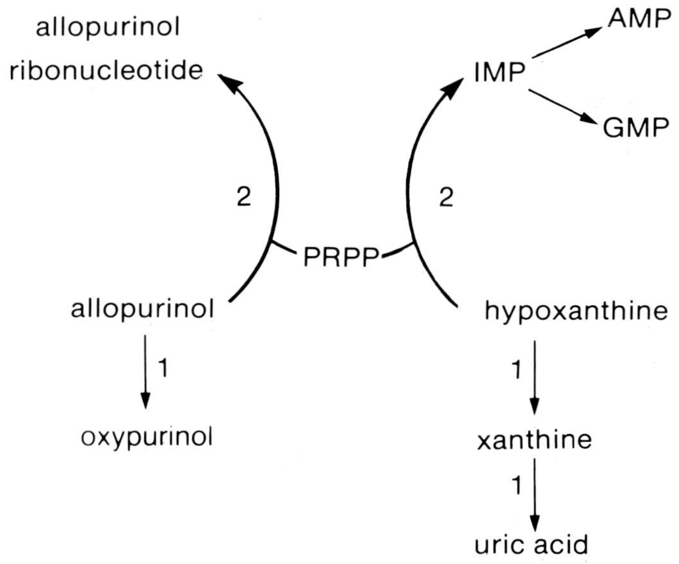

FIGURE 106–3. Abbreviated scheme of allopurinol and hypoxanthine metabolism. The inhibition of xanthine oxidase (enzyme 1) by allopurinol and oxypurinol lowers uric acid formation by blocking the conversion of hypoxanthine to xanthine and xanthine to uric acid. Xanthine oxidase inhibition also results in the accumulation of hypoxanthine and allopurinol, which are converted to their respective ribonucleotide monophosphates by the action of hypoxanthine-guanine phosphoribosyltransferase (HGPRTase, enzyme 2). The formation of these ribonucleotides further decreases uric acid production by diminishing de novo purine biosynthesis by three mechanisms: (1) inhibition of amidophosphoribosyltransferase activity by allopurinol ribonucleotide; (2) inhibition of both amidophosphoribosyltransferase and phosphopyrophosphate (PRPP) synthetase activity by inosine 5′-monophosphate (IMP), adenosine 5′-monophosphate (AMP), and guanosine 5′-monophosphate (GMP); and (3) depletion of phosphoribosylpyrophosphate. PRPP is not only a substrate for HGPRTase but also is an essential and rate-limiting substrate for de novo purine synthesis.

rare patients with Lesch-Nyhan syndrome,[88] lymphosarcoma,[89] and Burkitt's lymphoma.[90] Microcrystalline deposits of oxypurinol, as well as of hypoxanthine and xanthine, have been demonstrated in muscle biopsy specimens from gouty patients taking allopurinol.[91] No clinical sequelae are known to result from that deposition, however.

The overall incidence of side effects from allopurinol is 5 to 20%, but only half the affected patients consider these effects sufficient to warrant discontinuing the medication.[61,92] the most frequent side effects include skin rash, gastrointestinal distress, diarrhea, and headache.[93] The most common rash is a maculopapular erythema, but exfoliative dermatitis and toxic epidermal necrolysis have been reported.[94,95] A mild rash is not a contraindication for further use of allopurinol. The drug should be stopped, but it may be reinstituted once the rash has cleared. Desensitization with low doses may be required in some individuals.[96,97]

More serious adverse effects include alopecia, fever, lymphadenopathy, bone marrow suppression,[98] hepatic toxicity,[99] interstitial nephritis,[100] renal failure, hypersensitivity vasculitis, and death.[101,102] Some data also suggest that allopurinol may cause or may worsen existing cataracts.[103,104] Serious toxicity is fortunately rare, but it is most often seen in patients with renal insufficiency or in those taking thiazide diuretics.[82,101] Unfortunately, the majority of serious reactions and deaths have occurred in patients whose medical problems did not require allopurinol in the first place.[105]

Potentially important drug interactions must be considered when allopurinol is prescribed. Because 6-mercaptopurine and azathioprine are inactivated by xanthine oxidase, allopurinol prolongs the half-life of these agents and thus potentiates their therapeutic and toxic effects.[106] Cyclophosphamide toxicity may be enhanced,[107] and a threefold increase in the incidence of ampicillin- and amoxicillin-related skin rashes has been reported in patients taking allopurinol.[108] On the other hand, allopurinol can reduce the toxicity of 5-fluorouracil.[109]

Allopurinol and a uricosuric agent may be used simultaneously in the rare patient whose hyperuricemia cannot be controlled by a single medication.[110] Although uricosuric agents increase the urinary excretion of oxypurinol,[81] this effect is balanced because allopurinol increases the half-life of probenecid by inhibiting microsomal drug-metabolizing enzymes.[61] Clinically, the drugs can be used in combination without modifying the dosage schedule of either agent. The addition of a uricosuric drug to a therapeutic program including allopurinol usually increases the patient's urinary uric acid excretion and further lowers the serum urate concentration.

The use of allopurinol in acute uric acid nephropathy and in the hyperuricemic individual with nephrolithiasis has been discussed in previous sections. One additional indication for the use of this agent is in the treatment of 2,8-dihydroxyadenine kidney stones. Individuals with this condition have a homozygous deficiency of adenine phosphoribosyltransferase,[111] an enzyme that catalyzes the conversion of adenine to adenosine 5′-monophosphate. In the absence of this activity, adenine is converted by xanthine oxidase to the insoluble 2,8-dihydroxyadenine, which is excreted in the urine. Reports of 2,8-dihydroxyadenine stones are rare, most likely because of the chemical similarity between this compound and uric acid. X-ray powder diffraction analysis is necessary for correct identification. Stones of this type, however, may be more common than previously thought because the prevalence of the heterozygous state for this enzyme deficiency in the general population may be as high as 1%.[112]

REFERENCES

1. Hall, A.P. et al.: Epidemiology of gout and hyperuricemia: a long term population study. Am. J. Med., *42*:27–37, 1967.
2. Zalokar, J. et al.: Serum uric acid in 23,923 men and gout in a subsample of 4,257 men in France. J. Chronic Dis., *25*:305–312, 1972.
3. Paulus, H.E. et al.: Clinical significance of hyperuricemia in routinely screened hospitalized men. JAMA, *211*:277–281, 1970.
4. Mikkelsen, W.M., Dodge, H.J., and Valkenburg, H.: The distribution of serum uric acid values in a population unselected as to gout or hyperuricemia: Tecumseh, Michigan, 1959–1960. Am. J. Med., *39*:242–251, 1965.
5. Wortmann, R.L., and Fox, I.H.: Limited value of uric acid to creatinine ratios in estimating uric acid excretion. Ann. Intern. Med., *93*:822–825, 1980.
6. Seegmiller, J.E. et al.: Uric acid production in gout. J. Clin. Invest., *40*:1304–1314, 1961.
7. Campion, E.W., Glynn, R.J., and DeLabry, L.O.: Asymptomatic hyperuricemia. Risks and consequences in the normative aging study. Am. J. Med., *82*:421–426, 1987.
8. Klinenberg, J.R., Gonick, H.C., and Dornfield, L.: Renal function abnormalities in patients with asymptomatic hyperuricemia. Arthritis Rheum., *18*(Suppl.):725–730, 1975.
9. Liang, M.H., and Fries, J.F.: Asymptomatic hyperuricemia: The case for conservative management. Ann. Intern. Med., *88*:666–670, 1978.
10. Fessel, W.J.: Renal outcomes of gout and hyperuricemia. Am. J. Med., *67*:74–82, 1979.
11. Beck, L.H.: Requiem for gouty nephropathy. Kidney Int., *30*:280–287, 1986.
12. Yu, T.-F., and Talbott, J.H.: Changing trends of mortality in gout. Semin. Arthritis Rheum., *10*:1–9, 1980.
13. Yu, T.-F. et al.: Renal function in gout. V. Factors influencing the renal hemodynamics. Am. J. Med., *67*:766–771, 1979.
14. Yu, T.-F., and Berger, L.: Impaired renal function in gout: its association with hypertensive vascular disease and intrinsic renal disease. Am. J. Med., *72*:95–100, 1982.
15. Yu, T.-F.: Urolithiasis in hyperuricemia and gout. J. Urol., *126*:424–430, 1981.
16. Armstrong, W.A., and Greene, L.F.: Uric acid calculi with particular reference to determinations of uric acid content of blood. J. Urol., *70*:545–547, 1953.
17. Talbott, J.H.: Gout, New York, Grune & Stratton, 1957, p. 205.
18. Ettinger, B. et al.: Randomized trial of allopurinol in the prevention of calcium oxalate calculi. N. Engl. J. Med., *315*:1386–1389, 1986.
19. Noda, S., Hayashi, K., and Eto, K.: Oxalate crystallization in the kidney in the presence of hyperuricemia. Scanning Microsc., *3*:829–836, 1989.
20. Yu, T.-F., and Gutman, A.B.: Uric acid nephrolithiasis in gout. Predisposing factors. Ann. Intern. Med., *67*:1133–1148, 1967.
21. Levine, W. et al.: Serum uric acid and 1.5 year mortality of middle-aged women of the Chicago Heart Association Detection project in Industry. J. Clin. Epidemiol., *42*:257–267, 1989.
22. Reunanen, A. et al.: Hyperuricemia as a risk factor for cardiovascular mortality. Acta Med. Scand., *668*(Suppl.):49–59, 1982.
23. Fessel, W.J.: High uric acid as an indicator of cardiovascular disease: Independence from obesity. Am. J. Med., *68*:401–404, 1980.
24. Messerli, F.H. et al.: Serum uric acid in essential hypertension: An indicator of renal vascular involvement. Ann. Intern. Med., *93*:817–821, 1980.
25. Woolliscroft, J.O., Colfer, H., and Fox, I.H.: Hyperuricemia in acute illness: A poor prognostic sign. Am. J. Med., *72*:58–62, 1982.
26. Cebul, R.D., and Beck, J.R.: Biochemical profiles. Applications in ambulatory screening and preadmission testing of adults. Ann. Intern. Med., *106*:403–413, 1987.
27. Wallace, S.L., Berstein, D., and Diamond, H.: Diagnostic value of colchicine therapeutic trial. JAMA, *199*:525–528, 1967.
28. Diamond, H.S.: Control of crystal-induced arthropathies. Rheum. Dis. Clin. North Am., *15*:557–567, 1989.
29. Hench, P.S.: The diagnosis of gout and gouty arthritis. J. Lab. Clin. Med., *22*:48–55, 1936.
30. Boss, G.R., and Seegmiller, J.E.: Hyperuricemia and gout: Classification, complications and management. N. Engl. J. Med., *300*:1459–1468, 1979.
31. Nakayama, D.A. et al.: Tophaceous gout: A clinical and radiographic assessment. Arthritis Rheum., *27*:468–471, 1984.
32. Barthelemy, C.R. et al.: Gouty arthritis: A prospective radiographic evaluation of sixty patients. Skeletal Radiol., *11*:1–8, 1984.
33. Yu, T.-F.: The efficacy of colchicine prophylaxis in articular gout—A reappraisal after 20 years. Arthritis Rheum., *12*:256–264, 1982.
34. Kungl, R.W. et al.: Colchicine myopathy and neuropathy. N. Engl. J. Med., *316*:1562–1568, 1987.
35. Bull, P.W., and Scott, T.J.: Intermittent control of hyperuricemia in the treatment of gout. J. Rheumatol., *16*:1246–1248, 1989.
36. Ralston, S.H., Capell, H.A., and Sturrock, R.D.: Alcohol and response to treatment of gout. Br. Med. J., *296*:1641–1642, 1988.
37. Faller, J., and Fox, I.H.: Ethanol-induced hyperuricemia: Evidence for increased urate production and activation of adenine nucleotide turnover. N. Engl. J. Med., *307*:1598–1602, 1982.
38. Loebl, W.Y., and Scott, J.T.: Withdrawal of allopurinol in patients with gout. Ann. Rheum. Dis., *33*:304–307, 1974.
39. Gast, L.F.: Withdrawal of long-term antihyperuricemic therapy in tophaceous gout. Clin. Rheumatol., *6*:70–73, 1987.
40. McCarthy, G.M. et al.: Influence of anti-hyperuricemic therapy on the clinical and radiographic progression of gout. Arthritis Rheum., 34:1991.
41. Pak, C.Y.C. et al.: Is selective therapy of recurrent nephrolithiasis possible? Am. J. Med., *71*:615–622, 1981.
42. Pak, C.Y.C., Sakhaee, K., and Fuller, C.: Successful management of uric acid nephrolithiasis with potassium citrate. Kidney Int., *30*:422–428, 1986.
43. Conger, I.D.: Acute uric acid nephropathy. Med. Clin. North Am., *74*:859–71, 1990.
44. Smith, T.: Tumor lysis syndrome after steroid therapy for arraphylaxis. South. Med. J., *81*:415–416, 1988.
45. Kjellstrand, C.M. et al.: Hyperuricemic acute renal failure. Arch. Intern. Med., *133*:349–359, 1974.
46. Kelton, J., Kelley, W.N., and Holmes, E.W.: A rapid method for the diagnosis of acute uric acid nephropathy. Arch. Intern. Med., *138*:612–615, 1978.
47. Kelley, W.N. et al.: Acetazolamide in phenobarbital intoxication. Arch. Intern. Med., *117*:64–69, 1966.
48. Simmonds, H.A., Cameron, J.S., Morris, G.S., and Davies, P.M.: Allopurinol in renal failure and the tumor lysis syndrome. Clin. Chim. Acta, *160*:189–195, 1986.
49. Chua, C.C. et al.: Use of polyethylene glycol-modified uricase (PEG-uricase) to treat hyperuricemia in a patient with non-Hodgkin lymphoma. Ann. Intern. Med., *109*:114–117, 1988.
50. Talbott, J.H.: Solid and liquid nourishment in gout: selected historical excerpts, largely empiric or fashionable and current scientific(?) concepts in the management of gout and gouty arthritis. Semin. Arthritis Rheum., *11*:288–306, 1981.
51. Gutman, A.B., and Yu, T.-F.: Gout, a derangement of purine metabolism. Adv. Intern. Med., *5*:227–302, 1952.

52. Lieber, C.S. et al.: Interrelations of uric acid and ethanol metabolism in man. J. Clin. Invest., *41*:1863–1870, 1962.
53. MacLachlan, M.J., and Rodnan, G.P.: Effect of food, fast, and alcohol on serum uric acid and acute attacks of gout. Am. J. Med., *42*:38–57, 1967.
54. Levinson, D.J., and Sorensen, L.B.: Renal handling of uric acid in normal and gouty subjects: Evidence for a 4-component system. Ann. Rheum. Dis., *39*:173–179, 1979.
55. Gutman, A.B., and Yu, T.-F.: Protracted uricosuric therapy in tophaceous gout. Lancet, *2*:1258–1260, 1957.
56. Gutman, A.B., and Yu, T.-F.: Benemid (p-[di-n-propylsulfamyl] benzoic acid) as uricosuric agent in chronic gouty arthritis. Trans. Assoc. Am. Physicians. *64*:279–287, 1951.
57. Hansten, P.D.: Drug Interactions. 4th Ed. Philadelphia, Lea & Febiger, 1979, p. 255.
58. Wyngaarden, J.B.: Metabolic and clinical aspects of gout. Am. J. Med., *22*:819–824, 1957.
59. Talbott, J.H., Bishop, C., and Norcross, M.: The clinical and metabolic effects of Benemid in patients with gout. Trans. Assoc. Am. Physicians, *64*:372–377, 1951.
60. Dayton, P.G. et al.: The physiological disposition of probenecid, including renal clearance in man, studied by an improved method for its estimation in biological material. J. Pharmacol. Exp. Ther., *140*:278–286, 1963.
61. Tjandramaga, T.B. et al.: Observations on the disposition of probenecid on patients receiving allopurinol. Pharmacology, *8*:259–272, 1972.
62. Wyngaarden, J.B., and Kelley, W.N.: Gout and Hyperuricemia. New York, Grune & Stratton, 1976, pp. 430–438.
63. Reynolds, E.S. et al.: Fatal massive necrosis of the liver as a manifestation of hypersensitivity to probenecid. N. Engl. J. Med., *256*:592–596, 1957.
64. Ferris, T.F., Morgan, W.S., and Levitin, H.: Nephrotic syndrome caused by probenecid. N. Engl. J. Med., *256*:592–596, 1957.
65. Hertz, P., Yager, H., and Richardson, J.A.: Probenecid induced nephrotic syndrome. Arch. Pathol., *94*:241–243, 1972.
66. Dayton, P.G. et al.: Metabolism of sulfinpyrazone (Anturane) and other thio analogues of phenylbutazone in man. J. Pharmacol. Exp. Ther., *132*:287–290, 1961.
67. Gutman, A.B. et al.: A study of the inverse relationship between pK_a and rate of renal excretion of phenylbutazone analogs in man and dog. Am. J. Med., *29*:1017–1033, 1960.
68. Ali, M., and McDonald, W.D.: Effects of sulfinpyrazone on platelet prostaglandin synthesis and platelet release of serotonin. J. Lab. Clin. Med., *89*:868–875, 1977.
69. Emmerson, B.T.: A comparison of uricosuric agents in gout, with special reference to sulfinpyrazone. Med. J. Aust., *1*:839–844, 1963.
70. Sinclar, D.S., and Fox, I.H.: The pharmacology of hypouricemic effect of benzbromarone. J. Rheumatol., *2*:437–445, 1975.
71. Masbernard, A., and Giudicelli, C.P.: Ten year's experience with benzbromarone in the management of gout and hyperuricemia. S. Afr. Med. J., *59*:701–706, 1981.
72. Zollner, N., Griebsch, A., and Fink, J.K.: Uber die Wirkung von Benzbromarone auf den Serumharnsauerespiegel und die Harnsaureausscheidung des Gichtkranken. Dtsch. Med. Wochenschr., *95*:2405–2411, 1970.
73. Rundles, R.W.: Metabolic effects of allpurinol and alloxanthine. Ann. Rheum. Dis., *25*:615–620, 1966.
74. Lockard, O., Jr. et al.: Allergic reaction to allopurinol with cross-reactivity to oxypurinol. Ann. Intern. Med., *85*:333–335, 1976.
75. Delbarre, F. et al.: Treatment of gout with allopurinol: A study of 106 cases. Ann. Rheum. Dis., *25*:627–633, 1966.
76. Auscher, C. et al.: Allopurinol and thiopurinol: Effect in vivo on urinary oxypurine excretion and rate of synthesis of their ribonucleotides in different enzymatic deficiencies. Adv. Exp. Med. Biol., *41B*:657–662, 1974.
77. Rundles, R.W.: The development of allopurinol. Arch. Int. Med., *145*:1492–1503, 1985.
78. Feigelson, P., Davidson, J.K., and Robins, P.K. Pyrazolopyrimidines as inhibitors and substrates of xanthine oxidase. J. Biol. Chem., *226*:993–1000, 1957.
79. Massey, V., Komai, H., and Palmer, G.: On the mechanism of inactivation of xanthine oxidase by allopurinol and other pyrazolo(3,4-d)pyrimidines. J. Biol. Chem., *245*:2837–2844, 1970.
80. Hande, K., Reed, E., and Chabner, B.: Allopurinol kinetics. Clin. Pharmacol. Ther., *23*:598–605, 1978.
81. Elion, G.B. et al.: Renal clearance of oxypurinol, the chief metabolite of allopurinol. Am. J. Med., *45*:69–77, 1968.
82. Hande, K.R., Noone, R.M., and Stone, W.J.: Severe allopurinol toxicity. Description and guidelines for prevention in patients with renal insufficiency. Am. J. Med., *76*:47–56, 1984.
83. Wyngaarden, J.B., Rundles, R.W., and Metz, E.N.: Allopurinol in the treatment of gout. Ann. Intern. Med., *62*:842–847, 1965.
84. Klinenberg, J.R., Goldfinger, S.E., and Seegmiller, J.E.: The effectiveness of the xanthine oxidase inhibitor allopurinol in the treatment of gout. Ann. Intern. Med., *62*:639–647, 1965.
85. Edwards, N.L. et al.: Enhanced purine salvage during allopurinol therapy: An important pharmacologic property in humans. J. Lab. Clin. Med., *98*:673–683, 1981.
86. Kelley, W.N., and Beardmore, T.D.: Allopurinol: Alteration in pyrimidine metabolism in man. Science, *169*:388–390, 1970.
87. Yu, T.-F.: The effect of allopurinol in primary and secondary gout. Arthritis Rheum., *8*:905–906, 1965.
88. Kranen, S., Keough, D., Gordon, R.B., and Emmerson, B.T.: Xanthine-containing calculi during allopurinol therapy. J. Urol., *133*:658–659, 1985.
89. Band, P.R., Silverberg, D.S., and Henderson, J.F.: Xanthine nephropathy in a patient with lymphosarcoma treated with allopurinol. N. Engl. J. Med., *283*:354–357, 1970.
90. Albin, A. et al.: Nephropathy, xanthinuria, and orotic aciduria complicating Burkitt's lymphoma treated with chemotherapy and allopurinol. Metabolism, *21*:771–778, 1972.
91. Watts, R.W.E. et al.: Microscopic studies on skeletal muscle in gout patients treated with allopurinol. Q. J. Med., *40*:1–14, 1971.
92. McInnes, G.T., Lawson, D.H., and Jick, H.: Acute adverse reactions attributed to allopurinol in hospitalized patients. Ann. Rheum. Dis., *40*:245–249, 1981.
93. Yu, T.-F., and Gutman, A.B.: Effect of allopurinol (4-hydroxypyrazolo-(3,4-d) pyrimidine) on serum and urinary uric acid in primary gout. Am. J. Med., *37*:885–898, 1964.
94. Lang, P.G.: Severe hypersensitivity reactions to allopurinol. South. Med. J., *72*:1361–1368, 1979.
95. Stratigos, J.D., Bartsokas, S.K., and Capetanakis, J.: Further experience of toxic epidermal necrolysis incriminating allopurinol, pyrazoline, and derivatives. Br. J. Dermatol., *86*:564–567, 1972.
96. Fam, A.G., Paton, T.W., and Chaiton, A.: Reinstitution of allopurinol therapy for gouty arthritis after cutaneous reactions. Can. Med. Assoc. J., *123*:128–129, 1980.
97. Webster, E., and Panush, R.S.: Allopurinol hypersensitivity in a patient with severe, chronic, tophaceous gout. Arthritis Rheum., *28*:707–709, 1985.
98. Greenberg, M.S., and Zambrano, S.S.: Aplastic agranulocytosis after allopurinol therapy. Arthritis Rheum., *15*:413–416, 1972.
99. Tam, S., and Carroll, W.: Allopurinol hepatotoxicity. Am. J. Med., *86*:357–358, 1989.
100. Gelbart, D.R., Weinstein, A.B., and Fajardo, L.F.: Allopurinol-

induced interstitial nephritis. Ann. Intern. Med., *86*:196–198, 1977.

101. Young, J.L., Jr., Boswell, R.B., and Nies, A.S.: Severe allopurinol hypersensitivity: Association with thiazides and prior renal compromise. Arch. Intern. Med., *134*:553–558, 1974.
102. Lupton, G.P., and Odon, R.B.: The allopurinol hypersensitivity syndrome. J. Am. Acad. Dermatol., *1*:365–379, 1979.
103. Fraunfelder, F.T. et al.: Cataracts associated with allopurinol therapy. Am. J. Ophthalmol., *94*:137–140, 1982.
104. Lerman, S., Megaw J.M., and Gardner, K.: Allopurinol therapy and cataractogenesis in humans. Am. J. Ophthalmol., *94*:141–146, 1982.
105. Singer, J.Z., and Wallace, S.L.: The allopurinol hypersensitivity syndrome. Unnecessary morbidity and mortality. Arthritis Rheum., *29*:82–87, 1986.
106. Elion, G.B. et al.: Potentiation by inhibition of drug degradation: 6-substituted purines and xanthine oxidase. Biochem. Pharmacol., *12*:85–93, 1963.
107. Boston Collaborative Drug Surveillance Program: Allopurinol and cytotoxic drugs: Interactions in relation to bone marrow depression. JAMA, *227*:1036–1040, 1974.
108. Jick, H., and Porter, J.B.: Potentiation of ampicillin skin reactions by allopurinol or hyperuricemia. J. Clin. Pharmacol., *21*:456–458, 1981.
109. Howell, S.B. et al.: Modulation of 5-fluorouracil toxicity by allopurinol in man. Cancer, *48*;1281–1289, 1981.
110. Kelley, W.N.: Pharmacologic approach to the maintenance of urate homeostasis. Nephron, *14*:99–115, 1975.
111. Gault, M.H. et al.: Urolithiasis due to 2,8-dihydroxyadenine in an adult. N. Engl. J. Med., *305*:1570–1572, 1981.
112. Fox, I.H. et al.: Partial deficiency of adenine phosphoribosyltransferase in man. Medicine, *56*:515–526, 1977.

107

Pathogenesis and Treatment of Crystal-Induced Inflammation

ROBERT A. TERKELTAUB

The cellular and molecular mechanisms, and treatment of the inflammatory host response to several microcrystals implicated in human rheumatic diseases. Crystal species definitely identified in human joints are listed in Table 5–7, and arthropathies associated with these compounds are discussed in Chapters 106 and 109 to 111. Techniques useful for the identification of crystals in routine clinical practice and in experimental work are discussed in Chapters 5 and 111.

NUCLEATION, GROWTH, AND SHEDDING OF CRYSTALS

The nucleation and growth of the monosodium urate monohydrate (MSU) and calcium pyrophosphate dihydrate (CPPD) crystals serve as examples for this discussion.

DEPOSITION OF MSU CRYSTALS

Urate crystallizes and its monosodium salt in oversaturated tissue fluids. MSU crystals found in joint fluid at the time of the acute attack may derive from rupture of preformed synovial deposits (Fig. 107–1) or may have precipitated de novo, as exemplified in certain instances by the recognition of urate spherulites (Chapter 5). Arthroscopically, the earliest urate crystal deposits are apparently in the synovium, rather than in cartilage; they appear as white furuncles with an erythematous base. Investigators have found tophi in synovial membrane at the time of the first gouty attack.[1] In addition, in some individuals with gout, urate crystals can be found in asymptomatic metatarsophalangeal and knee joints that have never been involved in an acute attack of gout.[2] And individuals with asymptomatic hyperuricemia may have MSU crystals in metatarsophalangeal joint fluid.[3] These findings confirm that gout, like CPPD crystal deposition, can exist in a lanthanic (asymptomatic) state, as discussed below, and in Chapter 109.

Only a minority of individuals with sustained hyperuricemia develop tophi and gouty arthropathy. Though many factors are implicated in the tissue deposition of MSU crystals (Table 107–1), the reasons for the clinical selectivity of tophus formation are poorly understood at present.

The decreased solubility of sodium urate at the lower temperatures of peripheral structures such as the toes and ears may help explain why MSU crystals deposit in there areas.[4] The predilection for marked MSU crystal deposition in the first metatarsophalangeal joint may also relate to repetitive minor trauma at this articulation. Simkin has demonstrated that the rate of diffusion of urate molecules from synovial space to plasma is only half that of water.[5] Thus, the urate concentration in a small effusion in a dependent joint such as the great toe, could equilibrate with plasma urate during the day. Subsequently, as the effusion resorbed during recumbency, a localized increase in urate level would be expected. This phenomenon might help account for the usual nocturnal onset of acute gouty symptoms in a dependent joint. In addition, such a mechanism might help explain Schumacher's observation of rapid tophus formation at the site of a burn.[6]

The finding by Katz of threefold elevations of serum uronic acid levels in patients with articular gout but not in patients with hyperuricemia or other inflammatory diseases provides a clue to the possible specificity of MSU crystal deposition.[7] The normalization of these elevated levels by the usual therapeutic doses of colchi-

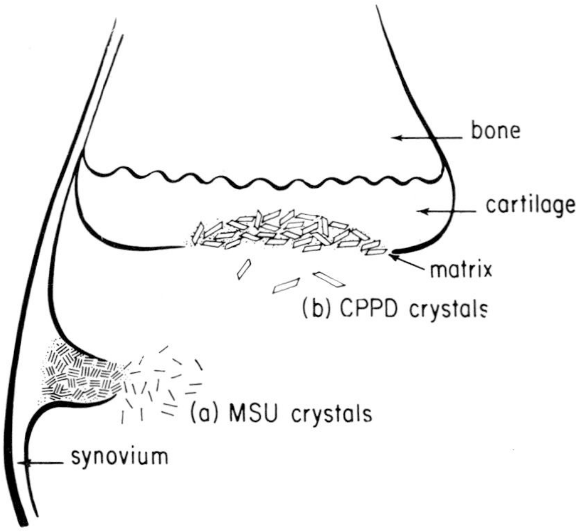

FIGURE 107–1. Autoinjection of monosodium urate (MSU) crystals (a) from preformed tophus in synovium into adjacent joint space. Autoinjection of calcium pyrophosphate dihydrate (CPPD) crystals (b) from preformed cartilaginous deposit into adjacent joint space, as a result of crystal shedding. Both concepts are still hypothetic and have only indirect supportive evidence. See text for details.

TABLE 107–1. FACTORS PROPOSED TO MODULATE TISSUE DEPOSITION OF MSU CRYSTALS

Temperature
pH
Trauma, tissue injury
Glycosaminoglycans and connective tissue turnover
Degenerative joint disease
Plasma proteins
Concentrations of other solutes (lead, calcium, sodium)
Urate secretion and sequestration within macrophage acini
Unknown factors

cine lends further credence to this finding and suggests that the prophylactic mechanism of colchicine may be different from that operating in the treatment of established acute gouty arthritis and might also relate to effects of colchicine on collagen metabolism or connective tissue turnover.[8] The observations that hemiplegia appears to have a sparing effect on the development of tophi and acute gout on the paretic side[9] and that tophi and acute gout occur in distal interphalangeal joints at the location of Heberden's nodes[10] direct further emphasis to the potential importance of focal connective-tissue structure and turnover. In this regard, urate is more soluble in aggregated proteoglycans than in nonaggregated proteoglycans.[11] Furthermore, chondroitin sulfate concentration influenced urate crystal formation in synovial fluids in vitro.[12]

Mononuclear phagocytes of variable maturity encircle deposited urate in many small tophi but not in some larger urate deposits.[13] Olecranon bursa tophi contained small acini of macrophages surrounding necrotic tissues that do not contain internal urate crystals. Palmer and colleagues have hypothesized[13] that macrophages may play an active role in urate deposition via their ability to transport (and potentially centripetally sequester) organic anions.[14]

Variable amounts of lipid debris have been observed in the intercrystalline matrix of tophi.[15] A similar physical association of lipids with cartilaginous deposits of CPPD crystals has also been described.[16] However, whether such deposits are a causative factor or a consequence of crystal deposition is unknown.

The role of plasma protein binding to uric acid in maintaining its solubility was postulated by Aakesson and Alvasker,[17] who found a partial deficiency of a uric acid-binding α-globulin in a kindred with gout.[18] Several studies, however, have concluded that uric acid binding to plasma proteins is generally weak and reversible and that plasma proteins have minimal effects on the distribution of uric acid in equilibrium dialysis.[19] Variable effects of albumin on MSU crystallization from supersaturated uric acid solutions have been reported.[20] In this regard, Perl-Treves and Addadi have demonstrated that human albumin greatly accelerates the nucleation at a pH higher than 7.5 but that the effects of albumin are minimal at pH 7.0. Albumin appears to interact selectively with one of the hydrophilic faces of urate crystals, and this interaction requires available protein carboxylate groups.[20] The potential role of plasma proteins in MSU crystal nucleation and growth in vivo is unresolved.

Lowering of pH may enhance urate nucleation in vitro by the formation of protonated solid phases.[21] The solubility of sodium urate, however, as opposed to that of uric acid, actually increased as pH decreased from 7.4 to 5.8, and measurements in gouty joints of both pH and buffering capacity have failed to demonstrate significant acidosis. Thus, acute pH changes are unlikely to significantly influence MSU crystal formation.

Critical urate supersaturation levels can be altered by the concentrations of a number of other solutes, including sodium and calcium in vitro.[4,22–24] In addition, lead at 100 μg/L, can effectively nucleate MSU from normal saline solution containing 10 mg/dL urate.[24] However, such high levels are found only in acute lead poisoning, making it unlikely that lead acts as a nucleating agent, even in saturnine gout. Whether relative changes in solute concentrations contribute to the well-documented lack of tophi in gout secondary to the hyperuricemia of renal disease is unknown.[25]

Interestingly, joint fluid supernatants from gouty joints enhanced MSU crystal formation in vitro.[23] Whether these effects are due to increased nucleation or an enhanced rate of crystal growth via the possible participation of ultramicrocrystals in the gouty fluids as "seeds" remains to be determined.

Acute attacks of gout in patients correlated with the *rate of change* of serum urate (either up or down) rather than with a steady-state level. Initial treatment with allopurinol commonly produces an abrupt decline in urate levels and precipitates acute attack of gout. Falling serum urate levels may promote the release of MSU crystals into the vascular synovial space from tophaceous deposits via a slight decrease in the size of crystals, loosening them from their organic matrix (crystal "shedding").

DEPOSITION AND SHEDDING OF CPPD CRYSTALS

The initial site of CPPD crystal formation is probably articular cartilages although precipitation de novo in synovial fluid or synovium has not been ruled out, CPPD crystals are frequently found in these sites as well as in extra-articular tendons, ligaments, and bursae.[26] In hyaline cartilage, such crystals often lie in a granular matrix,[27] which stains more densely than surrounding cartilage with periodic acid-Schiff (PAS), alcian blue, colloidal iron, and ruthenium red.[28] These features suggest the presence of abnormal proteoglycan.

The generation of inorganic pyrophosphate (PPi) by cartilage and the nucleation and growth of CPPD crystals from solution from gels are discussed in Chapter 109.

Assuming that the CPPD crystals lying in their cartilaginous mold of proteoglycan are the thermodynamic equilibrium with Ca^{++} and P_2O_7-4, the ions from which they were formed, conditions that either lower ionized calcium or reduce Ca^{++} and P_2O_7-4 should increase the solubility of these crystals and should free them from their mold. This still hypothetic phenomenon has been called "crystal shedding."[29] The marked effect of even small changes in ionized calcium level on crystal solubility in vitro, the onset of acute pseudogout after lavage of joints with solubilizers of CPPD crystals such as EDTA or Mg^{++}-containing buffers,[29] and the clinical correlation of acute arthritis with falling serum calcium concentrations[30] all support this hypothesis. Joint fluid PPi levels are lower during acute attacks of pseudogout, owing to a more rapid equilibration with the much lower ($\sim$2 μM) plasma PPi level. Thus, once an acute attack begins, the fall in ambient PPi that is due to increased synovial blood flow may further increase crystal solubility and shedding.

Other postulated mechanisms for the autoinjection of CPPD crystals presumed to precede acute pseudogout are summarized in Table 107–2. Mechanical disruption of cartilage accompanying subchondral microfracture was implicated in an acute attack developing for the first time in a knee joint with acute neuropathic changes,[31] and trauma is a common antecedent of acute pseudogout. "Enzymatic strip mining" of crystals from preformed cartilaginous deposits is reviewed in Chapters 109 and 110. Presumably, any significant intrasynovial discharge of inflammatory proteases might digest the components of the "mold," releasing crystals into the joint space. CPPD crystals were readily released from cartilage incubated in vitro with synovial cell collagenase, for example.[32] *Thus, the mere presence of CPPD or MSU crystals in joint fluid must be interpreted in the clinical context because they might be a result, as well as a cause, of joint inflammation.*

Finally, the reported association of silent CPPD crystal deposition and hypothyroidism with the onset of acute pseudogout after thyroid hormone therapy suggests that metabolically induced changes in cartilage matrix may also release crystals.[33]

PATHOGENESIS OF CRYSTAL-INDUCED INFLAMMATION

Gout was the first crystal deposition disease to be defined and studied in detail and will serve as a paradigm for the following discussion. Acute onset, severity, edema, and erythema extending beyond the joint margin, neutrophil influx, and systemic manifestations are the hallmarks of the articular inflammation in a gouty paroxysm. These features reflect the ability of MSU crystals to activate a remarkable number of humoral and cellular inflammatory mediator systems, some of which are depicted in Fig. 107–2. The other crystals found in arthritis have been less thoroughly studied but in many instances have been demonstrated to share the ability of MSU to activate pathways that generate inflammatory mediators.

GENERATION AND RELEASE OF INFLAMMATORY MEDIATORS

Complement Activation

MSU crystals activate the classic complement pathway in vitro.[34] They can bind and induce cleavage of purified macromolecular C1 in the absence of immunoglobu-

TABLE 107–2. PROPOSED MECHANISMS OF AUTOINJECTION OF CALCIUM PYROPHOSPHATE DIHYDRATE (CPPD) CRYSTALS FROM CARTILAGE TO VASCULAR JOINT TISSUE SPACE

TRIGGER	HYPOTHETIC MECHANISM	CLINICAL CIRCUMSTANCES OF ACUTE ATTACK
Fall in synovial fluid (Ca^{++}) or inorganic pyrophosphate level	Partial dissolution crystal shedding	Postoperatively or during acute medical illness
Mechanic disruption of cartilage architecture	Microfractures of subchondral bone	Trauma
Increased activity of enzymes degrading cartilage matrix	Crystal shedding as a result of removal of matrix by "enzymatic strip-mining"	Pseudogout superimposed on another type of arthritis; i.e., pyogenic infection, acute gout, or osteoarthritis
Hypothyroidism with treatment	Altered cartilaginous "mold" with crystal shedding	Joint symptoms after thyroid hormone replacement

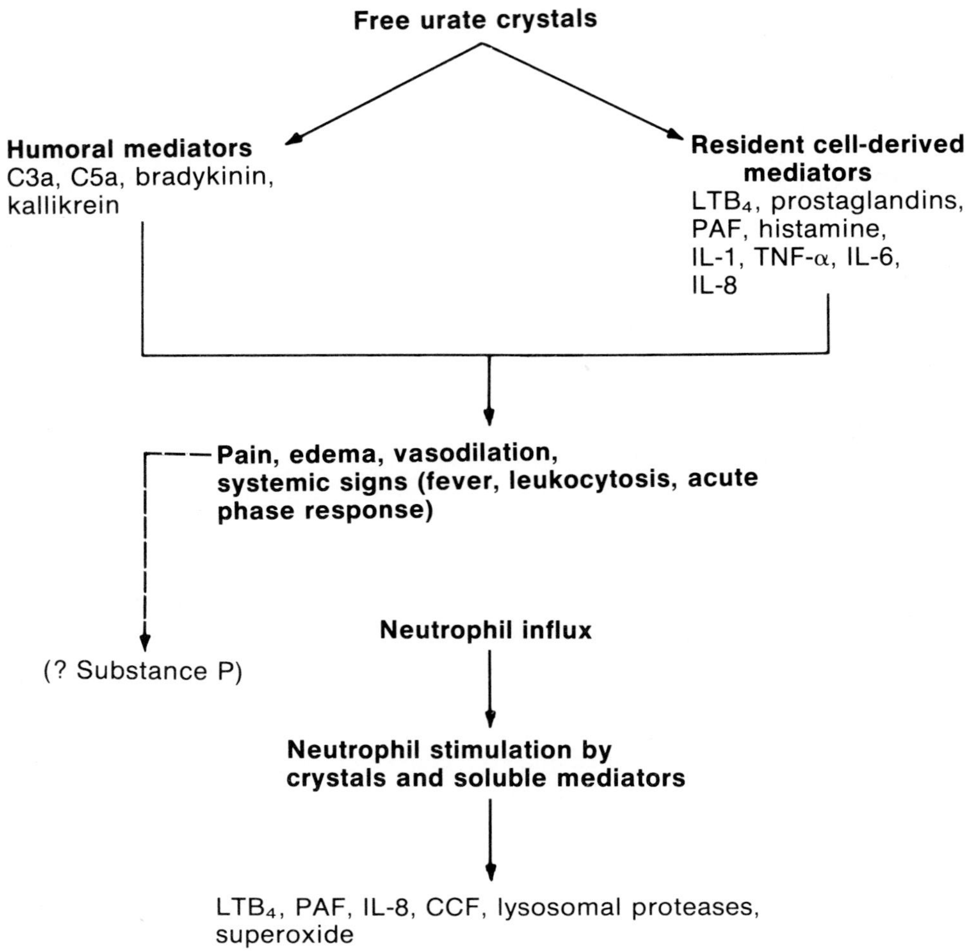

FIGURE 107–2. Hypothetical pathways involved in the development of acute gouty arthritis. CCF = crystal-induced chemotactic factor; IL-1 = interleukin-1; LTB_4 = leukotriene B_4; PAF = platelet-activating factor. (From Terkeltaub, R. *In* Uric Acid Deposition in Man and Its Clinical Consequences. Edited by U. Gresser and N. Zollner. New York, Springer-Verlag.)

lin.[34,35] In addition, classic pathway activation is amplified by IgG or C-reactive protein.[36] Alternative pathway activation also occurs in vitro at higher crystal concentrations when classic pathway activation is inhibited.[37] Direct cleavage of C5 to C5a and C5b is also effected via a stable C5 convertase formed on the crystal surface.[38] Complement activation occurs in many human gouty synovial fluids.[39] Though the amount of complement in normal joint fluid is low, C5a and C5a-des-arg are known to exert chemotactic effects at low concentrations.

Coagulation System Activation

Urate crystals activate Hageman factor (HF) and the contact system of coagulation in vitro, resulting in generation of kallikrein, bradykinin, plasmin, and other inflammatory mediators.[40] Joint fluids in both spontaneous acute gout and in synthetic urate crystal-induced inflammation contained substantial amounts of kinins.[41]

Neutrophil Activation

Neutrophils exposed to MSU crystals release lysosomal proteases,[42] superoxide,[43] and lipoxygenase-derived products of arachidonic acid, including leukotriene B_4 (LTB_4).[44] A chemotactic, 15-kilodalton (kd) protein[45] termed *crystal-induced chemotactic factor (CCF)*[46] also appears to be transcriptionally activated and secreted in neutrophils after phagocytosis of MSU and certain other particulates. Importantly, CCF has an amino acid composition distinct from that of interleukin-8 (IL-8),[47] which is also transcribed by activated neutrophils.[48] CCF caused neutrophil infiltration and synovitis in vivo. LTB_4 and a molecule resembling CCF have been identified in human acute gouty synovial fluids.[46,49]

Activation of Cells Other Than Neutrophils

MSU crystals interact physically with synovial lining cells and mononuclear phagocytes in gouty joints,[15] stimulating the release of a number of mediators, including collagenase, from fibroblasts in vitro. MSU crystals also stimulated the release of vasoactive prostaglandins, proteases, and a number of proinflammatory cytokines (including IL-1, tumor necrosis factor-α [TNF-x], IL-6, and IL-8)[50,51] from cultured monocytes and synoviocytes.

The participation of synovial mast cells, platelets, or both in acute gout is theoretically possible; platelets are among the earliest cells to mediate inflammatory responses (Chapter 22), and their interaction with urate crystals in vitro is well recognized.[52] Mast cells (Chapter 21) reside in the synovium, and stimulation of these cells in vitro by C3a, C5a, and IL-1 results in the release of a variety of inflammatory mediators, including histamine. In this regard, early articular swelling was diminished by antihistaminic drugs in experimental MSU crystal-induced inflammation.[53]

BASIC MECHANISMS OF MSU CRYSTAL-INDUCED CELLULAR ACTIVATION

Crystal-Induced Membrane Perturbation and Lysis

The considerable surface reactivity of the MSU crystal[54] imparts to it a high capacity to induce perturbation[55] and delayed lysis of plasma membranes and model liposomes.[56] Furthermore, rapid cellular responses not mediated by membrane lysis are prominent, including platelet serotonin secretion and neutrophil superoxide anion and lysosomal protease secretion.[57,58] Membrane cholesterol,[56] and MSU crystal-induced cross linking of mobile membrane proteins[59] have been proposed to be important factors in MSU crystal-induced membrane lysis.

Phagocytosis of MSU crystals by neutrophils is followed by rapid dissolution of the phagolysosomal membrane. This process has been termed "suicide sac formation" by Weissmann and co-workers, because internal release of lysosomal contents supervenes, followed by cellular swelling and death.[60–62] Protein-coated MSU crystals are stripped by enzymatic digestion within phagolysosomes. Because the protein coat of MSU crystals inhibits membrane injury,[63] its removal allows phagolysosome membrane lysis to proceed. Cell death following phagocytosis of membranolytic crystals may also depend on an influx of extracellular calcium into the damaged cell.[64]

Signal Transduction

The mechanisms whereby MSU crystals induce functional leukocyte responses are heterogeneous. Opsonization of the crystals is clearly unnecessary, though crystal-bound IgG enhances the capacity of MSU to stimulate neutrophils and a number of other cells.[58,63] MSU crystals appear to activate membrane G proteins (including Gi-α-2) in neutrophils.[65] Though MSU crystals can increase membrane permeability of lytic effects,[56] MSU crystals also induce rapid cytosolic calcium mobilization, modulated by phosphatidylinositol 4,5 bisphosphate (PIP2) hydrolysis and inositol 1,4,5-trisphosphate generation in neutrophils.[66] Unlike neutrophil activation induced by chemotactic factors, however, MSU crystal-induced PIP2 hydrolysis, cytosolic calcium mobilization, and functional responses do not require the activation of a pertussis toxin-sensitive G protein.[65,66]

PIP2 hydrolysis is not the sole indication of membrane phospholipase activation by MSU. For example, MSU crystals also induce direct phospholipase A2 activation and release of a phospholipase A2-activating protein in leukocytes.[67]

MSU crystal-induced leukocyte membrane activation events are likely modulated by both membrane perturbation and crystal surface reactivity, which gives it the ability to bind and potentially cross link and cluster membrane proteins, including adhesion molecules. For example, in platelets, the membrane integrin GpIIb/IIIa binds to urate crystals and modulates urate-induced platelet serotonin secretion.[52] Cross linking and clustering of freely mobile membrane proteins by multivalent ligands such as MSU crystals (as schematically depicted in Fig. 107–3) may be analogous to the effects on leukocytes of cross linking certain membrane proteins including Fc receptors[68] or solid-phase bound CD44 and

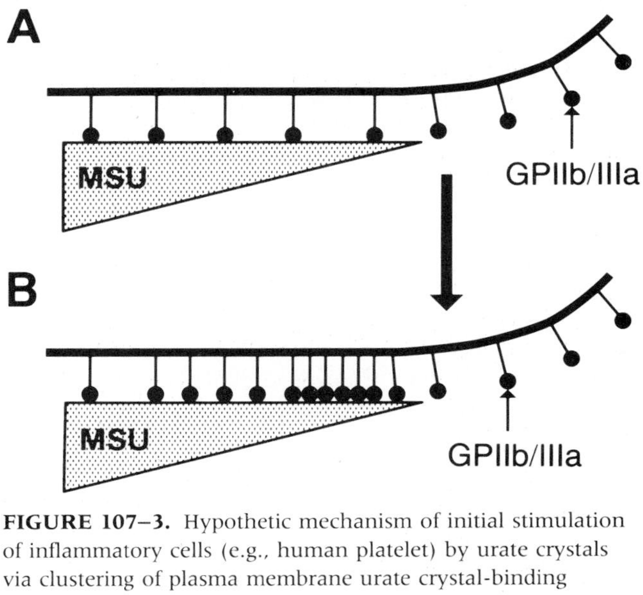

FIGURE 107–3. Hypothetic mechanism of initial stimulation of inflammatory cells (e.g., human platelet) by urate crystals via clustering of plasma membrane urate crystal-binding glycoproteins. *A*, Platelet-membrane GPIIb/IIIa is initially homogeneously distributed in the membrane. GPIIb/IIIa, in close proximity to the rigid crystal surface, binds to it, thereby immobilizing the glycoprotein in the plane of the membrane. *B*, Continued lateral diffusion of the unbound GPIIb/IIIa brings it to the junction zone, where it becomes immobilized by binding to the crystal surface.

CD45.[69] Such cross-linking events can result in pertussis toxin-insensitive cytosolic calcium mobilization[68] or cytokine induction.[69]

INITIATION AND PROPAGATION OF ACUTE GOUT

Hypothetical Sequence of Events

MSU crystals liberated from synovial microtophi, or precipitated de novo, are believed to activate the humoral and cellular mediator cascades described previously (Fig. 108–2). Early vasodilation, enhanced vascular permeability, and pain in gouty arthritis are likely mediated by vasoactive prostaglandins, kinins (which also potentiate prostaglandin synthesis via release of membrane arachidonate), complement peptides, and histamine. The role of prostaglandins as mediators of pain in gout is underlined by the strikingly complete suppression of tenderness (out of proportion to its effects on swelling, local heat, and volume of local effusion) in synovitis induced by MSU crystals in normal human volunteers pretreated with aspirin.[70] Pain signals may also theoretically mediate acute gout via the release from nociceptive afferent sensory nerve fibers of substance P, which has a number of proinflammatory functions.[71]

Neutrophil influx and neutrophil activation appear to be the central events in acute gouty arthritis. This is supported by the striking accumulation of these cells in both the joint fluid and synovial membrane, where they phagocytose crystals actively, and where they aggregate and degranulate in the microvasculature in areas remote from the joint space.[15] Second, Phelps and McCarty established that experimental urate crystal-induced synovitis is absent in neutrophil-depleted animals.[72] Third, a number of agents that suppress neutrophil function effectively prevent and/or terminate acute gouty inflammation.

Neutrophils are virtually absent in normal joint fluid (see Chapter 5). Humoral and resident cell-derived mediators (including LTB_4 and platelet-activating factor [PAF]) likely trigger initial neutrophil ingress into joints. MSU crystal-induced release of IL-1 and TNF-α from monocytes and synovial lining cells likely promotes neutrophil ingress via the induction of adhesion protein expression by the endothelial cells of postcapillary venules (Chapter 23). IL-1 and TNF-α are also known to induce the release of the neutrophil chemotactic/activating cytokine IL-8 from mononuclear phagocytes, fibroblasts, and many other cells.[47] In this regard, IL-8 is the major neutrophil chemotactic factor released from monocytes activated by MSU crystals in vitro, and it is abundant in acute gouty joint fluids.[73]

The release of neutrophil-derived mediators (e.g., CCF, LTB_4, lysosomal proteases) in response to contact with both intra-articular MSU crystals and fluid-phase mediators (e.g., LTB_4, C5a, kallikrein, TNF-α, IL-8) is believed to play a major role in gouty inflammation by establishing a self-amplifying cycle of further neutrophil ingress and neutrophil activation.

Systemic Manifestations and Chronic Inflammation

MSU crystals can directly (and indirectly) induce IL-1, TNF-α, IL-8, and IL-6 release from mononuclear phagocytes and synovial lining cells.[50,51,73] These cytokines are all enriched in acute gouty synovial fluid, and their escape into the circulation likely plays the critical role in the development of systemic manifestations (including low-grade fever, leukocytosis, and the hepatic acute-phase protein response). MSU crystal deposition can be associated not only with episodic acute inflammation but also with chronic synovitis, articular erosions, and cartilage and subchondral osseous destruction. The MSU crystal-induced release from resident mononuclear phagocytes and synovial lining cells of the previously mentioned cytokines and of proteases and biologic oxidants likely fuels chronic inflammation and connective tissue degradation. Thus, adequate and expeditious measures to reduce hyperuricemia and to promote resorption of crystals are imperative (Chapter 107). In this regard, articular destructive changes and deformities can progress despite uric acid-lowering therapy that adequately diminishes further episodes of acute gout.[74]

Inherent Redundancy of Crystal-Induced Inflammatory Mediator Expression

The inherent redundancy of the inflammatory reactions to MSU crystals (Fig. 108–2) suggests that no single mediator is absolutely necessary for MSU crystal-induced inflammation. This hypothesis has been addressed in several ways. First, the degree of urate crystal-induced inflammation has been reduced only minimally, at the most, by complement depletion in animal studies.[75,76] Second, acute gout occurs in humans with HF deficiency,[77,78] and an acute inflammatory response to injected MSU crystals is seen in chickens which lack HF.[79] Third, though dietary enrichment with fish oil or primrose oil (which provide alternative substrates to arachidonate for oxidative metabolism) do suppress inflammation in rats after injection of MSU crystals into subcutaneous air pouches,[80] MSU crystals are capable of inducing inflammation in subcutaneous rat air pouches (facsimile synovia) in animals effectively pretreated with 5-lipoxygenase inhibitors.[81] Last, clinical manifestations of gouty inflammation have been reported to occur in the absence of neutrophils in human synovial fluid.[82]

REGULATION OF THE INFLAMMATORY POTENTIAL OF THE MSU CRYSTAL

Self-Limitation of Acute Gouty Inflammation

The self-limitation characteristic of acute gout has been known since Hippocrates. Factors other than MSU crystal dissolution[83] or sequestration must play a role in terminating attacks, because free MSU crystals are often found in synovial fluid for many weeks after subsidence of an acute gouty paroxysm. Many factors are likely to contribute. Inactivation and clearance of mediators (e.g., ω-oxidation of LTB_4 and inactivation of bradykinin, C3a, and C5a by carboxypeptidases) are likely to be accompanied by tachyphylaxis to such mediators.[84,85] The latter mechanism is exemplified in vitro by stimulus-specific desensitization of neutrophils to chemotactic factors and inhibition of neutrophil phagocytosis of MSU by CCF.[46] Because of such mechanisms and the limited (days) normal functional life span of neutrophils,[86] continued recruitment of new neutrophils to the gouty site is probably necessary for the persistence of inflammation.[87]

Changes in the balance between molecules that exert pro- and anti-inflammatory effects during the course of acute crystal-induced inflammation are likely to modulate the clinical features. Activated inflammatory cells can release a variety of substances that are capable of dampening inflammation.[88] In gouty inflammation, these would be expected to first include the E-series prostaglandins, which inhibit IL-1 and TNF-α production, suppress neutrophil function, and suppress MSU crystal-induced inflammation in rat air pouches.[89] Second, transforming growth factor-β (TGF-β), though it has some proinflammatory activities, is a potent inhibitor of IL-1 receptor expression and IL-1–driven cellular responses.[90] TGF-β is known to be released from activated monocytes and from other cells, and it is abundant in some acute gouty synovial fluids.[91] Third, IL-6 can inhibit TNF-α release under certain conditions[92] and can, along with IL-1 induce central adrenocorticotropin hormone (ACTH) release with subsequent endogenous adrenal glucocorticoid release. Fourth, shedding of soluble Fc and TNF-α receptors by activated neutrophils[93,94] may inhibit phagocytosis, neutrophil priming, and other proinflammatory events.

Changes in the type of adsorbed proteins during the evolution of the gouty paroxysm may also modulate inflammation. Gordon and co-workers found that removal of proteins coating the surface of MSU crystals isolated from a quiescent tophus dramatically increased their capacity to activate neutrophils in vitro.[95] Binding of neutrophil lysosomal enzymes to MSU crystals displaced IgG from the crystal surface, decreasing the ability of MSU crystals to stimulate neutrophils in vitro.[96] Other mechanisms whereby molecules absorbed to MSU crystals surfaces might modulate the crystal's inflammatory potential are discussed in the following sections.

Crystals With and Without Inflammation

The lack of direct correlation between the number of urate crystals seen in joint fluid and the severity of acute gout is well accepted.[2,97] For example, large quantities of crystals ("joint milk") may be aspirated from joints that show little or no sign of inflammation.[98] In other patients, few crystals might be detected despite full-blown acute gouty arthritis. A striking absence of inflammation about subcutaneous deposits of urate crystals is the rule, and some patients with chronic tophaceous gout give no history of acute attacks.[99] A multitude of factors could account for such observations.

Possible Regulatory Factors

Host factors that may mediate MSU crystal-induced inflammation include renal failure and rheumatoid arthritis (RA). Patients with chronic renal insufficiency have diminished inflammatory responses to the subcutaneous injection of MSU crystals.[100] Gouty attacks may be less severe and less frequent in such individuals.[25,101] The high incidence of gouty arthritis in association with lead nephropathy seems paradoxic.

The coexistence of RA and gout is much rarer than expected statistically,[102] perhaps reflecting many factors, including hypouricemic and anti-inflammatory effects of many agents employed continuously in the treatment of RA.

Polymeric hyaluronic acid inhibited both neutrophil chemotactic mobility and phagocytosis of MSU crystals in a dose-dependent manner[103] and may thus regulate crystal inflammation. A fall in hyaluronate concentration as a result of development of an effusion—for example, following trauma—might dilute its inhibitory effect on crystal–cell interactions and render the crystals more inflammatory. Urate in solution suppressed protein adsorption by neutrophil plasma membranes and could result in increased crystal-induced membranolysis.[104] No correlation existed between crystal size, and the severity of MSU-induced inflammation.[105] Whether variations in the mechanism of MSU crystal formulation can alter their inflammatory potential remains to be determined.[20]

Inhibition of MSU Crystal-Induced Cell Activation by Crystal-Bound Proteins

Much attention has focused on the possibility that protein adsorbed to MSU crystal surfaces[35,106] could be a critical determinant of their inflammatory potential. MSU crystals incubated with whole serum are markedly less stimulatory for leukocytes,[63,73] which is due to the binding of apolipoprotein B-bearing lipoproteins.[63,107] Low-density lipoprotein (LDL), the predominant apo B lipoprotein, suppressed cellular responses to MSU by binding to the crystal surface, thereby physically inhibiting particle–cell interaction, phagocytosis, and membrane activation.[63,65] Apo B is both necessary and sufficient for this activity of LDL.[108]

MSU crystals in quiescent tophaceous synovial deposits are physically associated with variable amounts of surface proteins and lipids.[15,109] The lipids in tophi include cholesteryl esters, which are predominantly carried by plasma LDL. Furthermore, LDL binds to MSU crystals in vivo, particularly in the later stages of acute gout.[110] In addition, apolipoprotein E can be bound to MSU crystals in vivo, and at physiologic concentrations it blunts crystal-induced neutrophil activation in vitro.[111] Importantly, unlike apo B, apo E is synthesized within synovial joints by cells of the monocyte–macrophage lineage,[111] and thus it exemplifies a locally produced factor capable of markedly altering the inflammatory potential of MSU crystals.

THE GOUT PARADIGM AND INFLAMMATION CAUSED BY OTHER CRYSTALS

The range in intensity of acute synovitis associated with intra-articular crystals other than MSU is broad. Similarly, the pathogenesis of inflammation induced by other microcrystals appears complex. For example, acute pseudogout is associated with neutrophil leukocytosis in synovial fluid and with intracellular crystals. CPPD crystals activate complement[112] and trigger release of CCF from neutrophils,[46] but several studies with CPPD crystals suggest that their capacity to induce the release of a number of cytokines (including IL-1, and IL-6) from macrophages is much weaker than that of MSU crystals.[50,51,113]

Negativity of surface charge and surface irregularity appear to be important determinants of the inflammatory potential of crystals; that is, the crystal surfaces of more inflammatory membranolytic crystals (MSU, CPPD, the α-quartz form of silicon dioxide) are irregular and possess a high density of charged groups, whereas the surfaces of nonhemolytic noninflammatory crystals (e.g., diamond dust and the stishovite and anatase forms of silicon dioxide) are smooth.[54] Brushite and hydroxyapatite crystals present a lesser partial negatively charged surface atomic array than the more membranolytic CPPD crystals,[54] which may explain why these crystals are less frequently associated with acute inflammation.

Basic calcium phosphate (BCP) crystals have a remarkable tendency to form aggregates, the larger of which ("too big to swallow") may escape endocytosis. However carbonate-substituted hydroxyapatite and other BCPs directly stimulate both leukocytes and synoviocytes in vitro. They are phlogistic when injected into animals and are sometimes associated with severe acute articular and periarticular inflammation in humans. They are also associated with widespread articular inflammation in ank/ank mice.[114,115] Thus, other factors that account for the remarkable lack of acute articular inflammation and leukocytosis generally associated with the presence of intra-articular BCP crystals in humans require definition. Such factors may include the low complement-activating potential of BCP crystals relative to MSU;[112] the diminished ability of BCP crystals to stimulate the release of cytokines (e.g., IL-1) from human monocyte–macrophages[51,113] and chemotactic factors from neutrophils;[116] and, their inability, unlike MSU and silica crystals, to directly activate neutrophil membrane G proteins.[65] In addition, adsorbed molecules may attenuate the inflammatory potential of BCP crystals, as already demonstrated for MSU. For example, α-2 HS-glycoprotein, a serum protein produced by the liver that localizes to mineralizing bone, has been identified as a major specific inhibitor of neutrophil responses to BCP crystals in vitro.[117]

Acute synovitis associated with CPPD crystals is sometimes relatively long-lived and refractory to treatment. Ingested CPPD crystals (and BCP crystals) are relatively potent mitogens for synovial and other anchorage-dependent cells compared to MSU crystals. A heightened role of synovial proliferation in acute articular inflammation provoked by CPPD and other calcium-containing crystals is possible.

EXPERIMENTAL MODELS OF CRYSTAL-INDUCED ARTHRITIS

Although experimental model systems using synthetic crystals are only analogs of their natural counterparts, such model systems have been useful in the dissection of some critical features of the host response to crystals. Animal models of crystal-induced inflammation have used dog[72] bird,[79] and rabbit joints;[75,118] rat paws;[119] and rat pleural spaces[120] (reviewed in detail in reference 121). A rodent subcutaneous air pouch, lined by cells histologically similar to synoviocytes, created by repeated injection of sterile air, is also a useful model.[81,89] Such artificial "joints," however, do not contain hyaluronate-rich fluid, and it has been established that MSU crystal-induced inflammation in such tissue spaces is neutrophil dependent. Indomethacin treatment failed to suppress MSU crystal-induced neutrophil influx in this system.[122]

A useful, natural animal model of BCP crystal-induced inflammation is the progressive ankylosis disorder of ank/ank mice, characterized by the presence of BCP crystals in joint fluids, chronic inflammation, and joint fusion.[114,115]

Experimental crystal-induced inflammation in humans can be successfully used for testing for drug effectiveness.[70,123] For example, the intradermal injection of sterile MSU crystals in humans has reproducibly provoked a transient, self-limiting local response, with a systemic response detected by leukocytosis and a rise in serum amyloid A protein, the level of which peaks while the intradermal lesion is resolving.[123]

TREATMENT OF CRYSTAL-INDUCED INFLAMMATION

GOUT

The aims of therapy in gout are to alleviate pain, which is often excruciating, and to restore the inflamed joint to useful function. After protection of the joint by splinting and after administration of analgesics, a choice of many effective drugs is at hand.

Colchicine

Therapy of Acute Gout: Toxicities observed. Under most circumstances, colchicine has the poorest therapeutic benefit/toxicity ratio of drugs in the primary

TABLE 107–3. MANIFESTATIONS OF COLCHICINE TOXICITY

INTRAVENOUS	
Bone marrow depression producing peripheral thrombocytopenia and neutropenia (nadir of values about 3–6 days after drug is given; recovery in absence of additional drug in 4–7 days)	
Cellulitis or thrombophlebitis at injection site	
Alopecia	
Gastrointestinal—Abdominal pain, nausea, vomiting, diarrhea (rare)	
CNS dysfunction	
Peripheral neuropathy	
Myopathy (proximal weakness and elevated serum creatine kinase)	
Shock—Delayed and associated with oliguria, hematuria, weakness, paralysis, delirium, convulsions, and (often) death	
ORAL	
Gastrointestinal—Cramps, diarrhea (most common), nausea, vomiting	
Neuropathy	Uncommon
Myopathy	Uncommon
Alopecia	Uncommon
Bone marrow depression	Rare
Shock	Rare

treatment of acute gout[124,125] (Table 107–3). For this reason, colchicine use has justifiably been eclipsed by the use of other modalities. In particular, diarrhea is almost always provoked by oral colchicine: associated electrolyte imbalances in the elderly may be severe.

Colchicine is most effective when administered in the first 24 hours after onset of acute gout. The drug can be given orally, typically 0.5 mg every hour, until relief or side effects occur, or until a predetermined maximum total dose has been reached (up to 10 or 12 tablets in normal individuals, less in the elderly, or in those with renal insufficiency). Signs and symptoms of inflammation generally subside in 12 to 24 hours and pain is gone in 90% of patients in 24 hours.[126] A response to colchicine treatment is seen in a number of articular conditions other than gout[8] (including sarcoid arthritis, calcific tendinitis and pseudogout).[127,128] Thus, a response to colchicine alone is insufficient to confirm the diagnosis of acute gout.

Colchicine or nonsteroidal anti-inflammatory drugs (NSAIDs) cannot be given orally in certain persons with postoperative acute gout. Intravenous colchicine can be used in this instance: 1 mg, diluted in 20 ml of normal saline and administered slowly (over not less than 10 minutes) as a single dose is adequate for most attacks. Care is necessary to avoid extravasation because of the marked irritating proper ties of the drug. *No more than 2 mg of colchicine should be given in a single intravenous dose, and a total intravenous dose of greater than 4 mg and repeated intravenous administration beyond 24 hours for one attack of gout are inadvisable.* Furthermore, it has been recommended that patients should receive no more colchicine by any route for the first 7 days following intravenous colchicine therapy.[124,125]

Intravenous colchicine is not available in Britain and in many other countries. The infrequency of early gastrointestinal side effects with intravenous colchicine, as compared to oral colchicine, may have imparted the mistaken belief among practitioners in the United States that intravenous colchicine is harmless. However, the use of intravenous colchicine under most circumstances is questionable.[129,129a] Two deaths occurring in a 4-year period in a Boston teaching hospital were thought to represent 2% of patients treated with intravenous colchicine. One patient had renal insufficiency and the other was 91 years old: each had received the drug both orally and intravenously.

Manifestations of intravenous colchicine toxicity are listed in Table 107–3. Intravenous colchicine should only be used if strict precautions are followed (Table 107–4). First, because colchicine is excreted in urine and bile, patients with oliguria, severe renal insufficiency (creatinine clearance < 10 ml/min), and biliary tract obstruction should be treated with alternative agents. In patients with renal failure, fatal marrow suppression is a particular risk even with low doses. Second, individuals with significant renal, hepatic, and cardiac dysfunction, persons with depressed bone marrow function or those receiving cytotoxic chemotherapy, and those with severe infection have an elevated risk of colchicine toxicity, mandating a dose reduction and strong consideration of alternative therapy. Third, the maximum dose of intravenous colchicine should be decreased by 50% in the elderly. Fourth, intravenous colchicine should be avoided, or used only judiciously, in patients with a history of immediate prior use of therapeutic or daily, prophylactic oral colchicine.

Recent work has described a number of colchicine analogs with comparable anti-inflammatory activities in vivo, but less toxicity.[130,131] The possible use of these compounds to suppress human rheumatic disease remains to be explored.

Prophylactic Use. Acute gouty attacks are effectively prevented by small daily doses of colchicine. Doses of 0.5 to 1.8 mg daily are given; the average patient requires about 1 mg. Such doses either completely prevented attacks or greatly reduced their frequency in

TABLE 107–4. CONTRAINDICATIONS TO THE USE OF INTRAVENOUS COLCHICINE

ABSOLUTE
Pre-existing depressed bone marrow function
Creatinine clearance <10 mL/min
Extrahepatic biliary obstruction
Liver disease with bilirubin and/or alkaline phosphatase greater than twice the upper range of normal
Severe sepsis, bacteremia
RELATIVE
Immediate prior use of oral colchicine, either therapeutically or in daily prophylactic doses
Presence of borderline hepatic or renal function
Advanced age (decrease the dose by one half)
Localized infection

93% of a large series of gouty patients during many years of followup.[132] Only 4% had gastrointestinal toxicity, and many of these patients had underlying intestinal disease. Importantly, even with a standard daily prophylactic dose of up to 1 mg/day, renal failure or concomitant cytotoxic drug treatment may predispose to more serious toxicity, including a reversible proximal myopathy.[133,134,134a]

Acute attacks may be heralded by "twinges" in the target joint. If attacks are relatively infrequent (<3/year), the patient not on daily prophylactic colchicine doses can often abort an attack by taking 1 mg of colchicine at the first symptom and 0.5 mg every 2 hours thereafter (for less than 1 day or until symptoms are relieved).

Metabolism. After a single 2-mg intravenous dose of colchicine, the drug is still detectable in plasma days later by radioimmunoassay.[135] The drug is rapidly distributed into a space greater than that of total body water, which probably is due to its concentration in certain cells, as described later. Mean plasma half-life has been estimated to be 58 $\pm$ 20 minutes and peak plasma concentration at 2.9 $\pm$ 1.5 μg/dL under these conditions ($\sim 10^{-5}$M). In volunteers given a single 1-mg oral dose of colchicine, peak plasma levels of up to 0.6 μg/dL have been measured ($\sim 10^{-6}$M). However, the drug is concentrated in leukocytes at 10-fold or greater levels relative to plasma.[8] Although maximal urinary excretion occurs 2 hours after intravenous colchicine administration, the overall excretion of the drug is slow, and it has been detected in the urine 10 days after injection.

Mechanism of Action. The ability of colchicine to concentrate in leukocytes appears central to its efficacy and is probably related to the high content of labile microtubules in these cells. Colchicine binds irreversibly to tubulin dimers and prevents their assembly into microtubules.[8,131] This property makes colchicine, like other tubulin-binding plant alkaloids (e.g., vinblastine) a potent, and potentially lethal, antimitotic cell toxin.

Peak colchicine concentration in peripheral blood leukocytes after a standard intravenous dose can reach 1 to 2 $\times$ 10^{-5}M; at 72 hours after injection, leukocyte colchicine levels of 5 $\times$ 10^{-6}M are reported, and detectable drug levels can still be found in cells isolated from the blood 10 days later. At concentrations achievable therapeutically, colchicine suppresses many neutrophil functions, including random motility, adherence, chemotaxis, and chemotactic factor (CCF and leukotriene B_4) release; degranulation is inhibited in a ligand-specific manner, but superoxide release is unaffected.[8,44,46,136–139] In particular, neutrophil response to many soluble chemotactic agonists (including LTB_4, IL-8, and CCF) are markedly inhibited by colchicine. Weak inhibitory effects on phagocytosis of certain particulates are also produced.

The effects of colchicine on cells other than neutrophils may also be important. Colchicine and other related tubulin-binding agents, down-regulate TNF-α receptors (and TNF-α–driven responses) in macrophages and endothelial cells.[140] Neutrophil TNF-α receptors are unaffected under identical conditions. Colchicine also inhibits mast cell histamine release.[8]

Colchicine affects neutrophil inhibition by heterogeneous mechanisms. It directly elevates cyclic adenosine monophosphate (cAMP) levels, potentiating prostaglandin E-, and β-adrenergic-induced rises in neutrophil cAMP, probably by stimulating the guanine triphosphatase (GTPase) activity of tubulin.[8] Elevation of cAMP globally depresses neutrophil function. Intact microtubule function contributes to optimum expression of neutrophil 5- and 15-lipoxygenase activity, and colchicine markedly suppresses these activities in neutrophils.[137] Colchicine may also affect microtubule-mediated membrane distribution and cycling of specific receptors.[138] Colchicine may alter diacylglycerol generation, thus modulating certain stimulus–response coupling mechanisms.[138] Last, the stabilization, by colchicine, of labile microtubules normally needed for leukocyte motility may inhibit chemotaxis, phagocytosis, and adhesiveness.

The effects of colchicine on microtubules may not be the only reason for the drug's effectiveness. Colchicine also binds to leukocyte membrane proteins, which might be tubulin-like attachment points for microtubules.[141] Furthermore, certain colchicine analogs that do not effectively bind to tubulin and that are not metabolized to colchicine in humans have anti-inflammatory effects in animal model systems and in gouty patients.[130,131,142] Conversely, certain colchicine analogs that effectively bind tubulin have little anti-inflammatory activity.[130]

Fatal overdoses of colchicine are associated with infection accompanying severely depressed bone marrow function with neutropenia and/or with irreversible shock. There are no antidotes. Hemodialysis is ineffective, and therapy is strictly supportive.

Nonsteroidal Anti-inflammatory Agents

Many NSAIDs provide satisfactory therapy for acute gout.[127] The basis for the neutrophil-suppressive and anti-inflammatory activities of NSAIDs are reviewed in Chapters 19 and 32. Caution needs to be exercised in the elderly, and in other patient subsets (e.g., individuals with dehydration or renal insufficiency).

Indomethacin is an effective choice for acute gout (an adequate dose is generally 150 to 200 mg/day for 2 to 3 days, and then 75 to 100 mg daily over the next week, or until pain and inflammation subside). Naproxen, 750 mg as a single dose followed by maintenance doses (375 to 500 mg bid), is a reasonable alternative.[127] Phenylbutazone is as effective orally as colchicine is intravenously. However, because fluid retention, hypertension, gastritis, and marrow toxicity are common, this drug has fallen into disuse.

Azopropazone[143] and other NSAIDs that possess uricosuric effects (e.g., the fluorinated salicylate diflusinal)[144] are under investigation for the adequacy and safety of long-term prophylaxis of acute gout and for uric acid-lowering effectiveness.

Corticosteroids and ACTH

Thorough aspiration of the joint, often possible at the time of diagnostic arthrocentesis to obtain fluid for crystal identification, can be followed by local injection of microcrystalline adrenocorticosteroid esters. Such therapy is ideal in a single large joint; crystal-induced inflammation subsides predictably within 12 hours of treatment regardless of the prior duration of the acute attack.

Therapy with ACTH or systemic corticosteroids[145,146] should generally be reserved for polyarticular gout refractory to other agents, or for gout in settings where the approaches discussed previously are absolutely contraindicated (including renal failure, gastrointestinal bleeding, and certain postoperative states). ACTH may be administered by slow intravenous infusion of 25 IU, and this dose can be repeated (as often as q12h for 1 to 3 days in incomplete responders). In a recent therapeutic trial for monoarticular gout, ACTH, given as a single intramuscular injection of 40 IU, was consistently and rapidly effective (relief of pain in 3 hours), and tolerance was excellent.[146] ACTH is preferable to oral prednisone, which is effective for gout only at initial doses of 30 mg/day (tapering to less than 20 mg/day by 1 week, followed by continuing therapy for 1 to 3 weeks).[145] Intravenous methylprednisolone (individual doses of 50 to 150 mg) can be used in place of prednisone where necessary.

Acute gout can be observed in transplant patients receiving maintenance (~10mg/day) doses of prednisone[147] underscoring the lack of potency of systemic corticosteroids in acute crystal-induced inflammation. In addition, rebound can be observed after cessation of therapy with systemic steroids. Thus, adjunctive low-dose daily colchicine or an NSAID should generally be instituted as soon as possible in patients with acute gout treated with ACTH or systemic corticosteroids.

PSEUDOGOUT

Supportive measures are useful in treatment of pseudogout, as outlined previously. Thorough aspiration of a large joint often effectively controls acute inflammation even without local corticosteroid injection, presumably because of removal of sufficient crystals to control what may be a dose-related response. Concomitant use of local corticosteroid ester crystals is virtually 100% effective in control of acute pseudogout in a single large joint, although a postinjection flare has been implicated as a precipitating acute pseudogout, possibly resulting the enzymatic "strip-mining" mechanism already discussed.

NSAIDs are effective in large doses for the treatment of acute pseudogout. Colchicine effectiveness is less predictable for acute pseudogout when the drug is given orally. Intravenous colchicine (1 to 2 mg) more predictably controls acute pseudogout,[126] probably because it produces much higher intracellular levels, as outlined previously. The frequency of acute attacks of pseudogout can be diminished by the use of small daily prophylactic doses of colchicine, as used for gout.[148]

REFERENCES

1. Schumacher, H.R.: Pathogenesis of crystal-induced synovitis. Clin. Rheum. Dis., *3*:105–131, 1977.
2. Bomalaski, J.A., Lluberas, G., and Schumacher, H.R., Jr.: Monosodium urate crystals in the knee joints of patients with asymptomatic nontophaceous gout. Arthritis Rheum., *39*:1480–1484, 1986.
3. Rouault, T., Caldwell, D.S., and Holmes, D.W.: Aspiration of the asymptomatic metatarsophalangeal joint in gout patients and hyperuricemic controls. Arthritis Rheum., *25*:209–212, 1982.
4. Wilcox, W.R., and Khalaf, A.A.: Nucleation of monosodium urate crystals. Ann. Rheum. Dis., *34*:332–339, 1975.
5. Simkin, P.A.: The pathogenesis of podagra. Ann. Intern. Med., *86*:230–233, 1977.
6. Schumacher, H.R.: Bullous tophi in gout. Ann. Rheum. Dis. *36*:91–93, 1977.
7. Katz, W.A.: Deposition of urate crystals in gout. Arthritis Rheum. *18*:751–756, 1975.
8. Famaey, J.D.: Colchicine in therapy. State of the art and new perspectives for an old drug. Clin. Exp. Rheumatol., *6*:305–317, 1988.
9. Glynn, J.J., and Clayton, M.L.: Sparing effect of hemiplegia on tophaceous gout. Ann. Rheum. Dis., *35*:534–535, 1976.
10. Lally, E.V., Zimmerman, B., Ho, G., Jr., and Kaplan, S.R.: Urate-mediated inflammation in nodal osteoarthritis: Clinical and roentgenographic correlations. Arthritis Rheum., *32*:86–90, 1989.
11. Perricone, E., and Brandt, K.D.: Enhancement of urate solubility by connective tissue: 1. Effect of proteoglycan aggregates and buffer cation. Arthritis Rheum., *21*:453–460, 1978.
12. Burt, H.M., and Dutt, Y.C.: Growth of monosodium urate monohydrate crystals: Effect of cartilage and synovial fluid components on in vitro growth rates. Ann. Rheum. Dis., *45*:858–864, 1986.
13. Palmer, D.G., Highton, J., and Hessian, P.A.: Development of the gouty tophus: An hypothesis. Am. J. Clin. Pathol., *91*:190–195, 1989.
14. Steinberg, T.H., Newman, A.S., Swanson, J.A., and Silverstein, S.C.: Macrophages possess probenicid-inhibitable organic anion transporters that remove fluorescent dyes from the cytoplasmic matrix. J. Cell Biol., *105*:2695–2702, 1987.
15. Agudelo, C., and Schumacher, H.R.: The synovitis of acute gouty arthritis. A light and electron microscopic study. Hum. Pathol., *4*:265–269, 1973.
16. Ohira, T. et al.: Histologic localization of lipid in the articular tissues in calcium phosphate dihydrate crystal deposition disease. Arthritis Rheum., *31*:1057–1062, 1988.
17. Aakesson, I., and Alvasker, J.O.: The urate-binding alpha 1-2 globulin. Isolation and characterization of the protein from human plasma. Eur. J. Clin. Invest., *1*:281–287, 1971.
18. Alvasker, J.O.: Genetic studies in primary gout: Investigations on the plasma levels of the urate-binding alpha-globulin in individuals from two gouty kindred. J. Clin. Invest., *47*:1254–1261, 1968.
19. Hardwell, T.R., Manley, G., Braven, J., and Whitaker, M.: The binding of urate plasma proteins determined by four different techniques. Clin. Chim. Acta, *133*:75–83, 1983.

20. Perl-Treves, D., and Addadi, L.: A structural approach to pathological crystallizations. Gout: The possible role of albumin in sodium urate crystallization. Proc. R. Soc. Lond., *235*:145–159, 1988.
21. Lam-Erwin, C.Y., and Nancollas, G.H.: The crystallization and dissolution of sodium urate. J. Crystal Growth, *53*:214–223, 1981.
22. Tak, H.K., and Wilcox, W.R.: Crystallization of monosodium urate and calcium urate at 37°C. J. Coll. Int. Sci., *77*:195–201, 1980.
23. Tak, H.K., Cooper, S.M., and Wilcox, W.R.: Studies on the nucleation of monosodium urate at 37°C. Arthritis Rheum., *23*:574–580, 1980.
24. Tak, H.K., Wilcox, W.R., and Cooper, S.M.: The effect of lead upon urate nucleation. Arthritis Rheum., *24*:1291–1295, 1981.
25. Sorensen, J.B.: Gout secondary to chronic renal disease: Studies on urate metabolism. Ann. Rheum. Dis., *39*:424–430, 1980.
26. Gerster, J.C., Lagier, R., and Boivin, G.: Olecranon bursitis related to calcium pyrophosphate dihydrate crystal deposition disease. Clinical and pathologic study. Arthritis Rheum., *25*:989–996, 1982.
27. Reginato, A.S., Schumacher, H.R., and Martinez, V.A.: The articular cartilage in familial chondrocalcinosis: Light and electron microscopic study. Arthritis Rheum., *17*:997–992, 1974.
28. Schumacher, H.R.: Ultrastructural findings in chondrocalcinosis and pseudogout. Arthritis Rheum., *19*:413–425, 1976.
29. Bennett, R.M., Lehr, J.R., and McCarty, D.J.: Crystal shedding and acute pseudogout: An hypothesis based on a therapeutic failure. Arthritis Rheum., *19*:93–97, 1976.
30. O'Duffy, J.D.: Clinical studies of acute pseudogout attacks: Prevalence, predisposition and treatment. Arthritis Rheum., *19*:349–352, 1976.
31. Bennett, R.M., Mall, J.C., and McCarty, D.J.: Pseudogout in acute neuropathic arthropathy. A clue to pathogenesis? Ann. Rheum. Dis., *33*:563–567, 1974.
32. Halverson, P.B., Cheung, H.S., and McCarty, D.J.: Enzymatic release of microspheroids containing hydroxyapatite crystals from synovium, and of calcium pyrophosphage dihydrate crystals from cartilage. Ann. Rheum. Dis., *41*:527–531, 1982.
33. Dorwart, B.B., and Shumacher, H.R.: Joint effusion, chondrocalcinosis and other rheumatic manifestations in hypothroidism. Am. J. Med., *59*:780–789, 1975.
34. Giclas, P.C., Ginsberg, M.H., and Cooper, N.R.: Immunoglobulin G independent activation of the classical complement pathways by monosodium urate crystals. J. Clin. Invest., *63*:759–765, 1979.
35. Terkeltaub, R., Tenner, A.J., Kozin, F., and Ginsberg, M.H.: Plasma protein binding by monosodium urate crystals. Analysis by two-dimensional gel electrophoresis. Arthritis Rheum., *26*:775–783, 1983.
36. Russell, I.J. et al.: Effects of IgG and C-reactive protein on complement depletion by monosodium urate crystals. J. Rheumatol., *10*:425–433, 1983.
37. Fields, T.R. et al.: Activation of the alternate pathway of complement of monosodium urate crystals. Clin. Immunol. Immunopathol., *26*:249–257, 1983.
38. Russell, I.J., Mansen, C., Kolb, L.M., and Kolb, W.P.: Activation of the fifth component of human complement (C5) induced by monosodium urate crystals: C5 convertase assembly on the crystal surface. Clin. Immunol. Immunopathol., *24*:239–250, 1982.
39. Kim, H.J., McCarty, D.J., Kozin, F., and Koethe, S.: Clinical significance of synovial fluid total hemolytic complement activity. J. Rheumatol., *7*:143–152, 1980.
40. Ginsberg, M.H., Jaques, B., Cochrane, C.G., and Griffin, J.H.: Urate crystal-dependent cleavage of Hageman factor in human plasma and synovial fluid. J. Lab. Clin. Med., *95*:497–506, 1980.
41. Melmon, K.L., Webster, M.E., Goldfinger, S.E., and Seegmiller, J.E.: The presence of kinin in inflammatory synovial effusion from arthritides of varying etiologies. Arthritis Rheum., *10*:13–20, 1967.
42. Cheung, H.S., Bohon, S., and Kozin, F.: Kinetics of collagenase and neutral protease release by neutrophils exposed to microcrystalline sodium urate. Con. Tissue Res., *2*:79–85, 1983.
43. Bhatt, A., and Spilberg, I.: Purification of crystal induced chemotactic factor from human neutrophils. Clinical Biochem., *21*:341–345, 1988.
44. Serhan, C.N. et al.: Formation of leukotrienes and hydroxy acids by human neutrophils and platelets exposed to monosodium urate. Prostaglandins, *17*:563–581, 1984.
45. Abramson, S., Hoffstein, S.T., and Weismann, G.: Superoxide anion generated by human neutrophils exposed to monosodium urate. Arthritis Rheum., *15*:174–180, 1982.
46. Spilberg, I., and Mandell, B.: Crystal-induced chemotactic factor. *In* Advances in Inflammation Research. Edited by G. Weissmann. New York, Raven Press, 1982.
47. Baggiolini, M., Walz, A., and Kunkel, S.L.: Neutrophil-activating peptide-1/interleukin-8, a novel cytokine that activates neutrophils. J. Clin. Invest. *84*:1045–1049, 1989.
48. Streiter, R.M. et al.: Disparate gene expression of chemotactic cytokines by human mononuclear phagocytes. Biochem. Biophys. Res. Commun., *166*:886–891, 1990.
49. Rae, A.A., Davidson, E.M., and Smith, M.J.H.: Leukotriene B4, an inflammatory mediator in gout. Lancet, *2*:1122–1123, 1982.
50. Di Giovine, F.S., Malawista, S.E., Nuki, G., and Duff, G.W.: Interleukin-1 (IL-1) as a mediator of crystal arthritis: Stimulation of T cell and synovial fibroblast mitogenesis by urate crystal-induced IL-1. J. Immunol., *138*:3213–3218, 1987.
51. Geurne, P.A., Terkeltaub, R., Zuraw, B., and Lotz, M.: Stimulation of IL-6 production in human monocytes and synoviocytes by inflammatory microcrystals. Arthritis Rheum., *32*:1443–1452, 1989.
52. Jaques, B.C., and Ginsberg, M.H.: The role of cell surface proteins in platelet stimulation by monosodium urate crystals. Arthritis Rheum., *25*:508–521, 1982.
53. Webster, M.E. et al.: Urate crystal-induced inflammation in the rat: Evidence of the combined actions of kinins, histamine and components of complement. Immunol. Commun., *1*:185–198, 1972.
54. Mandel, N.S.: The structural basis of crystal-induced membranolysis. Arthritis Rheum., *19*:439–455, 1976.
55. Herring, F.G., Lam, E., and Burt, H.M.: A spin label study of the membranolytic effects of crystalline monosodium urate monohydrate. J. Rheumatol., *13*:623–630, 1986.
56. Weissmann, G., and Rita, G.A.: Molecular basis of gouty inflammation: Interaction of monosodium urate crystals with lysosomes and liposomes. Nature [New Biol.], *240*:167–172, 1972.
57. Ginsberg, M.H., and Kozin, F.: Mechanisms of cellular interaction with monosodium urate crystals. Arthritis Rheum., *21*:896–903, 1978.
58. Ginsberg, M.H. et al.: Mechanisms of platelet response to monosodium urate crystals. Am. J. Pathol., *94*:549–568, 1979.
59. Burt, H.M., and Jackson, J.K.: Role of membrane proteins in monosodium urate crystal-membrane interactions: 2. Effect of pretreatments of erythrocyte membranes with membrane permeable and impermeable protein crosslinking agents. J. Rheumatol. *17*:1359–1363, 1990.
60. Weissmann, G., Zurier, R.B., Speiler, P.J., and Goldstein, I.M.: Mechanisms of lysosomal enzyme release from leukocytes exposed to immune complexes and other particles. J. Exp. Med., *134*:149–165, 1971.

61. Hoffstein, S., and Weissmann, G.: Mechanisms of lysosomal enzyme release from leukocytes: 4. Interaction of monosodium urate with dogfish and human leukocytes. Arthritis Rheum., *18*:153–165, 1975.
62. Schumacher, H.R., and Phelps, P.: Sequential changes in human polymorphonuclear leukocytes after urate crystal phagocytosis. Arthritis Rheum., *14*:513–526, 1971.
63. Terkeltaub, R. et al.: Lipoproteins containing apoprotein B are a major regulator of neutrophil responses to monosodium urate crystals. J. Clin. Invest., *73*:1719–1730, 1984.
64. Kane, A.B. et al.: Dissociation of intracellular lysosomal rupture from the cell death caused by silica. J. Cell. Biol., *87*:643–651, 1980.
65. Terkeltaub, R., Sklar, L.A., and Mueller, H.: Neutrophil activation by inflammatory microcrystals of monosodium urate monohydrate utilizes pertussis toxin-insensitive and sensitive pathways. J. Immunol., *144*:2719–2724, 1990.
66. Onello, E., Traynor-Kaplan, A., Sklar, L., and Terkeltaub, R.: Mechanism of neutrophil activation by an unopsonized inflammatory particulate: Monosodium urate crystals induce pertussis toxin-insensitive hydrolysis of phosphatidylinositol 4.5-bisphosphate. J. Immunol., *146*:4289–4299, 1991.
67. Bomalaski, J.S., Baker, D.G., Brophy, L.M., and Clark, M.A.: Monosodium urate crystals stimulate phospholipase A2 enzyme activities and the synthesis of a phospholipase A2-activating protein. J. Immunol., *145*:3391–3397, 1990.
68. Kimberly, R.P., Ahlstrom, J.W., Click, M.E., and Edberg, J.C.: The glycosyl phosphatidylinositol-linked FcgammaRIII$_{PMN}$ mediates transmembrane signalling events distinct from Fcgamma-RII. J. Exp. Med., *171*:1239–1255, 1990.
69. Webb, D.S.A. et al.: LFA-3, CD44, and CD45: Physiologic triggers of human monocyte TNF and IL-1 release. Science, *249*:1295–1297, 1990.
70. Steele, A.D., and McCarty, D.J.: An experimental model of acute inflammation in man. Arthritis Rheum., *9*:430–442, 1966.
71. Lotz, M., Carson, D., and Vaughan, J.H.: Substance P activation of rheumatoid synoviocytes: Neural pathway in pathogenesis of arthritis. Science, *235*:893–895, 1987.
72. Phelps, P., and McCarty, D.J.: Crystal-induced inflammation in canine joints: 2. Importance of polymorphonuclear leukocytes. J. Exp. Med., *124*(1):150, 1966.
73. Terkeltaub, R. et al.: Monocyte-derived neutrophil chemotactic factor/IL-8 as a potential mediator of crystal-induced synovitis. Arthritis Rheum., *34*:894–903, 1991.
74. McCarthy, G.M., Barthelemy, C.R., Veum, J.A., and Wortmann, R.L.: Influence of antihyperuricemic therapy on the clinical and radiographic progression of gout. (Abstract.) Arthritis Rheum., *33*:S54, 1990.
75. Spilberg, I., and Osterland, C.K.: Anti-inflammatory effect of the trypsin-kallikrein inhibitor in acute arthritis induced by urate crystals in rabbits. J. Lab. Clin. Med., *76*:472–479, 1970.
76. Webster, M.E. et al.: Urate crystal-induced inflammation in the rat: Evidence for the combined actions of kinins, histamine and components of complement. Immunol. Commun., *1*:185–198, 1973.
77. Green, D., Arsever, C.L., Grumet, K.A., and Ratnoff, O.D.: Classic gout in Hageman factor (factor XII) deficiency. Arch. Intern. Med., *142*:1556–1557, 1982.
78. Londino, A.V., and Luparello, F.J.: Factor XII deficiency in a man with gout and angioimmunoblastic lymphadenopathy. Arch. Intern. Med., *133*:1497–1498, 1984.
79. Spilberg, I.: Urate crystal arthritis in animals lacking Hageman factor. Arthritis Rheum., *17*:143–148, 1974.
80. Tate, G. et al.: Suppression of monosodium urate crystal-induced acute inflammation by diets enriched with gamma-linolenic acid and eicosapentaenoic acid. Arthritis Rheum., *31*:1543–1551, 1988.
81. Forrest, M.J., Aammit, V., and Brooks, P.M.: Inhibition of leucotriene B4 synthesis by BW 755c does not reduce polymorphonuclear leucocyte accumulation induced by monosodium urate crystals. Ann. Rheum. Dis., *47*:241–246, 1988.
82. Ortel, R.W., and Newcombe, D.S.: Acute gouty arthritis and response to colchicine in the virtual absence of synovial fluid leukocytes. N. Engl. J. Med., *190*:1363–1364, 1974.
83. Howell, R.R., and Seegmiller, J.E.: Uricolysis by human leukocytes. Nature, *196*:482–483, 1962.
84.. Colditz, I.G., and Movat, H.Z.: Desensitization of acute inflammatory lesions to chemotaxins and endotoxin. J. Immunol., *133*:2163–2168, 1984.
85. Cybulsky, M.I., Colditz, I.G., and Movat, H.Z.: The role of interleukin-1 in neutrophil leukocyte emigration induced by endotoxin. Am. J. Pathol., *124*:367–372, 1986.
86. Savill, J.S. et al.: Macrophage phagocytosis of aging neutrophils in inflammation. Programmed cell death in the neutrophil leads to its recognition by macrophages. J. Clin. Invest., *83*:865–875, 1989.
87. Haslett, C. et al.: Cessation of neutrophil influx in C5a-induced acute experimental arthritis is associated with loss of chemoattractant activity from the joint space. J. Immunol., *142*:3510–3517, 1989.
88. Arend, W.P., and Dayer, J.M.: Cytokines and cytokine inhibitors or antagonists in rheumatoid arthritis. Arthritis Rheum., *33*:305–315, 1990.
89. Tate, G.A., Mandell, B.F., Schumacher, H.R., and Zurier, R.: Suppression of acute inflammation by 15-methylprostaglandin E_1. Lab Invest., *59*:192–199, 1988.
90. Dubois, C.M. et al.: Transforming growth factor beta is a potent inhibitor of Interleukin 1 (IL-1) receptor expression: Proposed mechanism of inhibition of IL-1 action. J. Exp. Med., *172*:737–744, 1990.
91. Fava, R. et al.: Active and latent forms of transforming growth factor beta activity in synovial effusions. J. Exp. Med., *169*:291–296, 1989.
92. Aderka, D., Le, J., and Vilcek, J.: IL-6 inhibits lipopolysaccharide-induced tumor necrosis factor production in cultured human monocytes, U937 cells, and in mice. J. Immunol., *143*:3517–3523, 1989.
93. Huizinga, T.W.J. et al.: Soluble Fc gamma Receptor III in human plasma originates from release by neutrophils. J. Clin. Invest., *86*:416–423, 1990.
94. Porteau, F., and Nathan, C.: Shedding of tumor necrosis factor receptors by activated human neutrophils. J. Exp. Med., *172*:599–607, 1990.
95. Gordon, T.P., and Roberts-Thompson, P.J.: Preliminary evidence for the presence of an inhibitor on the surface of natural monosodium urae crystals. Arthritis Rheum., *29*:1172–1173, 1986.
96. Rosen, M.S., Baker, D.G., Schumacher, H.R., Jr., and Cherian, P.V.: Products of polymorphonuclear cell injury inhibit IgG enhancement of monosodium urate-induced superoxide production. Arthritis Rheum., *29*:1473–1479, 1986.
97. Arnold, W.J., and Simmons, R.A.: Clinical variability of the gouty diathesis. Adv. Exp. Med. Biol., *122A*:33–46, 1980.
98. Horowitz, M.D., Abbey, L., Sirota, D.K., and Spiera, H.: Intraarticular noninflammatory free urate suspension (urate milk) in 3 patients with painful joints. J. Rheumatol., *17*:712–714, 1990.
99. Hollingworth, P., Scott, J.T., and Burry, H.C.: Nonarticular gout: Hyperuricemia and tophus formation without gouty arthritis. Arthritis Rheum., *26*:98–101, 1983.
100. Buchanan, W.W., Klinenberg, J.R., and Seegmiller, J.E.: The

inflammatory response to injected microcrystalline monosodium urate in normal, hyperuricemic, gouty and uremic subjects. Arthritis Rheum., *8*:361–367, 1965.
101. Emmerson, B.T., Stride, P.J., and Williams, G.: The clinical differentiation of primary gout from primary renal disease in patients with both gout and renal disease. Adv. Exp. Med. Biol., *122A*:9–13, 1980.
102. Wallace, D.J. et al.: Coexistent gout and rheumatoid arthritis. Case report and literature review. Arthritis Rheum., *22*:81–86, 1979.
103. Brandt, K.D.: The effect of synovial hyaluronate on the ingestion of monosodium urate crystals by leukocytes. Clin. Chim. Acta, *55*:307–315, 1974.
104. Malawista, S.E., Van Blaricom, G.V., Cretella, S.B., and Schwartz, M.L.: The phlogistic potential of urate in solution. Studies of the phagocytic process in human leukocytes. Arthritis Rheum., *22*:728–736, 1979.
105. Antommattei, O., Schumacher, H.R., Reginato, A.J., and Clyburne, G.: Prospective study of morphology and phagocytosis of synovial fluid monosodium urate crystals in gouty arthritis. J. Rheumatol., *2*:741–744, 1984.
106. Kozin, F., Ginsberg, M.H., and Skosey, J.: Polymorphonuclear leukocyte responses to monosodium urate crystals: Modification by adsorbed serum protein. J. Rheumatol., *6*:519–528, 1979.
107. Terkeltaub, R., Smeltzer, D., Curtiss, L.K., and Ginsberg, M.H.: Low density lipoprotein inhibits the physical interaction of phlogistic crystals and inflammatory cells. Arthritis Rheum., *29*:363–370, 1986.
108. Terkeltaub, Martin, J., Curtiss, L.K., and Ginsberg, M.H.: Apolipoprotein B mediates the capacity of low density lipoprotein to suppress neutrophil stimulation by particulates. J. Biol. Chem., *261*:15662–15667, 1986.
109. Sokoloff, L: The pathology of gout. Metabolism, *6*:230–243, 1957.
110. Ortiz-Bravo, E. et al.: Immunolabeling of proteins coating monosodium urate (MSU) crystals in sequential samples from acute gouty arthritis and MSU-induced inflammation in the rat subcutaneous air pouch. (Abstract.) Arthritis Rheum., *33*:S55, 1990.
111. Terkeltaub, R., Dyer, C., Martin, J., and Curtiss, L.K.: Apolipoprotein E (apo E) inhibits the capacity of monosodium urate crystals to stimulate neutrophils: Characterization of intraarticular apo E and demonstration of apo E binding to urate crystals in vivo. J. Clin. Invest., *87*:20–26, 1991.
112. Hasselbacher, P.: C3 activation by monosodium urate monohydrate and other crystalline material. Arthritis. Rheum., *22*:571–578, 1979.
113. Malawista, S.E. et al.: Crystal-induced endogenous pyrogen production. A further look at gouty inflammation. Arthritis Rheum., *28*:1039–1046, 1985.
114. Hakim, F.T. et al.: Hereditary joint disorder in progressive ankylosis (ank/ank) mice: 1. Association of calcium hydroxyapatite deposition with inflammatory arthropathy. Arthritis Rheum., *27*:1141–1420, 1984.
115. Hakim, F.T., Brown, K.S., and Oppenheim, J.J.: Hereditary joint disorder in progressive ankylosis (ank/ank) mice: 2. Effect of high-dose hydrocortisone treatment on inflammation and intraarticular calcium hydroxyapatite deposits. Arthritis Rheum., *29*:114–123, 1986.
116. Swan, A., Dularay, B., and Dieppe, P.: A comparison of the effects of urate, hydroxyapatite and diamond crystals on polymorphonuclear cells: Relationship of mediator release to the surface area and adsorptive capacity of different particles. J. Rheumatol., *17*:1346–1352, 1990.
117. Terkeltaub, R., Santoro, D., and Mandel, G.: Serum and plasma inhibit neutrophil stimulation by hydroxyapatite crystals: Evidence that serum alpha 2 HS-glycoprotein is a potent and specific crystal-bound inhibitor. Arthritis Rheum., *31*:1081–1089, 1988.
118. Spilberg, I., Rosenberg, D., and Mandell, B.: Induction of arthritis by purified cell-derived chemotactic factor. J. Clin. Invest., *59*:582–585, 1977.
119. Dieppe, P. et al.: Changes in monosodium urate crystals on heating or grinding. Arthritis Rheum., *24*:975–976, 1981.
120. Dieppe, P.A. et al.: Apatite deposition disease. Lancet, *1*:266–270, 1976.
121. McCarty, D.J.: Pathogenesis and treatment of crystal-induced inflammation. *In* Arthritis and Allied Conditions. 10th Ed. Edited by D.J. McCarty. Philadephia, Lea & Febiger, 1983.
122. Gordon, T.P., Kowasko, I.C., James, M., and Roberts-Thompson, P.J.: Monosodium urate crystal-induced prostaglandin synthesis in the rat subcutaneous air pouch. Clin. Exp. Rheumatol., *3*:291–295, 1985.
123. Hutton, C.W. et al.: Systemic response to local urate crystal induced inflammation in man: A possible model to study the acute phase response. Ann. Rheum. Dis., *44*:533–536, 1985.
124. Wallace, S.W., and Singer, J.Z.: Therapy in Gout. Rheum. Dis. Clin. North Am., *14*:441–458, 1988.
125. Wallace, S.L., an Singer, J.Z.: Review: Systemic toxicity associated with the intravenous administration of colchicine–Guidelines for use. J. Rheumatol., *15*:495–499, 1988.
126. Spilberg, I. et al.: Colchicine and pseudogout. Arthritis Rheum., *23*:1062–1063, 1980.
127. Wallace, S.L.: The treatment of the acute attack of gout. Clin. Rheum. Dis., *3*:133–143, 1977.
128. Meed, S.D., and Spilberg, I.: Successful use of colchicine in acute polyarticular pseudogout. J. Rheumatol., *8*:689–691, 1981.
129. Roberts, W.M., Liang, M.H., and Stern, S.H.: Colchicine in acute gout. JAMA, *257*:1920–1921, 1987.
129a. Moreland, L.W., and Ball, G.V. Editorial: Colchicine and gout. Arthritis Rheum., *34*:782–786, 1991.
130. Sugio, K. et al.: Separation of tubulin-binding and anti-inflammatory activity in colchicine analogs and congeners. Life Sci., *40*:35–39, 1987.
131. Brossi, A. et al.: Colchicine and its analogues: Recent findings. Med. Res. Rev., *8*:77–94, 1988.
132. Yu, T.F., and Gutman, A.B.: Efficiency of colchicine prophylaxis in gout. Ann. Intern. Med., *55*:179–192, 1961.
133. Neuss, M.N.: Long-term colchicine administration leading to colchicine toxicity and death. Arthritis Rheum., *29*:448–449, 1986.
134. Kuncl, R.W. et al.: Colchicine myopathy and neuropathy. N. Engl. J. Med., *316*:1562–1568, 1987.
134a. Wallace, S.L., Singer, J.Z., Duncan, G.J., et al.: Renal failure predicts colchicine toxicity: Guidelines for the prophylactic use of colchicine in gout. J. Rheumatol., *18*:264–269, 1991.
135. Ertel, N.H., Mittler, J.C., and Akgun, S.: Radioimmunoassay for colchicine in plasma and urine. Science, *193*:233–239, 1976.
136. Dallaverde, F., Fan, P.T., and Chang, Y.H.: Mechanism of action of colchicine: 5. Neutrophil adherence and phagocytosis in patients with acute gout treated with colchicine. J. Pharmacol. Exp. Ther., *223*:197–202, 1982.
137. Reibman, J. et al.: Colchicine inhibits ionophore-induced formation of leukotriene B4 of microtubules. J. Immunol., *136*:1027–1032, 1986.
138. Reibman, J., Haines, K.A., Gude, D., and Weissmann, G.: Differences in signal transduction between Fc gamma receptors (Fc gamma R II, Fc gamma R 111) and FMLP receptors in neutrophils. Effects of colchicine on pertussis toxin sensitivity and diacyglycerol formation. J. Immunol., *146*:988–996, 1991.
139. Djeu, J.Y. et al.: Functional activation of neutrophils by recom-

binant monocyte-derived neutrophil chemotactic factor/IL-8. J. Immunol., *144*:2205–2210, 1990.
140. Ding, A.H., Porteau, P., Sanchez, F., and Nathan, C.F.: Down-regulation of tumor necrosis factor receptors on macrophages and endothelial cells by microtubule depolymerizing agents. J. Exp. Med., *171*:715–727, 1990.
141. Stodler, J., and Franke, W.: Colchicine binding of proteins in chromatin and membranes. Nature, *237*:237–238, 1972.
142. Wallace, S.L.: Colchicine analogs in the treatment of acute gout. Arthritis Rheum., *2*:389–396, 1959.
143. Gibson, T. et al.: Azopropazone—A treatment for hyperuricemia and gout. Br. J. Rheumatol., *23*:44–51, 1984.
144. Emmerson, B.T., Hazelton, R.A., and Whyte, I.M.: Comparison of the urate lowering effects of allopurinol and diflusinal. J. Rheumatol., *14*:335–337, 1987.
145. Groff, G.D., Frank, W.A., and Raddatz, D.A.: Systemic steroid therapy for acute gout: A clinical trial and review of the literature. Semin. Arthritis Rheum., *19*:329–336, 1990.
146. Axelrod, D., and Preston, S.: Comparison of parenteral adrenocorticotrophic hormone with oral indomethacin in the treatment of acute gout. Arthritis Rheum., *31*:803–805.
147. Kahl, L.E., Thompson, M.E., and Griffith, B.P.: Gout in the heart transplant recipient: Physiologic puzzle and therapeutic challenge. Am. J. Med., *87*:289–294, 1989.
148. Alvarellos, A., and Spilberg, I.: Colchicine prophylaxis in pseudogout. J. Rheumatol., *13*:804–805, 1986.

108

Calcium Pyrophosphate Crystal Deposition Disease; Pseudogout; Articular Chondrocalcinosis

LAWRENCE M. RYAN
DANIEL J. McCARTY

Microscopic examination of wet preparations of synovial fluid under compensated polarized light has provided a rapid, specific, and sensitive method for identification of crystals in gout, which might be called monosodium urate (MSU) crystal deposition disease.[1] See Chapters 5 and 110 for a discussion of this and other techniques of crystal identification. Application of polarized light microscopic examination of synovial fluids led to the discovery of nonurate crystals in patients with a gout-like syndrome termed pseudogout.[2] These biaxial crystals were identified as calcium pyrophosphate dihydrate ($Ca_2P_2O_7 \cdot 2H_2O$, or CPPD)[3] (Fig. 108–1A). Like MSU crystals, CPPD exhibited monoclinic and triclinic dimorphism and frequently showed twinning. Polariscopically, they had a weakly positive birefringence and inclined extinction. Some crystals were isotropic under polarized light (nonrefractile). Urate crystals, on the other hand, were negatively birefringent under compensated polarized light and showed axial extinction. Fluid removed from acutely inflamed joints of patients with pseudogout invariably showed phagocytosed CPPD crystals (Fig. 108–1B).

Both MSU and CPPD crystals with morphologic features identical to natural crystals were synthesized.[4–6] Injection of such crystals into normal human and canine joints was followed by an acute inflammatory response. The phrase *crystal-induced synovitis* was coined to describe the tissue reaction provoked by either type of crystal,[7] and the responsible mechanisms are discussed in Chapter 108.

NOMENCLATURE

We initially termed the syndrome associated with CPPD deposition *pseudogout* because of the obvious parallel with true (urate) gout.[2] Many patients with symptomatic arthritis, however, do not have acute attacks, so this term should be reserved for the acute episodes associated with CPPD crystals. The term *chondrocalcinosis* was coined by Zitnan and Sitaj, based on the characteristic radiologic features.[8] Because subsequent analysis of cartilage calcifications showed at least three distinct mineral phases, this term is too broad and nonspecific, although it may suffice to indicate radiologic cartilage calcifications when crystal identification is lacking. *Pyrophosphate arthropathy* was coined in 1969 by H.L.F. Currey and is widely used in the United Kingdom.[9] No reason appears to justify blaming pyrophosphate for the arthropathy. Indeed, the calcium component of the crystal is responsible for most of its biologic effects (see Chapter 109). It appears most prudent to use the specific term *CPPD crystal deposition disease* unless some good reason can be found to abandon it.

EARLY REPORTS

Initially, seven patients were studied, using the presence of microcrystalline CPPD as a common denominator (see Fig. 108–1A). The radiographic appearance of calcification of fibroarticular and hyaline articular cartilage was noted (see Fig. 108–1C). Analysis of such deposits

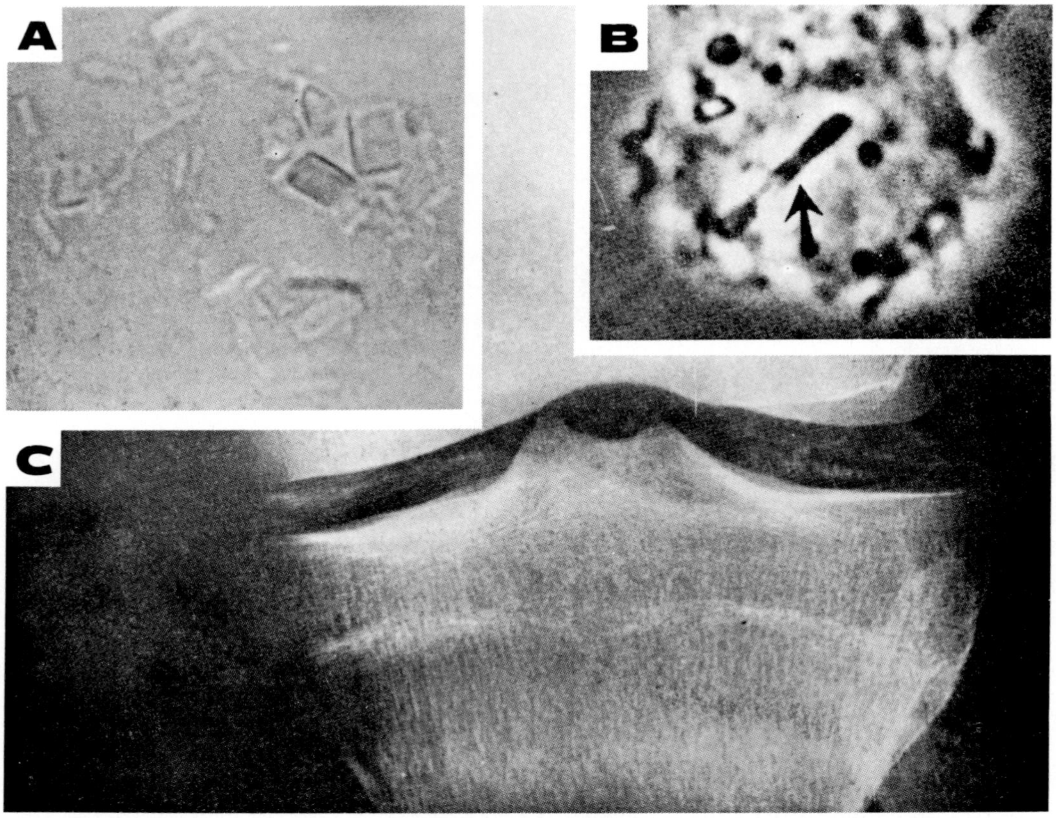

FIGURE 108–1. *A*, Weakly birefringent monoclinic and triclinic calcium pyrophosphate dihydrate (CPPD) microcrystals in synovial fluid removed from a chronically symptomatic knee (polarized light × 1250). *B*, Phagocytosed crystal (*arrow*) in a polymorphonuclear leukocyte (phase contrast × 1250). *C*, Anteroposterior roentgenogram of the knee showing typical punctate and linear deposits of CPPD in the menisci and articular hyaline cartilage.

showed CPPD crystals identical to those seen in joint fluid.

In addition to pseudogout attacks and a chronic degenerative arthropathy, other findings in this initial group of patients have been confirmed by subsequent separate reports. For example, a destructive arthropathy resembling Charcot joints, radiologic lesions resembling osteochondromas, hemorrhagic joint fluids, prominent subchondral cysts, and urate crystals associated with gouty arthritis were all documented at least once in our initial series. When the clinical and roentgenographic findings in this group were analyzed, a review of the literature revealed a similarity to chondrocalcinosis polyarticularis (familiaris), as described in 1958 by Zitnan and Sitaj.[8] These workers used the characteristic roentgenographic appearance as the unifying diagnostic feature. They pointed out that the menisci of the knee were most commonly involved (see Fig. 108–1C). These authors later reported 27 cases, 21 from 5 Hungarian families living in a single village in Slovakia.[10]

Perhaps the first report of CPPD deposition was made in 1903 by Bennett.[11] He described autopsy findings in an elderly man of mineral deposits in cartilages of the hips, shoulders, sternoclavicular joints, and temporomandibular joints. Chemical analysis indicated a substantial calcium and carbonate content, but no urates by the murexide test. The individual crystals were described as smaller than urate crystals and rhomboidal in shape under an ordinary light microscope. Other historical reports have been reviewed earlier.[12]

PREVALENCE

A summary of reported anatomic and radiologic studies of the prevalence of knee joint calcification has been presented earlier.[12] The study of elderly Jewish subjects by Ellman and Levin, using high-resolution film, is of particular interest.[13] Fully 27.6% of their ambulatory volunteers showed calcific deposits. Assuming that all were CPPD deposits, this finding implicated age as a factor in the expression of the condition. These findings have been confirmed by a report using standard radiograms of the knee in 108 women over 80 years of age.[14] Meniscal calcification was found in 16% of the 55 women aged 80 to 89 and in 30% of 53 women aged

89 to 99; 22 of 25 with chondrocalcinosis had deposits in other joints as well. A radiographic survey of patients admitted to a geriatric unit disclosed a 44% prevalence of chondrocalcinosis in patients over 84 years of age, when films of the hands and wrist, pelvis, and knees were examined.[15] The prevalence was 15% in patients between 65 and 74 years of age and 36% in those between 75 and 84 years.

X-ray diffraction powder patterns were obtained from at least one tissue deposit or from crystals harvested from synovial fluid in 51 of our first 80 cases; all were CPPD. A study of over 800 menisci from 215 anatomic cadavers was undertaken, using the CPPD crystal as a "marker."[16] At least one tiny deposit was seen in the type-M roentgenogram of 22% of excised menisci; most were too small to permit dissection, much less identification. Seven sets of menisci (3.2% of cadavers) showed linear and punctate deposits of CPPD; five sets (2.3% of cadavers) showed multiple punctate deposits of dicalcium phosphate dihydrate ($CaHPO_4 \cdot 2H_2O$, or DCPD); three single menisci (1.4% of cadavers) showed solitary deposits of "hydroxyapatite." Studies now suggest the term *basic calcium phosphate* (BCP) instead of hydroxyapatite (see Chapter 109). Four cadavers in this series had sodium urate deposits in the menisci.

A survey of a large number of pathologic nonarticular calcifications using crystallographic techniques showed no CPPD crystals and thus established their relative specificity for articular tissue.[17] Identification of crystals in aortic plaques, costal cartilages, pancreas, and pineal glands obtained from pseudogout patients at necropsy showed only "apatite." Periarticular deposits of crystallographically proved CPPD, however, have been reported in tendons, dura mater, ligamenta flava, and the olecranon bursa, as well as in isolated "tophi."[12]

JOINT FLUID FINDINGS

Nearly all fluids aspirated from inflamed joints showed phagocytosed CPPD microcrystals (Fig. 108–1B). Unlike urate crystals, they were often within phagolysosomes.[2] CPPD crystals are much more difficult to see by polarized light microscopy than are MSU crystals, and we routinely use phase-contrast in addition to polarized light at thousandfold magnification for crystal identification. Even using these sensitive techniques, ultramicrocrystals cannot be detected.[18,19] The number of crystals bears some relation to the acuteness of inflammation because pellets from joint fluid taken during acute attacks contained much more pyrophosphate on chemical analysis then did pellets from noninflamed joints.[12] Exceptions occur, however. Some fluids from inflamed joints have few CPPD crystals, and some fluids from noninflamed joints are milky because of the large number of crystals present. This same phenomenon has been noted in true gout. The mean leukocyte concentration in acute attacks is exactly the same as in urate gout, about 20,000/mm^3, with over 90% polymorphonuclear (PMN) cells. As already noted, the fluid in pseudogout may be tinged with blood, especially early in the acute episode.[12] In at least one case, such fluid was associated with subchondral bony fractures.[20] Synovial fluids containing CPPD crystals more often than not also contain BCP. Of 30 CPPD-containing knee fluids in one study, 22 showed BCP also.[21]

DIAGNOSTIC CRITERIA

A diagnostic classification, based on the premise that CPPD crystals are the specific feature of the disease,[7] has been modified to include radiographic clues suggested by Resnick[22] and Martel[23] (Table 108–1). A case is considered "definite" if CPPD crystals are demonstrated in tissues or synovial fluid by definitive means or if crystals compatible with CPPD are demonstrated by compensated polarized light microscopy and typical calcifications are seen on roentgenograms. If only one of these criteria is found, a "probable" diagnosis is made. The clinical findings or the radiologic clues given in Table 108–1 should alert the clinician to the possible presence of underlying CPPD crystal deposition disease.

CLINICAL FEATURES

In our series of over 1000 "definite" and "probable" cases, men predominate in a ratio of 1.5 : 1. A similar sex ratio was recorded at the Mayo Clinic.[24] Female predominance has been reported in other surveys of patients with symptomatic CPPD deposition.[25,26] Our patients' ages averaged 72 years at the time of diagnosis.

The various patterns of arthritis encountered clinically are summarized graphically in Figure 108–2. We regard CPPD deposition as a great mimic because it often superficially resembles not only gout, but also rheumatoid arthritis (RA), osteoarthritis, and other types of joint disease.[9,27]

TYPE A—PSEUDOGOUT

The pseudogout pattern is marked by acute or subacute arthritic attacks lasting from 1 day to 4 weeks. These episodes are self-limited and generally involve only one or a few appendicular joints. Such attacks can be as severe as those of true gout, but they usually take longer to reach peak intensity and are less painful and disabling. Inflammation may begin in a single "mother" joint with spread to involve other nearby "daughter" joints the so-called *cluster attack* of the crystal deposition diseases. Mild "petite" attacks also occur, as in urate gout, and these may often outnumber full-blown attacks. Such attacks produce local effusions, joint stiffness, and warmth of the overlying skin, but they are not painful. Leukocytosis is noted in the synovial fluid. Injection of CPPD crystals into the joints of volunteers confirms that the inflammatory response is dose related. Pain is the last symptom to appear and the first to disappear.

TABLE 108–1. DIAGNOSTIC CRITERIA FOR CALCIUM PYROPHOSPHATE DIHYDRATE CRYSTAL DEPOSITION DISEASE (PSEUDOGOUT)

Criteria

I. Demonstration of CPPD crystals, obtained by biopsy, necropsy, or aspirated synovial fluid, by definitive means; e.g., characteristic "fingerprint" by x-ray diffraction powder pattern or by chemical analysis.

II. A. Identification of monoclinic or triclinic crystals showing a weakly positive, or a lack of, birefringence by compensated polarized light microscopy.

B. Presence of typical calcifications on roentgenograms.*

III. A. Acute arthritis, especially of knees or other large joints, with or without concomitant hyperuricemia.

B. Chronic arthritis, especially of knees, hips, wrists, carpus, elbow, shoulder, and metacarpophalangeal joints, particularly if accompanied by acute exacerbations; the chronic arthritis shows the following features helpful in differentiating it from osteoarthritis.[22]

1. Uncommon site for primary osteoarthritis; e.g., wrist metacarpophalangeal joints, elbow, or shoulder.
2. Radiographic appearance; e.g., radiocarpal or patellofemoral joint space narrowing, especially if isolated (patella "wrapped around" the femur†); femoral cortical erosion superior to the patella on the lateral view of the knee.
3. Subchondral cyst formation.
4. Severe progressive degeneration, with subchondral bony collapse (microfractures), and fragmentation, with formation of intra-articular radiodense bodies.
5. Variable and inconstant osteophyte formation.
6. Tendon calcifications, especially of Achilles, triceps, and obturator tendons.
7. Involvement of the axial skeleton with subchondral cysts of apophyseal and sacroiliac joints, multiple levels of disc calcification and vacuum phenomenon, and sacroiliac vacuum phenomenon.

Categories

A. Definite—criteria I or II(A) and (B) must be fulfilled.

B. Probable—criteria IIA or IIB must be fulfilled.

C. Possible—criteria IIIA or B should alert the clinician to the possibility of underlying CPPD deposition.

CPPD = calcium pyrophosphate dihydrate (CPPD); DCPD = dicalcium phosphate dihydrate.

*Heavy punctate and linear calcifications in fibrocartilages, articular (hyaline) cartilages, and joint capsules, especially if bilaterally symmetric; faint or atypical calcifications may be due to DCPD ($CaHPO_4 \cdot 2H_2O$) deposits or to vascular calcifications; both are also often bilaterally symmetric.

† Also described as a feature of the arthritis of hyperparathyroidism.

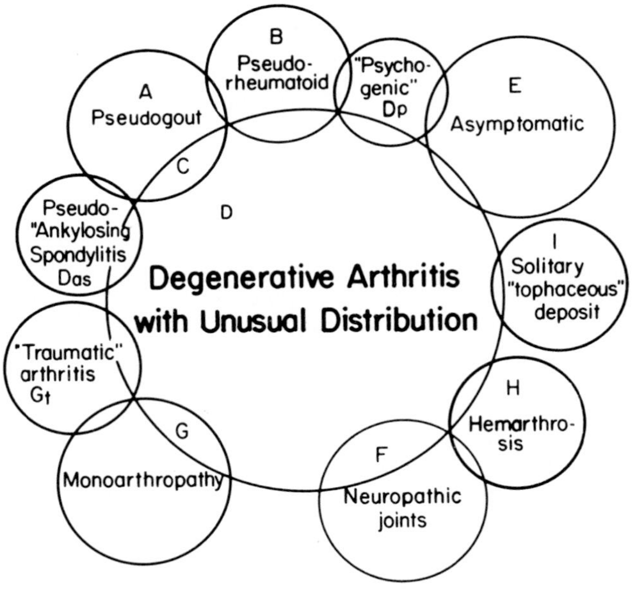

FIGURE 108–2. Diagrammatic representation of various clinical presentations of joint disease associated with calcium pyrophosphate dihydrate crystal deposition. (From McCarty, D.: The Heberden Oration, 1982. Crystals, joints, and consternation. Ann. Rheum. Dis., *42*:243–253, 1983.)

Provocation of acute episodes by a surgical procedure or by medical illness is common in both gout and pseudogout. One study reported that the percentage of patients with either disease who had at least a single episode after operation was virtually identical: 8.3% of 168 gouty patients and 9.4% of 106 patients with pseudogout.[27] Parathyroidectomy is particularly likely to precipitate acute arthritis.[24,28] Similarly, severe medical illness, particularly vascular occlusion such as stroke or myocardial infarction, provoked attacks in 20.3% of 167 gouty subjects, as opposed to 24% of 104 patients with pseudogout. Trauma may provoke acute arthritis in patients with either gout or pseudogout. Because both types of crystals are often found in the same subject and because either may cause self-limited attacks under identical clinical circumstances and may respond similarly to treatment, joint aspiration and specific crystal identification are essential for precise differential diagnosis.

The knee joint is to pseudogout as the bunion joint is to gout, and it is the site of over half of all acute attacks. At least 11 crystal-proved instances of first metatarsophalangeal joint involvement are known to us.

Although not nearly as predictably effective as in urate gout, oral colchicine may provide dramatic relief in pseudogout. The release of a chemotactic factor by PMN leukocytes after phagocytosis of either MSU or CPPD crystals[29] (see Chapter 107) is inhibited by colchicine in concentrations easily reached in serum by the usual therapeutic doses. The inhibition of urate crys-

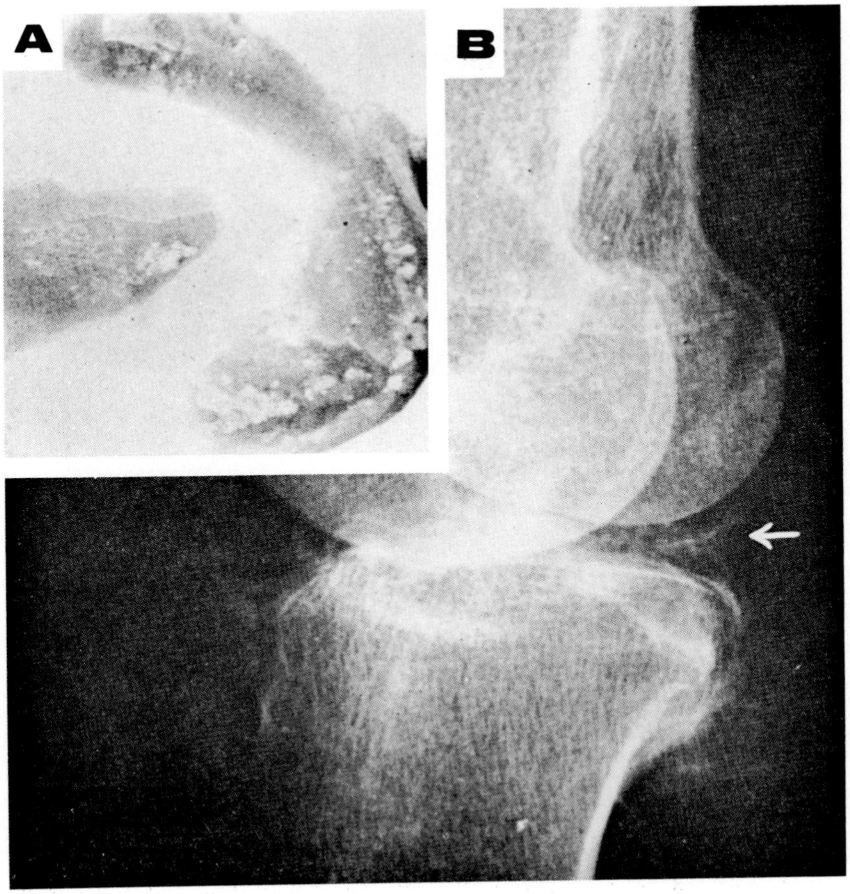

FIGURE 108–3. *A*, Meniscus excised at necropsy showing punctate and linear aggregates of calcium pyrophosphate dihydrate microcrystals; a wedge of articular cartilage from the tibial plateau shows similar deposits. *B*, Lateral roentgenogram of the knee showing the typical Y-shaped appearance of meniscal calcification (*arrow*).

tal–induced release was more predictable than the inhibition induced by CPPD crystals, which provides in vitro results parallel to the clinical experience in patients. Spilberg and associates found that colchicine, 1 to 2 mg, given intravenously predictably controls acute attacks of pseudogout.[30]

Approximately 20% of patients with CPPD deposits have hyperuricemia, and about 5% have MSU crystal deposits as well. About 25% of our series of patients show this gout-like, type A pattern. Men predominate. As in gout, the patients are usually completely asymptomatic between attacks. Radiographic evidence of CPPD deposits is found in most patients with this pattern of disease (Figs. 108–3A and B, and 108–4 and 108–5).

TYPE B—PSEUDORHEUMATOID ARTHRITIS

Approximately 5% of patients have multiple joint involvement with subacute attacks lasting 4 weeks to several months. Nonspecific symptoms of inflammation, such as morning stiffness and fatigue, are common; signs such as synovial thickening, localized pitting edema, limitation of joint motion that is due to inflammation or to flexion contractures, and elevated erythrocyte sedimentation rates are found. Such patients are often thought to have RA.[31] In addition, because about 10% of patients with CPPD-related arthritis have positive tests for rheumatoid factor (RF),[27] albeit usually in low titer, the opportunities for confusion abound. The presence of high titers of RF and typical radiographic erosions favor a diagnosis of "true" RA.[32] Interestingly, urate gout may also present with polyarticular involvement, RFs in 10% of cases, and symptoms mimicking those of RA.[33]

CPPD deposits have been described both histologically[34] and radiographically[35] in patients with presumably bona fide RA. By chance alone, at least 1% of patients with CPPD joint deposits would be expected to have RA. This figure agrees with the finding of nine cases of true RA in our series. A lower incidence (3%) of joint cartilage calcification in RA subjects was found in one study as compared to controls (14%), but the high incidence in the latter group, whose average age was 64.8 years, is more than is usually observed in an asymptomatic population.[36] This disparity may be due to the use as controls of patients presenting to the emergency unit with knee pain. Conversely, we have studied over 1000 cases of crystal-proved urate gout and only 1 showed a coincidence with RA. This patient had rheumatoid nodules, RF, hyperuricemia, and an ear tophus; the articular disease has unequivocally RA. The appar-

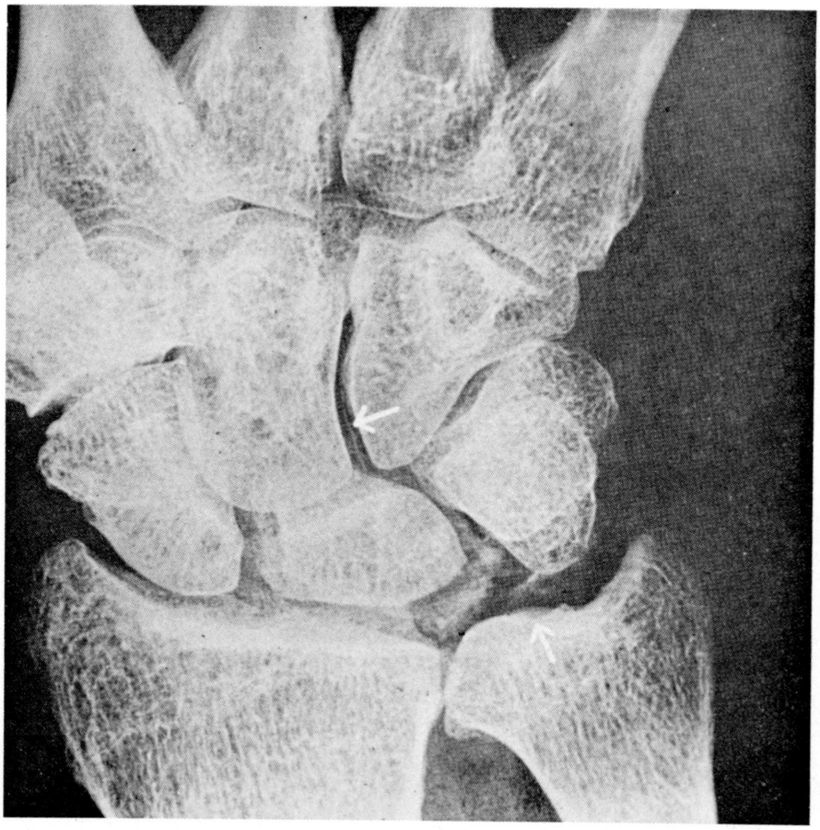

FIGURE 108–4. Anteroposterior roentgenogram of the wrist showing calcification of the fibrocartilaginous articular disc and a fine line of calcification parallel to the radiodensity of the underlying bone, indicative of articular cartilage calcification (*arrow*).

ent negative association of urate gout and RA probably does not hold for CPPD deposits and RA.

The type-B pattern is intended to apply only to patients (1) whose joints are inflamed "out of phase" with one another, as in gout, rather than "in phase," as in RA; (2) who form osteophytes; (3) who have CPPD crystals in joint fluid leukocytes; and (4) who do not have typical radiographic erosive disease. When RA and CPPD crystal deposition coexist, the typical radiographic appearance of the former is said to be atypical for RA.[36] Asymmetric disease, retained bone density, prominent osteophytes, well-corticated cysts, and paucity of erosions were found in 7 of 10 patients thought to have both diseases. It seems probable that those 7 patients actually had the *pseudorheumatoid* pattern of CPPD crystal deposition.

A variant of pseudorheumatoid arthritis (type B) can cause confusion clinically. The patient, usually elderly, has multiple acutely inflamed joints, marked leukocytosis, fever of 102 to 104° F, and mental confusion or disorientation.[37] Systemic sepsis is suspected by the attending physicians, and antibiotics have usually been prescribed despite negative cultures. The entire clinical picture reverses with anti-inflammatory drug therapy.

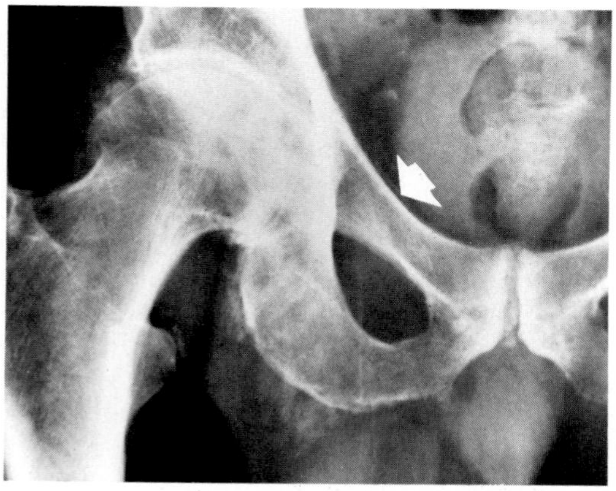

FIGURE 108–5. Calcific deposits in the symphysis pubis, the hyaline cartilage, and the acetabular labrum of the hip, the origin of the adductor tendons on the ischium and lesser trochanter, and Copper's ligament (arrow). (Courtesy of Dr. Harry K. Genant.)

TYPES C AND D—PSEUDO-OSTEOARTHRITIS

Approximately half of our patients have progressive degeneration of multiple joints (Figs. 108–6 to 108–8). Women predominate. The knees are most commonly affected, followed by the wrists, metacarpophalangeal joints, hips, spine, shoulder, elbows, and ankles. Involvement is generally bilaterally symmetric, although the degenerative process may be much further advanced on one side, especially in joints that have been

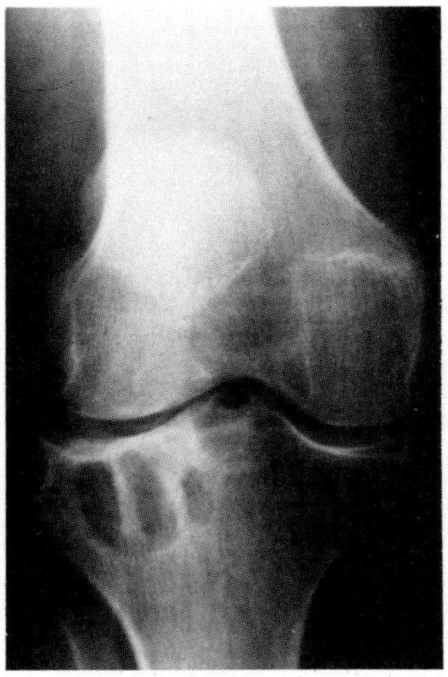

FIGURE 108–6. Subchondral bone cyst under the lateral tibial plateau in a patient with generalized calcium pyrophosphate dihydrate deposition and hyperparathyroidism.

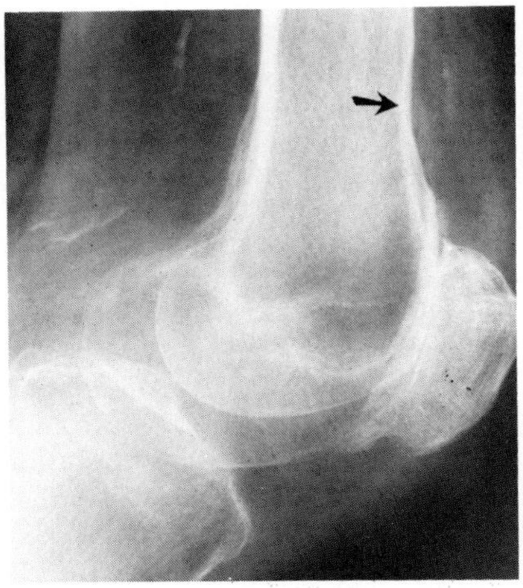

FIGURE 108–7. Lateral roentgenograms of the knee showing peculiar erosion of the femoral cortex superior to the patella (arrow). Note the patella "wrapped around" the femur. (Courtesy of Dr. Harry K. Genant.)

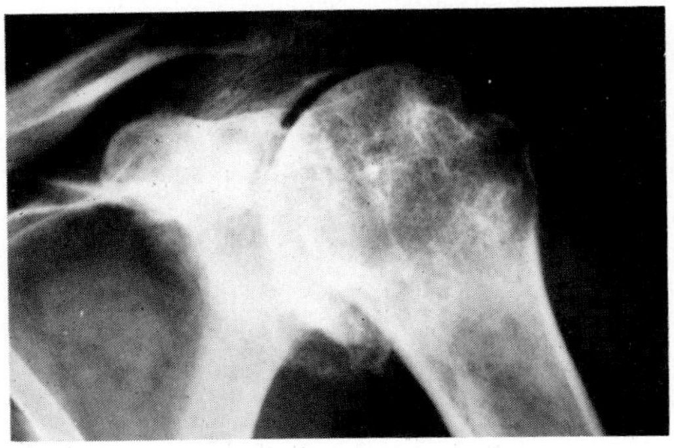

FIGURE 108–8. Anteroposterior roentgenogram of the shoulder showing neurotrophic joint appearance with extensive cystic bone lesions and powdered bony fragments in the synovial recesses inferiorly.

subjected to fracture or trauma. Flexion contractures of the involved joints are common. CPPD crystal deposition should be suspected in patients with bilateral or unilateral valgus deformity, or flexion contractures of the knees, especially if accompanied by osteophytes and flexion contractures of other joints not usually affected by primary osteoarthritis, such as the wrists, elbows, shoulders, and metacarpophalangeal joints.

About 25% of the total series, or about half of those with types C and D disease, have a history of episodic, superimposed acute attacks and have been classified as type C. Those without an apparent inflammatory component have been classified as type D.

Characteristic CPPD deposits may or may not be visible on radiographs of involved joints. CPPD crystals are often found in radiographically negative joints, especially those with extensive degenerative change. Serial radiographic studies by Zitnan and Sitaj contain examples of joints with obvious CPPD deposits at an early phase of the disease that may be difficult to discern when severe degeneration has supervened.[38] Fine-detail roentgenograms are helpful in the detection of small or faint deposits.[39]

Martel and co-workers,[40] as well as Hamilton and his colleagues,[41] have described squaring of bone ends, subchondral cystic changes, and hooklike osteophytes, especially in the metacarpophalangeal joints. Atkins and associates compared the radiographic features of metacarpophalangeal degeneration in sporadic CPPD crystal deposition disease with that associated with hemochromatosis; they found more severe changes in a greater proportion of patients with hemochromatosis-associated CPPD.[42]

Resnick and his colleagues have studied patients with CPPD deposition using age- and sex-matched control subjects. Useful diagnostic clues have been incorporated into the criteria outlined in Table 108–1. Axial skeleton involvement is frequent and is characterized by calcification of the anulus fibrosus, multiple levels of disc degeneration with vacuum phenomenon and subchondral erosions, and vacuum phenomena of the sacroiliac joints.[22,23]

The pattern of joint degeneration in types C and D (e.g., wrists, metacarpophalangeal joints, elbow, and shoulder) is clearly different from that of primary osteoarthritis (e.g., proximal and distal interphalangeal and first carpometacarpal joints). The knee is commonly affected in both conditions. Concomitant Heberden's and Bouchard's nodes, as well as other stigmata of primary osteoarthritis, often coexist with the pattern of joint involvement peculiar to CPPD crystal deposition, probably a chance association of two common conditions in elderly persons.

TYPE E—LANTHANIC (ASYMPTOMATIC) CALCIUM PYROPHOSPHATE DIHYDRATE CRYSTAL DEPOSITION

Type E CPPD crystal deposition may be the most common of all. Most joints with CPPD deposits plainly visible on roentgenograms are not symptomatic, even in patients with acute or chronic symptoms in other joints. Wrist complaints and genu varus deformities, but not acute joint inflammation, were more common in patients with CPPD deposits than in control subjects from the same population.[13]

TYPE F—PSEUDONEUROPATHIC JOINTS

One of the patients in our original report had a Charcot-like arthropathy of a knee in the absence of neurologic abnormality.[2] Subsequently, three of four cases of "neuropathic" arthritis of the knees associated with polyarticular CPPD deposition had mild tabes dorsalis; the fourth case also had late latent syphilis, but no neurologic abnormality.[43] One of these patients later developed an acute Charcot joint with hemorrhagic joint fluid and acute pseudogout.[20] Other reports of destructive arthropathy similar to neurotrophic arthropathy in patients with CPPD deposits and normal neurologic examinations underscore this association.[44–47] Severe degeneration of the neuropathic type has even been reported in the temporomandibular joints.[48]

Charcot knee joints develop in only 5 to 10% of patients with tabes dorsalis. Because our three cases were seen consecutively and because CPPD deposition affects about 5% of the adult population, the two conditions might be expected to coexist by chance alone in only 1 of 20 tabetics with Charcot joints. Thus, it was postulated that neurotrophic joints actually develop in the 5% of tabetic patients who have underlying CPPD crystal deposition.[43] That CPPD crystals alone can be associated with a destructive arthropathy, without the help of a neurologic deficit, reinforces this hypothesis (see Fig. 108–8).

OTHER PATTERNS OF CRYSTAL DEPOSITION

Multiple other patterns of disease have been described.[9] Stiffening of the spine that mimics ankylosing or diffuse idiopathic skeletal hyperostosis has been observed, particularly in familial CPPD deposition.[10,47] True bony ankylosis was observed in the Chilean series of familial cases, and none of the affected individuals were HLA-B27 positive.[49]

Neurologic presentations of CPPD crystal deposition are increasingly recognized. A syndrome of acute neck pain ascribed to CPPD or BCP deposits associated with a tomographic appearance of calcification surrounding the odontoid process has been termed the *"crowned dens" syndrome.*[50] At times neck pain has been accompanied by stiffness and fever so as to mimic meningitis.[51] Other patients have developed long tract signs and symptoms related to deposits of CPPD crystals and adjacent tissue hypertrophy in the cervical spine.[52–55] The ligamentum flavum has been the most regularly reported cervical site of CPPD crystal deposition (Fig. 108–9). Crystal deposits, ligament hypertrophy, and chondroid metaplastic growths all contribute to encroachment on the cord. Less frequent involvement of the posterior longitudinal ligament or facet joints has been reported.[56,57] Excised surgical samples have shown chondroid metaplasia, occasional matrix vesicles, and CPPD crystals. BCP crystals have also been noted. Surgical decompression has generally been effective.

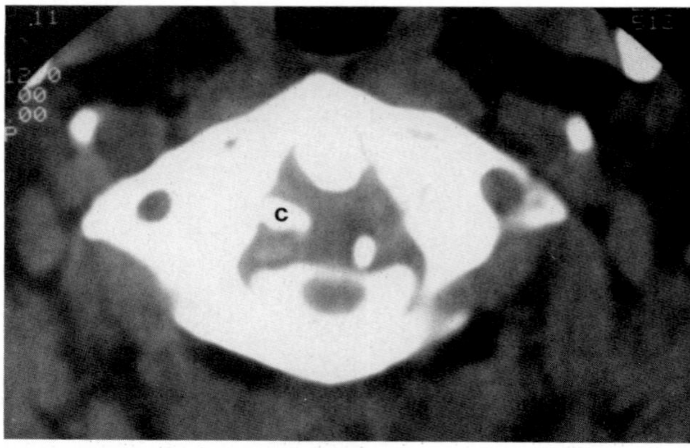

FIGURE 108–9. Excess calcification (C) at C_{1-2} level in a patient with chondrocalcinosis and long tract signs. Surgical specimen revealed crystal deposits in metaplastic fibrocartilage.

Monoarticular inflammation or degeneration may occur in CPPD secondary to trauma or attendant operations. This presentation is particularly common in the knee, years after meniscectomy,[58] after operations to remove osteochondral fragments in osteochondritis dissecans,[59] or in disc fibrocartilage after lumbar surgical procedures.[60,61]

The frequent finding (8%) of polymyalgia rheumatica in a series from the United Kingdom suggests that CPPD deposition may mimic the proximal stiffness, pain, and elevated erythrocyte sedimentation rate of polymyalgia rheumatica.[25] Rarely, a localized, progressively destructive, solitary, "tophaceous" mass of CPPD crystals occurs in synovial tissue with chondroid metaplasia. Seven cases have been reported, six in humans, and one in the paw of a 12-year-old golden retriever.[12]

It is clear from the long-term observations of the natural history of CPPD joint deposition in familial cases by Zitnan and Sitaj that a given patient may show one pattern of arthritis early in the course of the disease and a different pattern later; many type-A patients may eventually have pattern C, D, or F, for example.[38]

Systemic findings during an acute attack are frequent but not invariable.[2] These include a fever of 99 to 103° F, leukocytosis of 12 to 15,000/mm³ with a "left shift," and an elevated erythrocyte sedimentation rate and serum acute-phase reactants. Interleukin-6 may mediate some of these systemic effects.[62]

CALCIUM PYROPHOSPHATE DIHYDRATE DEPOSITS IN ANIMALS

CPPD crystals have been identified in the cartilages of a barbary ape in elderly rhesus monkeys and in dogs.[12] Calcifications in old rabbits have also been found, but were composed of BCP rather than of CPPD.

ETIOLOGIC CLASSIFICATION

A tentative classification is given in Table 108–2. The genetic aberrations responsible for each of the 10 largest reported series of *hereditary* cases probably differ. Table 108–3 lists the evidence. Most families show disease transmission as an autosomal dominant trait. The Hungarian group has an HLA association, no male-to-male transmission, and symptomatic heterozygotes. Five of the other series showed male-to-male transmission of disease, indicating autosomal inheritance. Because nearly half the offspring of a heterozygote in all series eventually developed radiographic evidence of CPPD crystal deposition, penetrance is nearly complete. "Associated" metabolic conditions, such as hyperparathyroidism, were rare in any of these kindreds. Phenotypic manifestations of the disease were severe in some kindreds and mild in others. The Hungarian homozygotes had severe disease, and the heterozygotes developed milder disease.

The so-called *sporadic* or idiopathic cases deserve comment. Generally, no systematic search for the condition had been conducted among blood relatives, and none of the putative metabolic disease associations had been found. We examined 1 or more relatives clinically and radiologically in 12 of the first 18 cases and found 3 examples of familial disease. Such a study is difficult in the United States in view of the extreme mobility of our citizens and the widespread psychologic resistance to submit to study because of possible discovery of abnormality. In Spain, a study of 46 apparently "sporadic" cases revealed a familial incidence in 5 (11%).[63] This finding could represent a coincidence of sporadic cases in aged subjects. Other surveys in Spain noted a 27 to 28% prevalence of familial CPPD deposition, defined as at least one other blood relative with evidence of CPPD deposits.[64,65] It is likely that a thorough study of "sporadic cases" would result in reclassification of many as either hereditary or as associated with metabolic disease.

TABLE 108–2. ETIOLOGIC CLASSIFICATION OF CALCIUM PYROPHOSPHATE DIHYDRATE CRYSTAL DEPOSITION DISEASE

I.	Hereditary (see Table 108–3)
II.	Sporadic (idiopathic)
III.	Associated with metabolic disease (see Table 109–4)
IV.	Associated with trauma or surgical procedures

ASSOCIATED DISEASES

A number of metabolic diseases and physiologic stresses, such as aging and trauma, have been associated with CPPD crystal deposition. Only aging and previous joint surgery have been statistically proved to be associated with CPPD deposition. Nonetheless, strong circumstantial evidence suggests that many of these associations are "true," and the converse has often been proved; that is, that radiographically evident chondrocalcinosis occurred more frequently in patients with several of these conditions, notably gout,[66] hemochromatosis,[67] and hyperparathyroidism,[68] than in age- and sex-matched control populations. Even when associations seem significant, however, a cause-and-effect relationship should not be inferred. If it is assumed that the putative associations are real, an immediate generalization is that all the metabolic diseases listed in Table 108–4 affect connective tissue metabolism in some way.

Reported associations must be interpreted with caution because CPPD deposits occur in about 5% of the adult population and are associated with nearly all diseases by chance alone. Pragmatically, the clinician is well advised to keep the diseases listed in Table 108–4 in mind when confronted with a case of CPPD crystal deposition disease. Unsuspected hyperparathyroidism, hypothyroidism, and other metabolic abnormalities have been found repeatedly when appropriate laboratory studies were performed in such patients. Conversely, when arthritis supervenes in a patient with one

TABLE 108–3. CHARACTERISTICS OF HEREDITARY CALCIUM PYROPHOSPHATE DIHYDRATE CRYSTAL DEPOSITION DISEASE

			ASSOCIATIONS		
SERIES	TYPE	MALE-TO-MALE TRANSMISSION	Arthritis	Onset	HLA Antigens
Slovakian (Hungarian gene)		No	Severe	Early	Yes
Chilean (Spanish gene)	Autosomal dominant	Yes	Severe	Early	No
French	Autosomal dominant	Yes	Severe	Early	No
Japanese	Autosomal dominant	Yes	Severe	Early	NA*
Swedish	Autosomal dominant	Yes	Severe	Early	No
Dutch	Autosomal dominant	Yes	Mild	Early	No
Mexican-American	Autosomal dominant	Yes	Mild	Early	No
French-Canadian	Autosomal dominant	?	Mild	Early	No
Spanish			Mild	Late	NA*
Jewish[69]	Autosomal dominant	No	Mild	Early	NA*

* NA = Not available.

TABLE 108–4. CONDITIONS PROBABLY ASSOCIATED WITH CALCIUM PYROPHOSPHATE DIHYDRATE CRYSTAL DEPOSITION

Hyperparathyroidism
Familial hypocalciuric hypercalcemia
Hemochromatosis
Hemosiderosis
Hypophosphatasia
Hypomagnesemia
Hypothyroidism
Gout
Neuropathic joints
Aging
Amyloidosis
Trauma, including surgery

of these metabolic conditions, the possibility of CPPD deposition disease should be considered in the differential diagnosis.

HYPERPARATHYROIDISM

Numerous reports of CPPD crystal deposition in patients with hyperparathyroidism have appeared,[68,70–72] and most series of patients with CPPD deposition show an incidence of 2 to 15%.[46,73,74] Conversely, 20 to 30% of patients with hyperparathyroidism have radiologic chondrocalcinosis.[68,75] Hyperparathyroid patients with CPPD deposits are older than those without such deposits. In most surgically treated cases, parathyroid adenomas rather than hyperplasia have been found. Acute attacks of pseudogout are common after parathyroidectomy.[24,28] During long-term postoperative followup study, the calcific deposits persist despite normal serum calcium levels.[75–77] An important effect of persistent hypercalcemia on the development of CPPD crystal deposits is reinforced by the reported associations of joint symptoms and radiologic chondrocalcinosis suggestive of CPPD crystal deposits in persons with a benign lifelong condition called hypocalciuric hypercalcemia.[78,79] A better rheumatologic analysis of such patients is needed.

HEMOCHROMATOSIS

The original report of arthritis in patients with hemochromatosis noted one example of articular cartilage calcification.[80] Many subsequent reports have documented this association.[81] Nearly half the patients with hemochromatosis have arthritis, and half of these have radiologic chondrocalcinosis.[82,83] Again, these are the older patients in the series.[83,84] CPPD deposition and related joint complaints are often present in patients with asymptomatic hemochromatosis. Involvement of metacarpophalangeal joints was more common in patients with hemochromatosis than in those with idiopathic chondrocalcinosis,[42] but the appearance of "squared off" bone ends, joint-space narrowing, and subchondral cysts in these joints was identical to that described by Martel and colleagues in patients with idiopathic chondrocalcinosis.[40] Adamson et al. pointed out more prevalent narrowing of the metacarpophalangeal joints, especially those in the fourth and fifth digits, peculiar hook-like osteophytes on the radial aspect of the metacarpal heads, and less prevalent scapholunate separation in CPPD crystal deposition.[85] Appropriate treatment of the iron overload did not prevent the development of new calcifications over a 10-year period.[67] Radiologic evidence of CPPD crystal deposition increased from 7 to 13 of the 18 patients followed.

That iron itself may be directly related to the calcific deposits is suggested by reports of CPPD deposition in patients with transfusion hemosiderosis.[81] Moreover, patients with hemophilia arthritis and chondrocalcinosis have been recorded.[12]

Just how tissue iron predisposes to CPPD crystal deposits is unclear. Ferrous, but not ferric, ions inhibited some inorganic pyrophosphatases;[86] ferric ions promoted CPPD crystal growth in vitro at lower inorganic pyrophosphate concentrations.[87] Synovial hemosiderosis slowed the metabolic clearance of radiolabeled CPPD crystals from rabbit joints by about 50%.[88] Finally, normocalcemic hyperparathyroidism may occur in 50% of patients with hemochromatosis.[89] Whether any of these mechanisms relate to the association of local tissue iron overload with CPPD crystals, however, is still conjectural.

OTHER DISORDERS

O'Duffy reported a patient with *hypophosphatasia* and CPPD deposits,[90] and subsequently several others have been described.[91,92] Inorganic pyrophosphate is a natural substrate of alkaline phosphatase, and as urinary and plasma inorganic pyrophosphate levels are elevated in hypophosphatasia,[93,94] it is not surprising that hypophosphatasia may be associated with CPPD crystal deposition. BCP deposition may also be common in this population.[95] Attempts at replacing alkaline phosphatase by infusing plasma from patients with Paget's disease of bone into a patient with infantile hypophosphatasia had no appreciable effect on the urinary excretion of inorganic pyrophosphate but may have improved the bony abnormalities.[96]

Hypomagnesemia associated with CPPD crystal deposition was first reported in 1974;[97] at least 10 cases have been recognized since.[12] This association makes sense teleologically, because magnesium increases the solubility of CPPD crystals[4] and is also an important cofactor for alkaline phosphatase[98] as well as for many inorganic pyrophosphatase.[86] In most reported instances, the defect appeared to be a failure of renal conservation of magnesium. In one case, magnesium replacement therapy decreased radiologic calcification.[99] A controlled study of oral magnesium therapy in patients with CPPD crystal deposits showed statistically significant beneficial effects on articular signs and symptoms but not on radiographic calcification.[100] CPPD deposition has also been reported in *Bartter's syndrome*,[12] perhaps secondary to the association hypomagnesemia. Abnormalities in urinary or serum magnesium, however, are not present in most patients with CPPD crystal deposition.[97]

Hypothyroidism is associated with asymptomatic CPPD deposits, with frequent onset of joint inflammation after treatment with thyroid hormone.[101] One survey reported that 11% of 105 consecutive patients with CPPD deposition were hypothyroid,[102] more than detected in comparative populations of patients with acute medical conditions or osteoarthritis. Nonetheless, studies of patients with hypothyroidism over 40 years of age have not shown an increased prevalence of radiographic knee chondrocalcinosis compared to a control euthyroid group.[103]

Periarticular and intra-articular *amyloid* deposits have been noted in association with CPPD deposition since the first report in 1976.[104] Four of five elderly patients with amyloid arthropathy, most of whom had carpal tunnel syndrome and pitting edema of the hands, had chondrocalcinosis.[105] Subsequent histologic studies have shown frequent amyloid deposits in cartilage and synovium, often in close proximity to the CPPD crystals.[81] Because most such patients are elderly, this association may represent the chance concurrence of two age-related processes. Amyloid is known to bind pyrophosphate analogues,[106] as well as calcium, however, and local sequestration could favor CPPD crystal formation. Amyloid has also been described in osteoarthritic cartilage[107,108] and has been reported in joints of senescent mice.[109]

Hyperuricemia, often accompanying mild azotemia, hypertension, or diuretic use, is common in the elderly population. The co-existence of pseudogout and *urate gout* varies from 2 to 8% in most reported series;[81] 5% of our series had both CPPD and MSU crystals. If the prevalence of MSU crystal deposition were 2% of the adult male population, as it might be,[16] then this association could be one of chance. Although 32% of a series of 31 gouty patients had radiologically evident chondrocalcinosis,[88] only 5% of another series of 43 gouty patients showed such deposits, a percentage no greater than in control subjects.[35] In carefully controlled prospective studies, the prevalence of chondrocalcinosis in patients with gout was 8 of 138; in age-matched normal control patients and in asymptomatic hyperuricemic patients, the prevalence was 0 of 142 and 1 of 84, respectively.[66,109] These results imply an association of CPPD with gout but not with hyperuricemia.

An association of chondrocalcinosis and spondyloepiphyseal dysplasia has been postulated.[110–112] This relationship has not been extensively investigated.

Ankylosing hyperostosis has been noted in serial studies of hereditary cases of CPPD deposition in Slovakia.[38] It appeared in one third of 18 Japanese patients,[113] and it was found in a number of hereditary cases studied in the Netherlands.[114] Conversely, CPPD deposits were found in 6% of 34 patients with ankylosing hyperostosis.

We suggest that *the routine examination of a newly diagnosed patient with CPPD deposition should include determinations of the following: serum calcium, magnesium, phosphorus, alkaline phosphatase, ferritin, iron and total iron-binding capacity, and thyroid-stimulating hormone*, with further metabolic study if abnormalities are found.

TRAUMA/SURGERY

Mounting evidence links CPPD deposition with antecedent joint trauma or surgical procedures. In 1942, Weaver discussed monarticular calcific deposition following trauma.[115] Arthroscopic findings in such joints have been described.[116] Radiographic chondrocalcinosis has been recognized in hypermobile joints,[117] unstable joints,[118] and neuropathic joints.[43] The most compelling evidence was presented by Linden and Nilsson[59] and Doherty et al.[58] In the former study, 25 of 42 knees previously treated operatively for osteochondritis dissecans of the femoral condyle developed chondrocalcinosis in the operated, but not the contralateral, knee. A control group of meniscectomy patients developed chondrocalcinosis in 14 of 41 operated knees. In the latter study of postmeniscectomy patients, knee radiographs were obtained a mean of 25 years after operation; at that time, 20% of operated, but only 4% of contralateral, knees showed chondrocalcinosis. A case of monarticular chondrocalcinosis following local radiation therapy has also been reported.[119]

ROENTGENOGRAPHIC FEATURES

Heavy CPPD crystal deposits in fibrocartilaginous structures, hyaline (articular) cartilage, ligaments, and joint capsules have a characteristic appearance that is diagnostically helpful. Punctate and linear radiodensities are most frequently seen in the fibrocartilaginous menisci of the knee and usually involve both menisci of both knees (see Figs. 108–1C and 108–3B). Other fibrocartilaginous structures often calcified in this miliary fashion are the articular discs of the distal radioulnar joint (see Fig. 108–4), the symphysis pubis (see Fig. 108–5), the glenoid and acetabular labra, and the anulus fibrosus of the intervertebral discs. The articular discs of the sternoclavicular joints are often involved, but those of the temporomandibular joint are usually spared.

Calcification of the hyaline articular cartilage is common; the deposits in the midzonal layer appear as a radiopaque line paralleling the density of the underlying bone (see Figs. 108–3B and 108–4). The larger joints show these deposits most frequently, although they have been observed in nearly every diarthrodial joint. Calcifications of articular capsules or synovium, especially of the elbow, shoulder, hip, and knee, are frequent; the deposits appear as a broader; more diffuse, faintly opaque line.

Calcification of bursae, tendons, and ligaments also occurs in CPPD deposition disease. This calcification may represent BCP crystal deposition in some patients, but crystal-proved CPPD deposits have been reported in all the aforementioned sites. Synovial deposits may be so large as to mimic synovial chondromatosis,[120] and ligamentous or tendinous deposits may produce local compressive symptoms, such as carpal tunnel syndrome[121] or myelopathy, as already outlined.

Subchondral bone cysts are common and can attain a large size. Histologic examination of the walls of the lesion shown in Fig. 108–6 confirmed that it was only a bone cyst. How such lesions are related to CPPD deposition disease is unknown, but they occur frequently enough to be a diagnostic clue.[22]

A number of distinct regional radiographic abnormalities may suggest CPPD deposition. A peculiar erosion of the femoral cortex superior to the patella has been reported.[122,123] This lesion appears to correlate with osteoarthritis of the patellofemoral compartment (see Fig. 108–7). Carpal instability reported in association with CPPD deposits resembles that of RA.[124] A particular propensity for radiocarpal involvement has been observed. Navicular-lunate dissociation is thought to result from degeneration of the ligamentous structures. Axial involvement has been described.[23] In the lumbar spine, multiple levels of anulus fibrosus calcification, vacuum disc phenomena, and disc narrowing are emphasized. A syndrome of acute neck pain associated with calcifications surrounding the odontoid process, the "crowned dens syndrome," has been described[50] (see Fig. 108–9). It has occurred in patients who have either BCP or CPPD crystal deposition in peripheral joints. Sacroiliac joint abnormalities include subchondral erosions, reactive sclerosis, and bilateral vacuum phenomena. Axial involvement is particularly prominent in uremic patients with secondary hyperparathyroidism.[75]

Features that may accompany CPPD crystal deposition include joint degeneration, tibial stress fractures, and avascular necrosis of the medial or lateral femoral condyle. Degenerative changes in joints not commonly involved in primary osteoarthritis, such as the metacarpophalangeal, radiocarpal, elbow, and shoulder joints may suggest underlying CPPD crystal deposition even in the absence of radiographic chondrocalcinosis. Subchondral cysts, bone and cartilage fragmentation, and variable osteophyte formation are characteristic (see Fig. 108–8). The best serial studies are those of the Hungarian familial cases.[38] CPPD deposits first appeared in radiographically normal cartilage, and degeneration inevitably followed. Tibial stress fractures were reported in five elderly patients with CPPD deposition and severe degenerative knee disease.[125] Because their knees were usually painful before the fractures, the source of increased pain was not readily apparent. Interestingly, 4 of 14 patients with osteonecrosis of the medial femoral condyle had CPPD knee deposits,[126] an association subsequently confirmed.[127]

An arthritic patient may be screened for CPPD deposition with four suitably exposed roentgenograms: (1 and 2) an anteroposterior view of each knee; (3) an anteroposterior view of the pelvis; and (4) a posteroanterior view of the wrists. If nothing diagnostic is seen on these films, a more extensive survey is unlikely to be helpful.

The chemical composition of the crystal deposits may be inferred with confidence from typical roentgenograms. Caution must be exercised when the calcifications are faint or atypical, however, because of the possibility of DCPD, BCP, or calcium oxalate crystal deposits or vascular calcifications, all of which are symmetric.[16]

PATHOLOGIC FEATURES

The joints of three cases at necropsy and seven anatomic cadavers were extensively examined.[19] The distribution of calcification generally paralleled that seen on radiogram. Joint capsules, especially in the hip and shoulder, and the hyaline articular cartilages, were often affected, but the heaviest deposits were in fibrocartilaginous structures. The menisci of the knee were involved in all cases (see Fig. 108–3A). Heavy deposits were often noted in tendons and in intra-articular ligaments, such as the cruciate ligaments in the knee. Microscopically, the deposits were composed of various-sized microcrystalline aggregates of CPPD (Fig. 108–10). Their diameters varied from 15 μm to 0.6 cm; the larger ones appeared grossly as white chalky deposits. It was difficult on gross inspection to distinguish these deposits (see Fig. 108–3A) from the white chalky lesions of true gout. These lesions are distributed diffusely in fibrocartilage, mainly in the midzonal or superficial areas of hyaline cartilage (Fig. 108–11).

The smallest, and presumably the earliest, crystals appeared at the lacunar margin of chondrocytes. When adjacent chondrocytes were damaged, pericellular matrix vesicles were often seen. Increased glycogen islands and rough endoplasmic reticulum were observed in the chondrocytes.[128] The surrounding matrix may appear normal or granular. Collagen fibril fragmentation in uncalcified areas of CPPD cartilage has been described in familial cases.[129] Larger superficial deposits occur in degenerative cartilages, usually at sites of surface ulcerations and fissuring and often associated with chondrocyte "cloning."

Cartilage sections from patients with acute pseudogout showed neutrophils migrating into the matrix.[130] CPPD crystals were observed within the cells. The superficial cartilage was eroded, and collagen fibers were degraded. Presumably, the neutrophils generated enzymes and free oxygen radical species harmful to adjacent matrix and cells.

Ishikawa and co-workers have shown convincing evidence of abnormal proteoglycan deposition within chondrocytes in the immediate vicinity of early CPPD crystal deposits. These "red cells," stained with safranin-0, were not seen if the tissue was first exposed to either papain or chondroitinase ABC, which confirms their proteoglycan nature. "Red cells" were a constant feature of evolving, but not of "mature," CPPD crystal deposits in fibrocartilage, hyaline cartilage, and synovium showing chondroid metaplasia.[131] They were seen in tissue from both sporadic and familial cases. Ishikawa

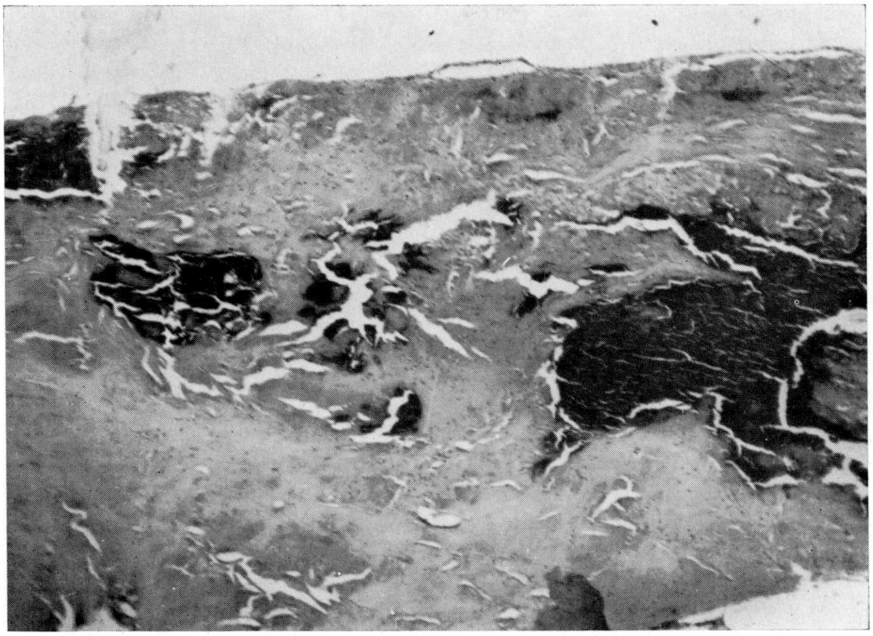

FIGURE 108–10. Photomicrograph of a section through the meniscus shown in Figure 108–3A, various-sized aggregates of calcified material are distributed throughout (hematoxylin and eosin stain, ×26).

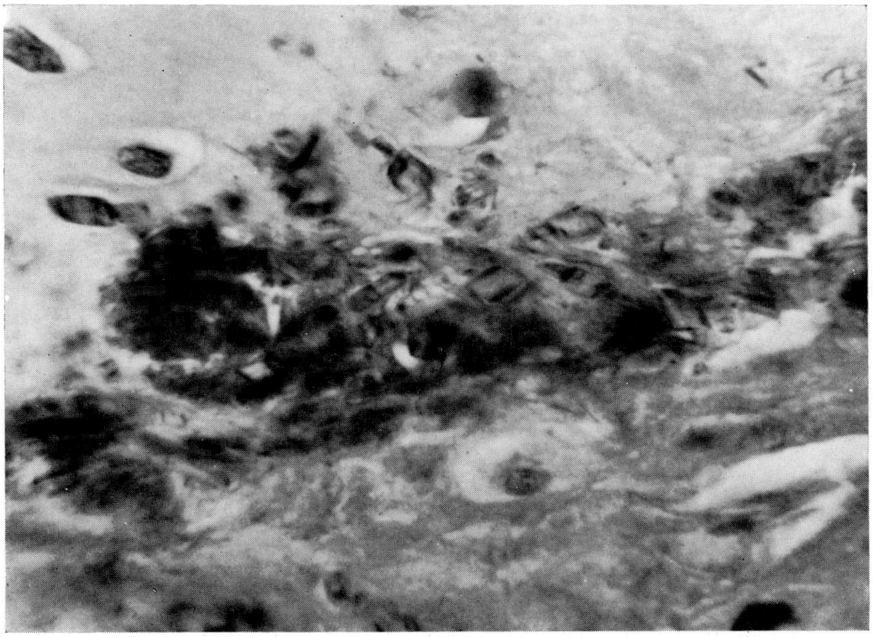

FIGURE 108–11. Photomicrograph of the smallest deposits found shows them surrounding the lacunae of the chondrocytes. This process begins in the midzonal layer of articular cartilage, more diffusely in fibrocartilage. Individual crystals of calcium pyrophosphate dihydrate are visible in this section (alazarin red, ×800; linear magnification ×3).

also found the following: (1) absence of normal safranin-0 staining in the matrix in areas of early crystal deposition; (2) "packing" of the proteoglycan-denuded collagen fibers in these same areas; (3) hypertrophy and mitotic activity of the red cells; (4) the appearance of CPPD crystals in empty chondrocyte lacunae; and (5) "mature" deposits were ringed with dense, proteoglycan-free collagen, but the crystals were coated with a thin film of proteoglycan. No collagen or cells could be identified within these crystal masses by light or electron microscopy. The surrounding matrix now contained normal-appearing cells and stained normally.

Ishikawa et al. speculated that the cell-associated proteoglycan may indicate faulty release from the chondrocytes after synthesis, or that it may enter these cells by endocytosis. Their findings deserve further exploration and, if confirmed, must be taken into account in any scheme of the pathogenesis of CPPD crystal deposition.

Ohira et al. reported that articular hyaline and fibrocartilage as well as synovium from patients with CPPD deposits contain excess lipid.[132] Sites of crystal deposits stained strongly with Sudan III. Adjacent metaplastic chondrocytes contained large Sudan III–positive granules. The lipid nature of this material was confirmed by extraction with chloroform/ethanol. The role of lipid in mineralization could not be elucidated, but lipid may bind calcium needed for CPPD formation. A calcium-binding protein, S-100, has also been immunolocalized to CPPD-containing articular tissues, but not CPPD-free tissues from patients with osteoarthritis.[133] Others, however, note increased S-100 protein in degenerative joints without crystals.[134]

In three patients, superficial amyloid deposits were adjacent to CPPD crystals.[107] Isolated descriptions of CPPD crystals within chondrocytes have been reported,[135–138] indicating that chondrocytes may phagocytose crystals with attendant biologic consequences (see Chapter 109).

In no case has a cause-and-effect relationship been established between crystal deposits and morphologic changes.

Synovial biopsy material obtained with the Polley-Bickel needle showed inflammatory and reparative changes consistent with the clinical state of the joint at the time of biopsy. Early in an acute attack, the edematous synovium was infiltrated with PMN leukocytes; later, mononuclear infiltration and fibroblastic proliferation were seen. Synovial proliferation and infiltration with chronic inflammatory cells in chronically symptomatic joints can resemble rheumatoid pannus. Crystals have been identified in the superficial synovium under polarized light and by electron microscopy.[137] In patients with pseudo-osteoarthritis undergoing knee replacement, synovial deposits were focal and concentrated in avascular areas.[138]

PATHOGENESIS

The cause of CPPD crystal deposition is unknown. Conceptually, formation of CPPD crystals in cartilage may result from elevated levels of either calcium or inorganic pyrophosphate (PPi), from changes in the matrix that promote crystal formation, or from combinations of these factors. Because CPPD crystal deposition is a clinically heterogeneous disorder, different factors probably predominate in individual cases, much as hyperuricemia preceding MSU crystal deposition may have different causes.

Bjelle favors the hypothesis that matrix changes antedate and predispose persons to CPPD crystal formation. In studies of Swedish patients with familial CPPD deposition, he found weakly staining midzonal matrix with decreased collagen content, some fragmentation of collagen fibers, and an abnormal hexosamine profile.[129] The proportions of keratan sulfate and chondroitin-6-sulfate were increased, and those of chondroitin-4-sulfate were decreased. A decrease in mucin-like oligosaccharides was found. Because these changes were independent of the amount of crystal deposits and because morphologically abnormal crystal-free areas in midzonal cartilage were seen by electron microscopy, Bjelle postulated a primary role of a matrix abnormality in promoting CPPD mineral phase. Alterations of matrix collagen and proteoglycan were reported by Masuda, Ishikawa, and Usuku in sporadic cases.[133]

The inorganic composition of matrix may also affect CPPD crystal formation. Ferrous ions inhibit some pyrophosphatases;[86] ferric ions lower the formation product for CPPD crystals in vitro[87] and slowed the intracellular degradation of CPPD crystals injected into rabbit joints.[88] Hypomagnesemia, both primary and secondary to Bartter's syndrome, has also been associated with chondrocalcinosis. Magnesium is a cofactor for many pyrophosphatases and increases the solubility of CPPD crystals.[4] Therefore, its deficiency may decrease hydrolysis of PPi and may slow crystal dissolution. Profound hypomagnesemia induced by dietary magnesium deprivation did not change the rate of CPPD crystal clearance from rabbit joints, however.[139] Elevations of inorganic phosphate have promoted CPPD crystal nucleation and growth in vitro and may act similarly in vivo.[140] The effect of inorganic phosphate in aqueous solution on CPPD crystal formation is most prominent in the 0.01 to 1.0 mM range.[141] That such an aberration may exist is suggested by the finding of elevated levels of inorganic phosphate in synovial fluid in pseudogout.[142]

Studies of crystal formation in gels provide indirect evidence that organic matrix components may be nucleating agents in CPPD crystal formation. In aqueous solutions, CPPD crystal synthesis occurred at acid pH or at high ionic concentrations.[5,141] In model collagen gels, however, crystals formed at neutral pH[143] and at PPi concentrations between 2 and 20 μM.[144] Formation of amorphous calcium pyrophosphate and orthorhombic calcium pyrophosphate tetrahydrate preceded formation of monoclinic and triclinic CPPD crystals identical to those observed in vivo.[145] These studies seem particularly relevant because cartilage is a gel. The modulatory effect of other organic matrix components, such as proteoglycans, on CPPD crystal formation has not been studied systematically.

No systematic study has been made of cartilage interstitial fluid calcium in patients with CPPD deposition. Clearly, some of these patients have hyperparathyroidism, usually due to adenoma, with associated hypercalcemia. CPPD deposition has also been noted in patients with familial hypocalciuric hypercalcemia,[78,79] further supporting a role for calcium in promoting CPPD deposition.

PPi is produced by most biosynthetic reactions in macromolecular synthesis.[93] The ubiquitous pyrophosphatases, hydrolyzing PPi into inorganic orthophosphate, drive these reactions in the direction of synthesis; but the intracellular enzymatic hydrolysis of PPi does not go to completion, and detectable amounts are measurable in cells, including fibroblasts and chondrocytes.[146]

The amount of PPi produced in the body is immense. It has been calculated that 30 g are made daily in the human liver as a by-product of the synthesis of albumin alone.[93] Only a small amount of that synthesized appears in the urine (approximately 10 to 100 μmol daily), where it acts as a powerful inhibitor of crystal nucleation and growth. The turnover rate of plasma PPi in dogs is only about 2 minutes, which further complicates the interpretation of plasma values. Neither the source nor the fate of plasma PPi is known.

Much PPi is adsorbed to bone mineral,[147,148] where it is thought to act as a regulator of mineralization. In addition to its effect on crystal precipitation, it retards the conversion of amorphous calcium phosphate into crystalline hydroxyapatite, inhibits crystal aggregation, and slows the dissolution rate of hydroxyapatite crystals. The diphosphonates, which have P-C-P bonds, instead of P-O-P bonds, are nonhydrolyzable analogues of PPi. These compounds have similar biologic effects and are used as therapeutic agents in various diseases of mineral metabolism and, coupled with tin and ^{99m}Tc, as bone-scanning agents.

Studies of PPi metabolism were stimulated by recognition of this substance as a constituent of the crystal deposits. Because urinary levels are much easier to quantify than those in plasma, these were measured earliest and were found to be normal in patients with CPPD deposition disease.[149,150] Blood levels of PPi were later measured; serum contained two to three times the concentration of plasma.[151] This increase resulted from the release of PPi by platelets during clotting. Plasma levels were higher in venous blood than in arterial blood, increased with systemic exercise, and spuriously elevated by application of a venous tourniquet before phlebotomy.[152,153] Plasma concentrations in sporadic cases of CPPD deposition were similar to those in osteoarthritic or normal control subjects.[149,153,154] In patients with hypophosphatasia, a disease associated with CPPD deposition, both urinary and plasma levels of PPi were elevated,[94,155] presumably as a result of decreased hydrolysis.

Abnormal local metabolism of PPi was suggested by reports of elevated levels in synovial fluids from patients with CPPD crystal deposition, although elevations were also observed in synovial fluids from patients with gout, osteoarthritis, and even RA. The highest joint fluid levels were found in the most severely degenerated joints, as judged radiographically.[142] PPi levels were lower during acute attacks and rose as the episode subsided,[142,156] probably because of increased synovial blood flow during acute attacks with more rapid equilibration with plasma PPi. The elevated synovial fluid levels could not be explained by dissolution of crystals in the fluid. The gradient between synovial fluid and plasma implied a local origin of PPi.[142,154] The site of the synovial fluid production was expected to be cartilage, based on the histologic observation that the smallest and presumably the earliest crystals are seen adjacent to chondrocytes. Subsequent studies indicated that articular hyaline and fibrocartilages in organ culture liberated PPi into the ambient media, whereas synovium, subchondral bone, and nonarticular (elastic) cartilages did not.[157,158] Extrapolation of the amount produced by incubated slices to the amount of cartilage in a whole knee joint yielded figures for local production of the same order of magnitude as estimated from in vivo kinetic experiments.[157,159] Thus, cartilage is the most likely source of locally elevated concentrations of PPi in CPPD deposition.

There is evidence for three pathways of extracellular PPi generation by chondrocytes: (1) extracellular generation by ectoenzymes (ectoenzyme hypothesis); (2) "leakage" or transport from chondrocytes containing excess PPi (secretion hypothesis); and (3) release of PPi together with matrix-destined synthetic products (coexport hypothesis) (Fig. 108–12). Whether each pathway is important in all patients or whether abnormal PPi generation occurs via different pathways in different patients is unknown. As in gout, the crystals represent a final common pathway of disease expression.

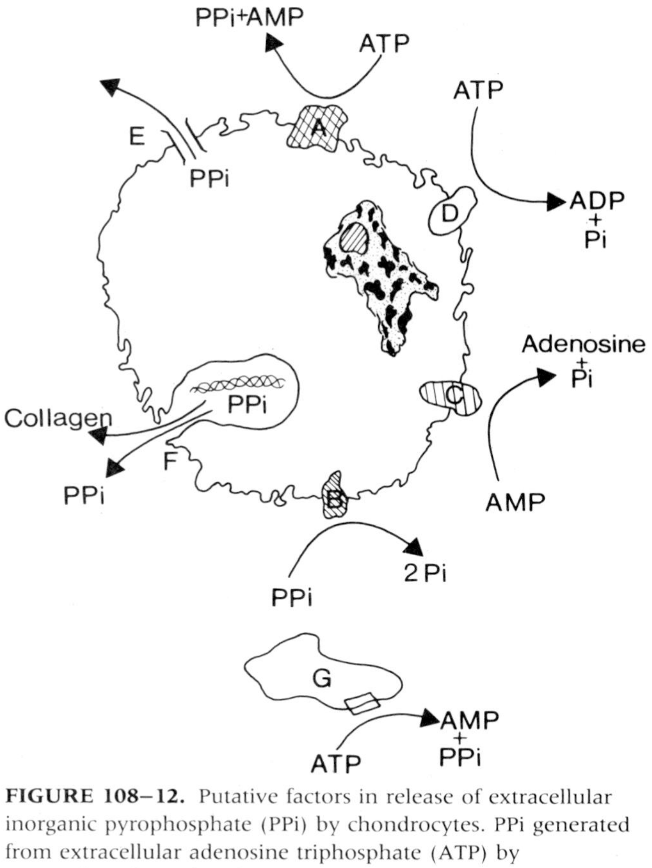

FIGURE 108–12. Putative factors in release of extracellular inorganic pyrophosphate (PPi) by chondrocytes. PPi generated from extracellular adenosine triphosphate (ATP) by ectonucleoside triphosphate pyrophosphohydrolose (ectoenzyme hypothesis) (A). Degradation of extracellular PPi by ecto- or extracellular PPiase (B). 5′-Nucleotidase degrades adenosine monophosphate (AMP), promoting reaction A (C). Ecto ATPase competes with reaction A for substrate (D). PPi leak or secretion from chondrocyte cytoplasm (E). Release of PPi together with matrix molecules (coexport hypothesis) (F). Vesicles derived from chondrocytes contain nucleoside triphosphate pyrophosphohydrolase and other enzymes (G).

Augmented PPi generation was found in the presence of adenosine triphosphate (ATP) by extracts of cartilages from patients with CPPD deposition, as compared with generation in extracts of osteoarthritic or normal cartilages, supporting the ectoenzyme hypothesis.[160] ATP was enzymatically hydrolyzed to adenosine monophosphate and PPi by ATP pyrophosphohydrolase. A similar activity had been described in calcifying sheep cartilage.[161] Subsequent reports have verified the presence of this enzyme in matrix vesicle fractions of epiphyseal cartilage,[162,163] where it may play a role in calcium pyrophosphate precipitation.[164,165] We have characterized this activity as a chondrocyte nucleoside triphosphate pyrophosphohydrolase with broad substrate reactivity and as an ectoenzyme.[166] The cell surface location of this enzyme has been confirmed by Howell et al.[167] and Caswell and Russell.[168]

Because CPPD crystals appear to form extracellularly adjacent to chondrocytes and because PPi does not passively cross cell membranes,[169] the external position of this enzyme might allow the generation of PPi at the site of crystal formation in the presence of suitable substrate. Levels of nucleoside triphosphate pyrophosphohydrolase activity were higher in the synovial fluid of patients with CPPD deposition and osteoarthritis than in fluids from patients with RA or gout.[156] Activity was also elevated in synovial fluids containing BCP crystals, implying a broader connection between NTPPPH and mineralization in general.[170] Enzyme activity correlated directly with the concentration of PPi in synovial fluid. In addition to elevated nucleoside triphosphate pyrophosphohydrolase activity in detergent extracts of cartilages with CPPD deposition, Tenenbaum et al. also described higher levels of 5′ nucleotidase activity and lower levels of alkaline phosphatase and PPiase activity than in osteoarthritic cartilages.[160] All these aberrations would favor the accumulation of PPi in the ectoenzyme system shown in Fig. 108–13. A naturally occurring extracellular substrate for nucleoside triphosphate pyrophosphohydrolase in cartilage has not yet been conclusively demonstrated, but preliminary studies found

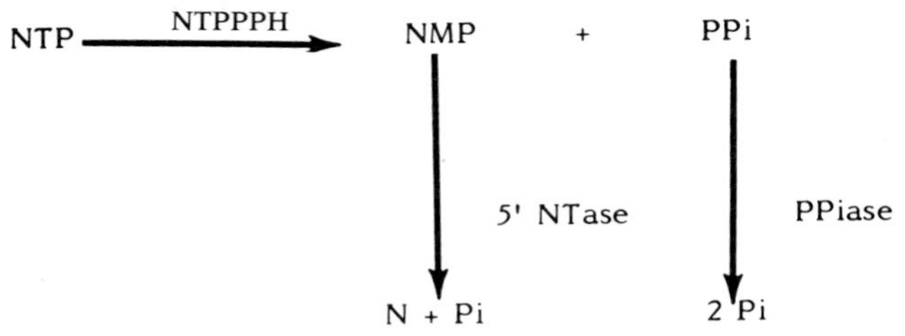

FIGURE 108–13. Postulated enzymatic cascade of inorganic pyrophosphate (PPi) production from nucleotide triphosphate (NTP). Elevated NTP pyrophosphohydrolase and 5′nucleotidase activities and decreased inorganic pyrophosphatase activity in chondrocalcinosic cartilages all favor PPi accumulation. 5′NTase = 5′nucleotidase; PPiase = inorganic pyrophosphatase; Pi = inorganic phosphate; N = nucleotide; NMP = nucleotide monophosphate.

concentrations of ATP in synovial fluid as high as 1 μM.[170] Alternatively, chondrocytes may discharge cellular nucleoside triphosphate pyrophosphohydrolase (NTP) substrates for their own ectoenzyme.

Vesicles, derived by collagenase digestion of articular cartilage and resembling matrix vesicles, are also rich in NTP. These structures promoted calcium mineral formation when incubated with ATP in defined media. The precipitates contained PPi derived from the ATP and positively birfringent crystals resembling monoclinic CPPD. These dissolved when incubated with yeast inorganic pyrophosphatase.[171] Fourier transform infrared spectroscopy identified peaks characteristic of P-P bonds in the mineral. X-ray diffraction has not yet been performed. Thus, ectoenzyme on cell-derived membrane particles as well as on intact cells may promote CPPD formation.

Support for the secretion hypothesis is derived from the work of Lust et al., who found intracellular PPi levels twice those of control subjects in cultured skin fibroblasts and in lymphoblasts obtained from affected members of a French kindred with familial CPPD deposition.[146,172] A generalized metabolic abnormality phenotypically expressed only in chondrocytes was postulated. The PPi total and releasable content of platelets in 5 patients with sporadic or familial CPPD deposition was similar to that of 17 control subjects,[173] but a significant positive correlation was found between platelet PPi content and the age of the donor.

PPi levels in cultured skin fibroblasts from patients with both sporadic and familial CPPD crystal deposition were significantly elevated compared to those from normal persons or subjects with osteoarthritis.[174] Activity of ectonucleoside triphosphate pyrophosphohydrolase was elevated in fibroblasts from sporadic, but not familial, CPPD crystal deposition.[174] Lastly, intracellular PPi levels and ectonucleoside triphosphate pyrophosphohydrolase activity were positively correlated in fibroblasts from each of the groups studied.

Last, the coexport of PPi, formed during synthesis of matrix-destined macromolecules, and its metabolic coproducts was investigated. Liberation of PPi correlated with release of uronic acid in one study,[158] but chondrocyte coexport of PPi and glycosaminoglycans has been disproven.[175,176] However, incubation of adult articular hyaline cartilage with ascorbate, which stimulates collagen synthesis, markedly increased PPi elaboration, an effect specifically reversed when ascorbate oxidase was added.[177] General protein synthesis inhibitors and more specific inhibitors of collagen production prevented ascorbate enhancement of PPi elaboration. Interestingly, cycloheximide, a nonspecific protein synthesis inhibitor, abrogated ascorbate-enhanced PPi production, but not basal PPi production, by unstimulated cells. This implies at least two modes of extracellular PPi elaboration, one independent of protein synthesis and the other cycloheximide inhibitable, possibly cosecretion of collagen and PPi.

Although these biochemical changes cannot yet be directly related to the pathogenesis of CPPD crystal deposition, they represent the earliest biochemical correlates of this metabolic arthropathy.

THERAPY

Acute attacks of pseudogout are readily treated by several methods, including (1) thorough aspiration of the joint to remove crystals; (2) administration of nonsteroidal anti-inflammatory drugs, such as indomethacin; (3) joint immobilization; and (4) local injection of microcrystalline corticosteroid esters. Intravenous colchicine works as well in pseudogout as it does in gout.[30] The prophylactic effectiveness of oral colchicine in patients who have recurrent attacks has been demonstrated.[178]

No known way exists to halt the progressive deposition of crystals or to remove those already deposited. Correction of associated metabolic disorders such as hyperparathyroidism, myxedema, and hemochromatosis has not resulted in the disappearance of radiographic cartilage calcification. New calcifications have developed in some such patients.[67] Attempts at lavage of affected joints with magnesium chloride were unsuccessful in removing significant amounts of crystal, but acute attacks were precipitated.[179] Several examples of spontaneous disappearance of calcific deposits have been reported. Wrist calcification disappeared in one case after immobilization and subsequent development of reflex sympathetic dystrophy.[180] The increased blood flow may have increased the clearance of pyrophosphate from the wrist. Another case associated with familial hypomagnesemia showed radiologic evidence of decreased meniscal calcification 2 years after institution of magnesium treatment.[99] In a double-blinded, placebo-controlled trial of magnesium carbonate treatment for sporadic CPPD crystal deposition, radiographic calcification did not change over 6 months, although symptoms improved significantly.[100] One group reported that repeated injections of glycosaminoglycan polysulfate (Arteparon) in 12 patients reduced pain and increased mobility in knees affected with chondrocalcinosis compared to contralateral untreated knees that also had chondrocalcinosis.[181] Radiographic calcification decreased after 2 to 7 weeks of treatment. This study needs confirmation.

Treatment of the frequently associated degenerative disease is the same as for osteoarthritis. Intra-articular injection with ^{90}Y was reported to ameliorate pain and stiffness and decrease the size of effusion in knee joints over a 6-month period.[182] Joint deformity and radiographic changes were not better than in the contralateral, uninjected knee, however.

Even if effective treatment were available, two problems would remain. First, no biochemical marker identifies those patients who will develop crystal deposition. We must await radiographic evidence of cartilage calcification or identification of crystals in joint fluids, both of which probably signal long-standing disease. Therapeutic interventions at this stage may be much less ef-

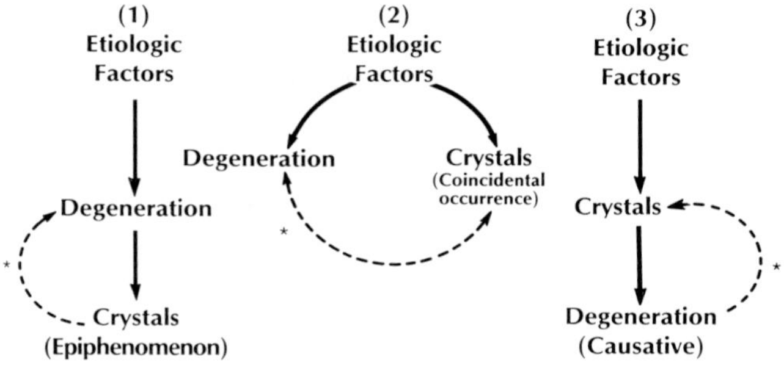

FIGURE 108–14. Prevention of crystal formation or dissolution of calcium pyrophosphate dihydrate crystals would have little effect on cartilage degeneration except in schema number 3 or if an amplification loop exists.
*amplification loop.[58]

fective. Second, although treatment of the crystal deposition would probably ameliorate or would prevent acute pseudogout attacks, it might have no effect on the much more significant degenerative joint disease. Fig. 108–14 illustrates three potential pathogenetic sequences relating degenerative disease to crystal deposition. Only in sequence 3, which is analogous to the pathogenesis of tophaceous gout, would removal or prevention of crystal formation affect cartilage degeneration. Doherty, Watt, and Dieppe have postulated that the biologic phenomena induced by crystals may act as an amplification loop, as shown by the hatched lines in sequences 1 and 2, which envision crystal formation as an epiphenomenon or as a coincidental phenomenon, respectively.[58] If an amplification loop exists, then prevention of crystal formation or crystal removal would both have a salutary effect. Perhaps each of the paradigms shown here actually occurs in patients with CPPD crystal deposition, with varying sequences in different patients. Because the clinical importance of CPPD crystals will rise as the population ages, these therapeutic considerations are of more than theoretic interest.

REFERENCES

1. McCarty, D.J., and Hollander, J.L.: Identification of urate crystals in gouty synovial fluid. Ann. Intern. Med., *54*:452–460, 1961.
2. McCarty, D.J., Kohn, N.N., and Faires, J.S.: The significance of calcium phosphate crystals in the synovial fluid of arthritis patients: The "pseudogout syndrome." I. Clinical aspects. Ann. Intern. Med., *56*:711–737, 1962.
3. Kohn, N.N. et al.: The significance of calcium phosphate crystals in the synovial fluid of arthritis patients: The "pseudogout syndrome." II. Identification of crystals. Ann. Intern. Med., *56*:738–745, 1962.
4. Bennett, R.M., Lehr, J.R., and McCarty, D.J.: Factors affecting the solubility of calcium pyrophosphate dihydrate crystals. J. Clin. Invest., *56*:1571–1579, 1975.
5. Brown, E.H. et al.: Preparation and characterization of some calcium pyrophosphates. J. Agr. Food Chem., *11*:214–222, 1963.

6. McCarty, D.J., and Faires, J.S.: A comparison of the duration of local anti-inflammatory effect of several adrenocorticosteroid esters: A bioassay technique. Curr. Ther. Res., *5*:284–290, 1963.
7. McCarty, D.J.: Crystal-induced inflammation: Syndromes of gout and pseudogout. Geriatrics, *18*:467–478, 1963.
8. Zitnan, D., and Sitaj, S.: Mnohopocentna familiarna kalcifikacin articularnych chrupiek. Bratisl. Lek. Listy, *38*:217–228, 1958.
9. McCarty, D.J.: The Heberden Oration, 1982. Crystals, joints, and consternation. Ann. Rheum. Dis., *42*:243–253, 1983.
10. Zitnan, D., and Sitaj, S.: Chondrocalcinosis articularis. Section I. Clinical and radiological study. Ann. Rheum. Dis., *22*:142–169, 1963.
11. Bennett, E.H.: Abnormal deposits in joints. Dublin J. Med. Sci., *65*:161–163, 1903.
12. Ryan, L., and McCarty, D.: Calcium pyrophosphate crystal deposition disease; pseudogout; articular chondrocalcinosis. *In* Arthritis and Allied Conditions. 11th Ed. Edited by D.J. McCarty. Philadelphia, Lea & Febiger, 1989.
13. Ellman, M.H., and Levin, B.: Chondrocalcinosis in elderly persons. Arthritis Rheum., *18*:43–47, 1975.
14. Memin, Y., Monville, C., and Ryckewaert, A.: La chondrocalcinose articulaire apres 80 ans. Rev. Rheum. Mal. Osteoartic, *45*:77–82, 1978.
15. Wilkins, E. et al.: Osteoarthritis and articular chondrocalcinosis in the elderly. Ann. Rheum. Dis., *42*:280–284, 1983.
16. McCarty, D.J. et al.: Studies on pathological calcifications in human cartilage. I. Prevalence and types of crystal deposits in the menisci of two hundred fifteen cadavera. J. Bone Joint Surg., *48A*:308–325, 1966.
17. Gatter, R.A., and McCarty, D.J.: Pathological tissue calcification in man. Arch. Pathol., *84*:346–353, 1967.
18. Bjelle, A., Crocker, P., and Willoughby, D.: Ultra-microcrystals in pyrophosphate arthropathy. Acta Med. Scand., *207*:89–92, 1980.
19. Parel, H., Reginato, A., and Schumacher, H.R.: Alizarin red S staining as a screening test to detect calcium compounds in synovial fluid. Arthritis Rheum., *26*:191–200, 1983.
20. Bennett, R.M., Mall, J.C., and McCarty, D.J.: Pseudogout in acute neuropathic arthropathy: A clue to pathogenesis. Arthritis Rheum. Dis., *33*:563–567, 1974.
21. Rachow, J.W., Ryan, L.M., McCarty, D.J., and Halverson, P.B.: Synovial fluid inorganic pyrophosphate concentration and nucleotide pyrophosphohydrolase activity in basic calcium phosphate deposition arthropathy and Milwaukee shoulder syndrome. Arthritis Rheum., *31*:408–413, 1988.
22. Resnick, D. et al.: Clinical, radiographic and pathologic abnormalities in calcium pyrophosphate dihydrate deposition disease (CPPD) pseudogout. Diagn. Radiol., *122*:1–15, 1977.
23. Martel, W. et al.: Further observations on the arthropathy of calcium pyrophosphate crystal deposition disease. Radiology, *141*:1–15, 1981.
24. O'Duffy, J.D.: Clinical studies of acute pseudogout attacks. Arthritis Rheum., *19*(Suppl.):349–353, 1976.
25. Dieppe, P.A. et al.: Pyrophosphate arthropathy: A clinical and radiological study of 105 cases. Ann. Rheum. Dis., *41*:371–376, 1982.
26. Fam, A.G. et al.: Clinical and roentgenographic aspects of pseudogout: A study of 50 cases and review. Can. Med. Assoc. J., *124*:545–550, 1981.
27. McCarty, D.J.: Diagnostic mimicry in arthritis: Patterns of joint involvement associated with calcium pyrophosphate dihydrate crystal deposits. Bull. Rheum. Dis., *25*:804–809, 1975.
28. Bilezikian, J.P. et al.: Pseudogout after parathyroidectomy. Lancet, *1*:445–449, 1973.
29. Phelps, P.: Polymorphonuclear leukocyte motility in vitro. IV. Colchicine inhibition of chemotactic activity formation after phagocytosis of urate crystals. Arthritis Rheum., *13*:1–9, 1970.
30. Spilberg, I et al.: Colchicine and pseudogout. Arthritis Rheum., *23*:1062–1063, 1980.
31. Moskowitz, R.W. et al.: Chronic synovitis as a manifestation of calcium crystal deposition disease. Arthritis Rheum., *14*:109–116, 1971.
32. Resnick, D. et al.: Rheumatoid arthritis and pseudorheumatoid arthritis in calcium pyrophosphate dihydrate crystal deposition disease. Radiology, *140*:615–621, 1981.
33. Wallace, S.L. et al.: Preliminary criteria for the classification of the acute arthritis of primary gout. Arthritis Rheum., *20*:895–900, 1977.
34. Bywaters, E.G.L.: Calcium pyrophosphate deposits in synovial membrane. Ann. Rheum. Dis., *31*:219–220, 1972.
35. Good, A.E., and Rapp, R.: Chondrocalcinosis of the knee with gout and rheumatoid arthritis. N. Engl. J. Med., *277*:286–290, 1967.
36. Doherty, M., Dieppe, P., and Watt, I.: Low incidence of calcium pyrophosphate dihydrate crystal deposition in rheumatoid arthritis, with modification of radiographic features in coexistent disease. Arthritis Rheum., *27*:1002–1009, 1984.
37. Bong, D., and Bennett, R.: Pseudogout mimicking systemic disease. JAMA, *246*:1438–1440, 1981.
38. Zitnan, D., and Sitaj, S.: Natural course of articular chondrocalcinosis. Arthritis Rheum., *19*(Suppl.):363–390, 1976.
39. Genant, H.K.: Roentgenographic aspects of calcium pyrophosphate dihydrate crystal deposition disease (pseudogout). Arthritis Rheum., *19*:307–328, 1976.
40. Martel, W. et al.: A roentgenologically distinctive arthropathy in some patients with pseudogout syndrome. AJR, *109*:587–605, 1970.
41. Hamilton, E.B.D., et al.: The arthropathy of idiopathic haemochromatosis. Q. J. Med., *37*:171–182, 1968.
42. Atkins, C.J., et al.: Chondrocalcinosis and arthropathy: Studies in haemochromatosis and in idiopathic chondrocalcinosis. Q. J. Med., *39*:71–79, 1970.
43. Jacobelli, S. G., et al.: Calcium pyrophosphate dihydrate crytal deposition in neuropathic joints: Four cases of polyarticular involvement. Ann. Intern. Med., *79*:340–347, 1973.
44. Gerster, J.C., Vischer, T.L., and Fallet, G.H.: Destructive arthropathy in generalized osteoarthritis with articular chondrocalcinosis. J. Rheumatol., *2*:265–269, 1975.
45. Hamilton, E.B.D., and Richards, A.J.: Destructive arthropathy in chondrocalcinosis articularis. Ann. Rheum. Dis., *33*:196–203, 1974.
46. Menkes, C.J., Simon, F., and Chourki, M.: Les arthropathies destructrices de la chondrocalcinose. Rev. Rhum. Mal. Osteoartic, *40*:115–123, 1973.
47. Reginato, A.J., et al.: Polyarticular and familial chondrocalcinosis. Arthritis Rheum., *13*:197–213, 1970.
48. Pritzker, K.P.H., et al.: Pseudotumor of temporomandibular joint: Destructive calcium pyrophosphate dihydrate arthropathy. J. Rheumatol., *3*:70–81, 1976.
49. Reginato, A.J., et al.: HLA antigens in chondrocalcinosis and ankylosing chondrocalcinosis. Arthritis Rheum., *22*:928–932, 1979.
50. Bouvet, J., et al.: Acute neck pain due to calcifications surrounding the odontoid process: The crowned dens syndrome. Arthritis Rheum., *28*:1417–1420, 1985.
51. LeGoff, P., Penunec, Y., and Youinou, P.: Signes cervicaux aigus pseudomeninge, relateurs de la chondrocalcinose articulaire. Sem. Hop. Paris, *56*:1515–1518, 1980.
52. Kawano, N. et al.: Calcium pyrophosphate dihydrate crystal deposition disease in the cervical ligamentum flavum. J. Neurosurg., *68*:613–620, 1988.

53. Berghausen, E.J. et al.: Cervical myelopathy attributable to pseudogout. Clin. Orthop. Rel. Res., *214*:217–221, 1987.
54. Gomez, H., and Chou, S.M.: Myeloradiculopathy secondary to pseudogout in the cervical ligamentum flavum. Neurosurgery, *25*:298–302, 1989.
55. Kawano, N. et al.: Cervical radiculomyelopathy caused by deposition of calcium pyrophosphate dihydrate crystals in the ligamenta flava. J. Neurosurg., *52*:279–283, 1980.
56. Parker, P.D., Jones, N.R., and Scott, G.: Cervical myelopathy in CPPD deposition disease. Australas Radiol., *34*:82–85, 1990.
57. Ciricillo, S.F., and Weinstein, P.R.: Foramen magnum syndrome from pseudogout of the atlanto-occipital ligament. J. Neurosurg., *71*:141–143, 1989.
58. Doherty, M., Watt, I., and Dieppe, P.A.: Localised chondrocalcinosis in post-meniscectomy knees. Lancet, *1*:1207–1210, 1982.
59. Linden, B., and Nilsson, B.E.: Chondrocalcinosis following osteochondritis dissecans in the femur condyle. Clin. Orthop., *130*:223–227, 1978.
60. Andres, T.L., and Trainer, T.D.: Intervertebral chondrocalcinosis: A coincidental finding possibly related to previous surgery. Arch. Pathol. Lab. Med., *104*:269–271, 1980.
61. Ellman, M.H., et al.: Calcium pyrophosphate dihydrate deposition in lumbar disc fibrocartilage. J. Rheumatol., *8*:955–958, 1981.
62. Guerne, P.A., Terkeltaub, R., Zuraw, B., and Lotz, M.: Inflammatory microcrystals stimulate interleukin-6 production and secretion by human monocytes and synoviocytes. Arthritis Rheum., *32*:1443–1452, 1989.
63. Rodriguez-Valverde, V. et al.: Hereditary articular chondrocalcinosis. Am. J. Med., *84*:101–106, 1988.
64. Fernandez Dapica, M., and Gomez-Reino, J.: Familial chondrocalcinosis in the Spanish population. J. Rheum., *13*:631–633, 1986.
65. Balsa, A. et al.: Familial articular chondrocalcinosis in Spain. Ann. Rheum. Dis., *49*:531–535, 1990.
66. Hollingworth, P., Williams, P.L., and Scott, J.T.: Frequency of chondrocalcinosis of the knees in asymptomatic hyperuricemia and rheumatoid arthritis: A controlled study. Ann. Rheum. Dis., *41*:344–346, 1982.
67. Hamilton, E.B.D., et al.: The natural history of arthritis in idiopathic haemochromatosis: Progression of the clinical and radiological features over ten years. Q. J. Med., *50*:321–329, 1981.
68. Rynes, R.I., and Merzig, E.G.: Calcium pyrophosphate crystal deposition disease and hyperparathyroidism: A controlled prospective study. J. Rheumatol., *5*:460–468, 1978.
69. Eshel, G. et al.: Hereditary chondrocalcinosis in an Ashkenazi Jewish family. Ann. Rheum. Dis., *49*:528–530, 1990.
70. Aitken, R.E., Kerr, J.L., and Lloyd, H.M.: Primary hyperparathyroidism with osteosclerosis with calcification in articular cartilage. Am. J. Med., *37*:813–820, 1964.
71. Bywaters, E.G.L., Dixon, A. St. J., and Scott, J.T.: Joint lesions of hyperparathyroidism. Ann. Rheum. Dis., *22*:171–187, 1963.
72. Zvaifler, N.J., Reefe, W.E., and Black, R.L.: Articular manifestations in primary hyperparathyroidism. Arthritis Rheum., *5*:237–249, 1962.
73. Currey, H.L.F., et al.: Significance of radiological calcification of joint cartilage. Ann. Rheum. Dis., *25*:295–306, 1966.
74. Skinner, M., and Cohen, A.S.: Calcium pyrophosphate dihydrate crystal deposition disease. Arch. Intern. Med., *123*:636–644, 1969.
75. Van Geertruyden, J. et al.: Effect of parathyroid surgery on cartilage calcification. World J. Surg., *10*:111–115, 1986.
76. Glass, J.S., and Grahame, R.: Chondrocalcinosis after parathyroidectomy. Ann. Rheum. Dis., *35*:521–525, 1976.
77. Pritchard, M.H., and Jessop, J.D.: Chondrocalcinosis in primary hyperparathyroidism. Ann. Rheum. Dis., *36*:146–151, 1977.
78. Marx, S.J., et al.: The hypocalciuric or benign variant of familial hypercalcemia: Clinical and biochemical features in fifteen kindreds. Medicine, *60*:397–412, 1981.
79. Marx, S.J., et al.: An association between neonatal severe primary hyperparathyroidism and familial hypocalciuric hypercalcemia in three kindreds. N. Engl. J. Med., *306*:257–263, 1982.
80. Schumacher, H.R.: Hemochromatosis and arthritis. Arthritis Rheum., 7:41–50, 1964.
81. Ryan, L., and McCarty, D.J.: Calcium pyrophosphate crystal deposition disease; pseudogout; articular chondrocalcinosis. *In* Arthritis and Allied Conditions. 10th Ed. Edited by D.J. McCarty. Philadelphia, Lea & Febiger, 1985.
82. Dorfmann, H., et al.: Les arthropathies des hemochromatoses: Resultats d'une enquete prospective portant sur 54 malades. Sem. Hop. Paris, *45*:416–523, 1969.
83. Dymock, I.W., et al.: Arthropathy of hemochromatosis. Ann. Rheum. Dis., *29*:469–476, 1970.
84. Hamilton, E.B.D.: Diseases associated with CPPD deposition disease. Arthritis Rheum., *19*(Suppl.):353–357, 1976.
85. Adamson, T.C., et al.: Hand and wrist arthropathies of hemochromatosis and calcium pyrophosphate deposition disease: Distinct radiographic features. Radiology, *146*:377–381, 1983.
86. McCarty, D.J., and Pepe, P.F.: Erythrocyte neutral inorganic pyrophosphatase in pseudogout. J. Lab. Clin. Med., *79*:277–284, 1972.
87. Hearn, P.R., Russell, R.G.G., and Elliott, J.C.: Formation product of calcium pyrophosphate crystals in vitro and the effect of iron salts. Clin. Sci. Mol. Med., *54*:29–33, 1978.
88. McCarty, D.J., Palmer, D.W., and Garancis, J.C.: Clearance of calcium pyrophosphate dihydrate crystals in vivo. III. Effects of synovial hemosiderosis. Arthritis Rheum., *24*:706–710, 1981.
89. Pawlotsky, Y., et al.: Histomorphometrie osseuse et manifestations osteo-articulares de l'hemochromatose idiopathique. Rev. Rheum., *46*:91–99, 1979.
90. O'Duffy, J.D.: Hypophosphatasia associated with calcium pyrophosphate dihydrate deposits in cartilage. Arthritis Rheum., *13*:381–388, 1970.
91. Earde, A.W., Swannell, A.J., and Williamson, N.R.: Pyrophosphate arthropathy in hypophosphatasia. Ann. Rheum. Dis., *40*:164–170, 1981.
92. Whyte, M.P., Murphy, W.A., and Fallon, M.D.: Adult hypophosphatasia with chondrocalcinosis and arthropathy: Variable penetrance of hypophosphatemia in a large Oklahoma kindred. Am. J. Med., *72*:631–641, 1982.
93. Russell, R.G.G.: Metabolism of inorganic pyrophosphate (PPi). Arthritis Rheum., *19*(Suppl.):463–478, 1976.
94. Russell, R.G.G., et al.: Inorganic pyrophosphate in plasma in normal persons and in patients with hypophosphatasia, osteogenesis imperfecta and other disorders of bone. J. Clin. Invest., *50*:961–969, 1971.
95. Chuck, A.J. et al.: Crystal deposition in hypophosphatasia: A reappraisal. Ann. Rheum. Dis., *48*:571–576, 1989.
96. Whyte, M.P., et al.: Infantile hypophosphatasia: Enzyme replacement therapy by intravenous infusion of alkaline phosphatase-rich plasma from patients with Paget's bone disease. J. Pediatr., *101*:379–386, 1982.
97. McCarty, D.J., et al.: Diseases associated with calcium pyrophosphate dihydrate crystal deposition: A controlled study. Am. J. Med., *56*:704–714, 1974.
98. McCarty, D.J., et al.: Inorganic pyrophosphate concentrations in the synovial fluid of arthritis patients. J. Lab. Clin. Med., *78*:216–229, 1971.
99. Runeberg, L., et al.: Hypomagnesemia due to renal disease of unknown etiology. Am. J. Med., *59*:873–881, 1975.

100. Doherty, M., and Dieppe, P.A.: Double blind, placebo controlled trial of magnesium carbonate in chronic pyrophosphate arthropathy. (Abstract.) Ann. Rheum. Dis., *42*(Suppl.):106–107, 1983.
101. Dorwart, B.B., and Schumacher, H.R.: Joint effusions, chondrocalcinosis and other rheumatic manifestations in hypothyroidism. Am. J. Med., *59*:780–789, 1975.
102. Alexander, G.M., et al.: Pyrophosphate arthropathy: A study of metabolic associations and laboratory data. Ann. Rheum. Dis., *41*:377–381, 1982.
103. Komatireddy, G.R., Ellman, M.H., and Brown, N.L.: Lack of association between hypothyroidism and chondrocalcinosis. J. Rheumatol., *16*:807–808, 1989.
104. Kaplinski, N., Biran, D., and Frankl, O.: Pseudogout and amyloidosis. Harefuah, *91*:59, 1976.
105. Ryan, L.M., Liang, G., and Kozin, F.: Amyloid arthropathy: Possible association with chondrocalcinosis. J. Rheumatol., *9*:273–278, 1982.
106. Yood, R.A., et al.: Soft tissue uptake of bone seeking radionuclide in amyloidosis. J. Rheumatol., *8*:760–766, 1981.
107. Egan, M.S., et al.: The association of amyloid deposits and osteoarthritis. Arthritis Rheum., *25*:204–208, 1982.
108. Ladefoged, C.: Amyloid in osteoarthritic hip joints: A pathoanatomical and histological investigation of femoral head cartilage. Acta Orthop. Scand., *53*:581–586, 1982.
109. Stockman, A., Darlington, L.G., and Scott, J.T.: Frequency of chondrocalcinosis of the knees and avascular necrosis of the femoral heads in gout: A controlled study. Ann. Rheum. Dis., *39*:7–11, 1980.
110. Hamza, M., and Bardin, T.: Camptodactyly, polyepiphyseal dysplasia and mixed crystal deposition disease. J. Rheumatol., *16*:1153–1158, 1989.
111. Sambrook, P.N. et al.: Synovial complications of spondyloepiphyseal dysplasia of late onset. Arthritis Rheum., *31*:282–287, 1988.
112. Kahn, M.F. et al.: Le rhumatisme chondrodyplasique. Sem. Hop. Paris, *46*:1938–1953, 1970.
113. Okazaki, T. et al.: Pseudogout: Clinical observations and chemical analyses of deposits. Arthritis Rheum., *19*:293–305, 1976.
114. VanderKorst, J.K., Geerards, J., and Driessens, F.C.M.: A hereditary type of idiopathic articular chondrocalcinosis. Am. J. Med., *56*:307–314, 1974.
115. Weaver, J.B.: Calcification and ossification of the menisci. J. Bone Joint Surg., *24*:873–882, 1942.
116. Altman, R.D.: Arthroscopic findings of the knee in patients with pseudogout. Arthritis Rheum., *19*:286–292, 1976.
117. Bird, H.A., Tribe, C.R., and Bacon, P.A.: Joint hypermobility leading to osteoarthrosis and chondrocalcinosis. Ann. Rheum. Dis., *37*:203–211, 1978.
118. Settas, L., Doherty, M., and Dieppe, P.: Localized chondrocalcinosis in unstable joints. Br. Med. J., *285*:175–176, 1982.
119. Collis, C.H., Dieppe, P.A., and Bullimore, J.A.: Radiation-induced chondrocalcinosis of the knee articular cartilage. Clin. Radiol., *39*:450–451, 1989.
120. Ellman, M., Krieger, M.I., and Brown, N.: Pseudogout mimicking synovial chondromatosis. J. Bone Joint Surg., *57A*:863–865, 1975.
121. Gerster, J.C. et al.: Carpal tunnel syndrome in chondrocalcinosis of the wrist. Arthritis Rheum., *23*:926–931, 1980.
122. Ahlgren, P.: Chondrocalcinois og knogleusurer. Nord. Med., *73*:309–313, 1965.
123. Lagier, R.: Case report: Rare femoral erosions and osteoarthritis of the knee associated with chondrocalcinosis. A histological study of this cortical remodeling. Virchows Arch. [A], *364*:215–223, 1974.
124. Resnick, D., and Niwyama, G.: Carpal instability in rheumatoid arthritis and calcium pyrophosphate deposition disease. Ann. Rheum. Dis., *36*:311–318, 1977.
125. Ross, D.J. et al.: Tibial stress fracture in pyrophosphate arthropathy. J. Bone Joint Surg., *65B*:474–477, 1983.
126. Houpt, J.B., and Sinclair, D.S.: Spontaneous osteonecrosis of the medial femoral condyle. (Abstract.) J. Rheumatol., *1*(Suppl.):117, 1974.
127. Watt, I., and Dieppe, P.: Medial femoral condyle necrosis and chondrocalcinosis: A causal relationship. Br. J. Radiol., *56*:7–22, 1983.
128. Ali, S.Y. et al.: Ultrastructural studies of pyrophosphate crystal deposition in articular cartilage. Ann. Rheum. Dis., *42*(Suppl.):97–98, 1983.
129. Bjelle, A.: Cartilage matrix in hereditary pyrophosphate arthropathy. J. Rheumatol., *8*:959–964, 1981.
130. Ishikawa, H. et al.: Interaction of polymorphonuclear leukocytes with calcium pyrophosphate dihydrate crystals deposited in chondrocalcinosis cartilage. Rheumatol. Int., *7*:217–221, 1987.
131. Ishikawa, K. et al.: A histological study of calcium pyrophosphate dihydrate crystal-deposition disease. J. Bone Joint Surg., *71-A*:875–886, 1989.
132. Ohira, T. et al.: Histologic localization of lipid in the articular tissues in calcium pyrophosphate dihydrate crystal deposition disease. Arthritis Rheum., *31*:1057–1062, 1988.
133. Masuda, I., Ishikawa, I., and Usuku, G.: A histologic and immunohistochemical study of calcium pyrophosphate dihydrate crystal deposition disease. Clin. Orthop., *263*:272–287, 1991.
134. Chen, F. et al.: The distribution of S-100 protein in articular cartilage from osteoarthritic joints. J. Rheumatol., *17*:1676–1681, 1990.
135. Boivin, G., and Lagier, R.: An ultrastructural study of articular chondrocalcinosis in cases of knee osteoarthritis. Virchows Arch. [A], *400*:13–29, 1983.
136. Mitrovic, D.: Pathology of articular deposition of calcium salts and their relationship to osteoarthritis. Ann. Rheum. Dis., *42*(Suppl.):19–26, 1983.
137. Schumacher, H.R.: The synovitis of pseudogout: electron microscopic observations. Arthritis Rheum., *11*:426–435, 1968.
138. Schumacher, H.R.: Articular cartilage in the degenerative arthropathy of hemochromatosis. Arthritis Rheum., *25*: 1460–1468, 1982.
139. McCarty, D.J., Palmer, D.W., and James, C.: Clearance of calcium pyrophosphate dihydrate crystals in vivo: II. Studies using triclinic crystals doubly labeled with ^{45}Ca and ^{85}Sr. Arthritis Rheum., *22*:1122–1131, 1979.
140. Hearn, P.R., Guilland-Cumming, D.F., and Russell, R.G.G.: Effect of orthophosphate and other factors on the crystal growth of calcium pyrophosphate. Ann. Rheum. Dis., *42*(Suppl.):101, 1983.
141. Cheng, P.T., and Pritzker, K.: Pyrophosphate, phosphate ion interaction: Effects on calcium pyrophosphate and calcium hydroxyapatite crystal formation in aqueous solution. J. Rheumatol., *10*:769–777, 1983.
142. Silcox, D.C., and McCarty, D.J.: Elevated inorganic pyrophosphate concentrations in synovial fluid in osteoarthritis and pseudogout. J. Lab. Clin. Med., *83*:518–531, 1974.
143. Pritzker, K.P.H. et al.: Calcium pyrophosphate dihydrate crystal formation in model hydrogels. J. Rheumatol., *5*:469–473, 1978.
144. Mandel, N.S., and Mandel, G.S.: Nucleation and growth of CPPD crystals and related species in vitro. *In* Calcium in Biological Systems. Edited by R.P. Rubin, G. Weiss, and J.W. Putner. New York, Plenum, 1985.
145. Mandel, N., Mandel, G., Carroll, D., and Halverson, P.: Calcium

pyrophosphate crystal deposition. An in vitro study using a gelatin matrix model. Arthritis Rheum., *27*:789–796, 1984.

146. Lust, G. et al.: Increased pyrophosphate in fibroblasts and lymphoblasts from patients with hereditary diffuse articular chondrocalcinosis. Science, *214*:809–810, 1981.
147. Jung, A., Bisaz, S., and Fleisch, H.: The binding of pyrophosphate and two diphosphonates by hydroxyapatite crystals. Calc. Tiss. Res., *11*:269–280, 1973.
148. McGaughey, C.: Binding of polyphosphates and phosphonates to hydroxyapatite, subsequent hydrolysis, phosphate exchange and effects on demineralization, mineralization, and microcrystal aggregation. Caries Res., *17*:229–241, 1983.
149. Russell, R.G.G., Bisaz, S., and Fleisch, H.: Inorganic pyrophosphate in plasma, urine and synovial fluid of patients with pyrophosphate arthropathy (chondrocalcinosis or pseudogout). Lancet, *2*:899–902, 1970.
150. Pflug, M., McCarty, D.J., and Kawahara, F.: Basal urinary pyrophosphate excretion in pseudogout. Arthritis Rheum., *12*:228–231, 1969.
151. Silcox, D.C., Jacobelli, S.G., and McCarty, D.J.: The identification of inorganic pyrophosphate in human platelets and its release on stimulation with thrombin. J. Clin. Invest., *52*:1595–1600, 1973.
152. Ryan, L.M., Kozin, F., and McCarty, D.J.: Quantification of human plasma inorganic pyrophosphatase: II. Biologic variables. Arthritis Rheum., *22*:892–895, 1979.
153. Ryan, L.M., Kozin, F., and McCarty, D.J.: Quantification of human plasma inorganic pyrophosphate: I. Normal values in osteoarthritis and calcium pyrophosphate dihydrate crystal deposition disease. Arthritis Rheum., *22*:886–891, 1979.
154. Altman, R.D. et al.: Articular chondrocalcinosis: Microanalysis of pyrophosphate (PPi) in synovial fluid and plasma. Arthritis Rheum., *16*:171–178, 1973.
155. Sorensen, S.A., Flodgaard, H., and Sorensen, E.: Serum alkaline phosphatase, serum pyrophosphatase, phosphoreylethanolamine, and inorganic pyrophosphate in plasma and urine: A genetic and clinical study of hypophosphatasia. Monogr. Hum. Genet., *10*:66–69, 1978.
156. Rachow, J., and Ryan, L.: Adenosine triphosphate pyrophosphohydrolase and neutral inorganic pyrophosphatase in pathologic joint fluids. Arthritis Rheum., *28*:1283–1288, 1985.
157. Howell, D.S. et al.: Extrusion of pyrophosphate into extracellular media by osteoarthritic cartilage incubates. J. Clin. Invest., *56*:1473–1480, 1975.
158. Ryan, L.M., Cheung, H.S., and McCarty, D.J.: Release of pyrophosphate by normal mammalian articular hyaline and fibrocartilage in organ culture. Arthritis Rheum., *24*:1522–1527, 1981.
159. Camerlain, M. et al.: Inorganic pyrophosphate pool size and turnover rate in arthritic joints. J. Clin. Invest., *55*:1373–1381, 1975.
160. Tenenbaum, J. et al.: Comparison of phosphohydrolase activities from articular cartilage in calcium pyrophosphate deposition disease and primary osteoarthritis. Arthritis Rheum., *24*:492–500, 1981.
161. Cartier, P., and Picard, J.: La mineralisation du cartilage ossifiable: III. Le mechanisme de la reaction atpasique du cartilage. Bull. Soc. Chim. Biol., *37*:1159–1168, 1955.
162. Hsu, H.: Purification and partial characterization of ATP pyrophosphohydrolase from fetal bovine epiphyseal cartilage. J. Biol. Chem., *258*:3463–3468, 1983.
163. Siegel, S.A., Hummel, C.F., and McCarty, R.P.: The role of nucleoside triphosphate pyrophosphohydrolase in vitro nucleoside triphosphate-dependent matrix vesicle calcification. J. Biol. Chem., *258*:8601–8607, 1983.
164. Hsu, H., and Anderson, H.: The deposition of calcium pyrophosphate and phosphate by matrix vesicles isolated from fetal bovine epiphyseal cartilage. Calcif. Tiss. Int., *36*:615–621, 1984.
165. Hsu, H., and Anderson, H.: The deposition of calcium pyrophosphate by NTP pyrophosphohydrolase of matrix vesicles from fetal bovine epiphyseal cartilage. Int. J. Biochem., *18*:1141–1146, 1986.
166. Ryan, L.M. et al.: Cartilage nucleoside triphosphate (NTP) pyrophosphohydrolase: I. Identification as an ectoenzyme. Arthritis Rheum., *27*:913–918, 1984.
167. Howell, D. et al.: NTP pyrophosphohydrolase in human chondrocalcinotic and osteoarthritic cartilage: II. Further studies on histologic and subcellular distribution. Arthritis Rheum., *27*:193–199, 1984.
168. Caswell, A., and Russell, R.G.G.: Identification of ecto-nucleoside triphosphate pyrophosphatase in human articular chondrocytes in monolayer culture. Biochim. et Biophys. Acta., *847*:40–47, 1985.
169. Felix, R., and Fleisch, H.: The effect of pyrophosphate and diphosphonates on calcium transport in red cells. Experientia, *33*:1003–1005, 1977.
170. Ryan, L., Rachow, J., and McCarty, D.J.: Synovial fluid ATP: A possible substrate for generation of inorganic pyrophosphate in calcium pyrophosphate dihydrate (CPPD) crystal deposition disease. J. Rheumatol., *18*:716–720, 1991.
171. Derfus, B.A., et al.: Articular cartilage vesicles form calcium pyrophosphate dihydrate-like crystals. Clin. Res., *39*:249A, 1991.
172. Lust, G. et al.: Evidence of a generalized metabolic defect in patients with hereditary chondrocalcinosis. Arthritis Rheum., *24*:1517–1521, 1981.
173. Ryan, L.M., Lynch, M.P., and McCarty, D.J.: Inorganic pyrophosphate levels in blood platelets from normal donors and patients with calcium pyrophosphate dihydrate crystal deposition disease. Arthritis Rheum., *26*:564–566, 1983.
174. Ryan, L. et al.: Pyrophosphohydrolase activity with inorganic pyrophosphate content of cultured human skin fibroblasts. J. Clin. Invest., *77*:1689–1693, 1986.
175. Pieter, A. et al.: Inorganic pyrophosphate release by rabbit articular chondrocytes in vitro. Arthritis Rheum., *29*:1485–1492, 1986.
176. Ryan, L.M. et al.: Cartilage inorganic pyrophosphate elaboration is independent of sulfated glycosaminoglycan synthesis. Arthritis Rheum., *33*:235–240, 1990.
177. Ryan, L.M., Kurup, I., and Cheung, H.S.: Stimulation of cartilage inorganic pyrophosphate elaboration by ascorbate. Matrix, (in press).
178. Alvarellos, A., and Spilberg, I.: Colchicine prophylaxis in pseudogout. J. Rheumatol., *13*:804–805, 1986.
179. Bennett, R.M., Lehr, J.R., and McCarty, D.J.: Crystal shedding and acute pseudogout: A hypothesis based on a therapeutic failure. Arthritis Rheum., *19*:93–97, 1976.
180. Fam, A.G., and Stein, G.: Disappearance of chondrocalcinosis following reflex sympathetic dystrophy. Arthritis Rheum., *24*:747–749, 1981.
181. Sarkozi, A.M., Nemeth-Csoka, M., and Bartosiewicz, G.: Effect of glycosaminoglycan polysulphate in the treatment of chondrocalcinosis. Clin. Exp. Rheumatol., *6*:3–8, 1988.
182. Doherty, M., and Dieppe, P.A.: Effect of intra-articular yttrium-90 on chronic pyrophosphate arthropathy of the knee. Lancet, *1*:1243–1246, 1981.

109

Basic Calcium Phosphate (Apatite, Octacalcium Phosphate, Tricalcium Phosphate) Crystal Deposition Diseases

PAUL B. HALVERSON
DANIEL J. McCARTY

There are innumerable reports of pathologic calcium phosphate mineral phase deposition in various human tissues. These reports are largely descriptive, and most present no clear pattern of disease. Basic calcium phosphate (BCP) crystals, formerly thought to be simply hydroxyapatite (HA), have long been associated with calcific periarthritis and tendonitis.[1] BCP crystals were later found in synovial fluid by scanning electron microscopy (SEM) or transmission electron microscopy (TEM).[2,3]

CRYSTAL IDENTIFICATION

The study of BCP crystal–associated arthritis has been relatively difficult because of the lack of a simple, reliable diagnostic test (see also Chapter 5). Heterogeneity of crystal species in periarticular shoulder joint calcifications was first established by Faure et al., who directly measured the interplanar spacings of individual apatite crystals using high-resolution TEM.[4] These crystals were largely carbonate-substituted, and other nonapatitic calcium phosphates were found. Intensive study of a subcutaneous calcification from a patient with scleroderma showed amorphous and poorly crystallized calcium phosphate in nodular aggregates with internodular apatite crystals.[5] Fourier transform infrared (FTIR) analysis of shoulder joint fluid crystals, of calcified rabbit synovium and of subcutaneous calcifications from dermatomyositis showed that each contained partially carbonate-substituted HA, octacalcium phosphate (OCP), and particulate collagens (Table 109–1).[6] Samples from one patient had tricalcium phosphate instead of OCP. BCP is therefore used generically here to designate these crystal mixtures. "BCP crystal deposition disease" proposed as the most appropriate term for the associated clinical syndromes.

Radiography. BCP crystal deposits are rounded or fluffy calcifications varying from a few millimeters to several centimeters in diameter. They may occur either as solitary nodules or as multiple deposits. Although radiography is a useful diagnostic tool, it is both relatively insensitive and nonspecific in the diagnosis of BCP crystal arthropathies.[7] Asymptomatic periarticular calcific deposits are frequently observed as incidental findings.

Synovial Fluid. Phase-contrast polarized light microscopy, invaluable for the detection of the larger monosodium urate monohydrate and calcium pyrophosphate dihydrate crystals, provides little help with BCP crystals, because their size is below the limits of resolution of optical microscopy. Although these crystals tend to aggregate, their orientation within an aggregate is usually random, and they are not birefringent. Rarely, birefringence is noted because thousands of ultramicroscopic crystals are oriented along the same axis.[8] Individual needle- or plate-shaped crystals are usually less than 0.1 μm long (Fig. 109–1). BCP crystal aggregates may be visible by light microscopy as shiny laminated "coins" (see Fig. 5–5B). Alizarin red S staining of synovial fluid pellets has been suggested as a screening technique for BCP crystals.[9] The method is sensitive to 0.005

TABLE 109–1. CHEMICAL FORMULAE AND MOLAR RATIOS OF CALCIUM (Ca) TO PHOSPHORUS (P) OF CALCIUM-CONTAINING CRYSTALS FOUND IN HUMAN SYNOVIAL FLUID, CARTILAGE, OR SYNOVIUM

CRYSTAL	FORMULA	Ca/P
BCP		
Hydroxyapatite (HA)	$Ca_5(PO_4)_3OH2H_2O$	1.67
Octacalcium phosphate (OCP)	$Ca_8H_2(PO_4)_65H_2O$	1.33
Tricalcium phosphate (TCP) (whitlockite)	$Ca_3(PO_4)_2$	1.5
OTHER		
Dicalcium phosphate dihydrate (brushite)	$CaHPO_42H_2O$	1.0
Calcium pyrophosphate dihydrate	$Ca_2P_2O_7H_2O$	1.0
Calcium oxalate	$CaC_2O_4H_2O$	∞

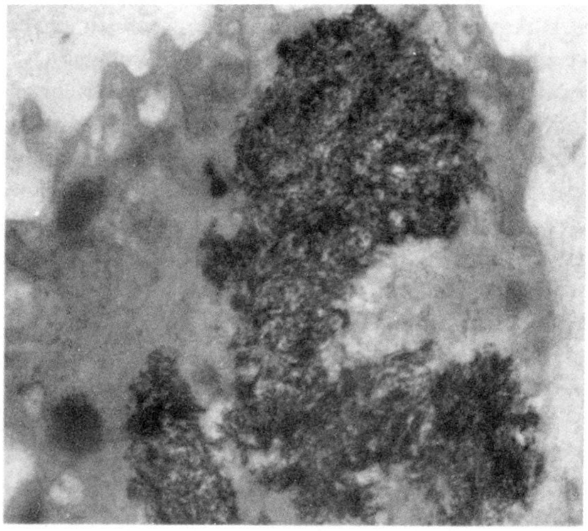

FIGURE 109–1. Aggregate of needle-shaped crystals within a synovial fibrocyte. No limiting membrane can be identified (×43,800). (Garancis, J.C., et al.: Milwaukee shoulder: Association of microspheroids containing hydroxyapatite crystals, active collagenase and neutral protease with rotator cuff defects. III. Morphologic and biochemical studies of an excised synovium showing chondromatosis. Arthritis Rheum., *24*:484–491, 1981.)

μg of HA standard per milliliter, but it is not specific for calcium phosphates and may provide many false-positive results.[10,11]

A semiquantitative technique using the binding of (^{14}C) ethane-1-hydroxy-1, 1-diphosphonate (EHDP) to BCP crystals has proved useful as a screening test and is sensitive to about 2 μg HA standard.[1,12] Diphosphonate binding in synovial fluid correlated strongly with the radiographic grade of osteoarthritis present (Fig. 109–2).[12,13] Synovial fluid pellets that bound EHDP were examined routinely by SEM. Microspheroidal aggregates approximately 1 to 19 μm in diameter were generally found (Fig. 109–3A). These aggregates were then further characterized by x-ray energy dispersive analysis.[14] The spectrum analyzed for calcium and phosphorus, and the relative molar amounts of each element were calculated using an on-line computer (Fig. 109–3B). Schumacher has suggested routine use of TEM,[15] which, while not quantitative, has the advantage of better definition of crystal morphology and location (e.g., in cells).

X-ray diffraction of BCP mineral by the powder method is relatively insensitive. Such small, poorly crystallized material yields broad diffraction minima that cannot differentiate between closely related calcium phosphate compounds. Electron diffraction, high-resolution TEM, and FTIR spectrophotometry are useful research tools but are not practical for everyday clinical use.

Direct chemical analysis for calcium and phosphorus of several pellets from joint fluid that bound (^{14}C) EHDP showed levels of 12 to 45 μg BCP mineral per milliliter.[14]

DISEASES

Several articular and periarticular conditions associated with BCP crystals have been described (Table 109–2). Calcific tendonitis and bursitis are discussed in Chapters 89 and 99, and calcinosis in Chapter 73. The secondary BCP arthropathies occur in conditions known to predispose to such crystal deposition (Table 109–2).

TABLE 109–2. BASIC CALCIUM PHOSPHATE CRYSTAL-ASSOCIATED JOINT DISEASE*

CALCIFIC PERIARTHRITIS
Unifocal
"Hydroxyapatite pseudopodagra"[16]
Multifocal
Familial[17]
CALCIFIC TENDONITIS AND BURSITIS[18]
INTRA-ARTICULAR BCP ARTHROPATHIES
Acute (gout-like) attacks
Milwaukee shoulder/knee syndrome[7]
(Idiopathic destructive arthritis; cuff tear arthropathy)
Erosive polyarticular disease
Mixed crystal deposition disease (BCP and CPPD)
SECONDARY BCP CRYSTAL ARTHROPATHIES/PERIARTHROPATHIES†
Chronic renal failure
"Collagen" disease (calcinosis)[19,20]
Sequel to severe neurologic injury
Postlocal corticosteroid injection
Other
TUMORAL CALCINOSIS
Hyperphosphatemic
Nonhyperphosphatemic

BCP = basic calcium phosphate; CPPD = calcium pyrophosphate dihydrate.

* See reference 1 for references to older publications.

† Mineral deposits may also occur in fibrous tissues remote from joints in these conditions.

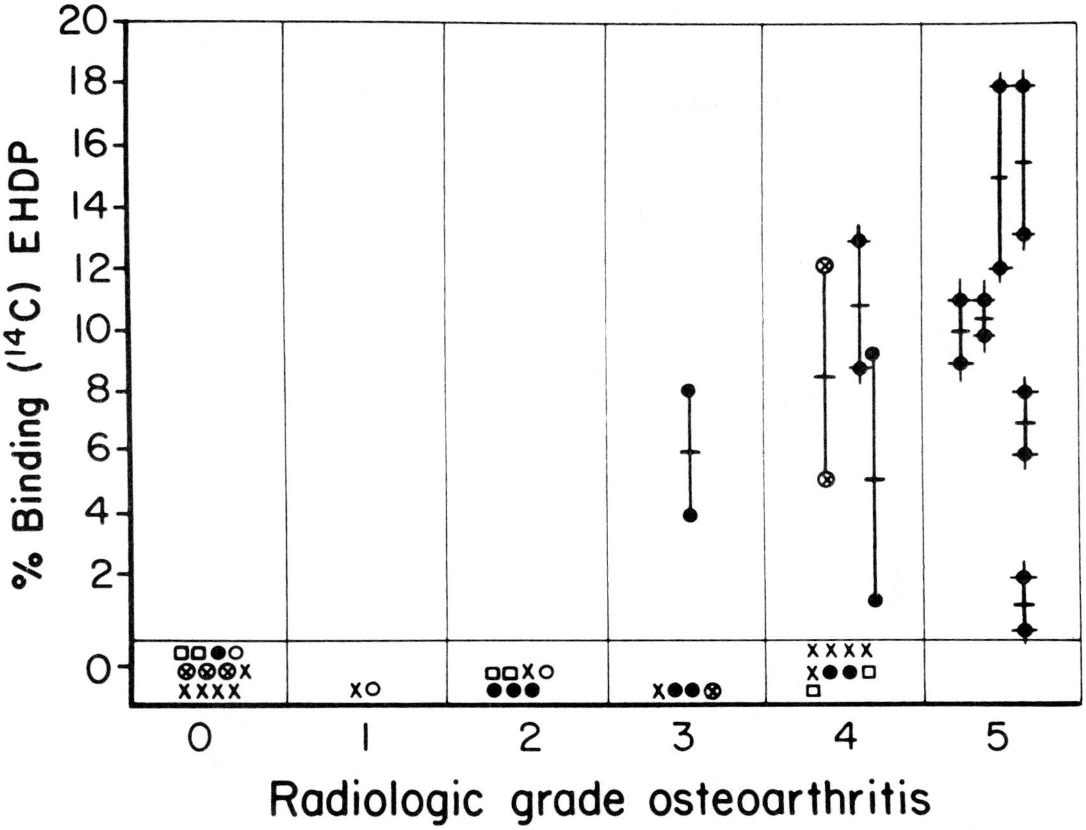

FIGURE 109–2. Fluids that bound (^{14}C) ethane-1-hydroxy-1, 1-diphosphonate (EHDP) generally were obtained from joints with advanced degenerative changes (radiologic grades 4 and 5). □ = internal derangement of knee; ● = osteoarthritis; ✦ = osteoarthritis with few calcium pyrophosphate deposition crystals in fluid; × = inflammatory arthritis with white blood cell (WBC) concentration >3,000 mm³; ⊗ = inflammatory arthritis with WBC concentration <3,000 mm³; ○ = miscellaneous arthritis. Positive results are shown in duplicate. (From Halverson, P.B., and McCarty, D.J.[12])

ROTATOR CUFF CALCIFICATIONS

In the shoulder, the location of rotator cuff calcifications has been related to etiopathogenesis, natural history, and prognosis.[21] Sarkar and Uhthoff found that calcifications at the tidemark of the rotator cuff insertion into the greater tuberosity of the humerus represented degenerative enthesopathy with *secondary calcifications.* These and the secondary calcification of the torn ends of a rotator cuff are irreversible. On the other hand, *"primary" calcification* in the rotator cuff, approximately 1.5 cm away from the tidemark in "Codman's critical area," occurred in metaplastic fibrocartilage. These deposits were associated with matrix vesicles and with crystal phagocytosis by macrophages and giant cells. *The natural history of such deposits is resorption.* Scalloping of the fluffy radiodense deposits on roentgenograms represents the radiologic correlate of cellular resorption of mineral.[21] Others have not found chondroid metaplasia or matrix vesicles in calcific tenosynovitis but found instead psammoma bodies and calcification within necrotic cells.[22]

CARTILAGE AND SYNOVIAL CALCIFICATIONS

Ali has presented electron microscopic evidence for pericellular matrix vesicles in normal articular cartilage, which he regards as a latent growth plate.[23] Vesicles were present at all levels of the cartilage but were most numerous near the tidemark adjoining the subchondral bone. Microcrystals within mineral nodules (0.6 μm in diameter) were noted in various stages of formation. Both vesicles and mineral were greatly increased in osteoarthritic cartilage; quantitatively, this increase was reflected by a marked increase (up to 30-fold) in alkaline phosphatase activity. Three distinct types of calcification in osteoarthritic cartilage were seen. In addition to the mineral nodules just discussed, dense cuboidal-shaped crystals resembling whitlockite morphologically, but with a molar Ca/P of 1.72, were found in

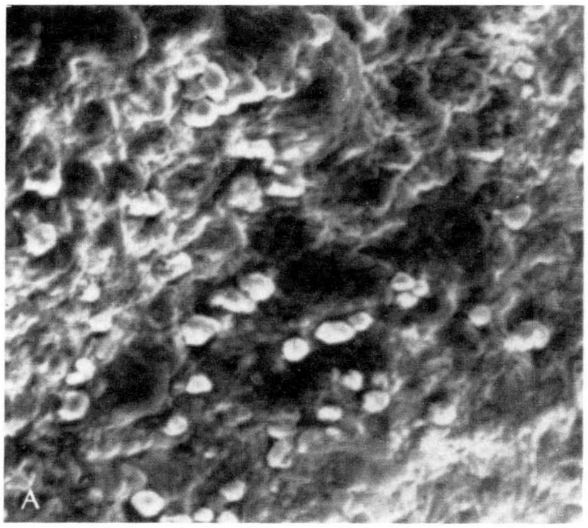

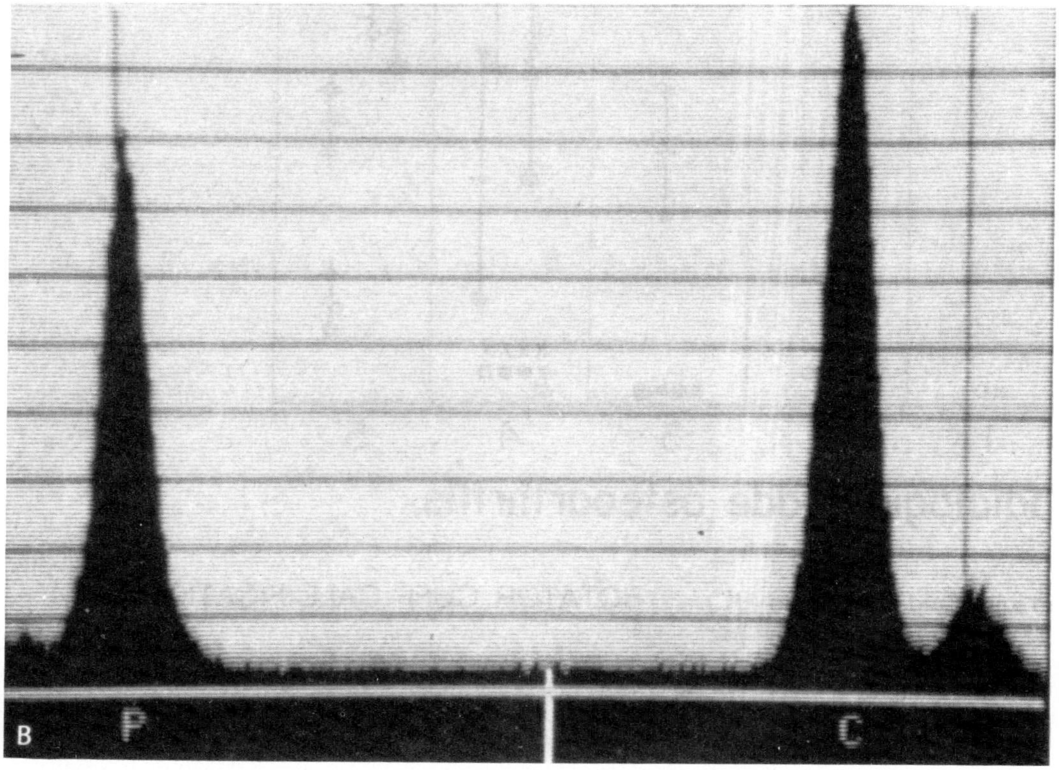

FIGURE 109–3. *A*, Scanning electron micrograph of synovial fluid sediment showing typical microspheroidal crystal aggregates (×525). (From Halverson, P.B., et al.[14]) *B*, Spectrograph from x-ray energy dispersive analysis showing peaks for phosphorus and calcium.

pericellular matrix around the surface chondrocytes. Fine needle-shaped crystal clusters were observed on the cartilage surface in the acellular amorphous zone (lamina splendens). These clusters had a molar Ca/P of 1.7 and resembled the crystals found in synovial fluid. Matrix vesicles and crystals were seen in rabbit fibrocartilage that had formed from autologous grafts of synovial tissue implanted into defects produced surgically in hyaline cartilage but not in sham-operated joints.[24]

A systematic study of articular cartilage from 28 patients with advanced osteoarthritis (OA) showed superficial HA-type needle-shaped crystals in 56%; calcified deposits were found in 36% in deeper repair-type fibrocartilage, and calcium pyrophosphate deposition (CPPD) crystals were seen in 11% of cases.[25] Overall, 75% of the cartilages had microcrystalline deposits of some kind. Synovium from the same joints all showed a patchy lining cell hyperplasia and giant cells, whether, or not calcific deposits were present in the area. Calcific deposits were present in 70% of synovial specimens. All were of the HA type, but four specimens also showed CPPD deposits. The pathologic prevalence of 70 to 75% synovial calcification is in accord with a radiologic survey of osteoarthritic knee joints, wherein 72% showed periarticular or intra-articular calcification.[26]

CALCIFIC PERIARTHRITIS

Periarticular calcifications are found most commonly around the shoulder but have been described near many other joints. Calcific scapulohumeral periarthritis was first described in 1870.[1] Roentgenographic demonstration of periarticular shoulder calcifications was accomplished in 1907,[1] and a classic review of 329 cases of peritendinitis calcarea was presented in 1938.[1] Calcium deposits were found in one or both shoulders of 138 of 5061 employees of a life insurance company.[1] More than 70% of patients were under age 40, and many remained asymptomatic, although large deposits usually caused acute painful inflammation eventually. Spontaneous resorption of some deposits, especially the smaller ones, occurred. Nearly half of these subjects had bilateral deposits.

Most cases of acute calcific periarthritis consist of a single attack in a single joint, frequently with localized warmth, erythema, swelling, and pain lasting up to a few weeks. The roentgenographic finding of periarticular calcification is useful as a confirmatory diagnostic aid (see Fig. 99–9).

Hydroxyapatite pseudopodagra is a term used by Fam and Rubenstein[16] to describe acute inflammation in the first metatarsal phalangeal joint usually in young women. Radiographs show periarticular calcific deposits, which later disappear. However, because the crystals are almost certainly a mixture of basic calcium phosphates and because podagra means "seizure in the foot," it is perhaps an unfortunate choice of words.

Recurrent attacks of calcific periarthritis occurring at multiple sites suggest a more generalized condition rather than a chance localized process with resultant calcification.[1] Several reports describe familial occurrences of calcific arthritis and periarthritis.[1,17]

Episodic attacks of calcific periarthritis have been treated successfully with a variety of nonsteroidal anti-inflammatory drugs (NSAIDs) and colchicine.[1] Needle aspiration of the paste-like calcific deposits with or without irrigation may be helpful.[1] Mechanical disruption and dispersion of the deposits may speed their removal by phagocytosis, as outlined by Sarkar and Uhthoff.[21] Surgical removal of large calcific deposits usually provides permanent symptomatic relief. Codman considered this procedure to be essential for symptomatic relief.[1]

BCP CRYSTAL–RELATED ARTHRITIS

BCP crystals may be found within joint fluid as well as in cartilage and synovium. Schumacher and associates have described both acute and chronic forms of arthritis.[3] Acute attacks of arthritis in relatively young persons occurred with pain, swelling, and erythema resembling gout. Crystals resembling BCP were found by TEM in synovial fluid pellets with significantly elevated synovial fluid leukocyte counts and normal joint roentgenograms. The phlogistic potential of BCP crystals was demonstrated by injecting them into rabbit joints. Persons with chronic degenerative arthropathy and three patients with erosive arthritis were also described.[1] Recurrent episodes of pain and swelling were associated with gradual erosion and destructive changes in metacarpophalangeal, proximal interphalangeal, and wrist joints. One of the three patients had chronic renal failure. Although all had radiographic evidence of periarticular calcific deposits, no synovial fluid was obtained; therefore, it remains unclear whether intrasynovial crystals were present.

In 1976, Dieppe et al. reported that synovial fluid from five patients with clinical evidence of osteoarthritis contained 0.15- to 0.8-μm crystals, which by x-ray energy dispersive analysis were compatible with apatite.[2] Other reports have established that crystals of the apatite family are found in approximately 30 to 60% of synovial fluid from patients with knee joint osteoarthritis.[13,27,28] Leukocyte levels in synovial fluid from osteoarthritic joints were no different if crystals were also present.[27] BCP and CPPD crystals were found more frequently together than separately in fluid from joints of patients with osteoarthritis of the knee; the presence of BCP crystals correlated with joint deterioration, whereas the finding of CPPD crystals correlated with patient age.[13] BCP and CPPD crystals were found together in soft tissues in association with carpal tunnel syndrome.[29]

MILWAUKEE SHOULDER/KNEE SYNDROME

We have studied 30 cases of a peculiar arthropathy, which we named *Milwaukee shoulder syndrome (MSS)*.[7] Robert Adams of Dublin was the first to describe this entity as *rheumatic arthritis of the shoulder* in 1857.[30,31,31a] Salient clinical, radiographic, and synovial fluid findings are listed in Table 109–3.

Adams and his colleague Smith described the regular disappearance of the rotator cuff and the intra-articular

TABLE 109–3. FEATURES OF MILWAUKEE SHOULDER/KNEE SYNDROME

CLINICAL FEATURES
Elderly, female predominance
Dominant shoulder usually affected but often bilateral
Symptoms variable—asymptomatic to severe pain at rest; mostly painful after use and at night. Glenohumeral joint stiffness or instability
ROENTGENOGRAPHIC FEATURES
Glenohumeral joint degeneration
Soft tissue calcification
Upward subluxation of the humeral head
SYNOVIAL FLUID
Low leukocyte counts; few to many erythrocytes
Basic calcium phosphate crystal aggregates
Particular collagens
Elevated protease activities in some fluids.

portion of the tendon of the long head of the biceps. Because the process was often bilateral and patients had no history of trauma, Adams and Smith attributed such massive loss of fibrous tissue to an intra-articular disease process and not to a traumatic cuff tear. They described upward subluxation of the humeral head with eburnation of its superior aspect as it formed a pseudo-articulation with the coricoacromial vault. Synovial hypertrophy with frequent formation of pedunculated loose bodies and separation of the acromion into two parts along the plane of the epiphysis was also clearly described.

Clinical Features. The primary findings include female predominance (80%), greater involvement of the dominant side, glenohumeral joint degeneration, and lysis of the rotator cuff. Others have described similar patients under a variety of descriptive terms. A summary of all reported studies is shown in Table 109–4. The average age of patients was 72 years with range of 50 to 90 years. The average duration of symptoms, when ascertainable, was 3.8 years, but the range was variable (1 to 10 years). The exact time of onset could not be determined in some cases. The syndrome appeared to evolve slowly over a span of years in most patients, with the exception of one woman in whom it was documented to occur in less than 1 year. She had suffered a traumatic rotator cuff tear from a motor vehicle accident. A surgical repair was attempted but broke down when the shoulder became infected. After resolution of sepsis, a large, noninflammatory effusion associated with chronic pain ensued. Symptoms also varied. Three patients with bilateral shoulder involvement had asymptomatic disease on the nondominant side. Most persons experienced mild to moderate pain, especially after use, but one patient had severe pain even at rest. Other symptoms included limitation of motion, stiffness, and pain at night. Examination showed reduced active range of motion in all affected shoulders, sometimes associated with pronounced joint instability. Crepitation and pain were often noted when the humerus was grated passively against the glenoid. Unusual features may include acromioclavicular joint cyst, acromial stress fracture, and formation of a sinus draining into the tissues of the anterior chest wall.[32–34]

Aspiration of the affected shoulder joints routinely yielded 3 to 40 mL of synovial fluid that was frequently blood tinged. Occasionally, hydrops of the shoulder yielding 130 mL or more of synovial fluid was encountered (Fig. 109–4). In two instances, hydrops was asso-

TABLE 109–4. SUMMARY OF REPORTS DESCRIBING 72 PATIENTS WITH SEVERE SHOULDER DEGENERATION*

N	MALE/ FEMALE	MEAN AGE (YEARS)	AGE RANGE	BILATERAL	(%)
72	13:59	72	(50–90)	46	(64)

* Data cited in refs. 1 and 7.

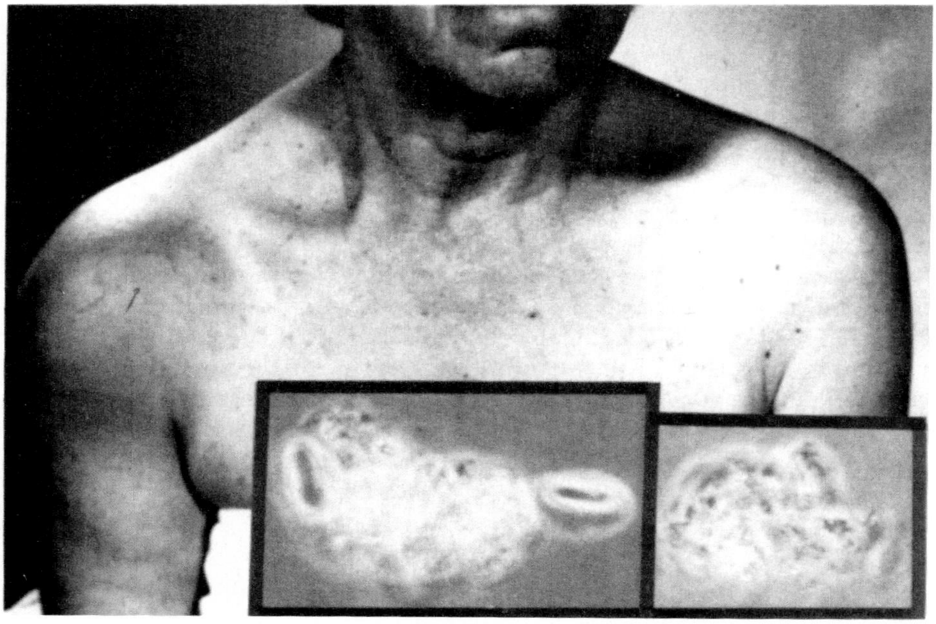

FIGURE 109–4. Photograph of a 62-year-old woman with grotesque swelling of the right shoulder. Inserts show two crystal masses found in a wet preparation of fresh joint fluid. Note the erythrocytes for size comparison (phase contrast × 1,000). (From McCarty, D.J. et al.: Milwaukee shoulder: Association of microspheroids containing hydroxyapatite crystals, active collagenase and neutral protease with rotator cuff defects: I. Clinical aspects. Arthritis Rheum., *24*:464–473, 1981.)

ciated with joint rupture and dissection of fluid onto the anterior chest wall.

Associated Factors. Several factors that may predispose to the development of MSS have been identified.[7] Trauma or overuse was observed in 9 of our 30 cases. Four patients had fallen on an outstretched hand, and one was involved in a motor vehicle accident. Two men had "traumatic" professions (jackhammer operation and professional wrestling), and two other men had experienced recurrent shoulder dislocations. Recurrent dislocation has been identified as a predisposing cause of shoulder arthropathy.[35] Two patients with paraparesis used their shoulders as weight-bearing joints while crutch-walking and later using wheelchairs—conditions described as the "impingement syndrome of paraplegia.[36] Another patient had a dysplastic left shoulder from birth and developed MSS on the opposite side. Eight patients were found to have BCP and CPPD crystals simultaneously and all but one of these also had symptomatic knee involvement. Three patients had severe neurologic disorders (syringomyelia in one and cervical radiculopathies in two). Thus, the shoulder disease was partially attributable to denervation resulting in neuropathic joints. One patient had chronic renal failure requiring hemodialysis. The remaining one third of patients, all of them women, had no identifiable contributing factor.

Milwaukee shoulder/knee syndrome may represent the final common pathway of several conditions, although other factors must also be involved because these "associated" conditions do not always progress to such severe joint destruction.

Roentgenographic Features. Glenohumeral joint degeneration was noted in 49 of 55 shoulders examined in our series of 30 cases. Soft tissue calcifications were present in 55% of shoulders. Upward subluxation of the humeral head or arthrographic evidence of rotator cuff defects was evident in 46 of 55 shoulders (Fig. 109–5). The distance from the superior rim of the humeral head to the acromion, measured on routine roentgenograms with the patient erect, was reduced to 2 mm or less in all but three patients in the series of 26 patients reported by Neer et al.[1] Erosion of the coracoid process, of the undersurface of the anterior third of the acromion, and of the acromioclavicular joint was common (Figs. 109–6 and 109–7); in many instances a rounding off of the greater tuberosity occurred with loss of the sulcus demarcating the anatomic neck of the humerus. Erosions, subchondral cysts, and roughening of the bony cortex over the greater tuberosity at the site of the insertion of the rotator cuff were also noted frequently.

Arthrograms or bursagrams were performed in all 26 of the patients studied by Neer et al.[4] Each showed a grossly defective rotator cuff with communication between the glenohumeral and acromioclavicular joints in 10 instances. Arthrograms of the contralateral shoulder were performed in 11 of the 26 patients, and all showed a complete tear of the rotator cuff, although only 5 had typical radiographic changes in the glenohumeral joint. Pseudarthrosis formation between the humeral head and the acromion and clavicle was common (see Fig. 109–6). Bony destruction of the humeral head was also common, whereas osteophyte formation was usually modest.[1] An area of collapse of the proximal aspect of

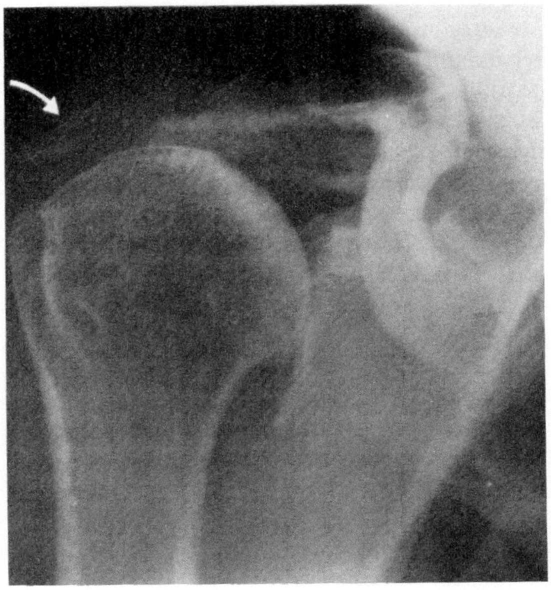

FIGURE 109–5. Anteroposterior roentgenogram of the right shoulder showing soft tissue calcifications (*arrow*) and superior subluxation and sclerosis of the humeral head.

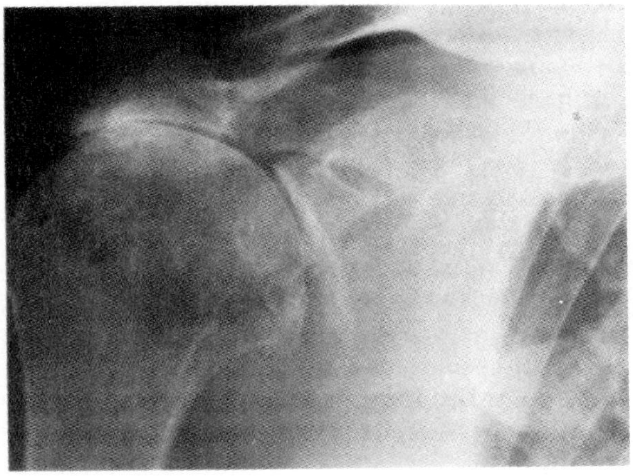

FIGURE 109–6. Anteroposterior roentgenogram of the right shoulder in a patient showing more advanced changes. Superior displacement of the humeral head has resulted in a pseudoarticulation with the acromion. Sclerosis, cystic changes, and irregularity of the humeral head are also present and (From McCarty, D.J. et al.: Milwaukee shoulder: Association of microspheroids containing hydroxyapatite crystals, active collagenase and neutral protease with rotator cuff defects: I. Clinical aspects. Arthritis Rheum., *24*:464–473, 1981.)

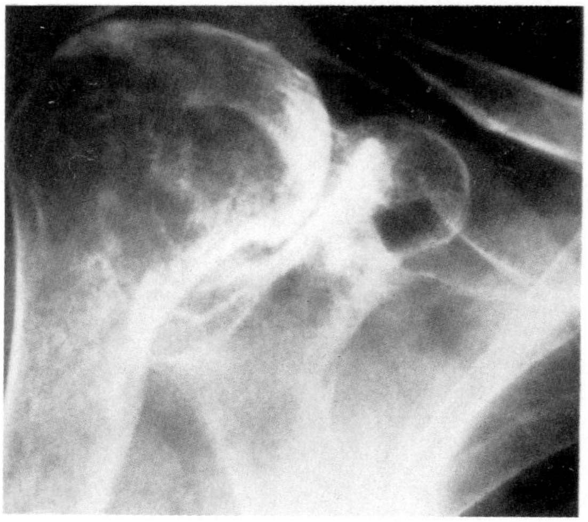

FIGURE 109–7. Anteroposterior roentgenogram of the right shoulder of another patient showing superior displacement of the humeral head and pseudoarticulation with the clavicle, acromion, and coracoid process. The humeral head is partly collapsed with eburnation only in its inferomedial articulating surface. Note the absence of osteophytes.

the humeral articular surface was present in all patients in the Neer series and was a requirement for the diagnosis. These changes are not those of OA of the shoulder where the rotator cuff remains intact with sclerosis of bone and prominent osteophytes.

Synovial Fluid Features. Synovial fluid leukocyte counts were usually less than 1000 per mm^3 (76 of 78 fluids). When the fluids were assayed for BCP crystals by (^{14}C) diphosphonate binding as described previously 73 of 78 fluids were positive. CPPD crystals were also seen in eight fluids. Crystal concentrations estimated serially in fluids from two shoulders were remarkably constant for nearly a year, suggesting that they were under homeostatic control. SEM detected microspheroidal aggregates in 33 of 46 fluids that bound (^{14}C) diphosphonate. The molar Ca/P of these aggregates ranged from 1.4 to 1.7 by x-ray energy dispersive analysis.[7]

Low levels of collagenolytic activity, either active or latent, were found in at least one synovial fluid supernatant from half our patients. Although the total protein concentration in these fluids was 3 to 4 g/dL, most was albumin. Low levels of α_2-macroglobulins, a natural inhibitor of collagenase, and α_1-antitrypsin were found. Synovial fluids also demonstrated types I, II, and III particulate collagens and elevated neutral protease activities.[14] FTIR analyses showed collagen as a constant feature in these joint fluid pellets.[6]

Knee Involvement. In our series of 30 patients with shoulder disease, 16 had symptomatic knee involvement. Lateral tibiofemoral compartment narrowing occurring in 14 of 36 patients (39%) (Figs. 109–8 and 109–9). as is often seen in CPPD crystal deposition disease (see Chapter 108), exceeded medial compartment narrowing in 11 of 36 patients (31%). This differed significantly from 56 patients (62 evaluable knees) with symptomatic OA of the knee without shoulder joint involvement ($p < 0.01$).[7] CPPD crystal deposition was detected either in synovial fluid or by radiographs in seven patients. One patient had osteochondromatosis, and another lateral femoral condylar osteonecrosis, both of which have also been associated with CPPD crystal deposition. Dieppe's patients also showed primarily hip and lateral compartment knee involvement.[1] Thus, the pattern of knee joint degeneration in patients with shoulder joint disease appears to differ from that of primary OA of the knee, where mediol tibiofemoral compartment predominates.

Other Joint Involvement. Two of our patients had severe degenerative arthritis of the hips, but because they already had prosthetic joint replacement, there was no fluid to study. Whether a similar process was involved in pathogenesis is unclear. We have also studied a man with bilateral elbow joint degeneration and synovial fluid findings consistent with those of MSS. The erosive arthropathy of wrists and small hand joints associated with periarticular calcific deposits described by Schumacher et al.[1] may share some of these features, although again, no fluid had been obtained for analysis.

Pathology. Synovial biopsies obtained at the time of operation from the shoulders of four patients demonstrated increased numbers of villi, focal synovial lining cell hyperplasia, a few giant cells, fibrin, and BCP crystal deposits (Fig. 109–10) (Table 109–5).[37] Electron microscopy showed crystals being engulfed by synovial lining cells and histiocytes (Fig. 109–11). Calcific deposits in synovial microvilli appeared to have access to the joint space through areas denuded of synovial lining cells (Fig. 109–12).

In the series of Neer et al., a large, complete cuff tear was found in each patient at operation.[1] The humeral head could be dislocated passively in 14 instances and was fixed in a dislocated position in the remaining 12 shoulders. The supraspinatus tendon was completely ruptured in all patients, and the infraspinatus tendon in

TABLE 109–5. MICROSCOPIC FEATURES OF SYNOVIAL MEMBRANE IN MILWAUKEE SHOULDER/KNEE SYNDROME

Villous hyperplasia
Focal synovial lining cell hyperplasia
Basic calcium phosphate crystal deposition (extracellular, intracellular)*
Fibrin deposition
Giant cells
Fibrosis
Vascular congestion
No inflammatory cells

* The only specific feature.

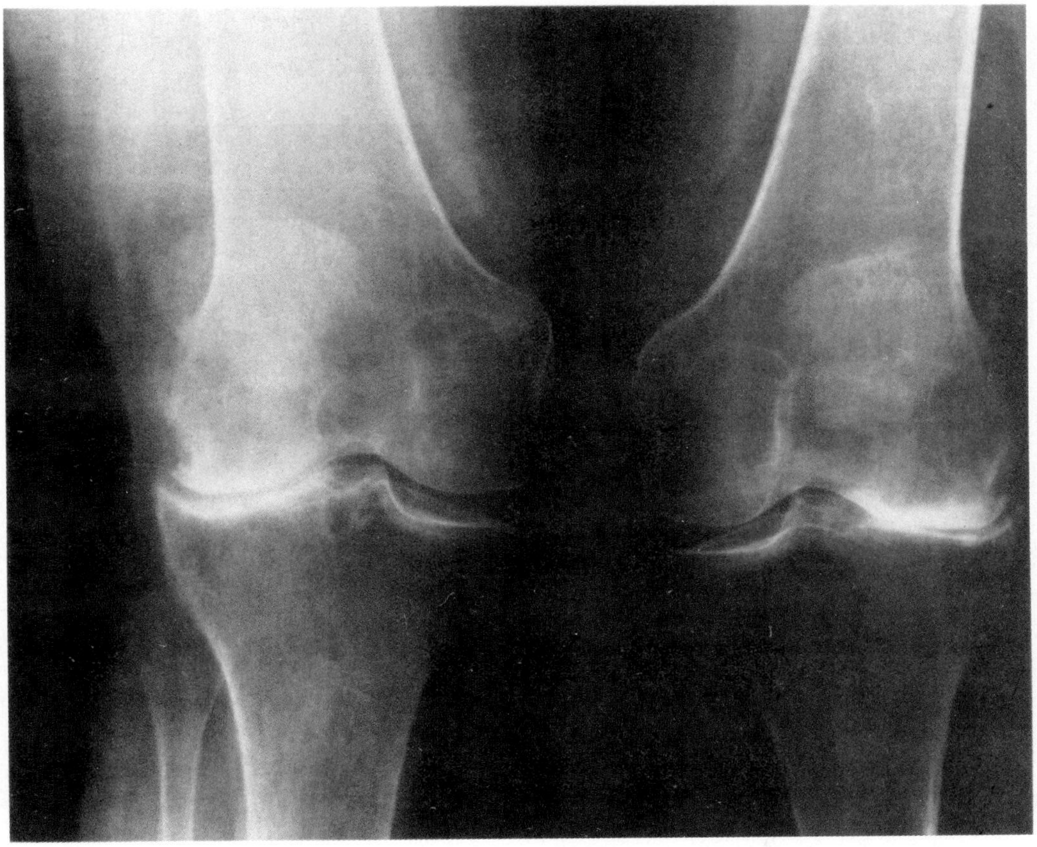

FIGURE 109–8. Standing anteroposterior roentgenogram of the knees from a patient with Milwaukee shoulder syndrome showing lateral tibiofemoral compartment narrowing and incongruity with subchondral bony sclerosis but minimal osteophyte formation.

all but one instance. The teres minor and subscapularis tendons were usually involved, but some vestiges remained in all patients. The tendon of the long head of the biceps was ruptured, dislocated, or frayed in 18, 3, and 5 patients, respectively. The subdeltoid bursa was thickened, forming a large loose pouch around the head of the biceps, and contained variable amounts of (often) sanguineous synovial fluid. The articular cartilage was pebble-like, and the collapsed articular surface, the major point of contact with the acromion, was eburnated and denuded of cartilage with small marginal osteophytes. The remainder of the humeral head was covered with degenerated cartilage and fibrous tissue. The subchondral bone could be indented easily with a finger. The anterior acromial epiphysis had failed to fuse in three patients, which may have contributed to subacromial impingement.

Histologically, the atrophic articular cartilage of the humeral head was covered to a variable degree with a fibrous membrane (pannus). In these areas, the adjacent bone was osteoporotic and hypervascularized with attempts at repair at points of bony collapse. At points of contact between the humeral head and scapula, the cartilage was completely denuded and the bone was sclerotic. Fragments of articular cartilage were found in the subsynovium. These fragments resembled those found in neuropathic joints, albeit less extensive.

In glenohumeral OA, the entire humeral head is sclerotic without large areas of softening[38] is enlarged by marginal osteophytes without collapse.[1] The rotator cuff is nearly always intact.[38]

Pathogenesis. The pathogenesis of this syndrome is not clear. A hypothesis was formulated (Fig. 109–13) in which BCP crystals and possibly particulate collagens are endocytosed by synovial lining cells. These cells are then stimulated to produce PGE_2 and enzymes such as collagenase, stromelysin, and perhaps other proteases. Although collagenase is not a constant finding in synovial fluids and was not identified by Dieppe et al. in any shoulder joint fluid,[39] the massive lysis of the rotator cuff and the intrasynovial portion of the long head of the biceps tendon is difficult to explain without implicating this enzyme. Synovial lining cells metabolize BCP crystals in acidic phagolysosomes. The release of calcium within the cell may contribute to synovial cell proliferation in which BCP crystals from eburnated bone, metaplastic synovium, and perhaps cartilage are proba-

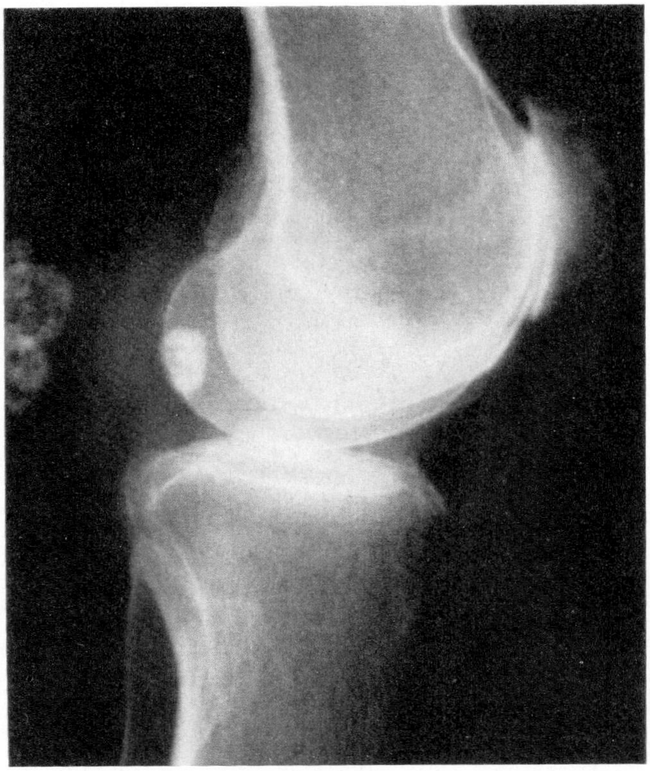

FIGURE 109–9. Lateral roentgenogram of the right knee of another patient showing isolated patellofemoral osteoarthritis (patella "wrapped around" the femur), femoral cortical defect, and chondrocalcinosis of the femoral articular cartilage. Osteochondromata can be seen in the posterior joint recess.

bly continually released by mechanical forces, and possibly by enzymatic "strip" mining as previously postulated for sodium urate and CPPD crystal release (see Chapters 107 and 108).

Werb and Reynolds demonstrated that particulates, such as latex beads, added to rabbit synovial cells in culture are phagocytized, stimulating increased secretion of proteases, including collagenase.[40] This increased secretion continued until the ingested particles were biodegraded, at which time it returned to baseline. Collagen also stimulated collagenase release from cultured human skin fibroblasts,[41] and synovial fluid "wear" particles released neutral proteases from cultured synovial cells.[42]

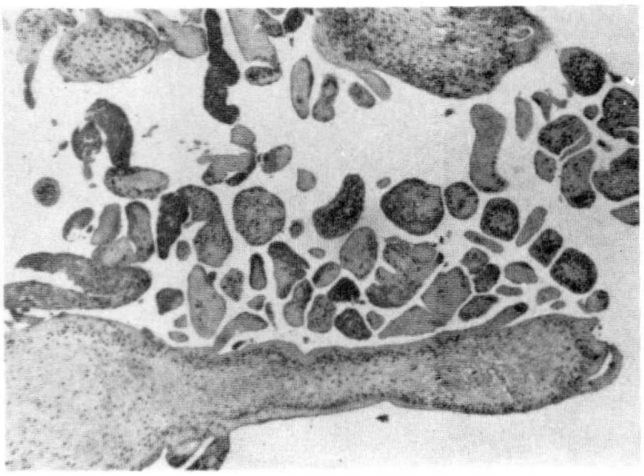

FIGURE 109–10. Light micrograph of synovium showing many villi and focal synovial cell hyperplasia. In cross section, the branching villi appear as free bodies. Some villi are partially covered with fibrin or contain fibrin in various stages of organization (×110).

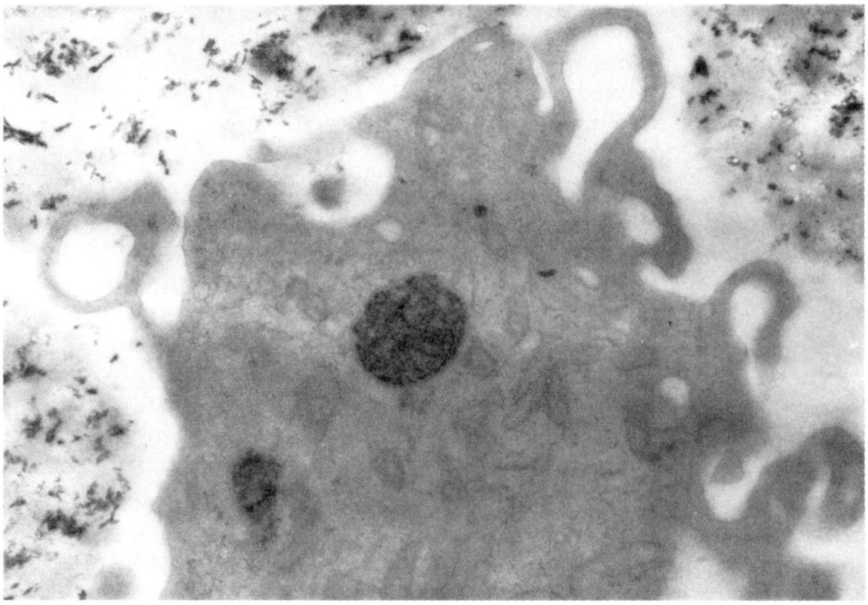

FIGURE 109–11. Electron micrograph of a hyperplastic synovial cell. Crystals within phagolysosomes are bounded by distinct limiting membranes. Many extracellular crystals are also present (×26,400).

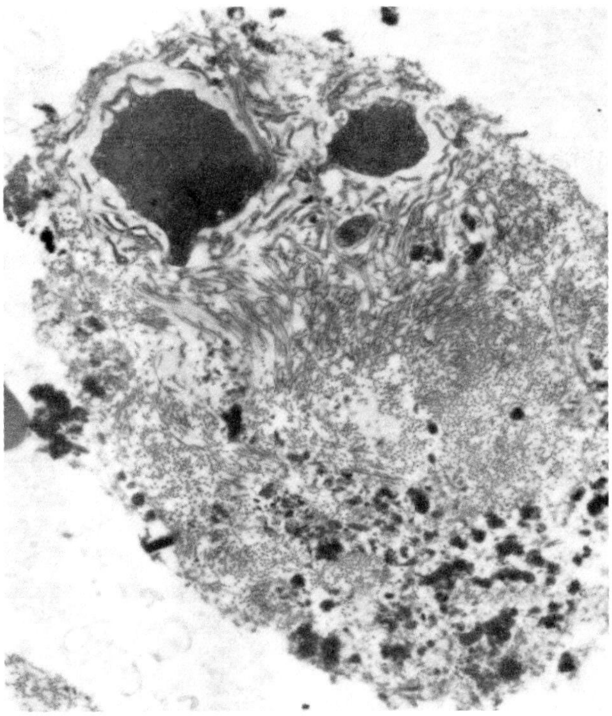

FIGURE 109–12. Electron micrograph showing a small villus in cross section. Synovial lining cells are absent. Crystal microaggregates are seen dispersed among collagen fibers, lying free on the surface and in the synovial space. Several fibrocytes are present (×6,400). (From Garancis, J.C., et al.: Milwaukee shoulder: Association of microspheroids containing hydroxyapatite crystals, active collagenase and neutral protease with rotator cuff defects: III. Morphologic and biochemical studies of an excised synovium showing chondromatosis. Arthritis Rheum., *24*:484–491, 1981.)

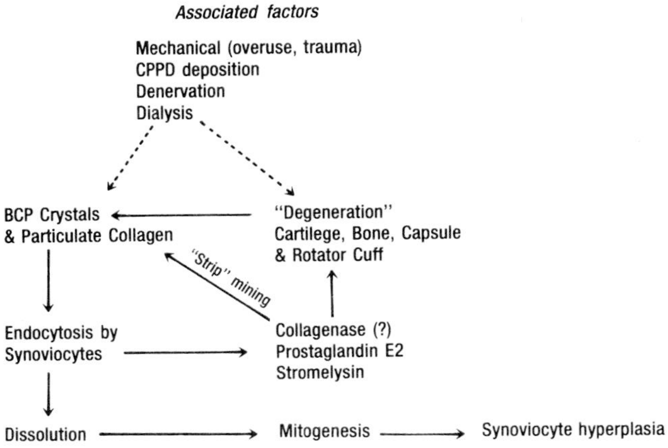

FIGURE 109–13. Hypothetical schema relating the various features of Milwaukee shoulder/knee syndrome.

This hypothesis was tested by adding natural or synthetic BCP, CPPD, and other crystals to cultured human or canine synovial cells.[43] Neutral protease (stromelysin) and collagenase secretion was augmented in a dose-related fashion approximately five to eight times over control cultures incubated without crystals. Collagenase and stromelysin message induction were later shown by Northern blot analysis in chondrocytes in primary culture as well.[44,45] Because crystals have been described within human chondrocytes,[46,47] it is possible that autolysis of cartilage may occur without crystal shedding into synovial fluid. Partially purified mammalian collagenase released BCP crystal microspheroidal aggregates from calcified synovial tissue in vitro.[48] The mean diameter and size ranges of the released aggregates were virtually identical to those observed in synovial fluids obtained from the same patient. Fluid obtained several weeks after synovectomy of the affected shoulder in this patient showed no mineral by (^{14}C) EHDP binding and greatly reduced protease activities.[14] Although degenerating articular cartilage can form mineral, as discussed previously, there is little doubt about the synovial origin of the crystals in this patient, who had synovial chondromatosis (chondrometaplasia of subsynovial fibroblasts).

In addition to the stimulation of relentless enzyme secretion, BCP or CPPD crystal endocytosis was associated with a massive genesis of prostaglandins, especially PGE_2.[49,50] All PGE_2 release occurred in the first few hours after crystals were added to the cells.[49] PGE_2 release and collagenase release have been found after exposure of macrophages or synovial cells to sodium urate crystals also and have been related to the hard tissue destruction in gout, (Chapter 107). CPPD crystal–stimulated prostaglandin and protease release may account for the destructive arthropathies associated with these crystals. PGE_2 was found in joint fluid from our patients[14] and was isolated from the periarticular calcium phosphate deposits from a patient with phalangeal osteolysis.[50]

This hypothesis is consistent with the concept of "crystal traffic" derived from studies of the fate of radiolabeled CPPD or BCP crystals injected intrasynovially. One half of a dose of CPPD crystals was cleared from human joints in 30 to 90 days and from rabbit joints in 16 to 20 days.[1] Clearance rates were inversely proportional to crystal size. Injected crystals were phagocytized by synovial cells, where virtually all dissolution appeared to take place. This phenomenon was evidenced by localization of all nuclide in synovial tissue, the finding of all crystals inside cells by electron microscopy, the lack of effect on clearance rate of extracellular magnesium depletion by dietary deprivation, the failure of joint lavage to remove significant radionuclide, and reduction of clearance rate by 65% in the presence of synovial cell hemosiderosis induced by injection of autologous blood.[1] Both CPPD crystals and hemosiderin were shown in the same cells by TEM and x-ray energy dispersive analysis. ^{85}Sr-labeled BCP crystals were cleared from rabbit joints with a half-life of about 6 days, about three times faster than CPPD crystals.[51]

The focal cell hyperplasia found in the four synovial membranes we examined[37] was described by Doyle as a constant feature of synovial membranes containing calcium crystals.[52] This finding might be related to their mitogenic properties. BCP, CPPD, calcium urate, calcium diphosphonate, and calcium carbonate, but not crystals or particulates without calcium (such as sodium urate, diamond, silicon dioxide, or latex beads), were capable of substituting for serum growth factors in certain cell systems.[53] Crystals must undergo endocytosis and dissolution by cells for mitogenesis to occur.[54,55] Calcium-containing crystals act as a "competence" factor, because they can substitute for growth factors found in serum (platelet-derived growth factor, PDGF); like PDGF, calcium-containing crystals require a progression factor, such as insulin-like growth factor-1 (somatomedin C) for full expression of mitogenic potency.[56] (^{45}Ca) BCP crystals added to cultured synovial cells, skin fibroblasts, or peripheral blood monocytes were phagocytized and degraded, probably by the adenosine triphosphatase (ATPase)-driven lysosomal proton pump.[57,58] Weak bases, such as chloroquine or NH_4^+, inhibited BCP crystal solubilization by all three cell types in a dose-dependent fashion.[55] Calcium crystal–induced mitogenesis was also reduced in a parallel dose-dependent fashion by these inhibitors but serum-stimulated mitogenesis was unaffected.[55]

BCP crystal stimulation of fibroblasts includes activation of protein kinase C and the induction of the protooncogenes c-*fos*, c-*myc*, and c-*jun*.[59] Messenger RNA for stromelysin, and probably gelatinase, is induced.[60] In addition to protein kinase C activation, mitogenesis required crystal dissolution and release of calcium within the cell as well as a progression factor. Inhibitors of BCP crystal dissolution block mitogenesis but not collagenase induction or secretion.

The stimulation of cytokines by BCP crystal has not been thoroughly studied. Available data suggest a very limited role if any. In culture, BCP crystals caused release of PGE_2 but not interleukin-1 (Il-1) from mouse macrophages.[61] In a study of synovial fluids from OA patients, levels of tumor necrosis factor-α (TNF-α) but not Il-1 were increased relative to RA.[61]

Although BCP crystals can elicit a major acute inflammatory response such as in "hydroxyapatite pseudopodagra,"[16] BCP crystals as found in OA synovial fluid do not stimulate a neutrophilic response very often. This may be related to a lesser phlogistic potential and/or to adsorbed surface proteins, which modulate crystal–cell interactions. BCP crystals generated reduced amounts of chemotactic factors from neutrophils, and these showed greater surface binding to BCP crystals in comparison to monosodium urate (MSU) crystals.[63] Further, other proteins adsorbed onto the surface of BCP crystals, such as α_2-HS glycoprotein, inhibited superoxide generation and chemiluminescence.[64]

Indirect evidence does suggest that BCP crystals contribute to low-grade joint inflammation. The severity of joint symptoms in OA correlated with the synovial fluid leukocyte count and with the presence of "hydroxyapatite" crystals and other particulates.[65] In patients wtih OA of the knee, synovial effusions were larger when BCP crystals were present.[66]

Neer et al. favor a pathogenesis based on disuse osteoporosis and mechanical instability.[1] The greater severity of symptoms, radiologic evidence of destruction, the higher joint fluid levels of crystals and enzymes in the shoulder on the dominant side, and the frequent history of overuse or trauma support a pathogenetic role of movement. But the finding of destructive arthropathies of the knee and possibly other joints in the same patients suggests that systemic metabolic effects might be operative. Biomechanical factors probably play a major role in the pathogenetic scheme outlined in Figure 109–13.

Treatment. The treatment of MSS is generally unsatisfactory. A conservative approach including NSAIDs, repeated shoulder aspirations, and decreased joint use has sometimes controlled symptoms satisfactorily. Surgical therapy is sometimes successful for relief of pain and restoration of some function, as described in Chapter 50.

At the time of diagnosis, advanced destructive changes are usually present, and may even be asymptomatic. Thus, there is no a priori way to identify persons at risk for this condition.

SECONDARY BCP ARTHROPATHIES

Several conditions, including chronic renal failure, the "collagen" diseases, and neurologic injury, have been associated with calcification that may occur in almost any tissue. In these conditions, BCP crystals have been found in periarticular soft tissues, in bursae, and within joints and are often associated with symptoms. For a more complete listing of conditions associated with calcinosis, see Chapter 73.

Soft-tissue calcifications involving the fibrous tissue in skin or muscle occur in the "collagen" diseases.[1] Rare cases of intra-articular calcification have been reported in scleroderma, one case with a chalky joint effusion,[1] polymyositis,[19] and mixed connective tissue syndrome.[20]

Heterotopic ossification mimicking arthritis has been described following neurologic catastrophes.[1] Such ossification tends to occur in periarticular tissues. The mechanisms are unknown. How synovial fluid leukocyte counts and high protein concentrations have been found.

Several miscellaneous causes of BCP crystal deposition have been described.[1] One patient had Laennec's cirrhosis, hypertrophic osteoarthropathy, and synovial calcifications in the knees probably related to vitamin D intoxication. A patient with "draft dodger's knee" developed calcifications around the knee many years after self-injection of olive oil.

The intra-articular injection of triamcinolone hexacetonide has been associated with the formation of periarticular calcifications along the injection tract, which may become apparent months after the injection.[1] Such calcifications may gradually be resorbed over a period of months to years.

Tumoral Calcinosis. This condition, consisting of massive, expanding calcific deposits in or near one or more large joints, is rare in North America and Europe, but nonhyperphosphatemic cases are relatively common in Africa. Phosphate deprivation constitutes definitive therapy for hyperphosphatemic cases, which are often familial.[1]

Arthropathy in Chronic Renal Failure Although patients with chronic renal failure are susceptible to virtually any type of arthritis, uremia and hemodialysis predispose to osteodystrophy, tendonitis, tendon rupture,[67] carpel tunnel syndrome, and several forms of arthritis and periarthritis (Table 109–6). Although metastatic soft tissue calcifications occur frequently in uremic patients with high calcium × phosphorus products (calciphylaxis?), greater attention to control of calcium and phosphorus plasma levels has reduced this complication.[1]

Musculoskeletal symptoms occur in 57 to 82% of patients receiving long-term dialysis.[68–70] One study of 80 patients showed that arthralgias were the most common complaint (74%), but radiographic evaluation disclosed erosive arthropathy of the fingers (8%) and spine (9%); bone cysts of the carpus (10%), humeral head (9%), and hip (11%); cervical spondylolisthesis (5%), and multiple diaphyseal lacunae (1%).[68]

In the small joints of the hands, erosive arthropathy has been ascribed to secondary hyperparathyroidism.[71] Erosive disease has also been observed in axial joints and large joints, especially the shoulder.[72–74] "Erosive azotemic arthropathy" described a subset of patients with erosive changes in large and small joints, "noninflammatory" synovial fluids, and renal osteodystrophy.[75] Histologic analysis of material found in bone cysts has shown amyloid composed of β_2-microglobulin.[76] Cases with carpal tunnel syndrome have consistently demonstrated this type of amyloid as well.[77] Amyloid has been detected in synovium, tenosynovium, capsule, and extra-articular locations.[78] The term dialysis myelopathy has ceased to describe a case of quadriparesis resulting from extradural amyloid deposition.[79]

TABLE 109–6. ARTHROPATHIES AND PERIARTHROPATHIES ASSOCIATED WITH CHRONIC RENAL FAILURE

PERIARTHRITIS
TENDONITIS
Tendon rupture
EROSIVE ARTHROPATHY
Hands (secondary hyperparathyroidism)
Large joints (especially shoulders)
Axial skeleton
"Erosive azotemic arthropathy" (large and small joints and renal osteodystrophy)
CRYSTAL DEPOSITION
Monosodium urate monohydrate
Calcium pyrophosphate dihydrate
Basic calcium phosphates
Calcium oxalate
Aluminum phosphate
β_2-MICROGLOBULIN AMYLOID
Carpal tunnel syndrome
Bone cysts

Crystal-induced arthritis appears to be common in uremia (Table 109–6). Hyperuricemia predisposes to acute gout, although attacks are less common than might be expected. BCP crystals are likely to form in or around joints and in other tissues in the milieu of excess phosphorus or calcium. CPPD crystal deposition has been associated with hyperparathyroidism.[1] Calcium oxalate has been found in the synovial fluid from patients receiving chronic hemodialysis,[80] especially in those receiving ascorbic acid supplementation.[81] Worcester et al. showed that uremic serum is supersaturated with respect to calcium oxalate.[82] Finally, aluminum phosphate has been demonstrated in the synovium of patients taking aluminum compounds by mouth to bind intestinal phosphate.[83,84]

Synovial fluid leukocyte counts are generally not increased, although leukocytosis was found in two of three inflamed shoulders in dialysis patients,[1] and BCP crystals were found in two of these.

Animal Models of BCP Crystal Deposition. Spontaneous periarticular calcinosis has been reported in dogs[85,86] and may be familial.[87] Reginato et al. successfully calcified rabbit synovium with vitamin D.[87] These deposits were composed of BCP crystals identical to those found in the synovial fluid of patients.[6]

Treatment. The identification of the calcium-binding amino acid GLA (γ-carboxyglutamic acid) in pathologic soft tissue calcification[88] provides a rationale for the use of warfarin therapy. Synthesis of GLA-containing proteins, such as prothrombin, is vitamin K–dependent. Reports of success, however,[89] must be viewed in the light of the natural tendency for spontaneous resorption as already discussed. Probenecid has been used successfully to treat patients with calcinosis, but the same caveat applies in the absence of suitable controls.[90]

UNANSWERED QUESTIONS

Many questions about BCP crystal arthropathies and periarthropathies remain to be answered. Such crystals have been described in the synovial fluid of patients with many different types of joint disease. Whether BCP crystals participate in the inflammation of RA and other diseases or merely represent an epiphenomenon is unknown. Dieppe and Watt have suggested that crystal deposition is not the primary event but occurs secondarily as an opportunistic event in damaged joints.[91] Crystal deposition may then contribute further to joint deterioration.

Campion et al. have found a considerable overlap in the features of patients with destructive shoulder arthritis resulting from different primary arthropathies. They refer to severe, destructive shoulder lesions unassociated with any other definable arthropathy as "idiopathic destructive arthritis of the shoulder" suggest that crystals are not related to any specific arthropathy,[92] a proposition with which we agree.

Perhaps the greatest mystery is the mechanism of pathologic calcification. Codman considered the formation of periarticular calcific deposits in the shoulder to be the result of necrosis,[1] but Sarkar and Uhthoff were unable to detect histologic evidence of necrosis.[21] They hypothesized that hypoxia induces the tendon to transform into fibrocartilage. BCP crystals then form in matrix vesicles generated by metaplastic chondrocytes, subsequently coalescing into larger deposits.[1] They suggest that vascular invasion and resorption of the calcific deposits follow, leaving a reconstituted vascularized tendon.

Anderson has presented a unified concept of pathologic calcification encompassing both metastatic and dystrophic forms. Matrix vesicles or mitochondria may serve as repositories for calcium and, on exposure to sufficient phosphate, mineralization begins.[93] The mechanism responsible for most pathologic calcifications occurring in the absence of hypercalcemia or hyperphosphatemia is unclear.

REFERENCES

1. Halverson, P.B., and McCarty, D.J.: Basic calcium phosphate (apatite, octacalcium phosphate, tricalcium phosphate) crystal deposition diseases. *In* Arthritis and Allied Conditions. 11th Ed. Edited by D.J. McCarty. Philadelphia, Lea & Febiger, 1989.
2. Dieppe, P.A., Crocker, P., Huskisson, E.C., and Willoughby, D.A.: Apatite deposition disease. A new arthropathy. Lancet, *1*:266–269, 1976.
3. Schumacher, H.R., Smolyo, A.P., Tse, R.L., and Maurer, K.: Arthritis associated with apatite crystals. Ann. Intern. Med., *87*:411–416, 1977.
4. Faure, G. et al.: Apatites in heterotopic calcifications. Scan. Electron Microsc., *4*:1624–1634, 1982.
5. Daculsi, G., Faure, G., and Kerebel, B.: Electron microscopy and microanalysis of a subcutaneous heterotopic calcification. Calcif. Tissue Int., *35*:723–727, 1983.
6. McCarty, D.J., Lehr, J.R., and Halverson, P.B.: Crystal populations in human synovial fluid. Identification of apatite, octacalcium phosphate, tricalcium phosphate. Arthritis Rheum., *26*:247–251, 1983.
7. Halverson, P.B., Carrera, G.F., and McCarty, D.J.: Milwaukee shoulder syndrome: Fifteen additional cases and a description of contributing factors. Arch. Intern. Med., *150*:677–682, 1990.
8. Schumacher, H.R., Rothfuss, S., Bertken, R., and Linder, J.: Unusual laminated birefringent arrays of apatite crystals in inflammatory arthritis. Arthritis Rheum., *30*:S106, 1987.
9. Paul, H., Reginato, A.J., and Schumacher, H.R.: Alizarin red S staining as a screening test to detect calcium compounds in synovial fluid. Arthritis Rheum., *26*:191–200, 1983.
10. Bardin, T., Bucki, B., Lansaman, J., et al.: Coloration par le rouge alizarine des liquides articulaires. Rev. Rhum. Mal. Osteoartic, *54*:149–154, 1987.
11. Gordon, C., Swan, A., and Dieppe, P.: Detection of crystals in synovial fluids by light microscopy: Sensitivity and reliability. Ann. Rheum. Dis., *48*:737–742, 1989.
12. Halverson, P.B., and McCarty, D.J.: Identification of hydroxyapatite crystals in synovial fluid. Arthritis Rheum., *22*:389–395, 1979.
13. Halverson, P.B., and McCarty, D.J.: Patterns of radiographic abnormalities associated with basic calcium phosphate and calcium pyrophosphate dihydrate crystal deposition in the knee. Ann. Rheum. Dis., *45*:603–605, 1986.
14. Halverson, P.B., Cheung, H.S., and McCarty, D.J.: "Milwaukee shoulder": Association of microspheroids containing hydroxyapatite crystals, active collagenase and neutral protease with rotator cuff defects: II. Synovial fluid studies. Arthritis Rheum., *24*:474–483, 1981.
15. Cherian, P.V., and Schumacher, H.R.: Diagnostic potential of rapid electron microscopic analysis of joint effusions. Arthritis Rheum., *25*:98–100, 1982.
16. Fam, A.G., and Rubenstein, J.: Hydroxyapatite pseudopodagra. Arthritis Rheum., *32*:741–747, 1989.
17. Caspi, D., Rosenbach, T.O., Yaron, M., et al.: Periarthritis associated with basic calcium phosphate crystal deposition and low levels of serum alkaline phosphatase—Report of three cases from one family. J. Rheumatol., *15*:823–828, 1988.
18. Uhthoff, H.K., Sarkar, K., and Maynard, J.A.: Calcifying tendonitis. Clin. Orthop. Rel. Res., *118*:164–168, 1976.
19. Kazmers, I.S., Scoville, C.D., and Schumacher, H.R.: Polymyositis associated apatite arthritis. J. Rheumatol., *15*:1019–1021, 1988.
20. Hutton, C.W., Maddison, P.J., Collins, A.J., and Berriman, J.A.: Intra-articular apatite deposition in mixed connective tissue disease: Crystallographic and technetium scanning characteristics. Ann. Rheum. Dis., *47*:1027–1030, 1988.
21. Sarkar, K., and Uhthoff, H.K.: Rotator cuff tendinopathies with calcification. *In* Calcium in Biological Systems. Edited by R.P. Rubin, G. Weiss, and J.W. Putney. New York, Plenum, 1984.
22. Gravanis, M.G., and Gaffney, E.F.: Idiopathic calcifying tenosynovitis. Histopathologic features and possible pathogenesis. Am. J. Surg. Pathol., 7:359–361, 1983.
23. Ali, S.Y., and Griffiths, S.: New types of calcium phosphate crystals in arthritis cartilage. Semin. Arthritis Rheum., *11*:124–126, 1981.
24. Stein, H., Bab, I.A., and Sela, J.: The occurrence of hydroxyapatite crystals in extracellular matrix vesicles after surgical manipulation of the rabbit knee joint. Cell Tissue Res., *214*:449–454, 1981.
25. Doyle, D.V., Dieppe, P.A., Crocker, P.R. et al.: Mixed crystal deposition in an osteoarthritic joint. J. Pathol., *123*:1–5, 1977.
26. Huskisson, E.C. et al.: Another look at osteoarthritis. Ann. Rheum. Dis., *38*:423–428, 1979.
27. Dieppe, P.A., Crocker, P.R., Corke, C.F. et al.: Synovial fluid crystals. Q. J. Med., *192*:533–553, 1979.
28. Gibilisco, P.A., Schumacher, H.R., Hollander, J.L., and Soper, K.A.: Synovial fluid crystals in osteoarthritis. Arthritis Rheum., *28*:511–515, 1985.
29. Lagier, R., Boivin, G., and Gerster, J.C.: Carpal tunnel syndrome associated with mixed calcium pyrophosphate dihydrate and apatite crystal deposition in tendon synovial sheath. Arthritis Rheum., *27*:1190–1195, 1984.
30. Adams, R.: A Treatise on Rheumatic Gout or Chronic Rheumatic Arthritis of All the Joints. 2nd Ed. Dublin, Fannin; London, John Churchill and Sons; Edinburgh, Maclachlan and Stewart; 1873, pp. 1–568.

31. Adams, R.: Illustration of the Effects of Rheumatic Joint in Chronic Rheumatic Arthritis of All the Articulations; with Descriptive and Explanatory Statements. London, John Churchill and Sons, 1857, pp. 1–31.
31a. McCarty, D.J.: Robert Adams' rheumatic arthritis of the shoulder: Milwaukee shoulder revisited. J. Rheumatol., *16*:668–670, 1989.
32. Craig, E.V.: The acromioclavicular joint cyst. Clin. Orthop. Rel. Res., *202*:189–192, 1986.
33. Dennis, D.A., Ferlic, D.C., and Clayton, M.D.: Acromial stress fracture associated with cuff-tear arthropathy. J. Bone Joint Surg., *68A*:937–940, 1986.
34. Klimaitis, A., Carroll, G., and Owen, E.: Rapidly progressive destructive arthropathy of the shoulder—A viewpoint on pathogenesis. J. Rheumatol., *15*:1859–1862, 1988.
35. Samilson, R.L., and Prieto, V.: Dislocation arthropathy of the shoulder. J. Bone Joint Surg., *65A*:456–460, 1983.
36. Bagley, J.D., Cochran, T.P., and Sledge, C.B.: The weight-bearing shoulder—The impingement syndrome in paraplegics. J. Bone Joint Surg., *69A*:676–678, 1987.
37. Halverson, P.B., Garancis, J.C., and McCarty, D.J.: Histopathologic and ultrastructural studies of Milwaukee shoulder syndrome—A basic calcium phosphate crystal arthropathy. Ann. Rheum. Dis., *43*:734–741, 1984.
38. Neer, C.S.: Replacement arthroplasty in glenohumeral osteoarthritis. J. Bone Joint Surg., *69A*:1232–1234, 1983.
39. Dieppe, P.A., Cawston, T., Mercer, E., et al.: Synovial fluid collagenase in patients with destructive arthritis of the elbow joint. Arthritis Rheum., *31*:882–890, 1988.
40. Werb, Z., and Reynolds, J.J.: Stimulation by endocytosis of the secretion of collagenase and neutral protease from rabbit synovial fibroblasts. J. Exp. Med., *140*:1482–1497, 1974.
41. Biswas, C., and Dayer, J.: Stimulation of collagenase production by collagen in mammalian cell cultures. Cell, *18*:1035–1041, 1979.
42. Evans, C.H., Means, D.C., and Cosgrove, J.R.: Release of neutral proteinase from mononuclear phagocytes and synovial cells in response to cartilaginous wear particles in vitro. Biochim. Biophys. Acta, *677*:287–294, 1981.
43. Cheung, H.S., Halverson, P.B., and McCarty, D.J.: Release of collagenase, neutral protease and prostaglandins from cultured synovial cells by hydroxyapatite and calcium pyrophosphate dihydrate. Arthritis Rheum. *24*:1338–1344, 1981.
44. Mitchell, P.G., McCarthy, G.M., and Cheung, H.S.: Basic calcium phosphate crystals stimulate cell proliferation and collagenase message accumulation in cultured adult articular chondrocytes. Arthritis Rheum., (in press), 1991.
45. McCarthy, G.M., Mitchell, P.G., and Cheung, H.S.: Basic calcium phosphate crystals cause coordinate induction and secretion of collagenase and stromelysin. Clin. Res., *39*:249A, 1991.
46. Boivin, G., and Lagier, R.: An ultrastructural study of articular chondrocalcinosis in cases of knee osteoarthritis. Virchows Arch. (A), *400*:13–19, 1983.
47. Mitrovic, D.R.: Pathology of articular deposition of calcium salts and their relationship to osteoarthritis. Ann. Rheum. Dis., *42*:519–526, 1983.
48. Halverson, P.B., Cheung, H.S., and McCarty, D.J.: Enzymatic release of microspheroids containing hydroxyapatite crystals from synovium and of calcium pyrophosphate dihydrate crystals from cartilage. Ann. Rheum. Dis., *41*:527–531, 1982.
49. McCarty, D.J., and Cheung, H.S.: Prostaglandin (PG)E_2 generation by cultured synovial fibroblasts exposed to microcrystals containing calcium. Ann. Rheum. Dis., *44*:316–320, 1985.
50. Caniggia, A. et al.: Prostaglandin (PGE_2): A possible mechanism for bone destruction in calcinosis circumscripta. Calcif. Tissue Res., *25*:53–57, 1978.
51. Palmer, D.W., and McCarty, D.J.: Clearance of ^{85}Sr labelled calcium phosphate (CP) crystals from normal rabbit joints. Arthritis Rheum., *27*:427–432, 1984.
52. Doyle, D.V.: Tissue calcification and inflammation in osteoarthritis. J. Pathol., *136*:199–216, 1982.
53. Cheung, H.S., Story, M.T., and McCarty, D.J.: Mitogenic effects of hydroxyapatite and calcium pyrophosphate on cultured mammalian cells. Arthritis Rheum., *27*:668–674, 1984.
54. Borkowf, A., Cheung, H.S., and McCarty, D.J.: Endocytosis is required for the mitogenic effect of basic calcium phosphate crystals in fibroblasts. Calcif. Tissue Int., *40*:173–176, 1987.
55. Cheung, H.S., and McCarty, D.J.: Mitogenesis induced by calcium containing crystals: Role of intracellular dissolution. Exp. Cell Res., *157*:63–70, 1985.
56. Cheung, H.S., Van Wyk, J.J., Russell, W.E., and McCarty, D.J.: Mitogenic activity of hydroxyapatite: Requirement for somatomedin C. J. Cell Physiol., *128*:143–148, 1986.
57. Evans, R.W., Cheung, H.S., and McCarty, D.J.: Cultured canine synovial cells solubilize ^{45}Ca labeled HA crystals. Arthritis Rheum., *27*:829–832, 1984.
58. Evans, R.W., Cheung, H.S., and McCarty, D.J.: Cultured human monocytes and fibroblasts solubilize calcium phosphate crystals. Calcif. Tissue Int., *36*:645–650, 1984.
59. Mitchell, P.G., Pledger, W.J., and Cheung, H.S.: Molecular mechanisms of basic calcium phosphate crystal-induced mitogenesis: Role of protein kinase. J. Biol. Chem., *264*:14071–14077, 1989.
60. McCarthy, G.M., Mitchell, P.G., and Cheung, H.S.: The mitogenic response to stimulation with basic calcium phosphate crystals is accompanied by induction and secretion of collagenase in human fibroblasts. Arthritis Rheum., *34*:1021–1030, 1991.
61. Alwan, W.H., Dieppe, P.A., Elson, C.J., and Bradfield, J.W.B.: Bone resorbing activity in synovial fluids in destructive osteoarthritis and rheumatoid arthritis. Ann. Rheum. Dis., *47*:198–205, 1988.
62. Westacott, C.I., Whicher, J.T., Barnes, I.C., et al.: Synovial fluid concentrations of five different cytokines in rheumatic diseases. Ann. Rheum. Dis., *49*:676–681, 1990.
63. Swan, A., Dularay, B., and Dieppe, P.: A comparison of the effects of urate, hydroxyapatite and diamond crystals on polymorphonuclear cells: Relationship of mediator release to the surface area and adsorptive capacity of different particles. J. Rheumatol., *17*:1346–1352, 1990.
64. Terkeltaub, R.A., Santoro, D.A., Mandel, G., and Mandel, N.: Serum and plasma inhibit neutrophil stimulation by hydroxyapatite crystals: Evidence that serum α2-HS glycoprotein is a potent and specific crystal-bound inhibitor. Arthritis Rheum., *31*:1081–1089, 1988.
65. Schumacher, H.R., Jr., Stineman, M., Rahman, M., et al.: The relationship between clinical and synovial fluid findings and treatment response in osteoarthritis (OA) of the knee. Arthritis Rheum., *33*:S92, 1990.
66. Carroll, G.J., Stuart, R.A., Armstrong, J.A., et al.: Hydroxyapatite crystals are a frequent finding in osteoarthritic synovial fluid, but are not related to increased concentrations of keratan sulfate or interleukin 1β. J. Rheumatol., *18*:861–865, 1991.
67. Lauerman, W.C., Smith, B.G., and Kenmore, P.I.: Spontaneous bilateral rupture of the extensor mechanism of the knee in two patients on chronic ambulatory peritoneal dialysis. Orthopedics, *10*:589–591, 1987.
68. Brown, E.A., Arnold, I.R., and Gower, P.E.: Dialysis arthropathy: Complication of long term hemodialysis. Br. Med. J., *292*:163–166, 1986.
69. Hardouin, P., Flipo, R.-M., Foissac-Gegoux, P., et al.: Current aspects of osteoarticular pathology in patients undergoing hemodialysis: Study of 80 patients: 1. Clinical and radiological analysis. J. Rheumatol., *14*:780–783, 1987.

70. Menery, K., Braunstein, E., Brown, M., et al.: Musculoskeletal symptoms related to arthropathy in patients receiving dialysis. J. Rheumatol., *15*:1848–1854, 1988.
71. Resnick, D.L.: Erosive arthritis of the hand and wrist in hyperparathyroidism. Radiology, *110*:263–269, 1974.
72. Kuntz, D. et al.: Destructive spondyloarthropathy in hemodialyzed patients: A new syndrome. Arthritis Rheum., *27*:369–375, 1984.
73. Goldstein, S. et al.: Chronic arthropathy in long-term hemodialysis. Am. J. Med., *78*:82–86, 1985.
74. McCarthy, J.T., Dahlberg, P.J., Krieghauser, J.S., et al.: Erosive spondyloarthropathy in long-term dialysis patients: Relationship to severe hyperparathyroidism. Mayo Clin. Proc., *63*:446–452, 1988.
75. Rubin, L.A. et al.: Erosive azotemic arthropathy. Arthritis Rheum., *27*:1086–1094, 1984.
76. Huaux, J., Noel, H., Malghem, J., et al.: Erosive azotemic osteoarthropathy: Possible role of amyloidosis. Arthritis Rheum., *28*:1075–1076, 1985.
77. Bardin, T. et al.: Synovial amyloidosis in patients undergoing long-term hemodialysis. Arthritis Rheum., *28*:1052–1058, 1985.
78. Bardin, T. et al.: Hemodialysis-associated amyloidosis and beta-2 microglobulin. Am J. Med., *83*:419–424, 1987.
79. Allain, T.J., Stevens, P.E., Bridges, L.R., and Phillips, M.E.: Dialysis myelopathy: Quadriparesis due to extradural amyloid of β2 microglobulin origin. Br. Med. J., *296*:752–753, 1988.
80. Hoffman, G.S., Schumacher, H.R., Paul, H., et al.: Calcium oxalate microcrystalline-associated arthritis in end-stage renal disease. Ann. Intern. Med., *97*:36–42, 1982.
81. Reginato, A. et al.: Arthropathy and cutaneous calcinosis in hemodialysis oxalosis. Arthritis Rheum., *29*:1387–1396, 1986.
82. Worcester, E., Nakagawa, Y., Bushinsky, D., and Coe, F.: Evidence that serum calcium oxalate supersaturation is a consequence of oxalate retention in patients with chronic renal failure. J. Clin. Invest., *77*:1888–1896, 1986.
83. Netter, P. et al.: Inflammatory effect of aluminum phosphate. Ann. Rheum. Dis., *42*:114, 1983.
84. Netter P., Kessler, M., Durnel, D., et al.: Aluminum in joint tissues of chronic renal failure patients treated with regular hemodialysis and aluminum compounds. J. Rheumatol., *11*:66–70, 1984.
85. Ellison, G.W., and Norrdin, R.W.: Multicentric periarticular calcinosis in a pup. J. Am. Vet. Med. Assoc., *177*:542–546, 1980.
86. Woodard, J.C. et al.: Calcium phosphate deposition disease in Great Danes. Vet. Pathol., *19*:464–485, 1982.
87. Reginato, A.J., Schumacher, H.R., and Brighton, C.T.: Experimental hydroxyapatite synovial and articular cartilage calcification: Light and electron microscopic studies. Arthritis Rheum., *25*:1239–1249, 1982.
88. Lian, J.B., Pachman, L.M., Gundberg, C.M., et al.: Gamma-carboxyglutamate excretion and calcinosis in juvenile dermatomyositis. Arthritis Rheum., *25*:1094–1100, 1982.
89. Berger, R.G., and Hadler, N.M.: Treatment of calcinosis universalis secondary to dermatomyositis or scleroderma with low dose warfarin. Arthritis Rheum., *26*:S11, 1983.
90. Skuterud, E., Sydnes, A.O., and Haavik, T.K.: Calcinosis in dermatomyositis treated with probenecid. Scand. J. Rheumatol., *10*:92–94, 1981.
91. Dieppe, P., and Watt, I.: Crystal deposition in osteoarthritis: An opportunistic event. Clin. Rheum. Dis., *11*:367–392, 1985.
92. Campion, G.V., McCrae, F., Alwan, W., et al.: Idiopathic destructive arthritis of the shoulder. Semin. Arthritis Rheum., *17*:232–245, 1988.
93. Anderson, H.C.: Calcific diseases—A concept. Arch. Pathol. Lab. Med., *107*:341–348, 1983.

110

Calcium Oxalate and Other Crystals or Particles Associated with Arthritis

ANTONIO J. REGINATO

Besides monosodium urate monohydrate (MSU), calcium pyrophosphate dihydrate (CPPD), and other calcium phosphates, other crystals have been found in synovial fluid of arthritic patients[1] (Table 110–1). Sufficient information is available to describe the clinical manifestations associated with calcium oxalate,[1–14] cholesterol,[14–17] lipid liquid crystals,[14,18–22] cryoglobulin crystals,[14,23–25] Charcot-Leyden crystals,[14,26–29] and synthetic corticosteroid crystals[1,30] (see also Chapter 5). Other crystals such as cystine,[14,31,32] hypoxanthine,[14,32–35] aluminum phosphate,[14,36–38] hemoglobulin,[14,39–41] hematoidin,[14,41,42] and other crystalline lipids[14] thought to be fatty acids have been described only in single case reports. In synovial fluid, synovium, muscle, or bone in single case reports. Other endogenous compounds such as bilirubin,[43,44] myoglobin,[45] porphyrins,[46] tyrosine,[47,48] orotic acid,[49] and a variety of proteins such as amyloid, α-1 antitrypsin,[51] adenosinetriphosphatase (ATPase),[52] and other less well-identified proteins secreted by different tumors or leukemia cells,[53–55] as well as drugs,[56–59] can also crystallize in various body fluids and tissues.

Conceivably, some of these crystals could play a role in the pathophysiology of the clinical manifestations associated with hemoglobinopathies, porphyria cutanea tarda, or drug toxicity, but this remains speculative.

Exogenous particles described in association with foreign-body synovitis also often have a crystalline structure.[60–63] Sea urchin spines, for example, are formed from calcium carbonate crystals,[60] and talcum powder consists of magnesium silicate crystals, or starch granules.[62] Also, other foreign bodies such as plant thorns or polyethylene and polymethylmethacrylate polymer particles have a paracrystalline or crystalline structure.[61,63]

CALCIUM OXALATE CRYSTAL DEPOSITION

The articular manifestations of both primary oxalosis and secondary oxalosis occurring in uremic patients managed with long-term hemodialysis have been confused with those of gout and pseudogout.[2–14] Such patients may present a variety of articular manifestations (Fig. 110–1) as well as life-threatening organ involvement, which includes devastating peripheral vascular insufficiency with gangrene,[14,64,65] cardiomyopathy,[66,67] complete heart block,[67] peripheral neuropathy,[68] and aplastic anemia.[69,70]

ACQUIRED OXALOSIS

Oxalic acid is the metabolic end product of glycine, serine, other amino acids, and ascorbic acid.[71,72] Large amounts are also found in certain foods such as spinach and rhubarb. Oxalate is readily absorbed after ingestion. It is removed from the body almost entirely by glomerular filtration and secretion in the proximal tubule. Hyperoxalemia, hyperoxaluria, oxalate kidney stones, and crystalline tissue deposits may be the result of several contributing factors that may affect oxalate metabolism[14,71–75] (Table 110–2). Excessive oxalate in the diet or increased absorption in patients with chronic inflammatory bowel disease, bowel resection, or intestinal bypass can lead to hyperoxalemia.[73] Methoxyflurane, ethyleneglycol, ascorbic acid, and xylitol are metabolized to oxalate.[71,72]

Thiamine and pyridoxine deficiencies may inhibit glyoxylate metabolism, increasing oxalate production.[71,72] Aspergillus niger can synthesize oxalic acid, which may crystallize in affected tissues and in aspergillomas.[71,76] Chronic renal failure can lead to serum oxa-

TABLE 110–1. CRYSTALS AND BIREFRINGENT PARTICLES UNCOMMONLY FOUND IN JOINT, MUSCLE, OR BONE

Calcium oxalate
Cholesterol
Lipid liquid crystals
Other crystalline lipids
Corticosteroid ester crystals
Cystine
Xanthine
Hypoxanthine
Cryoglobulins
Charcot-Leyden (lysophospholipase) crystals
Aluminum
Hemoglobulin
Hematoidin
Foreign bodies
Plant thorns
Sea urchin spines (calcium carbonate)
Polyethylene polymer
Methylmethacrylate polymer

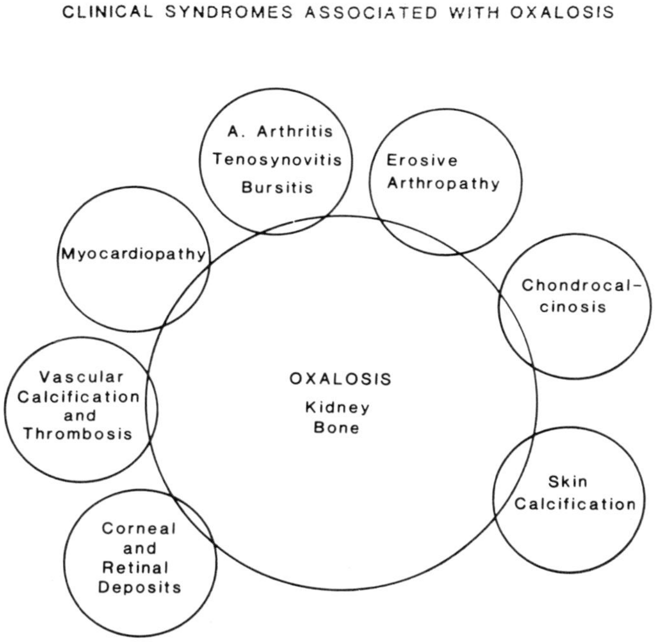

FIGURE 110–1. Clinical manifestations of oxalosis. A = acute.

TABLE 110–2. TYPES OF OXALOSIS

Primary or Familial
Type I: Glycolic aciduria
Type II: Glyceric aciduria
Acquired
Diet rich in oxalate, e.g., rhubarb
Increased ingestion of oxalate precursors, e.g., ascorbic acid, ethyleneglycol
Increased absorption, e.g., small bowel resection or bypass, inflammatory bowel disease
Increased production, e.g., deficiency thiamine or pyridoxine
Decreased renal excretion; uremia
Dystrophic: retinal damage

late levels four to eight times greater than normal.[77] Serum levels parallel creatinine, becoming saturated when levels of the latter reach 8 to 9 mg/dL.[77] (Primary oxalosis is discussed later.)

The formation of calcium oxalate crystals in biologic fluids and tissues results when the limits of solubility are exceeded.[77] In the urine, the degree of saturation of calcium oxalate expressed in terms of the ionic concentration of calcium and oxalic acid is the most important single factor in the formation of oxalate stones.[78] Similar mechanisms may operate in serum and other tissues.[77] Some tissues, such as kidney, myocardium, and retina, and aspergillus infections produce oxalic acid, so that local acid concentration may exceed those of serum.[75,79,80] This may account for calcium oxalate crystal formation in aspergillosis and in dystrophic retinal damage.[75,80]

PRIMARY OXALOSIS

Primary oxalosis is a rare, recessive disorder characterized by excretion of excessive amounts of oxalate in the urine.[2,71,72,81–83] Two types of enzymatic defects have been recognized.

In type 1 (glycolic aciduria), excessive amounts of glyoxylic and glycolic acids are found in the urine. The increased oxalate and glycolic acid synthesis is the result of a blockage of glyoxylate alternate pathways (Fig. 110–2). Dempure and Jennings demonstrated that the defect is in the peroxisomal enzyme, alanine glyoxylase aminotransferase[72,83] and this observation has been confirmed[84,85] (Fig. 110–2). This defect can be diagnosed using liver tissue obtained through needle biopsy. Immunoblot studies have provided evidence of genetic heterogeneity with some patients expressing normal-sized enzyme monomers, while others lacked the enzyme.[85,86] Assays of this enzyme activity may be useful in determining the prognosis and severity of the disease.[83]

Type-2 oxalosis (glyceric aciduria) is the result of a defect in hydroxypyruvate metabolism (see Fig. 110–2). Decreased activity of D glyceric acid dehydrogenase has been found in leukocytes of patients with this type of oxalosis.[72,86] Excessive hydroxypyruvate resulting from D glyceric dehydrogenase deficiency is reduced to L glycerate with a parallel increase in the oxidation of glyoxylate to oxalate in a coupled reaction catalyzed by lactic acid dehydrogenase.[86]

Oxalosis symptoms begin during early childhood with nephrolithiasis and nephrocalcinosis, leading to renal failure and death before age 20 in most patients.[81,82] Renal insufficiency is associated with rapid, progressive calcium oxalate crystal deposits in kidney, myocardium, skin, bone, and blood vessels. Oxalate crystals have been described in articular tissues at autopsies.[87] Over the past 50 years, tenosynovitis[88] and both acute and chronic arthritis have been described in these patients, but identification of crystals in synovial fluid or tissue has only rarely been possible.[4,82] As more patients with primary oxalosis are being managed with

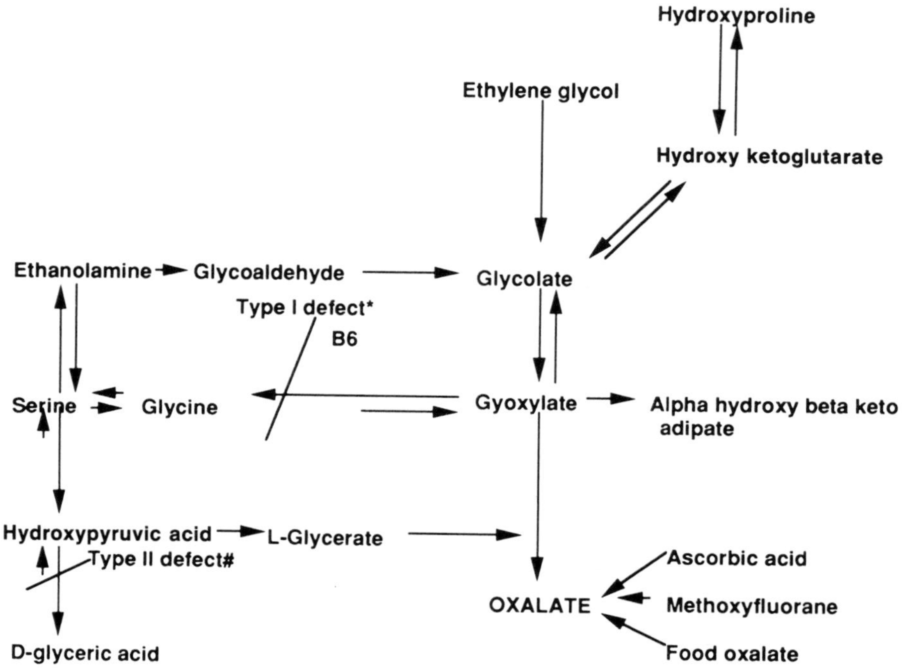

FIGURE 110–2. Glyoxylate and oxalate metabolism * = alanine glyoxylate aminotransferase deficiency. # = D-glyceric dehydrogenase deficiency. (Adapted from Ernest, D.L.: Enteric hyperoxaluria. Adv. Intern. Med., *24*:407, 1979.)

long-term hemodialysis, oxalate crystal deposition may become more important as a cause of morbidity.[89] Oxalate crystals have been identified in articular tissues of patients with primary oxalosis, older than 30 years at the time of diagnosis and managed with long-term hemodialysis.[4,7,12] One presented with severe hand arthropathy with bony erosions and cysts and with large subcutaneous calcium oxalate crystalline deposits around his phalanges and olecranon mimicking tophaceous gout[4] (Fig. 110–3A and B).

ROENTGENOLOGIC MANIFESTATIONS

The roentgenologic appearance of primary and secondary oxalosis is similar, characteristically involving the hands and feet, with skin, vascular, periarticular, and intra-articular calcifications (Figs. 110–4 and 110–5).[90,91] Rosette-like areas of bony sclerosis in hands and feet, metaphyseal sclerotic bands, pathologic fractures, and pseudarthrosis[90–92] may be seen alone or in combination with the bony changes of renal osteodystrophy.[92,93] Chondrocalcinosis of larger joints and periarticular calcified masses have been described (Figs. 110–5 and 110–6).

PATHOLOGIC STUDIES

Synovium

Most synovium has been obtained during chronic synovitis and has shown mild synovial cell hyperplasia with hyperemia and pleomorphic calcium oxalate crystals lying in a mildly fibrotic interstitium with scarce mononuclear cells and a few giant cells[5,6,14] (Fig. 110–7A). Clumps of closely packed crystals with intensely and weakly positive birefringence may be seen in the subsynovium without an inflammatory reaction (Fig. 110–7B).

Cartilage, Meniscus, and Bone

Few studies of articular cartilage in oxalosis have been performed.[3,5] Kinnet and Bullough[3] described erosion of articular cartilage by chronically inflamed synovium containing oxalate crystals, and Hoffman et al.[5] found oxalate crystals in a large cystic area of a meniscus of a patient with hemodialysis oxalosis. Cartilage and bone obtained from a first metatarsophalangeal joint did not reveal any crystals, although the synovium and capsule contained many.[6] However, bone histology in most patients with oxalosis shows oxalate crystal deposits surrounded by giant cells and bone marrow fibrosis. These deposits correlate with radiologic areas of subperiosteal resorption, endosteal erosion, pseudofractures, or localized osteosclerosis resulting from deposits of radiopaque calcium oxalate crystals in the bone marrow.[92–95] Massive oxalate crystal deposits in bone may cause a form of renal osteodystrophy in hemodialysis patients that is pathologically and radiologically similar to osteitis fibrose but without biochemical evidence of hyperparathyroidism.[96–98]

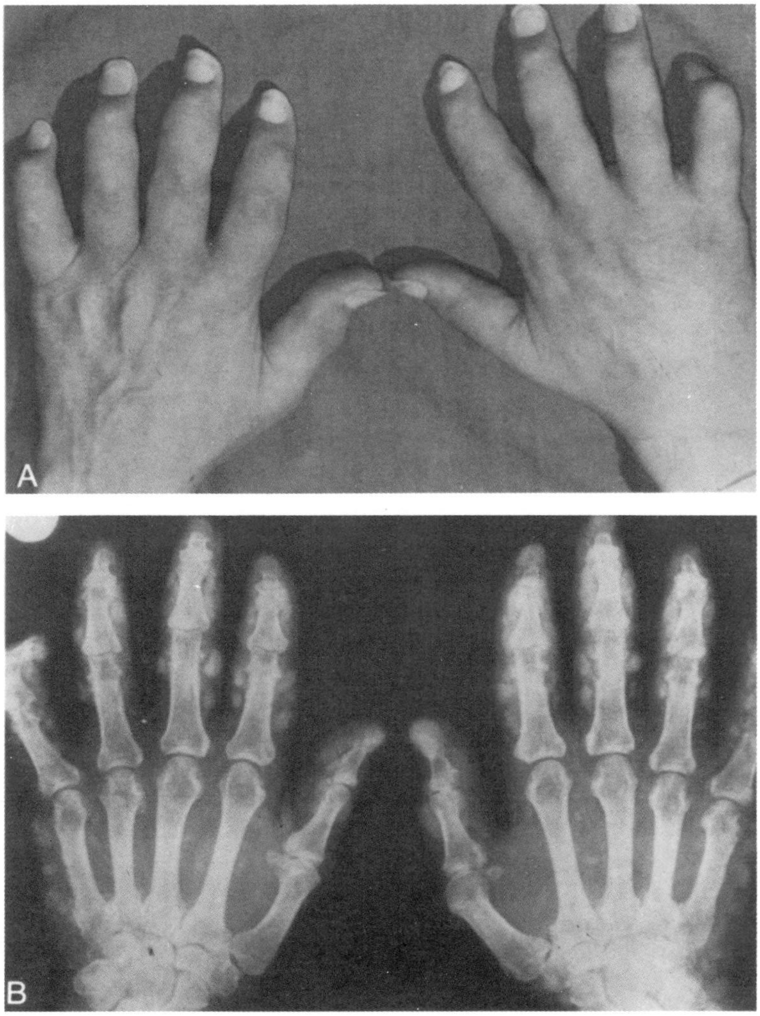

FIGURE 110–3. *A*, Hands of a patient with primary oxalosis mimicking gout or rheumatoid arthritis. *B*, Radiographs of the same hands, showing periarticular calcific deposits, bony erosions, and resorption of distal phalanges. (From Schmidt, K.L. et al.: Arthropathies bei primarer Oxalose-Krystallsynovitis oder Osteopathie. Dtsch. Med. Wochenschr., *106*:19, 1981.)

CRYSTALLOGRAPHIC FEATURES

Calcium oxalate crystals deposit in bone,[2,3,81,92–95] tendon,[88] articular cartilage,[3,5,87,94] menisci,[5] and synovium.[2,3,5,6] These sites are probably the source of crystals found in joint fluid. Two types of oxalate crystals have been identified: (1) characteristic dipyramidal crystals formed by calcium oxalate dihydrate (weddellite) (see Fig. 110–7C) and (2) polymorphic crystals composed of calcium oxalate monohydrate (whewellite). The latter appear as irregular squares, chunks, short rods, stretched ovals, dumb-bells, and even microspherules.[1,5,6] Sizes range from 5 to 30 μm. Some calcium oxalate crystals show strongly positive birefringence, but most exhibit a weakly positive birefringence or none at all. Most crystals showing no birefringence are simply too small and thin to retard sufficient light. Most of them stain with alizarin red S on fresh preparations,[99,100] and those in tissue deposits can also be recognized with Pizzolato's stain,[101,102] a modification of the von Kossa stain. Under transmission electron microscopy, they are electron dense with sharp margins and a foamy structure similar to that of CPPD crystals.[1,5,6] Both x-ray diffraction analysis and scanning electron microscopy have been helpful in determining which of the two types of oxalate crystal is present and to correlate crystallographic structure with optical morphology.[103,104] (Fig. 110–8A to C). As a result of their polymorphism and variable strength of birefringence, calcium oxalate crystals can easily be confused with CPPD crystals or even with apatite microspherules when synovial fluid is examined only by ordinary or compensated polarized light.[5,6] The phlogistic potency of calcium oxalate crystals is similar to that of MSU crystals or calcium phosphate crystals as assessed by injections of synthetic preparations into dog knees[105] or rat paws.[106] Crystalline calcium oxalate also stimulates synovial cells to synthesize and release latent collagenase and prostaglandins.[107] It seems possible that activation of synovial cells, fibroblasts, and osteoclasts by calcium oxalate crystals might play a role in inducing bone erosions, cysts, and even pathologic fractures like those seen in patients with bone and articular oxalosis.[5,6,92,93,107]

BIOCHEMICAL FEATURES

Serum oxalate levels have been measured in two of the three reports of articular oxalosis complicating long-term dialysis.[5,8,14] The levels ranged from 168 ± 36 mg/L, about eight times higher than normal. Synovial fluid oxalate levels in these patients were considerably higher than those found in fluid of patients with rheumatoid arthritis (RA), osteoarthritis (OA), or pseudogout.[5] Some patients had mild hypercalcemia and an increased calcium/phosphorous ratio that was due to secondary hyperparathyroidism and/or vitamin D administration.[6] Most patients with end stage renal disease had a low serum calcium level, although a few were hypercalcemic.[92,93]

Hypercalcemia could be a contributory factor in precipitating calcium oxalate crystals in tissues, but parathyroidectomy, performed in a few patients with bone oxalosis and end stage renal disease, was ineffective in correcting the elevated serum calcium or in decreasing crystal deposits.[93] Another possible explanation for the hypercalcemia seen in these patients is increased osteoclastic bone resorption at the site of oxalate deposits in bone.[92,93,96–98]

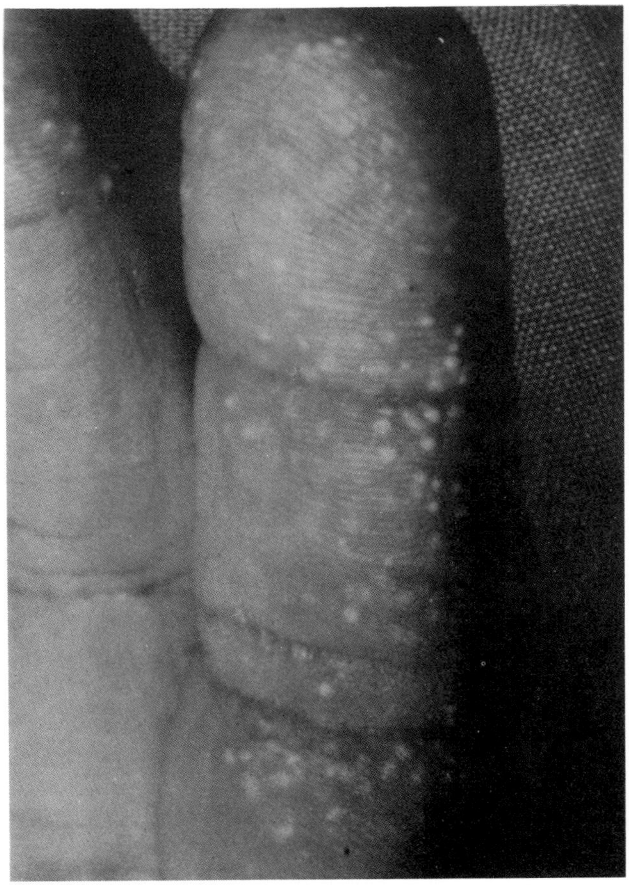

FIGURE 110–4. Miliary skin deposits in a patient with hemodialysis oxalosis. (From Reginato, A.J., et al.[6])

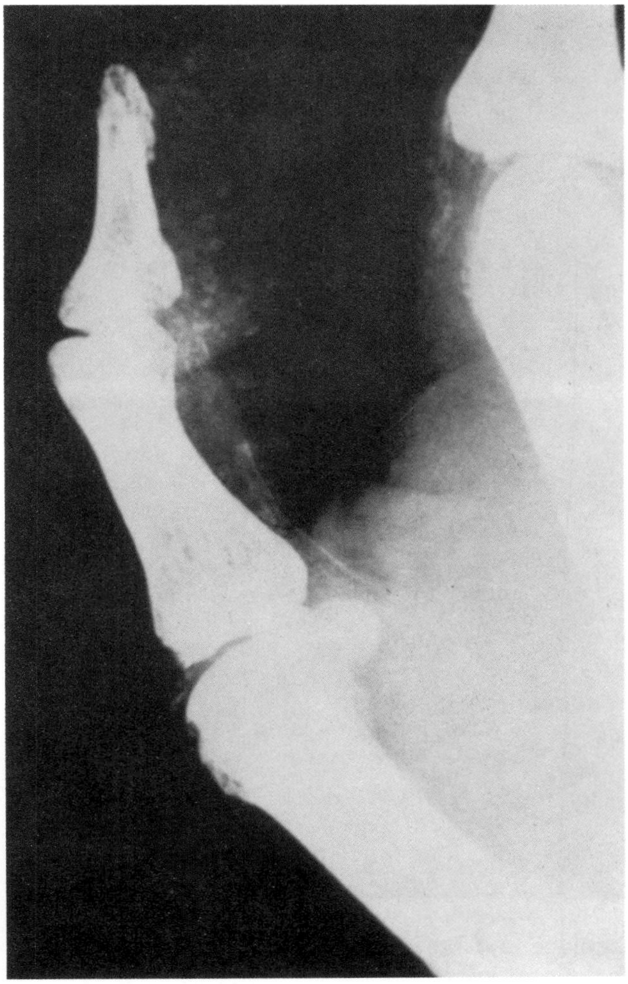

FIGURE 110–5. Radiograph of a patient with hemodialysis oxalosis, showing skin, vascular, periarticular calcifications, and chondrocalcinosis. (From Reginato, A.J., et al.[6])

Oxalate is removed by both hemodialysis and peritoneal dialysis, but neither procedure induces a negative balance that would result in effective removal of oxalate from tissues of patients with either primary oxalosis or end stage renal disease.[108–112] Autopsy series show that renal and bone oxalosis occur in about 90% of patients with end stage renal disease managed with long-term hemodialysis.[113,114] Because articular tissues have not been included in most of these studies, the frequency of articular oxalosis is unknown.[113,114] Several reports of articular oxalosis have implicated ascorbic acid administration in aggravating oxalate deposition.[5,6,8] In some dialysis protocols, ascorbic acid is added to dialysis solutions to neutralize chloramine and prevent hemolysis.[115] Because oxalate is a metabolic end product of ascorbic acid, large amounts given to patients receiving

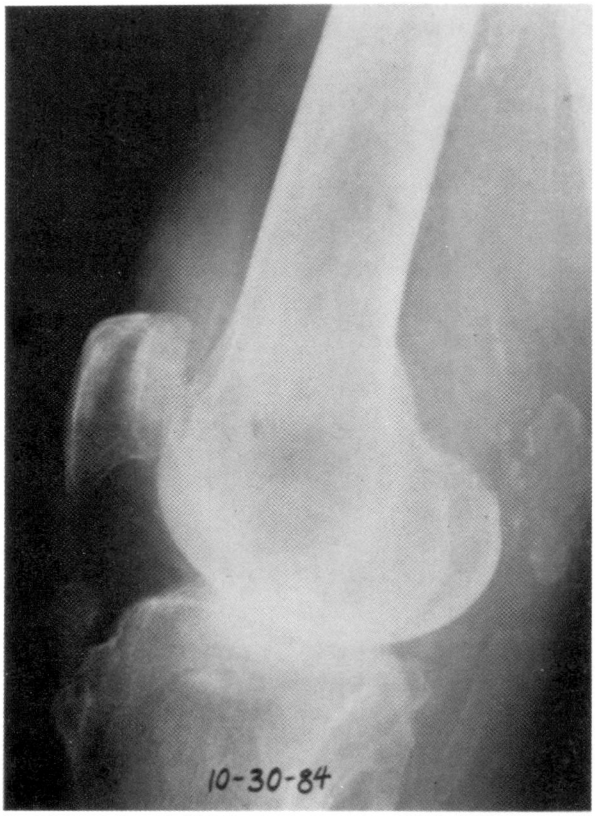

FIGURE 110–6. Knee radiograph of a patient with acquired oxalosis that was due to renal failure managed with chronic peritoneal dialysis and also to large calcified masses and arterial calcifications. (From Schumacher, J.R., Reginato, A.J., and Pullman, S.: Synovial fluid oxalate deposition complicating rheumatoid arthritis with amyloidosis and renal failure: Demonstration of intracellular oxalate crystals. J. Rheumatol., *14*:361, 1987.)

dialysis may result in higher serum oxalate levels and increased crystal deposition in tissues.[74,112,115,116] Most patients with articular oxalosis have received 500 to 1000 mg of ascorbic acid after each dialysis.[5,6,8,117]

CLINICAL MANIFESTATIONS

Symmetric proximal interphalangeal and metacarpophalangeal joints, acute arthritis, with or without flexor tenosynovitis, miliary calcific deposits of digits, and digital vascular calcification are the most characteristic clinical presentation[5,6,14,117] (see Figs. 110–3A to 110–5). Acute or chronic effusions of larger joints such as knees, elbows, or ankles may develop[5,6,8] (see Fig. 110–6). Podagra, Achilles tenosynovitis, and bursitis have been observed in single patients.[6,14] In most patients, the initial acute synovitis follows a chronic course, responding poorly to colchicine, nonsteroidal anti-inflammatory drugs (NSAIDs), intra-articular injections of corticosteroids, or even increased frequency of dialysis.[5,6] Synovial fluid from acute and chronic effusions has been clear or bloody with normal viscosity.[1,5,6,8] Leukocyte counts have been low, ranging from 150 to 2100 cells/μL with 60 to 90% of polymorphonuclear (PMN) cells in some samples[1,5,6] In others, a predominance of large mononuclear cells was observed.[5,6] Abundant clumps of crystals are usually seen, most of which are extracellular (see Fig. 110–7C), but intracellular crystals were found in fluid from three patients.[5,8,11]

MANAGEMENT

There is no effective medical therapy for either primary or secondary oxalosis.[118–120] Therapeutic methods that have been tried unsuccessfully for primary oxalosis include a low-oxalate diet,[118] allopurinol,[118] pyridoxine,[118–120] orthophosphate, magnesium administration; and renal transplantation with aggressive hemodialysis.[72,118–122] Because renal transplantation in patients with primary oxalosis and end stage renal disease is associated with only a 30% three-year survival, combined renal and liver transplantation have been performed to improve renal function and correct the enzymatic defect.[123–125] Preliminary results suggest that hepatic transplantation should be considered as a definite treatment before end stage renal failure develops.[125]

SYNDROMES ASSOCIATED WITH CHOLESTEROL CRYSTALS AND OTHER CRYSTALLINE LIPIDS

CHOLESTEROL CRYSTALS

Although cholesterol crystals are occasionally identified in rheumatoid joint fluid[1,14–17] or bursal effusions,[14] their possible contribution to either inflammation or joint deterioration is unclear.

Cholesterol crystals have also been observed (rarely) in synovial fluids from patients with osteoarthritis, chronic tophaceous gout, ankylosing spondylitis, and even systemic lupus erythematosus.[1,14,126] These crystals also have been found in pleural or pericardial effusions of patients with RA as well as effusions resulting from tuberculosis or a tumor.[14,126] Cholesterol crystals have been seen in rheumatoid nodules, tophi, unicameral bone cysts, and even as isolated granulomas or "cholesterol tophi" in the skin.[14,126] They have been demonstrated in bone granuloma, tosis (Erdhein Chester disease) and in the kidneys of patients with nephrotic syndrome.[14] The few studies performed on synovial fluid of patients with arthritis associated with hyperlipoproteinemias have failed to show cholesterol or other crystalline lipids.[14,127] Synovium from two such patients has not shown crystalline lipid deposits either,[128,129] but in one of these, MSU deposits were found,[128] and in the other, apatite-like crystals were found inside synovial cells.[128] Xanthomas often develop in the Achilles tendons and extensor tendon sheaths of

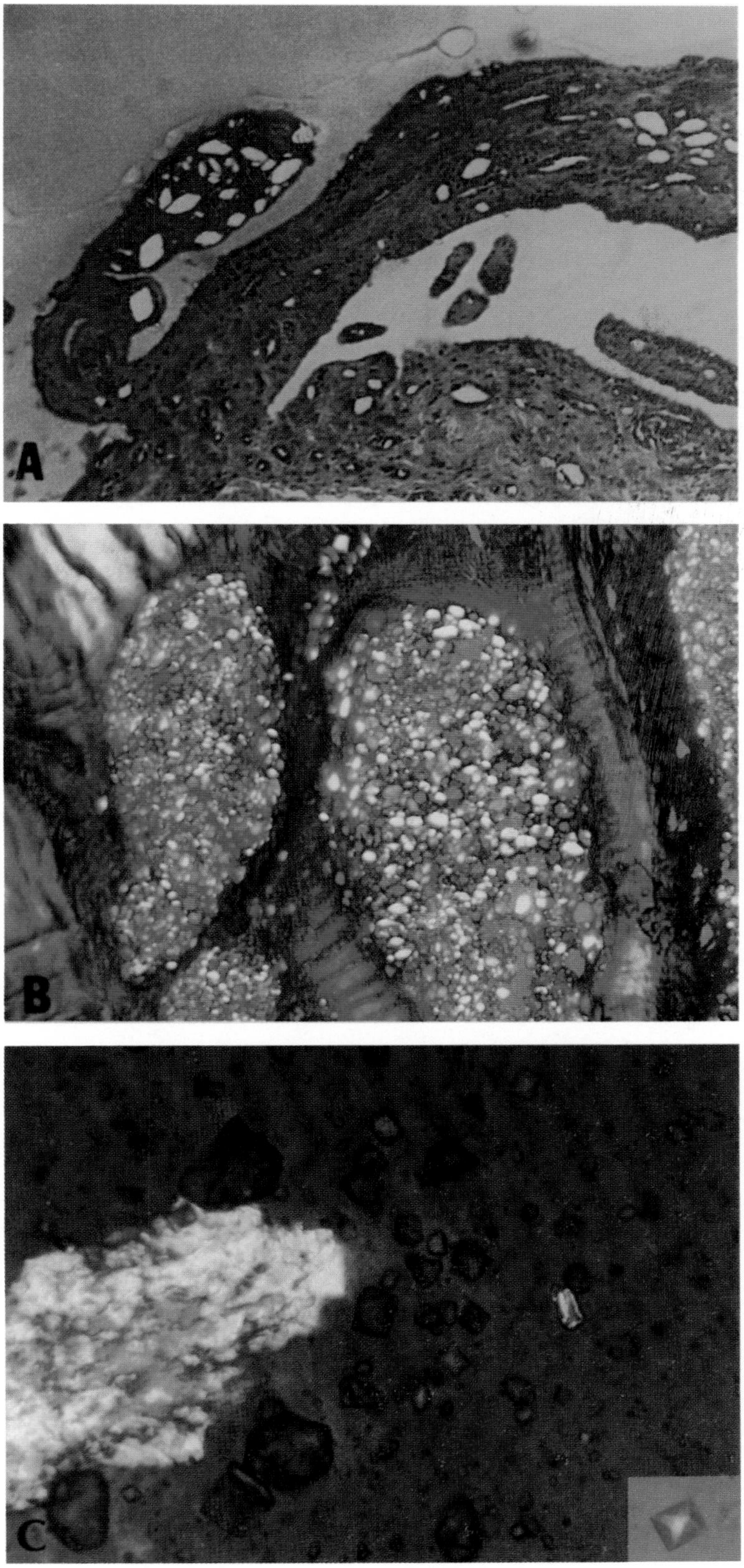

FIGURE 110–7. *A*, Isolated calcium oxalate crystals in the superficial synovium (hematoxylin and eosin stain ×180). *B*, Large clumps of birefringent crystals lying between collagen fibers. Compensated light microscopy (×180). *C*, Calcium oxalate crystals in synovial fluid. Pseudotophaceous deposits surrounded by abundant polymorphic and a few dipyramidal crystals showing no birefringence and weakly or intensely positive birefringence (insert). Compensated polarized (×400). (From Reginato, A.J. et al.[6])

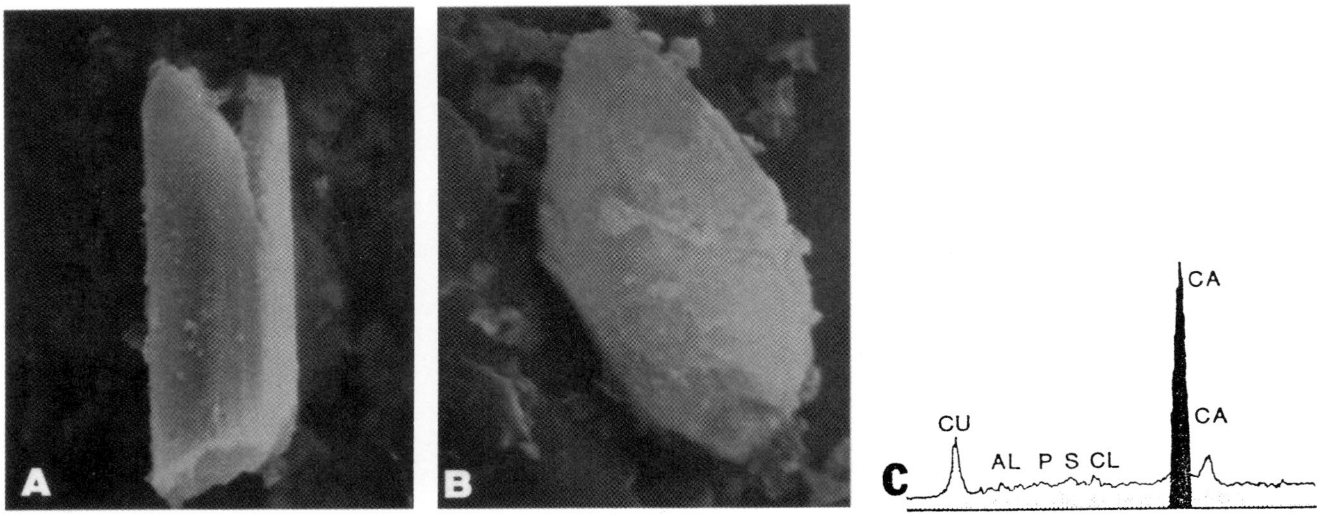

FIGURE 110–8. Scanning electron micrographs. *A*, Rod-shaped and, *B*, hexagonal-shaped crystals of calcium oxalate monohydrate in synovial fluid (×4000). *C*, Energy dispersive analysis, showing calcium but no phosphorus. (From Reginato, A.J. et al.[6])

the hands of patients with familial hypercholesterolemia.[130,131] Increased tendon size can produce pain and interfere with function, but tenosynovitis and tendon rupture occur rarely.[130,132] The syndrome of multiple cholesterol emboli may present a constellation of systemic manifestations mimicking necrotizing vasculitis[133,134] (see Chapter 75).

CRYSTALLOGRAPHIC FEATURES

Synovial fluid containing cholesterol crystals often has a golden-honey or yellow-brown color.[1,16] Cholesterol crystals in synovial fluid are extracellular but are often associated with intra- and extracellular birefringent "Maltese crosses" (Fig. 110–9A and B). Cholesterol crystals show two morphologic forms:[1,135] (1) highly birefringent, large, flat, rectangular plates with one or more notched corners, ranging from 8 to 100 μm (Fig. 110–10) and (2) rod or needle-shaped, strongly negative birefringent crystals ranging from 2 to 30 μm long (see Fig. 110–10, insert). Needle-shaped crystals are much more difficult to recognize and may be confused with MSU.[1,135] (See also Chapter 5.)

Under transmission electron microscopy, cholesterol crystals are electron dense and retain their plate-like morphology before beam damage occurs. Under scanning electron microscopy, they appear as notched plates covered by synovial exudate.[1,4] X-ray diffraction analysis of joint fluid crystals showed that both the needle and plate-like forms were anhydrous cholesterol,[135] but in studies of cholesterol crystals in bile, the plate-like crystals were identified as cholesterol monohydrate and the needle-shaped crystals as anhydrous cholesterol.[136] Small amounts of proteins and phospholipids may be entrapped in these crystals.[135]

Many factors are probably involved in the formation of cholesterol crystals in inflamed tissues including increased cholesterol synthesis,[137] in situ bleeding, lipid release from damaged cell membranes and organelles,[126] and abnormal intracellular transport of lipids resulting from chronic inflammation and/or infection.[126,138] The capability of synthetic cholesterol crystals to induce moderate acute and chronic inflammation in skin, subcutaneous tissue, and knee joint of rabbits has been demonstrated in studies performed by Bland et al.[16] Denko and Petricevic,[139] and Pritzker et al.[140] Cholesterol crystals have not been observed inside phagocytes, as occurs with MSU, CPPD, or basic calcium phosphate crystals. Because pyrogen contamination was not ruled out or similarity of crystal structure with that of natural cholesterol crystals was not shown in any of these studies, extrapolation to human disease states remains speculative. Although cholesterol crystals may activate serum complement,[141] which might potentiate inflammation and aggravate joint destruction in RA and even OA, there is no clinical evidence to support this concept.[140]

LIPID LIQUID CRYSTALS

As already noted, birefringent Maltese crosses occasionally have been found in synovial or bursal fluids of patients with RA.[14] These structures are usually associated with increased synovial fluid lipid content and with cholesterol crystals and have been called "fluid spherocrystals,"[142] liposomes,[143] smetic mesophases,[144–146] or lipid liquid crystals.[144–146] They were found in the synovial fluid of 13 patients with otherwise unexplained acute monoarthritis,[18,19,22] in 7 patients with acute olecranon bursitis, and in 1 patient with chronic unexplained symmetric polyarthritis[14,18–22] (see Fig. 110–9A to C).

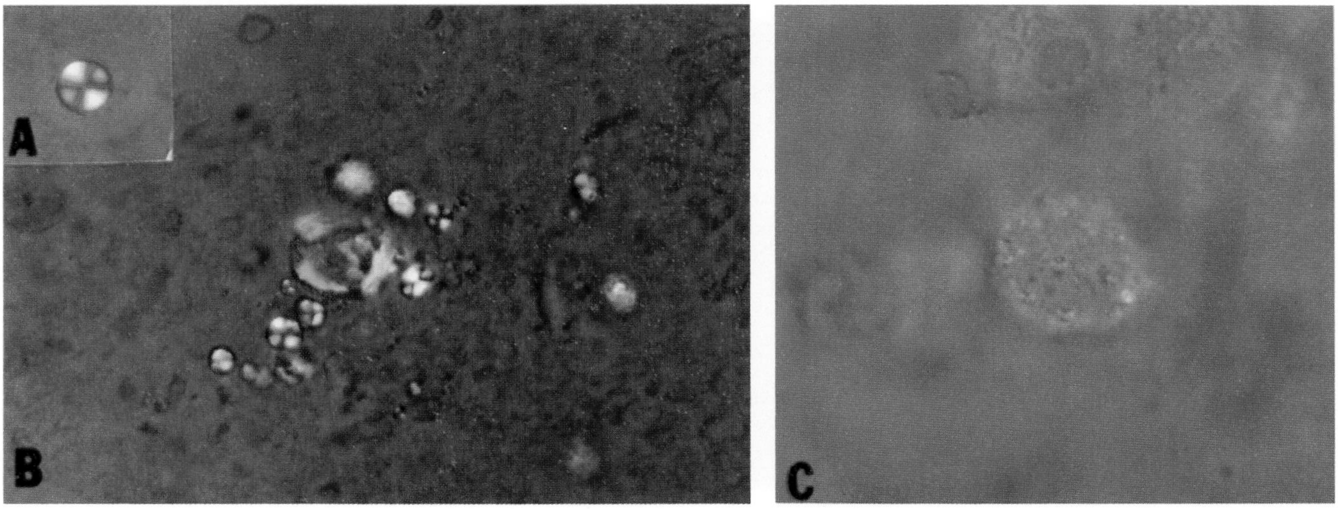

FIGURE 110–9. Lipid liquid crystals. *A*, Single, large, double-positive birefringent microspherule. *B*, Extracellular small microspherules. *C*, Abundant intracellular small microspherules. Compensated polarized light (×200). (With permission of Ann. Rheum. Dis. From Reginato, A.J., et al.[19])

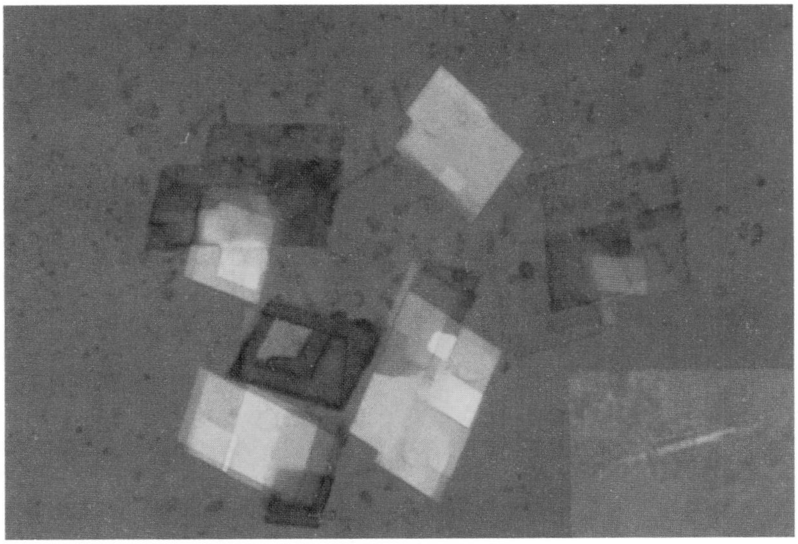

FIGURE 110–10. Characteristic highly birefringent plate-like cholesterol crystals and a needle-like cholesterol crystal (insert). Compensated polarized light (×200).

Lipid liquid crystals represent states of matter having characteristics of both liquid and solids.[143–145] They have some degree of order in their molecular arrangement but also some degree of fluidity. Molecules that form liquid crystals are longer than they are wide and have a polar or aromatic ring on the molecule.[144] The long shape and polar interactions permit molecular alignment in partially ordered *smetic* or *layered* arrays, similar to that of liposomes and in contrast to *nematic* arrays, in which the molecules are aligned side by side but not in mandatory layers.[144]

A liquid crystalline ordering of molecules has been described in both normal and pathologic biologic systems, for example, normal cell membranes and organelles, myelin, bile, serum lipoproteins,[144] atherosclerotic plaques,[143,146] adrenal glands,[144–146] nephrotic kidneys,[142,144] and lipid storage diseases.[143,146] Inclusions with similar ultrastructure can be seen in muscles, myocardium, lung, and nerve as a result of toxicity with different medications such as amiodarone,[56] chloroquine, hydroxychloroquine[147] and with some psychotherapeutic agents such as thioridazine and amitriptyline.[57] These inclusions are formed by phospholipids or by polar molecules of the drugs themselves, which can also be arranged as liquid crystals.[56–57]

CRYSTALLOGRAPHIC FEATURES

Under compensated polarized light, these microspherules have an intense double-positive birefringence (see Fig. 110–9A to C). Sizes range from 2 to 8 μm. Larger, irregularity birefringent plates (see Fig. 110–9B) probably represent transitional forms preceding the formation of cholesterol crystals.[1,144,146] In atherosclerotic plaques and in bile, these liquid lipid microspherules precede the formation of cholesterol crystals.[146] They are commonly seen inside cells, stain with Sudan black B, and are dissolved completely in 1:1 alcohol-ether.[1,19] Smaller microspherules may appear to be anisotropic (not birefringent). These positively birefringent Maltese crosses must be differentiated from the negatively birefringent MSU microspherules ("beachballs") rarely seen in patients with gout and from talcum powder crystals that may contaminate synovial fluids when gloves are used during arthrocentesis.[1,62] The latter are magnesium silicate or starch granules and show a positive birefringence, but their outlines are more irregular than MSU and lipid liquid crystal microspherules.

CLINICAL FEATURES

Acute Arthritis

All patients described have experienced the acute onset of monoarticular synovitis as often seen in other crystal-associated arthritis.[1,18–22] The knee is most commonly involved, although wrist involvement was noted in one instance.[19] Synovial fluid is inflammatory, with white cell counts ranging from 10,000 to 45,000/μL with 75 to 90% neutrophils. About 10 to 20% of these contain doubly birefringent microspherules (see Fig. 110–9A to C). Arthritis in all patients subsided completely within a week after NSAIDs were given. Synovium has been obtained in only two patients with acute synovitis;[14,20] mild inflammatory changes with rare lymphocytic, mononuclear, or PMN cell infiltrates were seen in both cases, and in one specimen, intracellular birefringent microspherules were seen inside mononuclear cells.[20] Because both the clinical presentation and the subsequent course were similar to those seen in patients with gout or pseudogout, it was suggested that these crystals might induce inflammation as has been proposed for solid crystals.[1,21]

Synthetic lipid liquid crystals injected into rabbit knees induced either acute or subacute synovitis.[148] The origin of these microspherules in articular tissues is unknown. In the few cases reported, associated diseases included sarcoidosis and alcoholic cirrhosis in one patient each, while two other patients had recent joint trauma and hemarthrosis.[14] Injection of autologous blood into rabbit knee joint was associated with formation of Maltese crosses.[149,150] Similar spherules seen in human joints may be formed by lipids derived from breakdown of membranes of platelets, erythrocytes, leukocytes, and even from serum lipids.[151]

Acute Bursitis

In one study, 7 of 18 bursal fluid samples contained positive birefringent microspherules.[14] One patient had gout, another had RA, while the remaining six had "traumatic" bursitis. Bursal fluid was inflammatory in all but the patient with gout.

Chronic Arthritis

The presence of lipid birefringent microspherules with chronic polyarthritis has been reported in one patient with otherwise unexplained symmetric polyarthritis resembling RA.[21]

Fabry's Disease

Fabry's disease, a sex-linked disorder affecting only males, is due to deposition of glycolipids in blood vessels, nerve, synovium, and kidney. Because of its unusual skin lesions, the disease is also known as angiokeratoma corporis universalis. Arthralgia and arthritis, usually exacerbated by warm weather, have been observed in patients with Fabry's disease.[152] Synovium and other tissues examined in these patients have shown glycolipidic inclusions with features of lipid liquid crystals.[152,153]

Other Crystalline Lipids

Other crystalline lipids, thought to be fatty acids, have been described in skin fat necrosis of newborns.[154] Identical structures have been observed in synovial fluid of patients with OA associated with large bone cysts in hemarthrosis and in synovial fluid examined several days after arthrocentesis.[155,156] Such crystals may have either a strongly positive or negative birefringence and may present with needle, plate, or rod shapes. Some may form clumps or rosettes. The rod- and needle-shaped crystals can be confused with CPPD or MSU crystals (Fig. 110–11).

CRYOGLOBULIN CRYSTALS

Paraproteins and cryoglobulins can crystallize within plasma cells of patients with multiple myeloma[14,23–25,157] (Fig. 110–12). These crystals are usually seen in areas of tumor in the bone marrow and, more rarely, in plasma cell infiltrates in different organs.[14,24] Similar crystals can be seen independent of plasma cells in the renal glomeruli, tubules, lungs, skin, liver, spleen, lymph nodes, adrenals, testis, and cornea.[1,14,24] These deposits can be associated with variable degrees of organ failure.[24,25] They may also occur in coronary and renal arteries and induce thrombosis and infarction.[24] Similar crystalline deposits have been observed in patients with essential cryoglobulinemia with purpuric and necrotic skin lesions[25] and in synovial fluid and synovium in association with arthritis.[14,23]

CRYSTALLOGRAPHIC FEATURES

Crystalline paraproteins are not associated with any particular type of heavy or light chains.[1,24] Their composition has been studied with trypsin digestion and immunofluorescent techniques.[24]

Paraprotein crystals are characterized by their large size, ranging from 3 to 60 μm or more, and their polymorphic shapes, which may vary with the cooling process used.[1,23,24] They usually appear as hexagonal, diamond-shaped, or polygonal crystals, but they may resemble squares, rectangles, rhomboids, or needles.[1,24] They may show either a strongly positive or a strongly negative birefringence. They stain with Giemsa and hematoxylin and eosin but not with Congo red or stains for lipids.[157] Under transmission electron microscopy, they are electron dense, with sharply demarcated borders and a homogenous structure; they stain with osmium and uranyl acetate.[156]

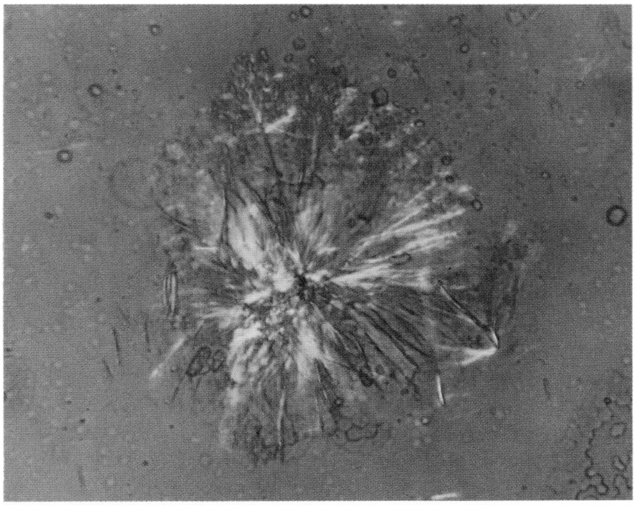

FIGURE 110–11. Lipid crystals of uncertain composition. Strongly negative birefringent needle-like lipid crystals in a patient with hemarthrosis. (Compensated polarized light ×400.) (From Reginato, A.J. and Kurnik, B.[14])

CLINICAL FEATURES

Episodic joint pain followed by an erosive, chronic, symmetric polyarthritis involving joints of the hands, feet, and one ankle have been observed in one patient with cryoprecipitable immunoglobulin G (IgG) in his serum and cryoglobulin crystals in joint fluid and synovium.[23] Synovial fluid was inflammatory with a white cell count of 30,000/μL with 90% neutrophils and abundant large rectangular and rhomboid cryoglobulin crystals. Synovium revealed a chronic inflammatory reaction and a few giant cells surrounding crystal deposits. These crystals were identical to those obtained from the serum cryoprecipitates. This patient also had crystalline corneal deposits. The arthritis failed to improve with administration of several NSAIDs, penicillamine, and plasmapheresis but was better controlled with cyclophosphamide. Similar improvement of eye symptoms, with dissolution of corneal crystalline deposits, has been observed in a few patients with multiple myeloma managed with chemotherapy.[159] Another patient with erosive polyarthritis and crystallizable monoclonal cryoglobulin also has been reported.[14] Two patients with multiple myeloma and corneal paraprotein crystalline deposits presented with foot arthritis, including podagra.[159] Arthritis associated with cryoglobulin-

FIGURE 110–12. Cryoglobulin crystals. Polygonal positive birefringent crystals of serum cryoprecipitate of a patient with multiple myeloma. Compensated polarized light (×200).

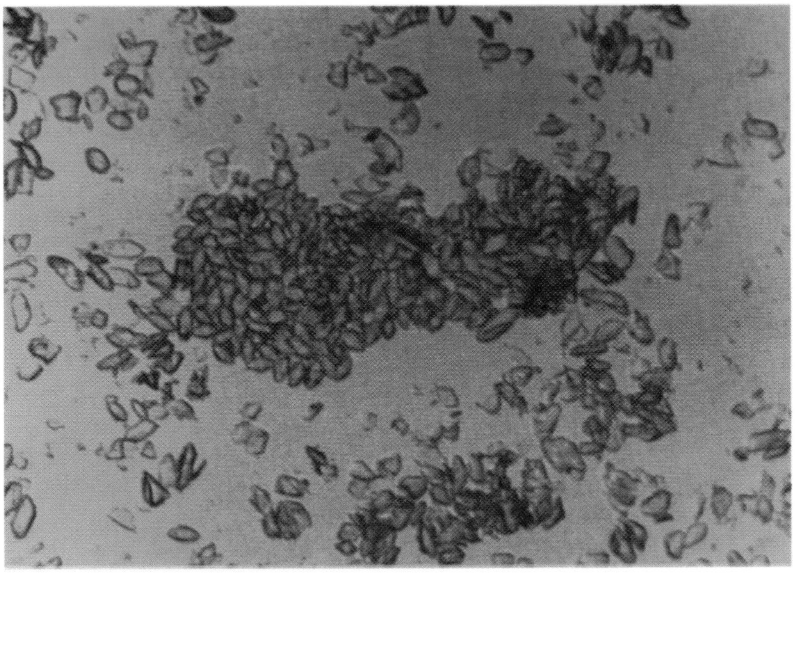

emia but without paraprotein crystals in synovial fluid has also been reported.[160,161]

CYSTINOSIS

Cystinosis is an autosomal recessive inborn error of metabolism characterized by excessive accumulation of cystine in reticuloendothelial cells of liver, spleen, lymph nodes, and bone marrow.[162] The basic defect is an impairment of normal carrier-mediated transport of cystine across the lysosomal membrane.[163] Three different types have been described. The most severe type is the infantile (nephrogenic), a milder type is seen in adolescents, and the most benign type is seen in adults.[162–164] The form is characterized for polydipsia, polyuria, crystalline deposits in renal tubule and glomeruli, Fanconi's syndrome, and progressive renal failure. These patients also present with conjunctivitis, retinopathy, and vitamin D-resistant rickets.

CRYSTALLOGRAPHIC FEATURES

Cystine crystals have a characteristic hexahedral shape with a weak-to-intense birefringence.[1,31,162] Typical crystals are rarely seen in tissue deposits, where they appear polymorphic, assuming square, rectangular, lozenge, and even acicular (needle-like) shapes.[31,162] Under transmission electron microscopy, they are surrounded by osmiophilic dense bodies and almost always appear within lysosomes inside cells.[164] Histochemical studies showed crystals surrounded by membrane-bound structures staining positively for alkaline phosphatase and binding ferritin.[165] These intracellular crystals may form in situ rather than by phagocytosis of preformed crystals.[162,166]

CLINICAL FEATURES

Patients with the infantile type of cystinosis present with vitamin D-resistant rickets, that is, with growth retardation, pseudofractures, and bone pain.[162] Hypothyroidism has accompanied cystine deposits in the thyroid gland.[166] Symptomatic crystal deposits in bone were described in a single patient and correlated with localized focal demineralization.[32] In another patient, cystinosis of bone was associated with acute knee and wrist synovitis and with polyarthralgias of larger joints,[31] but no cystine crystals were found in his synovial fluid. Radiographs revealed coarse bone trabeculation with diffuse demineralization and flattening of one of the metacarpal heads with punctiform periarticular calcific deposits. Cystine crystalline deposits in muscles have been described in a patient with long-standing cystinosis and generalized muscle weakness and wasting.[167] Also, patients with cystinosis and Fanconi's syndrome may develop plasma and muscle carnitine deficiency. Their muscles may show infiltration with fat droplets[168] (see Chapter 111).

Management of patients with cystinosis include adequate fluid intake and correction of metabolic acidosis, hypokalemia, and rickets.[162] End stage renal failure can be managed with dialysis or renal transplantation. Oral administration of cysteamine has been shown to stabilize renal function, improve growth, and decrease cystine crystalline corneal deposits.[168,169] Cysteamine or β-mercaptoethylamine is a free thiol with marked cystine-depleting activity.

XANTHINE CRYSTALS

Xanthinuria is an uncommon hereditary disorder of purine metabolism resulting from a deficiency of the enzyme xanthine oxidase.[170] It is characterized by hypouricemia, decreased uric acid excretion in the urine, and the presence of xanthinuria, hypoxanthinuria, and xanthine kidney stones. Hypoxanthine and xanthine crystals have been identified in the muscle of three patients with xanthinuria and tender muscles.[33–35,171] Muscle pain was crampy and increased by walking. Two other patients presented with acute arthritis mimicking gout; unfortunately no synovial fluid was obtained.[172] Xanthine, hypoxanthine, and oxipurinol crystals also have been identified in kidney stones and muscles of a patient with Lesch-Nyhan syndrome treated with allopurinol.[173,174] Similar deposits were found in kidneys of a patient with lymphosarcoma managed with aggressive chemotherapy and allopurinol.[175] Deposits of xanthine, hypoxanthine, and oxipuriol crystals have been found in skeletal muscle in absence of muscle pain or weakness of 10 patients with gout treated with allopurinol.[58]

CRYSTALLOGRAPHIC FEATURES

Xanthine crystals are plate-like or rhomboidal in shape, measure up to 2.5 μm, and are strongly birefringent.[1,35] Hypoxanthine crystals are more polymorphic, although they may also appear as large plates or rhomboidal crystals. They range in size from 9.5 and 50 μm and show strong negative birefringence. Exact identification of these crystals requires electron or x-ray diffraction analysis.[1,35]

CHARCOT-LEYDEN CRYSTALS

The formation of protein crystals within cytoplasm of human cells is infrequent, but Charcot-Leyden crystals represent an example of this phenomenon.[1,176] They are formed in the cytoplasm of disrupted eosinophils and are found in the sputum of asthmatic patients,[176] the tissue of patients with hypereosinophilia,[29] eosinophilic disease processes such as eosinophilic bone granuloma, hypereosinophilic syndrome,[29] the stool of patients with parasitic infections,[176] granulocytic leukemia,[176] and the synovial fluid of patients with eosinophilic synovitis.[1,14,26–28] Circulating Charcot-Leyden crystals have been observed in one patient with

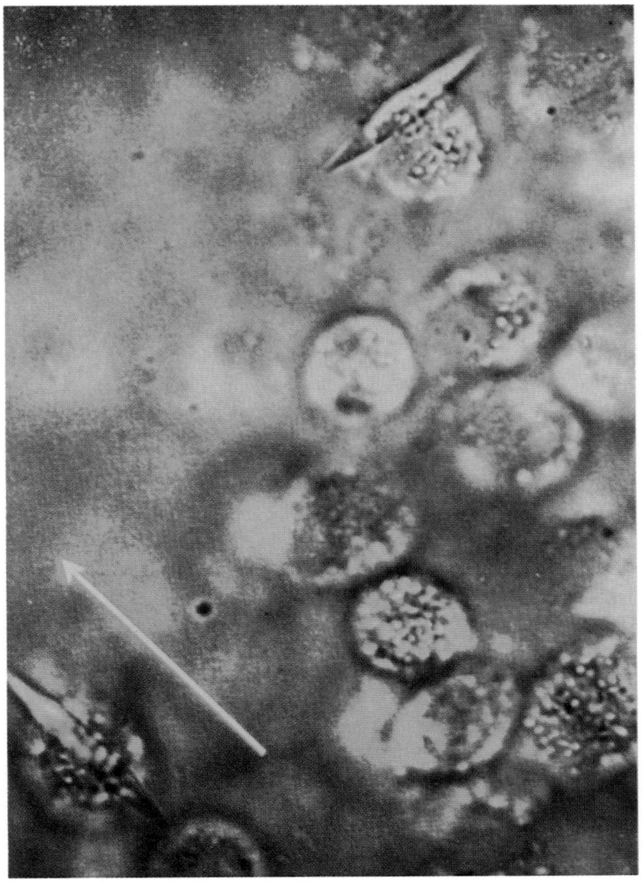

FIGURE 110–13. Charcot-Leyden crystals in synovial fluid of a patient with eosinophilic synovitis. Compensated polarized light (×350). Arrow indicates compensator axis. (Courtesy of Dr. R. De Medicis.[26])

hypereosinophilic syndrome and crystalline deposits in thrombosed vessels and in the renal glomeruli.[29]

CRYSTALLOGRAPHIC FEATURES

Charcot-Leyden crystals are bipyramidal hexagonal-shaped crystals formed by a lysophospholipase or phospholipase B[177,178] (Fig. 110–13). Crystal sizes range from 17 to 25 μm. With hematoxylin and eosin stain, they appear fairly eosinophilic; with Giemsa stain, they appear light purple or pink.[179] By transmission electron microscopy, these crystals are made of uniform, finely granular electron-dense material with a fine fibrillar pattern.[180,181] They may have a weakly positive birefringence,[26] but others have observed them to have a negative birefringence or a very weak birefringence.[1]

CLINICAL FEATURES

Eosinophilic synovitis associated with Charcot-Leyden crystals on wet synovial fluid preparations has been recently documented in seven patients with a history of allergic reactions and dermatographism.[26–28] These patients developed painless monoarthritis after minor trauma without concurrent allergic symptoms. Joint swelling was seen in the knee of seven patients and in the first metatarsophalangeal joint of another patient. Each episode subsided within 1 to 2 weeks without therapy; three patients had recurrent episodes. Synovial fluid was mildly inflammatory, with leukocyte counts of 10,850 ± 3,665/μL and up to 46% eosinophils. Charcot-Leyden crystals were seen inside cells on wet preparations. The in vitro formation of these crystals was facilitated by slight pressure on the coverslip and by overnight incubation at 4° C. It has been suggested that Charcot-Leyden crystals may be repository of human lysophospholipase by generating lysophospholipids and therefore possess a biologic function more significant than being solely a hallmark of an eosinophilic inflammatory process.[28,181]

ALUMINUM

In hemodialyzed patients, aluminum intoxication has been associated with a mineralization defect of bone matrix, resulting in osteomalacia, bone pain, and fractures.[37] Transmission electron microscopy and x-ray elemental microdispersive analysis have shown amorphous deposits of aluminum phosphate in mitochondria of bone cells and extracellular hexagonal crystals measuring 200 to 1000 Å at the mineralization front.[37] Aluminum levels in synovial fluid synovium, and articular cartilage of patients undergoing chronic dialysis are higher than normal.[36] A high proportion of dialysis patients may also have amyloid and iron deposits in the synovium, as well as secondary hyperparathyroidism.[182,183] It has been difficult to separate such conditions from possible articular manifestations associated with intra-articular aluminum deposition.[182,183] Intra-articular injections of crystalline and amorphous aluminum phosphate in rabbits induced acute and chronic synovitis,[184,185] but these results cannot be extrapolated directly to humans.

HEMOGLOBIN CRYSTALS

Hemoglobin crystals have been described in stored normal human blood,[39] the blood of patients with sickle cell anemia,[40] and the blood of rats, and white deer.[1,14] Hemoglobin and hematoidin crystals may be found occasionally in fresh pleural and spinal fluid, in synovial fluid of patients with hemarthrosis. They have been observed in gouty synovial fluid also.[41] Rat hemoglobin crystals injected in rat skin air pouches induced mild acute inflammation.[186]

CRYSTALLOGRAPHIC FEATURES

Human hemoglobin crystals are rectangular and measure 10 to 12 μm in length and are usually found inside red cells as well as extracellularly (Fig. 110–14). They are weakly birefringent with either positive or negative elongation.[1,14] Under transmission electron microscopy, hemoglobin crystals demonstrate a well-organized pattern typical of crystalline structure.[186] Elemental analysis of such crystals shows only the presence of iron.

HEMATOIDIN CRYSTALS

Hematoidin crystals, formed as a by product of hemoglobin degradation under reduced oxygen tension, have been found in hematomas, hemarthroses, and in uterine cervix exudates.[1,14,42,187] Possible hematoidin crystals have been found in the synovial fluid of four patients with hemarthrosis[41] and one patient with sickle cell disease and septic arthritis[188] and also as artifactual crystals in bloody fluid refrigerated for several weeks.[1,187]

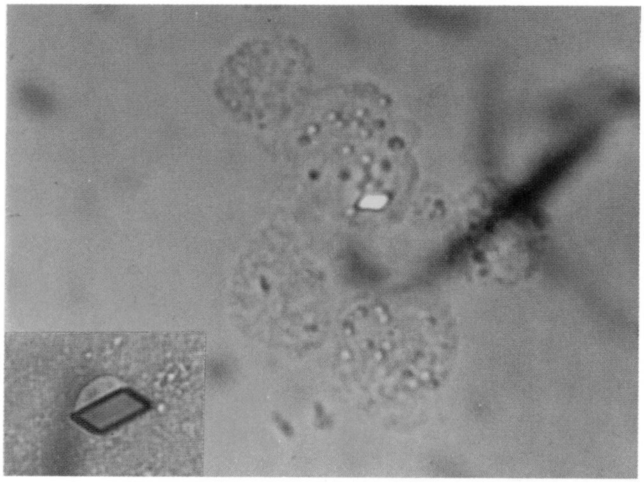

FIGURE 110–15. Rhomboid-suspected hematoidin crystal with negative elongation observed inside a macrophage-like cell. Under ordinary light, these crystals present a characteristic golden-brown color (insert). (Compensated polarized light ×600.) (From Tate, G. et al.[41])

CRYSTALLOGRAPHIC FEATURES

Hematoidin-like crystals described in synovial fluid are rhomboid, measure 8 to 10 μm in length and are bright gold or brown under ordinary light (Fig. 110–15). In other cytologic preparations, they may resemble needles forming cockleburr arrays of various sizes, ranging from 2 to 25 μm but occasionally reaching 100 μm. Under compensated polarized light they show intense birefringence with positive and negative elongation[1,187,188] (Fig. 110–15).

The role of these hemoglobin-derived crystals in inducing articular inflammation is uncertain, but knowledge of their presence in synovial fluid is important to avoid confusion with CPPD or other pathologic crystals.[1]

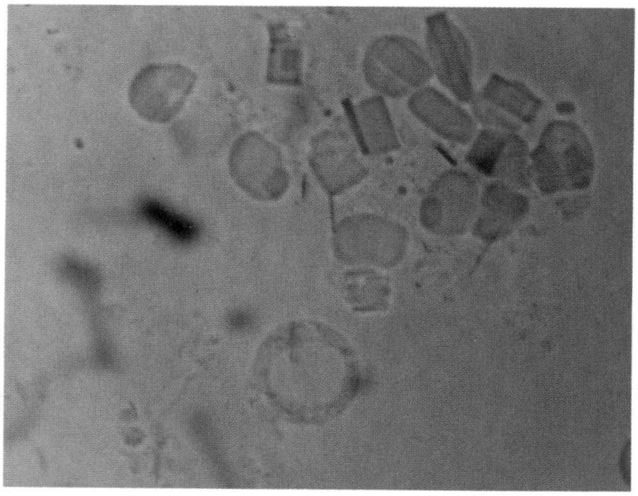

FIGURE 110–14. Weakly birefringent rectangular hemoglobin crystals and characteristic monosodium urate crystals in a patient with gout and bloody effusion. (Compensated polarized light ×400.) (From Tate, G., et al.[41])

FOREIGN-BODY SYNOVITIS

The introduction of hard penetrating particles into joints, tendon sheaths, and periarticular soft tissues, by causing infection or sterile inflammatory foreign-body reaction, can induce monoarticular synovitis, tenosynovitis, or cellulitis.[60,61,189] Those materials most commonly described with foreign-body synovitis include different vegetable particles such as plant thorns[60,61,189] and wood splinters,[61] which easily break inside the joint cavity (Table 110–3). Less often, sea urchin spines,[60,61] fish bone fragments,[61] chitin spine,[61,191] stones, gravel, and brick fragments,[190] plastic,[192] sea mouse spine[191] rubber,[190] fiberglass,[193] and glass[190] can also be introduced into joints. Similar chronic granulomatous reaction of synovium can be induced by wear particles from articular implants such as metals,[194] silicones,[195] polyethylene,[63,196] and methylmethacrylate.[196] Bullet fragments, when lodged inside major joints, may induce mild synovitis and cause systemic manifestations of lead toxicity.[197] High-pressure injection injury of fingers with paint or grease guns usually induces a delayed necrotizing dactylitis, which requires immediate emergency surgical drainage and debridement.[198]

TABLE 110–3. PARTICLES ASSOCIATED WITH FOREIGN-BODY SYNOVITIS

Vegetal	
	Plant thorns
	Date and sentinel plants
	Blackthorn bushes
	Roses, yuccas, hawthorns
	Mesquites, bougainvilles
	Ulex europeus (Tojo)
	Wood splinters
	Starch
Marine	
	Sea urchin spines
	Chitin spines (crab, seamouse)
	Fish bone
Minerals	
	Stone, gravel, silica
	Brick fragments
Metals	
	Vitalium
	Stainless steel
	Lead
Miscellaneous	
	Silicone
	Glass
	Fiberglass
	Polyethylene
	Methylmethacrylate
	Plastic
	Rubber

CLINICAL FEATURES

Clinical presentation of foreign-body synovitis is characterized by the sudden onset of pain at the site of the injury. Acute synovitis usually appears several days after the injury. Inflammation at the site of the penetrating injury may subside completely or become chronic with a steady or relapsing clinical course.[60,61,189] Frequently, the initial injury is forgotten by the patient or overlooked by the examiner. Joints most commonly involved are those of the hands and knees. Joint involvement is characterized by a variable degree of periarticular tender swelling and synovial thickening of small joints (Fig. 110–16), while larger joints may have large and persistent joint effusions. Fever, myalgias, lymph node enlargement, and synovitis of other noninjured joints have been observed in patients with sea urchin synovitis and subcutaneous silicone implants used for facial, breast, and small joint reconstruction.[60,61,199,200] In patients with high-pressure injection injury, the only initial clinical finding may be a painless puncture wound in the finger tip. After a few hours, however, signs of rapidly necrotizing dactylitis become apparent.[198]

Diving and other marine recreational activities, farming, and gardening are well-recognized risk factors.[61,191] Intravenous drug abuse also may be a possible risk factor.[61,201–203] Foreign-body synovitis must be differentiated from other conditions associated with acute, recurrent, or chronic monoarticular synovitis such as infectious arthritis, gout, pseudogout, and monoarticular juvenile RA,[201] or different causes of dactylitis.[61] These conditions include typical and atypical mycobacterial infections (tuberculous dactylitis or spina ventosa), erysipeloid, seal finger, sarcoidosis, psoriasis, tophaceous gout, and giant cell tumor of finger flexor tendon sheaths.

LABORATORY FINDINGS

White blood cell count and erythrocyte sedimentation rate are usually normal.[61] Synovial fluid can be cloudy or bloody; in those patients with detritic synovitis resulting from loose joint prostheses, it may be brownish and contain abundant debris.[1,194] Synovial fluid leukocyte counts range from 10,000 to 60,000/μL, with predominance of neutrophils.[61,201] Low-grade chronic infection is commonly seen in detritic synovitis associated with loose prostheses[63,194] Fresh preparation of synovial fluid may reveal birefringent fragments of plant thorns, polyethylene, or polymethylmethacrylate,[61,63] or nonbirefringent particles such as needle-shape fiberglass and metallic particles.[193,194] Metallic particles appear as black rods or dots.[194]

RADIOGRAPHIC FEATURES

Radiographs are useful to detect radiodense particles of metals, fish bones, and sea urchin spines, but wood, plastic, and plant thorn particles are usually missed. Radiographs may reveal soft tissue swelling only, when obtained early. In patients with a chronic or relapsing

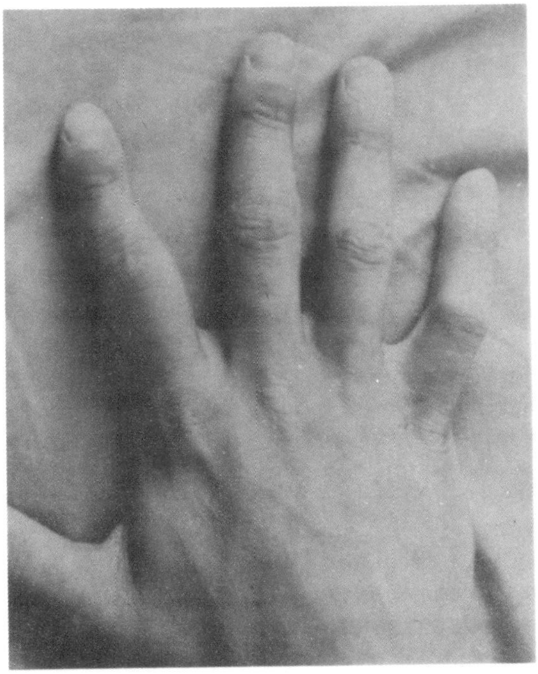

FIGURE 110–16. Dactylitis of index finger and proximal interphalangeal joint synovitis due to plant thorn. (Courtesy of Dr. J.L. Ferreiro.)

course, however, periarticular demineralization, areas of localized osteolysis, osteosclerosis, and periosteal new bone formation can be seen[61,189] (Fig. 110–17). These changes may mimic those of osteomyelitis or primary bone tumors.[61,203] Ultrasonography,[204] computed tomography (CT)[205,206] and nuclear magnetic resonance imaging[206] may be helpful in detecting small pieces of nonmetallic, wood, or plastic foreign bodies when radiographs are unrevealing.

PATHOLOGIC FEATURES

Excisional biopsy and bacteriologic studies of synovium, synovial fluid, and periarticular tissues are usually required for diagnosis and successful management of those with a chronic or relapsing course.[61,189,207] Synovium usually reveals synovial cell proliferation and diffuse infiltrates of lymphocytes and plasma cells with focal collections of PMN cells. Giant cell formation in synovium is usually striking in those patients in whom foreign bodies are found inside the joint, but it can be minimal or absent in patients in whom foreign particles are located in periarticular tissues or skin[61,201] (Fig. 110–18). Granulomas identical to those seen in sarcoidosis have been found in association with sea urchin synovitis.[61,208] Polarized light microscopy is useful in detecting birefringent fragments of plant thorn,[1,61] polyethylene, polymethylmethacrylate, and sea urchin spines (calcium carbonate crystals).[61] Elemental dispersive microprobe analysis may allow exact identification of metal particles, silica, silicon, and fiberglass.[1,193,207]

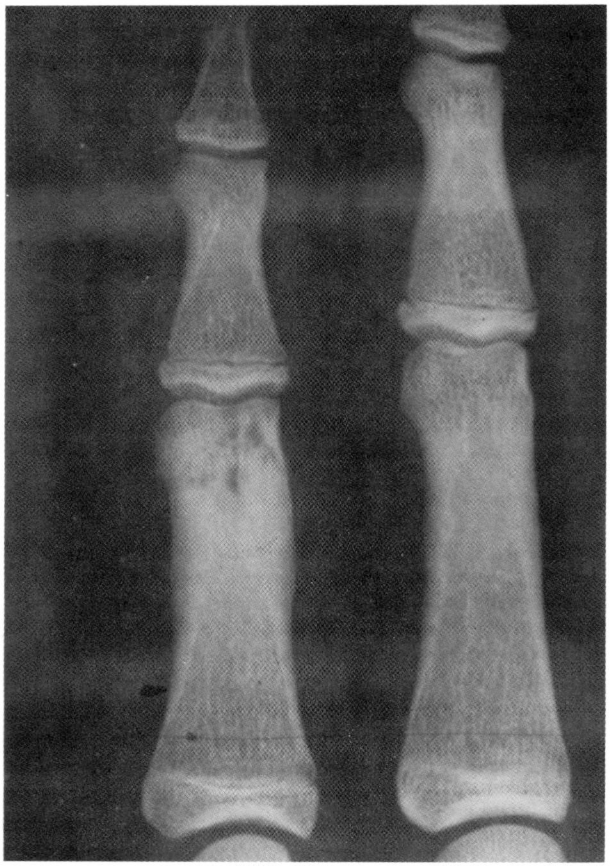

FIGURE 110–17. Plant thorn synovitis with localized area of osteolysis, osteosclerosis, and periosteal new bone formation. (Courtesy of Dr. J.L. Ferreiro.)

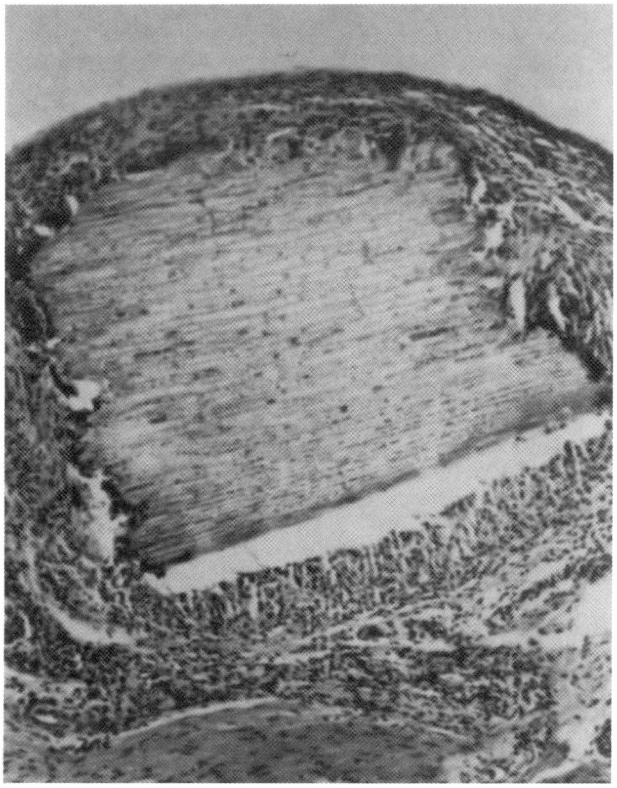

FIGURE 110–18. Foreign-body synovitis. Characteristic plant thorn fragment surrounded by mononuclear and giant cells. (Hematoxylin and eosin stain ×150.) (Courtesy of Dr. J.L. Ferreiro.)

MECHANISM OF INFLAMMATION

Mechanisms mediating foreign-body synovitis are not well understood, but several have been postulated: associated low-grade infection, presence of toxins, alkaloid, mitogens, or other proteins on the surface of foreign bodies, as well as crystalline or paracrystalline structures with a negative surface charge.[192,208] Few experimental studies of foreign-body effects on synovium and skin of animals and humans have been performed.[192,209] In one study, minimal acute flammation was induced by the injection of sterilized ground plant thorns or sea urchin spines into rabbit knees and the rat skin air pouch model of synovium,[209] but 1 to 4 weeks later, both synovium and skin showed prominent chronic inflammation with lymphocytes, plasma cells, and giant cells. Dieppe injected plant thorns into rat paws and human forearm skin, and correlated the intensity of the inflammatory reaction with the surface charge of the thorns.[192]

MANAGEMENT

In about one third of patients with foreign-body synovitis caused by exogenous particles, the inflammatory changes subside spontaneously. The remaining patients with a chronic or relapsing course usually require an excisional biopsy with synovectomy and articular lavage.[61,189,208] Occasionally, recurrent joint swelling with periosteal new bone formation can be seen after removal of the foreign body and synovectomy.

Arthroscopy has been performed in few patients with knee foreign-body synovitis but has failed to reveal suspected foreign bodies by direct visualization or by histologic studies of the small amount of synovium obtained.[61]

REFERENCES

1. Schumacher, H.R., and Reginato, A.J.: Atlas of Synovial Fluid and Crystal Analysis. 1st Ed. Philadelphia, Lea & Febiger, 1991.
2. Chisholm, G.D., and Heard, B.E.: Oxalosis. Br. J. Surg., *50*:78–92, 1962.
3. Kinnett, J.G., and Bullough, P.G.: Identification of calcium oxalate deposits in bone by electron diffraction. Arch. Pathol. Lab. Med., *100*:656, 1976.
4. Schmidt, K.L., Leber, H.W., and Schutterle, G.: Arthropathies bei primarer Oxalose-Kristallsynovitis oder Osteopathie? Dtsch. Med. Wochenschr., *106*:19–22, 1981.
5. Hoffman, G.S. et al.: Calcium oxalate micro-crystalline-associated arthritis in end stage renal disease. Ann. Intern. Med., 97:36–42, 1982.
6. Reginato, A.J. et al.: Arthropathy and cutaneous calcinosis in hemodialysis oxalosis. Arthritis Rheum., *29*:1387–1396, 1986.
7. Benhamou, C.L. et al.: Arthropathie microcristalline a oxalate de calcium au cours d'une oxalose primitive. Rev. Rhum. Med. Osteoartic., *52*:267–270, 1985.
8. Schumacher, H.R., Reginato, A.J., and Pullman, S.: Synovial fluid oxalate deposition complicating rheumatoid arthritis with amyloidosis and renal failure: Demonstration of intracellular oxalate crystals. J. Rheumatol., *14*:361–366, 1987.
9. Eade, A.W.T., Swannell, A.J., and Williamson, N.: Pyrophosphate arthropathy in hypophosphatasia. Ann. Rheum. Dis., *40*:164–170, 1981.
10. Simkin, P.A.: Articular oxalate crystals and the taxonomy of gout. JAMA, *260*:1285–1286, 1988.
11. Rosenthal, A., Ryan, L.M., and McCarty, D.J.: Arthritis associated with calcium oxalate crystals in an anephritic patient treated with peritoneal dialysis. JAMA, *260*:1290–1292, 1988.
12. Verbruggen, L.A., Bourgain, C., and Verbeelen, D.: Late presentation and microcrystalline arthropathy in primary hyperoxaluria. Clin. Exp. Rheumatol., *7*:631–633, 1989.
13. Coral, A., van Holsbeeck, M., and Hegg, C.: Secondary oxalosis complicating chronic renal failure (oxalate gout). Skel. Radiol., *19*:147–149, 1990.
14. Reginato, A.J., and Kurnik, B.: Calcium oxalate and other crystals associated with kidney disease and arthritis. Semin. Arthritis Rheum., *18*:198–224, 1989.
15. Ettlinger, E., and Hunder, G.G.: Synovial effusions containing cholesterol crystals. Report of 12 patients and review. Mayo Clin. Proc., *54*:366–374, 1979.
16. Bland, J.H., Gierthy, J.F., and Suhre, E.D.: Cholesterol in connective tissue of joints. Scand. J. Rheumatol., *3*:199–203, 1974.
17. Zuckner, J., Uddin, J., Gantner, G.E., and Dorner, R.W.: Cholesterol crystals in synovial fluid. Ann. Intern. Med., *60*:436–446, 1964.
18. Weinstein, J.: Synovial fluid leukocytosis associated with intracellular lipid inclusions. Arch. Intern. Med., *140*:560–561, 1980.
19. Reginato, A.J., Schumacher, H.R., Allan, D.A., and Rabinowitz, J.: Acute monoarthritis associated with lipid liquid crystals. Ann. Rheum. Dis., *44*:537–643, 1985.
20. Trostle, D.C., Schumacher, H.R., Medsger, T.A., and Kapoor, W.N.: Microspherule associated acute monoarticular arthritis. Arthritis Rheum., *29*:1166–1168, 1986.
21. Schlesinger, P.A., Stillman, M.T., and Peterson, L.: Polyarthritis with birefringent lipid within synovial fluid macrophages: Case report and ultrastructural study. Arthritis Rheum., *25*: 1365–1368, 1982.
22. Gardner, G.C., and Terkeltaub, R.A.: Acute monoarthritis associated with intracellular positively birefringent Maltese cross appearing spherules. J. Rheumatol., *16*:294–396, 1989.
23. Langlands, D.R. et al.: Arthritis associated with crystallizing cryoprecipitable IG paraprotein. Am. J. Med., *68*:461–465, 1980.
24. Dornan, T.L. et al.: Widespread crystallization of paraprotein in myelomatosis. Q. J. Med., *222*:659–667, 1985.
25. Stone, C. et al.: A vasculopathy with deposition of lambda light chain crystals. Ann. Intern. Med., *110*:275–276, 1989.
26. Menard, H.A., de Medicis, R., Lussier, A., and Brown, J.: Charcot-Leyden crystals in synovial fluid. (Letter.) Arthritis Rheum., *24*:1591–1593, 1981.
27. Dougados, M., Benhamod, L., and Amor, B.: Charcot-Leyden crystals in synovial fluid. Arthritis Rheum., *26*:1416, 1983.
28. Brown, J.P., Rola-Pleszcynski, M., and Menard, H.A.: Eosinophilic synovitis: Clinical observations on a newly recognized subset of patients with dermatographism. Arthritis Rheum., *29*:1147–1151, 1986.
29. Honsoon, P., Burton, T.J., and Van der Bel-Kahn, J.M.: Circulating Charcot-Leyden crystals in hypereosinophilic syndrome. Am. J. Clin. Pathol., *75*:236–242, 1981.
30. Kahn, C.B., Hollander, J.L., and Schumacher, H.R.: Corticosteroid crystals in synovial fluid. JAMA, *221*:807–809, 1970.
31. Stephan, J., Pitrova, S., and Pazderka, V.: Cystinosis with crystal-induced synovitis and arthropathy. Z. Rheumatol., *35*: 347–355, 1976.
32. Antoci, B., and Gherlinzoni, G.: Cystinosis of bone. Ital. J. Orthop. Traumatol., *1*:81–97, 1975.
33. Berman, L., and Salomon, L.: Xanthine gout, crystal deposition in skeletal muscle in a case of xanthinuria. Rheumatologie, *5*:253–256, 1975.
34. Isaacs, A., Heffron, I.H., and Berman, L.: Xanthine, hypoxanthine and muscle pain: Histochemical and biochemical observations. S. Afr. Med. J., *49*:1035–1038, 1975.
35. Chalmers, R.A., Watts, R.W.E., Bitenski, L., and Chayen, J.: Microscopic studies on crystals in skeletal muscle in two cases of xanthinuria. J. Pathol., *99*:45–65, 1969.
36. Netter, P. et al.: Aluminum in the joint tissues of chronic renal failure patients treated with regular hemodialysis and aluminum compounds. J. Rheumatol., *11*:66–70, 1984.
37. Plachot, J. et al.: Bone ultrastructure and x-rays microanalysis of aluminum-intoxicated hemodialyzed patients. Kidney Internat., *25*:796–803, 1984.
38. Netter, P.: Does aluminum have a pathogenic role in dialysis associated arthropathy? Ann. Rheum. Dis., *49*:573–575, 1990.

39. Ager, J.A.M., and Lehman, H.: Intra-erythrocytic hemoglobin crystals. J. Clin. Pathol., *10*:336–340, 1957.
40. Bessis, M., Normarski, G., Thiery, J.P., and Breton-Gorius, J.: Etudes sur la falciformation des globules rougess au microscope polarizant et au microscope electronique. II. L'interiur du globule: Comparison avec les cristaux intra-globulaires. Rev. Hemat., *13*:249–260, 1958.
41. Tate, G., Schumacher, H.R., Reginato, A.J., and Algeo, S.: Synovial fluid crystals derived from hemoglobin crystals. J. Rheumatol., (in press), 1991.
42. Zahaopoulos, P., Wong, J.Y., and Keagy, N.: Hematoidin crystals in cervicovaginal smears. Report of two cases. Acta Cytol., *29*:1029–1034, 1985.
43. Marwaha, N. et al.: Bilirubin crystal in peripheral blood smears from neonates with unconjugated hyperbilirubinemia. Med. Lab. Sci., *47*:278–281, 1990.
44. Sengupta, P.C. et al.: The bilirubin crystals in neutrophils of jaundiced neonates and infants. Acta Hematol., *70*:69–70, 1983.
45. Sussuki, T., Sugawara, Y., Sdatoh, Y., and Shikama, K.: Human oxymyoglobin: Isolation and characterization. J. Chromatogr., *195*:227–280, 1980.
46. Waldo, E.D., and Tobias, H.: Needle-like cytoplasmic inclusions in the liver in porphyria cutanea tarda. Arch. Pathol., *96*:368–371, 1973.
47. Thomas, K., and Hut, M.S.R.: Tyrosine crystals in salivary gland tumor. J. Clin. Pathol., *96*:368–371, 1983.
48. Campbell, W.G., Priest, R.E., and Weathers, D.R.: Characterization of two types of crystalloids in pleomorphic adenomas of minor salivary glands. A light microscopic, electron microscopic, and histochemical study. Am. J. Pathol., *118*:194–202, 1985.
49. McLeod, P., Mackenzie, S., and Scriver, C.R.: Partial ornithine carbamyl transferase deficiency: An inborn error of the urea cycle presenting as orotic aciduria in a male infant. Can. Med. Assoc. J., *107*:405–408, 1972.
50. Tischler, A.S., and Compagno, J.: Crystal-like deposits of amyloid in pancreatic islet cell tumors. Arch. Pathol. Lab. Med., *103*:247–251, 1979.
51. Ordonez, N.G., Manning, J.T., and Mackay, B.: Crystals and alpha 1-antitrypsin-reactive globoid inclusions in an islet cell tumor of the pancreas. Ultrastruct. Pathol., *8*:319–338, 1985.
52. Machinami, R., and Kikuchi, F.: Adenosine triphosphatase activity of crystalline inclusions in alveolar soft part sarcoma. An ultrahistochemical study of a case. Pathol. Res. Pract., *181*: 357–361, 1986.
53. Nesland, J.M., Langholm, R., and Marton, P.F.: Hexagonal crystals in the bone marrow in patients with myeloproliferative disease and preleukemia. Scand. J. Hematol., *32*:552–558, 1984.
54. Staven, P., and Bjorneklett, A.: A light green crystal in May-Grunwald and Giemsa-stained bone marrow macrophages in patients with myeloid leukemia. Scand. J. Haematol., *18*: 67–72, 1977.
55. Nagano, T., and Ohtsuki, I.: Reinvestigation of the fine structure of Reinke's crystals in human testicular interstitial cell. J. Cell. Biol., *51*:148–161, 1971.
56. Adams, P.C. et al.: Amiodarone pulmonary toxicity: Clinical and subclinical features. Q. J. Med., *229*:440–441, 1986.
57. Lullman, H., Lullman-Rauch, R., and Wasserman, O.: Drug induced phospholipidoses. CRC Crit. Rev. Toxicol., *4*:185–218, 1975.
58. Watts, R.W.E. et al.: Microscopic studies on skeletal muscle in gout patients treated with allopurinol. Q. J. Med., *157*:1–14, 1971.
59. Peterslund, N.A., Larsen, M.L., and Mygind, H.: Acyclovir crystalluria. Scand. J. Infect. Dis., *22*:225–228, 1988.
60. Cracchiolo, A., and Goldberg, L.: Local and systemic reactions to puncture injuries by the sea urchin spine and the date palm thorn. Arthritis Rheum., *20*:1206–1212, 1977.
61. Reginato, A.J. et al.: Clinical and pathologic studies of twenty-six patients with penetrating foreign body injury to the joints, bursae, and tendon sheaths. Arthritis Rheum., *33*:1753–1762, 1990.
62. Henderson, W.J. et al.: Identification of talc on surgeons gloves and in tissue from starch granulomas. Br. J. Surg., *62*:941–944, 1975.
63. Crugnola, A., Schiller, A., and Radin, E.: Polymeric debris in synovium after total joint replacement. Histological identification. J. Bone Joint Surg., *59A*:860–862, 1977.
64. Blackburn, W.E. et al.: Severe vascular complications in oxalosis after bilateral nephrectomy. Ann. Intern. Med., *82*:44–46, 1975.
65. Arbus, G.S., and Sniderman, S.: Oxalosis with peripheral gangrene. Arch. Pathol., *97*:107–110, 1974.
66. Lewis, R.D., Lowenstam, H.A., and Rossman, G.R.: Oxalate nephrosis and crystalline myocarditis. Case report with postmortem and crystallographic studies. Arch. Pathol. Lab. Med., *98*: 149–155, 1974.
67. West, R.R., Salyer, W.R., and Hutchins, G.M.: Adult onset primary oxalosis with complete heart block. Johns Hopkins Med. J. *133*:195–200, 1973.
68. Moorhead, P.J., Cooper, D.J., and Timperley, W.R.: Progressive peripheral neuropathy in a patient with primary hyperoxaluria. Br. Med. J., *2*:312–313, 1975.
69. McKenna, R.W., and Dehner, L.P.: Oxalosis: An unusual cause of myelophthisis in childhood. Am. J. Clin. Pathol., *66*: 991–997, 1976.
70. Hricik, D.E., and Hussain, R.: Pancytopenia and hepatosplenomegaly in oxalosis. Arch. Intern. Med., *144*:167–168, 1984.
71. Williams, H.E., and Smith, L.H.: Disorders of oxalate metabolism. Am. J. Med., *45*:715–735, 1968.
72. Hillman, R.E.: Primary hyperoxaluria. *In* The Metabolic Basis of Inherited Diseases: Primary Hyperoxalurias. Edited by C. R. Scriver. 6th Ed. New York, McGraw-Hill, 1989, pp. 933–944.
73. Earnest, D.L.: Enteric hyperoxaluria. Adv. Intern. Med., *24*:407–427, 1979.
74. Pru, C., Eaton, J.R., and Kjellstrand, C.: Vitamin C intoxication and hyperoxalemia in chronic hemodialysis patients. Nephron, *39*:112–116, 1985.
75. Louthrenco, W. et al.: Localized peripheral calcium oxalate crystal deposition caused by Aspergillus niger infection. J. Rheumatol., *17*:407–412, 1990.
76. Nime, F.A., and Hutchins, G.M.: Oxalosis caused by Aspergillus infection. Johns Hopkins Med. J., *133*:183–184, 1973.
77. Worcester, E.M., Nakagawa, Y., Bushinsky, D.A., and Coe, F.L.: Evidence that serum calcium oxalate supersaturation is a consequence of oxalate retention in patients with chronic renal failure. J. Clin. Invest., *77*:1888–1896, 1986.
78. Weber, D.V. et al.: Urinary saturation measurements in calcium nephrolithiasis. Ann. Intern. Med., *90*:180–184, 1979.
79. Hautman, R.A. et al.: Intrarenal distribution of oxalic acid, calcium, sodium, and potassium in man. Eur. J. Clin. Invest., *10*:173–176, 1980.
80. Cogan, D.G. et al.: Calcium oxalate and calcium phosphate crystals in detached retinas. Arch. Ophthalmol., *60*:366–371, 1958.
81. Dunn, H.G.: Oxalosis. Am. J. Dis. Child., *90*:58–80, 1955.
82. Hockaday, T.D.R., Clayton, J.E., Frederick, E.W., and Smith, L.H.: Primary hyperoxaluria. Medicine, *43*:315–345, 1964.
83. Danpure, C.J., Jennings, P.R., and Watts, R.W.E.: Enzymological diagnosis of primary hyperoxaluria by measurement of hepatic alanine: Glyoxylate aminotransferase activity. Lancet, *1*:289–293, 1987.

84. Wander, R.J.A. et al.: Alanine-glyoxylate aminotransferase and the urinary excretion of oxalate and glycolate in hyperoxaluria type 1 and the Zellweger syndrome. Clin. Chim. Acta, *165*: 229–311, 1987.
85. Wise, P.J., Dampure, C.J., and Jennings, P.R.: Immunological heterogeneity of hepatic alanine-glyoxylate aminotransferase in primary hyperoxaluria type 1. FEBS Lett., *222*:17–20, 1987.
86. Williams, H.E., and Smith, L.H., Jr.: L-Glyceric aciduria, a new genetic variant of primary oxaluria. N. Engl. J. Med., *278*: 233–239, 1968.
87. Scowen, E.F., Stansfeld, A.G., and Watts, R.W.E.: Oxalosis and primary oxaluria. J. Pathol. Bacteriol., *77*:195–205, 1959.
88. Cohen, H., and Reid, J.B.: Tenosynovitis crepitans associated with oxaluria. Liverpool Med. Chirurg. J., *43*:193–199, 1935.
89. Morris, M.C. et al.: Oxalosis in infancy. Arch. Dis. Child., *57*:224–228, 1982.
90. Nartijn, A., and Thijn, C.J.P.: Radiologic findings in primary oxaluria. Skeletal Radiol., *8*:21–24, 1982.
91. Halifa, G., Dossans, B., Gagnadoux, M.F., and Sauvegrain, J.: Aspect radiologiques de l'oxalose. J. Radiol., *60*:45–49, 1979.
92. Milgram, J.W.: Chronic renal failure. Recurrent secondary hyperparathyroidism. Multiple metaphyseal infractions, and secondary oxalosis. Bull. Hosp. Joint Dis., *35*:118–144, 1974.
93. Gherardi, G. et al.: Bone oxalosis and renal osteodystrophy. Arch. Pathol. Lab. Med., *104*:105–111, 1980.
94. Mathews, M. et al.: Bone biopsy to diagnose hyperoxaluria in patients with renal failure. Ann. Intern. Med., *90*:777–779, 1979.
95. Milgran, J.W., and Salyer, W.R.: Secondary oxalosis of bone in chronic renal failure. A histopathological study of three cases. J. Bone Joint Surg., *56*:387–395, 1974.
96. Canavese C. et al.: Primary oxalosis mimicking hyperparathyroidism diagnosed after long-term hemodialysis. Am. J. Nephrol., *10*:344–349, 1990.
97. Brady, H.R. et al.: Oxalate bone disease—An emerging form of renal osteodystrophy. Int. J. Artif. Organ., *12*:715–719, 1989.
98. Julian, B.A. et al.: Oxalosis in bone causing a radiographical mimicry of renal osteodystrophy. Am. J. Kidney Dis., *9*: 438–440, 1987.
99. Paul, H., Reginato, A.J., and Shumacher, H.R.: Alizarin red S stain as screening test to detect calcium compounds in synovial fluid. Arthritis Rheum., *26*:191–201, 1983.
100. Prioa, A.D., and Brinn, N.T.: Identification of calcium oxalate crystals using alizarin red S stain. Arch. Pathol. Lab. Med., *109*: 186–190, 1985.
101. Chaplin, A.J.: Histopathologic occurrence and characterization of calcium oxalate. A review. J. Clin. Pathol., *30*:800–811, 1977.
102. Pizzolato, P.: Histochemical recognition of calcium oxalate. J. Histochem. Cytochem., *12*:333–336, 1969.
103. Khan, S.R., Finlayson, B., and Hackett, R.: Scanning electron microscopy of calcium oxalate crystal formation in experimental nephrolithiasis. Lab. Invest., *41*:504–510, 1979.
104. Siew, S.: Investigation of crystallosis of the kidney by means of polarization, scanning transmission and high voltage electron microscopy. Isr. J. Med. Sci., *15*:698–710, 1979.
105. Faires, J.S., and McCarty, D.J., Jr.: Acute synovitis in normal joints of man and dog produced by injections of microcrystalline sodium urate, calcium oxalate and corticosteroid esters. (Abstract.) Arthritis Rheum., *5*:95, 1962.
106. Denko, C.W., and Whitehouse, M.W.: Experimental inflammation induced by naturally occurring microcrystalline calcium salts. J. Rheumatol., *3*:54–62, 1976.
107. Hasselbacher, P.: Stimulation of synovial fibroblasts by calcium oxalate and monosodium urate monohydrate. A mechanism of connective tissue degradation in oxalosis and gout. J. Lab. Clin. Med., *100*:977–981, 1982.
108. Op de Hock, C.T. et al.: Oxalosis in chronic renal failure. Proc. Eur. Dial. Transplant Assoc., *17*:730–735, 1980.
109. Zarembski, P.M., Hodgekinson, A., and Parson, F.M.: Elevation of the concentration of plasma oxalic acid in renal failure. Nature, *212*:511–512, 1966.
110. Ramsay, A.G., and Reed, R.G.: Oxalate removal by hemodialysis stage renal disease. Am. J. Kidney Dis., *4*:123–127, 1984.
111. Borland, W.W., Payton, C.D., Simpson, K., and Macdougall, A.I.: Serum oxalate in chronic renal failure. Nephron, *45*:119–121, 1987.
112. Balcke, P. et al.: Ascorbic acid aggravates secondary hyperoxalemia in patients on chronic hemodialysis. Ann. Intern. Med., *10*:344–345, 1984.
113. Fayemi, A.O., Ali, M., and Braun, E.V.: Oxalosis in hemodialysis patients: A pathologic study of 80 cases. Arch. Pathol. Lab. Med., *103*:58–62, 1977.
114. Salyer, W.R., and Keren, D.: Oxalosis as a complication of chronic renal failure. Kidney Int., *4*:61–67, 1973.
115. Sullivan, J.P., and Eisenstein, A.B.: Ascorbic acid depletion during hemodialysis. JAMA, *226*:1697–1699, 1972.
116. Ott, S.W., Andress, D.L., and Sherrard, D.J.: Bone oxalate in long term hemodialysis patients who ingested high doses of vitamin C. Am. J. Kidney Dis., *113*:450–454, 1986.
117. Abuelo, G., and Reginato, A.J.: Cutaneous and articular dialysis oxalosis. Archivos Int. Med. (In press).
118. Scheimman, J.L.: The management of primary hyperoxaluria. Kidney, *17*:13–17, 1984.
119. Watts, R.W.E. et al.: Primary hyperoxaluria (type I) attempted treatment with combined hepatic and renal transplantation. Q. J. Med., *57*:697–703, 1986.
120. Watts, R.W.E.: Studies of some possible biochemical treatments of primary hyperoxaluria. Q. J. Med., *48*:259–271, 1979.
121. Will, E.J., and Bijvoet, O.L.M.: Primary oxalosis: Clinical and biochemical response to high dose pyridoxine therapy. Metabolism., *28*:542–548, 1979.
122. Katz, A. et al.: Long-term follow up of kidney transplantation in children with oxalosis. Transplant. Proc. *21*:2033–2035, 1989.
123. Broyer, M.: Kidney transplantation in primary oxalosis from the EDTA registry. Nephrol. Dial. Transplant., *5*:332–336, 1990.
124. McDonald, J.C.: Reversal of liver transplantation of the complications of primary hyperoxaluria. N. Engl. J. Med., *321*: 1100–1103, 1989.
125. Watts, W.E. et al.: Combined hepatic and renal transplantation in primary hyperoxaluria type I: Clinical report of 9 cases. Am. J. Med., *90*:179–187, 1991.
126. Wise, C.M., White, R.E., and Agudelo, C.: Synovial fluid lipid abnormalities in various disease states; review and classification. Semin. Arthritis Rheum., *16*:222–230, 1987.
127. Kieffer, D. et al.: Manifestations articulaires ou cours des dyslipedemies. A propos de deux observations personelles. Rev. Rhum. Mal. Osteoartic., *48*:569–573, 1981.
128. Delbarre, F., Laoussadi, S., Kahan, A., and Aubony, G.: Le rhumatisme des thesaurismoses a lipides. Atteinte articulaire au cours de hyperdyslipidemie de type II. Presence de microcristaux dans les mitochondries des synoviocytes. C.R. Acad. Sci. Paris, *288*:181–184, 1979.
129. Zoppini, A., Teodori, S., and Tacari, E.: Valeur de la biopsie synoviale dans le diagnostic de arthropathies associees aux hyperlipoproteinemies. Rev. Rhum. Mal. Osteoartic., *47*:111–115, 1980.
130. Shapiro, J.R. et al.: Achilles tendinitis and tenosynovitis. A diagnostic manifestation of familial Type II hyperlipoproteinemia in children. Am. J. Dis. Child., *128*:486–490, 1974.

131. Kruth, H.S.: Lipid deposition in human tendon xanthoma. Am. J. Pathol., *121*:311–315, 1985.
132. Schumacher, H.R., and Michaelis, R.: Recurrent tendinitis and Achilles tendon nodule with positive birefringent crystals in a patient with hyperlipoproteinemia. J. Rheumatol., *16*: 1387–1389, 1989.
133. Smith, M.C., Chose, M.K., and Henry, A.R.: The clinical spectrum of renal cholesterol embolization. Am. J. Med., *11*:174–180, 1981.
134. Young, D.K., Burton, M.F., and Herman, J.: Multiple cholesterol emboli simulating systemic necrotizing vasculitis. J. Rheumatol., *13*:423–426, 1986.
135. Nye, W.H.R., Terry, R., and Rosenbaum, D.L.: Two forms of crystalline lipid in "cholesterol" effusions. Am. J. Clin. Pathol., *49*:718–728, 1968.
136. Sutor, D.J., and Gaston, P.J.: Anhydrous cholesterol: A new crystalline form in gallstones. Gut, *13*:64–65, 1972.
137. Newcombe, S.S., and Cohen, A.S. Chylous effusion in rheumatoid arthritis. Am. J. Med., *39*:134–156, 1965.
138. Fabricant, C.G., Krock, L., and Gillespe, J.H.: Virus-induced cholesterol crystals. Science, *181*:566–567, 1973.
139. Denko, C.W., Petricevic, M.: Modification of cholesterol induced inflammation. Agents Actions, *10*:353–357, 1980.
140. Pritzker, K.P.H., Fam, A.G., Omar, S.A., and Gertbein, S.D.: Experimental cholesterol crystal arthropathy. J. Rheumatol., *8*:281–290, 1981.
141. Hasselbacher, P., and Hahn, J.L.: Activation of the alternative pathway of complement by microcrystalline cholesterol. Arteriosclerosis, *37*:239–245, 1980.
142. Zimmer, J.G., Dewey, R., Waterhouse, C., and Terry, R.: The origin and nature of anisotropic urinary lipids in the nephrotic syndrome. Ann. Intern. Med., *54*:205–214, 1961.
143. Bangham, A.D.: Development of the liposome concept. *In* Liposomes in Biological Systems. Edited by G. Gregoriadis and A. C. Allison. New York, Wiley, 1980.
144. Small, D.M.: Liquid crystals in living and dying systems. J. Colloid. Interface Sci., *58*:581–602, 1977.
145. Ferguson, J.L.: Liquid crystals. Sci. Am., *211*:77–85, 1964.
146. Small, D.M., and Shipley, G.G.: Physical chemical basis of lipid deposition in atherosclerosis. Science, *175*:222–229, 1974.
147. Ratliff, N.B. et al.: Diagnosis of chloroquine cardiomyopathy by endomyocardial biopsy. N. Engl. J. Med., *316*:191–193, 1977.
148. Choi, S.J., Schumacher, H.R., Clayburne, G., and Rothfuss, M.S.: Liposome-induced synovitis in rabbits. Arthritis Rheum., *29*:889–896, 1986.
149. Roy, S., and Ghadially, F.N.: Pathology of experimental hemoarthrosis. Ann. Rheum. Dis., *26*:402–415, 1966.
150. Choi, S.J. et al.: Experimental haemarthrosis produces mild inflammation associated with intracellular Maltese crosses. Ann. Rheum. Dis., *45*:1025–1028, 1986.
151. Baldassare, J.J. et al.: Reconstitution of platelet proteins into phospholipid vesicles. Functional proteoliposomes. J. Clin Invest., *75*:35–39, 1985.
152. Sheth, K.J., and Bernhard, G.C.: The arthropathy of Fabry's disease. Arthritis Rheum., *22*:781–783, 1979.
153. Delbarre, F. et al.: Le rhumatisme des thesuriamoses a lipides. Arthropathies au cours de la carence en alpha-galactosidase A (maladie de Fabry). Etude ultrastructurale de la membrane synoviale avec mise en evidences de micro-cristaux dans les mitrochondries des synoviocytes. C.R. Acad. Sci. Paris, *288*:579–582, 1979.
154. Black, M.M.: Panniculitis. J. Cutan. Pathol., *12*:366–380, 1985.
155. Reginato, A.J. et al.: Unusual birefringent crystals in synovial fluid of patients with osteoarthritis and subchondral bone cysts and in hemarthrosis. (Abstract.) Arthritis Rheum., *29*:S15, 1986.
156. Freemon, A.J., and Denton, J.: Synovial fluid findings early in traumatic arthritis. J. Rheumatol., *15*:881–882, 1988.
157. Neuman, V.: Multiple plasma cell myeloma with crystalline deposits in the tumor cells and in the kidneys. J. Pathol. Bacteriol., *61*:165–169, 1949.
158. Stoebner, P. et al.: Ultrastructural study of human IgG–IgM crystalcryoglobulins. Am. J. Clin. Pathol., *71*:404–410, 1979.
159. Klintworth, C.K., Brodehoeft, S.J., and Reed, J.W.: Analysis of corneal crystalline deposits in multiple myeloma. Am. J. Ophthalmol., *86*:303–313, 1978.
160. An, H.S., Namey, T.C., Kim, K.: Essential cryoglobulinemia with intense and persistent synovitis of the knee. Clin. Orthop. Rel. Res., *215*:173–178, 1987.
161. Weinberger, A., Berlinger, S., and Pinkhas, J.: Articular manifestations of essential cryoglobulinemia. Semin. Arthritis Rheum., *10*:224–230, 1981.
162. Gahl, W.A. et al.: Lysosomal transport disorders. *In* The Metabolic Basis of Inherited Diseases. 6th Ed. Edited by C. R. Scriver et al. New York, McGraw-Hill, 1989, pp. 2619–2648.
163. Gahl, W.A. et al.: Defective cystine exodus from isolated lysosome-rich fractions of cystinotic leucoytes. J. Biol. Chem., *257*: 9570–9575, 1982.
164. Lietman, P.S. et al.: Adult cystinosis. A benign disorder. Am. J. Med., *40*:511–540, 1966.
165. Korn, D.: Demonstration of cystine crystals in peripheral white blood cells in patient with cystinosis. N. Engl. J. Med., *262*:545–548, 1960.
166. Koizumi, F. et al.: Cystinosis with marked atrophy of the kidney and thyroid. Histological and ultrastructure studies in an autopsy case. Acta Pathol. Jpn., *35*:145–150, 1985.
167. Gahl, W.A. et al.: Myopathy and cystine storage in muscles in a patient with nephropathic cystinosis. N. Engl. J. Med., *319*: 1461–1464, 1988.
168. Gahl, W.A. et al.: Cystinosis progress in a prototypic disease. Ann. Intern. Med., *109*:557–569, 1988.
169. Kaiser-Kupfer, M.I. et al.: A randomized placebo-controlled trial of cysteamine eye drops in nephropathiccystinosis. Arch. Opthalmol., *108*:689–693, 1990.
170. Felicitas, A. et al.: Hereditary xanthinuria. Evidence for enhanced hypoxanthine salvage. J. Clin. Invest., *79*:847–852, 1987.
171. Holmes, E.W., and Wyngaarden, J.B.: Hereditary xanthinuria. *In* The Metabolic Basis of Inherited Diseases. 6th Ed. Edited by C. R. Scriver et al. New York, McGraw-Hill, 1989, pp. 1085–1094.
172. Delbarre, F. et al.: Acces de goutte chez un xanthinurique. Nouv. Presse Med., *2*:2465–2466, 1973.
173. Bradford, M.J. et al.: Study of purine metabolism in a xanthinuric female. J. Clin. Invest., *47*:1325–1332, 1968.
174. Greene, M.L., Fujimoto, W.Y., and Seegmiller, J.E.: Urinary xanthine stones. A rare complication of allopurinol therapy. N. Engl. J. Med., *280*:426–428, 1969.
175. Band, P.R. et al.: Xanthine nephropathy in a patient with lymphosarcoma treated with allopurinol. N. Engl. J. Med., *283*:354–360, 1970.
176. Thompson, J.H., and Paddock, F.K.: The significance of Charcot-Leyden crystals. N. Engl. J. Med., *223*:936–939, 1940.
177. Weller, P.F., Bach, D., and Austen, K.F.: Human eosinophil lysophospholipase: The sole protein component of Charcot-Leyden crystals. J. Immunol., *128*:1346–1349, 1982.
178. Weller, P.F., Goetzl, E.J., and Austen, K.F.: Identification of human eosinophil lysophospholipase as the constituent of Charcot-Leyden crystals. Proc. Natl. Acad. Sci. USA, *77*: 7440–7448, 1980.
179. Dawes, C.J., and Williams, W.L.: Histochemical studies of Charcot-Leyden crystals. Anat. Rec., *116*:53–71, 1953.

180. Welsh, R.A.: The genesis of the Charcot-Leyden crystal in the eosinophilic leukocyte of man. Am. J. Pathol., *35*:1091–1103, 1959.
181. Samter, M.: Charcot-Leyden crystals: A study of the conditions necessary for their formation. Allergy, *18*:221–230, 1947.
182. Benhamou, C.L. et al.: Arthropathies des membres chez les insuffisants renaux dialyses. Presse Med., *16*:119–122, 1987.
183. Cary, N.R.B. et al.: Dialysis arthropathy: amyloid or iron? Br. Med. J., *293*:1392–1394, 1986.
184. Netter, P. et al.: Inflammatory effect of aluminum phosphate. Ann. Rheum. Dis., *42*:114, 1983.
185. Royer, D. et al.: Inflammatory effect of aluminum phosphate on rat paws. Pathol. Biol., *30*:211–215, 1982.
186. Tate, G. et al.: Inflammation following blood injection into synovial-like spaces is result of the cellular component rather than the plasma. J. Rheumatol., *15*:1686–1692, 1988.
187. Kerolus, G., Clayburne, G., and Schumacher, H.R.: It is mandatory to examine synovial fluid promptly after arthrocentesis. Arthritis Rheum., *37*:271–275, 1989.
188. Pappu, R., Reginato, A.J.: Hematoidin-like crystals in the synovial fluid of a patient with sickle cell and septic polyarthritis. Manuscript submitted to J. Rheumatol.
189. Kelly, J.J.: Blackthorn inflammation. J. Bone Joint Surg., *48B*:474–478, 1966.
190. Goodnough, C.P., and Frymore, J.W.: Synovitis secondary to non-metallic foreign bodies. J. Trauma, *15*:960–969, 1975.
191. Wilson, G.E. et al.: Severe granulomatous arthritis due to spinous injury by a "sea mouse" annelid worm. J. Clin. Pathol., *43*:291–294, 1990.
192. Dieppe, P.: Miscellaneous crystals and particles. *In* Crystals and Joint Disease. Edited by P. Calvert. London, Chapman and Hall, 1983.
193. Cleland, I.G., Vernon-Roberts, B., and Smith, K.: Fibre-glass induced synovitis. Ann. Rheum. Dis., *43*:530–534, 1984.
194. Kitridou, R.C., Schumacher, H.R., Sbarbaro, J.L., and Hollander, J.L.: Recurrent hemarthrosis after prosthetic knee arthroplasty: Identification of metal particles in the synovial fluid. Arthritis Rheum., *12*:520–523, 1969.
195. Rosenthal, D.F., Rosenberg, A.E., Schiller, A.L., and Smith, R.J.: Destructive arthritis due to silicone: A foreign body reaction. Radiology, *149*:69–72, 1983.
196. Kaufman, R.L., Tong, I., and Beardmore, T.D.: Prosthetic synovitis: Clinical and histologic characteristics. J. Rhematol., *12*:1066–1074, 1985.
197. Windler, E.C., Smith, R.B., Bryan, W.J., and Woods, G.W.: Lead intoxication and traumatic arthritis of hip secondary to retained bullet fragments. A case report. J. Bone Joint Surg., *60A*:254–255, 1978.
198. Conolly, W.B.: Color atlas of hand conditions. High pressure injection injury. 1st Ed. Chicago, Year Book Medical Publishers, 1980.
199. Christie, A.J., Weinberger, K.A., and Dietrich, M.: Silicone lymphadenopathy and synovitis. Complications of silicone elastomer finger joint prosthesis. JAMA, *237*:1463–1464, 1977.
200. Kumagai, Y., Shiokawa, Y., Medsger, T.A., and Rodnan, G.P.: Clinical spectrum of connective tissue disease after cosmetic surgery. Observation on eighteen patients and a review of the Japanese literature. Arthritis Rheum., *27*:1–12, 1984.
201. O'Connor, C.R., Reginato, A.J., and DeLong, W.: Foreign body reaction simulating acute septic arthritis. (Submitted for publication.)
202. Kiburz, D.: Intra-articular drug abuse. J. Bone Joint Surg., *66A*:1469–1470, 1984.
203. Maylahn, D.J.: Thorn-induced "tumors" of bone. J. Bone Joint Surg., *34A*:386–389, 1952.
204. Little, C.L. et al.: The ultrasonic detection of soft tissue foreign bodies. Invest. Radiol., *21*:275–277, 1986.
205. Bauer, A.R., and Yutani, D.: Computed tomography localization of wooden foreign bodies in children's extremities. Arch. Surg., *118*:1084–1086, 1983.
206. Russel, R.C. et al.: Detection of foreign body in the hand. J. Hand Surg. [Am], *16A*:2–11, 1991.
207. Lazaro, M.A. et al.: Lymphadenopathy secondary to silicone hand joint prosthesis. Clin. Exp. Rheumatol., *8*:17–22, 1990.
208. Sugarman, M. et al.: Plant thorn synovitis. Arthritis Rheum., *20*:1125–1128, 1977.
209. Kinmont, P.D.C.: Sea urchin sarcoidal granulomas. Br. J. Dermatol., *77*:336–343, 1965.
210. Reginato, A.J., Ferreiro, S.J.L., Clayburne, G., and Sieck, M.: Experimentally induced foreign body synovitis. Light and transmission electron microscopic studies. Arthritis Rheum., *31*:R3, 1988.

111

Metabolic Diseases of Muscle

ROBERT L. WORTMANN

A wide variety of conditions can be classified as metabolic diseases of muscle. These have in common an underlying abnormality in muscle glycogen, lipid, or adenosine triphosphate (ATP) metabolism. The study of metabolic muscle disease is relatively new. Myophosphorylase deficiency, the first described metabolic myopathy, was predicted in 1951[1] and the biochemical defect identified in 1959.[2] Subsequently, additional defects of glycogen metabolism and disorders of lipid and purine metabolism in muscle have been recognized. Other metabolic diseases of muscle assuredly await discovery. Clinically, these conditions must be considered in the differential diagnosis of individuals with proximal muscle weakness, myoglobinuria, or exercise intolerance as a result of fatigue, myalgias, or cramps. The evaluation of such patients requires an awareness of potential diagnoses, an understanding of energetics in normal muscle, and an acceptance that much remains to be learned about this general area before successful therapies will be available.

SKELETAL MUSCLE FIBERS

Skeletal muscle contains multinucleated cells called *fibers* (Fig. 111–1), functionally grouped in *motor units*. A motor unit is composed of all the fibers innervated by an individual *motor neuron*. The fibers within each motor unit have common histochemical and electrophysiologic properties and can be classified based on those characteristics (Table 111–1). Type 1 (red) fibers respond to stimulation slowly but are relatively resistant to fatigue. They are rich in lipids, mitochondria, and oxidative enzymes. In contrast, type 2B (white) fibers respond to stimulation briskly, with greater force, but fatigue rapidly. Their glycogen content and myophosphorylase activity are greater. The properties of type 2A fibers share some properties with each of the other types and respond to stimulation in an intermediate fashion. Individual human muscles are composed of mixtures of all fiber types.

CONTRACTION AND RELAXATION

Muscular activity can be initiated by electric, chemical, and mechanical stimulation to produce an *action potential* transmitted along the cell membrane. An action potential moves down the motor neuron to the *presynaptic nerve terminal*, where depolarization causes the release of acetylcholine, which diffuses to the postsynaptic membrane on a muscle cell and binds to specific receptors. Such binding causes conformational changes, opening channels permeable to sodium and potassium. As a consequence, sodium moves into the cell and potassium moves out, depolarizing the muscle fiber and generating a signal called an *end plate potential*. As the wave of depolarization spreads, the resting state of the membrane is restored and maintained, in part by an active sodiumpotassium exchanger (Na-K-dependent ATPase). The wave of depolarization spreads from the membrane to the interior of the muscle fiber through the system of T tubules, connecting the cell surface with the sarcoplasmic reticulum (Fig. 111–1). When the signal reaches the sarcoplasmic reticulum, calcium is released from the lateral sacs to diffuse among the fibrils, initiating *contraction*.

Contraction in muscle occurs as a consequence of a magnesium-dependent actomyosin ATPase. The activity of that enzyme results in the formation of *cross bridges between actin and myosin* and the *sliding of filaments*. At rest, actomyosin ATPase is inhibited and there are no cross bridges between the thick filaments (myosin) and thin filaments (troponin, tropomyosin, and actin). Tro-

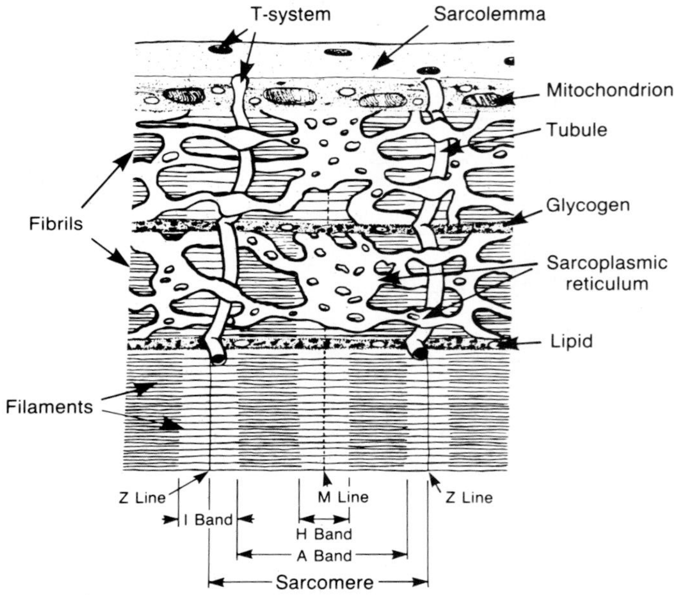

FIGURE 111–1. Structure of a skeletal muscle fiber. Each muscle fiber is a multinucleated cell composed of fibrils that contain filaments of contractile proteins surrounded by a plasma membrane, the sarcolemma. Communication between the plasma membrane and fibrils is provided by the T system of tubules that runs along the border of the sarcomeres and connects to the sarcoplasmic reticulum that invests the fibrils. The varying refractile indices of the filaments give skeletal muscle its characteristic cross-striated appearance by electron microscopy. The functional contractile unit of the muscle cell is the sarcomere and is defined as the area between two Z lines. The A band is composed of the thick filaments (myosin), and the M line is due to bulges in the centers of the thick filaments. At rest, the I band is the area occupied by thin filaments (troponin, tropomyosin, and actin) not overlapped by myosin. With contraction, cross bridges are formed between thick and thin filaments, Z lines move toward the M line, and the I bands become smaller.

ponin, along with tropomyosin, and protein that connects troponin to actin, inhibits the interaction of actin and myosin. As calcium concentrations around myofibrils increase, calcium binds to troponin causing conformational changes that release the inhibition of the enzyme. With the hydrolysis of ATP, actin-containing filaments bridge with and slide along myosin, shortening the fiber.

Muscle fiber relaxation is also the result of an active process. Shortly after calcium is released, it is pumped back into the sarcoplasmic reticulum by a calcium-dependent ATPase. Once the concentration of calcium around the fibrils is lowered, calcium is displaced from troponin and the interaction between actin and myosin stops, cross-links are broken, and fiber lengthening occurs.

ENERGY METABOLISM IN SKELETAL MUSCLE

Energy necessary for muscle contraction is provided by the *hydrolysis of ATP*. Intracellular concentrations of ATP are maintained by the action of enzymes such as creatine phosphokinase (CPK), adenylate cyclase, and myoadenylate deaminase. The energy needed to replenish ATP when it is consumed during muscle contraction is provided by the *intermediary metabolism of carbohydrate and lipid* by the pathways of glycosis, the Krebs (tricarboxylic acid) cycle, β-oxidation, and oxidative phosphorylation.

The immediate source of energy for skeletal muscle during work is found in preformed organic compounds containing high-energy phosphate such as ATP and creatine phosphate. At rest, the terminal phosphate of ATP is transferred to creatine, forming creatine phosphate and adenosine diphosphate (ADP) in a reaction catalyzed by CPK. Creatine phosphate thus acts as a reservoir of high-energy phosphate immediately available to reform ATP, and CPK acts to buffer cytoplasmic changes in ATP concentration.[3] CPK and its products, creatine

TABLE 111–1. PROPERTIES OF MUSCLE FIBER TYPES

FIBER TYPE DESIGNATION	1	2A	2B
	Red	Red	White
	SO	FOG	FG
	S	FR	FF
Motor unit properties			
Twitch speed	Slow	Intermediate	Fast
Tetanic force	Small	Large	Largest
Fatigue resistance	Highest	High	Low
Histochemical properties			
ATPase (pH 4.4)	High	Low	Low
ATPase (pH 10.6)	Low	High	High
Glycogen	Low	High	High
Lipid	High	Variable	Low
Myophosphorylase	Low	High	High
NADH dehydrogenase	High	Intermediate	Low

ATPase = adenosine triphosphatase; NADH = reduced nicotinamide adenine dinucleotide.

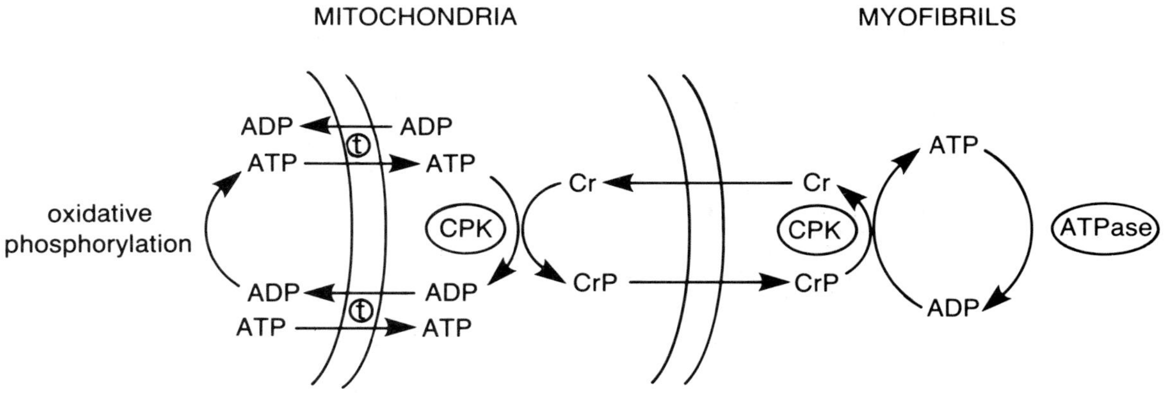

FIGURE 111–2. Scheme of the creatine–creatine phosphate shuttle. CPK is located on the inner mitochondrial membrane, on myofibrils, and in the cytoplasm. It provides a buffer mechanism for maintaining homeostatic concentrations of intracellular adenine nucleotides and plays an important role in the energy transfer within the cell after ATP is produced in mitochondria. CPK also buffers ADP and inorganic phosphate levels. The cytosolic ADP concentration is an important metabolic regulator of mitochondrial respiration, and inorganic phosphate is a regulator of glycolysis. ADP = adenosine diphosphate; ATP = adenosine triphosphate; Cr = creatinine; CrP = creatine phosphate; CPK = creatine phosphokinase; t = adenine nucleotide translocase.

and creatine phosphate, also play a significant role in the transport of energy from mitochondria to myofibrils. This latter action is referred to as the *creatine–creatine phosphate shuttle* (Fig. 111–2).

During rest and less strenuous exercise, the activity of CPK renders the concentration of ATP within cells constant at the expense of creatine phosphate. When metabolic requirements such as those that occur during prolonged contraction and muscle fatigue exceed the capacity of oxidative phosphorylation to regenerate ATP, creatine phosphate is used to replenish ATP. When approximately 50% of the creatine phosphate has been converted to creatine, ATP levels begin to fall and inosine monophosphate (IMP) accumulates. ATP is hydrolyzed to ADP and then to adenosine monophosphate (AMP) by adenylate kinase, and the AMP is converted to IMP by myoadenylate deaminase. During recovery from exercise, IMP is converted back to AMP by a two-step process. The conversion of AMP to IMP and back to AMP has been called the *purine nucleotide cycle* (Fig. 111–3). The reactions of the purine nucleotide cycle (1) reduce AMP levels, which are inhibitory to ATP generating reactions; (2) generate ammonia, which stimulates glycolysis; and (3) release fumarate, an intermediate of the Krebs cycle and promoter of oxidative phosphorylation.[8,9]

The majority of cellular energy is produced in mitochondria by degradation of metabolites through the pathways of the Krebs cycle and respiratory (cytochrome) chain. Products of the aerobic degradation of carbohydrate (pyruvate) and fatty acids enter the Krebs cycle, generating reducing equivalents. The respiratory chain, a series of enzymes and coenzymes that function as hydrogen carriers, transfers reducing equivalents to molecular oxygen (Fig. 111–4 and Table 111–2). The large amount of free energy released is captured and conserved in the form of ATP by a process called *oxidative phosphorylation*. Factors that influence the relative amounts of carbohydrate and lipids used for ATP production include the oxygen concentration of blood and muscle blood flow, the number of mitochondria and glycogen stores in muscle, and plasma free fatty acid levels.

Intracellular glycogen stores provide the major source of carbohydrate available for energy production in skeletal muscle. Most glucose entering the fibers from the blood is converted to glycogen, although glucose itself can be metabolized directly to pyruvate under certain conditions. On demand, glucose units are enzymatically split from glycogen and are degraded through a series of reactions to pyruvate (Fig. 111–5). Under aerobic conditions, pyruvate enters the Krebs cycle and is metabolized by that cycle and by oxidative phosphorylation to carbon dioxide and water. In the process, large amounts of energy are liberated to form ATP. The metabolism of one molecule of glucose by aerobic glycolysis yields a net gain of 38 molecules of ATP.

However, during exercise of short duration and high intensity, the major source of energy is glycogen, not glucose. Glycogen, a branched homopolymer of glucose, is the major storage form of carbohydrate in the body and is distributed evenly between slow- and fast-twitch muscle fibers at rest. Although glycogen products can enter the aerobic pathways previously described they can also be metabolized anaerobically. In *anaerobic glycolysis*, pyruvate does not enter the Krebs cycle but is converted to lactate instead. This process produces smaller quantities of ATP (2 ATP per molecule of glu-

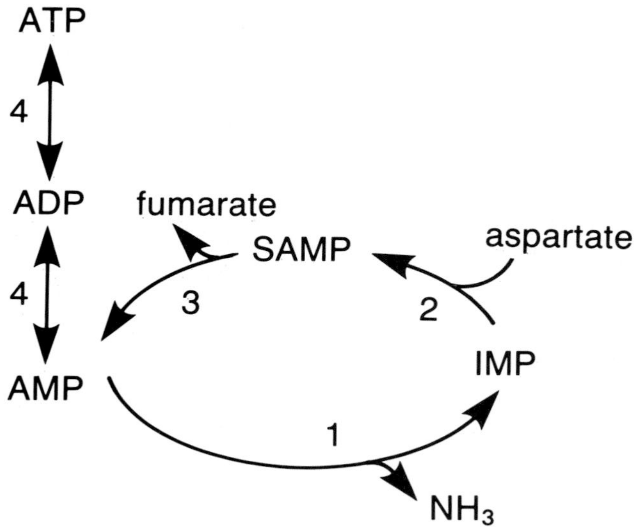

FIGURE 111–3. The purine nucleotide cycle. When muscle contraction is sufficient to exceed the buffering capacity of creatine phosphate and deplete ATP, ADP and AMP are formed by the activity of adenylate kinase. Under these conditions, glycolysis becomes the major route for regeneration of ATP, and the enzymes of the purine nucleotide cycle play a critical regulatory role. The conversion of AMP to IMP by myoadenylate deaminase causes ammonia release and changes in nucleotide concentrations that stimulate glycolysis.[8] IMP accumulates until muscle activity decreases and recovery occurs. Oxidative conditions are restored and AMP is regenerated by a two-step process with the liberation of fumarate. Fumarate is converted to malate, which is an intermediate in the Krebs cycle. The increased levels of malate drive the Krebs cycle, causing efficient resynthesis of ATP by oxidative phosphorylation.[9] 1 = myoadenylate deaminase; 2 = adenylsuccinate synthetase; 3 = adenylsuccinate lyase; 4 = adenylate kinase; ADP = adenosine diphosphate; AMP = adenosine monophosphate; ATP = adenosine triphosphate; IMP = inosine monophosphate; NH_3 = ammonia; SAMP = adenylsuccinate.

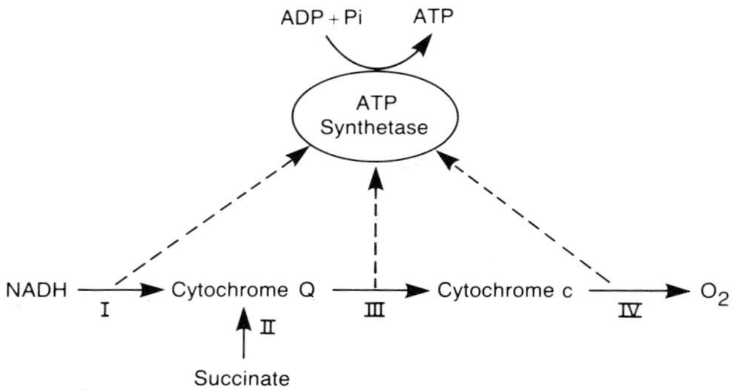

FIGURE 111–4. Scheme of respiratory chain-linked oxidative phosphorylation. The respiratory chain takes reducing units from NADH and succinate derived from the Krebs cycle and passes them through a sequence of enzymes and coenzymes to molecular oxygen. In the process, the energy released is transferred to ATP by the action of ATP synthetase I, II, III, and IV = respiratory chain complexes with enzymatic activity; cytochrome Q is also called *ubiquinone*. ADP = adenosine diphosphate; ATP = adenosine triphosphate; NADH = reduced nicotinamide adenine dinucleotide.

cose or 3 ATP per glucose unit from glycogen) compared to aerobic metabolism.

Lipids in the form of fatty acids (FAs) constitute the major, substrates for energy production for muscles at rest, during contraction, and during recovery. Plasma free fatty acids provide the largest source of lipids; intracellular stores provide very small contributions. Long-chain fatty acids move through the bloodstream from adipose tissues bound to albumin. These, plus smaller fatty acids, move across endothelial cells and into muscle cells, where they are available for energy production storage, or synthesis into membrane components. Each of these processes requires activation of the fatty acids to acyl-CoA derivatives. The resulting activated fatty acids can undergo oxidation following carnitine-mediated transport into mitochondria catalyzed by carnitine palmitoyltransferase (CPT) activities (Fig. 111–6) or esteri-

TABLE 111–2. COMPOSITION OF RESPIRATORY CHAIN COMPLEXES

	COMPLEX (ACTIVITY)	MAJOR COMPONENTS
I	(NADH dehydrogenase)	Flavin mononucleotide (FMN) Iron-sulfur
II	(Succinate dehydrogenase)	Flavin adenine dinucleotide (FAD) Cytochrome b Iron-sulfur
III	(Cytochrome Q dehydrogenase)	Cytochrome b Cytochrome c_1 Iron-sulfur Q-binding protein Antimycin A-binding protein
IV	(Cytochrome oxidase)	Cytochrome a Cytochrome a_3 Heme a Copper

NADH = reduced nicotinamide adenine dinucleotide.

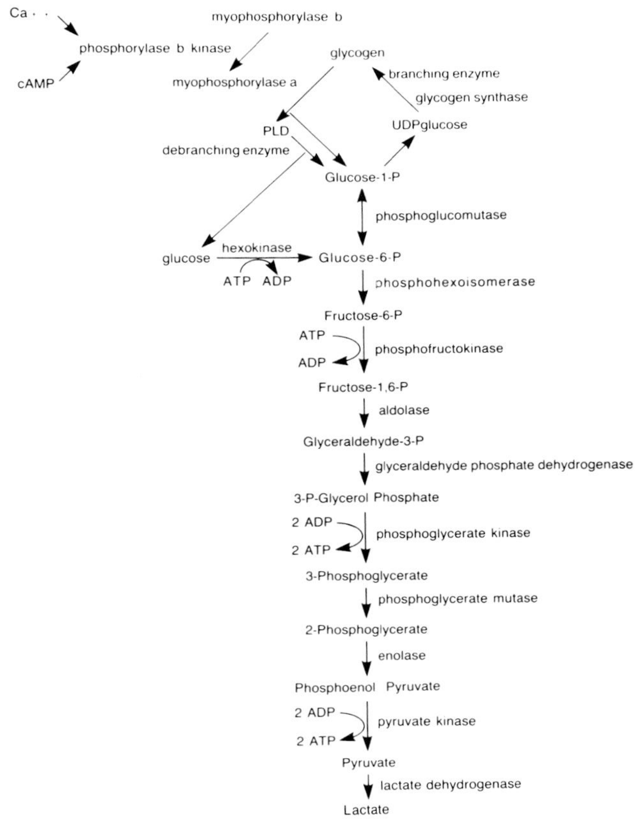

FIGURE 111–5. Pathways for glycogen metabolism and glycolysis. Aided by insulin, glucose moves across the sarcoplasmal membrane into the cell, where it is immediately phosphorylated by the activity of hexokinase. The resulting glucose-6-phosphate is then converted to glucose-1-phosphate by phosphoglucomutase and then to UDPglucose by UDPglucose pyrophosphorylase. Glycogen synthesis then proceeds by a combination of reactions catalyzed by glycogen synthase, transferring glucose molecules from UDPglucose to a pre-existing polymeric chain of other glucose molecules, which are linked by α-1,4-glucosidic bonds in a linear fashion, and branching enzyme, which results in the formation of new outer side chains by forming α-1,6-glucosyl bonds.

Glycogen remains in the cell in reserve until metabolic demands lead to the activation of myophosphorylase (glycogen phosphorylase), degrading glycogen to glucose-1-phosphate, which can enter the glycolytic pathway, and degrading phosphorylase limit dextran (PLD). Myophosphorylase exists in active (phosphorylase a) and inactive (phosphorylase b) forms. Conversion of the inactive to the active form is regulated by the enzyme phosphorylase b kinase, which is stimulated either by calcium release from the sarcoplasmic reticulum after electric stimulation or by activity of cAMP-dependent protein kinase, which in turn is activated by β-adrenergic agonists such as epinephrine or glucagon.

Active phosphorylase can degrade only about 35% of a glycogen molecule to glucose-1-phosphate. In the process, it leaves PLDs, containing terminal α-1,6-glucosidically bound glucose units each covered by three α-1,4-glucosidically bound units. Further degradation of PLD requires the action of debranching enzyme (amylo-1,6-glucosidase), which rearranges the exposed 1,4-linked units to sites where they are accessible to myophosphorylase action and hydrolyzes the 1,6-linked units as well.

The glucose-1-phosphate formed is then available for entry into the glycolytic pathway. Under anaerobic conditions it is converted in ten steps of lactate. For each glucose unit entering the pathway, one ATP molecule is hydrolyzed but four ATP molecules are generated and two lactate molecules result. Under aerobic conditions, the end product of glycolysis is pyruvate. Pyruvate molecules can enter the Krebs cycle and proceed through oxidative phosphorylation. Rate-limiting steps in glycolysis are those catalyzed by phosphofructokinase, glyceraldehyde phosphate dehydrogenase and phosphoglycerate kinase.

ADP = adenosine diphosphate; ATP = adenosine triphosphate; cAMP = cyclic adenosine monophosphate.

fication leading to the formation of cytosolic triglyceride droplets that provide a depot of lipid for future use. Once in the mitochondria, fatty acyl-CoA units are converted to acetyl-CoA by the process of β-oxidation, and acetyl-CoA is processed through the Krebs cycle. Although intracellular concentrations of free fatty acids play a role in determining the overall rate of fatty acid oxidation, the predominant regulating factor is the rate of ADP formation in working muscle.

DISORDERS OF GLYCOGEN METABOLISM

The discovery in 1959 of myophosphorylase deficiency in muscle was the first report of a biochemical abnormality in an inherited myopathy.[2] This observation occurred 8 years after McArdle had deduced that "a gross failure of the breakdown in muscle of glycogen to lactic acid" was responsible for lifelong exercise intolerance in a 30-year-old man.[1] Subsequently, additional inborn errors of glycogen metabolism associated with muscle symptoms have been reported (Table 111–3), and undoubtedly more remain to be described. Individuals with a glycogen storage disease are well at rest and perform mild exercise without difficulty, because free fatty acids are the major source of energy under those conditions. The enzymatic block that interferes with the use of carbohydrate to generate ATP causes problems only when exercise reaches a level that produces anaerobic conditions. The inability to replenish depleted high-energy phosphate stores then results in pain, contracture, and muscle necrosis.

DEFECTS OF GLYCOGENOLYSIS

Myophosphorylase Deficiency (McArdle's Disease)

The cardinal clinical manifestation of myophosphorylase deficiency is *exercise intolerance* associated with pain, fatigue, stiffness, or weakness. The degree of exercise intolerance varies among affected individuals. Symp-

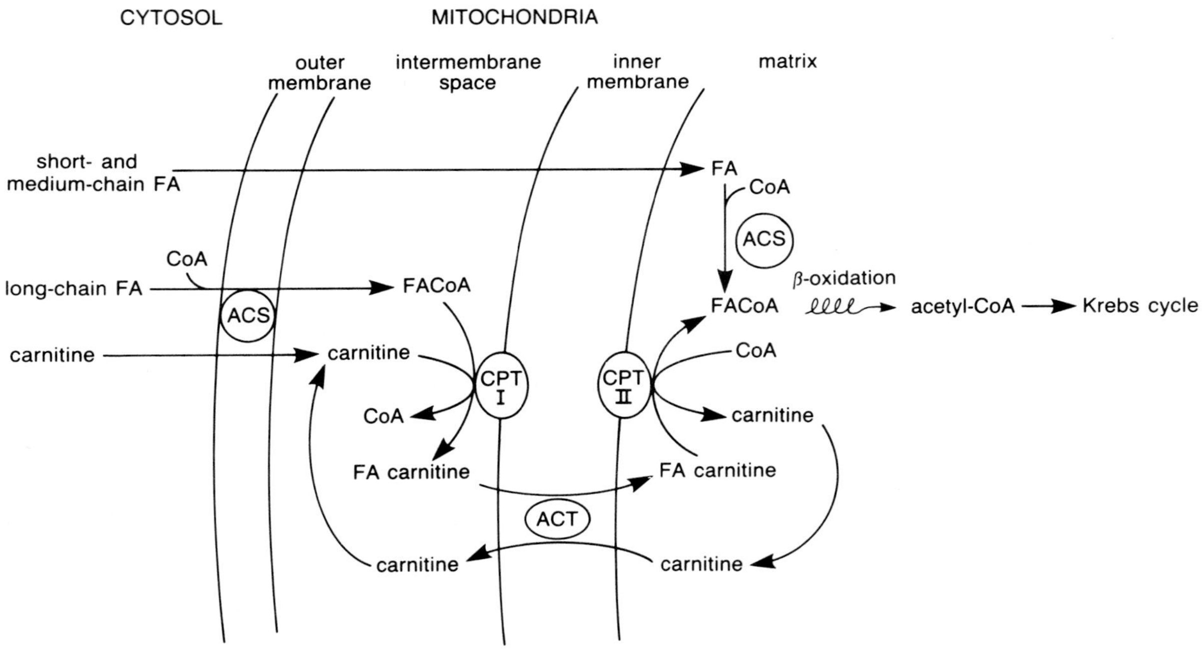

FIGURE 111–6. Scheme of fatty acid metabolism in mitochondria. Short- and medium-chain fatty acids cross the mitochondrial membrane by diffusion but the process for long-chain fatty acids is more complex requiring four steps. First, the long-chain fatty acids must be activated, a reaction catalyzed by ACS in the outer mitochondrial membrane. The acyl-CoA products formed are substrate for the second step, the formation of acylcarnitine by the action of CPT I. L-carnitine is ubiquitous and has the primary function of transfering long-chain fatty acids across the inner mitochondrial membrane. Next, acylcarnitine is transported across the inner mitochondrial membrane by ACT. Finally, the long-chain acylcarnitine is converted to the corresponding acyl-CoA structure by CPT II, which is located on the matrix side of the inner mitochondrial membrane. Once in the mitochondrial matrix, the fatty acids are converted to acetyl-CoA by a repetitive process called β-oxidation. The β-oxidation process nets 5 molecules of adenosine triphosphate for each acetyl-CoA molecule generated, and each acetyl-CoA molecule formed is available for combustion through the Krebs cycle. Accordingly, the degradation of 1 molecule of palmityl-CoA requires seven β-oxidation cycles, yields 8 acetyl-CoA molecules, and produces 131 molecules of ATP. ACS = acyl-CoA synthetase; ACT = acylcarnitine translocase; CPT I = carnitine palmitoyltransferase 1; CPT II = carnitine palmitoyltransferase 2; FA = fatty acid.

TABLE 111–3. INBORN ERRORS OF GLYCOGEN METABOLISM THAT AFFECT MUSCLE

ENZYME DEFICIENCY	EPONYM	SYMPTOMS
Acid maltase	Pompe's disease	Proximal weakness
Brancher enzyme	Andersen's disease	Hypotonia, weakness
Debrancher enzyme	Cori-Forbes' disease	Proximal weakness
Phosphorylase b kinase	—	Exercise intolerance, cramps, myoglobinuria
Myophosphorylase	McArdle's disease	Exercise intolerance, cramps, myoglobinuria
Phosphofructokinase	Tarui's disease	Exercise intolerance, cramps, myoglobinuria
Phosphoglycerate kinase	—	Exercise intolerance, myoglobinuria
Phosphoglycerate mutase	—	Exercise intolerance, myoglobinuria
Lactate dehydrogenase	—	Exercise intolerance, cramps, myoglobinuria

toms can follow activities of high intensity and short duration or those that require less intense effort for longer intervals but always resolve with rest. In fact, at-rest affected individuals function well, provided they adjust their activities to a level below their individual threshold for symptoms. When they exceed their exercise tolerance, they become symptomatic. In addition to stiffness and weakness, painful muscle cramps are sometimes associated with muscle necrosis, myoglobinuria, and potentially reversible renal failure.[10] Some individuals experience a "second wind" phenomenon; if they stop their activities at the onset of myalgia or stiffness and rest briefly, they can then resume exercising with increased tolerance. This ability to tolerate gradually increasing workloads is probably due to the combination of increased blood flow in exercising muscles and mobilization of fatty acids.[11]

Although the onset of symptoms is usually noted in childhood, symptoms are often overlooked and recognized only in retrospect. For unknown reasons, severe cramps and myoglobinuria are rare before adolescence. The late development of significant symptoms accounts for the rarity of the diagnosis before age 10. Another possible reason is the clinical heterogeneity of the disease. Some individuals only complain of being tired and having poor stamina, but others develop progressive muscle weakness that tends to be proximal and may initially be misdiagnosed as polymyositis.[12] Rarely, symptoms develop so insidiously that the diagnosis is not made until after age 75.[13]

Elevated levels of serum CPK are a common finding in myophosphorylase deficiency, helping to distinguish it from the other significant metabolic myopathy that causes myoglobinuria, namely CPT deficiency. Electromyographic (EMG) studies are usually normal unless myoglobinuria is present, although nonspecific abnormalities including increased insertional activity and an increased number of polyphasic potentials, as well as evidence of muscular irritability with fibrillations and positive waves (changes that can also be seen in inflammatory muscle disease), have been reported. The cramps that follow voluntary activity or ischemic exercise are electrically silent.[1]

A useful, but nonspecific, tool used to study individuals suspected of being myophosphorylase deficient is the forearm ischemic exercise test (Table 111–4). This test exploits the abnormal biochemistry that results in the absence of myophosphorylase activity. Normal muscle generates lactate from the degradation of glycogen when it exercises intensely under ischemic or anaerobic conditions (Fig. 111–5). This pathway is blocked when myophosphorylase activity is absent, and consequently no lactate is released into the circulation under anaerobic conditions. In addition, ammonia, inosine, and hypoxanthine concentrations increase significantly compared to providing evidence of excessive purine nucleotide breakdown.[14] Similarly, other defects in the glycogenolytic and glycolytic pathways can interfere with lactate production during ischemic exercise and provide similar results.

TABLE 111–4. PROTOCOL FOR FOREARM ISCHEMIC EXERCISE TESTING

1. A blood sample for analysis of baseline lactate and ammonia concentrations is drawn through an indwelling needle in an antecubital vein preferably without use of a tourniquet.
2. A sphygmomanometer cuff is placed on the upper arm and inflated to, and maintained at, a level at least 20 mm Hg above systolic pressure while the subject squeezes a tennis ball, or like object, vigorously at a rate of one squeeze every 2 seconds for 90 seconds.
3. After 90 seconds, the cuff is deflated and additional venous samples are obtained 1, 3, 5, and 10 minutes thereafter.

In normal individuals, lactate and ammonia concentrations increase at least threefold from baseline values. The major reason for a false-positive result is insufficient work by the subject while exercising.[24] More work is required to increase ammonia levels than lactate levels.[15] When an abnormal result is obtained, the putative diagnosis should always be confirmed by muscle biopsy.

In normal individuals, venous lactate levels increase three to sixfold shortly after ischemic exercise; in myophosphorylase-deficient individuals, levels do not change (Table 111–5).[1] The test can be painful if performed correctly. Some normal individuals cannot exercise more than a minute under ischemic conditions and find they are unable to fully flex or extend their fingers. The pain completely clears, and full function is regained immediately after restoring the circulation. Painful persistent cramping, contracture, and even myoglobinuria can occur in an individual with McArdle's disease. The major limitation of the test is that some individuals cannot or will not exercise with enough intensity to raise lactate concentrations above baseline, and thus given false-positive results.[15] Thus, if lactate concentrations do rise after ischemic exercise, myophosphorylase deficiency is excluded but if lactate levels do not rise after ischemic exercise, the diagnosis is still a possibility.

The definitive diagnosis is made by analysis of muscle tissue. Classic changes observed with light microscopy include thick deposits of glycogen at the periphery and thinner, linear deposits within cells (Fig. 111–7). The amount of variation is wide, and in milder cases deposits may not be obvious, even with periodic acid-Schiff (PAS) staining. The deposition is readily appreciated using the electron microscope (Fig. 111–8). Specific histochemical staining for myophosphorylase activity secures the diagnosis.[16] False-positives can only be seen in patients with low residual activity[17] or when they are regenerating fibers after rhabdomyolysis. Regenerating fibers an immature muscle cells express a different isoenzyme.

Other Defects in Glycogen Metabolism

Deficiencies of *brancher and debrancher enzymes* have been reported but are rare. *Brancher enzyme* deficiency causes fatal hepatic failure in childhood, which can be

TABLE 111–5. RESULTS OF FOREARM ISCHEMIC EXERCISE TESTING

SAMPLE	NORMAL		MYOPHOSPHORYLASE DEFICIENCY		MYOADENYLATE DEAMINASE DEFICIENCY	
	Lactate*	NH_3*	Lactate	NH_3*	Lactate	NH_3*
Baseline	0.8	15	0.9	20	1.2	26
1 minute	5.9	106	0.8	94	3.8	26
3 minute	3.8	91	0.9	82	2.4	29
5 minute	2.0	45	0.9	40	1.6	30
10 minute	1.2	30	0.9	25	1.4	27

* Lactate in mEq/L; NH_3 (ammonia) in μmol/L.

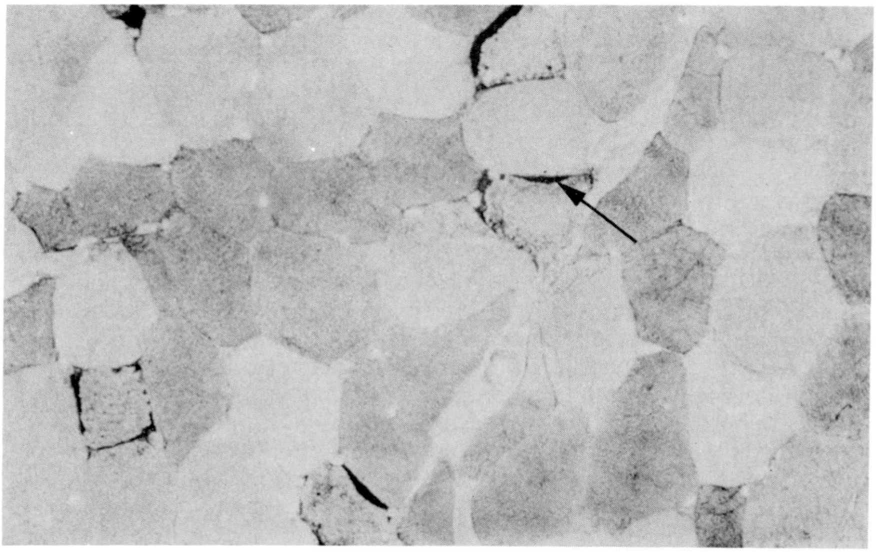

FIGURE 111–7. Muscle biopsy specimen from a patient with myophosphorylase deficiency. The periodic acid-Schiff–positive material (arrow) seen at the periphery of the cells and as lines within the cells, is excess glycogen.

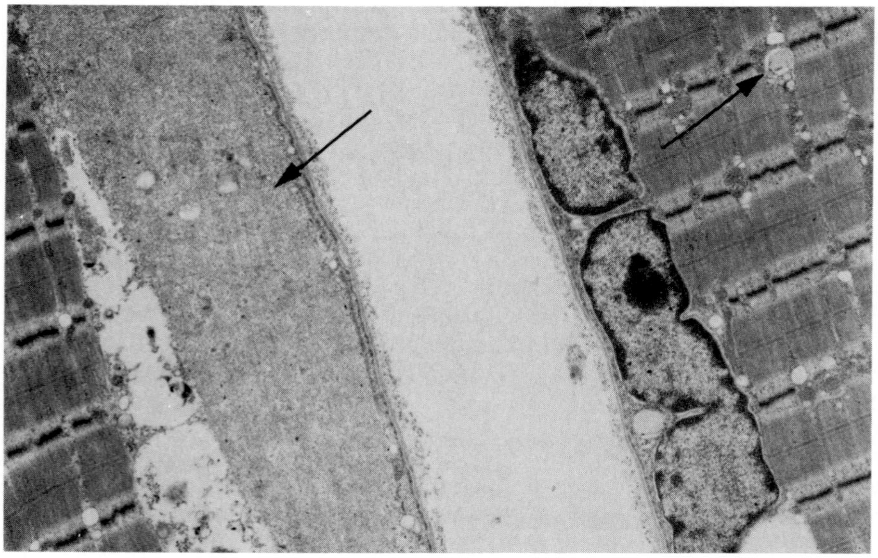

FIGURE 111–8. Electron micrograph demonstrating increased glycogen deposition beneath the sarcolemma and between filaments (arrows). These changes could be seen in all glycogen storage diseases.

associated with hypotonia and contracture[18] or exercise intolerance and cardiopathy.[19] It is characterized histologically by deposition of an abnormal PAS-positive polysaccharide. Deficiency of *debrancher enzyme* results in phosphorylase limit dextran (PLD) accumulation and deposition in muscle, liver, and blood cells. This deficiency can cause hepatomegaly, fasting hypoglycemia, and failure to thrive in childhood, however, the first recognized manifestation of the disease may be slowly progressive muscle weakness sometimes associated with distal muscle wasting, beginning after age 20.[20] These individuals have elevated CPK levels and fail to generate lactate after forearm ischemic exercise. More recently, deficiency of muscle phosphorylase b kinase has been described.[21] This can cause a myopathy in childhood[22] or mimic McArdle's disease in adulthood.[23]

DEFECTS IN GLYCOLYSIS

Phosphofructokinase Deficiency (Tauri's Disease)

The clinical manifestations of *phosphofructokinase* (PFK) *deficiency* can be identical to McArdle's disease.[24,25] Almost all patients are diagnosed as adults but in retrospect report having had problems with either exercise intolerance or cramps in their youth. PFK-deficient individuals differ from myophosphorylase-deficient individuals in that the "second wind" phenomenon may be less common[26] and exercise intolerance is likely to be associated with nausea and vomiting. About one third develop myoglobinuria, and most have elevated serum CPK levels at rest. EMG is either normal or provides nonspecific results, suggesting myopathy or inflammation. Predictably, these patients' venous lactate levels fail to increase after forearm ischemic exercise, and the test can initiate a prolonged contracture. Histochemical analysis of muscle tissue is needed to confirm the diagnosis. In addition to increased glycogen deposition and decreased PFK activity, deficient muscle also contains an abnormal polysaccharide similar to that seen in brancher enzyme deficiency.[27]

PFK deficiency can also cause hemolytic anemia.[25] This may be seen with or without myopathy, depending on the genetic defect. Isoenzymes of PFK vary in subunit composition. Generally, the muscle enzyme is composed of M subunits, and the erythrocyte enzyme contains M and L subunits. Defects in the L subunit cause only hemolysis, but defects involving M subunits can affect both muscle and red cells. Much heterogeneity exists. The hemolysis associated with myopathic disease may be subclinical, causing only an increased reticulocyte count, or severe, causing jaundice and gallstones. Hyperuricemia and gout are common in these individuals, perhaps because of the high levels of purines released with hemolysis and during exercise.[14,28]

Other Defects in Glycolysis

Deficiencies of phosphoglycerate kinase,[29] phosphoglycerate mutase,[30] and lactate dehydrogenase (LDH)[31] have been described in individuals whose problems began during adolescence or later and included exercise-induced myoglobinuria. These genetic defects all cause a failure of lactate release after ischemic exercise and require histochemical studies for diagnosis.

ACID MALTASE DEFICIENCY

Acid maltase is an enzyme, found in lysosomes, that catalyzes the release of glucose from maltose, oligosaccharides, and glycogen. Its precise role in cellular metabolism is not known. Deficiency of this enzyme is transmitted by autosomal recessive inheritance and produces three clinical syndromes that differ in age of presentation, organ involvement, and prognosis.[32] The *infantile* form causes symptoms of muscle weakness, hypotonia, and congestive heart failure that begin shortly after birth and progress to death within the first 2 years of life.[33] This form is characterized by massive glycogen deposits in cardiac, hepatic, neural, and muscular tissues. The second variety presents in *early childhood* with muscle weakness that is more proximal than distal and may affect respiratory muscles.[34] It tends not to involve the heart or liver and progresses slowly. Death, usually a result of respiratory failure, occurs before age 30.

The *adult* form causes few problems before age 20 and typically manifests as muscle weakness beginning in the third or fourth decade.[35] Although diaphragmatic involvement and respiratory failure dominate the clinical picture in about a third of cases,[36] most develop a slowly progressive myopathy that is easily confused with polymyositis or limb-girdle muscular dystrophy.[37] The weakness tends to occur in proximal muscles and the torso. Individual muscles or even parts of muscles can be affected, but craniobulbar muscles are spared. CPK is usually elevated but can be normal or only slightly increased. EMG is always abnormal, though variably. The characteristic changes include an unusually intense electrical irritability in response to movement of the needle electrode and myotonic discharges in the absence of clinical myotonia.[32] In some individuals, however, the changes are indistinguishable from those observed in some cases of polymyositis. Acid maltase–deficient subjects have no block in anaerobic glycolysis or nonlysosomal glycogenolysis because venous lactate concentrations increase normally after forearm ischemic exercise. This difference readily distinguishes them from individuals with other recognized forms of glycogen storage disease.

Acid maltase deficiency causes a vacuolar myopathy.[38] The vacuoles have a high glycogen content and stain for acid phosphatase. Small foci of acid phosphatase activity may also be found in muscle fibers that do not contain vacuoles. Glycogen is readily seen in involved muscle by electron microscopy, but the excess glycogen is not confined just to vacuolar structures. It is unclear why this nonlysosomal glycogen collects and why it is not degraded by cytosolic enzymes, nor is it clear what causes the muscular symptoms, because the pathways of glycogen and glucose metabolism for energy production are intact. The clinical heterogeneity is also not understood.

Biochemical studies are necessary to prove the diagnosis. Although characteristic EMG changes in the presence of typical vacuolar changes on biopsy from a patient with weakness involving respiratory muscles are strongly suggestive, they are not specific. Furthermore, these abnormalities tend to be less widespread and less striking in many adult cases. Assay of acid maltase in muscle, lymphocytes, cultured fibroblasts, or urine can be used to confirm the diagnosis.[39,40]

MANAGEMENT OF DISORDERS OF GLYCOGEN METABOLISM

Although no specific treatments are available for these inborn errors of metabolism, knowledge of the correct diagnosis is helpful in managing affected individuals. Patients and their families can be given a prognosis and counseled to avoid levels of activity and conditions that might provoke symptoms. They should also be advised concerning means of recognizing and getting immediate treatment for signs of rhabdomyolysis and myoglobinuria.

Dietary manipulation may be beneficial to some but not all patients. A high-protein diet has been reported to be remarkably effective in some patients with McArdle's disease,[41] debrancher disease,[42] and acid maltase deficiency[43] but to have no immediate or long-term benefit in others with the same diseases.[44,45] In addition, dietary supplementation with polyunsaturated fatty acids, medium-chain triglycerides, or ribose has enhanced short-term exercise performance in some individuals.[44,46]

DISORDERS OF LIPID METABOLISM

Plasma free fatty acids are the major source of energy while fasting, at rest, and exercising at low intensity and for long duration. Abnormalities involving the processing of long-chain fatty acids for energy lead to lipid storage myopathies, conditions in which the predominant pathologic alteration is the accumulation of abnormal amounts of lipid droplets between myofibrils (Fig. 111–6). Carnitine deficiency is the classic example of such a myopathy. CPT deficiency is the other major biochemical defect in the use of fatty acids for energy that causes human disease.

CARNITINE DEFICIENCY STATES

L-carnitine is essential for the transfer of long-chain fatty acids across the inner mitochondrial membrane and helps regulate CoA/acyl-CoA ratios in mitochondria.[47] Sources of carnitine include the diet, with red meat and dairy products containing large quantities, and de novo synthesis from lysine and methionine in liver, brain, and kidney. Carnitine is transported from the blood by an active saturable process into muscle, which contains 98% of the body stores. The major route of elimination from the body is in the urine.

In 1973, Engel and Angelini reported the first recognized case of muscle carnitine deficiency in an individual with lipid storage myopathy.[48] One year later, Karpati reported another form of carnitine deficiency, a systemic variety.[49] Carnitine deficiencies are now classified as either *primary* or *secondary*. Primary deficiencies have a genetic basis and can be further divided between *myopathic* and *systemic* forms. Secondary deficiencies are those that result from other disorders or that result from genetic defects in other pathways of intermediary metabolism.

Primary Carnitine Deficiencies

The syndrome of myopathic carnitine deficiency is characterized by progressive muscle weakness that, with some exceptions, begins in childhood.[50,51] The weakness is of the limb-girdle variety, but facial and pharyngeal muscle involvement is observed. Less common features are exertional myalgias, myoglobinuria, and cardiomyopathy. Half or more of patients have high CPK levels, and most have myopathic changes (polyphasic motor unit potentials of small amplitude and short duration) on EMG. Serum carnitine concentrations are usually normal, a finding consistent with the evidence indicating that a defect in carnitine transport into muscle cells underlies this form of the disease.[52] The only histologic abnormality in muscle is the nonspecific finding of increased lipid (Fig. 111–9). Similar changes can occur with ischemia and obesity. The diagnosis is made by biochemical analysis of muscle tissue.[53]

The first reported patient with systemic carnitine deficiency was an 11-year-old boy with progressive muscle weakness and a history of recurrent attacks that resembled Reye's syndrome.[49] The attacks began with vomiting and were followed by coma, hepatomegaly, liver function abnormalities, and hypoglycemia. Onset of this form is almost always in early childhood, with the attacks preceding the onset of muscle weakness in the majority of cases. The weakness is more proximal than distal and can affect cervical musculature, resulting in loss of head control.[54,55] Cardiac muscle involvement, manifested by congestive heart failure, can occur. Carnitine concentrations are reduced in skeletal muscle, heart, liver, and serum. A renal leak in carnitine is at least partially responsible for the deficiency in some patients, but the mechanism in other patients is unknown.[56]

Secondary Carnitine Deficiencies

Carnitine deficiency can be secondary to genetic defects in other reactions in intermediary metabolism or to other disorders. Attacks resembling Reye's syndrome occur in *acyl-CoA dehydrogenase deficiency* states,[55,57] and exercise intolerance occurs with defects in oxidative phosphorylation (see Mitochondrial Myopathies, following). The histologic features of lipid storage myopa-

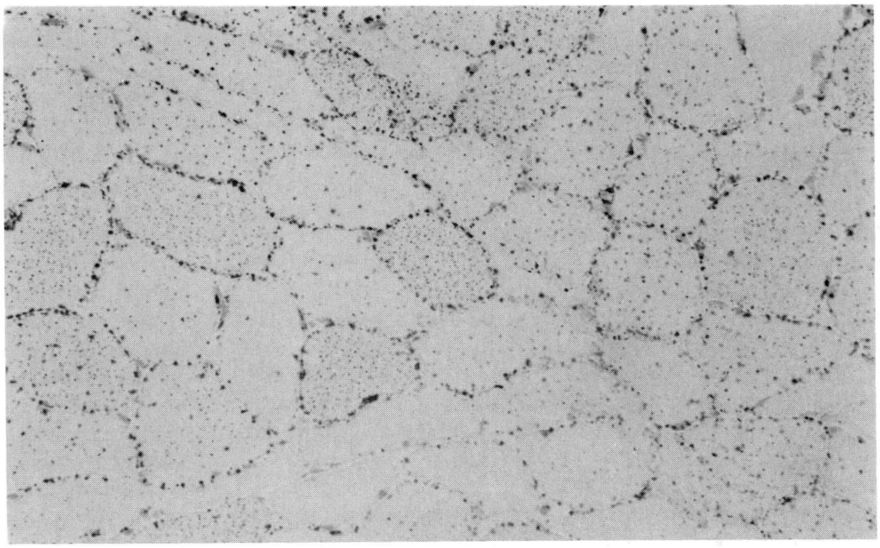

FIGURE 111–9. Muscle tissue stained with oil red O. Lipid droplets of varying size are deposited between myofibrils. Large collections appear as vacuoles. The increased staining is typical of lipid storage myopathy but by itself is a nonspecific finding.

thy are present in these inborn errors of metabolism. Other disorders in which carnitine deficiency has been observed include renal failure requiring chronic hemodialysis (but not chronic peritoneal dialysis),[58,59] end-stage cirrhosis with cachexia,[60] valproic acid therapy for seizure disorders,[61] myxedema, adrenal insufficiency, hypopituitarism,[62,63] and pregnancy.[64]

Therapy

In theory, treatment of all types of carnitine deficiency should be effective with L-carnitine supplementation of the diet. In reality, however, the response to that therapy is variable. Attempts at treatment must include a diet rich in carbohydrates and medium-chain fatty acids and avoidance of fasting. During acute attacks, therapy should be designed to prevent hypoglycemia and to correct any electrolyte and acid–base imbalances that develop.

Dietary supplementation with L-carnitine has sometimes been successful in improving each form of deficiency.[65,66] The dose for children is 100 mg/kg/day,[67] adults require 2 to 4 g in divided doses. Preparations containing the D-isomer of carnitine should not be used, because it is not effective and can actually cause muscle weakness. Some patients benefit from steroid therapy[69] or propranolol.[70] Intravenous infusion of L-carnitine (20 mg/kg) at the end of dialysis treatment decreases postdialysis symptoms, improves exercise capacity and sense of well-being, and possibly increases muscle mass in patients requiring chronic hemodialysis.[71] In addition, treatment with riboflavin alone or in combination with L-carnitine has proven beneficial to individual patients with low acyl-CoA dehydrogenase activities,[72] complex I–deficient mitochondrial myopathy,[73] and carnitine palmitoyltransferase deficiency.[74]

CARNITINE PALMITOYLTRANSFERASE DEFICIENCY

DiMauro and Melis-DiMauro in 1973 first reported a deficiency of *carnitine palmitoyltransferase* in two brothers with recurrent myoglobinuria.[75] It is transmitted by autosomal recessive inheritance.[76] The clinical syndrome associated with CPT deficiency invariably includes attacks of exertional myalgias and muscular weakness associated with myoglobinuria. CPT is necessary for transport of long-chain fatty acids into mitochondria for energy production. Because long-chain fatty acids provide the major source of cellular energy during prolonged exercise and in the fasting state, it is not surprising that attacks usually develop with prolonged exercise and fasting. Cold exposure and infection may also be important contributing and precipitating factors.[77] An episode of rhabdomyolysis culminating in respiratory failure followed initiation of ibuprofen therapy in one patient.[78] Mild attacks may be experienced in childhood, but severe attacks usually do not occur until the teenage years or later. About 25% of individuals develop renal failure with episodes of myoglobinuria,[79] but this is reversible. Respiratory failure may result during severe attacks. Between attacks, CPT-deficient individuals feel and function well and have no abnormalities on physical examination.

The clinical picture of CPT differs in several ways from that of the glycogen storage diseases that also cause myoglobinuria. First, CPT-deficient patients do not experience severe cramping, and fixed proximal muscle weakness is rare. CPK is usually normal, except during episodes of rhabdomyolysis, or with prolonged fasting, and the increase in serum lactate concentration after forearm ischemic exercise is normal. Electrophysiologic studies and muscle tissue are entirely normal between attacks. Lipid accumulation is rarely observed in CPT-deficient muscle, and the diagnosis is made by measuring CPT activity in muscle.[80] Based on the known biochemistry, it could be predicted that CPT deficiency and carnitine deficiency would cause similar abnormalities, but this is not the case. Why the clinical and histologic features of these diseases differ is not understood.

Management consists primarily of education, although the combination of oral supplementation L-carnitine and riboflavin may be of some benefit.[74] Avoidance of both prolonged strenuous exercise and fasting will prevent most attacks. Infection may not be preventable, but the need for adequate rest during an infection must be emphasized. Myoglobinuria constitutes a medical emergency. Interestingly, the development of renal failure does not correlate well with the amount of myoglobin in the urine. Treatment consists of hydration and use of an osmotic diuretic, such as mannitol, to force excretion of a dilute urine.[81] Alkalinizing the urine may also be prudent, but its efficacy has not been clearly established.

MITOCHONDRIAL MYOPATHIES

Mitochondrial myopathy is a term applied to cases of muscle disease in which the major morphologic abnormalities are alterations in the number, size, and structure of mitochondria. These changes are nonspecific and are associated with widely varying clinical syndromes. Perhaps it is more meaningful to consider mitochondrial myopathies to be disorders in muscle energetics caused by a defect in mitochondrial function that may be associated with structural changes. Defects in transport of pyruvate, fatty acids, and ketones into mitochondria as well as defects in the processing of these chemicals for energy to regenerate ATP are included in this category. Carnitine and CPT deficiency should be considered mitochondrial myopathies because of the biochemical defects, but they are not usually included under that classification because there are no associated changes in mitochondrial structure.

The most typical morphologic change in these diseases is the "ragged-red" fiber,[82] a distorted-appearing fiber that contains large peripheral and intermyofibrillar aggregates of abnormal mitochondria (Fig. 111–10). These appear as red deposits with the modified Gomori trichrome stain. An occasional ragged-red fiber is not diagnostic of a mitochondrial myopathy, but presence of these fibers does indicate the possibility of one of those diseases. On the other hand, many diseases that result from mitochondrial defects do not manifest this change. Additional changes, such as increased amounts of lipid or glycogen, intramitochondrial inclusions, or changes in mitochondrial size and/or shape, can be seen at the ultrastructural level.[83]

Mitochondrial myopathies recognized to data are associated with a variety of clinical manifestations. In general they can be divided into syndromes that cause limb myopathy with or without ophthalmoplegia and those in which central nervous system manifestations predominate.[84] The former cause problems primarily affecting muscle, with manifestations such as exercise intolerance, muscle weakness that may have limb-girdle or facioscapulohumeral distributions, or extraocular muscle dysfunction with or without bulbar and limb muscle involvement. Hypermetabolism, salt craving, and peripheral neuropathy are reported in other cases, indicating extreme heterogeneity. Although some of these diseases affect infants, many cause symptoms in childhood that are recognized as the result of a disease only retrospectively, after the diagnosis is made later in life (Table 111–6[85–90]).

To date, over 25 different biochemical defects have been described in individuals with mitochondrial myopathies.[86] These defects can occur in nutrient transport into mitochondria, in the use of substrates such as pyruvate and fatty acids, in β-oxidation and the respiratory

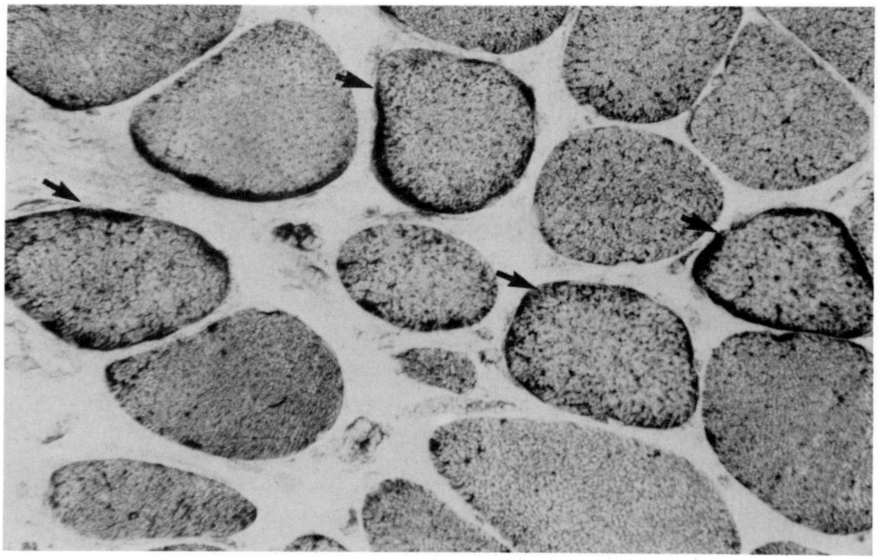

FIGURE 111–10. Typical-appearing ragged-red fiber is strongly suggestive, but not diagnostic, of a mitochondrial myopathy.

TABLE 111–6. EXAMPLES OF MITOCHONDRIAL MYOPATHIES DIAGNOSED IN ADULTS

DEFICIENCY	AGE	SYMPTOMS
Enzyme of β-oxidation[85]	33	Exercise intolerance, progressive weakness
NADH-CoQ reductase[86]	20–49	Exercise intolerance, progressive weakness
CoQ-cytochrome bc, reductase[87]	40, 43	Exercise intolerance, oculoskeletal myopathy
Cytochrome b[88]	38	Exercise intolerance, lacticacidemia
Cytochrome bc_1[89]	20	Exercise intolerance
Mitochondrial ATPase[90]	37	Nonprogressive weakness

ATPase = adenosine triphosphatase; NADH = reduced nicotinamide adenine dinucleotide.

chain, or in energy conservation. There is little correlation between the biochemical defect, morphologic changes, and clinical picture. Precisely how these defects cause muscle fatigue and weakness is still not well understood.[91]

The biochemical defects that cause mitochondrial syndromes result from a variety of changes at the molecular level. The Kearnes-Sayre syndrome, Pearson's syndrome, and the syndrome of chronic progressive external ophthalmoplegia are associated with a variety of defects effecting all respiratory chain complexes (Fig. 111–4) and attributed to large deletions of mitochondrial DNA.[92,93] Mitochondrial myopathy, lactic acidosis, and stroke-like (MELAS) syndrome and the myoclonus epilepsy, ragged red fiber (MERRF) disease are caused by single mutations of mitochondrial genes.[94] In contrast, mutations at a single loci on nuclear genes that encode for proteins in complex I or IV underlie syndromes of pure limb myopathies and fulminant infantile lactic acidosis.[95] Whereas the diseases described here are inherited, acquired mitochondrial syndromes can also occur. Mitochondrial myopathy has resulted from toxic effects of zidovudine (AZT) therapy in patients infected with the human immunodeficiency virus (HIV).[96]

DISORDERED PURINE METABOLISM

Myoadenylate Deaminase Deficiency

Myoadenylate deaminase (MADA), a distinct isoenzyme of adenylate deaminase found only in skeletal muscle, catalyzes the irreversible deamination of AMP to IMP and plays an important role in the purine nucleotide cycle (Fig. 111–3).[97] In 1978, Fishbein reported the first cases of MADA deficiency.[98] This deficiency is probably the most common metabolic myopathy recognized today. Approximately 2% of a large series of muscle biopsy specimens were deficient in MADA activity.[99,100] The diagnosis has been made at ages ranging from 7 to over 70 years.

MADA deficiency exists in both primary (inherited) and secondary (acquired) forms.[101] Patients with a primary deficiency complain of exercise intolerance due to fatigue with postexertional cramps and myalgias. Symptoms are typically mild early in the course but gradually become more severe, leading to increased disability over time. The secondary deficiencies are associated with a wide variety of other neuromuscular diseases including periodic paralysis, influenza-like illness, Kugelberg-Welander syndrome, amyotrophic lateral sclerosis, spinal muscular atrophy, facial and limb-girdle myopathies, polymyositis, dermatomyositis, systemic lupus erythematosus, systemic sclerosis, diabetes, hyperthyroidism, and gout.[102] In primary deficiency, MADA activity is the only protein affected. It is attributed to homozygosity for a common point mutation in the gene that encodes for the enzyme.[103] This mutation results in normal abundance of MADA transcript but deficient (generally less than 2% of normal) enzyme protein. In contrast, higher residual activities of immunoreactive enzyme protein occur in the secondary deficiencies, and reductions occur in other muscle enzymes such as CPK and adenylate kinase.[101] Furthermore the reduction in enzyme activity occurs in conjunction with a parallel decrease in MADA messenger RNA.[104] The factors responsible for the molecular changes underlying the secondary deficiency states are not understood, although myonecrosis appears to play a significant role in the secondary MADA deficiency associated with polymyositis.[105]

The precise relationship between MADA deficiency and muscular symptoms is unknown. The low exercise tolerance of these individuals is accompanied by rapid depletion of ATP in skeletal muscle, and the time required to replenish ATP to normal concentrations is prolonged compared to normals.[106] The response to forearm ischemic exercise is also abnormal in MADA deficiency (Table 111–5). Although the expected rise in venous lactate occurs, a corresponding change in ammonia concentration is not present. In addition, generation of the purine nucleotide degradation products adenosine, inosine, and hypoxanthine is diminished with exercise.[15,107]

Serum enzymes such as the CPK and aldolase are usually normal in primary MADA deficiency and vary according to the associated condition in secondary deficiencies. Results of EMG are also normal or nonspecific. The measurement of venous lactate and ammonia concentrations following forearm ischemic exercise is effective for screening for MADA deficiency. However, submaximal exercise performance because of weakness, pain, or poor effort can be responsible for false-positive results.[15] Consequently, failure to generate ammonia after exercise does not indicate MADA deficiency unless an adequate effort is documented. An abnormal result from forearm ischemic exercise testing should be followed by a muscle biopsy to confirm the putative enzyme deficiency. The structure of muscle tissue is usually normal. Histochemical techniques are useful in establishing the deficiency state.[108]

ENDOCRINE MYOPATHIES

A variety of endocrine diseases can cause symptoms of neuromuscular dysfunction. These include disorders of either hyperfunction or hypofunction of the adrenal, parathyroid, pituitary, and thyroid glands. A major mechanism responsible for the symptoms involves electrolyte imbalance.[109] This should not be surprising because muscle contraction requires transmembrane shifts in sodium, potassium, and calcium; inorganic phosphate is critical to the maintenance of high-energy compounds; and magnesium is an essential cofactor for ATPase activity. Thus, any hormonal change (or disease, drug, or other factor) that raises or lowers the concentrations of these ions can cause myopathic symptoms by altering surface membrane excitability, excitation–contraction coupling, or actin–myosin bridging. Endocrine disorders also cause skeletal muscle dysfunction through the effects of hormones on protein and carbohydrate metabolism.[110] The rheumatic aspects and myopathic syndromes of endocrinopathies are discussed in Chapter 114.

CLINICAL EVALUATION

The evaluation of patients with suspected metabolic muscle disease begins with a careful history and a thorough physical examination. Myopathies typically cause weakness, exercise intolerance as a result of fatigue, and postexertional myalgias, cramps, and stiffness. The weakness develops insidiously and is therefore ignored until it becomes truly limiting. The actual onset of the symptoms is often difficult to determine even in retrospect. Everyone experiences cramps, stiffness, and pain after certain exercise. Thus, the patient may deny the significance of his problems, and others, including physicians, may disregard the patient's complaints for many years. Distinguishing between "normal" and "abnormal" exercise intolerance can truly be difficult.

The problem of diagnosing a metabolic muscle disease is confounded because at rest, patients are often completely asymptomatic and have no abnormal physical findings. The most significant complaints are severe, prolonged cramps and red wine–colored urine indicating myoglobinuria. Although these findings can hardly be ignored, special attention and questioning are required to determine the significance of the less dramatic symptoms. *The weakness of a metabolic myopathy is proximal and symmetrically distributed.* Initial complaints include difficulty climbing stairs or reaching a top shelf. Physical examination may be entirely normal and at most may show only weakness of a limb-girdle distribution. The prime importance of the physical examination in a neuromuscular disease may be to rule out evidence of a "neuro" component.

Measurement of muscle enzymes and electrodiagnostic studies follow if the patient's complaints are suspicious for myopathy or severe enough to alter his lifestyle. Increased levels of CPK, aldolase, serum glutamic-oxaloacetic transaminase (SGOT), serum glutamic-pyruvic transaminase (SGPT), and lactic dehydrogenase (LDH) may be observed in the blood of patients with muscle disease. Of these, the CPK is the most sensitive. However, in metabolic diseases of muscle, the presence of an elevated CPK is variable. Levels are usually increased in patients with glycogen storage diseases but are usually normal with the other diseases such as CPT or MADA deficiency. An isolated elevation of the CPK should be interpreted with caution. In normal individuals, spurious elevations can result from fever, blunt trauma, intramuscular injection, aerobic exercise, EMG, muscle biopsy, and the use of medications such as morphine and barbiturates, which retard the excretion of the enzyme in the urine.[111,112] The patient's race and sex must also be considered in the interpretation of CPK levels. CPK values are significantly higher in healthy asymptomatic blacks than in whites or Hispanics and in males compared to females.[113,114] CPK levels are always raised in patients who have rhabdomyolysis. The MB isoenzyme fraction, which is usually considered as derived from cardiac muscle, may be increased under these conditions because regenerating skeletal muscle also produces this form.

Nerve conduction studies are entirely normal in metabolic myopathies. Finding normal nerve conduction in a patient with symptoms of muscle dysfunction defines the process as a myopathy by exclusion. EMG may also provide normal results in these individuals. Exceptions are in deficiencies of acid maltase, debrancher enzyme, and carnitine. But even in those conditions, the findings of abnormal motor unit potential and fibrillations are variable and nondiagnostic. The electromyogram, however, may be useful in clearly demonstrating myopathic changes and indicating preferential sites for muscle biopsy on the opposite side of the body.

Measurement of venous lactate and ammonia before and after forearm ischemic exercise provides a useful tool for ruling out MADA deficiency and all myopathic forms of glycogen storage disease except acid maltase deficiency. Individuals with MADA deficiency produce little ammonia compared to normal amounts of lactate under these conditions, whereas patients with the glycogenic and glycolytic defects produce the opposite result (Tables 111–4 and 111–5). Valid results from the forearm ischemic exercise test require an appropriate exercise effort on the part of the individual because false-positive results can result from poor subject performance.[15,115] A positive result must be confirmed by tissue analysis.

A muscle biopsy produces the most important diagnostic

information in the evaluation of a patient with a metabolic muscle disease. It is, however, the final step in the clinical evaluation and should not be performed until a preliminary diagnosis has been made. Selection of the muscle for biopsy is important. A clinically weak muscle that has not been traumatized (by intramuscular injection, EMG needle, or previous biopsy) is ideal. If weakness is not obvious, the biopsy site may be guided by EMG abnormalities on the opposite side of the body. Severely involved muscle, as seen acutely in rhabdomyolysis, should be avoided. The tissue can be severely distorted, and the biochemical features of regenerating muscle can provide confusing information. Magnetic resonance imaging provides a noninvasive means of identifying the patterns of distribution and severity of muscle involvement and may also be used to determine a biopsy site.[116,117]

Routine histology can be helpful primarily in ruling out other conditions that can cause symptoms of muscle dysfunction such as inflammatory muscle disease and muscular dystrophies. *Histochemical studies* can provide the important information. The increased glycogen storage of disorders of glycogen metabolism can be detected with PAS staining (Fig. 111–7). Increased lipid accumulation, indicative of lipid storage myopathy, can be identified with Sudan or oil red O stains (Fig. 111–9). The Gomori modified trichrome stain reveals changes in mitochondria and the ragged-red fiber (Fig. 111–10). Acid phosphatase stains will demonstrate increased lysosomal enzyme activity indicative of acid maltase deficiency. Abnormal staining with reduced nicotinamide adenine dinucleotide (NADH) dehydrogenase, and other oxidative enzyme stains, suggests mitochondrial defects. Specific enzyme defects can be diagnosed with stains for myophosphorylase, PFK, LDH, cytochrome oxidase, and MADA (Fig. 111–11). Carnitine concen-

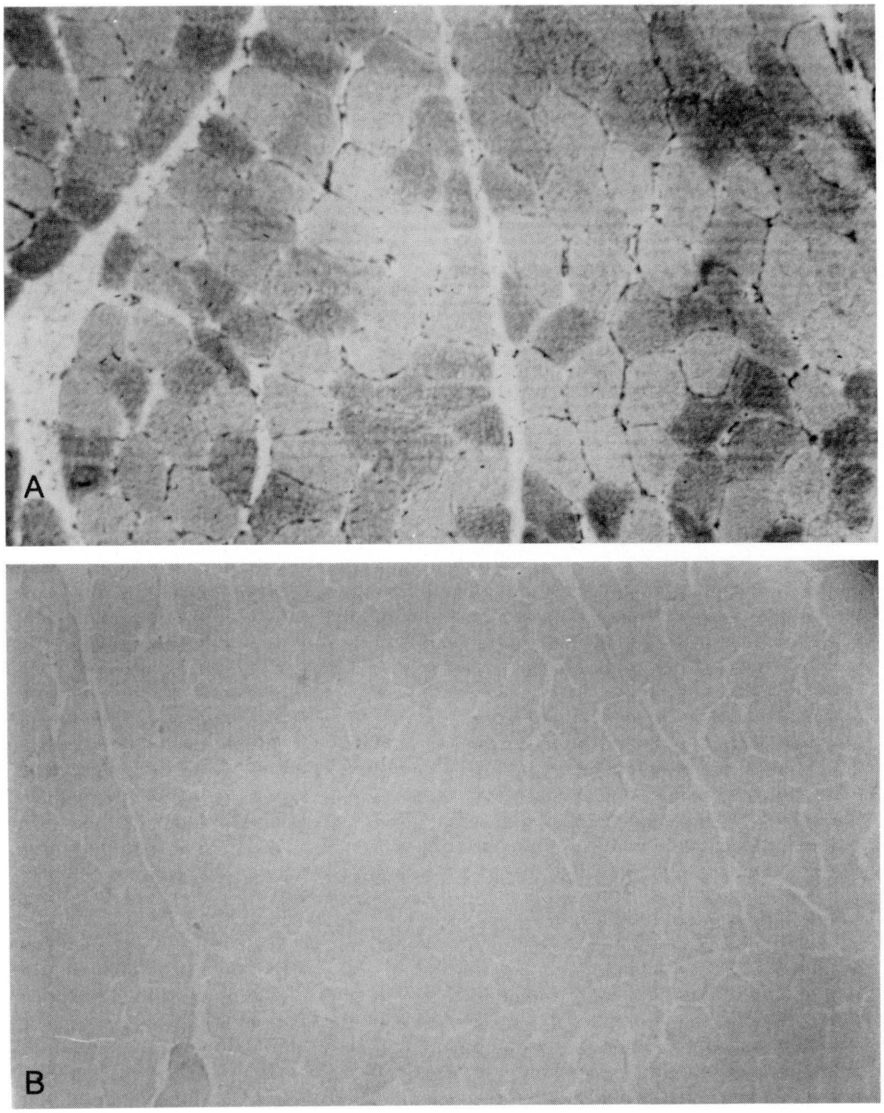

FIGURE 111–11. *A,* Muscle stained for myoadenylate deaminase activity with normal results. *B,* Muscle from an individual with myoadenylate deaminase deficiency stained by the same method as the tissue in *A.*

tration and CPT activity can be determined on muscle homogenate by radiochemical techniques.

Ultrastructural analysis by electron microscopy is clearly more sensitive than light microscopy in identifying glycogen (Fig. 111–8) and lipid deposition and reveals morphologic changes in mitochondria, membranes, and sarcoplasmic reticulum. This technique will play an increased role in the evaluation of metabolic muscle diseases.

In the future, the evaluation of patients with symptoms of muscle dysfunction will include *^{31}P magnetic resonance spectroscopy*. Presently, this technique is used primarily for research purposes. Magnetic resonance spectroscopy can be used to measure tissue contents of ATP, creatine phosphate, and inorganic phosphate. This technique can be used to follow the shifts in these metabolites during exercise and to determine the pH of the tissue studied. It is noninvasive and harmless. Magnetic resonance spectroscopy has been applied to patients with McArdle's disease.[118] and PFK deficiency,[119] confirming the predicted rapid decreases in creatine phosphate and lack of pH change during ischemic exercise. At least four different patterns of metabolic change have been identified in muscle of patients with mitochondrial myopathies.[120] Additional studies with this technique will help elucidate normal patterns of muscle metabolism and detect altered states in various diseases and will provide a valuable tool in following the effects of therapies.

REFERENCES

1. McArdle, B.: Myopathy due to a defect in muscle glycogen breakdown. Clin. Sci., *24*:13–36, 1951.
2. Mommaerts, W.F.H.M. et al.: A functional disorder of muscle associated with the absence of phosphorylase. Proc. Natl. Acad. Sci. USA, *45*;791–797, 1959.
3. Williamson, J.R.: Mitochondrial function in the heart. Ann. Rev. Physiol., *41*:485–506, 1979.
4. Bessman, S.P., and Geiger, P.J.: Transport of energy in muscle: The phosphorylcreatine shuttle. Science., *211*:448–452, 1981.
5. Kushmerick, M.J.: Patterns in mammalian muscle energetics. J. Exp. Biol., *115*:165–177, 1985.
6. Lowenstein, J.M.: Ammonia production in muscle an other tissues: The purine nucleotide cycle. Physiol. Rev., *52*:382–414, 1972.
7. Meyer, R.A., and Terjung, R.L.: AMP deamination and IMP reamination in working skeletal muscle. Am. J. Physiol., *239*(Cell Physiol. 8):C32–C38, 1980.
8. Wy, T-F.L., and Davis, E.J.: Regulation of glycolytic flux in an energetically controlled cell-free system: The effects of adenine nucleotide ratios, inorganic phosphate, pH, and citrate. Arch. Biochem. Biophys., *209*:85–99, 1981.
9. Aragon, J.J., and Lowenstein, J.M.: The purine nucleotide cycle. Comparisons of the levels of citric acid intermediates with the operation of the purine nucleotide cycle in rat skeletal muscle during exercise and recovery from exercise. Eur. J. Biochem., *110*:371–377, 1980.
10. DiMauro, S., and Bresolin, N.: Phosphorylase deficiency., *In* Myology. Edited by A.G. Engel and B.Q. Banker. New York, McGraw-Hill Book Company, 1986.
11. Pernow, B.B., Havel, R.J., and Jennings, D.B.: The second wind phenomenon in McArdle's syndrome. Acta Med. Scand., *472*(Suppl.):294–307, 1967.
12. Wortmann, R.L.: Myositis or myopathy. J. Rheumatol., *16*:1525–1527, 1989.
13. Pourmand, R., Sanders, D.B., and Corwin, H.M.: Late-onset McArdle's disease with unusual electromyographic findings. Arch. Neurol., *40*:374–377, 1983.
14. Mineo, I. et al.: Myogenic hyperuricemia. A common pathophysiologic feature of glycogenosis types III, V, and VII. N. Engl. J. Med., *317*:75–80, 1987.
15. Valen, P.A. et al.: Myoadenylate deaminase deficiency and forearm ischemic exercise testing. Arthritis Rheum., *30*:661–668, 1987.
16. Engel, W.K., Eyerman, E.L., and Williams, H.E.: Late-onset type of skeletal muscle phosphorylase deficiency. A new familial variety with completely and partially affected subjects. N. Engl. J. Med., *268*:135–137, 1963.
17. Mitsumoto, H.: McArdle's disease: Phosphorylase activity in regenerating muscle fibers. Neurology, *29*:258–262, 1979.
18. Fernandes, J., and Huijing, F.: Branching enzyme-deficiency glycogenosis: Studies in therapy. Arch. Dis. Child., *43*:347–352, 1968.
19. Sernella, S. et al.: Severe cardiopathy in branching enzyme deficiency. J. Pediatr., *111*:51–56, 1987.
20. Brunberg, J.A., McCormick, W.F., and Schochet, S.S.: Type III glycogenosis. An adult with diffuse weakness and muscle wasting. Arch. Neurol., *25*:171–178, 1971.
21. Lederer, B., Van de Werve, G., De Barsy, T., and Hers, H.G.: The autosomal form of phosphorylase kinase deficiency in man: Reduced activity of the muscle enzyme. Biochem. Biophys. Res. Commun., *92*:169–174, 1980.
22. Ohtani, Y. et al.: Infantile glycogen storage myopathy in a girl with phosphorylase kinase deficiency. Neurology, *32*:833–838, 1982.
23. Abarbanel, J.M. et al.: Adult muscle phosphorylase "b" kinase deficiency. Neurology, *36*:560–562, 1986.
24. Tarui, S. et al.: Phosphofructokinase deficiency in skeletal muscle. A new type of glycogenosis. Biochem. Biophys. Res. Commun., *19*:517–523, 1965.
25. Rowland, L.P., DiMauro, S., and Layzer, R.B.: Phosphofructokinase deficiency. *In* Myology. Edited by A.G. Engle and B.Q. Banker. New York, McGraw-Hill Book Company, 1986.
26. Haller, R.G., and Lewis, S.F.: Glucose-induced exertional fatigue in muscle phosphofructokinase deficiency. N. Engl. J. Med., *324*:364–369, 1991.
27. Danon, M.J. et al.: Late-onset muscle phosphofructokinase (PFK) deficiency. Neurology, *35*(Suppl.):207, 1985.
28. Kono, N. et al.: Increased plasma uric acid after exercise in muscle phosphofructokinase deficiency. Neurology, *36*: 106–108, 1986.
29. DiMauro, S., Dalakas, M., and Miranda, A.F.: Phosphoglycerate kinse (PGK) deficiency: Another cause of recurrent myoglobinuria. Ann. Neurol., *13*:11–19, 1983.
30. DiMauro, S. et al.: Muscle phosphoglycerate mutase deficiency. Neurology, *32*:584–591, 1982.
31. Kanno, T. et al.: Hereditary deficiency of lactate dehydrogenase M-subunit. Clin. Chim. Acta, *108*:267–276, 1980.
32. Engel, A.G., Gomez, M.R., Seybold, M.E., and Lambert, E.H.: The spectrum and diagnosis of acid maltase deficiency. Neurology, *23*:95–106, 1973.
33. Hogan, G.R. et al.: Pompe's disease. Neurology, *19*:894–900, 1969.
34. Nakagawa, M. et al.: Muscle type acid maltase deficiency: An intermediate case between childhood type and adult type. Clin. Neurol. (Tokyo), *22*:54–57, 1982.

35. Hudgson, P. et al.: Adult myopathy from glycogen storage disease due to acid maltase deficiency. Brain, *91*:435–462, 1968.
36. Keunen, R.W.M., Lambregts, P.C.L.A., Op de Coul, A.A.W., and Joosten, E.M.G.: Respiratory failure as initial symptom of acid maltase deficiency. J. Neurol. Neurosurg. Psychiatry, *47*:549–552, 1984.
37. Engel, A.G.: Acid maltase deficiency in adults: Studies in four cases of a syndrome which may mimic muscular dystrophy or other myopathies. Brain, *93*:599–616, 1970.
38. Hudgson, P., and Fulthorpe, J.J.: The pathology of type II skeletal muscle glycogenosis: A light and electron-microscopic study. J. Pathol., *116*:139–147, 1975.
39. Taniguchi, N. et al.: Alpha-glucosidase activity in human leucocytes: Choice of lymphocytes for the diagnosis of Pompe's disease and the carrier state. Clin. Chim. Acta, *89*:293–299, 1978.
40. Schram, A.W. et al.: Use of immobilized antibodies in investigating acid alpha-gluocosidase in urine in relation to Pompe's disease. Biochim. Biophys. Acta, *567*:370–383, 1979.
41. Slonim, A.E., and Goans, P.J.: Myopathy in McArdle's syndrome: Improvement with a high-protein diet. N. Engl. J. Med., *312*:355–359, 1985.
42. Slonim, A.E. et al.: Reversal of debrancher deficiency myopathy by use of high-protein nutrition. Ann. Neurol., *11*:420–422, 1982.
43. Issacs, H., Savage, N., Badenhorst, M., and Whistle, T.: Acid maltase deficiency: A case study and review of the pathophysiological changes and proposed therapeutic measures. J. Neurol. Neurosurg. Psychiatry, *49*:1011–1018, 1986.
44. Hopewell, R., Yeater, R., and Ullrich, I.: The effect of three test meals on exercise tolerances of an individual with McArdle's disease. J. Am. Coll. Nutr., *7*:485–489, 1989.
45. Kushner, R.F., and Berman, S.A.: Are high-protein diets effective in McArdle's disease? Arch. Neurol., *47*:383–384, 1990.
46. Wagner, D.R., and Zollner, N.: McArdle's disease: Successful symptomatic therapy by high dose oral administration of ribose. Klin. Wochenschr., *69*:92, 1991.
47. Bremer, J.: Carnitine-metabolism and functions. Physiol. Rev., *63*:1420–1480, 1983.
48. Engel, A.G., and Angelini, C.: Carnitine deficiency of skeletal muscle associated with lipid storage mypathy: A new syndrome. Science, *179*:899–902, 1973.
49. Karpati, G. et al.: The syndrome of systemic carnitine deficiency: Clinical, morphologic, biochemical and pathophysiologic features. Neurology, *25*:16–24, 1975.
50. Carrier, H.M., and Berthillier, G.: Carnitine levels in normal children and adults and in patients with diseased muscle. Muscle Nerve, *3*:326–334, 1980.
51. Rebouche, C.J., and Paulson, D.J.: Carnitine metabolism and function in humans. Annu. Rev. Nutr., *6*:41–66, 1986.
52. Treem, W.R. et al.: Primary carnitine deficiency due to a failure of carnitine transport in kidney, muscle, and fibroblasts. N. Engl. J. Med., *319*:1331–1336, 1988.
53. McGarry, J.D., and Foster, D.W.: An improved and simplified radioisotope assay for the determination of free and esterified carnitine. J. Lipid Res., *17*:277–281, 1976.
54. Chapoy, P.F. et al.: Systemic carnitine deficiency: A treatable inherited lipid-storage disease presenting as Reye's syndrome. N. Engl. J. Med., *303*:1389–1394, 1980.
55. Rowe, P.C., Valle, D., and Brusilow, S.W.: Inborn errors of metabolism referred with Reye's syndrome. A changing pattern. JAMA *260*:3167–3170, 1988.
56. Rebouche, C.J., and Engel, A.G.: Carnitine transport in cultured muscle cells and skin fibroblasts from patients with primary systemic carnitine deficiency. In Vitro, *18*:495–500, 1982.
57. Engel, A.G.: Carnitine deficiency syndromes and lipid storage myopathies. *In* Myology. Edited by A.G. Engel and B.Q. Banker. New York, McGraw-Hill Book Company, 1986.
58. Savica, V. et al.: Plasma and muscle carnitine levels in haemodialysis patients with morphological-ultrastructural examination of muscle samples. Nephron, *35*:232–236, 1983.
59. Moorthy, A.V., Rosenblum, M., Rajaram, R., and Shug, A.L.: A comparison of plasma and muscle carnitine levels in patients on peritoneal or hemodialysis for chronic renal failure. Am. J. Nephrol., *3*:205–208, 1983.
60. Rudman, D., Sewell, C.W., and Ansley, J.D.: Deficiency of carnitine in cachetic cirrhotic patients. J. Clin. Invest., *60*:716–723, 1977.
61. Laub, M.C., Paetzke-Brunner, I., and Jaeger, G.: Serum carnitine during valproic acid therapy. Epilepsia, *27*:559–562, 1986.
62. Maebashi, M. et al.: Urinary excretion of carnitine in patients with hyperthyroidism and hypothyroidism: Augmentation by thyroid hormone. Metabolism, *26*:351–356, 1977.
63. Maebashi, M. et al.: Urinary excretion of carnitine and serum concentrations of carnitine and lipids in patients with hypofunctional endocrine diseases: Involvement of adrenocorticoid and thyroid hormones in ACTH-induced augmentation of carnitine and lipid metabolism. Metabolism, *26*:357–361, 1977.
64. Cederblad, G., Fahraeus, L., and Lindgren, K.: Plasma carnitine and renal-carnitine clearance during pregnancy. Am. J. Clin. Nutr., *44*:379–383, 1986.
65. Prockop, L.D., Engel, W.K., and Shug, A.L.: Nearly fatal muscle carnitine deficiency with full recovery after replacement therapy. Neurology, *33*:1629–1631, 1983.
66. Carroll, J.E. et al.: Carnitine "deficiency": Lack of response to carnitine therapy. Neurology, *30*:618–626, 1980.
67. Strumpf, D.A., Parker, W.D., and Angelini, C.: Carnitine deficiency, organic acidemias, and Reye's syndrome. Neurology, *35*:1041–1045, 1985.
68. Keith, R.E.: Symptoms of carnitinelike deficiency in a trained runner taking DL-carnitine supplements. JAMA, *255*:1137, 1986.
69. VanDyke, D.H., Griggs, K.R.C., Markesbery, W., and DiMauro, S.: Hereditary carnitine deficiency of muscle. Neurology, *25*:154–159, 1975.
70. Issacs, H. et al.: Weakness associated with the pathological presence of lipid in skeletal muscle: A detailed study of a patient with carnitine deficiency. J. Neurol. Neurosurg. Psychiatry, *39*:1114–1123, 1976.
71. Ahmed, S. et al.: Multicenter trial of L-carnitine in maintenance hemodialysis patients: II. Clinical and biochemical effects. Kidney Int., *38*:912–918, 1990.
72. Turnbull, D.M. et al.: Lipid storage myopathy associated with low acyl-CoA dehydrogenase activities. Brain, *111*:815–828, 1988.
73. Bersen, P.L. J.A. et al.: Successful treatment of pure myopathy, associated with complex I deficiency, with riboflavin and carnitine. Arch. Neurol., *48*:334–338, 1991.
74. Lindsley, H.B., Kepes, J.J., Tekkanat, K.K., and Wortmann, R.L.: Treatment of carnitine palmityltransferase (CPT) deficiency with L-carnitine and riboflavin. Arthritis Rheum., *33*(Suppl.):S70, 1990.
75. Dimauro, S., and Melis-DiMauro, P.: Muscle carnitine palmitoyltransferase deficiency and myoglobinuria. Science, *182*: 929–931, 1973.
76. Angelini, C. et al.: Carnitine palmitoyltransferase deficiency: Clinical variability, carrier detection, and autosomal recessive inheritance. Neurology, *31*:883–886, 1981.
77. DiMauro, S., and Papadimitriou, A.: Carnitine palmitoyltransferase deficiency. *In* Myology. Edited by A.G. Engel and B.Q. Banker. New York, McGraw-Hill Book Company, 1986.
78. Ross, N.S., and Hoppel, C.L.: Partial muscle carnitine palmitoyl-

transferase-A deficiency. Rhabdomyolysis associated with transiently decreased muscle carnitine content after ibuprofen therapy. JAMA, *257*:62–65, 1987.

79. DiDonato, S. et al.: Heterogeneity of carnitine-palmitoyltransferase deficiency. J. Neurol. Sci., *50*:207–215, 1981.
80. Zierz, S., and Engel, A.G.: Regulatory properties of a mutant carnitine palmitoyltransferase in human skeletal muscle. Eur. J. Biochem., *149*:207–214, 1985.
81. Gabow, P.A., Kaehny, W.D., and Kelleher, S.P.: The spectrum of rhabdomyolysis. Medicine, *61*:141–152, 1982.
82. Olson, W., Engel, W.K., Walsh, G.O., and Einaugler, R.: Oculocraniosomatic neuromuscular disease with "ragged-red" fibers: Histochemical and ultrastructural changes in limb muscles of a group of patients with idiopathic progressive external ophthalmoplegia. Arch. Neurol., *26*:193–211, 1972.
83. Carpenter, S., and Karpati, G.: Pathology of Skeletal Muscle. 1st ed. New York, Churchill Livingstone, 1984.
84. Byrne, E.: Mitochondrial myopathies and myoencephalopathies. Curr. Opin. Rheumatol., *2*:889–895, 1990.
85. Willner, J.H. et al.: Muscle carnitine deficiency. Genetic heterogeneity. J. Neurol. Sci., *41*:235–246, 1979.
86. Morgan-Hughes, J.A.: The mitochondrial myopathies. *In* Myology. Edited by A.G. Engel and B.Q. Banker. New York, McGraw-Hill Book Company, 1986.
87. Karpati, G. et al.: The Kearns Shy syndrome. A multisystem disease with mitochondrial abnormality demonstrated in skeletal muscle and skin. J. Neurol. Sci., *19*:133–151, 1973.
88. Land, J.N., Morgan-Hughes, J.A., and Clark, J.B.: Mitochondrial myopathy studies revealing a deficiency of NADH-cytochrome b reductase activity. J. Neurol. Sci., *50*:1–13, 1981.
89. Hayes, D.J. et al.: A new mitochondrial myopathy: Biochemical studies revealing a deficiency in the cytochrone-bc_1 complex (complex III) of the respiratory chain. Brain, *107*:1165–1177, 1984.
90. Schotland, D.L. et al.: Neuromuscular disorder associated with a defect in mitochondrial energy supply. Arch. Neurol., *33*:475–479, 1976.
91. Wilke, D.R.: Shortage of chemical fuel as a cause of fatigue: Studies by nuclear magnetic resonance and bicycle ergometry. *In* Human Muscle Fatigue: Physiological Mechanisms, Ciba Foundation Symposium 82. Edited by R. Porter and J. Whelan. London, Pitman Medical, 1981.
92. Mores, C.T. et al.: Mitochondrial DNA deletions in progressive external ophthalmoplegia and Kearnes-Sayre syndrome. N. Engl. J. Med., *320*:1293–1299, 1989.
93. Holt, I.J. et al.: Mitochondrial myopathies: Clinical, biochemical features of 30 patients with major deletions of muscle mitochondrial DNA. Ann. Neurol., *26*:699–708, 1989.
94. Shoffner, J.M. et al.: Myoclinic epilepsy and ragged red fibre disease (MERRF) is associated with a mitochondrial DNA t-RNA^{LYS} mutation. Cell, *61*:931–937, 1990.
95. Zheng, X. et al.: Evidence of a lethal infantile mitochondrial diseases for a nuclear mutation affecting respiratory complexes I and IV. Neurology, *39*:1203–1209, 1989.
96. Dalakas, M.C. et al.: Mitochondrial myopathy caused by long-term zidovudine therapy. N. Engl. J. Med., *322*:1098–1105, 1990.
97. Lowenstein, J.M., and Goodman, M.N.: The purine nucleotide cycle in muscle. Fed. Proc., *37*:2308–2312, 1978.
98. Fishbein, W.N., Armbrustmacher, V.W., and Griffen, J.L.: Myoadenylate deaminase deficiency: A new disease of muscle. Science, *200*:545–548, 1978.
99. Shumate, J.B. et al.: Myoadenylate deaminase deficiency. Muscle Nerve, *2*:213–216, 1981.
100. Kar, N.C., and Pearson, C.M.: Muscle adenylate deaminase deficiency. Arch. Neurol., *38*:279–281, 1981.
101. Fishbein, W.N.: Myoadenylate deaminase deficiency: Inherited and acquired forms. Biochem. Med., *33*:158–169, 1985.
102. Sabina, R.L., Swain, J.L., and Holmes, E.W.: Myoadenylate deaminse deficiency. *In* The Metabolic Basis of Inherited Disease. 6th ed. Edited by C. Scriver, A.L. Beaudet, W. Sly, and D. Valle. New York, McGraw-Hill Book Company, 1989, pp. 1077–1084.
103. Gross, M., Morisaki, H., Morisaki, T., and Holmes, E.: A common point mutation is responsible for AMP deaminase deficiency. Int. J. Purine Pyrimidine Res., *2*(Suppl.):50, 1991.
104. Sabina, R.L. et al.: Molecular analysis of the myoadenylate deaminase deficiencies. Neurology, (in press), 1991.
105. Sabina, R.L., Sulaiman, A.R., and Wortmann, R.L.: Molecular analysis of acquired myoadenylate deaminase deficiency in polymyositis (idiopathic inflammatory myopathy). Adv. Exp. Biol. Med., (in press), 1991.
106. Sabina, R.L. et al.: Disruption of the purine nucleotide cycle: A potential explanation for muscle dysfunction in myoadenylate deaminase deficiency. J. Clin. Invest. *66*:1419–1423, 1980.
107. Sinkeler, S.P.T. et al.: Ischaemic exercise test in myoadenylate deaminase deficiency and McArdle's disease: Measurement of plasma adenosine, inosine and hypoxanthine. Clin. Sci., *70*:399–401, 1986.
108. Fishbein, W.N., Griffen, J.L., and Armbrustmacher, V.M.: Stain for skeletal muscle adenylate deaminase: An effective tetrazolium stain for frozen biopsy specimens. Arch. Pathol. Lab. Med., *104*:482–486, 1980.
109. Knochel, J.P.: Neuromuscular manifestations of electrolyte disorders. Am. J. Med., *72*:521–535, 1982.
110. Goldberg, A.L., Tischler, M., DeMartino, G., and Griffith, G.: Hormonal regulation of protein degradation and synthesis in skeletal muscle. Fed. Proc., *39*:31–36, 1980.
111. Kagen, L.J.: Approach to the patient with myopathy. Bull. Rheum. Dis., *33*:1–8, 1983.
112. Hood, D., Van Lente, F., and Estes, M.: Serum enzyme alterations in chronic muscle disease. A biopsy-based diagnostic assessment. A.J.C.P., *95*:402–407, 1991.
113. Black, H.R., Quallich, H., and Gareleck, C.B.: Racial differences in serum creatine kinase levels. Am. J. Med., *81*:479–487, 1986.
114. Worrall, J.G., Phongsathorn, V., Hooper, R.J.L., and Paice, E.W.: Racial variation in serum creatine kinase unrelated to lean body mass. Br. J. Rheumatol., *29*:371–373, 1990.
115. Sinkeler, S.P.T. et al.: The relation between blood lactate and ammonia in ischemic handgrip exercise. Muscle Nerve, *8*:523–527, 1985.
116. Lamminen, A.E.: Magnetic resonance of diseased skeletal muscle: Combined T_1 measurement and chemical shift imaging. Br. J. Radiol., *63*:591–596, 1990.
117. Lamminen, A.E.: Magnetic resonance imaging of primary skeletal muscle diseases: Patterns of distribution and severity of involvement. Br. J. Radiol., *63*:946–950, 1990.
118. Ross, B.D. et al.: Examination of a case of suspected McArdle's syndrome by ^{31}P nuclear magnetic resonance. N. Engl. J. Med., *304*:1338–1342, 1981.
119. Chance, B. et al.: ^{31}P NMR studies of control of mitochondrial function in phosphofructokinase-deficiency human skeletal muscle. Proc. Natl. Acad. Sci. USA, *79*:7714–7718, 1982.
120. Matthews, P.M. et al.: In vivo muscle magnetic resonance spectroscopy in the clinical investigation of mitochondrial disease. Neurology, *41*:114–120, 1991.

112

Ochronosis, Hemochromatosis, and Wilson's Disease

H. RALPH SCHUMACHER, JR.

ALKAPTONURIA AND OCHRONOSIS

Alkaptonuria is a hereditary disorder characterized by homogentisic acid in the urine, which, when oxidized, imparts a brownish black color to the urine. The term *alkaptonuria,* denoting an avidity for oxygen in alkaline solution, was coined by Boedeker in 1859 and is derived from fusion of an Arabic word meaning "alkali" and a Greek word (*kaptein*), meaning "to suck up avidly." When the freshly passed urine is alkalinized, polymerization of homogentisic acid is accelerated, and the urine turns black. Ochronosis denotes a bluish black pigmentation of connective tissue in patients with alkaptonuria, usually apparent clinically in the cartilage of the ear, in the skin, and in the sclera. This term was originated by Virchow in 1866, who described the microscopic appearance of this pigmentation as "ochre" or dark yellow.

Alkaptonuria itself is a symptomless condition. Clinical signs and symptoms develop when pigment is deposited in cartilage and other connective tissues (ochronosis). The relationship between alkaptonuria and ochronosis was first recognized in 1902 by Albrecht. Table 112–1 lists factors in the diagnosis of these and related conditions.

HISTORY

The earliest clinical observation, that of a boy who passed dark urine, was made by Scribonius in 1584. Boedeker, in 1859, was the first to isolate homogentisic acid from the urine of a patient with alkaptonuria. Wolkow and Bauman in 1891 established the chemical structure of this compound as 2,5-dihydroxyphenylacetic acid and named it homogentisic acid. LaDu and his collaborators in 1958 demonstrated the absence of the enzyme homogentisic acid oxidase in the liver of a patient with alkaptonuria, ochronotic spondylosis, and peripheral arthropathy.[1]

NATURE OF THE BIOCHEMICAL LESION

Alkaptonuria is the result of a defect in the metabolic pathway for the aromatic amino acid tyrosine. Normally, the benzene ring of homogentisic acid is broken by the enzyme homogentisic acid oxidase, and maleylacetoacetic acid is formed. LaDu, et al. assayed liver homogenates from ochronotic patients and control subjects and demonstrated that the pattern of enzyme activities of the alkaptonuric liver was essentially the same as in the control liver, except with respect to homogentisic acid oxidase activity, which was completely missing in the alkaptonuric patient.[1] Of interest is the presence of the enzyme maleylacetoacetic acid isomerase in the alkaptonuric liver despite the apparent absence of the substrate maleylacetoacetic acid, which could be derived only from the metabolism of homogentisic acid. The presence of this enzyme in the absence of its substrate demonstrates that the genetic mechanism that controls the synthesis of this enzyme is not regulated by the substrate.

GENETIC FACTORS

Alkaptonuria is felt to be transmitted by a single recessive autosomal gene. The occasional occurrence of this disorder in successive generations of certain families may be the result of consanguineous marriages in which homozygotes mate with heterozygotes. The present concept of the mode of transmission of alkaptonuria,

TABLE 112–1. DIAGNOSTIC FEATURES OF ALKAPTONURIA, OCHRONOSIS, OCHRONOTIC SPONDYLITIS, AND PERIPHERAL ARTHROPATHY

ALKAPTONURIA
- Urine turns black:
  - On alkalinization
  - On standing
  - When tested for sugar by Benedict's reagent; in addition, yellow-orange precipitate forms
- Positive family history

OCHRONOSIS
- Pigmentation of cartilage and skin:
  - Pinna of ear, eardrum, and cerumen
  - Sclera
  - Skin over malar area, nose, axilla, groin
- Prostatic calculi

OCHRONOTIC SPONDYLOSIS
- Calcification and ossification of intervertebral discs
- Disproportionately little osteophytosis
- Sacroiliac joints not fused and no "bamboo" spine
- Loss of lumbar lordosis
- Spine rigid and stooped, knees flexed, stance typical

OCHRONOTIC PERIPHERAL ARTHROPATHY
- Knees, shoulders, and hips most commonly affected
- Synovial fluid contains small amounts of homogentisic acid and is noninflammatory, except with occasional calcium pyrophosphate crystal—associated inflammation
- Brittle cartilage fragments and pigmented "chards" in the synovium
- Osteochrondral joint bodies common
- Small joints of hands and feet usually not affected

originally advanced by Garrod, and challenged at times, has been substantiated by several careful family studies in which complete pedigrees were available.[2] One family had HLA-B27 in 8 of 10 members with alkaptonuria.[3]

LABORATORY ASPECTS OF ALKAPTONURIA

The freshly passed urine of an alkaptonuric patient is of normal color and does not darken at once unless it is alkaline or contains less than a normal concentration of vitamin C or other reducing agents. On standing, it may turn brownish black as the homogentisic acid becomes oxidized. If Benedict's reagent is used in testing the urine for sugar, the yellowish orange precipitate that is formed because homogentisic acid reduces the copper can be misinterpreted as indicating glucosuria. The color of the supernatant solution in these cases is always brownish black, which is diagnostic for alkaptonuria.

With the use of copper-reduction tablets (Clinitest), a black supernatant may also be seen in patients with malignant melanoma and after intravenous urography with sodium diatrizoate (Hypaque) and other x-ray contrast media.[4] Specific glucose oxidase tapes (Clinistix) may not detect urine glucose in diabetics with ochronosis because of interference with the peroxidase-indicator chromagen reaction by homogentisic acid.[5] Spuriously increased serum and urinary uric acid determinations have been described in ochronosis when colorimetric methods were used, but values were normal by the uricase spectrophotometric technique.[5] Homogentisic acid in the urine may also falsely elevate creatinine levels when measured by Jaffé's reaction.

DIAGNOSTIC TESTS FOR ALKAPTONURIA

Several presumptive, nonspecific tests for alkaptonuria are available. These tests are color reactions based on the reducing properties of homogentisic acid. Thus, in the Briggs tests, molybdate is reduced and a deep blue color is obtained. When a drop of urine is placed on photographic paper, a black spot indicates reduction of silver. When sodium hydroxide is added to the freshly passed urine, homogentisic acid is rapidly oxidized, and the urine properly darkens. A specific enzymatic method for quantitative determination of homogentisic acid in urine and blood has been developed.[6] Thin-layer chromatography can also be used.

PATHOLOGIC FEATURES OF OCHRONOSIS

The lesions of ochronosis result from the intercellular or intracellular deposition of pigment in many organs or structures. The exact chemical composition of the pigment has not yet been defined, although it is believed to be a polymer derived from homogentisic acid. Benzoquinoneacetic acid may be an intermediate compound that, when bound to connective tissue, may participate in a polymerization process leading to the final pigment formation.[7] Homogentisic acid is concentrated preferentially by connective tissue, but this process is reversible until after polymerization.[7] Homogentisic acid has been shown to inhibit hydroxylysine formation in vitro.[8] The predilection of ochronosis for cartilage that contains hydroxylysine-rich collagen may be in part related to this. Recent studies have documented the deleterious effect of homogentisic acid on cultured chondrocytes.[9] The typical pathologic findings include granules of insoluble, melanin-like pigment, which are usually found in the skin and subcutis, the cartilage of joints, the intervertebral discs, including the anulus fibrosus as well as the nucleus pulposus, the tracheal cartilages, the epithelial cells of the renal tubules, and the islets of the pancreas. Pigment granules impregnate the walls of large and medium-sized arteries and arterioles, including the aorta and the pulmonary, coronary, and renal arteries.

CLINICAL PICTURE OF OCHRONOSIS

Patients with alkaptonuria who live to the fourth decade almost invariably develop ochronosis. The cartilage of the ear, especially the concha and anthelix, is frequently involved and takes on a slate blue discoloration while becoming irregularly thickened and inflexible. When the pinna is transilluminated, the opaque pigmented area stands out prominently. The cerumen in the external canal is often black, and the periphery of the tympanic membrane is grayish black. Many patients with long-standing ochronosis have impaired hearing. Pigmentation of the sclera is usually localized to a small area midway between the limbus of the cornea and the inner or outer canthus. The skin over the malar areas, nose, axilla, and groin is often pigmented.

Deposition of pigment in the intervertebral discs and articular cartilages of the large joints leads to spondylosis and peripheral arthropathy.

Loud cardiac murmurs, mostly systolic, have been noted in about 15 to 20% of patients with ochronosis.[10] Pigment deposits in the mitral and aortic valves may be associated with deformity of the leaflets or cusps. Clinically significant aortic stenosis has been successfully treated by aortic valve replacement.[11]

Prostatic calculi occur in a large proportion of men with ochronosis and are readily palpable on rectal examination. Dysuria and frequency of urination may be present, and a prostatic operation may be necessary. Calculi may be passed spontaneously or removed surgically. These calculi have a characteristic black color and contain ochronotic pigment and calcium phosphate salts.

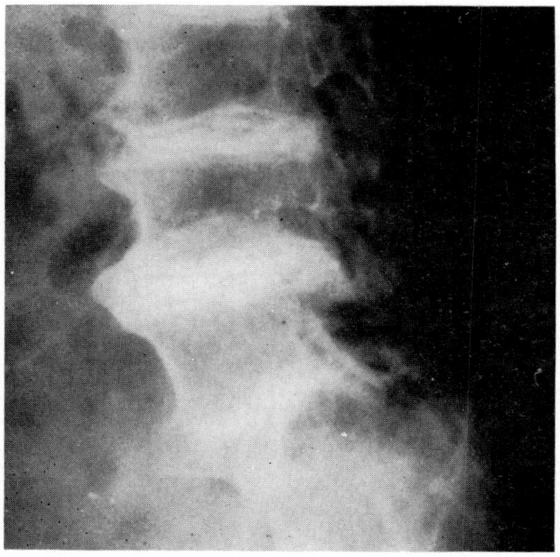

FIGURE 112–1. Roentgenogram of the lumbar spine of a 55-year-old man with ochronotic spondylosis. Note the calcification of intervertebral discs. The osteophytes are of only moderate size.

OCHRONOTIC SPONDYLOSIS

The majority of patients with ochronosis past the age of 30 develop spondylosis. Symptoms usually consist of stiffness and discomfort in the lower back. In about 10 to 15% of patients with ochronosis, the onset of spondylosis occurs with herniation of a nucleus pulposus.[10] In such instances, the symptoms and signs are indistinguishable from those in typical cases of herniated disc without alkaptonuria. The earliest site of spondylosis is the lumbar spine; years later, the dorsal and finally the cervical spine become involved. Stiffness of the lower back slowly progresses to rigidity and obliteration of normal lumbar lordosis. In many cases, lumbar kyphosis develops. Symptoms may be minimal despite prominent roentgenographic changes.

The earliest change apparent in roentgenograms of the spine consists of a wafer of calcification, and actual ossification, in the intervertebral disc of the lumbar spine (Fig. 112–1). Crystallographic study has shown the calcium in these discs to be hydroxyapatite.[12] Radiographic evidence of calcified intervertebral discs in adults is characteristic of ochronosis, but it is not diagnostic because similar changes can also be seen in pseudogout, in hemochromatosis, in chronic respiratory paralytic poliomyelitis, in spinal fusion of any origin, and occasionally in other disorders or without detectable associated disease. Secondary narrowing of the intervertebral spaces occurs. Osteophytes are usually small. Splits in disc material appear to account for radiolucencies in the discs that have been termed "vacuum discs."[13] In contrast to ankylosing spondylitis, the sacroiliac joints in ochronotic spondylosis are not fused, although they may show degenerative changes, the interfacetal articulations retain a normal radiographic appearance, and annular ossification with a "bamboo" pattern does not appear. The marked narrowing of multiple intervertebral spaces results in a loss of several inches in height. The spinal deformity and forward stoop cause the patient to stand with knees flexed and on a broad base. This posture imparts to the patient with ochronotic spondylosis a stance and gait similar to that of a patient with ankylosing spondylitis (Fig. 112–2).

OCHRONOTIC PERIPHERAL ARTHROPATHY

A degenerative arthritis of the peripheral joints also occurs, although it is less frequent and develops later than spondylosis. The joints most commonly affected are the knees, shoulders, and hips, in descending order of frequency. The knees are involved in the majority of cases of peripheral arthritis. Pain, stiffness, crepitation, flexion contractures, and limitation of motion are the most common features. In the peripheral joints, symptoms often antedate any visible roentgenographic changes. Effusion occurs in about half these cases. Synovial fluid is generally clear, viscous, and yellow, without darkening on exposure to alkali. Although homogentisic acid can be demonstrated, its concentration is much lower than in the urine. Occasionally, black specks of ochronotic cartilage are seen floating in the fluid.[14,15] Leukocyte counts in a large series by Huttl ranged from 112 to 700/mm^3 with predominantly mononuclear cells.[16] Occasional cells have dark inclusions that appear to be phagocytized cartilage containing ochronotic pigment (Fig. 112–3). Synovial effusions or membrane can contain calcium pyrophosphate crystals without inflammation,[15–18] or the patient may have typical acute episodes of pseudogout with increased synovial fluid leukocyte counts.[19]

Pigmentation of the articular cartilage occurs initially in the deeper layers, with relative sparing of the surface.

It is seen predominantly in the matrix of the tangential zone but also in chondrocytes. Necrosis of chondrocytes occurs. Pigment appears by electron microscopy to be associated with the surface of collagen fibers in cartilage but not in synovium.[17,20] The pigmented articular cartilage is brittle; minute fragments are broken off and are displaced into the synovial tissue (Fig. 112–4). Shards can be phagocytized[21] and may evoke a foreign-body reaction and new formation of bone tissue called *osteochondral bodies* (Fig. 112–5).[22] These bodies may be sev-

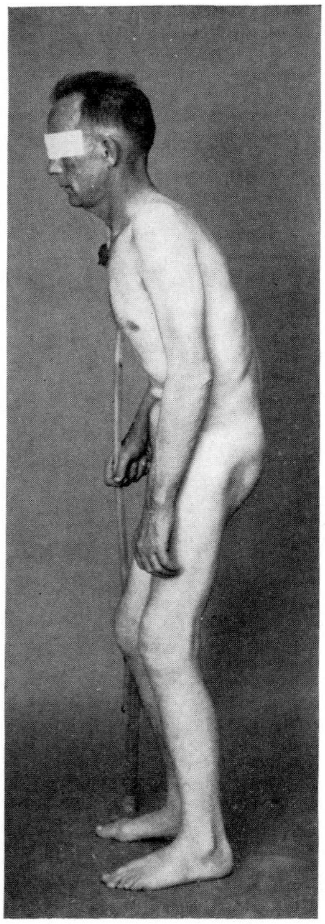

FIGURE 112–2. Typical posture and stance of a patient with ochronotic spondylosis: forward stoop, loss of lumbar lordosis, flexed hips and knees, wide-based stance. This 40-year-old man lost 6 inches in height.

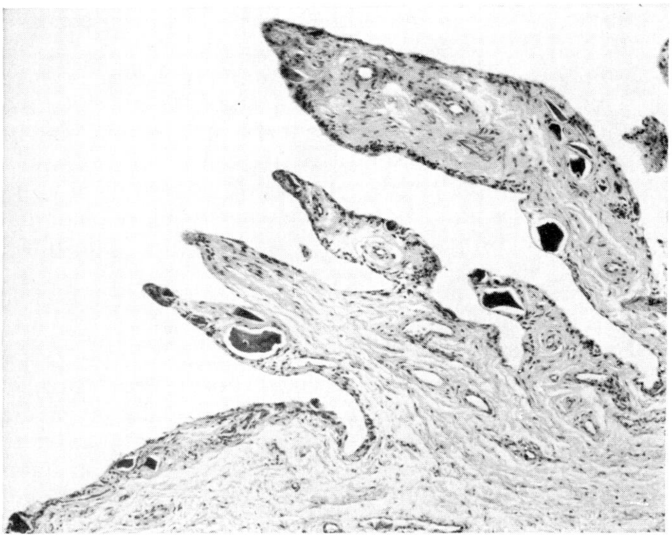

FIGURE 112–4. Synovial tissue in ochronotic arthropathy. Minute fragments of darkly pigmented cartilage lie within the superficial portion of the tissue. The sharp edges of the "shards" are characteristic. A foreign-body cell reaction is present at the margins of a few and is accompanied by mild synovial fibrosis. Associated infiltration of lymphocytes and plasma cells may also be present (hematoxylin and eosin stain ×90).

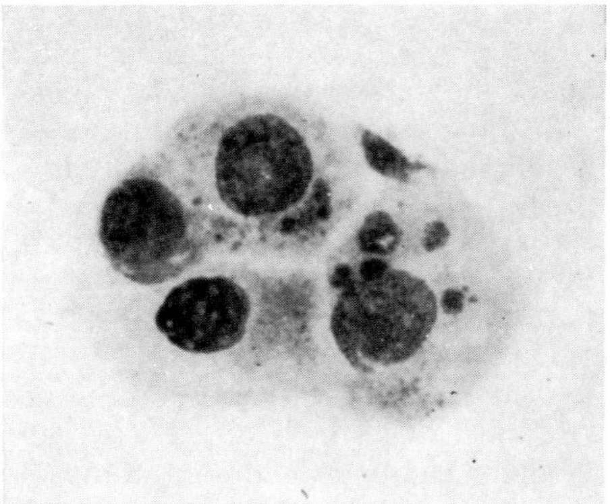

FIGURE 112–3. Synovial fluid mononuclear cells in ochronotic arthropathy. The dark cytoplasmic inclusions appear to be phagocytized pigmented debris (Giemsa stain ×1250). (Courtesy of S. Huttl and Acta Rheum. Baln. Pistiniana.)

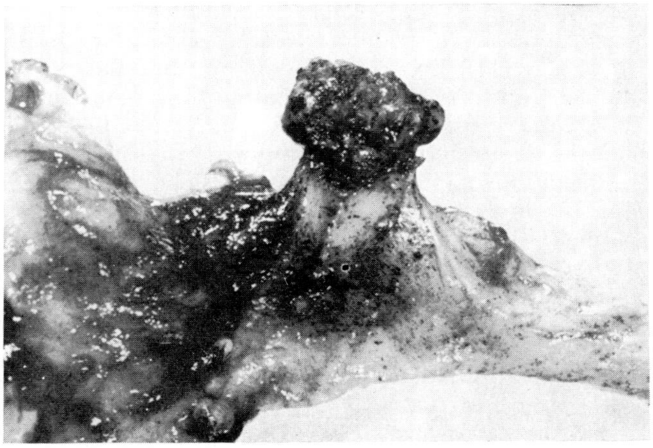

FIGURE 112–5. Synovial tissue in ochronotic arthropathy. Numerous pigmented deposits are present. A polypoid nodule has formed in the central portion as an osteochondroid reaction of the displaced cartilage fragments.

eral centimeters in diameter and are readily palpable in and around the knee joint. They are often not tender and may be freely movable. Surgical removal may be necessary when the bodies interfere with motion.

The radiographic appearance of the large peripheral joints in ochronotic arthritis, virtually indistinguishable from that of primary osteoarthritis, demonstrates narrowing of the joint space, small marginal osteophytes, and eburnation. Rarely the diagnosis is first suggested at knee arthroscopy or surgery when the black pigmentation is encountered unexpectedly.[23] Protrusio acetabuli may be seen.[17] Ossification or calcification of the ligaments and tendons near the joints may be present.[24] Rupture of deeply pigmented ochronotic Achilles tendons has been reported.

In contrast to rheumatoid arthritis (RA) and osteoarthritis, the small joints of the hands and feet are rarely affected in ochronosis.

EXPERIMENTAL AND NONALKAPTONURIC PRODUCTION OF OCHRONOSIS

Rats fed with 8% L-tyrosine for 18 to 24 months develop pigment deposition in joint capsules and cartilages and a degenerative arthritis similar to that of spontaneous human alkaptonuria.[25] The cartilage pigment is melanin-like and includes phenolic bodies as in homogentisic acid or its metabolite benzoquinoneacetic acid.

A grossly bluish black connective tissue pigmentation associated with degenerative arthritis has also been described following prolonged administration of quinacrine in the absence of alkaptonuria. Ochronosis-like skin pigmentation attributed to enormous elastotic fibers has occurred in some blacks using hydroquinone bleaching creams.[26] Application of phenol dressings has been reported to produce ochronosis with alkaptonuria and arthropathy. Cartilage pigmentation does not occur in metastatic malignant melanoma.

TREATMENT

It is not yet feasible to use gene therapy or to compensate for the enzymatic deficiency of homogentisic acid oxidase. Attempts have been made to treat patients with a diet low in phenylalanine and tyrosine that is, unfortunately, unpalatable. Urinary excretion of homogentisic acid can be decreased, but clinical change was minimal in patients with advanced joint disease. Initiation of this diet at an early age before massive ochronosis develops has not been tried. Reduced protein intake can also decrease urine homogentisic acid levels, but this regimen is impractical for routine treatment. Although high doses of ascorbic acid do not decrease total urine homogentisic acid levels, they have been reported to reduce binding to connective tissue in experimental alkaptonuria of rats and to reverse homogentisic acid-induced chondrocyte growth inhibition in vitro.[27] Despite this, long-term use of ascorbic acid has not been useful in limited trials in human ochronosis.

Symptomatic measures are of most practical value. Analgesics, braces, a program limiting joint overuse, and weight reduction have all provided some help. Adrenal corticosteroids, x irradiation, tyrosinase, insulin, various vitamins, and phenylbutazone are among the measures tried without benefit. Total joint replacements have been successful at hips and knees.[28]

HEMOCHROMATOSIS

Hemochromatosis is a chronic disease first recognized by Trousseau in 1865 and characterized pathologically by excessive iron deposition and fibrosis in many organs and tissues with ultimate functional impairment in untreated patients. This disorder occurs in a clinically detectable form in at least 1 in 7000 people in various populations of European origin. Clinical disease occurs five times more often in men than in women. Frequent clinical manifestations are hepatomegaly and cirrhosis, skin pigmentation, mostly from increased melanin, diabetes, other endocrine dysfunction, and heart failure.[29,30] Sicca syndrome has been reported, possibly adding to confusion with other rheumatic diseases.[31] Arthropathy occurs in 20 to 40% of patients. Hemochromatosis is often idiopathic, with a definite increased familial incidence first recognized by Sheldon in 1935.[30] It is inherited as an autosomal recessive trait. That patients have an increased frequency of HLA-A3 and HLA-B7 or HLA-B14 antigens suggests a hemochromatosis locus tightly linked to the HLA region on chromosome 6.[32] Because HLA haplotypes linked to the hemochromatosis alleles differ from family to family, HLA typing is best used after an index case has been identified in a family. Hemochromatosis can also be a late result of alcoholic cirrhosis or occasionally of multiple transfusions, refractory anemia, and long-term excessive oral iron ingestion. In all instances, iron absorption is excessive. Significant overload occurs only after many years, so the onset of symptoms is most common between 40 and 60 years. A form of hemochromatosis occurring before age 30 is often associated with hypogonadism and cardiac involvement. This is not obviously familial but may be associated with arthropathy as occurs in older patients.[33] Tables 112–2 and 112–3 list diagnostic features of hemochromatosis and its related arthropathy.

TABLE 112–2. DIAGNOSTIC FEATURES OF HEMOCHROMATOSIS

Cirrhosis with iron deposition, predominantly in parenchymal cells
Iron deposition in other organs causing cardiomyopathy, diabetes, or other endocrine deficiencies
Increased skin pigmentation, largely by melanin
Elevated serum iron concentration and saturated iron-binding capacity

TABLE 112–3. DIAGNOSTIC FEATURES OF ARTHROPATHY OF HEMOCHROMATOSIS

Degenerative arthropathy
Prominent involvement of metacarpophalangeal and proximal and distal interphalangeal joints, hips, and knees
Chondrocalcinosis
Iron deposition in synovial lining cells

PATHOLOGIC FEATURES AND PATHOGENESIS

Iron as hemosiderin can be identified histologically in all the symptomatically affected tissues, as well as elsewhere. The largest iron deposits are in the liver, and diagnosis is most frequently established by liver biopsy. Large amounts of hemosiderin are seen in parenchymal cells in the liver and in other organs. Iron confined to reticuloendothelial tissues is termed *hemosiderosis* and does not produce the clinical picture seen in hemochromatosis. Although suspected, the iron has not been proved to be the cause of the tissue damage. Organ fibrosis, as in hemochromatosis, has not yet been produced by experimental iron overload alone. Iron may act in an additive fashion with nutritional deficiencies, alcohol, or other, still unidentified, hereditary factors.

DIAGNOSIS

The most important simple diagnostic laboratory tests is the determination of serum iron concentration and the percentage of saturation of iron-binding capacity. Both values are elevated in hemochromatosis, but they can also be elevated in hemolytic anemia and other situations. Greater than 50% saturation of iron-binding capacity should raise consideration of hemochromatosis. Serum ferritin concentrations are often elevated but may be normal in precirrhotic disease.[34] Magnetic resonance imaging showing reduced signal intensity can suggest liver iron overload.[35] Liver biopsy is needed to determine the extent of tissue iron deposition and the degree of tissue damage. One case of hemochromatosis with associated hypoxanthine-guanine phosphoribosyltransferase deficiency has been recorded where serum-iron concentrations and transferrin saturation were normal.[36]

OSTEOPENIA

Diffuse demineralization of bone can be seen, but its frequency and relationship to the hemochromatosis are difficult to ascertain. A diffuse osteopenia of the hands, without the periarticular demineralization as seen in RA, is most common. Hypogonadism is probably an important contributing factor.[37] Serum calcium, phosphorus, and alkaline phosphatase levels are normal. Biopsy specimens have shown osteoporosis rather than osteomalacia. Experimental acute iron overload can produce iron deposits in osteoblasts and trabeculae with decreased osteoblast numbers and activity.[38] Because osteopenia is also seen in alcoholic cirrhosis, a direct relation to the defect in iron metabolism is not always necessary.

DEGENERATIVE ARTHROPATHY AND CHONDROCALCINOSIS

An arthropathy associated with hemochromatosis was first described in 1964,[39] and since then more than 300 cases have been reported.[40–44] The most frequent joint involvement is degenerative, occurring in 20 to 50% of patients with hemochromatosis.[42] The age of onset varies from 20 to 70, but it is most common in the sixth decade. The onset of arthropathy is usually close in time to the onset of other symptoms of hemochromatosis, but joint symptoms and findings may antedate other clinical manifestations of hemochromatosis and may thus be the first clue to diagnosis.[41,45] Joint symptoms occasionally are first noted many years later, even after completion of phlebotomy therapy.

Hands, knees, and hips are most frequently involved, although other joints including the feet can be affected. Characteristic hand findings are a firm, only mildly tender, enlargement of the metacarpophalangeal and the proximal and distal interphalangeal joints. The second and third metacarpophalangeal joints are most often affected (Fig. 112–6). These joints are stiff and have limited motion but no increased warmth or erythema. Ulnar deviation is not seen. Involvement is generally symmetric. Pain, when present, is accentuated on use. Morning stiffness usually lasts less than half an hour. This arthropathy is gradually progressive. Acute inflammation has occasionally been described, and whether it is always due to associated chondrocalcinosis and crystal-induced synovitis is not certain. Test results for rheumatoid factor are typically negative. Sedimentation rates are only occasionally elevated. Serum uric acid levels are generally normal and occasionally low.[36]

Roentgenograms often show the characteristic involvement of the metacarpophalangeal, proximal, and distal interphalangeal joints. Narrowing of the joint space, subchondral cysts, joint-space irregularity, subchondral sclerosis, and moderate bony proliferation with frequent hook-like osteophytes are seen[39,46] (Fig. 112–7). In 30 to 60% of those with arthropathy, especially older patients, chondrocalcinosis is also seen. Roentgenograms of other joints show changes similar to those in the hands and are often indistinguishable from degenerative arthritis and idiopathic chondrocalcinosis. Involvement of metacarpophalangeal joints 4 and 5 is rare in idiopathic chondrocalcinosis and is most suggestive of underlying hemochromatosis.

Synovial fluid is usually noninflammatory, with low leukocyte counts and predominantly mononuclear cells, adequate viscosity, and a pale yellow color. Iron measurements on synovial fluid are comparable to serum levels.[43] Synovial tissue shows a striking deposition of iron, mostly in the synovial lining cells, but also in some deeper cells. On hematoxylin and eosin stain-

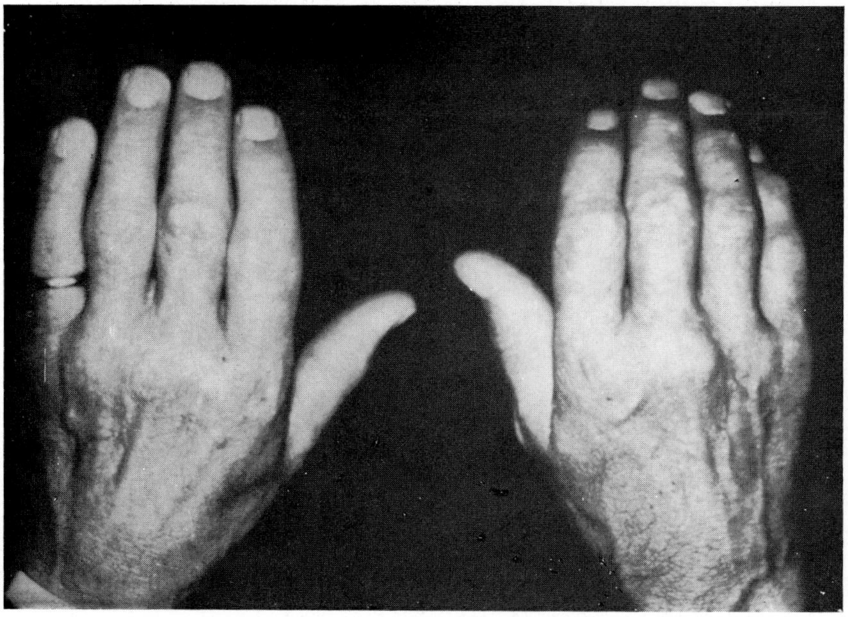

FIGURE 112–6. Photograph of the hands of a 45-year-old man with hemochromatosis. Note the knobby enlargement at the metacarpophalangeal, proximal interphalangeal, and distal interphalangeal joints. He is unable to extend these joints fully.

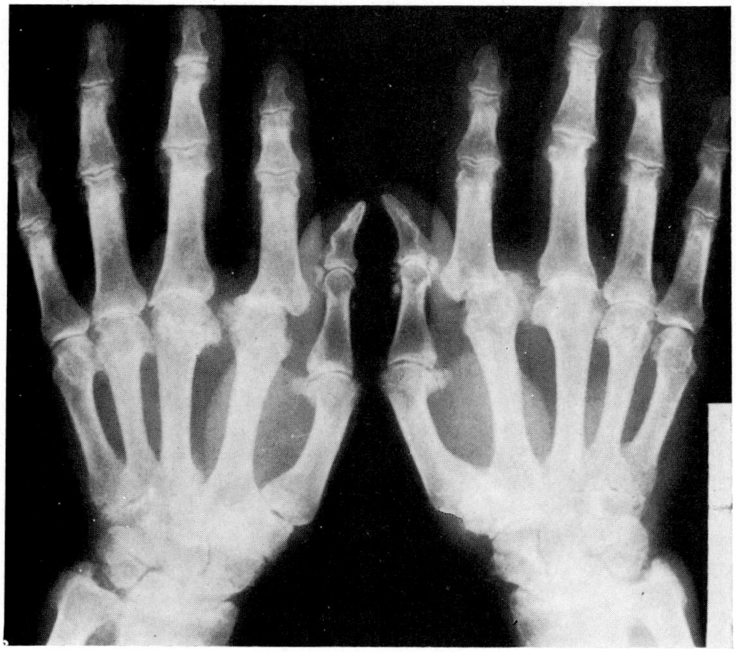

FIGURE 112–7. Roentgenogram of hands showing involvement of the metacarpophalangeal and the proximal and distal interphalangeal joints, with characteristic joint-space narrowing, cystic subchondral lesions, joint-space irregularity, subluxation, some osteophytosis, and areas of bony sclerosis. Multiple periarticular calcifications are also present in the interphalangeal joint of the left thumb, and probable chondrocalcinosis is seen at the right ulnocarpal joint. Osteopenia is minimal in these hands.

ing, golden brown hemosiderin granules are seen. The iron can also be stained blue by Prussian blue (Fig. 112–8). By electron microscopy, the iron is principally seen in type B or synthetic lining cells (Fig. 112–9).[47] This distribution of synovial iron differs from that in hemarthrosis, RA, and other diseases in which iron is presumably derived from gross or microscopic bleeding into the joint. In these conditions, the iron is mostly found in deeper cells and macrophages. In addition to the iron, most synovial membranes in hemochromatosis show only mild lining-cell proliferation, fibrosis, and scattered chronic inflammatory cells. Biopsies of synovium during bouts of acute inflammation have not been reported.

Chondrocalcinosis with hemochromatosis, although usually associated with degenerative arthropathy, can also be an isolated joint finding.[45] Calcification is most commonly detected in menisci and articular cartilages at the knee, but it can also be seen at the wrists, fingers, elbows, shoulders, hips, ankles, toes, symphysis pubis,

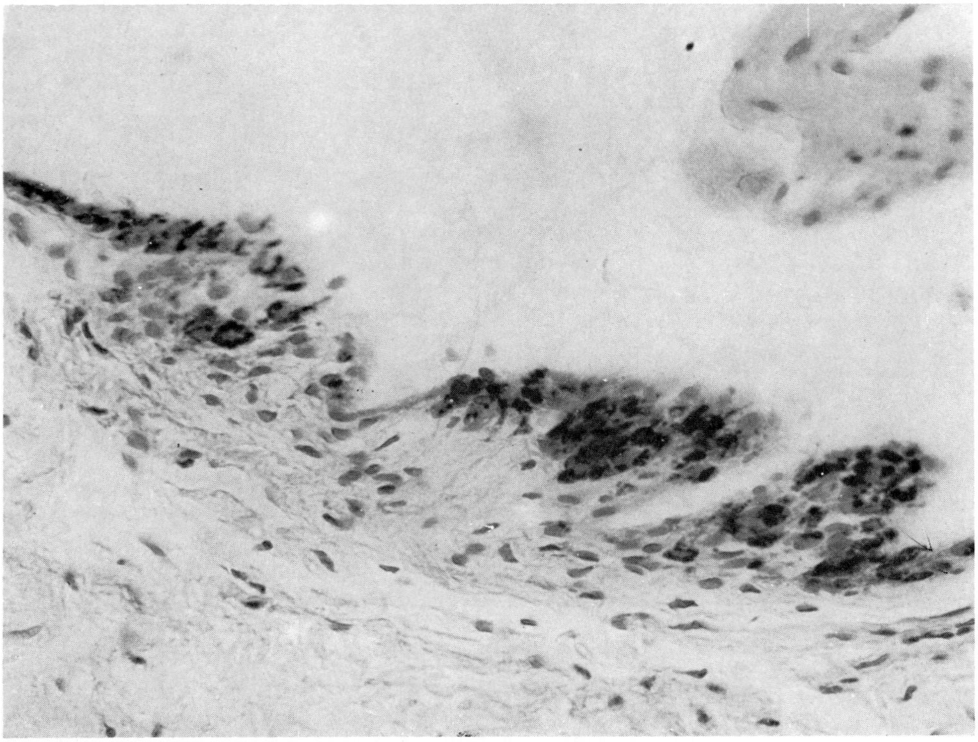

FIGURE 112–8. Synovium in hemochromatosis with dark Prussian blue—stained iron granules in the synovial lining cells (×400).

intervertebral discs, and the periarticular soft tissues and bursae.

Iron staining of cartilage has also been noted, but this characteristic is seen in chondrocytes and at the line of ossification, not at the crystal deposits.[47,48] Similarly, x-ray diffraction and chemical studies have shown no iron at the sites of cartilage calcification.[42,48] Periarticular and bursal calcifications have not been studied to determine the type of calcium salt. Crystals resembling hydroxyapatite have been identified in hemochromatotic synovium and cartilage by electron microscopy.[47,48] Even when no calcification is radiographically visible, cartilage calcium pyrophosphate crystals or apatite are often identifiable by light and electron microscopy.[48]

POSSIBLE MECHANISMS FOR ARTHROPATHY

It is attractive to speculate that the iron directly or indirectly causes the osteoarthropathy, but such has not been demonstrated. Arthropathy has only occasionally been reported in patients with transfusion siderosis;[49,50] this finding suggests that factors other than iron deposition are required. Patients with spherocytosis appear to develop iron overload only when they are also heterozygous for the hemochromatosis gene.[51] Many patients with iron-loading anemias do not survive long enough to develop tissue damage. Aseptic necrosis and osteopenia, but no other arthropathy, have been reported so far in Bantu siderosis. That experimental iron loading of rabbits produces cartilage degeneration only when initiated early in life suggests the importance of early initiation of the toxic effect of iron.[52] Localized predominantly in synthetic-type cells in cartilage or synovium, iron might cause joint damage by altering the protein polysaccharide or collagen produced by such cells. Iron can injure chondrocytes or other cells by lipid peroxidation of membranes. Several possible ways that iron or transferrin saturation can affect the immune system have been reviewed.[53] Ferric ion can irreversibly oxidize ascorbic acid and can impair hydroxylation of proline and thus allow deficient collagen formation.[52] Iron might produce damage by binding to connective tissue protein polysaccharides as it does in vitro in the Hale stain for protein polysaccharide. Some iron is present in lysosomes, and it could increase the release of lysosomal enzymes.

Iron in vitro inhibits pyrophosphatase and might in this manner help to allow the deposition of the calcium pyrophosphate of chondrocalcinosis.[54] Experimental synovial siderosis also inhibited clearance of calcium pyrophosphate crystals from rabbit joints.[55] The primary site of joint damage is not established. The cartilage is most suspect in this degenerative process, but subchondral bone or synovial involvement may also be important because cartilage depends on both these areas for nutrition. No correlation has been found between the presence of advanced liver disease, general-

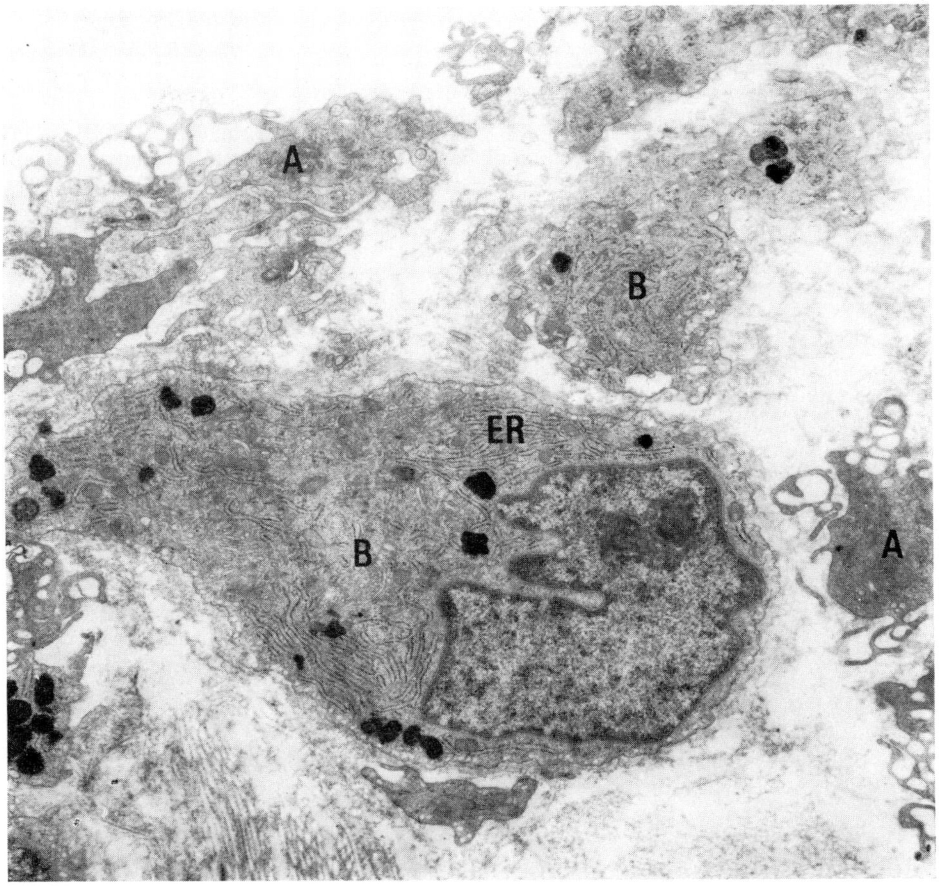

FIGURE 112–9. Electron micrograph of electron-dense iron deposits in Type B synovial lining cells (B) in hemochromatosis. Type-B cells are primarily synthetic in function and have profuse rough endoplasmic reticulum (ER). The type-A cells (A) often have prominent filopodia and vacuoles and are believed to be more active in phagocytosis. Here they contain no identifiable iron (× 13,000).

ized osteopenia, diabetes, or other endrocrine disease and the arthropathy. Classic RA has been reported to coexist in several cases, so the arthropathy is not an iron-altered rheumatoid disease.

TREATMENT

Present therapy of hemochromatosis is directed at prompt removal of the excess iron by phlebotomy, and this approach appears to reverse cardiac failure, to improve liver function, and to ameliorate diabetes. Improvement depends largely on the amount of existing tissue damage. Prevention certainly would be preferable, so serum iron concentrations of relatives should be checked, and prophylactic phlebotomy should be considered. Phlebotomy of 450 mL per week, until the development of mild iron deficiency anemia or demonstrable depletion of liver iron, is usual. Maintenance phlebotomy every 2 to 3 months is usually needed. Alcohol and excessive vitamin C ingestion can increase iron absorption and should be avoided. Supportive treatment of the diabetes, liver disease, and heart failure is pursued as needed. Phlebotomy has not had any beneficial effect on the arthritis; arthritis and chondrocalcinosis may progress[42] and clinical arthritis has even developed after therapeutic phlebotomy. One recent in vitro study showed that ferrous iron inhibited de novo formation of calcium pyrophosphate crystals and suggested that depletion of ferrous ions by phlebotomy could remove an inhibitor of calcium pyrophosphate crystal formation.[56] Irreversible connective tissue and joint change may well become established long before arthritis can be clinically or radiographically detected. Treatment of the arthritis is symptomatic; analgesics, nonsteroidal anti-inflammatory drugs, and systematic range-of-motion exercises are most helpful. Prosthetic hip and knee arthroplasties have been successfully performed in patients with advanced disease, although further breakdown after 18 months has occurred in a knee after prosthetic arthroplasty.

WILSON'S DISEASE

Hepatolenticular degeneration (Wilson's disease), described by Wilson in 1912,[57] is an uncommon familial disease characterized by a ring of golden brown pigment at the corneal margin, known as the Kayser-Fleischer ring, sometimes visible only on slit-lamp examination, basal ganglion degeneration, and cirrhosis. The condition is inherited as an autosomal recessive trait. Symptoms may first appear between the ages of 4 and 50.

TABLE 112–4. BONE AND JOINT CHANGES IN WILSON'S DISEASE

Bone demineralization
Occasionally, rickets or osteomalacia attributable to renal tubular disease
Premature degenerative arthritis with prominent subchondral bone fragmentation
Prominent involvement of wrists, knees, and, less often, other joints
Periarticular calcifications and bone fragments

Neurologic symptoms are usually earliest and include tremor, rigidity, dysarthria, incoordination, or personality change. Liver involvement can mimic chronic hepatitis or can cause fulminant hepatic failure. Many patients also develop renal tubular disease manifested by aminoaciduria, proteinuria, glucosuria, renal stones, phosphaturia, defective urine acidification, or uricosuria. Uricosuria often results in low serum uric acid levels. Hemolytic anemia can occur. Untreated disease is invariably fatal.[58]

Characteristic disorders of copper metabolism are present.[59] Copper concentrations are increased in liver, brain, and other tissues; urine copper excretion is increased; and the serum copper-binding protein, ceruloplasmin, as well as total serum copper are almost always decreased. Measurement of the hepatic copper concentration appears to be the most reliable test. Although the basic underlying defect is not known, increased absorption of copper can be demonstrated. Copper may cause the tissue damage. Mobilization of copper from the body seems to produce an improvement in many patients. Although seen in at least 95% of patients, Kayser-Fleischer rings are not entirely specific and may be seen in other diseases.[60] Table 112–4 lists osseous and articular changes in Wilson's disease.

OSTEOPENIA

Radiographic evidence of demineralization of bone has long been recognized as part of Wilson's disease and is described in 25 to 50% of patients.[61,62] Osteopenia is seen at all ages and usually is asymptomatic. Occasional patients have pathologic fractures. Others have definite rickets,[63] or osteomalacia that can be attributed to the renal tubular disease.

ARTHROPATHY

Boudin, et al. first described articular alterations in Wilson's disease in 1957.[64] Joint changes are rare in childhood but are seen in up to 50% of adults. Most patients studied have been 20 to 40 years old. Articular involvement ranges from premature osteoarthritis with pronounced symptoms to asymptomatic radiographic findings.[61,62,65–69] Scattered subchondral bone fragmentations, cortical irregularity, and sclerosis at the margin of wrist, hand, elbow, shoulder, hip, and knee joints are seen (Fig. 112–10). The cartilage space is also often narrowed. Early age of onset and prominent involvement of wrists suggest a difference from the usual osteoarthritis. Tiny periarticular cysts,[62] vertebral wedging and marginal irregularity,[69] osteochrondritis dissecans, and chondromalacia patellae[65] have been seen in several patients and may be related to Wilson's disease. Periarticular calcifications are common; many such calcifications occur in ligaments, tendons, and capsule insertions. Other calcifications seem to represent bone fragments. There is occasional radiographic evidence of chondrocalcinosis.[65,66,69] The cause of the chondrocalcinosis has not been well studied. Although copper could be identified in some cartilages by elemental analysis, calcium crystals were not found in one recent light and electron microscopic study.[68] Calcium pyrophosphate crystals were reported earlier in an intervertebral disc.[69a] Joint effusions are usually small, with clear, viscous fluid and 200 to 300 cells/mm^3, predominantly mononuclear cells.[65,67] Synovial fluid copper and ceruloplasmin levels have not been studied. Only mild lining-cell hyperplasia and small numbers of chronic inflammatory cells have been noted on synovial biopsies.[67]

No correlation has been found between the severity of the disease, spasticity and tremors, osteopenia, liver or renal disease and the arthropathy. The primary defect may occur in the cartilage or subchondral bone, but no histologic or chemical studies of these tissues have been conducted. Although the joint involvement in Wilson's disease is generally milder, an analogy can be made with that of hemochromatosis. In both diseases, the metal excess is a possible mechanism for direct or indirect production of the arthropathy. Short-term experimental copper loading has not produced arthropathy. McCarty and Pepe have shown in vitro inhibition of inorganic cytosolic pyrophosphatase by cupric as well as by ferrous ions and have suggested this inhibition as a possible mechanism for deposition of calcium pyrophosphate producing chondrocalcinosis in Wilson's disease and hemochromatosis.[54]

TREATMENT

Penicillamine, 1 to 4 g/day orally, is the most successful chelating agent for mobilizing copper from the tissue and has produced definite clinical improvement in mental and neurologic changes in many patients. Treatment must be continued for life. Low-copper diets and potassium sulfide may also be used to decrease copper absorption. Symptomatic disease may be preventable by early D-penicillamine treatment of asymptomatic persons with biochemical abnormalities only.[70] Occasional patients treated with penicillamine still develop arthropathy. Whether early and long-term treatment will decrease the bone and joint disease is not yet known. Occasionally, penicillamine appears to cause polymyositis or lupus-like syndromes. Acute polyarthritis complicated penicillamine therapy in five patients with Wilson's disease.[66] There is some

FIGURE 112–10. Arthropathy in a 30-year-old woman with Wilson's disease. *A,* Wrist. Note the bony ossicles (*arrow*) suggested to be a result of cortical fragmentation. Some sclerosis is also present at the distal radius. *B,* Knee. Ossicles are seen near the tibiofibular articulation. Significant chondromalacia patellae with spurs is present on the posterior surface of the patella. The articular cortex of the lateral femoral condyle is irregular, with a suggestion of fragmentation (*arrow*).

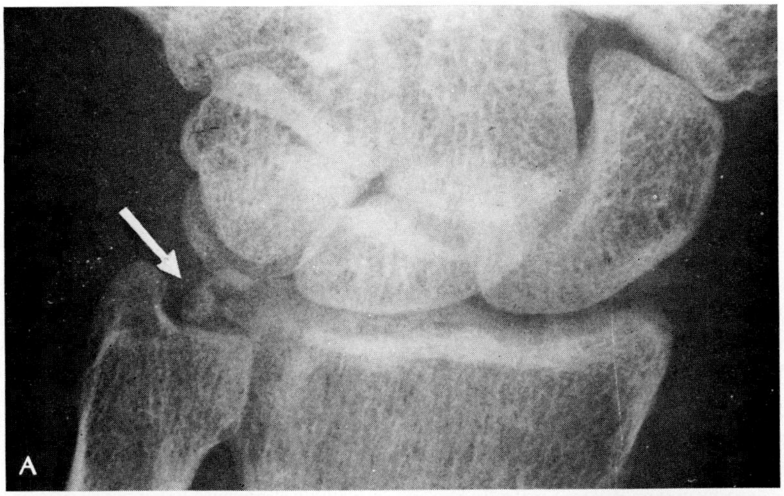

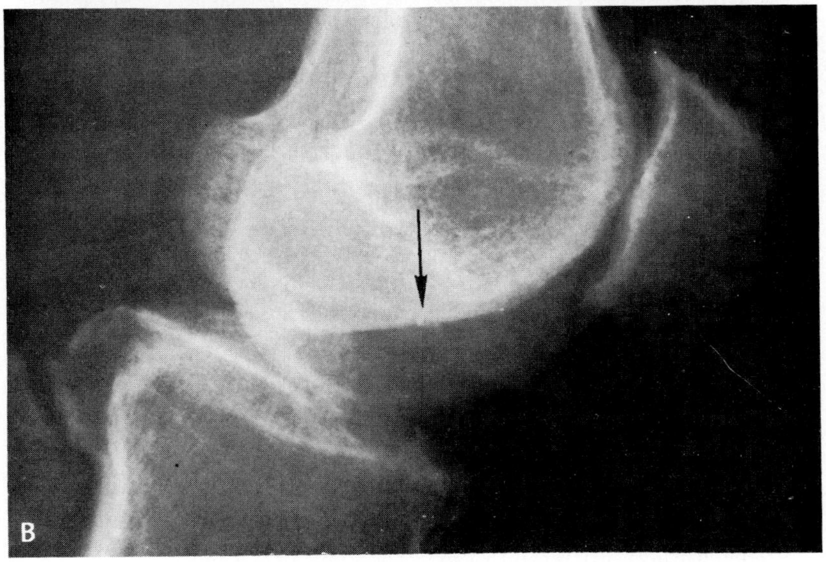

controversy about the safety of penicillamine in pregnancy.[71,72] Zinc[73] trientine, a newer chelating agent,[72] or tetrathiomolybdate[74] may be considered as alternative therapies in patients who cannot tolerate penicillamine. Liver transplants have been used successfully.

REFERENCES

1. LeDu, B.N., Zannoni, V.G., Laster, L., and Seegmiller, J.E.: The nature of the defect in tyrosine metabolism in alcaptonuria. J. Biol. Chem., *230*:251–260, 1958.
2. Knox, W.E.: Sir Archibald Garrod's inborn errors of metabolism. II. Alkaptonuria. Am. J. Hum. Genet., *10*:95–124, 1958.
3. Gaucher, A. et al.: HLA antigens and alkaptonuria. J. Rheumatol., *3*(Suppl.):97–100, 1977.
4. Lee, S., and Schoen, I.: Black copper reduction reaction simulating alkaptonuria—occurrence after intravenous urography. N. Engl. J. Med., *275*:266–267, 1966.
5. Kelley, W.N. et al.: Significant laboratory artifacts in alkaptonuria. Arthritis Rheum., *12*:673, 1969.
6. Seegmiller, J.E. et al.: An enzymatic spectrophotometric method for the determination of homogentisic acid in plasma and urine. J. Biol. Chem., *236*:774–777, 1961.
7. Zannoni, V.G., Malawista, S.E., and LaDu, B.N.: Studies on ochronosis. II. Studies on benzoquinoneacetic acid, a probable intermediate in the connective tissue pigmentation of alcaptonuria. Arthritis Rheum., *5*:547–556, 1962.
8. Murray, J.C., Lindberg, K.A., and Pinnell, S.R.: In vitro inhibition of chick embryo lysyl hydroxylase by homogentisic acid. J. Clin. Invest., *59*:1071–1079, 1977.
9. Angeles, A.P., Badger, R., Gruber, H., and Seegmiller, J.E.: Chondrocyte growth inhibition induced by homogentisic acid and its partial prevention with ascorbic acid. J. Rheum., *16*:512, 1989.
10. O'Brien, W.M., LaDu, D.N., and Bunim, J.J.: Biochemistry pathologic and clinical aspects of alcaptonuria, ochronosis and ochronotic arthropathy. Am. J. Med., *34*:813–838, 1963.
11. Levine, H.D. et al.: Aortic valve replacement for ochronosis of the aortic valve. Chest, *74*:466–467, 1978.
12. Bywaters, E.G.L., Dorling, J., and Sutor, J.: Ochronosis densification. (Abstract.) Arthritis Rheum. Dis., *29*:563, 1970.
13. Deeb, Z., and Frayha, R.: Multiple vacuum disks, an early sign

of ochronosis: Radiologic findings in 2 biopsies. J. Rheumatol., *3*:82–87, 1976.
14. Hunter, T., Gordon, D.A., and Ogryzlo, M.A.: The ground pepper sign of synovial fluid: A new diagnostic feature of ochronosis. J. Rheumatol., *1*:45–53, 1974.
15. Reginato, A.J., Schumacher, H.R., and Martinez, V.A.: Ochronotic arthropathy with calcium pyrophosphate crystal deposition. Arthritis Rheum., *16*:705–714, 1973.
16. Huttl, S.: Synovial effusion. A nosographic and diagnostic study. Part I. Acta Rheum. Baln. Pistiniana, *5*:1–100, 1970.
17. Schumacher, H.R., and Holdsworth, D.E.: Ochronotic arthropathy. 1. Clinicopathologic studies. Semin. Arthritis Rheum., *6*:207–246, 1977.
18. McClure, J., Smith, P.S., and Gramp, A.A.: Calcium pyrophosphate dihydrate (CPPD) deposition in ochronotic arthropathy. J. Clin. Pathol., *36*:894–902, 1983.
19. Rynes, R.J., Sosman, J.L., and Holdsworth, D.E.: Pseudogout in ochronosis: Report of a case. Arthritis Rheum., *18*:21–25, 1975.
20. Mohr, W., Wessinghage, D., and Lendschaw, E.: Die Ultrastruktur von Hyalinem Knorpel und Gelenkkapsel-gewebe bei der alkaptonurischen Ochronose. Z. Rheumatol., *39*:55–73, 1980.
21. Gaines, J.J., Tom, G.D., and Khankhaniam, N.: An ultrastructural and light microscopic study of the synovium in ochronotic arthropathy. Hum. Pathol., *18*:1160–1164, 1987.
22. O'Brien, W.M., Banfield, W.G., and Sokoloff, L.: Studies on the pathogenesis of ochronotic arthropathy. Arthritis Rheum., *4*:137–152, 1961.
23. Lurie, D.P., and Musil, D.: Knee arthropathy in ochronosis: Diagnosis by arthroscopy with ultrastructural features. J. Rheumatol., *11*:101–103, 1984.
24. MacKenzie, C.R., Major, P., and Hunter, T.: Tendon involvement in a case of ochronosis. J. Rheumatol., *9*:634–636, 1982.
25. Blivaiss, B.B., Rosenberg, E.F., Katuzov, H., and Stoner, R.: Experimental ochronosis: Induction in rats by long-term feeding of L-tyrosine. A.M.A. Arch. Pathol., *82*:45–53, 1966.
26. Horshaw, R.A., Zimmerman, K.G., and Menter, A.: Ochronosis-like pigmentation from hydroquinone bleaching creams in American Blacks. Arch. Dermatol., *121*:105–108, 1985.
27. Lustberg, T.J., Schulman, J.D., and Seegmiller, J.E.: Decreased binding of ^{14}C-homogentisic acid induced by ascorbic acid in connective tissue of rats with experimental alcaptonuria. Nature, *222*:770–771, 1970.
27a. Forslind, K., Wollheim, F.A., Akeeson, B., et al.: Alkaptonuria and ochronosis in 3 siblings. Ascorbic acid treatment monitored by urinary HGA excretion. Clin. Exp. Rheum., *6*:289–292, 1988.
28. Carrier, D.A., and Harris, C.M.: Bilateral hip and bilateral knee arthroplasties in a patient with ochronotic arthropathy. Orthop. Rev., *19*:1005–1009, 1990.
29. Finch, S.C., and Finch, C.A.: Idiopathic hemochromatosis: An iron storage disease. Medicine, *34*:381–430, 1955.
30. Sheldon, J.H.: Haemochromatosis. London, Oxford University Press, 1935.
31. Blandford, R.L. et al.: Sicca syndrome associated with idiopathic hemochromatosis. Br. Med. J., *1*:1323, 1979.
32. Cartwright, G.E., Edwards, C.Q., and Kravitz, K.: Hereditary hemochromatosis: Phenotypic expression of the disease. N. Engl. J. Med., *301*:175–179, 1979.
33. Goldschmidt, H., et al.: Idiopathic hemochromatosis presenting as arthropathy and amenorrhea in a young woman. Am. J. Med., *82*:1057–1059, 1987.
34. Wands, J.R. et al.: Normal serum ferritin concentrations in precirrhotic hemochromatosis. N. Engl. J. Med., *294*:302–305, 1976.
35. Murphy, F.B., and Bernardino, M.E.: MR imaging of focal hemochromatosis. J. Comput. Assist. Tomogr., *10*:1044–1046, 1986.
36. Rosner, I.A. et al.: Arthropathy, hypouricemia, and normal serum iron studies in hereditary hemochromatosis. Am. J. Med., *70*:870–874, 1981.
37. Diamond, T., Stiel, D., and Posen, S.: Osteoporosis in hemochromatosis; iron excess, gonadal deficiency or other factors. Ann. Intern. Med., *110*:430–436, 1989.
38. deVernejoul, M.C., et al.: Effects of iron overload on bone remodelling on pigs. Am. J. Pathol., *116*:377–383, 1984.
39. Schumacher, H.R.: Hemochromatosis and arthritis. Arthritis Rheum., *7*:41–50, 1964.
40. Delbarre, F.: Les manifestations ostéo-articulaires de l'hémochromatose. Presse Med., *72*:2973–2978, 1964.
41. Dymock, I.W., et al.: Arthropathy of hemochromatosis. Ann. Rheum. Dis., *29*:469–476, 1970.
42. Hamilton, E.B. et al.: The natural history of arthritis in idiopathic hemochromatosis: Progression of the clinical and radiological features over 10 years. Q. J. Med., *50*:321–329, 1981.
43. Kra, S.J., Hollingsworth, J.W., and Finch, S.C.: Arthritis with synovial iron deposition in a patient with hemochromatosis. N. Engl. J. Med., *272*:1268–1271, 1965.
44. Mitrovic, D. et al.: Etude histologique et histoclinique des lésion articulaires de la chondrocalcinose survenant au cous d'une hémochromatose. Arch. Anat. Pathol., *14*:264–270, 1966.
45. Gordon, D.A., Clarke, P.V., and Ogryzlo, M.A.: The chondrocalcific arthropathy of iron overload. Arch. Intern. Med., *134*:21–28, 1974.
46. Adamson, T.C. et al.: Hand and wrist arthropathies of hemochromatosis and calcium pyrophosphate deposition disease: Distinct radiographic features. Radiology, *147*:377–381, 1983.
47. Schumacher, H.R.: Ultrastructural characteristics of the synovial membrane in idiopathic hemochromatosis. Ann. Rheum. Dis., *31*:465–473, 1972.
48. Schumacher, H.R.: Articular cartilage in the degenerative arthropathy of hemochromatosis. Arthritis Rheum., *25*:1460–1468, 1982.
49. Abbott, D.F., and Gresham, D.F.: Arthropathy in transfusional hemosiderosis. Br. Med. J., *1*:418–419, 1972.
50. Sella, E.J., and Goodman, A.H.: Arthropathy secondary to transfusion hemochromatosis. J. Bone Joint Surg., *55A*:1077–1081, 1973.
51. Mohler, D.N., and Wheby, M.S.: Case report: Hemochromatosis heterozygotes may have significant iron overload when they also have hereditary spherocytosis. Am. J. Med. Sci., *292*:320–324, 1986.
52. Brighton, C.T., Bigley, E.C., and Smolenski, B.I.: Iron induced arthritis in immature rabbits. Arthritis Rheum., *13*:849–857, 1970.
53. DeSousa, M., Breedvelt, F., Dynesius-Trentham, R., et al.: Iron, iron binding proteins and immune system cells. Ann. NY Acad. Sci., *526*:310–322, 1988.
54. McCarty, D.J., and Pepe, P.F.: Erythrocyte neutral inorganic pyrophosphatase in pseudogout. J. Lab. Clin. Med., *79*:277–284, 1972.
55. McCarty, D.J., Palmer, D.W., and Garancis, J.C.: Clearance of calcium pyrophosphate dihydrate crystals in vivo. III. Effects of synovial hemosiderosis. Arthritis Rheum., *24*:706–710, 1981.
56. Cheng, P.T., and Pritzker, K.P.: Ferrous but not ferric ions inhibit de novo formation of calcium pyrophosphate dihydrate crystals: Possible relationships to chondrocalcinosis and hemochromatosis. J. Rheum., *15*:321–324, 1988.
57. Wilson, S.A.K.: Progressive lenticular degeneration: A familial nervous disease associated with cirrhosis of the liver. Brain, *34*:295–509, 1912.
58. Dobyns, W.B., Goldstein, N.P., and Gordon, H.: Clinical spectrum of Wilson's disease. Mayo Clin. Proc., *54*:35–42, 1979.
59. Perman, J.A. et al.: Laboratory measurements of copper metabo-

lism in the differentiation of chronic active hepatitis and Wilson disease in children. J. Pediatr., *94*:564–568, 1979.

60. Weinberg, L.M., Brasitus, T.A., and Leskowitch, J.H.: Fluctuating Kayser-Fleischer-like rings in a jaundiced patient. Arch. Intern. Med., *142*:246–247, 1981.
61. Finby, N., and Bearn, A.G.: Roentgenographic abnormalities of the skeletal system in Wilson's disease (hepatolenticular degeneration). Am. J. Roentgenol., *79*:603–611, 1958.
62. Mindelzun, R. et al.: Skeletal changes in Wilson's disease: A radiological study. Radiology, *94*:127–132, 1970.
63. Cavallino, R., and Grossman, H.: Wilson's disease presenting with rickets. Radiology, *90*:493–494, 1968.
64. Boudin, G. et al.: Relapsing meningeal tuberculosis, cisternal blocking with symptoms similar to lethargic encephalitis (somnolence, ptosis, extrapyramidal syndromes). Bull. Soc. Med. Hop. Paris, *73*:559–561, 1957.
65. Feller, E., and Schumacher, H.R.: Osteoarticular changes in Wilson's disease. Arthritis Rheum., *15*:259–266, 1972.
66. Golding, D.N., and Walshe, J.M.: Arthropathy of Wilson's disease: Study of clinical and radiological features in 32 patients. Ann. Rheum. Dis., *36*:99–111, 1977.
67. Kaklamanis, P., and Spengos, M.: Osteoarticular change and synovial biopsy findings in Wilson's disease. Ann. Rheum. Dis., *32*:422–427, 1973.
68. Menerey, K. et al: The arthropathy of Wilson's disease. J. Rheum., *15*:331–337, 1988.
69. Zakraoui, L. et al.: Les atteintes articulaires au cours de la maladie de Wilson. Rev. Rhum., *53*:345–348, 1986.

69a. McClure, J., and Smith, P.S.: Calcium pyrophosphate dihydrate deposition in the intervertebral discs in a case of Wilson's disease. J. Clin. Pathol., *36*:764–768, 1983.

70. Sternlieb, I., and Scheinberg, I.H.: Prevention of Wilson's disease in asymptomatic patients. N. Engl. J. Med., *278*:352–359, 1968.
71. Endres, W.: D-Penicillamine in pregnancy—To ban or not to ban. Klin. Wochenschr., *59*:535–537, 1981.
72. Walshe, J.M.: The management of pregnancy in Wilson's disease treated with trientine. Q. J. Med., *58*:81–87, 1986.
73. Brewer, G.J. et al.: Treatment of Wilson's disease with oral zinc. Clin. Res., *29*:578A, 1981.

113

Osteopenic Bone Diseases

BEVRA HANNAHS HAHN

Diseases of bone constitute a major cause of pain and disability, especially in individuals over the age of 50. Many disorders and drug therapies can reduce bone mass until it is inadequate to withstand ordinary mechanical stresses. Disability results from fractures, from bone pain, and from increasing dorsal kyphosis with decreasing lung volumes. The physiologic and histologic features of normal bone, the differential diagnosis of osteopenias, and methods of preventing and treating the most common metabolic bone diseases are the subjects of this chapter.

PHYSIOLOGY OF NORMAL BONE

Bone has two major functions in humans: It provides a means of support, locomotion, and protection, and it serves as a reservoir of ions necessary to multiple body functions including calcium, phosphorus, magnesium, sodium, and carbonate. As with other body tissues, continual turnover (remodeling) occurs; during this process, rates of formation and rates of resorption are normally in equilibrium. The essential role of bone in maintaining normal ion and buffer concentrations in the extracellular fluid takes precedence over the supportive role when formation and resorption rates become uncoupled.

COMPOSITION OF BONE

Bone is composed of connective tissue that becomes mineralized. Collagen is the major component of the connective tissue, accounting for approximately 70% of the dry weight of bone and 95% of the protein.[1] Bone collagen is predominantly type I and is composed of 3 polypeptide chains (two $\alpha 1(I)$ and one $\alpha 2(I)$ chain). The peptide sequence of each chain contains glycine-X-Y in repeating trimers; the glycines permit winding into a mature triple helix. X and Y are most frequently hydroxyproline or hydroxylysine. Hydroxyproline stabilizes the helix by forming interchain hydrogen bonds. The collagen helices form fibrils, which cross-link. Those fibrils are the structural core in and around which minerals deposit. Abnormalities of collagen (e.g., in osteogenesis imperfecta) or of mineralization (e.g., in rickets) result in bone with inadequate strength.

The mineral phase consists primarily of hydroxyapatite, a microcrystal of $Ca_{10}(PO_4)_6(OH)_2$.[2] In addition to calcium and phosphate, the crystals contain sodium, carbonate, potassium and magnesium.

Noncollagenous proteins form about 5% of the protein matrix and probably play essential roles in normal remodeling.[2,3] The most frequent of these proteins is osteocalcin (also called *bone Gla protein* [BGP]), which interacts with the hydroxyapatite crystal and may prevent mineralization. Matrix Gla protein (MGP) probably acts as osteocalcin does. Osteonectin, found in mineralized bone, also binds to hydroxyapatite crystals and collagen and probably permits mineralization to occur. The sialoglycoproteins of bone affect the rate of formation and final size of collagen fibrils. Precursors of collagen—procollagens I and III—are found in bone matrix.

Polypeptides that are synthesized by bone cells and act as local growth or inhibition factors are also part of bone matrix. These are discussed in a subsequent section.

STRUCTURE AND REMODELING OF BONE

During fetal life and early childhood, bones are formed from cartilaginous growth plates, which form the epiphysis and metaphysis of long bones and most of the mass of short bones such as vertebrae. The cortex of long bones derives from periochondral areas of new bone deposition. Until puberty, bone formation exceeds bone resorption. Bone growth is regulated by mechanical stimuli such as physical activity and weight bearing, which help to shape bone, and by the stimulus of several hormone systems including growth hormone and somatomedins. In adults, bone modeling has stopped, as has bone growth, and changes in bone are called *remodeling*.

The two major forms of mature mineralized bone are compact cortical bone, which forms the largest portion of long bones of the appendicular skeleton, and transverse interwoven trabecular bone, which forms the majority of bone in vertebral bodies and the flat bones of the skull and pelvis. Compact cortical bone is laid down around the haversian systems in ellipses or circles; the structure is more archlike in trabecular bone. The mechanical relationship of these types of bone and the direction in which they are laid down can be as important in determining skeletal strength as the total quantity of mineralized bone. Consider, for example, the high fracture rate in patients with Paget's disease, in whom the quantity of bone may be large in a given area, but in which structure is mechanically weak.

In both cortical and trabecular bone, the process of remodeling is continuous. Remodeling occurs from three "envelope" areas: from the Haversian envelope (Fig. 113–1); from the periosteal envelope; and from the endosteal envelope. The Haversian envelope occurs within and consists of tunneling canals in which bone is initially resorbed and then reformed.

The endosteal envelope covers the inner surface of the cortex and the trabecular bone surface and separates bone from bone marrow. During adult life, the endosteal surface has a higher rate of resorption than formation; the bone marrow cavity consequently expands at the expense of the thickness of cortical and trabecular bone.

BONE CELLS AND THEIR CONTROL OF REMODELING

Three types of cells occupy bone: osteoblasts, osteocytes, and osteoclasts.[4] Osteoblasts can be derived from precursor cells that exist in several body compartments (bone marrow, endosteal envelopes), if acted on by the correct differentiation signals. They synthesize most of the proteins found in bone, including collagen, osteocalcin, osteonectin, and alkaline phosphatase.[3] The unmineralized collagen-rich matrix they make is called *osteoid*. Osteocytes are sessile and are probably derived from osteoblasts; their function is unclear. Osteoclasts are probably derived from bone marrow or circulating macrophages, which are functionally activated in Haversian canals or Howship's lucunae; they are macro phage-like cells that resorb mineralized bone. The actions of osteoblasts and osteoclasts are closely linked. Hormones that activate the osteoclast (1,25$(OH)_2$vitamin D, parathyroid hormone) probably deliver their initial signals to the osteoblast, which then sends activating signals to the osteoclast.

Frost[4] suggested the concept of bone modeling units, called *basic multicellular units* (Fig. 113–2). He suggested that two types of such units exist: one in which resorption is the major activity and one in which bone formation is the major activity. These units occur on each skeletal envelope. In each basic multicellular unit, the following sequence of events occurs: (1) The unit is activated; (2) osteoclasts appear and begin to resorb bone—a process that takes on the average 2 weeks; (3) osteoblasts then synthesize osteoid, a process that takes approximately 6 weeks; and (4) mineralization of the new bone occurs. This entire process requires 3 to 5 months. In health, a steady state exists between rates of bone formation and resorption in the basic multicellular unit. Several factors can upset this balance, however, including change in the "birth rate" of new multicellular units, an uncoupling of rates of resorption and for-

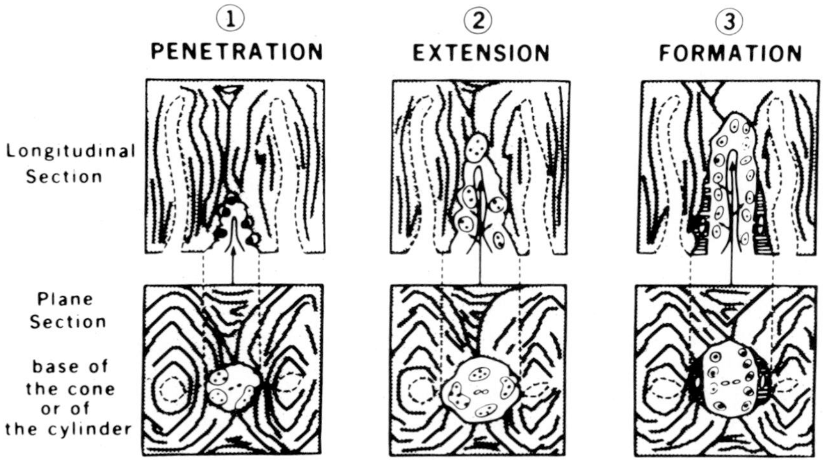

FIGURE 113–1. A model of the sequential events in the formation of a new Haversian system in cortical bone. (From Rasmussen, H., and Bordier, P.: The Physiological and Cellular Basis of Metabolic Bone Disease. Baltimore, Williams & Wilkins, 1974.)

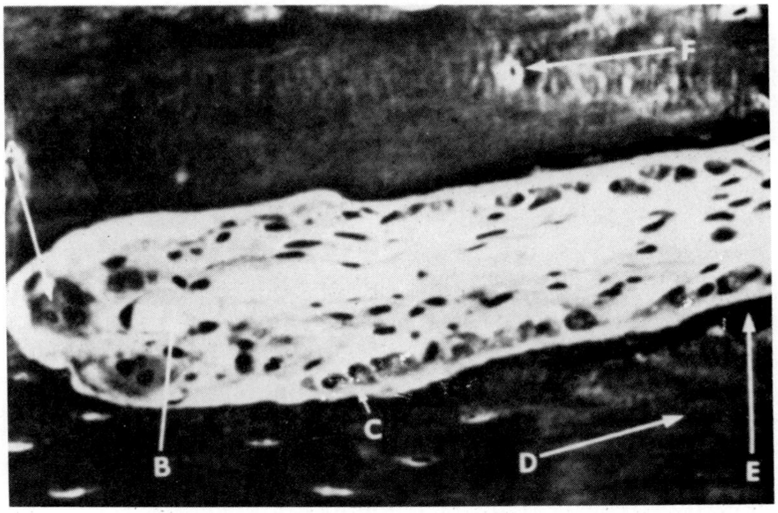

FIGURE 113–2. A basic multicellular unit of bone; longitudinal section through an evolving Haversian system. At the front, the osteoclasts (A) are drilling a tunnel through the bone (D) from right to left, to make a temporary space filled by blood vessels and loose connective tissue (B). Further behind, the osteoblasts (C) lined up along the osteoid seam (E) are refilling the tunnel. (From Parfitt, A.M.: Mineral Electrolyte Metab., 3:277, 1980; reprinted with permission of the publisher.)

mation in multiple units, and failure to mineralize the osteoid that has been formed.

Adults have a wider variation in birth rates of basic multicellular units in the Haversian and endosteal envelopes than in the periosteal envelope; loss of trabecular and cortical bone on the endosteal surface and loss of intracortical bone are more common than losses of subperiosteal bone. In cortical bone, remodeling caused by basic multicellular units occurs predominantly in the Haversian system; in trabecular bone, remodeling occurs predominantly in Howship's lacunae. In most metabolic bone diseases in adults, the rate of remodeling determines whether total formation remains in equilibrium with resorption, or whether bone is lost as the rates are uncoupled. Most current therapeutic interventions for osteopenia are designed to control bone remodeling. *There is a strong stimulus toward equilibrium; therefore when an intervention suppresses one (usually resorption), the other usually becomes suppressed a few weeks or months later.*[2,5]

HORMONAL AND GROWTH FACTOR INFLUENCES ON BONE REMODELING

SYSTEMIC HORMONAL (ENDOCRINE) INFLUENCES

The movement of calcium and phosphorus ions in and out of the mineral phase of bone is under the control of three major hormones: parathyroid hormone, the active metabolites of vitamin D, and calcitonin. Parathyroid hormone[6] maintains the level of ionized calcium in the extracellular fluid by stimulating bone resorption, increasing resorption of calcium in the renal tubules, and increasing intestinal calcium absorption by stimulating metabolism of vitamin D into its most active form, $1,25(OH)_2D$. Parathyroid hormone in small quantities can increase the synthesis of bone collagen; in larger quantities it decreases that synthesis.

Vitamin D is formed in the skin from the conversion of 7-dehydrocholesterol to vitamin D_3 (cholecalciferol).[7] Cholecalciferol is hydroxylated to 25 OH D (calcifediol) in the liver and is further hydroxylated to $1,25(OH)_2D$ (calcitriol) in the kidney. Calcitriol is a potent stimulant of intestinal absorption of calcium and phosphorus. When this process is operating normally, calcitriol promotes bone growth and bone formation by providing adequate levels of mineral. When dietary intake of minerals is low, however, calcitriol can directly resorb calcium and phosphate from the skeleton.

Calcitonin, which is made in the thyroid gland, inhibits the resorption of calcium from bone[8] and thus reduces the concentrations of serum calcium. It acts directly on osteoclasts, inhibiting their capacity to resorb bone; this activity is the basis of its use in therapy of high-turnover forms of metabolic bone disease.

With age, the concentration of parathyroid hormone rises and the concentrations of $1,25(OH)_2D$ and calcitonin fall.

Several other hormones also influence bone. Thyroid hormone is necessary for normal bone growth and remodeling, and excessive levels of thyroxin can stimulate bone resorption and a rapid birth rate of basic multicellular units, with net bone loss.[9] Sex hormones, including estrogens, androgens, and progestins also affect bone.[5,10,11] The decline in estrogen levels that occurs at the time of menopause is associated with rapid bone loss. Estrogens probably have direct effects on osteoblasts, which have receptors for that hormone. The major physiologic effect of estrogen, is to reduce bone resorption; estrogenic stimulation of the osteoblast probably results in a signal to osteoclasts that reduces their activity. Androgens also reduce bone resorption and may have anabolic effects as well.[11] As discussed in detail later, adrenal glucocorticoids also play an important role in skeletal remodeling.[12] Pharmacologic levels decrease the intestinal absorption of calcium, the conversion of precursor cells to osteoblasts, and the formation of osteoid by differentiated osteoblasts. Physiologic levels are probably important in maintaining normal bone formation and resorption rates. Through its effects on somatomedins (insulin-like growth factor 1 [IGF1]), growth hormone stimulates collagen synthesis and cell replication in adult bone as well as growth in children. In parallel to this action, insulin stimulates osteoblasts to synthesize collagen.

LOCAL GROWTH FACTOR INFLUENCES (AUTOCRINE AND PARACRINE)

Several polypeptides synthesized in bone also influence local remodeling; some may mediate the effects of systemic hormones on bone.[13] These factors may be synthesized by bone cells or by cells in nearby tissues such as cartilage and bone marrow. Polypeptides synthesized by bone cells and/or found in matrix include bone cell derived growth factor (BDGF), platelet-derived growth factor (PDGF), somatomedin C IGF1, skeletal growth factor (IGF-2),[14] transforming growth factor-β (TGF-β), acidic and basic fibroblast growth factors (aFGF and bFGF), and bone morphogenic protein (BMP).[15] Growth factors synthesized by nonbone cells include IGF-1, FGF, interleukin-1 (IL-1), tumor necrosis factors-α and -β (TNF-α and -β), PDGF, macrophage-derived growth factors, and interferon-γ (INF-γ).

Osteoblasts are stimulated to proliferate and synthesize collagen by (1) IGF-1 and -2, (2) TGF-β, (3) BDGF, (4) PDGF, and possibly, (5) BMP. FGF has proliferative effects on osteoblasts but can inhibit their function under certain conditions. Osteoclasts are stimulated by IL-1 and TNFs (probably via osteoblast-mediated signals). Interleukin-1, however, can stimulate replication of osteoclasts or osteoblasts and in low quantities can stimulate synthesis of bone collagen. In high quantities it decreases collagen production. TNF-α and -β stimulate both osteoblast replication and osteoclastic bone resorption but inhibit collagen production. INF-γ is antiproliferative and thus inhibits bone resorption and collagen synthesis. Prostaglandins, also found in bone, can mediate either formation or resorption, depending on co-stimulatory factors. The ability of individuals to make granulocyte-monocyte colony-stimulating factor 1 (GM-CSF-1) is apparently essential to normal osteoclast function. Mice with genetic defects in CSF-1 have osteopetrosis—a disorder in which osteoclasts fail to resorb bone.[16]

Some of these polypeptides can have dual effects.[17] For example, IL-1 reduces DNA synthesis by osteoblast-like cells in vitro, unless prostaglandins are inhibited, in which case mitogenesis is increased.

PHYSICAL INFLUENCES

Mechanical and electrical stimuli also play a role in development of normal skeleton and in bone remodeling. It is known that mechanical stimulation of bone, probably modulated by the generation of small electrical currents, enhances bone formation.

SUMMARY OF BONE REMODELING

The net results of interaction of the various endocrine, paracrine and autocrine factors, mechanical stresses, and the components of the basic multicellular units at all three remodeling envelopes is that bone is in a constant dynamic equilibrium. Bone turnover rates in children can be as high as 20% per year; in adults, those rates fall to 3 to 5% annually. To maintain normal bone, an adequate quantity of tropocollagen must be formed and arranged in the correct configuration to permit mineralization. Furthermore, adequate mineral must be available, and mineralization must be mechanically sound to maintain normal tensile strength. When any one of these factors or any combination of them becomes abnormal, metabolic bone disease results.

HISTOLOGIC FEATURES OF BONE

The morphologic results of bone remodeling can be seen histomorphometrically by examining stained, undecalcified bone biopsy sections, usually obtained from the iliac crest.[18,19] A model of sequential events in a basic multicellular unit and the resultant histologic picture is shown in Fig. 113–2. Osteoclasts, which can be clearly identified in this figure, form a "cutting cone," that is, a tunnel through cortical bone. Behind the osteoclasts are blood vessels and connective tissue, and farther behind is a line of osteoblasts forming osteoid, which appears as the dark area in Fig. 113–2.

In the series of color plates in Fig. 113–3, osteoid stains bright orange-pink and mineralized bone stains blue-black (von Kossa stain). The osteoblasts and osteoclasts can be differentiated by their morphologic features. From similar bone biopsies, one can measure the quantity of osteoid per unit of bone, the width of the osteoid seam (a wide seam suggests lack of mineralization and osteomalacia), the quantity of trabecular bone, and the number of osteoclasts and resorbing surfaces or cavities. All these factors give a picture of the dynamic turnover of bone at the time of biopsy.

The *rate* of bone formation can be estimated more accurately by the technique of double tetracycline labeling first developed by Frost. Before biopsy, two short courses of tetracycline are administered 7 to 14 days apart. Tetracycline forms fluorescent bands (Fig. 113–3G) after deposition at the mineralization front of bone. The distance between those fluorescent bands divided by the time interval between the midpoints of tetracycline administration is called the mean mineral apposition rate and is a measure of osteoblast function, rates of bone formation, and mineralization.

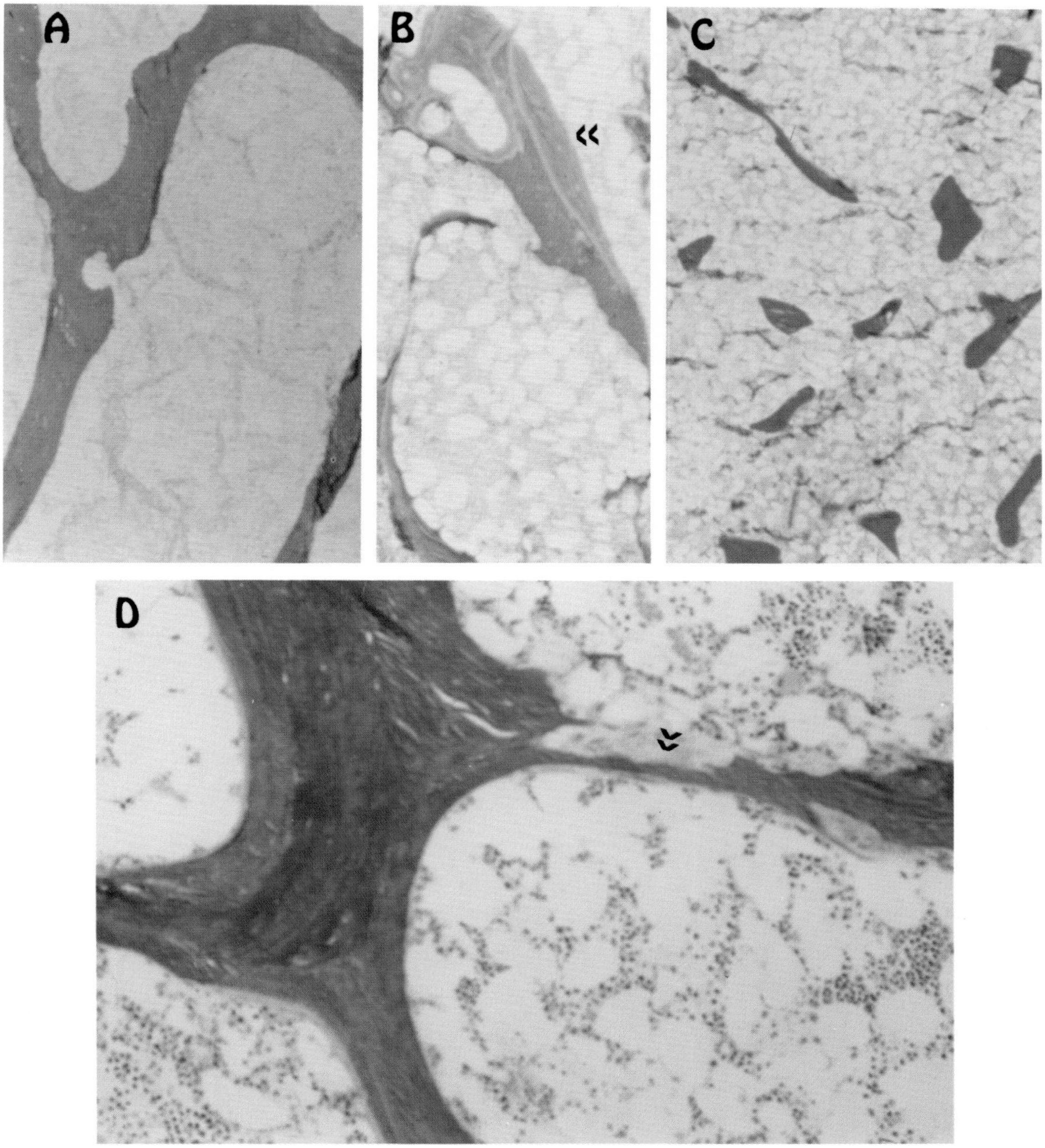

FIGURE 113–3. Histologic specimen of bone obtained from iliac crest biopsies. Sections are undemineralized and are stained with the von Kossa stain. Mineralized bone stains blue-black; undemineralized osteoid stains pink-orange. *A* Normal bone histologic specimen from a core biopsy of the iliac crest (× 10). *B*, Osteomalacia; note the large quantities of orange-staining undemineralized osteoid (arrows) laid down along all areas of previously mineralized bone (blue) (× 10). *C*, Low-turnover osteoporosis; note the small total quantities of mineralized bone. The absence of areas of osteoid formation and of resorption indicates a low rate of turnover (× 10). *D*, High-turnover osteoporosis; note the large area of resorption of a bone trabecula (arrows) and formation of osteoid (pink). This patient has osteoporosis with a high rate of turnover (× 100).

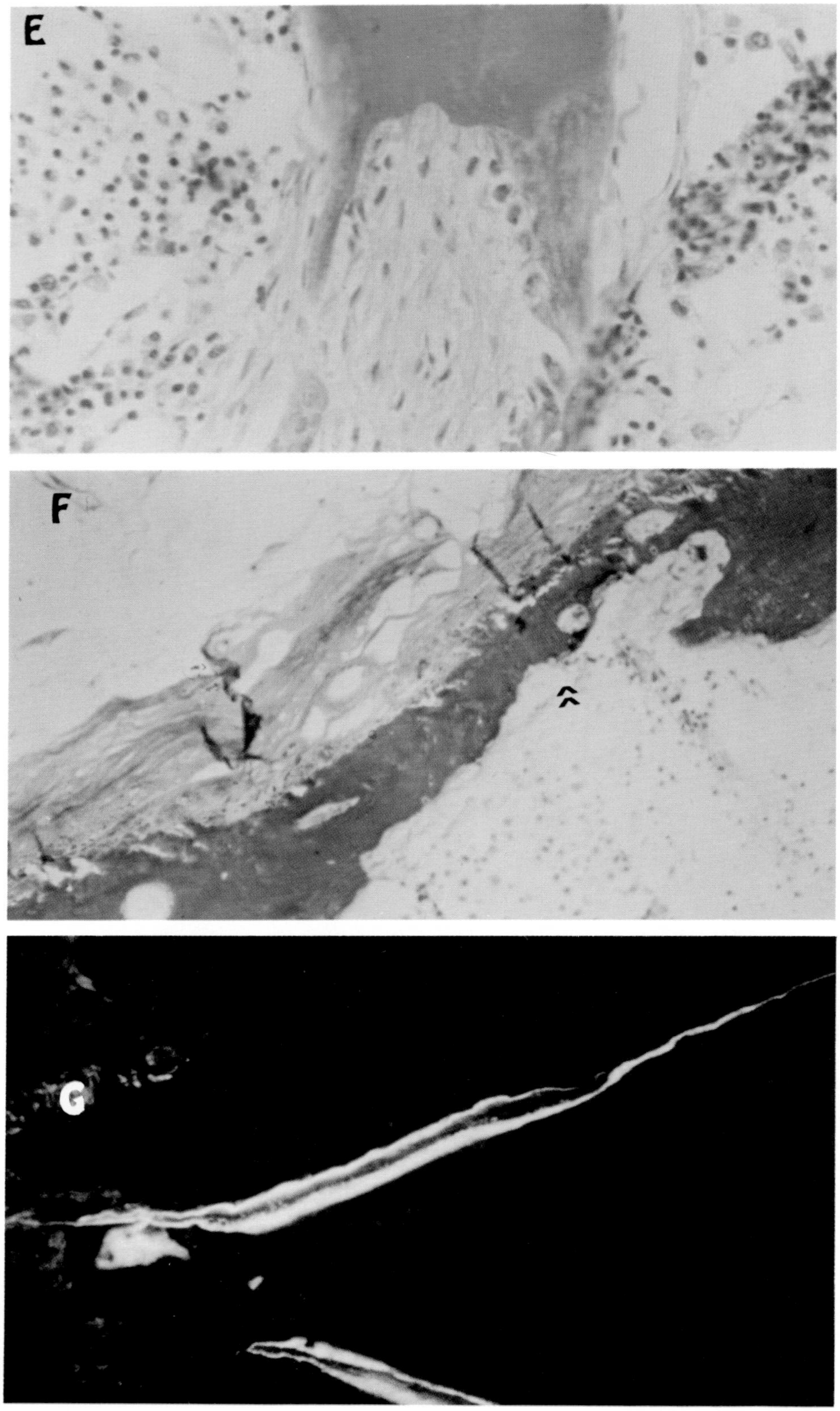

(Legend appears on Facing Page)

METHODS OF MEASURING BONE MASS

Methods of measuring bone mass are reviewed in Chapter 7.

DIAGNOSIS AND DIFFERENTIAL DIAGNOSIS OF OSTEOPENIA

Several different signs and symptoms should alert the physician to the possible diagnosis of osteopenia. These include bone fractures after minor trauma or in the absence of trauma, loss of height, increasing dorsal kyphosis, and bone pain. In addition, some patients with osteomalacia or hyperparathyroidism have muscle symptoms, including stiffness and weakness, that can be confused with inflammatory myopathies. Some patients have no symptoms, but the diagnosis is suspected because of osteopenia seen on roentgenograms obtained for another reason.

The differential diagnosis of generalized osteopenia in adults is shown in Table 113–1. The disorders include osteoporosis, glucocorticoid-induced osteopenia, osteo-

TABLE 113–1. DIFFERENTIAL DIAGNOSIS OF OSTEOPENIA IN ADULTS

DISORDER	POSSIBLE CAUSES AND CHARACTERISTICS
OSTEOPOROSIS	
Involutional or Senile Form	Associated with aging, genetics, leanness, lifetime low calcium intake. Fractures of hip dominate and often occur after age 70.
Postmenopausal Form	Associated with menopause, especially before age 45. Fractures of vertebrae, ribs, radius (bones with high trabecular content) dominate, in women in the sixth and seventh decades.
Hypogonadal Form	Associated with low luteinizing hormone or androgen levels in men.
Idiopathic Form	No obvious predisposing factors.
Disuse of Immobilization Forms	
GLUCOCORTICOID-INDUCED OSTEOPOROSIS	
Iatrogenic Form	
Spontaneous Form (Cushing's Syndrome)	
OSTEOMALACIA	
Vitamin D Deficiency	Inadequate intake, intestinal malabsorption, drug-induced accelerated catabolism of vitamin D.
Phosphate-Wasting Syndromes	Acquired renal tubular defects with phosphate loss, renal tubular acidosis, antacid abuse.
Aluminum Bone Disease	Dialysis, total parenteral nutrition (TPN)
Hypophosphatasia	
OSTEITIS FIBROSA (HYPERPARATHYROIDISM)	
Primary Hyperparathyroidism (Adenoma)	
Secondary Hyperparathyroidism	Vitamin D-deficiency states, decreased intestinal calcium absorption with age, chronic renal failure
HYPERTHYROIDISM	High-turnover osteoporosis
MALIGNANCIES	Replacement of bone by tumor
GENETIC DEFECTS	Osteogenesis imperfecta, sickle cell disease, lipid storage disorders

FIGURE 113–3 (*Continued*) *E*, Osteitis fibrosa of hyperparathyroidism. A line of osteoclasts has resorbed a large area along a trabecula. The space is being replaced by fibrous tissue. At the leading edge of resorption osteoid is being laid down (× 400). *F*, Glucocorticoid-induced osteopenia. Osteoclasts have been activated and have resorbed part of the cortical bone at the endosteal surface (arrows). In contrast to *E*, however, no osteoid is forming (× 100). *G*, Bone biopsy viewed under ultraviolet light after tetracycline labeling; tetracycline deposits at the mineralizing front of new bone. This patient received 3 days of tetracycline therapy twice, with a 2-week interval between doses. The distance between the two fluorescent bands of tetracycline is a measure of the rate of bone formation; the label of the bone indicates osteoid has been formed and mineralized. (Illustrations kindly provided by Steven Teitelbaum, M.D., Professor of Pathology, Washington University/Jewish Hospital of St. Louis.)

malacia, osteitis fibrosa, and other diseases such as hyperthyroidism, diffuse malignancies involving bone, and osteogenesis imperfecta tarda.

A complete evaluation of osteopenia should consist of medical history and physical examination; routine roentgenograms of affected portions of the skeleton; sensitive measurements of bone mass (x-ray–based dual-energy densitometry or quantitative computerized tomography measurements of axial and appendicular skeletal bone mass—see Chapter 7), and several measurements of fasting serum levels of calcium, phosphorus, and alkaline phosphatase. Routine tests measuring thyroid, hepatic, and renal function are recommended. Measuring 24-hour excretion of calcium is useful to identify patients who malabsorb calcium (total excretion in 24 hours less than 100 mg), or patients with high urinary levels of calcium (greater than 250 mg) in whom therapy with calcium and/or vitamin D or its metabolites might be hazardous. If hyperparathyroidism is suspected on the basis of the initial blood and urine tests, serum levels of parathyroid hormone (PTH) should be measured. If tests suggest malabsorption are observed, serum levels of 25 OH D are useful.

Once the diagnosis of osteopenia is established and conditions such as a diffuse malignant osteolytic disease and hyperthyroidism are ruled out, one must establish the basis of the metabolic bone disorder. A good starting point is measurement of fasting serum calcium, phosphorus, and alkaline phosphatase levels. These determinations should be performed on fasting serum because postprandial rises in serum calcium and phosphorus can obscure mild abnormalities in basal levels. Most currently available PTH assays can readily detect the marked increase in serum levels occurring in primary hyperparathyroidism and renal osteodystrophy, but these tests are less likely to detect the usual minor elevations found in states of mild secondary hyperparathyroidism, such as vitamin D deficiency and glucocorticoid-induced osteopenia. An elevated serum PTH, in combination with other confirmatory data, is useful in establishing a diagnosis. Serum for PTH determinations should also be drawn in the fasting state to increase the likelihood of detecting a minimally elevated basal level. Serum 25 OH D measurements provide a sensitive means of assessing vitamin D status. The normal ranges for a center in the Midwestern United States was 10 to 25 ng/mL in the winter and 14 to 40 ng/mL in the summer.[80] Values at or below normal limits indicate a deficiency state and warrant further evaluation for intestinal malabsorption, drug-induced osteomalacia, and other disorders. Malabsorption syndromes are best defined by determining 72-hour fecal fat excretion and D-xylose absorption.

Determination of 24-hour urinary calcium excretion is a simple and useful, albeit indirect, means of detecting abnormalities in calcium metabolism. With the patient on a 600- to 800-mg calcium diet for 1 or 2 weeks (the average white American diet provides that amount), normal urinary calcium excretion is 100 to 250 mg/24 hours. Values below 100 mg on several determinations suggest intestinal calcium malabsorption with a decreased filtered calcium load, or a secondary PTH elevation that promotes renal tubular calcium retention. Use of diuretics alters these values; thiazides decrease urine calcium excretion to 50 to 60% of basal values, and furosemide increases urinary calcium. An elevated urine calcium excretion and hyperchloremic acidosis suggest acquired distal renal tubular acidosis. This diagnosis can be confirmed by recording urine pH values for 2 to 3 consecutive days and by failure of urine pH to fall below 5.3 following NH_4Cl loading in the form of 0.1 mg/kg body weight in four divided doses. Other useful tests include fasting 4-hour tubular resorption of phosphate to detect renal phosphate wasting in hyperparathyroidism or renal tubular phosphate "leak" syndromes and measurement of serum cortisol levels in suspected cases of excessive endogenous glucocorticoid production.

Some experts measure additional parameters of bone turnover, including osteocalcin, 2-hour urinary calcium/creatinine ratios, and urinary excretion of hydroxyproline. Osteocalcin is made only by osteoblasts. High serum levels, along with high levels of osteoblast-derived alkaline phosphatase, are associated with activation and/or proliferation of osteoblasts and should indicate high rates of bone synthesis. Measurements of osteocalcin have been useful in indicating changes in activation of osteoblasts in some large population studies evaluating treatment of osteoporosis, but use of serial measurements in individual patients has been disappointing because of insensitivity. An elevated ratio of calcium/creatinine excretion in a 2-hour urine specimen collected after an overnight fast may reflect active bone resorption (in the absence of other causes of hypercalciuria) and identify patients with high rates of bone turnover or resorption. The convenience of a 2-hour collection makes patients compliance good. In the management of individuals with osteoporosis, however, the large variation in results (which are quite dependent on recent dietary intake and state of hydration) reduce the usefulness of this test. I prefer 24-hour urine collections for measurement of total calcium excretion, with the patient receiving his normal diet. Results of that assay also vary considerably. Because hydroxyproline is found only in collagen, elevated levels in 24-hour urine collections should reflect active bone resorption. This test is influenced by the protein content of the diet. Accurate measurements require strict dietary control for a period of 3 to 5 days—making this test impractical for office practice. Because most therapeutic interventions for osteoporosis suppress bone resorption (sex hormones, calcitonin, bisphosphonates) and the pathology of osteoporosis may involve either high resorption and high turnover states, or low resorption with low turnover states, it would be desirable to have measures that would accurately identify individuals with high or low bone turnover rates. Theoretically, high serum levels of osteocalcin and alkaline phosphatase coupled with high urinary excretion of calcium and hydroxyproline would identify those individuals with high turn-

TABLE 113–2. LABORATORY FINDINGS IN OSTEOPENIAS

	SERUM						URINE			
DISORDER	Ca	PO_4	Alkaline Phosphatase	Osteocalcin (BGP)	iPTH	25 OH D	Ca	PO_4	Hydroxy-proline	**OTHER**
OSTEOPOROSIS-IDIOPATHIC										
High turnover	N	N	⇈	⇈	N	N	⇈	N	⇈	Bone biopsy discriminates high and low turnover
Low turnover	N	N	N	N	N	N	N	N	N	
OSTEOPOROSIS										
Glucocorticoid induced	N	N	N	⇊	↑	N	N	N	⇊, N, ↑	
OSTEOMALALIA										
Vitamin D deficiency	⇊	⇊	↑	N	↑	⇊	⇊	⇊	N	Bone biopsy diagnostic of osteomalacia
Phosphate depletion	N	⇊	↑	N	N	N	↑	↑, N	N	
PRIMARY HYPERPARATHYROIDISM	↑	⇊	N, ↑	↑	↑	N	↑	↓	↑	
RENAL OSTEODYSTROPHY	N, ⇊, ↑	↑, N	↑, N	↑	↑	N	↓	↓	↑	Serum creatinine elevated
METASTATIC BONE DISEASE	N, ↑	N	↑, N	↑, N, ⇊	N, ⇈	N	N, ↑	N	↑	Bone scans, routine x-rays show metastases. Some tumors make PTH-like hormones, which may be detected in PTH assays. Those patients usually have hypercalcemia, not osteoporosis
HYPERTHYROIDISM	N	N	N, ↑	↑	N	N	N, ↑	N	↑	TSH low, T_4/T_3 high, includes iatrogenic hyperthyroidism

Symbols: N = normal; ⇈ = levels higher than normal; ⇊ = levels lower than normal; ↑ = levels slightly higher than normal.
BGP = bone Gla protein (osteocalcin); iPTH = parathyroid hormone.

over, who might be most likely to respond to antiresorptive therapies. Unfortunately, none of the tests or test combinations currently available allow this type of discrimination.

Finally, in individuals in whom osteopenia is present but the diagnosis is not clear after the tests discussed previously are completed, or in individuals who fail to respond to therapeutic interventions, analysis of quantities and turnover of bone in an iliac crest bone biopsy is often useful. Interpretation of bone histomorphometry has already been discussed.

The interpretation of laboratory results in patients with osteopenia for the purpose of differential diagnosis is reviewed in Table 113–2.

OSTEOPOROSIS

DEFINITION

The term *osteoporosis* refers to the parallel loss of both mineral and matrix that renders residual quantities of mineralized bone inadequate to withstand minor trauma without fracture. The term is confusing because it has been used to refer to the physiologic loss of bone that occurs with aging as well as to the syndromes of accelerated or early bone loss that occur with inactivity, in menopausal or early postmenopausal women, and in men in late middle age. Thus, the terms *idiopathic osteoporosis, postmenopausal osteoporosis, involutional osteoporosis, senile osteoporsis, disuse osteoporosis*, and *osteopenia* are all in use, with some confusion as to their exact meanings. I agree with the view, expressed by Riggs et al.,[20] that parallel loss of cortical and trabecular bone is physiologic and after many decades results in enough loss of mineralized bone to predispose a person to fractures. This phenomenon should be referred to as *senile or involutional osteoporosis or osteopenia*. In contrast, individuals with rapid loss of bone mass have another form of osteoporosis. In women with rapid loss in the perimenopausal period, with perhaps a disproportionate loss of trabecular as compared to cortical bone and a high risk for vertebral or Colles fractures, the diagnosis of postmenopausal osteoporosis is appropriate. Some experts use the term *osteopenia* to refer to individuals with low bone mass by roentgenographic or densitometric techniques and the term *osteoporosis* to refer to individuals with low bone mass who have experienced bone fractures.

INCIDENCE

Data regarding the rate of bone loss as individuals age have been obtained from weighing bones at autopsy, from the various radiographic techniques discussed in Chapter 7, and from histomorphometry.[2,5,20–22] Rates of bone loss vary with age, race, sex, and the region of the skeleton measured.

Males have a greater bone mass than females. In both

sexes, after age 40 to 50, bone mass is lost from *appendicular* bone at an average annual rate of .5%. In women during the decade following menopause, however, that rate increases to approximately 1% per year, leveling off to the slower rate after age 60 to 65. Parallel to this accelerated postmenopausal appendicular bone loss is an increase in the negative calcium balance that occurs after age 40 and almost doubles after menopause.[21] The patterns of bone loss from the midradius in women and in men are shown in Fig. 113–4A and B. Loss of bone from the *axial* skeleton may occur in a different pattern and at a different rate from loss in the appendicular skeleton. In vertebrae, bone loss may begin as early as 20 years of age, and it proceeds steadily at a high rate in women, approximately 7% per decade, and at a much slower rate in men, under 2% per decade (Fig. 113–4C and D). Total loss of bone mass in normal women and men over a lifetime, as estimated by the studies of Riggs and colleagues[20,22] is shown in Table 113–3. If bone loss occurs at different rates in different areas of the skeleton, it is difficult to interpret changes in density or histologic features at a single location as measurement of the impact of a therapeutic intervention.

The incidence of vertebral, hip, and distal radial fractures undoubtedly increases with age. Osteoporosis probably occurs in 15 to 20 million women over the

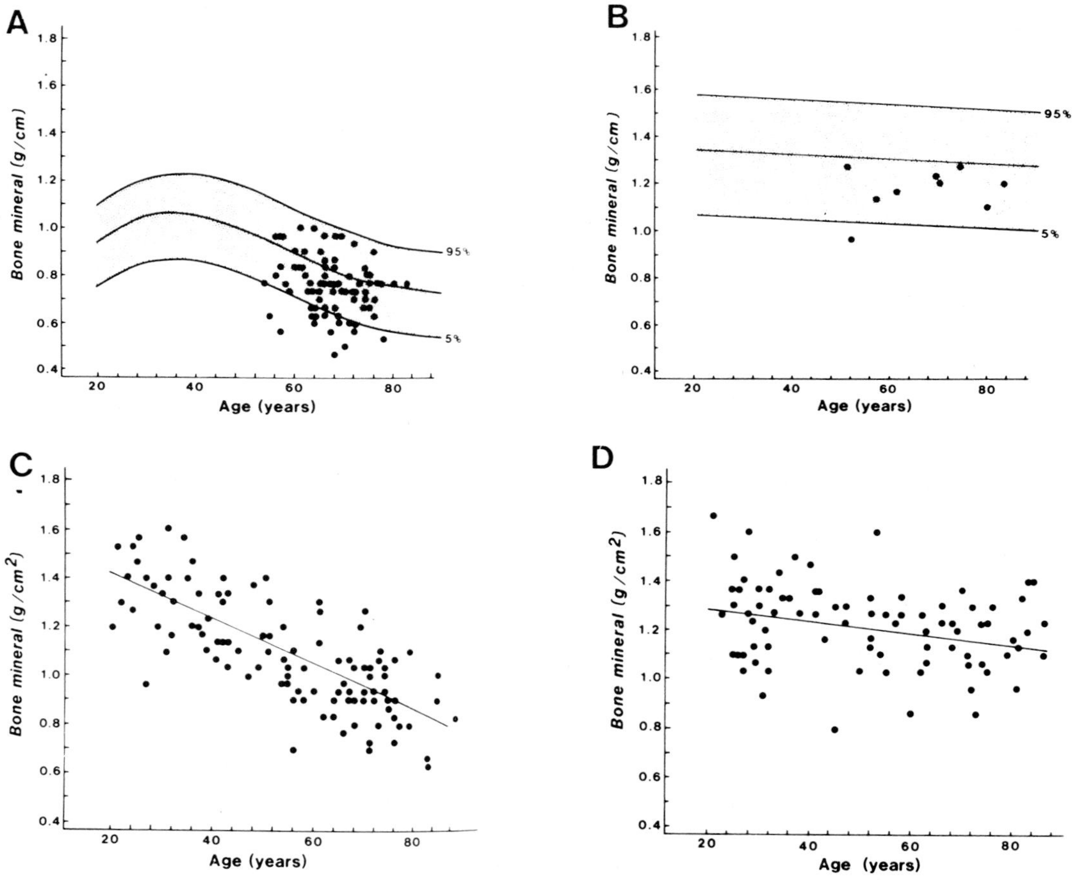

FIGURE 113–4. Loss of bone mass with advancing age as determined by single and dual photon absorptiometry. *A,* Loss of bone mass from the midradius in normal United States women. Loss begins at age 35 to 40, accelerates around the time of menopause, and slows in rate after age 65. The center line represents the mean density for normal women; the shaded area encloses two standard deviations; dots are the bone mass in women who have osteoporosis and have had one or more vertebral fractures. *B,* Loss of bone mass from the midradius in normal United States men. The rate of loss is lower than in women. *C,* Loss of bone mass from lumbar vertebrae in normal United States women. The pattern is different from the pattern in the midradius. Bone mass begins to fall at age 20 and declines at a rapid rate unchanged by menopause. Dots represent bone mineral content in normal women. *D,* Loss of bone mass from lumbar vertebrae in United States men. The rate is much slower than in women. Dots represent values for normal men. (From Riggs, B.L. et al.,[20] with permission of the publishers.)

TABLE 113–3. LOSS OF BONE MASS IN NORMAL INDIVIDUALS OVER LIFETIME

LOCATION	TOTAL LOSS IN WOMEN (%)	TOTAL LOSS IN MEN (%)
Lumbar vertebrae	42–47	13
Midradius	30	5
Distal radius	39	11
Neck of femur	58	36
Intertrochanteric femur	53	35

age of 45 in the United States. Approximately 250,000 osteoporosis-related hip fractures occur in the United States per year.[2,5] Hip fractures in the elderly are associated with a mortality rate of 12 to 20% in 6 months,[23] and costs of short- and long-term care for these problems constitute a major expenditure in our society.

PATHOGENESIS

Although bone turnover rates decrease progressively with age, bone formation is decreased to a slightly greater degree than is resorption, probably because resorption rates increase. The result is a gradual net loss of bone. A variety of hypotheses regarding the nature of this pattern have been suggested, including relative osteoblast failure, calcium and vitamin D deficiencies related to dietary change, decreased efficiency of intestinal calcium absorption and renal calcium retention, and falling levels of calcitonin and estrogen in the face of rising levels of PTH. Thus, physiologic involutional osteopenia has multiple etiologic factors. Pathologic osteopenia has additional etiologies and different phenotypic expressions in different individuals. For example, biopsies from men or women with mid-life symptomatic osteoporosis can contain a spectrum of changes, with some individuals showing inactive bone remodeling and others showing very high turnover rates.[24]

Diminished absorption of calcium by the intestine is a physiologic consequence of aging, although the reasons are unknown.[25] In some women, this malabsorption becomes severe enough to add a component of hyperparathyroidism to their osteoporosis. Estrogen loss after menopause probably enhances bone resorption; androgenic hormones and some progestins, levels of which also decline with time, may have positive effects on bone mass. Premature menopause, occurring before the age of 45, is associated with rapid bone loss in some women.[26] Early menopause may be caused by the use of cytotoxic drugs in young women. Dimunution in physical activity, in sunlight exposure, and in dietary intake of calcium and vitamin D probably play important roles in the osteopenia of aging.

Racial and genetic factors are important in predisposing individuals to symptomatic osteoporosis. In a study of Californians of different racial backgrounds,[27] the incidence of vertebral and hip fractures was significantly higher in whites than in any other race. This was true for both men and women. Asian Americans had significantly lower rates than whites, but significantly higher than Hispanic or black Americans. Fracture rates in Hispanics and blacks were similar, and were the lowest. Certain populations have a high incidence of osteoporosis, including Scandinavians and Eskimos.[28] Identical twins have a higher concordance for low bone mass than do dizygotic twins.[29,30] Daughters of women with symptomatic postmenopausal osteoporosis have significantly lower bone density in their lumbar spines than daughters of postmenopausal women without osteopenia.[31]

Peak bone mass is probably quite important in determining risk for symptomatic osteoporosis at a later age.[32,33] Bone mass in older individuals is determined by the rate of loss from peak bone mass, which occurs between ages 20 and 35. Some evidence indicates genetic influences on peak bone mass, and nutritional factors are undoubtedly quite important. The most effective preventive strategies for involutional and postmenopausal osteoporosis might be in enabling young people to attain their maximum possible peak bone mass. Individuals who are "small boned" have low bone mass; osteoporosis is positively correlated with thinness and is negatively correlated with obesity.[32,34]

Total immobilization results in severe bone loss, as much as 20% over 4 months.[35] Health habits other than nutrition and exercise also play a role in predisposing individuals to osteoporosis. Alcohol ingestion, smoking, and coffee drinking probably have deleterious effects on bone mass. Many medications, including prostaglandin inhibitors, glucocorticoids, and methotrexate, reduce rates of bone turnover and may reduce mass. The factors that predispose persons to osteoporosis are listed in Table 113–4.

DIAGNOSIS

The clinical diagnosis of idiopathic, postmenopausal, or involutional osteoporosis is essentially one of exclusion. A middle-aged or elderly individual complains of loss of height, increasing dorsal kyphosis, or back pain. Fractures may have occurred. In general, patients with involution osteoporosis are 70 years of age or older; hip fractures are the most common manifestation of the disease; many patients are men, although fractures are more common in women.[22] Patients with postmenopausal osteoporosis are women aged 50 to 65 and are more likely to have vertebral, rib, or radial fractures than hip fractures. Radiologic osteopenia, measured either by routine roentgenograms or by more sensitive techniques, is evident. Serum studies show normal levels of calcium, phosphate, alkaline phosphatase, PTN, and 25 OH D. Urine calcium may be low (less than 100 mg/24 hours) but is usually normal. Other causes of metabolic bone disease should be ruled out, including hyperthyroidism, malignancies, hypercortisolism, hyperparathyroidism, and osteomalacia. Once a diagnosis of osteoporosis is established, baseline studies of bone

TABLE 113–4. FACTORS THAT PREDISPOSE TO INVOLUTIONAL, POSTMENOPAUSAL, AND IDIOPATHIC OSTEOPOROSIS

GENERAL	SPECIFIC
AGING	Reduced intestinal calcium absorption, rise in parathyroid hormone, decline in calcitonin, senescence of bone multicellular units
GENETICS	Increased susceptibility of certain populations, low peak bone mass, small body build (especially leanness), concordance in monozygotic twins and mothers–daughters
RACE	Osteoporosis incidence in whites > Asians > hispanics > blacks
MENOPAUSE	Declining levels of estrogens and progestins; especially severe if decline is sudden, as in oophorectomy
DRUGS	Glucocorticoids, methotrexate
IMMOBILIZATION	Any inactivity or weightlessness
ADVERSE HEALTH HABITS	Low intake of calcium, little sunlight exposure, cigarette smoking, alcohol abuse, little physical activity

density should be obtained. This is a somewhat controversial point, because correlations between low bone mass and subsequent fracture, although statistically significant, are not perfect. Disagreements exist regarding the cost-effectiveness of initial and serial measurements of bone mass using modern methods of x-ray based densitometry or quantitative computed tomography (CT) scanning.[36] My opinion is that no other risk factors correlate as well with fracture as does low bone density. Therefore, baseline and serial measurements of bone mass are the only current quantitative methods available to estimate need for or results of therapeutic interventions, and I recommend them. If patients continue to experience fractures after 1 or 2 years of therapy, bone biopsies are useful in designing new interventions. Also, some patients with what looks like ordinary midlife osteoporosis by all other parameters actually have elements of osteomalacia on bone biopsies, which indicates need for interventions that address mineralization defects. An additional benefit of bone biopsy is the ability to accurately classify a patient as having low-turnover or high-turnover osteoporosis, which may influence therapy.

PREVENTION OF OSTEOPOROSIS

It is difficult, perhaps impossible, to restore large quantities of bone once that mass is lost. Therefore, it is appealing to construct programs that prevent osteoporosis, rather than to treat symptomatic disease. To this end, several studies have evaluated the benefits of physical exercise, dietary calcium supplementation, and hormonal replacement in perimenopausal women. Because peak bone mass is important in determining predisposition to osteoporosis, it may be effective to optimize exercise programs and ensure adequate calcium intake in children and adolescents, as well as introducing later interventions. To evaluate the effect of any intervention, it is most desirable to demonstrate prevention of bone fractures, because that is the single-most important outcome. Such data, however, are not available for some interventions, in which case, quantities of bone mass in selected areas of the skeleton, or of whole body calcium (99% of which is in bone), have been used as outcome measures.

Several types of *exercise* help maintain bone mass in adults.[35] Several cross-sectional studies have shown that adolescents and young women who exercise regularly have higher bone mass than those who do not. Among adolescent athletes, heavy exercise leads to an increase in bone mass. Perimenopausal women who performed 3 hours a week of the President's Council on Fitness exercises increased their total body calcium.[37,38] Optimal results seem to require skeletal weight bearing and muscle activity. This includes walking, jogging, and standing while exercising. Optimal results also require adequate calcium intake, and maintenance of the exercise. All benefits to bone mass are apparently lost after exercise is discontinued. On the other hand, some exercises are probably undesirable. One prospective study suggested that weight-lifting that loaded the spine was associated with elevations in PTH and loss of lumbar spine mass. Women who exercise to the point of amenorrhea lose bone rapidly.[39] Exercise must be chosen carefully to be appealing and free of adverse musculoskeletal side effects. In women at high risk for osteoporosis (between 50 and 70 years of age), walking for 30 to 60 minutes, three or four times a week, is probably effective in maintaining bone mass, provided that other factors are optimal. Elderly individuals often experience hip fracture after a fall; exercises that strengthen muscle as well as bone are highly desirable. No firm data show that stimulation of bone formation by exercise translates into lower fracture rates. Thus, moderate exercise programs remain a logical, but unproven, prevention strategy.

Certain nutritional modifications may influence bone mass. High intakes of sodium, phosphates, protein, caffeine, and alcohol have negative effects. High intakes of *calcium* have a positive effect.[33,40,41] Positive calcium balance correlates directly with increasing calcium intake. The average intake of calcium in the white North American diet is 500 to 700 mg daily. To maintain positive calcium balance, most men and premenopausal white females require 800 to 1000 mg of elemental calcium a day; postmenopausal women and men over age 55 require 1500 mg daily.[21] A lifetime of high calcium intake is associated with a significantly lower fracture risk; differences between populations with high or low intake begin to appear at approximately age 40.[33] The value of introducing supplemental calcium tablets in perimenopausal women has been controversial, because some studies were unable to show a significant difference in appendicular or axial bone mass after as much as 2 years supplementation.[42,43] However, a meta-analysis of 49 studies[40] concluded that (1) a positive correlation exists between calcium intake and bone mass in women (especially during premenopausal years), and (2) 1000 mg/day of calcium supplement in early postmenopausal women can prevent about 1% loss of bone mass per year in all bone sites except vertebrae; a decrease of that quantity is probably enough to translate into decreased fracture rates. Several studies have shown decreased fracture rates (hip and vertebrae) in postmenopausal women with osteoporosis who received several years of calcium supplementation.[33,44]

Physicians and the public should give attention to the form in which supplemental calcium is provided.[45] All supplements do not have equal bioavailability, which depends on solubility, availability of calcium as an ion, and acidic pH of the stomach. Calcium tablets are not regulated in the same way that drugs are, so there is considerable variation between commercial products in disintegration times; some do not dissolve at all. Patients should test their preparations by being sure a tablet dissolves in a glass of vinegar within 30 minutes at room temperature. Calcium carbonate, phosphate, and citrate are well absorbed; absorption is maximized if tablets are taken with a meal and with 6 to 8 ounces of liquid. Individuals who are achlorhydric should receive calcium citrate salts. The bioavailability of calcium in foods is also not uniform. For example, the calcium in spinach is not bioavailable; the calcium in milk is. An 8-ounce glass of milk contains approximately 300 mg of calcium.

In summary, addition of calcium supplements to the dietary intake of pre- and perimenopausal women at risk for osteoporosis is probably effective in helping maximize peak bone mass and in slowing loss that occurs with menopause and with aging. Preparations used for supplementation—tablet or dietary—should be carefully chosen. Calcium supplementation is generally safe—hypercalcemia occurred in 1% of a population treated with calcium supplements; 1000 mg of supplemental calcium increased urinary calcium by only 70 mg/24 hours.

It is clear that, although increased calcium intake is helpful in maintaining bone mass, the intervention is not as potent as sex hormone replacement.[42,44,46] Therefore, *providing estrogen within 5 years of menopause is a much more effective intervention than increasing calcium intake.*

Strong evidence shows that estrogens, and probably low doses of some progestins and androgens, also prevent or slow the rate of bone loss from both appendicular and axial skeleton in perimenopausal women. In individuals who have premature menopause (before age 45), estrogen replacement clearly slows bone loss, is effective for at least 8 to 10 years, and cannot be discontinued without rapid bone loss.[26,47] Most authorities recommend that all women with premature menopause be treated with estrogen replacement, in cyclic form, at least .625 mg of conjugated estrogens 25 days out of 30, unless a specific contraindication exists. Alternatively, estrogens can be administered percutaneously, also in a cyclic regimen. Another alternative is to administer estrogens daily, rather than cyclically, balanced each day by administration of low doses of progesterone, to prevent the endometrial hyperplasia caused by estrogen.

Stabilization of bone mass, as well as a small increase (2 to 5%) in bone density, can be achieved by administration of estrogen to women after a natural menopause, especially in those who are within 5 years of cessation of menses. Such replacement therapy is associated with a significantly reduced incidence of hip fractures.[48] In fact, 4 or more years of estrogen use is associated with a relative risk for fractures of 0.5, making this a highly effective preventive strategy. The studies of Ettinger, Genant, and Cann[42] and of Riis et al.[49] showed that administration of estrogen for 2 years to women within 3 years of menopause maintained stable bone mass in the radius and spine, whereas treatment with calcium alone, or no treatment, did not. In the Ettinger study, the effective dose of estrogen was 0.3 mg/day of conjugated estrogen orally, with 1000 mg of calcium carbonate; this was given cyclically 25 days of 30, with a progestogen added from day 16 to 25.[42] In the Riis study, estrogen was administered percutaneously as 3 mg daily of 17 β-estradiol plus 2000 mg of calcium carbonate 24 of 28 days; some patients received progesterone on days 13 to 24.[49] Therefore, cyclic administration of estrogen balanced by progesterone, which is considered to be the safest method of administering estrogen to postmenopausal women, is effective in maintaining bone mass for at least a few years if initiated shortly after menopause begins. Daily administration of unopposed estrogen is associated with increased risks for endometrial hyperplasia and carcinoma, hypertension, migraine headaches, and hypercoagulable states. The risk of uterine malignancy is *not* increased if administration of estrogen and cyclic and progestogens are also used. The use of transcutaneous estradiol may decrease the incidence of undesirable side effects of estrogen, which depend on increased synthesis of certain polypeptides by the liver, such as renin precursors.[50]

Many women who might benefit from estrogen replacement do not wish to take it.[51] A substantial portion of those who begin replacement therapy do not continue it. A major disincentive for continuing cyclic therapy is the return of regular menses. I often administer conjugated estrogen 0.625 mg daily and progesterone 2.5 to 5 mg daily without interruption. On this regimen, endometrial hyperplasia does not occur, and fewer than 20% of women experience bleeding.[52,53] Another disincentive is fear of breast cancer. There is controversy regarding associations between estrogen replacement therapy and carcinoma of the breast,[54–56] with some studies showing no increase in risk. Several long-term studies, however, suggest that women who use replacement therapy for long periods of time (10 to 20 years), even if the therapy is cyclic, have a statistically signifi-

TABLE 113–5. PREVENTION OF OSTEOPOROSIS IN SUBJECTS AT HIGH RISK

PROVIDE ADEQUATE CALCIUM INTAKE	Ensure intake of 800–1500 mg calcium* daily. May supplement with dissolvable calcium carbonate, citrate, or maleate given with meals.
ENSURE ADEQUATE VITAMIN D INTAKE	400–800 IU vitamin D daily. If urine calcium consistently 100 mg/24 hours add 50,000 units once a week and titrate to urine calcium of 150–250 mg/24 hours.
REGULAR EXERCISE REGIMEN	Exercise* against gravity: 3 to 4 hours a week of walking, jogging, tennis, etc.
SEX HORMONE REPLACEMENT IN WOMEN WITHIN 5 YEARS OF MENOPAUSE	Regimens: Estrogen plus Progestin **1.** Conjugated estrogens: 0.3–1.25 mg qd, plus calcium 500 mg qd, plus provera 2.5–5 mg qd **2.** Conjugated estrogens: 0.3–1.25 mg on days 1–25, plus calcium 500 mg qd, plus provera 10 mg on days 15–25 **3.** Transcutaneous estradiol: 100-μg patch cyclically or daily with high or low doses of provera as in 1 or 2
ALTERNATIVES TO SEX HORMONE REPLACEMENT When contraindicated or when ineffective as determined by serial measurements of bone density	**1.** Etidronate: 400 mg qd for 2 weeks then rest 13 weeks (supply calcium during that period). Repeat cycle. **2.** Calcitonin*: 50–100 MRC units three to seven times a week, subcutaneous. **3.** Thiazide*: 25–50 mg daily.

* Intervention less effective than estrogen replacement therapy.

cant increase in breast cancer. The risk is small—on the order of a relative risk of 1.5 to 1.8. Because the risk of hip fracture (with its attendant high mortality) and of ischemic heart disease are both reduced about 50% by estrogen replacement therapy, most authorities continue to recommend estrogen–progestin replacement therapies in the perimenopausal period for women at increased risk for osteoporosis.

Several studies have shown that estrogen therapy is effective in stabilizing bone mass even if introduced in elderly individuals who are 10 or more years past menopause.[53,57] Of course, at that time bone loss has often been great, so those individuals continue to be at risk for fracture. In elderly women, return of menses is particularly unacceptable, so daily therapy balanced by progesterone is recommended.

In summary, cyclic estrogen–progestin therapy, or daily therapy with estrogen and a progestin, should be considered for postmenopausal women who are at risk for osteoporosis, if there are no contraindications to its use. Data have been obtained primarily in white women, and risk factors have been identified in that group. Selecting women who should be treated can be difficult. Risk factors can be used to identify candidates for treatment, or the physician can rely on measurements of bone density, choosing to treat only women who are one standard deviation or greater below the mean bone mass for sex-, age-, and race-matched controls. Alternatively, some physicians prefer to treat all perimenopausal white women because of benefits not only on bone but on climacteric symptoms and cardiovascular disease. For detail, see the regimens listed in Table 113–5.

Androgens and some progestogens have effects similar to estrogens in maintaining bone mass in postmenopausal women.[10,11,58] Androgens may be useful in men with osteoporosis; estrogens are preferable in women.

Chronic use of thiazide diuretics is associated with higher bone mass in men and women, compared to matched controls who have not used thiazides.[59] The differences are statistically significant but require years to reach that level and are lost over a period of several months after thiazides are discontinued. I consider the use of thiazides an effective but relatively weak intervention to prevent osteoporosis.

OSTEOPOROSIS IN MEN

The differential diagnosis for osteoporosis in men is similar to that for women, with hypogonadism being an important component in some cases.[60] In one series, long-standing testosterone deficiency was found in 30% of men presenting with spinal fractures and osteoporosis, most of whom were in their 50s. Hypogonadism can result from idiopathic hypogonadotropic hypogonadism, hemochromatosis, hyperprolactinemia, Klinefelter's syndrome, anorexia nervosa, and other causes of primary testicular failure of hypothalamic pituitary dysfunction. As in postmenopausal women, deficiency of sex hormone—be it androgen or estrogen—is associated with loss of trabecular bone and spinal osteoporosis. However, there is also evidence that serum testosterone levels are subnormal in the majority of men who experience hip fractures. Many men with hypogonadism are capable of sexual function and do not have testicular atrophy. Therefore, it is a good policy to measure serum levels of luteinizing hormone and testosterone in all men with osteoporosis. Some with hypogonadism have high luteinizing hormone and normal testosterone.

Other causes of osteoporosis should be considered, including osteomalacia, hyperparathyroidism, hyperthyroidism, Cushing's syndrome, neoplasms, and collagen disorders such as osteogenesis imperfecta and Ehlers-Danlos syndromes. In men receiving chronic glucocorticoid therapy, risk for fractures is particularly high after age 50.[61] Involutional bone loss occurs in men, although at a slower rate than in women.

With regard to therapy, good responses can be expected to androgens in hypogonadal patients. Long-acting esters (testosterone cypionate or enanthate) in doses of 200 to 300 mg intramuscularly every 2 to 3 weeks are recommended. Oral androgens are less desirable because of potential hepatotoxicity. Patients so treated should be monitored for development of prostatic hypertrophy and carcinoma. Androgen therapy can increase bone mass; effects on fracture rates have not been reported. Additional therapies are similar to those used in women: calcium supplementation, calcitonin, bisphosphonates, and possibly fluoride.

TREATMENT OF SYMPTOMATIC OSTEOPOROSIS

Therapy of symptomatic osteoporosis can be frustrating to both patient and physician because of the uncertainty that any interventions will increase bone mass enough to reduce pain and fractures.

Calcium

As discussed earlier, a high intake of calcium in childhood and adolescence probably increases peak bone mass,[32,33] and supplementing intake later probably has measurable although relatively small benefit.[40] Calcium has many effects on bone. It is required for mineralization, and a positive calcium balance helps maintain bone mass. Calcium also suppresses bone turnover by slowing remodeling. Riggs and colleagues[44] initially reported that recurrent episodes of vertebral fractures were diminished by approximately 50% if postmenopausal osteoporotic women were treated with calcium carbonate (1500 to 2500 mg daily) for more than a year. This benefit was seen with or without pharmacologic doses of vitamin D. However, the use of calcium as a sole agent to treat symptomatic osteoporosis is a relatively weak intervention.

Estrogens

The use of estrogens in perimenopausal women and androgens in hypogonadal men has been discussed.[42,44,48–57,60] Estrogens act primarily as suppressors of bone resorption and thus reduce the rate of remodeling. As a preventive measure, estrogen therapy reduces bone loss and fracture rates in postmenopausal women. Androgens also suppress bone resorption; they may also have anabolic effects that promote bone formation.[11,58] Their administration to women or men is effective in slowing loss of bone, and some studies have reported gains in bone mass, both axial and appendicular, of 5 to 20% over the first 2 years of treatment. Data showing decreased fracture rates are not available for androgens. Androgens have potential adverse hepatic effects (peliosis, tumors, obstructive jaundice) especially if given orally: they have potential adverse effects on lipids; and their virilizing side effects are unpopular with women.

With regard to treatment of symptomatic osteoporosis with estrogen, Recker, Saville, and Heaney[46] demonstrated that the combination of calcium and estrogen maintained bone mass in symptomatic postmenopausal women better than did calcium alone. In the studies of Riggs et al.,[44] the combination resulted in vertebral fracture rates significantly lower than those in women receiving calcium alone. Although this intervention is effective when started within 5 years of menopause, introduction in osteoporotic women in their 60s is also effective in stopping decline in bone mass and probably in producing a net gain in bone during the first year or two.[53,57] Patients with symptomatic osteoporosis who are treated with estrogen should receive cyclic therapy or daily therapy balanced with daily progestins, as discussed previously in the section on prevention of osteoporosis.

Vitamin D and Its Metabolites

Vitamin D and its metabolites are advocated by some authorities as therapy for osteoporosis, to ensure maximal absorption of dietary calcium and to maintain positive calcium balance. Several studies, however, have failed to demonstrate a reduction in fracture rates or an increase in bone mass accompanying vitamin D therapy for osteoporosis.[5,62] Hypercalciuria, defined as a urine calcium level greater than 300 mg/24 hours, and hypercalcemia are complications of vitamin D therapy occurring in approximately 25% of patients, especially with 25 OH D and 1,25 $(OH)_2D$ regimens. Currently, I use supraphysiologic doses of vitamin D or its metabolites only in osteoporotic individuals who have urine calcium levels less than 100 mg/24 hours. For most patients, vitamin D supplementation of 400 to 800 IU/day is adequate.

Etidronate

Studies of etidronate, a form of bisphosphonate available in the United States, suggest that cyclic administration is highly effective in maintaining bone mass and in reducing fracture rates in women with symptomatic osteoporosis.[63–65] Bisphosphonates bind to apatite crystals and thus inhibit the ability of osteoclasts to resorb bone. If suppressive effects are then removed by discontinuing the drug, the units should refill with osteoid and mineralize. Women who had experienced vertebral fractures were treated with 400 mg of etidronate daily for 2 weeks, followed by daily calcium (500 mg) alone for 10 to 13 weeks. This cycle was repeated for 2 to 3 years. Patients receiving etidronate, compared to women on placebo or phosphate followed by placebo (1) increased their vertebral bone mass by a mean of 5% and (2) reduced their incidence of new vertebral fractures by 50 to 90%. Used in this cyclic regimen, etidronate was associated with no adverse side effects during the first two years of treatment. However, long-term safety and efficacy have not been established.

When used daily for several months, etidronate can shut off osteoblast as well as osteoclast activity, with net bone loss. The cyclic regimens minimize that problem, at least for the first two years. Furthermore, newer preparations available outside the United States have minimal effects on osteoblasts and may be even better therapeutic agents than etidronate. For now, the cyclic etidronate regimen seems to be a safe intervention (for use over two years) that should be particularly effective in the treatment of high turnover osteoporosis.

Calcitonin

Calcitonin is approved by the Food and Drug Administration (FDA) for use in osteoporosis. It acts directly on osteoclasts to suppress their activity, thus reducing bone resorption.[8] It is effective therapy in some cases of Paget's disease and tumor-induced hypercalcemia. Several studies have shown that subcutaneous administration of 50 to 100 units three to seven times weekly prevents loss of bone mass in perimenopausal women and results in a gain of up to 15%. Patients with high-turnover osteoporosis are most responsive, especially in vertebral mass.[66] However, no long-term studies of effect on fracture rate are available, the drug must be injected subcutaneously (a nasal spray form is available in Europe), and higher doses are associated with nausea and flushing. Therefore, estrogen and etidronate are easier to use and of established efficacy with regard to decreasing fracture rates and are probably preferable to calcitonin at this time. Calcitonin has some analgesic effect and may be useful in therapy of patients with acute fractures and bone pain.

All of the strategies discussed—calcium, estrogen, bisphosphonates, calcitonin—exert their primary effects on bone remodeling by diminishing bone resorption. Thus, all should be effective in patients with high-turnover osteoporosis. A substantial subset of individuals (those with low-turnover osteoporosis who have little osteoclastic activity in bone) cannot be expected to respond to these interventions. A therapy that can activate osteoblasts and increase bone formation is badly needed. The only currently available drug that has this capacity is fluoride, and its use in osteoporosis is quite controversial.[67,68] It is generally agreed that 70 to 80% of individuals who receive 50 to 75 mg of sodium fluoride daily will increase vertebral bone density dramatically—as much as 20 to 35%; the therapy does not increase bone mass as much in the femoral trochanter or neck, nor does the mass of the radius increase. Therefore, it seems logical that fracture rates in vertebra would diminish but hip fracture rates would not. A beneficial effect on fracture rate depends on denser bone being stronger bone, and that is not clearly the case. Some evidence indicates that fluoride incorporated into the bone mineral crystal renders it more brittle. However, some studies have shown that vertebral fracture rates diminish in symptomatic postmenopausal women treated with fluoride.[44,67] In contrast, another study reported that treatment of women (with previous vertebral fractures) with 75 mg of sodium fluoride daily for 4 years resulted in no dimunition of vertebral fracture rates compared to women treated with placebo. Furthermore, women receiviing fluoride had a *higher* rate of extravertebral fractures.[68] Some authorities suggest that 75 mg daily for 4 years is too high a dose for too long a period and recommend cyclical therapy with lower doses, such as 50 mg daily for 3 month periods. Sodium fluoride has a relatively high incidence of undesirable side effects, with gastrointestinal discomfort (including peptic ulcers) and lower leg pain being the major problems. The leg pain is poorly understood but may reflect stress fractures. Both gastrointestinal symptoms and bone pain resolve after discontinuation of the drug. Gastrointestinal symptoms are considerably less with time-release preparations. In summary, fluoride therapy is the only intervention that can activate osteoblasts and increase bone formation. However, it probably is not effective in preventing hip fractures, and its effectiveness in diminishing vertebral fractures is unclear. It has not been approved by the FDA for use in osteoporosis. I still use it in patients with low-turnover osteoporosis who are continuing to experience vertebral or rib fractures after standard therapeutic interventions, but I give no more than 50 mg daily for no more than 3 months at a time. If fluoride is used, it should be given with supplemental calcium and vitamin D to ensure mineralization of the new osteoid formed.[44,67,68]

Additional therapies, which should be considered experimental, include PTH and ADFR. Parathyroid hormone in intermittent low doses stimulates osteoblasts; it may have anabolic effects on bone.[69] Convenient preparations of proven utility are not yet available in the United States. ADFR is cyclical therapy designed to control the bone multicellular units:[70] A = activate the unit, D = depress the unit, F = free the unit of stimuli, R = repeat the cycle. The unit could be activated by PTH or phosphate, then depressed by calcitonin or calcium or sex hormone administration, then freed of therapy. To date, studies employing the ADFR approach have not had greater success than some of the interventions already discussed.[64,67]

Finally, there may be a role for multiple therapies. At least one study suggest that use of calcium, estrogen, and fluoride together is more effective than any single intervention alone.[44] This should be considered in patients who continue to experience fractures after optimal interventions, such as calcium plus estrogen in the perimenopausal period.

Therapy of symptomatic osteoporosis is reviewed in Table 113–6.

GLUCOCORTICOID-INDUCED OSTEOPENIA

DEFINITION

Bone loss associated with glucocorticoid therapy is another state in which the rate of bone resorption exceeds the rate of bone formation. The uncoupling of formation and resorption caused by supraphysiologic glucocorti-

TABLE 113–6. THERAPY OF SYMPTOMATIC OSTEOPOROSIS (WITH FRACTURES)

1. Measure serum and urine calcium levels.
   If both are normal: Add calcium 1000 mg qd, vitamin D 400 IU qd.
   If urine calcium <120 mg/24 hours: Add calcium 1000 mg qd, Vitamin D 50,000 units one to three times per week
   MONITOR SERUM AND URINE CALCIUM LEVELS EVERY 4 MONTHS.
   If serum calcium is abnormal: Evaluate for another metabolic bone disease.
2. Establish appropriate exercise program if tolerated.
3. Add one of the following, which have been shown to reduce fracture rates in individuals with osteoporotic fractures:
   Estrogen plus progestin therapy in women after menopause (See regimens in Table 113–5)
   Etidronate in Women (See regimen in Table 113–5)
   Note: These interventions decrease bone resorption but do not have major effects on increasing bone formation. Net bone gain occurs in the first several months of treatment, but that plateaus when bone formation rates decrease as they become coupled to reduced resorption rates.
4. If new fractures occur after 1 year of these interventions, or if the interventions are contraindicated or not tolerated, consider adding or substituting one of the following interventions, none of which has been proven to lower fracture rates:
   Androgens in Hypogonadal Men: Testosterone cypionate or enanthate, 200–300 mg IM every 2–3 weeks.
   Etidronate in Men: See regimen in Table 113–5
   Calcitonin: See regimen in Table 113–5. May be particularly useful in immediate postfracture period because it has analgesic properties.
   Fluoride: Consider administration of 40–50 mg daily for 3-month periods, 3-month rest, then repeat. Some data suggest extravertebral fracture rates may increase on high doses for sustained periods.[68] Give supplemental calcium and vitamin D throughout therapy (see Table 113–5 for selection of doses).
   Androgens in Women: Nandrolone 50 mg IM every 3–4 weeks.

Note: Physicians should read the text and appropriate references before instituting any of these therapies for full understanding of benefits and risks.

coid levels has two mechanisms: reduction of formation and increase of resorption.[12,71,72] As in many other metabolic bone diseases, bone with a large surface area available for endosteal osteoclastic resorption is lost at a faster rate than compact cortical bone. Therefore, bones with high trabecular content, such as vertebrae and ribs, are at a high risk for fracture—a fact recognized for decades in both spontaneous and iatrogenic Cushing's syndrome (Fig. 113–5). Fracture rates are also high in bones of the appendicular skeleton in individuals with rheumatic diseases treated chronically with glucocorticoids. Several studies of bone mass in patients receiving long-term glucocorticoids for pulmonary or rheumatic diseases have shown rapid loss of trabecular bone in the first year of treatment. These include estimations of trabecular mass in iliac crest bone biopsies, and osteodensitometric or CT measurements of bone mass in areas of the skeleton with relatively high trabecular mass—the distal end of the radius or vertebrae. Trabecular mass can decrease 20 to 27% over the initial 12-month period of glucocorticoid therapy.[73] One study showed that bone mass at the metaphyseal site of the radius falls rapidly with predisone use, with approximately a 4% loss after 6 months and a 30% loss after 100 months.[74]

MECHANISMS

The mechanisms by which supraphysiologic levels of gluococorticoids cause bone loss are fairly well understood.[12,71,72] Multiple actions of these hormones cause rates of bone resorption to increase while rates of formation decrease.

Effect on Osteoblasts. Glucocorticoids in supraphysiologic amounts decrease the maturation of pre-osteoblastic cells to osteoblasts. In addition, proliferation, RNA synthesis, and synthesis of collagen and noncollagenous proteins by mature osteoblasts are reduced. Very little new bone is made. Administration of a single dose of 10 mg of prednisone decreases serum osteocalcin by 50 to 80% in healthy young men.[75]

Effect on Osteoclasts. Initially, osteoclasts are activated by exogenous administration of glucocorticoids. This may be partly a direct effect, but secondary hyperparathyroidism is probably the major stimulus for osteoclast activation.

Effect on Intestinal Absorption of Calcium. Absorption is decreased. This is probably due to the ability of glucocorticoids to suppress calcium-binding protein in intestinal epithelial cells.

Effect on Renal Excretion of Calcium. This increases. Tubular resorption of calcium is reduced, probably by suppression of the calcium-binding protein of renal tubular epithelial cells. Secondary hyperparathyroidism results primarily from the decrease in ionized serum calcium, which occurs in response to decreased intestinal absorption and increased urinary loss.

Effect on Polypeptides Influencing Bone. These are numerous. Many of the local growth factors are reduced in quantity during glucocorticoid therapy. Prostaglandin synthesis is also suppressed; prostaglandin mediates some actions of growth factors. The mechanisms by which glucocorticoids cause bone loss are reviewed in Table 113–7.

INCIDENCE

Fractures of both axial and appendicular skeleton in patients receiving glucocorticoid therapy remain a major clinical problem. Such fractures occur in highest

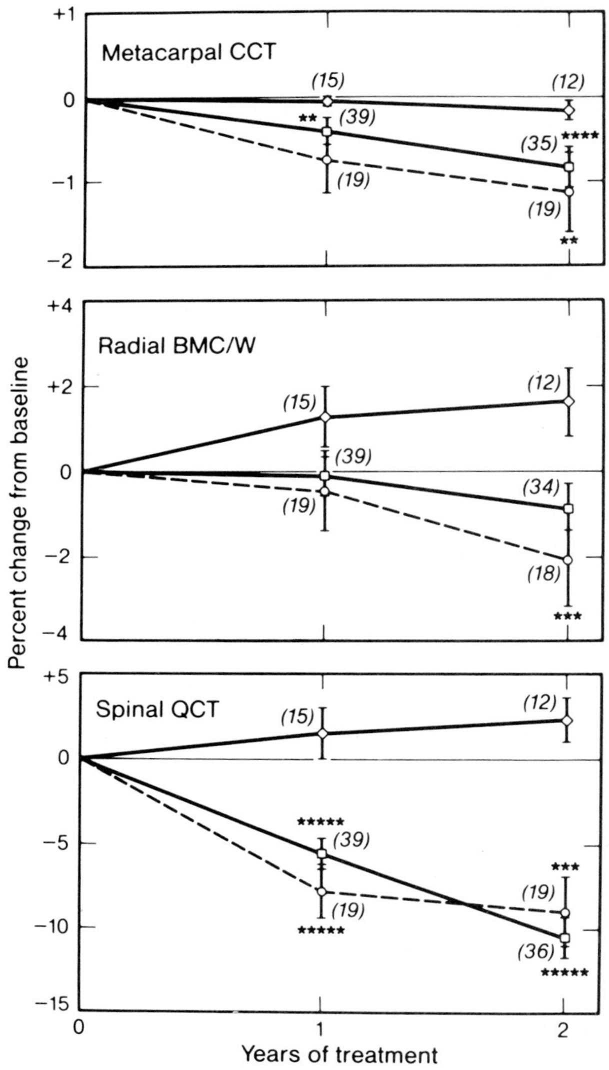

FIGURE 113–5. These data illustrate: (1) the increased effectiveness of estrogen compared to calcium alone in preserving bone mass in women within 3 years of menopause; (2) different rates of bone loss in different areas of the skeleton; and (3) use of multiple different methods to measure bone mass. Numbers in parenthesis are the number of women entered into each treatment group. *Open circles* represent women who were not treated; *open squares* represent women treated with 1000 to 1500 mg of oyster shell calcium daily; *open diamonds* represent women treated with conjugated estrogen, .3 mg daily 25 days out of 30 (with a progestogen added from day 16 through 25) plus 1000 to 1500 mg of calcium daily. Bone mass was well maintained in all skeletal areas studied only in the groups that received estrogen; bone mass declined, especially in the spine, in the group receiving calcium alone. Bone loss was most marked in the lumbar spine compared to the radius or metacarpal bones. Metacarpal mass was measured as combined cortical thickness, radial mass as bone density by single photon absorptiometry, and spinal mass by quantitative computed tomography scanning. (Reproduced from Ettinger, B. et al.,[42] with permission of the author and the publisher.)

TABLE 113–7. MECHANISMS OF GLUCOCORTICOID-INDUCED OSTEOPENIA

SUPPRESSION OF BONE FORMATION
Reduced conversion of precursor cells to osteoblasts
Reduced synthesis of osteoid by mature osteoblasts
Suppression of local bone growth factors
ENHANCEMENT OF BONE RESORPTION
Reduced intestinal absorption of calcium
Reduced renal tubular resorption of calcium with increased urinary loss
Secondary hyperparathyroidism resulting from calcium malabsorption and renal loss
Activation of osteoclasts secondary to parathyroid hormone signals
NET RESULT: RATE OF RESORPTION > RATE OF FORMATION

frequency in older individuals; therefore, glucocorticoid osteopenia is usually an insult added to bone loss resulting from age, the postmenopausal state, or decreased physical activity. We have seen vertebral fractures as early as 3 months after the institution of glucocorticoid therapy in older individuals.

The incidence of glucocorticoid osteopenia is not clear because of variations in definition and in populations studied. In studies in which bone mass was measured by direct weight of bones at autopsy or by calculation of trabecular bone volume from iliac crest biopsies, 85 to 90% of patients treated with glucocorticoids had significantly less bone mass than age-, sex-, and race-matched normal individuals.[19] We studied 161 patients with rheumatic disease treated for more than 6 weeks with various doses of daily or alternate-day prednisone.[61] Bone density was measured by single photon absorptiometry at two sites in the radius—metaphyseal and diaphyseal. The metaphyseal area has more trabecular bone than the diaphyseal, and it is lost at a faster rate during glucocorticoid therapy. The incidence of glucocorticoid osteopenia, defined as abnormally low metaphyseal mass, varied from 23 to 78%, depending on the cumulative dose of prednisone (Table 113–8). More than 80% of individuals who had received more than 30 g of prednisone had either low trabecular (metaphyseal) mass or fractures. Most individuals receiving glucocorticoid therapy on a long-term basis clearly will lose bone to the extent that their risk for fracture is increased.

The prevalence of bone fractures in the group of rheumatic disease patients we[61] studied is shown in Table 113–8. The data suggest that such patients have a twofold to threefold increase in prevalence of axial or appendicular bone fractures if they are receiving long-term glucocorticoid therapy.

Risk Factors

Factors that may influence risk include sex, age, race, body habitus, type of rheumatic disease, duration of disease, glucocorticoid dose, duration of therapy, con-

TABLE 113–8. INCIDENCE OF FRACTURES IN RHEUMATIC DISEASE PATIENTS RECEIVING LONG-TERM GLUCOCORTICOID THERAPY

	FRACTURES		
	Vertebral (%)	Extravertebral (%)	All (%)
Patients never receiving systemic glucocorticoid therapy	5–8	6	9
Patients receiving long-term glucocorticoid therapy	12–18	19	30

TABLE 113–9. RISK FACTORS FOR GLUCOCORTICOID-INDUCED OSTEOPENIA*

DEFINITE RISK FACTORS

High Cumulative Dose of Glucocorticoids

Total Dose (g)	Elevated DM/MM (%)	Fractures (%)	p
<10	18/77 (23)	10/45 (22)	
10–30	25/61 (40)	10/33 (33)	< .03
>30	18/23 (78)	8/15 (53)	< .01

Increasing Age

Individuals over age 50, men or women, have increased risk for fractures.

Postmenopausal State

PROBABLE RISK FACTORS

Increasing Duration of Glucocorticoid Therapy

High Daily Doses of Glucocorticoids

Age <15 Years

Small Body Size

Especially leanness (presteroid habitus)

White Race

Female Sex (before menopause)

* Data are based on studies reported in reference 61.

comitant therapies, level of activity, nutritional status (especially vitamin D and calcium intake), and amount of exposure to sunlight.

Table 113–9 summarizes the factors that increase the risk of trabecular (metaphyseal) bone loss and of fractures; data are based on our study.[61] An increasing cumulative glucocorticoid dose was the strongest risk factor, with the highest positive correlation with loss of trabecular (metaphyseal) bone. Daily prednisone dose and duration of therapy did not correlate as strongly but were obviously related to total cumulative doses. Therefore, the duration of glucocorticoid therapy probably correlates inversely with bone mass, with most of the loss occurring early in the course of therapy.[73] This suggests that interventions to combat osteopenia should be started shortly after introduction of glucocorticoids. Some investigators have suggested that there is a "safe" dose of glucocorticoids—that doses of 10 mg daily or less are not associated with impairment of intestinal calcium absorption or with loss of bone mass.[76] However, in our studies, we detected loss of metaphyseal bone on doses of prednisone as low as 10 mg of prednisone every other day,[61,77] and administration of a single dose of 10 mg reduced serum levels of osteocalcin in healthy individuals,[75] so I doubt that there is an exogenous low dose of glucocorticoids that does not affect bone adversely. Our data also show that alternate-day glucocorticoid regimens cause bone loss similar to that of daily regimens.[77] On the other hand, low daily doses are obviously safer than high doses.

The second strongest risk factor correlating positively with increasing loss of trabecular bone mass and increasing fracture rates was increasing age. Individuals over age 50 had significantly higher incidence of fracture than did younger individuals; these findings were similar to those reported by others. Postmenopausal women, including those with premature menopause, had a significantly higher fracture rate than did premenopausal women. Before age 50, the fracture rate was much lower in men than in women, but thereafter the rates were essentially the same in both sexes. This is not surprising, because glucocorticoid-osteopenia in adults is often added to postmenopausal, involutional, or inactivity-related osteoporosis. Children, with their rapidly growing bones, are also at high risk.

Individuals of small body size, especially those who are lean, may be at greater risk for glucocorticoid osteopenia. We showed a significant negative correlation between increasing body surface area (presteroid) and abnormal bone mass; however, we could not demonstrate a difference in fracture rates.[61]

Interestingly, no correlations were noted between type of rheumatic disease and either trabecular bone loss or fracture rates when data were corrected for age. Clinically, we suspect that older individuals (especially whites with polymyalgia rheumatica are at high risk for glucocorticoid-related fractures, individuals with rheumatoid arthritis (RA) are at moderate risk, and those with systemic lupus erythematosus are at lower risk. This could be primarily based on the average age of those populations. Several studies,[76] however, have shown that patients with RA who never received glucocorticoids had significantly lower bone mass than age-, sex-, and race-matched healthy control subjects; the degree of disability correlated best with low bone mass.

We were not able to show significant differences in the prevalence of glucocorticoid osteopenia when we compared black individuals to white, but our numbers were relatively small.[61] Data are too few to comment about the relative risks in whites compared to any other ethnic groups for glucocorticoid-induced osteopenia.

Diagnosis

As discussed previously, no inexpensive, simple techniques are widely available to confirm a specific diagnosis of glucocorticoid-induced osteopenia. The clinician can only suspect its presence in most individuals who have received daily or alternate-day doses of glucocorticoids for several months. If routine roentgenograms, especially of vertebrae, show osteopenia, the patient is probably at high risk for fracture. For practical purposes, the diagnosis of glucocorticoid-induced osteopenia can be made in any patient with vertebral (or other high trabecular content bone) bone mass reduced below the mean for age-, race-, and sex-matched controls who is receiving daily or alternate-day therapy with supraphysiologic quantities of glucocorticoids for more than a month. Simple screening tests should be done to rule out other conditions, including hyperparathyroidism, hyperthyroidism, osteomalacia, and malignancies in bone. Serum levels of calcium and phosphate are almost always normal in untreated glucocorticoid osteopenia. Alkaline phosphatase is usually normal but may be mildly elevated, especially if recent fracture has occurred. If any of these tests are abnormal, alternate etiologies for osteopenia should be sought.

Treatment

The best therapy for glucocorticoid-induced osteopenia is complete withdrawal of the glucocorticoids. I have observed exuberant new bone formation in iliac crest bone biopsies obtained from patients with rheumatic disease 3 to 6 months after discontinuation of prednisone therapy; similar findings have been reported in patients after surgery for Cushing's disease.[78] Unfortunately, in patients with chronic allergic, inflammatory, or rheumatic conditions, it is often undesirable to discontinue glucocorticoids, so other strategies are used, always with the goal of administering the smallest possible dose of this agent.

Two additional strategies might be employed. First, a glucocorticoid less toxic to bone might be given, and second, additional strategies might be added to diminish the adverse effects of glucocorticoids. Comparisons of the different types of glucocorticoid currently available in the United States have been made. At equivalent anti-inflammatory doses, they all had similar adverse effects on calcium balance. One molecule currently designated deflazacort (formerly oxazacort) in which an oxazoline ring has been added to the prednisolone molecule has been developed in Europe. In short-term studies in healthy volunteers and longer term studies in patients with RA, less calcium wasting was seen with deflazacort than with equivalent doses of prednisone or betamethasone.[79,80] The drug is currently undergoing testing in the United States, and additional studies to confirm its calcium-sparing effect are in progress.

For the present, only the second strategy, that is, one designed to counteract the adverse effects of glucocorticoids on bone, is practical (Table 113–10).

Many such strategies have been tested in short-term trials; several have been shown to reduce the rate of bone loss and/or to increase bone mass; none have been shown to reduce fracture rates. Two approaches are desirable: one that suppresses the excessive bone resorption characteristic of early glucocorticoid osteopenia and one that stimulates formation of bone.

As for other forms of osteoporosis, only antiresorptive approaches are readily available. These include calcium, vitamin D and 25 OH D, estrogen, modified androgens, calcitonin, and bisphosphonates. Some evidence indicates that supplemental calcium is useful in prevention. One study showed diminution of urinary hydroxyproline and calcium excretion in glucocorticoid-treated patients receiving 1 g of calcium daily for 2 months, suggesting suppression of bone resorption.[81] Two studies showed that control groups receiving 500 mg of calcium daily did not lose bone as rapidly as groups receiving no supplement; however, in both those studies, additional interventions (vitamin D or bisphosphonates) were more effective than calcium alone in maintaining bone mass.[82,83] Therefore, calcium supplementation alone appears to have some effect in preserving bone mass, but this effect is relatively weak. I recommend it for all patients receiving chronic glucocorticoid treatment, unless a contraindication is present.

The use of vitamin D or its metabolites to prevent or to treat glucocorticoid osteopenia is somewhat controversial because of the risk of hypercalciuria and hypercalcemia. Treatment with vitamin D, 25 OH D, or $1,25(OH)_2D$ can partially overcome the intestinal malabsorption of calcium induced by glucocorticoids.[82,84] The treatment is usually associated with an increase in urinary calcium excretion, so regular monitoring of serum and urine calcium levels is required. Patients

TABLE 113–10. STRATEGIES TO MINIMIZE BONE LOSS DURING CHRONIC GLUCOCORTICOID THERAPY

1. Maintain patient on minimal quantities of glucocorticoid required for disease control. Withdraw drug if possible.
2. Encourage regular exercise against gravity when possible.
3. Consider prophylactic therapy for all patients. Therapy should be initiated as soon as possible after starting glucocorticoids—as soon as disease is stable and hypercalciuria has subsided.
  a. Measure serum Ca, PO4, alkaline phosphatase, and urine Ca levels.
  b. Introduce following therapies:

Serum studies normal *Urine Ca > 120 mg/24 hours*	Serum studies normal *Urine Ca < 120 mg/24 hours* *No Nephrolithiasis*	*Serum studies abnormal*
Add Ca 500–1000 mg qd Monitor serum/urine Ca every 6 months.	**Add Ca 500–1000 mg qd** **Add vitamin D 50,000 un one to five times a week.** Or **25 OH D 20 μg qd.** Monitor serum and urine calcium every 3–4 months.	Evaluate for another bone disease.

4. In patients at high risk for fracture, or in patients who develop fractures on this regimen, consider adding the following interventions:
  a. Sex hormone replacement in hypogonadal women or men. (See Tables 113–5 and 113–6 for appropriate regimens.)
  b. Etidronate (See Table 113–5 for regimen.)
  c. Calcitonin (See Table 113–5 for regimen.)
  d. Thiazide diuretic (See Table 113–5 for regimen.)
  e. Fluoride (See Table 113–6 for regimen).

Note: None of these interventions have been shown to reduce fracture rates in patients with glucocorticoid-induced osteopenia. All have been shown to help maintain or increase bone mass in areas of the skeleton with high trabecular bone content. Physicians should read the text and appropriate references before instituting any of these regimens to maximize knowledge of efficacy and toxicity.

with past or present evidence of nephrolithiasis should be excluded from such therapy. Our studies in rheumatic disease patients with trabecular bone loss receiving glucocorticoids demonstrated a significant increase of 8 to 15% in metaphyseal bone mass after 12 months of therapy with vitamin D (50,000 units three times a week) or 25 OH D (20 to 40 μg daily).[84] In patients receiving 25 OH D, we found increased intestinal absorption of calcium, reduced serum PTH levels, and reduced resorption surfaces and osteoclast numbers on iliac crest biopsies. Bone formation rates, judged by tetracycline labeling, were unchanged or increased. In contrast, an 18-month trial of $1,25(OH)_2D$ resulted in improved calcium absorption and reduced PTH levels, but metaphyseal mass did not increase.[82] This probably resulted from suppression of osteoblastic osteoid, as well as suppression of osteoclasts. In summary, *I recommend addition of vitamin D or 25 OH D to the therapeutic regimen of any patient with rheumatic disease receiving chronic glucocorticoid therapy, if the 24-hour urinary excretion of calcium is less than 120 mg, which suggests intestinal malabsorption of calcium.* The vitamin D preparation of choice is 25 OH D, because it is eliminated more quickly than vitamin D. Rapid elimination is desirable if hypercalciuria or hypercalcemia occur. Vitamin D, however, is cheaper and more widely available, and it is effective. The use of $1,25(OH)_2D$ is probably contraindicated in this particular form of osteoporosis. *Caution: patients receiving any forms of vitamin D are prone to hypercalcemia, especially during periods of intercurrent illness that require bed rest. Careful monitoring of serum and urine calcium must be performed at regular intervals to ensure safety.* We do not permit patient's 24-hour urine calcium excretion to exceed 350 mg.

Several other antiresorptive therapies have been tested. A bisphosphonate known as ADP, available in New Zealand, has been studied by Reid and colleagues.[71,83,85] Two years of treatment with ADP led to increased mass in the cortex of metacarpal bones. Sequential studies showed early suppression of urinary hydroxyproline levels (after 6 weeks of treatment) followed later by suppression of serum osteocalcin and alkaline phosphatase (at 3 to 6 months). Therefore, bone resorption was suppressed early, and bone formation was suppressed later as equilibrium between formation and suppression was restored. Net bone gain occurred in the interval and was sustained for 2 years. Whether etidronate, the bisphosphonate available in the United States, will be as useful remains to be seen. It probably should be adminsitered only in cyclic regimens, because prolonged daily use is deleterious to osteoblasts. Estrogen should be provided to perimenopausal and postmenopausal women on chronic glucocorticoid therapy if not contraindicated by their particular rheumatic disease or by other health concerns. Short-term studies have shown that estrogen or androgen (nandrolone) can maintain bone mass in women receiving glucocorticoids.[71,72] A 6-month prospective study in similar subjects treated with calcitonin showed maintenance of bone mass.[86] Thiazide diuretics diminish urinary calcium loss induced by glucocorticoids and may be useful in reducing bone loss; they constitute a relatively weak intervention in postmenopausal osteoporosis compared to the effects of estrogen, and their utility in glucocorticoid-induced bone disease has not been evaluated.

Finally, fluoride preparations[87] or *nandrolone* (an anabolic steroid with mild virilizing properties)[88] might increase the low bone formation rates caused by glucocorticoids. Fluoride can increase trabecular bone volume in iliac crest biopsies of glucocorticoid-treated patients.[87] In our experience, most patients show increased density of vertebral bone after this intervention. Because no data are available regarding the effect of fluoride on fracture rates in such patients, we cannot be sure it is helpful. Nandrolone in short-term trials maintains bone mass.[88]

In summary, most agents that benefit other forms of osteoporosis are probably helpful in glucocorticoid-induced osteopenia. I maintain all patients on supplemental calcium, 500 to 1000 mg/day, and add vitamin D 50,000 units one to three times a week if 24-hour urine calcium levels are less than 120 mg. The intervention should be started within weeks of institution of glucocorticoids—as soon as the patient's medical condition permits. If measures of bone density indicate rapid bone loss, or fractures occur after 6 to 12 months of this regimen, I introduce an additional agent, which may be sex hormone, calcitonin, bisphosphonate, or fluoride. All these approaches should be considered experimental until data regarding their impact on fracture rates become available.

OSTEOMALACIA

Osteomalacia[89,90] is a pathologic loss of mineralized bone caused by reduction of calcium phosphate levels to below that required for normal mineralization of bone matrix. As a result, the ratio of bone mineral to matrix is reduced, undecalcified matrix (osteoid) accumulates, and bone strength declines. The most common causes of osteomalacia beginning after early childhood are reduced vitamin D absorption that is due to biliary, proximal small-bowel mucosal, or ileal disease; increased vitamin D catabolism as a result of drug-induced increases in liver oxidase enzymes; and acquired renal tubular defects with renal phosphate wasting. This third group includes acquired renal tubular phosphate leaks (adult-onset vitamin D-resistant rickets), Fanconi's syndrome, and renal tubular acidosis of the variety seen with the chronic dysproteinemias associated with Sjögren's syndrome, systemic lupus erythematosus, monoclonal gammopathies, and heavy metal poisoning. Additionally, an occasional patient with peptic ulcer disease develops phosphate depletion because of chronic magnesium-aluminum gel antacid use; large amounts of these substances convert dietary phosphate to insoluble complexes in the intestine.

CLINICAL AND DIAGNOSTIC FEATURES

Clinically, patients with osteomalacia have many of the symptoms commonly associated with the rheumatic diseases, including generalized aching and fatigability, proximal myopathy, periarticular tenderness, and sensory polyneuropathy. When osteomalacia is treated, these symptoms all remit rapidly. Radiographs may show only mild generalized demineralization, or they may reveal multiple old rib fractures with poor callus formation, or pathognomonic pseudofractures, termed *Looser's zones* (Fig. 113–6).

Characteristics of vitamin D deficiency osteomalacia are a low-normal to decreased calcium level, hypophosphatemia, an elevated bone alkaline phosphatase level, a mild PTH elevation, and decreased 25 OH D levels. In the renal phosphate leak syndromes, levels of serum calcium and 25 OH D are normal, but serum phosphate levels are low. A mild hyperchloremic acidosis is compatible with severe vitamin D deficiency and secondary hyperparathyroidism leading to proximal tubular bicarbonate wasting. Marked hyperchloremic hypokalemic acidosis suggests renal tubular acidosis, a diagnosis that can be confirmed by inadequate urine acidification after an ammonium chloride load. Vitamin D deficiency decreases urine calcium excretion. In the renal phosphate leak syndrome, urine calcium excretion is generally normal or, in renal tubular acidosis, elevated. In both varieties of osteomalacia, tubular reabsorption of phosphate is appropriately low for the level of serum phosphate.

Bone biopsy in patients with vitamin D deficiency shows changes of both osteomalacia and osteitis fibrosa. In pure phosphate deficiency, osteomalacia predominates.

The differential diagnosis of osteomalacia caused by vitamin D deficiency includes severe dietary deprivation, intestinal fat malabsorption syndromes, and drug-induced acceleration of hepatic vitamin D catabolism. The diagnosis of dietary deficiency can be established by a careful history, and the patient can be treated with vitamin D (or its metabolites), 50,000 IU three times weekly, in addition to calcium supplementation, until serum chemistries and urinary calcium excretion return to normal. At that point, an adequate diet with a 400-IU supplement of vitamin D daily is sufficient. Intestinal fat malabsorption may be readily apparent by the patient's medical history but is more often occult, as in smoldering ileitis. An adequate evaluation should include appropriate radiologic studies, quantitation of intestinal fat absorption, assessment of mucosal function by D-xylose uptake, and jejunal biopsy, if indicated. Proper treatment involves both control of the primary intestinal disorder and replenishment of body vitamin D and mineral stores. Depending on the severity of the malabsorption syndrome and the degree of vitamin D depletion, one should administer vitamin D, 50,000 units three to seven times per week and calcium, 1000 mg/day. In patients with unusually severe malabsorption, even higher doses may be required.

Therapeutic response can be assessed by following levels of serum calcium, phosphorus, alkaline phosphatase, and 25 OH D as well as 24-hour urine calcium excretion. Several months or longer may be required before these parameters return to normal. At that point, doses of vitamin D and calcium can be reduced to maintain normal serum and urine calcium levels. In these disorders especially, it is essential to monitor patients'

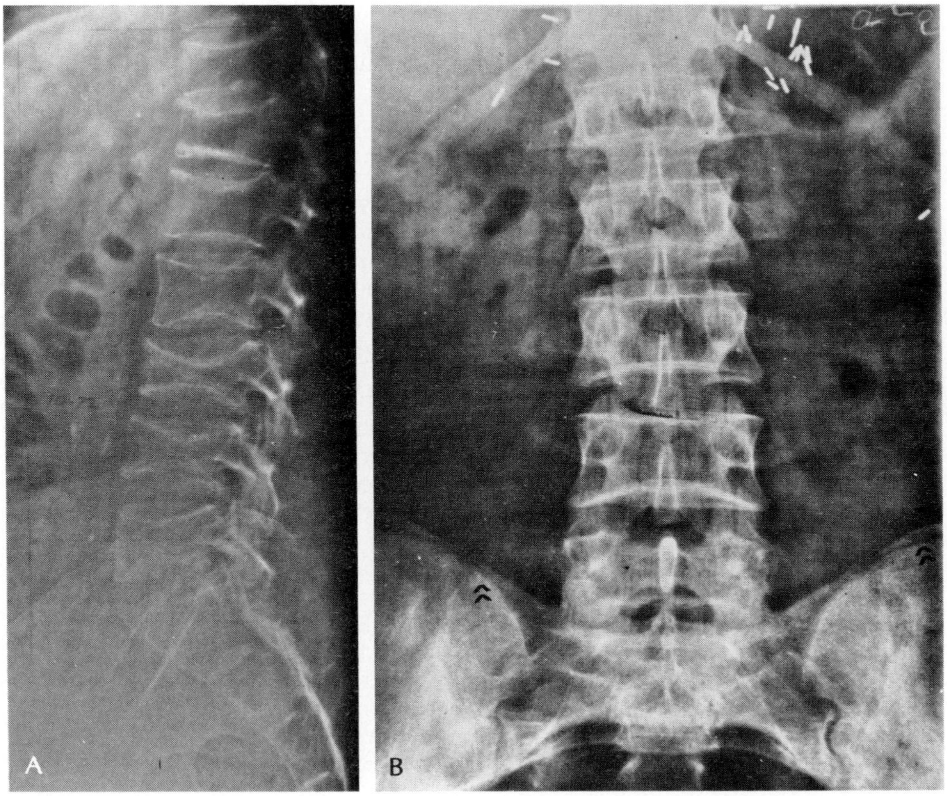

FIGURE 113–6. Roentgenograms of patients with glucocorticoid-induced osteopenia. *A*, Multiple vertebral compression fractures in a middle-aged woman with rheumatoid arthritis treated for several years with 10 to 15 mg prednisone daily. Note the anterior wedging of thoracic vertebrae (T12) in contrast to the central collapse of lumbar vertebrae (L1–L5). Similar radiographic findings occur in idiopathic or postmenopausal or senile osteoporosis. *B*, Lumbar spine and pelvis in a 24-year-old man treated for 10 years with prednisone to suppress glomerulonephritis. Note the mottled appearance of bone in the lumbar vertebrae and ilia indicating bone loss and the failure of the epiphyses of the ilia to close (arrows). (Courtesy of Richard H. Gold, M.D., Professor of Radiology, University of California, Los Angeles.)

serum and urine calcium levels frequently because improved intestinal absorption following treatment of the primary disease can lead to vitamin D intoxication if the dose is not adjusted promptly.

In the renal tubular phosphate leak syndromes, therapy is directed toward reversing the acidosis, if present, compensating for renal phosphate wasting, and maintaining normal calcium absorption with supplemental vitamin D. In the case of an isolated tubular phosphate leak, one should prescribe vitamin D 50,000 IU three times weekly, and phosphate 1.8 to 2.4 g/day in two to four divided doses. In patients with Fanconi's syndrome, it is important to correct the acidosis with bicarbonate or Shol's solution because the acidosis itself impairs bone mineral content. It is essential to supplement with calcium and vitamin D in renal tubular acidosis because alkali therapy alone may precipitate tetany in a severely osteomalacic patient. When healing has occurred, vitamin D supplementation should be discontinued; relapse does not usually occur if the acidosis is controlled.

The active metabolites of vitamin D—25 OH D or $1,25(OH)_2D$—may be substituted for vitamin D in the treatment of osteomalacia. Both metabolites have a shorter half-life than vitamin D; therefore, toxicity will disappear more quickly. Because $1,25(OH)_2D$ is the final metabolite, however, it may not be associated with feedback control; hypercalciuria and hypercalcemia are more frequent with $1,25(OH)_2D$ than with other forms of vitamin D. For a more detailed discussion of osteomalacia and its treatement, the reader is referred to recent reviews.[89–91]

OSTEITIS FIBROSA

Osteitis fibrosa is a histologic diagnosis based on the findings of increased osteoclast numbers and resorption sites with replacement of bone by fibrous tissue. The sole basis of these changes is increased secretion of PTH, either as a primary process or as a secondary response to a prolonged hypocalcemic stimulus, such as calcium malabsorption.[92–94]

PRIMARY HYPERPARATHYROIDISM

The initial manifestations of primary hyperparathyroidism occasionally include generalized osteopenia with vertebral compression or long-bone fractures. Associated clinical findings are weakness and easy fatigability, weight loss, muscular aches and proximal muscle weakness, arthralgias, morning stiffness, or pseudogout,[94] as well as the more classic symptoms of epigastric pain and renal colic. Hypertension and proximal myopathy may be observed on physical examination; band keratopathy is an infrequent finding. Radiologic clues include subperiosteal bone resorption, especially in the phalanges (Fig. 113–7), occasional brown tumors appearing as smooth, sharply demarcated, cystlike lesions in any part of the skeleton, and renal calculi. Subperiosteal resorption is the most consistent radiologic finding. Occasionally, erosive and sclerotic changes in the sacroiliac joints mimic ankylosing spondylitis (Fig. 113–8). *Most frequently, the diagnosis is made in individuals with asymptomatic hypercalcemia.*

The diagnosis can be readily established by demonstrating consistently elevated serum levels of calcium and PTH, and a low serum level of phosphate. The bone fraction of serum alkaline phosphatase is usually elevated in patients with bone disease. Hyperuricemia is frequent. Whereas urinary calcium excretion may be normal or low because of the renal calcium-retaining effects of PTH, patients with significant bone disease usually have an elevated urinary calcium excretion because of the increased filtered load.

The only curative treatment of osteopenia caused by primary hyperparathyroidism is parathyroidectomy, following which, some return of bone mass occurs. In patients who are not operative candidates, serum and urine calcium levels may be reduced by the administration of phosphates. The resultant elevation of urinary phosphate excretion increases the risk of calcium-phosphate stone formation, however, and the increased (calcium × phosphate) product make metastatic soft-tissue calcification more likely.

Ectopic tumor production of PTH or similar molecules

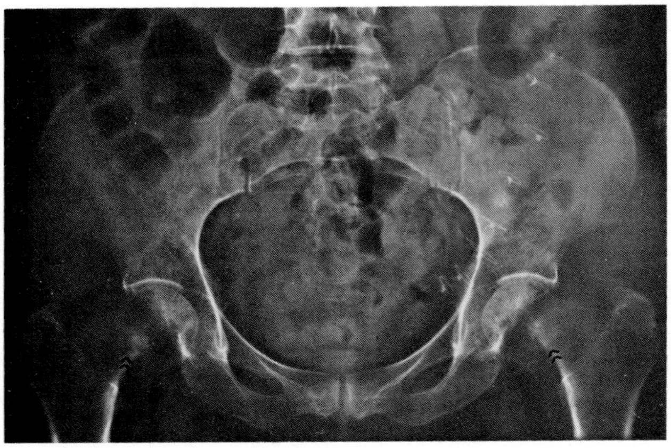

FIGURE 113–7. Roentgenogram of the pelvis and hips of a patient with osteomalacia. Note the generalized osteopenia and symmetric pseudofractures in both femoral necks (arrows). (Courtesy of Richard H. Gold, M.D., Professor of Radiology, University of California, Los Angeles.)

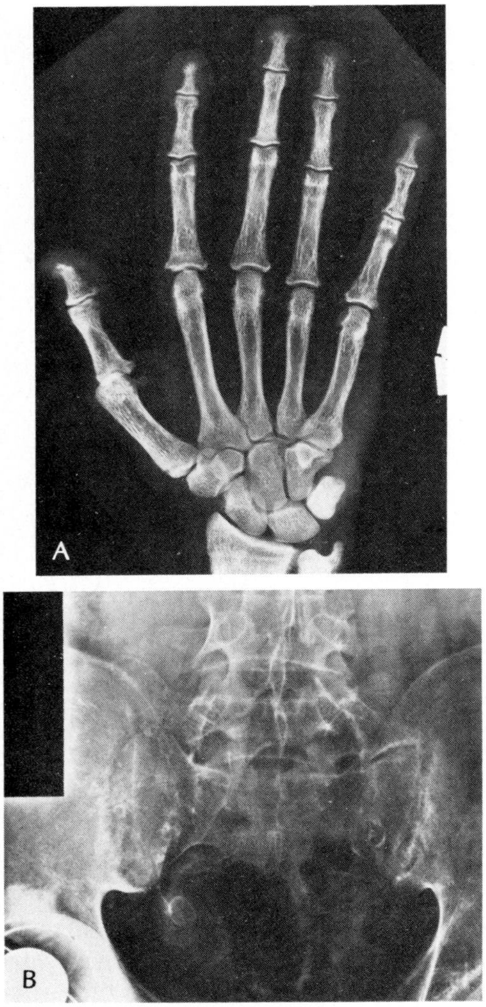

FIGURE 113–8. Roentgenograms of patients with hyperparathyroidism. *A*, Hand film from a middle-aged woman with long-standing primary hyperparathyroidism. Note erosions and resorption of digital tufts, subperiosteal resorption of shafts of the proximal and middle phalanges, and bony erosions at the second and fifth metacarpophalangeal joints. *B*, Bilateral erosive changes in the sacroiliac joints in a young man with severe secondary hyperparathyroidism resulting from chronic renal failure. The right femoral head has been replaced because of ischemic necrosis. (Courtesy of Richard H. Gold, M.D., Professor of Radiology, University of California, Los Angeles.)

accounts for about 15% of cases of hypercalcemic (autonomous) hyperparathyroidism in adults,[95] but because of rapid progression of the malignantt process, osteopenia is rarely observed. Approximately 90% of PTH-producing tumors occur in the lung, kidney, or urogenital tract.

SECONDARY HYPERPARATHYROIDISM

Hyperparathyroidism may be secondary to disorders that decrease intestinal calcium absorption. The most common of these are vitamin D-deficiency states and the idiopathic reduction in intestinal calcium absorption seen occasionally in older individuals. In cases of vitamin D deficiency, fatigability and myopathic symptoms are common. Diagnostic findings include low-normal to mildly reduced serum calcium levels, reduced serum phosphate levels, a mild PTH elevation, and much-reduced urinary calcium excretion. Treatment consists of restoring intestinal calcium absorption to normal (see the sections on osteoporosis and osteomalacia in this chapter).

Although severe secondary hyperparathyroidism is common in chronic renal disease, the histologic bone picture is generally mixed and can include osteomalacia, osteitis fibrosa, osteoporosis, and even patchy osteosclerosis. The osteitis fibrosa component responds to therapy with $1,25(OH)_2D$ or 1 α-OH D, which is metabolized to $1,25(OH)_2D$, and most patients with bone pain and myopathy benefit. The response of the osteomalacic component to this treatment is variable, however. At least some of the osteomalacia in patients undergoing renal dialysis is due to aluminum toxicity rather than to a deficiency of vitamin D. The management of the bone disease associated with renal failure, and dialysis is complex and beyond the scope of this chapter; the reader is referred to reviews of the subject.[96–98]

HYPERTHYROIDISM

The bone disease of hyperthyroidism is high-turnover osteoporosis.[9] Patients may have bone pain and fracture, in addition to other features of hyperthyroidism. Although the disease is often endogenous, significant osteoporosis can clearly be caused by the exogenous administration of thyroid replacement therapy, especially after decades of treatment. Radiographs usually show diffuse osteopenia; occasionally, abnormal striations of cortical bone are seen. Biochemical parameters usually include slight elevations in serum calcium levels and elevated serum levels of alkaline phosphatase. Urinary studies often show high levels of calcium and hydroxyproline.

The mechanisms of this disease is probably direct stimulation of bone resorption by excessive levels of thyroid hormone. This process reduces the levels of serum PTH and thereby causes renal retention of phosphate and mild elevations of serum phosphate. Both low PTH levels and high serum phosphate levels lead to reduced activity of renal 1-α-hydroxylase with a subsequent decrease in serum levels of $1,25(OH)_2D$ and an increase of $24,25(OH)_2D$. In spite of low $1,25(OH)_2D$ levels, bone biopsies rarely show osteomalacia. Typical findings include a high rate of bone turnover, characterized by an increase of osteoclasts and osteoclastic surfaces and increased osteoid formation surfaces, involving cortical as well as trabecular bone; mineralization is normal. Increased porosity of cortical bone is typical.

The treatment of this disorder is correction of the hyperthyroid state. Special attention should be given to correct adjustment of supplemental thyroid hormone therapies.

OSTEOGENESIS IMPERFECTA

Occasionally, an adult with multiple fractures, especially in the long bones of the legs, and radiographic osteopenia, actually has osteogenesis imperfecta.[99] This group of disorders is characterized by a genetically determined inability to form quantitatively or qualitatively normal collagen. To date, different mutations in the gene for type I procollagen have been identified in several variants of osteogenesis imperfecta; all result in formation of unstable collagen helices.[100] Most patients develop bone fractures in childhood. One prenatal form is lethal. Some of these individuals are deaf or have blue sclerae, but others have only osseous manifestations. If the disease begins in childhood, bones may grow abnormally. Extremities are short, legs are bowed, and saber shins occur. Pectus excavatum or carinatum can appear, as well as a dome-shaped forehead and lateral widening of the skull. Some individuals have lax joints, bruise easily, and have small, misshapen, discolored teeth. Fractures usually diminish in frequency at puberty but increase in the perimenopausal period in women and at a similar age in men.

If none of the phenotypic characteristics of osteogenesis imperfecta are present except for fragile bones, the diagnosis can be difficult. A positive family history and a history of multiple fractures in childhood are helpful in establishing the diagnosis. Radiographs show thinning of cortical and trabecular areas of bones indistinguishable from that seen in other osteopenias. Platybasia of the skull and bone islands in the cranium suggest osteogenesis imperfecta. Bone biopsy shows diminished quantities of osteoid with replacement by a blue-staining material. Therapy with sodium fluoride or with sex hormones has been advocated, but it is not clear whether any interventions reduce fracture rates. For a discussion of the different types of this disorder, the reader is referred to a recent review[99] and to Chapters 12 and 85.

REFERENCES

1. Seyer, J.M., and Kang, A.H.: Collagen and Elastin. *In* Textbook of Rheumatology. 3rd Ed. Edited by W. Kelley, E. Harris, S. Ruddy, and C. Sledge. Philadelphia, W.B. Saunders, 1989.

2. Raisz, L.G., and Rodan, G.A.: Cellular basis for bone turnover. *In* Metabolic Bone Disease and Clinically Related Disorders. 2nd Ed. Edited by L. Avioli and S. Krane. Philadelphia, W.B. Saunders, 1990.
3. Epstein, S.: Serum and urinary markers of bone remodeling: Assessment of bone turnover. Endocr. Rev., *9*:437–449, 1988.
4. Frost, H.M.: The pathomechanics of osteoporosis. Clin. Orthop., *200*:198–225, 1985.
5. Raicz, L.: Osteoporosis. Annu. Rev. Med., *40*:251–267, 1989.
6. Stewart, A.F. and Broadus, A.E.: Parathyroid hormone-related proteins: Coming of age in the 1990s. J. Clin. Endocrinol. Metabol., *71*:1410–1414, 1990.
7. Mawer, E.B., Blackhouse, J., and Holman, C.: The distribution and storage of vitamin D and its metabolites in man. Clin. Sci., *43*:413–420, 1972.
8. Wallach, S., Carstens, J.B. Jr., and Avioli, L.V.: Calcitonin, osteoclasts, and bone turnover. Calcif. Tissue Int., *47*:388–391, 1990.
9. Moskilde, L., Eriksen, E.F., and Charles P.: Effects of thyroid hormones on bone and mineral metabolism. Endocrinol. Metab. Clin. North Am., *19*:35–63, 1990.
10. Prior, J.C., Progesterone as a bone-trophic hormone. Endocr. Rev., *1*:386–398, 1990.
11. Need, A.G., Horowitz, M., Walker, C.J., et al.: Cross-over study of fat-corrected forearm mineral content during nandrolone decanoate therapy for osteoporosis. Bone, *10*:3–6, 1989.
12. Mitchell, D.R. and Lyles, K.W.: Glucocorticoid-induced osteoporosis: Mechanisms for bone loss; evaluation of strategies for prevention. J. Gerontol., *45*:153–158, 1990.
13. Canalis, E., McCarty, T., Centrell, M.: Growth factors and the regulation of bone remodeling. J. Clin. Invest., *81*:277–281, 1988.
14. Hauschka, P.B., Chen, T.L., and Mavrakos, A.E.: Polypeptide growth factors in bone matrix. Ciba Found. Symp., *136*:207–225, 1988.
15. Reddi, A.H., and Cunningham, N.S.: Bone induction by osteogenin and bone morphogenetic proteins. Biomaterials, *11*:33–34, 1990.
16. Wiktor-Jedrzejczak, W., Bartocci, A., Ferrante, A.W. Jr., et al.: Total absence of colony-stimulating factor 1 in the macrophage-deficient osteopetrotic (op/op) mouse. Proc. Natl. Acad. Sci. USA, *87*:4828–4832, 1990.
17. Canalis, E.: Interleukin-1 has independent effects on deoxyribonucleic acid and collagen synthesis in cultures of rat calvariae. Endocrinology, *118*:74–81, 1986.
18. Melson, F., and Mosekilde, L.: The role of bone biopsy in the diagnosis of metabolic bone disease. Orthop. Clin. North Am., *12*:571–602, 1981.
19. Meunier, P.G. and Bressot, C.: Endocrine influence on bone cells and bone remodeling evaluated by clinical histomorphometry. *In* The Endocrinology of Calcium Metabolism. Edited by J.A. Parson. New York, Raven Press, 1982.
20. Riggs, B.L., Wahner, H.W., Dunn, W.L., et al.: Differential changes in bone mineral density of the appendicular and axial skeleton with aging: Relationship to spinal osteoporosis. J. Clin. Invest., *67*:328–335, 1981.
21. Heaney, R.P., Recker, R.R. and Saville, P.D.: Menopausal changes in calcium balance performance. J. Lab. Clin. Med., *92*:953–963, 1978.
22. Riggs, B.L., Wahner, H.W., Seeman, E., et al.: Changes in the bone mineral density of the proximal femur and spine with aging: Difference between the postmenopausal and senile osteoporosis syndromes. J. Clin. Invest., *70*:716–723, 1982.
23. Jensen, J.S., and Tondevold, E.: Mortality after hip fractures. Acta Orthop. Scand., *50*:161–167, 1979.
24. Whyte, M.P., Bergfeld, M.A., Murphy, W.A., et al.: Postmenopausal osteoporosis. A heterogeneous disorder as assessed by histomorphometric analysis of iliac crest bone from untreated patients. Am. J. Med., *72*:193–201, 1982.
25. Avioli, L.V., McDonald, J.E., and Lee, S.W.: The influence of age on the intestinal absorption of ^{47}calcium in women and its relation to ^{47}calcium absorption in postmenopausal osteoporosis. J. Clin. Invest., *44*:1960–1967, 1965.
26. Aitken, J.M., Hart, D.M. and Lindsay, R.: Osteoporosis after oophorectomy for non-malignant disease in premenopausal women. Br. Med. J., *2*:325–328, 1973.
27. Silverman, A.L. and Madison, R.E.: Decreased incidence of hip fracture in hispanics, blacks, and asians. Am. J. Public Health, *78*:1482–1483, 1988.
28. Mazess, R.B., and Mather, W.E.: Bone mineral content in Canadian Eskimos. Hum. Biol., *47*:45–63, 1975.
29. Pocock, N.A., Eisman, J.A., Hopper, J.L., et al.: Genetic determinants of bone mass in adults: a twin study. J. Clin. Invest., *80*:706–710, 1987.
30. Dequeker, J., Nijs, J., Verstraeten, A., et al.: Genetic determinants of bone mineral content at the spine and radius: a twin study. Bone, *8*:207–209, 1987.
31. Seeman, E., Hopper, J.L., Bach, L.A., et al.: Reduced bone mass in daughters of women with osteoporosis. N. Engl. J. Med., *320*:554–558, 1989.
32. Ott, S.M.: Editorial: Attainment of peak bone mass. J. Clin. Endocrinol. Metab., *71*:1082A–1082C, 1990.
33. Matkovic, V., Fontana, D., Tominac, C., et al.: Factors that influence peak bone mass formation: a study of calcium balance and the inheritance of bone mass in adolescent females. Am. J. Clin. Nutr., *52*:878–888, 1990.
34. Liel, Y., Edwards, J., Shary, J., et al.: The effects of race and body habitus on bone mineral density of the radius, hip and spine in premenopausal women. J. Clin. Endocrinol. Metab., *66*:1247–1250, 1988.
35. Birge, S.J. and Dalsky, G.: The role of exercise in preventing osteoporosis. Public Health Rep., *104*(Suppl.):54–58, 1989.
36. Melton, L.J. III: Epidemiology of osteoporosis: Predicting who is at risk. Ann. NY Acad. Sci., *592*:295–306, 1990.
37. Aloia, J., Cohn, S.H., Ostuni, J.A., et al.: Prevention of involutional bone loss by exercise. Ann. Intern. Med., *89*:356–358, 1978.
38. President's Council on Physical Fitness: Adult Physical Fitness: A program for Men and Women. Washington, D.C., United States Government Printing Office, 1965.
39. Prior, J.C., Vigna, Y.M., Schechter, M.T., and Burgess, A.E.: Spinal bone loss and ovulatory disturbances. N. Engl. J. Med., *323*:1221–1227, 1990.
40. Cumming, R.G.: Calcium intake and bone mass: A quantitative review of the evidence. Calcif. Tissue Int., *47*:194–201, 1990.
41. Dawson-Hughes, B., Dallal, G.E., Krall, E.A., et al.: A controlled trial of the effect of calcium supplementation on bone density in postmenopausal women. N. Engl. J. Med., *323*:878–883, 1990.
42. Ettinger, B., Genant, H.K., and Cann, C.E.: Postmenopausal bone loss is prevented by treatment with low-dosage estrogen with calcium. Ann. Intern. Med., *106*:40–45, 1987.
43. vanBeresteijn, E.C.H., van 't Hof, M., Schaafsma, G., et al.: Habitual dietary calcium intake and cortical bone loss in perimenopausal women: A longitudinal study. Calcif. Tissue Int., *47*:338–344, 1990.
44. Riggs, B.L., Seeman, E., Hodgson, J.F., et al.: Effect on the fluoride calcium regimen on vertebral fracture occurrence in postmenopausal osteoporosis: Comparison with conventional therapy. N. Engl. J. Med., *107*:923–925, 1982.
45. Shangraw, R.F.: Factors to consider in the selection of a calcium supplement. Public Health Rep., *104*(Suppl.):46–50, 1989.

46. Recker, R.R., Saville, P.D., and Heaney, R.P.: Effect of estrogens and calcium carbonate on bone loss in postmenopausal women. Ann. Intern. Med., *87*:649–655, 1987.
47. Lindsay, R., Hart, D.M., and Baird, C.: Prevention of spinal osteoporosis in oophorectomized women. Lancet, *2*:1151–1157, 1980.
48. Paganini-Hill, A., Ross, R.K., Gerkins, V.R., et al.: Menopausal estrogen therapy and hip fractures. Ann. Intern. Med., *95*:28–31, 1981.
49. Riis, B.J., Thomsen, K., Strom, V., and Christiansen, C.: The effect of percutaneous estradiol and natural progesterone on postmenopausal bone loss. Am. J. Obstet. Gynecol., *156*:61–65, 1987.
50. Chetkowski, R.J., Meldrum, D.R., Steingold, K.A., et al.: Biologic effects of transdermal estradiol. N. Engl. J. Med., *314*:1615–1620, 1986.
51. Cauley, J.A., Cummings, S.R., Black, D.M., et al.: Prevalence and determinants of estrogen replacement therapy in elderly women. Am. J. Obstet. Gynecol., *163*:1438–1444, 1990.
52. Williams, S.R., Frenchek, B., Speroff, T., and Speroff, L.: A study of combined continuous ethinyl estradiol and norethindrone acetate for postmenopausal hormone replacement. Am. J. Obstet. Gynecol., *162*:438–446, 1990.
53. Christiansen, C., and Riis, B.J.: 17-beta-estradiol and continuous norethisterone: A unique treatment of established osteoporosis in elderly women. J. Clin. Endocrinol. Metab., *71*:836–841, 1990.
54. Barrett-Connor, E.L.: The risks and benefits of long-term estrogen replacement therapy. Public Health Rep., *104* (Suppl.):62–65, 1989.
55. Colditz, G.A., Stampfer, M.J., Willett, W.C., et al.: Prospective study of estrogen replacement therapy and risk of breast cancer in postmenopausal women. JAMA, *264*:2648–2653, 1990.
56. Bergkvist, L., Adami, H., Persson, I., et al.: The risk of breast cancer after estrogen and estrogen-progestin replacement. N. Engl. J. Med., *321*:293–297, 1989.
57. Lindsay, R., and Tohme, J.F.: Estrogen treatment of patients with established postmenopausal osteoporosis. Obstet. Gynecol., *72*:290–295, 1990.
58. Need, H.G., Horowitz, M., Bridges, A., et al.: Effects of nandrolone decanoate and antiresorptive therapy on vertebral density in osteoporotic postmenopausal women. Arch. Intern. Med., *149*:57–60, 1989.
59. Wasnich, R.D., Benfante, J., Yano, K., et al.: Thaizide effect on the mineral content of bone. N. Engl. J. Med., *309*:344–347, 1983.
60. Jackson, J.A. and Kleerekoper, M.: Osteoporosis in men: Diagnosis, pathophysiology, and prevention. Medicine, *69*: 137–148, 1990.
61. Dykman, T.R., Gluck, O.S., Murphy, W.A., et al.: Evaluation of factors associated with glucocorticoid-induced osteopenia in patients with rheumatic diseases. Arthritis Rheum., *28*: 361–368, 1985.
62. Ott, S.M., and Chesnut, C.H. III: Calcitriol treatment is not effective in postmenopausal osteoporosis. Ann. Intern. Med., *4*:267–274, 1989.
63. Storm, T., Thamsborg, G., Steiniche, T., et al.: Effect of intermittent cyclical etidronate therapy on bone mass and fracture rate in women with postmenopausal osteoporosis. N. Engl. J. Med., *322*:1265–1271, 1990.
64. Watts, N.B., Harris, S.T., Genant, H.K., et al.: Intermittent cyclical etidronate treatment of postmenopausal osteoporosis. N. Engl. J. Med., *323*:73–79, 1990.
65. Etidronate for osteoporosis. Medical Letter, *32*:111–112, 1990.
66. Civitelli, R., Gonnelli, S., Zacchei, F., et al.: Bone turnover in postmenopausal osteoporosis: Effect of calcitonin treatment. J. Clin. Invest., *82*:1268–1274, 1988.
67. Pak, C.Y.C., Sakhaee, K., Zerwekh, J.E., et al.: Safe and effective treatment of osteoporosis with intermittent slow release sodium fluoride: Augmentation of vertebral bone mass and inhibition of fractures. J. Clin. Endocrinol. Metab., *68*:150–159, 1989.
68. Riggs, B.L., Hodgson, S.F., O'Falon, M., et al.: Effect of fluoride treatment on the fracture rate in postmenopausal women with osteoporosis. N. Engl. J. Med., *322*:802–809, 1990.
69. Gera, I., Dobrolet, N., and Hock, J.M.: Intermittent but not continuous PTH (hPTH 1-34) increases bone mass independently of resorption. J. Bone Min. Res., *4*:5303–5308, 1989.
70. Shulman, L.E.: Panel summary on prevention and treatment of osteoporosis. Public Health Rep., *104*(Suppl.):59–62, 1989.
71. Reid, J.R.: Steroid osteoporosis. Calcif. Tissue Int., *45*:63–67, 1989.
72. Lukert, B.P. and Raicz, L.G.: Glucocorticoid-induced osteoporosis: pathogenesis and management. Ann. Intern. Med., *112*:352–364, 1990.
73. LoCascio, V., Bonucci, E., Imbimbo, B., et al.: Bone loss after glucocorticoid therapy. Osteoporosis, *37*:1044–1046, 1987.
74. Caniggia, A., Nuti, R., Lore, F. and Vattimo, A.: Pathophysiology of the adverse effects of glucoactive corticosteroids on calcium metabolism in man. J. Steroid Biochem., *15*:153–161, 1981.
75. Godschalk, M.G. and Downs, R.W.: Effect of short-term glucocorticoids on serum osteocalcin in healthy young men. J. Bone Min. Res., *3*:113–115, 1988.
76. Sanbrook, P.N., Eisman, J.A., Yeates, M.F.G., et al.: Osteoporosis in rheumatoid arthritis: safety of low dose corticosteroids. Ann. Rheum. Dis., *45*:950–953, 1986.
77. Gluck, O.S., Murphy, W.A., Hahn, T.J. and Hahn, B.H.: Bone loss in adults receiving alternate day glucocorticoid therapy. Arthritis Rheum., *24*:892–898, 1981.
78. Pocock, N.A., Eismen, J.A., Dunstan, C.R., et al.: Recovery from steroid-induced osteoporosis. Ann. Intern. Med., *107*:319–323, 1987.
79. LoCascio, V., Bonnucci, E., Imbimbo, B., et al.: Bone loss after glucocorticoid therapy. Calcif. Tissue Int., *36*:435–438, 1984.
80. Hahn, T.J., Halstead, L.R., Strates, B., et al.: Comparison of subacute effects of oxazacort and prednisone on mineral metabolism in man. Calcif. Tissue Int., *31*:109–115, 1980.
81. Reid, I.R. and Ibbertson, H.K.: Calcium supplements in the prevention of steroid-induced osteoporosis. Am. J. Clin. Nutr., *44*:287–290, 1986.
82. Dykman, T.R., Haralson, K.M., Gluck, O.S., et al.: Effect of oral 1,25 dihydroxyvitamin D and calcium on glucocorticoid-induced osteopenia in patients with rheumatic diseases. Arthritis Rheum., *27*:1336–1343, 1984.
83. Reid, I.R., King, A.R., Alexander, C.J., and Ibbertson, H.K.: Prevention of steroid-induced osteoporosis with (3-amino-1-hydroxypropylidene)-1,1-bisphosphonate (APD). Lancet, *1*:143–146. 1988.
84. Hahn, T.J., Halstead, L.R., Teitelbaum, S.L., and Hahn, B.H.: Altered mineral metabolism in glucocorticoid-induced osteopenia: Effect of 25-hydroxyvitamin D administration. J. Clin. Invest., *64*:655–665, 1979.
85. Reid, I.R., Schooler, B.A., and Stewart, A.: Prevention of glucocorticoid-induced osteoporosis. J. Bone Min. Res., *5*:619–623, 1990.
86. Ringe, J.D. and Welzel, D.: Salmon calcitonin in the therapy of corticoid-induced osteoporosis. Eur. J. Clin. Pharmacol. *33*:35–39, 1987.

87. Meunier, P.J., Briancon, D., Chavassieux, P. et al.: Treatment with fluoride: bone histomorphometric findings. *In* Osteoporosis 1987. Edited by C. Christiansen et al. Copenhagen, Osteopress Aps., 1987.
88. Need, A.G.: Corticosteroids and osteoporosis. Aust. NZ J. Med., *17*:267–272, 1987.
89. Mankin, H.J.: Rickets, osteomalacia, and renal osteodystrophy. An update. Orthop. Clin. North Am., *21*:81–96, 1990.
90. Bontoux, D., and Alcalay, M.: Clinical disorders of vitamin D, renal osteodystrophy, and hypophosphatasia. Curr. Opin. Rheumatol., *2*:12–29, 1990.
91. Davies, M.: High dose vitamin D therapy: indications, benefits and hazards. Int. J. Vitam. Nutr. Res., *30*(Suppl.):81–86, 1989.
92. Parisien, M., Silverberg, S.J., Shane, E. et al.: Bone disease in primary hyperparathyroidism. Endocrinol. Metab. Clin. North Am., *19*:19–34, 1990.
93. Potts, J.T. Jr.: Management of asymptomatic hyperparathyroidism. J. Clin. Endocrinol. Metab., *70*:1489–1493, 1990.
94. Bhalla, A.K.: Musculoskeletal manifestations of primary hyperparathyroidism. Clin. Rheum. Dis., *12*:691–705, 1986.
95. Muggia, F.M.: Overview of cancer-related hypercalcemia: epidemiology and etiology. Semin. Oncol., *17*:3–9, 1990.
96. Malluche, H. and Faugere, M.C.: Renal bone disease 1990: an unmet challenge for the nephrologist. Kidney Int., *38*:193–211, 1990.
97. Tzamaloukas, A.H.: Diagnosis and management of bone disorders in chronic renal failure and dialyzed patients. Med. Clin. North Am., *74*:961–974, 1990.
98. Slatapolsky, E., Lopez-Hilker, S., Dusso, A., et al.: Renal osteodystrophy: past and future. Contrib. Nephrol., *78*:38–45, 1990.
99. Whyte, M.P.: Heritable metabolic and dysplastic bone diseases. Endocrinol. Metab. Clin. North Am., *19*:133–173, 1990.
100. Prockop, D.J., Baldwin, C.T. and Constantinou, C.D.: Mutations in type I procollagen genes that cause osteogenesis imperfecta. Adv. Hum. Genet., *19*:105–132, 1990.

114

Rheumatic Aspects of Endocrinopathies

MARY E. CRONIN

Hormonal excess or deprivation can lead to a variety of syndromes with musculoskeletal manifestations. Their recognition is important because they are often treatable. Awareness of these features can suggest the appropriate diagnosis. Such states of altered hormonal balance, including pregnancy, have shed light on the pathogenesis of some rheumatic disorders and promise new insights into their treatment. These relationships are described here.

The role of the neuroendocrine system in immunity is a relatively new area of research, but it is now well recognized that the neuroendocrine system has direct and indirect regulatory functions affecting the immune system. The study of the clinical implications of these systems to rheumatic diseases is just beginning but merits close attention.

ACROMEGALY

Pituitary adenomas may produce excessive quantities of growth hormone, like anabolic effects of which can lead to significant changes in connective tissues. Such tumors usually occur in older persons, in whom epiphyseal closure has already taken place, and *acromegaly* results. Excessive growth hormone production before puberty results in *gigantism.* Although many anabolic influences derive from the direct action of this hormone, stimulation of chondroitin sulfate and collagen synthesis by articular chondrocytes are due to insulin-like growth factors induced by growth hormone.[1] Insulin-like growth factor I (IGF-I), also known as somatomedin C, and IGF-II (somatomedin A) are synthesized predominantly in the liver but also in chondrocytes, kidney, muscle, pituitary, and the gastrointestinal tract. IGF-I in particular is a potent stimulus to cellular proliferation and is further discussed in Chapter 13.[1]

Growth hormone and IGF-I act synergistically to stimulate the proliferation of soft tissues including bursae, joint capsules, synovium, cartilage (Fig. 114–1), and bone. Soft-tissue changes include coarse, thickened digits; bursal thickening caused by noninflammatory fibrous hyperplasia, particularly of the prepatellar, olecranon, and subacromial bursae; and joint capsular hypertrophy and laxity permitting hypermobility. Synovial thickening, villous and usually noninflammatory, is due to increased adipose and fibrous tissue rather than to synoviocyte hyperplasia. An abnormally thickened heel pad can be found in 35% of acromegalic patients.

Most endochondral tissues are not as susceptible to growth hormone in adults as they are in the prepubertal state, but some cartilage remains responsive, as in the mandibular condyle, in which the jaw may actually lengthen, and in the costochondral junctions, in which fusiform enlargement may take place leading to a beading pattern and rib lengthening. This process results in an increased anteroposterior diameter of the chest. Cartilaginous overgrowth may even occur in the larynx, interfering with speech and, rarely, with respiratory function. Bony thickening results in a thickened calvarium, an enlarged mandible, and *hyperostosis frontalis interna.* Another characteristic finding is widening of the distal ungual tufts, seen in 67% of patients.[2] This can lead to an appearance of the hands similar to that of clubbing. The sesamoid bones are enlarged in approximately half these patients, and even the stapedial footplate of the ear may be affected, causing auditory symptoms.

The rheumatologic manifestations of acromegaly listed in Table 114–1 are found frequently if sought by careful medical history, physical examination, and laboratory testing. Their presence correlates more with the duration of disease than with absolute levels of

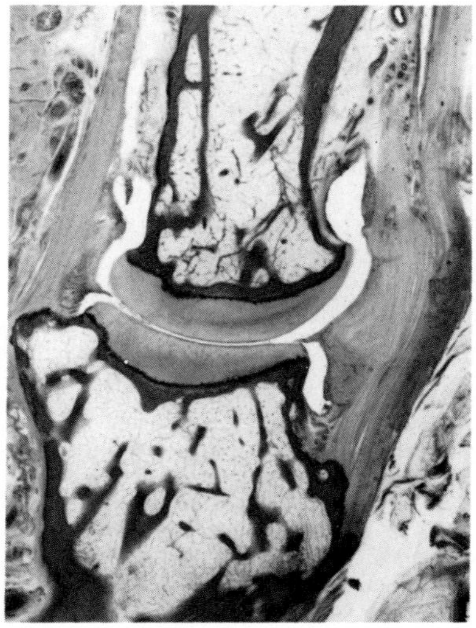

FIGURE 114–1. Midsagittal section through the distal toe of a 50-year-old acromegalic man; irregular hypertrophy and hyperplasia of the cartilage, and bony overgrowth at the joint margins with sparse, thickened trabeculae has occurred. Courtesy of R.T. McCluskey, M.D., Department of Pathology, Massachusetts General Hospital, Boston.

TABLE 114–1. RHEUMATIC MANIFESTATIONS OF ACROMEGALY

Tissue overgrowth	Bursal hyperplasia Capsular thickening Synovial proliferation and edema Cartilage hyperplasia Bony proliferation
Arthropathy	Hypermobility of joints Cartilage degeneration Bony remodeling with osteophytosis and periosteal reaction Intermittent (crystal-induced?) synovitis
Muscle abnormalities	Increased muscle mass Proximal weakness, fatigue, myalgias, cramps
Neuropathy	Palpable peripheral nerves Peripheral neuropathy Carpal tunnel syndrome
Others	Back pain and hypermobility Kyphosis Raynaud's phenomenon

growth hormone. Rheumatic complaints, however, may arise early in the disease and can be the presenting manifestation. With the exception of soft-tissue thickening, carpal tunnel symptoms, and paresthesias, many of these rheumatologic consequences of prolonged exposure to growth hormone may not remit with ablative pituitary therapy, but earlier recognition and treatment of this endocrine disorder may change this pessimistic view.[3,4]

ARTHROPATHY

The usual manifestations of acromegalic arthropathy resemble those of osteoarthritis, with cartilaginous thickening and hypermobility as important distinguishing features. Involvement of large and small peripheral joints may occur in as many as 75% of patients. The arthropathy may consist of a noninflammatory proliferation of articular and periarticular structures, with osteophytosis and degenerative changes of the articular cartilage. The arthropathy has been divided into an early form consisting of hypermobility, recurrent effusions, and widened joint spaces, and an advanced form with bony hypertrophy, loss of motion, and deformities. Human necropsy studies and animal experimentation using exogenous growth hormone to produce polyarticular lesions have shed light on the pathogenesis of these changes.[5] The cartilaginous matrix, although massively thickened in acromegaly, is laid down in a random manner, and degenerative changes arise in the middle and basal layers, leading to friability, fissuring, and ulceration. Joint hypermobility caused by capsular hypertrophy and redundancy accelerate this degenerative process.

Such osteoarthritis-like changes may be monoarticular or polyarticular, and can affect the knees, shoulders, hips, or hands; the elbows and ankles are involved less frequently. Some patients develop intermittent painful episodes lasting weeks or months. The exact mechanism responsible for these episodes and the possible role of CPPD crystals remain to be determined.[5] Less commonly, patients complain initially of joint pain and morning stiffness. This presentation, together with the elevated erythrocyte sedimentation rate seen in some patients, can cause confusion with rheumatoid arthritis (RA).

Physical examination often reveals many of the characteristics of osteoarthritis, but the pronounced degree of joint crepitation, attributed to cartilaginous thickening and joint hypermobility, help to differentiate acromegalic arthropathy from primary osteoarthritis. Palpable dorsal phalangeal ridging just distal to the proximal interphalangeal joints may also be useful diagnostically. Thickened synovium and periarticular tissues may have a swollen appearance, but effusions are relatively rare, and when present are noninflammatory, contain no crystals, and have low leukocyte counts just as in osteoarthritis.

The radiographic features of acromegaly include widened cartilage spaces, enlarged bones with periosteal remodeling and increased density along the shaft, marginal osteophyte formation, and calcified tendinous and capsular insertions.[5] The cartilage space in the bones can be easily quantitated by measuring the second metacarpophalangeal joint space on an anteroposterior radiogram. The normal space in men is less than 3 mm and in women is less than 2 mm. Approximately one third of acromegalic individuals have increased joint spaces.[2] Exostoses at the sites of ligamentous attachments produce a "squared-off" appearance at the bone

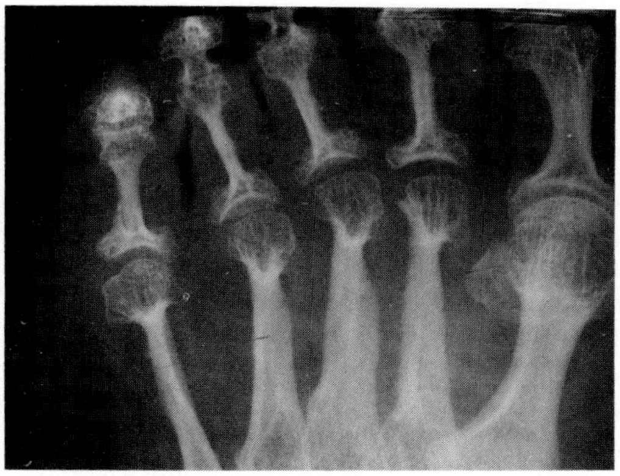

FIGURE 114–2. Radiograph of an acromegalic foot showing widened joint spaces, periosteal proliferation, dense diaphyses with pipe-stem configuration, and thickened and widely spaced trabeculae giving a porotic appearance of the metatarsal heads.

ends. Although thickening of the trabeculae at the epiphyses occurs, their simultaneous widening may lead to an osteoporitic appearance while the diaphyses remain dense; this is especially common at the metacarpal and metatarsal heads (Fig. 114–2). The humeral and femoral heads may develop a mushroom configuration along with joint-space widening. Hypertrophic spurring with flaring of the femoral and tibial condyles may be found in knee films.

Troublesome symptoms can be treated with nonsteroidal anti-inflammatory agents and other conservative measures, as in osteoarthritis (see Chapter 104). Although intra-articular corticosteroids are reported to be ineffective, no controlled studies are available. Advanced degenerative changes may be treated surgically; a preoperative corticosteroid may be required in a previously treated acromegalic patient with pituitary insufficiency.

MYOPATHY

Up to 50% of acromegalic patients with long-standing disease develop a proximal myopathy. Growth hormone preferentially increases proximal muscle mass in experimental animals but the muscle is functionally inefficient. Muscle biopsies from patients with acromegaly have shown both hypertrophic and atrophic changes occurring separately or concurrently. Type I fiber hypertrophy and type IIa and type IIb muscle fiber atrophy predominate. The atrophy is not that of disuse, which primarily affects type I fibers. Disease duration, but not growth hormone levels, correlated with biopsy findings.[6] Ultrastructurally, glycogen and lipofuscin deposits, coiled membranous bodies (probably phospholipid), and pleomorphic mitochondria with abnormal cristae and vacuolization has been found, consistent with the known influence on glycogen uptake in skeletal muscle by growth hormone and its stimulation of ribonucleic acid (RNA) turnover.[7] But a causal relationship between the mitochondrial disruption and the decreased muscle strength noted clinically has not been established.

Proximal weakness and decreased exercise tolerance are the usual complaints, followed by myalgias, cramps, and muscle twitching. The muscles may feel flabby, with weakness out of proportion to muscle mass.

The serum creatine kinase and aldolase levels, although usually normal, may be increased as a reflection of patchy necrosis. The electromyogram is abnormal in most untreated acromegalic patients with myopathy, even those without demonstrable weakness, but the findings of low-amplitude, short-duration, and polyphasic potentials are nonspecific myopathic findings.[8] In treated patients the electromyograms (EMGs) and creatine kinase (CK) levels are usually normal though muscle biopsies might still show myopathic changes.[9]

Return of normal strength after pituitary ablative therapy is gradual and may be incomplete even after 2 years.[8]

NEUROPATHY

As noted in Table 114–1, several forms of neuropathy are associated with acromegaly. These neuropathies do not correlate with increased growth hormone levels, may be independent of carpal tunnel syndrome, and may occur without concomitant diabetes mellitus. Their pathogenesis is varied and consists of the following: (1) possible metabolic effects on the neuron directly or indirectly related to growth hormone; (2) compression of the spinal cord secondary to bony (foramen magnum, vertebral body) and paraspinal connective tissue overgrowth; and (3) ischemic neuropathy secondary to proliferation of endoneural and perineural tissues. Vague paresthesias involving several peripheral nerves may be the earliest symptoms and these resolve after treatment. Five of eleven acromegalic patients had palpable enlargement of the ulnar or popliteal nerves with paresthesias, decreased or absent deep tendon reflexes, distal wasting, and even footdrop.[10] Decreased vibratory and position sense has also been described. Microscopic studies of peripheral nerves revealed a decrease in both myelinated and unmyelinated fibers, with segmental demyelination and remyelination and occasional axonal degeneration. The supporting neural tissues were increased, with significant proliferation, particular in the hypertrophic form.[10]

Typical carpal tunnel syndrome, usually bilateral, develops in as many as 50% of patients with acromegaly.[5] Although encroachment on the carpal tunnel by enlarging bone and soft tissue is a major part of the pathogenesis of this disorder, local swelling and hypertrophy of the median nerve itself may also contribute. Edema has been observed beneath the transverse carpal ligament at operation. The disappearance of this soft-tissue swelling after pituitary therapy can account for the rapid improvement in symptoms after surgery but the return to normal of nerve conduction velocities is more prolonged.

BACK PAIN

Nearly half of acromegalic patients complain of back pain during the course of their disease. Although most symptoms are in the lumbosacral spine, cervical and thoracic involvement may also occur. In spite of severe pain and sometimes advanced radiographic changes, such patients may show hypermobility of the spine. This striking finding may be a key in distinguishing between this and other spinal disorders and is presumably due to the enlarged intervertebral discs, which retain their resiliency and turgor.[5] Such mobility may accelerate spinal degeneration and osteophyte formation. Radiographically, disc spaces are normal or increased, and occasionally calcified. Hypertrophic spurring develops at the anterior vertebral margin mimicking diffuse idiopathic skeletal hyperostosis. Posteriorly, the exaggeration of the normal concavity of the vertebral body is probably caused by remodeling or pressure from paraspinal tissues. Kyphosis is frequently observed, possibly secondary to the barrel-chest deformity related to rib elongation.

RAYNAUD'S PHENOMENON

Raynaud's phenomenon occurred in 14 to 25 acromegalic patients in one series. Although the exact mechanism is uncertain, thickening of the blood vessel walls may contribute to its development.

GIGANTISM

The accelerated endochondral ossification and lengthening of tubular bone occurring in prepubertal patients with a pituitary adenoma is termed gigantism. The disorder is rare and the true incidence of rheumatic manifestations is not known; the arthropathy, myopathy, and hypertrophic neuropathy noted in acromegaly may also occur in gigantism. The incidence of carpal tunnel syndrome may be less frequent. Bony and soft tissue growth occur in tandem, and thus the carpal tunnel may not be compromised.

HYPOTHYROIDISM

In primary hypothyroidism, hyaluronic acid and other mucoproteins deposit in many organs and tissues. Many of the numerous rheumatic syndromes associated with this disorder are probably secondary to such deposits in connective tissues and basement membranes (Table 114–2). The stimulus for the synthesis of the excess hyaluronic acid could be thyroid-stimulating hormone.[11] If this hypothesis is correct, it would account for the apparent paucity of musculoskeletal syndromes in secondary hypothyroidism, in which concentrations of thyroid-stimulating hormone are low. Other reasons for the infrequency of rheumatologic problems in secondary hypothyroidism include its rarity and its association with other endocrine deficiencies, which might mask musculoskeletal symptoms.

NEUROPATHY

Neurologic features, although frequent in myxedema, are easily overlooked. Hypothyroid patients have few spontaneous complaints, and the neurologic examination is difficult to perform, owing to the patient's inability to cooperate. Several authors have emphasized the generalized nature of the *peripheral neuropathy.*[12,13] Originally believed to be caused by nerve compression by mucinous deposits, it is now thought to be due to a neuronal metabolic dysfunction secondary to the hypothyroid state. Segmental demyelination of nerve fibers has been detected with a proliferation of Schwann cells, together with mucinous infiltration of the endoneurium and perineurium. The neuropathy is primarily sensory; slowed sensory conductive velocities have been found in the ulnar, median, and posterior tibial nerves. Abnormalities of conduction in the motor fibers have been found also although the reported frequency is variable.

All 25 patients with myxedema in one series complained of paresthesias, and 60% had diminished peripheral sensation. Sensory loss primarily involved pain and light touch; decreased vibratory sensation was less common. One of the best recognized neurologic complications of hypothyroidism is *carpal tunnel syndrome.* Approximately 10% of all patients with carpal tunnel syndrome have myxedema. Conversely, median nerve compression can be documented in from 5 to 80% of those with hypothyroidism. Symptoms of carpal tunnel syndrome can occur before clinical hypothyroidism is apparent. This association is important because treatment by thyroid replacement is followed by complete relief of the neuropathy, thus avoiding surgery.

In addition to the effects of hypothyroidism on pe-

TABLE 114–2. RHEUMATIC MANIFESTATIONS OF THYROID DISORDERS

Hypothyroidism	Peripheral neuropathy—carpal tunnel syndrome
	Arthropathy—noninflammatory viscous effusions, chondrocalcinosis (calcium pyrophosphate crystals), Charcot-like joint destruction, hyperuricemia and gout, flexor tenosynovitis, epiphyseal dysplasia
	Myopathy—aches, pain, stiffness, cramping, weakness, myoedema, hypertrophy
Hyperthyroidism	Thyroid acropachy—clubbing, periosteal proliferation, soft tissue swelling, pretibial myxedema, exophthalmos, LATS (long-acting thyroid stimulator)
	Periarthritic osteoporosis
	Myopathy—atrophy, exophthalmic ophthalmoplegia, myasthenia gravis, periodic paralysis
Autoimmune (Hashimoto's) thyroiditis	Fibrositis syndrome
	Chest-wall pains
	Association with connective tissue diseases

ripheral nerves, the cerebral cortex, cerebellum, and cranial nerves may also be involved. In hypothyroid patients, the cerebral spinal fluid protein concentration averages 115% above normal, with γ-globulin levels over 3 times normal.[13] With rare exceptions, all neurologic manifestations of hypothyroidism disappear completely after treatment.

ARTHROPATHY

The initial studies of Bland and Frymoyer,[11] and the subsequent clinical pathologic study by Dorwart and Schumacher,[14] have defined a joint disorder distinctive for myxedema whose characteristic features are listed in Table 114–2. Joint involvement usually develops concurrently with the onset of hypothyroidism, but occasionally antedates the development of clinical myxedema. Approximately one third of hypothyroid patients have symptomatic synovial effusions. Inflammation is neither common nor severe, with minimal pain and tenderness and only slight warmth and erythema. The arthritis is usually bilateral, most often affecting the knees; the ankles, metacarpophalangeal joints, and small joints of the hands and feet are less frequently involved. Periarticular tissues appear thickened, and the increased intra-articular fluid is reflected in a sluggish "bulge" sign. This finding, caused by hyperviscosity, is secondary to an increased concentration of synovial fluid hyaluronic acid.[14] The synovial fluid otherwise is generally noninflammatory, with a leukocyte count less than 1000/mm^3.

Radiographs are characteristically normal except for signs of effusions. Occasionally, a hypothyroid patient will present with an erosive arthropathy of the fingers that might be responsive to therapy with thyroxine.[15]

In addition, although Frymoyer and Bland excluded patients with hyaline cartilage calcification from their series, they did comment that radiographs in three cases showed destructive lesions of the tibial plateau and what appeared to be pathologic compression fractures. Because a Charcot-like destructive arthropathy has been associated with chondrocalcinosis (see Chapter 108), these three patients may have had associated calcium pyrophosphate dihydrate (CPPD) crystal deposition. Dorwart and Schumacher found chondrocalcinosis of the knee in 7 of 12 myxedematous patients; 9 patients had knee effusions, with calcium pyrophosphate crystals demonstrable in 6.[14] Conversely, an increased incidence of hypothyroidism (10.5%) was found in a study of 105 patients with chondrocalcinosis.[16] Both intraleukocytic and extracellular calcium pyrophosphate and sodium urate crystals were noted, but *without* an associated inflammatory response. Others have not demonstrated an association between the two.[17,18]

The frequent failure of patients with myxedema to manifest intense inflammatory joint effusions in response to either sodium urate or calcium pyrophosphate crystals is of interest. Two findings may provide the explanation. First, neutrophil functions are reduced in hypothyroidism, an abnormality corrected after treatment with thyroxine.[19] Second, the high intrinsic viscosity and elevated concentration of hyaluronic acid in synovial fluid impedes the chemotactic movement of leukocytes and diminishes the rate of crystal endocytosis.[20] After treatment with thyroid hormone, several patients developed typical crystal-induced inflammatory joint attacks, in contrast to the resolution of noncrystal-related joint pain and effusions.

Asymptomatic hyperuricemia often occurs in hypothyroid men, but not women.[21] The increased incidence of clinical myxedema in patients with gout is small but significant.[22] The contributions of obesity and the influence of thyroid hormone on renal urate excretion remain unclear, and as a result, the association of gout and hypothyroidism remains controversial.

Wrist flexor tenosynovitis associated with hypothyroidism[14] was reported not to respond to thyroid therapy, but to subside promptly after injections of corticosteroid into the tendon sheaths. Although biopsies were not performed, hyaluronate deposition was believed to be responsible for the thickened, tender, and boggy palmar sheaths.

Ligamentous laxity occurs in approximately one third of patients with myxedema. The synovial effusions with edematous, lax joint capsules, ligaments, and tendons resemble the changes seen in an animal model of hypothyroidism thought to be due to increased concentrations of hyaluronate in the involved tissues. Myxedematous joint disease has been described only in primary hypothyroidism, in which levels of thyroid-stimulating hormone are increased. This hormone may increase synovial synthesis of hyaluronate, which may result in the changes described.[23]

Both the congenital and the acquired forms of hypothyroidism in children can delay epiphyseal closure and can retard maturation and ossification. This phenomenon, most often seen in the femoral head, may cause slipped capital femoral epiphysis. Helpful diagnostic features in such children include hip pain, limping, and an elevated serum creatine kinase level.[24]

MYOPATHY

Myopathic features may accompany many different endocrinopathies, but numerically their occurrence in hypothyroidism is probably the most important. Besides the slow movement and the delayed muscle contraction and relaxation classically seen in hypothyroidism, about half these patients complain of *weakness* and *muscle cramps, aches* and *pains*, or *stiffness*.[25] Muscle hypertrophy occurs in about 12% of patients. Pain and stiffness may be present during rest and are exacerbated on exposure to cold, thus resembling primary fibrositis. Such muscular symptoms may be the presenting complaints in many patients without overt clinical hypothyroidism. Like the neuropathy and arthropathy, myopathy can antedate the diagnosis of hypothyroidism by several months. The various muscle symptoms of hypothyroidism probably constitute a continuous spectrum, beginning with aches and pains and progressing to muscle cramping, proximal weakness, and even hypertrophy in association with severe, long-standing hypothyroidism. A case of rhabdomyolysis with hypothyroidism has been reported.[26]

On physical examination, weakness usually is not severe. The proximal muscles are principally affected. Muscle contraction and relaxation are slowed, owing more often to muscle disease than to altered nerve conduction or to defective neuromuscular transmission. Direct percussion of the muscle with a reflex hammer leads to an interesting sign, termed the "mounding phenomenon" or *myoedema*. This transient focal ridging seen in response to striking or pinching the muscle persists for several seconds and can also be present in patients with hypoalbuminemia. Muscles are usually of normal bulk; atrophy is rare in hypothyroidism. Generalized hypertrophy of muscles, when observed in infants and children, is called the *Kocher-Debre-Semelaigne syndrome*, and in adults, *Hoffman's syndrome*. This unusual finding, producing an athletic or "Herculean" appearance, disappears with therapy. Percussion of these hypertrophic muscles produces prolonged contractions resembling myotonia, although electromyographic studies have shown these muscle responses to be electrically silent.

The activities of most "muscle" enzymes are increased in the serum of patients with hypothyroidism.[25] Creatine kinase has been best studied and its concentrations correlate well with the severity of hypothyroidism. The exact contribution of the cardiac muscle isoenzyme to the serum creatine kinase level in hypothyroidism remains to be resolved. The creatine kinase level returns to normal within 2 months after restoration of the euthyroid state. In the few studies of patients with hypopituitarism and secondary hypothyroidism, myopathy was not a clinical feature, and serum creatine kinase levels were normal suggesting a role of thyroid-stimulating hormone in the pathogenesis of hypothyroid myopathy.

Electromyographic changes are independent of muscle bulk. Approximately half the patients demonstrate increased needle insertional activity and hyperirritability. An equal number manifest polyphasic motor unit action potentials. Frequently, chains of repetitive discharges are observed after reflex motion. These changes are nonspecific indicators of a myopathy and not pathognomonic of hypothyroid muscle disease.

Although biopsies may be normal, light microscopy reveals evidence of muscle degeneration in many patients as well as areas of focal necrosis, regeneration, and basophilia with vacuolization of fibers. Fiber size varies, and the sarcolemmal nuclei are numerous, enlarged, and centrally positioned. Mucoprotein deposits, widespread in multiple organs in hypothyroidism, are found in the muscles of one third of patients. Histochemical staining has demonstrated a decrease in type II fibers proportional to the severity of the hypothyroidism. This lower percentage of type II fibers correlates with the severity of the disease and with the elevation of creatine kinase levels. With treatment, the ratios of the fiber types return to normal.[27] The pathophysiology of myopathy in hypothyroidism is poorly understood. A study of the effects of L-thyroxine on muscle bioenergetics in humans and rodents using ^{31}P magnetic resonance spectroscopy suggests a hormone-dependent mitochondrial disorder that is reversible with therapy. Such changes were not present in patients or rodents with hyperthyroidism.[28]

Although most cases of connective tissue disease have occurred in patients with autoimmune thyroiditis, a case of hypothyroidism secondary to panhypopituitarism with Raynaud's phenomenon has been reported; all symptoms resolved after thyroid hormone replacement.[29]

OSTEOPOROSIS ASSOCIATED WITH L-THYROXINE TREATMENT

Thyroid hormone activates osteoclasts and accelerates remodeling of bone. Excess hormone, whether endogenous or exogeneous, causes more rapid resorption than formation of bone with resulting osteoporosis.[30] A number of studies have measured bone mineral density in women with Grave's disease or receiving replacement therapy for hypothyroidism. All of these revealed a loss of bone mineral density as great as 9% or more as compared to age-matched control patients without thyroid disease.[31,32] Some studies have suggested that osteoporosis might be accelerated in patients with low serum concentrations of thyroid-stimulating hormone (TSH) indicating overreplacement despite clinical euthyroidism; others have not found this correlation. The association between TSH levels and osteoporosis remains ill defined thus far, but all information available argues for replacement therapy with the lowest adequate dose possible of L-thyroxine in the hope of preventing accelerated rates of bone loss.

HYPERTHYROIDISM

THYROID ACROPACHY

This extraordinary rheumatic manifestation of hyperthyroidism usually follows treatment for thyrotoxicosis.[33] Thyroid acropachy, or thickening of small parts, occurs in approximately 1% of patients with past or present thyroid disease and usually develops approximately 1 year after either thyroidectomy or radioablation. The fingers and toes become *clubbed*, and patients develop *periostitis* of the digits and distal extremities with swelling of soft tissues. Usually, these patients also have *exophthalmos* and *pretibial myxedema*. These features, in addition to the presence in the serum of long-acting thyroid stimulator (LATS), help to differentiate thyroid acropachy from other causes of hypertrophic osteoarthropathy. When this syndrome appears, patients are often clinically hypothyroid. Signs of inflammation are not prominent, although the syndrome is *painful*, especially on palpation over the periosteal new bone. Partial improvement, with incomplete resolution of pains in the extremities and digits and subsidence of the periosteal new bone proliferation, occurs in some patients after treatment with thyroid hormone or prednisone (see also Chapter 88).

Immune factors appear to participate in the pathogenesis of Graves' disease and possibly in its extrathyroidal manifestations, including acropachy.[34] Patients with Graves' disease have circulating thyroid-stimulating immunoglobulins, considered to be antibodies to the thyroid-stimulating hormone receptor on thyroid cell membranes. The presence of other thyroid autoantibodies suggests a close relationship between Graves' disease and Hashimoto's thyroiditis. Evidence indicates cell-mediated immunity in both diseases, with the finding of T-lymphocytes sensitized to a thyroid antigen.[34] It has been postulated that local interferon production induces Ia-like antigens on the surface of thyroid cells with a subsequent immune response to the tissue adjacent to the Ia molecule.[35] Additional evidence linking these disorders includes the development of acropachy in both, their occurrence in the same families, and their histopathologic coexistence within the same thyroid gland. The significant excess of the histocompatibility antigens HLA-B8 and HLA-DR3 in patients with Graves' disease is evidence of a genetic association. The exact role of organ-specific autoantibodies or sensitized leukocytes in the production of either of these thyroid disorders or of the acropachy remains unclear.

Another rheumatic association of uncertain pathogenesis is periarthritis of the shoulder, which is said to coexist with hyperthyroidism and to respond to restoration of the euthyroid state.[36] Marked osteoporosis, with subsequent fractures, is also frequently seen in thyrotoxicosis and is due to bone resorption stimulated by thyroid hormone, possibly by osteoclast activating factor (OAF), or interleukin-1, with subsequent elevation of serum calcium and phosphorus levels. Both parathyroid hormone and 1,25 dihydroxyvitamin D_3 concentrations are decreased.[30] This osteoporosis is also reversible when the thyroid disorder is treated.

THYROTOXIC MYOPATHY

Clinical evidence of weakness can be found in almost all thyrotoxic patients.[25] The myopathy of thyrotoxicosis can be mild, characterized by weakness, fatigability, and minimal atrophy, or it can be extreme, characterized by proximal wasting and severe weakness, resembling polymyositis. Unlike polymyositis, acute inflammatory changes are not evident, and laryngeal and pharyngeal muscles are usually not involved. Atrophy and infiltration by fat cells and lymphocytes occur. "Muscle" enzymes are generally not increased in the serum, although creatinuria is present. Electromyographic abnormalities include short-duration motor unit potentials and an increased percentage of polyphasic potentials. Full recovery of muscle strength occurs as patients become euthyroid. There is controversy over the possible beneficial effect of β blockade on thyrotoxic myopathy.[37]

Three other forms of myopathy are less common. *Exophthalmic ophthalmoplegia* usually parallels the severity of exophthalmos. Associated findings include swelling of the eyelid and conjunctiva and sometimes of the optic nerve head. A second form is the coexistence of Graves' disease in 5% of patients with *myasthenia gravis*. The association of these disorders has a distinct female sex preponderance. Patients respond to prostigmine, but improvement is incomplete, owing to the thyrotoxicosis. *Thyrotoxic periodic paralysis* is the third of the rarer forms of skeletal muscle involvement in thyrotoxicosis. It is similar to the periodic paralysis of primary hypokalemia. This syndrome has the cardinal features of flaccid paralysis of the extremities, with absent reflexes and diminished electrical excitability. Precipitating factors are thought to be exercise, a high carbohydrate intake, and the administration of insulin or epinephrine. This disorder is rare in whites and is more common in Oriental males. Serum potassium concentrations are usually low, and the administration of potassium salts can prevent or abort attacks. Restoration of the euthyroid state leads to resolution of the paralytic attacks.

AUTOIMMUNE (HASHIMOTO'S) THYROIDITIS

Early in the course of autoimmune thyroiditis, as the thyroid gland gradually enlarges, most patients are euthyroid and some are hyperthyroid. But with progressive lymphocytic infiltration, fibrosis, and obliteration of thyroid follicles nearly half of these patients develop hypothyroidism. This common cause of diffuse goiter, with a female predilection, is frequently associated with musculoskeletal symptoms. The most common rheumatic syndrome resembles *fibrositis;* patients complain of stiffness of the joints and muscles, exacerbated by cold or dampness and worse on arising in the morning or after any period of immobility. This syndrome resembles that seen in hypothyroidism and can be present in autoimmune thyroiditis even in the absence of thyroid deficiency. Another rheumatic symptom is *unusual chest-wall pains* of intermittent nature. Described in 12% of patients with Hashimoto's disease, these thoracic and shoulder-girdle pains, lasting for several minutes to hours, are relieved by changes of position or by mild exercises.[38] Half the patients with Hashimoto's disease have an *elevated erythrocyte sedimentation rate,* with or without rheumatic symptoms.

Most patients with Hashimoto's disease have high serum titers of *thyroid antibodies,* both to thyroglobulin and to microsomal antigens. Cellular immunity may also be important in the pathogenesis of the disease.[34] Biologic false-positive tests for syphilis, rheumatoid factors, and antinuclear antibodies are also common. Hashimoto's disease coexists with other autoimmune disorders, especially pernicious anemia and hemolytic anemia, and possibly with RA, systemic lupus erythematosus (SLE), and Sjögren's syndrome. These disorders appear in family members of patients with autoimmune thyroiditis too often to be coincidental.

The frequency of thyroid disease in patients with

rheumatic disorders has also been examined. Although patients with connective tissue diseases, notably systemic lupus erythematosus and RA, have a high incidence of antibodies to thyroid antigens, the majority are euthyroid and do not have detectable goiters. A prospective study showed frequent thyroid function test abnormalities, including elevated thyroid-stimulating hormone, in patients with SLE without clinically evident thyroid disease. The most common abnormalities were consistent with incipient or true hypothyroidism. Mild to moderate hypothyroidism may be missed because of the similarity of some of its symptoms with those of SLE.[39] Despite this and other uncontrolled series, the coexistence of either hyperthyroidism or hypothyroidism with RA, polymyositis, scleroderma, or systemic lupus erythematosus may be coincidental and deserves further investigation. Two other situations associated with thyroid disorders are known: (1) the administration of antithyroid drugs may be followed by syndromes resembling either RA or systemic lupus erythematosus, especially in children[40]; and (2) falsely low values of serum thyroxine can be seen in patients treated either with salicylates or with corticosteroid hormones.

PARATHYROID DISORDERS

A number of rheumatic findings are associated with parathyroid hormone excess (Table 114–3). A more detailed discussion of the osseous consequences of increased levels of this hormone, including osteitis fibrosa cystica, may be found in Chapter 113.

Most patients are diagnosed with hyperparathyroidism before the development of osteitis fibrosa cystica because of findings of hypercalcemia by automated biochemical screening tests. These patients can have varying degrees of osteoporosis that can improve after surgical removal of the adenoma. These patients, however, never achieve normal bone mineral density after their operations and might require further medical management of osteoporosis.[41,42]

The resorptive effects of parathyroid hormone on bone may lead to the characteristic *subperiosteal erosive* radiographic appearance, particularly at the radial aspect of the middle phalanges, the medial aspect of the proximal femur or tibia, and the inferior aspect of the distal third of the clavicle. *Erosions* may also occur in juxta-articular sites, especially at the interphalangeal, metacarpophalangeal, carpal, and acromioclavicular joints. These lesions can be found in the absence of subperiosteal resorption, can be symmetric, and can be associated with morning stiffness, thus mimicking RA. Several features distinguish parathyroid disorders: (1) the erosions may have a shaggy appearance; (2) they often occur at the distal interphalangeal joints and spare the proximal interphalangeal joints; (3) joint-space narrowing in association with these erosions is uncommon because parathyroid hormone does not directly induce inflammatory synovitis or cartilage dissolution; and (4) concurrent articular calcification is common.

Parathyroid hormone increases collagenase activity, which may account for the *laxity of capsular and ligamentous structures* seen in this disorder. *Tendon ruptures and avulsions* have been reported.[43] Tendon rupture in patients with systemic lupus erythematosus can also be associated with hyperparathyroidism. These patients almost invariably have chronic renal failure and elevated levels of parathyroid hormone.[44] *Vertebral subluxation* occurs, especially in the cervical spine; *dorsal kyphosis* is present, with anterior bowing of the sternum; the lumbar spine is *hypermobile*. Additional changes include *sacroiliac erosions* and *intervertebral disc calcifications*. The laxity leads to joint abuse, which contributes to the back pain, disc protrusion, and degenerative joint changes seen in hyperparathyroidism.

Chondrocalcinosis has been reported in 18 to 25% of patients with hyperparathyroidism[44,45] (see also Chapter 108). Calcium pyrophosphate dihydrate (CPPD) crystal deposition may cause attacks of pseudogout, which can precede the recognition of parathyroid hormone excess and may thus be an initial manifestation of this disease. *Pseudogout* attacks may flare within 2 to 3 days of parathyroidectomy, or they may occur later, often coincident with the postoperative nadir of the serum calcium level.[46] Once chondrocalcinosis is present, it usually persists in spite of parathyroidectomy, and the frequency of episodes of pseudogout continues unabated or even increases. Bywaters and co-workers have described subchondral cyst formation with subsequent destructive joint changes in 15 of 19 patients with hyperparathyroidism.[47] More than half their patients had chondrocalcinosis. Because similar joint changes with severe destruction and the development of Charcot-like joints have been described in association with chondrocalcinosis per se, the relative contribution of CPPD crystals and parathyroid hormone to this type of arthropathy remains to be elucidated. The presence of

TABLE 114–3. RHEUMATIC MANIFESTATIONS OF PARATHYROID DISORDERS

Hyperparathyroidism	Asymptomatic hypercalcemia and osteoporosis
	Osteitis fibrosa cystica
	Subperiosteal resorption
	Bony erosions
	Joint laxity
	Tendon avulsions/ruptures
	Back abnormalities
	Degenerative arthritis
	Chondrocalcinosis and pseudogout
	Charcot-like joints
	Hyperuricemia and gout
	Ectopic calcifications
	Neuromyopathy
Hypoparathyroidism and pseudohypoparathyroidism	Subcutaneous calcifications; myopathy
	Paraspinal ligament calcifications (spondylitis without sacroiliitis)

severe osteoarthritis should prompt a search for CPPD crystals, and if these are found, for the metabolic diseases associated with them, including hyperparathyroidism.

The persistently elevated serum calcium levels in primary hyperparathyroidism may result in nephrocalcinosis and a nephropathy characterized by an impaired tubular-concentrating mechanism. Some hyperparathyroid patients have a decreased uric acid clearance, which may explain the finding of hyperuricemia. The incidence of actual gouty attacks by hyperparathyroidism varies from 3 to 45%.[21] Because hyperuricemia and gout do not seem to occur without underlying renal changes, they may persist after parathyroidectomy. Elevated levels of parathyroid hormone were found in about 70% of patients with CPPD crystal deposits and in age- and sex-matched control subjects with osteoarthritis of the knee.[17] Chemical hyperparathyroidism occurred in patients in both groups. Serum levels of parathyroid hormone correlated directly with serum calcium levels, female patients having the most severe osteoarthritis, and with bone density. These findings have not been confirmed.

In secondary hyperparathyroidism, as well as in other disorders in which metastatic calcifications are found, deposits of amorphous and crystalline basic calcium phosphate salts may occur in periarticular or articular tissues. Their presence can induce a local inflammatory reaction with pain and swelling (see also Chapter 110). Treatment consists of prophylaxis with aluminum hydroxide gels and the use of antiinflammatory agents or intra-articular corticosteroids during acute episodes.

Fatigue, generalized weakness, and other neuromuscular complaints occur in the majority of patients with primary or secondary hyperparathyroidism. Weakness is usually in the *proximal muscles*, often only in the lower extremities. This symptom is most commonly secondary to a *peripheral neuropathic process.*[48,49] Other neurologic findings include abnormalities of the cranial nerves, long-tract signs, and decreased vibratory sensation. Muscle enzyme levels are not elevated, and nerve conduction velocities are reported normal despite other electromyographic findings suggesting a neuropathic process. Muscle biopsy reveals neurogenic atrophy of both fiber types, with type II atrophy predominating.[49] Parathyroidectomy usually rapidly reverses these abnormalities. Other causes of neuromuscular symptoms in hyperparathyroid patients are a polymyositis-like myopathy[50] and an ischemic myopathy caused by intravascular calcifications[51] that occurs in the secondary hyperparathyroidism associated with uremia.

Hypoparathyroidism. In addition to the bony features of hypoparathyroidism, pseudohypoparathyroidism, and pseudopseudohypoparathyroidism, *subcutaneous* and *ectopic calcifications* may be seen. *Spondylitis without sacroiliitis*, with extensive paraspinal calcifications in hypoparathyroidism and pseudohypoparathyroidism, has been reported.[52] *Myopathy*, in association with elevated serum levels of creatine kinase and normal muscle biopsy has also been seen in hypoparathyroidism.[53]

DIABETES MELLITUS

The musculoskeletal complications of diabetes mellitus, both articular and periarticular, are listed in Table 114–4. Some of these, such as destructive arthropathy, reflex sympathetic dystrophy, carpal tunnel syndrome, interosseous muscle wasting, and proximal weakness, may be primarily the result of neuropathic changes. Ischemic vascular disease may also contribute to their genesis. Complications that appear to be related to a proliferation of fibrous tissue include the increased incidence of capsulitis of the shoulder, Dupuytren's contractures and flexor tenosynovitis in adults, and flexion contractures in juvenile-onset diabetics. The collagen from skin and tendon samples of young diabetics is stiff and stabilized, similar to samples from normal control subjects 50 to 65 years older. Possible reasons for the excessive fibrosis and accelerated aging of collagen is discussed in Chapter 96.

The association between diabetes and hyperuricemia or gout remains controversial. Joslin, et al. reported only one case of gout in 1500 diabetic patients,[54] and studies of patients with hyperuricemia compared with age- and weight-matched controls showed no difference in results of glucose tolerance tests. Nonobese, type II, diabetic patients have no greater incidence of gout than the normal population. Similarly, there is a consensus that there is no increase in the incidence of diabetes in gout.[21] Less clearly defined is the putative association with ankylosing hyperostosis.[55] Controlled studies have failed to support an association of diabetes mellitus (see Chapter 108) with CPPD crystal deposition.

TABLE 114–4. RHEUMATIC MANIFESTATIONS OF DIABETES MELLITUS

Neuropathy	Distal sensory and sensorimotor disorders
	Mononeuropathy multiplex
	Diabetic amyotrophy
	Radiculopathy
	Autonomic neuropathy
Neuroarthropathy	Osteolysis
	Osteoporosis
	Charcot joint
	Coexistent osteomyelitis
	Periarthritis of the shoulder (adhesive capsulitis)
Other Associations	Hyperuricemia and gout?
	Ankylosing hyperostosis
	Flexion contractures (Dupuytren's contractures, limited joint mobility)
	Tenosynovitis

NEUROPATHY

Diabetic neuropathy may take several forms: (1) a peripheral symmetric sensory or sensorimotor loss; (2) a mononeuropathy multiplex with an increased frequency of cranial nerve involvement; (3) a neuropathy resulting in proximal muscle weakness, termed diabetic amyotrophy; (4) a radiculopathy leading to lancinating pains in a dermatomal distribution; (5) an autonomic neuropathy; and (6) carpal tunnel syndrome. With *peripheral neuropathic* involvement, patients frequently have a stocking-glove distribution of sensory loss, with decreased vibratory and position sense and decreased or absent deep-tendon reflexes. Wasting of the interosseous muscles of the hands and feet may give a claw-hand or hammer-toe appearance.

Mononeuropathies most commonly affect the third and sixth cranial nerves, and occasionally the fourth and seventh as well. Mononeuropathy involving the motor supply of the proximal hip and leg muscles, and less often of the upper extremities, occurs more in men, often in those with only mild diabetes. This so-called *diabetic amyotrophy* is usually bilateral but asymmetric. Muscle biopsy shows a predominance of type I fibers, with type II atrophy and no evidence of significant necrosis or inflammation. Muscle enzyme levels are normal, and the electromyogram shows some fibrillation potentials. The weakness may spontaneously remit. Evidence also indicates that control of hyperglycemia contributes to recovery.[56] *Diabetic radiculopathy* may occur secondary to infarction of a nerve root, with resultant lancinating pains. These pains are sometimes confused with the symptoms of a herniated disc. When proprioceptive loss and ataxia accompany this shooting pain, it is called "diabetic pseudotabes."

Involvement of the *autonomic nervous system* results in orthostatic hypotension, impotence, dyshidrosis, and diarrhea. Autonomic dysfunction may be related to the unilateral or bilateral reflex dystrophy and to the apparently increased shoulder pain seen in diabetes. *Periarthritis (adhesive capsulitis) of the shoulder,* often bilateral, was found in 11% of a large group of diabetic patients.[57] Conversely, in another study, approximately 25% of patients with periarthritis were diabetic.[58] This entity occurs more commonly in women on the nondominant side of the body and produces aching with limitation of shoulder motion. Calcific bursitis and tendinitis may be present. The natural course of the disorder varies, but spontaneous remissions may occur. Physical therapy, anti-inflammatory drugs, and local corticosteroid injections are helpful. Although 5 to 17% of patients with carpal tunnel syndrome have diabetes, systematic, controlled observations have not demonstrated a significant association.[59]

ARTHROPATHY

As a consequence of sensory neuropathy, severe arthropathy with Charcot-like changes develops in approximately 0.1% of long-standing diabetes.[60] The tarsometatarsal and metatarsophalangeal joints are by far the most common sites of involvement, but changes may rarely affect joints above the ankle. A combination of microfragmentation from trauma, ischemia from small blood vessel disease, and superimposed infection can contribute to the clinical and radiographic changes of neuroarthropathy. All patients with diabetic neuroarthropathy have peripheral neuropathy. In advanced disease, the longitudinal arch of the foot collapses, leading to an unstable gait and a "rocker-sole" appearance. Ulcerations and plantar callosites occur over hypoesthetic pressure points. Osteolysis of bone can develop, with periosteal reaction and remodeling, whittling of the metatarsal bones, cupping deformities, and telescoping of the phalanges.[60] Fractures may be the initial lesion in a Charcot joint or may simply contribute to more extensive joint damage. In all involved joints, the discrepancy between pain, which is minimal or absent, and the destructive radiographic appearance, which is severe, is striking. The mainstay of therapy is rest of the involved area, attention to care of the feet including proper shoes, treatment of concomitant osteomyelitis, and amputation if required (see Chapter 83).

A group of disorders of more obscure pathogenesis has in common excessive proliferation of fibroblastic tissue. *Fibrous palmar nodules* with subsequent Dupuytren's contractures have been reported in as many as 21% of diabetic patients; diabetes was found in 10% of those with Dupuytren's contractures (see Chapter 96).[61] Diabetes has also been described in 10 to 30% of all adult cases of trigger finger or flexor tenosynovitis.[62] In addition, reports exist of interphalangeal flexion deformities (cheiroarthropathy or limited joint mobility), initially described in insulin-dependent, juvenile-onset diabetic patients.[63] Noninsulin-dependent adult-onset diabetics have deformities as severe as juvenile-onset diabetics.[64] This progressive stiffness has been seen only in the hands and is not related to Dupuytren's contractures or flexor tenosynovitis. The stiffness and limited mobility appear to be related to a thick, tight, waxy skin. A simple screening test for limited joint mobility consists of asking the patient to place both hands on a table palm down with fingers fanned. The entire palmar surface of the fingers makes contact in normal persons.[63] Rosenbloom et al. showed that, in patients who had had diabetes for an average of 16 years, the presence of stiff joints increased the risk of retinal and renal complications from 25 to 83%.[65] The clinical signs and the presence of microvascular disease are reminiscent of scleroderma, but nailfold capillaroscopy is normal.[66]

Type B insulin-resistant diabetes mellitus secondary to insulin receptor antibodies has been associated with multiple rheumatic complaints suggestive of systemic lupus erythematosus, Sjögren's syndrome, or progressive systemic sclerosis.[67,68] Fourteen such patients developed features of an autoimmune disease; 8 of the 14 met the American Rheumatism Association criteria for systemic lupus erythematosus, and 4 developed glomerulonephritis histologically consistent with lupus nephritis.[69] Whenever a patient has extremely insulin-resistant diabetes mellitus and features of a systemic rheumatic disease, the possibility of circulating antibodies to insulin receptors should be considered.

CORTICOSTEROID EXCESS AND DEFICIENCY

Corticosteroid excess due to adrenal hyperproduction or secondary to exogenous administration can profoundly affect the musculoskeletal system. Generalized osteoporosis, osteonecrosis* of the humeral and femoral heads, and pathologic fractures are consequences in bone. Changes in the vertebral column can cause severe pain, kyphosis, and loss of height. In children, growth is retarded, and, if not corrected, results in permanently short stature. A polyarthropathy associated with Cushing's disease has been reported in a single patient.[72] A noninflammatory proximal myopathy may progress from the pelvic to the shoulder girdle and, ultimately, to the distal musculature. Serum muscle enzyme levels are usually normal in states of corticosteroid excess, but urinary creatine excretion is increased.[70] Following correction of hypercortisolism, creatinuria subsides. This dissociation between serum and urine laboratory tests may help to differentiate corticosteroid-related from inflammatory myopathies. The electromyogram in corticosteroid myopathy has yielded confusing results and is not helpful diagnostically. Muscle biopsy reveals a type II atrophy without inflammatory change. Although some recovery of muscle strength occurs within days after reduction of corticosteroid dose, complete resolution usually takes 1 to 4 months.

Adrenal insufficiency after corticosteroid withdrawal may be associated with constitutional symptoms of weakness, fatigue and lassitude, and arthralgias. Addison's disease is generally associated with weakness, but flexion contractures caused by progressive stiffening of the pelvic girdle and thigh muscles can occur. This painful condition, also seen in patients with hypopituitarism, responds to therapy with corticosteroids but not mineralocorticoids.[71] A number of articles have reported an association between Addison's disease and antiphospholipid antibodies as well as the development of hypoadrenalism secondary to thrombosis, hemorrhage, or both in patients with primary antiphospholipid antibody syndrome. The possibility of a clotting disorder related to these antibodies should not be overlooked in patients presenting with acute adrenal insufficiency.[73]

CARCINOID ARTHROPATHY

Distinctive rheumatologic findings occur in at least 10% of carcinoid patients. Arthralgias of the wrists and hands, constant stiffness and pain on movement, and marked intensification of pain after a sustained grip are characteristic complaints. Because the arthralgias can be rapidly reversed with parachlorophenylalanine, which blocks serotonin synthesis, serotonin is believed to be responsible for these symptoms. Bradykinin and histamine may also be involved. One may detect juxta-articular demineralization and erosions at the metacarpophalangeal joints and at the proximal and distal interphalangeal joints, with subchondral cystic changes.[74]

ECTOPIC HORMONAL SYNDROMES

Tumor cells can synthesize polypeptide hormones, such as adrenocorticotropic hormone, growth hormone, thyroid-stimulating hormone, and parathyroid hormone, with structural and functional characteristics similar or identical to those of normal hormones.[75] Because the bony, myopathic, and neuropathic changes associated with endocrinopathies require prolonged hormonal exposure, these syndromes are not seen with ectopic hormone production by malignant tissues. Several cases of *hypertrophic pulmonary osteoarthropathy* have been reported in patients with *acromegalic* physical features and increases in growth hormone or similar substances that resolved when the tumor was removed, suggesting a possible relationship.[76] The periosteal proliferation seen in this osteoarthropathy may resemble the periosteal remodeling of acromegaly, but further clarification is needed to determine whether any humeral substance mediates this syndrome.

PREGNANCY

The symptoms of RA frequently remit during pregnancy. Since Hench's description in 1938 of the beneficial action of pregnancy,[77] improvement has been reported in numerous other rheumatic disorders as well (Table 114–5).[78] Many of these reports have dealt with a few patients or even a single patient, however, and with rare exception, the observations have been retrospective and anecdotal.

The most complete data have been accumulated on the course of RA during gestation and in the postpartum period.[79] Improvement of disease was not noted in all pregnancies. Only 74% had some degree of subsidence of arthritis activity during gestation. Fifty percent of patients with RA had some degree of improvement of disease activity during the first trimester of pregnancy. Thereafter, an additional 24% experienced relief of symptoms throughout the second and third trimesters, some even waiting until the last month of gestation for improvement. In 26% of published cases, patients failed to note an amelioration of arthritis. Some even had more severe symptoms; still others experienced the onset of their disease during pregnancy. There are no factors to predict a patient's response to pregnancy including presence or absence of rheumatoid factor, dis-

* *Editor's note.* Paradoxically, osteonecrosis in natural Cushing's disease or syndrome is exceedingly uncommon although the other bony changes noted with exogenous corticosteroid use are frequent. The reason for this is a conundrum.

TABLE 114–5. DISORDERS REPORTED TO BE AMELIORATED BY PREGNANCY

Rheumatoid arthritis	Sarcoidosis
Psoriatic arthropathy (and psoriasis)	Raynaud's phenomenon
Fibrositis	Gout (possibly)
Intermittent hydrathrosis	Cutaneous anaphylaxis
Erythema nodosum	Angioneurotic edema
Experimental Animal Diseases	
Experimental vasculitis (dogs)	Carrageenan inflammation (rats)
Adjuvant arthritis (rats)	Allergic thyroiditis (guinea pigs)
Disorders with Variable Course	
Systemic lupus erythematosus	Ankylosing spondylitis
Scleroderma	Polyarteritis nodosa
Myasthenia gravis	Polymyositis/dermatomyositis
Inflammatory bowel diseases	Behçet's disease
Necrotizing cutaneous vasculitis	

ease duration, and functional class, but whatever response the patient had with her first pregnancy is predictive for the following one.

After delivery, the symptoms of RA recurred in more than 90% of patients, although complete data are not available. Information has been published on the postpartum experience of only 128 patients.[79] All had an exacerbation following parturition; 64% noted a return of symptoms by the eighth week after delivery. Thirty-six percent had no joint inflammation until more than 8 weeks postpartum. These data indicate that the benefits of pregnancy are temporary, lasting an average of 6 weeks after delivery. The return of symptoms can be abrupt or insidious and is not related to the resumption of menstruation or to the termination of lactation. A careful quantitation of disease activity has not been performed, but it is generally stated that postpartum RA is at least as severe as prior to gestation.

There are few studies of the effect of rheumatoid arthritis on fertility or on the fetus. One retrospective study found that the fertility rate of patients with rheumatoid arthritis was normal although the rate of spontaneous abortion was slightly higher, but in general rheumatoid arthritis patients have successful pregnancies with normal babies.[78]

Another disorder in which a considerable clinical experience during pregnancy has been accumulated is systemic lupus erythematosus.[78] Most authors have noted a high spontaneous abortion rate in pregnancies occurring before the onset of their first recognizable manifestation of this disease, as well as in pregnancies after the onset of clinical disease. Spontaneous abortions may be related to antiphospholipid antibodies, particularly antibodies to cardiolipin.[81] The possibility of heart block in offspring of mothers with systemic lupus erythematosus is now well known[82] and is related to anti-Ro (SSA) antibody.[82] Mothers of babies born with complete heart block should be monitored for signs of lupus because the diagnosis may not be known before delivery. One mother did not develop the disease until 16 years after the birth of the first three children with congenital heart block.[83] Neonatal lupus has also been described in the infants of women with antibodies to U_1RNP.[84]

Less certain is the relationship between disease activity and pregnancy, including the progression of renal or other organ dysfunction. As with RA, exacerbations of systemic lupus have been documented frequently in the postpartum period. Less frequent exacerbations, usually of minor consequence, have been noted in more recent studies. Renal function deterioration is not frequent and usually reversible.[85,86] These results may be due to more aggressive therapy and/or differences in the definition of a lupus flare. It can be difficult to differentiate changes caused only by pregnancy from true disease exacerbation. Serum hemolytic complement levels may be helpful, because these are usually high in normal pregnancies. Because of these uncertainties, a number of investigators have suggested that pregnancies be delayed in these patients until their disease has been inactive for 6 months or more prior to conception.[86] The same risks during pregnancy have been reported in patients with mixed connective tissue disease[87] (see also Chapters 67 and 71).

FACTOR RESPONSIBLE FOR AMELIORATION

The factors responsible for improvement of rheumatoid arthritis during pregnancy is not yet known. The increased susceptibility of pregnant women to certain infectious diseases and the specific suppression of normal immune responses during pregnancy might be relevant. During gestation, women are believed to suffer increased morbidity and mortality from certain infectious agents, chiefly viruses and fungi.[88] The virulence of these intracellular micro-organisms may be related to impaired cell-mediated immunity. Skin-graft rejection is delayed and in vitro T-lymphocyte responses are depressed, effects believed to be mediated by the serum or plasma of pregnancy.[89] The ameliorating substance may be responsible for all the clinical alterations associated with gestation.

Because the concentration of blood cortisol increases during pregnancy, it has been related to the suppression of rheumatoid activity.[90] Subsequent studies have shown, however, that the increased corticosteroid concentrations alone were not fully responsible for the observed improvement.[78] Measurement of plasma cortisol levels did not correlate with disease activity during pregnancy. Plasma cortisol levels fall to normal by 48 hours after delivery, and yet RA remains suppressed post partum for more than 6 weeks in 50% of patients. The hormone is mostly transcortin-bound during gestation and is therefore not biologically active. Thus, despite the original enthusiasm for cortisol, other factors responsible for improvement during gestation have been sought.

A variety of other products of pregnancy, including placental extracts, umbilical cord serum, and blood or urine fractions, have been used to treat RA without reproducible improvement. The concentrations of many plasma proteins are increased during gestation, including: (1) the carrier proteins, such as transcortin, thyroxin-binding globulin, testosterone-binding globulin, estrogen-binding globulin, transferrin, and ceruloplasmin; (2) the coagulation proteins, including fibrinogen and factors VII, VIII, and IX; (3) plasminogen; (4) α_2-macroglobulin; (5) C-reactive protein and other so-called "acute phase" proteins; and (6) the pregnancy-associated plasma proteins.[91]

Of these proteins, studies on the biologic activities of the pregnancy-associated α_2-glycoprotein have been the most promising. This glycoprotein is found at low concentrations in the serum of women who are not pregnant and increases during gestation in most individuals.[92] Following delivery, the level falls at a slower rate than the other pregnancy-associated plasma proteins. The timing of changes in the concentration of plasma pregnancy-associated α_2-glycoprotein paralleled both the remissions and the postpartum exacerbations of RA. Additionally, approximately 25% of women have only minimal elevations of this protein in their plasma during gestation; this finding may explain the failure of this percentage of patients to experience clinical improvements.[88] This substance affects a variety of in vitro parameters of inflammation and acts on the membranes of isolated organelles, polymorphonuclear leukocytes, and lymphocytes as well.[88] Unlike previous observations using corticosteroid hormones, pregnancy-associated α_2-glycoprotein is effective in vitro in physiologic concentrations.

The dramatic changes in the metabolism of the sex hormones during pregnancy are well known. Estrogens reduce the metabolic activity of neutrophils, alter delayed skin-test reactivity in experimental animals, and suppress the development and severity of adjuvant arthritis in rats. Progesterone has also been shown in vitro to suppress leukocyte functions. Most of these effects have resulted from large, nonphysiologic amounts of these sex hormones, however.[89] Despite original enthusiasm, the beneficial effects of sex hormones on patients with RA have not been substantiated by clinical trials, but carefully controlled studies have not been performed. Because estrogenic hormones are known to induce a variety of serum protein changes similar to those in pregnancy, their effect on serum concentrations of pregnancy-associated α_2-glycoprotein has been studied. Significant increases in this protein were observed during the administration of either combinations of estrogen and progesterone or of estrogen alone. Serum concentrations of pregnancy-associated α_2-glycoprotein induced by exogenous sex hormone administration reached only one tenth the levels usually found during pregnancy,[88] however, and this factor may account for the failure of estrogens to produce the clinical response observed during gestation. Thus, sex hormones, corticosteroids, and pregnancy-associated α_2-glycoprotein protein, the plasma constituents increased during pregnancy, have been demonstrated in vitro and in some animal models to possess anti-inflammatory activity. Other potential ameliorating factors in patients with rheumatoid arthritis include (1) the carbohydrate composition of immunoglobulin G molecules, which is altered in RA and partially compensated in the pregnant state,[93] (2) a defect in suppressor T-lymphocytes, and (3) antibodies to HLA-DR molecules that inhibit a cell-mediated reaction in RA.[94]

SEX HORMONES IN AUTOIMMUNE DISORDERS

Many autoimmune diseases are more common in women than in men. In systemic lupus erythematosus (SLE), the best example, the female to male ratio can be as high as 15:1. The ratio does vary with age. In premenarcheal or postmenopausal women, the ratio falls to 2:1. This change in ratio suggests hormonal influence. Oral contraceptive agents either may exacerbate latent SLE or may induce the formation of antibodies to nuclear antigens. In a series of eight patients with antinuclear antibodies believed secondary to oral contraceptive use, all had rheumatic complaints of arthralgias, myalgias, and morning stiffness, and two had synovitis.[95] A subsequent prospective study by the same investigators confirmed the development of autoantibodies in response to these agents, but other investigators were unable to find either rheumatic symptoms or autoantibodies in large groups of women using oral contraceptives.[96] Studies using the newer low-dose estrogen contraceptives in SLE have not been done. These preparations may be a safe, effective alternative for contraception in women with SLE.

In addition to the exacerbating effects of estrogens, it is postulated that androgens play a protective role in autoimmune disease. Indeed, there is a higher incidence of SLE in patients with Klinefelter's syndrome. Treatment of these patients with testosterone may have a therapeutic effect on their autoimmune disease as well.[97] The effect of androgen therapy in RA is controversial. An uncontrolled study of seven male patients showed a favorable response with such therapy.[98]

The effects of sex steroid hormones on autoimmune disease have been studied in murine lupus models. Androgens suppressed murine lupus, and estrogens accelerated the disease. Estrogen receptor-like binding has been found in mouse thymus tissue, and estrogens may inhibit the clearance of immune complexes; these findings reflect the probable influence of sex hormones on the immune system by means of thymus epithelium and the reticuloendothelial system. Thymic hormones are also influenced by sex hormones. T cells, however, appear to be the primary target for hormones. Hormonal manipulation has a profound effect on T cells, with effects on B cells probably orchestrated through the T cells.[99] Additionally, that androgens have preserved interleukin-2 activity in some mice with lupus suggests a relationship between interleukin-2 and sex hormones.[100]

Metabolism of estrogens and androgens in patients with lupus has been investigated. Patients with SLE showed an elevation of 16 hydroxylated metabolites with increased estrogenic activity. First-degree relatives of these patients also had higher levels of 16 hydroxylated metabolites; a genetic predisposition to altered estrogen metabolism is implied.[98]

Expression of class II major histocompatibility antigen on "nontraditional" antigen-presenting cells such as thyroid epithelium or pancreatic islet cells has been proposed as a mechanism of autoimmunity involving these organs. Interferon-γ produced by T-lymphocytes can upregulate major histocompatibility antigens on a variety of cell types and might contribute to autoimmunity in general. Other cytokines such as tumor necrosis factor-α could be involved as well. Sex hormones might modulate some of these cytokines. Subsets of T-cells have estrogen receptors; mice treated with estrogens have produced an increased level of interleukin-1. Interleukin-1 is also elevated during the luteal phase of the menstrual cycle. Estrogen stimulation of T-lymphocytes from female mice resulted in a greater production of interferon-γ. The promoter for the interferon-γ gene in transgenic mice can be upregulated by estrogen and is probably the normal control mechanism. Interleukin-2 production by lymphocytes is diminished by treatment with estrogens. All of these changes could have profound effects on autoimmunity.[101]

The results of these and other studies suggest an important role for hormonal modulation of the immune system in autoimmune disorders, in particular systemic lupus erythematosus, and may lead to novel therapeutic techniques (see Chapters 37 and 38).

AUTOIMMUNITY AND THE HYPOTHALAMIC-PITUITARY ADRENAL AXIS

The role of the central nervous system (CNS) and the hypothalamic-pituitary-adrenal (HPA) axis in autoimmunity has not been defined, but the observation that RA does not develop on the affected side after a cerebral vascular accident or polio has been noted for years. Stress has long been clinically associated with exacerbations of autoimmune diseases and suspected as a component in their initiation, but there are no objective data to support these observations. New information about the interactions between the CNS, HPA axis, and immune system includes the observation that cytokines elaborated by immune cells have direct effects on the HPA axis. Interleukin-1 can stimulate the hypothalamus to secrete corticotropin-releasing factor (CRF), which triggers the whole HPA axis with the end result of secretion of adrenal corticosteroids. Interleukin-2 stimulates the pituitary to release ACTH and thus also stimulating the adrenal glands. Corticosteroids have many immunomodulating effects, including inhibition of the secretion of both interleukin-1 and -2 thus providing feedback inhibition of the immune system as well as of the HPA axis. Interleukin-6 has been found to have similar activities.[102,103]

Cells of the immune system have receptors for ACTH and endorphins as a possible link to the HPA axis. They also secrete a number of neuropeptides including ACTH, endorphins, thyrotropin, prolactin, and others. These substances are secreted in response to virus infections or mitogens, and to hypothalamic-releasing factor.[103]

A few studies have had more direct implications for autoimmune diseases. Sternberg and colleagues found that a strain of rats considered "high-stress" do not develop streptococcal cell wall–induced arthritis unless treated with a corticosteroid-receptor antagonist, whereas "low-stress" Lewis rats do develop arthritis. The Lewis rats have smaller adrenal glands and treatment of them with low doses of corticosteroids decreased the intensity of the arthritis.[104] Studies of adjuvant-induced arthritis in rats revealed higher concentrations of substance P in the joints that become inflamed. Through immunohistochemical staining a decreased level of substance P was detected in rheumatoid versus normal synovium. Substance P might be involved in the onset of disease and might be depleted at later times.[105] Substance P has direct in-vitro effects, including increased synoviocyte proliferation and increased release of prostaglandin E2 and collagenase, all of which could have profound effects on the development of pannus and cartilage destruction.[106]

It is obvious from these and many other studies that the interactions between the immune and the central neuroendocrine systems are being explored diligently. Future studies will undoubtedly have important effects on our knowledge of the pathogenesis of autoimmune states and on treatment strategies to interrupt or modulate the process.

REFERENCES

1. Melmed, S.: Acromegaly, N. Engl. J. Med., *322*:966–977, 1990.
2. Anton, H.C.: Hand measurements in acromegaly. Clin. Radiol., *23*:445–450, 1972.
3. Lacks, S., and Jacobs, R.P.: Acromegalic arthropathy: A reversible rheumatic disease. J. Rheumatol., *13*:634–636, 1986.
4. Layton, M.W., Fudman, E.J., Barker, A., et al.: Acromegalic arthropathy. Characteristics and response to therapy. Arthritis Rheum., *31*:1022–1027, 1988.
5. Bluestone, R., et al.: Acromegalic arthropathy. Ann. Rheum. Dis., *30*:243–258, 1971.
6. Nagulesparen, M., et al.: Muscle changes in acromegaly. Br. Med. J., *2*:914–915, 1976.
7. Revel, J.P., Ito, S., and Fawcett, D.W.: Electron micrographs of

phospholipids simulating intercellular membranes. J. Biophys. Biocytol., *4*:495–498, 1958.
8. Pickett, J.B.E., III et al.: Neuromuscular complications of acromegaly. Neurology, *25*:638–645, 1975.
9. Khaleeli, A.A., Levy, R.D., Edwards, R.H.T., et al.: The neuromuscular features of aromegaly. A clinical and pathological study. J. Neurol. Neurosurg. Psychiatry, *47*:1009–1015, 1984.
10. Low, P.A., et al.: Peripheral neuropathy in acromegaly. Brain, *97*:139–152, 1974.
11. Bland, J.H., and Frymoyer, J.W.: Rheumatic syndromes of myxedema. N. Engl. J. Med., *282*:1171–1174, 1970.
12. Rao, S.N., et al.: Neuromuscular status in hypothyroidism. Acta Neurol. Scand., *61*:167–177, 1980.
13. Swanson, J.W., Kelly, J.D., and McConahey, W.M.: Neurologic aspects of thyroid dysfunction. Mayo Clin. Proc., *56*:504–512, 1981.
14. Dorwart, B.B., and Schumacher, H.R.: Joint effusions, chondrocalcinosis and other rheumatic manifestations in hypothyroidism. A clinicopathologic study. Am. J. Med., *59*:780–790, 1975.
15. Neeck, G., Riedel, W., and Schmidt, K.L.: Neuropathy myopathy and destructive arthropathy in primary hypothyroidism. J. Rheumatol., *17*:1697–1700, 1990.
16. Dieppe, P.A., et al.: Pyrophosphate arthropathy: A clinical and radiological study of 105 cases. Ann. Rheum. Dis., *41*:371–376, 1982.
17. McCarty, D.J., et al.: Diseases associated with calcium pyrophosphate dihydrate crystal deposition: A controlled study. Am. J. Med., *56*:704–714, 1974.
18. Komatireddy, G.R., Ellman, M.H., and Brown, N.L.: Lack of association between hypothyroidism and chondrocalcinosis. J. Rheumatol., *16*:807–808, 1989.
19. Farid, N.R., et al.: Polymorphonuclear leukocyte function in hypothyroidism. Horm. Res., *7*:247–253, 1976.
20. Brandt, K.D.: The effect of synovial hyaluronate on the ingestion of monosodium urate crystals by leukocytes. Clin. Chim. Acta, *55*:307–315, 1974.
21. Newcombe, D.S.: Endocrinopathies and uric acid metabolism. Semin. Arthritis Rheum., *2*:281–300, 1973.
22. Durward, W.F.: Gout and hypothyroidism in males. Arthritis Rheum., *19*:123, 1976.
23. Newcombe, D.S., Ortel, R.W., and Levey, G.S.: Activation of synovial membrane adenylate cyclase by thyroid stimulating hormone. Biochem. Biophys. Res. Commun., *48*:201–214, 1972.
24. Hirano, T., et al.: Association of primary hypothyroidism and slipped capital femoral epiphysis. J. Pediatr., *93*:262–264, 1978.
25. Ramsey, I.D.: Thyroid Disease and Muscle Dysfunction. London. Whitefriars Press, 1974.
26. Halverson, P.B., et al.: Rhabdomyolysis and renal failure in hypothyroidism. Ann. Intern. Med., *91*:57–58, 1979.
27. McKeran, R.O., et al.: Muscle fibre type changes in hypothyroid myopathy. J. Clin. Pathol., *28*:659–663, 1975.
28. Argov, Z., Rehshaw, P.F., Boden, B., et al.: Effects of thyroid hormones on skeletal muscle bioenergetics. In vivo phosphorus-31 magnetic resonance spectroscopy study of humans and rats. J. Clin. Invest., *81*:1695–1701, 1988.
29. Shagan, B.P., and Friedman, S.A.: Raynaud's phenomenon and thyroid deficiency. Arch. Intern. Med., *140*:831–832, 1980.
30. Auwerx, J., and Bouillon, R.: Mineral and bone metabolism in thyroid disease. A review. Q. J. Med., *60*:737–752, 1986.
31. Ross, D.S., Neer, R.M., Ridgway, E.C., and Daniels, G.H.: Subclinical hyperthyroidism and reduced bone density as a possible result of prolonged suppression of the pituitary-thyroid axis with L-thyroxine. Am. J. Med., *82*:1167–1170, 1987.
32. Stall, G.M., Harris, S., Sokoll, L.J., and Dawson-Hughes, B.: Accelerated bone loss in hypothyroid patients overtreated with L-thyroxine. Ann. Intern. Med., *113*:265–269, 1990.
33. Gimlette, T.M.D.: Thyroid acropachy. Lancet, *1*:22–24, 1960.
34. Volpé, R.: The role of autoimmunity in hypoendocrine and hyperendocrine function: With special emphasis on autoimmune thyroid disease. Ann. Intern. Med., *87*:86–99, 1977.
35. Londei, M., et al.: Epithelial cells expressing aberrant MHC class II determinants can present antigen to cloned human T cells. Nature, *312*:639–641, 1984.
36. Wohlgethan, J.R.: Frozen shoulder in hyperthyroidism. Arthritis Rheum., *30*:936–939, 1987.
37. Miller, J.L., Ismail, F., Waligora, J.K., and Gevers, W.: Modulating influence of D,L-propranolol on triiodothyronine-induced skeletal muscle protein degradation. Endocrinology, *117*:869–871, 1985.
38. Becker, K.L., Ferguson, R.H., and McConahey, W.M.: The connective tissue diseases and symptoms associated with Hashimoto's thyroiditis. N. Engl. J. Med., *268*:277–280, 1963.
39. Miller, F.W., Moore, G.F., Weintraub, B.D., and Steinberg, A.D.: Prevalence of thyroid disease and thyroid function test abnormalities in patients with systemic lupus erythematosus. Arthritis Rheum., *30*:1124–1131, 1987.
40. Cassorla, F.G., et al.: Vasculitis, pulmonary cavitation and anemia during antithyroid drug therapy. Am. J. Dis. Child., *137*:118–122, 1983.
41. Wishart, J., Horowitz, M., Need, A., and Nordin, B.E.C.: Relationship between forearm and vertebral mineral density in postmenopausal women with primary hyperparathyroidism. Arch. Intern. Med., *150*:1329–1331, 1990.
42. Martin, P., Bergmann, P., Gillet, C., et al.: Long-term irreversibility of bone loss after surgery for primary hyperparathyroidism. Arch. Intern. Med., *150*:1495–1497, 1990.
43. Preston, E.T.: Avulsion of both quadriceps tendons in hyperparathyroidism. JAMA, *221*:406–407, 1972.
44. Babini, S.M., Maldonado Cocco, J.A., de la Sota, M., et al.: Tendinous laxity and Jaccoud's Syndrome in patients with systemic lupus erythematosus. Possible role of secondary hyperparathyroidism. J. Rheumatol., *16*:494–498, 1989.
45. Hamilton, E.B.D.: Diseases associated with CPPD deposition disease. Arthritis Rheum., *19*:353–357, 1976.
46. Bilezikian, J.P., et al.: Pseudogout after parathyroidectomy. Lancet, *1*:445–446, 1973.
47. Bywaters, E.G.L., Dixon, A. St. J., and Scott, J.T.: Joint lesions of hyperparathyroidism. Ann. Rheum. Dis., *22*:171–184, 1963.
48. Mallette, L.E., Patten, B.M., and Engel, W.K.: Neuromuscular disease in secondary hyperparathyroidism. Ann. Intern. Med., *82*:474–483, 1975.
49. Patten, B.M., et al.: Neuromuscular disease in primary hyperparathyroidism. Ann. Intern. Med., *80*:182–193, 1974.
50. Frame, B., et al.: Myopathy in primary hyperparathyroidism: Observations in three patients. Ann. Intern. Med., *68*:1023–1027, 1968.
51. Richardson, J.A., et al.: Ischemic ulcerations of skin and necrosis of muscle in azotemic hyperparathyroidism. Ann. Intern. Med., *77*:129–138, 1969.
52. Chaykin, L.B., Frame, B., and Sigler, J.W.: Spondylitis: A clue to hypoparathyroidism. Ann. Intern. Med., *70*:995–1000, 1969.
53. Kruse, K., et al.: Hypocalcemic myopathy in idiopathic hypoparathyroidism. Eur. J. Pediatr., *138*:280–282, 1982.
54. Treatment of Diabetes Mellitus. 9th Ed. Edited by E.P. Joslin, H.F. Root, P. White, and A. Marble. Philadelphia, Lea & Febiger, 1952.
55. Julkunen, H., Heinonen, O.P., and Pyörälä, K.: Hyperostosis of the spine in an adult population: Its relation to hyperglycaemia and obesity. Ann. Rheum. Dis., *30*:605–612, 1971.

56. Locke, S., Lawrence, D.G., and Legg, M.A.: Diabetic amyotrophy. Am. J. Med., *34*:775–785, 1963.
57. Bridgeman, J.E.: Periarthritis of the shoulder and diabetes mellitus. Ann. Rheum. Dis., *31*:69–71, 1972.
58. Lequesne, M., et al.: Increased association of diabetes mellitus with capsulitis of the shoulder and shoulder hand syndrome. Scand. J. Rheumatol., *6*:53–56, 1977.
59. Pastan, R.S., and Cohen, A.S.: The rheumatologic manifestations of diabetes mellitus. Med. Clin. North Am., *62*:829–839, 1978.
60. Sinha, S., Munichoodappa, C.S., and Kozak, G.P.: Neuropathy (Charcot joints) in diabetes mellitus. Medicine, *51*:191–210, 1972.
61. Viljanto, J.A.: Dupuytren's contracture—a review. Semin. Arthritis Rheum., *3*:155–176, 1973.
62. Strom, L.: Trigger finger in diabetes. J. Med. Soc. N.J., *74*:951–954, 1977.
63. Grgic, A., et al.: Joint contracture—common manifestation of childhood diabetes mellitus. J. Pediatr., *88*:584–588, 1976.
64. Campbell, R.R., Hawkins, S.J., Maddison, P.J., and Reckless, J.P.D.: Limited joint mobility in diabetes mellitus. Ann. Rheum. Dis., *44*:93–97, 1985.
65. Rosenbloom, A.L., et al.: Limited joint mobility in childhood diabetes mellitus indicates increased risk for microvascular disease. N. Engl. M. Med., *305*:191–194, 1981.
66. Trapp, R.G., Soler, N.G., and Spencer-Green, G.: Nailfold capillaroscopy in type I diabetes with vasculopathy and limited joint mobility. J. Rheumatol., *13*:917–920, 1986.
67. Hardin, J.G., and Siegal, A.M.: A connective tissue disease complicated by insulin resistance due to receptor antibodies: Report of a case with high titer nuclear ribonucleoprotein antibodies. Arthritis Rheum., *25*:458–463, 1982.
68. Weinstein, P.S., et al.: Insulin resistance due to receptor antibodies: A complication of progressive systemic sclerosis. Arthritis Rheum., *23*:101–105, 1980.
69. Tsokos, G.C., et al.: Lupus nephritis and other autoimmune features in patients with diabetes mellitus due to autoantibody to insulin receptors. Ann. Intern. Med., *102*:176–181, 1985.
70. Askari, A., Vignos, P.J., and Moskowitz, R.W.: Steroid myopathy in connective tissue disease. Am. J. Med., *61*:485–492, 1976.
71. Ebinger, G., Six, R., Bruyland, M., and Somers, G.: Flexion contractures: A forgotten sympton in Addison's disease and hypopituitarism. Lancet, *2*:858, 1986.
72. Kingsley, G.H., and Hickling, P.: Polyarthropathy associated with Cushing's disease. Br. Med. J., *292*;1363, 1986.
73. Asherson, R.A., and Hughes, G.R.V.: Hypoadrenalism, Addison's disease and antiphospholipid antibodies. J. Rheumatol., *18*:1–3, 1991.
74. Plonk, J.W., and Feldman, J.M.: Carcinoid arthropathy. Arch. Intern. Med., *134*:651–654, 1974.
75. Odell, W.D., and Wolfsen, A.R.: Humoral syndromes associated with cancer. Annu. Rev. Med., *29*:379–406, 1978.
76. DuPont, B., et al.: Plasma growth hormone and hypertrophic osteoarthropathy in carcinoma of the bronchus. Acta Med. Scand., *188*:25–30, 1970.
77. Hench, P.S.: The ameliorating effect of pregnancy on chronic atrophic (infectious rheumatoid) arthritis, fibrositis and intermittent hydrarthrosis. Mayo Clin. Proc., *13*:161–167, 1938.
78. Cecere, F.A., and Persellin, R.H.: The interaction of pregnancy and the rheumatic diseases. Clin. Rheum. Dis., *2*:747–768, 1981.
79. Neely, N.T., and Persellin, R.H.: Activity of rheumatoid arthritis during pregnancy. Tex. Med., *73*:59–63, 1977.
80. Kaplan, D.: Fetal wastage in patients with rheumatoid arthritis. J. Rheumatol., *13*:875–877, 1986.
81. Lockshin, M.D. et al.: Antibody to cardiolipin as a predictor of fetal distress or death in pregnant patients with systemic lupus erythematosus. N. Engl. J. Med., *313*:152–156, 1985.
82. Ramsey-Goldman, R., et al.: Anti-SSA antibodies and fetal outcome in maternal systemic lupus erythematosus. Arthritis Rheum., *29*:1269–1273, 1986.
83. Kasinath, S.B., and Katz, A.I.: Delayed maternal lupus after delivery of offspring with congenital heart block. Arch. Intern. Med., *142*:2317, 1982.
84. Provost, T.T., Watson, R., Gammon, W.R., et al.: The neonatal lupus syndrome associated with u1 RNP (nRNP) antibodies. N. Engl. J. Med., *316*:1135–1138, 1987.
85. Lockshin, M.D., Reinitz, E., Druzen, M.L., et al.: Lupus pregnancy, case-control prospective study demonstrating absence of lupus exacerbation during or after pregnancy. Am. J. Med., *77*:893–898, 1984.
86. Mintz, G., and Rodriguez-Alvarez, E.: Systemic lupus erythematosus. Rheum. Clin. North Am., *15*:255–274, 1989.
87. Kaufman, R.L., and Kitridou, R.C.: Pregnancy in mixed connective tissue disease: Comparison with systemic lupus erythematosus. J. Rheumatol., *9*:549–555, 1982.
88. Persellin, R.H.: Inhibitors of inflammatory and immune responses in pregnancy serum. Clin. Rheum. Dis., *7*:769–780, 1981.
89. Schiff, R.I., Mercier, D., and Buckley, R.H.: Inability of gestational hormones to account for the inhibitory effects of pregnancy plasmas on lymphocyte responses in vitro. Cell. Immunol., *20*:69–80, 1975.
90. Hench, P.S.: Potential reversibility of rheumatoid arthritis. Mayo Clin. Proc., *24*:167–178, 1949.
91. Lin, T.M., Halbert, S.P., and Spellacy, W.N.: Measurement of pregnancy-associated plasma proteins during human gestation. J. Clin. Invest., *54*:576–582, 1974.
92. Von Schoultz, B.: A quantitative study of the pregnancy zone protein in the sera of pregnant and puerperal women. Am. J. Obstet. Gynecol., *119*:792–797, 1974.
93. Pekelharing, J.M., Hepp, E., Kamerling, J.P., et al.: Alterations in carbohydrate composition of serum IgG from patients with rheumatoid arthritis and from pregnant women. Ann. Rheum. Dis., *47*:91–95, 1988.
94. Combe, B., Cosso, B., Clot, J., et al.: Human placenta-eluted gammaglobulins in immunomodulating treatment of rheumatoid arthritis. Am. J. Med., *78*:920–928, 1985.
95. Bole, G.G., Friedlander, M.H., and Smith, G.K.: Rheumatic symptoms and serological abnormalities induced by oral contraceptives. Lancet, *1*:323–326, 1969.
96. Tarzy, B.J., et al.: Rheumatic disease, abnormal serology and oral contraceptives. Lancet, *2*:501–502, 1972.
97. Bizzaro, A., et al.: Influence of testosterone therapy on clinical and immunological features of autoimmune diseases associated with Klinefelter's syndrome. J. Clin. Endocrinol. Metab., *64*:32–36, 1987.
98. Cutolo, M., Balleari, E., and Guisti, M.: Androgen replacement therapy in male patients with rheumatoid arthritis. Arthritis Rheum., *34*:1–5, 1991.
99. Ansar Ahmed, S., Penhale, W.J., and Talal, N.: Sex hormones, immune responses, and autoimmune diseases. Mechanisms of sex hormone action. Am. J. Pathol., *12*:531–551, 1985.
100. Lahita, R.G., et al.: Abnormal estrogen and androgen metabolism in the human with systemic lupus erythematosus. Am. J. Kidney Dis., *2*:206–211, 1982.
101. Sarvetnick, N., and Fox, H.S.: Interferon-gamma and the sexual dimorphism of autoimmunity. Mol. Biol. Med., *7*:323–331, 1990.

102. Carr, D.J.J., and Blalock, J.E.: From the neuroendocrinology of lymphocytes toward a molecular basis of the network theory. Horm. Res., *31*:76–80, 1989.
103. Bateman, A., Singh, A., Kral, T., and Solomon, S.: The immune-hypothalamic-pituitary-adrenal axis. Endocr. Rev., *10*:92–112, 1989.
104. Sternberg, E.M., Hill, J.M., Chrousos, G.P., et al.: Inflammatory mediator-induced hypothalamic-pituitary-adrenal axis activation is defective in streptococcal cell wall arthritis-susceptible Lewis rats. Proc. Natl. Acad. Sci. U.S.A., *86*:2374–2378, 1989.
105. Pereira da Silva, J.A., and Carmo-Fonseca, M.: Peptide containing nerves in human synovium: Immunohistochemical evidence for decreased innervation in rheumatoid arthritis. J. Rheumatol., *17*:1592–1599, 1990.
106. Lotz, M., Carson, D.A., and Vaughan, J.H.: Substance P activation of rheumatoid synoviocytes: Neural pathway in pathogenesis of arthritis. Science, *235*:893–895, 1987.

SECTION XI

Infectious Arthritis

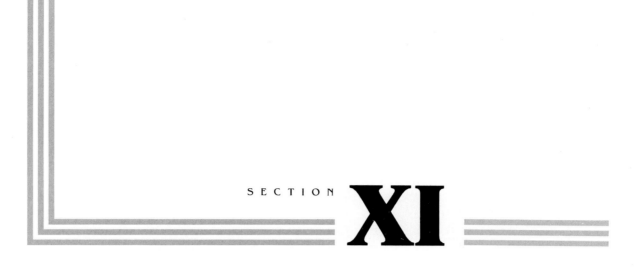

115

Principles of Diagnosis and Treatment of Bone and Joint Infections

FRANK R. SCHMID

Bone and joint infections are curable if antimicrobial drugs active against the invading microorganisms are given early, and if retained necrotic material is drained. Application of these principles eradicates the infectious inflammatory response and, if initiated in a normal host before irreversible tissue damage has occurred, complete restoration of joint function can be expected (Table 115-1).

PATHOGENESIS OF BONE AND JOINT INFECTIONS

SEPTIC ARTHRITIS, BURSITIS, AND TENDINITIS

Except in cases of direct penetration by instrumentation or trauma,[1,2] invasion of the joint cavity by microorganisms occurs most often from the blood and usually reflects the culmination of a series of successive failures of the host's elaborate defense mechanisms. A primary focus of infection is first established at a portal of entry, usually remote from the joint. Microorganisms escaping from this beachhead enter the circulation, where they must resist serum bactericidal activity,[3] as well as elude an active reticuloendothelial system in sufficient numbers and for an adequate time to allow colonization of synovial tissue or juxta-articular bone. Finally, the joint cavity itself must be breeched from this periarticular location to permit the full-blown expression of acute septic arthritis. In normal circumstances, therefore, the joint is a privileged sanctuary. For each example of overt sepsis, countless instances of failure to infect must occur, considering the low incidence of infectious arthritis in comparison with the much higher incidence of systemic infectious diseases and bacteremia.[4]

Thus, the likelihood of infectious arthritis is greater if host resistance is impaired by genetic defects[5,6] or by prior disease[7,8] or by treatment with drugs that interfere with defense mechanisms, such as corticosteroids or immunosuppressive agents.[9–11] Although sepsis may develop in normal joints, particularly with gonococcal and staphylococcal infections, previous damage by trauma or by another arthritic disease predisposes a joint to infection.[9,12–15] The characteristic monoarticular presentation of septic arthritis suggests that local factors, even within an apparently "normal" joint, favor its colonization over that of other joints equally traversed by the same blood-borne agent.

As microorganisms penetrate the joint cavity, a rapid series of events occurs. Although studies of the inflammatory process in septic arthritis are sparse,[16] the process is similar to that produced by other phlogistic stimuli. The synovial microvasculature dilates, subsynovial tissue becomes edematous, and the volume of synovial fluid increases dramatically with a rise in intra-articular pressure.[17,18] Marked elevation of pressure induces tamponade of subsynovial vessels. Such microvascular injury may cause intravascular thrombosis and ischemia, leading to microabscess formation and, in adjacent bone, ischemia and foci of avascular necrosis.[19] Concentrations of macromolecules, such as immunoglobulins and complement proteins in joint fluid, approach those in plasma.[20]

Because hematogenous dissemination usually occurs at least several days after the infection has become established at a primary site, lymphocyte activation and antibody production against the microorganisms ordinarily will have begun. Thus, immune complexes can form between the antibody and the microorganism or its antigenic fragments, some of which may have become fixed within the cartilage matrix; this both favors

TABLE 115–1. GUIDELINES FOR MANAGEMENT OF A PATIENT WITH INFECTIOUS ARTHRITIS

INITIAL EVALUATION

Objective: Develop support for diagnosis of infectious arthritis

1. Historical and physical data
   —Primary site of infection
   —Septicemia: fever, chills, skin rash, polyarthralgia, other metastatic sites of infection
   —Host defense impairment
   —Pre-existing joint damage
2. Initial joint fluid examination
   —Joint fluid analysis: order of priority if amount of joint fluid is limited; smear and culture (or antigen detection); microscopy of wet-mount preparation, cell count, glucose measurement
3. Joint visualization
   —Radiographs of affected and contralateral joint
   —Radioisotope joint scan, especially for deep-seated joints

INITIAL THERAPEUTIC DECISIONS

Objective: Selection of antibiotic for the most probable infecting microorganism and initiation of joint drainage

1. Identification of suspected microorganism
   —Clinical clues: age, geography, environment, primary site of infection
   —Bacteriologic smear of joint fluid
2. Selection of antibiotic(s)
   —Route for administration: intravenous or intramuscular, usually
   —Dosage
3. Institution of joint drainage
   —Needle aspiration and lavage
   —Arthrotomy: reserved initially for such special circumstances as infancy, some deep-seated joint infections, or grossly contaminated wounds
4. Joint immobilization, analgesia

REAPPRAISAL: 27–72 HOURS

Objective: Reassessment of initial antibiotic choice and decision concerning joint drainage

1. Confirmation of antibiotic choice
   —Culture report and sensitivity of invading microorganism to antibiotic drugs
   —Review of dosage requirements: bacterial assay of synovial fluid if adequacy of drug levels in doubt
2. Repeat joint drainage, if indicated.
3. Monitoring treatment response
   —Systemic findings and primary site of infection
   —Infected joint(s): appearance and size; synovial fluid appearance, volume, white blood cell count, glucose, culture

REAPPRAISAL: 5–8 DAYS

Objective: Assessment of efficacy of joint drainage and antibiotic treatment

1. Assessment of frequency and type of joint drainage
   —Review clinical and laboratory data from monitoring system
   —Criteria for arthrotomy/arthroscopy: microorganism, treatment response, radiographic changes
2. Problems associated with antibiotic usage
   —Inability to detect an invading microorganism
   —Hypersensitivity to initial drug choice
   —Decision for duration and dosage: microorganism, treatment response
   —Postinfectious synovitis
3. Passive or active range-of-motion exercises

REAPPRAISAL: 2–8 WEEKS

Objective: Planning out-patient care

1. Need for continued antibiotic use: route, dosage, and duration
2. Joint assessment
   —Sequential monitoring to maximal improvement
   —Radiologic comparison with initial films
   —Joint use and weight-bearing

REAPPRAISAL: 3–6 MONTHS OR LONGER

Objective: Planning corrective surgical procedure or supportive measures for patients with incomplete restoration of joint function or structure

1. Joint assessment
   —Evaluation of residual inflammation, motion, and structural integrity of joint
   —Radiologic comparison with previous films
2. Decision for surgical reconstruction

its destruction and acts as a reservoir to prolong the inflammation of the entire joint.[21] These complexes can induce such complement-mediated events in the joint as histamine release, chemotaxis, and phagocytosis.[18,22] Bacterial products alone, even in the absence of antibody, can trigger complement activation through the alternate pathway.[23]

A major difference between an infection within the joint space and one dispersed throughout the fibrillar scaffolding of connective tissue, such as cellulitis, is the slower rate of exchange of its fluid contents with the surrounding vascular and lymphatic spaces. Solutes in synovial fluid must diffuse across the synovial lining, often tamponaded by increased pressure,[24] in contrast to the rapid access of molecules in interstitial tissues to and from nearby capillary networks. Diffusion of solutes between joint fluid and blood, although slowed, finally reaches equilibrium, but only after several hours.[25] Thus, the diminished effectiveness of antibiotics against bacteria in a closed-space infection is not because of suboptimal local concentrations of the drug. Rather, the slowed diffusion from the joint of metabolic by-products of the infection retards bacterial cell growth.[26–31] *Bacteria remain dormant under these conditions and survive in the presence of otherwise bactericidal drug concentrations.* For this reason, the time-honored principle of relief of pressure and removal of infected contents by drainage of pus is a critical component of an effective therapeutic program.

Other synovial tissues, such as bursae and tendon sheaths, share the same pathogenetic mechanism for infection as described for the joint synovium with a few exceptions. Direct penetration of microorganisms from the skin is a more common means of infection of superficial sacs, such as the olecranon and prepatellar bursae.[32,33] Also, because bursae lack the restraining capsule of the joint, intrabursal fluids diffuse easily into surrounding connective tissues, often presenting as cellulitis.

Structures at risk for injury by the infectious process are those lying within the confines of the synovial-lined capsule or sheath, although surrounding soft tissues outside this space are sometimes involved in rare instances of rupture or sinus formation. Damage to the synovium of a bursa is reversible, but tendons within synovial sheaths are vulnerable to the effects of the inflammatory process and can rupture. Even more vulnerable is articular cartilage. Chondrolysis is readily demonstrated in the presence of pus,[16,24,34–36] and destroyed hyaline cartilage cannot be totally or effectively replaced. These anatomic considerations influence the need for drainage, which is obviously even more critical for joints and tendons than for bursae.

OSTEOMYELITIS

Bone becomes infected from the blood or from a site of contiguous infection. Hematogenous osteomyelitis most often involves rapidly growing bone, characteristically the metaphysis of long bones in children.[37,38] In adults, the vertebrae are more commonly involved.[39] Osteomyelitis from an adjacent area of infection may result from trauma, open wounds, compound fractures, or an operative infection.[39,40] In recent years, problems relative to infection of joint prostheses have been of great importance.[41]

The acquisition and spread of such infections are tied closely to differences in the microvascular anatomic structures of growing and of mature bone[39] (Fig. 115-1). Between the age of 1 year and puberty, osteomyelitis usually starts in the metaphyseal sinusoidal vein. This site is favored because the afferent loop of the metaphyseal capillary lacks phagocytic lining cells and the efferent loops are frequently multiple, with a broad diameter in which blood flow becomes slow and more turbulent. Furthermore, the capillary loops adjacent to the epiphyseal growth plate are nonanastomotic, so necrosis can result from obstruction caused by microbial emboli and vascular thrombosis.[16] The metaphyseal infection does not cross the epiphyseal growth plate in children, but spreads laterally, perforating the cortex and lifting the loose periosteum to cause a subperiosteal abscess (route 4, Fig. 115-1). In some joints, such as the hip and shoulder, the synovial reflection reaches beyond the epiphyseal growth plate, so infection penetrates directly into the joint through cortical bone (route 1, Fig. 115-1). In the infant less than a year old, capillaries perforate the growth plate, and the infection may thereby spread into the epiphysis and, by further extension, into the joint, with destruction of the epiphyseal growth center (route 3, Fig. 115-1). An analogous situation can occur in the adult.[42] After resorption of the growth cartilage, anastomoses form between the metaphyseal and the epiphyseal blood vessels and allow the spread of infection from the epiphyseal portion of bone to the joint cavity (route 2, Fig. 115-1).

Once microorganisms have colonized the perivascular bone, edema, cellular infiltration, and accumulation of products of inflammation develop in much the same manner as in septic arthritis and contribute to the necrotic breakdown of bone trabeculae and loss of matrix and mineral. The part played by vascular obstruction is even more important in bone infection. Large segments of bone devoid of blood supply can separate to form sequestra. In cross section, the infected bone shows a core of necrosis with fibrin deposits and massive polymorphonuclear cell infiltration surrounded by an area with granulation tissue containing lymphocytes and plasma cells, and finally an outer layer of fibrous tissue in which new bone is formed. When the infection ruptures beneath the periosteum, more common in children than in adults, the periosteum overgrows to form an involucrum. Cortical destruction can predispose such a patient to fractures.[39]

The vertebral body is the most common site of hematogenous osteomyelitis in the adult. This infection spreads readily along the adjacent ligaments by means of freely anastomosing venous channels, thus commonly involving two adjacent vertebral bodies. The disc between each vertebra loses its vascular supply early in life, but it can be infected by direct extension from the vertebral abscess. The infection can also extend centrally into the spinal canal under the dura mater, with resulting spinal cord compression, or externally to paraspinal soft tissues. In the cervical region, osteomyelitis can cause a retropharyngeal abscess or mediastinitis; in the thoracic spine, mediastinitis, empyema, or pericarditis; and in the lumbar spine, peritonitis or an abscess

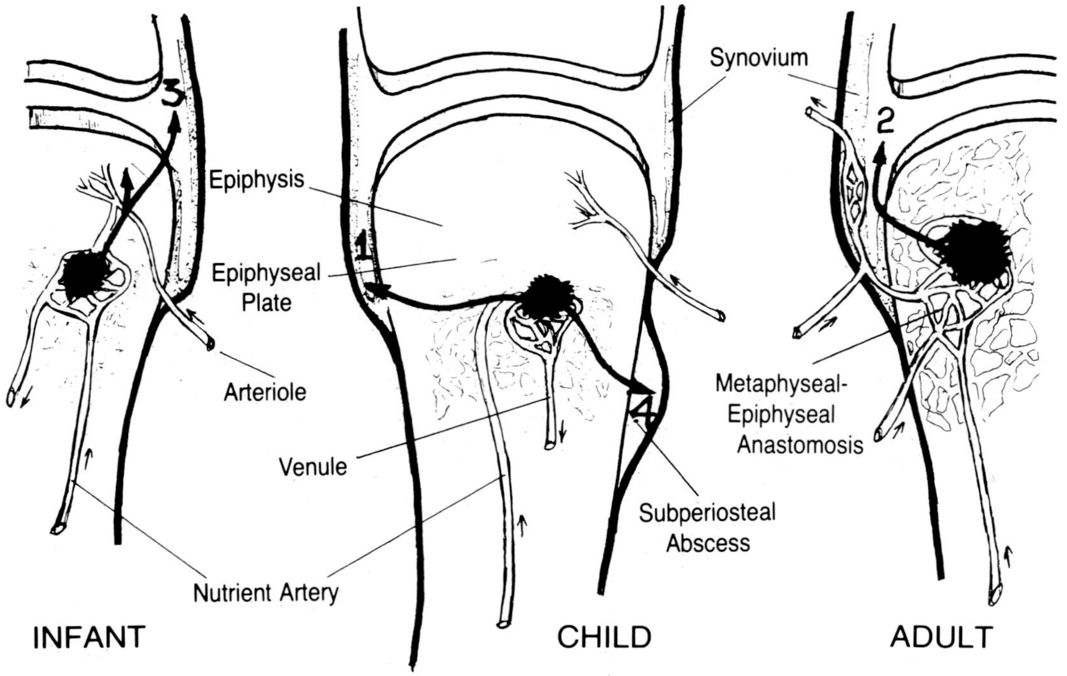

FIGURE 115–1. Schematic representation of the vascular supply to the bone and joint in the infant, the child, and the adult. Blood-borne microbial emboli reach the metaphysis where conditions favor their lodgment. The bone abscess that forms can spread in several directions, depending on the age of the patient. In children older than1 year, the epiphyseal growth plate blocks extension of the infection, so the abscess penetrates laterally to the subperiosteum (route 4) or to the joint, in the case of the shoulder, in which the synovial reflection extends beyond the epiphysis to the metaphysis (route 1). In the infant, small capillaries cross the epiphyseal growth plate and thus permit extension of the infection to the epiphysis and subsequently to the joint (route 3). In the adult, osteomyelitis can spread by the anastomotic metaphyseal-epiphyseal vessels to the subperiosteum and then to the joint (route 2). Adapted from Waldvogel, F.A., Medoff, G., and Schwartz, M.[39] and from Atcheson, S.G. and Ward, J.R.[42]

beneath the diaphragm or along fascial planes of the iliopsoas muscle.

An infection established in any soft tissue or viscus may spread directly to adjacent bone. The source may be exogenous, as in sepsis introduced into a postsurgical or post-traumatic wound, or it may be an already infected neighboring tissue, such as a nasal sinus, tooth, or abdominal organ. The propensity for bone to become infected in these instances appears to be enhanced by concomitant arterial disease. In diabetic feet or in the extremities of patients with rheumatoid vasculitis, an infection in necrotic tissue may involve the underlying bone.[39]

MICROORGANISMS RESPONSIBLE FOR BONE AND JOINT INFECTIONS

Almost any microorganism can cause infectious arthritis, but most infections are caused by a few common agents (Table 115-2). In children who have a high incidence of pyogenic arthritis,[43] Staphylococcus aureus and other cocci are often found, but Haemophilus influenzae is most frequent in the younger child,[37,44,45] probably as a result of an immature immune system. In those under age 2, the absence of antibody has been linked to vulnerability to H. influenzae. Even gonococcal arthritis, although rare, occurs in children.[46] In adults, gonococci and staphylococci cause the majority of joint infections.[5,8,47–49] In endemic areas, infection by Borrelia burgdorferi, the causative agent of Lyme disease, presents a common diagnostic challenge (see Chapter 120).[50,51]

Gram-positive cocci are also the most frequent invaders of bone in hematogenous osteomyelitis (Table 115-2). Gram-negative bacilli are next, but Neisseria species are rare. In some settings, as in osteomyelitis in heroin addicts, infection with Pseudomonas aeruginosa or Serratia species stands out,[52] in patients with sickle cell disease, Salmonella species are prominent;[39,53] and in the neonate, group B streptococci.[54] Although fungi and mycobacteria are only occasionally the cause of musculoskeletal infections (see Chapter 118), they have a propensity to localize in bone. Diagnosis is especially

TABLE 115–2. ESTIMATE OF THE INCIDENCE OF MICROORGANISMS COMMONLY RESPONSIBLE FOR ACUTE PYOGENIC ARTHRITIS AND OSTEOMYELITIS

	SEPTIC ARTHRITIS		HEMATOGENOUS OSTEOMYELITIS	
MICROORGANISM	Adults (%)	Children* (%)	Adults (%)	Children* (%)
Gram-positive cocci				
Staphylococcus aureus	35	27	65	75
Streptococcus pyogenes, S. pneumoniae, viridans-group streptococci	10	16	10	15
Gram-negative cocci				
Neisseria gonorrhoeae and meningitidis	50	8	—	—
Haemophilus influenzae†	<1	40	—	5
Gram-negative bacilli				
Escherichia coli, Salmonella sp., Pseudomonas, etc.	5	9	20	5
Mycobacteria, fungi	<1	<1	<5	<1

* Data of Fink, C.W., and Nelson, J.D.[37]

† H. influenzae are actually coccobacilli, but are listed under "cocci" because they are frequently mistaken on smears for cocci.

difficult unless the bone lesion can be aspirated and the material from the lesion cultured. These microorganisms should always be considered whenever routine cultures are sterile. Occasionally, infection may be caused by several microorganisms, as, for example, septic arthritis of the hip after perforation of an abdominal organ,[2] or osteomyelitis from a contiguous infection. Both aerobic and anaerobic bacteria may be present in a polymicrobial infection.[55,56]

The microorganisms that usually infect bone and joint tissues are not the most common causes of clinical septicemia. Gram-negative bacilli, other than Haemophilus species, are common causes of septicemia, but they invade osseous or synovial tissue usually only when the tissue has suffered previous damage,[7,57] or when the host has become immunocompromised. Thus, the staphylococcus and other cocci may thus have a special affinity for bone and synovial structures.

MICROBE-HOST INTERACTION

Hematogenous infections of bones and joints almost always occur after the host has had sufficient time to mount an immune response. As part of that response, committed lymphocytes and plasma cells respond to the various products made by the infecting microbial agents or to portions of its structure.[58] Immune complexes that form between these antigens and specific antibody or human cells that are cytolytic for antibody-coated or other target tissues can induce inflammation even in the absence of viable microorganisms. Furthermore, host tissues that cross-react with microbial antigens may also participate in this response. Thus, a pathogenic spectrum varying, on the one hand, from an inflammatory process generated mainly by virulence factors of the actively metabolizing microbe, to sterile inflammation generated by the host's immune system, on the other hand, may account to varying degrees for the signs of inflammation seen in different patients infected by the same agent or seen at various times during the course of the disease in a single patient[18] (Fig. 115-2).

Well-known examples of inflammation associated with immune complexes are found in patients with the disseminated gonococcal syndrome.[59] (see Chapter 117), with hepatitis[60] and rubella[61] virus infections (see Chapter 119), and Lyme disease[62] (see Chapter 120). In each instance, viable bacteria, viruses, and spirochetes have been cultured from the inflamed joint, and im-

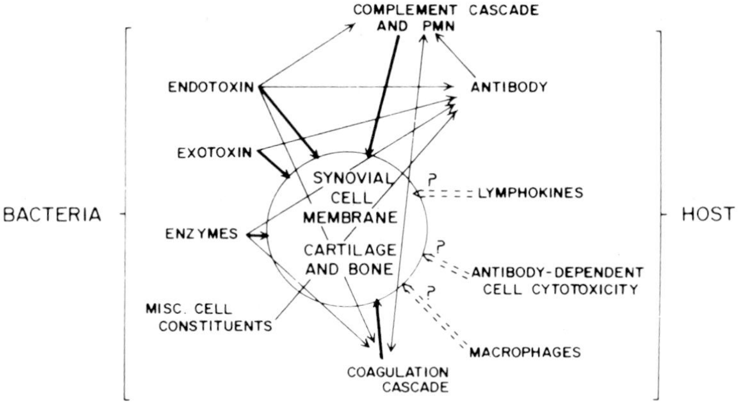

FIGURE 115–2. Interaction of bacterial and host factors in the inflammatory process of septic arthritis. A thick arrow indicates a final and direct pathway of tissue damage; a thin arrow represents the interaction of one component with another leading to induction of synovial inflammation; and an interrupted arrow signifies a possible, but insufficiently documented, host effect. PMN = Polymorphonuclear leukocytes. From Tesar, J.T., and Dietz, F.[18]

mune complexes have been detected in the plasma or joint fluid. When both are present at the same time, the relative contribution of either to the inflammation cannot be determined. When cultures of synovial fluid or tissue are sterile, the cause of the inflammation may be attributed to the host's immune response. Yet even in such patients, special culture techniques may be necessary to uncover the presence of a viable agent. For example, spirochetes were recovered from the skin and joints of patients with Lyme disease only after a long search,[50] and rubella virus was "rescued" from the peripheral blood lymphocytes of an arthritic patient who had received live rubella vaccine 2 years earlier.[63] The implications of these observations for therapy are discussed later in the section of this chapter on postinfectious synovitis.

A unique illustration of the effects of both infectious and noninfectious inflammation in the same patient may be the development of sterile, so-called *sympathetic* effusions in a bursa or joint adjacent to a primary site of septic arthritis or osteomyelitis. No explanation is known for these effusions, but it is assumed to be the result of inflammatory mediators that are transported from the infected region to the nearby sac.

A few observations have been made about the immune response in osteomyelitis. Antibodies to a staphylococcal cell-wall constituent, teichoic acid, have been found mainly in the serum of patients with bone infections.[64] Rheumatoid factors develop, but less commonly in staphylococcal osteomyelitis than in staphylococcal endocarditis.[65] The possible relevance of these serologic findings to the pathogenesis of the bone disease is not known.

The pathogenesis of reactive arthritis, that is sterile inflammation in the joints of patients with infectious involvement at extraarticular sites, is even more elusive. Examples are streptococcal pharyngitis in patients with rheumatic fever (see Chapter 79), enteritis resulting from Salmonella, Shigella, or Yersinia species, urethritis resulting from Mycoplasma agents in patients with Reiter's syndrome (see Chapter 60), or bowel lesions related to parasitic infections,[66] and to bacterial residues in patients with Whipple's disease (see Chapter 62). The type of immune or other response that induces the arthritis in these cases is not known. Pathogenetic immune complexes either have not been found or, if found, do not correlate with the disease process. CD4 T-helper cells are likely to be of less importance because AIDS patients with diminished numbers of these cells develop Reiter's syndrome and psoriatic arthritis.[67] In some cases, success attends eradication of the triggering infecting agent by administration of appropriate drugs, although most often this approach fails to control the arthritis.

CLINICAL PRESENTATIONS

Infectious arthritis may become manifest in a variety of ways, both typical and atypical.

TYPICAL PRESENTATION

Pyogenic arthritis affecting single or, less commonly, two or more joints is usually of acute onset.[7,8,37] A migratory polyarthritis may precede this phase, especially in gonococcal and meningococcal arthritis.[68–71] Large joints, such as the knee and hip, are involved most often, but articular structures of any size or location, including the sacroiliac and spinal joints, may be affected. The infected joint is typically warm, painful, and distended with fluid. Because bacterial entry into a joint is most often hematogenous, the patient may have fever with chills.[48] Signs and symptoms of a primary infection should be sought. Careful examination may reveal pneumonia as a source of pneumococci or a carbuncle as a source of staphylococci. A history of urethritis, pharyngitis, or prostatitis suggesting gonococcal infections might be obtained. In staphylococcal or streptococcal joint disease, and less often in gram-negative bacillary arthritides, a primary site of infection may not be found, however.[7]

ATYPICAL PRESENTATIONS

Unfortunately, septic arthritis may present in an atypical fashion. In a joint damaged by prior disease, superimposed infection may not be obvious because the new process may become "lost" among other painful, chronically swollen joints.[9,14] Careful questioning usually reveals that the infected joint has become more symptomatic than it was before, however. Some elderly patients, or those under treatment with immunosuppressive or corticosteroid drugs, are more vulnerable to superimposed infection and may show less evidence of inflammation than other patients. A wide range of rheumatic diseases develop in patients with AIDS, including septic arthritis, osteomyelitis, and pyomyositis.[72] Some locations may be overlooked, such as a popliteal cyst,[73] the sternoclavicular or sternomanubrial joints,[52,74] or the hip joints.[75] Infected superficial bursae such as the prepatellar and olecranon bursae are sometimes mistaken for the adjacent knee and elbow joints, respectively.[2,33,76]

Infection of the deeply situated axial joints of the body, such as the hip, shoulder, pubic, and sacroiliac joints, can present major difficulties in diagnosis and treatment because evidence of inflammation may be masked, or, if present, may be ascribed to noninfectious causes until the process is far advanced.[75,77–80] This situation is of particular concern in the evaluation of acute shoulder pain. Delay in diagnosis may result in severe joint destruction and loss of motion.[77]

JOINT INFECTIONS IN CHILDREN

Septic arthritis most often resulting from Staphylococcus aureus, group B streptococci and gram-negative bacilli, in neonates 1 to 28 days of age may induce signs and symptoms of septicemia, such as lethargy, fever, tachycardia, and hypotension. Decreased spontaneous movement of the involved extremity, even in the absence of pain and swelling, helps to locate the infection. Multiple joints may be involved. Although bacteria can gain access into the joint directly by lodging in subsynovial vessels, more commonly they do so from a region of adjacent osteomyelitis (see route 3, Fig. 115–1). Predisposing factors are a low birth weight and perinatal complications that necessitate instrumentation, such as fetal monitoring or exchange transfusions.[37,54,81]

In older children, the clinical appearance of septic arthritis more closely parallels that observed in adults.

Diagnostic problems are magnified in children, especially those with an infection of the hip. This joint is affected more often than any other except the knee, particularly in children below the age of 6 months.[43] Unless treatment is started promptly, irreversible destruction can occur within days.[82,83,84] Increased intraarticular pressure and purulent fluids destroy cartilage and bone. Hematogenous dissemination of microorganisms from a primary portal of entry to the joint or adjacent bone is usual, and prior joint disease or associated illness predisposes the child to infection in the hip, just as in other joints.[85] Direct penetration may occur as a complication of femoral venipuncture,[86] or it may result from infection extending from an abdominal abscess into the retroperitoneal space near the iliopsoas muscle.[2]

Symptoms of sepsis in the hip include pain in the groin, lateral upper thigh, or buttocks. Referred pain along the obturator nerve to the knee is common.[87] The thigh is usually held in flexion, adduction, and internal rotation, and pain permits only a few degrees of motion. In adults, external signs of inflammation are rare, but in children, the massive increase in the volume of joint fluid may distend the capsule, obliterating the inguinal crease and causing generalized edema of the thigh. Marked tenderness may be elicited by local pressure.

INFECTIONS OF BONE

Hematogenous osteomyelitis commonly affects rapidly growing bones in children, frequently the metaphysis of the tibia or the femur. In a large series, more than 80% of the cases were found in children below age 10, and almost 60% below age 5.[37] In recent years, the prevalence of bone infections in adults has increased, especially in the vertebral bodies.[39]

Most patients have fever, with or without chills, constitutional symptoms such as weight loss and fatigue, and symptoms referable to the local site of bony involvement. Thus, osteomyelitis of the long bones of the lower extremity may be associated with local pain, sometimes accompanied by swelling and erythema, a limp, or in a young child, refusal to walk. Vertebral osteomyelitis may be associated with back pain and local tenderness, spasm of paraspinal or psoas muscles, and limitation of motion. Pelvic osteomyelitis may cause abdominal pain or pain referred to the hip or lower extremities.[88] Findings in patients with spinal or pelvic osteomyelitis may be so subtle that infection in these regions should be considered in any individual who only has systemic signs of inflammation, such as a fever of unknown origin.[89] In such patients, a positive blood culture increases the likelihood of deep-seated osteomyelitis. Sepsis of the sacroiliac joint should be considered in the differential diagnosis of low-back or hip pain, particularly when unilateral sacroiliac disease is noted on a radiograph or scintiphotograph.[90,91]

Chronic recurrent multifocal osteomyelitis is an uncommon, apparently noninfectious bony lesion of children, more common in girls than boys, that needs to be differentiated from bacterial osteomyelitis, which can occasionally also be multifocal. An obscure relationship exists with lesions of the skin (psoriasis, pustulosis palmaris plantaris, acne fulminans, and possibly histiocytosis). Laboratory tests show only an elevated sedimentation rate. Chronic inflammation, occasionally with granulomas, marks the histopathology. The disease is self-limited.[92,93]

INFECTED JOINT PROSTHESES

Infection following a joint implant is a serious complication. Rates of infection initially were greater than 10%, but with extensive experience, they have dropped to only a few percent in most large centers.[41] Although most infections occur during the early postoperative months, some appear several years later.[94] Rheumatoid patients are predisposed to this risk. They had an infection rate of 2.2% at one large institution, compared to an overall rate of 1.6%; male rheumatoid patients had a higher rate (4.0%) than females (1.7%).[95]

In the postoperative period, systemic signs such as fever may be falsely attributed to other complications such as pneumonia or a urinary tract infection. Persistent joint pain may be the only finding that suggests the real cause of the problem. Its character helps to distinguish mechanical loosening of the prosthesis from infection. With infection, pain is generally dull, is present also at night, is described as deep gnawing or throbbing, and may diminish after the use of antibiotics. Pain with loosening is related to motion or weight-bearing, and may be accentuated by sharp movement.[94] If purulent material drains from the wound, and if the infection does not respond to antibiotics, a deep infection around the prosthesis rather than a superficial wound infection should be considered, and exploration of the operative site may be required. Staphylococcus aureus or S. epidermidis are the most common causes of an infected joint prosthesis; gram-negative bacilli and anaerobic and other bacteria are less common.[41,56,94] Anaerobic organisms have fastidious growth requirements, and their presence must be looked for carefully by appropriate culture techniques when the routine cultures are sterile and the index of suspicion for infection is high.[41]

DIAGNOSTIC STUDIES

DIFFERENTIAL DIAGNOSIS OF SEPTIC ARTHRITIS

Other acute arthritic disorders, such as gout, pseudogout, palindromic rheumatism, rheumatic fever, trauma, and the oligoarticular syndromes associated with the spondyloarthropathies or with juvenile rheumatoid arthritis (RA), may be confused with infectious arthritis. Constitutional symptoms, such as high fever or chills and marked leukocytosis, are uncommon in these conditions. Even when a noninfectious form of arthritis is actually present, an added infectious process must be excluded by bacteriologic examination of synovial fluid. An unusual but distressing example is infection superimposed on crystal-induced synovitis. The previous deposition of urate or calcium pyrophosphate crystals in the joint predisposes the patient to sepsis.[12,13,15,96] Subsequent cartilage breakdown by septic inflammation may even release pre-existing crystal deposits, a phenomenon aptly termed "enzymatic strip mining"[15,97] (see Chapter 107). Patients with RA have a high incidence of joint infection, usually due to staphylococci.[9,14] Therefore, suspicion of joint sepsis should be heightened whenever a primary site of infection or evidence of septicemia is recognized in any arthritic patient.

DIFFERENTIAL DIAGNOSIS OF BONE INFECTION

Infections of the vertebral body, disc, or sacroiliac joint may be overlooked because symptoms and signs can mimic other conditions, such as post-traumatic thinning of a disc, congenital absence of a disc, osteochondritis of a disc, metastatic carcinoma, Paget's disease, or Charcot arthropathy.[39] Ankylosing spondylitis or the spondyloarthropathy associated with Reiter's disease, psoriasis, or bowel disease may present problems in the differential diagnosis of sacroiliac joint disease; these conditions usually affect both sacroiliac joints, however, whereas infection is almost always unilateral.[78] Correct diagnosis may require identification or exclusion of an infecting microorganism by aspiration under fluoroscopic control or rarely by surgical exploration.[98,99]

GENERAL STUDIES

A complete medical history and physical examination are essential, with special attention to the portals of entry for infection: skin, nasal passages, including sinuses and the middle ear, lungs, rectum, urethra, and pelvis.

Initial studies in a patient with acute septic arthritis or hematogenous osteomyelitis may reveal leukocytosis with an increased percentage of immature leukocytes, but the absence of leukocytosis does not rule out sepsis, particularly in a debilitated individual. Anemia is not likely to be present early, unless an underlying disease antedates the infectious process. The erythrocyte sedimentation rate and other acute-phase reactants, such as C-reactive protein and the serum precursor of amyloid protein AA (SAA),[100] are elevated both in infectious arthritis and in noninfectious inflammatory states. That elevated C-reactive protein levels failed to identify infection in patients with systemic lupus erythematosus dashed a hope raised by an earlier study.[101,102] The form of α_1-acid glycoprotein that reacts with concanavalin A can be measured in the serum and may offer real promise in deciding whether an infection has occurred, however. Lupus patients who became infected had significantly higher values for this acute-phase reactant than did noninfected lupus patients.[103] Serum calcium, phosphorus, and alkaline phosphatase levels are usually normal in osteomyelitis. At least two blood cultures for aerobic and anaerobic organisms should be taken within the first several hours in every suspected case of pyogenic arthritis or osteomyelitis. A single positive blood culture may be difficult to interpret because of possible contamination during collection. Two blood cultures containing the same organism virtually rule out contamination. Cultures should also be made of any exudate or secretion at a suspected portal of entry.

RADIOLOGIC EXAMINATION

Several weeks are usually needed before cartilaginous or bony abnormalities can be detected in previously normal bone or joints. In septic arthritis, rarefaction of subchondral bone develops first, followed by erosion of juxta-articular bone and narrowing of the joint space[104] resulting from destruction of articular cartilage (Fig. 115-3). When superimposed on a diseased joint, changes caused by infection may be indistinguishable from those already present. The decalcification resulting from infection is particularly troublesome in children, in whom skeletal immaturity already makes significant bony structures radiolucent.

In osteomyelitis, bone is destroyed locally, but this change does not become visible for 2 to 3 weeks when 30 to 50% of bone mineral has been removed. New bone also forms, but about a month is required for the deposition of mineral to be sufficient to be detected. Thus, areas of lysis and increased bone density appear at about the same time radiographically, although soft-tissue swelling and periosteal elevation may be seen earlier. For the same reason, radiologic evidence of healing of osteomyelitis also lags behind clinical improvement and actual bone reconstruction.[39]

Within a few weeks of the onset of vertebral disc or bone infection, thinning of the involved disc and destruction of vertebral bone may occur. Tomograms may more clearly outline lesions that are obscure on standard films (Fig. 115-4). Lesions may heal by fusion. Most infections of the sacroiliac joint are unilateral, in contradistinction to bilateral involvement by the sterile spondylitic syndromes.

In deep-seated joints, such as the hip, soft-tissue changes resulting from joint-space distension may be helpful in diagnosis. The *obturator sign*, a widening and curving of the border of the obturator internus tendon adjacent to the capsule of the hip joint, may be helpful if positive. A radiolucent *air sign* is an unusual finding in lesions produced by some gas-forming microorganisms. This sign was noted in the disc space of a patient with vertebral osteomyelitis and in joints of patients with septic arthritis resulting from Clostridium per-

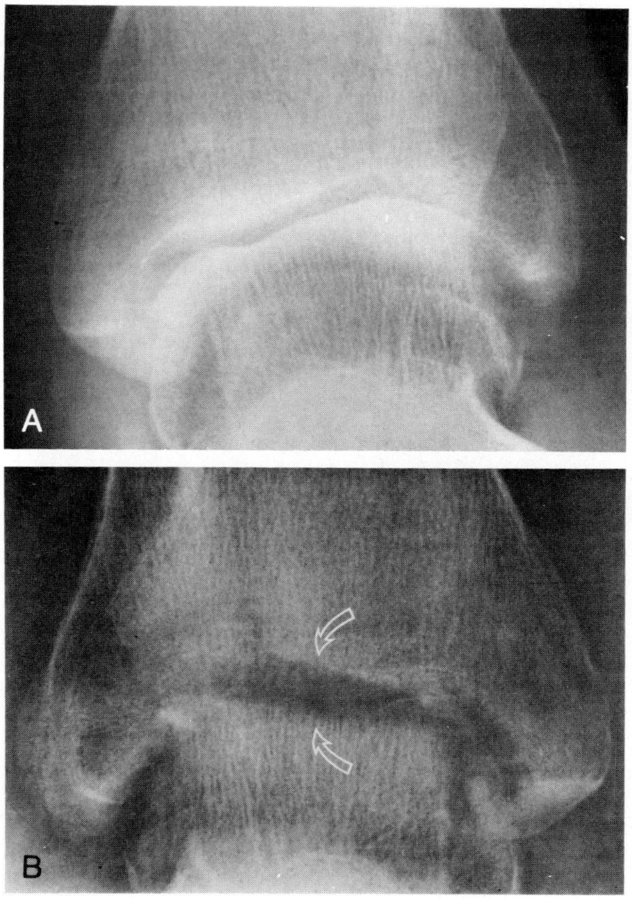

FIGURE 115–3. *A,* Ankle joint of a 36-year-old man 3 weeks after it was injected for pain. Pseudomonas aeruginosa grew from the culture of synovial fluid. The joint space is normal and the white line of the articular cortical margin is normal. *B,* Same ankle joint 5 weeks later. The white line of the articular margin (*open arrows*) is destroyed on both sides of the joint. Underlying bone trabeculae are bare and irregularly destroyed, causing the fuzzy appearance of the bone margins. From Hendrix, R.W., and Fisher, M.R.[104]

fringens,[105,106] Streptococcus milleri, anaerobic bacteria, and gram-negative bacilli.[107]

Although evidence of sepsis may not be evident, films taken early document the extent of prior damage and permit an estimate of the degree to which function might ultimately be restored. Comparison with radiographs of the contralateral bone and joint may reveal subtle changes in the involved side. Sequential films are helpful to monitor treatment (see Table 115-1).

ARTHROGRAPHY

In addition to determining placement of structures within the joint, arthograms may reveal capsular or ligamentous damage. The contrast material does not exacerbate the infectious process, nor does it interfere with antibiotic treatment. Rupture of the rotator cuff, with or without superior subluxation of the humeral head,[77] and delineation of the position and integrity of the femoral head, especially in children,[108–110] are often detectable by arthrography. Synovial fluid obtained should be examined for microorganisms by staining and culture before the contrast dye is injected.

COMPUTED TOMOGRAPHY (CT)

This procedure is most valuable when the anatomic structures are complex, as in the spine, or when the involved areas are surrounded by bone; it is less valuable in examining peripheral joints and the neck (see Chapter 92).[111] Osteomyelitis in a long bone increases the density of medullary tissues, presumably because of vascular congestion and edema, even before bone destruction becomes apparent. Later, just as on standard radiographs and conventional tomograms, CT scanning can be used to document bone destruction, cavitation, and sequestration.[112] In the spine, this technique permits identification of a soft-tissue abscess.[104] Swelling and effusion can be recognized in a deep-seated area such as the sacroiliac joint.[113]

MAGNETIC RESONANCE IMAGING

Magnetic resonance imaging (MR) can demonstrate, in superb anatomic detail, soft-tissue structures of the musculoskeletal system with striking differentiation between muscles, fibrous structures, and blood vessels. These structures on the CT scan have an almost indistinguishable appearance.[104,111] Articular cartilage and, in children, growth cartilage can be depicted. In the knee, the fibrous cartilage of the meniscus is seen as a very low intensity structure distinctly different from the articular cartilage. Extension of infection into adjacent soft tissue can be clearly delineated. The increased anatomic visualization afforded by MR can be compared to the findings on standard radiographs and CT scans in the case of an infected hip joint (Fig. 115-5) and in the case of osteomyelitis of the spine in a child (Fig. 115-6).

RADIOISOTOPIC SCINTIGRAPHY

^{99m}Technetium (^{99m}Tc) diphosphonate and ^{67}gallium (^{67}Ga) citrate scintigraphy may detect the presence of infection at an early stage; these techniques are particularly useful in examining deep joints such as the hip, shoulder, and spine.[104,111,114] Positive results by either isotope are not specific for infection because other inflammatory or even degenerative joint diseases can create the same image.[115] Specificity for bone and joint infection, however, may be enhanced by giving more weight to a positive ^{67}Ga citrate scintigram than to a positive ^{99m}Tc scintigram,[116] for osteomyelitis, one may perform a three-phase study, consisting of the radionuclide angiogram, the immediate postinjection "blood pool" image, and the 2- to 3-hour delayed image, to

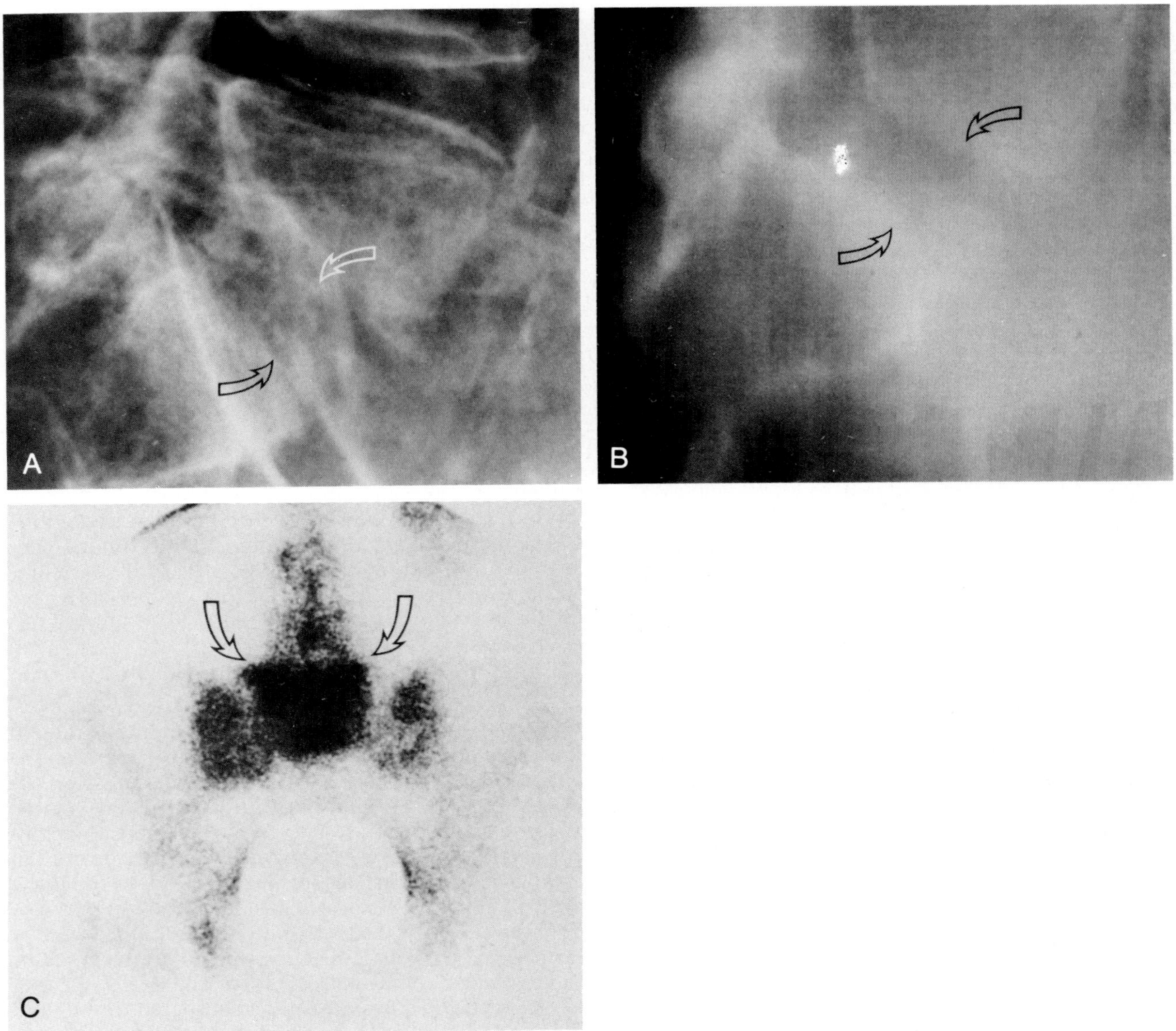

FIGURE 115–4. *A,* The vertebral end-plates at L5-S1 of a 58-year-old woman are indistinct (*open arrows*) because of destruction by a disc space-vertebral infection by Staphylococcus aureus. *B,* A conventional tomogram demonstrates this indistinctness more clearly (*open arrows*). *C,* A ^{99m}Tc-disphosphonate bone scintigram shows increased activity at the L5-S1 level (*open arrows*). The greater activity in the left sacroiliac compared to the right is a result of patient rotation; the left sacroiliac joint is closer to the crystal detector of the gamma camera. From Hendrix, R.W., and Fisher, M.R.[104]

distinguish bone infection from soft-tissue infection and from noninfectious skeletal disease.[117] Using these techniques, the pathologic process can be localized to a joint rather than to overlying tissue, as in cellulitis. This feature has been particularly useful in evaluating disease in the sacroiliac joint.[90,114]

In acute osteomyelitis, ^{99m}Tc-diphosphonate often fails to demonstrate a high-uptake lesion in the neonate, in contrast to the expected greater yield of abnormal images in the slightly older infant or child.[118] Even in older children, however, fulminant osteomyelitis may escape detection. Instead, a focal decrease in nuclide accumulation occurs, considered to be a result of thrombosis in the microcirculation[16] or of intraosseous pressure on the nutrient artery.[119]

Radionuclide studies should always be interpreted together with findings revealed by the standard radiograph because the detailed anatomic information provided by the radiograph often complements the functional information provided by scintigraphy.

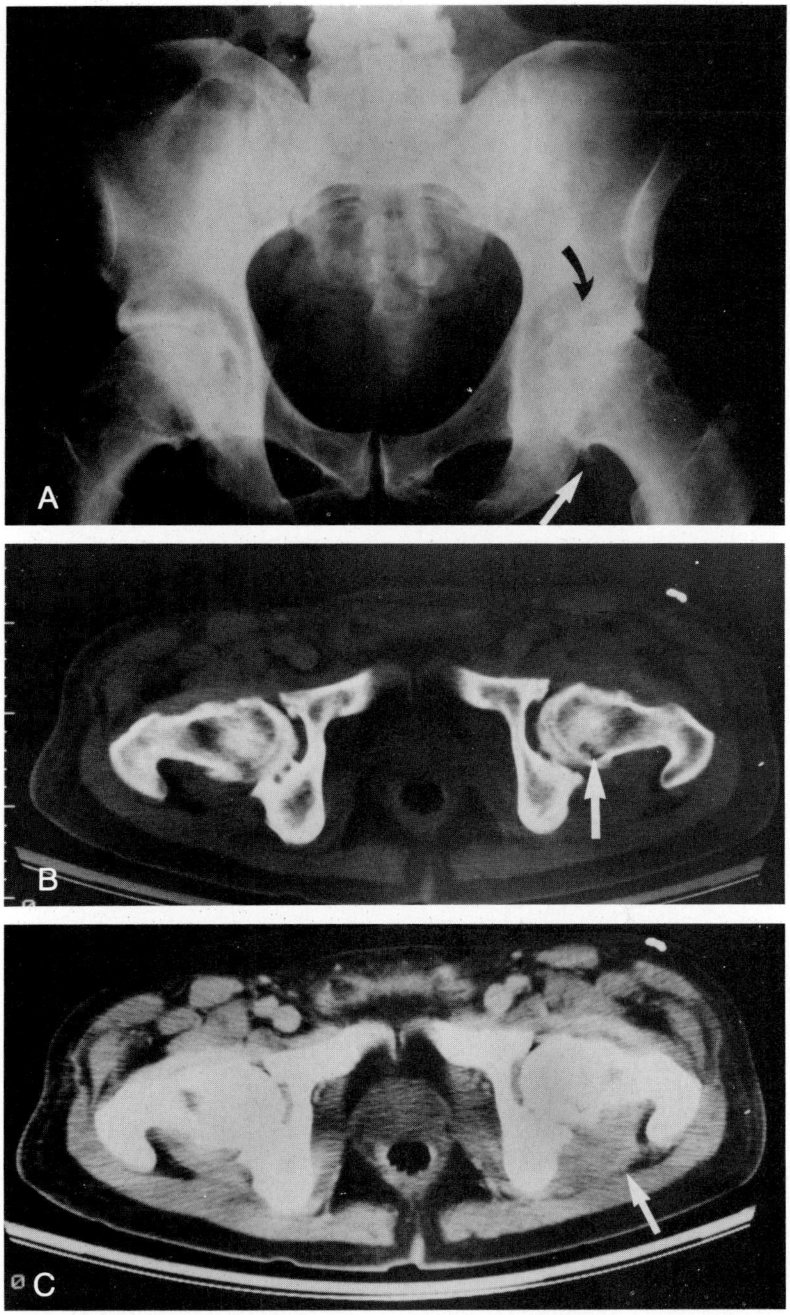

FIGURE 115–5. Infectious arthritis of the left hip in a 53-year-old drug-addicted patient. *A,* In the conventional radiograph, narrowing of the joint space is greater on the left than the right, with associated evidence of prior osteoarthritis (*straight arrow showing osteophytes*). The ill-defined left acetabular margin (*curved arrow*) is suspicious for infection. *B,* CT at the level of the hip joints with a bone window setting shows minimal differences between the bone density and joint space of the left and right hip, except for a vague area (*arrow*) of decreased bone density along the posterior aspect of the left femoral head; *C,* CT with a soft-tissue window setting showing enlargement of the surrounding musculature (*arrow*).

RADIOLOGY OF AN INFECTED JOINT PROSTHESIS

Several weeks or months may elapse before conventional radiographs indicate changes compatible with infection in an endoprosthesis. These changes include the formation of a radiolucent zone at the bone-cement interface, scalloping of the cortical margin, a periosteal reaction resembling lamination, and regions of increased bone density and radiolucency typical of osteomyelitis (Fig. 115-7). Early and minor alterations are not recognizable without a comparison with previous films. Arthrograms are not helpful for the diagnosis of infection itself, but they can demonstrate the extent and location of soft tissue involvement, such as a sinus tract. If a sinus tract has perforated to the exterior, a sinogram can be done. Subtraction technique is essential to verify details when radiopaque cement is present. ^{99m}Tc-diphosphonate uptake may fail to distinguish mechanical loosening from infection; as mentioned earlier, imaging by ^{67}Ga citrate may be more specific for infection.[120] Scintigraphy using ^{111}In-labeled leukocytes, like other forms of scintigraphy, is

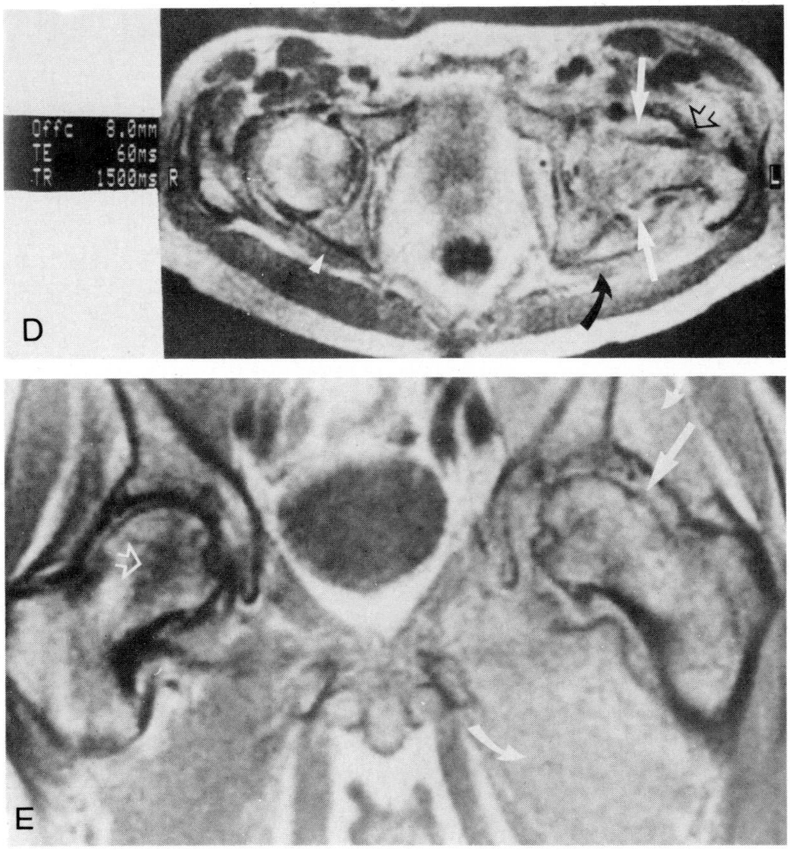

FIGURE 115–5. (*Continued*) *D,* A transverse MRI at a similar level shows an abnormal collection of material (*closed straight arrows*) within the left hip joint displacing the joint capsule (*open arrow*) outward. The signal intensity within the surrounding musculature (*curved arrow*) is increased on the left compared to the opposite normal side (*arrowhead*). The left femoral head and neck have a nonhomogeneous signal intensity. *E,* In a coronal MRI through the hip joints, the abnormal collection within the joint (*closed arrow*) and the enlarged adjacent musculature with an increased intensity (*curved arrows*) are shown. The low-intensity line on the right femoral neck is the site of normal trabecular thickening (*open arrow*). From Hendrix, R.W., and Fisher, M.R.[104]

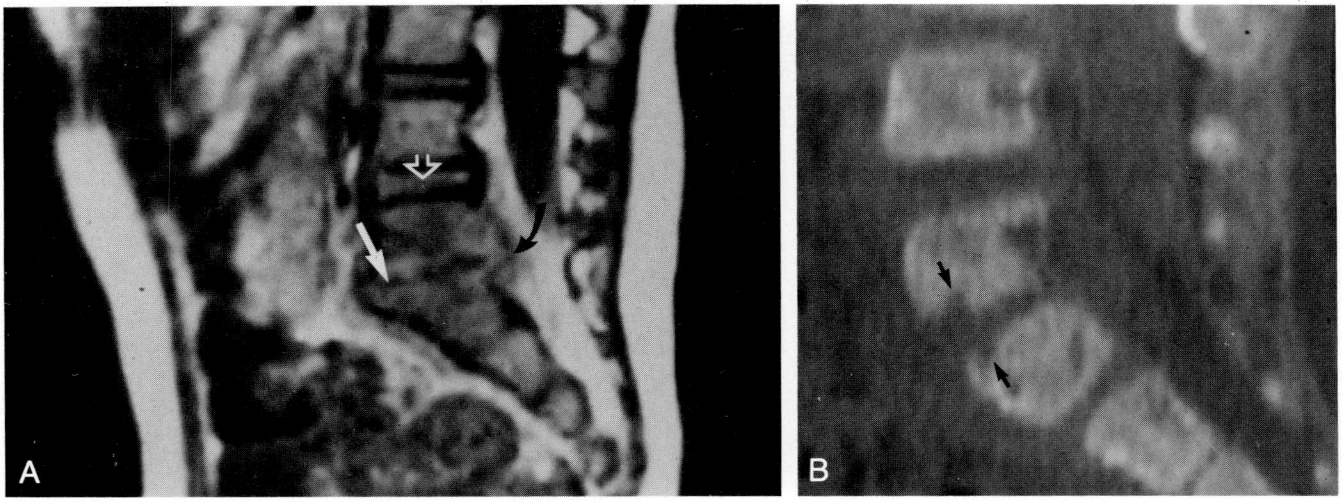

FIGURE 115–6. Osteomyelitis of the spine in a child. *A,* A sagittal MRI through the lumbosacral region demonstrates decreased signal intensity of the involved L5 and S1 vertebral bodies and disc. Note disc space narrowing (*closed straight arrow*) compared to the high intensity of normal disc material (*open arrow*). The extension into the epidural space is well visualized (*curved arrow*). *B,* The same view by CT demonstrates irregularity of the L5-S1 end-plates (*arrows*) and loss of disc height. The degree of bone involvement and extension into the spinal canal is not as well delineated as with MRI. From Hendrix, R.W., and Fisher, M.R.[104]

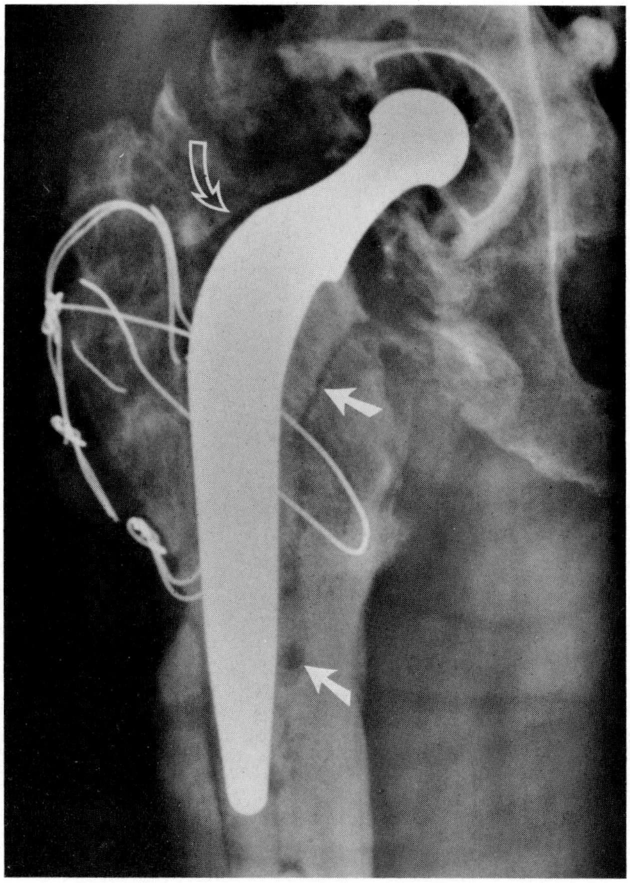

FIGURE 115–7. Infected total hip replacement resulting from Staphylococcus aureus 18 months after insertion shows well-defined cement-metal (*open arrow*) and bone-cement (*closed arrows*) lucent zones. From Hendrix, R.W., and Fisher, M.R.[104]

highly sensitive, but like ^{67}Ga citrate is only moderately specific.[121]

JOINT FLUID EXAMINATION

Aspiration and examination of joint fluid are mandatory whenever infection is considered. These procedures must be done immediately and must not be deferred.

Arthrocentesis requires strict asepsis. Inadvertent introduction of infection from skin, blood, or a para-articular focus into a joint cavity represents a serious, albeit rare hazard of joint aspiration. For this reason, a careful examination of the area is required to define anatomically the exact site of infection. The needle should be introduced into the joint through uninvolved subcutaneous tissue.

An arthrocentesis tray should contain sterile culture tubes. If indicated, joint fluid should be inoculated into these tubes as well as into tubes for chemical determinations and tubes with heparin or ethylene diamine tetracetate anticoagulant for cell examination. These culture samples should be taken directly to a laboratory by the physician. Lacking such tubes, the syringe into which the joint fluid was aspirated can be refitted with a new capped, sterile needle and carried to the laboratory where its contents can be distributed, first for smears and cultures and then for other studies. Some even recommend bedside inoculation of the fluid onto media when infection with fastidious microorganisms, such as the gonococcus, are anticipated, but this additional precaution rarely seems necessary. If only one or two drops of synovial fluid can be obtained, they should be cultured, and any remaining fluid should be smeared onto a slide for Gram's staining. Rank order priority for studies on joint fluid are given in Table 115-1.

Additional studies of joint fluid are regularly performed (Table 115–3). The total leukocyte count can be determined manually or with an automated cell counter *using physiologic saline solution as a diluent.* The acid diluents used for blood leukocyte counts coagulate the hyaluronate of synovial fluid and trap leukocytes, so counts are falsely low. Although fluids in septic arthritis often appear grossly purulent and have elevated cell counts, predominantly of polymorphonuclear leukocytes, high white blood cell counts containing many polymorphonuclear cells can appear in noninfected fluids obtained from some patients with acute gout, pseudogout, or RA.[122] In a few immobilized patients unable to turn, layering of cells and debris has occurred in a joint such as the knee to such an extent that the initial aspirate is much less turbid than the final aspirate.[123]

The *fasting* synovial fluid glucose value is usually reduced to less than half the blood glucose value obtained simultaneously.[122] Reductions of this magnitude, however, can occur in inflammatory joint fluids of nonseptic origin, in infectious arthritis resulting from viruses, and in gonococcal arthritis. Similarly, the synovial fluid lactate level is higher in patients with bacterial arthritis than in those with noninfectious inflammatory states. Lactate values are often just barely elevated, however, in gonococcal arthritis and in partially treated cases of infectious arthritis.[26,122,124] Lactate, along with other metabolites, such as succinic acid,[26] may be measured by gas-liquid chromatography, which detects end-products of bacterial and host-tissue metabolism, but the method is laborious. A simpler and quicker technique makes use of the enzymatic oxidation of lactate to pyruvate.[125]

Although measurements of synovial fluid glucose and lactate levels provide information in the diagnosis of joint sepsis, their diagnostic utility is limited in many instances.[122]

Other characteristics of septic synovial fluids appear to offer promise in distinguishing septic from nonseptic conditions. In children, values for tumor necrosis factor α (TNFα) and interleukin-1β (IL-1β) were often elevated in infected fluids but barely detectable or not present at all in noninfected fluids. Concentrations of these cytokines correlated with synovial fluid leukocyte counts. These dramatic results are preliminary and need confirmation in larger numbers of patients and controls.[126]

TABLE 115–3. SYNOVIAL FLUID FINDINGS IN ACUTE PYOGENIC ARTHRITIS (SEE ALSO CHAPTER 5)

JOINT FLUID EXAMINATION	NONINFLAMMATORY FLUIDS	INFLAMMATORY FLUIDS	
		Noninfectious	Infectious
Color	Colorless, pale yellow	Yellow	Yellow
Turbidity	Clear, slightly turbid	Turbid	Turbid, purulent
Viscosity	Not reduced	Reduced	Reduced
Mucin clot	Tight clot	Friable	Friable
Cell count (per mm^3)	200 to 2000	3000 to >30,000	10,000 to >100,000
Predominant cell type	Mononuclear	PMN*	PMN*
Synovial fluid/blood glucose ratio	0.8–1.0	0.5–0.8	<0.5
Lactic acid	Same as plasma	Higher than plasma	Often very high
Gram's stain for organism	None	None	Positive†
Culture	Negative	Negative	Positive†

* PMN = polymorphonuclear leukocyte
† In some cases, especially in gonococcal infection, no organisms may be demonstrated.

Inflammation from any cause increases the vascular permeability of the fenestrated synovial capillaries and augments the influx of serum proteins with a larger proportion of macromolecules, such as the complement proteins. In infectious arthritis, the level of these proteins in synovial fluid does not approach that found in serum because they are consumed intra-articularly in the inflammatory process. Complement proteins of both the classic and the alternative pathways are involved. Therefore, the ratio of fluid C3 to total protein concentration of joint fluid is lower than the ratio of serum C3 to total serum protein.[127] A similar reduction is well recognized in RA, but not in other inflammatory arthritides, such as gout, pseudogout, and seronegative spondyloarthropathy. Thus, decreased joint fluid complement levels are of interest in understanding the pathogenesis of sepsis, but they have a minor role in its diagnosis.

SYNOVIAL OR BONE BIOPSY

Tissue may be required to confirm a diagnosis of sepsis in patients whose synovial fluid has not yielded a positive culture. In some cases, this procedure may prove helpful because the quantity of bacteria may be greater in tissue,[128] and in other cases, such as in tuberculous and fungal infections, because microbial growth, even on appropriate culture media, is slow and thus may delay diagnosis and appropriate treatment. Tissue can be obtained by a blind synovial biopsy or under direct vision at arthroscopy or arthrotomy. Bone biopsy can be performed either with a needle or surgically. The fresh tissue specimen should be transported to the laboratory in a sterile container or in a sterile sponge moistened with saline solution. In addition to the appropriate bacteriologic studies, a portion of the tissue should be fixed and submitted for histologic examination.

BACTERIOLOGIC STUDIES

Blood agar should be used routinely for culturing all synovial fluid or tissue specimens, with chocolate agar used in addition when Neisseria gonorrhoeae or Haemophilus infection is suspected. The medium designed by Thayer and Martin is suitable for gonococcal isolation, but it contains vancomycin and colistin methanesulfonate because it was designed to isolate gonococci from the mixed flora of the female genital tract.[129] Therefore, many other bacteria such as Haemophilus species do not grow on Thayer-Martin media. Media of higher ionic strength have been advocated to culture gonococcal protoplasts. In one patient with gonococcal arthritis, standard cultures were negative, but growth occurred on such hypertonic media.[130] Haemophilus species can easily be isolated on peptic digest of blood agar, which is prepared from commercially available products. Placement of about 1 ml of synovial fluid in thioglycolate broth allows recovery of many anaerobic and aerobic bacteria. Many microaerophilic bacteria actually grow more rapidly after primary inoculation in thioglycolate broth than on solid media.

Isolation of strict anaerobes may require special anaerobic techniques. Fungal media, such as Sabouraud agar, should be inoculated in most instances. If fungal media are not inoculated, fungi may be recovered from the blood agar plates after incubation for as long as 2 weeks at room temperature. Drying of ordinary blood agar plates can be retarded by sealing the plate with paraffin tape. Culture of Mycobacterium species is best done with at least two kinds of media, an egg-glycerol-potato medium, such as A.T.S. medium, and a synthetic medium, such as Middlebrook 7H10 agar. If a large volume of synovial fluid is available, it should be concentrated by centrifugation before inoculating mycobacterial cultures. Because of improvements in culture media, one no longer needs to use guinea pig inoculation as a means of recovering M. tuberculosis; results in the guinea pig are rarely positive when mycobacterial cultures are negative.[131] Furthermore, atypical Mycobacterium species, which also infect joints, are nonpathogenic for guinea pigs (see also Chapter 118).

After inoculation of joint fluid into all appropriate media, smears are prepared on glass slides, which are air dried, and Gram's stain, Wright's stain, and appropriate stains for acid-fast and fungal organisms are applied.

Examination of such slides provides the necessary information to begin treatment.

DETECTION OF MICROBIAL RESIDUES

Countercurrent immunoelectrophoresis has been used to identify soluble bacterial antigens in various body fluids.[132,133] The method has been particularly helpful to detect the antigens of microorganisms such as the pneumococcus, meningococcus, and Haemophilus influenzae, and of viruses such as hepatitis B. Results, available within several hours, provide a quantitative measurement of the amount of antigen within body fluids. In studies of cerebrospinal and pleural fluids, the quantity of antigen has borne a direct relation to the severity of the infection and to prognosis.[134]

A technique employed by molecular biologists, the polymerase chain reaction, has the potential to amplify almost infinitesimal amounts of genetic material into quantities that can be precisely analyzed. When the method becomes adapted to the clinical laboratory, nonviable microbial nucleic acid fragments can be identified in circumstances in which current culture methods are inadequate or in which prior antibiotic therapy has eradicated viable microorganisms. Results are promising in Lyme disease[135,136] and in parvovirus infection.[137]

ANTIBODY AND OTHER TESTS

Detection of specific antibody to an infecting microorganism indicates a prior immune response by the host. However, a positive test does not reveal whether the exposure to the microorganism is current or remote, although an IgM antibody response usually means that the infection is recent. The laboratory diagnosis of Lyme disease illustrates this confounding situation. Not only does great variability exist among commercial laboratories,[138] but about 20% of the population in endemic areas, most of whom have no active disease, possess antibodies to Borrelia. Were any of these to develop another inflammatory illness, the positive Lyme antibody test could prove misleading.[139]

Teichoic acid antibodies to staphylococci have been found in the serum of many patients with osteomyelitis, but only infrequently in the serum of patients with septic arthritis resulting from this organism.[64] The value of this test as a diagnostic procedure seems marginal because staphylococci can be readily cultured from infected fluids and tissues. When the culture is negative or when material for culture is unavailable, the detection of such antibodies may complement the information obtained from the clinical, radiologic, and scanning examinations.

Assays using limulus amebocyte lysate to detect endotoxin in body fluids have not been able to distinguish septic arthritis, not even that owing to gram-negative organisms, from noninfectious inflammatory arthritis.[140]

The nitroblue-tetrazolium (NBT) reduction test is useless in confirming the presence of infection in joint fluids. The test depends on the conversion of a soluble, colorless compound into an insoluble, blue granule on phagocytosis by polymorphonuclear or other phagocytic cells. Synovial fluid polymorphonuclear cells usually show a positive reaction, whether they come from infected or noninfected joints. The study of peripheral blood polymorphonuclear cells also does not discriminate between infectious and noninfectious inflammation.[141]

ANTIBIOTIC TREATMENT

IMMEDIATE MANAGEMENT

Antibiotics should be given in cases of clear-cut or strongly suspected bone and joint infections, even before an exact identification of the infecting microorganism is made. When the microorganism has been identified and its sensitivity to antimicrobial drugs has been assayed, the choice and dose of antibiotic can be reconsidered. If no microorganism is recovered from the bone or joint, further decisions about drug treatment will depend on the use of other, albeit nonspecific, laboratory tests and on the clinical course.

Antibiotic treatment for septic arthritis should begin within the first few hours after the patient's admission to the hospital. A preliminary estimate of the type of infecting microorganism can be made on the basis of the findings noted on the Gram's-stained smear of synovial fluid, which may show gram-positive cocci, gram-negative cocci or coccobacilli, gram-negative bacilli, or no microorganisms.

If no organism is detected in an otherwise healthy young or middle-aged adult, I treat with cephazolin or cephtriaxone intravenously (Table 115–4), which is adequate for most infections caused by pneumococci, gonococci, penicillin G–susceptible staphylococci, and several less-common bacteria. Gonococcal arthritis in the adult is frequently accompanied by a negative Gram's-stained smear, despite clinically convincing evidence of infection.[68–71] Improvement, often in 4 to 7 days of treatment with these extended spectrum cephalosporins, may be dramatic. Resistant gonococcal strains are appearing more frequently and retain their invasiveness despite a tendency for gonococci associated with arthritis to be sensitive to penicillin.[142] In an ill or elderly patient, particularly with reduced renal function, in whom gram-negative bacillary infection is suspected, I use a third-generation cephalopsorin or a monobactam. Management for the patient with either proven or suspected Lyme disease is given in Chapter 120. Initial treatment in the newborn in whom infection owing to staphylococci, group B streptococci, or coliform organisms might occur should be a penicillinase-resistant penicillin or vancomycin plus an aminoglycoside.[37] Beyond the neonatal period and until 4 to 5 years of age when β-lactamase-positive strains of Haemophilus influenzae are a common cause of septic arthritis, chloramphenicol has been recommended,[143] but cefuroxime may be as effective without the bone marrow toxicity associated with chloramphenicol.[37] If β-lactamase-negative microorganisms are found later on culture, ampicillin can be substituted.[143]

Initial antibiotic treatment for acute hematogenous osteomyelitis is usually a penicillinase-resistant penicillin. If gram-negative sepsis is suspected, an aminoglycoside is added. In nonhematogenous osteomyelitis, which may be a result of a polymicrobic infection, dual antibiotic therapy is appropriate, as in the case of gram-negative sepsis.

During the acute phase of the illness, antibiotics should be given parenterally. If the drug is administered intravenously, the daily dose should be divided into fractions, and a fractional dose should be given every 6 to 8 hours over a span of 30 to 60 minutes into a constant infusion. This "piggyback" technique is preferred to continual delivery of the drug by intravenous infusion, to avoid loss owing to interruption of flow that might result from subcutaneous infiltration or blockage of the needle or tubing.

When a specific bacterium is seen on the Gram's-stained smear, one may attempt a closer approximation to definitive antibiotic therapy. Types and doses of drugs currently recommended for several different kinds of infection are listed in Table 115-4. Infections caused by gram-negative bacilli such as Escherichia coli and Pseudomonas require a more aggressive approach, usually with two antibiotics.

Suggestions for antibiotic therapy given here provide only general guidelines. Such information quickly becomes outdated as more effective drugs are discovered or changing patterns of drug resistance emerge in some strains of bacteria. For these reasons, the therapist must have access to current knowledge concerning antibiotics. Knowledge of drug toxicity is also essential. The dosage of antibiotic must be appropriately reduced in a patient with diminished renal function. Blood levels of antibiotic determined by the tube-dilution technique provide the necessary information.

TRANSPORT OF ANTIBIOTICS INTO SYNOVIAL FLUID

Antibiotics diffuse readily from the circulation into infected and uninfected inflamed joints.[25,144–149] Early studies of synovial fluid concentrations of pencillin showed inadequate amounts of this drug in the joint, but the dose was much lower than currently recommended. Effective synovial fluid concentrations of a number of common antibiotics were measured in a study of 75 paired samples of synovial fluid and blood obtained from 29 adult patients with a presumptive diagnosis of infectious arthritis.[149] Parenteral administration of penicillin G, phenoxymethyl penicillin (penicillin V), nafcillin, cloxacillin, cephaloridine, tetracycline, erythromycin, and lincomycin in conventional doses produced bactericidal fluid concentrations within the joint (Fig. 115-8). Similar results have been reported in infants and children for ampicillin, methicillin, penicillin G, and cephalothin.[147] Knowledge of such effective concentrations in infected joints obviates the need for direct instillation of antibiotics into the joint space and thus reduces the risk of introducing a new infectious agent, as well as the risk of producing a "chemical syno-

TABLE 115–4. ANTIBIOTIC SELECTION BASED ON PATIENT'S AGE AND GRAM'S-STAIN FINDINGS

AGE (YEARS)	GRAM-NEGATIVE BACILLI	GRAM-NEGATIVE COCCI	GRAM-POSITIVE COCCI	NO ORGANISM SEEN
<½	Ceftazidime and aminoglycoside (Enterobacteriaceae or Pseudomonas aeruginosa)*	Extended-spectrum cephalosporin (Neisseria gonorrhoeae)	Penicillinase-resistant penicillin OR vancomycin (staphylococci or streptococci)	Penicillinase-resistant penicillin AND aminoglycoside (staphylococci, group B streptococci, or coliforms)
½ to 2–4	Extended-spectrum cephalosporin (Haemophilus influenzae)	As above	As above	Extended-spectrum cephalosporin (Haemophilus influenzae or streptococci)
2–4 to 14	Ceftazidime and aminoglycoside (Enterobacteriaceae or Pseudomonas aeruginosa)	As above	As above	Penicillinase-resistant penicillin OR vancomycin (staphylococci or streptococci)
15 to 59	As above	As above	As above	Extended-spectrum cephalosporin (Neisseria gonorrhoeae and staphylococci)
>60	Extended-spectrum cephalosporin and ciprofloxacin (Enterobacteriaceae or Pseudomonas aeruginosa)	As above	As above	Extended-spectrum cephalosporin AND vancomycin (staphylococci, coliforms)

* Presumed identity of pathogenetic microorganism in parentheses. If other microorganisms are suspected, consult appropriate sources for alternative antibiotic selection.

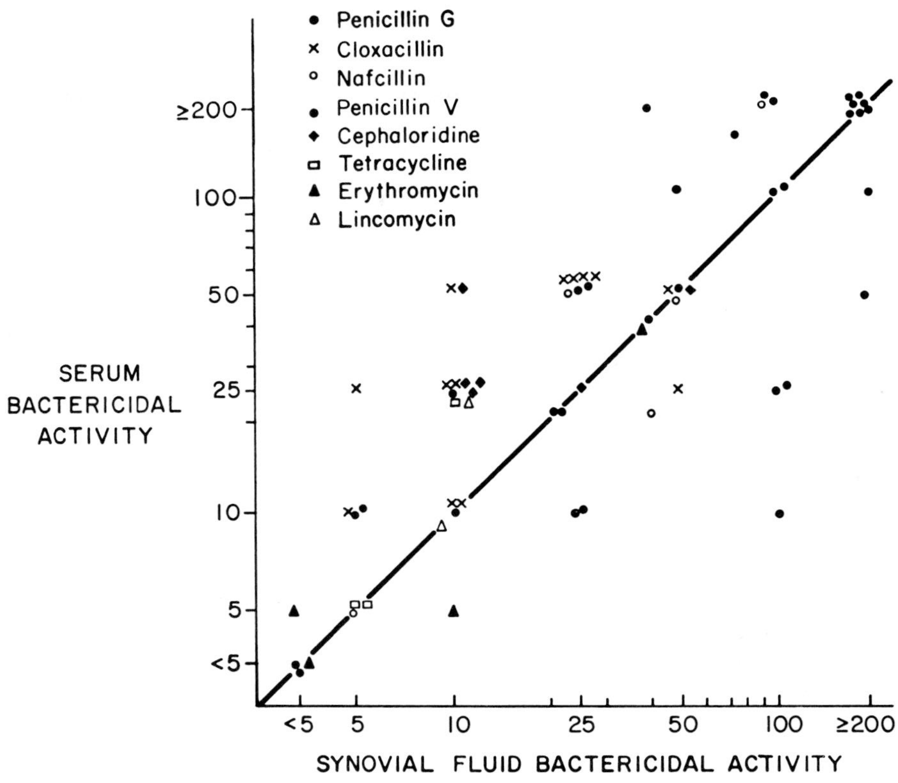

FIGURE 115–8. Comparison of the bactericidal activity of 75 paired specimens of serum and synovial fluid obtained from 29 patients during systemic antibiotic therapy. Points on the diagonal line indicate pairs with equal activity. Bactericidal activity is expressed as the reciprocal of the maximum dilution showing this activity. From Parker, R.H., and Schmid, F.R.[149]

vitis" from local irritation by excessively high local concentrations of some drugs.[145]

Protein binding of the antibiotic and the degree of the inflammatory response influence the rate of diffusion of serum constituents into the joint. When the diffusion of nafcillin, which is strongly bound to serum protein, was compared to another penicillin analogue, ampicillin, which shows little protein binding, comparable, effective joint fluid levels of both drugs were found at 4 hours, although the rate of entry of ampicillin was initially more rapid than that of nafcillin (Fig. 115-9). Thus, protein binding does not impair the entry into the joint or the efficacy of an antibiotic administered extra-articularly.[25] *The general rule in the use of antibiotics in infectious arthritis is that most drugs reach therapeutic levels in the synovial fluid if adequate amounts are given systemically.*

Information on newly marketed antibiotics may be unavailable. Therefore, until such data are provided, adequate transport of these drugs can be documented by studies in the patient in which they are used. If diffusion of the drug is inadequate, an unlikely event, local instillation into the joint might be done once or twice a day, or another antibiotic known to enter the joint more readily can be substituted. Finally, aminoglycoside effectiveness decreases by an order of magnitude at pH 6.5. Thus, effective removal of purulent exudate, which correlates with low pH, is especially important when this antibiotic is used.[97]

TRANSPORT OF ANTIBIOTICS INTO BONE

Although measurement of antibiotics in bone poses more difficulties than in synovial fluid,[150] most studies indicate that, as in synovial fluid, adequate concentrations of antibiotics are reached when bactericidal doses have been administered systemically. Problems in interpreting drug levels in bone are the use of normal, uninfected bone for the assay, usually from uninfected patients undergoing elective operations, the variations in porosity of cancellous and cortical bone, destruction of the test antibiotic by the heat generated by the pulverization process used to grind the bone, and contamination of the specimen by plasma not removed in the washing process. Therefore, only approximate drug levels can be measured. These levels are usually far below those obtained in plasma, yet they are often greater than the concentration needed to achieve bacterial inhibition and killing. Some data are available on most penicillins, cephalosporins, erythromycin, lincomycin, and clindamycin, but few data are available on aminoglycosides.[151]

DEFINITIVE MANAGEMENT OF INFECTIOUS ARTHRITIS

As soon as the exact identity of the microorganism and its susceptibility to antibiotics are known, definitive therapy can be planned. Details of such management

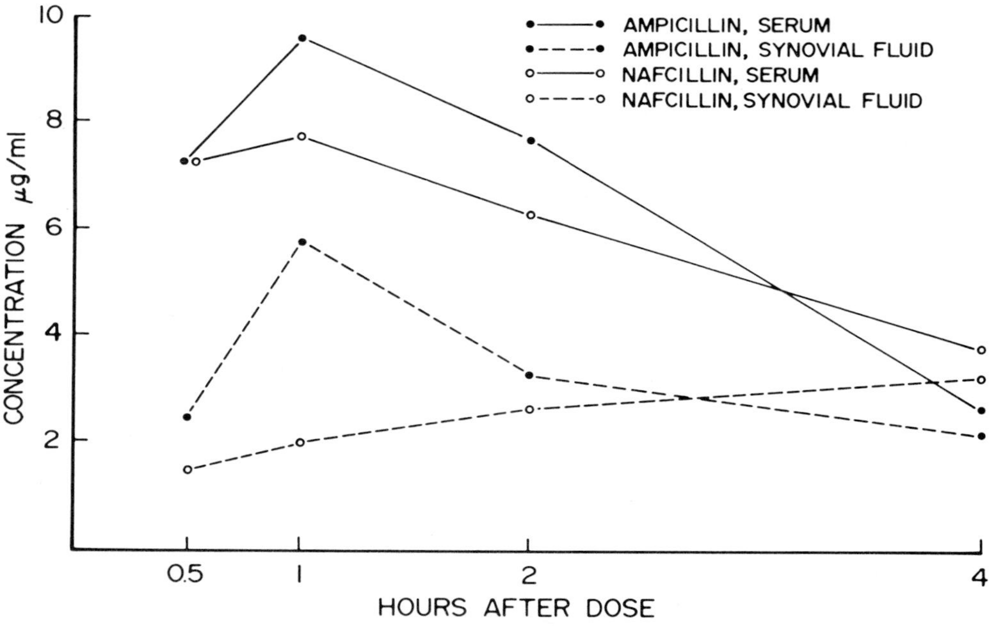

FIGURE 115–9. Comparison of serum and synovial fluid concentrations of ampicillin and nafcillin in 6 patients receiving a single dose of each drug, 500 mg intramuscularly, in a cross-over study. From Parker, R.H., Birbara, C., and Schmid, F.R.[25]

are provided in Chapters 116 through 120. Either the initial antibiotic is continued at the same or modified dose, or a more appropriate antibiotic is selected. Proof that the intravenous antibiotic is actually entering the joint in bactericidal concentrations can be obtained by determining antibacterial activity in paired samples of synovial fluid and serum. A simple tube-dilution technique can be performed in most clinical bacteriologic laboratories, using either the bacterium isolated from the patient or a bacterial species with identical antibiotic susceptibility.[149] Test results indicate the limiting dilution of serum and synovial fluid that still retains bacteriostatic or bactericidal activity. A margin of bactericidal effect ten or more times than found in undiluted synovial fluid provides sufficient antibiotic for antimicrobial action. One should rely on a regimen that produces bactericidal, not just bacteriostatic, activity. If this end has not been achieved, the dose of antibiotic should be increased until adequate bactericidal activity is reached, or else another antibiotic should be substituted. An excellent correlation exists between this simple tube-dilution test and the more quantitative agar-diffusion technique.[149]

Parenteral antibiotic administration should be maintained until clinical signs of active synovitis and inflammatory changes in the joint fluid begin to revert toward normal.[152] Synovial fluid should be recultured repeatedly during the initial stages of therapy to demonstrate sterility. if prolonged use of an antibiotic is anticipated, intravenous administration can be attempted with the placement of a subcutaneous reservoir that feeds into a large central vein, such as the subclavian vein. An external pump can be attached to deliver a constant amount of the antibiotic through a needle inserted into the reservoir. Use of this type of device allows treatment for a protracted infection to be carried out at home. When one is certain that the infection is controlled, the antibiotic may be given orally. The oral route is unreliable in early treatment because patients with sepsis often have nausea, vomiting, and other gastrointestinal disturbances. Sterility and a progressive decline in total joint fluid leukocyte concentration are signs of a good prognosis; conversely, continued bacterial growth and a steady or rising leukocyte level suggest the need to reassess the treatment regimen.

Infections caused by the gonococcus and certain other coccal organisms, such as the pneumococcus and the streptococcus, generally respond rapidly to appropriate antibiotic management. In patients with such infections, the duration of therapy might be expected to be brief, perhaps 2 weeks or less. Infections caused by staphylococci and gram-negative bacteria respond more slowly to treatment.[7,44,57] A satisfactory explanation for these differences is not available. Local factors may play a role, but a change in the drug sensitivity of the microorganisms present within the joint fluid is not likely to be a factor. In most cases, the strain of organism infecting the joint remains constant and is not replaced by another drug-resistant, variety unless a contaminating strain is carried into the joint inadvertently during arthrocentesis. This finding contrasts with the changing bacterial flora noted during the treatment of "open" infections in bone in which a sinus tract has formed, or during the open drainage and suction sometimes carried out after arthrotomy. In addition, staphylococci do not usually show spontaneous mutation in their patterns of drug sensitivity. Thus, a strain of Staphylococcus aureus sensitive to penicillin G at the outset remains sensitive to this drug during treatment.

DEFINITIVE MANAGEMENT OF OSTEOMYELITIS

In patients with osteomyelitis, plasma bactericidal levels of antibiotics are an indication of the adequacy of the drug dose. If this information is correlated with the sensitivity of the microorganism obtained either from blood or an aspirate of the bone lesion, an informed decision can be made. How long to continue drug therapy is contingent on an evaluation of the clinical response, which, although less quantitative than the assessment of synovitis and joint fluid changes, provides useful evidence of the effects of treatment.

SERUM SICKNESS FROM ANTIMICROBIAL AGENTS

Serum sickness is a well-known but unusual complication of drug therapy. Almost any antibiotic, acting as a hapten, can induce this reaction. When symptoms of fever, rash, and flare of arthritis develop during the course of treatment of infectious arthritis, one must distinguish between a relapse of the primary joint disease and the onset of the polyarthritis of serum sickness.

Careful examination of the bacterial status of the inflamed joint is mandatory and, if necessary, one must use an unrelated drug. In the interval between stopping the original drug and giving the new antibiotic, the joint fluid should be tested for the presence of microorganisms by smear and culture, along with cell count and glucose level. Pending the results of these tests, antibiotic treatment can be administered with a drug to which the patient is not known to be sensitive.

POSTINFECTIOUS SYNOVITIS

Tissue injury in septic arthritis is caused directly by toxic factors produced by viable microorganisms and indirectly by the host's response to microbial antigens. The killing of microorganisms by the action of antibiotics does not remove microbial products. Such materials may persist within the joint for prolonged periods, either in loculated areas or possibly embedded in articular cartilage. The retention of these substances may thereby contribute to persistence of the inflammatory response.

Such postinfectious synovitis leads to confusion about the adequacy of antibiotic treatment. Because viable microorganisms may still be present in tissues even after synovial fluid cultures have become sterile, antibiotics are usually not discontinued. Instead, a nonsteroidal anti-inflammatory drug is added, but only after several days or more of antibiotic drug treatment. If the combination of antibiotic and anti-inflammatory therapy controls the inflammatory process, both drugs can be continued until all signs of active disease have disappeared. It is not advisable to initiate nonspecific anti-inflammatory drug use earlier because such drugs are also antipyretic; the patient's initial response to the antibiotic alone provides reassurance that the infection is coming under control. A rapid response, particularly in the case of a gonococcal infection, provides added weight for the diagnosis, especially in bacteriologically unproved cases.

In carefully selected patients in whom the inflammatory response in the joint persists for several weeks despite negative cultures and in whom arthrotomy or arthroscopy is not advisable, intra-articular injection of a corticosteroid drug may be considered. Its use should be restricted to instances in which the microorganism is known to be sensitive to the antibiotic and antibiotic coverage is maintained in the post-injection interval until all signs of synovitis have ceased. Under these circumstances, I have treated two patients with complete resolution of inflammation in a few days.

ANTIBIOTIC PROPHYLAXIS FOR PATIENTS WITH JOINT PROSTHESES

Infection is the most feared complication of total joint replacement, and removal of the prosthesis is often necessary to eradicate the septic process successfully. Thus, during the perioperative period, ways to avoid infection are emphasized. Attention is also directed to the prevention of a late infection, particularly in situations that might favor bacteremia.

PERIOPERATIVE PROPHYLAXIS

In addition to the use of scrupulously sterile technique, special operative clothing, avoidance of unnecessary personnel or traffic in the operating room, and sometimes, laminar air-flow systems at the operating table, almost all patients undergoing total joint replacement receive antibiotics (usually antistaphylococcal agents such as oxacillin or vancomycin) prior to and during the procedure and for a number of days postoperatively.[41,94,95,153,154] The rationale for the use of systemic antibiotics is that, despite precautions, most wounds may become contaminated during the course of a long operation. In most centers, the rate of infection has dropped as surgical experience has grown and as the operative time has been shortened. Transient bacteremia with hematogenous seeding of microorganisms is also a possibility. For this reason, any known focus of infection elsewhere in the body is treated aggressively prior to the operation.

Antibiotic-impregnated cement has also been used; the idea is that a drug reservoir can be maintained at the operative site from which an antibiotic, such as gentamicin, can diffuse throughout the wound.[155] Evidence for its added value to an otherwise exemplary surgical program is not clear; some are concerned that the antibiotic might weaken the mechanical properties of the cement.

PROPHYLAXIS AGAINST LATE BACTEREMIA

A few well-placed prostheses become infected months after operation, most likely by hematogenous seeding of bacteria to the implant area.[41,94,95,156] For this reason, antibiotics have been used prophylactically in circumstances in which bacteremia is known to occur (Table 115–5).[157] A recommended regimen after oropharyngeal, bronchial, gastrointestinal, and urologic procedures is listed in Table 115–6.[157]

DRAINAGE OF INFECTED BONE AND JOINTS

DRAINAGE OF SYNOVIAL FLUID

Except for infants with septic arthritis of the hip, who require open surgical drainage as soon as the diagnosis is made,[85,158–160] drainage can be accomplished by needle aspiration in almost all cases of uncomplicated infectious arthritis. Patients with a prosthetic joint infection or an infection secondary to prior trauma or surgery may require early surgical drainage. All possible fluid and debris are removed on a regular basis, sometimes daily, or even more frequently if needed. Because some material always remains in the joint and may be compartmentalized by fibrinous adhesions, some clinicians suggest lavage of the joint cavity with sterile physiologic saline or Ringer's solution.[161] At each aspiration, the volume, cell count, culture, and, at appropriate intervals, the fasting glucose or lactate levels should be determined (see Table 115–1).

In the deep-seated joint of the older child or adult, the decision whether to perform open surgical drainage or needle drainage poses a problem because of the difficulty associated with repeated aspiration. If sepsis is recognized early, and if the organism recovered from the joint is sensitive to antibiotics, particularly if it is a gonococcus or another nonstaphylococcal coccus, then needle drainage is still preferred because it prevents the conversion of a closed-space infection into an open wound. If recognition of sepsis is delayed, however, or if sepsis is a result of "difficult" organisms, such as staphylococci or gram-negative bacilli, or if the infected joint is the result of extension of infection from a periarticular site, such as a contiguous bone or soft tissue, then open drainage may be needed.[162,163] Open drainage is indicated if needle aspiration fails to decompress the joint adequately.

TABLE 115–5. DENTAL OR SURGICAL PROCEDURES FOR WHICH ANTIBIOTIC PROPHYLAXIS IS RECOMMENDED*

Dental procedures known to induce gingival or mucosal bleeding, including professional cleaning
Tonsillectomy, adenoidectomy, or both
Surgical operations that involve intestinal or respiratory mucosa
Bronchoscopy with a rigid bronchoscope
Sclerotherapy for esophageal varices
Esophageal dilation
Gall bladder surgery
Cystoscopy
Urethral dilatation
Urethral catheterization if urinary tract infection is present†
Urinary tract surgery if urinary tract infection is present†
Prostatic surgery
Incision and drainage of infected tissue†
Vaginal hysterectomy
Vaginal delivery in the presence of infection†

* This table lists selected procedures but is not meant to be all-inclusive. It is adapted from recommendations of the American Heart Association for prevention of bacterial endocarditis.[157]

† In addition to the recommended prophylactic regimen for genitourinary procedures (Table 115–6), antibiotic therapy should be directed against the most likely bacterial pathogen.

SURGICAL DRAINAGE

Except for the foregoing circumstances, surgical drainage is withheld unless one sees little or no clinical or laboratory evidence of improvement during the first 4 to 7 days of treatment. This time interval is arbitrary. I would still continue to treat a slowly responding gonococcal infection by needle aspiration for another 4 to 7 days. On the other hand, infections owing to staphylococci or to gram-negative bacilli, unrelenting synovitis present a week after treatment is begun call for arthrotomy or arthroscopy. No adequately controlled study to support this opinion is available, although almost all large series in which this question is

TABLE 115–6. RECOMMENDED STANDARD PROPHYLACTIC REGIMEN FOR ADULT PATIENTS WITH PROSTHETIC JOINT IMPLANTS*

A. For dental, oral, or upper respiratory tract procedures	
Amoxicillin	3 g orally 1 h before procedure; then 1.5 g 6 h after initial dose
B. For genitourinary/gastrointestinal procedures	
Ampicillin, clindamicin, and amoxicillin	Intravenous or intramuscular administration of ampicillin (2 g) plus gentamicin (1.6 mg/kg, not to exceed 80 mg) 30 min before procedure; followed by amoxicillin (1.5 g orally) 6 h after initial dose; alternatively, the parenteral regimen may be repeated once 8 h after initial dose

* Adapted from recommendations of the American Heart Association for prevention of bacterial endocarditis. Alternative regimens for patients allergic to the standard recommendation or presenting special risks and dosing regimens for infants and children are provided in the original source.[157]

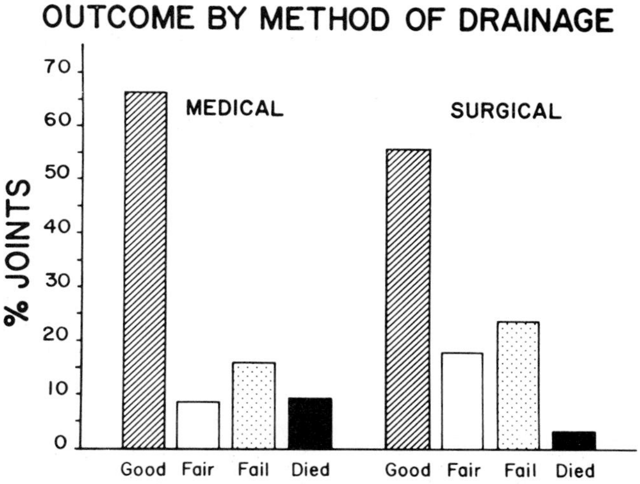

FIGURE 115–10. The outcome of joint function in 242 joints that received needle aspiration and in 125 that received either arthrotomy or arthroscopy. From Broy, S.B., and Schmid, F.R.[161]

examined have failed to demonstrate an advantage of initial open drainage over deferred open drainage (Fig. 115–10).[158,161,164,165]

ARTHROSCOPY

This technique offers the prospect of inspecting the joint cavity and the opportunity to lavage its contents and to remove fibrotic or necrotic tissue, some of which might be further examined by culture and histologic study for evidence of persisting infection.[166,167] Morbidity is much lower with arthroscopy than with open drainage. The procedure can be repeated at a later stage if further local debridement is required. Its limitations need to be recognized, however, because current models of arthroscopes are used only for the knee and for a few other large joints, such as the shoulder or ankle. Smaller bore instruments now are being introduced that should make arthroscopy more widely applicable. However, when adjacent osteomyelitis is extensive, open drainage and debridement may still be needed.

DEBRIDEMENT IN OSTEOMYELITIS

For hematogenous osteomyelitis, the prognosis for recovery of function is good with suitable antibiotic therapy. Little or no disability is apt to result, even with spontaneous vertebral fusion, and surgical debridement is not necessary. A diagnostic aspiration of exudate from the body of the vertebra or from the disc space can be done, if necessary, to identify the microorganism and its drug sensitivities. If an abscess or spinal cord compression develops, however, surgical drainage and debridement of the infected area are indicated.

DEBRIDEMENT OF AN INFECTED JOINT PROSTHESIS

If an infection occurs during the immediate postoperative period after insertion of the prosthesis, surgical drainage of an infected hematoma and antibiotic therapy can frequently eradicate the infectious process and salvage a functional arthroplasty. With an established infection, however, the prosthetic device and associated acrylic bone cement almost always must be removed. Three surgical approaches are then possible: (1) immediate reconstruction during the same surgical procedure—a one-stage exchange arthroplasty; (2) delayed reconstruction at a future date—a two-stage arthroplasty; and (3) if the bone stock is insufficient, a new approach with debridement followed by a bone grafting procedure in 6 months and a reconstructive arthroplasty 12 to 18 months after debridement—a three-stage arthroplasty. The one-stage procedure with gentamicin-impregnated cement may provide short-term success, but long-term results are less favorable. The two-stage procedure, however, can usually be successfully performed 3 months after resection arthroplasty for infections from which streptococci other than enterococci, methicillin-susceptible staphylococci, and gram-positive bacilli were isolated. For all other agents, reconstruction should be delayed for 12 months.[94,95,168]

GENERAL SUPPORTIVE MEASURES

The affected joint must be kept at rest during the acute phases of the illness. A splint helps to reduce pain and, by immobilization, to control inflammation. A posterior resting splint of the leg or arm is usually sufficient. In an experimental model of infectious arthritis in the rabbit, use of continuous passive motion (CPM) for the infected joint was associated with less articular cartilage damage.[169] Therefore, the use of a CPM device in a patient with sepsis of the knee might prove effective in much the same way such a device improves function in the patient who receives a total knee replacement. Patients in the acute phase of infectious spondylitis should be treated by bed rest. If a danger of subluxation exists, the spine should be immobilized in a plaster shell or brace.

As the inflammatory process subsides, one should attempt to restore range of motion and to increase muscle strength gradually. Passive exercises, followed by graded active exercises, are begun with the assistance of a physical therapist. Weight-bearing should be deferred until signs of acute inflammation have disappeared.

In addition to treatment of the joint, efforts are needed to control the primary infection that led to the arthritis, to supply fluids and nutrition, and to control pain. Anti-inflammatory drugs, including aspirin, should be withheld for several days or longer until the response of the joint to the antibiotic can be correctly assessed. Codeine or propoxyphene, which have no anti-inflammatory properties, can be used to control pain.

ONGOING EVALUATION OF THE TREATMENT PROGRAM

Clinical and laboratory studies are used to monitor the outcome of infectious arthritis.

ACUTE STAGE OF INFECTIOUS ARTHRITIS

The response of the infection to treatment is assessed by changes in tenderness, heat, swelling, and range of motion of the affected joint. The frequency of aspiration is reduced as the volume and the inflammatory character of the fluid decrease. If one is uncertain whether effective bactericidal levels have been achieved because of a change in the type, dose, or route of administration of an antibiotic drug, a tube-dilution assay of paired serum and synovial fluid should be performed. If joint fluid is no longer obtainable, assay of antibiotic concentrations of blood alone provides an acceptable approximation of the drug concentration in the joint. The results of this continuous monitoring should be charted chronologically, so the effectiveness of the treatment program can be accurately determined.

Antibiotic therapy is ordinarily continued for about a week after all systemic or local findings of inflammation have subsided. In staphylococcal and in some gram-negative bacillary infections, which respond more slowly, this period is extended to several weeks. The patient should be observed for another few weeks after cessation of antibiotic therapy for any sign of relapse. If the infection is slow to improve or if it worsens during any phase of the treatment period, one must review all aspects of the program. The following questions should be asked: Was the joint fluid rendered sterile? Were bactericidal levels of antibiotic in the joint fluid achieved? Was needle aspiration successful in decompressing the joint? Answers to these questions dictate the appropriate change in the type or the dosage of antibiotic administered or in the method of drainage. Consultation from the outset with an infectious-disease specialist and with an orthopedic surgeon is invaluable in planning a co-ordinated approach.

ILLUSTRATIVE CASE

A patient with RA with a chronic effusion of the knee developed septic arthritis of that joint. Because it was possible to sample synovial fluid repeatedly, the response to treatment could be monitored periodically (Fig. 115–11). Gram-positive cocci, subsequently proved to be Staphylococcus aureus, were identified in the smear of fluid obtained from the knee. Penicillin G was given intravenously. On the second day of treatment, bactericidal levels of antibiotic against the staphylococcus recovered from the joint were present, but the patient developed an intense allergic response that required the substitution of lincomycin. Again, suitable bactericidal drug concentrations were achieved. As the patient improved, smaller amounts of fluid were obtained by needle aspiration from the joint. For the balance of the treatment schedule, erythromycin was given. Initially by the intravenous route and later orally, bactericidal levels of drug were noted. After the patient's discharge from the hospital after 29 days, oral medica-

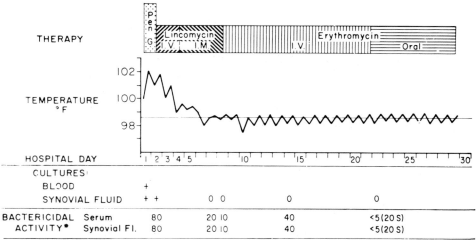

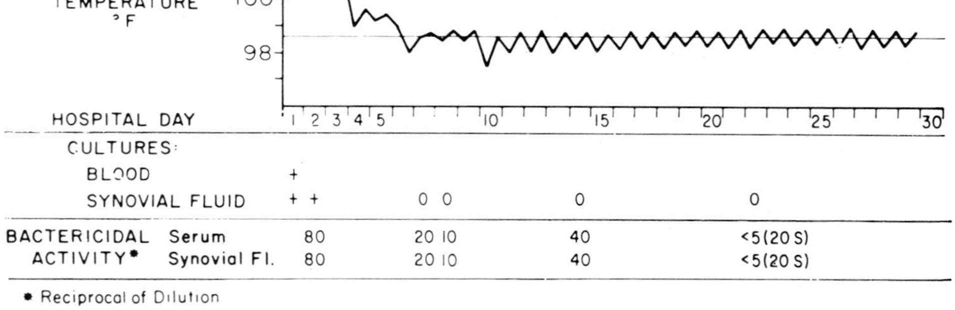

FIGURE 115–11. Response of a 56-year-old white male patient with septic arthritis to antibiotic treatment. Comparable bactericidal drug levels were achieved in the joint fluid and blood for each drug. I.V. = intravenous; I.M. = intramuscular.

tion was continued for another 2 weeks. Although this patient had developed septic arthritis in a joint already damaged by RA, prompt diagnosis and therapy prevented further loss of joint function.

LATE OUTCOMES OF INFECTIOUS ARTHRITIS

Any septic joint untreated or inadequately treated for more than 1 or 2 weeks may develop some of the pathologic changes of a chronic infection. These manifestations include damage to cartilage and bone, increased fibrosis, and ultimately, destruction of the normal joint mechanism.[159] Fortunately, the number of such complications has decreased since the introduction of antibiotic therapy. In one large clinic, the number of cases of bacterial arthritis decreased approximately by half from 1952 to 1957, when compared to two periods extending, respectively, from 1939 to 1945 and from 1946 to 1951. This reduction occurred in the number of patients with chronic, rather than acute, disease.[43]

In patients with chronic disease, a major effort should be directed toward analysis of the factor(s) responsible for the failure of the therapeutic regimen. The bacterial status of the joint should be reevaluated by a synovial fluid culture obtained several days after withdrawal of all antibiotics and again a week or two later if active synovitis persists.

Open arthrotomy or arthroscopy may be required for adequate drainage and excision of necrotic bone and soft tissue, including sinuses.[162,164,166] Tissue should be obtained for culture as well as for histologic examination. Culture of synovial tissue may be positive when the synovial fluid is sterile. Care must be taken to inoculate a wide range of culture media to facilitate the recovery of fungi or mycobacteria, agents that may have eluded earlier detection. Moreover, during inspection of the joint, a nonradiopaque foreign body, such as a plant thorn, that had allowed the inflammatory process to persist may be found and removed.

Antibiotics, such as the penicillins and cephalosporins, that inhibit bacterial cell-wall synthesis may induce the formation of cell-wall-free bacteria or protoplasts. Little evidence suggests that these crippled bacteria are pathogenic.[47,130] In one case familiar to me, such forms of bacteria, as well as native bacterial forms of Staphylococcus aureus, were cultured from the necrotic remnants of a patient's patella after several months of continuous penicillin therapy. In the postoperative period, this patient was treated successfully with erythromycin because this drug influences bacterial metabolism by means other than the inhibition of cell-wall synthesis.

The prognosis for the complete recovery of function in a previously normal joint infected with antibiotic-sensitive bacteria is generally excellent when treatment is begun within a few days of the onset of infection. Delayed diagnosis is directly related to a poorer outcome. The prognosis may be difficult to judge at the outset.[37] In one study, the predictability of good results was not completely ascertained until many months later.[159] Thus, long-term observation is necessary to determine the end result.

RECONSTRUCTION OF DAMAGED JOINTS

If a joint has been damaged, reconstructive procedures may be considered, but the operation should be deferred until all evidence of infection has been absent for several months. Arthroplasty or fusion of a joint may be indicated.[170,171] However, prosthetic replacement to restore normal joint function is now widely accepted.[172–174] Guidelines for this procedure generally follow those that were given previously for the insertion of a new prosthesis into the site of a prior infected joint prosthesis.[94,95,168] The possibility of re-exacerbating a dormant infection, however, must always be considered, particularly in patients with tuberculosis. Nevertheless, prosthetic replacement of a damaged hip, knee, and other joint has been undertaken with satisfactory results.

LATE OUTCOMES OF OSTEOMYELITIS

The therapeutic program for patients with osteomyelitis needs closer monitoring than that for patients with septic arthritis. Clinical findings at the site of the bone infection and serial radiologic and scintiphotographic examinations are used to determine whether the infection has been eradicated. In hematogenous osteomyelitis of a long bone or a vertebra, antibiotics are given orally for several weeks after initial intravenous use; in chronic osteomyelitis, most often when secondary to continuous infection, long-term oral therapy has been successful.[40] Surgical treatment of osteomyelitis is largely empiric and is based on concepts that have gained wide acceptance, some with and others without scientific documentation. Included are drainage of infected areas, excision of necrotic bone, and removal of sequestra and foreign material, such as cement and prostheses.[40]

The likelihood of only partial eradication of the infection is greater in osteomyelitis than in septic arthritis. Reactivation has been recognized many years after the implantation of the original infection. The late outcome of acute hematogenous osteomyelitis in children between 1947 and 1976 was failure to cure or recurrence in almost 20% of cases, most often in the first year. Half of these patients had more than a single recurrence. With the more effective use of antibiotics, especially in those over age 16, the failure rates were lower.[175] Treatment of a recurrence requires extended antibiotic administration, usually for months.[176] For staphylococcal osteomyelitis, a penicillinase-resistant penicillin can be given orally or, in some cases, intravenously by a pump mechanism that delivers the antibiotic into a subcutaneously implanted reservoir. At the same time, the involved bone needs to be evaluated by the surgeon for possible osteotomy to remove residual necrotic materials. Persistent treatment almost always eradicates the infection.

REFERENCES

1. Chusid, M.J., Jacobs, W.M., and Sty, J.R.: Pseudomonas arthritis following puncture wounds of the foot. J. Pediatr., *94*:429–431, 1979.
2. Smith, W.S., and Ward, R.M.: Septic arthritis of the hip complicating perforation of abdominal organs. JAMA, *195*:1148–1150, 1966.
3. Schoolnick, G.K., Ochs, H.O., and Buchanan, T.M.: Immunoglobulin class responsible for gonococcal bactericidal activity of normal human sera. J. Immunol., *122*:1771–1779, 1979.
4. Cluff, L.E., et al.: Staphylococcal bacteremia and altered host resistance. Ann. Intern. Med., *69*:859–873, 1968.
5. Spickett, G.P., Misbah, S.A., and Chapel, H.M.: Primary antibody deficiency in adults. Lancet, *337*:281–284, 1991.
6. Petersen, B.H., et al.: Neisseria meningitidis and Neisseria gonorrhoeae bacteremia associated with C6, C7, or C8 deficiency. Ann. Intern. Med., *90*:917–920, 1979.
7. Goldenberg, D.L., and Cohen, A.S.: Acute infectious arthritis: a review of patients with nongonococcal joint infections (with emphasis on therapy and prognosis). Am. J. Med., *60*:369–377, 1976.
8. Willkens, R.F., Healey, L.A., and Decker, J.L.: Acute infectious arthritis in the aged and chronically ill. Arch. Intern. Med., *106*:354–364, 1960.
9. Kellgren, J.H., et al.: Suppurative arthritis complicating rheumatoid arthritis. Br. Med. J., *1*:1193–1200, 1958.
10. Mills, L.C., et al.: Septic arthritis as a complication of orally given steroid therapy. JAMA, *164*:1310–1314, 1957.
11. Vincenti, F.: Septic arthritis following renal transplantation. Nephron, *30*:253–256, 1982.
12. Heinicke, M.: Crystal arthropathy as a complication of septic arthritis. J. Rheumatol., *8*:529–531, 1981.
13. McConville, J.H., et al.: Septic and crystalline joint disease: a simultaneous occurrence. JAMA, *231*:841–842, 1975.
14. Gardner, G.C., and Weisman, M.H.: Pyarthrosis in patients with rheumatoid arthritis: A report of 13 cases and a review of the literature for the past 40 years. Am. J. Med., *88*:503–511, 1990.
15. Smith, J.R., and Phelps, P.: Septic arthritis, gout, pseudogout and osteoarthritis in the knee of a patient with multiple myeloma. Arthritis Rheum., *15*:89–96, 1972.
16. Mahowald, M.L.: Animal models of infectious arthritis. Clin. Rheum. Dis., *12*:403–421, 1986.
17. Reginato, A.J., et al.: Synovitis in secondary syphilis: clinical, light, and electronmicroscopic studies. Arthritis Rheum., *22*:170–176, 1979.
18. Tesar, J.T., and Dietz, F.: Mechanisms of inflammation in infectious arthritis. Clin. Rheum. Dis., *4*:51–61, 1978.
19. Mahowald, M.L., et al.: Experimental septic arthritis in rabbits with antigen induced arthritis following intra-articular injection of *Staphylococcal aureus*. J. Infect Dis., *154*:273–282, 1986.
20. Kushner, I., and Somerville, J.A.: Permeability of human synovial membrane to plasma proteins: relationship to molecular size and inflammation. Arthritis Rheum., *14*:560–570, 1971.
21. Bobechko, W.P., and Mandell, L.: Immunology of cartilage in septic arthritis. Clin. Orthop. Res., *108*:84–89, 1975.
22. Hadler, N.M.: Phlogistic properties of microbial debris. Semin. Arthritis Rheum., *8*:1–16, 1978.
23. Ward, P.A., et al.: Generation by bacterial proteinases of leukotactic factors from human serum and human C3 and C5. J. Immunol., *111*:1003–1006, 1973.
24. Phemister, D.B.: The effect of pressure on articular surfaces in pyogenic and tuberculous arthritides and its bearing on treatment. Ann. Surg., *80*:481–500, 1924.
25. Parker, R.H., Birbara, C., and Schmid, F.R.: Passage of nafcillin and ampicillin into synovial fluid. *In* Staphylococci and Staphylococcal Diseases. Edited by J. Jeljaszewicz. Stuttgart, New York, Gustav Fischer Verlag, pp. 1151–1123, 1976.
26. Borenstein, D.G., Gibbs, C.A., and Jacobs, R.P.: Gas-liquid chromatographic analysis of synovial fluid: succinic acid and lactic acid as markers for septic arthritis. Arthritis Rheum., *25*:947–953, 1982.
27. Eagle, H.: Experimental approach to the problem of treatment failure with penicillin. I. Group A streptococcal infection in mice. Am. J. Med., *13*:389–399, 1952.
28. Harris, E.D., Jr., and Krane, S.M.: Collagenases. N. Engl. J. Med., *291*:605–609, 1974.
29. McCarty, D.J., Jr., Phelps, P., and Pyenson, J.: Crystal-induced inflammation in canine joints. I. An experimental model with quantification of the host response. J. Exp. Med., *124*:99–114, 1966.
30. Steere, A.C., et al.: Elevated levels of collagenase and prostaglandin E_2 from synovium associated with erosion of cartilage and bone in a patient with chronic Lyme arthritis. Arthritis Rheum., *23*:591–599, 1980.
31. Yaron, M., et al.: Stimulation of prostaglandin E production by bacterial endotoxins in cultured human synovial fibroblasts. Arthritis Rheum., *23*:921–925, 1980.
32. Canoso, J.J., and Sheckman, P.R.: Septic subcutaneous bursitis: report of sixteen cases. J. Rheumatol., *6*:96–102, 1979.
33. Ho, G., Jr., and Tice, A.D.: Comparison of nonseptic and septic bursitis: further observations on the treatment of septic bursitis. Arch. Intern. Med., *139*:1269–1273, 1979.
34. Curtiss, P.H., and Klein, L.: Destruction of articular cartilage in septic arthritis. J. Bone Joint Surg., *45A*:797–806, 1963.
35. Roy, S., and Bhawan, J.: Ultrastructure of articular cartilage in pyogenic arthritis. Arch. Pathol., *99*:44–47, 1975.
36. Ziff, M., Gribetz, H.J., and LoSpalluto, J.: Effect of leukocyte and synovial membrane extracts on cartilage mucoprotein. J. Clin. Invest., *39*:405–412, 1960.
37. Fink, C.W., and Nelson, J.D.: Septic arthritis and osteomyelitis in children. Clin. Rheum. Dis., *12*:423–435, 1986.
38. Peterson, S.: Acute haematogenous osteomyelitis and septic arthritis in childhood: a 10 year review and follow-up. Acta Orthop. Scand., *51*:451–457, 1980.
39. Waldvogel, F.A., Medoff, G., and Schwartz, M.N.: Osteomyelitis: a review of clinical features, therapeutic considerations and unusual aspects. N. Engl. J. Med., *282*:198–206, 260–266, 316–322, 1970.
40. Waldvogel, F.A., and Vasey, H.: Osteomyelitis: the past decade. N. Engl. J. Med., *303*:360–370, 1980.
41. Brause, B.D.: Infection associated with prosthetic joints. Clin. Rheum. Dis., *12*:523–536, 1986.
42. Atcheson, S.G., and Ward, J.R.: Acute hematogenous osteomyelitis progressing to septic synovitis and eventual pyarthrosis: the vascular pathway. Arthritis Rheum., *21*:968–971, 1978.
43. Newman, J.H.: Review of septic arthritis throughout the antibiotic era. Ann. Rheum. Dis., *35*:198–205, 1976.
44. Borrela, L., et al.: Septic arthritis in childhood. J. Pediatr., *62*:742–747, 1963.
45. Nelson, J.D.: The bacterial etiology and antibiotic management of septic arthritis in infants and children. Pediatrics, *50*:437–440, 1972.
46. Fink, C.W.: Gonococcal arthritis in children. JAMA, *194*:237–238, 1965.
47. Garcia-Kutzbach, A., et al.: Identification of Neisseria gonorrhoeae in synovial membrane by electron microscopy. J. Infect. Dis., *130*:183–186, 1974.
48. Rosenthal, J., Bole, G.G., and Robinson, W.D.: Acute nongonococcal infectious arthritis. Arthritis Rheum., *23*:889–897, 1980.
49. Sharp, J.T., et al.: Infectious arthritis. Arch. Intern. Med., *139*:1125–1130, 1979.

50. Steere, A.C.: Lyme Disease. N. Engl. J. Med., *321*:586–596, 1989.
51. Sigal, L.H.: Summary of the first 100 patients seen at a Lyme disease referral center. Am. J. Med., *88*:577–581, 1990.
52. Roca, R.P., and Yoshikawa, T.T.: Primary skeletal infections in heroin users: clinical characterization, diagnosis and therapy. Clin. Orthop., *144*:238–248, 1979.
53. Ebong, W.W.: Septic arthritis in patients with sickle-cell disease. Br. J. Rheum., *26*:99–102, 1987.
54. Memon, I.A., et al.: Group B streptococcal osteomyelitis and septic arthritis: its occurrence in infants less than two months old. Am. J. Dis. Child., *133*:921–923, 1979.
55. Dodd, M.J.: Pyogenic arthritis due to Bacteroides complicating rheumatoid arthritis. Ann. Rheum. Dis., *41*:248–249, 1982.
56. Fitzgerald, R.H., Jr.: Anaerobic septic arthritis. Clin. Orthop., *164*:141–148, 1982.
57. Goldenberg, D.L., et al.: Acute arthritis caused by gram negative bacilli: a clinical characterization. Medicine, *53*:197–208, 1974.
58. Aaskov, J.G., Fraser, J.R.E., and Dalglish, D.A.: Specific and non-specific immunological changes in epidemic polyarthritis patients. Aust. J. Exp. Biol. Med. Sci., *59*:599–608, 1981.
59. Manicourt, D.H., and Orloff, S.: Gonococcal arthritis-dermatitis syndrome: study of serum and synovial fluid immune complex levels. Arthritis Rheum., *25*:574–578, 1982.
60. Dienstag, J.L., et al.: Circulating immune complexes in non-A, non-B hepatitis. Lancet, *1*:1265–1267, 1979.
61. Chantler, J.K., Tingle, A.J., and Petty, R.E.: Persistent rubella virus infection associated with chronic arthritis in children. N. Engl. J. Med., *313*:1117–1123, 1985.
62. Hardin, J.A., Steere, A.C., and Malawista, S.E.: Immune complexes and the evolution of Lyme arthritis: dissemination and localization of abnormal Clq-binding activity. N. Engl. J. Med., *301*:1358–1363, 1979.
63. Chantler, J.K., Ford, D.K., and Tingle, A.J.: Rubella-associated arthritis: rescue of rubella virus from peripheral blood lymphocytes two years postvaccination. Infect. Immun., *32*: 1274–1280, 1981.
64. Tuazon, C.U.: Teichoic acid antibodies in osteomyelitis and septic arthritis caused by Staphylococcus aureus. J. Bone Joint Surg., *64A*:762–765, 1982.
65. Williams, R.C., Jr., and Kunkel, H.G.: Rheumatoid factor, complement and conglutinin aberrations in patients with subacute bacterial endocarditis. J. Clin. Invest., *41*:666–675, 1962.
66. Bocanegra, T.S., et al.: Reactive arthritis induced by parasitic infestation. Ann. Intern. Med., *94*:207–209, 1981.
67. Winchester, R., Bernstein, D.H., Fisher, H.D., et al.: The cooccurrence of Reiter's syndrome and acquired immunodeficiency. Ann. Intern. Med., *106*:19–26, 1987.
68. Brandt, K.D., Cathcart, E.S., and Cohen, A.S.: Gonococcal arthritis: clinical features correlated with blood, synovial fluid, and genitourinary cultures. Arthritis Rheum., *17*:503–510, 1974.
69. Garcia-Kutzbach, A., Dismuke, S.E., and Masi, A.T.: Gonococcal arthritis: clinical features and results of penicillin therapy. J. Rheumatol., *1*:210–221, 1974.
70. Keefer, C.S., and Spink, W.W.: Gonococcic arthritis: pathogenesis, mechanism of recovery and treatment. JAMA *109*: 1448–1453, 1937.
71. Keiser, H., Ruben, F.L., and Wolinsky, E.: Clinical forms of gonococcal arthritis. N. Engl. J. Med., *279*:234–240, 1968.
72. Ruskila, D., and Gladman, D.: Musculoskeletal manifestations of infection with human immunodeficiency virus. Rev. Infect. Dis., *12*:223–235, 1990.
73. Richards, A.J.: Ruptured popliteal cyst and pyogenic arthritis. Br. Med. J., *282*:1120–1121, 1981.
74. Nitsche, J.F.: Septic sternoclavicular arthritis with Pasteurella multocida and Streptococcus sanguis. Arthritis Rheum., *25*:467–469, 1982.
75. Kelly, P.J., Martin, W.J., and Coventry, M.B.: Bacterial arthritis of the hip in the adult. J. Bone Joint Surg., *47A*:1005–1018, 1965.
76. Ho, G., Jr., and Mikolich, D.J.: Bacterial infection of the superficial subcutaneous bursae. Clin. Rheum. Dis., *12*:437–457, 1986.
77. Gelberman, R.H., et al.: Pyogenic arthritis of the shoulder in adults. J. Bone Joint Surg., *62A*:550–553, 1980.
78. Gordon, G., and Kabins, S.A.: Pyogenic sacroiliitis. Am. J. Med., *69*:50–56, 1980.
79. Schaad, U.B., McCracken, G.H., and Nelson, J.D.: Pyogenic arthritis of the sacroiliac joint in pediatric patients. Pediatrics, *66*:375–379, 1980.
80. Sequeira, W., et al.: Pyogenic infections of the pubic symphysis. Ann. Intern. Med., *96*:604–606, 1982.
81. Morrissy, R.T.: Bone and joint infection in the neonate. Pediatr. Ann., *18*:33–44, 1989.
82. Fielding, J.W., and Lieber, W.A.: Septic dislocation of hip joint in infancy: follow-up of fifteen years. N.Y. State J. Med., *61*:3916–3917, 1961.
83. Lunseth, P.A., and Heiple, K.G.: Prognosis in septic arthritis of the hip in children. Clin. Orthop., *139*:81–85, 1979.
84. Stetson, J.W., DePonte, R.J., and Southwick, W.O.: Acute septic arthritis of the hip in children. Clin. Orthop., *56*:105–116, 1968.
85. Morrey, B.F., Bianco, A.J., and Rhodes, K.H.: Suppurative arthritis of the hip in children. J. Bone Joint Surg., *58A*:388–392, 1976.
86. Asnes, R.S., and Arendar, G.M.: Septic arthritis of the hip: a complication of femoral venipuncture. Pediatrics, *38*:837–841, 1966.
87. Flatman, J.G.: Hip disease with referred pain to the knee. JAMA, *234*:967–968, 1975.
88. Morrey, B.F., Bianco, A.J., and Rhodes, K.H.: Hematogenous osteomyelitis at uncommon sites in children. Mayo Clin. Proc., *53*:707–713, 1978.
89. Bernard, T.N., Jr., and Haddad, R.J.: Fever of undetermined etiology masks vertebral osteomyelitis. Orthop. Rev., *9*:63–71, 1982.
90. Coy, J.T., III, et al.: Pyogenic arthritis of the sacro-iliac joint: long-term follow-up. J. Bone Joint Surg., *58A*:845–849, 1976.
91. Delbarre, F., et al.: Pyogenic infection of the sacro-iliac joint: report of thirteen cases. J. Bone Joint Surg., *57A*:819–825, 1975.
92. Howe, R.S., Starshak, R.J., and Chusid, M.J.: Chronic recurrent multifocal osteomyelitis: Case report and review of the literature. Clin. Pediatr., *28*:54–59, 1989.
93. Petty, R.E.: Septic arthritis and osteomyelitis in children. Curr. Opin. Rheumatol., *2*:616–621, 1990.
94. Ross, A.C.: Infection complicating orthopedic procedures and arthroplasties. Curr. Opin. Rheumatol., *2*:628–634, 1990.
95. Wilson, M.G., Kelley, K., and Thornhill, T.S.: Infection as a complication of total knee replacement arthroplasty. J. Bone Joint Surg. [A], *72*:878–883, 1990.
96. Hamilton, M.E., et al.: Simultaneous gout and pyarthrosis. Arch. Intern. Med., *140*:917–919, 1980.
97. McCarty, D.J.: Joint sepsis: a chance for cure: (Editorial.) JAMA, *247*:835, 1982.
98. Miskew, D.B., Block, R.A., and Witt, P.F.: Aspiration of infected sacro-iliac joints. J. Bone Joint Surg., *61A*:1071–1072, 1979.
99. Hendrix, R.W., Lin, P.P., and Kane, W.J.: Simplified aspiration or injection technique for the sacroiliac joint. J. Bone Joint Surg., *64A*:1249–1252, 1982.
100. Scheinberg, M.A., and Benson, M.D.: SAA amyloid protein levels in amyloid-prone chronic inflammatory disorders: lack of

association with amyloid disease. J. Rheumatol., *7*:724–726, 1980.
101. Honig, S., Gorevic, P., and Weissmann, G.: CRP in SLE patients: an aid in diagnosing superimposed infections. Arthritis Rheum., *20*:121, 1977.
102. Zein, N., Ganuza, C., and Kushner, I.: Significance of serum C-reactive protein elevations in patients with systematic lupus erythematosus. Arthritis Rheum., *21*:605, 1978.
103. Mackiewicz, A., et al.: Marcinkowska-Pieta, R., Ballou, S., Mackiewicz, S., and Kushner, I.: Microheterogeneity of alpha$_1$-acid glycoprotein in the detction of intercurrent infection in systemic lupus erythematosus. Arthritis Rheum., *30*:513–518, 1987.
104. Hendrix, R.W., and Fisher, M.R.: Imaging of septic arthritis. Clin. Rheum. Dis., *12*:459–487, 1986.
105. Pate, D., and Katz, A.: Clostridia discitis: a case report. Arthritis Rheum., *22*:1039–1040, 1979.
106. Schiller, M., et al.: Clostridium perfringens septic arthritis. Report of a case and review of the literature. Clin. Orthop., *139*:92–96, 1979.
107. Lever, A.M.L., Owen, T., and Forsey, J.: Pneumoarthropathy in septic arthritis caused by Streptococcus milleri. Br. Med. J., *285*:24, 1982.
108. Crawford, A.H., and Carothers, T.S.: Hip arthrography in the skeletally immature. Clin. Orthop., *162*:54–60, 1982.
109. Glassberg, G.B., and Ozonoff, M.B.: Arthrographic findings in septic arthritis of the hip in infants. Radiology, *128*:151–155, 1978.
110. Schwartz, A.M., and Goldberg, M.J.: Medial adductor approach to arthrography of the hip in children. Radiology, *132*:483, 1979.
111. Mitchell, M., Howard, B., Haller, J., et al.: Septic arthritis. Radiol. Clin. North Am., *26*:1295–1313, 1988.
112. Azouz, E.M.: Computed tomography in bone and joint infections. J. Can. Assoc. Radiol., *32*:102–106, 1981.
113. Morgan, G.J., Jr.: Early diagnosis of septic arthritis of the sacroiliac joint by use of computed tomography. J. Rheumatol., *8*:979–982, 1981.
114. Majd, M., and Frankel, R.S.: Radionuclide imaging in skeletal inflammatory and ischemic disease in children. AJR, *126*: 832–841, 1976.
115. Coleman, R.E.: Imaging with Tc-99m MDP and Ga-67 citrate in patients with rheumatoid arthritis and suspected septic arthritis. J. Nucl. Med., *23*:479–482, 1982.
116. Lisbona, R., and Rosenthall, L.: Observations on the sequential use of ^{99m}Tc-phosphate complex and ^{67}Ga imaging in osteomyelitis, cellulitis, and septic arthritis. Radiology, *123*:123–129, 1977.
117. Maurer, A.H.: Utility of three-phase skeletal scintigraphy in suspected osteomyelitis. J. Nucl. Med., *22*:941–949, 1981.
118. Ash, J.M., and Gilday, D.L.: The futility of bone scanning in neonatal osteomyelitis. J. Nucl. Med., *21*:417–420, 1980.
119. Murray, I.P.C.: Photopenia in skeletal scintigraphy of suspected bone and joint infection. Clin. Nucl. Med., *7*:13–20, 1982.
120. LaManna, M.M., et al.: An assessment of technetium and gallium scanning in the patient with painful total joint arthroplasty. Orthopedics, *6*:580–582, 1983.
121. Magnuson, J.E., Brown, M.L., Hauser, M.F., et al: In-111-labeled leukocyte scintigraph in suspected orthopedic prosthesis infection: Comparison with other imaging modalities. Radiology, *168*:235–240, 1988.
122. Shmerling, R.H., Delbanco, T.L., Tosteson, A.N.A., and Trentham, D.E.: Synovial fluid tests. What should be ordered? JAMA, *264*:1009–1014, 1990.
123. Hasselbacher, P., Passero, F.C., and Ludvico, C.L.: Sedimentation of leukocytes within the joint space. Pennsylvania Med., *81*:54–55, 1978.
124. Riordan, T.: Synovial fluid lactic acid measurement in the diagnosis and management of septic arthritis. J. Clin. Pathol., *35*:390–394, 1982.
125. Behn, A.R., Matthews, J.A., and Phillips, I.: Lactate UV-system: a rapid method for diagnosis of septic arthritis. Ann. Rheum. Dis., *40*:489–492, 1981.
126. Saez-Llorens, X., Mustafa, M.M., Ramilo, O., et al.: Tumor necrosis factor alpha and interleukin 1 beta in synovial fluids of infants and children with suppurative arthritis. Am. J. Dis. Child, *144*:353–356, 1990.
127. Bunch, T.W., et al.: Synovial fluid complement determination as a diagnostic aid in inflammatory joint diseases. Mayo Clin. Proc., *49*:715–720, 1974.
128. Wofsy, D.: Culture-negative septic arthritis and bacterial endocarditis: diagnosis by synovial biopsy. Arthritis Rheum., *23*:605–607, 1980.
129. Thayer, J.D., and Martin, J.E.: Improved medium selective for cultivation of N. gonorrhoeae and N. meningitidis. Public Health Rep., *81*:559–562, 1966.
130. Holmes, K.K., et al.: Recovery of Neisseria gonorrhoeae from "sterile" synovial fluid in gonococcal arthritis. N. Engl. J. Med., *284*:318–320, 1971.
131. Klein, S.J., Craggs, E., and Konwaler, B.E.: Guinea pig inoculation versus culture for isolation of M. tuberculosis. Am. Rev. Respir. Dis., *87*:451, 1963.
132. Dorff, G.J., Ziokowski, J.S., and Rytel, M.W.: Detection by counterimmunoelectrophoresis of pneumococcal antigen in synovial fluid from septic arthritis. Arthritis Rheum., *18*:613–615, 1975.
133. Merritt, K., et al.: Counter immunoelectrophoresis in the diagnosis of septic arthritis caused by Haemophilus influenzae. J. Bone Joint Surg., *58A*:414–415, 1976.
134. Rytel, M.W.: Rapid diagnostic methods in infectious diseases. Adv. Intern. Med., *20*:37–60, 1975.
135. Schwan, T.G., and Rosa, P.A.: A specific and sensitive assay for the Lyme disease spirochete Borrelia burgdorferi using the polymerase chain reaction. J. Infect. Dis., *160*:1018–1029, 1989.
136. Nielsen, S.L., Young, K.K., and Barbour, A.C.: Detection of Borrelia burgdorferi DNA by the polymerase chain reaction. Mol. Cell. Probes, *4*:73–79, 1990.
137. Salimans, M.M., Holsappel, S., van de Rijke, F.M., et al.: Rapid determination of human parvovirus B19 DNA by dot blot hybridization and the polymerase chain reaction. J. Virol Methods, *23*:19–28, 1989.
138. Schwartz, B.S., Goldstein, M.D., Ribecro, J.M., et al.: Antibody testing in Lyme disease. JAMA, *262*:3431–3434, 1989.
139. Kaell, A.T., Volkman, D.J., Gorevic, P.D., and Dattwyler, R.J.: Positive Lyme serology and subacute bacterial endocarditis. A study of four patients. JAMA, *264*:2916–2918, 1990.
140. Spagna, V.A., and Prior, R.B.: The limulus amebocyte lysate assay. Am. Fam. Physician, *22*:125–128, 1980.
141. Steigbigel, R.T., Johnson, P.K., and Remington, J.S.: The nitroblue tetrazolium reduction test versus conventional hematology in the diagnosis of bacterial infection. N. Engl. J. Med., *290*:235–238, 1974.
142. Rinaldi, R.Z., Harrison, W.O., and Fan, P.T.: Penicillin-resistant gonococcal arthritis: a report of four cases. Ann. Intern. Med., *97*:43–45, 1982.
143. Chang, M.J., Contron, G., and Rodriguez, W.J.: Ampicillin-resistant Hemophilus influenzae type B septic arthritis in children. Clin. Pediatr., *20*:139–141, 1981.
144. Drutz, D.J., et al.: The penetration of penicillin and other anti-

microbials into joint fluid: three case reports with a reappraisal of the literature. J. Bone Joint Surg., *49A*:1415–1421, 1967.
145. Hirsch, H.L., Feffer, H.L., and O'Neil, C.B.: A study of the diffusion of penicillin across the serous membranes of joint cavities. J. Lab. Clin. Med., *31*:535–543, 1946.
146. Latif, R., et al.: Pharmacokinetic and clinical evaluation of moxalactam in infants and children. Rev. Pharmacol. Ther., *3*:222–231, 1981.
147. Nelson, J.D.: Antibiotic concentrations in septic joint effusions. N. Engl. J. Med., *284*:349–353, 1971.
148. Pancoast, S.J., and Neu, H.C.: Antibiotic levels in human bone and synovial fluid used in the evaluation of antimicrobial therapy of joint and skeletal infections. Orthop. Rev., *9*:49–61, 1980.
149. Parker, R.H., and Schmid, F.R.: Antibacterial activity of synovial fluid during therapy of septic arthritis. Arthritis Rheum., *14*:96–104, 1971.
150. Quinlan, W.R., Hall, B.B., and Fitzgerald, R.H., Jr.: Fluid spaces in normal and osteomyelitic canine bone. J. Lab. Clin. Med., *102*:78–87, 1983.
151. Smith, B.R., et al.: Bone penetration of antibiotics. Orthopedics, *6*:187–193, 1983.
152. Ho, G., Jr.: Therapy for septic arthritis. JAMA, *247*:797–800, 1982.
153. Carlsson, A.S., Lidgren, L., and Lindberg, H.: Prophylactic antibiotics against early and late deep infection after total hip replacement. Acta Orthop. Scand., *48*:405–410, 1977.
154. Hirschmann, J.V., and Inui, T.S.: Antimicrobial prophylaxis: a critique of recent trials. Rev. Infect. Dis., *2*:1–23, 1980.
155. Wahlig, H., et al.: The release of gentamicin from polymethylmethacrylate beads. J. Bone Joint Surg., *60B*:270–275, 1978.
156. D'Ambrosia, R.D., Shoji, H., and Heater, R.: Secondarily infected total joint replacements by hematogenous spread. J. Bone Joint Surg., *58A*:450–453, 1976.
157. Dajani, A.S., Bisno, A.L., Chung, K.J., et al.: Prevention of bacterial endocarditis. Recommendations by the American Heart Association. JAMA, *264*:2919–2922. 1990.
158. Dunkle, L.M.: Towards optimum management of serious focal infections. The model of suppurative arthritis. Pediatr. Infect. Dis. J., *8*:195–196, 1989.
159. Howard, J.B., Highgenboten, C.L., and Nelson, J.D.: Residual effects of septic arthritis in infancy and childhood. JAMA, *236*:932–935, 1976.
160. Samilson, R.L., Bersani, F.A., and Watkins, M.B.: Acute suppurative arthritis in infants and children. The importance of early diagnosis and surgical drainage. Pediatrics, *21*:798–803, 1958.
161. Broy, S.B., and Schmid, F.R.: A comparison of medical drainage (needle aspiration) and surgical drainage (arthrotomy or arthroscopy) in the initial treatment of infected joints. Clin. Rheum. Dis., *12*:501–522, 1986.
162. Ballard, A., et al.: Functional treatment of pyogenic arthritis of the adult knee. J. Bone Joint Surg., *57A*:1119–1123, 1975.
163. Kawashima, M., et al.: The treatment of pyogenic bone and joint infections by closed irrigation-suction. Clin. Orthop., *148*:240–244, 1980.
164. Goldenberg, D.L., et al.: Treatment of septic arthritis: comparison of needle aspiration and surgery as initial modes of joint drainage. Arthritis Rheum., *18*:83–90, 1975.
165. Mielants, H.: Long-term functional results of the non-surgical treatment of common bacterial infections of joints. Scand. J. Rheumatol., *11*:101–105, 1982.
166. Jarrett, M.P., et al.: The role of arthroscopy in the treatment of septic arthritis. Arthritis Rheum., *24*:737–739, 1981.
167. Broy, S.B., Stulberg, S.D., and Schmid, F.R.: The role of arthroscopy in the diagnosis and management of the septic joint. Clin. Rheum. Dis., *12*:489–500, 1986.
168. Fitzgerald, R.H., Jr.: Problems associated with the infected total hip arthroplasty. Clin. Rheum. Dis., *12*:537–554, 1986.
169. Salter, R.B.: The protective effect of continuous passive motion on living articular cartilage in acute septic arthritis: an experimental investigation in the rabbit. Clin. Orthop., *159*:223–247, 1981.
170. Price, C.T.: Thompson arthrodesis of the hip in children. J. Bone Joint Surg., *62A*:1118–1123, 1980.
171. Tuli, S.M.: Excision arthroplasty for tuberculous and pyogenic arthritis of the hip. J. Bone Joint Surg., *63B*:29–32, 1981.
172. Jupiter, J.B., et al.: Total hip arthroplasty in the treatment of adult hips with current or quiescent sepsis. J. Bone Joint Surg., *63A*:194–200, 1981.
173. McLaughlin, R.E., and Allen, J.R.: Total hip replacement in the previously infected hip. South. Med. J., *70*:573–575, 1977.
174. Salvati, E.A.: Total hip replacement in current or recent sepsis. Orthop. Rev., *9*:97–102, 1980.
175. Gillespie, W.J.: The management of acute haematogenous osteomyelitis in the antibiotic era: a study of the outcome. J. Bone Joint Surg., *63B*:126–131, 1981.
176. Black, J., Hunt, T.L., Godley, P.H., and Matthew, E.: Oral antimicrobial therapy for adults with osteomyelitis or septic arthritis. J. Infect. Dis., *155*:968–972, 1987.

116

Bacterial Arthritis

GEORGE HO, JR.

The general principles of septic arthritis are discussed in Chapter 115. Characteristics of the host and the microorganisms and the clinical setting in which bacterial arthritis occurs are the subject of this chapter.

BACTERIAL ARTHRITIS IN CHILDREN

The largest American study of septic arthritis in children comes from Dallas. Fink and Nelson reviewed a series of 591 cases collected over 30 years and concluded that there was no significant increase in the incidence of septic arthritis between 1955 and 1984.[1] The mean proportion of their cases wherein a specific pathogen was identified has remained fairly constant at 66%. Table 116–1 summarizes the data from five series, with 865 patients available for analysis. The percentages of cases with bacteriologic confirmation varied from 64 to 100%, in part reflecting the nonuniform inclusion criteria used by the different authors. Overall, 611 of 865 children with septic arthritis (71%) had an identified bacterial etiology.

Cultures of the synovial fluid were positive in only 70 to 97% of the cases of septic arthritis with bacteriologic confirmation (Table 116–1). When antibiotic treatment had been instituted before joint aspiration, the yield of positive synovial fluid cultures dropped to 36%.[4] Similarly, the likelihood of identifying microorganisms on the Gram-stained smear of the synovial fluid was higher in those who had not received antibiotic therapy (54%) than in those who had (19%).[4] Approximately one-third of all Gram-stained smears of infected synovial fluid in children were positive for bacteria.[1]

Blood cultures were positive in 33 to 46% of children with septic arthritis, and were often the only clue in identifying the responsible pathogen. The importance of obtaining blood cultures as well as cultures of other extra-articular sites of infection cannot be overemphasized because positive results enhance the yield of bacteriologic confirmation and aid in planning specific antimicrobial drug therapy.

In children, septic arthritis might be secondary to a contiguous acute osteomyelitis where the metaphysis is intracapsular. These areas include the hip, proximal humerus, proximal radius, and distal tibia. In the neonate, infection of bone with joint involvement is especially common because of the proximity of the joint capsule to the metaphysis.[6] Bony tenderness near the affected joint is an important clue to diagnosis.

Age is an important determinant of the susceptibility of a child to a given pathogen. Whether the infection is community-acquired or nosocomial also influences which organism is most likely to be the cause. The most common bacteria in childhood septic arthritis are Hemophilus influenzae and Staphylococcus aureus. In children between 6 months and 2 years of age, Hemophilus influenzae is most common.[1,2,5] Among children over 5 years old, and in neonates or infants less than 6 months old, Staphylococcus aureus is the major pathogen.

The bacteria that cause septic arthritis in the neonatal and early infancy periods can be further subdivided according to where the infection was acquired.[7] Pathogens in community-acquired joint infections include group B streptococcus (52%), staphylococcus (25%), gonococcus (17%), and gram-negative bacilli (5%). In sharp contrast, the relative frequencies of the hospital-acquired pathogens are staphylococcus (62%), Candida (17%), gram-negative enteric bacilli (13%), and streptococcus and Hemophilus influenzae (4% each). Group B streptococcus is frequently found in the birth canal and is the most frequent agent causing bone and joint infection in the neonate.[6] Candida skeletal infection occurs in the context of the debilitated neonate with a

TABLE 116–1. SEPTIC ARTHRITIS IN CHILDREN

	FINK AND NELSON, 1986[1]	SEQUEIRA ET AL., 1985[2]	WILSON AND DIPAOLA, 1986[3]	SPEISER ET AL., 1985[4]	WELKON ET AL., 1986[5]
Duration of study (years)	1955–1984	1972–1981	1972–1981	1974–1983	1975–1985
Location	Dallas	Chicago	Glasgow	St. Louis	Philadelphia
Total cases	591	32	61	86	95
Percentage of patients with confirmed bacterial diagnosis	66	100	92	84	64
Among those with proven bacterial cause (%)					
Positive Gram's stain of synovial fluid	33	—	—	19–54*	—
Positive culture of synovial fluid	79	97	71–80†	36–70*	84
Positive blood culture	33	—	41	46	46
Site of infection (%)					
Knee	40	37	29	30	49
Hip	23	27	40	29	27
Ankle	13	15	22	17	17
(Total)	76	79	91	76	93
More than 1 affected joint	7	—	5	7	8
Infecting Agent (%)					
Staphylococcus aureus	17	25	44	37	13
Hemophilus influenzae	25	37	16	17	29
Others	25	38	32	29	22
Culture-negative specimens	33	—	8	16	36

* The lower percentages reflect results of studies of patients receiving antibiotics; the higher values are from studies of patients not treated with antibiotics.

† Arthrotomy yielded a 71% positivity rate, vs. 80% for aspirated samples.

central venous catheter who is receiving hyperalimentation and prolonged antibiotic therapy.[6]

The need to determine the local pattern of bacterial causes of septic arthritis is of utmost importance, because the selection of the initial antimicrobial drugs might depend solely on this information. Knowledge about the antibiotic sensitivities of the local bacterial isolates is also crucial. For example, in the Dallas study 18% of the Hemophilus influenzae were β-lactamase–positive and resistant to ampicillin.[1] Similarly, there are regions where methicillin-resistant Staphylococcus aureus is prevalent, especially metropolitan Detroit.[8] Neisseria gonorrhoeae remains a possible cause of septic arthritis in the adolescent and in the young infant, especially when the disease is polyarticular. Gonococcal joint disease in children is polyarticular in 50% of cases, whereas all the other common bacteria cause monoarticular disease (93%) rather than polyarticular disease (7%).[1] In the neonate, who is immunologically immature and whose inflammatory response to infection is weak, bone and joint infection is commonly multifocal.[6]

Joint infections in children favor the large joints of the lower extremities. In a review of infections in 1023 joints, 39% affected the knee, 26% the hip, and 13% the ankle.[1] These three joint sites accounted for 79% of the joint infections in 948 patients. Data from other studies (Table 116–1) confirm this general distribution of joint involvement. Aspiration of both hips of any neonate who has a bone or joint infection at another site has been recommended for the following reasons: in the neonate, the hip is a difficult joint to examine, it is the most common joint to be infected, multifocal skeletal infection is common, and the sequelae of a missed hip infection are severe.[6]

THERAPY

The age-dependent vulnerability to a specific pathogen, the circumstances under which the joint infection is acquired, the knowledge of the regional trends in the bacterial causes of septic arthritis, and the local antibiotic susceptibility patterns, in addition to the fact that approximately 30% of the cases of presumed bacterial arthritis in children have not been bacteriologically confirmed, must all be taken into account when planning drug treatment. The most efficacious, specific, least toxic, and least expensive drug should be chosen. A positive Gram-stained smear of the synovial fluid and the results of the laboratory investigation on extra-articular sites of infection (i.e., cerebral spinal fluid, sputum, and urine) are used to determine the most appropriate antibiotic treatment before culture confirmation. When the Gram-stained smear shows no microorganisms, the initial empirically chosen antimicrobial agent or agents should be broad-spectrum with optimal activity against the most likely pathogens. For example, in the neonate with hospital-acquired bacterial arthritis, the antibiotic regimen must be directed at Staphylococcus aureus as well as gram-negative enteric bacilli. Empiric treatment of community-acquired infection should be directed against group B streptococcus, staphylococcus, and gonococcus. In children between 6 months and 5 years of age in whom Hemophilus influenzae is suspected but

Staphylococcus aureus cannot be ruled out, initial treatment should be chloramphenicol and a penicillinase-resistant penicillin[9] or cefuroxime alone.[4] In the child over age 5 years and in the adolescent, the initial antibiotic treatment should be directed at S. aureus for monoarticular joint disease. Vancomycin should be chosen as the initial antistaphylococcal drug in areas where the prevalence of methicillin resistance is high. Polyarticular disease in a sexually active adolescent deserves treatment directed at Neisseria gonorrhoeae.

The duration of antibiotic therapy and the mode of joint drainage have not been studied in a controlled, prospective fashion. Recommendations on the duration of antibiotic treatment vary between 2 to 4 weeks for uncomplicated bacterial arthritis caused by less virulent pathogens and 4 to 6 weeks for joint sepsis caused by Staphylococcus aureus or gram-negative bacilli and for joint infections complicated by osteomyelitis. The length of hospitalization may be reduced by the use of home intravenous therapy[10,11] or the substitution of oral antibiotic treatment[12,13] in carefully controlled situations.

General agreement regarding the drainage of an infected joint in the child includes the prompt surgical decompression of hip infections and the need for open drainage when repeated needle aspirations show the persistence of infection or when they cannot be carried out satisfactorily because of technical difficulty. The morbidity associated with arthrotomy must be weighed against the benefit gained by initial open drainage. One study showed that infections of joints other than the hip had an excellent chance of responding to nonoperative treatment when there was minimal delay in diagnosis and treatment.[14]

The outcome of treated bacterial arthritis in children is a function of the patient's age, the joint infected, the infecting microorganism, and the promptness of diagnosis and treatment. Overall, about 25% of children with bacterial arthritis had some degree of residual abnormality on long-term follow-up.[15,16] Infants, especially those with infected hips, showed poorer results.[3] Hip infection in general had a less favorable outcome than that of the knee and ankle.[15,16] Of the two most common causes of childhood septic arthritis, Staphylococcus aureus was more likely to lead to residual impairment than was Hemophilus influenzae,[4] although this finding was not invariable.[16] Finally, delay in diagnosis and treatment was certainly detrimental to the outcome of treatment.[14]

BACTERIAL ARTHRITIS IN THE ELDERLY

In 1900 barely 4% of the total American population, or 3 million people, were 65 years and older. Today 12% of the population in the United States, or 28 million people, are 65 or older. By the year 2000, 35 million Americans will be 65 and over.[17] Although the incidence of septic arthritis in adults has not changed significantly over the last several decades,[18] a British study spanning 30 years showed that the percentage of patients older than 60 had increased from 19% between 1954 and 1963 to 45% in the following decade.[19] These observations suggest that although the number of cases of acute bacterial arthritis will increase proportionally to the growth of the population, a larger percentage will come from the geriatric population. An analysis of 402 adults with septic arthritis reported from 1960 to 1986 found that 163 (41%) were more than 60 years old.[20]

Systemic factors impairing the ability of the host to combat infections are numerous. The more prevalent illnesses among adults with septic arthritis are diabetes mellitus, cirrhosis, chronic renal failure, rheumatoid arthritis (RA), and neoplastic disease.[21] Two other major risk factors for infectious complications are associated with the management of these chronic illnesses. One is the employment of invasive diagnostic procedures and surgical interventions, and the other is the lowering of host resistance with immunosuppressive drugs. Even in the absence of overt systemic illness, aging itself can lead to the decline of immune function and increased susceptibility to infectious diseases.[22]

Table 116–2 summarizes data from five retrospective studies examining nongonococcal bacterial arthritis in 89 elderly patients.[23,24–27] The mean age of the 89 patients was 70.3 years. The prevalence of underlying joint disease ranged from 23 to 71% (mean 61%). Osteoarthritis and RA were the most common of these diseases, but gout, lupus erythematosus, and hemophiliac arthropathy were also noted. Many patients had a history of joint trauma that subsequently became infected. The knee joint was most often affected, followed by the hip, shoulder and wrist.

Finding the presence of monosodium urate or calcium pyrophosphate dihydrate crystals in inflammatory fluids does not preclude the coexistence of a septic process. The simultaneous occurrence of septic arthritis and crystal-induced arthritis is especially common in the geriatric population (see Septic Arthritis Associated with Crystal-Induced Arthritis below).

The microbiology of acute bacterial joint infection in the elderly is not different from that of nongonococcal septic arthritis in adults in general. Staphylococcus aureus was the predominant microorganism, responsible for 43 to 67% of the cases of septic arthritis in the elderly (Table 116–2). Other less common gram-positive coccal causes included various streptococci, pneumococci, and Staphylococcus epidermidis, in that order. Neisseria gonorrhoeae was much less frequent in the elderly, but when it occurred its features were similar to those in a younger person with gonococcal arthritis (see Chapter 117).[28,29]

Gram-negative bacilli have emerged as a significant cause of septic arthritis in the last two decades[30] because of the increased incidence of bacteremia caused by gram-negative bacillary organisms in general[31] and because of the septic arthritis caused by Pseudomonas aeruginosa[32] and Serratia marcescens[33] in intravenous drug abusers. The latter situation is much less likely in a geriatric population than in young adults. The per-

TABLE 116–2. SEPTIC ARTHRITIS IN THE ELDERLY

	VINCENT AND AMIRAULT, 1990[23]	COOPER AND CAWLEY, 1986[24]	MCGUIRE AND KAUFFMAN, 1985[25]	HO AND SU, 1982[26]	WILLKENS ET AL., 1960[27]
Study period	1979–88	1973–82	1973–83	1975–80	1954–59
No. of patients	21	21	23	11	13
Mean age	72.3	73.8	67.1	66.7	69.9
Age range	60–92	60–85	60–87	60–78	60–82
With underlying joint disease	71%	71%	65%	55%	23%
With knee infections	38%	48%	43%	55%	54%
Next most-frequent site of infection	Shoulder (24%)	Hip (38%)	Wrist (17%)	Shoulder (27%)	Shoulder (38%)
Infected with Staphylococcus aureus	67%	43%	52%	64%	62%
Infected with gram-negative bacilli	—	14%	35%	18%	—
In-hospital mortality	29%	33%	22%	9%	—
Poor functional outcome	—	52%	—	40%	46%

centages of the elderly with septic arthritis caused by gram-negative bacilli were 14%, 18%, and 35% in three series (Table 116–2). These figures are similar to the overall rate of 23% reported from the Boston University Medical Center experience of 97 adults between 1965 and 1982.[21]

THERAPY

Treatment of septic arthritis in these five series of elderly patients was examined retrospectively. It did not differ significantly in principle from the current general recommendations on antibiotic treatment[34] and drainage[35] of an infected joint. The outcome of treatment was generally disappointing, with mortality ranging from 9 to 33% (overall 25%) (Table 116–2). Such high mortality was not due solely to the infectious disease that affected the joint. Nosocomial pseudomonas infection contributed significantly in one series.[25] Other age-related chronic diseases contributed to the demise of some of these patients, although the contribution of pre-existing conditions was often difficult to assess. Among survivors, functional outcome was poor in approximately half (Table 116–2); the rate of complications such as osteomyelitis and secondary osteoarthritis was 73% in one series.[23] These results compare unfavorably with the mortality (9%) and morbidity (34%) of adult nongonococcal septic arthritis in general.[36] Factors portending a poor outcome included delay in diagnosis, underlying joint disease (especially RA with polyarticular infection[36]), gram-negative bacillary septic arthritis, involvement of the hip joint, and serious chronic debilitating illnesses such as cancer and liver disease and their associated treatments.

SEPTIC ARTHRITIS COMPLICATING RHEUMATOID ARTHRITIS

Bacterial infection of a joint already affected by RA is "dangerous, not only to limb but to life."[37] That a joint previously damaged by RA is prone to bacterial invasion was recognized in the 1958 report by Kellgren and associates[38] and confirmed by others.[39–47] This serious complication of RA was reviewed comprehensively in 1989[48] and in 1990.[49] The therapeutic use of corticosteroids, cytotoxic drugs, or both, as well as other defects in RA patients such as decreased chemotaxis[50] and phagocytosis of synovial fluid neutrophils,[51] depressed hemolytic complement levels, and decreased bacteriolytic activity of synovial fluid,[52] impair normal host defenses. Which factor is most responsible for the increased susceptibility to joint infection is unclear, but septic arthritis in a patient with RA can have catastrophic results, especially when the diagnosis is delayed.

Typically, the patient is older with long-standing seropositive disease and significant functional impairment and debility (Table 116–3). Nearly half of the patients (45%) were receiving systemic corticosteroids. Thus, the clinical expression of joint infection can be blunted with an onset that is insidious rather than abrupt. The usual signs of fever and toxicity might be absent (Table 116–3); only 56% of cases had peripheral blood leukocytosis. Increased pain in one or more joints can easily be mistaken for an RA flare. The true diagnosis is delayed, and the patient then is treated at a more advanced stage of infection. A high index of suspicion must be maintained and joint fluid must be studied if septic arthritis complicating RA is suspected. One series of cases showed periarticular manifestations (e.g., sinus tract formation, concomitant septic bursitis, and infected synovial cysts) associated with joint infection.[49]

Table 116–3 provides the relative frequencies of the various bacteria found in infections of the rheumatoid joint. Gram-positive cocci caused 89% of the infections, and Staphylococcus aureus was the major pathogen. Gram-negative bacilli were responsible for the remaining cases, with Enterobacteriaceae accounting for most of them. Polymicrobial infection was extremely rare.[40] The spectrum of bacterial causes continues to broaden

TABLE 116–3. BACTERIAL ARTHRITIS IN RHEUMATOID ARTHRITIS PATIENTS*

Number of patients	116
Patient characteristics	
Mean age in years (range)	56 (27–82)
Mean duration of RA in years (range)	14 (1–55)
Systemic corticosteroid therapy	45% (51 ÷ 113)
Clinical features	
Fever	76% (62/82)
Leukocytosis >10,000 cells/mm^3	56% (43/77)
Polyarticular infection	25% (22/89)
Microbiology of 109 bacterial isolates†	
Gram-positive cocci	89% (97/109)
Staphylococcus aureus	77%
Staphylococcus epidermidis	2%
Hemolytic streptococcus	7%
Streptococcus pneumoniae	3%
Gram-negative bacilli	11% (12/109)
Escherichia coli	6%
Proteus mirabilis	1%
Morganella morganii	1%
Salmonella spp.	1%
Pseudomonas aeruginosa	1%
Hemophilus influenzae	1%
Fusobacterium necrophorum	1%
Outcome	
Deaths	25% (29/116)
Range of mortality rates	0–88%
Survivors with good outcome	50% (25/50)

*Analysis of 89 cases taken from references 39 through 47 published between 1966 and 1986 plus 27 cases from 1958 to 1964 reviewed in reference 39.

† See text for other bacteria responsible for septic arthritis in RA patients.

**1% each for Proteus mirabilis, Morganella morganii, Salmonella spp., Pseudomonas aeruginosa, Hemophilus influenza, and Fusobacterium necrophorum.

with reports of cases caused by uncommon and opportunistic pathogens, including Plesiomonas shigelloides,[53] Pasteurella multocida,[54] Kingella kingae,[55] Listeria monocytogenes,[56] Micrococcus luteus,[57] Bacteroides melaninogenicus,[58] and Bacteroides fragilis.[58] Polyarticular infections occurred in 25% of cases. Some microorganisms have a predilection to infect multiple joints, for example, Bacteroides fragilis,[59] pneumococcus,[60] and group G streptococcus.[61] Rheumatoid damage occurs often in multiple joints, and this can predispose to polyarticular localization of infection. Large joints, especially the knee, are affected most commonly but unusual sites such as the temporomandibular joint[62] and the cricoarytenoid joint can be involved.[63]

THERAPY

Treatment of septic arthritis superimposed on RA adheres to the principles of therapy for acute bacterial arthritis in general. Systemic antibiotic administration and adequate drainage of the purulent synovial fluid are necessary. Whether the infected rheumatoid joint is better served by immediate open surgical drainage and debridement is debatable.[42,49] Open drainage, however, might be indicated because the diagnosis of infection is often delayed and rheumatoid joints are often difficult to aspirate completely because of intrasynovial adhesions and debris (rice bodies). The deleterious effect of delayed diagnosis on outcome is illustrated by a study showing that patients with full recovery had an average delay of 6.6 days between onset of symptoms to diagnosis, whereas in those with a poor outcome the average delay was 18.0 days.[47]

The mortality of 25% in patients with RA complicated by acute septic arthritis (Table 116–3) is much higher than the rate of 9% in adults with nongonococcal septic arthritis.[36] This is due in part to the extremely poor outcome (mortality of 56%) of rheumatoid patients with polyarticular septic arthritis.[36] Only half of surviving patients recovered their preinfection level of function. Thus, septic arthritis is a serious complication of RA that requires early diagnosis and aggressive treatment.

BONE AND JOINT INFECTIONS ASSOCIATED WITH INTRAVENOUS DRUG ABUSE

The rheumatic manifestations of diseases associated with illicit substance abuse have been reviewed.[64] Infectious complications of parenteral drug abuse include viral infections such as hepatitis B and human immunodeficiency virus infection, bacterial infections such as skin abscesses or endocarditis, and fungal infections such as candidemia. Bacterial infections of the skeletal system include osteomyelitis and septic arthritis. The pathogenesis is believed to involve hematogenous dissemination of bacteria injected into the bloodstream with the illicit drug. Staphylococcus aureus infections often come from the patient. The carrier rate of S. aureus in the nose and throat and on the skin of parenteral drug abusers is very high.[65] Contamination of shared dirty needles and syringes serves as a reservoir for Pseudomonas aeruginosa.[66] The predilection for such infections to involve the bones of the vertebral column and the fibrocartilaginous joints of the pelvis and the sternum has been noted by some authors,[32,67] but less frequently by others.[68]

The relative frequencies of the different sites of skeletal infection were analyzed from 158 reported cases.[32,67] Most common was the lumbar vertebral column (49%), followed by the cervical and thoracic vertebral columns.[67] The least common sites were the large peripheral diarthrodial joints (17%). The fibrocartilaginous articulations were involved in 33% of cases, including the sacroiliac joint (9 to 20%),[69] the symphysis pubis (3 to 9%),[70] the ischium (3 to 9%), [67] the sternoclavicular joint (6 to 10%),[71] and the other sternoarticulations (8%). The latter included the sternocostal[71] and sternomanubrial joints.[72]

The bacteriology of these skeletal infections primarily reflects pathogens contaminating the blood. In one review, 78% of the infections were caused by Pseudomonas aeruginosa, 11% were due to gram-positive cocci including staphylococci and streptococci, and the remainder were due to the Klebsiella (3%), Enterobacter

(4%), and Serratia (5%) groups of gram-negative microorganisms.[67] The prevalence of the different bacterial pathogens varied from region to region. In a series of 45 patients from Detroit, staphylococci and streptococci were the predominant microorganisms (82%).[68] Another report from Detroit illustrated the changing trends by comparing an experience from 1966 to 1977 with one from 1981 to 1982.[8] They found an increased incidence of bacterial arthritis, an increased number of drug addicts among their patients with septic arthritis, a decreased number of cases caused by Pseudomonas, and an increased number of cases resulting from methicillin-resistant Staphylococcus aureus.

Infections of the axial skeleton caused by gram-negative bacilli in addicts had a more insidious clinical presentation with less toxicity[32] and a longer duration of symptoms[67] than did acute staphylococcal infection of a peripheral joint. Similarly, physical findings in patients with axial skeleton involvement were less obvious than in those with peripheral joint infection. Bone scintigraphy was useful in localizing skeletal infections when plain radiographs were unrevealing. Once the site of suspected infection is localized, the bacterial cause can and should be sought aggressively. Aspiration of synovial fluid, needle biopsy of the synovium, aspiration under fluoroscopic guidance, or open biopsy and culture of affected bone or joint tissue are used as needed.

THERAPY

Antimicrobial treatment is directed at the isolated bacteria according to in-vitro antibiotic sensitivities. Against Pseudomonas, the combination of an aminoglycoside and an antipseudomonal penicillin is recommended. The duration of antibiotic treatment is usually 4 to 6 weeks. Surgical decompression, drainage, or debridement is necessary in patients with epidural or paravertebral abscess complicating vertebral infection, with osteomyelitis or retrosternal abscess accompanying sternoarticular disease, with abscess or sequestra in periarticular osteomyelitis of the sacroiliac joint or the symphysis pubis, and with hip infection or infection of another peripheral joint that fails to respond to repeated needle aspirations and adequate systemic antibiotic therapy. The immediate outcome of treatment of these skeletal infections in drug addicts is generally favorable. Long-term results in this population are rarely available.[68]

BACTERIAL INFECTION OF PROSTHETIC JOINTS

Bacterial infection occurring in a prosthetic joint is an extremely grave and costly complication of total joint replacement. A conservative estimate of the cost of treating infected joint prostheses in the United States alone is between 40 and 80 million dollars per year.[73] Besides the expense of medical care, there is the agony of the return of symptoms, loss of function, and risk of uncontrolled infection resulting in the loss of limb or life. However, millions have benefited from joint replacement for advanced arthritis of the hip, knee, and other joints. Because the need for these operations is greatest in people over 60 years old[74] and the aging population in the United States is enlarging,[17] the number of people undergoing prosthetic joint replacement will continue to rise.

Under optimal conditions, the overall infection rate of total joint replacement is probably close to 1%,[75,76] which is below the 2% for total hip replacement and 4% for total knee replacement cited in a 1983 review.[77] The experience with prostheses for the shoulder, elbow, or ankle is more limited in both number and duration of follow-up. Reported infection rates for total elbow replacement are as high as 6%[76] and 9%.[78] Such figures are similar to the higher infection rates for hip or knee prostheses when these were first performed.[77]

There are two ways to classify prosthetic joint infections: (1) by the route of bacterial invasion, that is, direct introduction at the time of surgery versus hematogenous seeding from an extra-articular site, and (2) by the time of occurrence of infection after implantation of the prosthesis, that is, early or acute (usually within 12 weeks), delayed or subacute (up to 12 months), and late (greater than 1 year). Neither classification is totally satisfactory. For the former, accurate categorization is difficult because the source of the bacteria is often obscure. In the latter classification, the subdivisions have been criticized as being arbitrary. Early infections are mostly related to postoperative wound infection and respond to prompt aggressive treatment; retention of the original prosthesis is more likely. Late infections usually result from hematogenous dissemination of bacteria and are more common in RA patients.[79,80] The relative frequencies are 36 to 50% for early, 23 to 45% for delayed, and 15 to 27% for late infections.[77,80–82] Hematogenous seeding seems to be responsible for 20 to 40% of all cases of prosthetic joint infection.[83]

Certain patients are at greater risk. Many factors predispose to infection, including impairment of host defense, the surgical technique employed, the duration of the operation, and the material and design of the prosthesis. RA confers a higher risk of prosthetic joint infection, especially the late hematogenous type.[76,79,80] Revision arthroplasty is technically more difficult than primary joint replacement and often prolongs the operation. Increased operation time contributes to the increased infection rate in joints that have undergone previous surgery.[76,84] In one study, changing from a posterior to a posterolateral surgical approach in total elbow replacement was thought to have lowered the rate of infection from 6% to 2.5%.[76] The less constrained design of knee joint prostheses, allowing for natural multiaxial movement, might have reduced the incidence of both septic and aseptic failures.[76]

Pain most commonly (95% of the time) heralds infection in a joint prosthesis; fever (43%), swelling (38%), and drainage through the skin (32%) occur less commonly.[83] Presentation can be acute and fulminant or it can be indolent, with a gradual onset of pain in a previously painless prosthesis. The virulence of the causative bacteria influences the acuteness and the severity of the clinical presentation. The possibility of infection must always be entertained when the site of a prosthetic joint becomes painful, when there are signs of local inflammation or drainage, or when there is progressive radiographic evidence of loosening.

Aspiration of joint fluid for the isolation of the bacterial pathogen is the most specific means of establishing the diagnosis. The Gram-stained smear of the joint aspirate is positive for microorganisms in approximately 30% of cases.[83] Estimates of culture-negative joint aspirates vary between 2 to 15%[83] and 7 to 15%,[77] and the diagnosis of prosthetic infection in these instances is made at the time of surgery when periprosthetic specimens are examined bacteriologically and histologically.

Prosthetic joint infection can be caused by aerobic gram-positive cocci (75 to 80%), aerobic gram-negative rods (10 to 20%), and anaerobic microorganisms (5 to 10%).[82,83] Staphylococci account for 75 to 90% of the gram-positive coccal infections. Staphylococcus epidermidis might be more common than S. aureus in prosthetic joint infections,[83] in contrast with septic arthritis in natural joints, in which S. aureus predominates and S. epidermidis is extremely uncommon. The presence of a foreign body might play a permissive role in infections caused by the less virulent microorganisms.[85] The other gram-positive cocci found in infected prosthetic joints are the various streptococci including groups A, B, G, and D (enterococci),[61,86,87] as well as Streptococcus pneumoniae.[88] Among the gram-negative bacilli, Escherichia coli, Proteus mirabilis, and Pseudomonas aeruginosa are the major culprits.[89] The less common gram-negative pathogens include Enterobacter aerogenes, Pasteurella multocida, Moraxella, Klebsiella, Salmonella, and Serratia.[79,81,89,90] Anaerobic bacteria, accounting for 5 to 10% of infections, include Peptococcus species, Peptostreptococcus species, Clostridium perfringens, and Bacteroides fragilis.[86,91] Other rare causes are corynebacteria (aerobic diphtheroides), Propionibacterium acnes (anaerobic diphtheroides),[78] Hemophilus influenzae,[76] Listeria monocytogenes,[81] Aeromonas hydrophila,[79] Pseudomonas pyocyanea,[80] and Mycoplasma hominis.[92] Infections caused by mixed microorganisms, or polymicrobial disease, range from 6%[86] to 25%,[76] and these are usually early infections.

THERAPY

Antibiotics directed at the isolated pathogen(s) and surgical debridement or removal of the infected prosthesis are essential steps in management. A review on the outcome of treatment of prosthetic joint infections in the elderly revealed generally poor results.[93] The best chance for retention of the prosthesis is in the patient with early, postoperative infection that is diagnosed promptly and treated aggressively.[94] The Mayo Clinic experience with 73 infected total knee prostheses from 1973 to 1984 resulted in retention of the prosthesis by early debridement for acute infection in 10 patients but, 2 developed recurrences after an average follow-up +of 6.5 years.[94] For chronic infections, attempted arthrodesis in 43 patients resulted in a solid fusion in 33 (success rate of 77%). The 10 patients whose treatment failed had painful pseudarthrosis. Resection arthroplasty was carried out in five patients with successful control of the infection, but 80% of the patients were dissatisfied with the result because of persistent pain and instability. Early reimplantation was done in 15 patients with a 33% success rate.[94] A 90% success rate for chronically infected total knee replacement has been reported from the Cleveland Clinic employing the following sequence: isolation of the infecting microorganism(s), complete removal of the infected prosthesis and cement, systemic antibiotic administration guided by culture results and antibiotic sensitivity data, use of antibiotic-impregnated spacer, followed by reimplantation with antibiotic-impregnated cement when all signs of infection have been eradicated.[95] At the Hospital for Special Surgery, a two-stage revision arthroplasty protocol with 6 weeks of parenteral antibiotic therapy guided by quantitative in-vitro sensitivity testing before reimplantation had a 97% success rate for infected total knee prostheses and 90% success rate for infected total hip prostheses.[83,96,97]

One-stage revision for infected total hip prostheses with[98,99] and without[100] antibiotic-impregnated cement had success rates of 90 to 91% and 86%, respectively. The success of the latter approach could lie in the utilization of an antibiotic regimen consisting of three agents followed by prolonged oral treatment.[100] A review on antibiotic-impregnated cement concluded that it is "not known whether the combination of systemically delivered antibiotics and antibiotic-impregnated cement might be superior to either used separately" in the management of infected total hip prosthesis.[101] A two-stage reconstruction of infected total hip replacement is recommended when the microorganism is virulent.[102] Prolonged antibiotic treatment (of more than 28 days) and delayed reimplantation (more than 1 year after complete removal of the infected prosthesis) reduced the rate of recurrent infection.[102]

Excision arthroplasty or Girdlestone's pseudarthrosis is an alternative treatment for infected total hip prostheses if reimplantation is not feasible, but poor functional outcome is expected.[103] A final option in the treatment of an infected total joint replacement might be chronic suppressive antibiotic therapy in very selected patients: (1) the retained prosthesis must not be loose, (2) the pathogen has to be of low virulence, exquisitely sensitive to the oral antibiotic agent used, or both, and (3) the patient must be able to tolerate the long-term antibiotic program. Even with these rigid criteria, the success rate is only 50%.[83]

A survey of 1112 total joint replacements, with an average follow-up of 6 years, found an overall incidence of 0.27% for late hematogenous infections or an annual incidence of only 0.04%.[80] No matter how small this risk of hematogenous infection might be, antibiotic prophylaxis against transient bacteremia associated with certain diagnostic and therapeutic procedures might be warranted to avoid the disastrous consequences of an infected total joint replacement. This is especially applicable to high-risk patients, such as those with RA or others who are predisposed to bacterial infections. An appropriate prophylactic regimen parallels the recommendations for patients with prosthetic cardiac valves.[104] However, data on the efficacy of such practices are not available, and issues surrounding the cost-effectiveness of antibiotic prophylaxis are controversial.[105]

SEPTIC ARTHRITIS ASSOCIATED WITH CRYSTAL-INDUCED ARTHRITIS

The simultaneous occurrence of septic arthritis and crystal-induced arthritis is relatively uncommon, but undiagnosed infection in the presence of acute gout or pseudogout can result in delayed treatment and poor outcome. Furthermore, inappropriate treatment for joint sepsis in acute arthritis caused by crystals without infection can lead to serious side effects associated with antibiotic administration.[106] Coexistent septic and crystal-induced arthritis is often a disease of the elderly. The mean age of the 31 patients reported to date was 73 years, ranging from 42 to 94 years.[107–109] The knee was the most commonly affected joint. Monoarticular disease was more common than polyarticular involvement. When infection is found in a joint affected by crystal disease, other inflamed joints in the same patient must also be examined for the presence of infection.

Of these 31 patients 29 had bacterial causes; Mycobacterium marinum[110] and Candida albicans[111] were responsible for one case each. Mixed bacterial infection caused by Pasteurella multocida and Pseudomonas aeruginosa was present in only one case.[112] Gram-positive and gram-negative organisms were isolated in 16 and 14 patients, respectively. Staphylococcus, streptococcus, and pneumococcus caused the gram-positive infections, whereas the gram-negative microorganisms included bacilli (e.g., Escherichia coli, Serratia marcescens, and Pseudomonas aeruginosa), coccobacilli (e.g., Hemophilus influenzae and Pasteurella multocida), and cocci (e.g., Neisseria meningitidis and N. gonorrhoeae).

Experimental evidence suggests that the presence of infection promotes crystal "shedding" and precipitates acute crystal arthritis superimposed on sepsis.[109] Conversely, a joint previously damaged by crystals might be more susceptible to infection during bacteremia. Thus, the coexistence of septic and crystal arthritis might be more than a mere coincidence. Synovial fluid analysis of highly inflammatory or purulent-appearing joint fluid should include examination for crystals and microbiologic studies, especially if the arthritis is resistant to usual nonsteroidal anti-inflammatory drugs or colchicine.

SEPTIC ARTHRITIS OF THE FIBROCARTILAGINOUS JOINTS IN THE AXIAL SKELETON

The sternomanubrial joint and the symphysis pubis are midline fibrocartilaginous joints of the axial skeleton that lack a synovial membrane. Various diseases can affect these sites.[113,114] Primary bacterial infection rarely affects these joints. Staphylococcus aureus infections of the sternomanubrial joint have been reported in association with systemic lupus erythematosus,[115] heroin abuse,[72] and normal health.[116] Pseudomonas pseudomallei was cultured from the sternomanubrial joint of a 49-year-old Vietnam veteran.[117]

Bacterial infections of the symphysis pubis occur in children, in elderly debilitated patients, and in parenteral drug abusers.[118] Staphylococcus aureus is the major pathogen in children, whereas Pseudomonas aeruginosa is most common in adults. In the elderly, infection of the symphysis pubis is often related to diseases of the genitourinary system and their treatment. The susceptibility of drug abusers to bone and joint infections, especially the fibrocartilaginous articulations of the axial skeleton, has already been discussed. The clinical features of pyogenic osteitis pubis (septic arthritis of the symphysis pubis) in drug addicts have been reviewed with an emphasis on the difficulty of diagnosis because of the poorly localized pain, the potentially misleading physical findings suggesting hip disease, and the (often) normal radiographs.[70] Bone scintigraphy is useful to confirm inflammation in the symphysis pubis. Attempts to establish a bacterial cause should include open biopsy of the joint, adjacent bone, or both.

The sternoclavicular and sacroiliac joints, paired fibrocartilaginous joints of the axial skeleton with synovial lining, are also affected by a variety of diseases,[119,120] including bacterial infections. Unilateral involvement is the rule. Predispositions to sternoclavicular joint infection include previous damage by underlying arthritis and contamination of the bloodstream through venous channels, for example, a subclavian catheter, hemodialysis, or intravenous drug abuse.[121] The diagnosis of a shoulder joint problem is often mistakenly made because the pain is diffuse and the motion of the shoulder is limited. Delay in diagnosis and frequent (20% of the time) abscess formation as a complication have been emphasized in a review on the subject.[122] Computed tomography is most helpful in defining the destructive arthritis and in detecting abscess formation, associated osteomyelitis, or both.[122,123]

Infections of the sternoclavicular joint have been caused by Staphyloccus aureus, Streptococcus pneumoniae, other streptococci, Pseudomonas, Salmonella, Brucella, Escherichia coli, Hemophilus influenzae, Bacteroides species, Neisseria meningitidis, and Neisseria gonorrhoeae.[119] Other bacterial causes include Streptococcus milleri,[121,124] group B streptococcus,[125] Serratia marcescens,[126] Acinetobacter anitratus,[71] and a case of mixed infection due to Streptococcus sanguis and Pasteurella multocida.[127]

Infection of the sacroiliac joint is an uncommon cause of sacroiliitis.[69,128–131] It is usually seen in young adults who present with acute or subacute pain in the buttock, hip, or flank associated with inability to bear weight because of pain. Mistaken diagnosis of intrinsic hip, back, intra-abdominal, or retroperitoneal disease and delayed therapy can accompany unfamiliarity with this entity and misleading physical findings. Pressure over the joint or any maneuver that distracts or compresses the joint reproduces the pain.[120] Blood cultures are positive in about one-third of the cases.[69,132] The affected joint is best aspirated under the guidance of fluoroscopy[133] or computed tomography.[128]

The bacteriology of pyogenic sacroiliitis reflects the primary site of infection that seeds the joint through the blood. Staphylococcus aureus is isolated most frequently in both children[134–136] and adults.[129–132] Skin infections are the most common primary source. Tonsillitis, dental manipulation, and an infected tooth impaction were responsible for cases of pyogenic sacroiliitis resulting from group A,[129] group B,[69] and group G[137] streptococcus, respectively. Urinary tract infections were associated with Escherichia coli and enterococcus sacroiliitis,[130] upper respiratory tract infection with Branhamella catarrhalis,[69] enteritis with Salmonella schwarzengrund,[129] and cervical carcinoma with group B streptococcus.[69] Intravenous drug abuse has led to sacroiliitis from Pseudomonas aeruginosa, Serratia marcescens, Staphylococcus, and Enterobacter aerogenes.[69,138] Fusobacterium necrophorum,[139] Clostridium septicum, and Peptostreptococcus[140] are anaerobic microorganisms that have been found in sacroiliac joint infections. Brucellar sacroiliitis is discussed later under "Microorganisms Acquired From Animals."

Rapid improvement follows early diagnosis and appropriate antibiotic treatment, but antibiotic treatment of bacterial infections affecting the fibrocartilaginous joints must often be prolonged because osteomyelitis of the adjacent bone is frequently present. Surgical exploration and drainage is indicated when a juxta-articular abscess is present or when sequestrectomy is necessary.[71,114,115,122,129,130]

OTHER PREDISPOSITIONS TO SEPTIC ARTHRITIS

Two uncommon underlying joint diseases that can provide fertile soil for superimposed septic arthritis are hemophiliac arthropathy and Charcot (neuropathic) joints. Staphylococcus aureus has caused infection of a "target" joint of hemophiliacs where recurrent intra-articular bleedings have previously occurred.[141] Many hemophiliacs are infected by the human immunodeficiency virus (HIV), which can further increase the risk of developing septic arthritis.[142] Traumatic hemarthrosis in elderly patients with osteoarthritis can become secondarily infected by S. aureus.[143] Charcot joints caused by tabes dorsalis, syringomyelia, or congenital insensitivity to pain have been sites of bacterial infection. Gram-positive cocci have caused this infectious complication in the knee,[144,145] shoulder,[145,146] and ankle.[147]

Other specific examples of increased host susceptibility to bacterial infections of bone and joint are illustrated by patients with chronic renal failure,[148,149] renal transplant,[150] and sickle cell anemia.[151,152] Bacterial infections are a major cause of morbidity and mortality among patients with sickle cell anemia.[153] These patients and those with related hemoglobinopathies are at increased risk of bacterial meningitis, pneumococcal bacteremia, and Salmonella osteomyelitis. The musculoskeletal manifestations of sickle cell disease are protean and result from different pathogenic mechanisms ranging from ischemic necrosis of the bone to synovitis, hemarthrosis, and secondary gout.[154] The predilection of Salmonella species to cause osteomyelitis, and of Streptococcus pneumoniae to cause septic arthritis, are noteworthy.[151,152] The differentiation of ischemic bone infarcts from multifocal bacterial osteomyelitis is often difficult, and the exclusion of a bacterial cause of inflammatory joint fluid must be made.

A report from a renal unit detailed the varied presentations and the difficulties in diagnosis and management of serious bone and joint infections among patients with chronic renal failure.[149] Extradural abscess in the lumbar region and diskitis with vertebral osteomyelitis and paravertebral abscess of the thoracic spine were commonly caused by Staphylococcus aureus. Infections of the sternoclavicular joint, and the large peripheral joints and long bones by Staphylococcus aureus, Pseudomonas, Serratia, and Proteus species, are reminiscent of the skeletal infections seen in intravenous drug abusers (see above). Bomalaski et al. reviewed the spectrum of infectious arthritis among renal transplant patients.[150] In addition to Staphylococcus aureus and the more common gram-negative bacilli, other causes included Nocardia asteroides, Cryptococcus neoformans, Mycobacterium tuberculosis, M. chelonei, M. fortuitum, M. kansasii, M. scrofulaceum, M. gordonae, and cytomegalovirus. Immunosuppression against transplant rejection leaves the patient vulnerable to bacterial agents and opportunistic microorganisms. Another example of profound depression of normal immunity is the acquired immunodeficiency syndrome (AIDS). Rheumatic manifestations in HIV-infected patients are being more frequently recognized and characterized.[155–157] Arthritis in AIDS has many different causes. Among the infectious causes, common bacteria such as Staphylococcus aureus[158] and Neisseria gonorrhoeae,[157] as well as opportunistic agents such as Sporothrix schenckii,[159] Cryptococcus neoformans,[160] Mycobacterium haemophilum,[161] and Mycobacterium avium[162] have been reported.

POLYARTICULAR SEPTIC ARTHRITIS

Although acute bacterial arthritis is most often monoarticular, polyarticular infection occurs in 5 to 8% of pediatric cases (see Table 116–1) and in 10 to 19% of nongonococcal adult cases.[36,163] Polyarticular infection is a function of the bacteria as well as the host.[36] Bacteria that have a predilection for polyarticular involvement are Neisseria gonorrhoeae,[21] Bacteroides fragilis,[59] Streptococcus pneumoniae, group G streptococcus, and Hemophilus influenzae.[36] But the most common microorganism recovered in cases of septic polyarthritis is Staphylococcus aureus. Prior disease in multiple joints predisposes to polyarticular septic involvement; 18[36] to 35%[164] of patients with RA and superimposed joint infections have polyarticular involvement. Of the RA patients reviewed in Table 116–3, 25% had polyarticular septic arthritis. Patients with septic arthritis superimposed on gout often had polyarticular disease, compared with the predominantly monoarticular infections among patients with concomitant pseudogout.[107–109] The importance of polyarticular septic arthritis is at least twofold. First, knowledge of its relative frequency might help one to avoid misdiagnosis or delayed diagnosis. Second, its poor outcome (23% mortality) is primarily due to the subgroup of patients with antecedent RA who had a 56% mortality.[36]

POLYMICROBIAL SEPTIC ARTHRITIS

Polymicrobial septic arthritis (two or more bacterial species) is rare in a normal joint unless penetrating trauma has occurred or surgery has been recently performed. Combinations of gram-positive, gram-negative, mixed gram-positive and gram-negative, aerobic, and anaerobic microorganisms have all been encountered.[165,166] Most instances of polymicrobic infection involve two different microorganisms, but cases with three or four microbes have been reported.[165,166] In one review, hip infections were most common among the 12 adults, many resulting from a communication of a retroperitoneal or pelvic abscess directly with the hip.[165] In prosthetic joint infections, 6 to 25% of the cases were polymicrobic,[76,86] and the early postoperative wound infections accounted for most of these infections.

PATHOGENS CAUSING BACTERIAL ARTHRITIS

ANAEROBIC BACTERIA

Anaerobic bacteria are probably responsible for less than 1% of all cases of acute hematogenous septic arthritis affecting native joints. Finegold's review included data from the preantibiotic era, and found that over one-third of 180 anaerobic joint infections were caused by Fusobacterium necrophorum.[167] Anaerobic cocci, Bacteroides fragilis, and other Fusobacterium, Bacteroides, and Clostridium species accounted for most of the other cases.

Anaerobes are found more frequently (5 to 10% of the time) in infected joint prostheses.[82,83] The Mayo Clinic experience noted two different clinical settings where anaerobic bacteria caused joint infection[168]; most cases occurred after joint surgery, 53% after reconstructive surgery, and 28% after trauma. In these postoperative infections, anaerobic cocci, such as Peptococcus and Peptostreptococcus species, were the major pathogens. But Bacteroides fragilis was the most frequent cause of a second type of infection (19%), occurring in patients with chronic illnesses such as inflammatory bowel disease, rheumatoid arthritis, psoriatic arthritis, and chronic osteomyelitis. The anaerobic bacteria seeding the joints by the bloodstream arose from intra-abdominal sources or decubitus ulcers. Another route of infection was the extension of chronic osteomyelitis into the adjacent joint. The patients with anaerobic septic arthritis not related to surgery had 50% mortality; the poor outcome was attributed to their debilitated antecedent condition.

GRAM-POSITIVE COCCI

The gram-positive cocci of the Micrococcaceae and Streptococcaceae families are responsible for the great majority (50 to 90%) of all cases of nongonococcal bacterial arthritis.[169–173] Staphylococcus species, predominantly Staphylococcus aureus and occasionally coagulase-negative staphylococci, and rarely Micrococcus species,[57] represent the Micrococcaceae family. The Streptococcaceae family includes the various species of hemolytic streptococci, the different groups of viridans streptococci including pneumococcus, and Aerococcus species.

Staphylococci are the major cause of septic arthritis among the gram-positive cocci. In the elderly, Staphylococcus aureus causes 43 to 64% of all cases (see Table 116–2). In RA patients, 77% of joint infections were due to S. aureus (see Table 116–3). In prosthetic joint infections, 75 to 90% of the gram-positive microorganisms are staphylococci, although S. epidermidis might be more common than S. aureus. In the neonate, staphylococci are responsible for 25% of the community-acquired joint infections and 62% of the nosocomial cases of septic arthritis. Overall, 13 to 44% of all cases of childhood septic arthritis are due to S. aureus (see Table 116–1), a low estimate because many cases are not bacteriologically confirmed (30%), and Hemophilus influenzae is another predominant pathogen among young children.

Staphylococcus aureus can cause septic diskitis (Fig. 116–1). Computed tomography, radionuclide scintigraphy, or both are often positive early in the course of the condition when plain films are negative. Needle aspiration of the disc under fluoroscopic guidance using an image intensifier or direct open biopsy should be done for precise diagnosis.

The microbiologic, clinical, therapeutic, and preventive aspects of diseases caused by Staphylococcus aureus have been reviewed.[174] Special therapeutic consideration against methicillin-resistant staphylococci includes the empiric use of vancomycin in areas where resistant microorganisms are prevalent[8] while culture and anti-

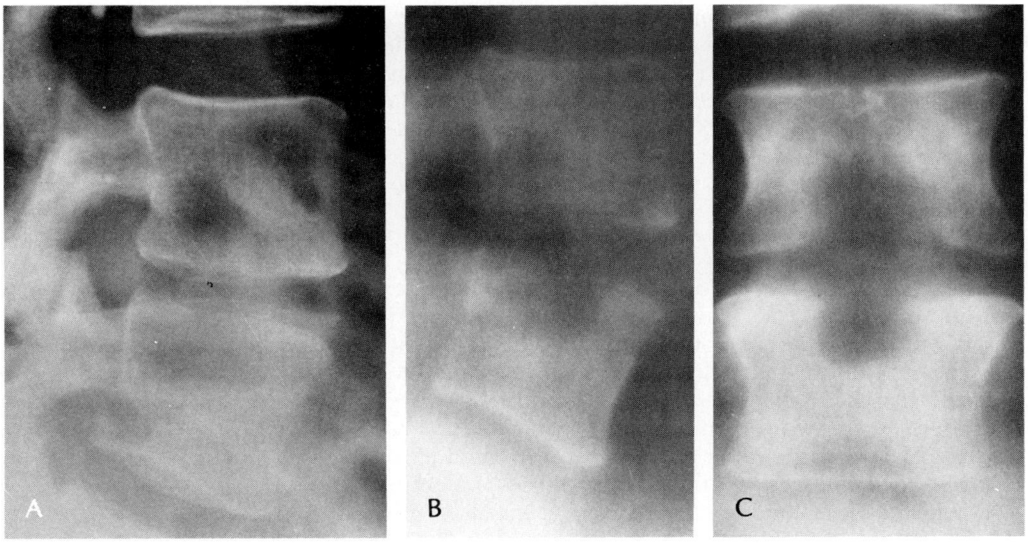

FIGURE 116–1. Septic discitis on the spine due to staphylococci. *A,* Conventional lateral radiograph demonstrates mild disc-space narrowing and dissolution of the vertebral end plate. The extensive destruction of the cancellous bone can only be detected tomographically, as shown in lateral *(B)* and anteroposterior *(C)* projections.

biotic-sensitivity results are pending. Vancomycin resistance has been reported in coagulase-negative staphylococci isolated from the peritoneal fluid of a diabetic patient undergoing continuous ambulatory peritoneal dialysis.[175] The fluoroquinolones are active in vitro against methicillin-resistant S. aureus, as well as multiple antibiotic-resistant gram-negative bacilli and β-lactamase–producing Neisseria gonorrhoeae.[176] Use of this class of antimicrobial agents might be considered in patients with serious infections caused by methicillin-resistant staphylococci when vancomycin cannot be used, or when β-lactams or aminoglycosides are contraindicated.[177]

Streptococci account for 15 to 30% of all nongonococcal causes of bacterial arthritis and are second only to staphylococci. Most cases are due to Streptococcus pyogenes group A. Joint infections caused by group B (S. agalactiae) and group G streptococci have been further elucidated. Diabetes mellitus causes a major predisposition to group B streptococcal septic arthritis.[87,178] Among adults with group B streptococcal joint infection, 20% have polyarticular disease,[36,179] and involvement of the joints of the axial skeleton[178] and prosthetic joints[87] is common. The disease can be aggressive, leading to functional loss and significant morbidity and mortality.[87,178] Group B streptococcus is also a major pathogen of community-acquired septic arthritis in neonates.[7]

Serious group G streptococcal infection occurs in patients with neoplastic disease, alcoholism, and diabetes mellitus.[180] Septic arthritis caused by group G streptococcus was often polyarticular (25% of 36 cases).[61] More than one-third of the patients had underlying RA, and over one-fourth of the infections affected a prosthetic joint. Polymicrobial infection, frequently associated with Staphylococcus aureus, probably indicates the skin as the common portal of entry.[61,180] Prepatellar bursitis caused by group G streptococcus was noted in 8% of 38 cases.[61]

Streptococcus pneumoniae has remained an uncommon cause of joint infection. Predispositions include alcoholism, hypogammaglobulinemia,[181] underlying joint disease such as RA,[60] gout,[182] and joint prostheses.[88] Often, the primary pneumococcal infection is meningitis, pneumonia, or rarely endocarditis, with secondary seeding of the joint, but one or more joints can be the primary and only site(s) of infection.[181] Polyarticular pneumococcal infection is common,[36] possibly reflecting impairments in host defense such as decreased serum chemotactic factors[183] or RA.[60]

Septic arthritis caused by group C streptococcus is rare. Polyarticular infection (in 4 of 10 patients), high mortality (3 of 10), and poor functional outcome (4 of 7) were characteristic of the 10 reported cases.[184] Group D enterococcus is another rare cause of septic arthritis. Zwillich et al. reported two adults, one with a knee infection and another with RA and enterococcal infection in a hip prosthesis.[185] The first patient required an above-knee amputation because of recurrence and osteomyelitis, and the second underwent a Girdlestone excision arthroplasty. Unlike other streptococcal joint infections for which penicillin is the drug of choice, enterococcal disease requires a combined regimen of ampicillin and gentamicin similar to that used in enterococcal endocarditis.[185] A woman with septic arthritis of a hip caused by Aerococcus viridans responded to treatment with penicillin and open drainage.[186] This microorganism is similar to other viridans streptococci, but can be confused with enterococci. Other viridans streptococci that have caused septic arthritis include Streptococcus sanguis,[127] S. milleri,[124] S. anginosus-constellatus,[121] and S. mitis.[187]

GRAM-POSITIVE BACILLI

Gram-positive bacillary septic arthritis is extremely rare. Listeria monocytogenes can cause meningitis and bacteremia in hosts who are compromised by hematologic or lymphoproliferative malignancy, renal transplantation or other nonmalignant disease requiring corticosteroid therapy, or alcoholism.[188] Louthrenoo and Schumacher reviewed the bone and joint infections due to L. monocytogenes.[189] Septic arthritis caused by L. monocytogenes has been reported in patients with RA,[56,190] gout,[191] prosthetic joints and RA,[192–194] and prosthetic joints associated with another systemic disease such as renal transplantation[195] or diabetes mellitus.[196] Other gram-positive bacilli that have caused septic arthritis include Corynebacterium pyogenes,[197] C. kutscheri,[198] Bacillus cereus,[199] and other Bacillus species.[200] Propionibacterium acnes, an anaerobic gram-positive rod, can cause septic arthritis in joint prosthesis[78] and in joints affected by RA.[201]

GRAM-NEGATIVE COCCI AND COCCOBACILLI

The two most important gram-negative cocci that infect joints are Neisseria gonorrhoeae and N. meningitidis, as discussed in Chapter 117. Other members of the family Neisseriaceae that have caused joint infection include Branhamella, Moraxella, and Kingella species. Moraxella (Branhamella) catarrhalis was implicated in pyogenic sacroiliitis in a 15-year-old girl with an upper respiratory tract infection[69] and in septic arthritis of the hip in a 23-year-old Navajo man.[202]

Joint infections caused by Moraxella or Kingella species are uncommon, usually following an indolent course because of their low pathogenicity.[203] Morphologic resemblance to Hemophilus influenzae and Neisseria gonorrhoeae has been noted.[203,204] Infants and young children (under 4 years) appear especially vulnerable to bone and joint infections caused by Kingella kingae.[203,205] Adult cases of K. kingae septic arthritis include a 49-year-old alcoholic,[206] a 51-year-old woman with RA and Felty's syndrome,[55] and a 76-year-old man with chronic lung disease.[207]

Hemophilus influenzae is an aerobic, pleomorphic, gram-negative coccobacillus. Of the typeable strains, type B is the major pathogen in humans. In adults, it is an important cause of pneumonia, meningitis, epiglottitis, and acute sinusitis.[208] Rarely it infects a diarthrodial joint, accounting for fewer than 1% of all bacterial causes of septic arthritis in adults.[172] In children, the spectrum of disease caused by H. influenzae includes bacteremia, meningitis, pneumonia, epiglottitis, arthritis, cellulitis, osteomyelitis, and pericarditis.[209] Septic arthritis accounts for about 8% of all H. influenzae infections in children.[209] Among bacterial causes of septic arthritis in children, H. influenzae is a major pathogen that rivals Staphylococcus aureus (see "Bacterial Arthritis in Children").

Peak vulnerability to Hemophilus influenzae arthritis is between the ages of 6 months and 2 years. Children under 3 months and over 5 years old are much less likely to experience H. influenzae joint infection. The disease in children is usually monoarticular, affecting predominantly the large joints of the lower extremity.[1] Joint infection often follows an upper respiratory tract infection or otitis media with bacteremia.[209,210] It can be associated with concurrent meningitis (8 to 30%) and osteomyelitis (12 to 22%).[209,210]

The much rarer adult disease has some different clinical features. A systemic or local predisposition to infection was present in two-thirds of 25 cases.[211] Infection was monoarticular in 12 (48%), polyarticular in 6 (24%), and accompanied by tenosynovitis, bursitis, or both in 7 (28%). Five of the six patients reported since 1983[212–214] had a systemic predisposition to infection.[212,214] Four had polyarticular infection,[213,214] one had septic olecranon bursitis without joint involvement,[212] and the other had an infected hip prosthesis.[214] Thus, Hemophilus influenzae arthritis in an adult can mimic the polyarthritis and tenosynovitis of gonococcal infection, resemble septic olecranon bursitis most commonly caused by Staphylococcus aureus,[215] or involve a prosthetic joint. Although ampicillin is the drug of choice against *sensitive* Hemophilus influenzae, the initial antibiotic agent directed at suspected H. influenzae infection should be chloramphenicol or cefuroxime because of possible ampicillin resistance.

GRAM-NEGATIVE BACILLI

Gram-negative bacilli account for 7 to 26% of cases of adult nongonococcal septic arthritis.[30,216] Ruthberg and Ho noted that 17% of 412 cases of septic arthritis in adults recorded between 1934 and 1980 had been caused by these microorganisms.[217] Analysis of data from three periods (pre-1960, the 1960s, and the 1970s) showed frequencies of gram-negative bacillary arthritis of 6%, 14%, and 27%, respectively. This trend could reflect the progressively increasing frequency of gram-negative bacteremia in general.[31] Among the elderly with septic arthritis, 24% of cases were due to gram-negative bacilli (see Table 116–2). Among RA patients, the percentage was 11%. Intravenous drug abusers are especially prone to bone and joint infections from Pseudomonas,[32,218] Serratia,[33,138] and Staphylococcus. Gram-negative bacilli were responsible for less than 10% of joint infections among children over 2 years of age, but children under 2 years old were more susceptible to gram-negative bacillary joint infection (28%),[216] and these bacilli were also more prevalent in nosocomial than in community-acquired infections among neonates.[7] Of prosthetic joint infections, 10 to 20% were due to aerobic gram-negative rods.

Two series of cases highlight the major features of the two ends of the spectrum of gram-negative bacillary joint infections.[30,219] Host factors determine many of the clinical features including the microbiology, the site of the joint infection, and the outcome of treatment. The 1974 series of 13 patients from Boston University is characteristic of an older population (mean age 56 years) with serious underlying systemic diseases, preexisting joint disease, or both.[30] These patients developed Escherichia coli or Proteus mirabilis septic arthritis secondary to hematogenous spread from the urinary or biliary tract. Less commonly, Serratia marcescens, Pseudomonas aeruginosa, and Salmonella species caused joint infection. The patients often had been receiving antibiotics, corticosteroids, or both, and the infection was monoarticular, most commonly affecting a knee. Many patients failed to respond to medical treatment alone and required subsequent surgical debridement. Mortality was high and the cure rate low. In contrast, the 1977 series of 21 patients from UCLA is representative of a younger patient population (mean age 29 years) whose primary predisposition was intravenous drug abuse.[219] Otherwise healthy, many of the patients had infections localized to the sternal articulations caused by Pseudomonas aeruginosa. Escherichia coli and Proteus mirabilis were less commonly encountered, with single cases due to Enterobacter aerogenes, E. liquefaciens, Klebsiella pneumoniae, Eikenella corrodens, Acinetobacter anitratus, and Bacteroides fragilis. Despite the frequent occurrence of juxta-articular osteomyelitis, periarticular abscess requiring surgery, or both, the cure rate was 90% and the mortality only 5%. The Geisinger Medical Center of Danville, Pennsylvania also reported on an elderly population (mean age 61 years).[220] The 22 patients were infected with a range of bacilli comparable to that in the Boston series, but the mortality was only 5% and good outcomes were achieved in 68%. Prompt diagnosis, early treatment, and more-effective antibiotics might have been responsible for the better results.

Among the members of the Enterobacteriaceae family, Escherichia coli and Proteus mirabilis are the most frequent causative agents of septic arthritis followed by Klebsiella, Enterobacter, Serratia, and Morganella species. Salmonella species,[221,222] Arizona hinshawii,[223] Yersinia enterocolitica,[224,225] and Campylobacter fetus[226] have been isolated from synovial fluids, but reactive arthritis following gastrointestinal infection by Salmonella, Yersinia, Shigella flexneri, or Campylobacter jejuni is a more common problem associated with these pathogens (see Chapter 60).[227,228]

Pseudomonas aeruginosa, a member of the Pseudomonadaceae family, is an important cause of gram-negative septic arthritis in chronically debilitated older patients with serious systemic illnesses as well as in younger parenteral drug abusers (see "Bone and Joint Infections Associated with Intravenous Drug Abuse"). It is also the most common etiologic agent associated with osteochondritis of the foot from puncture wounds seen in children[229] and in adults.[230] Besides adequate debridement and drainage of the infected site, an aminoglycoside and an antipseudomonal semisynthetic penicillin are used for 4 to 6 weeks.[34] One exception, a knee infected with Pseudomonas aeruginosa, failed to respond to gentamicin and azlocillin,[231] but responded to ceftazidime given intravenously and intra-articularly. Other reported exceptions include a septic knee caused by Pseudomonas cepacia[232] and a case of osteochondritis of the foot caused by P. maltophilia.[233] Typically resistant to aminoglycosides, antipseudomonal penicillins, and first- and second-generation cephalosporins, these Pseudomonas species proved difficult to eradicate even with third-generation cephalosporins.

The spectrum of gram-negative bacillary septic arthritis is constantly expanding with reports of new isolations. Examples of such occurrences include joint infections caused by Capnocytophaga ochracea,[234] Plesiomonas shigelloides,[53] and Aeromonas hydrophila.[79,235,236]

MICROORGANISMS ACQUIRED FROM ANIMALS

Pasteurella Multocida

This small, aerobic, facultatively anaerobic, gram-negative coccobacillus is found in the normal oral flora of many domestic and wild animals.[237] Human infections can result from casual contact with cats or dogs or more commonly from their bites and scratches. Of 446 cases of human infection by Pasteurella multocida, 48% affected the skin, 14% the oral and respiratory tract, 13% the cardiovascular system, 13% the skeletal and articular system, 5% the central nervous system, 4% the gastrointestinal tract, 2% the genitourinary tract, 1% the eye.[237] The bone and joint infections separate into three distinct categories: osteomyelitis, septic arthritis with osteomyelitis, and septic arthritis alone.[238] *Osteomyelitis* can result from soft-tissue wound infection with extension to adjacent bone or by direct inoculation of P. multocida into the periosteum by a bite. Common sites are the forearm, leg, hand, and wrist. Almost all the cases of *septic arthritis with osteomyelitis* affect the small joints and bones of the hand after cat bites. Few patients had underlying systemic illness predisposing to bacterial infection.

In sharp contrast, *septic arthritis* caused by P. multocida without osteomyelitis rarely occurs in a host who is not immunocompromised or in a joint not previously damaged. Chronic RA receiving corticosteroid treatment is the most common underlying joint disease. Here bacterial dissemination is hematogenous rather than due to local extension or direct penetration. Bacteremia and polyarticular infection might be noted,[90,239,240] but the infection is usually monoarticular, affecting the knee most commonly. Almost a third of the reported cases have involved total knee replacements,[238] perhaps reflecting the increased susceptibility to infection of a patient with RA of long duration. However, P. multocida infection of bilateral knee prostheses in a patient with osteoarthritis has been reported also.[90] Joint infection with P. multocida has been reported in association with Staphylococcus aureus in a prosthetic knee,[241] with Streptococcus sanguis in a sternoclavicular joint,[127] and with Pseudomonas aeruginosa in a patient with bilateral knee prostheses.[90]

Penicillin is the agent of choice for treatment of Pasteurella multocida septic arthritis. Drainage of the infected joint is necessary. Some patients with infected knee prostheses were able to retain the artificial joint,[239,242] but others required its eventual removal.[90,241]

Rat-bite Fever

Two microorganisms, Streptobacillus moniliformis, a pleomorphic gram-negative rod, and Spirillum minus, a spirochete, can cause rat-bite fever. Both are normal flora in the oropharynx of many rodents. Streptobacillus infection presents with fever, morbilliform or petechial rash, and polyarticular pain 2 to 10 days after a rodent bite. Rarely, streptobacilli have been isolated from joint fluid.[243–245] Spirillum minus causes a febrile illness after an incubation period of over 10 days. Joint symptoms are rare, but regional adenopathy draining the site of the bite is common. Treatment is with penicillin for both causative agents.

Brucellosis

Brucellosis has a worldwide distribution, but the pathogenic species depends on the geographic location. The four species causing human disease are Brucella melitensis, B. abortus, B. suis, and B. canis. The clinical manifestations and the severity of disease vary according to the responsible species and the host.[246,247] Humans acquire the disease from infected animals. Ingestion of raw milk or dairy products made from unpasteurized milk, inhalation of aerosolized bacteria, or contact with contaminated animals through broken skin or conjunctiva are the known routes of infection. The spectrum of organ system involvement by brucellosis has been reviewed by Young.[246] Examples of ingestion-acquired, laboratory-acquired, and abatoir-acquired disease are well illustrated. A comprehensive review of 304 cases of human infection by B. melitensis from Lima, Peru found joint involvement in a third (33.8%) of patients.[247] Sacroiliitis (46.6%), peripheral arthritis (38.8%), or a combination of the two (7.8%) accounted for 93.2% of musculoskeletal involvement, and tended to occur in young patients with acute infection. *Spondylitis* (6.8%) was most common in the lumbosacral region, generally affecting older patients with more chronic infection. Its pathogenesis is believed to represent a septic discitis with contiguous involvement of the adjacent vertebral body and eventual vertebral osteomyelitis. Paraspinal abscesses can complicate vertebral brucellosis and can be the cause of antibiotic resistance until found and drained.[248] *Sacroiliitis* is usually unilateral and nondestructive, and responds to antibiotic treatment. *Peripheral arthritis* also responds to antibiotic treatment, but can remit spontaneously, raising the possibility of a reactive form of brucellar arthritis.[247] Recovery of the microorganism from the sacroiliac joint, sternoclavicular joint, or other peripheral joints is uncommon but well documented.[246–247,249–250]

In the United States, Brucella melitensis infections are uncommon relative to B. abortus and B. suis. Brucella canis has been responsible for at least two cases of septic arthritis in children.[246,251] A popular antibiotic regimen against brucellosis consists of tetracycline plus streptomycin, but trimethoprim-sulfamethoxazole, rifampin, and third-generation cephalosporins have all been used with some success.[246,251,252]

SPIROCHETES

Spirillum minus is a rare cause of rat-bite fever in the United States. Lyme arthritis, first described by Steere and Malawista, is caused by Borrelia burgdorferi and is the subject of Chapter 120 and 121. Another spirochete, Treponema pallidum, is responsible for syphilitic joint disease.[253] Arthritis as a result of primary or secondary syphilis is rare. In tertiary syphilis, arthritis can result from gummata deposited in the juxta-articular tissue, cartilage, or bone. Large, usually painless effusions with little evidence of limitation of motion are characteristic of gummatous arthritis. Syphilitic spondylitis is an osteitis caused by the invasion of bone and periosteum by Treponema pallidum. Charcot's joint secondary to lues occurs in 5% of patients with tabes dorsalis and primarily involves the weight-bearing articulations (see Chapter 83).

Congenital syphilis has been associated with several musculoskeletal syndromes. *Parrot's pseudoparalysis* is an osteochondritis affecting the epiphysis and articular cartilage of the humerus or the tibia of neonates and infants within the first 3 months of life. *Clutton's joint* is a late sequela of congenital syphilis manifested by chronic hydrarthrosis of one or both knees in children between 6 and 16 years old.

MYCOPLASMA

Mycoplasmas as agents of human disease have been reviewed by Cassell and Cole.[254] Septic arthritis has resulted from infection by Mycoplasma hominis, M. pneumoniae, and Ureaplasma urealyticum. Some patients with hypogammaglobulinemia develop polyarthritis resembling RA, and from their joint fluids mycoplasmas and ureaplasmas have been cultured.[255,256] Mycoplasma joint disease is responsive to antibiotic treatment; tetracycline or erythromycin are used most frequently. Prosthetic joint infection with Mycoplasma hominis has been reported in two patients with RA[92,257] and in another patient with systemic lupus erythematosus.[258] All three patients retained their joint prostheses

TABLE 116–4. SUMMARY FOR PRINCIPLES FOR DIAGNOSIS AND MANAGEMENT OF SEPTIC ARTHRITIS CAUSED BY BACTERIA[263]

1. Suspect septic arthritis in a patient (1) with debilitating disease, especially neoplastic or hepatic disease, (2) who is taking corticosteroids or immunosuppressive agents, (3) who has infection elsewhere, even if receiving antibiotics, or (4) who has pre-existing joint damage from another type of arthritis.
2. Diagnose septic arthritis by synovial fluid smear and culture, or by counterimmunoelectrophoresis for bacterial antigens. High fluid concentrations of lactate and other organic acid (especially succinate), fluid glucose levels 40 mg/dl or more below plasma glucose levels (after fasting), and poor mucin clot suggest bacterial sepsis. Fluid leukocyte concentrations are usually high; neutrophils predominate >90%).
3. Splint the affected joint initially, give an analgesic, and mobilize the joint as inflammation subsides with antibiotic treatment.
4. Treat with parenteral antibiotics after obtaining synovial fluid and blood cultures but before obtaining the results; time is important. A direct correlation exists between the duration of symptoms before treatment and the time needed to sterilize joint fluid once treatment is begun.[26] Prescribe an empiric antibiotic regimen using clinical clues as to the probable causative agent. Do not inject antibiotics into the joint because they are irritants and can confuse the clinical picture. Aminoglycoside effectiveness decreases by an order of magnitude at pH 6.5; synovial fluid pH correlates with local leukocyte concentration.[264] Hence adequate drainage of exudate is very important.
5. Decompress joint by daily needle drainage, which gives better results than open drainage, except in infections of long duration and in deeply situated joints, where needle drainage is technically difficult.
6. Follow daily joint fluid leukocyte count and cultures for prognosis. A serial fall in the leukocyte count and sterile fluid correlate with good outcome.[26]

with antibiotic treatment and joint drainage, debridement, or both.

NOCARDIA

Nocardia are aerobic, gram-positive, partially acid-fast bacteria that form branching filaments. Nocardia asteroides and N. brasiliensis are the major pathogens causing human disease. Septic arthritis from either organism is rare. The reported cases are usually in compromised hosts receiving corticosteroids or other immunosuppressive drugs.[259–261] However, a case of Nocardia olecranon bursitis in a healthy 44-year-old man has been described.[262] Trimethoprim and sulfamethoxazole appear to be the antibiotic combination of choice. Treatment duration is usually prolonged, from months to a year.

THERAPY

Suggested antimicrobial therapy has been discussed in the sections dealing with specific organisms. The principles for diagnosis and management are summarized in Table 116–4. Draining with repeated needle aspiration must produce repeated success in decompressing local pus accumulation. A serial fall in the total joint fluid leukocyte count and sterility of aspirate are good omens, correlating with a good outcome.[26]

A summary of recommended antimicrobials and alternative drugs is provided in Table 116–5 for most of the microorganisms causing bacterial arthritis. Drug dosages and duration of treatment must be determined for each case.

TABLE 116–5. ANTIBIOTIC THERAPY REGIMENS FOR BACTERIAL ARTHRITIS*

MICROORGANISM	ANTIBIOTIC OF CHOICE	ALTERNATIVE DRUGS
Staphylococcus aureus	Nafcillin	Cefazolin Vancomycin Clindamycin
Methicillin-resistant staphylococcus	Vancomycin	
Streptococcus	Penicillin G	Cefazolin Vancomycin Clindamycin
Enterococcus	Penicillin or ampicillin plus gentamicin	Vancomycin plus an aminoglycoside
Neisseria gonorrhoeae	A third-generation cephalosporin (ceftriaxone) or ampicillin (if organism is penicillin-sensitive)	Spectinomycin Ciprofloxacin Erythromycin
Hemophilus influenzae	Ampicillin	A third-generation cephalosporin Cefuroxime Chloramphenicol
Enterobacteriaceae	A third-generation cephalosporin (cefotaxime, ceftizoxime, or ceftriaxone)	Imipenem Aztreonam Ampicillin An aminoglycoside (not alone)
Pseudomonas aeruginosa	Antipseudomonal penicillin plus an aminoglycoside	An aminoglycoside plus ceftazidime, imipenem, or aztreonam
Bacteroides fragilis	Metronidazole	Clindamycin

* Table prepared with the assistance of John M. Boyce, M.D. and Antone A. Medeiros, M.D. of the Division of Infectious Diseases at the Miriam Hospital.

REFERENCES

1. Fink, C.W., and Nelson, J.D.: Septic arthritis and osteomyelitis in children. Clin. Rheum. Dis., *12*:423–435, 1986.
2. Sequeira, W., Swedler, W.I., and Skosey, J.L.: Septic arthritis in childhood. Ann. Emerg. Med., *14*:1185–1187, 1985.
3. Wilson, N.I.L., and Di Paola, M.: Acute septic arthritis in infancy and childhood: 10 years' experience. J. Bone Joint Surg., *68B*:584–587, 1986.
4. Speiser, J.C., et al.: Changing trends in pediatric septic arthritis. Semin. Arthritis Rheum., *15*:132–138, 1985.
5. Welkon, C.J., Long, S.S., Fisher, M.C., and Alburger, P.D.: Pyogenic arthritis in infants and children: A review of 95 cases. Pediatr. Infect. Dis., *5*:669–676, 1986.
6. Morrissy, R.T.: Bone and joint infection in the neonate. Pediatr. Ann., *18*:33–34,36–38,40,42–44, 1989.
7. Dan, M.: Septic arthritis in young infants: Clinical and microbiologic correlations and therapeutic implications. Rev. Infect. Dis., *6*:147–155, 1984.
8. Ang-Fonte, G.Z., Rozboril, M.B., and Thompson, G.R.: Changes in nongonococcal septic arthritis: Drug abuse and methicillin-resistant Staphylococcus aureus. Arthritis Rheum., *28*:210–213, 1985.
9. Scoles, P.V., and Aronoff, S.C.: Antimicrobial therapy of childhood skeletal infections. J. Bone Joint Surg., *66A*:1487–1492, 1984.
10. Poretz, D.M., et al.: Intravenous antibiotic therapy in an outpatient setting. JAMA, *248*:336–339, 1982.
11. Rehm, S.J., and Weinstein, A.J.: Home intravenous antibiotic therapy: A team approach. Ann. Intern. Med., *99*:388–392, 1983.
12. Tetzlaff, T.R., McCracken, G.H., Jr., and Nelson, J.D.: Oral antibiotic therapy for skeletal infections of children. II. Therapy of osteomyelitis and suppurative arthritis. J. Pediatr., *92*:485–490, 1978.
13. Syrogiannopoulos, G.A., and Nelson, J.D.: Duration of antimicrobial therapy for acute suppurative osteoarticular infections. Lancet, *1*:37–40, 1988.
14. Herndon, W.A., Knauer, S., Sullivan, J.A., and Gross, R.H.: Management of septic arthritis in children. J. Pediatr. Orthop., *6*:576–578, 1986.
15. Gillspie, R.: Septic arthritis in childhood. Clin. Orthop., *96*:152–159, 1973.
16. Howard, J.B., Highgenboten, C.L., and Nelson, J.D.: Residual effects of septic arthritis in infancy and childhood. JAMA, *236*:932–935, 1976.
17. U.S. Senate Special Committee on Aging: Size and growth of the older population. *In* Aging America. Trends and Projections. 1985–86 Edition. U.S. Govt. Printing Office, 1986.
18. Kelly, P.J.: Bacterial arthritis in the adult. Orthop. Clin. North Am., *6*:973–981, 1975.
19. Newman, J.H.: Review of septic arthritis throughout the antibiotic era. Ann. Rheum. Dis., *35*:198–205, 1976.
20. Lalley, E.V., et al.: Rheumatologic disorders in the elderly. *In* Contemporary Geriatric Medicine. Vol. III. Edited by S.R. Gambert. New York, Plenum Medical Book Company, 1988, pp. 189–198.
21. Goldenberg, D.L., and Reed, J.I.: Bacterial arthritis. N. Engl. J. Med., *312*:764–771, 1985.
22. Schneider, E.L.: Infectious diseases in the elderly. Ann. Intern. Med., *98*:395–400, 1983.
23. Vincent, G.M., and Amirault, J.D.: Septic arthritis in the elderly. Clin. Orthop., *251*:241–245, 1990.
24. Cooper, C., and Cawley, M.I.D.: Bacterial arthritis in the elderly. Gerontology, *32*:222–227, 1986.
25. McGuire, N.M., and Kauffman, C.A.: Septic arthritis in the elderly. J. Am. Geriatr. Soc., *33*:170–174, 1985.
26. Ho, G., Jr., and Su, E.Y.: Therapy of septic arthritis. JAMA, *247*:797–800, 1982.
27. Willkens, R.F., Healey, L.A., and Decker, J.L.: Acute infectious arthritis in the aged and chronically ill. Arch. Intern. Med., *106*:354–364, 1960.
28. Geelhoed-Duyvestijn, P.H.L.M., et al.: Disseminated gonococcal infection in the elderly patients. Arch. Intern. Med., *146*:1739–1740, 1986.
29. Straus, S.E., Vest, J.V., and Glew, R.H.: Gonococcal arthritis in the elderly. South. Med. J., *71*:214–215, 1978.
30. Goldenberg, D.L., Brandt, K.D., Cathcart, E.S., and Cohen, A.S.: Acute arthritis caused by gram-negative bacilli: A clinical characterization. Medicine (Baltimore), *53*:197–208, 1974.
31. Kreger, B.E., Craven, D.E., Carling, P.C., and McCabe, W.R.: Gram-negative bacteremia. III. Reassessment of etiology, epidemiology and ecology in 612 patients. Am. J. Med., *68*:332–343, 1980.
32. Miskew, D.B., Lorenz, M.A., Pearson, R.L., and Pankovich, A.M.: Pseudomonas aeruginosa bone and joint infection in drug abusers. J. Bone Joint Surg., *65A*:829–832, 1983.
33. Donovan, T.L., Chapman, M.W., Harrington, K.D., and Nagel, D.A.: Serratia arthritis: Report of seven cases. J. Bone Joint Surg., *58A*:1009–1011, 1976.
34. Schmid, F.R.: Routine drug treatment of septic arthritis. Clin. Rheum. Dis., *10*:293–311, 1984.
35. Broy, S.B., and Schmid, F.R.: A comparison of medical drainage and surgical drainage in the initial treatment of infected joints. Clin. Rheum. Dis., *12*:501–522, 1986.
36. Epstein, J.H., Zimmermann, B., and Ho, G., Jr.: Polyarticular septic arthritis. J. Rheumatol., *13*:1105–1107, 1986.
37. Septic arthritis in rheumatoid disease. Leading article. Br. Med. J., *2*:1089–1090, 1976.
38. Kellgren, J.H., Ball, J., Fairbrother, R.W., and Barnes, K.L.: Suppurative arthritis complicating rheumatoid arthritis. Br. Med. J., *1*:1193–1200, 1958.
39. Rimoin, D.L., and Wennberg, J.E.: Acute septic arthritis complicating chronic rheumatoid arthritis. JAMA, *196*:617–621, 1966.
40. Karten, I.: Septic arthritis complicating rheumatoid arthritis. Ann. Intern Med., *70*:1147–1158, 1969.
41. Myers, A.R., Miller, L.M., and Pinals, R.S.: Pyarthrosis complicating rheumatoid arthritis. Lancet, *2*:714–716, 1969.
42. Gristina, A.G., Rovere, G.D., and Shoji, H.: Spontaneous septic arthritis complicating rheumatoid arthritis. J. Bone Joint Surg., *56A*:1180–1184, 1974.
43. Resnick, D.: Pyarthrosis complicating rheumatoid arthritis. Radiology, *114*:581–586, 1975.
44. Mitchell, W.S., Brooks, P.M., Stevenson, R.D., and Buchanan, W.W.: Septic arthritis in patients with rheumatoid disease: A still underdiagnosed complication. J. Rheumatol., *3*:124–133, 1976.
45. Gelman, M.I., and Ward, J.R.: Septic arthritis: A complication of rheumatoid arthritis. Radiology, *122*:17–23, 1977.
46. Kraft, S.M., Panush, R.S., and Longley, S.: Unrecognized staphylococcal pyarthrosis with rheumatoid arthritis. Semin. Arthritis Rheum., *14*:196–210, 1985.
47. Blackborn, W.D., Jr., Dunn, T.L., and Alarcon, G.S.: infection versus disease activity in rheumatoid arthritis: Eight years' experience. South Med. J., *79*:1238–1241, 1986.
48. Goldenberg, D.L.: Infectious arthritis complicating rheumatoid arthritis and other chronic rheumatic disorders. Arthritis Rheum., *32*:496–502, 1989.
49. Gardner, G.C., and Weisman, M.H.: Pyarthrosis in patients with rheumatoid arthritis: a report of 13 cases and a review of the

literature from the past 40 years. Am. J. Med., *88*:503–511, 1990.

50. Mowat, A.G., and Baum, J.: Chemotaxis of polymorphonuclear leukocytes from patients with rheumatoid arthritis. J. Clin. Invest., *50*:2541–2549, 1971.
51. Turner, R.A., Shumacher, H.R., and Myers, A.R.: Phagocytic function of polymorphonuclear leukocytres in rheumatic diseases. J. Clin. Invest., *52*:1632–1635, 1973.
52. Pruzanski, W., Leers, W.D., and Wardlaw, A.C.: Bacteriolytic and bactericidal activity of sera and synovial fluids in rheumatoid arthritis and in osteoarthritis. Arthritis Rheum., *17*:207–218, 1974.
53. Gordon, D.L., Philpot, C.R., and McGuire, C.: Plesiomonas shigelloides septic arthritis complicating rheumatoid arthritis. Aust. N.Z. J. Med., *13*:275–276, 1983.
54. Barth, W.F., Healey, L.A., and Decker, J.L.: Septic arthritis due to Pasteurella multocida complicating rheumatoid arthritis. Arthritis Rheum., *11*:394–399, 1968.
55. Lewis, D.A., and Settas, L.: Kingella kingae causing septic arthritis in Felty's syndrome. Postgrad. Med. J., *59*:525–526, 1983.
56. Wilson, A.P.R., Prouse, P.J., and Gumpel, J.M.: Listeria monocytogenes septic arthritis following intra-articular yttrium-90 therapy. Ann. Rheum. Dis., *43*:518–519, 1984.
57. Wharton, M., Rice, J.R., McCallum, R., and Gallis, H.A.: Septic arthritis due to Micrococcus luteus. (Letter.) J. Rheumatol., *13*:659–660, 1986.
58. Dodd, M.J., Griffiths, I.D., and Freeman, R.: Pyogenic arthritis due to bacteroides complicating rheumatoid arthritis. Ann. Rheum. Dis., *41*:248–249, 1982.
59. Rosenkranz, P., Lederman, M.M., Gopalakrishna, K.V., and Ellner, J.J.: Septic arthritis caused by Bacteroides fragilis. Rev. Infect. Dis., *12*:20–30, 1990.
60. Good, A.E., Gayes, J.M., Kauffman, C.A., and Archer, G.L.: Multiple pneumococcal pyarthrosis complicating rheumatoid arthritis. South. Med. J., *71*:502–504, 1978.
61. Gaunt, P.N., and Seal, D.V.: Group G streptococcal infection of joints and joint prostheses. J. Infect., *13*:115–123, 1986.
62. Trimble, L.D., Schoenaers, J.A.H., and Stoelinga, P.J.W.: Acute suppurative arthritis of the temporomandibular joint in a patient with rheumatoid arthritis. J. Maxillofac. Surg., *11*:92–95, 1983.
63. Berger, A.J., and Calcaterra, V.E.: Septic cricoarytenoid arthritis. Otolaryngol. Head Neck Surg., *91*:211–213, 1983.
64. Lohr, K.M.: Rheumatic manifestations of diseases associated with substance abuse. Semin. Arthritis Rheum., *17*:90–111, 1987.
65. Tuazon, C.U., and Sheagren, J.N.: Increased rate of carriage of Staphylococcus aureus among narcotic addicts. J. Infect. Dis., *129*:725–727, 1974.
66. Rajashekaraiah, K.R., Rice, T.W., and Kallick, C.A.: Recovery of Pseudomonas aeruginosa from syringes of drug addicts with endocarditis. J. Infect. Dis., *144*:482, 1981.
67. Roca, R.P., and Yoshikawa, T.T.: Primary skeletal infections in heroin users: A clinical characterization, diagnosis and therapy. Clin. Orthop., *144*:238–248, 1979.
68. Chandrasekar, P.H., and Narula, A.P.: Bone and joint infections in intravenous drug abusers. Rev. Infect. Dis., *8*:904–911, 1986.
69. Gordon, G., and Kabins, S.A.: Pyogenic sacroiliitis. Am. J. Med., *69*:50–56, 1980.
70. Magarian, G.J., and Reuler, J.B.: Septic arthritis and osteomyelitis of the symphysis pubis (osteitis pubis) from intravenous drug use. West. J. Med., *142*:691–694, 1985.
71. Bayer, A.S., Chow, A.W., Louie, J.S., and Guze, L.B.: Sternoarticular pyoarthrosis due to gram-negative bacilli. Arch. Intern. Med., *137*:1036–1040, 1977.
72. Lopez-Longo, F.J., et al.: Primary septic arthritis of the manubriosternal joint in a heroin user. Clin. Orthop. *202*:230–231, 1986.
73. Salvati, E.A., et al.: Infections associated with orthopedic devices. *In* Infections associated with prosthetic devices. Edited by B. Sugarman and E.J. Young. Boca Raton, FL, CRC Press, 1984, pp. 181–218.
74. Melton, L.J., III, Stauffer, R.N., Chao, E.Y.S., and Ilstrup, D.M.: Rates of total hip arthroplasty: A population-based study. N. Engl. J. Med., *307*:1242–1245, 1982.
75. Total hip joint replacement in the United States. (Consensus Conferences.) JAMA, *248*:1817–1821, 1982.
76. Poss, R., et al.: Factors influencing the incidence and outcome of infection following total joint arthroplasty. Clin. Orthop., *182*:117–126, 1984.
77. Gristina, A.G., and Kolkin, J.: Total joint replacement and sepsis. J. Bone Joint Surg., *65A*:128–134, 1983.
78. Morrey, B.F., and Bryan, R.S.: Infection after total elbow arthroplasty. J. Bone Joint Surg., *65A*:330–338, 1983.
79. Stinchfield, F.E., et al.: Late hematogenous infection of total joint replacement. J. Bone Joint Surg., *62A*:1345–1350, 1980.
80. Ainscow, D.A.P., and Denham, R.A.: The risk of haematogenous infection in total joint replacements. J. Bone Joint Surg., *66B*:580–582, 1984.
81. Grogan, T.J., Dorey, F., Rollins, J., and Amstutz, H.C.: Deep sepsis following total knee arthroplasty. J. Bone Joint Surg., *68A*:226–234, 1986.
82. Hunter, G., and Dandy, D.: The natural history of the patient with an infected total hip replacement. J. Bone Joint Surg., *59B*:293–297, 1977.
83. Brause, B.D.: Infections associated with prosthetic joints. Clin. Rheum. Dis., *12*:523–536, 1986.
84. Hofammann, D.Y., Keeling, J.W., and Meyer, R.D.: Total hip arthroplasty: Comparison of infection rates in a VA and a University hospital. South Med. J., *79*:1252–1255, 1986.
85. Gristina, A.G., Costerton, J.W., Hobgood, C.D., and Webb, L.X.: Bacterial adhesion, biomaterials, the foreign body effect, and infection from natural ecosystems to infections in man: A brief review. Contemp. Orthop., *14*:27–35, 1987.
86. Inman, R.D., et al.: Clinical and microbial features of prosthetic joint infection. Am. J. Med., *77*:47–53, 1984.
87. Small, C.B., et al.: Group B streptococcal arthritis in adults. Am. J. Med., *76*:367–375, 1984.
88. Mallory, T.H.: Sepsis in total hip replacement following pneumococcal pneumonia. J. Bone Joint Surg., *55A*:1753–1754, 1973.
89. Prince, A., and Neu, H.C.: Microbiology of infections of the prosthetic joint. Orthop. Rev., *8*:91–96, 1979.
90. Orton, D.W., and Fulcher, W.H.: Pasteurella multocida: Bilateral septic joint prostheses from a distant cat bite. Ann. Emerg. Med., *13*:1065–1067, 1984.
91. Eftekhar, N.S.: Wound infection complicating total hip joint arthroplasty. Orthop. Rev., *8*:49–64, 1979.
92. Sneller, M., Wellborne, F., Barile, M.F., and Plotz, P.: Prosthetic joint infection with Mycoplasma hominis. (Letter.) J. Infect. Dis., *153*:174–175, 1986.
93. Powers, K.A., Terpenning, M.S., Voice, R.A., and Kauffman, C.A. Prosthetic joint infections in the elderly. Am. J. Med., *88*:5-9N–5-13N, 1990.
94. Morrey, B.F., et al.: Long-term results of various treatment options for infected total knee arthroplasty. Clin. Orthop., *248*:120–128, 1989.
95. Wilde, A.H., and Ruth, J.T.: Two-stage reimplantation in infected total knee arthoplasty. Clin. Orthop., *236*:23–35, 1988.
96. Insall, J.N., Thompson, F.M., and Brause, B.D.: Two-stage reimplantation for the salvage of infected total knee arthroplasty. J. Bone Joint Surg., *65A*:1087–1098, 1983.

97. Brause, B.D.: Infections with prostheses in bones and joints. *In* Principles and Practice of Infectious Diseases. 3rd Ed. Edited by G.L. Mandell, R.G. Douglas Jr. and J.E. Bennett. New York, Churchill Livingstone, 1990, pp. 919–922.
98. Buchholz, H.W., et al.: Management of deep infection of total hip replacement. J. Bone Joint Surg., *63B*:342–353, 1981.
99. Wroblewski, B.M.: One-stage revision of infected cemented total hip arthroplasty. Clin. Orthop., *211*:103–107, 1986.
100. Turner, R.H., Miley, G.D., and Fremont-Smith, P.: Septic total hip replacement and revision arthroplasty. *In* Revision Total Hip Arthoplasty. Edited by R.H. Turner and A.D. Schiller. New York, Grune & Stratton, 1982.
101. Trippel, S.B.: Antibiotic-impregnated cement in total joint arthroplasty. J. Bone Joint Surg., *68A*:1297–1302, 1986.
102. McDonald, D.J., Fitzgerald, R.H., and Ilstrup, D.M.: Two-stage reconstruction of a total hip arthroplasty because of infection. J. Bone Joint Surg. [A], *71*:828–834, 1989.
103. McElwaine, J.P., and Colville, J.: Excision arthroplasty for infected total hip replacements. J. Bone Joint Surg., *66B*:168–171, 1984.
104. Dajani, A.S., et al.: Prevention of bacterial endocarditis, recommendations by the American Heart Association. JAMA, *264*:2919–2922, 1990.
105. Blackburn, W.D. Jr., and Alarcon, G.S.: Prosthetic joint infections, a role for prophylaxis. Arthritis Rheum., *34*:110–117, 1991.
106. Radcliffe, K., Pattrick, M., and Doherty, M.: Complications resulting from misdiagnosing pseudogout as sepsis. Br. Med. J., *293*:440–441, 1986.
107. Baer, P.A., Tenebaum, J., Fam., A.G., and Little, H.: Coexistent septic and crystal arthritis. Report of four cases and literature review. J. Rheumatol., *13*:604–607, 1986.
108. Brancos, M.A., et al.: Septic arthritis and pseudogout. (Letter.) J. Rheumatol., *12*:1021–1022, 1985.
109. Gordon, T.P., Reid, C., Rozenbilds, M.A.M., and Ahern, M.: Crystal shedding in septic arthritis: Case reports and in vivo evidence in an animal model. Aust. N.Z. J. Med., *16*:336–340, 1986.
110. Zyskowski, L.P., Silverfield, J.C., and O'Duffy, J.D.: Pseudogout masking other arthritides. J. Rheumatol., *10*:449–453, 1983.
111. Ide, A., Jacobelli, S., and Zenteno, G.: Candida arthritis associated with positive birefringent crystals without chondrocalcinosis. (Letter.) J. Rheumatol., *4*:327–328, 1977.
112. Heinicke, M., Gomez-Reino, J.J., and Gorevic, P.D.: Crystal arthropathy as a complication of septic arthritis. J. Rheumatol. *8*:529–531, 1981.
113. Parker, V.S., Malhotra, C.M., Ho, G., Jr., and Kaplan, S.R.: Radiographic appearance of the sternomanubrial joint in arthritis and related conditions. Radiology, *153*:343–347, 1984.
114. Sequeira, W.: Diseases of the pubic symphysis. Semin. Arthritis Rheum., *16*:11–21, 1986.
115. Gruber, B.L., Kaufman, L.D., and Gorevic, P.D.: Septic arthritis involving the manubriosternal joint. J. Rheumatol., *12*:803–804, 1985.
116. Glushakow, A.S., Carlson, D., and DePalma, A.F.: Pyarthrosis of the manubriosternal joint. Clin. Orthop., *114*:214–215, 1976.
117. Borgmeier, P.J., and Kalovidouris, A.E.: Septic arthritis of the sternomanubrial joint due to Pseudomonas pseudomallei. Arthritis Rheum., *23*:1057–1059, 1980.
118. Sequeira, W., et al.: Pyogenic infections of the pubic symphysis. Ann. Intern. Med., *96*:604–606, 1982.
119. Yood, R.A., and Goldenberg, D.L.: Sternoclavicular joint arthritis. Arthritis Rheum., *23*:232–239, 1980.
120. Bellamy, N., Park, W., and Rooney, P.J.: What do we know about the sacroiliac joint? Semin. Arthritis Rheum., *12*:282–313, 1983.
121. Hynd, R.F., Klofkorn, R.W., and Wong., J.K.: Streptococcus anginosus-constellatus infection of the sternoclavicular joint. J. Rheumatol., *11*:713–715, 1984.
122. Wohlgethan, J.R., Newberg, A.H., and Reed, J.I.: The risk of abscess from sternoclavicular septic arthritis. J. Rheumatol., *15*:1302–1306, 1988.
123. Alexander, P.W., and Shin, M.S.: CT manifestation of sternoclavicular pyarthrosis in patients with intravenous drug abuse. J. Comput. Assist. Tomogr., *14*:104–106, 1990.
124. Seviour, P.W., and Dieppe, P.A.: Sternoclavicular joint infection as a cause of chest pain. Br. Med. J., *288*:133–134, 1984.
125. Tabatabai, M.F., Sapico, F.L., Canawati, H.N., and Harley, H.A.J.: Sternoclavicular joint infection with group B streptococcus. (Letter.) J. Rheumatol., *13*:466, 1986.
126. Watanakunakorn, C.: Serratia marcescens osteomyelitis of the clavicle and sternoclavicular arthritis complicating infected indwelling subclavian vein catheter. Am. J. Med., *80*:753–754, 1986.
127. Nitsche, J.F., Vaughan, J.H., Williams, G., and Curd, J.G.: Septic sternoclavicular arthritis with Pasteurella multocida and Streptococcus sanguis. Arthritis Rheum., *25*:467–469, 1982.
128. Kerr, R.: Pyogenic sacroiliitis. Orthopedics, *8*:1030–1034, 1985.
129. Shanahan, M.D.G., and Ackroyd, C.E.: Pyogenic infection of the sacroiliac joint. J. Bone Joint Surg., *67B*:605–608, 1985.
130. Delbarre, F., et al.: Pyogenic infection of the sacro-iliac joint. J. Bone Joint Surg., *57A*:819–825, 1975.
131. Hodgson, B.F.: Pyogenic sacroiliac joint infection. Clin. Orthop., *246*:146–149, 1989.
132. Iczkovitz, J.M., Leek, J.C., and Robbins, D.L.: Pyogenic sacroiliitis. J. Rheumatol., *8*:157–160, 1981.
133. Miskew, D.B., Block, R.A., and Witt, P.F.: Aspiration of infected sacroiliac joints. J. Bone Joint Surg., *61A*:1071–1072, 1979.
134. Schaad, U.B., McCracken, G.H., and Nelson, J.D.: Pyogenic arthritis of the sacroiliac joint in pediatric patients. Pediatrics, *66*:375–379, 1980.
135. Reilly, J.P., Gross, R.H., Emans, J.B., and Yngve, D.A.: Disorders of the sacroiliac joint in children. J. Bone Joint Surg. [A], *70*:31–40, 1988.
136. Moyer, R.A., Bross, J.E., and Harrington, T.M.: Pyogenic sacroiliitis in a rural population. J. Rheumatol., *17*:1364–1368, 1990.
137. Quevedo, S.F., Mikolich, D.J., Humbyrd, D.E., and Fisher, A.E.: Pyogenic sacroiliitis caused by group G streptococcus. (Letter.) Arthritis Rheum., *30*:115, 1987.
138. Ross, G.N., Baraff, L.J., and Quismorio, F.P.: Serratia arthritis in heroin users. J. Bone Joint Surg., *57A*:1158–1160, 1975.
139. Ziment, I., Davis, A., and Finegold, S.M.: Joint infection by anaerobic bacteria. Arthritis Rheum., *12*:627–635, 1969.
140. Longoria, R.R., and Carpenter, J.L.: Anaerobic pyogenic sacroiliitis. South. Med. J., *76*:649–651, 1983.
141. Scott, J.P., Maurer, H.S., and Dias, L.: Septic arthritis in two teenaged hemophiliacs. J. Pediatr., *107*:748–751, 1985.
142. Ragni, M.V., and Hanley, E.N.: Septic arthritis in hemophilic patients and infection with human immunodeficiency virus. (Letter.) Ann. Intern. Med., *110*:168–169, 1989.
143. Helliwell, M.: Staphylococcus aureus infection complicating haemarthroses in elderly patients. Clin. Rheumatol., *4*:90–92, 1985.
144. Martin, J.R., Root, H.S., Kim, S.O., and Johnson, L.G.: Staphylococcus suppurative arthritis occurring in neuropathic knee joints. Arthritis Rheum., *8*:389–402, 1965.
145. Rubinow, A., Spark, E.C., and Canoso, J.J.: Septic arthritis in a charcot joint. Clin. Orthop., *147*:203–206, 1980.
146. Goodman, M.A., and Swartz, W.: Infection in a charcot joint. J. Bone Joint Surg., *67A*:642–643, 1985.
147. Ascuitto, R., Drennan, J., and Fitzgerald, V.: Group C strepto-

coccal arthritis an osteomyelitis in an adolescent with a hereditary sensory neuropathy. Pediatr. Infect. Dis., *4*:553–554, 1985.
148. Mathews, M., Shen, F.H., Lindner, A., and Sherrard, D.J.: Septic arthritis in hemodialyzed patients. Nephron, *25*:87–91, 1980.
149. Spencer, J.D.: Bone and joint infection in a renal unit. J. Bone Joint Surg., *68B*:489–493, 1986.
150. Bomalaski, J.S., Williamson, P.K., and Goldstein, C.S.: Infectious arthritis in renal transplant patients. Arthritis Rheum., *29*:227–232, 1986.
151. Mallouh, A., and Talab, Y.: Bone and joint infection in patients with sickle cell disease. J. Pediatr. Orthop., *5*:158–162, 1985.
152. Syrogiannopoulos, G.A., McCracken, G.H., and Nelson, J.D.: Osteoarticular infections in children with sickle cell disease. Pediatrics, *78*:1019–1096, 1986.
153. Barrett-Connor, E.: Bacterial infection and sickle cell anemia. Medicine, *50*:97–112, 1971.
154. Espinoza, L.R., Spilberg, I., and Osterland, C.K.: Joint manifestations of sickle cell disease. Medicine, *53*:295–305, 1974.
155. Espinoza, L.R., et al.: Rheumatic manifestations associated with human immunodeficiency virus infection. Arthritis Rheum., *32*:1615–1622, 1989.
156. Kaye, B.R.: Rheumatologic manifestations of infection with human immunodeficiency virus. Ann. Intern. Med., *111*:158–167, 1989.
157. Rowe, I.F., et al.: Rheumatologic lesions in individuals with human immunodeficiency virus infection. Q. J. Med., *73*:1167–1184, 1989.
158. Zimmermann, B., Erickson, A.D., and Mikolich, D.J.: Septic acromioclavicular arthritis and osteomyelitis in a patient with acquired immunodeficiency syndrome. Arthritis Rheum., *32*:1175–1178, 1989.
159. Lipstein-Kresch, E., et al.: Disseminated Sporothrix schenckii infection with arthritis in a patient with acquired immunodeficiency syndrome. J. Rheumatol., *12*:805–808, 1985.
160. Ricciardi, D.D., et al.: Cryptococcal arthritis in a patient with acquired immune deficiency syndrome. Case report and review of the literature. J. Rheumatol. *13*:455–458, 1986.
161. Rogers, P.L., et al.: Disseminated Mycobacterium haemophilum infection in two patients with the acquired immunodeficiency syndrome. Am. J. Med., *84*:640–642, 1988.
162. Blumenthal, D.R., Zucker, J.R., and Hawkins, C.C.: Mycobacterium avium complex-induced septic arthritis and osteomyelitis in a patient with the acquired immunodeficiency syndrome. (Letter.) Arthritis Rheum., *33*:757–758, 1990.
163. Smith, J.W.: Infectious arthritis. *In* Principles and Practice of Infectious Diseases. Edited by G.L. Mandell, R.G. Douglas, Jr., and J.E. Bennett. 2nd Ed. New York, John Wiley & Sons, 1985, Chapter 83.
164. Wolski, K.P.: Staphylococcal and other Gram-positive coccal arthritides. Clin. Rheum. Dis., *4*:181–196, 1978.
165. Esposito, A.L., and Gleckman, R.A.: Acute polymicrobic septic arthritis in adult: Case report and literature review. Am. J. Med. Sci., *267*:251–254, 1974.
166. Petty, B.G., Sowa, D.T., and Charache, P.: Polymicrobial polyarticular septic arthritis. JAMA, *249*:2069–2072, 1983.
167. Finegold, S.M.: Anaerobic Bacteria in Human Disease. New York, Academic Press, 1977, pp. 443–454.
168. Finegold, R.H., Jr., Rosenblatt, J.E., Tenney, J.H., and Bourgault, A.: Anaerobic septic arthritis. Clin. Orthop., *164*:141–148, 1982.
169. Goldenberg, D.L., and Cohen, A.S.: Acute infectious arthritis. A review of patients with nongonococcal joint infections (with emphysis on therapy and prognosis). Am. J. Med., *60*:369–377, 1976.
170. Rosenthal, J., Bole, G.G., and Robinson, W.D.: Acute nongonococcal infectious arthritis. Evaluation of risk factors, therapy, and outcome. Arthritis Rheum., *23*:889–897, 1980.
171. Manshady, B.M., Thompson, G.R., and Weiss, J.J.: Septic arthritis in a general hospital 1966–1977. J. Rheumatol., *7*:523–530, 1980.
172. Sharp, J.T., Lidksy, M.D., Duffy, J., and Duncan, M.W.: Infectious arthritis. Arch. Intern. Med., *139*:1125–1130, 1979.
173. Cooper, C., and Cawley, M.I.D.: Bacterial arthritis in an English health district: A 10 year review. Ann. Rheum. Dis., *45*:458–463, 1986.
174. Sheagren, J.N.: Staphylococcus aureus. The persistent pathogen. N. Engl. J. Med., *310*:1368–1373, 1437–1442, 1984.
175. Schwalbe, R.S., Stapleton, J.T., and Gilligan, P.H.: Emergence of vancomycin resistance in coagulase-negative staphylococci. N. Engl. J. Med., *316*:927–931, 1987.
176. Wolfson, J.S., and Hooper, D.C.: The fluoroquinolones: Structures, mechanisms of action and resistance, and spectra of activity in vitro. Antimicrob. Agents Chemother., *28*:581–586, 1985.
177. Hooper, D.C., and Wolfson, J.S.: The fluoroquinolones: Pharmacology, clinical uses, and toxicities in humans. Antimicrob. Agents Chemother., *28*:716–721, 1985.
178. Pischel, K.D., Weisman, M.H., and Cone, R.O.: Unique features of Group B streptococcal arthritis in adults. Arch. Intern. Med., *145*:97–102, 1985.
179. Laster, A.J., and Michels, M.L.: Group B streptococcal arthritis in adults. Am. J. Med., *76*:910–915, 1984.
180. Vartian, C., Lerner, P.I., Shlaes, D.M., and Gopalakrishna, K.V.: Infections due to Lancefield group G streptococci. Medicine, *64*:75–88, 1985.
181. Kauffman, C.A., Watanakunakorn, C., and Phair, J.P.: Pneumococcal arthritis. J. Rheumatol., *3*:409–419, 1976.
182. Edwards, G.S., Jr., and Russell, I.J.: Pneumococcal arthritis complicating gout. J. Rheumatol., *7*:907–910, 1980.
183. Andersen, B.R., Mayer, M.E., Geiseler, P.J., and Niebel, J.R.: Multi-joint pneumococcal pyarthrosis in a patient with a chemotactic defect. Arthritis Rheum., *26*:1160–1162, 1983.
184. Ike, R.W.: Septic arthritis due to group C streptococcus: Report and review of the literature. J. Rheumatol., *17*:1230–1236, 1990.
185. Zwillich, S.H., Hamory, B.H., and Walker, S.E.: Enterococcus: An unusual cause of septic arthritis. Arthritis Rheum., *27*:591–595, 1984.
186. Taylor, P.W., and Trueblood, M.C.: Septic arthritis due to Aerococcus viridans. J. Rheumatol., *12*:1004–1005, 1985.
187. Catto, B.A., Jacobs, M.R., and Shlaes, D.M.: Streptococcus mitis, a cause of serious infection in adults. Arch. Intern. Med., *147*:885–888, 1987.
188. Nieman, R.E., and Lorber, B.: Listeriosis in adults: A changing pattern. Rev. Infect. Dis., *2*:207–227, 1980.
189. Louthrenoo, W., and Schumacher, H.R. Jr.: Listeria monocytogenes osteomyelitis complicating leukemia: Report and literature review of listeria osteoarticular infections. J. Rheumatol., *17*:107–110, 1990.
190. Newman, J.H., Waycott, S., and Cooney, L.M., Jr.: Arthritis due to Listeria monocytogenes. Arthritis Rheum., *22*:1139–1140, 1979.
191. Breckenridge, R.L., Jr., Buck, L., Tooley, E., and Douglas, G.W.: Listeria monocytogenes septic arthritis. Am. J. Clin. Pathol., *73*:140–141, 1980.
192. Curosh, N.A., and Perednia, D.A.: Listeria monocytogenes septic arthritis, a case report and review of the literature. Arch. Intern. Med., *149*:1207–1208, 1989.
193. Booth, L.V., et al.: Listeria monocytogenes infection in a prosthetic knee joint in rheumatoid arthritis. Ann. Rheum. Dis., *49*:58–59, 1990.
194. Massarotti, E.M., and Dinerman, H.: Septic arthritis due to Lis-

teria monocytogenes: Report and review of the literature. J. Rheumatol., *17*:111–113, 1990.

195. Abadie, S.M., Dalovisio, J.R., Pankey, G.A., and Cortez, L.M.: Listeria monocytogenes arthritis in a renal transplant recipient. (Letter.) J. Infect. Dis., *156*:413–414, 1987.

196. Weiler, P.J., and Hastings, D.E.: Listeria monocytogenes, an unusual cause of late infection in a prosthetic hip joint. J. Rheumatol., *17*:705–707, 1990.

197. Norenberg, D.D., Bigley, D.V., Virata, R.L., and Liang, G.C.: Corynebacterium pyogenes septic arthritis with plasma cell synovial infiltrate and monoclonal gammopathy. Arch. Intern. Med., *138*:810–811, 1978.

198. Messina, O.D., et al.: Corynebacterium kutscheri septic arthritis. (Letter.) Arthritis Rheum., *32*:1053, 1989.

199. Robinson, S.C.: Bacillus cereus septic arthritis following arthrography. Clin. Orthop., *145*:237–238, 1979.

200. Morrison, V.A., and Chia, J.K.S.: Septic arthritis due to Bacillus. South. Med. J., *79*:522–523, 1986.

201. Kooijmans-Coutinho, M.F., Markusse, H.M., and Dijkmans, B.A.C.: Infectious arthritis caused by Propionibacterium acnes: A report of two cases. Ann. Rheum. Dis., *48*:851–852, 1989.

202. Craig, D.B., and Wehrle, P.A.: Branhamella catarrhalis septic arthritis. J. Rheumatol., *10*:985–986, 1983.

203. Patel, N.J., Moore, T.L., Weiss, T.D., and Zuckner, J.: Kingella kingae infectious arthritis: case report and review of literature of Kingella and Moraxella infections. Arthritis Rheum., *26*:557–559, 1983.

204. Feigin, R.D., San Joaquin, V., and Middelkamp, J.N.: Septic arthritis due to Moraxella osloensis. J. Pediatr., *75*:116–117, 1969.

205. deGroot, R., et al.: Bone and joint infections caused by Kingella kingae: Six cases and review of the literature. Rev. Infect. Dis., *10*:998–1004, 1988.

206. Vincent, J., Podewell, C., Frankin, G.W., and Korn, J.H.: Septic arthritis due to Kingella (Moraxella) kingii. J. Rheumatol., *8*:501–503, 1981.

207. Salminen, I., Von Essen, R., Koota, K., and Nissinen, A.: A pitfall in purulent arthritis brought out in Kingella kingae infection of the knees. Ann. Rheum. Dis., *43*:656–657, 1984.

208. Hirschmann, J.V., and Everett, E.D.: Haemophilus influenzae infections in adults: Report of nine cases and a review of the literature. Medicine (Baltimore), *58*:80–94, 1979.

209. Dajani, A.S., Asmar, B.I., and Thirumoorthi, M.C.: Systemic Hemophilus influenzae disease: An overview. J. Pediatr., *94*:355–364, 1979.

210. Rotbart, H.A., and Glode, M.P.: Haemophilus infuenzae type b septic arthritis in children: Report of 23 cases. Pediatrics, *75*:254–259, 1985.

211. Ho, G., Jr., Gadbaw, J.J., Jr., and Glickstein, S.L.: Hemophilus influenzae septic arthritis in adults. Semin. Arthritis Rheum., *12*:314–321, 1983.

212. Knisely, G.K., Gibson, G.R., and Reichman, R.C.: Hemophilus influenzae bursitis and meningitis in an adult. Arch. Intern Med. *143*:1465–1466, 1983.

213. Cohen, M.A., Levy, I.M., and Habermann, E.T.: Multiple joint sepsis by Hemophilus influenza in an adult. Clin. Orthop., *209*:198–201, 1986.

214. Borenstein, D.G., and Simon, G.L.: Hemophilus influenzae septic arthritis in adults. A report of four cases and a review of the literature. Medicine (Baltimore), *65*:191–201, 1986.

215. Ho, G., Jr., Tice, A.D., and Kaplan, S.R.: Septic bursitis in the prepatellar and olecranon bursae. Ann. Intern. Med., *89*;21–27, 1978.

216. Goldenberg, D.L., and Cohen, A.S.: Arthritis due to Gram-negative bacilli. Clin. Rheum. Dis., *4*:197–210, 1978.

217. Ruthberg, A.D., and Ho, G., Jr.: Nongonococcal bacterial arthritis. *In* Orthopedic Infections. Edited by R.D. D'Ambrosia and R.L. Marier. Thorofare, NJ, Slack, Inc., 1989, pp. 213–231.

218. Gifford, D.B., Patzakis, M., Ivler, D., and Swezey, R.L.: Septic arthritis due to Pseudomonas in heroin addicts. J. Bone Joint Surg., *57A*:631–635, 1975.

219. Bayer, A.S., et al.: Gram-negative bacillary septic arthritis: Clinical, radiographic, therapeutic, and prognostic features. Semin. Arthritis Rheum., *7*;123–132, 1977.

220. Newman, E.D., Davis, D.E., and Harrington, T.M.: Septic arthritis due to gram negative bacilli: Older patients with good outcome. J. Rheumatol., *15*:659–662, 1988.

221. David, J.R., and Black, R.L.: Salmonella arthritis. Medicine, *39*:385–403, 1960.

222. Brodie, T.D., and Ehresmann, G.R.: Salmonella dublin arthritis: An initial case presentation. J. Rheumatol., *10*:144–146, 1983.

223. Quismorio, F.P., Jr., et al.: Septic arthritis due to Arizona hinshawii. J. Rheumatol., *10*:147–150, 1983.

224. Spira, T.J., and Kabins, S.A.: Yersinia enterocolitica septicemia with septic arthritis. Arch. Intern. Med., *136*:1305–1308, 1976.

225. Taylor, B.G., Zafarzai, M.Z., Humphreys, D.W., and Manfredi, F.: Nodular pulmonary infiltrates and septic arthritis associated with Yersinia enterocolitica bacteremia. Am. Rev. Resp. Dis., *116*:525–529, 1977.

226. Kilo, C., Hagemann, P.O., and Marzi, J.: Septic arthritis and bacteremia due to Vibrio fetus. Am. J. Med., *38*:962–971, 1965.

227. Aho, K., Leirisalo-Repo, M., and Repo, H.: Reactive arthritis. Clin. Rheum. Dis., *11*:25–40, 1985.

228. Ford, D.K.: Reactive arthritis: A viewpoint rather than a review. Clin. Rheum. Dis., *12*:389–401, 1986.

229. Jacobs, R.F., McCarthy, R.E., and Elser, J.M.: Pseudomonas osteochondritis complicating puncture wounds of the foot in children: A 10 year evaluation. J. Infect. Dis., *160*:657–661, 1989.

230. Siebert, W.T., Dewan, S., and Williams, T.W.: Pseudomonas puncture wound osteomyelitis in adults. Am. J. Med. Sci., *283*:83–88, 1982.

231. Walton, K., Hilton, R.C., and Sen, R.A.: Pseudomonas arthritis treated with parenteral and intra-articular ceftazidime. Ann. Rheum. Dis., *44*:499–500, 1985.

232. Matteson, E.L., and McCune, W.J.: Septic arthritis caused by treatment resistant Pseudomonas cepacia. Ann. Rheum. Dis., *49*:258–259, 1990.

233. Baltimore, R.S., and Jenson, H.B.: Puncture wound osteochondritis of the foot caused by Pseudomonas maltophilia. Pediatr. Infect. Dis. J., *9*:143–144, 1990.

234. Winn, R.E., Chase, W.F., Lauderdale, P.W. and McCleskey, F.K.: Septic arthritis involving Capnocytophaga ochracea. J. Clin. Microbiol., *19*:538–540, 1984.

235. Dean, H.M., and Post, R.M.: Fatal infection with Aeromonas hydrophila in a patient with acute myelogenous leukemia. Ann. Intern. Med., *66*:1177–1179, 1967.

236. Chmel, H., and Armstrong, D.: Acute arthritis caused by Aeromonas hydrophila: Clinical and therapeutic aspects. Arthritis Rheum., *19*:169–172, 1976.

237. Weber, D.J., Wolfson, J.S., Swartz, M.N., and Hooper, D.C.: Pasteurella multocida infections. Report of 34 cases and review of the literature. Medicine (Baltimore), *63*:133–154, 1984.

238. Ewing, R., et al.: Articular and skeletal infections caused by Pasteurella multocida. South. Med. J., *73*:1349–1352, 1980.

239. Mellors, J.W., and Schoen, R.T.: Pasteurella multocida septic arthritis. Conn. Med., *48*:221–223, 1984.

240. Baker, G.L., Oddis, C.V., and Medsger, T.A.: Pasteurella multocida polyarticular septic arthritis. J. Rheumatol., *14*:355–357, 1987.

241. Sugarman, M., Quismorio, F.P., and Patzakis, M.J.: Joint infection by Pasteurella multocida. Lancet, *2*:1267, 1975.

242. Griffin, A.J., and Barber, H.M.: Joint infection by Pasteurella multocida. Lancet, *1*:1347–1348, 1975.
243. Mandel, D.R.: Streptobacillary fever. An unusual cause of infectious arthritis. Cleve. Clin. Q., *52*:203–205, 1985.
244. Anderson, D., and Marrie, T.J.: Septic arthritis due to Streptobacillus moniliformis. (Letter.) Arthritis Rheum., *30*:229–230, 1987.
245. Holroyd, K.J., Reiner, A.P., and Dick, J.D.: Streptobacillus moniliformis polyarthritis mimicking rheumatoid arthritis: An urban case of rat bite fever. Am. J. Med., *85*:711–714, 1988.
246. Young, E.J.: Human brucellosis. Rev. Infect. Dis., *5*:821–842, 1983.
247. Gotuzzo, E., et al.: Articular involvement in human brucellosis: A retrospective analysis of 304 cases. Semin. Arthritis Rheum., *12*:245–255, 1982.
248. Ariza, J., et al.: Brucellar spondylitis: A detailed analysis based on current findings. Rev. Infect. Dis., *7*:656–664, 1985.
249. Porat, S., and Shapiro, M.: Brucella arthritis of the sacro-iliac joint. Infection, *12*:205–207, 1984.
250. Baranda, M.M., et al.: Sternoclavicular septic arthritis as first manifestation of brucellosis. (Letter.) Br. J. Rheumatol., *25*:322, 1986.
251. Tosi, M.F., and Nelson, T.J.: Brucella canis infection in a 17-month-old child successfully treated with moxalactam. J. Pediatr., *101*:725–727, 1982.
252. Gomez-Reino, F.J., Mateo, I., Fuertes, A., and Gomez-Reino, J.J.: Brucellar arthritis in children and its successful treatment with trimethoprim-sulphamethoxazole. Ann. Rheum. Dis. *45*:256–258, 1986.
253. Clark, G.M.: Syphilitic joint disease. *In* Arthritis and Allied Conditions. 8th Ed. Edited by J.L. Hollander and D.J. McCarty, Jr. Philadelphia, Lea & Febiger, 1972, pp. 1255–1259.
254. Cassell, G.H., and Cole, B.C.: Mycoplasma as agents of human disease. N. Engl. J. Med., *304*:80–89, 1981.
255. Taylor-Robinson, D., Gumpel, J.M., Hill, A., and Swannell, A.J.: Isolation of Mycoplasma pneumoniae from synovial fluid of a hypogammaglobulinemic patient in a survey of patients with inflammatory polyarthritis. Ann. Rheum. Dis., *37*:180–182, 1978.
256. Vogler, L.B., et al.: Ureaplasma urealyticum polyarthritis in agammaglobulinemia. Pediatr. Infect. Dis., *4*:687–691, 1985.
257. Madoff, S., and Hooper, D.C.: Nongenitourinary infections caused by Mycoplasma hominis in adults. Rev. Infect. Dis., *10*:602–613, 1988.
258. Nylander, N., Tan, M., and Newcombe, D.S.: Successful management of Mycoplasma hominis septic arthritis involving a cementless prosthesis. Am. J. Med., *87*:348–352, 1989.
259. Boudoulas, O., and Camisa, C.: Nocardia asteroides infection with dissemination to skin and joints. Arch. Derm., *121*:898–900, 1985.
260. Cons, F., Trevino, A., and Lavelle, C.: Septic arthritis due to Nocardia brasiliensis. (Letter.) J. Rheumatol., *12*:1019–1021, 1985.
261. Rao, K.V., O'Brien, T.J., and Andersen, R.C.: Septic arthritis due to Nocardia asteroides after successful kidney transplantation. Arthritis Rheum., *24*:99–101, 1981.
262. Chowdhary, G., Wormser, G.P., and Mascarenhas, B.R.: Nocardia bursitis. J. Rheumatol., *15*:139–140, 1988.
263. McCarty, D.J.: Joint sepsis: A chance for cure. (Editorial.) JAMA, *247*:835, 1982.
264. Ward, T.T., and Steigbigel, R.T.: Acidosis of synovial fluid correlated with synovial fluid leukocytosis. Am. J. Med., *64*:933–936, 1978.

117

Gonococcal Arthritis and Other Neisserial Infections

DON L. GOLDENBERG

MICROBIOLOGY AND EPIDEMIOLOGY OF NEISSERIA GONORRHOEAE

To understand the clinical and therapeutic aspects of disseminated gonococcal infection (DGI), the microbiologic characteristics of Neisseria gonorrhoeae must be understood. The molecular basis of N. gonorrhoeae infections has probably been more intensively studied than that of any other bacterial infection during the past two decades. Complicated, integrated mechanisms that determine microbial virulence in local and systemic gonococcal infections have been unraveled (Table 117–1).

The cell surface structure of N. gonorrhoeae is complex and intimately related to the pathogenesis of infections. Important cell wall structural components include the pili and the trilaminar outer membrane containing proteins I, II, III, as well as lipopolysaccharide (LPS) and peptidoglycan. Gonoccal pili facilitate attachment to epithelial cells.[1] Once attached to the mucosal surface, endocytosis allows the gonococci to pass through epithelial cells where they are released to supepithelial tissues. Pili also impede phagocytosis by polymorphonuclear leukocytes (PMNs).[2] Gonococcal morphology in culture correlates with virulence.[1] Small, sharply bordered colonies, termed P+ or P++ colony types, are more virulent than larger colonies, and this morphologic characteristic is associated with the presence of surface pili. Pili from different strains are antigenically different, and single gonococcal strains can produce antigenically variant pili.

TABLE 117–1. IMPORTANT MICROBIAL-HOST VIRULENCE FACTORS

MICROBIAL VIRULENCE FACTORS
Gonococcal pili (P+, P++ colony morphology)
Outer membrane protein 1A
Nutritional requirements (AHU$^-$ strains)
Resistance to bactericidal effects of normal human sera
Antimicrobial resistance
HOST VIRULENCE FACTORS
High-risk sexual practices including number of partners, prostitutes, previous antibiotics
State of endocervix, urethra, such as pH
Complement deficiency

Protein I is the predominant outer membrane protein and is important in attachment and endocytosis.[3] Protein I is genetically stable and therefore used for gonococcal serotyping. There are three distinct protein I serogroups—A, B, and C—which correspond to WI, WII, and WIII, as determined by coagglutination serotyping.[4] Protein II also is important in gonococcal attachment, intergonococcal adhesion, and susceptibility to the bactericidal activity of normal human sera.[2] Protein III is closely associated with protein I and also is important in determining virulence. Gonococcal LPS is active in local cytotoxicity and in systemic toxicity, including fever.[2] Gonococci also produce IgA protease, which cleaves IgA secretory immunoglobulins.

Gonococcal serotyping has led to a greater understanding of virulence factors and clinical manifestations of DGI. The presence of protein IA correlates with the ability of gonococcal strains to disseminate, and the outer membrane antigenic variation is a critical factor in microbial virulence.[5] However, other typing characteristics such as nutritional requirements, plasmid content, and antibiotic sensitivity help determine disease potential. For example, the stable nutritional requirements for growth (termed auxotype) of gonococcal colonies isolated from DGI patients differ from those of colonies isolated from patients with uncomplicated gonorrhea.[6] Strains requiring arginine, hypoxanthine, and uracil for growth, designated AHU strains, are more commonly isolated from DGI patients. Protein I serotyping combined with auxotyping has been especially helpful in revealing clinical and epidemiologic patterns.[7]

The ability of a gonococcal strain to disseminate is associated with its resistance to the bactericidal action of normal human sera.[8] The precise mechanism of gonococcal serum resistance is unclear but is strongly associated with protein IA and with the AHU auxotype.[7,8] These three risk factors for DGI are interrelated. Variations in the in-vitro serum susceptibility of gonococcal strains isolated from patients with DGI based on the patient's clinical manifestations were noted in one study.[9] Seventy-five percent of the N. gonorrhoeae isolates from patients with tenosynovitis and dermatitis were resistant to the bactericidal activity of normal human sera, whereas only 47% of strains isolated from patients with suppurative arthritis were resistant. Sixty-nine percent of patients with suppurative arthritis, but only 17% of those with dermatitis-tenosynovitis, developed a significant rise in serum bactericidal antibody activity. Thus, microbial phenotypic characteristics can not only determine virulence and ability to disseminate but can also influence the clinical features of DGI.

Host factors that predispose to gonorrhea and DGI include high-risk sexual practices such as multiple partners and prostitution, and prior antibiotics.[8] Women with localized gonococcal infections early in pregnancy or at certain phases of their menstrual cycle harbor strains that are more resistant to killing by normal human sera and have transparent colonial morphology.[6–10] The gonococcus can antigenically vary the pilus and outer membranes to evade host defense mechanisms that can change according to local environment, such as the pH of the endocervix.[8]

Congenital or acquired complement deficiencies also predispose patients to neisserial infections.[10,11] Congenital deficiencies of late complement components are especially important. There have been more meningococcal than gonococcal infections reported in such patients.[10] Patients with systemic lupus erythematosus (SLE) are especially susceptible to neisserial infections. A report combining four cases from one medical center with 7 others already described in the literature revealed that 9 of 11 cases were due to N. meningitidis.[11] The under-representation of DGI might represent a reporting bias (Table 117–2). Seven of the eight patients had low CH50 levels and two had congenital C2 deficiency. Most patients presented with septicemia or meningitis; three of 11 died. In addition to the prominent complement deficiency in SLE, other risk factors for neisserial infection include asplenia or functional reticuloendothelial dysfunction and use of immunosuppressive medications.

The emergence of antibiotic resistance is of utmost importance in the treatment of DGI. Until recently there were few reports of DGI strains that were resistant to antibiotics, and most DGI strains have been more sensitive to penicillin than strains isolated from local infections.[8] However, the epidemic of antibiotic resistant strains and the growing number of reports of such strains associated with DGI has been alarming.[12] Antibiotic resistance is controlled by genes on either plasmid or chromosome. A β-lactamase plasmid produces β-lactamase, which chiefly affects β-lactam antibiotics. Chromosomally mediated antibiotic resistance is generally related to multiple chromosomal mutations and affects many antibiotics including β-lactams, tetracyclines, erythromycin, and spectinomycin.[13] The mechanism of antimicrobial resistance can involve decreased cell wall permeability, decreased affinity of the penicillin-binding proteins for β-lactam antibiotics, and increased concentration of penicillin-binding proteins.[13] Testing for penicillinase-producing strains of N. gonorrhoeae is simple, inexpensive, and widely available. However, the other types of antimicrobial resistance can be detected only with expensive and

TABLE 117–2. NEISSERIAL INFECTIONS IN SLE PATIENTS

Patient	1	2	3	4	5	6	7	8	9	10	11
Age (yrs)	19	19	18	15	43	17	16	14	20	23	14
Disease Duration (yrs)	2	2	5	2	NA	0	NA	NA	1.5	10	NA
Renal Involvement	Y	N	Y	Y	NA	N	Y	Y	Y	Y	NA
Steroid Rx (mg)	MP	—	P	P	—	—	P	DM	—	NA	P
	4		20	30			10	11			7.5
C3 (mg/dl)	76	78	59	55	37	35	NA	98	54	NA	NA
C4 (mg/dl)	9	12	9	6	9	4	NA	39	8	NA	NA
CH 50 (% of control)	NA	28	20	NA	100	NA	NA	NA	NA	70	5
Congenital complement deficiency	—	C2	—	—	C2	—	—	—	—	—	—
Azathioprine (mg/d)	—	—	—	—	—	—	100	100	—	—	—
Infecting organism	NM	NG	NM	NG	NM	NM	NM	NM	NM	NM	NM
Presenting mode	S	S	M	S	M	A	M	M	M	S	NA
Outcome	D	R	R	R	R	R	D	R	R	D	NA

Rx = treatment; MP = methylprednisolone; P = prednisone; DM = dexamethasone; NM = *N. meningitis*; NG = *N. gonorrhea*; A = arthritis; M = meningitis; S = septicemia; D = died; R = recovered; NA = not available.

Complement: C3, normals > 85 mg/dl; C4, normals > 15 mg/dl

Modified from Mitchell, S.R., Nguyen, P.Q., and Katz, P.[11]

technically difficult methods and are often not well standardized. Of 6204 isolates of N. gonorrhoeae from 21 clinic sites in the United States treating patients with gonorrhea between September 1987 and December 1988, 21% were resistant to penicillin, tetracycline, cefoxitin, or spectinomycin.[12] Two percent of isolates were penicillin-producing. A plasmid-mediated resistance to tetracycline was found in 1% of strains. Seventeen percent of the isolates had chromosomally mediated resistance.

Thus, the incidence of gonorrhea has decreased since 1975, but the incidence of antibiotic resistant infections has increased. This antimicrobial resistance and other microbial virulence factors are important in the epidemiology of gonorrhea and of DGI. DGI is much less common in the United Kingdom than in the United States or Scandinavia,[14] as is the presence of protein 1A and AHU-gonococcal strains. Furthermore, most gonococci isolated from patients in sexually-transmitted disease clinics in England are susceptible to penicillin, whereas antibiotic-resistant strains are the rule in Africa, Southeast Asia, and the Pacific.[14] Because of the emergence of antibiotic resistant strains of N. gonorrhoeae, the Centers for Disease Control revised their recommended treatment for all gonococcal infections, including DGI, in 1989.[15] Uncomplicated gonorrhea should be treated with a single dose of ceftriaxone, 250 mg intramuscularly (IM), combined with doxycycline 100 mg orally twice daily for 7 days. Alternative regimens include spectinomycin, 2 g IM, followed by doxycycline, or ciprofloxacin 500 mg orally followed by doxycycline.

Factors that can predict antimicrobial resistance include increased number of sexual partners, prostitute contact, recent travel history, and prior antibiotic use.[16] The widespread use of tetracycline to treat potential coexistent chlamydial infection might have promoted the emergence of resistant gonococci.[13,16] Of 6204 isolates of gonococci, all were sensitive to ceftriaxone and only three were resistant to spectinomycin.[12] However, ceftriaxone- and spectinomycin-resistant strains are being reported. Such resistance will probably increase as it has for penicillins and for tetracycline.[17]

The definitive diagnosis of neisserial infections requires identification with Gram's stain, in-vitro culture, or both. The characteristic intracellular gram-negative diplocci seen on Gram's stain smears of genitourinary exudates or synovial fluid are highly predictive of a positive culture.[2] However, the reliability of Gram's stain smear depends on the clinical setting. For example, in asymptomatic men, the reliability of Gram's stain smear of urethral exudates drops to 60%, and in women cervical Gram's stains have a 40 to 70% sensitivity.[2] Furthermore, atypical organisms or bacteria seen outside leukocytes are less predictive of positive cultures.

Optimal culture yield requires rapid transfer of specimens to the microbiology laboratory and incubation in a moist environment of 5% CO_2 atmosphere at 34 to 36°C. Specimens from normally sterile sites including synovial fluid and blood should be inoculated on chocolate agar. However, specimens from sites with normal bacteria flora such as the cervix, rectum, and pharynx should be inoculated on selective media that incorporate antibiotics to suppress the growth of the normal flora but not of N. gonorrhoeae. The initial Thayer-Martin medium incorporated vancomycin, colistin, and nystatin into chocolate agar, but there are now other selective media including modified Thayer-Martin, Martin-Lewis, and New York media.

N. gonorrhoeae can be differentiated from other Neisseria species by its ability to utilize glucose but not maltose, sucrose, or lactose and by its ability to reduce nitrates. Commercially available immunologic methods based on monoclonal antibodies have been used to distinguish N. gonorrhoeae from other Neisseria organisms and other diplococci.[18] However, serologic diagnosis of gonorrhea has not been sensitive or specific enough to be used diagnostically in the absence of a positive culture.[2] A solid phase enzyme immunoassay has been the most widely used nonculture method.[19]

Gonococcal isolates should be tested for β-lactamase routinely. If therapy with appropriate antibiotics does not quickly eradicate the infection, antimicrobial susceptibility testing of the gonococcal isolates must be carried out.

CLINICAL MANIFESTATIONS OF DGI

Most patients with DGI do not report symptomatic genitourinary infections. Therefore, DGI generally develops following untreated mucosal infections. It is estimated that 0.5 to 3% of such untreated infections will disseminate.[8] Only about 25% of our DGI patients had a history of urethritis or cervicitis, and only 5% of our DGI patients with a positive pharyngeal or rectal culture reported a history of any local infectious symptoms at those mucosal surfaces.[8] DGI is more common in women, a finding that might relate to a greater frequency of asymptomatic mucosal infection. Reports of last sexual encounter to the onset of the initial symptoms of DGI have varied from 1 day to weeks. Because there are 1 million cases of gonorrhea yearly in the United States, there should be 10,000 cases of DGI expected per year.

The initial most common symptoms in DGI are migratory polyarthralgias, tenosynovitis, dermatitis, and fever (Table 117–3). Tenosynovitis is an important clue

TABLE 117–3. INITIAL SYMPTOMS AND SIGNS IN DGI.

SYMPTOM, SIGN	PERCENTAGE
Migratory polyarthralgia	70
Tenosynovitis	67
Dermatitis	67
Fever	63
Purulent arthritis	42
(Monoarthritis)	(32)
(Polyarthritis)	(10)
Genitourinary symptoms	25

From O'Brian, J.P., Goldenberg, D.L., and Rice, P.A.[8]

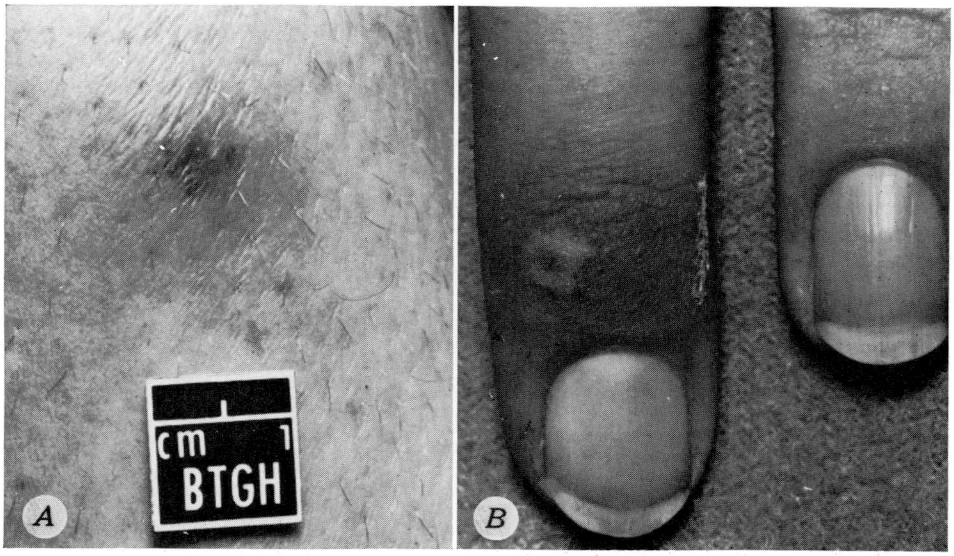

FIGURE 117–1. Skin lesions characteristic of septicemia due to Neisseria gonorrhoeae, N. meningitidis, Streptobaccillus moniliformis, and Hemophilus influenzae. *A*, Hemorrhagic spot 5 to 6 mm in diameter on the upper arm; the gray area 1 to 2 mm in diameter in the center indicates necrosis. *B*, Pustulovesicular lesion on the finger of the same patient; the necrotic center is evident as a dark gray area.

for the diagnosis of DGI because it is rare in most other forms of septic arthritis. Often multiple tendons are simultaneously inflamed, especially around the dorsum of the wrists, fingers, ankles, and toes. The concurrent presence of dermatitis and tenosynovitis, which has been designated the acute arthritis-dermatitis syndrome,[20] is highly suggestive of disseminated neisserial infection.[21]

Dermatitis occurs in two-thirds of patients with DGI (Table 117–3). Skin lesions are usually multiple and are most often found on the extremities or on the trunk, but rarely on the face, palms, or soles (Fig. 117–1). These lesions are often painless, and patients might be unaware of their existence, although some skin lesions are painful. The most common skin lesions are hemorrhagic macules or papules, but pustules, vesicles, bullae, erythema nodosum, and erythema multiforme have also been described. New skin lesions can develop during the initial 24 to 48 hours of antibiotic therapy.

Frank, purulent arthritis occurs in 40 to 50% of patients.[8] Usually more than one joint is involved, and the knees, wrists, and ankles are affected most commonly. Sometimes a relatively transient effusion with unimpressive synovial fluid leukocytosis is present, but most often the clinical and synovial fluid characteristics are similar to that of other forms of bacterial arthritis. The mean synovial fluid leukocyte count in gonococcal arthritis is about 50,000 cells/mm^3. Although chronic gonococcal arthritis was common in the pre-antibiotic era, it is now rare, but should still be included in the differential diagnosis of inflammatory arthritis lasting several weeks or even several months.[22] Unusual presentations of gonococcal arthritis include hip monoarthritis,[23] calcaneocuboid infection,[24] and carpal tunnel syndrome.[25]

Most patients are febrile, although the temperature is usually only moderately elevated. A modest peripheral blood leukocytosis is common. Transiently elevated liver function studies have been described, probably representing subclinical hepatitis during bacteremia.[8,20] Additionally, a perihepatitis, termed the Fitz-Hugh–Curtis syndrome, can occur in women secondary to adhesions between the surfaces of the liver and the peritoneum as a result of intraperitoneal spread of infection. Gonococcal meningitis and endocarditis are rarely reported today. A presumed immune-mediated glomerulonephritis secondary to DGI has been reported.[26] Gonococcal pericarditis with tamponade has also been reported in association with gonococcal arthritis.[27,28]

Some investigators have proposed that DGI progresses sequentially from a bacteremic phase, characterized by chills, tenosynovitis, and skin lesions, to a joint-localized phase manifested by purulent arthritis.[20*] The diagnostic utility of such a classification is suspect, however, because of the significant clinical overlap and the inconsistent temporal sequence of the articular manifestations.

The clinical manifestations of DGI caused by antibiotic-resistant strains of N. gonorrhoeae can differ from those of penicillin-sensitive cases (Table 117–4).[29–35] Antibiotic-resistant cases can be more difficult to eradi-

**Editor's note:* Observations made before the antibiotic era might best reflect the natural history of DGI. Philip Hench thought that the migratory tenosynovitis or joint lesions flitted on and off stage like a *corps de ballet* to be eventually eclipsed by a fixed septic monoarthritis—the "ballerina."

cate, therefore causing chronic synovitis and possible irreversible joint destruction. Unusual joint presentations and failure to initiate appropriate antibiotics has resulted in treatment delays in such situations. In one series from France, 4 of 15 cases of gonococcal arthritis in a 1-year period were due to penicillinase-producing N. gonorrhoeae (PPNG).[34] These patients had a prominence of monoarthritis, male predominance, and delayed diagnosis. Eventual joint destruction was not uncommon.

PATHOGENESIS

Suppurative arthritis caused by N. gonorrhoeae is generally considered secondary to bacteremic spread of the organisms to the synovium, with replication of bacteria and the subsequent release of proteolytic enzymes from synovial lining cells and from neutrophils. Eventually, cartilage is destroyed as in most other types of bacterial arthritis. Gonococcal bacteremia is more likely to cause arthritis or tenosynovitis than infection with pneumococci or other common bacteria. Microscopically, the synovial membrane initially reveals lining-cell hyperplasia and neutrophilic infiltration. Gram's-stained smears of the synovial membrane are sometimes initially positive. If a second synovial membrane specimen is obtained 5 to 7 days after treatment, most of the acute infiltrate will have cleared, but chronic inflammatory cells are prominent. Rarely, a chronic synovitis persists despite appropriate antibiotic therapy.[36] This sterile synovitis might be responsible for persistent pain and joint effusions despite eradication of the organism, a phenomenon termed "postinfectious" arthritis.

Although the synovial membrane and fluid characteristics of acute gonococcal arthritis are generally similar to those of arthritis caused by other bacteria, DGI rarely destroys cartilage or bone. Even in the preantibiotic era, untreated gonococcal arthritis rarely caused permanent joint destruction,[22] although reports of joint destruction in cases of antibiotic-resistant N. gonorrhoeae have been described (Table 117–4).

Clinical and laboratory evidence indicates that the arthralgias, tenosynovitis, dermatitis, and the "sterile" arthritis associated with DGI could be due to immune-mediated mechanisms or hypersensitivity. The initial presentation of DGI often resembles that of serum sickness, with tenosynovitis and migratory polyarthralgias that are usually transient and often disappear without antimicrobial therapy. Similar musculoskeletal symptoms are common in immune complex–related infections such as hepatitis, but they are absent in non-neisserial bacterial arthritis. Furthermore, N. gonorrhoeae organisms recovered from fewer than 50% of purulent synovial effusions, in contrast with nongonococcal bacterial arthritis.[8,20] Positive blood cultures are found in fewer than one-third of patients with DGI. Positive blood and synovial fluid cultures were mutually exclusive in our study (Table 117–5). Investigators have attributed the frequent absence of positive blood and synovial fluid cultures to the fastidious growth requirements of N. gonorrhoeae, yet the organisms are easily recovered from the genitourinary tract or other local sites in most cases of DGI. Therefore, some investigators have questioned the role of immune-mediated phenomena or hypersensitivity in the synovitis and dermatitis associated with DGI.

The dermatitis associated with DGI is almost always sterile, and the cause of the skin lesions does not seem to be secondary to embolic spread of viable organisms.[37] Erythema nodosum, erythema multiforme, and vasculitis all have been associated with DGI, suggesting immune-mediated or hypersensitivity reactions. Although viable N. gonorrhoeae organisms are rarely recovered from these skin lesions, immunofluorescent evidence suggests the presence of gonococcal cell-wall components, gonococcal antibody, and complement.[37] Circulating immune complexes have also been detected in patients with DGI, especially early in the clinical course. These could cause a sterile synovitis that might promote the later entrance of bacteria into the joint.[38]

In animal models of gonococcal arthritis, intra-articular injections of nonviable N. gonorrhoeae or gonococcal cell-wall lipopolysaccharide caused an initially acute and then chronic persistent synovitis.[39] A lipopolysaccharide concentration as low as 5 μg (10^{-6} g dry weight) caused arthritis, whereas much larger concentrations of another gonococcal antigenic component, the outer membrane protein, did not cause synovitis. Both clinical and laboratory evidence suggest that the synovitis, tenosynovitis, and dermatitis associated with DGI does not necessarily require viable N. gonorrhoeae.

DIAGNOSIS

The diagnosis of DGI should be suspected in any young, sexually active patient with acute arthritis and dermatitis. Although tenosynovitis can occur with other types of arthritis, the presence of tenosynovitis or arthritis in association with a skin rash is sufficient clinical grounds for a presumptive diagnosis of DGI. Most patients are febrile, with peripheral blood leukocytosis, an elevated erythrocyte sedimentation rate and other acute phase reactants, but such nonspecific findings are not always present. If synovial fluid can be aspirated, the leukocyte count is generally 30,000 to 100,000 cells/mm^3, although the range is wider than the range in the joint effusions of nongonococcal bacterial arthritis, and some fluids are relatively acellular. A Gram's-stained smear of concentrated synovial fluid is positive in fewer than 25% of purulent joint effusions, in contrast with other forms of bacterial arthritis. In most recent series, genitourinary cultures provided the best yield of N. gonorrhoeae, whereas blood and skin cultures were rarely positive (Table 117–5). The urethra should be swabbed to obtain a specimen for culture because most men do not have a urethral discharge. In women, a specimen should be obtained directly from the cervix. Rectal and pharyngeal cultures should be obtained, particularly the

TABLE 117–4. REPRESENTATIVE CASES OF DGI CAUSED BY ANTIBIOTIC-RESISTANT ORGANISMS

SEX	AUTHOR	YEAR	JOINT(S)	TYPE OF ANTIBIOTIC RESISTANCE	ANTIBIOTIC	OUTCOME/COMMENTS
F	CDC	1987	Knee	PPNG	Ceftriaxone	Despite 10 days of antibiotics, surgical drainage was required
F	CDC	1987	Knee, ankle tenosynovitis	PPNG	Cefotaxime	Complete, rapid recovery
F	CDC	1987	Wrist, PIP	PPNG	Ceftriaxone	Complete rapid recovery
F	Saraux[30]	1987	Hip	PPNG	Cefotaxime	10 days of antibiotics, made a complete recovery. Unusual joint
M	Saraux[30]	1987	Knees, ankles, wrists, PIP, MCP, vertebrae	PPNG PPNG	Cefotaxime and gentamicin	X-ray destruction of wrist and development of spondylodiscitis at T_2–T_3. 15 days of antibiotics
F	Bush and Boscia[31]	1987	Wrist	PPNG	Ceftriaxone	Good results
F	Bush and Boscia[31]	1987	MCP	PPNG	Ceftriaxone	Good results
F	Bush and Boscia[31]	1987	Shoulder	PPNG	Ceftriaxone	Good results
F	Pritchard and Berney[32]	1988	Knee, ankle	PPNG	Cefotaxime	Good results
F	Venkatesh[33]	1988	Knee	PPNG	Cefotaxime	Complete, rapid recovery
F	Livneh	1988	Ankle, wrist, shoulder	PPNG	2 million, then 24 million units of penicillin	Responded to high-dose penicillin
F	Liote	1990	Hip	PPNG	Ceftriaxone	Hip cartilage narrowing, erosions
F	Liote	1990	Knee	PPNG	Ceftriaxone	Complete, rapid recovery
M	Strader et al.[35]	1986	Knee	Chromosomal	Penicillin for 14 days then ceftriaxone	Did not respond to 2 weeks of penicillin and daily arthrocentesis. Quickly responded to ceftriaxone
M	Strader et al.[35]	1986	Knee, both wrists	Chromosomal	Cefoxitin for 5 days, penicillin for 6 days, then tetracycline for 7 days	Did not respond until the addition of tetracycline
M	Liote et al.[34]	1989	Wrist, MCP, ankles	Chromosomal	Standard penicillin dose for 7 days then 20 million units per day and probenecid	Very high doses of penicillin were required for recovery

CDC = Centers for Disease Control; PIP = proximal interphalangeal; MCP = metacarpal; PPNG = penicillinase-producing Neisseria gonorrhoeae

TABLE 117–5. *NEISSERIA GONORRHOEAE* CULTURE POSITIVITY IN DGI

SITE	% ISOLATION
Genitourinary area	80
Synovial fluid	27
Rectum	21
Pharynx	10
Blood	5
Skin	0

From O'Brien, J.P., Goldenberg, D.L., and Rice, P.A.[8]

latter, because pharyngeal gonorrhea can lead to disseminated infection.

Until the recent emergence of antibiotic-resistant cases of DGI, a rapid therapeutic response to penicillin or other antibiotics was of diagnostic significance. Rapid response to antibiotics will not be present in cases caused by antibiotic-resistant strains, however. An antibiotic regimen might have to be adjusted after susceptibility testing is determined. Because N. gonorrhoeae organisms are recovered from joint fluid or blood in only about one-third of patients with DGI (Table 117–5), the diagnosis is often presumptive. A positive genitourinary culture and a characteristic clinical presentation is usually sufficient.

The most important conditions to differentiate from

DGI are other forms of bacterial arthritis; meningococcal arthritis is the most difficult to distinguish (see below). However, most other forms of bacterial arthritis occur in young children, elderly patients, or patients with compromised host-defense mechanisms or prior arthritis who present with acute monoarthritis. Tenosynovitis and dermatitis are rare in non-neisserial bacterial arthritis.

Other differential diagnostic considerations include prodromal hepatitis B, Reiter's syndrome, acute rheumatic fever, bacterial endocarditis, other bacteremias, and connective tissue diseases. Polyarthritis, tenosynovitis, and a skin rash are common in hepatitis; the rash and arthritis generally occur in the anicteric phase. The skin rash is usually urticarial, and the synovial fluid leukocyte count is usually lower than it is in DGI. The most helpful diagnostic features are elevated hepatocellular enzymes normal erythrocyte sedimentation rate, and the identification of hepatitis surface antigen (HB_SAg) in the blood, with negative blood and synovial fluid cultures. Reiter's syndrome can also cause arthritis, tenosynovitis, and urethritis. In classic Reiter's syndrome, the urethritis is not due to N. gonorrhoeae, but rather is nongonococcal in origin (ureaplasma and chlamydia). Other helpful clinical features include conjunctivitis, characteristic painless mucosal ulcers, circinate balanitis, and keratoderma blennorrhagicum. Clinical and radiologic evidence of sacroiliitis and the presence of HLA-B27 are also characteristic of Reiter's syndrome. Acute rheumatic fever can cause polyarthritis in young adults without carditis, chorea, or subcutaneous nodules. Some investigators have termed this disorder *poststreptococcal arthritis* rather than acute rheumatic fever. If a skin rash is present, it usually is transient (erythema marginatum). The diagnosis relies on evidence of a recent streptococcal throat infection, confirmed by culture or by serologic testing of blood, and a rapid response to salicylates or another nonsteroidal anti-inflammatory agent.

Many bacteremias or other systemic infections can cause musculoskeletal and dermatologic manifestations that mimic DGI. Bacterial endocarditis is especially important to differentiate from DGI. Purulent arthritis is not common in bacterial endocarditis unless hematogenous spread to the synovium occurs, such as is occasionally seen in endocarditis caused by Staphylococcus aureus. Myalgias, arthralgias, tendonitis, and back pain are common musculoskeletal manifestations associated with bacterial endocarditis, particularly subacute disease that has been present for several weeks. Viral diseases including measles and rubella, as well as various arboviral infections not commonly seen in the United States, can also cause skin lesions and arthritis. Rarely, infections caused by herpesviruses are accompanied by a skin rash and arthralgias. The characteristic rash and evolution of clinical manifestation of Lyme disease differ from those of DGI.

As described above, patients with SLE can be predisposed to neisserial infections. Therefore, it is important to consider DGI or meningococcal infection in a lupus patient presenting with an acute febrile illness that can mimic an exacerbation of SLE itself.

TREATMENT

The recent emergence of PPNG strains and chromosomally mediated antibiotic-resistant strains of *Neisseria gonorrhoeae* has dramatically altered treatment recommendations. In the past nearly all N. gonorrhoeae strains that caused DGI were not only sensitive to penicillin but were sensitive to much lower concentrations than were strains isolated from patients with pelvic inflammatory disease.[8] Antibiotic-resistant strains often cause a more chronic arthritis that requires hospitalization for appropriate susceptibility testing and for a longer course of parenteral antibiotics and joint drainage. Older treatment recommendations using low or moderate doses of multiple antibiotics including outpatient oral regimens might no longer be appropriate.

The initial drug of choice in all local gonococcal infections is now ceftriaxone, 250 mg IM as a single dose, followed by doxycycline, 100 mg orally 2 times daily for 7 days. Prolonged parenteral therapy is recommended for DGI; 1 to 2 g per day of ceftriaxone or comparable doses of ceftizoxime or cefotaxime are given intravenously until signs and symptoms resolve. Patients should be hospitalized and joint effusions should be drained by repeated needle aspiration. Although open surgical drainage or arthroscopy is rarely required, any joint not responding adequately must be evaluated for more aggressive drainage. Once symptoms are largely resolved, daily outpatient therapy for 7 more days with 250 mg ceftriaxone daily intramuscularly or an oral regimen as defined by in-vitro susceptibility should follow. Alternative antibiotics include spectinomycin, ciprofloxacin, and norfloxacin. If the strain isolated is not PPNG, parenteral penicillin or ampicillin may be used. Despite the emergence of antibiotic-resistant DGI strains, most patients should make a rapid and complete recovery, provided appropriate antibiotics and joint drainage are instituted (Table 117–4).

MENINGOCOCCAL ARTHRITIS

N. meningitidis can be differentiated from N. gonorrhoeae microbiologically because the former ferments both dextrose and maltose whereas the latter ferments only dextrose.[40] Only N. meningitidis has an immunizing polysaccharide capsule. However, most other microbial characteristics are identical. Although traditionally N. meningitidis has been acquired via the respiratory tract and N. gonorrhoeae via the genitourinary tract, either organism can cause disease by venereal transmission, and be recovered from joint fluid, blood, cerebrospinal fluid, conjunctiva, or pharynx.[40]

The articular and dermatologic manifestations of disseminated meningococcal infection are virtually identical to those of DGI.[40–42] Arthritis occurs in 2 to 10%

of acute meningococcal infections. Three distinct types have been described: (1) an acute polyarthritis, usually associated with acute meningococcemia and meningitis, (2) a monoarthritis or oligoarthritis that usually begins 5 to 7 days after septicemia, and (3) a primary acute pyogenic arthritis, not associated with meningitis or classic signs of meningococcemia.[41,42] However, as noted in DGI, the notion of distinct articular syndromes can be alternatively interpreted as an evolution from one phase to the next. The proposed pathogenesis of the articular manifestations of meningococcal arthritis is also similar to that of DGI. Direct bacterial invasion of the synovium and recovery of N. meningitidis from synovial fluid is most common in chronic, primary meningococcal arthritis.[42] In most cases of acute polyarticular arthritis associated with meningococcemia, however, the synovial fluid is sterile. A "postinfectious" arthritis or immune-mediated synovitis have been postulated to account for this disorder.[43] In one study, purified meningococcal polysaccharide caused an acute synovitis when injected into the knee of rabbits previously sensitized by parenteral injections of heat-killed meningococci.[43] Classic meningococcal purpura associated with severe meningococcemia might be present, but the dermatitis often resembles that of DGI. Tenosynovitis is common, especially tenosynovitis associated with acute polyarthritis.

Until recently, the acute arthritis-dermatitis syndrome of meningococcal infections was rare in the United States and was more often described in Africa. In 151 consecutive patients with acute arthritis or arthralgias in Seattle from 1970 to 1972, N. gonorrhoeae was isolated from blood or synovial fluid in 30 cases and N. meningitidis in only two cases.[21] However, in 62 patients seen with acute arthritis from 1980 to 1983, N. gonorrhoeae was recovered in nine and N. meningitidis in five. A separate analysis of blood culture results revealed a decline in the number of cases of gonococcemia from 1970 to 1984 but a shift to a relatively greater number of cases due to N. meningitidis. The clinical manifestations of the 39 patients with DGI and the seven with arthritis-dermatitis associated with meningococcemia were similar (Table 117–6). More than 100 skin lesions were present more often in patients with N. meningitidis infection. The median peripheral blood leukocyte count was also higher in those patients. These data strengthen the case for hospitalization of all patients with the arthritis-dermatitis syndrome.[21] Treatment includes antimeningococcal antibiotics and joint drainage when necessary.

TABLE 117–6. SELECTED CLINICAL AND LABORATORY FINDINGS AMONG PATIENTS WITH ACUTE ARTHRITIS OR ARTHRALGIA

CHARACTERISTICS	PROVEN INFECTION: DISSEMINATED GONOCOCCAL (N = 39)	PROVEN INFECTION: MENINGOCOCCAL (N = 7)
Clinical		
Male sex	16/39	7/7
Age in years		
Median	25	32
Range	16–57	20–59
Temperature, °C		
Median	38.3	38.5
Range	36.4–39.9	36.5–39.8
Synovial effusion, no. (%) of patients	17/39 (44)	3/7 (43)
Skin lesions		
Present, no. (%) of patients	26/39 (67)	4/7 (57)
>100 lesions, no. (%) of patients	5/26 (19)	4/4 (100)*
Range	1 to 100	1 to 100
White blood cell count/mm³ (x 10^9/L)		
Median	9800	17,400†
Range	4700–17,100	6400–23,500
Site of isolation no. (%) of positive cultures/total cultures		
Blood	20/33 (61)	5/6 (83)
Synovial fluid	20/25 (80)	2/3 (66)
Urethra or cervix	21/36 (58)	0/7 (0)
Rectum	7/28 (25)	0/1 (0)
Throat	4/26 (15)	3/5 (60)

* $p < .01$ by Fisher's exact test.
† $p < .05$ by Mann-Whitney rank sum test.
From Rompalo, A.M., et al.[21]

OTHER NEISSERIAL INFECTIONS

Nongonococcal, nonmeningococcal Neisseria rarely causes joint disease.[45] These organisms are often saprophytic inhabitants of the upper respiratory tract and are usually considered nonpathogenic. Thus, positive cultures may be considered contaminants. Many of these organisms are resistant to penicillin, and therapy should be guided by the results of antimicrobial susceptibility tests.

REFERENCES

1. Heckels, J.E.: Molecular studies on the pathogenesis of gonorrhoeae. J. Med. Microbiol., *18*:293, 1984.
2. Dallabetta, G., and Hook, E.W. III: Gonococcal infections. Infect. Dis. Clin. North Am., *1*:25, 1987.
3. Blake, M.S., and Gotschlich, E.C.: Purification and partial characterization of the opacity-associated proteins of *Neisseria gonorrhoeae*. J. Exp. Med., *159*:452, 1984.
4. Sandstrom, E.G., Chen, E.C.S., and Buchanan, T.M.: Serology of *Neisseria gonorrhoeae* coagglutination serogroups WI and WII/WIII correspond to different outer membrane protein I molecules. Infect. Immun. *38*:462, 1982.
5. Cannon, J.G., Buchanan, T.M., Sparling, P.F.: Confirmation of association of protein I serotype of *Neisseria gonorrhoeae* with ability to cause disseminated infection. Infect. Immun., *40*:816, 1983.
6. Bohnhoff, M., Morello, J.A., and Lerner, S.A.: Auxotypes, penicillin susceptibility, and serogroups of *Neisseria gonorrhoeae* from

disseminated and uncomplicated infections. J. Infect. Dis., *154*:225, 1986.
7. Morello, J.A., and Bohnhoff, M.: Serovars and serum resistance of *Neisseria gonorrhoeae* from disseminated and uncomplicated infections. J. Infect. Dis., *160*:1012, 1989.
8. O'Brien, J.P., Goldenberg, D.L., and Rice, P.A.: Disseminated gonococcal infection: A prospective analysis of 49 patients and a review of the pathophysiology and immune mechanisms. Medicine, *62*:395, 1983.
9. Rice, P.A., and Goldenberg, D.L.: Clinical manifestations of disseminated infection caused by *Neisseria gonorrhoeae* are linked to differences in bactericidal reactivity of infecting strains. Ann. Intern. Med., *95*:175, 1981.
10. Ross, S.C., and Densen, P.: Complement deficiency states and infection. Medicine, *63*:243, 1984.
11. Mitchell, S.R., Nguyen, P.Q., and Katz, P.: Increased risk of Neisserial infections in systemic lupus erythematosus. Semin. Arthritis Rheum., *20*:174, 1990.
12. Schwarcz, S.K., et al.: National surveillance of antimicrobial resistance in *Neisseria gonorrhoeae*. JAMA, *264*:1413, 1990.
13. Easmon, C.S.F.: Gonococcal resistance to antibiotics. J. Antimicrob. Chemother., *16*:409, 1985.
14. Easmon, C.S.F.: The changing pattern of antibiotic resistance of *Neisseria gonorrhoeae*. Genitourin. Med., *66*:55, 1990.
15. Centers for Disease Control. 1989 Sexually transmitted diseases treatment guidelines. MMWR, *38*:21, 1989.
16. Hook, E.W. III, et al.: Risk factors for emergence of antibiotic resistant *Neisseria gonorrhoeae*. J. Infect. Dis., *159*:900, 1989.
17. Boslego, J.W., Tramont, E.C., and Takafuji, E.T.: Effect of spectinomycin use on the prevalence of spectinomycin-resistant and of penicillinase-producing *Neisseria gonorrhoeae*. N. Engl. J. Med., *317*:272, 1987.
18. Cavicchini, S., and Alessi, E.: Monoclonal antibody direct immunofluorescence for the identification of *Neisseria gonorrhoeae* strains grown on selective culture media. Sex. Transm. Dis., *16*:195, 1989.
19. Hossain, A., Bakir, T.M.F., Siddiqui, M., and DeSilva, S.: Enzyme immunoassay in the rapid diagnosis of gonorrhoeae. J. Hyg. Epidemiol. Microbiol. Immunol., *32*:425, 1988.
20. Holmes, K.K., Counts, G.W., and Beaty, H.N.: Disseminated gonococcal infection. Ann. Intern. Med., *74*:979, 1971.
21. Rompalo, A.M., et al.: The acute arthritis-dermatitis syndrome. Arch. Intern. Med., *147*:281, 1987.
22. Livneh, A., Sewell, K.L., and Barland, P.: Chronic gonococcal arthritis. J. Rheumatol., *16*:115, 1983.
23. Rubinow, A.: Septic arthritis of the hip caused by *Neisseria gonorrhoeae*. Clin. Orthop., *181*:115, 1983.
24. Grippo, G.N., Genovese, M.N., and Piccora, R.: Monoarthric gonococcal arthritis involving the calcaneocuboid joint. J. Am. Podiatr. Med. Assoc., *80*:91, 1990.
25. DeHertogh, D., Ritland, D., and Green, R.: Carpal tunnel syndrome due to gonococcal tenosynovitis. Orthopedics, *11*:199, 1988.
26. Ebright, J.R., and Komorowski, R.: Gonococcal endocarditis associated with immune complex glomerulonephritis. Am. J. Med., *68*:793, 1980.
27. Coe, M.D., et al.: Gonococcal pericarditis with tamponade in a patient with systemic lupus erythematosus. Arthritis Rheum., *33*:1438, 1990.
28. Wilson, J., Zaman, A.G., and Simmons, A.V.: Gonococcal arthritis complicated by acute pericarditis and pericardial effusion. Br. Heart J., *63*:134, 1990.
29. Disseminated gonorrhea caused by penicillinase-producing *Neisseria gonorrhoeae* in Wisconsin, Pennsylvania. MMWR, *36*:161, 1987.
30. Saraux, J.L., et al.: Disseminated gonococcal infection caused by penicillinase-producing organisms in patients with unusual joint involvement. J. Infect. Dis., *155*:154, 1987.
31. Bush, L.M., and Boscia, J.A.: Disseminated multiple antibiotic-resistant gonococcal infection: Needed changes in antimicrobial therapy. Ann. Intern. Med., *107*:692, 1987.
32. Pritchard, C., and Berney, S.N.: Septic arthritis caused by penicillinase producing *Neisseria gonorrhoeae*. J. Rheumatol., *15*:719, 1988.
33. Venkatesh, S., et al.: Disseminated infection caused by penicillin-resistant gonococci in two Jamaicans. West Indian Med. J., *37*:240, 1988.
34. Liote, F., et al.: Infectious arthritis due to penicillinase producing *Neisseria gonorrhoeae*. Arthritis Rheum., *32*(Suppl.):114, 1989.
35. Strader, K.W., Wise, C.M., Wasilauskas, B.L., and Salzer, W.L.: Disseminated gonococcal infection caused by chromosomally medicated penicillin-resistant organisms. Ann. Intern. Med., *104*:365, 1986.
36. Goldenberg, D.L.: "Post-infectious" arthritis: A new look at an old concept with particular attention to disseminated gonococcal infection. Am. J. Med., *74*:925, 1983.
37. Scherer, R., and Braun-Falco, O.: Alternative pathway complement activation: A possible mechanism inducing skin lesions in benign gonococcal sepsis. Br. J. Dermatol., *95*:303, 1976.
38. Shiel, W.C., et al.: Immune complexes in synovial fluid and serum from patients with disseminated gonococcal infection: Evidence for local immune complex formation within the joint. Ann. Rheum. Dis., *45*:816, 1986.
39. Goldenberg, D.L., Reed, J.I., and Rice, P.A.: Arthritis in rabbits induced by killed *Neisseria gonorrhoeae* and gonococcal lipopolysaccharide. J. Rheumatol., *11*:3, 1984.
40. Mitchell, S.R., and Katz, P.: Disseminated neisserial infection in pregnancy: The empress may have a change of clothing. Obstet. Gynecol. Surv., *44*:780, 1989.
41. Christensen, C.: Meningococcal arthritis. Scand. J. Rheumatol., *16*:451, 1987.
42. Anderson, S., and Krook, A.: Primary meningococcal arthritis. Scand. J. Infect. Dis., *19*:51, 1987.
43. Greenwood, B.M., Mohammed, I., and Whittle, H.C.: Immune complexes and the pathogenesis of meningococcal arthritis. Clin. Exp. Immunol., *59*:513, 1985.
44. Degan, T.J., Rand, J.A., and Morrey, B.F.: Musculoskeletal infection with nongonococcal Neisseria species not associated with meningitis. Clin. Orthop., *176*:206, 1983.
45. Izraeli, S., et al.: *Branhamella catarrhalis* as a cause of suppurative arthritis. Pediatr. Infect. Dis. J., *8*:256, 1989.

118

Arthritis Due to Mycobacteria, Fungi, and Parasites

RONALD P. MESSNER

MYCOBACTERIA

Tuberculous, mycotic, and parasitic infections are relatively rare causes of arthritis. They are important because they are potentially curable. Proper diagnosis requires awareness of their clinical presentations together with identification of the organism in synovial fluid or tissue. Certain immunologic tests are helpful but do not replace the need to examine material directly from the involved joints. Constitutional symptoms and radiographic evidence of extra-articular involvement are often absent. These infections should be sought in the evaluation of patients with chronic monoarticular arthritis and should be considered in various other situations, including spondylitis, tendonitis, and erythema nodosum (Table 118–1).

TUBERCULOSIS

The incidence of new cases of tuberculosis of all types has decreased dramatically in the United States in the last 40 years. In 1932 there were 77 new cases per 100,000 population, and in 1984 only 9.4 per 100,000. The incidence is highest in congested cities. Tuberculosis affects nonwhites six times more frequently than whites, and males twice as often as females. Immigrants from developing countries, elderly nursing home patients, and hemodialysis patients appear to be at increased risk. Approximately 15% of cases involve extrapulmonary sites,[1] and 1 to 3% of patients have bone and/or joint tuberculosis.[2,3] The rarity of bone and joint tuberculosis has lowered the index of suspicion in the medical community, often resulting in unfortunate delays in diagnosis.[4] There is evidence that the number of newly reported cases of extrapulmonary tuberculosis remained constant throughout the last decade.[5] On a global scale, there are an estimated 10 million new cases of all types of tuberculosis per year, and one half of the world's population has been infected with this organism.[6]

In the nonimmune host, primary tuberculosis begins in the lungs. It is characterized by rapid multiplication of tubercle bacilli and dissemination by way of blood and lymph to all parts of the body. The disease usually resolves coincident with development of delayed hypersensitivity and cellular immunity. In a few patients, it progresses and may result in disseminated tuberculosis or progressive disease limited to one or two organ systems. In contrast, tuberculosis in the immune person is characterized by a vigorous tissue response with local necrosis but relative containment of the infection. Dissemination does not occur unless a bronchus or blood vessel is eroded. Tuberculosis of bone can develop in three ways: by hematogenous spread, by lymphatic spread from chronic pleural, renal, or lymph node foci, or by reactivation of latent infection at sites seeded in the primary illness.[7] Involvement of joints may be direct by the hematogenous route or may occur secondary to osseous infection. Articular tuberculosis is often a combination of osteomyelitis and arthritis.[2] The inflammatory reaction in the synovium is followed by formation of granulation tissue, effusion, and production of a pannus. Cartilage destruction begins in the periphery of the joint and proceeds slowly compared with pyogenic infections. Ultimately, the process results in severe destruction of bone, cold abscesses, and sinus tract formation.

Fifty percent of cases of skeletal tuberculosis occur in the spine. The next most common sites are large weight-bearing joints. The hip and knee are each affected in

TABLE 118–1. TYPICAL CLINICAL PRESENTATIONS OF ARTHRITIS DUE TO TUBERCULOSIS OR MYCOSES

Tuberculosis	Spondylitis; monoarticular disease of large weight-bearing joints.
Atypical tuberculosis	Tendonitis in hand or wrist.
Leprosy	Polyarthritis with erythema nodosum leprosum; destruction of small bones and joints of hands and feet; neuropathic wrists or ankles.
Coccidioidomycosis	Polyarthritis with erythema nodosum; monoarticular arthritis of knee.
Blastomycosis	Monoarticular arthritis of large weight-bearing joints associated with lung and skin involvement; spondylitis.
Cryptococcosis	Monoarticular arthritis secondary to osseous infection; spondylitis.
Histoplasmosis	Polyarthritis with erythema nodosum.
Sporotrichosis	Monoarticular arthritis of knee, wrist, or hand; polyarthritis with disseminated skin lesions.
Candidiasis	Monoarticular arthritis of the knee in patient with serious concurrent illness.
Actinomycosis	Spondylitis.

about 15% of cases and the ankle or wrist in 5 to 10% of cases. Involvement of non–weightbearing joints including the shoulder is more common in the elderly. Skeletal infection often occurs in the absence of active or even inactive pulmonary disease. The incidence of coexistent active pulmonary infection varies from 10 to 50% in various series.[7–9] Evidence of previous infection has been found in up to 40% of patients and other extrapulmonary disease in about 20% of patients. Multiple skeletal lesions are more common in children but occur in only 5 to 15% of all patients.

Tuberculosis of the Spine. In developing countries, spinal tuberculosis (Pott's disease) is seen primarily in children and young adults. In the United States and Europe, cases in which the patients are in the first decade of life have almost disappeared, and most patients are over 40. Typically, the infection starts in the margins of the vertebral bodies and invades the disc space early. The disc space narrows, destruction of bone leads to vertebral collapse with kyphosis or gibbous deformity, and a cold paraspinous abscess forms. The midthoracic to upper lumbar area is usually affected.[7,10] Skip areas with radiographically normal vertebrae in-between occur in about 10% of patients. Paraspinous abscesses are common (50 to 96%) and may dissect for long distances up or down the spine or out along the ribs to point in the neck, groin, chest wall, or sternum.[7,10] The most common symptom is back pain. Muscle spasm, local tenderness, kyphosis, and referred pain from root compression complete the typical clinical picture. Neurologic symptoms caused by cord compression (Pott's paraplegia) occur in 10 to 25% of patients with spinal tuberculosis.[8] Kyphosis, which is more common in paraplegic patients, is associated with destructive vertebral lesions in the thoracic area more often than in the lumbar area. Altered sensation is present below the level of the lesion. Lower motor neuron weakness caused by coexistent root compression is sometimes observed. Cerebral spinal fluid examination reveals a partial or complete block and increased protein with normal cell count and sugar.

Another complication of spinal tuberculosis is a mycotic aneurysm of the aorta, usually created when a paraspinous abscess penetrates the vessel wall. The resulting hematoma walls off to form a false aneurysm. Penetration of the abscess into the arterial blood may lead to secondary hematogenous spread and miliary disease.[11] Other notable frequent sites of tuberculosis of the axial skeleton are the sacroiliac joints and the ribs. Rib lesions are often associated with a local soft-tissue mass and pain. They generally occur in patients with other skeletal involvement, particularly in the spine. Sacroiliac joint involvement, usually unilateral, occurs in about 7% of patients with skeletal tuberculosis.

Tuberculosis of Peripheral Joints. Articular tuberculosis presents as chronic monoarticular disease in approximately 85% of patients. Involvement of three or more joints is rare. Though it may occur at any age, peripheral arthritis is now rare in patients in the first decade of life in developed countries. The peak incidence is in the fourth and fifth decades. The incidence in males and nonwhites is twice that in females and whites. In the hip, tubercle bacilli may localize in the synovium, acetabulum, or proximal femur. Bony destruction is seen most commonly in the acetabulum. The femoral neck and capital and trochanteric epiphyses are also frequent sites of involvement. Symptoms include mild to moderate pain in the groin, knee, or thigh, and limitation of motion. A limp is the most common presenting complaint in children. Atrophy of the gluteal muscles and tenderness in the groin are often present. At rest, the hip is held in flexion and abduction. Later severe destruction of the femoral neck and acetabulum occurs with formation of a cold abscess and sinus tract, which usually points to the outer thigh.

In the knee, pain is the first symptom of tuberculosis in 70% of patients. It is insidious in onset and may persist for years before the patient seeks medical attention. About 20% of patients describe swelling, and 10% have stiffness as the initial complaint.[12] Localized heat and muscular wasting are usually present on examination. A limp, synovial swelling, and limitation of motion are common. Although pure synovial infection does occur, most patients have involvement of both synovium and bone.[12] Symptoms in other joints are similar to those described in the hip and knee: chronic low-grade pain, swelling, and stiffness with slowly progressive loss of function and eventual abscess formation. Tuberculosis involving tendons in the hand and wrist may cause a carpal tunnel syndrome.[13] Infection of the trochanteric bursa has also been reported. A rare patient with visceral or pulmonary tuberculosis will develop acute polyarthritis without evidence of tuberculous infection of the joints (Poncet's disease). In these patients, joints are normal radiographically, and articular symptoms resolve several weeks after initiation of antituberculous drugs.[14]

Radiographic Signs. There are no pathognomonic roentgenographic signs of skeletal tuberculosis. In general, tuberculosis causes destruction of bone without stimulating much reactive new bone formation. Destructive osseous lesions adjacent to joints[8] are often oval with clear margins and no periosteal reaction (Fig. 118–1). As they expand and erode the cortex, some periosteal reaction occurs. Sequestra formation is rare. When the joint itself is involved, local osteopenia and soft-tissue swelling are early signs. Later small subchondral erosions appear at the margins of the joint (Fig. 118–2). The cartilage space tends to be preserved until extensive destruction of adjacent cortical bone has occurred (Fig. 118–3). With advanced disease, total destruction of the joint can occur. Destruction is not accompanied by osteophyte formation, but the shadow of a cold abscess may be seen.

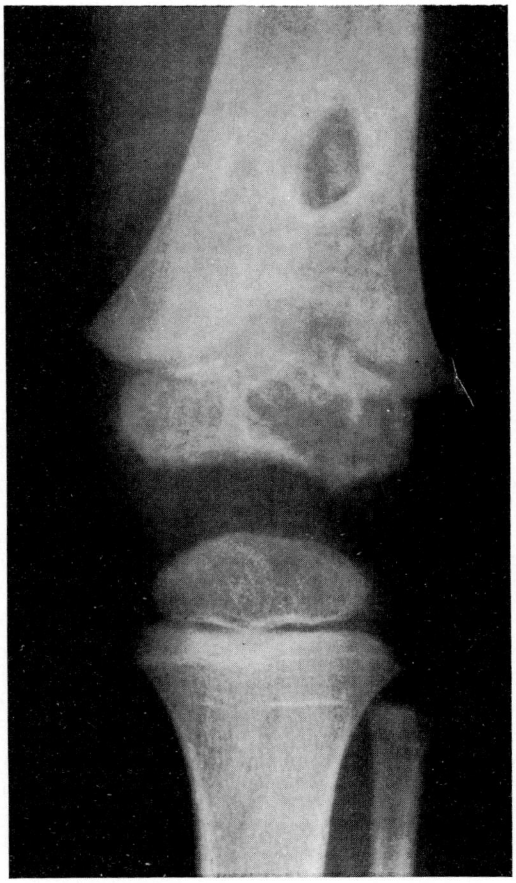

FIGURE 118–1. Tuberculosis of the knee and femur in a child.

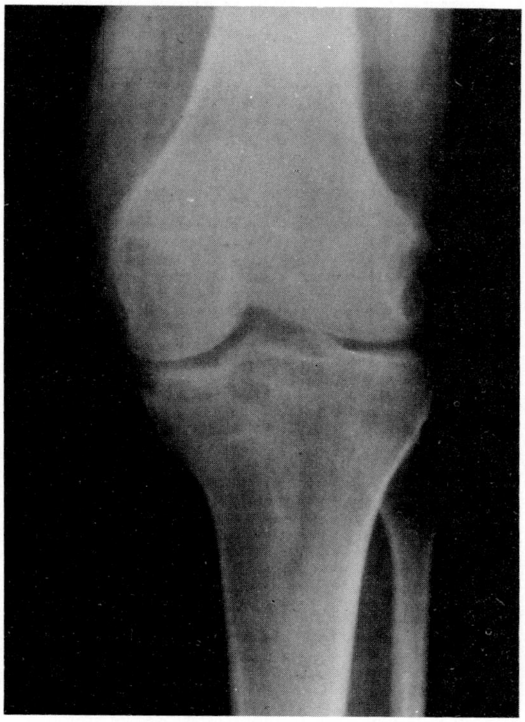

FIGURE 118–2. Tuberculosis of the knee in an adult. Courtesy of Donald Resnick, M.D.

In the spine, the classic picture is narrowing of the disc space with vertebral collapse and a paraspinous abscess. Scalloping of the anterior vertebral surface is common.[10] Occasional infection of the central portion of the vertebrae may cause extensive bone destruction without disc space invasion. In about 10% of patients productive or sclerotic changes, which are difficult to see radiographically, may occur in infected vertebrae. Computerized tomographic scanning or magnetic resonance imaging is helpful in determining the extent of the involvement.[15]

Diagnostic Tests. Diagnosis of tuberculous arthritis requires an index of suspicion and a willingness to obtain material for histologic examination and culture. The quickest and most reliable method of diagnosis is biopsy. A positive diagnosis can be made by either histology or culture of synovial tissue in over 90% of specimens. Synovial fluid culture is positive in approximately 80% of cases and smear in 20% of cases.[7,16,17] Synovial fluid protein is always elevated, whereas 60% of patients have fluid with low glucose levels. The synovial white blood cell count varies widely but is usually between 10,000 and 20,000/mm^3. Polymorphonuclear leukocytes may account for 90% of the total white cell count. In the case of spinal disease, ma-

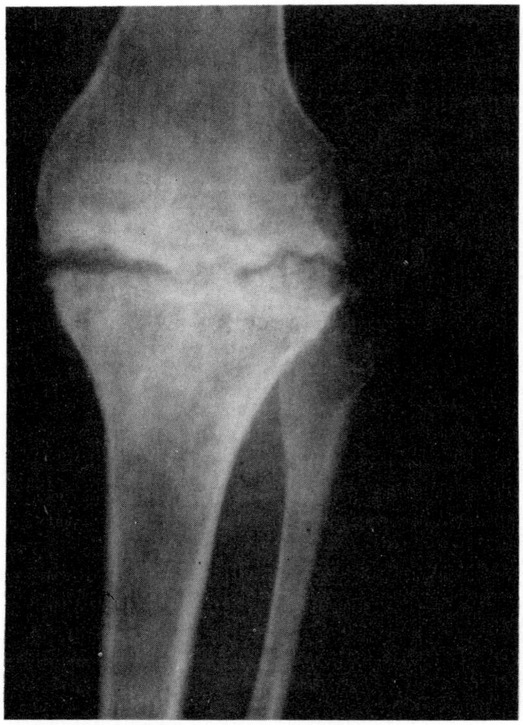

FIGURE 118–3. Advanced tuberculosis of the knee. Courtesy of Donald Resnick, M.D.

terial for culture is best obtained with a needle biopsy guided by fluoroscopy or computed tomography (CT). The Mantoux test with stabilized purified protein derivative (PPD-S) is positive in most cases of skeletal tuberculosis. In advanced disease or old age, anergy may be present. Anergy may be nonspecific or it may be specific for PPD-S.

Treatment. The keystone of treatment of skeletal tuberculosis is the use of combinations of chemotherapeutic agents. Because skeletal infection is rare compared with pulmonary involvement, the bulk of information on therapy comes from experience with pulmonary disease. The recommended initial combination is isoniazid (5 mg/kg, up to 300 mg orally daily) and rifampin (10 mg/kg, up to 600 mg orally daily) and pyrazinamide (15 to 30 mg/kg, up to 2 g daily). Pyrazinamide should be discontinued after 2 months. Ethambutol, 15 mg/kg daily, should be added until drug sensitivity is confirmed if the patient has emigrated from an area with a known high level of initial drug resistance or has a history of previous antituberculosis chemotherapy.[18] The optimum duration of treatment of skeletal tuberculosis has not been defined. Short-course therapy using isoniazid and rifampin for 9 months has proved equal or superior to other regimens in initial treatment of pulmonary disease. It is suggested that this form of treatment is also adequate for extrapulmonary disease, but the response to treatment must be evaluated in each case. The major contraindication to the combined use of isoniazid and rifampin is the presence of active liver disease. If alternative drug combinations are used, treatment must be continued for 18 to 24 months.

The role of surgery is more controversial, but some general guidelines can be drawn. In articular disease with absent or minimal bone involvement, drug therapy alone is effective. If bone involvement is extensive, debridement of the foci of bone infection may hasten healing. Synovectomy with curettage may be important in children with hip disease. When destruction is extensive in weight-bearing joints, arthrodesis has been the procedure of choice. In developing countries where sitting cross-legged and squatting are important, Girdlestone excision arthroplasty has been used effectively for hip disease.[19] Total hip replacement may be successful if the active infection is controlled.[20]

A series of reports from around the world on spinal tuberculosis indicate that chemotherapy is as successful alone as when combined with surgery.[9,21] Immobilization offers no benefit, and debridement procedures are indicated only when material for culture cannot be obtained by needle biopsy. In Pott's paraplegia the role of surgery is more controversial. Some evidence suggests that surgery may not be needed unless there is severe neurologic dysfunction at presentation or progressive neurologic deterioration occurs on adequate chemotherapy, but recent advances in technique might yield better surgical results.[22,23]

Atypical Tuberculosis. Atypical mycobacteria are ubiquitous, generally saprophytic organisms that have low pathogenicity for man.[24] Surveys with skin tests have shown that up to 48% of healthy young adults have developed delayed hypersensitivity to various members of this group. In addition to producing pulmonary disease resembling typical tuberculosis, these mycobacteria can infect joints, tendons, and bursae. Patients with arthritis rarely have active pulmonary disease. Approximately 50% of patients with articular disease have involvement of tendon sheaths or joints in the hand and wrist, while 20% have infection of the knee.[25] Infection of the hip, elbow, ankle, and prepatellar and olecranon bursae, as well as periarticular tissue simulating arthritis, have also been described. Several patents with flexor tendonitis at the wrist have had carpal tunnel syndrome. Polyarticular disease has occurred in about 15% of patients. A history of prior trauma or operation has been obtained in 45% of patients, and 36% have had prior intra-articular injection of corticosteroids. About one quarter of these patients have an underlying illness, most commonly another form of arthritis, such as degenerative joint disease, rheumatoid arthritis, or systemic lupus. The group I photochromogens Mycobacterium kansasii and M. marinum are the most frequent offenders, followed by the group III nonphotochromogen M. intracellularis. The Mycobacterium avium complex is now the most common cause of systemic mycobacterial infection associated with acquired immunodeficiency syndrome (AIDS) and can cause septic arthritis and osteomyelitis in these patients.[26]

Skin testing with PPDs prepared from atypical mycobacteria correlates well with culture results in children. In adults, cross-reactivity between various PPDs can lead to confusion. Microscopic examination of synovial fluid or biopsy material may reveal granuloma and acid-fast bacilli, but definitive diagnosis of the type of infection requires culture. Although data are not as plentiful on atypical infections, it appears that the yield of positive cultures from biopsies and synovial fluid will be similar to that obtained with M. tuberculosis. Treatment should be based on in-vitro sensitivity testing because these organisms are often resistant to the standard antituberculosis drug regimen. A combination of four or five drugs and/or synovectomy may be necessary.[27]

LEPROSY

Joint involvement was noted as a prominent symptom of leprosy in the Chinese medical writings of the *Nei Ching* in 600 BC.[28] The "stiff joints" described by these ancient physicians may occur in several ways. The indolent course of leprosy is punctuated by reactions. In *lepromatous leprosy*, these reactions take the form of erythema nodosum leprosum, in which inflamed subcutaneous nodules develop in crops. This condition may be accompanied by fever and arthralgia, by pitting edema of the hands from the metacarpal joints to the midforearm, or by a frank polyarthritis that involves knees, ankles, and small joints of the hands.[29] Synovial biopsy reveals an acute inflammatory reaction.[30] In most patients, lepra organisms are not detected in the synovium, and the synovial fluid is a transudate.[31] It has been postulated that this form of arthritis has an immunologic basis. However, group III fluid, which contains lepra cells with ingested organisms and high synovial fluid complement values, has been found, suggesting that the synovitis in some patients is due to infection.[32] Reactions in *tuberculoid* or *borderline leprosy* may also be accompanied by symmetric polyarthritis. Another type of symmetric polyarthritis has been described that occurs independently of the type of leprosy.[33] This arthritis begins insidiously months to years after the first symptoms of leprosy and involves the wrists, small joints of the hands and feet, and the knees. It is associated with morning stiffness and erosions on radiograph. It responds poorly to nonsteroidal anti-inflammatory drugs but improves with treatment of the underlying disease.

The most common joint deformities in leprosy occur secondary to disease in the peripheral nerves. Neurotrophic changes lead to absorption of bones, especially in the distal ends of the metatarsals. Sensory loss and repeated trauma are responsible for degenerative changes and aseptic necrosis of bone. These changes, accompanied by infection in soft tissue and bone, are responsible for loss of terminal digits and severe deformities of the hands and feet.[33] The claw hand that occurs secondary to nerve damage can further compound the disability. True neuropathic joints with complete disorganization of the weight-bearing surfaces and supporting bone may also occur. Charcot joints are most frequently seen at the wrist and ankle. Another form of arthritis occurs secondary to bone disease. *Direct infection of bone* occurs most commonly in the distal ends of the phalanges. During a reaction, subchondral bone may collapse and cause destruction of the adjacent joint.[30,34] In addition to arthritis, a necrotizing vasculitis, the Lucio phenomenon, may occur in the lower legs.[29]

The diagnosis of leprosy rests on demonstration of acid-fast bacilli in skin smears and histologic evidence of lepra organisms, with involvement of peripheral nerves on skin biopsy. From a clinical standpoint, the cardinal sign is anesthesia of the skin. Typically, thermal and tactile senses are lost before the ability to sense pain and pressure. The ulnar and peroneal nerves frequently are involved early.

Treatment of leprosy requires a coordinated effort that includes attention to the social needs of the patient as well as specialized drug therapy and physical measures to protect the skin and joints and to reduce contractures. In response to the increasing incidence of primary and secondary dapsone resistance, the World Health Organization now recommends the use of three drugs in combination for patients with multibacillary disease: dapsone, rifampin, and clofazimine. Dapsone and rifampin are recommended for those with paucibacillary disease.[35] In the United States, patients with leprosy are entitled to treatment by the US Public Health Service.

FUNGI

COCCIDIOIDOMYCOSIS

Coccidioidomycosis is caused by a fungus found in the soil throughout the lower Sonoran life zone. This zone includes the semiarid areas of southern California, Arizona, and New Mexico as well as western Texas and northern Mexico. It is characterized by hot summers, moderately wet winters, and infrequent freezes. The fungus multiplies in the soil after the winter rains, resulting in a higher incidence of disease in the summer months. Primary infection occurs 1 to 3 weeks after inhalation of spores. Clinical signs, which are usually self-limited, include fever, malaise, cough, chest pain, and erythema nodosum. A chronic pulmonary infection closely resembling tuberculosis occurs in about 2% of patients, whereas 0.2% develop widely disseminated disease. Dissemination is more common in black and Filipino males. Patients with collagen vascular diseases or lymphomas who are taking corticosteroids may be at greater risk, and acquired immunodeficiency syndrome (AIDS) patients appear to be particularly susceptible.[36,37]

Arthritis occurs in both the benign primary illness and the chronic disseminated form. In primary disease, it is usually associated with erythema nodosum and clears without residual deformity. In chronic disseminated disease, arthritis may occur alone or secondary to bone infection. Bayer and Guze have reviewed 57 cases of coccidioidal arthritis.[38] The most common presentation was a chronic monoarticular arthritis of the knee. The mean age was 36 years, and males outnumbered females by 4 to 1. Patients were otherwise in good health. Only one patient had a major underlying illness. A history of antecedent arthritis or joint injury was rare and only 6 patients (10%) had evidence of coccidioidal infection in extraarticular sites. If the organisms seeded directly to synovium, symptoms of an indolent synovitis with effusion, stiffness, and mild pain dominated the early course. If infection began in adjacent bone with later penetration into the joint, the early signs were pain and loss of motion without effusion. In either case, untreated synovial infection gradually progressed to villous hypertrophy and pannus formation, which often led to bony erosive changes later in the course. The indolent nature of this process is reflected in the long interval from onset of symptoms to diagnosis, a mean of 4.5 years. Its destructive nature is clear; 11 of 26 (42%) of patients whose initial radiographic examination was available showed destructive changes and/or adjacent osteomyelitis at diagnosis. The knee was involved in 39 (70%) of cases, and the wrist, hand, and the ankle were the next most commonly affected sites.

Infection of bone occurs in 10 to 20% of patients with disseminated disease. Sites most often involved are the ends of the long bones, the skull, vertebrae, and ribs. Metacarpals, metatarsals, the tibial tubercle, the malleoli, and the acromial process also appear to be favorite sites of localization. Approximately 60% of patients have involvement of a single site, while 15 to 20% have infection in three or more sites. Multiple bone lesions are associated with rapid dissemination and a poor prognosis. In the more indolent forms of disseminated disease, solitary bone lesions are common. The course of these solitary lesions is one of slow destruction of bone that may progress to involve adjacent joints.

Most joint infections are diagnosed by culture or histologic examination of synovial tissue. Fewer than 5% of synovial fluid cultures have been positive. In purulent material, the characteristic spherules are best seen after digestion with 20% potassium hydroxide. Coccidioides immitis can be cultured on Sabouraud's agar. It is important to notify the bacteriology laboratory if coccidioidomycosis is suspected because the spore-forming mycelial cultures are highly infectious. Although most patients with disseminated coccidioidomycosis are anergic, 80% of those with coccidioidal arthritis have a positive skin test to coccidioidin. Serologic tests may also be helpful. The tube precipitation test is useful for detecting early primary disease. It is positive within 1 to 3 weeks of infection in 80% of cases, reverts to negative after 6 months, but becomes positive again with relapse or reinfection. In disseminated disease, complement fixation (CF) and immunodiffusion tests are usually positive. Ninety percent of patients with coccidioidal arthritis have positive CF tests. Circulating immune complexes containing coccidioidin antigen have been found in most patients with active disease. It has been suggested that these complexes or free anticoccidioidin antibodies may play a role in the depressed T-lymphocyte responses that may accompany progressive disease.[39]

If the diagnosis is made prior to bone involvement, the development of villonodular synovitis, or pannus formation, treatment with amphotericin B alone may be effective. If any of these events have occurred, drug treatment should be combined with surgery. Intraarticular amphotericin B has been used with success for a few patients.[40] Ketoconazole, a broad-spectrum fungistatic agent with relatively low toxicity, can be given orally and requires gastric acid for absorption. About 80% of patients with osteoarticular disease have shown a good initial response. Unfortunately, 40% have relapsed while still taking the drug or after it has been discontinued.[41,42] It should thus be considered second choice to amphotericin B.

BLASTOMYCOSIS

In the continental United States, blastomycosis occurs primarily in the Ohio and Mississippi river valleys and Middle Atlantic States. Peak incidence is in the 20- to 50-year age group. The organism exists in the soil, apparently in geographically restricted microfoci.[43] Males are affected 10 times more often than females, presumably owing to their greater exposure through outdoor activities.[44] There is only one documented case of human-to-human transmission. Despite the unique susceptibility of dogs to infection, dog-to-human transmission has been documented in only one instance of a bite from an infected animal. Infection, which begins in the lungs after inhalation of spores, may produce a variety of results ranging from an asymptomatic or acute self-limited illness to acutely or insidiously progressive disease. Extrapulmonary infection spreads from the lungs by lymphatic or hematogenous routes. Skin and bone are the most frequent sites. Skeletal involvement occurs in one half of patients, and approximately 5% will present with joint pain.[45,46]

Articular blastomycosis usually presents as an acute monoarticular synovitis in a patient who is systemically ill with pulmonary and multifocal extrapulmonary disease. Fully 90% of these patients have active lung infections, and 70% have cutaneous abscesses. The knee is the most frequently involved joint, followed by the ankle and elbow. In approximately 70% of patients, joint infection results from hematogenous seeding to synovium; in 30% it is a consequence of extension of an underlying osteomyelitis. Osseous blastomycosis is most common in the vertebrae, ribs, tibia, tarsus, and skull, although involvement of almost every site in bone has been reported. Direct extension into the joint is most often seen at the knee. Spinal infection is associated with destruction of disc spaces, erosion of anterior vertebral bodies, proximal rib development of paraspinal soft tissue, and dissection of the infection beneath the anterior longitudinal ligament. Vertebral infection usually occurs in the thoracic and/or lumbar areas, but is rare in the cervical spine.

Blastomyces dermatitidis organisms are usually seen on potassium hydroxide-treated smears of synovial fluid, sputum, or material from abscesses. Cytologic analysis may reveal the organisms when routine smears are negative.[46] Definitive diagnosis is made on culture. An immunodiffusion test using the A and B antigens of the yeast phase of the organism has a sensitivity of 80%. The drug of choice for treatment of blastomycotic arthritis is amphotericin B. Ketoconazole is an effective alternative in patients with mild to moderate disease.[47] Although the role of operative treatment has not been fully defined, debridement of devitalized bone or synovium may benefit patients who fail to respond to antifungal drugs.

CRYPTOCOCCOSIS

Infection with Cryptococcus neoformans begins in the lungs with inhalation of spores and spreads to other organs, especially the central nervous system. Predisposing factors for susceptibility to this disease include lymphoma, Hodgkin's disease, diabetes mellitus, sarcoidosis, and corticosteroid treatment.[48,49] The organism is widely distributed in nature. The most dangerous source of infection appears to be pigeon droppings. Bone infection occurs in only about 10% of patients and follows a slowly progressive course.[50] Radiologic changes consist of lytic lesions with sharply scalloped margins and little reaction in adjacent bone or periosteum. These lesions may be found in the metaphyses of long bones, in the flat bones or vertebrae, the ribs, tarsal bones, or carpal bones. Vertebral infection resulting in paraspinal abscess formation can mimic tuberculosis. Only a few detailed reports of cryptococcal arthritis exist in the literature.[51,52] One half involved the knee and three quarters were monoarticular. About three quarters of these patients were immunosuppressed or had an identifiable underlying illness. The synovial fluid of some patients was grossly purulent, whereas others had a relatively low white blood cell count of about 2000 cells/mm^3.

Serologic tests for antibody to cryptococcal antigens are positive in fewer than 50% of proved cases. Cryptococcal antigens in sera or synovial fluid have been detected by agglutination of latex particles coated with rabbit anticryptococcal antibody. Rheumatoid factors can react with rabbit IgG and give a false-positive test. Amphotericin B given in combination with 5-fluorocytosine is the recommended treatment. Although debridement of joints may also be advisable, the data are insufficient to conclude whether medical or combined medical-surgical treatment is more effective.

HISTOPLASMOSIS

Histoplasma capsulatum grows in mycelial form in soil, where it produces spores that infect humans when inhaled. It thrives in ground contaminated with chicken, bird, or bat excreta. The highest incidence of positive histoplasmin skin tests occur in persons from states adjacent to the confluence of the Mississippi and Ohio rivers. In this area, 60 to 90% of young men are positive. Fortunately, both primary infection and reinfection are usually benign, self-limited diseases. Symptoms range from a transient pneumonitis to more generalized disease characterized by fever, malaise, chest pain, dyspnea, and weight loss. An acute polyarthritis may occur alone or in association with erythema nodosum, and polyarthritis or an additive polyarthralgia may be the presenting symptom of primary histoplasmosis.[53–55] Both types of joint involvement clear without residual deformity.

Progressive disease occurs in only 5% of infected persons. The most common form is a localized pulmonary infection in middle-aged white men. Disseminated histoplasmosis occurs in fewer than 0.1% of infections, usually in older or immune-compromised persons. Its manifestations are protean, and prognosis is poor. In the chronic form of disease, arthritis is truly an unusual clinical problem. Chronic infection of the knee (both unilateral and bilateral) and of the wrist have been reported.[51] The diagnosis depends on demonstration of Histoplasma capsulatum in histologic sections or culture of involved tissues. Immunologic tests play a minor role in diagnosis. In sensitized persons, the hisotplasmin skin test may induce antibodies that will influence serologic tests drawn more than a few days after the skin test. The complement fixation test is positive in 50% of patients with disseminated disease and may also be positive in other fungal diseases. These tests must be interpreted with caution.[56]

SPOROTRICHOSIS

Sporotrichosis is a rare cause of chronic granulomatous arthritis. The organism is a ubiquitous fungus that lives on plants or in the soil. Infection with this organism is usually limited to the skin, where it begins as a painful red nodule at the site of a scratch or a thorn prick. Cutaneous sporotrichosis may spread proximally by the lymphatics to form multiple necrotic secondary satellite lesions, or it may penetrate directly into adjacent tissues. Only a small percentage of people exposed to the fungus develop the systemic form of infection.

Systemic sporotrichosis occurs primarily in men 40 years of age or older. It has been associated with outdoor occupations or hobbies, alcohol abuse, and diseases or drugs that compromise the immune system.[57,58] In many patients, however, it develops without a history of predisposing factors. Two forms of the disease have been described, unifocal and multifocal.[59] Unifocal systemic sporotrichosis most commonly affects the lungs as cavitary disease of the upper lobes closely resembling tuberculosis. The other common presentation is as a chronic monoarthritis or oligoarthritis. Morning stiffness and fever are absent, but synovial thickening and effusions are found in the involved joints. A history of transient improvement with intra-articular steroids but poor response to oral steroids or aspirin may be obtained. The knee is most often involved, followed in decreasing frequency by the wrist, small joints of the hand, ankle, and elbow. Tenosynovitis may occur in the hand or wrist.

Multifocal systemic sporotrichosis typically involves the skin, joints, and bones. These patients are more likely to have a compromised immune system than those who develop unifocal disease. Skin lesions differ from those in cutaneous sporotrichosis. Dusty red nodules up to several centimeters in diameter develop randomly any place on the body except the palms and soles. The lesions eventually ulcerate and may heal while new ones appear. The skin around joints, on the face, and on the scalp is most often involved.[61] Skin lesions usually precede joint symptoms. In this form of the disease, the arthritis is poly-articular in about two thirds of patients. As in the unifocal form, tendonitis may be present, and fistulas may develop after surgical procedures on the joints if proper antifungal therapy is not given. Infection of bones spares the vertebrae, ribs, and jaw, but involves long bones near the joints. Joint infection is rarely related to extension of osseous infection. Pulmonary involvement occurs in fewer than 20% of patients with multifocal disease. It differs from unifocal lung disease in that nodules are smaller and do not cavitate. Central nervous system involvement is rare.

Diagnosis of sporotrichosis arthritis rests on culture of Sporothrix schenckii from joint fluid or synovial tissue. Both have yielded positive results, but the percentage of positives appears to be higher with cultures of tissue. The best yield occurs with culture of both tissue and fluid. The organisms are difficult to see in tissue sections. The sedimentation rate is elevated, but peripheral white blood cell counts are normal. Joint fluid shows the pattern of low-grade inflammation with cell counts of 8,000 to 20,000/mm^3, a fair to good mucin clot, and decreased glucose concentration.[60,61] Two serologic tests are available for diagnosis, a latex slide test and an enzyme-linked immunosorbent assay (ELISA). Both tests can be used for diagnosis and to follow treatment because titers fall with effective therapy. Titers of 1:4 or greater are presumptive evidence of active disease. Soft-tissue swelling, osteoporosis, decreased joint space, and erosions similar to those occurring in rheumatoid arthritis may be seen radiographically.

Treatment consists of amphotericin B alone or in combination with surgical debridement of infected joints. Intra-articular amphotericin B has also been used successfully in some cases.[60] In a patient unable to tolerate amphotericin B, iodide therapy plus surgical debridement may be a reasonable alternative. Ketoconazole does not appear effective in this disease.[62] Results of treatment of unifocal disease are usually excellent. The main cause of poor results is a long delay between onset of disease and diagnosis. The outcome of multifocal sporotrichosis is less certain. In one report, 11 deaths occurred in 37 patients with this form of disease.[61]

CANDIDAL ARTHRITIS

Arthritis caused by Candida species has been reported with increasing frequency in the past several years. An underlying illness or direct predisposing cause has been present in all patients. Two thirds of the adults were hospitalized with a serious illness, such as cancer, renal failure, sepsis, or a connective tissue disease. Most were receiving antibiotics, chemotherapy, or immunosuppressive treatment and often had indwelling intravenous catheters.[63] The remainder of the adults were ambulatory. In these instances, predisposing causes included rheumatoid arthritis, osteoarthritis with repeated corticosteroid injections, recent joint surgery, and previous joint infection.[64] A similar pattern is seen with candidal osteomyelitis.[65] Heroin addiction has also been noted as a predisposing cause. A distinctive syndrome of follicular and nodular lesions of the scalp, beard, and pubis with ocular infection or osteoarticular lesions of the intervertebral discs, knee, or chondrocostal junctions has been noted in this group of individuals.[66] Ninety percent of children with candidal arthritis have been less than 1 year old. All have had a serious underlying illness, and most were critically ill from other causes at the time the arthritis was diagnosed. As in adults, antibiotics, immunosuppression, and catheters were frequently implicated as predisposing causes. Candidal arthritis may occur in as many as 2% of infants receiving hyperalimentation.[67] Only one case has been reported in association with chronic mucocutaneous candidiasis.

In both adults and children, the knee is involved in 75% of cases. The hip and shoulder are the next most frequently involved joints. Small joint involvement is rare. Multiple joint infections occur about twice as often in infants as in adults (35% vs. 15%), and coexistent osteomyelitis is more common in infants. Infection seeds from the blood to the synovium and may follow fungal septicemia by intervals of 2 to 12 weeks. Symptoms include pain, tenderness, synovial thickening, and effusion, but red hot joints are infrequent. Isolated candidal arthritis following direct injection of organisms into the joint by trauma or arthrocentesis follows a more indolent course. It is not associated with systemic symptoms and is usually caused by less virulent strains of Candida species.[68]

The synovial fluid contains a mean of 38,000 leukocytes/mm^3 with 80% polymorphonuclear leukocytes, but lower counts may be found in patients with leukemia.[64] Synovial fluid glucose levels have been low in 70% of reported cases. Culture of synovial fluid is a highly reliable method for identifying Candida species. Gram's stain is not reliable, however, being negative in 80% of culture-positive samples. Candida albicans is the most frequent offender followed by C. tropicalis. Serologic tests for serum antibodies to C. albicans antigens may show a rising titer with dissemination of infection, but these tests do not clearly differentiate heavy colonization of systemic disease.

The relatively small number of reported cases makes

it difficult to draw firm conclusions regarding optimum treatment. Amphotericin B alone has resulted in eradication of the infection in about 60% of cases in which it has been used. The failure rate appears to be somewhat less if it is combined with surgical operation or 5-fluorocytosine. The latter drug alone is not a good choice. A few reports on the successful use of ketoconazole have appeared.[69] Overall, 60% of adults and 40% of infants have recovered with normal joint function. Twenty percent of patients in both groups have died of Candida sepsis or of the underlying disease. The remainder have survived with significant disability resulting from destruction of the joint.

ACTINOMYCOSIS

Actinomycosis is caused by an anaerobic bacteria-like obligate parasite, Actinomyces israelii, which is a normal resident of the human mouth. Infection occurs through the gastrointestinal tract, particularly after dental procedures or injury to the mouth and jaw. It may also follow aspiration into an atelectatic portion of the lung. Abscesses form in the neck, jaw, lung, or abdomen. Bone involvement is frequent in the jaw and spine, and is usually secondary to abscesses in adjacent tissues. Infection of the spine typically involves several vertebrae, but not the intervening discs. Adjacent pedicles, transverse processes, and the heads of contiguous ribs may be eroded. In the vertebrae, channels of infection surrounded by sclerotic bone cause a "honeycomb" or "soap bubble" radiographic appearance. Long, dense, longitudinal spurs and sclerotic changes in the lateral portions of the vertebrae are sometimes seen when infection spreads from the abdomen to the spine by way of the psoas muscle. Dense trabeculae and sclerosis make vertebral collapse uncommon.[70] Any level of the spine may be affected. Symptoms vary from mild local pain to severe restriction of motion, radicular pain, or weakness. Extension of the infection into the spinal canal may result in meningitis. Diagnosis is made by identification of sulfur granules on Gram's stain of pus from the abscesses and is confirmed by growth of the organism in anaerobic culture. Blood cultures are rarely positive. No serologic test is currently available for actinomycosis. Treatment with tetracycline has been successful, but penicillin is the drug of choice.

MYCETOMA (MADUROMYCOSIS, MADURA FOOT)

Mycetoma is an indolent tumor-like infection found in tropical and semitropical climates. It is caused by a variety of actinomycetes or fungi that gain entrance through the skin. Allescheria boydii is the most common cause in North America, whereas Nocardia brasiliensis is the usual cause in Central and South America. Mycetoma commonly involves the foot, where it invades subcutaneous tissue, bone, and ligaments.[71] In long-standing cases, swelling, sinus formation, and clubbing with pronounced deformity may occur. A similar process may involve the hand. Systemic symptoms and regional lymphadenopathy are uncommon. Effective treatment requires accurate identification of the infecting organism, prolonged high-dose administration of the appropriate antimicrobial agent, and surgical debridement. Prognosis depends to some extent on the causative organism and is better with actinomycotic than with true fungal mycetoma. In some cases, amputation may be necessary.

PARASITES

Parasitic infections may cause arthritis by direct invasion of the joints or through secondary immune mechanisms. They may also involve periarticular tissues and produce nonarticular or soft-tissue rheumatic syndromes (Table 118–2). These mechanisms are not mutually exclusive. Joint involvement is relatively rare in these diseases but a very large number of people in developing countries are involved. For example, 600 million people are estimated to have schistosomiasis or filariasis. Thus even a low incidence of arthritis may result in significant morbidity in these populations.

FILARIASIS

The lymphatic-dwelling filarial parasite Wuchereria bancrofti is transmitted by mosquitoes and is found in tropic and subtropic areas. The adult worms live in the lymphatics where they cause first reversible and then irreversible damage to lymph flow, resulting in brawny edema and elephantiasis. An acute inflammatory arthritis of the knee may occur associated with fever and inguinal lymphadenopathy. The initial episode typically lasts only 7 to 10 days but recurrent, less inflammatory effusions may follow. The synovial fluid in these cases is chylous and devoid of parasites. Lymphangiographic studies suggest the presence of a fistula between the abnormal lymphatics and the synovial space.[72] In other instances an acute or chronic monoarthritis or oligoarthritis of large joints, usually involving the knee, occurs with a nonchylous effusion and few if any constitutional symptoms. In these persons the sedimentation rate is often normal, and the rheumatoid factor is usually negative. Resolution of the arthritis with treatment of the underlying filariasis provides the most convincing

TABLE 118–2. TYPICAL RHEUMATOLOGIC SYNDROMES ASSOCIATED WITH PARASITES

Filariasis	Chylous effusion of the knee Monoarthritis or oligoarthritis of large joints
Trichinosis	Myositis
Cisticercosis	Myalgia, skin and muscle nodules
Echinococcosis	Bone cysts
Schistosomiasis	Low back, thigh, knee, and heel pain; polyarthritis
Giardiasis	Seronegative arthritis of knees, ankles, and feet

evidence for a causal relationship between the arthritis and the helminthic infection.[73]

Infection with the guinea worm Dracunculus medinensis can involve the joints by several mechanisms. The adult female worm, which infects millions of people on the Indian subcontinent and in West Africa, migrates into the subcutaneous tissues usually of the lower leg, ankle, or foot where it emerges from the base of a cutaneous ulcer to discharge its larvae. A septic arthritis may occur secondary to bacterial infection of periarticular ulcers. In other cases a mild synovitis occurs in joints adjacent to deep-seated worms. The most dramatic form of arthritis occurs when the worm enters the synovial space and discharges its larvae. An intense inflammation results, probably from the toxic effects of the uterine secretions. The synovial fluid is exudative and the diagnosis can be confirmed by the finding of the larvae in the fluid. Surgical removal of the worm and irrigation of the joint cavity results in prompt relief of symptoms.[74] Other filaria may cause arthritis through direct invasion of the joint. In both *loa loa* and *onchocerciasis*, microfilaria have been found in the synovial fluid of patients with inflammatory arthritis of the knee. In the latter disease a symmetric polyarthritis, possibly caused by deposition of immune complexes, has also been described.

Diofilaria species are animal parasites than can infect man but do not survive to complete their life cycle in humans. Clinically these infections usually present as a subcutaneous nodule or solitary pulmonary nodule. An associated self-limited, intermittent, olgoarticular arthritis has been reported. The duration of symptoms can be shortened by surgical removal of the subcutaneous nodule containing the worm.[75]

TRICHINOSIS

Trichinella spiralis is a tissue-dwelling round worm that is transmitted directly from host to host by eating contaminated meat. The adult worm causes few if any symptoms in the intestine, but systemic invasion by the larvae, which occurs about 2 weeks after infection, typically results in myositis, with myalgia, weakness and swelling associated with fever, periorbital edema, and headache. Muscle enzymes are elevated in the serum but the erythrocyte sedimentation rate is usually normal. Frequent involvement of the extraocular muscles and eosinophilia help to distinguish trichinosis from polymyositis. A definitive diagnosis can be made with serologic testing.

SCHISTOSOMIASIS

Schistosomes are blood flukes that parasitize the venous channels of the human host. They are endemic in Africa, Asia, South America, and the Caribbean islands. Infection is usually acquired in childhood. Like other helminths, schistosomes do not multiply in man. They do, however, produce eggs that release enzymes to facilitate their exit from the body. The immune response to the eggs and their products results in granuloma formation and subsequent disruption of the function of the tissues in which they lie. Two types of arthritis have been described: one is pauciarticular, associated with enthesiopathy, and thought to be a form of reactive arthritis; the other is polyarticular and might be immune complex–mediated. Some patients show features of both.[77] The reactive type usually presents as low-back, thigh, knee, or heel pain. In one series of 124 patients with joint complaints, radiographs of the sacroiliac joints and heels were each abnormal in 40% of the cases.[76] None of the patients had morning stiffness or symptoms in the hands. Tests for rheumatoid factors were negative. In 3 of 11 biopsies of the knee, ova were identified in the synovium; but the other biopsies showed chronic synovitis with lymphocytic plasma cell infiltrates and no ova or adult worms. The polyarticular form is symmetric, and often involves the metacarpophalangeal and metatarsophalangeal joints, the wrists, the knees, and the ankles. It is associated with morning stiffness and gelling.[77] This type of arthritis often begins within days of the onset of systemic symptoms of schistosomiasis, and resolves within a month of initiation of treatment of the underlying disease.

CESTODE INFECTION

Infection with the pork tapeworm Taenia solium may cause fever, eosinophilia, and myalgia during the invasive phase. Late in the disease, cysticerci are frequently found in subcutaneous tissue or muscle, where they form painless nodules. Actual joint involvement is extremely rare. In echinococcosis the embryos are freed from the eggs in the intestine and enter the bloodstream, where they are usually filtered out in the capillary beds of the liver or lung. Occasionally they may lodge in bone, where the formation of the bladder-like cyst results in an enlarging mass that may cause chronic bone pain or spontaneous fracture. Rarely the cyst may involve a joint.[76]

OTHER HELMINTHIC INFECTIONS

Reactive arthritis or "parasitic rheumatism" has been described with Strongyloides stercoralis, Taenia saginata, and Toxocara canis infections.[79] Patients have presented with symmetric polyarthritis, asymmetric oligoarthritis, and also muscle pain and stiffness reminiscent of polymyalgia rheumatica. Most, but not all, have had eosinophilia. The sedimentation rate is usually elevated and the rheumatoid factor is often negative. In all reported cases the joint symptoms have resolved with treatment of the underlying infection. In most cases synovial biopsies or synovial fluid analysis has failed to reveal the organism. Immune complexes were found in serum and synovial fluid in two patients, and in one case immunoglobulin and complement deposits were found in the synovium. These cases may represent a reactive arthritis or immune complex-mediated disease, but in one instance direct joint infection was documented through the identification of S. stercoralis worms in the joints.[80]

PROTOZOAN INFECTION

A seronegative arthritis involving primarily the knees, ankles, and feet may occur in children infected with Giardia lamblia. In some children the arthritis is associated with fever, abdominal pain, diarrhea, and headache, while in a few it is the only symptom. More than one course of treatment with metronidazole may be needed to eliminate the parasite and thus alleviate the joint symptoms. This syndrome is also thought to represent a reactive arthritis.

REFERENCES

1. Glassworth, J., Robins, A.B., and Snider, D.E.J.: Tuberculosis in the 1980's. N. Engl. J. Med., *302*:1441–1450, 1980.
2. Davidson, P.T., and Horowitz, I.: Skeletal tuberculosis. Am. J. Med., *48*:77–84, 1970.
3. Enarsen, D.A., et al.: Bone and joint tuberculosis: A continuing problem. Can. Med. Assoc. J., *120*:139–145, 1979.
4. Evanchick, C.C., Davis, D.E., and Harrington, T.M.: Tuberculosis of peripheral joints: An often missed diagnosis. J. Rheumatol., *13*:187–189, 1986.
5. Alvarez, S., and McCabe, W.R.: Extrapulmonary tuberculosis revisited: A review of experience at Boston City and other hospitals. Medicine, *63*:25–55, 1984.
6. Ellner, J.J.: Immune dysregulation in human tuberculosis. J. Lab. Clin. Med., *108*:142–149, 1986.
7. Garrido, G., et al.: A review of peripheral tuberculous arthritis. Semin. Arthritis Rheum., *18*:142–149, 1988.
8. Nathanson, L., and Cohen, W.: A statistical and roentgen analysis of two hundred cases of bone and joint tuberculosis. Radiology, *36*:550–567, 1941.
9. Fancourt, G.J., et al.: Bone tuberculosis: Results and experience in Leicestershire. Br. J. Dis. Chest, *80*:265–272, 1986.
10. Bailey, H.L., et al.: Tuberculosis of the spine in children: Operative findings and results in one hundred consecutive patients. J. Bone Joint Surg., *54*:1633–1657, 1972.
11. Felson, R., et al.: Mycotic tuberculous aneurysm of the thoracic aorta. J.A.M.A., *237*:1104–1108, 1977.
12. Key, L.A.: Tuberculosis of the knee joint in adults. Br. Med. J., *1*:408, 1940.
13. Kofkorn, R.W., and Steigerwald, F.C.: Carpal tunnel syndrome as the initial manifestation of tuberculosis. Am. J. Med., *60*:583–586, 1976.
14. Southwood, T.R., et al.: Tuberculous rheumatism (Poncet's Disease) in a child. Arthritis Rheum., *31*:1311–1313, 1988.
15. Sharif, H.S., et al.: Granulomatous spinal infections: MR imaging. Radiology, *177*:101–107, 1990.
16. Berney, S., Goldstein, M., and Bishko, F.: Clinical and diagnostic features of tuberculous arthritis. Am. J. Med., *53*:36–42, 1972.
17. Wallace, R., and Cohen A.S.: Tuberculous arthritis: A report of two cases with review of biopsy and synovial fluid findings. Am. J. Med., *61*:277–282, 1976.
18. American Thoracic Society: Treatment of tuberculosis and tuberculosis infection in children and adults. Am. Rev. Respir. Dis., *134*:355–363, 1986.
19. Tulis, M., and Mukherjee, S.K.: Excision arthroplasty for tuberculosis and pyogenic arthritis of the hip. J. Bone Joint Surg., *63B*:29–32, 1981.
20. Laforgia, R., Murphy, J.C.M., and Redfern, T.R.: Low friction arthroplasty for old quiescent infection of the hip. J. Bone Joint Surg. [Br.] *70*:373–376, 1988.
21. Martini, M., Adjrad, A., and Boudjemaa, A.: Tuberculous osteomyelitis: A review of 125 cases. Int. Orthop., *10*:201–207, 1986.
22. Pattisson, P.R.M.: Pott's paraplegia: An account of the treatment of 89 consecutive patients. Paraplegia, *24*:77–91, 1986.
23. Louw, J.A.: Spinal tuberculosis with neurological deficit: Treatment with anterior vascularised rib grafts, posterior oseotomies, and fusion. J. Bone Joint Surg. [Br.] *72*:686–693, 1990.
24. Woods, G.L., and Washington, J.A.: Mycobacteria other than *Mycobacterium tuberculosis*: Review of microbiological and clinical aspects. Rev. Infect. Dis., *9*:275–294, 1987.
25. Travis, W.E., et al.: The histopathologic spectrum in *Mycobacterium marinum* infection. Arch. Pathol. Lab. Med., *109*:1109–1113, 1985.
26. Blumenthal, D.R., Zucker, J.R., and Hawkins, C.C.: Letters: Mycobacterium avium complex-induces septic arthritis and osteomyelitis in a patient with the acquired immunodeficiency syndrome. Arthritis Rheum., *33*:757–758, 1990.
27. Horsburgh, C.R.: Mycobacterium avium complex infection in the acquired immunodeficiency syndrome. N. Engl. J. Med., *324*:1332–1338, 1991.
28. Cochrane, R.G., and Davey, T.F.: Leprosy in Theory and Practice. Baltimore, Williams & Wilkins, 1964, p. 3.
29. Chavez-Legaspi, M., Gomez-Vazquez, A., and Garcia-DeLa Torre, I.: Study of rheumatoid manifestations and serologic abnormalities in patients with lepromatous leprosy. J. Rheumatol., *12*:738–741, 1985.
30. Karat, A.B.A., et al.: An exudative arthritis in leprosy-rheumatoid arthritis-like syndrome in association with erythema nodosum leprosum. Br. Med. J., *3*:770–772, 1967.
31. Modi, T.H., and Lele, R.D.: Acute joint manifestations in leprosy. J. Assoc. Physicians India, *17*:247–254, 1969.
32. Louie, J.S., and Glovsky, M.: Complement determinations in the synovial fluid and serum of a patient with erythema nodosum leprosum. Int. J. Lepr., *43*:252–255, 1975.
33. Atkin, S.L., et al.: Clinical and laboratory studies of arthritis in leprosy. Br. Med. J., *298*:1423–1425, 1989.
34. Paterson, D.E., and Job, C.K.: Leprosy in Theory and Practice. Baltimore, Williams & Wilkins, 1964, p. 425.
35. Shepard, C.C.: Leprosy today. N. Engl. J. Med., *307*:1640–1641, 1982.
36. Johnson, W.M., and Gall, E.P.: Fatal coccidiomycosis in collagen vascular diseases. J. Rheumatol., *10*:79–84, 1983.
37. Bronnimann, D.A., et al.: Coccidiomycosis in the acquired immunodeficiency syndrome. Ann. Int. Med., *106*:372–379, 1987.
38. Bayer, A.S., and Guze, L.B.: Fungal arthritis II. Coccidioidal synovitis: Clinical, diagnostic, therapeutic and prognostic considerations. Semin. Arthritis Rheum., *8*:200–211, 1979.
39. Yoshinoza, S., Cox, R.A., and Pope, R.M.: Circulating immune complexes in coccidioidomycosis. J. Clin. Invest., *66*:655–663, 1980.
40. Bried, J.M., and Galgiani, J.N.: *Coccidioides immitis* infection in bones and joints. Clin. Orthop. Rel. Res., *211*:235–243, 1985.
41. Catanzaro, A., et al.: Treatment of coccidiodomycosis with ketoconazole: An evaluation utilizing a new scoring system. Am. J. Med., *74*:64–69, 1983.
42. Stevens, D.A., et al.: Experience with ketoconazole in three major manifestations of progressive coccidioidomycosis. Am. J. Med., *74*:58–63, 1983.
43. Klein, B.S., et al.: Isolation of *Blastomyces dermatitidis* in soil associated with a large outbreak of blastomycosis in Wisconsin. N. Engl. J. Med., *314*:529–534, 1986.
44. Tenebaum, J.J., Greenspan, J., and Kerkering, T.M.: Blastomycosis. CRC Crit. Rev. Microbiol., *9*:139–163, 1982.

45. Cooperative Study of the Veterans Administration: Blastomycosis: A review of 198 collected cases in Veterans Administration hospitals. Am. Rev. Respir. Dis., *89*:659–672, 1964.
46. George, A.L., Hays, J.T., and Graham, B.S.: Blastomycosis presenting as monoarticular arthritis: The role of synovial fluid cytology. Arthritis Rheum., *28*:516–521, 1985.
47. National Institute of Allergy and Infectious Disease Mycoses Study Group: Treatment of blastomycosis and histoplasmosis with ketoconazole: Results of a prospective randomized clinical trial. Ann. Intern. Med., *103*:861–872, 1985.
48. Lewis, J.L., and Rabinovich, S.: Wide spectrum of cryptococcal infections. Am. J. Med., *53*:315–322, 1972.
49. Prefect, R.F., Durack, D.T., and Gallis, H.A.: Cryptococcemia. Medicine, *62*:98–109, 1983.
50. Collins, V.P.: Bone involvement in cryptococcosis (torulosis). Am. J. Roentgenol., *63*:102, 1950.
51. Ricciardi, D.D., et al.: Cryptococcal arthritis in a patient with acquired immune deficiency syndrome: Case report and review of the literature. J. Rheumatol., *13*:455–458, 1986.
52. Stead, K.J., Klugman, K.P., Painter, M.L., and Koornhof, H.J.: Septic arthritis due to Cryptococcus neoformans. Br. J. Infect., *17*:139–145, 1988.
53. Wheat, L.J., et al.: A large urban outbreak of histoplasmosis: Clinical features. Ann. Intern. Med., *94*:331–337, 1981.
54. Thornberry, D.R., et al.: Histoplasmosis presenting with joint pain and hilar adenopathy. Arthritis Rheum., *25*:1396–1402, 1982.
55. Rosenthal, J., et al.: Rheumatic manifestations of histoplasmosis in a recent Indianapolis epidemic. Arthritis Rheum., *26*:1065–1070, 1983.
56. Dratz, D.J., and Graybill, J.R.: Infectious disease. *In* Basic and Clinical Immunology. Edited by D.P. Stites, J.D. Stobo, and J.V. Wells. Norwalk, CT, Appleton and Lange, 1987, pp. 534–581.
57. Gullberg, R.M., et al.: Sporotrichosis: Recurrent cutaneous, articular and central nervous system infection in a renal transplant recipient. Rev. Infect. Dis., *9*:369–375, 1987.
58. Lipstein-Kresch, E., et al.: Disseminated *Sporothrix schenckii* infection with arthritis in a patient with acquired immune deficiency syndrome. J. Rheumatol., *12*:805–808, 1985.
59. Wilson, D.E., et al.: Clinical features of extracutaneous sporotrichosis. Medicine, *46*:265–279, 1967.
60. Downs, N.J., Daniel, R.H., Mhatre, V.R., and Liu, C.: Intra-articular amphotericin B treatment of sporothrix schenckii arthritis. Arch. Intern. Med., *149*:954–955, 1989.
61. Lynch, P.J., Voorhees, J.J., and Harrell, E.R.: Systemic sporotrichosis. Ann. Intern. Med., *73*:23–30, 1970.
62. Dismukes, W.E., et al.: Treatment of systemic mycosis with ketoconazole: Emphasis on toxicity and clinical response in 52 patients. Ann. Intern. Med., *98*:13–20, 1983.
63. Bayer, A.S., and Guze, L.B.: Fungal arthritis. Part I. Candida arthritis. Semin. Arthritis Rheum., *3*:142–150, 1978.
64. Campen, D.H., Kaufman, R.L., and Beardmore, T.D.: Candida septic arthritis in rheumatoid arthritis. J. Rheumatol., *17*:86–88, 1990.
65. Gathe, J.C., Jr., et al.: Candida osteomyelitis: Report of five cases and review of the literature. Am. J. Med., *82*:927–937, 1987.
66. Dupont, B., and Drouket, E.: Cutaneous, ocular, and osteoarticular candidiasis in heroin addicts: New clinical and therapeutic aspects in 38 patients. J. Infect. Dis., *152*:577–591, 1985.
67. Yousefzadeh, D.K., and Jackson, J.H.: Neonatal and infantile candidal arthritis with or without osteomyelitis: A clinical and radiographic review of 21 cases. Skeletal Radiol., *5*:77–90, 1980.
68. Katzenstein, D.: Isolated Candida arthritis: Report of a case and definition of a distinct clinical syndrome. Arthritis Rheum., *28*:1421–1424, 1985.
69. Duquesnoy, B., et al.: Ketoconazole for treatment of Candida arthritis. J. Rheumatol., *11*:105–107, 1984.
70. Crank, R.N., Sundaram, M., and Shields, J.B.: Case report 197. Skeletal Radiol., *8*:164–167, 1982.
71. Mariat, F., Destembes, P., and Segretain, G.: The mycetomas: Clinical features, pathology and epidemiology. Contrib. Microbiol. Immunol., *4*:1–39, 1977.
72. Das, G.C., and Sen, S.B.: Chylous arthritis. Br. Med. J., *2*:27–29, 1968.
73. Salfield, S.: Filarial arthritis in the Sepik district of Papua New Guinea. Med. J. Aust., *1*:264–267, 1975.
74. Sivaramappa, M., et al.: Acute guinea worm synovitis of the knee joint. J. Bone Joint Surg., *51A*:1324–1330, 1969.
75. Corman, L.C.: Acute arthritis occurring in association with subcutaneous dirofilaria tenuis infection. Arthritis Rheum., *30*:1431–1434, 1987.
76. Bassiouni, M., and Kamel, M.: Bilharzial arthropathy. Ann. Rheum. Dis., *43*:806–809, 1984.
77. Atkin, S.L., et al.: Schistosomiasis and inflammatory polyarthritis: A clinical, radiological, and laboratory study of 96 patients infected by S. mansoni with particular reference to the diarthrodial joint. Q. J. Med., *229*:479–487, 1986.
78. Naaseh, G.A.: Hydatid disease in bone and joint. J. Trop. Med. Hyg., *79*:243–244, 1975.
79. Bocanegra, T.S., et al.: Reactive arthritis induced by parasitic infestation. Ann. Intern. Med., *94*:207–209, 1981.
80. Akoglu, T., et al.: Parasitic arthritis induced by Stronglyoides stercoralis. Ann. Rheum. Dis., *43*:523–525, 1984.
81. Woo, P., and Panayi, G.: Reactive arthritis due to infection with *Giardia lamblia*. J. Rheumatol., *11*:79, 1984.

119

Viral Arthritis

STEVEN R. YTTERBERG

Arthritis can follow infection with several viral agents (Table 119–1). Additionally, a viral cause has been considered for many chronic rheumatic diseases, although this has been difficult to prove. This chapter focuses on the agents known to be associated with arthritis. Viral arthritis generally is acute in onset and of short duration, but infection with several of these agents may result in chronic joint symptoms (Table 119–2).

TABLE 119–1. VIRAL INFECTIONS ASSOCIATED WITH ARTHRITIS

VIRAL INFECTIONS OFTEN ASSOCIATED WITH ARTHRITIS
Parvovirus B19
Hepatitis B virus
Rubella virus and vaccine
Alphaviruses
Ross River virus
Chikungunya virus
O'nyong-nyong virus
Mayaro virus
Sindbis virus
Ockelbo virus
Mumps
VIRAL INFECTIONS OCCASIONALLY ASSOCIATED WITH ARTHRITIS
Adenoviruses
Herpesviruses
Cytomegalovirus
Epstein-Barr virus
Herpes simplex virus type 1
Varicella-zoster virus
Enteroviruses
Coxsackieviruses
Echoviruses
Hepatitis A virus
Lymphocytic choriomeningitis virus
Smallpox virus (Variola) and vaccinia virus

Most information about the relationship of viruses and arthritis comes from epidemiologic studies or case reports of arthritis associated with specific viral infections. Studies evaluating patients with arthritis of recent onset have also led to consideration of interesting relationships with viral infection, including possible etiologic roles for parvovirus B19,[1,2] coxsackieviruses,[3] and Epstein-Barr virus (EBV).[4] Most patients evaluated for recent-onset arthritis have no specific diagnosis, of course. Such illnesses may have an as yet unidentified viral cause. Study of the specific viruses that induce arthritis provides an opportunity to understand inflammatory joint diseases, which might lead to more specific treatment.

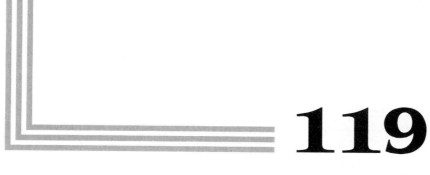

The mechanisms leading to arthritis are reasonably well understood in a few of these diseases, but remain unknown in many others (Table 119–3).[5,6] First, tissue damage may result directly from the viral infection. This may result from lysis of infected cells by virus or by persistent infection with loss of specialized cell function without cell lysis.[7] Second, disease may result from the effects of the normal host immune response to the virus. Virus-infected cells may be lysed by cytotoxic T cells, natural killer cells, or antibody plus complement. Furthermore, cytokines and other humoral mediators may exert pathologic effects distant from the site of the infection. Immune complexes of the virus and antiviral antibody may deposit in certain organs, causing disease.[8] Last, a viral infection may alter its host immune system and cause disease. Some viruses cause immune suppression by infecting cells of the immune system or by altering their function. Other viruses induce autoantibody formation via a variety of mechanisms including generation of new antigens, exposure of antigens, formation of antibodies that are cross reactive with host antigens as a result of molecular mimicry, polyclonal B-

TABLE 119–2. MUSCULOSKELETAL MANIFESTATIONS OF VIRAL ARTHRITIS

VIRUS	FREQUENCY OF ARTHRITIS	JOINT INVOLVEMENT	DURATION
Parvovirus B19	50% adults (women 60%, men 30%) 5% children	Symmetric polyarticular Small and large joints	Arthritis ≤2 weeks Arthralgia ≤4 weeks Recurrence or persistence in up to 10%
Hepatitis B virus	Arthritis 10%; arthralgia 25%	Symmetric usually, migratory in some Small and large joints	1–3 weeks; usually improves with onset of jaundice
Rubella virus	15–30% adult women; children and men less often	Symmetric polyarticular Small and large joints Tendonitis, neuritis, carpal tunnel syndrome	1–28 days
Rubella vaccine	15% adult women 1–5% children	Symmetric polyarticular Large and small joints Tendonitis, neuritis	1–46 days Chronicity or recurrences occur
Alphavirus	Most adults with clinical infection	Symmetric, oligo- or polyarticular Small and large joints	7–28 days Arthralgias or arthritis may persist
Mumps virus	0.4%; males > females	Arthralgia alone or migratory polyarticular arthritis or monoarticular arthritis of large joint	<1 to 4 weeks
Adenovirus	Case reports	Symmetric or asymmetric Large and small joints	7–30 days May persist in immunocompromised
Cytomegalovirus	Case report	Knee	>30 days
Epstein-Barr virus	Case reports	Monoarticular—knee or ankle Oligoarticular—knees Polyarticular	7–130 days
Herpes simplex virus type 1	Case reports	Monoarticular—knee or ankle	<14 days
Varicella-zoster virus	Case reports	Monoarticular—knee or ankle	2–6 days
Lymphocytic choriomeningitis virus	Case reports	Polyarticular—small joints of hands	Unknown
Coxsackieviruses	Case reports combined enterovirus 0.13%	Symmetric polyarticular Large and small joints Systemic features like Still's disease	Months to years with recurrences
Echoviruses	Case reports	Symmetric polyarticular or monoarticular—knees	2–9 days
Hepatitis A virus	Case reports Arthralgia 11%		
Smallpox virus	0.25–0.5% 2–5% children	Monoarticular—elbows or other large joints	≤60 days

EBV = Epstein-Barr virus; VZV = varicella zoster virus.

cell stimulation, or generation of anti-idiotypic antibodies (Table 119–3).[9]

Most cases of virus-induced arthritis are short-lived, but chronic or recurrent arthropathy occasionally develops. Chronicity might be explained by persistent or latent viral infection. This occurs with many viruses, including many that induce acute arthritis.[6,10] Episodes of viral reactivation might cause recurrent disease episodes as a result of direct effects of the virus and/or the host response. Chronic articular manifestations have been associated with the human retroviruses human immunodeficiency virus-1 (HIV-1)[11] and human T-cell lymphotropic virus-I (HTLV-1) (See chapters 123 and124).[12]

VIRAL INFECTIONS OFTEN ASSOCIATED WITH ARTHRITIS

PARVOVIRUSES

The parvoviruses are one of the three genera of the family Parvoviridae, small single-stranded DNA viruses.[13] Although first identified in human sera in only 1975,[14] they represent one of the most frequent causes of virus-induced arthritis in humans. Consistent with their name, they have a diameter of only 23 nm.[14] Two parvoviruses have been described in humans. The human parvovirus designated B19 was first detected in the serum of asymptomatic blood donors.[14] The only identified cell type supporting B19 replication in vitro is the

TABLE 119–3. POTENTIAL MECHANISMS OF VIRUS-INITIATED RHEUMATIC DISEASE

Direct effect of viral infection
- Lysis of infected cells with resultant tissue damage
- Loss of specialized cell functions resulting from nonlytic infection

Immunologically mediated tissue damage from normal immune responses
- Lysis of infected cells—cytotoxic T cells, natural killer cells, or antibody and complement
- Cytokine-mediated tissue damage
- Deposition of immune complexes consisting of viral antigens and antibody

Alteration of normal host immune response
- Virus-induced immune suppression
- Autoantibody formation
  - Neoantigen induction by viral infection
  - Molecular mimicry with formation of cross-reactive antibodies
  - Polyclonal B-cell stimulation
  - Anti-idiotype antibody generation

TABLE 119–4. CLINICAL SYNDROMES ASSOCIATED WITH PARVOVIRUS B19 INFECTION

Febrile illness
Erythema infectiosum (fifth disease)
Aplastic crisis in patients with hemoglobinopathy or hemolytic anemia
Intrauterine infection with spontaneous abortion or stillbirth
Arthritis
Vasculitis

erythroid progenitor. A second parvovirus-like agent, designated RA-1, was demonstrated in the synovium of a patient with rheumatoid arthritis (RA) but not in controls with osteoarthritis (OA).[15] The particles found were immunologically distinct from B19,[16] but little else is known about this agent.

Clinical Disease. The role of parvovirus in human disease has been summarized.[13,17,18] B19 infection usually causes acute disease, but it may persist in immunocompromised patients.[19] About 70% of B19 infections occurs in children 5 to 15 years of age.[17] Boys and girls are affected equally, while in adults, clinically evident disease occurs more often in women. Most infections occur in late winter or spring; respiratory spread is presumed, but cases following transfusion of infected blood products have been reported. Previous infection with B19, as demonstrated by the presence of viral-specific IgG antibodies, is present in 30 to 60% of adults.[17] B19 can cause several clinical illnesses (Table 119–4),[13,17,18] the most common of which is erythema infectiosum (EI).

Erythema Infectiosum. Erythema infectiosum, or "fifth disease," is usually a mild acute childhood disease. A rash or a prodrome of 1 to 4 days including headache, coryza, and low-grade fever may be the presenting feature.[17,20,21] The characteristic rash may be accompanied by gastrointestinal (GI) symptoms, cough, and/or conjunctivitis. The classic "slapped cheek" rash is brightly erythematous on the malar eminences, sparing the bridge of the nose. On the extremities and trunk, a maculopapular lacy rash may appear. The rashes tend to come and go, being enhanced by exercise, bathing, or exposure to sunlight. Pruritus is common in adults but not in children. The rash usually fades within 10 days but may persist or recur for weeks.[20] An erythematous or macular enanthem may occur. Arthralgias occur in about 7% of children with EI.

In adults, the illness is similar but has two major differences: (1) Rash is less frequent, and when present, it does not look like a "slapped cheek," and (2) joint manifestations are more frequent. A week after infection, viremia and respiratory shedding of virus occur, accompanied by a mild illness with fever, malaise, myalgia, and pruritus.[22] A second phase of illness begins 17 to 18 days after infection, including arthralgia and rash.

Joint Symptoms. The features of parvovirus B19-associated arthritis are summarized in Table 119–5. Arthralgia and arthritis occur in up to 80% of adults with EI.[20,21,23] The association of B19 infection with arthritis has become clear from studies of arthritis following community-based[24,25] and hospital-based[26] epidemics, and clinical suspicion of individual cases of arthritis of recent onset.[1,2,27] The frequency of adult infection with B19 and subsequent joint involvement has been well documented.[25] Serologic evidence of recent B19 infection was found in 12% of adult contacts of schoolchildren after a school-based outbreak of EI; 70% of exposed adults had pre-existing immunity to B19. Of the newly infected adults, 26% remained asymptomatic, while 74% became ill with manifestations including rash, flulike illness, GI symptoms, and acute arthritis. Arthritis developed in 48%, including 30% of infected men and 59% of infected women. Based on these figures, B19 arthritis must be presumed to be a common cause of arthritis in adults. It is estimated that 20 to 30% of the population seroconvert to B19 as adults and that

TABLE 119–5. CLINICAL FEATURES OF PARVOVIRUS B19-ASSOCIATED ARTHRITIS

Arthralgia: 7% children, 80% adults
Arthritis: 5% children, 50% adults
Female predominance in adult disease
Biphasic illness
- Fever, malaise, myalgia, headache, coryza—1 week after infection
- Rash arthritis—17–18 days after infection

Symmetric, polyarticular; small joints of hands and knees most often affected
Arthritis usually improves in 2 weeks, arthralgias in 4 weeks
Occasional patients with persistent or recurrent arthritis but no destructive changes
Synovial fluid mildly inflammatory

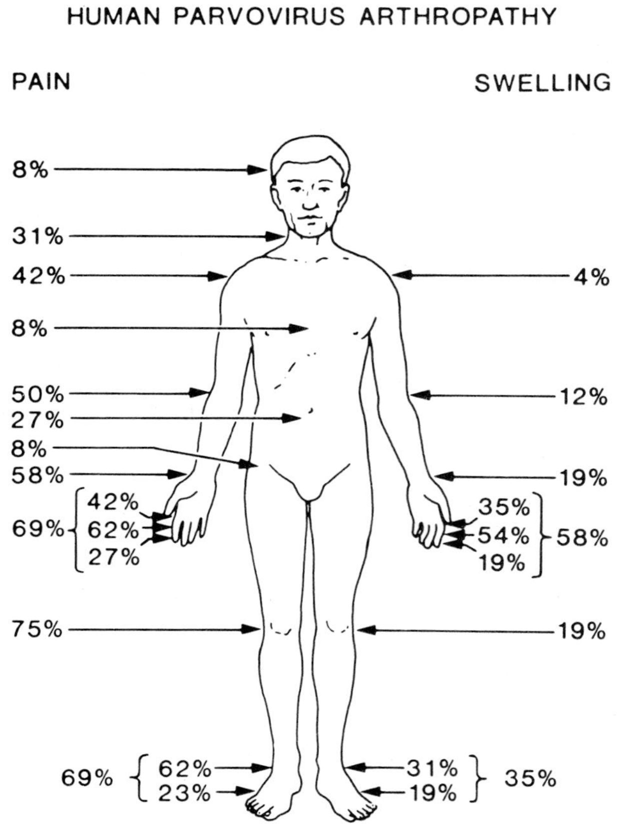

FIGURE 119–1. Pattern of joint involvement and swelling in adults with acute parvovirus B19 infection. (From Smith, C.A., Woolf, A.D., and Lenci, M.: Parvoviruses: Infections and arthropathies. Rheum. Dis. Clin. North Am., *13*:249, 1987.)

up to 60% of infected women develop arthritis, which persists in up to 10%.

The typical pattern of joint involvement induced by B19 is an acute onset, symmetric polyarticular arthritis,[1,2,24–27] as depicted in Fig. 119–1. Small joints of the hands and the knees are the most frequently involved and initially involved joints. Within a few days, the wrist, ankle, feet, elbow, shoulder, and hip joints may become symptomatic. Spinal joint involvement also has been described.[1,27] Pain is the most frequent complaint, but it is usually mild. Joint swelling is often present, and morning stiffness may occur.[2,25] Joint involvement may precede the rash of EI but usually follows it by 1 to 6 days. Many adults with B19 infection do not develop rash, and even if they do, it is often subtle. Lymphadenopathy is present in about one half of patients.[2,26,27] Adults, predominantly women, of any age can be affected. Arthritis usually improves within 2 weeks, arthralgias within 4 weeks, but some patients have persistent symptoms for months or years. Recurrence of rash and/or arthritis and complaints of lethargy are common for protracted periods. Even with persistent symptoms, no case with joint tissue destruction or functional loss has been reported. The differential diagnosis includes rubella arthritis, RA, and Lyme disease.

Nonsteroidal anti-inflammatory drugs (NSAIDs) are effective for most patients, although corticosteroids were ineffective in a patient with chronic symptoms.[2]

Laboratory Tests. The diagnosis is made by demonstration of serum IgM antibodies to B19. These are present by the time arthritis develops. Titers begin to fall 1 to 2 months after the onset of illness and are undetectable by 2 to 3 months.[17]

Anemia may be present as a result of a temporary arrest of hematopoesis. This effect is minimal in normal persons, but severe aplastic crises may develop in patients with hemolytic anemia or hemoglobinopathy. Leukopenia has been reported. The erythrocyte sedimentation rate (ESR) is usually normal but may be elevated. Rheumatoid factor tests may be positive during acute arthritis,[1,27] returning to normal on followup.[28] Antinuclear antibodies[27] as well as antibodies to single-stranded and double-stranded DNA and cytotoxic IgM antilymphocyte antibodies[29] have been found. Circulating immune complexes have been identified in patients with B19-associated acute arthritis[1] but have not been looked for during the time of chronic joint symptoms. Studies of human leukocyte antigen (HLA) associations with B19 arthritis showed an increased incidence of HLA-DR4 in one series[30] and a decreased incidence of HLA-DR1 in another.[25]

Synovial fluids are moderately inflammatory, with leukocyte counts ranging from 3,400 to 12,000/mm^3;[31–33] differential leukocyte counts varied in the few reports of joint fluid examination. Synovial biopsy from a patient with arthritis of 2 weeks' duration showed normal synovial cells with increased vascularity and edema; another biopsy from a patient with joint symptoms of 23 months' duration was normal.[1]

Pathogenesis. The mechanism of arthritis following B19 infection is not clear. Because of the presence of circulating immune complexes and low levels of serum C4 demonstrated in some patients with B19-associated arthritis,[1] immunologic mechanisms have been implicated. A direct effect of the virus also has been considered. Infectious virus has not been recovered from either synovium or synovial fluid, but B19 DNA has been detected using molecular hybridization techniques in synovial fluid[32] and synovial fluid cells.[33] As B19 arthritis develops after viremia has waned,[22] the presence of viral genome in joints most likely represents local persistence not contamination.

HEPATITIS B VIRUS

Hepatitis B virus (HBV) is the prototype hepadnavirus.[34] Its genome is mostly double-stranded, circular DNA. The virion is known as the *Dane particle.* Important antigenic determinants are the surface antigen (HBsAg) on the outer envelope, the core antigen (HBcAg) on the inner core or nucleocapsid, and the e

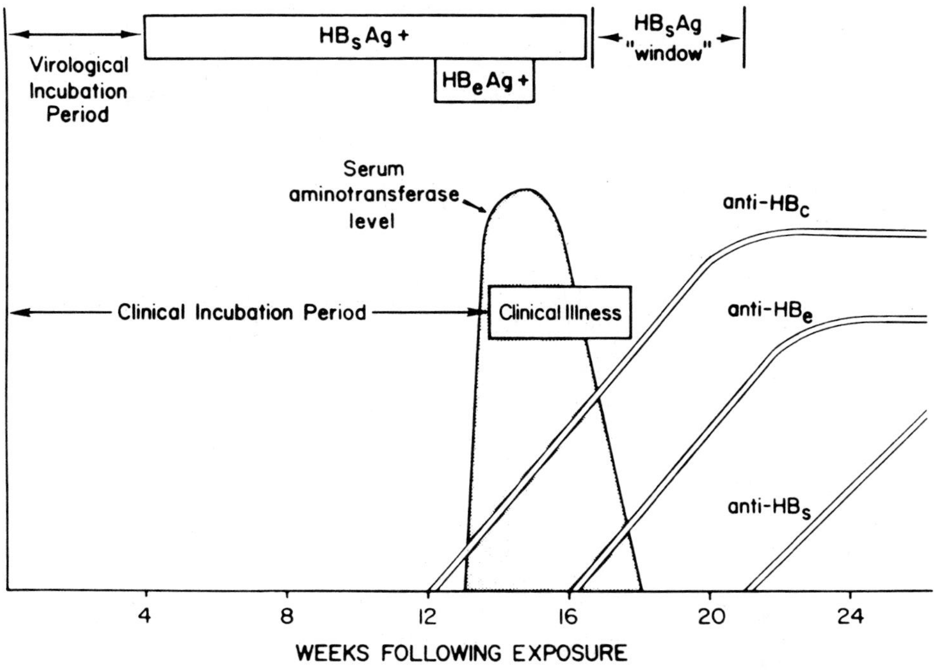

FIGURE 119–2. Time course of appearance of specific antigens and antibodies following hepatitis B virus infection. (From Lutwick, L.I.: Hepatitis B virus. *In* Textbook of Human Virology. Edited by R.B. Belshe. Littleton, MA, PSG Publishing Co., 1984, pp. 729–756.)

antigen (HBeAg), which is derived from the viral core. The time of appearance of each antigen and their antibodies during infection is depicted in Fig. 119–2.

Clinical Infection. The incubation period of HBV ranges from 60 to 180 days.[35] Early symptoms of infection include malaise and fatigue, with or without mild GI distress or fever. Serum sickness-like symptoms of arthralgia or arthritis and rash occur often, typically subsiding as jaundice and symptoms of anorexia, nausea, vomiting, and right upper quadrant abdominal pain develop, usually during the first week (Fig. 119–3). Approximately 50% of patients remain anicteric. Most patients improve within 4 weeks with normalization of liver function tests and clearance of HBsAg from the blood.

Rheumatic Syndromes. HBV infection has been associated with several rheumatic syndromes.[36] The most common is the serum sickness-like arthritis–dermatitis syndrome, occurring during the prodromal phase of the illness. HBV infection may also be associated with polyarteritis nodosa,[37,38] which occurs in about 1% of patients with HBsAg persistence[39] or with essential mixed cryoglobulinemia.[40] Other rheumatic syndromes sporadically reported to occur coincidentally with HBV infection include dermatomyositis and polymyositis, Raynaud's phenomenon, and RA.[36]

Arthritis. The features of HBV-associated arthritis are summarized in Table 119–6. Although the occurrence of arthritis and hives as prodromal features of jaundice was reported by Michael Graves in the nineteenth century, only since the 1970s has the association been recognized formally.[38,41–46] Joint symptoms typically begin abruptly, 1 day to 12 weeks after the onset of prodromal symptoms of malaise, sore throat, anorexia, and nausea.[38] Rash, which may be maculopapular or urticarial, frequently accompanies joint manifestations, although joint or skin involvement may occur alone.[47] Arthralgia occurs in about 25% of patients[46,48] and is usually symmetric and generalized but may be localized to specific small or large joints. Frank arthritis develops in approximately 10% of patients,[36,46,49] occasionally migratory but more often fixed, symmetric, and often polyarticular, involving, in order of frequency, small joints of the hands, knees, ankles, shoulders, and elbows.[36,49] Morning stiffness may be present. Symptoms usually decline as jaundice develops but may continue for several weeks or even months in some patients. Persistence of arthritis has been reported with development of chronic hepatitis,[43] but no joint deformity has ever been reported. Arthritis in anicteric hepatitis may mimic early RA or other systemic rheumatic disease.[47,50] Treatment does not shorten the duration of arthritis, but improvement has been reported with salicylates.[38]

Other causes of viral hepatitis, including hepatitis A virus (see following discussion), and non-A, non-B hepatitis, can be associated with joint symptoms at least as frequently as HBV.[51]

Laboratory Findings. The diagnosis is made by testing for HBV antigens or antibody. Generally, HBsAg can be detected in the serum, without anti-HBsAg, when arthritis is present (Fig. 119–2), although several samples may have to be tested. The titers of HBsAg fall as jaundice begins. Transaminases are often abnormal while joint symptoms are present.

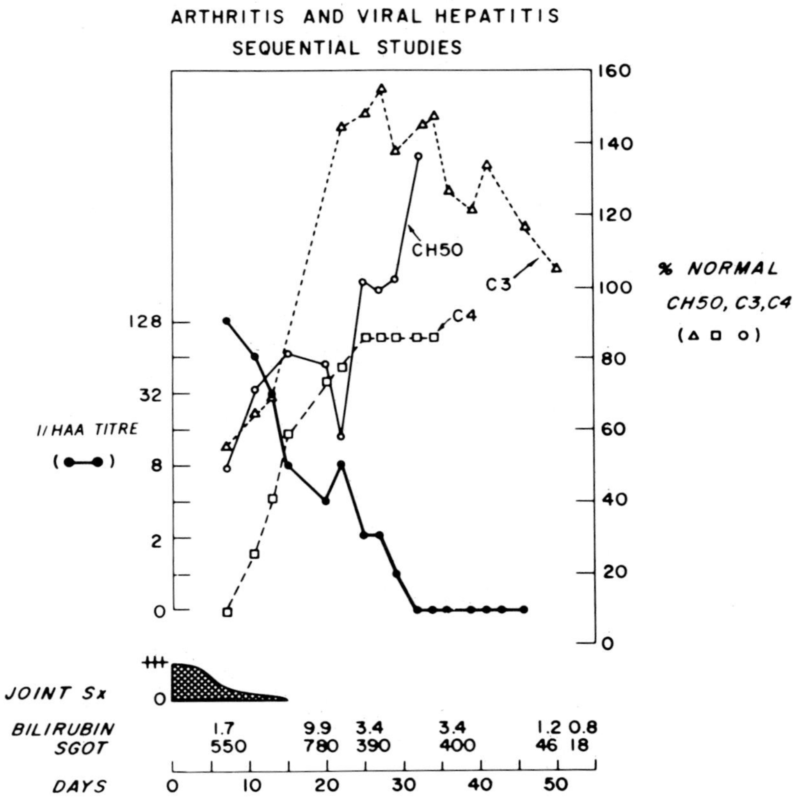

FIGURE 119–3. Changes in CH_{50}, C3, and C4 serum concentrations and hepatitis B surface antigen (HBsAg) (HAA) titers referred to as hepatitis associated antigen, HAA during the course of hepatitis B virus-associated arthritis preceding hepatitis. HBsAg is present, and complement components are depressed when the joints are active. The arthritis resolves as clinical hepatitis becomes apparent. (From Alpert, E., Schur, P.H., and Isselbacher, K.J.: Sequential changes of serum complement in HAA related arthritis. N. Engl. J. Med., *287*:103, 1972.)

TABLE 119–6. CLINICAL FEATURES OF HEPATITIS B ARTHRITIS

Arthralgias in about 25%; arthritis in 10%
Slight male predominance (male/female = 1.5:1)
Arthritis onset sudden
Morning stiffness in some patients
Symmetric polyarticular arthritis; most frequently involving small joints of hands, knees, and ankles
Rash in 40%
Erythematous, pruritic maculopapular, or urticarial
Systemic symptoms
Anorexia, and malaise in most, fever in 50%
Arthritis and dermatitis last 2–6 weeks; resolve with onset of jaundice; may persist or recur for weeks to months in a few patients
HBsAg is positive and liver function tests are abnormal in most patients at the time of arthritis
Synovial fluid inflammatory or noninflammatory, with predominance of either mononuclear cells or neutrophils

HBsAg = hepatitis B surface antigen.

Cryoproteins representing immune complexes are found frequently in serum from patients with HBV infection, with or without arthritis.[52,53] Complement levels may be depressed,[38] which is due to activation of the classic or alternate pathways,[52,54] but this is not invariable.[45] C4 and CH50 are most often depressed,[38,41,43,44,47,55]

Synovial fluid is usually inflammatory.[38,41,42,45] Reported cell counts ranged from 145 to 90,000/mm^3; polymorphonuclear cells usually predominate. Synovial fluid has been found to contain HBsAg and depressed hemolytic complement levels in some patients.[38,41,42,46] Synovial biopsy in two patients showed mild synovial hyperplasia and vascular damage but little inflammation.[55]

Pathogenesis. Strong evidence supports the role of immune complex deposition in the pathogensis of HBV-associated arthritis. Arthritis and dermatitis occur as prodromal features when the HBsAg is in excess of anti-HBsAg. Immune complexes are found in the serum of patients with HBV infection.[52,53] Hemolytic complement levels may be depressed in both serum and synovial fluid and return to normal as arthritis subsides or remain normal in patients with acute hepatitis without arthritis.[44] Serum cryoproteins contain HBsAg, anti-HBsAb, and complement.[52,53] Cryoproteins have been found in HBV-infected patients without arthritis, but unlike those from patients with arthritis, these do not contain complement. The IgG isotypes of patients with HBV arthritis are predominantly complement-fixing IgG1 and IgG3. HBsAg, immunoglobulin, and complement have been identified in synovium.[55]

A direct cytopathic effect of HBV in synovium has also been suggested by the finding of HBsAg in synovium and particles consistent with HBsAg within vessels, synovial lining cells, and other deep synovial cells.[55] Necrosis of many of these cells containing virus-like particles, despite the lack of inflammatory cells in synovium, supports the notion of a direct viral cytopathic effect. The occurrence of arthritis in a surgical team exposed at surgery to infected blood suggests the occurrence of arthritogenic strains of virus.[45]

RUBELLA VIRUS

Rubella virus is a member of the Togaviridae family and the only member of the genus Rubrivirus.[56,57] It is a single-stranded positive-sense RNA virus, closely related to the Alphaviruses (see following discussion) but without the need of an insect vector.

Traditionally, rubella infects children 5 to 9 years of age.[56–58] Since the introduction of rubella vaccination in the United States in 1969, the usual age at infection has risen; small outbreaks of rubella continue to occur in groups of susceptible adults.[58] Three live, attenuated vaccine strains of rubella were introduced initially: HPV77-DK12, grown in dog kidney cells; HPV77-DE5, grown in duck embryo cells; and the Cendehill strain.[59] The strain available currently in the United States is another live, attenuated strain, RA27/3.

Clinical Disease. Rubella, or "German measles," is typically a mild, self-limited disease characterized by constitutional symptoms, rash, and lymphadenopathy.[56,57,60] Infection causes subclinical illness in 25 to 50%. The incubation period averages 16 to 18 days, with a range of 12 to 23 days. Patient age is the major factor determining severity of illness following rubella virus infection. Congenital rubella can cause a variety of problems ranging from premature delivery to congenital deformities or fetal death. Postnatally acquired rubella is usually a mild disease, causing more symptoms in adults than children.

A prodrome is usually not noticed in children, but in adolescents and adults, malaise, fever, and anorexia may be present for several days. The characteristic rash begins on the face and neck and spreads rapidly to the trunk and extremities within 1 to 2 days. The rash, which is maculopapular, pale pink to red in color, lasts 3 to 5 days. Pruritus may be present, and skin may desquamate. Low-grade fever occurs in about half of cases, usually beginning with the rash and lasting 1 day. Lymphadenopathy usually involves the posterior auricular, posterior cervical, and suboccipital nodes; splenomegaly may occur. Patients are most contagious when the rash is erupting but may shed virus from 10 days before to 15 days after the rash begins.[57]

Rheumatic Manifestations. The features of rubella associated arthritis are summarized in Table 119-7. Arthritis and arthralgias have been reported in about a third of patients with natural rubella infection.[61–63] Joint involvement occurs more frequently in adults than in children, although arthritis has been reported in a 14-month-old child.[64] The female/male ratio is about 5:1.[65–67] Joint symptoms usually begin suddenly, 2 to 3 days after the onset of rash, but may occur from 6 days before to a week after the rash. Pain is the most common symptom, but swelling, stiffness, and other signs of inflammation are frequent. Small joints of the fingers and the knees are most often involved, followed by wrists, elbows, ankles, hip, and toes. Joint manifestations usually last about 7 days (range 1 to 28 days), with complete resolution, but occasional patients have intermittent arthralgias for a year or more.[68,69] Tenosynovitis,[70] carpal tunnel syndrome,[65,71–73] and brachial neuritis[74–76] have also been reported as complications of rubella infection. Treatment is symptomatic; aspirin may provide relief;[73,77,78] corticosteroids have been used for more severe cases.[72,77]

TABLE 119–7. CLINICAL FEATURES OF RUBELLA VIRUS ARTHRITIS

Arthralgias in a third following natural infection, an eighth following vaccination with RA27/3
Arthritis more common in adults than children
Female predominance (female/male ratio about 5:1)
Sudden onset 2–3 days after rash
Involvement of small joints of hands, knees, wrists, elbows, ankles, hips, toes; knees most common after vaccination
Arthritis usually lasts about 1 week; some patients have chronic symptoms
Neuropathic syndromes
Synovial fluid inflammatory, usually with mononuclear cell predominance
Virus frequently recovered from peripheral blood and synovial fluid

Rheumatic Manifestations After Rubella Vaccination. As the incidence of natural rubella infection has fallen, the importance of rubella vaccination as a cause of joint symptoms has risen. RA27/3 is the only rubella vaccine strain available in the United States. It induces antibody titers that are higher and similar to those following natural infection, including the presence of secretory antibody.[79] This enhanced immunogenicity is not associated with an increased frequency of side effects. The frequency of reactions after RA27/3, HPV77-DE5, and Cendehill are similar, whereas HPV77-DK12 had a higher frequency of side effects, particularly involving joints.[59] A mild rubella-like illness occurs 10 to 20 days after vaccination in about 10 to 15% of recipients of rubella vaccination.[58] As with natural rubella, viremia occurs after immunization.

Joint manifestations were recognized shortly after the introduction of rubella vaccination.[77,78,80–82] HPV77-DK12 was removed early because of its high frequency of joint manifestations, especially in children.[78,83–86] Arthralgias or arthritis occur in women after vaccination with the following frequencies: HPV77-DK12 49%, HPV77-DE5 30%, Cendehill 9%, and RA27/3 14%.[87] Joint manifestations are less frequent in children than in adolescents or adults.[82,88] In adults, females are preferentially affected, while among children, boys are affected as often as girls.[78] Joint manifestations generally begin 8 to 21 days after vaccination and last 3 to 5 days, with a range of 1 to 46 days. Knees are affected more often than following natural infection. Small joints of the hands are also frequently involved, followed by wrists, elbows, neck, ankles, shoulders, hips, and toes.

Chronic or recurrent arthropathy has been recognized infrequently, occurring in 1 to 4% of vaccinees.[69,89–96] Chronic symptoms occurred most often after vaccination with HPV77-DK12.[90,91] In children, recurrent attacks of arthritis most often involve the knee, occurring at intervals of 1 to 3 months and lasting 1 to 7 days, with complete clearing between attacks.[90,91] The intervals between attacks gradually increase and then cease. A potential relationship of rubella virus with juvenile RA (JRA) has been suggested, because virus has been recovered from peripheral blood and synovial fluid mononuclear cells from children with JRA.[93] In adults, continuous or recurrent monoarticular, oligoarticular, or polyarticular arthralgia or arthritis may develop.[69,94–96]

Two neuropathic syndromes also have been described after rubella vaccination.[97] Carpal tunnel syndrome may appear 10 to 62 days after vaccination and last an average of 14 days (range, 2 to 35 days).[97] The other syndrome is *knee pain and a crouching gait* referred to as the *"catcher's crouch."*[97,98] This syndrome occurs with an estimated incidence of 2.2/1000 following vaccination with HPV77-DK12 and 0.1/1,000 with HPV77-DE5. It begins 29 to 70 days after vaccination and lasts 6.5 days (range, 2 to 14 days).[97] The cause of the catcher's crouch has been attributed to neuropathy[98] or to arthropathy.[92] Episodic recurrence of catcher's crouch may occur.[99] Chronic recurrent neuropathy associated with arthritis has been reported in adults as well.[95]

Laboratory Findings. The diagnosis is made serologically with demonstration of elevated titers of rubella antibody, usually by hemagglutination inhibition or enzyme-linked immunosorbent assay (ELISA). Nonserologic laboratory tests are generally not helpful. The white blood cell (WBC) count may be low or normal.[72,73] ESRs have ranged from 1[68] to 53.[73] Rheumatoid factor tests have been positive in about 22% of patients, with individual series ranging from 0 to 90% positive.[68,72,73,93,100,101] Antinuclear antibody tests have been positive in a few patients.[93,94] Moderately inflammatory synovial fluid is usually present,[72,73,94,102] with total leukocyte counts ranging from 1,900 to 60,000/mm^3. Typically, mononuclear cells predominate, but occasional fluids contain mostly neutrophils. Synovial biopsies after rubella virus infection[73,102] or vaccination[92,94] have shown synovial cell hypertrophy and hyperplasia, lymphocytic (plasma cells in some cases[94]) infiltration, and increased vascularity.

Pathogenesis. Rubella virus has been isolated frequently from synovial fluid after natural infection from patients with either acute[64,102] or chronic arthritis[103,104] and after vaccination from patients with acute[77] or chronic arthritis.[89,93] Rubella virus can be cultivated in synovial cells in vitro.[105] Thus, arthritis may result from infection of synovial cells with direct tissue damage. Rubella virus has also been recovered from peripheral blood lymphocytes from patients with chronic rubella-associated arthritis[69,93,95,106] and from patients previously diagnosed as having RA or JRA.[93,94,103] The mechanism by which viral persistence in lymphocytes might induce acute or chronic arthritis remains unclear.

Immune complexes can be found in serum after natural infection[107,108] or vaccination.[108,109] When studied sequentially, complexes peak within 3 weeks of the rash,[107] at a time when joint manifestations are common. Patients without joint manifestations, however, have immune complexes just as often and at similar levels as those of patients with arthritis.[108,109]

No association with any particular HLA antigen has been detected.[93,110]

ALPHAVIRUSES

Several athropod-borne viruses (arboviruses) can cause arthritis, including Ross River, chikungunya, O'nyong-nyong, Mayaro, Sindbis, and Ockelbo viruses. These agents are classified as members of the α-virus genus of the family Togaviridae.[111,112] All are single-stranded, positive-sense RNA viruses.[111] Although their geographic distributions and specific vectors differ (Table 119–8), they are morphologically and antigenically very similar, are all spread by mosquitoes, and cause nearly identical diseases in humans characterized by fever, arthritis, and rash.[113]

ROSS RIVER VIRUS

Epidemic polyarthritis, caused by Ross River virus (RRV), is the best characterized and understood of the arthropod-borne viral illnesses that cause arthritis. Following the initial description of epidemic polyarthritis by Nimmo in 1928, descriptions of similar epidemics appeared from military installations in Australia and nearby islands during World War II.[114,115] The disease occurs in endemic[116] as well as epidemic fashion in Australia and has spread to other Pacific islands.[117,118] Approximately 600 cases of epidemic polyarthritis occur annually in Queensland, Australia, and it is presumed from serologic data that 50 to 100 times as many subclinical infections occur.[119]

Clinical Disease. Joint involvement is one of the cardinal manifestations of RRV infection,[114–116,120,121] resulting in its description as epidemic polyarthritis.[115] Clinical disease is more common in adults than children, with most cases occurring between ages 20 and 40.[116,122] The female/male ratio is about 1.6:1.[123] The incubation time may be as short as 3 days but is usually 7 to 11 days.[120,124] Constitutional symptoms occur in most patients, notably including fatigue, which may persist after other symptoms have improved.[125] Low-grade fever, myalgias, headache, nausea, vomiting, diarrhea, and lymphadenopathy may

TABLE 119–8. COMPARISON OF ALPHAVIRUSES CAUSING ARTHRITIS

VIRUS	MOSQUITO VECTOR	RESERVOIR	GEOGRAPHIC DISTRIBUTION
ROSS RIVER	Aedes vigilax Other Aedes species Culex annulirostris Mansonia	Mammals	Australia, South Pacific
CHIKUNGUNYA	Aedes aegypti Aedes africanus Aedes furcifer	Monkeys Human	Sub-Saharan Africa, India, Southeast Asia
O'NYONG-NYONG	Anopheles funestus Anopheles gambiae	?	East Africa
MAYARO	Haemogogus Culex spp. Mansonia Psorophora	Mammals	South America, Carribean
SINDBIS	Culex univittatus Culex annulirostris Culex tritaeniorhynchus	Mammals, birds	Africa, Asia, Australia, Middle East
OCKELBO	Aedes communis Culiseta spp.	?	Northern Europe

(Data from Craven, R.B.,[112] and Tesh, R.B.[113])

occur.[114–116,121,125] Rash is frequently, but not invariably, present, occurring from 11 days before to 15 days after the onset of arthritis.[115,116,120,121,125] The rash may be subtle. An erythematous maculopapular eruption on the limbs and trunk that may also involve the palms, soles, fingers, and face is usual. Nodules, vesicles, and purpura occur less frequently. Enanthems are unusual. The rash usually resolves in 1 to 10 days, sometimes leaving light-brown staining and desquamation.

Arthritis. Arthralgias are most common but arthritis is also seen, most often beginning acutely.[114–116,120,121] Symmetric involvement, typically involving two or more joints, is usual. The small joints of the hands and feet, ankles, wrists, and knees are most often involved. Tendon involvement is frequent, involving Achilles tendonitis, plantar fasciitis, epicondylitis, or patellar tendonitis. Morning stiffness is present in some patients. Transient paresthesias involving the hands, similar to carpal tunnel syndrome, or feet have been reported, similar to those observed in rubella.[114–116,121] Improvement is generally within 1 to 2 weeks,[114,115] but persistent symptoms may last for months.[115,116,121,125] Despite this, no destructive changes or deformity have been reported. Treatment with analgesics or NSAIDs is usually successful.[115,121,123] Intra-articular steroids have been used.[119]

Laboratory Findings. The diagnosis is made by demonstrating elevated IgM antibody to RRV by hemagglutination inhibition or ELISA.[125] Routine laboratory testing is generally unrewarding in establishing the diagnosis. The complete blood cell count (CBC) is usually normal, but atypical lymphocytes may be seen. The ESR is frequently elevated during the first few weeks but may be normal. Synovial fluids are highly viscous, with cell counts ranging from 1,500 to 14,200/mm^3.[126–128] The cells are virtually all mononuclear; highly vacuolated macrophages are frequent, and mitotic figures are seen occasionally. Synovial biopsy has been reported from one patient 21 days after the onset of symptoms. A hyperemic synovium with mononuclear cell infiltration, synovial cell hyperplasia, and fibrin deposition was noted.[128]

Pathogenesis. The mechanism by which RRV causes arthritis is unclear. Viral antigens have been detected in synovial fluid macrophages by immunofluorescence.[127] RRV has not been cultured from joint tissue or fluid,[126–128] but it can be found in serum[117,118,129] and can infect primary synovial cell cultures in vitro.[130] Firm evidence for the pathogenetic mechanism is equally lacking. Immune complexes and alterations of serum or synovial fluid complement have not been reported.[125–127] Biopsies of skin lesions in RRV infection showed no immunoglobulin or complement deposition; perivascular mononuclear cells, predominantly CD8-positive T cells and a few macrophages, were found.[131] RRV antigen was identified in skin, but the virus could not be grown. Natural killer cell activity was found to be decreased during the early stages of illness, but the significance of this is unclear.[132] An increased frequency of the major histocompatibility complex (MHC) class II antigen DR7 was found in one study of patients with epidemic polyarthritis.[133]

CHIKUNGUNYA VIRUS

The name *chikungunya* comes from a word meaning "that which binds up," used to describe the sudden onset of joint pain present in an epidemic or a new febrile illness in Tanzania in 1952.[134] The epidemic was attributed to a dengue-like disease because of its abrupt onset and clinical features of fever, arthralgia, and rash.[134–136] The explosive onset and severity of the joint symptoms, however, were unlike dengue. During this epidemic, a new virus was isolated from mosquitoes and the serum of infected patients.[136] Outbreaks of chikungunya have been reported from other areas of Africa,[137,138] India,[139,140] and Southeast Asia.[141,142]

Clinical Features. As in epidemic polyarthritis caused by RRV, arthritis is the key clinical feature of chikungunya.[134,137–142] The incubation period of chikungunya is from 1 to 6 days.[112] Usually, there is no prodrome, and the illness begins abruptly with intense joint pain involving one or more joints that can incapacitate patients within minutes.[134] Severe headache, myalgia, backache, malaise, facial flushing, conjunctivitis, pharyngitis, GI symptoms, and fever often follow. The fever is usually biphasic, with an initial temperature up to 105°F for 1 to 6 days, an afebrile period of 1 to 3 days, and a second febrile period with temperatures up to 101°F. Lymphadenopathy may be present.[139,141] Rash, which is present in 60 to 80% of patients, usually begins several days after the joints symptoms but may occur before arthritis.[134,141,142] It is usually macular or maculopapular, located on the trunk or extensor surfaces of the limbs. Petechiae have been observed in a few cases.[139,141]

Arthritis. Joint involvement is less frequent in children than adults.[137,139,140] Males and females are equally affected. Arthralgia associated with morning stiffness occurs in most patients, usually involving all joints during the acute illness. Frank arthritis has been reported in 3[134] to 70%.[141] Arthritis most often involves the small joints of the hands, wrists, feet, and ankles, but larger joints may be involved as well.[134,138,139,141] Joint symptoms are generally severe,[134] but milder symptoms have been reported.[140,141]

Joint involvement of chikungunya often subsides within a week, but chronic migratory joint pain can last for months,[134,138,139] simulating RA.[141] Persistent joint pain and stiffness, with or without swelling, was reported by 5.6% of patients with serologically proven chikungunya.[143] Erosive arthritis following chikungunya infection has been reported rarely.[138,144] Treatment usually consists of rest and analgesics including morphine. Chloroquine was useful for chronic joint symptoms in an open-label study.[145]

Laboratory Studies. The diagnosis is made by viral isolation or serologic testing. Patients with chikungunya develop hemagglutination-inhibiting (HI), complement-fixing, and neutralizing (NT) antibodies, with presence HI and NT antibodies occurring 2 weeks after the onset of illness.[112] Leukopenia or leukocytosis may be present.[134,141] The ESR is usually normal or moderately elevated[141] but has been as high as 94 mm/hour.[139] Serum complement levels are normal, and an occasional patient may have a positive rheumatoid factor.[138] There have been no reports of synovial fluid findings or isolation of chikungunya virus from joint fluid.

O'NYONG-NYONG VIRUS

O'nyong-nyong has many similarities to chikungunya. It was first characterized during an epidemic of a dengue-like illness in Africa in 1959 with manifestations of fever, arthritis, and rash.[146,147] The name *O'nyong-nyong* is derived from an Acholi tribe description of the illness and means "joint-breaker."[112] O'nyong-nyong occurs in sporadic epidemics. During the epidemic of 1959 to 1962, attack rates ranged over 70% in some villages, affecting all age groups.[147] Females were affected more commonly than males.

Clinical Disease. The incubation period of O'nyong-nyong is over 8 days.[147] The disease begins suddenly, with fever, rigor, and joint pain. The biphasic temperature curve of chikungunya is not present in O'nyong-nyong, and the peak temperature is lower, exceeding 101°F in only a third. Headache is present in virtually all patients, often with retro-orbital pain.[147] Other common systemic manifestations include backache, anorexia, conjunctivitis, pharyngitis, stomatitis, dry cough, and coryza. Occasional patients have edema of the eyelids, photophobia, or colicky abdominal pain. Cervical lymphadenopathy is frequent. Rash occurs in two thirds of patients, typically beginning on the fourth day, but ranging from a few hours to 1 week after the onset of joint symptoms. The rash is morbilliform, most frequently papular or maculopapular, with discrete lesions tending to become confluent; it is characteristically described as "irritating." It normally begins on the face and extends to trunk and extremities. Appearance of the rash is often followed by general improvement. Skin lesions usually last 4 to 7 days before fading. Joint pain is usually symmetric, often involving all joints.[147] In order of frequency, knees, elbows, wrists, fingers, and ankles are involved. The frequency of synovitis has not been reported. The average duration of disease is 5 days, but joint pain may often be protracted. Leukopenia is reported in 40% of patients.[147] The diagnosis of O'nyong-nyong has been made by viral isolation from blood but is usually made serologically.[148]

MAYARO VIRUS

Mayaro virus was isolated in Mayaro county, Trinidad,[149] but has also been found in Brazil, Bolivia, Colombia, and Surinam.[113] Like the syndromes caused by the other arthropod-borne alphaviruses, clinical illness is characterized by fever, arthritis, and rash.

The incubation time is less than 6 days.[150] Fever and arthralgia occur in all patients from whom virus is isolated from blood, whereas rash is present in two thirds. The clinical illness begins abruptly, with fever as high as 104°F, dizziness, chills, and headache. Other symptoms include nausea, vomiting, diarrhea, and mild photophobia. Inguinal lymphadenopathy is present in half the patients. Polyarticular arthralgia, frequently incapacitating, is prominent. Wrists, fingers, ankles, and toes are most often involved, although elbows and knees are also often reported. Joint swelling occurs in one fourth of patients. Joint symptoms usually improve within 7 days, but some patients have persistent arthralgias. Maculopapular rash, most prominent on the chest, back, arms, and legs, with face and hands less commonly affected, usually appears on the fifth day and lasts 3 days. Leukopenia with moderate lymphocytosis is present during the first week. Viremia lasts up to 4 days.

SINDBIS VIRUS

Sindbis virus was first isolated from mosquitoes in the Nile delta of Egypt in 1952.[112] The first description of illness associated with Sindbis virus was of a patient with headache, tenosynovitis of the hands and feet, rash, and low-grade fever.[151] A series of 11 patients with serologically proven Sindbis virus infection has been reported.[152] The incubation period is 3 to 6 days.[112] Illness usually begins abruptly with low-grade fever, lassitude, headache, joint pain, and generalized body ache. Pruritic skin rash involves the trunk, buttocks, and limbs primarily, lasting up to 10 days. Lesions are usually maculopapular, with some vesicles, occurring in crops. Small oral ulcers may be present. Lassitude and fatigue usually persist through convalescence. Muscle pain, joint tenderness, and pain in small joints of the hands and feet are present in all; larger joints may also be affected. Tendon pain in hands and Achilles tendons as well as paresthesias in the hands may occur. In most patients, symptoms disappear within 10 days, but fatigue, tendon pain, and arthritis may last several weeks. Blood counts are normal within the first 10 days.[152] The ESR is elevated in about half the cases.

OCKELBO VIRUS

Ockelbo disease[153] is a presumed viral illness that is strikingly similar to infections caused by other alphaviruses. Because of geographic proximity and clinical similarities, *Pogosta disease* in Finland,[154] and *Karelian fever* in the Soviet Union[155] are presumed to be the same disease. No virus has been isolated from patients, but viruses closely related to Sindbis virus have been isolated from mosquitoes in endemic areas.[155,156]

Ockelbo disease occurs annually in central Sweden, with a peak incidence in August.[153] Males and females are equally affected. Although patients of any age may be affected, the majority are between 30 and 60. Virtually all patients have joint symptoms and rash; low-grade fever is present in only a third. In nearly equal numbers of patients, joint symptoms precede, follow, or are concurrent with rash. The rash is maculopapular, with some vesicles. Joint pain commonly affects ankles, wrists, knees, and hips, with small joints of the hands, shoulders, elbows, and toes less frequently involved. Joint swelling is found in over half the patients. Articular symptoms subside within 2 weeks in half the patients, but persistence is common. Joint pain persisting for more than 24 months has been found in almost a third of patients with serologically confirmed Ockelbo disease.[157]

Immune complexes have been found in patients with Pogosta disease, but levels do not correlate the severity of arthritis, and no changes in serum complement levels have been found.[154] Thus, these complexes may not be pathogenic, but their presence may represent normal clearance of viral antigens.

MUMPS VIRUS

Mumps virus is a paramyxovirus, related to parainfluenza, measles, and Newcastle disease viruses.[158] Its genome is a single-stranded, negative-sense RNA. Mumps has a worldwide distribution and is endemic in urban areas. In the United States, the incidence of mumps infection rises during the winter and peaks in March and April.[158,159]

The peak incidence for mumps is between ages 5 and 9.[159] The incubation period is usually 16 to 18 days but ranges from 12 to 25 days.[158,159] Subclinical illness follows infection in about a third of patients. A prodrome including fever, anorexia, myalgia, and malaise usually precedes parotitis by 1 to 7 days. Parotitis typically lasts a week or less. Common complications of infection include meningitis, encephalitis, orchitis, oophoritis, or pancreatitis.

Arthritis is estimated to follow mumps infection in 0.44% of patients, based on observations during the epidemic in Paris in 1923 to 1924.[160,161] In contrast to the usual childhood age peak, mumps arthritis has a peak incidence in the third decade, with a range of 5 to 47 years. Arthritis affects men are more often than women, and there is a higher incidence of mumps orchitis among postpubertal men with arthritis (60 to 70%) than among mumps-infected men without arthritis.[160] Arthritis has not been reported as a complication of mumps vaccination.

Arthritis usually begins 1 to 3 weeks after the onset of parotitis and may be associated with low-grade fever.[160] Several cases of arthritis without clinical parotitis have been reported,[162,163] necessitating a high index of suspicion to seek the diagnosis serologically. Three patterns of joint involvement have been described with mumps: (1) arthralgias alone; (2) polyarticular arthritis, usually migratory, with knee effusions; and (3) monoarticular arthritis of a knee, hip, or ankle.[161] Cricoarytenoid joint involvement has been described.[164] Arthritis is usually self-limited, lasting a few days to 4 weeks, but persistent symptoms may last up to 6 months.[161] Treatment is symptomatic. Salicylates have been found to be ineffective,[160,161] but NSAIDs[162,165] and corticosteroids[163,166] provide relief.

The WBC often shows leukocytosis with a left shift.[160,161] The ESR is typically elevated and may be over 100 mm/hour.[161] Positive rheumatoid factor tests have been reported, which revert to negative after several months.[162,167] Synovial fluids, examined in two cases, were described as clear and yellow, with one noted to contain numerous polymorphonuclear leukocytes.[166] Assays for circulating immune complexes have been negative.[163] Mixed cultures of synovial cells and chondrocytes supported the replication of mumps virus and become persistently infected for 2 to 3 months,[168] but virus has not been recovered from synovial fluid or tissue from cases of mumps arthritis.

VIRAL INFECTIONS OCCASIONALLY ASSOCIATED WITH ARTHRITIS

ADENOVIRUSES

Adenoviruses, members of the Adenoviridae family containing a double-stranded DNA genome,[169] can have at least three different effects on cells: (1) lytic infection; (2) latent or chronic infection, usually of lymphoid cells; and (3) oncogenic transformation.[169] Adenoviruses are ubiquitous. Primary infection usually occurs in the first few years of life, causing respiratory illness. They are also associated with epidemics of penumonitis in military recruits.

Both acute and chronic arthritis have been associated with adenovirus infection. Acute arthritis was reported in a 19-year-old military recruit who developed arthralgias of hands and wrists, arthritis of the knees, respiratory symptoms, pharyngitis, nuchal rigidity, myalgia, and fevers resulting from adenovirus type 7.[170] Three women developed symmetric symptoms of large and small joints within 1 week of an adenoviral upper respiratory infection.[171] Improvement occurred after 1 to 4 weeks. Symptomatic treatment with aspirin was effective. Synovial fluid analyses have shown total leukocyte counts ranging from less than 4,000 to 24,800/mm^3, with a predominance of either polymorphonuclear or mononuclear leukocytes. A biopsy in one case showed an inflammatory synovitis with negative viral cultures.[170] Cryoglobulins and immune complexes containing adenovirus antigen were found in blood and synovial fluid.[171] Depressed levels of serum complement also have been noted.[170,171] These findings suggest immune complex involvement in the pathogenesis of arthritis.

Chronic arthritis that is due to adenovirus infection has also been described. Adenovirus type 7 was isolated from pericardial fluid of a child with fever, rash, pericarditis, and polyarthralgia.[3] She experienced recurrent episodes of oligoarticular arthritis over the next 2 years but no subsequent flares during 8 more years of followup. Persistence of adenovirus in joints was demonstrated in a patient with acquired hypo-γ-globulinemia who had seronegative, erosive RA.[172] Adenovirus type 1 was recovered from synovial tissue samples obtained 16 months apart. The humoral immune deficiency in this patient may have allowed wide viral dissemination with arthritis because of direct tissue damage.

Herpes Viruses

The Herpesviridae family includes over 80 members.[173] Four of the six viruses capable of infecting humans are rare causes of arthritis: cytomegalovirus, EBV, herpes simplex virus type 1, and varicella-zoster virus. The Herpesviridae are large (150 to 250 nm), enveloped viruses containing a double-stranded DNA genome. All members of this family can cause life-long latency in their hosts.

Cytomegalovirus

Cytomegalovirus (CMV) is a ubiquitous agent that infects most individuals at sometime during their life. The major clinical syndromes associated with CMV infection include cytomegalic inclusion disease in neonates, heterophile antibody–negative mononucleosis in healthy individuals, and pneumonitis in immunocompromised hosts.[174]

Acute arthralgias involving the knees, hips, ankles, sacroiliiac joints, and wrists may occur for 1 to 2 days in renal transplant patients with CMV infection.[175] Acute arthritis with CMV infection has been reported in a woman who developed hip and knee pain with fevers and chills 2 months after renal transplantation.[176] After 2 weeks of arthritis, the synovial fluid leukocyte count was 1,200/mm^3, with 93% neutrophils; CMV was isolated from the fluid. Two weeks later, synovial fluid leukocyte count was 37,000/mm^3, with a similar differential. A potential relationship of CMV to chronic arthritis was suggested by the isolation of CMV from synovial cells of a patient with a 17-year history of classic RA who had not received immunosuppressive agents.[177] It remains unclear if CMV was pathogenic in this case, however.

Epstein-Barr Virus

Infection with EBV is common, usually occurring in childhood as subclinical infection or in adolescents and young adults as heterophile antibody-positive infectious mononucleosis, an acute illness characterized by sore throat, fever, and lymphadenopathy.[178]

Arthralgias occur in about 2% and myalgias in 20% of patients with infectious mononucleosis.[178] Cases of acute arthritis have been reported rarely.[49,179–183] Joint symptoms appeared within a week of the onset of infectious mononucleosis symptoms; involvement was either polyarticular, of a single ankle or knee, or of both knees. Symptoms then abated in 8 days to 4.5 months. ESR ranged from 10 to 110 mm/hour. Inflammatory synovial fluids, with total leukocyte counts ranging from 18,000 to 80,000/mm^3, predominantly polymorphonuclear cells, have been recorded. Cryoglobulins were found in one patient,[182] and immune complex assays were negative in another.[183]

In a survey of patients with a recent onset of arthritis, four of nine with polyarticular arthritis had serologic evidence of a recent EBV infection.[4] Although one patients developed intermittent arthralgias, the others had no sequelae.

Herpes Simplex Virus Type 1

Herpes simplex virus (HSV) infections are extremely common.[184] HSV 1 is transmitted primarily by contact with oral secretions and causes primarily gingivostomatitis and labial infection, with cutaneous lesions in some patients. HSV 2 is transmitted by contact with genital secretions and causes genital infections. Arthritis has been associated with HSV 1 infection[176,185] including one patient who had undergone splenectomy.[186] Arthritis has involved a single knee or ankle in all patients, beginning 3 to 4 days after the onset of cutaneous or oral lesions. ESRs as high as 128 mm/hour have been reported.[176] Resolution of arthritis occurs within 2 weeks, although in one case, symptoms persisted for "several months,"[176] and this patient later developed a syndrome suggestive of systemic lupus erythematosus.

Varicella-zoster Virus

Varicella-zoster virus (VZV) causes two distinct diseases. Varicella, or chickenpox, is a common infection of childhood. Herpes simplex, or shingles, is due to reactivation of VZV that has been latent in dorsal root ganglia and most commonly occurs in elderly or immunocompromised persons. The incubation period for chickenpox is generally 14 to 15 days, with a range of 10 to 20 days,[187] and is recognized by its classic exanthem. Illness is usually benign; serious complications include encephalitis, cerebellar ataxia, meningitis, and pneumonitis.

In addition to aseptic arthritis, pyogenic arthritis has been reported in association with chickenpox[188–191] due to staphylococci or streptococci presumably originating in the skin. Because the presentation is identical to the presentation of aseptic arthritis associated with chickenpox, synovial fluid analysis is mandatory for proper diagnosis.

Aseptic arthritis has been reported as a complication of chickenpox in 10 children between the ages of 2 and 11 years—8 girls and 2 boys.[191–199] Arthritis usually begins several days after the onset of skin rash and lasts 2 to 6 days. Typically, a single knee is inflamed. Other patients have had involvement of one ankle,[196] both knees,[195] two metatarsophalangeal (MTP) joints;[199] and one patient had polyarticular disease.[193] Synovial fluid leukocyte counts have ranged from 3,600 to 51,700/mm^3, predominantly mononuclear cells. The ESR is usually only slightly elevated but has been as high as 107 mm/hour.[193] All cases showed complete resolution of arthritis, and no patient had associated serious systemic complications such as central nervous system, lung, or liver involvement.

A single case of acute arthritis of both knees in a patient with herpes zoster has been reported.[200] Arthritis began 6 days before the development of the typical skin rash. Synovial fluid from the knees contained 2200 and 9000 WBC/mm^3, with a predominance of polymorphonuclear cells.

VZV was recovered from the synovial fluid of a patient with chickenpox,[197] and VZV antigen was detected in synovial fluid macrophages of the patient with arthritis and herpes zoster.[200] Local viral proliferation may be responsible for the arthritis, although viral antigen presence might be due to simply macrophage ingestion of virus-containing immune complexes.

LYMPHOCYTIC CHORIOMENINGITIS VIRUS

Lymphocytic choriomeningitis virus (LCMV), a single-stranded, negative-sense RNA virus, is the prototype member of the family Arenaviridae. Clinical disease from LCMV infection usually includes a flulike illness with fever, myalgia, retro-orbital headache, lassitude, weakness, and anorexia.[201] After a week of illness, a remission of a day or two is often followed by a second or third wave of fever. Some patients develop chills, sore throat, chest pain, cough, vomiting, or photophobia. Aseptic meningitis, encephalitis, orchitis, or parotitis may occur. Arthralgias are common during the acute disease and convalescence. Arthritis was described in 10 patients infected with LCMV by exposure to infected hamsters.[202] All patients had arthralgias during the convalescent phase of illness, and two developed arthritis 2 weeks after the acute disease, affecting primarily the metacarpophalangeal and proximal interphalangeal joints. The outcome of the arthritis was not reported.

ENTEROVIRUSES

Enteroviruses, one of the major genera of the Picornaviridae family, are small, nonencapsulated viruses containing single-stranded, positive-sense RNA.[203] Members of the genus include the polioviruses, group A and B coxsackieviruses, echoviruses, and enteroviruses. Hepatitis A virus is an enterovirus.[34] Coxsackieviruses, echoviruses, and hepatitis A virus have been associated with arthritis. Enteroviral infections occur primarily during childhood, usually during the late summer months. Rheumatic complications are rare. Of 7075 reports of nonpolio enteroviral infections over 5 years, only 9 patients (0.13%) had rheumatic symptoms, most commonly arthritis but including myositis in two patients.[204]

Coxsackieviruses

Coxsackieviruses can cause a variety of clinical manifestations ranging from asymptomatic infection to epidemic pleurodynia, myocarditis, pericarditis, aseptic meningitis, or encephalitis.[205] Infection is usually self-limited but has been associated with chronic diseases including cardiomyopathy, polymyositis, and diabetes.

Systemic illness with fever, serositis, and rash, similar to Still's disease, is the most common presentation in patients with arthritis associated with coxsackievirus infection.[3,206,207] Group B coxsackieviruses have been implicated in each case. The patients reported have included seven men and four women, with an age range of 16 to 45 years. The arthritis is usually symmetric and polyarticular, involving both large and small joints. In one case, sacroiliitis was present in a patient who was HLA-B27 positive.[206] The arthritis tends to persist for several months or to recur, sometimes for years. Because of the chronicity of the arthritis, patients have been treated with corticosteroids, azathioprine,[207] or gold.[3,206] ESRs are often elevated, with some values over 100 mm/hour. Antinuclear antibodies, rheumatoid factor, immune complexes assays, and complement levels have been normal. The diagnosis is made by the demonstration of elevated antibody titers.

Echoviruses

The echoviruses produce a broad spectrum of disease, usually infecting children and young adults.[208] The usual pattern of disease is biphasic. After an incubation period of 5 to 10 days, mild illness with fever, anorexia, vomiting, and sore throat occur. This is followed by a short asymptomatic period and then more severe illness with fever, headache, nausea, vomiting, myalgia, and rash.

Arthritis infrequently complicates echovirus infection.[208–211] It lasted 2 to 9 days with symmetric polyarthritis in two cases,[208,209] and monoarticular knee involvement occurred in one.[210] A child with X-linked a-γ-globulinemia had bilateral knee effusions for 2 years from which echovirus was recovered on several occasions.[211] The arthritis in this case resolved after treatment with intravenous and intra-articular injections of γ-globulin. Treatment in the other cases has been symptomatic. Synovial fluid cell counts ranged from 2,250 to 46,900/mm^3, with mononuclear cells predominating. Synovial biopsy in one case revealed occasional perivascular lymphocytes and vascular occlusion but no synovial cell proliferation or plasma cells.[209] The diagnosis is made by serologic testing, although virus has been recovered from synovial fluid.[210,211]

Hepatitis A Virus

Hepatitis A virus (HAV) is transmitted from human to human usually, with an incubation period of about 4 weeks and a range of 14 to 40 days.[212] Anicteric cases occur about twice as frequently as do icteric cases. In symptomatic individuals, a prodrome of fever, fatigue, headache, nausea, vomiting, and abdominal discomfort often lasts a week. The icteric phase then develops, with abnormal liver functions lasting for a few days to weeks, the duration being correlated directly with age. Protracted cases may occur.

Studies of "infectious hepatitis," before the availability of serologic testing for hepatitis B surface antigen (HBsAg), suggested that arthralgias occurred in 30% of patients and arthritis in 11%,[213] but it is unknown how many of these patients actually had hepatitis B infection. In patients negative for HBsAg, arthralgia occurred in up to 11%.[51,214] Arthritis can occur with HAV infection but is infrequent.[215] A serum sickness-like syndrome, with maculopapular or urticarial rash and arthralgia, similar to that seen in hepatitis B infection, may occur.[214] Elevated transaminases and bilirubin are usually present during the period of joint symptoms.[215] Synovial fluid obtained in one case was noninflammatory.[215] The diagnosis is made by demonstration of IgM anti-HAV or by detection of HAV antigen in stool.[212]

Cryoglobulinemia occurs during the acute phase of HAV infection, with the cryoproteins containing HAV and IgM anti-HAV.[216] Arthritis and vasculitis have been reported in two patients with cryoglobulinemia during relapsing HAV infection.[217] Involved joints included knees and ankles in one patient and ankles, subtalar joints, and MTPs in the other.

SMALLPOX AND VACCINIA VIRUSES

Smallpox (variola) and vaccinia viruses belong to the Orthopoxvirus genus of the family Poxviridae.[218] The pox viruses are the largest of all viruses and contain a single linear molecule of double-stranded DNA as genome. Variola and vaccinia viruses have similar chemical and physical structures and share common antigens.

Smallpox was an important human disease until the end of the 1970s, when it was eradicated by the World Health Organization through a massive immunization effort.[218] Two forms of joint involvement were recognized in smallpox—pyogenic infection, spread hematogenously from secondary infection of skin lesions, and nonsuppurative osteomyelitis, termed *osteomyelitis variolosa*.[219] The incidence of joint involvement was 0.25 to 0.5%, affecting children primarily. Elbows were most frequently involved, followed by wrists, hands, ankles, feet, and knees. Joint involvement was usually symmetric and included more than one site in over half the patients. The onset was usually 10 to 28 days after the onset of rash. Radiographs showed osteomyelitis. Elementary bodies of variola were found in synovial fluid. Joint involvement was due to viremic seeding of the metaphyseal ends of the long bones. The course of the illness was one of recovery of the lesions over the course of a few months, without treatment. Unlike most other forms of viral arthritis, significant deformity was frequent, with interruption of normal bone growth resulting from epiphyseal damage.

Arthritis rarely complicates vaccination with vaccinia virus.[220–222] The onset of joint symptoms is 7 to 10 days after vaccination. The typical presentation is pain with or without swelling of a single knee. Synovial fluid has been reported in two cases, with a total leukocyte count of 44,000/mm^3 in one[220] and "many WBC" in the other[221]; in both, polymorphonuclear cells predominated. ESRs were moderately elevated, ranging up to 51 mm/hour. Virus can be recovered from synovial fluid.[220] The arthritis presumably arises from direct virus replication in the joint.

REFERENCES

1. White, D.G., Woolf, A.D., Mortimer, P.P., et al.: Human parvovirus arthropathy. Lancet, *1*:419–421, 1985.
2. Naides, S.J., Scharosch, L.L., Foto, F., and Howard, E.J.:

Rheumatologic manifestations of human parvovirus B19 infection in adults. Initial two-year clinical experience. Arthritis Rheum., *33*:1297–1309, 1990.

3. Rahal, J.J., Millian, S.J., and Noriega, E.R.: Coxsackie and adenovirus infection. Association with acute febrile and juvenile rheumatoid arthritis. JAMA, *235*:2496–2501, 1976.
4. Ray, C.G., Gall, E.P., Minnich, L.L., et al.: Acute polyarthritis associated with active Epstein-Barr virus infection. JAMA, *248*:2990–2993, 1982.
5. Sissons, J.G.P., and Borysiewicz, L.K.: Viral immunopathology. Br. Med. Bull., *41*:34–40, 1985.
6. Southern, P., and Oldstone, M.B.A.: Medical consequences of persistent viral infection. N Engl. J. Med., *314*:359–367, 1986.
7. Oldstone, M.B.A.: Virus can alter cell function without causing cell pathology: Disordered function leads to imbalance of homeostasis and disease. *In* Concepts in Viral Pathogenesis. Edited by A.L. Notkins and M.B.A. Oldstone. New York, Springer-Verlag, 1984, pp. 269–276.
8. Casali, P., and Oldstone, M.B.A.: Immune complexes in viral infection. Curr. Top. Microbiol. Immunol., *104*:7–48, 1983.
9. Notkins, A.L., Onodera, T., and Prabhakar, B.: Virus-induced autoimmunity. *In* Concepts in Viral Pathogenesis. Edited by A.L. Notkins and M.B.A. Oldstone. New York, Springer-Verlag, 1984, pp. 210–215.
10. Oldstone, M.B.A.: Viral persistence. Cell, *56*:517–520, 1989.
11. Kaye, B.R.: Rheumatologic manifestations of infection with human immunodeficiency virus (HIV). Ann. Intern. Med., *111*:158–167, 1989.
12. Kitajima, I., Maruyama, I., Maruyama, Y., et al.: Polyarthritis in human T-lymphotropic virus type-1-associated myelopathy. Arthritis Rheum., *32*:1342–1344, 1989.
13. Anderson, M.J., and Pattison, J.R.: The human parvovirus. Arch. Virol., *82*:137–148, 1984.
14. Cossart, Y.E., Field, A.M., Cant, B., and Widdows, D.: Parvovirus-like particles in human sera. Lancet, *1*:72–73, 1975.
15. Simpson, R.W., McGinty, L., Simon, L., et al.: Association of parvoviruses with rheumatoid arthritis of humans. Science, *223*:1425–1428, 1984.
16. Stierle, G., Brown, K.A., Rainsford, S.G., et al.: Parvovirus associated antigen in the synovial membrane of patients with rheumatoid arthritis. Ann. Rheum. Dis., *46*:219–223, 1987.
17. Anderson, L.J.: Role of parvovirus B19 in human disease. Pediatr. Infect. Dis. J., *6*:711–718, 1987.
18. Smith, C.A., Woolf, A.D., and Lenci, M.: Parvoviruses: Infections and arthropathies. Rheum. Dis. Clin. North Am., *13*:249–263, 1987.
19. Kurtzman, G.J., Cohen, B.J., Field, A.M., et al.: Immune response to B19 parvovirus and an antibody defect in persistent viral infection. J. Clin. Invest., *84*:1114–1123, 1989.
20. Ager, E.A., Chin, T.D.Y., and Poland, J.D.: Epidemic erythema infectiosum. N. Engl. J. Med., *275*:1326–1331, 1966.
21. Feder, H.M., and Anderson, I.: Fifth disease. A brief review of infections in childhood, in adulthood, and in pregnancy. Arch. Intern. Med., *149*:2176–2178, 1989.
22. Anderson, M.J., Higgins, P.G., Davis, L.R., et al.: Experimental parvoviral infection in humans. J. Infect. Dis., *152*:257–265, 1985.
23. Anderson, M.J., Lewis, E., Kidd, I.M., et al.: An outbreak of erythema infectiosum associated with human parvovirus infection. J. Hyg. (Lond.), *93*:85–93, 1984.
24. Reid, D.M., Reid, T.M.S., Brown, T., et al.: Human parvovirus-associated arthritis: A clinical and laboratory description. Lancet, 1:422–425, 1985.
25. Woolf, A.D., Campion, G.V., Chishick, A., et al.: Clinical manifestations of human parvovirus B19 in adults. Arch. Intern. Med., *149*:1153–1156, 1989.
26. Bell, L.M., Naides, S.J., Stoffman, P., et al.: Human parvovirus B19 infection among hospital staff members after contact with infected patients. N. Engl. J. Med., *321*:485–491, 1989.
27. Rowe, I.F., Deans, A.C., Midgley, J., et al.: Parvovirus infection in hospital practice. Br. J. Rheumatol., *26*:13–16, 1987.
28. Naides, S.J., and Field, E.H.: Transient rheumatoid factor positivity in acute human parvovirus B19 infection. Arch. Intern. Med., *148*:2587–2589, 1988.
29. Soloninka, C.A., Anderson, M.J., and Laskin, C.A.: Anti-DNA and antilymphocyte antibodies during acute infections with human parvovirus B19. J. Rheumatol., *16*:777–781, 1989.
30. Klouda, P.T., Corbin, S.A., Bradley, B.A., et al.: HLA and acute arthritis following human parvovirus infection. Tissue Antigens, *28*:318–319, 1986.
31. Semble, E.L., Agudelo, C.A., and Pegram, P.S.: Human parvovirus B-19 arthropathy in two adults after contact with childhood erythema infectiosum. Am. J. Med., *83*:560–562, 1987.
32. Dijkmans, B.A.C., van Elsacker-Niele, A.M.W., Salimans, M.M.M., et al.: Human parvovirus B19 DNA in synovial fluid. Arthritis Rheum., *31*:279–281, 1988.
33. Kandolf, R., Kirschner, P., Hofschneider, P.H., and Vischner, T.L.: Detection of parvovirus in a patient with "reactive arthritis" by in situ hybridization. Clin. Rheumatol., *8*:398–401, 1989.
34. Melnick, J.L.: Classification of hepatitis A virus as enterovirus type 72 and of hepatitis B virus as hepadnavirus type 1. Intervirology, *18*:105–106, 1982.
35. Robinson, W.S.: Hepatitis B virus and hepatitis delta virus. *In* Principles and Practice of Infectious Diseases. 3rd Ed. Edited by G.L. Mandell, R.G. Douglas, Jr., and J.E. Bennett. New York, Churchill Livingstone, 1990, pp. 1204–1231.
36. Inman, R.D.: Rheumatic manifestations of hepatitis B infection. Semin. Arthritis Rheum., *11*:406–420, 1982.
37. Sergent, J.S., Lockshin, M.D., Christian, C.L., and Gocke, D.J.: Vasculitis and hepatitis B antigenemia: Long-term observations in nine patients. Medicine, *55*:1–18, 1976.
38. Duffy, J., Lidsky, M.D., Sharp, J.T., et al.: Polyarthritis, polyarteritis, and hepatitis B. Medicine, *55*:19–37, 1976.
39. Drüeke, T., Barbanel, C., Jungers, P., et al.: Hepatitis B antigen-associated periarteritis nodosa in patients undergoing long-term hemodialysis. Am. J. Med., *68*:86–90, 1980.
40. Levo, Y., Gorevic, P.D., Kassab, H.J., et al.: Association between hepatitis B virus and essential mixed cryoglobulinemia. N. Engl. J. Med., *296*:1501–1504, 1977.
41. Onion, D.K., Crumpacker, C.S., and Gilliland, B.C.: Arthritis of hepatitis associated with Australia antigen. Ann. Intern. Med., *75*:29–33, 1971.
42. McKenna, P.J., O'Brian, J.T., Scheinman, H.Z., et al.: Hepatitis and arthritis with hepatitis-associated antigen in serum and synovial fluid. Lancet, *2*:214–215, 1971.
43. Alpert, E., Isselbacher, K.J., and Schur, P.H.: The pathogenesis of arthritis associated with viral hepatitis. Complement-component studies. N. Engl. J. Med., *285*:185–189, 1971.
44. Alpert, E., Schur, P.H., and Isselbacher, K.J.: Sequential changes of serum complement in HAA related arthritis. N. Engl. J. Med., *287*:103, 1972.
45. McCarty, D.J., and Ormiste, V.: Arthritis and HB Ag-positive hepatitis. Arch. Intern. Med., *132*:264–268, 1973.
46. Alarcon, G.S., and Townes, A.S.: Arthritis in viral hepatitis: Report of two cases and review of the literature. Johns Hopkins Med. J., *132*:1–15, 1973.
47. Shumaker, J.B., Goldfinger, S.E., Alpert, E., and Isselbacher, K.J.: Arthritis and rash. Clues to anicteric viral hepatitis. Arch. Intern. Med., *133*:483–485, 1974.
48. Lewis, J.H., Brandon, J.M., Gorenc, T.J., and Maxwell, N.G.:

Heptitis B. A study of 200 cases positive for the hepatitis B antigen. Am. J. Dig. Dis., *18*:921–927, 1973.
49. Sauter, S.V.H., and Utsinger, P.D.: Viral arthritis. Clin. Rheum. Dis., *4*:225–240, 1978.
50. Stevens, D.P., Walker, J., Crum, E., et al.: Anicteric hepatitis presenting as polyarthritis. JAMA, *220*:687–689, 1972.
51. Bamber, M., Thomas, H.C., Bannister, B., and Sherlock, S.: Acute type A, B, and non-A, non-B hepatitis in a hospital population in London: Clinical and epidemiological features. Gut, *24*:561–564, 1983.
52. Wands, J.R., Mann, E., Alpert, E., and Isselbacher, K.J.: The pathogenesis of arthritis associated with acute hepatitis-B surface antigen-positive hepatitis. Complement activation and characterization of circulating immune complexes. J. Clin. Invest., *55*:930–936, 1975.
53. McIntosh, R.M., Koss, M.N., and Gocke, D.J.: The nature and incidence of cryoproteins in hepatitis B antigen (HbsAg) positive patients. Q. J. Med., *45*:23–38, 1976.
54. Dienstag, J.L., Rhodes, A.R., Bhan, A.K., et al.: Urticaria associated with acute viral hepatitis type B. Studies of pathogenesis. Ann. Intern. Med., *89*:34–40, 1978.
55. Schumacher, H.R., and Gall, E.P.: Arthritis in acute hepatitis and chronic active hepatitis. Pathology of the synovial membrane with evidence for the presence of Australia antigen in synovial membranes. Am. J. Med., *57*:655–664, 1974.
56. Lamprecht, C.L.: Rubella virus. *In* Textbook of Human Virology. 2nd Ed. Edited by R.B. Belshe. St. Louis, MO: Mosby Year Book, 1991, pp. 675–698.
57. Gershon, A.A.: Rubella virus. *In* Principles and Practice of Infectious Diseases. 3rd Ed. Edited by G.L. Mandell, R.G. Douglas, Jr., and J.E. Bennett. New York, Churchill Livingstone, 1990, pp. 1242–1260.
58. Horstmann, D.M.: Rubella. *In* Viral Infections of Humans. Epidemiology and Control. 3rd Ed. Edited by A.S. Evans. New York, Plenum Medical Book Co., 1989, pp. 617–631.
59. Preblud, S.R., Serdula, M.K., Frank, J.A., Jr., et al.: Rubella vaccination in the United States: A ten-year review. Epidemiol. Rev., *2*:171–194, 1980.
60. Smith, C.A., Petty, R.E., and Tingle, A.J.: Rubella virus and arthritis. Rheum. Dis. Clin. North Am., *13*:265–274, 1987.
61. Geiger, J.C.: Epidemic of German measles in a city adjacent to an army cantonment and its probable relation thereto. JAMA, *70*:1818–1820, 1918.
62. Hope Simpson, R.E.: Rubella and polyarthritis. Br. Med. J., *1*:830, 1940.
63. Loudon, I.S.L.: Polyarthritis in rubella. Br. Med. J., *1*:1388, 1953.
64. Hildebrandt, H.M., and Maassab, H.F.: Rubella synovitis in a one-year-old patient. N. Engl. J. Med., *274*:1428–1430, 1966.
65. Fry, J., Dillane, J.B., and Fry, L.: Rubella, 1962. Br. Med. J., *2*:833–834, 1962.
66. Smith, D., and Guzowska, J.: Arthritis complicating rubella. Med. J. Aust., *1*:845–847, 1970.
67. Lee, P.R., Barnett, A.F., Scholer, J.F., et al.: Rubella arthritis. A study of twenty cases. Calif. Med., *93*:125–128, 1960.
68. Kantor, T.G., and Tanner, M.: Rubella arthritis and rheumatoid arthritis. Arthritis Rheum., *5*:378–383, 1962.
69. Chantler, J.K., Ford, D.K., and Tingle, A.J.: Persistent rubella infection and rubella-associated arthritis. Lancet, *1*:1323–1325, 1982.
70. Johnson, I.N.L.: Complications of rubella. Br. Med. J., *2*:414, 1962.
71. Heathfield, K.W.G.: Carpal-tunnel syndrome. Br. Med. J., *2*:58, 1962.
72. Chambers, R.J., and Bywaters, E.G.L.: Rubella synovitis. Ann. Rheum. Dis., *22*:263–268, 1963.
73. Yanez, J.E., Thompson, G.R., Mikkelsen, W.M., and Bartholomew, L.E.: Rubella arthritis. Ann. Intern. Med., *64*:772–777, 1966.
74. Harrison, B.L.: Neuritis following rubella. Br. Med. J., *1*:637, 1940.
75. Hodges, G.M.W.: Brachial neuritis following rubella. Br. Med. J., *1*:548, 1940.
76. Moylan-Jones, R.J., and Penny, P.T.: Complications of rubella. Lancet, *2*:355, 1962.
77. Weibel, R.E., Stokes, J.J., Buynak, E.B., and Hilleman, M.R.: Rubella vaccination in adult females. N. Engl. J. Med., *280*:682–685, 1969.
78. Thompson, G.R., Ferreyra, A., and Brackett, R.G.: Acute arthritis complicating rubella vaccination. Arthritis Rheum., *14*:19–26, 1971.
79. Plotkin, S.A., Farquhar, J.D., and Ogra, P.L.: Immunologic properties of RA27/3 rubella virus vaccine. A comparison with strains presently licensed in the United States. JAMA, *225*:585–590, 1973.
80. Horstmann, D.M., Liebhaber, H., and Kohorn, E.I.: Post-partum vaccination of rubella-susceptible women. Lancet, *2*: 1003–1006, 1970.
81. Rowlands, D.F., and Freestone, D.S.: Vaccination against rubella of susceptible schoolgirls in Reading. J. Hyg. (Lond.), *69*:579–586, 1971.
82. Swartz, T.A., Klingberg, W., Goldwasser, R.A., et al.: Clinical manifestation according to age, among females given HPV-77 duck embryo vaccine. Am. J. Epidemiol., *94*:246–251, 1971.
83. Austin, S.M., Altman, R., Barnes, E.K., and Doughterty, W.J.: Joint reactions in children vaccinated against rubella. Study I: Comparison of two vaccines. Am. J. Epidemiol., *95*:53–58, 1972.
84. Barnes, E.K., Altman, R., Austin, S.M., and Dougherty, W.J.: Joint reactions in children vaccinated against rubella. Study II: Comparison of three vaccines. Am. J. Epidemiol., *95*:59–66, 1972.
85. Spruance, S.L., and Smith, C.B.: Joint complications associated with derivatives of HPV-77 rubella virus vaccine. Am. J. Dis. Child., *122*:105–111, 1971.
86. Grand, M.G., Wyll, S.A., Gehlbach, S.H., et al.: Clinical reactions following rubella vaccination. A prospective analysis of joint, muscular, and neuritic symptoms. JAMA, *220*:1569–1572, 1972.
87. Polk, B.F., Modlin, J.F., White, J.A., and DeGirolami, P.C.: A controlled comparison of joint reactions among women receiving one of two rubella vaccines. Am. J. Epidemiol., *115*:19–25, 1982.
88. Fogel, A., Moshkowitz, A., Rannon, L., and Gerichter, C.B.: Comparative trials of RA 27/3 and Cendehill rubella vaccines in adult and adolescent females. Am. J. Epidemiol., *93*:392–398, 1971.
89. Ogra, P.L., and Herd, J.K.: Arthritis associated with induced rubella infection. J. Immunol., *107*:810–813, 1971.
90. Spruance, S.L., Klock, L.E., Jr., Bailey, A., et al.: Recurrent joint symptoms in children vaccinated with HPV-77DK12 rubella vaccine. J. Pediatr., *80*:413–417, 1972.
91. Thompson, G.R., Weiss, J.J., Shillis, J.L., and Brackett, R.G.: Intermittent arthritis following rubella vaccination. A three-year follow-up. Am. J. Dis. Child., *125*:526–530, 1973.
92. Spruance, S.L., Metcalf, R., Smith, C.B., et al.: Chronic arthropathy associated with rubella vaccination. Arthritis Rheum., *20*:741–747, 1977.
93. Chantler, J.K., Tingle, A.J., and Petty, R.E.: Persistent rubella virus infection associated with chronic arthritis in children. N. Engl. J. Med., *313*:1117–1123, 1985.
94. Grahame, R., Armstrong, R., Simmons, N., et al.: Chronic ar-

thritis associated with the presence of intrasynovial rubella virus. Ann. Rheum. Dis., *42*(1):2–13, 1983.

95. Tingle, A.J., Chantler, J.K., Pot, K.H., et al.: Postpartum rubella immunization: Association with development of prolonged arthritis, neurological sequelae, and chronic rubella viremia. J. Infect. Dis., *152*:606–612, 1985.
96. Tingle, A.J., Allen, M., Petty, R.E., et al.: Rubella-associated arthritis: I. Comparative study of joint manifestations associated with natural rubella infection and RA 27/3 rubella immunisation. Ann. Rheum. Dis., *45*:110–114, 1986.
97. Kilroy, A.W., Schaffner, W., Fleet, W.F., Jr., et al.: Two syndromes following rubella immunization. Clinical observations and epidemiological studies. JAMA, *214*:2287–2292, 1970.
98. Gilmartin, R.C., Jr., Jabbour, J.T., and Duenas, D.A.: Rubella vaccine myeloradiculoneuritis. J. Pediatr., *80*:406–412, 1972.
99. Schaffner, W., Fleet, W.F., Kilroy, A.W., et al.: Polyneuropathy following rubella immunization. A follow-up study and review of the problem. Am. J. Dis. Child., *127*:684–688, 1974.
100. Gupta, J.D., and Peterson, V.: Rubella and rheumatoid arthritis. Lancet, *2*:781, 1970.
101. Johnson, R.E., and Hall, A.P.: Rubella arthritis. Report of cases studied by latex tests. N. Engl. J. Med., *258*:743–745, 1958.
102. Fraser, J.R.E., Cunningham, A.L., Hayes, K., et al.: Rubella arthritis in adults. Isolation of virus, cytology and other aspects of the synovial reaction. Clin. Exp. Rheumatol., *1*:287–293, 1983.
103. Ford, D.K., da Roza, D., Reid, G., et al.: Synovial mononuclear cell responses to rubella antigen in rheumatoid arthritis and unexplained persistent knee arthritis. J. Rheumatol., *9*:420–423, 1982.
104. Chantler, J.K., DaRoza, D.M., Bonnie, M.E., et al.: Sequential studies on synovial lymphocyte stimulation by rubella antigen, and rubella virus isolation in an adult with persistent arthritis. Ann. Rheum. Dis., *44*:564–568, 1985.
105. Grayzel, A.I., and Beck, C.: The growth of vaccine strains of rubella virus in cultured human synovial cells. Proc. Soc. Exp. Biol. Med., *136*:496–498, 1971.
106. Chantler, J.K., Ford, D.K., and Tingle, A.J.: Rubella-associated arthritis: Rescue of rubella virus from peripheral blood lymphocytes two years postvaccination. Infect. Immun., *32*: 1274–1280, 1981.
107. Ziola, B., Lund, G., Meurman, O., and Salmi, A.: Circulating immune complexes in patients with acute measles and rubella virus infections. Infect. Immun., *41*:578–583, 1983.
108. Singh, V.K., Tingle, A.J., and Schulzer, M.: Rubella-associated arthritis: II. Relationship between circulating immune complex levels and joint manifestations. Ann. Rheum. Dis., *45*:115–119, 1986.
109. Coyle, P.K., Wolinsky, J.S., Buimovici-Klein, E., et al.: Rubella-specific immune complexes after congenital infection and vaccination. Infect. Immun., *36*:498–503, 1982.
110. Griffiths, M.M., Spruance, S.L., Ogra, P.L., et al.: HLA and recurrent episodic arthropathy associated with rubella vaccination. Arthritis Rheum., *20*:1192–1197, 1977.
111. Calisher, C.H., Shope, R.E., Brandt, W., et al.: Proposed antigenic classification of registered arboviruses: I. Togaviridae, Alphavirus. Intervirology, *14*:229–232, 1980.
112. Craven, R.B.: Togaviruses. *In* Textbook of Human Virology, 2nd Ed. Edited by R.D. Belshe. St. Louis, MO, Mosby Year Book, 1991, pp. 663–674.
113. Tesh, R.B.: Arthritides caused by mosquito-borne viruses. Annu. Rev. Med., *33*:31–40, 1982.
114. Halliday, J.H., and Horan, J.P.: An epidemic of polyarthritis in the Northern Territory. Med. J. Aust., *2*:293–295, 1943.
115. Dowling, P.G.: Epidemic polyarthritis. Med. J. Aust., *1*:245–246, 1946.
116. Clarke, J.A., Marshall, I.D., and Gard, G.: Annually recurrent epidemic polyarthritis and Ross River virus activity in a coastal area of New South Wales: I. Occurrence of the disease. Am. J. Trop. Med. Hyg., *22*:543–550, 1973.
117. Tesh, R.B., McLean, R.G., Shroyer, D.A., et al.: Ross River virus (Togaviridae: Alphavirus) infection (epidemic polyarthritis) in American Samoa. Trans. R. Soc. Trop. Med. Hyg., *75*:426–431, 1981.
118. Rosen, L., Gubler, D.J., and Bennett, P.H.: Epidemic polyarthritis (Ross River) virus infection in the Cook Islands. Am. J. Trop. Med. Hyg., *30*:1294–1302, 1981.
119. Hazelton, R.A.: Ross River virus infection and epdemic polyarthritis. Aust. Fam. Physician, *16*(2):130, 1987.
120. Anderson, S.G., and French, E.L.: An epidemic exanthem associated with polyarthritis in the Murray Valley, 1956. Med. J. Aust., *2*:113–117, 1957.
121. Seglenieks, Z., and Moore, B.W.: Epidemic polyarthritis in South Australia: Report of an outbreak in 1971. Med. J. Aust., *2*:552–556, 1974.
122. Mudge, P.R., and Aaskov, J.G.: Epidemic polyarthritis in Australia, 1980–1981. Med. J. Aust., *2*(6):269–273, 1983.
123. Mudge, P.: Epidemic polyarthritis in South Australia. Med. J. Aust., *2*:823, 1974.
124. Fraser, J.R.E., and Cunningham, A.L.: Incubation time of epidemic polyarthritis. Med. J Aust., *1*:550–551, 1980.
125. Fraser, J.R.: Epidemic polyarthritis and Ross River virus disease. Clin. Rheum. Dis., *12*:369–388, 1986.
126. Clarris, B.J., Doherty, R.L., Fraser, J.R.E., et al.: Epidemic polyarthritis: A cytological, virological, and immunochemical study. Aust. N.Z. J. Med., *5*:450–457, 1975.
127. Fraser, J.R.E., Cunningham, A.L., Clarris, B.J., et al.: Cytology of synovial effusions in epidemic polyarthritis. Aust. N.Z. J. Med., *11*:168–173, 1981.
128. Hazelton, R.A., Hughes, C., and Aaskov, J.G.: The inflammatory response in the synovium of a patient with Ross River arbovirus infection. Aust. N.Z. J. Med., *15*(3):336–339, 1985.
129. Aaskov, J.G., Ross, P.V., Harper, J.J., and Donaldson, M.D.: Isolation of Ross River virus from epidemic polyarthritis patients in Australia. Aust. J. Exp. Biol. Med. Sci., *63*(5):587–597, 1985.
130. Cunningham, A.L., and Fraser, J.R.E.: Ross River virus infection of human synovial cells in vitro. Aust. J. Exp. Biol. Med. Sci., *63*:197–204, 1985.
131. Fraser, J.R.E., Ratnamohan, V.M., Dowling, J.P.G., et al.: The exanthem of Ross River virus infection: Histology, location of virus antigen and nature of inflammatory infiltrate. J. Clin. Pathol., *36*:1256–1263, 1983.
132. Aaskov, J.G., Dalglish, D.A., Harper, J.J., et al.: Natural killer cells in viral arthritis. Clin. Exp. Immunol., *68*:23–32, 1987.
133. Fraser, J.R.E., Tait, B., Aaskov, J.G., and Cunningham, A.L.: Possible genetic determinants in epidemic polyarthritis caused by Ross River virus infection. Aust. N.Z. J. Med., *10*:597–603, 1980.
134. Robinson, M.D.: An epidemic of virus disease in southern province, Tanganyika territory, in 1952–53: I. Clinical features. Trans. R. Soc. Trop. Med. Hyg., *49*:28–32, 1955.
135. Lumsden, W.H.R.: An epidemic of virus disease in southern province, Tanganyika territory, in 1952–53: II. General description and epidemiology. Trans. R. Soc. Trop. Med. Hyg., *49*:33–57, 1955.
136. Ross, R.W.: The Newala epidemic: III. The virus: Isolation, pathogenic properties and relationship to the epidemic. J. Hyg. (Camb.), *54*:177–191, 1956.
137. Moore, D.L., Reddy, S., Akinkugbe, F.M., et al.: An epidemic of chikungunya fever in Ibadan, Nigeria, 1969. Ann. Trop. Med. Parasitol., *68*:59–68, 1974.
138. Kennedy, A.C., Fleming, J., and Solomon, L.: Chikungunya

viral arthropathy: A clinical description. J. Rheumatol., *7*:231–236, 1980.
139. de Ranitz, C.M., Myers, R.M., Varkey, M.J., et al.: Clinical impressions of chikungunya in Vellore gained from study of adult patients. Ind. J. Med. Res., *53*:756–763, 1965.
140. Jadhav, M., Namboodripad, M., Carman, R.H., et al.: Chikungunya disease in infants and children in Vellore: A report of clinical and hematological features of virologically proved cases. Ind. J. Med. Res., *53*:764–776, 1965.
141. Deller, J.J., Jr., and Russell, P.K.: Chikungunya disease. Am. J. Trop. Med. Hyg., *17*:107–111, 1968.
142. Nimmannitya, S., Halstead, S.B., Cohen, S.N., and Margiotta, M.R.: Dengue and Chikungunya virus infection in man in Thailand. 1962–1964: I. Observations on hospitalized patients with hemorrhagic fever. Am. J. Trop. Med. Hyg., *18*:954–971, 1969.
143. Brighton, S.W., Prozesky, O.W., and De la Harpe, A.L.: Chikungunya virus infection. A retrospective study of 107 cases. S. Afr. Med. J., *63*:313–315, 1983.
144. Brighton, S.W., and Simson, I.W.: A destructive arthropathy following Chikungunya virus arthritis—A possible association. Clin. Rheumatol., *3*(2):253–258, 1984.
145. Brighton, S.W.: Chloroquine phosphate treatment of chronic Chikungunya arthritis. An open pilot study. S. Afr. Med. J., *66*(6):217–218, 1984.
146. Haddow, A.J., Davies, C.W., and Walker, A.J.: O'nyong-nyong fever: An epidemic virus disease in East Africa: 1. Introduction. Trans. R. Soc. Trop. Med. Hyg., *54*:517–522, 1960.
147. Shore, H.: O'nyong-nyong fever: An epidemic virus disease in East Africa: III. Some clinical and epidemiological observations in the northern province of Uganda. Trans. R. Soc. Trop. Med. Hyg., *55*:361–373, 1961.
148. Williams, M.C., Woodall, J.P., and Gillett, J.D.: O'nyong-nyong fever: An epidemic virus disease in East Africa: VII. Virus isolations in man and serological studies up to July 1961. Trans. R. Soc. Trop. Med. Hyg., *59*:186–197, 1965.
149. Anderson, C.R., Downs, W.G., Wattley, G.H., et al.: Mayaro virus: A new human disease agent: II. Isolation from blood of patients in Trinidad, B.W.I. Am. J. Trop. Med. Hyg., *6*:1012–1016, 1957.
150. Pinheiro, F.P., Freitas, R.B., Travassos da Rosa, J.F., et al.: An outbreak of Mayaro virus disease in Belterra, Brazil: I. Clinical and virological findings. Am. J. Trop. Med. Hyg., *30*:674–681, 1981.
151. Malherbe, H., Strickland-Cholmley, M., and Jackson, A.L.: Sindbis virus infection in man. Report of a case with recovery of virus from skin lesions. S. Afr. Med. J., *37*:547–552, 1963.
152. McIntosh, B.M., McGillivray, G.M., Dickinson, D.B., and Malherbe, H.: Illness caused by Sindbis and West Nile viruses in South Africa. S. Afr. Med. J., *38*:291–294, 1964.
153. Espmark, A., and Niklasson, B.: Ockelbo disease in Sweden: Epidemiological, clinical and virological data from the 1982 outbreak. Am. J. Trop. Med. Hyg., *33*:1203–1211, 1984.
154. Julkunen, I., Brummer-Korvenkontio, M., Hautanen, A., et al.: Elevated serum immune complex levels in Pogosta disease, an acute alphavirus infection with rash and arthritis. J. Clin. Lab. Immunol., *21*:77–82, 1986.
155. Lvov, D.K., Berezina, L.K., Yakovlev, B.I., et al.: Isolation of Karelian fever agent from Aedes communis mosquitoes. Lancet, *2*:399–400, 1984.
156. Niklasson, B., Espmark, A., LeDuc, J.W., et al.: Association of a Sindbis-like virus with Ockelbo disease in Sweden. Am. J. Trop. Med. Hyg., *33*:1212–1217, 1984.
157. Niklasson, B., Espmark, A., and Lundström, J.: Occurrence of arthralgia and specific IgM antibodies three to four years after Ockelbo disease. J. Infect. Dis., *157*(4):832–835, 1988.
158. Tolpin, M.D.: Mumps virus. *In* Textbook of Human Virology. 2nd Ed. Edited by R.B. Belshe. St. Louis, MO, Mosby Year Book, 1991, pp. 351–366.
159. Feldman, H.A.: Mumps. *In* Viral Infections of Humans. Epidemiology and Control. 3rd Ed. Edited by A.S. Evans. New York, Plenum Medical Book Co., 1989, pp. 471–491.
160. Caranasos, G.J., and Felker, J.R.: Mumps arthritis. Arch. Intern. Med., *119*:394–398, 1967.
161. Gordon, S.C., and Lauter, C.B.: Mumps arthritis: A review of the literature. Rev. Infect. Dis., *6*:338–344, 1984.
162. Solem, J.H.: Mumps arthritis without parotitis. Scand. J. Infect. Dis., *3*:173–175, 1971.
163. Gordon, S.C., and Lauter, C.B.: Mumps arthritis: Unusual presentation as adult Still's disease. Ann. Intern. Med., *97*:45–47, 1982.
164. Bryer, D., and Rounthwaite, F.J.: Cricoarytenoid arthritis due to mumps. Laryngoscope, *83*:372–375, 1973.
165. Ghosh, S.K., and Reddy, T.A.: Arthralgia and myalgia in mumps. Rheumatol. Rehabil., *12*:97–99, 1973.
166. Appelbaum, E., Kohn, J., Steinman, R.E., and Shearn, M.A.: Mumps arthritis. Arch. Intern. Med., *90*:217–223, 1952.
167. Tracey, J.P., and Riggenbach, R.D.: Mumps arthritis associated with positive latex fixation reaction. South. Med. J., *63*:1122, 1126, 1970.
168. Huppertz, H.I., and Chantler, J.K.: Restricted mumps virus infection of cells derived from normal human joint tissue. J. Gen. Virol., *72*:339–347, 1991.
169. Baum, S.G.: Adenovirus. *In* Principles and Practice of Infectious Diseases. 3rd Ed. Edited by G.L. Mandell, R.G. Douglas, Jr., and J.E. Bennett. New York, Churchill Livingstone, 1990, pp. 1185–1191.
170. Panush, R.S.: Adenovirus arthritis. Arthritis Rheum., *17*: 534–536, 1974.
171. Utsinger, P.D.: Immunologic study of arthritis associated with adenovirus infection. (Abstract.) Arthritis Rheum., *20*:138, 1977.
172. Fraser, K.J., Clarris, B.J., Muirden, K.D., et al.: A persistent adenovirus type 1 infection in synovial tissue from an immunodeficient patient with chronic, rheumatoid-like polyarthritis. Arthritis Rheum., *28*:455–458, 1985.
173. Strauss, S.E.: Introduction of Herpesviridae. *In* Principles and Practice of Infectious Diseases. 3rd Ed. Edited by G.L. Mandell, R.G. Douglas, Jr., and J.E. Bennett. New York, Churchill Livingstone, 1990, pp. 1139–1144.
174. Naraqi, S.: Cytomegaloviruses. *In* Textbook of Human Virology. 2nd Ed. Edited by R.B. Belshe. St. Louis, MO, Mosby Year Book, 1991, pp. 889–924.
175. Fiala, M., Payne, J.E., Berne, T.V., et al.: Epidemiology of cytomegalovirus infection after transplantation and immunosuppression. J. Infect. Dis., *132*:421–433, 1975.
176. Friedman, H.M., Pincus, T., Gibilisco, P., et al.: Acute monarticular arthritis caused by herpes simplex virus and cytomegalovirus. Am. J. Med., *69*:241–247, 1980.
177. Hamerman, D., Gresser, I., and Smith, C.: Isolation of cytomegalovirus from synovial cells of a patient with rheumatoid arthritis. J. Rheumatol., *9*:658–664, 1982.
178. Schooley, R.T., and Dolin, R.: Epstein-Barr virus (infectious mononucleosis). *In* Principles and Practice of Infectious Diseases. 3rd Ed. Edited by G.L. Mandell, R.G. Douglas, Jr., and J.E. Bennett. New York, Churchill Livingstone, 1990, pp. 1172–1185.
179. Bernstein, A.: Infectious mononucleosis. Medicine, *19*:85–159, 1940.
180. Adebonojo, F.O.: Monarticular arthritis: An unusual manifestation of infectious mononucleosis. Clin. Pediatr., *11*:549–550, 1972.
181. Pollack, S., Enat, R., and Barzilai, D.: Monarthritis with hetero-

phil-negative infectious mononucleosis. Case of an older patient. Arch. Intern. Med., *140*:1109–1111, 1980.

182. Urman, J.D., and Bobrove, A.M.: Acute polyarthritis and infectious mononucleosis. West J. Med., *136*:151–153, 1982.
183. Sigal, L.H., Steere, A.C., and Niederman, J.C.: Symmetric polyarthritis associated with heterophile-negative infectious mononucleosis. Arthritis Rheum., *26*:553–556, 1983.
184. Hirsh, M.S.: Herpes simplex virus. *In* Principles and Practice of Infectious Diseases. 3rd Ed. Edited by G.L. Mandell, R.G. Douglas, Jr., and J.E. Bennett. New York, Churchill Livingstone, 1990, pp. 1144–1153.
185. Remafedi, G., and Muldoon, R.L.: Acute monarticular arthritis caused by herpes simplex virus type 1. Pediatrics, *72*:882–883, 1983.
186. Naraqi, S., Jackson, G.G., and Jonasson, O.M.: Viremia with herpes simplex type I in adults. Four nonfatal cases, one with features of chicken pox. Ann. Intern. Med., *85*:165–169, 1976.
187. Whitley, R.J.: Varicella-zoster virus. *In* Principles and Practice of Infectious Diseases. 3rd Ed. Edited by G.L. Mandell, R.G. Douglas, Jr., and J.E. Bennett. New York, Churchill Livingstone, 1990, pp. 1153–1159.
188. Slowick, F.: Purulent infection of the hip joint. N. Engl. J. Med., *212*:672–676, 1935.
189. Buck, R.: Pyarthrosis of the hip complicating chickenpox. JAMA, *206*:135–136, 1968.
190. Sethi, A., and Schloff, I.: Purulent arthritis complicating chickenpox. Clin. Pediatr., *13*:280, 1974.
191. Atkinson, L.S., Halford, J.G., Jr., Burton, O.M., and Moorhead, S.R., Jr.: Septic and aseptic arthritis complicating varicella. J. Fam. Pract., *12*:917–925, 1981.
192. Ward, J.R., and Bishop, B.: Varicella arthritis. JAMA, *242*:1954–1956, 1970.
193. Friedman, A., and Naveh, Y.: Polyarthritis associated with chickenpox. Am. J. Dis. Child., *122*:179–180, 1971.
194. Mulhern, L.M., Friday, G.A., and Perri, J.A.: Arthritis complicating varicella infection. Pediatrics, *48*:827–829, 1971.
195. Brook, I.: Varicella arthritis in childhood. Reports of 2 cases and 4 others found in the literature. Clin. Pediatr., *16*:1156–1157, 1977.
196. DiLiberti, J.H., Bartel, S.J., Humphrey, T.R., and Pang, A.W.: Acute monoarticular arthritis in association with varicella. Clin. Pediatr., *16*:663–664, 1977.
197. Priest, J.R., Urick, J.J., Groth, K.E., and Balfour, H.H., Jr.: Varicella arthritis documented by isolation of virus from joint fluid. J. Pediatr., *93*:990–992, 1978.
198. Pascual-Gomez, E.: Identification of large mononuclear cells in varicella arthritis. Arthritis Rheum., *23*:519–520, 1980.
199. Shuper, A., Mimouni, M., Mukamel, M., and Varsano, I.: Varicella arthritis in a child. Arch. Dis. Child., *55*:568–569, 1980.
200. Cunningham, A.L., and Fraser, J.R.E.: A study of synovial fluid and cytology in arthritis associated with herpes zoster. Aust. N.Z. J. Med., *9*:440–443, 1979.
201. Peters, C.J.: Arenaviruses. *In* Textbook of Human Virology. 2nd Ed. Edited by R.B. Belshe. St. Louis, MO, Mosby Year Book, 1991, pp. 541–570.
202. Baum, S.G., Lewis, A.M.J., Rowe, W.P., and Huebner, R.J.: Epidemic nonmeningitic lymphocytic-choriomeningitis-virus infection. An outbreak in a population of laboratory personnel. N. Engl. J. Med., *274*:934–936, 1966.
203. Modlin, J.F.: Picornaviridae. Introduction. *In* Principles and Practice of Infectious Diseases. 3rd Ed. Edited by G.L. Mandell, R.G. Douglas, Jr., and J.E. Bennett. New York, Churchill Livingstone, 1990, pp. 1352–1359.
204. Morens, D.M., Zweighaft, R.M., and Bryan, J.M.: Non-polio enterovirus disease in the United States. Int. J. Epidemiol., *8*:49–54, 1979.
205. Modlin, J.F.: Coxsackieviruses, echoviruses, and newer enteroviruses. *In* G.L. Mandell, R.G. Douglas, Jr., and J.E. Bennett. Principles and Practice of Infectious Diseases. 3rd Ed. New York, Churchill Livingstone, 1990, pp. 1367–1383.
206. Hurst, N.P., Martynoga, A.G., Nuki, G., et al.: Coxsackie B infection and arthritis. Br. Med. J., *286*:605, 1983.
207. Roberts-Thomson, P.J., Southwood, R.T., Moore, B.W., et al.: Adult onset Still's disease or coxsackie polyarthritis? Aust. N.Z. J. Med., *16*:509–511, 1986.
208. Sanford, J.P., and Sulkin, S.E.: The clinical spectrum of ECHO-virus infection. N. Engl. J. Med., *261*:1113–1122, 1959.
209. Blotzer, J.W., and Myers, A.R.: Echovirus-associated polyarthritis. Report of a case with synovial fluid and synovial histologic characterization. Arthritis Rheum., *21*:978–981, 1978.
210. Kujala, G., and Newman, J.H.: Isolation of echovirus type 11 from synovial fluid in acute monocytic arthritis. Arthritis Rheum., *28*:98–99, 1985.
211. Ackerson, B.K., Raghunathan, R., Keller, M.A., et al.: Echovirus 11 arthritis in a patient with X-linked agammaglobulinemia. Pediatr. Infect. Dis. J., *6*:485–488, 1987.
212. Frösner, G.: Hepatitis A virus. *In* Textbook of Human Virology. 2nd Ed. Edited by R.B. Belshe. St. Louis, MO, Mosby Year Book, 1991, pp. 498–516.
213. Klemola, E., and Torma, S.: Arthralgia and arthritis caused by infectious hepatitis. Ann. Med. Intern. Fenn., *38*:161–166, 1949.
214. Routenberg, J.A., Dienstag, J.L., Harrison, W.O., et al.: Foodborne outbreak of hepatitis A: Clinical and laboratory features of acute and protracted illness. Am. J. Med. Sci., *278*:123–137, 1979.
215. Fernandez, R., and McCarty, D.J.: The arthritis of viral hepatitis. Ann. Intern. Med., *74*:207–211, 1971.
216. Shalit, M., Wollner, S., and Levo, Y.: Cryoglobulinemia in acute type-A hepatitis. Clin. Exp. Immunol., *47*:613–616, 1982.
217. Inman, R.D., Hodge, M., Johnston, M.E.A., et al.: Arthritis, vasculitis, and cryoglobulinemia associated with relapsing hepatitis A virus infection. Ann. Intern. Med., *105*:700–703, 1986.
218. Baxby, D.: Poxviruses. *In* Textbook of Human Virology. 2nd Ed. Edited by R.B. Belshe. St. Louis, MO, Mosby Year Book, 1991, pp. 930–946.
219. Cockshott, P., and MacGregor, M.: Osteomyelitis variolosa. Q. J. Med., *27*:369–387, 1958.
220. Silby, H.M., Farber, R., O'Connell, C.J., et al.: Acute monoarticular arthritis after vaccination. Report of a case with isolation of vaccinia virus from synovial fluid. Ann. Intern. Med., *62*:347–350, 1965.
221. Holtzman, C.M.: Postvaccination arthritis. N. Engl. J. Med., *280*:111–112, 1969.
222. Nitzkin, J.L., Anderson, L., Skaggs, J.W., and Hernandez, C.: Complications of smallpox vaccination in Kentucky in 1968. Results of a statewide survey. J. Ky. Med. Assoc., *69*:184–190, 1971.

120

Lyme Disease

DANIEL W. RAHN
STEPHEN E. MALAWISTA

Lyme disease is a tick-borne immune-mediated inflammatory disorder caused by a spirochete, Borrelia burgdorferi. Its clinical hallmark is an early expanding skin lesion, *erythema chronicum migrans* (*ECM*), which can be followed weeks to months later by neurologic, cardiac, or joint abnormalities. Symptoms refer to any one of these four systems alone or in combination. All stages of Lyme disease can respond to antibiotics, but treatment of early disease is the most successful. Foci of Lyme disease are widely distributed within the United States and Europe.

HISTORY

"Lyme arthritis" was recognized in November, 1975 because of an unusual geographic cluster of children with inflammatory arthropathy in the region of Lyme, Connecticut.[1] Its early elucidation—natural history,[1–6] immunopathogenesis,[7–11] epidemiology,[12–15] pathology,[2,4,11] and therapy[16–19]—was carried out primarily at Yale University by Steere and Malawista and their colleagues. It soon became clear that this was a multisystem disorder (Lyme *disease*[2–6]) occurring at any age, in both sexes, and often preceeded by a characteristic expanding skin lesion, ECM (Afzelius, 1909[20]). In Europe ECM had been associated with the bite of the sheep tick, Ixodes ricinus,[21] and with tick-borne meningopolyneuritis (Garin-Bujadoux, 1922;[22] Bannwarth, 1941 and 1944[23]); these syndromes are now often subsumed under the names Lyme disease or Lyme borreliosis. In the Lyme region, a closely related deer tick, I. dammini (a member of the so-called I. ricinus complex), was implicated as the principal disease vector on epidemiologic grounds.[12–15]

In 1982, Burgdorfer and associates isolated the spirochete that now bears his name from I. dammini collected on Shelter Island, New York, and linked it serologically to patients with Lyme disease.[24] Within months of its discovery this organism was cultured from blood, skin, and cerebrospinal fluid (CSF) of Lyme disease patients, and specific IgM and IgG antibody responses were delineated.[25,26] Because it is infectious in origin but inflammatory or "rheumatic" in expression, Lyme disease, beyond its intrinsic interest as a new nosologic entity, presents a unique human model of an infectious etiology of rheumatic disease.[27]

PATHOGENESIS

The Lyme disease spirochete has been classified as a Borrelia rather than a Leptospire or Treponeme, the other two spirochetes pathogenic for man. All clinical isolates to date have belonged to a single species: Borrelia burgdorferi (Fig. 120–1),[28] although variation in the antigenic structure of surface proteins[29] and plasmid composition of different isolates[30,31] has been described. This organism also causes an early skin lesion, benign lymphocytoma,[32] and a late one, *acrodermatitis chronica atrophicans*,[32,33] both seen thus far primarily in Europe.

Recovery of B. burgdorferi is straightforward from infected ticks (see below) but generally difficult from patients, perhaps because of a paucity of organisms present during human infection. An exception is the culture of infecting organisms from ECM biopsy specimens in improved media: for example, 6 of 14 in one study;[34] 9 of 13 in another.[33] Nevertheless, B. burgdorferi has been cultured from involved tissues during all stages of the illness—from blood (early),[25,26,35] secondary annular lesions,[33] meningitic cerebrospinal fluid,[25]

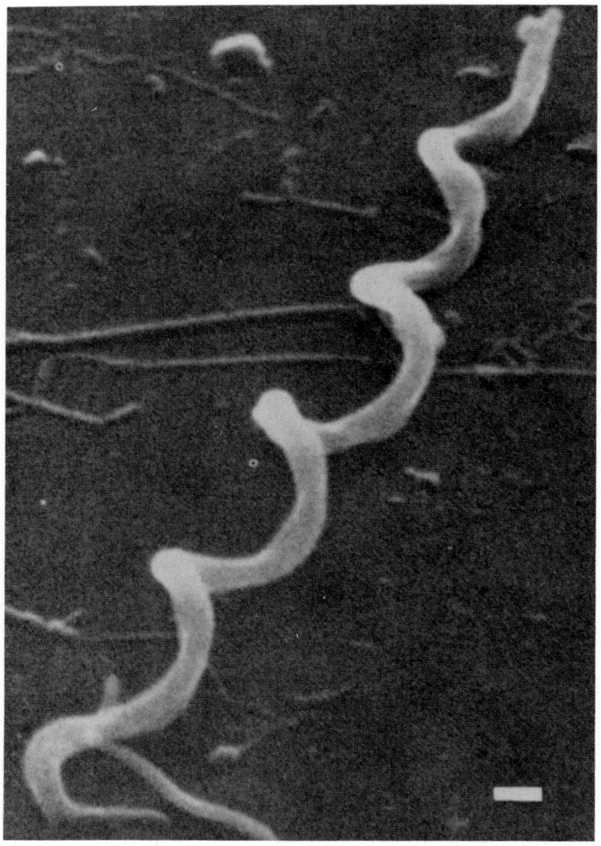

FIGURE 120–1. Scanning electron micrograph of Borrelia burgdorferi isolated from the spinal fluid of a patient with meningoencephalitis[25] whose Lyme disease had begun 2½ months earlier with erythema chronicum migrans. Bar = 0.5 μm. From Johnson, R.C., Hyde, F.W., and Rumpel, C.M.: Taxonomy of the Lyme disease spirochetes. Yale J. Biol. Med., 57:529–537, 1984.

joint fluid,[36] and even from an acrodermatitis chronica atrophicans that had been present for over 10 years.[33] Spirochetes have been identified by silver stain or by immunofluorescence in histologic sections of ECM,[37] and rarely of secondary annular lesions,[38] synovium,[39] brain,[40] eye,[41] heart,[42,43] spleen,[44] liver,[45] kidney, bone marrow,[46] and skeletal muscle.[47]

From these data, combined with the known clinical and epidemiologic features of Lyme disease (see below), the following pathogenetic sequence is likely. Borrelia burgdorferi is transmitted to the skin of the host via the tick vector. After an incubation period of 3 to 32 days,[6] the replicating organisms migrate outward in the skin (ECM), and disseminate hematogenously to secondary skin sites (secondary annular lesions) and other organs (e.g., central nervous system, liver, spleen, eye, skeletal muscle, and heart). Maternal-fetal transmission can occur, albeit rarely.[48,49] Later, chronic manifestations have been largely limited to the nervous system,[3,50–54] joints,[55,56] and skin.[33] It is not yet clear whether live spirochetes persist throughout the course of Lyme disease in all circumstances.[56] Evidence favoring persistence includes the response of most patients to antibiotics (see below), the rare sightings of spirochetes in affected tissues and fluids (see above), the antigen-specific proliferation of T-lymphocytes from affected organs,[57,58] and the expansion of the antibody response to include additional spirochetal antigens over time.[59]

Lyme disease is associated with characteristic immune abnormalities.[7–10] At disease onset (ECM), almost all patients have evidence of circulating immune complexes.[9,10] At that time, the findings of elevated serum IgM levels and cryoglobulins containing IgM predict subsequent nervous system, heart, or joint involvement[7,8]—that is, early humoral findings have prognostic significance. These abnormalities tend to persist during neurologic or cardiac involvement. Later in the illness, when arthritis is present, serum IgM levels are more often normal; immune complexes, often no longer detectably elevated in serum, are elevated uniformly in joint fluid,[10] where titers correlate positively with the local concentrations of polymorphonuclear leukocytes.[60] Microscopic examination of the synovial lesion of individuals with active Lyme arthritis reveals a dense infiltrate of lymphocytes and plasma cells, presumably responding to local spirochetal antigens.[2] Local production of antibody in the CSF is a hallmark of chronic neurologic involvement.[52,54] Thus, an initially disseminated, immune-mediated inflammatory disorder becomes in some patients localized and propagated in joints or in the central nervous system. (Inflammatory mediators are noted below under Arthritis.)

Individuals with the class II human leukocyte antigens (HLAs) DR4, DR2, or both are more likely to develop chronic arthritis refractory to antibiotic therapy.[4,56] Thus, a patient's immunogenetic background can determine what kind of immune response to antigens from the Lyme spirochete he or she might experience, which in turn determines the clinical pattern of disease.

EPIDEMIOLOGY

Although Lyme disease occurs in wide distribution, most cases in the United States occur in three distinct pockets of endemicity: the Northeast from Massachusetts to Maryland, the Midwest in Wisconsin and Minnesota, and the West in California and southern Oregon.[14,46] In 1989 there were more than 7000 new cases nationally reported to the Centers for Disease Control; the vast majority of new cases occurred in those three endemic areas.[61] However, the illness has been reported in 43 states as well as throughout Europe and the Soviet Union, and in China, Japan, and Australia.[62–66] The earliest known U.S. cases occurred on Cape Cod in 1962 and in Lyme, Connecticut in 1965,[14] but studies utilizing the polymerase chain reaction have indicated the presence of the Lyme spirochete in museum specimens of ticks from the region of Montauk, Long Island, New York as early as the 1940s.[67] Total cases reported in the United States now exceed 20,000. Disease can occur at any age and in either sex but there tends to be an increase in incidence in children under age 15 and in middle-aged adults, probably related to activities that place them at higher risk for contact with an infected tick vector.[15] Onset of illness is generally between May 1 and November 30 in temperate climates,with the peak in June and July.[6]

The primary vectors of Lyme disease are tiny hard-bodied ticks of the Ixodes ricinus complex: major foci of disease correspond to the distribution of I. dammini (Northeast and Midwest),[14,62] I. pacificus (West),[14,62] I. ricinus (Europe and Western Soviet Union),[62–64]and I. persulcatus (Soviet Union, China, and Japan[65]). However, Australia has Lyme disease but lacks ticks of the I. ricinus complex,[66] and other vectors, including the lone star tick, Amblyomma americanum, are likely to some areas of the Untied States.[68,69] Biting insects are possible secondary vectors.[70,71]

In one U.S. study, 31% of 314 patients recalled a tick bite at the skin site where ECM developed days to weeks later; most patients, therefore, were unaware of having been bitten.[6] The six ticks that were saved were all nymphal I. dammini, whose peak questing period is May through July, and which is the primary vector responsible for transmission of the infecting organism to humans.[72] This tick has a life cycle (larva, nymph, and adult) spanning 2 years.[72] Both larvae and nymphs feed preferentially on a variety of small mammals, especially the white-footed mouse (Peromyscus leukopus), which appears to be the most important reservoir of Borrelia burgdorferi.[13,72,73] Infected nymphs feed on and transmit spirochetes to mice from which previously uninfected larval ticks subsequently acquire infection (Fig. 120–2). Adult I. dammini feed primarily on larger mammals, especially white-tailed deer.[74] In areas endemic for Lyme disease, the prevalence of B. burgdorferi

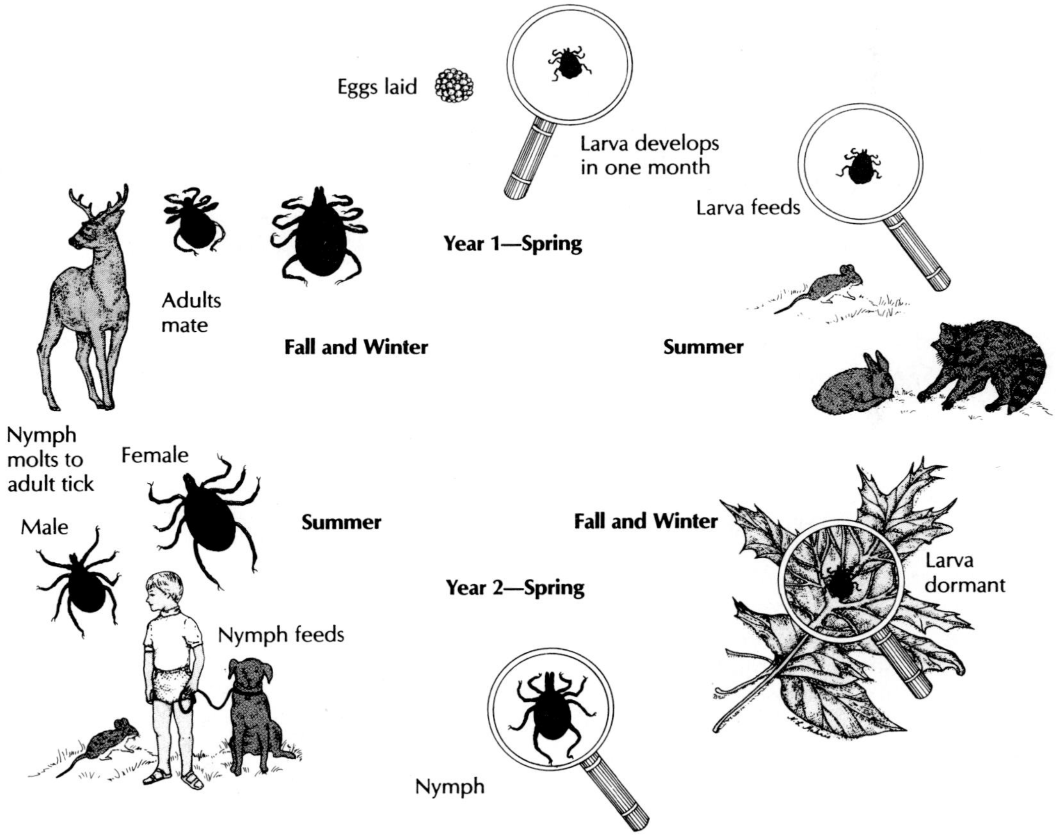

FIGURE 120–2. Life cycle of Ixodes dammini spans 2 years. In the spring of the first year (top), eggs hatch and six-legged larvae develop. In the summer, the larvae feed once. From their preferred host, the white-footed mouse, they acquire Borrelia burgdorferi, the spirochete that causes Lyme disease. Next spring (bottom), the larvae molt into eight-legged nymphs, which feed once. Again, mice are the preferred host; humans to whom the ticks transmit Lyme disease are not necessary for maintenance of the ticks' life cycle. The nymphs molt into adult male and female ticks. Mating often occurs while the female is feeding on a deer. The male might remain on the deer; the female drops off and subsequently lays her eggs. This figure is based on research by Andrew Spielman and colleagues. From Rahn, D.W., and Malawista, S.E.: Clinical judgment in Lyme disease. Hosp. Pract., *25*:39–56, 1990.

in nymphal Ixodes dammini ranges from about 20% to over 60%.[24,25,69] This can be compared with an infection rate of 0.9 to 2% in I. pacificus, which feeds preferentially on lizards that are incompetent reservoirs of Borrelia burgdorferi.[75]

The organism has been isolated, or specific antibody has been found, in blood and tissues of a wide variety of large and small animals, including domestic dogs, which can develop arthritis, and birds, which provide a natural means of distributing infected and uninfected ticks to new locales.[76–80] Indiscriminate feeding on a variety of animals by infected immature Ixodes dammini might favor the spread of infection.

CLINICAL CHARACTERISTICS

Lyme disease progresses through a series of clinical stages from early, localized, cutaneous involvement (ECM) or a flu-like illness (stage 1), through a period weeks to months later during which cardiac and nervous system inflammation predominate (stage 2), to a third, chronic stage primarily involving joints (stage 3). Chronic neurologic and skin involvement can also occur years after onset. This staging system is somewhat arbitrary, however, and time course and clinical expression vary considerably among different patients. Stages can overlap or be skipped entirely; in fact, seroconversion can occur without any symptoms having been recognized.[81,82]

EARLY MANIFESTATIONS

Erythema chronicum migrans, the unique clinical marker for Lyme disease, begins as a red macule or papule at the site of a tick bite.[2,6] Only a minority of affected individuals are aware of having been bitten, however. After an incubation period of a few days to a month, the area of redness expands to 15 cm or so (range, 3 to 68 cm), usually with partial central clearing (Fig. 120–3). The outer border is red, generally flat, and without scaling. The center is occasionally indurated, vesicular, or necrotic. Variations can occur—multiple rings, for example. The thigh, groin, and axilla are particularly common sites. The lesion is warm to touch but no often sore, and easily missed if out of sight. Routine histology is nonspecific: a heavy dermal infiltrate of mononuclear cells without epidermal change except at the site of the tick bite.

Within days of onset of ECM, half of U.S. patients develop multiple annular secondary lesions signaling early dissemination of the spirochete (Fig. 120–3; Table 120–1). Secondary lesions resemble ECM itself, but are generally smaller, migrate less, and lack indurated centers. Individual lesions can come and go, and their borders sometimes merge. Other less common skin lesions are noted in Table 120–1. In addition, benign lymphocytoma cutis has been reported in Europe.[32] ECM and secondary lesions fade even without treatment in 3 to 4 weeks (range, 1 day to 14 months) but can recur.

TABLE 120–1. EARLY SIGNS OF LYME DISEASE

SIGNS	NO. OF PATIENTS N = 314	(%)
Erythema chronicum migrans*	314	(100)
Multiple annular lesions	150	(48)
Lymphadenopathy		
Regional	128	(41)
Generalized	63	(20)
Pain on neck flexion	52	(17)
Malar rash	41	(13)
Erythematous throat	38	(12)
Conjunctivitis	35	(11)
Right upper quadrant tenderness	24	(8)
Splenomegaly	18	(6)
Hepatomegaly	16	(5)
Muscle tenderness	12	(4)
Periorbital edema	10	(3)
Evanescent skin lesions	8	(3)
Abdominal tenderness	6	(2)
Testicular swelling	2	(1)

* Erythema chronicum migrans was required for inclusion in this study.

From Steere, A.C., et al.: The early clinical manifestations of Lyme disease. Ann. Intern. Med., 99:79, 1983.

TABLE 120–2. EARLY SYMPTOMS OF LYME DISEASE

SYMPTOMS	NO. OF PATIENTS N = 314	(%)
Malaise, fatigue, and lethargy	251	(80)
Headache	200	(64)
Fever and chills	185	(59)
Stiff neck	151	(48)
Arthalgias	150	(48)
Myalgias	135	(43)
Backache	81	(26)
Anorexia	73	(23)
Sore throat	53	(17)
Nausea	53	(17)
Dysesthesia	35	(11)
Vomiting	32	(10)
Abdominal pain	24	(8)
Photophobia	19	(6)
Hand stiffness	16	(5)
Dizziness	15	(5)
Cough	15	(5)
Chest pain	12	(4)
Ear pain	12	(4)
Diarrhea	6	(2)

From Steere, A.C., et al.: The early clinical manifestations of Lyme disease. Ann. Intern. Med., *99*:79, 1983.

ECM is often accompanied by acute, flu-like symptoms—malaise and fatigue, headache, fever and chills, myalgia, and arthralgia (Table 120–2).[2,6] Some patients have brief (hours in duration) episodic attacks of excruciating headache, difficulty in concentrating, and neck pain, stiffness, or pressure suggesting meningeal irritation or mild encephalopathy, but spinal fluid pleocytosis is uncommon within the first few weeks of illness.[3] Except for fatigue and lethargy, which are often constant,

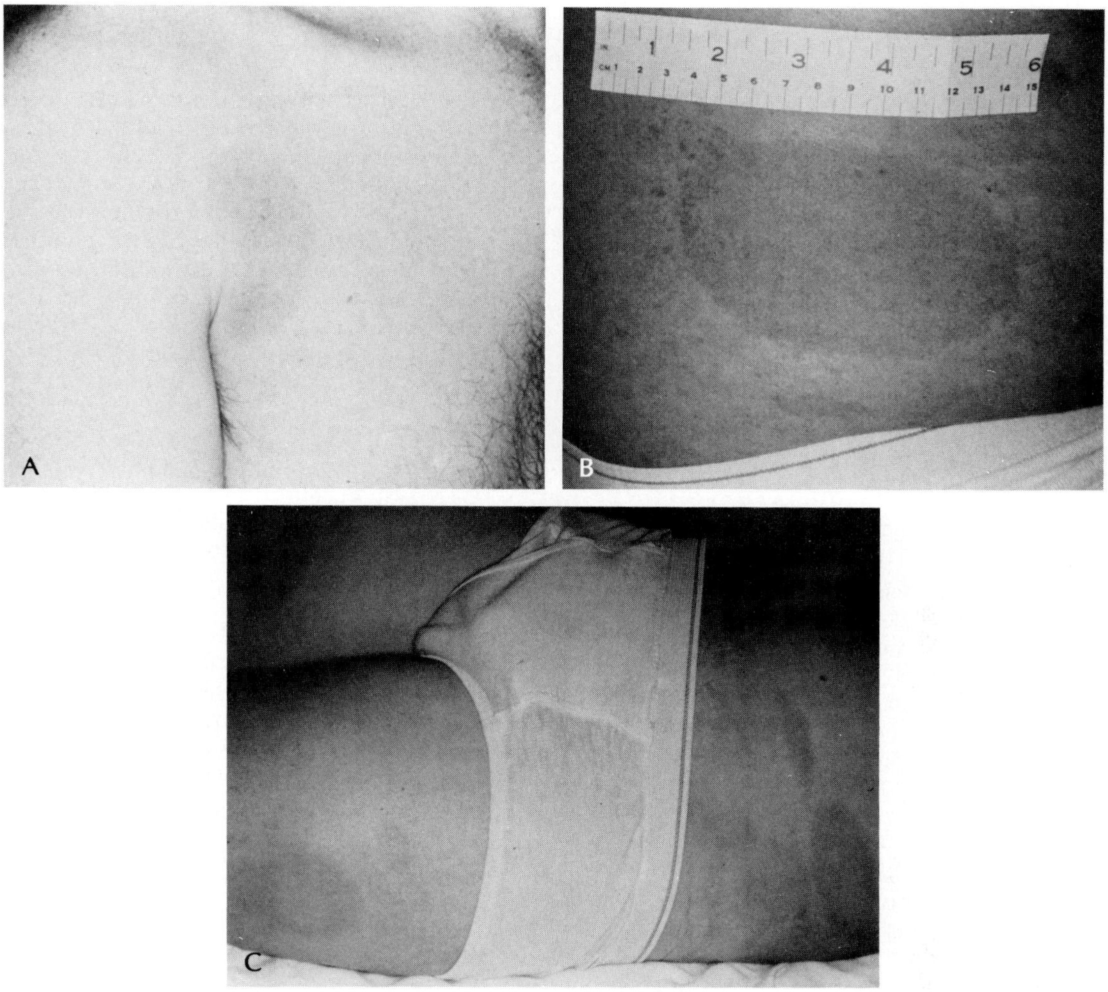

FIGURE 120–3. Dermatologic manifestations of Lyme disease. *A,* Erythema chronicum migrans (ECM). An early lesion is seen 4 days after detection. *B,* In a 10-day lesion of ECM, the red outer ring has expanded and central clearing is beginning. *C,* Eight days after onset of ECM, similar secondary lesions have appeared, and several of their borders have merged. From Steere, A.C., et al.: The early clinical manifestations of Lyme disease. Ann. Intern. Med., *99*:76–82, 1983.

the early signs and symptoms are typically intermittent and changing. A patient might have headache and neck stiffness for several days, to be replaced by migratory musculoskeletal pain involving one to a few joints (generally without swelling), tendons, bursae, muscles, or bone. Pain can last a few hours to several days in a given location. These systemic symptoms can occur several days before ECM appears (or without it) and last for months (especially fatigue and lethargy) after the skin lesions have disappeared.

In Europe, untreated ECM more commonly has a prolonged, indolent course, and is less commonly associated with multiple annular lesions, pronounced generalized symptoms, laboratory abnormalities, or subsequent arthritis.[83]

LATER MANIFESTATIONS

Neurologic Involvement. Within several weeks to months of the onset of illness, a minority of patients (15% in one series[3]) develop definite neurologic abnormalities. Manifestations variously involve either the central[51,52] or peripheral nervous system.[53] The commonest early abnormalities are meningitis with or without accompanying encephalopathy, cranial neuritis (most commonly involving the facial nerve, which can be affected bilaterally[84]), and motor or sensory radiculoneuritis (Fig. 120–4).[3,50] Less common conditions, which can occur much later in disease, have included chorea, focal demyelinating encephalopathy or myelopathy, chronic encephalopathy, peripheral polyneu-

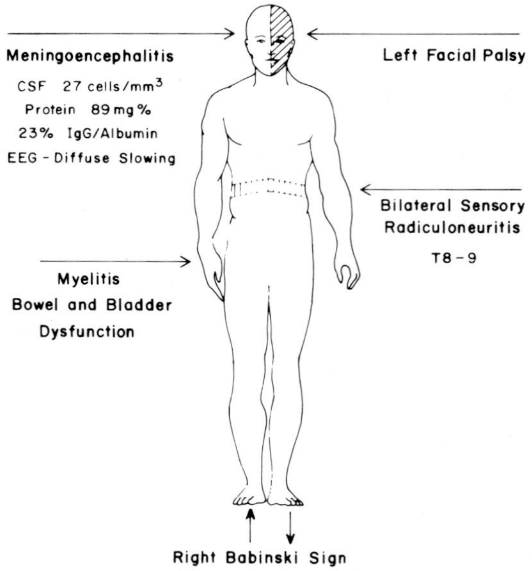

FIGURE 120–4. Neurologic abnormalities of Lyme disease that occurred in a 58-year-old man. Three weeks after the onset of erythema chronicum migrans, the patient developed meningoencephalitis, left facial palsy, and bilateral sensory radiculoneuritis. Although long-tract signs are unusual in Lyme disease, this patient had bowel and bladder dysfunction and a right Babinski sign, suggestive of myelitis.

ropathy, and transverse myelitis.[3,52–54,85] Any of these manifestations can occur *alone.*[50]

Lyme meningitis is characterized by lymphocytic pleocytosis (about 100 cells per mm^3), mild protein elevation, and normal glucose in cerebrospinal fluid. Headache sometimes is excrutiating and frequently fluctuates from day to day or even hour to hour. However, the neck is rarely stiff except on extreme flexion; Kernig's and Brudzinski's signs are absent. Encephalopathy is usually subtle with mild impairment of mentation or memory and diffuse slowing on electroencephalogram. These relatively acute neurologic manifestations will resolve spontaneously but often only after persisting for months.[3]

Chronic neurologic disease can first appear years after onset of disease, is typically subtle and difficult to diagnose definitively, and does not remit spontaneously.[54,86] Cognitive deficits and sensory polyneuropathy with distal paresthesias and abnormalities on electromyography or nerve conduction testing are both recently recognized late neurologic manifestations of Lyme disease.[52–54] Although "progressive Borrelia encephalomyelitis"[87] is currently seen more frequently in Europe than in the United States, this could be due to the more recent appearance of Lyme disease on this continent. Central nervous system manifestations are usually associated with local synthesis of immunoglobulin within the cerebrospinal fluid resulting in oligoclonal bands or hyperconcentration of specific antibody (see below), findings that can be useful diagnostically.[52,54]

Cardiac Involvement. Carditis occurs within weeks to months of onset in up to 8% of patients.[12] The commonest clinical manifestation is fluctuating atrioventricular block (first degree, Wenckebach, or complete heart block). Occasionally the heart is affected more diffusely with electrocardiographic changes compatible with acute myopericarditis, radionuclide evidence of contractile dysfunction, or rarely, cardiomegaly.[5,88] Biopsy-proven endomyocarditis[43,88] and, in one fatal case, spirochete-positive pancarditis[42] have been reported. No patients have had significant valvular lesions (compare with acute rheumatic fever).[5] Carditis is usually brief and self-limited (3 days to 6 weeks). Although clinical manifestations are usually limited to the conduction system, subclinical involvement can be more extensive.[43] Carditis, like other symptoms of disseminated disease, can be the presenting manifestation of Lyme disease.[89]

Arthritis. From weeks to as long as 2 years after the onset of illness, about 60% of patients develop frank arthritis,[2,4,11] usually characterized by intermittent attacks of asymmetric joint swelling and pain primarily in large joints, especially the knee, one or two joints at a time. The onset of overt arthritis is sometimes preceeded by months of migratory myalgias and arthralgias. Attacks typically begin suddenly; effusions can be massive and lead to the formation of Baker's cysts, which can dissect into the calf and rupture. However, both large and small joints can be affected, and a few patients have had symmetric polyarthritis. Attacks of arthritis, which generally last from weeks to months, typically recur for several years but decrease in frequency by 10 to 20% per year.[55] Fatigue commonly accompanies active joint involvement, but fever or other systemic symptoms are unusual. Joint fluid white cell counts vary widely from 500 to 110,000 cells/mm^3 and average about 25,000 cells/mm^3 with a predominance of polymorphonuclear leukocytes.[2] Total protein has ranged from 3 to 8 g/dl. C3 and C4 levels are usually greater than one-third, and glucose levels usually greater than two-thirds that of serum. Tests for rheumatoid factor and antinuclear antibody are generally negative.

In about 10% of patients with arthritis, especially those with HLA class II antigen DR4 or DR2, involvement in large joints can become chronic, with pannus formation and erosion of cartilage and bone (Fig. 120–5A).[4,11,55,56] The chronic synovial lesion mimics rheumatoid arthritis, with surface deposits of fibrin, villous hypertrophy, vascular proliferation, and a heavy infiltration of mononuclear cells (Fig. 120–5B).[2,4,11] In addition, there may be an obliterative endarteritis and (rarely) demonstrable spirochetes.[39] Borrelia burgdorferi potently stimulates mononuclear phagocytes to produce interleukin-1, which is found in synovial fluids.[90] Synovium from one patient with chronic Lyme arthritis, when grown in tissue culture, produced large amounts

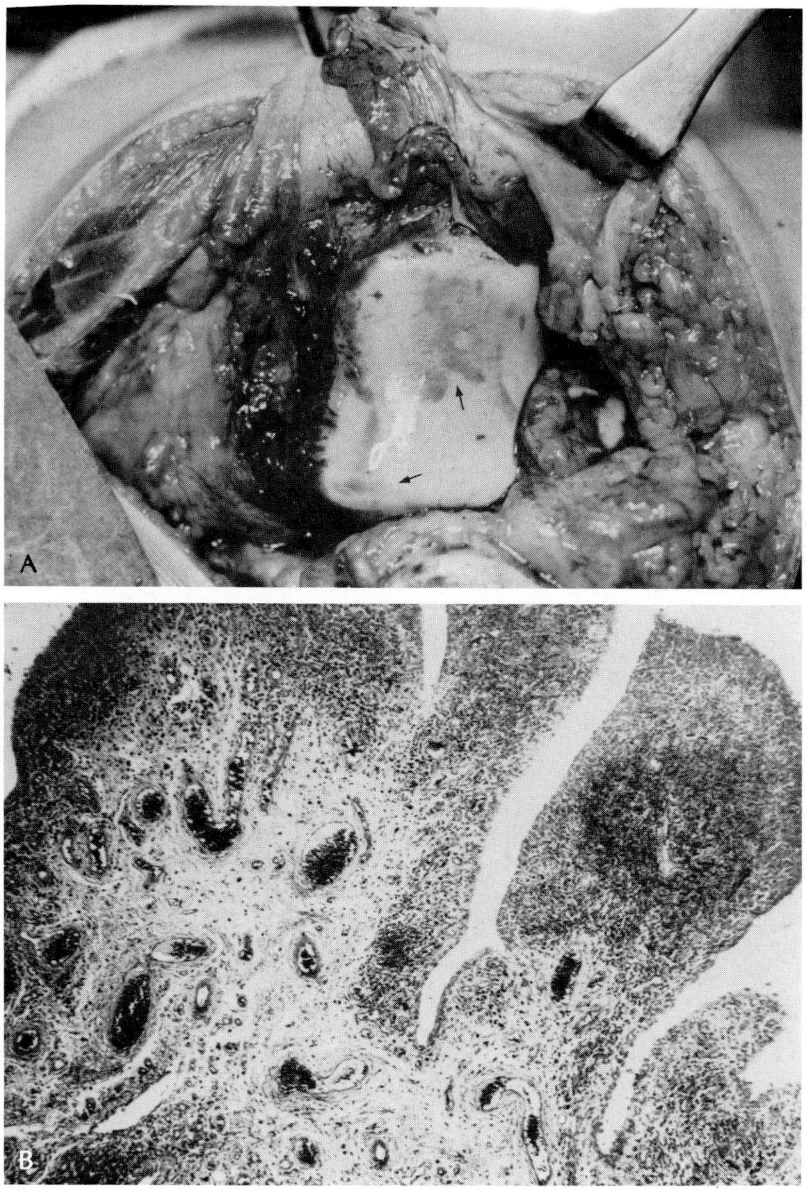

FIGURE 120–5. *A*, The knee of a patient with Lyme disease at the time of synovectomy. The patient had typical erythema chronicum migrans in June, 1974, followed by intermittent migratory polyarthritis. Two years later, he developed persistent swelling of the right knee. After 7 months, he underwent synovectomy. The articular surface of the femur can be seen; the arrows indicate what was the advancing border of pannus, now stripped away from the underlying eroded cartilage. *B*, Tissue structure of affected synovium. Individual polypoid stalks show central edema and vascular proliferation. Surrounding this central core is a rim of predominantly; mononuclear cells. In one area an aggregate resembling a lymphoid follicle is seen. From Steere, A.C., et al.: Erythema chronicum migrans and Lyme arthritis: the enlarging clinical spectrum. Ann. Intern. Med., *86*:693, 1977.

of collagenase and prostaglandin E_2.[11] Thus, in chronic Lyme arthritis the joint fluid cell counts, the immune reactants (except for rheumatoid factor), the synovial histology, the amounts of inflammatory mediators released, and the resulting destruction of cartilage and bone can be similar to those in rheumatoid arthritis.[91]

Another late finding (one seen after years) associated with this infection is a chronic skin lesion—acrodermatitis chronica atrophicans[32,33]—well known in Europe but still rare in the United States.[92] Lesions begin as violaceous infiltrated plaques or nodules, especially on extensor surfaces of acral areas of extremities. Eventually epidermal and dermal atrophy develop. There can be underlying joint changes.

LABORATORY TESTS

Determination of specific antibody titers is the most helpful diagnostic test for Lyme disease. Culture of B. burgdorferi from patients permits definitive diagnosis, but is rarely successful except from skin.[25,33,34] Similarly, spirochetes are not often seen by direct examination of blood, plasma, plasma pellets, or skin transudate specimens of ECM,[25] and special tissue staining techniques[37–39] are low-yield and not readily available.

When determined by immunofluorescence or enzyme-linked immunosorbent assay (ELISA), specific IgM antibody titers against B. burgdorferi usually reach a peak between the third and sixth week after the onset

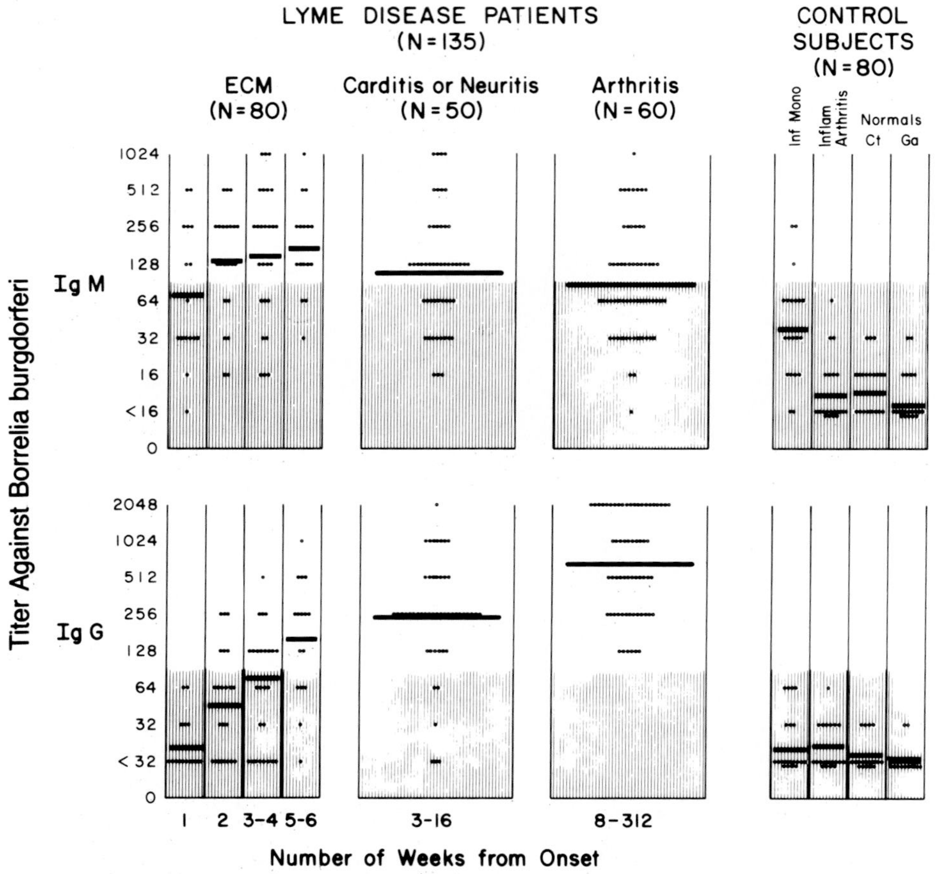

FIGURE 120–6. Antibody titers against Borrelia burgdorferi in serum samples from 135 patients with different clinical manifestations of Lyme disease, from 40 control patients with infectious mononucleosis or inflammatory arthritis, and from 40 normal control subjects, as determined by indirect immunofluorescence. The heavy bar shows the geometric mean titer for each group; the shaded areas indicate the range of titers generally observed in control subjects. Note that all patients with Lyme arthritis have elevated IgG antibody titers. From Steere, A.C., et al.: The spirochetal etiology of Lyme disease. N. Engl. J. Med., *308*:733–740, 1983.

of disease; specific IgG antibody titers rise more slowly and are generally highest months later when arthritis is present (Fig. 120–6).[25,93] Antibody titers against B. burgdorferi are particularly useful in differentiating Lyme *arthritis* from other rheumatic syndromes, especially when ECM is missed, forgotten, or absent. Borrelia burgdorferi contains epitopes that are cross-reactive with other spirochetes, including Treponema pallidum, but patients with Lyme disease do not have positive results with the Venereal Disease Research Laboratory (VDRL) test.[6,93] Low-titer false positivity is and will remain a problem until antibody tests for the Lyme spirochete have been standardized; at present Lyme titers can only be properly interpreted in the appropriate clinical context.[94–96] A few cases of true seronegative Lyme disease have been reported,[97] but this is a rare phenomenon with carefully-performed assays. Tests of T-cell blastogenic response to Borrelia burgdorferi antigens have demonstrated that a cell-mediated immune response occurs early after onset of infection, but such tests have not been useful in routine clinical practice because of the rarity with which T-cell tests are positive when routine serologies are negative.[97,98]

The determination of cerebrospinal fluid antibody levels is a useful adjunct in the diagnosis of neurologic involvement with Lyme disease.[52,54] When infection involves the central nervous system (CNS), specific antibody is secreted within the CNS by local B-cells, leading to an increased concentration of antibody in the CSF compared with simultaneous levels in serum (when corrected for total IgG). Such hyperconcentration of specific antibody is the best laboratory evidence of CNS Lyme disease.[99]

The most common nonspecific laboratory abnormalities, particularly early in the illness, are a high erythrocyte sedimentation rate, an elevated serum IgM level, and a transiently increased serum glutamic oxaloacetic transaminase (SGOT) level (Table 120–3).[2,7] Patients

TABLE 120–3. LABORATORY FINDINGS IN EARLY LYME DISEASE

LABORATORY TEST	NO. OF PATIENTS WITH ABNORMAL VALUES N = 314	(%)	MEDIAN (RANGE) OF ABNORMAL VALUES
Hematology			
Hematocrit	37	(12)	35 (36–81)
Leukocytes >10 cells × 10^3/mm^3	24	(8)	12 (11–18)
ESR >20 mm/hour	166	(53)	35 (21–58)
Immunoglobulins			
IgM >250 mg/dl	104	(33)	310 (252–930)
IgG >1500 mg/dl	10	(3)	1550 (1520–1760)
IgA >400 mg/dl	12	(4)	440 (410–580)
Liver Function			
SGOT >35 U/ml	59	(18)	71 (36–251)
SGPT >32 U/ml*	47	(15)	125 (42–491)
LDH >600 U/ml*	49	(16)	775 (608–1080)
Renal Function			
Microscopic hematuria (red cells/hpl)	18	(6)	15 (10–25)

* Tested only in the 55 patients with abnormal SGOT; CPK was normal in all these patients.
From Steere, A.C., et al.: The early clinical manifestations of Lyme disease. Ann. Intern. Med. *99*:80, 1983.

can be mildly anemic early in the illness and occasionally have elevated white cell counts with shifts to the left in the differential count. A few patients have had microscopic hematuria, sometimes with mild proteinuria (dipstick); values for creatinine and blood urea nitrogen have been normal. Throughout the illness, serum C3 and C4 levels are generally normal or elevated. Tests for rheumatoid factor and antinuclear antibodies are usually negative.

DIFFERENTIAL DIAGNOSIS

Erythema chronicum migrans is the unique herald lesion of Lyme disease (Fig. 120–3). When present in its classic form, there is little else that might be confused with it. However, some patients are not aware of having had ECM, and in others its appearance is atypical. Secondary lesions might suggest *erythema multiforme,* but blistering, mucosal lesions and involvement of the palms and soles are not features of Lyme disease. Malar rash can suggest systemic lupus erythematosus. Rarely patients develop an urticarial rash which may be confused with hepatitis B infection or serum sickness. Evanescent blotches and circles sometimes resemble *erythema marginatum,* but those of Lyme disease do not expand.

Early flu-like symptoms (fever, mycologia, arthralgia) can be misleading, especially when ECM is absent or missed or is not the first manifestation. Severe headache and stiff neck can suggest aseptic meningitis; abdominal symptoms, hepatitis; and generalized tender lymphadenopathy and splenomegaly, infectious mononucleosis. As in the last infection, profound fatigue in Lyme disease can be a major and persistent complaint.

In later stages Lyme disease can mimic other immune-mediated disorders. Like rheumatic fever, Lyme disease can be associated with sore throat followed by migratory polyarthritis and carditis, but without evidence of valvular involvement or of a preceding streptococcal infection. Migratory pain in tendons and joints can also suggest disseminated gonococcal disease. An isolated facial weakness can mimic other causes of Bell's palsy. Late neurologic involvement might suggest multiple sclerosis (transverse myelitis), Guillain-Barré syndrome (symmetric peripheral neuropathy), primary psychosis, or brain tumor. Chronic fatigue alone is not a manifestation of active Lyme disease. In adults with Lyme arthritis the large knee effusions can resemble those in Reiter's syndrome, and the occasional symmetric polyarthritis, that of rheumatoid arthritis. In children, the attacks of arthritis, although generally shorter, can be identical to those seen in the oligoarticular form of juvenile rheumatoid arthritis, but without iridocyclitis. Although fibromyalgia occasionally occurs as a sequel to Lyme disease, it is not an indication of persistent infection.[100,101]

TREATMENT

STAGE 1

Early Lyme disease responds promptly to oral antibiotic therapy, particularly when localized to a single skin lesion with minimal or no associated systemic symptoms. Erythema chronicum migrans resolves in days and subsequent major sequelae (myocarditis, meningoencephalitis, or recurrent arthritis) are prevented.[17,102,103] Signs of early dissemination (multiple secondary skin lesions, myalgias, arthralgias, fever, headache, stiff neck, or photophobia) might reflect more-pervasive infection (disseminated stage 1) with a greater likelihood of recurring after oral antibiotics, particularly when neurologic symptoms are present.[17,103] Prompt treatment is therefore important prior to dissemination. Patients treated early can be susceptible to reinfection.[104] For adults, preferred regimens include oral doxycycline 100 mg twice daily or amoxicillin 500 mg three times a day, to which some authors recommend the addition of probenecid 500 mg three times daily[102,105] (pediatric dose: 30 mg/kg per day) each for 10 to 20 days, depending on the severity of illness at presentation and rapidity of response; in general, patients with early dissemination should be given a longer course of therapy.[105,106] In the case of penicillin allergy, erythromycin 250 mg four times a day is the current alternative for pregnant or lactating women with early localized infection or children younger than 9 years (pediatric dose: 30 mg/kg per day, in divided doses), but outcomes with this agent have been less satisfactory than with the previous two antibiotics.[17]

Rare, isolated instances of maternal-fetal transmission of Borrelia burgdorferi infection have occurred when maternal Lyme disease has been untreated[46] or inadequately treated[49] during pregnancy. Epidemiologic surveys have failed to demonstrate congenital anomalies clearly attributable to maternal Lyme disease, however,[107] and there is no evidence of risk to a developing fetus ascribable to maternal seropositivity alone in the absence of clinical evidence of active infection.[108] Nevertheless, the available data provide additional impetus for early treatment with amoxicillin or erythromycin for localized early Lyme disease occurring during pregnancy, and consideration of intravenous therapy for more-advanced stages of infection.

About 10% of patients experience a Jarisch-Herxheimer–like reaction (higher fever, redder rash, or greater pain) during the first 24 hours of therapy.[17] Regardless of which drug is selected and the duration of administration, nearly half of patients with disseminated early disease have brief (lasting hours or days) recurrent episodes of headache or pain in joints, tendons, bursae, or muscles, often with ongoing fatigue, which can continue for 3 months or longer after completion of antibiotic therapy.[17,102] These symptoms seem not to reflect continuing infection and do not respond to further antibiotic therapy (they might reflect the persistence of residual undegraded antigen); they eventually resolve spontaneously in almost all cases.[100]

STAGE 2

Meningitis, cranial neuropathies, and radiculoneuritis respond to intravenous penicillin G, 20 million units a day in six divided doses for 10 days,[18] although longer courses (minimum of 14 days) are how generally recommended.[106] Ceftriaxone[109] and cefotaxime[110] have both been found effective when given intravenously for 14 days, and might be superior to penicillin.[109] Meningitic symptoms usually begin to subside by the second day of therapy and disappear by 7 to 10 days. Radicular pain and motor deficits frequently require 7 to 8 weeks for recovery and do not always resolve completely.[18] Optimal duration of antibiotic therapy for neurologic manifestations of Lyme disease is under study; courses longer than 4 weeks have not been examined systematically. Doxycycline 100 mg twice daily for 14 days has been used successfully in Europe for the treatment of radiculoneoropathy,[111] but has not been studied in the United States.

Chronic neurologic manifestations, including encephalopathy and peripheral neuropathy, are less uniformly responsive to antibiotic therapy but usually respond, albeit slowly, to 2 weeks of intravenous ceftriaxone.[52–54] Not unexpectedly, some patients have persistent, nonprogressive deficits after antibiotic therapy.

Carditis responds rapidly (in days) to intravenous antibiotic therapy with one of the above agent,[89] but has also been treated successfully with oral antibiotics, salicylates, or glucocorticoids.[5] Because carditis appears to result from direct myocardial invasion by spirochetes,[43] all cases should be treated with antibiotics. Prednisone, 40 to 60 mg a day in divided doses, produced a rapid resolution of heart block[5] but might interfere with attempts to cure the illness definitively, and for this reason should perhaps be avoided (in any case, spontaneous resolution is the rule). For patients who are allergic to penicillin and cephalosporins, doxycycline 100 mg twice a day for 30 days is reasonable but unevaluated. Temporary pacing might be required; permanent pacing, rarely.[5,89]

STAGE 3

For established Lyme arthritis, even with unremitting involvement, oral doxycycline (100 mg twice daily for 4 weeks) or amoxicillin and probenecid (500 mg each four times daily) cure a majority of patients.[112] Intravenous ceftriaxone is probably as effective when given for 2 weeks and might be superior.[109,112] Parenteral penicillin is curative in some patients.[19] Antibiotic failures occur with all regimens, particularly in individuals of HLA DR4 phenotype.[56] During treatment, the affected joint should be rested, and accumulated fluid should be removed by needle aspirations.[19] Optimal therapy for arthritis, as for the alter neurologic complications of Lyme disease, is not yet clear. In difficult cases longer periods of the highest-tolerated oral doses of amoxicillin (with probenecid), a tetracycline, or longer intravenous therapy with ceftriaxone or penicillin should be considered but require study at present. Synovectomy can be useful for treatment failures, particularly those involving the knee.[113]

Although rarely seen in the United States, the infiltrative lesions of acrodermatitis chronica atrophicans are usually cured by 3 weeks of oral phenoxymethyl penicillin, 2 to 3 g daily in divided doses.[114]

REFERENCES

1. Steere, A.C., Malawista, S.E., Snydman, D.R., et al.: Lyme arthritis: An epidemic of oligoarticular arthritis in children and adults in three Connecticut communities. Arthritis Rheum., *20*:7–17, 1977.
2. Steere, A.C., Malawista, S.E., Hardin, J.A., et al.: Erythema chronicum migrans and Lyme arthritis: The enlarging clinical spectrum. Ann. Intern. Med., *86*:685–698, 1977.
3. Reik, L., Steere, A.C., Bartenhagen, N.H., et al.: Neurologic abnormalities of Lyme disease. Medicine, *58*:281–294, 1979.
4. Steere, A.C., Gibofsky, A., Pattarroyo, M.E., et al.: Chronic Lyme arthritis: Clinical and immunogenetic differentiation from rheumatoid arthritis. Ann. Intern. Med., *90*:286–291, 1979.
5. Steere, A.C., Batsford, W.P., Weinberg, M., et al.: Lyme carditis: Cardiac abnormalities of Lyme disease. Ann. Intern. Med., *93*:8–16, 1980.
6. Steere, A.C., Bartenhagen, N.H., Craft, J.E., et al.: The early clinical manifestations of Lyme disease. Ann. Intern. Med., *99*:76–82, 1983.
7. Steere, A.C., Hardin, J.A., and Malawista, S.E.: Erythema chronicum migrans and Lyme arthritis. Cryoimmunoglobulins and clinical activity of skin and joints. Science, *196*:1121–1122, 1977.
8. Steere, A.C., Hardin, J.A., Ruddy, S., et al.: Lyme arthritis: Correlation of serum and cryoglobulin IgM with activity and serum IgG with remission. Arthritis Rheum., *2*:471–483, 1979.
9. Hardin, J.A., Walker, L.C., Steere, A.C., et al.: Circulating immune complexes in Lyme arthritis: Detection of the ^{125}I-Clq binding, Clq solid phase and Raji cell assays. J. Clin. Invest., *63*:468–477, 1979.
10. Hardin, J.A., Steere, A.C., and Malawista, S.E.: Immune complexes and the evolution of Lyme arthritis: Dissemination and localization of abnormal Clq binding activity. N. Engl. J. Med., *301*:1358–1363, 1979.
11. Steere, A.C., Brinckerhoff, C.E., Miller, D.J., et al.: Elevated levels of collagenase and prostaglandin E2 from synovium associated with erosion of cartilage and bone in a patient with chronic Lyme arthritis. Arthritis Rheum., *23*:591–599, 1980.
12. Steere, A.C., Broderick, T.E., and Malawista, S.E.: Erythema chronicum migrans and Lyme arthritis: Epidemiologic evidence for a tick vector. Am. J. Epidemiol., *108*:312–321, 1978.
13. Wallis, R.C., Brown, S.E., Kloter, K.O., and Main, A.J. Jr.: Erythema chronicum migrans and Lyme arthritis: Field study of ticks. Am. J. Epidemiol., *108*:322–327, 1978.
14. Steere, A.C., and Malawista, S.E.: Cases of Lyme disease in the Untied States: Locations correlated with distribution of Ixodes dammini. Ann. Intern. Med., *91*:730–733, 1979.
15. Steere, A.C., and Malawista, S.E.: The epidemiology of Lyme disease. *In* Current Topics in Rheumatology: Epidemiology of the Rheumatic Diseases. Proceedings of the Fourth International Conference. Edited by R.C. Lawrence and L.E. Schulman. New York, Gower Medical Publishing, 1983, pp. 33–42.
16. Steere, A.C., Malawista, S.E., Newman, J.H., et al.: Antibiotic therapy in Lyme disease. Ann. Intern. Med., *93*:1–8, 1980.
17. Steere, A.C., Hutchinson, G.J., Rahn, D.W., et al.: Treatment of the early manifestations of Lyme disease. Ann. Intern. Med., *99*:22–26, 1983.
18. Steere, A.C., Pachner, A.R., and Malawista, S.E.: Neurologic abnormalities of Lyme disease: Successful treatment with high-dose intravenous penicillin. Ann. Intern. Med., *99*:767–772, 1983.
19. Steere, A.C., Green, J., Schoen, R.T., et al.: Successful parenteral antibiotic therapy of established Lyme arthritis. N. Engl. J. Med., *312*:869–874, 1985.
20. Afzelius, A.: Verhandlungen der Dermatologischen Gesellschaft zu Stockholm on October 29, 1909. Arch. Dermatol. Syph., *101*:404, 1910.
21. Thone, A.W.: *Ixodes ricinus* and Erythema chronicum migrans (Afzelius). Dermatologica, *136*:57–60, 1968.
22. Garin-Bujadoux, C.: Paralysie par les tiques. J. Med. Lyon, *71*:765–767, 1922.
23. Bannwarth, A.: Zur Klink und Pathogenese der "chronischen lymphozytaren Meningitis." Arch. Psychiat. Nervenkr., *117*:161–185, 1944.
24. Burgdorfer, W., Barbour, A.G., Hayes, S.F., et al.: Lyme disease—A tick-borne spirochetosis? Science, *216*:1317–1319, 1982.
25. Steere, A.C., Grodzicki, R.L., Kornblatt, A.N., et al.: The spirochetal etiology of Lyme disease. N. Engl. J. Med., *308*:733–740, 1983.
26. Benach, J.L., Bosler, E.M., Hanrahan, J.P., et al.: Spirochetes isolated from the blood of two patients with Lyme disease. N. Engl. J. Med., *308*:740–742, 1983.
27. Malawista, S.E., Steere, A.C., and Hardin, J.A.: Lyme disease: a unique human model for an infectious etiology of rheumatic disease. Yale J. Biol. Med., *57*:473–477, 1984.
28. Johnson, R.C., Schmid, G.P., Hyde, F.W., et al.: *Borrelia burgdorferi* sp. nov.: Etiologic agent of Lyme disease. Int. J. Syst. Bacteriol., *34*:496–497, 1984.
29. Barbour, A.G., Heiland, R.A., and Howe, T.R.: Heterogeneity of major proteins in Lyme disease Borrelia: A molecular analysis of North American and European isolates. J. Infect. Dis., *152*:478–484, 1985.
30. Schwan, T.G., Burgdorfer, W., and Garon, C.: Changes in infectivity and plasmid profile of the Lyme disease spirochete, Borrelia burgdorferi, as a result of in vitro cultivation. Infect. Immun., *56*:1831–1836, 1988.
31. Barbour, A.G.: Plasmid analysis of *Borrelia burgdorferi*, the Lyme disease agent. J. Clin. Microbiol., *26*:475–478, 1988.
32. Weber, K., Schierz, G., Wilske, B., and Preac-Mursic, V.: European erythema migrans disease and related disorders. Yale J. Biol. Med., *57*:463–471, 1984.
33. Asbrink, E., and Hovmark, A.: Successful cultivation of spirochetes from skin lesions of patients with erythema chronicum migrans Afzelius and acrodermatitis chronica atrophicans. Acta Pathol. Microbiol. Immunol. Scand. [B], *93*:161–163, 1985.
34. Berger, B.W., Kaplan, M.H., Rothenberg, I.R., and Barbour, A.G.: Isolation and characterization of the Lyme disease spirochete from the skin of patients with erythema chronicum migrans. J. Am. Acad. Dermatol., *3*:444–449, 1985.
35. Nadelman, R.B., Pavia, C.S., Magnarelli, L.A., and Worsmer, G.P.: Isolation of *Borrelia burgdorferi* from the blood seven patients with Lyme disease. Am. J. Med., *88*:21, 1990.
36. Snydman, D.R., Schenkein, D.P., Berardi, V.P., et al.: *Borrelia burgdorferi* in joint fluid in chronic Lyme arthritis. Ann. Intern. Med., *104*:798–800, 1986.
37. Berger, B.W., Clemmensen, O.J., and Ackerman, A.B.: Lyme disease is a spirochetosis: A review of the disease and evidence for its cause. Am. J. Dermatopathol., *5*:111–124, 1983.
38. Berger, B.W.: Erythema chronicum migrans of Lyme disease. Arch. Dermatol., *120*:1017–1021, 1984.
39. Johnston, Y.E., Duray, P.H., Steere, A.C., et al.: Lyme arthritis: Spirochetes found in synovial microangiopathic lesions. Am. J. Pathol., *118*:26–34, 1985.
40. MacDonald, A.B.: Borrelia in the brains of patients dying with dementia. (Letter.) JAMA, *256*:2195–2196, 1986.
41. Steere, A.C., Duray, P.H., Kauffman, D.J., and Wormser, G.P.: Unilateral blindness caused by infection with the Lyme disease spirochete, *Borrelia burgdorferi.* Ann. Intern. Med., *103*: 382–384, 1985.
42. Marcus, L.C., Steere, A.C., Duray, P.H., et al.: Fatal pancarditis

in a patient with coexistent Lyme disease and babesiosis. Demonstration of spirochetes in the myocardium. Ann. Intern. Med., *103*:374–376, 1985.

43. de Koning, J., Hoogkamp-Korstanje, J.A.A., van der Linde, M.R., and Crijns, H.J.G.M.: Demonstration of spirochetes in cardiac biopsies of patients with Lyme disease. J. Infect. Dis., *160*:150–152, 1989.
44. Rank, E.L., Dias, S.M., Hasson, J., et al.: Human necrotizing splenitis caused by *Borrelia burgdorferi.* Am. J. Clin. Pathol., *91*:493–498, 1989.
45. Goellner, M.H., Agger, W.A., Burgess, J.H., and Duray, P.H.: Hepatitis due to recurrent Lyme disease. Ann. Intern. Med., *108*:707–708, 1988.
46. Schlesinger, P.A., Duray, P.H., Burke, B.A., and Steere, A.C.: Maternal-fetal transmission of the Lyme disease spirochete, *Borrelia burgdorferi.* Ann. Intern. Med., *103*:67–68, 1985.
47. Atlas, E., Novak, S.N., Duray, P.H., and Steere, A.C.: Lyme myositis: Muscle invasion by *Borrelia burgdorferi.* Ann. Intern. Med., *109*:245–246, 1988.
48. MacDonald, A.B.: Human fetal borreliosis, toxemia of pregnancy, and fetal death. Zentralbl. Bakteriol. Mikrobiol. Hyg. [A], *263*:189–200, 1986.
49. Weber, K., Bratzke, H.J., and Neubert, U.: *Borrelia burgdorferi* in a newborn despite oral penicillin for Lyme borreliosis during pregnancy. Pediatr. Infect. Dis. J., *7*:286–289, 1988.
50. Pachner, A.R., and Steere, A.C.: The triad of neurologic manifestations of Lyme disease: Meningitis, cranial neuritis, and radiculoneuritis. Neurology, *35*:47–53, 1985.
51. Pachner, A.R., Duray, P., and Steere, A.C.: Central nervous system manifestations of Lyme disease. Arch. Neurol., *46*: 790–795, 1989.
52. Halperin, J.J., Luft, B.J., Anand, A.K., et al.: Lyme neuroborreliosis: Central nervous system manifestations. Neurology, *39*:753–759, 1989.
53. Halperin, J.J., Little, B.W., Coyle, P.K., and Dattwyler, R.J.: Lyme disease: Cause of a treatable peripheral neuropathy. Neurology, *37*:1700–1706, 1987.
54. Logigian, E.L., Kaplan, R.F., and Steere, A.C.: Chronic neurologic manifestations of Lyme disease. N. Engl. J. Med., *323*:1438–1444, 1990.
55. Steere, A.C., Schoen, R.T., and Taylor, E.: The clinical evolution of Lyme arthritis. Ann. Intern. Med., *107*:725–731, 1987.
56. Steere, A.C., Dwyer, E., and Winchester, R.: Association of chronic Lymne arthritis with HLA-DR4 and HLA-DR2 alleles. N. Engl. J. Med., *323*:219–223, 1990.
57. Sigal, L., Steere, A.C., Freeman, D.H., and Dwyer, J.M.: Proliferative responses of mononuclear cells in Lyme disease. Arthritis Rheum., *29*:761–769, 1986.
58. Pachner, A.R., Steere, A.C., Sigal, L.H., and Johnson, C.J.: Antigen-specific proliferation of CSF lymphocytes in Lyme disease. Neurology, *35*:1642–1644, 1985.
59. Craft, J.E., Fischer, D.K., Shimamoto, G.T., and Steere, A.C.: Antigens of *Borrelia burgdorferi* recognized during Lyme disease: Appearance of a new immunoglobulin M response and expansion of the immunoglobulin G response late in the illness. J. Clin. Invest., *78*:934–939, 1986.
60. Hardin, J.A., Steere, A.C., and Malawista, S.E.: The pathogenesis of arthritis in Lyme disease: Humoral immune responses and the role of intra-articular immune complexes. Yale J. Biol. Med., *57*:589–593, 1984.
61. Tsai, T.F., Bailey, R.E., Miller, G.L., et al.: National surveillance of Lyme disease, 1987–1988. IV International conference on Lyme borreliosis, Stockholm, Sweden, 1990. (Abstract.) P. 13.
62. Schmid, G.P.: The global distribution of Lyme disease. Rev. Infect. Dis., *7*:41–50, 1985.
63. Stanek, G., Flamm, H., Barbour, A.G., and Burgdorfer, W. (eds.): Lyme borreliosis: Proceedings of the second international symposium on Lyme disease and related disorders, Vienna 1985. Stuttgart and New York, Gustav Vischer Verlag, 1987.
64. Dekonenko, E.J., Steere, A.C., Berardi, V.P., and Kravchuk, L.H.: Lyme borreliosis in the Soviet Union: A cooperative US-USSR report. J. Infect. Dis., *158*:748–753, 1988.
65. Burgdorfer, W.: Vector/host relationships of the Lyme disease spirochete, Borrelia burgdorferi. Rheum. Dis. Clin. North Am., *15*:775–787, 1989.
66. Fraser, J.R.E.: Lyme disease challenges Australian clinicians. The implications of Australia's first reported case of Lyme arthritis. Med. J. Aust., *1*:101–102, 1982.
67. Persing, D.H., Telford, S.R. III, Rys, P.N., et al.: Detection of *Borrelia burgdorferi* DNA in museum specimens of *Ixodes dammini* ticks. Science, *249*:1420–1423, 1990.
68. Schulze, T.L., Bowen, G.S., Bosler, E.M., et al.: *Amblyoma americanum:* A potential vector of Lyme disease in New Jersey. Science, *224*:601–603, 1984.
69. Magnarelli, L.A., Anderson, J.F., Apperson, C.S., et al.: Spirochetes in ticks and antibodies to *Borrelia burgdorferi* in white-tailed deer from Connecticut, New York State, and North Carolina. J. Wildlife Dis., *22*:178–188, 1986.
70. Magnarelli, L.A., Anderson, J.F., and Barbour, A.G.: The etiologic agent of Lyme disease in deer flies, horse flies, and mosquitoes. J. Infect. Dis., *154*:355–358, 1986.
71. Luger, S.W.: Lyme disease transmitted by a biting fly. N. Engl. J. Med., *322*:1752, 1990.
72. Spielman, A., Wilson, M.L., Levine, J.F., and Piesman, J.: Ecology of *Ixodes dammini*–borne human babesiosis and Lyme disease. Annu. Rev. Entomol., *30*:439–460, 1985.
73. Mather, T.N., Wilson, M.L., Moore, S.I., et al.: Comparing the relative potential of rodents as reservoirs of the Lyme disease spirochete (*Borrelia burgdorferi*). Am. J. Epidemiol., *130*: 143–150, 1989.
74. Steere, A.C., Malawista, S.E., Craft, J.E., et al. (eds.): First international symposium on Lyme disease. Yale J. Biol. Med., *57*:445–713, 1984.
75. Burgdorfer, W., Lane, R.S., Barbour, A.G., et al.: The western bleck-legged tick, *Ixodes pacificus:* A vector of *Borrelia burgdorferi.* Am. J. Trop. Med. Hyg., *34*:925–930, 1985.
76. Bosler, E.M., Coleman, J.L., Benach, J.L., et al.: Natural distribution of the *Ixodes dammini* spirochetes. Science, *220*:321–322, 1983.
77. Magnarelli, L.A., Anderson, J.F., Burgdorfer, W., and Chappell, W.A.: Parasitism by *Ixodes dammini* (Acari: Ixodidae) and antibodies to spirchetes in mammals at Lyme disease foci of Connecticut, U.S.A. J. Med. Entomol., *21*:52–57, 1984.
78. Anderson, J.F., Johnson, R.C., Magnarelli, L.A., and Hyde, F.W.: Identification of endemic foci of Lyme disease: Isolation of *Borrelia burgdorferi* from feral rodents and ticks (*Dermacentor variabilis*).
79. Kornblatt, A.N., Urband, P.H., and Steere, A.C.: Arthritis caused by *Borrelia burgdorferi* in dogs. J. Am. Vet. Med. Assoc., *186*:960–964, 1985.
80. Anderson, J.F., Johnson, R.C., Magnarelli, L.A., and Hyde, F.W.: Involvement of birds in the epidemiology of the Lyme diseae agent *Borrelia burgdorferi.* Infect. Immun., *51*:394–396, 1986.
81. Hanrahan, J.P., Benach, J.L., Colemen, J.L., et al.: Incidence and cumultive frequency of endemic Lyme disease in a community. J. Infect. Dis., *150*:489–496, 1984.
82. Steere, A.C., Taylor, E., Wilson, M.W., et al.: Longitudinal assessment of the clinical and epidemiological features of Lyme disease in a defined population. J. Infect. Dis., *154*:295–300, 1986.
83. Åsbrink, E., and Olsson, I.: Clinical manifestations of erythema

chronicum migrans Afzelius in 161 patients. A comparison with Lyme disease. Acta Derm. Venereol. (Stockh.), *65*:43–52, 1985.

84. Clark, J.R., Carlson, R.D., Casaki, C.T., et al.: Facial paralysis in Lyme disease. Laryngoscope, *95*:1341–1345, 1985.
85. Ackerman, R., Rehse-Kupper, B., Gollmer, E., and Schmidt, R.: Chronic neurologic manifestations of erythema migrans *borreliosis*. Ann. N. Y. Acad. Sci., *539*:16–23, 1988.
86. Reik, L. Jr., Smith, L., Khan, A., and Nelson, W.: Demyelinating encephalopathy in Lyme disease. Neurology, *35*:267–269, 1985.
87. Ackermann, R., Gollmer, E., and Rehse-Kupper, B.: Progressive Borrelien-Enzephalomyelitis. Chronische Manifestation der Erythema-chronicum-migrans-Krankheit am Nervensystem. Dtsch. Med. Wochenschr., *26*:1039–1042, 1985.
88. Stanek, G., Klein, J., Bittner, R., and Glogar, D.: Isolation of *Borrelia burgdorferi* from the myocardium of a patient with longstanding cardiomyopathy. N. Engl. J. Med., *322*:249–252, 1990.
89. McAlister, H.F., Klementowicz, P.T., Andrews, C., et al.: Lyme carditis: An important cause of reversible heart block. Ann. Intern. Med., *110*:339–345, 1989.
90. Habicht, G.S., Beck, G., Benach, J.L., et al.: Spirochetes induce human and murine interleukin-1 production. J. Immunol., *134*:3147–3154, 1985.
91. Zvaifler, N.J.: Etiology and pathogenesis of rheumatoid arthritis. *In* Arthritis and Allied Conditions, 12th Ed. Edited by D.J. McCarty and W.J. Koopman. Malvern, Lea & Febiger, 1993.
92. Kaufman, L.D., Gruber, B.L., Phillips, M.E., and Benach, J.L.: Late cutaneous Lyme diseae: *Acrodermatitis chronica atrophicans*. Am. J. Med., *86*:828–830, 1989.
93. Craft, J.E., Grodzicki, R.L., and Steere, A.C.: The antibody response in Lyme disease: Evaluation of diagnostic tests. J. Infect. Dis., *149*:789–795, 1984.
94. Schwartz, B.S., Goldstein, M.D., Ribeiro, J.M.C., et al.: Antibody testing in Lyme disease. JAMA, *262*:3431–3434, 1989.
95. Luger, S.W., and Krauss, E.: Serologic tests for Lyme disease: Interlaboratory variability. Arch. Intern. Med., *150*:761–763, 1990.
96. Magnarelli, L.A., Miller, J.N., Anderson, J.F., and Riviere, G.R.: Cross-reactivity of nonspecific treponemal antibody in serologic tests for Lyme disease. J. Clin. Microbiol., *28*:1276–1279, 1990.
97. Dattwyler, R.J., Volkman, D.J., Luft, B.J., et al.: Dissociation of specific T- and B-lymphocyte responses to *Borrelia burgdorferi*. N. Engl. J. Med., *319*:1441–1446, 1989.
98. Dressler, F., Yoshinari, N.H., and Steere, A.C.: The T cell proliferative assay in the diagnosis of Lyme disease. Ann. Intern. Med. *115*:533–539, 1991.
99. Halperin, J.J., Krupp, L.B., Golightly, M.G., and Volkman, D.J.: Lyme *borreliosis*-associated encephalopathy. Neurology, *40*: 1340–1343, 1990.
100. Sigal, L.H.: Summary of the first 100 patients seen at a Lyme disease referral center. Am. J.Med., *88*:577–581, 1990.
101. Dinerman, H., and Steere, A.C.: Fibromyalgia following Lyme disease: Association with neurologic involvement and lack of response to antibiotic therapy. (Abstract.) Arthritis Rheum., *33*(Suppl.):136, 1990.
102. Dattwyler, R.J., Volkman, D., Conaty, S., et al.: Amoxicillin plus probenecid compared to doxycycline for the treatment of erythema migrans (EM). Lancet, *337*:241–244, 1990.
103. Massarotti, E., Luger, S.W., Rahn, D.W., et al.: A multicenter randomized trial of doxycycline, amoxicillin/probenecid, and azithromycin for the treatment of early Lyme disease. (Abstract.) Arthritis Rheum., *33*(Suppl.):37, 1990.
104. Shrestha, M., Grodzicki, R.L., and Steere, A.C.: Diagnosing early Lyme disease. Am. J. Med., *78*:235–240, 1985.
105. Luft, B.J., and Dattwyler, R.J.: Treatment of Lyme *borreliosis*. Rheum. Dis. Clin. North Am., *15*:747–756, 1990.
106. Rahn, D.W., and Malawista, S.E.: Lyme disease: Recommendations for diagnosis and treatment. Ann. Intern. Med., *4*:472–481, 1991.
107. Markowitz, L.E., Steere, A.C., Benach, J.L., et al.: Lyme disease during pregnancy. JAMA, *255*:3394–3396, 1986.
108. Williams, C.L., Benach, J.L., Curran, A.S., et al.: Lyme disease during pregnancy: A cord blood serosurvey. Ann. N. Y. Acad. Sci., *539*:504–506, 1988.
109. Dattwyler, R.J., Volkman, D.J., Halperin, J.J., and Luft, B.J.: Treatment of late Lyme borreliosis—Randomized comparison of ceftriaxone and penicillin. Lancet, *1*:1191–1194, 1988.
110. Pfister, H.-W., Preac-Mursic, V., Wilske, B., and Einhaup, K.M.: Cefotazime versus penicillin G for acute neurologic manifestations in Lyme borreliosis: A prospective randomized study. Arch. Neurol., *46*:1190–1194, 1989.
111. Dotevall, L., Alestig, K., Hanner, P., et al.: The use of doxycycline in nervous system *Borrelia burgdorferi* infection. Scand. J. Infect. Dis., *53*:74–79, 1988.
112. Liu, N.Y., Dinerman, H., Levin, R.E., et al.: Randomized trial of doxycycline versus amoxicillin/probenecid for the treatment of Lyme arthritis: Treatment of non-responders with iv penicillin or ceftriaxone. (Abstract.) Arthritis Rheum., *32*(Suppl.):32, 1989.
113. Schoen, R.T., Aversa, J.M., Rahn, D.W., and Steere, A.C.: Treatment of refractory chronic Lyme arthritis with arthroscopic synovectomy. Arthritis Rheum., *34*:1056–1060, 1991.
114. Åsbrink, E., Hovmark, A., and Hederstedt, B.: Serological studies of erythema chronicum migrans Afzelius and acrodermatitis chronica atrophicans with indirect immunofluorescence and enzyme-linked immunosorbent assays. Acta Derm. Venereol. (Stockh.), *65*:509–514, 1985.

121

Basic Biology of Lyme Borreliosis

RUSSELL C. JOHNSON, Ph.D.

Lyme borreliosis is a term that encompasses Lyme disease and related disorders such as acrodermatitis chronica atrophicans and benign lymphocytoma cutis. As described in the preceding chapter, this is a multisystemic and chronic tick-borne disease of world-wide distribution. Both the diagnosis and evaluation of treatment of Lyme borreliosis are problematic because of the spirochete's latency and intermittent patterns of exacerbations and remissions in the natural history of untreated disease. The lack of a laboratory test to judge treatment effectiveness adds to the difficulties in the assessment of therapy for this illness. Knowledge of the basic biology of Borrelia burgdorferi should provide insight as to possible mechanisms of pathogenicity, approaches for therapy, and understanding of the immune response in this disease.

ETIOLOGIC AGENT

Borrelia burgdorferi is a very flexible, thin (0.2 to 0.25 μm × 8 to 30 μm) helical bacterium that has the same basic structural features of other spirochetes. The protoplasmic cylinder, consisting of the peptidoglycan layer, cytoplasmic membrane, and cytoplasmic contents, is enclosed by a highly fluid and fragile outer membrane. The periplasmic flagella are located between the outer membrane and the underlying peptidoglycan layer.[1] The unusual internal location of the flagella endow the borreliae with a unique type of motility. This motility, combined with their helical morphology and narrow diameter, allows them to move very efficiently in viscous environments equivalent to the matrix of tissue ground substance[2] and might play a major role in the highly invasive nature of this spirochete.[3] Organization of the extrachromosomal DNA of Borrelia is different from that of other bacteria. In addition to circular plasmids, Borrelia contain linear plasmids, a form of DNA present in eukaryotic cells. Genes for two major outer-surface proteins are present on a 49-kd linear plasmid,[1] and other plasmids have been associated with virulence of the spirochete.[4]

Borrelia burgdorferi is a microaerophilic, slow-growing spirochete with an in-vitro generation time of 12 to 24 hours at 35°C.[5] Unlike Treponema pallidium it will survive in blood at refrigerator temperature for weeks to months. The Borrelia are nutritionally fastidious, and some isolates are difficult to maintain in culture. *Borrelia* burgdorferi can be readily isolated from ticks and rodents but is more difficult to culture from patients. The erythema migrans is the best source of spirochetes on biopsy, followed by the spinal fluid. Only a few isolates have been made from the synovium and synovial fluid. Recently, B. burgdorferi was isolated from a biopsy of an enlarged heart.[6]

PATHOGENESIS

Borrelia burgdorferi is transmitted to the mammalian host via the infectious saliva of the feeding ixodid tick.[7] The interaction of the spirochete with the host dermal tissue results in the formation of an expanding annular erythematous rash, erythema migrans (EM). This occurs at the site of the tick bite within a few days to a month in 60 to 80% of patients. The spirochete is highly invasive, which could be due in part to its ability to move rapidly through hyaluronic acid, the viscous cement substance of tissues. When injected into the tail vein of a rat B. burgdorferi will penetrate the central nervous system within 24 hours.[3] The spirochete has also been shown to interact with and migrate through endothelial monolayers.[8,9] The spirochetemia of early Lyme borreliosis is of a low level and of short duration.

Borrelia burgdorferi can be disseminated to most tissues, but multiplication is apparently limited because only a few spirochetes will be present. Nevertheless, the disease manifestations, whether they are in the acute or chronic form of the illness, are associated with the presence of living spirochetes. This correlation is supported by the response of the disease to anti-microbial therapy.

Borrelia burgdorferi elicits an inflammatory response primarily consisting of mononuclear cells with the exception of the synovial fluid, where granulocytes predominate. Purified proteins from this spirochete are chemotactic for human leukocytes.[10] The histologic pattern present in the periphery of the EM is a superficial and deep perivascular and interstitial infiltrate largely composed of lymphocytes with some plasma cells. The epi- and trans-myocarditis of Lyme borreliosis is also associated with an interstitial infiltrate of lymphocytes and plasma cells. Patients manifesting the varying forms of meningopolyradiculitis usually have lymphoplasmacellular infiltration of the meninges, ganglia, and peripheral nerves. The arthritis is characterized by hypertrophic synovitis, frequently with fibrinaceous deposits and synovial vascular occlusion. The inflammatory infiltrate of the synovium consists of lymphocytes, plasma cells, mast cells, and macrophages. The chronic skin lesion acrodermatitis chronica atrophicans has a similar cellular infiltrate.[11]

The mechanism or mechanisms by which B. burgdorferi causes disease in the host is unknown. The only toxin associated with this spirochete is a putative lipopolysaccharide that was reported to have endotoxin-like activity in one study.[12] However, the lipid A characteristic of classic lipopolysaccharide was not detected in another study.[13]

Major tissue injury due to B. burgdorferi interacting directly with host cells by adhesion or penetration is unlikely because relatively few spirochetes are associated with the pathology of Lyme borreliosis. Accordingly it is plausible that the spirochete possesses some mechanism for amplifying its pathogenicity. The induction and release of the cytokines, interleukins, tumor necrosis factor, or g-interferon from host cells is a reasonable possibility. Interleukin-1 possesses diverse biologic properties and has been detected in the synovial fluid of patients with Lyme arthritis. It was produced by cells isolated from human synovium and exposed to B. burgdorferi.[14] Many of the destructive changes occurring in the joint could be correlated with interleukin-1 production in response to the presence of B. burgdorferi. The synovial fluids of Lyme borreliosis patients contain, in addition to interleukin-1, tissue necrosis factor. The report that B. burgdorferi will activate complement in the absence or presence of antibody provides another potential mechanism of pathogenicity.[15] Activation of complement results in the production of chemotactic factors, mediators of inflammation, and other biologically active substances that could contribute to the associated inflammatory response. Other mediators of injury in Lyme borreliosis such as immune complexes[16] and autoimmune phenomena[17–19] have been proposed.

Some insight concerning the role of cellular and humoral immune responses in the pathogenesis of Lyme disease has been provided through studies with severe combined immunodeficient (scid) mice.[20] After inoculation with virulent (low-passage tick isolate) but not avirulent B. burgdorferi, these mice with severely impaired T-cell and B-cell functions develop a multisystemic disease with a preponderance for polyarthritis and carditis. These disease manifestations do not occur in mice with a mature immune system, indicating immunologic control of the pathogenic activity of this spirochete. This hypothesis is supported by the induction of a more-severe arthritis in neonatal rats as compared to adult animals[21] and in irradiated hamsters versus nonirradiated animals.[22] A study of mice of selected genotypes and ages demonstrated that the severity of Lyme borreliosis is age- and genotype-dependent.[23] This is confirmatory evidence for the observation that Lyme arthritis in humans has an immunogenetic basis. Patients with human leukocyte antigens (HLAs) DR2 and DR4 are prone to develop progressive, destructive arthritis that is refractory to antibiotic therapy.[24] It is unlikely that the arthritis, carditis, nephritis, and hepatitis observed in the scid mice were due to inflammatory cell wall products of B. burgdorferi or were caused by circulating immune complexes or antigen-specific T-cells, because neither inactivated or avirulent spirochetes induced disease, and the scid mice lacked mature lymphocytes. The tissue injury in the scid mice could be due to spirochetes binding to and activating macrophages, resulting in the release of cytokines.[20]

IMMUNOGENICITY OF BORRELIA BURGDORFERI

Because B. burgdorferi can be isolated from patients who have a high titer of circulating antibodies, the protective activity of these antibodies was questioned. In-vitro assays were used to investigate the functional activity of these antibodies. Borrelia burgdorferi was found to be resistant to the nonspecific bactericidal activity of normal serum in spite of activating complement by both the alternative and classic pathways.[15] The addition of human anti–B. burgdorferi IgG to normal human serum resulted in the rapid killing of the spirochete through activation of complement by the classic pathway. Examination of the mechanism of serum resistance indicated that the bactericidal activity mediated by IgG was not due to increasing the rate or amount of complement deposition. Rather, it was due to antibody altering the structure of the outer membrane of B. burgdorferi, facilitating the insertion of the membrane attack complex of complement.[25] Antibodies also function as opsonins. The phagocytosis of B. burgdorferi by human polymorphonuclear cells and monocytes[26,27] and rabbit and mouse peritoneal exudate cells[28] is enhanced by antibody, primarily mediated by the Fc receptor.[29] The results of these in-vitro studies suggested that antibodies could have protective activity in the host.

Passive immunization investigations using the hamster as the experimental animal demonstrated that antibodies provide a high level of protection to experimental infection if administered prior to challenge.[30] No protection was observed if antibodies were administered several days post infection.[31] Thus, in this animal model, antibodies will prevent infection but have little or no anti–B. burgdorferi activity once the spirochetes are established in the hosts' tissues. This observation explains why it is possible to isolate spirochetes from patients with chronic Lyme borreliosis in spite of a high titer of serum antibodies. Also, it indicates that the specific immune responses that are detectable in patients with Lyme borreliosis develop too slowly or are not adequate to protect against illness. Accordingly, a vaccine against B. burgdorferi should be an important means of preventing this disease. The feasibility of vaccination was demonstrated with the hamster model. A vaccine preparation consisting of whole inactivated B. burgdorferi provided 80 to 100% protection from experimental infection.[32] Studies of one of the major outer surface proteins (Osp) of this spirochete, OspA, have shown that it is immunogenic in mice[33] and that monoclonal antibodies specific for OspA are protective.[34] Interestingly, when OspA is introduced by natural infection, specific antibodies are only detected late in the disease. In contrast, vaccinated animals have an early antibody response to OspA, facilitating the eradication of the invading spirochetes.

ANTIMICROBIAL SUSCEPTIBILITY OF *BORRELIA* BURGDORFERI

Antimicrobials are effective in the treatment of most cases of Lyme borreliosis, especially if given early in the illness. However, the most efficacious antimicrobial agents, dosage, optimal route of administration, and length of treatment have not been determined. Knowledge of the inherent antimicrobial susceptibility of B. burgdorferi is a major consideration in selecting an appropriate agent for the treatment of this disease. Standard methods have not been established for determining the in-vitro antimicrobial susceptibility of slow-growing bacteria such as B. burgdorferi (generation time of 12 to 24 hours). Accordingly, the antimicrobial susceptibility of this spirochete was determined by a number of investigators using a variety of protocols.[35–42] In spite of this diversity, there is general agreement on the in-vitro activity of the most commonly used antimicrobials. Borrelia burgdorferi was susceptible to the macrolides, tetracyclines, semisynthetic penicillins, and late second- and third-generation cephalosporins; moderately sensitive to penicillin G and chloramphenicol; and resistant to the aminoglycosides, trimethoprim sulphamethoxazole, ciprofloxin, and rifampicin. First-generation cephalosporins generally had a low level of activity against this spirochete.

We used a macrodilution broth procedure for determining the minimum bactericidal concentration (MBC) for a number of antimicrobials (Table 121–1). Isolates of B. burgdorferi from ticks, animals, and humans from diverse geographic areas were assayed by this procedure. All isolates had a similar level of sensitivity,[41] and isolates from patients who did not respond well to antimicrobial therapy did not display resistance to any of the antimicrobials used.[43] Because hydroxchloroquine is used to treat some forms of arthritis, we evaluated its in-vitro and anti-B. burgdorferi activity and found it to be lacking at concentrations as high as 100 μg/ml (unpublished data).

Antimicrobials of interest were further evaluated for the treatment of experimentally infected hamsters.[37,41,42] Hamsters were infected 2 weeks prior to treatment, which consisted of daily subcutaneous injections of one-fifth of the total dose for 5 days. Hamsters were sacrificed and spleen, kidney, and bladder were cultured 2 weeks after the final treatment. When comparing the efficacy of antimicrobial therapy of experimentally infected hamsters (Table 121–2) and Lyme borreliosis in humans, it is important to remember that in the hamster we are assaying for the elimination of

TABLE 121–1. IN VITRO ANTIMICROBIAL SUSCEPTIBILITY OF BORRELIA BURGDORFERI

ANTIMICROBIAL AGENT	MINIMUM BACTERICIDAL CONCENTRATION (μg/ml) GEOMETRIC MEAN
Penicillin G	17.5
Amoxicillin	1.5
Cefuroxime	1.0
Cefotaxime	0.5
Cefoxitin	0.5
Ceftriaxone	0.08
Tetracycline	1.0
Doxycycline	3.3
Erythromycin	0.13
Azithromycin	0.03
Ciprofloxicin	4.0

TABLE 121–2. IN VIVO ANTIMICROBIAL SUSCEPTIBILITY OF BORRELIA BURGDORFERI

ANTIMICROBIAL AGENT	50% CURATIVE DOSE (mg/kg)
Penicillin G	93.9, >197.5
Amoxicillin	45.0
Cefuroxime	28.6
Ceftriaxone	24.0
Tetracycline	15.6, 28.0
Doxycycline	36.5
Erythromycin	122.2, 235.2
Azithromycin	3.7

Data from references 37, 41, and 42.

spirochetes, whereas in humans the adequacy of treatment is based on the resolution of signs and symptoms of the disease. Also, to establish a relationship between the results of animal studies with human disease it is important to include agents that have poor as well as good efficacy in the treatment of clinical Lyme borreliosis. Therapy with tetracycline was much more effective than erythromycin both in experimentally infected hamsters and human disease.[44] The results with penicillin G are less straightforward. It has been used successfully for the treatment of many cases of Lyme borreliosis, whereas in the hamster[37,42] and the gerbil,[38] it is not very effective. The animal studies are supported by a report that patients who apparently failed to respond to penicillin G therapy were successfully treated with ceftriaxone.[45] This antimicrobial had good activity in hamster and gerbil.

REFERENCES

1. Barbour, A.G., and Hayes, S.F.: Biology of *Borrelia* species. Microbiol. Rev., *50*:381–400, 1986.
2. Kimsey, R.B., and Spielman, A.: Motility of Lyme disease spirochetes in fluids as viscous as the extracellular matrix. J. Infect. Dis., *162*:1205–1208, 1990.
3. Garcia-Monco, J.C., Fernandez-Villar, B., Allen, J.C., and Benach, J.L.: *Borrelia burgdorferi* in the central nervous system: Experimental and clinical evidence for early invasion. J. Infect. Dis., *161*:1187–1193, 1990.
4. Schwan, T., Burgdorfer, W., and Garon, C.F.: Changes in infectivity and plasmid profile of the Lyme disease spirochete, *Borrelia burgdorferi*, as a result of *in vitro* cultivation. Infect. Immun., *56*:1831–1836, 1988.
5. Barbour, A.G.: Isolation and cultivation of Lyme disease spirochetes. Yale J. Biol. Med., *57*:521–525, 1984.
6. Stanek, G., Klein, J., Bittner, R., and Glogar, D.: Isolation of *Borrelia burgdorferi* from the myocardium of a patient with longstanding cardiomyopathy. N. Engl. J. Med., *322*:249–252, 1990.
7. Ribeiro, J.M., Mather, T.N., Piesman, J., and Spielman, A.: Dissemination and salivary delivery of Lyme disease spirochetes in vector ticks (Acari:Ixodes). J. Med. Entomol., *24*:201–205, 1987.
8. Comstock, L.E., and Thomas, D.D.: Penetration of endothelial cell monolayers by *Borrelia burgdorferi*. Infect. Immun., *57*:1626–1628, 1989.
9. Szczepanski, A., Furie, M.B., Benach, J.L., et al.: Interaction between *Borrelia burgdorferi* and endothelium *in vitro*. J. Clin. Invest., *85*:1637–1647, 1990.
10. Benach, J.L., Coleman, J.L., Garcia-Monco, J.C., and DePonte, P.C.: Biological activity of *Borrelia burgdorferi* antigens. Ann. N. Y. Acad. Sci., *539*:115–125, 1988.
11. Duray, P.H., and Steere, A.C.: Clinical pathologic correlations of Lyme disease by stage. Ann. N. Y. Acad. Sci., *539*:65–79, 1988.
12. Beck, G., Habicht, G.S., Benach, J.L., and Coleman, J.L.: Chemical and biologic characterization of a lipopolysaccharide from the Lyme disease spirochete (*Borrelia burgdorferi*). J. Infect. Dis., *152*:108–117, 1985.
13. Takayama, K., Rothenberg, R.J., and Barbour, A.G.: Absence of lipopolysaccharide in the Lyme disease spirochete, *Borrelia burgdorferi*. Infect. Immun., *55*:2311–2313, 1987.
14. Habicht, G.S., Beck, G., Benach, J.L., et al.: Lyme disease spirochetes induce human and murine IL-1 production. J. Immunol., *134*:3147–3154, 1985.
15. Kochi, S.K., and Johnson, R.C.: Role of immunoglobulin G in killing of *Borrelia burgdorferi* by the classical complement pathway. Infect. Immun., *56*:314–321, 1988.
16. Hardin, J.A., Steere, A.C., and Malawista, S.E.: Immune complexes and the evolution of Lyme arthritis. N. Engl. J. Med., *301*:1358–1363, 1979.
17. Aberer, E., Brunner, C., Suchanek, G., et al.: Molecular mimicry and Lyme borreliosis: Shared antigenic determinant between *Borrelia burgdorferi* and human tissue. Ann. Neurol., *26*:732–737, 1989.
18. Sigal, L.H., and Tatum, A.H.: Lyme disease patient serum contains IgM antibodies to *Borrelia burgdorferi* that cross react with neuronal antigens. Neurology, *38*:1439–1442, 1988.
19. Martin, R., Ortlauf, J., Sticht-Groh, V., and Bogdahn, U.: *Borrelia burgdorferi* specific and autoreactive T cell lines from cerebrospinal fluid in Lyme radiculomyelitis. Ann. Neurol., *24*:509–516, 1988.
20. Schaible, U.E., Kramer, M.D., Museteanu, C., et al.: The severe combined immunodeficiency (scid) mouse: A laboratory model for the analysis of Lyme arthritis and carditis. J. Exp. Med., *170*:1427–1432, 1989.
21. Barthold, S.W., Moody, K.D., Terwilliger, G.A., et al.: Experimental Lyme arthritis in rats infected with *Borrelia burgdorferi*. J. Infect. Dis., *157*:842–846, 1988.
22. Schmitz, J.L., Schell, R.F., Hejka, A.G., and England, D.M.: Passive immunization prevents induction of Lyme arthritis in LSH hamsters. Infect. Immun., *58*:144–148, 1990.
23. Barthold, S.W., Beck, D.S., Hansen, G.M., et al.: Lyme borreliosis in selected strains and ages of laboratory mice. J. Infect. Dis., *162*:133–138, 1990.
24. Steere, A.C., Dwyer, E., and Winchester, R.: Association of chronic Lyme arthritis with HLA-DR4 and HLA-DR2 alleles. N. Engl. J. Med., *323*:219–223, 1990.
25. Kochi, S.K., Johnson, R.C., and Dalmasso, A.P.: Complement-mediated killing of the Lyme disease spirochete *Borrelia burgdorferi*. Role of antibody in formation of an effective membrane attack complex. J. Immunol., *146*:3964–3970, 1991.
26. Peterson, P.K., Clawson, C.C., Lee, D.A., et al.: Human phagocyte interactions with the Lyme disease spirochete. Infect. Immun., *46*:608–611, 1984.
27. Georgilis, K., Steere, A.C., and Klempner, M.S.: Infectivity of *Borrelia burgdorferi* correlates resistance to elimination by phagocytic cells. J. Infect. Dis., *163*:150–155, 1991.
28. Benach, J.L., Habicht, G.S., Gocinski, B.L., and Coleman, J.L.: Phagocytic cell responses to *in vivo* and *in vitro* exposure to the Lyme disease spirochete. Yale J. Biol. Med., *57*:599–605, 1984.
29. Benach, J.L., Fleit, H.B., Habicht, G.S., et al.: Interactions of phagocytes with the Lyme disease spirochete: role of the Fc receptor. J. Infect. Dis., *150*:497–507, 1984.
30. Johnson, R.C., Kodner, C., and Russell, M.: Passive immunization of hamsters against experimental infection with *Borrelia burgdorferi*. Infect. Immun., *53*:713–714, 1986.
31. Johnson, R.C., Kodner, C., Russell, M., and Duray, P.H.: Experimental infection of the hamster with *Borrelia burgdorferi*. Ann. N. Y. Acad. Sci., *539*:258–263, 1988.
32. Johnson, R.C., Kodner, C., and Russell, M.: Active immunization of hamsters against experimental infection with *Borrelia burgdorferi*. Infect. Immun., *54*:897–898, 1986.
33. Fikrig, E., Barthold, S.W., Kantor, F.S., and Flavell, R.A.: Protection of mice against the Lyme disease agent by immunizing with recombinant OspA. Science, *250*:553–556, 1990.
34. Schaible, U.E., Kramer, M.D., Eichmann, K., et al.: Monoclonal antibodies specific for the outer surface protein A (OspA) of *Borrelia burgdorferi* prevent Lyme borreliosis in severe combined immunodeficiency (scid) mice. Proc. Natl. Acad. Sci. U.S.A., *87*:3768–3772, 1990.
35. Johnson, S.E., Klein, G.C., Schmid, G.P., and Feeley, J.C.: Sus-

ceptibility of the Lyme disease spirochete to seven antimicrobial agents. Yale J. Biol. Med., *57*:549–553, 1984.

36. Berger, B.W., Kaplan, M.H., Rothenberg, I.R., and Barbour, A.G.: Isolation and characterization of the Lyme disease spirochete from the skin of patients with erythema chronicum migrans. J. Am. Acad. Dermatol., *13*:444–449, 1985.
37. Johnson, R.C., Kodner, C., and Russell, M.: *In vitro* and *in vivo* susceptibility of the Lyme disease spirochete, *Borrelia burgdorferi*, to four antimicrobial agents. Antimicrob. Agents and Chemotherapy., *31*:164–167, 1987.
38. Preac-Mursic, V.P., Wilske, B., Schierz, G., et al.: *In vitro* and *in vivo* susceptibility of *Borrelia burgdorferi*. Eur. J. Clin. Microbiol. Infect. Dis., *6*:424–426, 1987.
39. Luft, B.J., Volkman, D.J., Halperin, J.J., and Dattwyler, R.J.: New chemotherapeutic approaches in the treatment of Lyme borreliosis. Ann. N. Y. Acad. Sci., *539*:352–361, 1988.
40. Preac-Mursic, V., Wilske, B., Schlerz, G., et al.: Comparative antimicrobial activity of the new macrolides against *Borrelia burgdorferi*. Eur. J. Clin. Microbiol. Infect. Dis., *8*:651–653, 1989.
41. Johnson, R.C., Kodner, C., Russell, M., and Girard, D.: *In vitro* and *in vivo* susceptibility of *Borrelia burgdorferi* to azithromycin. J. Antimicrob. Chemother., *25*(Suppl. A):33–38, 1990.
42. Johnson, R.C., Kodner, C.B., Jurkovich, P.J., and Collins, J.J.: Comparative *in vitro* and *in vivo* susceptibilities of the Lyme disease spirochete *Borrelia burgdorferi* to cefuroxime and other antimicrobial agents. Antimicrob. Agents Chemother., *34*:2133–2136, 1990.
43. Berger, B.W., and Johnson, R.C.: Clinical and microbiologic findings in six patients with erythema migrans of Lyme disease. J. Am. Acad. Dermatol., *21*:1188–1191, 1989.
44. Steere, A.C., Malawista, S.E., Newman, J., et al.: Antibiotic therapy in Lyme disease: Ann. Intern. Med., *93*:1–8, 1980.
45. Dattwyler, R.J., Halperin, J.J., Volkman, D.J., and Luft, B.J.: Treatment of late Lyme borreliosis—Randomized comparison of ceftriaxone and penicillin. Lancet, *1*:1191–1194, 1988.

122

Retrovirus-associated Rheumatic Syndromes

LUIS R. ESPINOZA

In 1981, an unprecedented number of young men, all active homosexuals, presented with Pneumocystis pneumonia, Kaposi's sarcoma, constitutional symptoms including fever, weight loss, anorexia, lymphadenopathy, and other infections such as oral candidiasis, cytomagalovirus (CMV), cryptococcosis, mycobacterium, and other polybacterial sepsis. Further investigation revealed a profound disturbance of cellular immune function with lymphopenia, diminished T-cell numbers, depressed lymphocyte proliferation, and inversion of the T-helper to suppressor/cytotoxic lymphocyte ratio.[1–5] The term "acquired immunodeficiency syndrome" (AIDS) was eventually coined,[5,6] and its viral etiology was determined.[7,8] Two independent reports almost simultaneously identified a retrovirus, now named human immunodeficiency virus (HIV), as the responsible etiologic agent.[7,8]

The Centers for Disease Control (CDC) now estimates that approximately 1 million individuals in the United States are currently infected with HIV,[9] and the World Health Organization estimates that from 5 to 10 million people worldwide are infected.[10,11] As of March 1, 1991, 161,288 cases of AIDS in the United States had been reported to the CDC, and 62.8% of these patients are now dead.[12] Worldwide 199,237 cases of AIDS had been reported (including the United States).[12]

A wide spectrum of clinical manifestations have been described in association with HIV infection, ranging from acute infection, which can be asymptomatic or associated with an infectious mononucleosis or influenza-like syndrome, to full-blown AIDS characterized by a severe state of immunosuppression. Every organ system can be affected by HIV, and there have been multiple reports describing neurologic, pulmonary, gastrointestinal, renal, cardiac, dermatologic, hematologic, endocrinologic, and ocular involvement.[13–26] The development of rheumatic complications during the course of HIV infection is now well established and of great interest. Since the initial report by Winchester et al. of Reiter's syndrome in patients with AIDS,[27] several other rheumatic disorders have been described. These include psoriatic arthritis, oligo and polyarthritis, undifferentiated spondyloarthropathy, myositis, Sjögren's syndrome, and vasculitis.[28–35]

ETIOPATHOGENIC MECHANISMS

HIV is a retrovirus composed of RNA and associated proteins. It was originally called human T-lymphotropic virus (HTLV)-III, lymphadenopathy associated virus (LAV), or AIDS-associated retrovirus (ARV).[36] It belongs to the family Retroviridae (or retrovirus), and to the subfamily Lentivirinae. Other members of this group are the simian immunodeficiency virus, the caprine arthritis-encephalitis virus, the visna and maedi viruses that cause infection in sheep, the equine infectious anemia virus, the feline immunodeficiency virus, and the bovine immunodeficiency virus.[36] All retroviruses share a common set of proteins physically contained within the virion or virus particle. The three main proteins are the gag, pol, and env proteins. The gag proteins are the structural components of the core of the virion (i.e., p24), which is surrounded by a bilipid membrane approximately 100 mm in diameter. There are two env proteins: a transmembrane protein spans the lipid bilayer and anchors the second protein, the outer membrane protein. This is the viral glycoprotein (gp-120) that recognizes the receptor for the virus on target cells and is the usual target for neutralizing antibodies. The

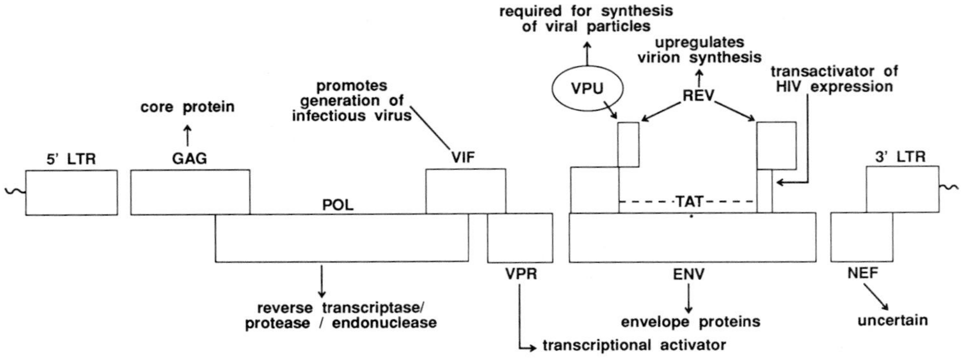

FIGURE 122–1. Schematic representation of the genomic structure of HIV-1. The functions of each of the nine known genes are summarized.

TABLE 122–1. PATHOGENIC MECHANISMS IN RETROVIRUS-RELATED RHEUMATIC CONDITIONS

Direct effect of retrovirus infection
Indirect effect of retrovirus infection
Cytokines
Retrovirus-derived growth factors
Reactive immune mechanisms
Autoimmunity
Circulating immune complexes
Anticardiolipin antibodies
Other anti-cell antibodies (i.e., anti-platelet)
Opportunistic infections: Arthritogenic organisms
Genetic factors: HLA-B27
Retrovirus antigens

pol gene products are centrally located in the core of the virion and function to replicate the viral genomic RNA, which is reverse-transcribed into double-stranded DNA by the viral DNA polymerase.[36,37]

The retrovirus proviral genome is well characterized. It is approximately 10 Kilobases (Kb) long and comprises the flanking long terminal repeat sequences that contain regulatory segments for viral replication as well as the gag, env, and pol genes that code for the core proteins, the internal and external envelope glycoproteins, and the reverse transcriptase-protease-endonuclease, respectively. HIV also has at least six additional genes, including tat, rev, nef, vpr, vif, and vpu, and all are expressed during infection. Their function, however and their contribution to pathogenesis, are defined only to a variable and incomplete degree (Fig. 122–1).

The CD4 receptor, expressed predominately by T-helper/inducer lymphocytes and, to a lesser extent, by monocytes and macrophages, has a high affinity for the gp-120 glycoprotein antigen of the envelope membrane of HIV. Consequently, in HIV infection, there is immune dysregulation caused by a quantitative and a qualitative defect of T-helper/inducer lymphocytes. Depletion and dysfunction of these lymphocytes leads to the occurrence of opportunistic infections and to neoplasias.[38]

The pathogenic mechanisms underlying the development of rheumatic syndromes in retrovirus infection remain unknown. Some possibilities are summarized in Table 122–1.

DIRECT EFFECT OF RETROVIRUS INFECTION

The direct role of retrovirus in associated rheumatic manifestations has not been proven conclusively. Most investigators have been unable to isolate HIV from synovial fluid or synovial membrane. In an extensively studied animal model of retrovirus related arthritis due to caprine arthritis-encephalitis virus (CAEV), the titers of coculturable CAEV in the synovial fluid and synovial fluid cells had disappeared by 8 months post infection.[39,40] The onset of clinical inflammatory articular disease rarely occurs before 12 months have elapsed following infection. Occasional reports have described the isolation of HIV from synovial fluid aspirates, however.[30,41,42] HTLV-I has also been demonstrated in muscle from a patient with polymyositis who was infected with both HIV and HTLV-I.[43] Furthermore, Dalakas et al. reported that polymyositis developed in 50% of monkeys infected with simian immunodeficiency virus;[44] here the retrovirus was isolated from affected muscle tissue.

INDIRECT EFFECT OF RETROVIRUS INFECTION

An important role for an indirect effect or effects of retrovirus infection in the pathogenesis of the associated rheumatic manifestations is likely, however. Increased production of cytokines such as interleukin-1, tumor necrosis factor, α-interferon, and γ-interferon (γ-IFN) have been demonstrated in both animal models and human retroviral infection.[45–47] Furthermore, γ-IFN enhances the expression of class II major histocompatibility complex (HLA) antigens in cells including Langerhans' cells in the epidermis, synovial, and muscle cells.[48–50] In this regard, changes observed in class II HLA gene expression in retroviral infections resemble those seen in idiopathic connective tissue disorders.[50]

The development of an HTLV-I transgenic mouse that develops a spontaneous inflammatory joint disorder should help to provide further insight into pathogenesis.[47] Data obtained from this model so far support an important role for cytokines. HIV-derived growth factors might play a role in the pathogenesis of Kaposi's sarcoma, which is a frequent complication of HIV infection.[51] Whether similar growth factors play a role in the pathogenesis of HIV-associated rheumatic manifestations is unknown.

REACTIVE IMMUNE MECHANISMS

The variable presence of synovial hyperplasia and subsynovial infiltration of mononuclear cells is characteristic in both animals and humans with retrovirus-related rheumatic disorders. In HIV infection these abnormalities occur despite a profound qualitative and quantitative deficiency of CD4 lymphocytes, suggesting a potential pathogenetic role for other T-cell subclasses including CD8 suppressor/oxtotoxic and γ-δ T-cells.[49,52]

AUTOIMMUNITY

The role of autoimmune mechanisms leading to the rheumatic manifestations of HIV-infected patients is not convincing. In general, no autoantibodies to nuclear or cytoplasmic antigens have been found in these patients.[53] Low titers of antinuclear antibodies has been reported rarely in HIV-infected patients,[54] but antiphospholipid antibodies including VDRL, anticardiolipin, and lupus anticoagulant are frequently seen in HIV patients. However, clinical complications including thrombosis do not correlate with the presence of these antibodies. Rather, these antibodies and circulating immune complexes might be related to the opportunistic infection in the HIV-infected population.[55,56]

OPPORTUNISTIC INFECTIONS

Hypothetically, repeated infections due to opportunistic or other organisms related to HIV-induced immunodeficiency could trigger a reactive form of arthritis. This is of particular relevance in Reiter's syndrome affecting black Zimbabwean patients, in whom there is no association with HLA-B27 positivity.[57–59] The prevalence of HLA-B27 in HIV-infected caucasians with Reiter's syndrome is similar to that of patients with the idiopathic form of the disease.

Data showing that coinfection with Mycoplasma fermentans (incognitus strain) enhances the ability of HIV to induce cytopathic effects on human T-lymphocytes in vitro[60] suggests that the modification of the biologic properties of HIV by coinfection with mycoplasma (or perhaps other microorganisms) could be involved in the pathogenesis of AIDS, including its rheumatic manifestations.

HIV ANTIGENS

Several antigens, including p24, gp-41, and gp-120, have been demonstrated in several tissues of HIV patients by immunohistochemical techniques and electron microscopy. HIV antigen p24 was shown in the synovial membrane of five HIV-infected patients, three of whom had HIV-associated arthritis and two of whom had HIV-associated psoriatic arthritis.[49] HIV antigens p24, gp-41, and gp-120 have been demonstrated in $CD4^+$ cells, macrophages, and degenerated muscle cells of patients with HIV-associated myositis.[50,61–64] All of these tissues have immune effector cells capable of reacting to inciting antigenic stimuli. An immune reaction and eventual tissue damage can result from stimulation of these cells by HIV antigens. Also, tissue inflammation is induced by cytokines in response to viral surface antigens in animal models.[65–67]

It is likely that complex interactions between environmental factors—the retrovirus, opportunistic and other infectious organisms genetic factors such as HLA-B27, and humoral and cell-mediated immune responses—participate in the pathogenesis of rheumatic disorders related to HIV or HTLV-I.

EPIDEMIOLOGIC CONSIDERATIONS

The prevalence of inflammatory musculoskeletal manifestations in patients with retrovirus infection, particularly HIV, is uncertain. Few prospective studies are available, but without exception, these have demonstrated a high frequency of arthritis, myositis, or both. We studied a large number of HIV patients prospectively to ascertain the frequency and clinical spectrum of associated rheumatic manifestations. Reiter's syndrome was found in 9.9% of 101 HIV-infected patients, psoriatic arthritis was found in 1.9%, and an HIV-associated arthropathy was found in 11.9%.[29] Also, 2.8% of this group presented other rheumatic syndromes, including polymyositis and vasculitis. Arthralgias were the most common complaint in these patients. Similar findings were reported by Bruskila et al. in a study of 52 HIV-infected patients (50 men and 2 women).[68] Arthralgias were the most common complaint, the characteristics of which were identical to those of our patients.[29] Reiter's syndrome was found in 3.8% of patients, psoriatic arthritis in 5.7%, and undifferentiated spondyloarthropathy in 9.5%. Sjögren's syndrome, Behçet's disease, and myositis were each seen in one patient.

A cross-sectional study of 65 individuals seen consecutively in an HIV clinic in New York City showed a prevalence of 4.6% for Reiter's syndrome, 3% for psoriatic arthritis, 8% for undifferentiated spondyloarthropathy, and 20% for psoriasis.[69] A study in London concluded that HIV infection was a risk factor for the development of seronegative arthritis and other rheumatic lesions.[70] Inflammatory joint disease was found in 29.2% of 123 HIV patients (34 men and 2 women) referred to a rheumatology clinic. These patients were not further classified, although psoriasis was seen in

12 instances, and several other patients presented with extra-articular clinical manifestations associated with Reiter's syndrome, undifferentiated spondyloarthropathy, or both. Arthralgias/myalgias were seen in 20 patients, and myalgias/myositis were seen in 13. Another prospectively designed study found Reiter's syndrome in 1.7%, psoriatic arthritis in 1.7%, and polyarthritis-oligoarthritis in 11.1% of patients.[71] Myalgias or myositis were seen in 6.8%, and myalgias/myositis plus symptoms placing patients in one of the arthritic groups occurred in an additional 4.3% of patients. Berman et al. studied two Argentinean populations prospectively with the usual risk factors for HIV infection (homosexual activity and intravenous drug use).[72] Reiter's syndrome was seen in 11.2% of those infected with HIV and in 2.5% of individuals with the risk factors but not infected with HIV ($p < 0.0001$). Psoriatic arthritis was found in 1.1% and an undifferentiated spondyloarthropathy occurred in 6.7% of HIV patients and in none of the HIV-negative individuals ($p < 0.001$). Myalgias and myositis were presented in 15.7%, septic arthritis in 1.1%, and a lupus-like syndrome in 1.1% of the HIV patients, compared to none in the control population.

All of the described studies were prospective with careful rheumatologic examination. The rheumatologic examination is important in view of the often subtle nature of the clinical findings.[29,68,71,74] The rheumatic complaints tend to occur in the later stages of HIV infection when patients are usually overwhelmed by many various severe clinical problems. In this setting a sausage digit or a mildly swollen joint is of little concern for patient or physician, and is often overlooked. Data obtained with questionnaires can miss many of these subtle findings. Thus a questionnaire study conducted in San Francisco found frequencies of 0.3 to 0.5% for Reiter's syndrome among a large cohort of homosexual men, with patients with Reiter's syndrome equally distributed between HIV-positive and HIV-negative individuals.[75] Another such study from Baltimore found Reiter's syndrome in 0.5% of 375 HIV-positive individuals, a prevalence not different than that found among 776 HIV-negative homosexuals.[76] It is possible that most patients capable of completing a questionnaire in these retrospective epidemiologic studies were in earlier stages of disease, in contrast with HIV patients with a rheumatic disorder. The findings of Solinger and Hess, who found a prevalence rate of less than 1% for Reiter's syndrome and psoriatic arthritis in more than 1000 HIV-infected individuals, are more difficult to explain.[77] Perhaps there are regional differences in some of the clinical manifestations of HIV infection. A reactive arthropathy usually affecting the larger joints of the lower extremities with no other clinical features of a connective tissue disease was described in black Africans, as was a second rheumatic disorder—complete or incomplete Reiter's syndrome.[57] The development of a rheumatic disorder in these patients was not associated with HLA-B27, which is virtually nonexistent in this population.

It can be concluded based on relatively few prospective epidemiologic studies that HIV-infected individuals can develop a variety of inflammatory musculoskeletal disorders including seronegative spondyloarthropathies (Table 122–2).

TABLE 122–2. PREVALENCE FOR REITER'S SYNDROME, PSORIATIC ARTHRITIS, AND UNDIFFERENTIATED SPONDYLOARTHROPATHY IN HIV-POSITIVE POPULATIONS

LOCATION	PREVALENCE (%)	REFERENCE
REITER'S SYNDROME		
Buenos Aires	11.2	72
Tampa, FL	9.9	29
New York, NY	4.6	69
Toronto	3.8	68
Cleveland, OH	1.7	71
Cincinnati, OH	<1.0	77
Baltimore, MD	0.5	76
San Francisco, CA	0.3	75
PSORIATIC ARTHRITIS		
Toronto	5.7	68
New York, NY	3.0	69
Tampa, FL	1.9	29
Cleveland, OH	1.7	71
Buenos Aires	1.1	72
Cincinnati, OH	<1.0	77
UNDIFFERENTIATED SPONDYLOARTHROPATHY		
Cleveland, OH	11.1	71
New York, NY	8.0	69
Toronto	5.7	68
Buenos Aires	2.2	72
INFLAMMATORY JOINT DISEASE*		
London	29.2	70

* No further classification made.

TABLE 122–3. RHEUMATIC MANIFESTATIONS ASSOCIATED WITH HIV INFECTION

Articular
Arthralgias
Reactive arthritis:
Reiter's syndrome
Psoriatic arthritis
Undifferentiated spondyloarthropathy
HIV-Arthritis
Muscular
Myalgias
Polymyositis-dermatomyositis
Myopathy (HIV-induced and AZT-induced)
Sjögren's syndrome
Septic arthritis
Other connective tissue disorders
Miscellaneous
Fibromyalgia
Hypertrophic osteoarthropathy
Bone avascular necrosis
Soft tissue lesions (i.e., bursitis)

CLINICAL MANIFESTATIONS

The clinical spectrum of rheumatic manifestations associated with HIV infection ranges from arthralgias to reactive arthritis to more severe conditions such as systemic necrotizing vasculitis (Table 122–3).[78–80]

ARTHRALGIAS

Every prospective study has described arthralgia as the most common rheumatic manifestation associated with HIV infection.[29,45,68,70,72] Arthralgias occur at any stage of HIV infection in approximately 25 to 35% of cases, and are usually of moderate intensity, intermittent, and oligoarticular. The knees, shoulders and elbows are involved must frequently, although any joint can be affected.[29,45,81] Up to 10% of patients may develop severe arthralgias, the "painful articular syndrome," which is characterized by severe, sharp articular pain of short duration (2 to 24 hours).[29] Here joint pains are excruciating and debilitating, and require emergency care or hospitalization. Intravenous narcotics are needed in more than half of these patients. None show evidence of inflammation, and tests including magnetic resonance imaging, computed tomography, electromyography, bone scan, and muscle biopsy are uniformly negative. No association with clubbing, hyperhidrosis, or dystrophic changes in the extremities has been found. A similar syndrome has been described in long bones by Winchester.[74]

REACTIVE ARTHRITIS—REITER'S SYNDROME

Reiter's syndrome (see also Chapter 60) was the first rheumatic disorder described in association with HIV infection.[27] Subsequent reports have confirmed this association.[29,30,45,52,57–59,68–73,77–81]

The onset of Reiter's syndrome may precede by as much as 2 years, occur concomitantly with, or (most commonly) follow the appearance of clinical evidence of immunodeficiency. The diagnosis of HIV infection should be considered in every individual with Reiter's syndrome who belongs to a high-risk group for HIV infection. This association is important when considering the use of immunosuppressive therapy for the symptoms of Reiter's syndrome because both AIDS and fulminant Kaposi's sarcoma have occurred shortly after the initiation of such therapy (steroids, methotrexate, and phototherapy).[27,82,83]

Most patients with HIV infection and Reiter's syndrome have developed its incomplete form.[29,45,84,85] The presentation is characterized by the typical articular pattern and several other extraarticular clinical features of Reiter's syndrome, but with *absence* of urethritis and conjunctivitis.[86] Some patients do present the classic triad of arthritis, urethritis, and conjunctivitis, however. The usual articular symptoms are asymmetric arthritis of the large joints, most commonly the knees, enthesopathy, and other extra-articular manifestations, such as circinate balanitis, keratoderma blennorrhagica, stomatitis, and uveitis. Clinical and radiologic evidence of spinal or sacroiliac joint involvement can occur. HLA-B27 antigen positivity is found in 63 to 75% of cases. In patients with Reiter's syndrome who have unusual clinical manifestations, a high index of suspicion for the diagnosis of HIV infection is needed. For example, one patient developed a malar rash that was diagnosed as seborrheic dermatitis, commonly seen in HIV infection, which prompted the correct diagnosis.[87] Other unusual findings for Reiter's syndrome such as oral thrush, hairy leukoplakia, persistent generalized lymphadenopathy, prominent constitutional features, and rapid progression of articular complaints with disabling deformities as well as leukopenia or lymphopenia, are clinical manifestations that should raise the possibility of underlying HIV infection. The clinical course of HIV-associated Reiter's syndrome is variable, from mild and transient to a rapidly deforming, disabling, and incapacitating course refractory to conventional anti-inflammatory medications (Figs. 122–2 and 122–3). The extra-articular manifestations usually respond to symptomatic therapy including local corticosteroid injection in patients with enthesitis and topical steroids in patients with uveitis.

The association of HIV infection and Reiter's syndrome in blacks from Zimbabwe[57–59] is of particular interest because both Reiter's syndrome and HLA-B27 antigen were extremely uncommon, but have become relatively common since the HIV epidemic.

PSORIATIC ARTHRITIS

The increased prevalence of psoriasis and related psoriatic arthritis (see also Chapter 61) in association with HIV infection is clearly established.[28–30] Johnson et al. first suggested that psoriasis in high-risk individuals should alert physicians to the possibility of HIV infection.[82] They reported three homosexual patients in whom the development of extensive erythrodermic psoriasis coincided with the appearance of AIDS. These

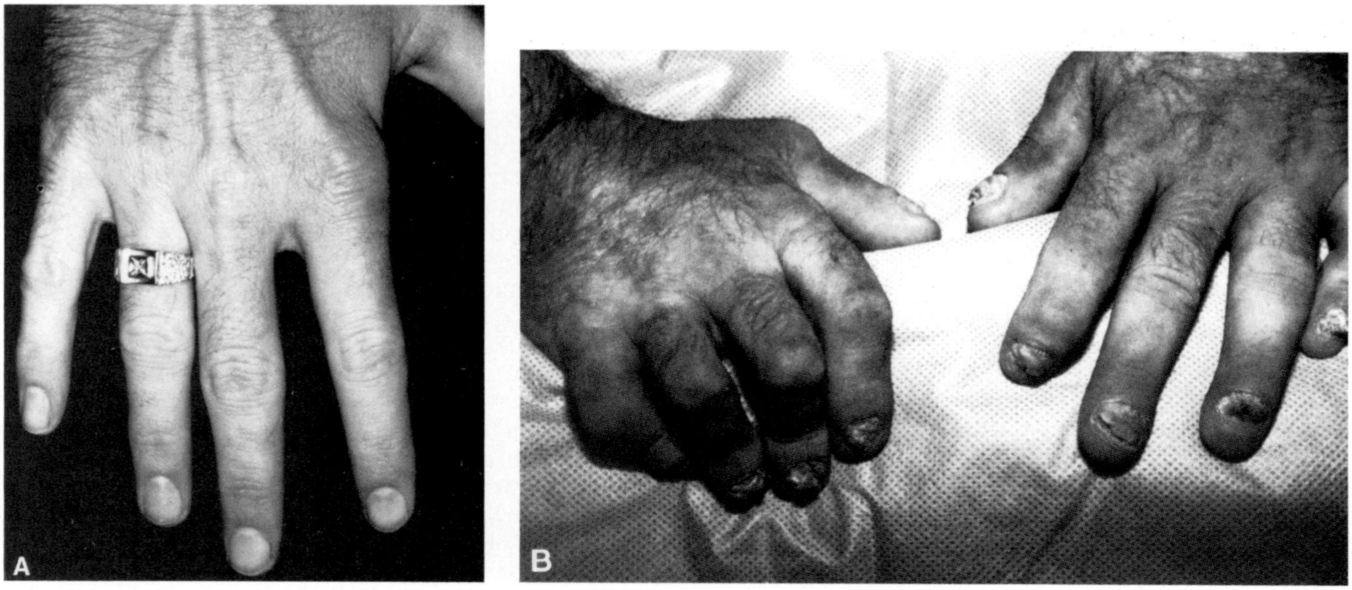

FIGURE 122–2. *A*, Right hand of a patient with Reiter's syndrome, showing mild erythema and swelling of second and third metacarpophalangeal joints. *B*, Ten months later, severe joint deformities and nail dystrophy are present.

authors subsequently described 13 patients with severe psoriasis that either flared or occurred de novo at the onset of AIDS. Four patients went on to develop Reiter's syndrome.[83] A variety of psoriatic manifestations can accompany HIV infection, including vulgaris, guttate, sebopsoriasis, pustules, and exfoliative erythroderma.[83] Single or combined expressions can occur in a given individual. Typical changes are common and range from nail pitting to severe onycholysis. Nail involvement occurs in most patients who present with inflammatory articular involvement. At times, nail involvement is confused with fungal infection or pyogenic paronychia, but potassium hydroxide (KOH) staining and cultures facilitate diagnosis. Psoriasis and psoriatic arthritis can precede or follow the clinical onset of immunodeficiency. The articular pattern is most frequently polyarticular and symmetric, but sacroiliac or spinal involvement can occur, as can enthesopathy and dactylitis.[88]

The course of psoriasis and related arthritis during HIV infection is variable but tends to progress and to be refractory to conventional therapy; erosions and crippling deformities develop in a relatively short period. The presence of psoriasis is a sign of a poor prognosis in HIV-positive individuals.[83,89]

HIV-ASSOCIATED ARTHRITIS

The existence of an arthropathy associated with HIV has been suggested.[29–31] This type of arthritis tends to be oligoarticular in approximately half of affected patients, and equally monoarticular and polyarticular in the others. Polyarthritis is asymmetric, involving large, weight-bearing joints such as knees and ankles. An occasional patient develops a polyarticular symmetric pattern re-

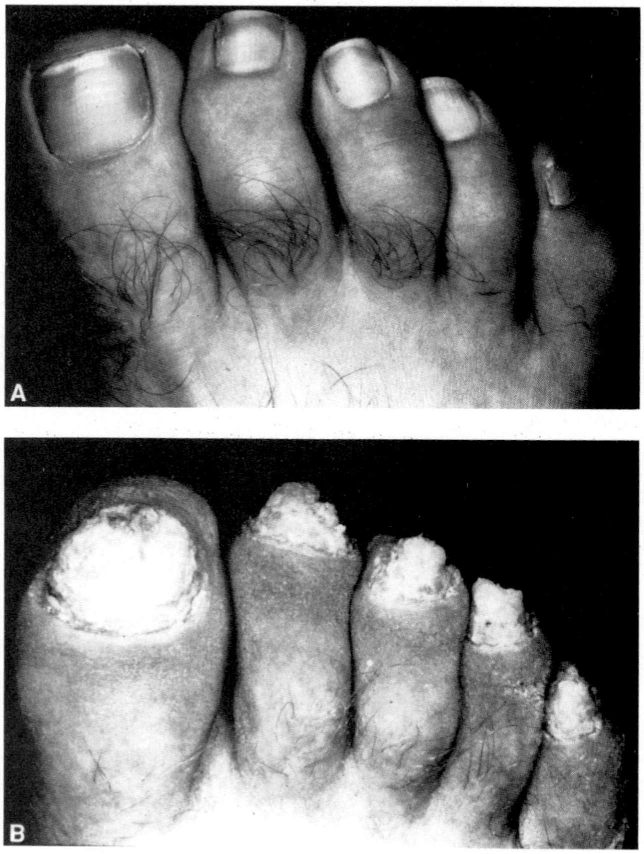

FIGURE 122–3. *A*, Right foot of same patient as in Figure 122–2 with Reiter's syndrome, showing mild sausage-like toes. *B*, Ten months later, there are persistent sausage-like deformities, accompanied by severe nail dystrophy.

sembling rheumatoid arthritis but with negative tests for rheumatoid factor. None of the patients with HIV-associated arthritis exhibit any extraarticular manifestations suggestive of Reiter's syndrome, psoriatic arthritis, or any other form of spondyloarthropathy. HLA-B27 is absent, and HLA-DR typing has not revealed any increased prevalence of a particular antigen. As in HIV-associated spondyloarthropathy, the majority of patients are in the late stages of infection. The average duration of arthritis is approximately 4 weeks.

UNDIFFERENTIATED SPONDYLOARTHROPATHY

The association of HIV infection with undifferentiated spondyloarthropathy has been recognized.[69–72] Affected patients characteristically do not develop enough clinical manifestations for their condition to be classified as Reiter's syndrome, psoriatic arthritis, or ankylosing spondylitis. Enthesitis, oligoarthritis, dactylitis, onycholysis, conjunctivitis, sacroilitis, and spondylitis are seen most commonly. Tests for antinuclear antibody (ANA) and rheumatoid factor are consistently negative.

MUSCLE INVOLVEMENT

Several types of muscle involvement are associated with HIV infection. Myalgias, usually generalized but occasionally localized, are most common but are transient and recurrent and readily respond to analgesics. Muscle atrophy, multifactorial and related to neurologic, nutritional, and infectious disorders, is also common.[29,45] The association of polymyositis with HIV infection is well established.[29,50] A subacute onset of proximal muscle weakness months or years after the development of immunodeficiency is usual. Proximal muscle weakness can be the presenting feature[90] or the only manifestation[64] of HIV infection. Clinical findings, elevated serum creatine kinase, and electromyographic findings are indistinguishable from those of idiopathic polymyositis. Various degrees of inflammatory necrosis, fibrosis, and mononuclear cell infiltration composed of CD8 suppressor lymphocytes, CD4 helper/inducer lymphocytes, and B lymphocytes are seen in muscle biopsy specimens.

A second histologic pattern of muscle involvement is characterized by abundant nemaline rod bodies and muscle fiber necrosis without inflammatory changes.[91–93] Nemaline rods can occur in a primary form of myopathy in adults in the fifth or sixth decades of life, and also can be seen occasionally in patients with polymyositis.[81] Simpson and Bender found nemaline rods in 3 of 11 patients with HIV-associated myopathy.[91] Whether the two histologic patterns reported in HIV-associated myopathy represent distinct entities or different aspects of one disorder is unclear.

Proximal muscle weakness in an HIV-infected patient most commonly follows zidovudine (AZT) therapy.[94–99] This myopathy is distinct from that associated with HIV and rapidly responds to drug withdrawal. A toxic myopathy with the appearance of "ragged-red" fibers, indicative of abnormal mitochondria with paracrystalline inclusions, is responsible for this disorder. The manifestations of AZT-associated myopathy are indistinguishable from those induced by HIV and can coexist with it. Myopathy in an HIV-infected patient on AZT can be due either to the HIV infection or to the AZT. Muscle biopsy can be valuable in differential diagnosis. Both conditions respond to corticosteroid therapy.[100,101]

Dermatomyositis can be associated with HIV infection also; it follows a course identical to that of the polymyositis.[62]

Other types of myopathy associated with HIV infection include microsporidiosis of the muscle,[102] myositis ossificans,[103] subclinical myopathy,[104] and *pyomyositis*.[105–110] Pyomyositis is a purulent infection of skeletal muscle common in the tropics and rare in temperate climates. With the advent of HIV infection an increasing number of cases are being recognized even in temperate climates. It can present in an indolent fashion in HIV-infected patients, delaying prompt diagnosis and treatment. It is characterized by muscle swelling, usually the quadriceps or gluteus, which becomes increasingly indurated (woody induration). It can be accompanied by fever, malaise, anemia, leukocytosis, and elevated erythrocyte sedimentation rate. Staphylococcus aureus is the causative organism in 95% of cases. This organism was cultured in drained pus in most cases associated with HIV infection. Once the diagnosis is suspected, needle aspiration of the area with ultrasonic guidance for identification of bacteria is recommended. Treatment consists of drainage of pus and administration of appropriate antibiotics.

SJÖGREN'S SYNDROME

Xerophthalmia, xerostomia, and parotid gland enlargement can be associated with HIV infection.[111,112] In contrast to the idiopathic form, HIV-associated Sjögren's syndrome (see also Chapter 78) is characterized by its predominance in men, the prominence of parotid gland swelling or large neck masses, the absence of arthritis, the prominence of extrasalivary lymphocyte infiltration, the absence of autoantibodies such as anti-Ro(SS-A), anti-La(SS-B), and rheumatoid factor, and a predominance of $CD8^+$ lymphocytes in the inflammatory infiltrate.[34] Itescu et al. coined the term "diffuse infiltration lymphocytosis syndrome" (DILS) to describe this disorder.[34] HLA-DR5 was highly prevalent in black patients, suggesting that DILS reflects a distinctive host immune response to HIV associated with a major histocompatibilty complex class II antigen. Participation of a retrovirus in the etiology of the idiopathic form of Sjögren's syndrome has been suggested by Talal et al., who found serum antibodies against HIV p24 antigen in 14 of 47 patients with primary Sjögren's syndrome, with relative absence of anti-Ro(SS-A) and anti-La(SS-B) antibodies.[113] On the other hand, Garry and coworkers detected a human intracisternal A-type retroviral particle in two of four patients with Sjögren's syndrome that was antigenically related (but distinguishable by several criteria) to HIV in lymphoblastoid cells exposed to salivary tissue homogenate.[114] The precise role of retrovirus infection in idiopathic Sjögren's syndrome is unclear.

VASCULITIS

Vasculitic syndromes (see also Chapter 75) are associated with HIV infection.[71] Most patients have a polyarteritis nodosa–like disease with involvement of medium-sized blood vessels to skin, nerve, and muscle. Viral antigens within vascular endothelial cells have been identified.[115,126] Mononeuritis multiplex is a frequent finding in HIV infection.[29,25,116,117] Such neuropathies either resolve spontaneously or progress to a sensorimotor polyneuropathy. Sural nerve biopsies show multifocal lesions with axonal degeneration, endoneurium infiltrates, and necrotizing vasculitis. Other associated vasculitic syndromes include primary angiitis of the central nervous system,[118,119] eosinophilic vasculitis presenting as temporal arteritis,[120] leukocytoclastic vasculitis (Henoch-Schönlein purpura),[121] lymphomatoid granulomatosis,[122–125] benign lymphocytic angiitis,[35] and angiocentric lymphoma.[35]

SEPTIC ARTHRITIS/OSTEOMYELITIS

HIV infection predisposes patients to joint infection with opportunistic as well as common pathogens. The profound state of immunosuppression with marked qualitative and quantitative deficiency in CD4 helper/inducer cells is associated with increased risk of fungal and mycobacterial infection. Isolated cases of septic arthritis have been reported, including Cryptococcus neoformans in the knee,[127] Sporothrix schenckii in a metacarpophalangeal and a proximal interphalangeal joint,[128] Mycobacterium haemophilium in the wrist,[129] M. avium in the wrist,[130] Campylobacter fetus in both knees and an ankle,[27] Ureaplasma urealyticum oligoarthritis,[131] Histoplasma capsulatum in the knee,[80] and septic acromioclavicular arthritis and osteomyelitis caused by Staphylococcus aureus.[132]

HIV-infected hemophilic patients are considered to be at especially high risk of septic arthritis because of their propensity for intra-articular bleeding.[133,134] HIV-infected intravenous drug users are also at risk for septic arthritis.[135]

Two cases of *septic olecranon bursitis* caused by S. aureus in HIV-infected homosexual men were refractory to conservative management.[136] A persistent clinical course of septic bursitis in the absence of other contributing factors should suggest the possibility of HIV infection.

Early detection of *septic arthritis* is important because specific antibiotic therapy can prevent severe irreversible joint damage. Identification of these infections is often difficult because most are caused by unusual organisms and because subtle clinical presentation with minimal inflammation is common.

Osteomyelitis can be present alone or can coexist with septic arthritis.[137,138] The spine and long bones can be affected.[139]

HIV ASSOCIATED WITH OTHER CONNECTIVE TISSUE DISORDERS

HIV infection is a systemic disorder that can mimic connective tissue diseases including systemic lupus erythematosus (SLE), rheumatoid arthritis, and polymyositis.[45,99] Moreover, false-positive HIV antibody test results are sometimes seen in SLE patients.[140,141]

The course of patients with idiopathic connective tissue diseases who subsequently become HIV infected is fascinating. Three patients with SLE and subsequent HIV infection showed lessened disease activity when $CD4^+$ lymphocyte depletion developed. Lupus activity reappeared when treatment with AZT was started.[42,43] Similar findings have been reported in patients with rheumatoid arthritis and dermatomyositis.[144] These observations support a central role for the $CD4^+$ cell population in the pathogenesis of the systemic rheumatic diseases. In contrast, vasculitis progressed in a patient with cryoglobulinemia despite profound HIV-related immunosuppression.[143]

MISCELLANEOUS RHEUMATIC DISORDERS

Other rheumatic disorders have been described in patients with HIV infection. Fibromyalgia was found in 29% of HIV patients in one study, compared with 24% of patients with psoriatic arthritis, and 57% of patients with rheumatoid arthritis.[145] Hypertrophic osteoarthropathy (HOA) has been reported with isolated pain on long bones or with the characteristic clubbing, arthritis, and periositis. HOA resolved in one patient after an pneumocystic pneumonia was treated with pentamidine.[146,147] Multiple osteonecrosis has been reported in HIV-infected patients,[148] as has soft tissue involvement including Dupuytren's contracture, adhesive capsulitis of the shoulder, rotator cuff lesions, tennis elbow, carpal tunnel syndrome, and osteochondritis.[149,150] These soft tissue lesions, with the exception of Dupuytren's contracture and adhesive capsulitis, were not more prevalent than the general population, however.[70]

MUSCULOSKELETAL MANIFESTATIONS ASSOCIATED WITH HTLV-I

Human T-cell lymphotropic virus type I (HTLV-I) is the etiologic agent of adult T-cell leukemia,[151] and is endemic in parts of Japan. There is a documented association between HTLV-I and a subset of chronic progressive myelopathy, HTLV-I–associated myelopathy/tropical spastic paraparesis (HAM/TSP),[152] alveolitis,[153] Sjögren's syndrome,[154] polymyositis,[43] and polyarthritis.[155,156]

The clinical picture of polymyositis associated with HTLV-I is identical to that seen in idiopathic or HIV-associated disease.

Patients with arthropathy associated with HTLV-I present with chronic persistent oligoarthritis affecting large weight-bearing joints, particularly the knees. Flare-ups occur only occasionally throughout a clinical course measured in years. A few patients present with polyarthritis that preferentially involves large joints including the shoulder, wrist, and knee. On examination mild to moderate synovitis is found. The erythrocyte sedimentation rate is elevated in most patients, and rheumatoid factor is positive in approximately half of patients. A polyclonal hypergammaglobulinemia is present in half of patients; C-reactive protein is elevated in 40% of patients. Antinuclear antibodies are sometimes found. Neither leukemia nor AIDS develops in these patients. Anti–HTLV-I antibodies are detected in both sera and synovial fluid in all patients.

Lymphocytes constituted approximately 45% of synovial fluid cells. Medium-sized atypical lymphocytes with characteristic nuclear indentations and resembling adult T-cell leukemia cells are frequently identified (Fig. 122–4). These flower cells constitute about 12% of synovial fluid lymphocytes. The majority of these atypical lymphocytes express CD2 and HLA-DR surface antigens. Radiologic findings can include narrowing of the joint space, small bony erosions, and minimal osteoporosis. Mild to moderate proliferation of the synovial lining cells and of subsynovial vascular endothelium occurs along with fibrinoid necrosis of collagen fibers, edematous synovial villi, and atypical lymphocytes with nuclear indentation. $CD4^+$ and $CD8^+$ T-cells, B-cells, and cells expressing HLA-DR antigens were found.[155] HTLV-I proviral DNA is integrated into the DNA of cells in the synovium and synovial fluid.[157,158] HTLV-I transgenic mice have spontaneously developed arthritis similar to human rheumatoid arthritis, but never leukemia.[47] These findings strongly support the notion that HTLV-I plays an important role in the pathogenesis of the associated inflammatory musculoskeletal complications, although the exact mechanism or mechanisms remain to be elucidated.[158]

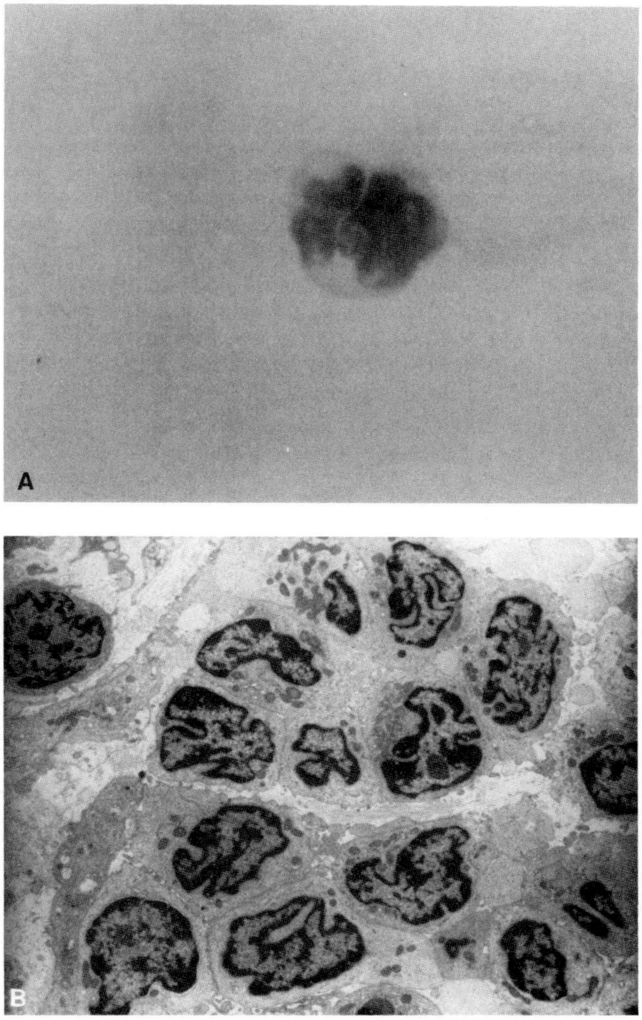

FIGURE 122–4. *A*, "Flower" cell on atypical lymphocyte present in synovial fluid from patients with HTLV-1 arthropathy (× 1000). Courtesy of Dr. K. Nishioka. *B*, Electron microscopic appearance of atypical lymphocytes (× 3000). Courtesy of Dr. K. Nishioka.

RHEUMATIC MANIFESTATIONS RELATED TO HIV-II

Boissier et al. described a 26-year-old female native of Cabo Verde, Africa who had been living in France since the age of 20 was asymptomatic although she was known to be HIV-II seropositive by ELISA and specific Western blotting.[159] No coinfection with another human retrovirus was detected. Twenty months after diagnosis she developed myalgias and severe pain in her feet that worsened upon walking or ascending stairs; the pain was found to be due to enthesitis at the Achilles and triceps tendon insertions. The authors speculated that HIV-II might have been responsible for the observed enthesitis.

LABORATORY FINDINGS

Many abnormal laboratory findings are present in patients with HIV infection. Polyclonal hypergammaglobulinemia is the most common abnormality,[160] with levels similar to those found in SLE and other systemic connective tissue diseases. A few cases of hypogammaglobulinemia or agammaglobulinemia also have been associated with HIV infection.

Circulating immune complexes, especially those containing IgA, are found in approximately 50 to 70% of patients.[161–163] Low-grade complement activation is present in some HIV patients, but hypocomplementemia is rare.[29] Low titers of ANA and rheumatoid factor are found in a few patients.[53] Antiphospholipid antibodies, particularly IgG anticardiolipin antibodies are found in 23 to 84% of HIV-infected patients,[55,56,164,165] compared to 2% in healthy young populations.[166] Small (5 to 10 ml) effusions are present in about one-third of patients. Such fluids are clear yellow with normal or slightly decreased viscosity, mild to moderate elevations of protein, normal glucose levels, and total leukocyte counts ranging from 2000 to 14,500 per cm^3 (predominantly neutrophils). Nonspecific proliferative synovitis accompanies increased vascularity of the subsynovial space (Fig. 122–5). Immunohistochemical staining yields positive results for HIV p24 antigen in synoviocytes and mononuclear sybsynovial cells[49]

Radiologic changes include soft tissue swelling, joint-space narrowing, erosions, whittling, osteolytic lesions, periostitis, sacroiliac joint space widening and erosions, and syndesmophyte formation (Fig. 122–6).[28,167] Changes characteristic of ankylosing spondylitis have

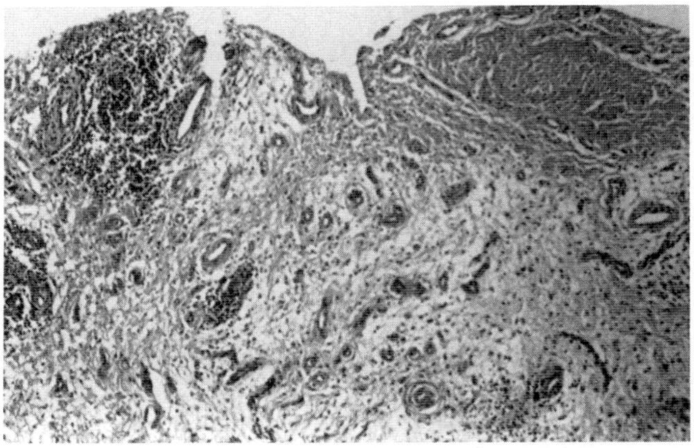

FIGURE 122–5. Synovium from a patient with HIV-associated Reiter's syndrome showing mild synovial cell hyperplasia, hypervascularity, and moderate inflammatory cell infiltrate in the subsynovial space (hematoxylin = eosin, × 100).

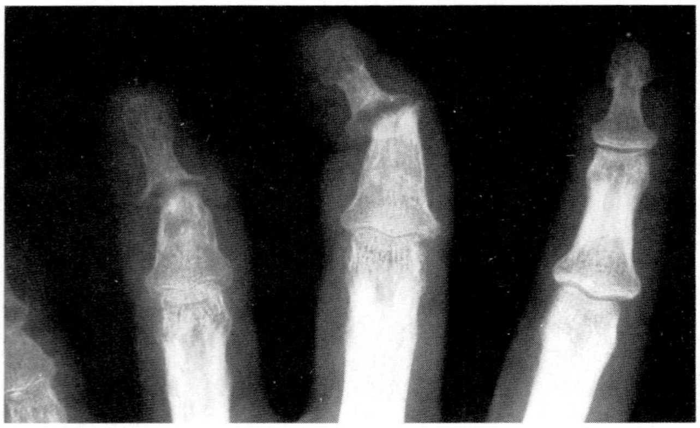

FIGURE 122–6. Severe erosive changes of distal interphalangeal joints leading to an appearance of "cup and saucer" in a patient with HIV-associated psoriatic arthritis.

not been reported, perhaps because HIV patients do not live long enough to develop them.

MANAGEMENT

Treatment of the rheumatic manifestations of retrovirus infection is ill-defined.[168] In general, patients presenting with arthralgias, myalgias, and reactive arthritis respond to a combination of analgesics and nonsteroidal anti-inflammatory drugs (NSAIDs). Immunosuppressive therapy should be given cautiously because of the strong possibility of worsening the immunodeficiency state as well as the possible development of Kaposi's sarcoma and overt AIDS. Some patients have benefited from the use of methotrexate and cyclosporin A.

Local steroid injections are useful to treat severely inflamed joints. Septic arthritis has not been reported in AIDS patients as a complication of this therapy. Prednisone, alone or in combination with methotrexate, AZT, or both, is useful in the management of polymyositis. Doses ranging from 30 to 60 mg daily are effective and have not been associated with the development of Kaposi's sarcoma or the precipitation of AIDS. Improvement of psoriasis and psoriatic arthritis has been reported with the use of AZT[169,170] or antibiotic treatment (trimethaprin/sulfamethoxazole or co-trimoxazole).[171] Improvement of associated Reiter's syndrome has been reported with the use of etretinate.[172]

A cure for HIV infection and its complications is not imminent, but therapy has been improving rapidly. As treatment prolongs life, the focus of management will likely shift to the management, prevention, and rehabilitation of patients' disabilities, including rheumatic ones.[173]

REFERENCES

1. Centers for Disease Control. Pneumocystis pneumonia. MMWR, *30*:250–253, 1981.
2. Kaposi's sarcoma and pneumocystis pneumonia among homosexual men. MMWR, *30*:305–308, 1981.
3. Gottlieb, M.S., Schroff, R., Schanker, H.M., et al.: Pneumocystis carinii pneumonia and mucosal candidiasis in previously healthy homosexual men. Evidence of a new acquired cellular immunodeficiency. N. Engl. J. Med., *305*:1425–1431, 1981.
4. Masur, H., Michelis, M.A., Greene, J.B., et al.: An outbreak of community acquired Pneumocystis carinii pneumonia. Initial manifestation of cellular immune dysfunction. N. Engl. J. Med., *305*:1431–1438, 1981.
5. Siegal, F.P., Lopez, C., Hammer, G.S., et al.: Severe acquired immunodeficiency in male homosexuals, manifested by chronic perianal ulcerative herpes simplex lesions. N. Engl. J. Med., *305*:1439–1444, 1981.
6. Brennan, T.A.: The acquired immunodeficiency syndrome (AIDS) as an occupational disease. Ann. Intern. Med., *107*:581–583, 1987.
7. Barrè-Sinoussi, F., Chermann, J.C., Rey, F., et al.: Isolation of a T-lymphocyte retrovirus from a patient at risk for acquired immunodeficiency syndrome (AIDS). Science, *220*:868–871, 1983.

8. Gallo, R.C., Salahuddin, S.Z., Popivic, M., et al.: Frequent detection and isolation of cytopathic retro virus (HTLV-III) from patients with AIDS and at risk of AIDS. Science, *224*:500–503, 1984.
9. HIV prevalence estimates and AIDS case projections for the United States: Report based upon a workshop. MMWR, *39*:1–31, 1990.
10. Up-date acquired immunodeficiency syndrome-United States. MMWR, *36*:522–526, 1987.
11. Fauci, A.S.: AIDS: immunopathogenic mechanisms and research strategies. Clin. Res., *35*:503–510, 1987.
12. Statistic from the World Health Organization and the Centers for Disease Control. AIDS, *5*:471–475, 1991.
13. Gabuzda, D.H., and Hirsh, M.S.: Neurologic manifestations of infection with human immunodeficiency virus-clinical features and pathogenesis. Ann. Intern. Med., *107*:383–391, 1987.
14. Levy, R.M., and Berger, J.R.: Neurologic complications of HIV infection: Diagnosis, therapy, and functional considerations. *In* Rehabilitation for Patients with HIV Disease. Edited by Jon Mukand. New York, McGraw-Hill, 1991, pp. 55–76.
15. Donath, J., and Hkhan, F.A.: Pulmonary infections in AIDS. Compr. Ther., *13*:49–58, 1987.
16. Santangelo, W.C., and Krejs, G.J.: Gastrointestinal manifestations of the acquired immunodeficiency syndrome. Am. J. Med. Sci., *292*:328–334, 1986.
17. Sreepada Rao, T.K., Friedman, E.A., and Nicastri, A.D.: The types of renal disease in the acquired immunodeficiency syndrome. N. Engl. J. Med., *316*:1062–1068, 1987.
18. Cammarosano, C., and Lewis, E.: Cardiac lesions in acquired immunodeficiency syndrome (AIDS). J. Am. Coll. Cardiol., *5*:703–706, 1985.
19. Cohen, I.S., Anderson, D.W., Virmani, R., et al.: Congestive cardiomyopathy in association with the acquired immunodeficiency syndrome. N. Engl. J. Med., *315*:628–630, 1986.
20. Friedman-Kien, A.F.: Disseminated Kaposi's sarcoma-like syndrome in young homosexual men. J. Am. Acad. Dermatol., *5*:468–472, 1981.
21. Penney, N.S.: Skin Manifestations of AIDS. Philadelphia, Lippincott, 1990, pp. 149–182.
22. Karpatkin, S.: Immunologic thrombocytopenic purpura in HIV-seropositive homosexuals, narcotic addicts and hemophiliacs. Semin. Hematol., *25*:219–231, 1988.
23. Rarick, M.H.: Hematologic abnormalities in HIV infection. *In* Rehabilitation for Patients with HIV Disease. Edited by Jon Mukand. New York, McGraw-Hill, 1991, pp. 21–32.
24. LoPresti, J.S., Fried, J.C., Spencer, C.A., and Nicoloff, J.T.: Unique alterations of thyroid hormone indices in the acquired immunodeficiency syndrome (AIDS). Ann. Intern. Med., *110*:970–975, 1989.
25. Shuman, J.S., Orellana, J., Friedman, A.H., and Teich, S.A.: Acquired immunodeficiency syndrome (AIDS). Surv. Ophthalmol., *31*:384–410, 1987.
26. Pomerantz, R.J., Kuritzes, D.R., DeLa Monte, S.M., et al.: Infection of the retina by human immunodeficiency virus type I. N. Engl. J. Med., *317*:1643–1647, 1987.
27. Winchester, R., Bernstein, D.H., Fischer, A.D., et al.: The co-occurrence of Reiter's syndrome and acquired immunodeficiency. Ann. Intern. Med., *106*:19–26, 1987.
28. Espinoza, L.R., Berman, A., Vasey, F.B., et al.: Psoriatic arthritis and acquired immunodeficiency syndrome. Arthritis Rheum., *31*:1034–1040, 1988.
29. Berman, A., Espinoza, L.R., Diaz, J.D., et al.: Rheumatic manifestations of human immunodeficiency virus infection. Am. J. Med., *85*:59–64, 1988.
30. Forster, S.M., Seifert, M.H., Keat, A.C., et al.: Inflammatory joint disease and human immunodeficiency virus infection. Br. Med. J., *296*:1625–1627, 1988.
31. Rynes, R.I., Goldenberg, D.L., Digiacomo, R., et al.: Acquired immunodeficiency syndrome–associated arthritis. Am. J. Med., *84*:810–816, 1988.
32. Aguilar, J.L., Berman, A., and Espinoza, L.R.: Artritis asociada a la infeccion por el virus de immunodeficiencia humana. Rev. Mexicana Reumatol., *3*:109–113, 1988.
33. Snider, W.D., Simpson, D.M., Nielsen, S., et al.: Neurological complications of acquired immunodeficiency virus: Analysis of 50 patients. Ann. Neurol., *14*:403–418, 1983.
34. Itescu, S., Brancato, L.J., Buxbaum, J., et al.: CD8 lymphocytosis syndrome in human immunodeficiency virus (HIV) infection: A host immuno response associated with HLA-DR5. Ann. Intern. Med., *112*:3–10, 1990.
35. Calabrese, L.H., Estes, M., Yen-Liebermann, B., et al.: Systemic vasculitis in association with human immunodeficiency virus infection. Arthritis Rheum., *32*:569–576, 1989.
36. Greene, W.C.: The molecular biology of human immunodeficiency virus type I infection. N. Engl. J. Med., *324*:308–317, 1991.
37. Michaels, F.H., Banks, K.L., and Reitz, M.S.: Lessons from caprine and ovine retrovirus infection. Rheum. Dis. Clin. North Am., *17*:5–23, 1991.
38. Fauci, A.S.: The human immunodeficiency virus: Infectivity and mechanisms of pathogenesis. Science, *239*:617–622, 1988.
39. Klevjer-Anderson, P., Adams, D.S., Anderson, L.W., et al.: A sequential study of virus expression in retrovirus induced arthritis of goats. J. Gen. Virol., *65*:1519–1526, 1984.
40. Straub, O.C.: Caprine arthritis encephalitis—A model for AIDS. Intervirology, *30*:45–50, 1989.
41. Withrington, R.H., Cornes, P., Harris, J.R.W., and Seifert, M.H.: Isolation of human immunodeficiency virus from synovial fluid of a patient with reactive arthritis. Br. Med. J., *294*:484–486, 1987.
42. Hughes, R.A., Macatonia, S.E., Rowe, J.F., et al.: The detection of human immunodeficiency virus DNA in dendritic cells from the joints of patients with aseptic arthritis. Br. J. Rheumatol., *29*:166–170, 1990.
43. Wiley, C.A., Nerenberg, M., Cross, D., and Soto-Aguilar, M.C.: HTLV-I polymyositis in a patient also infected with the human immunodeficiency virus. N. Engl. J. Med., *320*:992–995, 1989.
44. Dalakas, M.C., Gravell, M., and London, W.T.: Morphological changes of an inflammatory myopathy in Rhesus monkeys with simian acquired immunodeficiency syndrome. Proc. Soc. Exp. Biol. Med., *185*:368–376, 1987.
45. Espinoza, L.R., Aguilar, J.L., Berman, A., et al.: Rheumatic manifestations associated with human immunodeficiency virus infection. Arthritis Rheum., *32*:1615–1622, 1989.
46. Jutila, M.A., and Banks, K.L.: Increased macrophage division in the synovial fluid of goats infected with caprine arthritis-encephalitis virus. J. Infect. Dis., *157*:1193–1198, 1988.
47. Iwakura, Y., Tosu, M., Yoshida, E., et al.: Induction of inflammatory arthropathy resembling rheumatoid arthritis in mice transgenic for HTLV-I. Science, *253*:1026–1028, 1991.
48. Gottieb, A.B., Fu, S.M., Carter, D.M., and Fotino, M.: Marked increased in the frequency of psoriatic arthritis in psoriasis patients with HLA-DR^{+} keratinocytes. Arthritis Rheum., *30*:901–907, 1987.
49. Espinoza, L.R., Aguilar, J.L., Espinoza, C.G., et al.: HIV Associated arthropathy: HIV antigen demonstration in the synovial membrane. J. Rheumatol., *17*:1195–1201, 1990.
50. Illa, I., Nath, A., and Dalakas, M.: Immunocytochemical and virological characteristics of HIV-associated inflammatory myopathies: Similarities with seronegative polymyositis. Ann. Neurol., *29*:474–481, 1991.
51. Nakamura, S., Salahuddin, S.Z., Biberfield, P., et al.: Kaposi's

sarcoma cells long-term culture with growth factor from retrovirus-infected $CD4^+$ cells. Science, *242*:426–430, 1988.

52. Itescu, S., Dalton, J., Brancato, L.B., et al.: Increased circulating gamma-delta cells in HIV infection and in Reiter's syndrome. Clin. Res., *38*:230A, 1990.
53. Aguilar, J.B., Berman, A., Espinoza, L.R., et al.: Autoimmune phenomena in human immunodeficiency virus infection. Am. J. Med., *85*:283–284, 1988.
54. Kopelman, R.C., and Zola-Pazner, S.: Association of human immunodeficiency virus infection and autoimmune phenomena. Am. J. Med., *84*:82–87, 1988.
55. Cohen, A.J., Philips, T.M., and Kessler, C.M.: Circulating coagulation inhibitors in the acquired immunodeficiency syndrome. Ann. Intern. Med., *104*:178–180, 1986.
56. Canosa, R.T., Zon, L.I., and Groopman, J.E.: Anticardiolipin antibodies associated with HTLV-III infection. Br. J. Haematol., *65*:495–498, 1987.
57. Davis, P., Stein, M., Latif, A.S., and Emmanuel, J.: Acute arthritis in Zimbabwean patients: Possible relationship to human immunodeficiency virus infection. J. Rheumatol., *16*:346–348, 1989.
58. Stein, M., and Davis, P.: HIV and arthritis—Causal or casual acquaintances. J. Rheumatol., *16*:1267–1290, 1989.
59. Davis, P., and Stein, M.: Human immunodeficiency virus–related connective tissue diseases: A Zimbabwean perspective. Rheum. Dis. Clin. North Am., *17*:89–97, 1991.
60. Lo, S.-C., Tsai, S., Benish, J.R., et al.: Enhancement of HIV-I cytocidal effects in CD4 lymphocytes by the AIDS-associated mycoplasma. Science, *251*:1074–1076, 1991.
61. Bentin, J.B., Feremans, W., Pateels, J.-L., et al.: Chronic acquired immunodeficiency syndrome–associated arthritis: A synovial ultrastructural study. Arthritis Rheum., *33*:268–273, 1990.
62. Gresh, J.P., Aguilar, J.L., and Espinoza, L.R.: Human immunodeficiency virus (HIV) infection–associated dermatomyositis. J. Rheumatol., *16*:1397–1398, 1989.
63. Chad, D.A., Smith, T.W., Blumefeld, A., et al.: Human immunodeficiency virus (HIV)-associated myopathy: Immunocytochemical identification of an HIV antigen(gp41) in muscle macrophages. Ann. Neurol., *28*:579–582, 1990.
64. Dalakas, M., Wichman, A., and Sever, J.: AIDS and the nervous system. JAMA, *261*:2396–2399, 1989.
65. Narayan, O., and Cork, L.C.: Lentivirial disease of sheep and goats: Chronic pneumonia leukoencephalomyelitis and arthritis. Rev. Infect. Dis., *7*:89–98, 1985.
66. Crawford, T.B., Adams, D.S., Cheevers, W.P., and Cork, L.C.: Chronic arthritis in goats caused by retrovirus. Science, *30*:1046–1053, 1988.
67. Banks, K.L., Jacobs, C.A., Michaels, F.H., and Cheevers, W.P.: Lentivirus infection augments concurrent antigen-induced arthritis. Arthritis Rheum., *30*:1046–1053, 1987.
68. Buskila, D., Gladman, D.D., Langevitz, P., et al.: Rheumatologic manifestations of infection with the human immunodeficiency virus (HIV). Clin. Exp. Rheumatol., *8*:567–573, 1990.
69. Winchester, R., Brancato, L., Itescu, S., and Solomon, G.: Implications from the occurrence of Reiter's syndrome and related disorders in association with advanced HIV infection. Scand. J. Rheum. Suppl., *74*:89–93, 1988.
70. Rowe, I.F., Forster, S.M., Seifert, M.H., et al.: Rheumatological lesions in individuals with human immunodeficiency virus infection. Q. J. Med., *73*:1167–1184, 1989.
71. Calabrese, L.H., Kelley, D.M., Myers, A., et al.: Rheumatic symptoms and human immunodeficiency virus infection: The influence of clinical and laboratory variable in a longitudinal cohort study. Arthritis Rheum., *34*:257–263, 1991.
72. Berman, A., Reboredo, G., Spindler, A., et al.: Rheumatic manifestations in populations at risk for HIV infection. J. Rheumatol., *10*, 1991.
73. Buskila, D., and Gladman, D.: Musculoskeletal manifestations of infection with human immunodeficiency virus. Rev. Infect. Dis., *12*:223–235, 1990.
74. Winchester, R.: AIDS and the rheumatic diseases. Bull. Rheum. Dis., *39*:1–10, 1990.
75. Clark, M., Kinsolving, M., and Chernoff, D.: The prevalence of arthritis in two HIV-infected cohorts. Arthritis Rheum., *32*:585A, 1989.
76. Hochberg, M.C., Fox, R., and Nelson, K.R.: Reiter's syndrome is not associated with HIV infection. Arthritis Rheum., *33*:R16A, 1990.
77. Solinger, A.M., and Hess, E.V.: Rheumatic diseases and AIDS. Arthritis Rheum., *33*:87A, 1990.
78. Winchester, R., and Solomon, G.: Reiter's syndrome and acquired immunodeficiency. *In* Infections in the Rheumatic Diseases. Edited by L.R. Espinoza, D. Goldenberg, F. Arnett, and G. Alarcon. Orlando, Grune & Stratton, 1988, pp. 343–347.
79. Kaye, B.R., Rheumatologic manifestations of infection with human immunodeficiency virus (HIV). Ann. Intern. Med., *111*:158–167, 1989.
80. Calabrese, L.H.: The rheumatic manifestations of infection with the human immunodeficiency virus. Semin. Arthritis Rheum., *18*:225–239, 1989.
81. Silveira, L.H., Seleznick, M.J., Jara, L.J., et al.: Musculoskeletal manifestations of human immunodeficiency virus infection. J. Intensive Care Med., *6*:106–116, 1991.
82. Johnson, T.M., Duvic, M., and Rapini, R.P.: AIDS exacerbates psoriasis. N. Engl. J. Med., *313*:1415, 1985.
83. Duvic, M., Johnson, R.M., Rapini, R.P., et al.: Acquired immunodeficiency syndrome–associated psoriasis and Reiter's syndrome. Arch. Dermatol., *123*:1622–1632, 1987.
84. Lin, R.Y.: Reiter's syndrome and human immunodeficiency virus infection. Dermatologica, *176*:39–42, 1988.
85. Reveille, J.D., Conant, M.A., and Duvic, M.: Human immunodeficiency virus–associated psoriasis, psoriatic arthritis and Reiter's syndrome: A disease continuum? Arthritis Rheum., *33*:1574–1578, 1990.
86. Arnett, F.C., McCkluskey, E., Schacter, B.Z., and Lordon, R.E.: Incomplete Reiter's syndrome: Discriminating features and HL-AW27 in diagnosis. Ann. Intern. Med., *84*:8–12, 1976.
87. Buskila, D., Langevitz, P., Tenenbaum, J., and Gladman, D.D.: Malar rash in a patient with Reiter's syndrome—A clue for the diagnosis of human immunodeficiency virus infection. J. Rheumatol., *17*:843–845, 1990.
88. Gutierrez, F.J., Martinez-Osuna, P., Seleznick, M.J., and Espinoza, L.R.: Rheumatologic rehabilitation for patients with HIV. *In* Rehabilitation for Patients with HIV Disease. Edited by Jon Mukand. New York, McGraw Hill, 1991, pp. 77–94.
89. Arnett, F.C., Reveille, J.D., and Duvic, M.: Psoriasis and Psoriatic arthritis associated with human immunodeficiency virus infection. Rheum. Dis. Clin. North Am., *17*:59–78, 1991.
90. Dalakas, M.C., and Pezeshkpour, G.H.: Neuromuscular diseases associated with human immunodeficiency virus infection. Ann. Neurol., *23*:538–548, 1988.
91. Simpson, D.M., and Bendes, A.M.: Human immunodeficiency-virus–associated myopathy: Analysis of seven patients. Ann. Neurol., *24*:79–84, 1988.
92. Olney, R.K., Gonzalez, M.F., and So, Y.T.: Subacute myopathy with selective loss of thick filaments: A new muscle disease associated with HIV seropositivity. Neurology, *37*:206A, 1987.
93. Dalakas, M.C., Pezeshkpour, G.H., and Flakerty, M.: Progressive nemaline (rod) myopathy associated with HIV infection. N. Engl. J. Med., *317*:1602–1603, 1987.

94. Panegyres, P.K., Tan, N., Kakulas, B.A., et al.: Necrotizing myopathy and zidovudine. Lancet, *1*:1050–1052, 1988.
95. Bessen, I.J., Greene, J.B., Louie, E., et al.: Severe polymyositis-like syndrome associated with zidovudine therapy of AIDS and ARC. N. Engl. J. Med., *318*:708, 1988.
96. Espinoza, L.R., Berman, A., and Aguilar, J.L.: Myalgias in human immunodeficiency virus-infected patients. Am. J. Med., *86*:511, 1989.
97. Gertner, E., Thurn, J.R., Williams, D.W., et al.: Zidovudine-associated myopathy. Am. J. Med., *86*:814–818, 1989.
98. Till, M., and MacDonell, K.B.: Myopathy with human immunodeficiency virus type I (HIV-I) infection: HIV-I or zidovudine? Ann. Intern. Med., *113*:492–494, 1990.
99. Espinoza, L.R., Aguilar, J.L., Espinoza, C.G., et al.: Characteristics and pathogenesis of myositis in human immunodeficiency virus infection-distinction from azidothymidine-induced myopathy. Rheum. Dis. Clin. North Am., *17*:117–130, 1991.
100. Arnaudo, E., Dalaka, M., Shaske, S., et al.: Depletion of muscle mitochondrial DNA in AIDS patients with zidovudine-induced myopathy. Lancet, *337*:508–510, 1991.
101. Mhiric, C., Baudrimont, M., Bonne, G., et al.: Zidovudine myopathy: A distinctive disorder associated with mitochondrial dysfunction. Ann. Neurol., *29*:606–614, 1991.
102. Ledford, D.K., Overman, M.D., Gonzalvo, A., and Lockey, R.: Microsporidiosis myositis in a patient with the acquired immunodeficiency syndrome. Ann. Intern. Med., *102*:628–630, 1985.
103. Drane, W.E., and Tipler, B.M.: Heterotopic ossification (myositis ossificans) in acquired immunodeficiency syndrome. Detection by Gallium scintigraphy. Clin. Nucl. Med., *12*:433–435, 1987.
104. Comi, G., Medaglini, S., Galardi, G., et al.: Subclinical neuromuscular involvement in acquired immune deficiency syndrome. Muscle Nerve, *9*:665A, 1986.
105. Watts, R.A., Hoffbrand, B.I., Paton, D.F., and David, J.C.: Pyomyositis associated with human immunodeficiency virus infection. Br. Med. J., *294*:1524–1525, 1987.
106. Vartian, C., and Ceptimus, E.J.: Pyomyositis in an intravenous drug user with human immunodeficiency virus. Arch. Intern. Med., *148*:2689, 1988.
107. Victor, G., Branley, J., Opal, S.M., and Mayer, K.H.: Pyomyositis in a patient with the acquired immunodeficiency syndrome. Arch. Intern. Med., *149*:704–709, 1989.
108. Raphael, S.A., Wolfson, B.J., Parker, P., et al.: Pyomyositis in a child with acquired immunodeficiency syndrome. Patient report and brief review. Am. J. Dis. Child., *143*:779–781, 1989.
109. Widrow, C., Kelle, S., Salzman, B., et al.: Pyomyositis in HIV infected patients. Sixth International AIDS Conference. San Francisco, California, 1990, p. 367.
110. Schwartzman, W.A., Lambertus, M.W., Kennedy, C.A., and Bidwell Goetz, M.: Staphylococcal pyomyositis in patients infected by the human immunodeficiency virus. Am. J. Med., *90*:595–600, 1991.
111. Couderc, L.J., D'Agay, M.F., Danon, F., et al.: Sicca complex and infection with human immunodeficiency virus. Arch. Intern. Med., *147*:898–901, 1987.
112. DeClerck, L.S., Couthenye, M.M., De Broe, M.E., and Stevens, W.J.: Acquired immunodeficiency syndrome mimicking Sjögren's syndrome and systemic lupus erythematosus. Arthritis Rheum., *31*:272–275, 1988.
113. Talal, N., Dauphinee, M.J., Dang, H., et al.: Detection of serum antibodies to retroviral proteins in patients with primary Sjögren's syndrome (autoimmune exocrinopathy). Arthritis Rheum., *33*:774–781, 1990.
114. Garry, R.F., Fermin, C.D., Hart, D.J., et al.: Detection of a human intracisternal A-type retroviral particle antigenically related to HIV. Science, *250*:1127–1129, 1990.
115. Bardin, T., Gaudouen, C., Kuntz, D., et al.: Necrotizing vasculitis in human immunodeficiency virus infection. Arthritis Rheum., *30*:S105, 1987.
116. Calabrese, L.H.: Vasculitis and infection with the human immunodeficiency virus. Rheum. Dis. Clin. North Am., *17*:131–148, 1991.
117. Weber, C.A., Figueroa, J.P., Calabro, J.J., et al.: Co-occurrence of the Reiter's syndrome and acquired immunodeficiency. Ann. Intern. Med., *107*:112–113, 1987.
118. Yanker, B.A., Skolnik, P.R., Shoukimas, G.M., et al.: Cerebral granulomatous angiitis associated with isolation of human T-lymphotropic virus type III from the central nervous system. Ann. Neurol., *20*:362–364, 1986.
119. Frank, Y., Lim, W., Kahn, E., et al.: Cerebral granulomatous angiitis causing multiple ischemic cerebrovascular accidents in a child with acquired immunodeficiency syndrome. Ann. Neurol., *22*:452–453, 1987.
120. Schwartz, N.D., So, Y.T., Hollander, H., et al.: Eosinophilic vasculitis leading to amaurosis fugax in a patient with acquired immunodeficiency syndrome. Arch. Intern. Med., *146*:2059–2060, 1986.
121. Velji, A.M.: Leukocytoclastic vasculitis associated with positive HTLV-III serological findings. JAMA, *256*:2196–2197, 1986.
122. Montilla, P., Dronda, F., Moreno, S., et al.: Lymphomatoid granulomatosis and the acquired immunodeficiency syndrome. Ann. Intern. Med., *106*:166–167, 1987.
123. Vinters, H.V., and Anders, K.H.: Lymphomatoid granulomatosis and the acquired immunodeficiency syndrome (AIDS). Ann. Intern. Med., *107*:945, 1987.
124. Guillon, J.M., Fouret, P., Mayaud, C., et al.: Extensive T8 positive lymphocytic visceral infiltration in a homosexual man. Am. J. Med., *82*:655–661, 1987.
125. Anders, K.H., Latta, H., Chang, B.S., et al.: Lymphomatoid granulomatosis and malignant lymphoma of the central nervous system in the acquired immunodeficiency syndrome. Hum. Pathol., *20*:326–334, 1989.
126. Valeriano, J., Lolita, B., and Kerr, L.D.: HIV-associated polyarteritis modosa (PAN) diagnosed by rectal biopsy: A case report. J. Rheumatol., *17*:1091–1093, 1990.
127. Ricciardi, D.D., Sepkowitz, D.V., Berkowitz, L.B., et al.: Cryptococcal arthritis in a patient with acquired immunodeficiency syndrome: Case report and review of the literature. J. Rheumatol., *13*:455–458, 1986.
128. Lipstein-Kresch, E., Isenberg, H.D., Singer, C., et al.: Disseminated Sporothrix schenckii infection with arthritis in a patient with acquired immunodeficiency syndrome. J. Rheumatol., *12*:805–808, 1985.
129. Rogers, P.L., Walker, R.E., Lane, H.C., et al.: Disseminated Mycobacterium haemophilum infection in two patients with the acquired immunodeficiency syndrome. Am. J. Med., *84*:640–642, 1988.
130. Blumenthal, D.R., Zucker, J.R., and Hawkins, C.C.: Mycobacterium avium complex–induced septic arthritis and osteomyelitis in a patient with the acquired immunodeficiency syndrome. Arthritis Rheum., *33*:757–758, 1990.
131. Kraus, V.B., Baraniuk, J.N., Hill, G.B., and Allen, N.B.: Ureaplasma urealyticum septic arthritis in hypogammaglobulinemia. J. Rheumatol., *15*:369–371, 1988.
132. Zimmerman, B. III, Erickson, A.D., and Mikolich, D.J.: Septic acromioclavicular arthritis and osteomyelitis in a patient with acquired immunodeficiency syndrome. Arthritis Rheum., *32*:1175–1178, 1989.
133. Ragni, M.V., and Hanley, E.N.: Septic arthritis in hemophilic

patients and infection with human immunodeficiency virus. Ann. Intern. Med., *110*:168–169, 1989.

134. Pappo, A.S., Buchanan, G.R., and Johnson, A.: Septic arthritis in children with hemophilia. Am. J. Dis. Child., *143*:1226–1228, 1989.
135. Guyot, D.R., Manoli, A. II, and King, G.A.: Pyogenic sacroiliitis in IV drug abusers. Am. J. Radiol., *149*:1209–1211, 1987.
136. Buskila, D., and Tennenbaum, J.: Septic bursitis in human immunodeficiency virus infection. J. Rheumatol., *16*:1374–1376, 1989.
137. Jacobson, M.A., Gellerman, H., and Chambers, H.: Staphylococcus aureus bacteremia nad recurrent staphylococcal infection in patients with acquired immunodeficiency syndrome and AIDS-related complex. Am. J. Med., *85*:172–176, 1988.
138. Goh, B.T., Jawad, A.S.M., Chapman, D., et al.: Osteomyelitis presenting as a swollen elbow in a patient with the acquired immune deficiency syndrome. Ann. Rheum. Dis., *47*:695–696, 1988.
139. Goldberg, D.L.: Septic arthritis and other infections of rheumatological significance. Rheum. Dis. Clin. North Am., *17*:149–156, 1991.
140. Naher, H., Tilgen, W., Tilz, G., and Petzoldt, D.: False positive results in the detection of anti-LAV/HTLV III antibodies by enzyme immunoassay. Hautarzt, *37*:338–340, 1986.
141. Morales, J., Moreno-Maldonado, S., Hernandez-Ochoa, C., and Orozco-Martinez, M.E.: Falsas positivas anti-HIV en lupus eritematoso sistemico. Rev. Mex. Reum., *3*:114–117, 1988.
142. Furie, R., Kaell, A., Petrucci, R., et al.: Systemic lupus erythematosus complicated by infection with human immunodeficiency virus. Arthritis Rheum., *31*:R4, 1988.
143. Furie, R.A.: Effects of human immunodeficiency virus infection on the expression of rheumatic illness. Rheum. Dis. Clin. North Am., *17*:177–188, 1991.
144. Bijlsma, J.W.J., Derksen, R.W.H.M., Huber-Pruning, O., and Borleffs, J.C.C.: Does AIDS "cure" rheumatoid arthritis? Ann. Rheum. Dis., *47*:350–352, 1988.
145. Buskila, D., Gladman, D.D., Langevitz, P., et al.: Fibromalgia in human immunodeficiency virus infection. J. Rheumatol., *17*:1202–1206, 1990.
146. Harris, P.J.: Hypertrophic pulmonary osteoarthropathy and human immunodeficiency virus (HIV). Ann. Intern. Med., *109*:250, 1988.
147. Bhat, S., Heurich, A.E., Vaquer, R.A., et al.: Hypertrophic osteoarthropathy associated with Pneumocystis carinii pneumonia in AIDS. Chest, *96*:1208–1209, 1989.
148. Gerster, J.C., Camus, J.P., Chave, J.P., et al.: Multiple site avascular necrosis in HIV infected patients. J. Rheumatol., *18*:300–302, 1991.
149. Bower, M., Nelson, M., and Gazzard, B.G.: Dupuytren's contractures in patients infected with HIV. Br. Med. J., *300*:164–165, 1990.
150. French, P.D., Kitchen, V.S., and Harris, J.R.W.: Prevalence of Dupuytren's contracture in patients infected with HIV. Br. Med. J., *301*:967, 1990.
151. Uchiyama, T., Yodoi, J., Sagawa, K., et al.: Adult T cell leukemia: Clinical and hematological features of 16 cases. Blood, *50*:481–482, 1977.
152. Osame, M., Usuku, K., Izumo, S., et al.: HTLV-I associated myelopathy, a new clinical entity. Lancet, *1*:1013–1014, 1986.
153. Sugimoto, M., Nakashima, H., Matsumoto, M., et al.: Pulmonary involvement in patients with HTLV-I-associated myelopathy: Increased soluble IL-2 receptors in bronchoalveolar lavage fluid. Am. Rev. Respir. Dis., *139*:1329–1335, 1989.
154. Vernant, J.C., Buisson, G., Magdeleine, J., et al.: T-lymphocyte alveolitis tropical spastic paresis and Sjögren's syndrome. Lancet, *1*:177, 1988.
155. Kitajima, I., Maruyama, I., Maruyama, Y., et al.: Polyarthritis in human T lymphotropic virus type-I associated myelopathy. Arthritis Rheum., *32*:1342–1344, 1989.
156. Nishioka, K., Maruyama, I., Sato, K., et al.: Chronic inflammatory arthropathy associated with HTLV-I. Lancet, *1*:441, 1989.
157. Sato, K., Maruyama, I., Maruyama, Y., et al.: Arthritis in patients infected with human T lymphotropic virus type-I. Arthritis Rheum., *34*:714–721, 1991.
158. Kitajima, I., Yamamoto, K., Sato, K., et al.: Detection of HTLV-I proviral DNA and its gene expression in synovial cells in chronic inflammatory arthropathy. J. Clin. Invest., (in press).
159. Boissier, M.-C., Lefrere, J.-J., and Freyfus, P.: Rheumatic manifestations in a patient with human immunodeficiency virus type 2 infection. Arthritis Rheum., *34*:790, 1991.
160. Fauci, A.S., Macher, A.B., Longo, D.L., et al.: Acquired immunodeficiency syndrome epidemiologic, clinical, immunologic and therapeutic considerations. Ann. Intern. Med., *100*:92–106, 1984.
161. Euler, H.H., Kern, P., and Loffler, H.: Precipitable immune complexes in healthy homosexual men, acquired immune deficiency syndrome, and the related lymphadenopathy syndrome. Clin. Exp. Immunol., *59*:267–275, 1985.
162. Mayer-Siuta, R., Keil, L.B., and DeBari, V.A.: Autoantibodies and circulating immune complexes in subjects infected with human immunodeficiency virus. Med. Microbiol. Immunol., *177*:189–194, 1988.
163. Jackson, S., Dawson, L.M., and Kotler, D.P.: IgAI is the major immunoglobulin component of immune complexes in the acquired immunodeficiency syndrome. J. Clin. Immunol., *8*:64–68, 1988.
164. Bernard, C., Exquis, B., Reber, G., and deMoerlosse, P.: Determination of anticardiolipin and other antibodies in HIV-I-infected patients. J. AIDS, *3*:536–539, 1990.
165. Bloom, E.J., Abrams, D.I., and Rogers, G.: Lupus anticoagulant in the acquired immunodeficiency syndrome. JAMA, *256*:491–493, 1986.
166. Fields, R.A., Toubbeh, H., Searles, R.P., and Bankhurst, A.D.: The presence of anticardiolipin antibodies in a healthy elderly population and its association with antinuclear antibodies. J. Rheumatol., *16*:623–625, 1989.
167. Rosenberg, Z.S., Norman, A., and Solomon, G.: Arthritis associated with HIV infection: radiographic manifestations. Radiology, *173*:171–176, 1989.
168. Espinoza, L.R., Aguilar, J.L., and Berman, A.: Drug selection for rheumatic manifestations of acquired immunodeficiency syndrome. Am. J. Med., *85*:894–896, 1988.
169. Feeney, G.F., and Frazer, I.: AIDS-associated psoriasis responds to azidothymidine. Med. J. Aus., *48*:155, 1988.
170. Kaplan, M.H., Sadick, N.S., and Wieder, J.: Antipsoriatic effects of zidovudine in human immunodeficiency virus-associated psoriasis. J. Am. Acad. Dermatol., *20*:76–82, 1989.
171. Rasokat, H.: Psoriasis in AIDS-remission with dosage co-trimoxazole therapy. Z. Hautkr., *61*:1991, 1986.
172. Belz, J., and Breneman, D.L.: Successful treatment of a patient with Reiter's syndrome and acquired immunodeficiency syndrome using Etretinate. J. Am. Acad. Dermatol., *20*:898–903, 1989.
173. Mukand, J.: Rehabilitation for patients with HIV disease. New York, McGraw-Hill, 1991.

Index

Page numbers in *italics* indicate illustrations; page numbers followed by "t" indicate tables.